W9-AAX-355

TOURO COLLEGE LIBRARY
Bay Shore Campus

WITHDRAWN

PAIN MANAGEMENT

A Practical Guide for Clinicians

SIXTH EDITION

Editor Richard S. Weiner

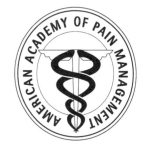

AMERICAN ACADEMY OF PAIN MANAGEMENT

WITHDRAWN
TOURO COLLEGE LIBRARY
Bay Shore Campus

CRC PRESS

Boca Raton   London   New York   Washington, D.C.

BS

The publishers, the authors, and the American Academy of Pain Management cannot assume responsibility for the validity of all materials contained in this book or for the consequences of their use. Some of the content represents an emerging area of study. As new information becomes available, changes in treatment and in the use of drugs may be necessary. The reader is advised to consult his or her healthcare practitioner before changing, adding, or eliminating any treatment. The reader is also advised to carefully consult the instruction and information material included in the package insert of each drug or therapeutic agent before administration. The publisher, authors, and the American Academy of Pain Management disclaim any liability, loss, injury, or damage incurred as a consequence, directly or indirectly, of the use and application of any of the contents of this volume.

Library of Congress Cataloging-in-Publication Data

Pain management : a practical guide for clinicians / executive editor, Richard S. Weiner.—6th ed.
       p. ; cm.
    Includes bibliographical references and index.
    ISBN 0-8493-0926-3 (alk. paper)
    1. Pain—Treatment. 2. Analgesia.   I. Weiner, Richard S., Ph.D.
    [DNLM: 1. Pain—therapy. 2. Chronic Disease—therapy. 3. Disability Evaluation. 4.
    Pain—diagnosis. 5. Patient Care Management. WL 704 P14656 2001]
    RB127 .P33233   2001
    616′.0472—dc21   2001037442

This book contains information obtained from authentic and highly regarded sources. Reprinted material is quoted with permission, and sources are indicated. A wide variety of references are listed. Reasonable efforts have been made to publish reliable data and information, but the author and the publisher cannot assume responsibility for the validity of all materials or for the consequences of their use.

Neither this book nor any part may be reproduced or transmitted in any form or by any means, electronic or mechanical, including photocopying, microfilming, and recording, or by any information storage or retrieval system, without prior permission in writing from the publisher.

All rights reserved. Authorization to photocopy items for internal or personal use, or the personal or internal use of specific clients, may be granted by CRC Press LLC, provided that $.50 per page photocopied is paid directly to Copyright clearance Center, 222 Rosewood Drive, Danvers, MA 01923 USA. The fee code for users of the Transactional Reporting Service is ISBN 0-8493-0926-3/02/$0.00+$1.50. The fee is subject to change without notice. For organizations that have been granted a photocopy license by the CCC, a separate system of payment has been arranged.

The consent of CRC Press LLC does not extend to copying for general distribution, for promotion, for creating new works, or for resale. Specific permission must be obtained in writing from CRC Press LLC for such copying.

Direct all inquiries to CRC Press LLC, 2000 N.W. Corporate Blvd., Boca Raton, Florida 33431.

Trademark Notice: Product or corporate names may be trademarks or registered trademarks, and are used only for identification and explanation, without intent to infringe.

Visit the CRC Press Web site at www.crcpress.com

© 2002 by CRC Press LLC

No claim to original U.S. Government works
International Standard Book Number 0-8493-0926-3
Library of Congress Card Number 2001037442
Printed in the United States of America   1 2 3 4 5 6 7 8 9 0
Printed on acid-free paper

03-03-03

Table of Contents

SECTION IX Behavioral, Social, and Spiritual Concerns and Aspects of Pain Management

Dedication

Pain and suffering is an issue that has affected society throughout the ages. Its impact has led healthcare professionals throughout the world to aggressively explore methods to reduce and eliminate the pain that afflicts thousands annually. Numerous attempts have been made to discover effective methods to diagnose and treat the problem time and again, yet the condition continues to exist. Throughout our research and treatments we have learned more about this topic by integrating multiple disciplines and cultures into our quest for answers. By incorporating this broad base of knowledge and experience, we are led to believe that our continuous contribution to this effort gives each of us an opportunity to make a difference in the study of pain management.

This book is dedicated to those who can and do make a difference in the lives of others. Special recognition goes to Barbara E. Norwitz, Publisher, CRC Press, Tiffany Lane, Editorial Assistant, Barry E. Cole, M.D., M.P.A., Kathryn A. Weiner, Ph.D., and the Board, Staff, and Members of the American Academy of Pain Management.

Preface

Significant advances in our understanding of pain and suffering, clinical and laboratory reports, and concepts for multidisciplinary team interaction, combined with a renewed desire to understand the whole patient delivery system require updating and further documenting the new information provided in this 6th edition of *Pain Management: A Practical Guide for Clinicians*. Interest in the field of pain management has grown dramatically since the 1970s. This has been attributable to the outstanding contribution of pioneers, who provided leadership in this field, such as Dr. John Bonica, Dr. Benjamin Crue, Mme. Abel Fessard, Dr. Burtram Wolf, Dr. John Leibskind, Drs. Richard and Kathryn Weiner, and so many others, leading to the current global, exponential, informational avalanche. To bring together this enormous amount of new and refined knowledge and data, the original two volumes have been reorganized and expanded several times.

So universal has this interest become, it can be likened to a pebble in the pond starting a propagation wave. Interest has grown exponentially; knowledge and wisdom constantly unfold. Quality pain management originally generated from a relatively small group of specialized experts forming a dynamic epicenter. These early leaders initiated a spread of integrated knowledge, team care, and multidisciplinary responses with many other health professionals, starting from basic neuroscience, which has blossomed to where we now encompass the special interest of many disciplines. Knowledge travels in many directions and today we have many primary care practices able to integrate tools and philosophies refined by pain management over the years. Many pain patients find care with a growing cadre of alternative and integrated disciplines. The primary care physician and clinician are often gate keepers because they are most frequently the first health professionals to see individuals with significant clinical problems and must decide to manage or seek referral from an appropriate specialist. Proper assessment and treatment planning are especially important for complex pain syndromes as they often are present with overlapping preexisting comorbidity. The needs of the patient must be best served when a "cure" is not possible. Chronicity complicates management for the health practitioner and patient. An integrated mind–body–spirit concept provides a fuller understanding for the complaint of pain. This holistic view in turn manifests complex interactive emotional and physical factors. Treatment programs must be individualized. Many pain syndromes are acute, chronic, and/or cancer related; one size does not fit all!

New chapters, advances in diagnosis employing new clinical testing methods, increase our scientific perspective and aid in our ability to evaluate the interpretation of many co-existing psychological, physical, functional, pathological, and structural impairments. When they indeed need to be separated or correlated for patient care within managed care agencies and medical–legal communities, we must remember that treatment decisions impact the whole fabric of a person's life. An appreciation of a "systems" view facilitates change. Clinically applied, this knowledge and experience can better guide treatments that are more cost effective. The clinician must be able to differentiate physiological signs associated with range of motion, reflex, proprioception, and other responses. Activities of daily living, body habits and age-related changes must be evaluated in terms of related impairments and measured for quality of life. How do you evaluate preexisting and comorbid conditions that may overlap in personal injury cases and may be associated with situations where life style matters? How do we factor weight, diabetes, and postoperative failed back syndrome, superimposed on congenital spinal changes and reactive depression? Not a simple matter; only a careful, knowledgeable, and experienced assessment, supported by laboratory data, will be convincing to third party reimbursement programs, and credible for the medical–legal community. When are such tests really necessary? Are there alternatives?

A clinical practitioner can choose from more than 8000 laboratory tests. Which are reasonable and necessary to verify injury or disease? There is also the responsibility of the clinician to consider laboratory tests that may have false positive or false negative reports. Relevant, reflective, clinical correlation is required to develop a credible conclusion. Furthermore, the clinician must exercise judgment about when to order a special study. Corroborating or repeating serial tests, whose initial results are felt not to be consistent with clinical findings, may provide valuable information. In certain delivery systems, authorization for a service may be difficult to obtain. Often administrative or clinical denial sets the tone for clinical practice at the new millennium. Test selection is especially important in view of rapidly advancing technology. For example, how do you compare varying magnetic radiation imaging test results between 0.5, 1.0, and 1.5 tesla resolution. When do your order 3-D reconstruction or tomograms? When are vitamins, nutritional, or other tests appropriate? It is exceedingly important to consider the fact that abnormal anatomic or structural tests can be misleading. There is no substitute for talking with the patient and often other persons for additional information. Frequently, patients who have injuries that remain unresolved come to involve a medical–legal setting. The inclusion of the judiciary provides an additional interactive issue based on an adversarial approach. The clinician may provide retrospective medical evaluations, declarations of permanent status, and need for future medical and vocational considerations, as well as describe how preexisting or comorbid factors influence rehabilitation. Regional pain syndrome (RPS) that causes functional impairments may be difficult to evaluate.

Reimbursement and cost shifting delays often impact care. Today, the astute clinician must understand his or her discipline to be able to work within a multidisciplinary team, document and justify opinions, and handle myriad tasks, that were far less demanding in years gone by. Authors will address these complex issues.

Today, there is an unprecedented need to justify treatment. There are barriers facing today's clinician, namely the highly interpretative rule and documentation to demonstrate necessity and reasonableness of care. Standards have frequently not been defined by statute. Experienced authors will address these issues. Moreover, third party payers are with greater frequency introducing a relatively new type of evolving medical management that could be called "contract medicine." Access to care is subject to wide interpretations. Disputes arise and this increases the frequency and involvement of the legal community with resultant adversity, which can be protracted and costly. State statutes or rules have long recognized that if there is a dispute, reimbursement may not be paid for extended periods of time, if at all. Practice management must be part of today's clinician's repertoire, as the dynamics of health policy and economics change. These issues will be reviewed in this new edition.

New and significant pharmacologic advances and treatment with respect to classes of drugs known as analgesics, anti-inflammatories, and receptor-specific forms of intervention are being discovered and re-emphasized. How do we keep up with this enormous growth in the ever expanding annual physician desk reference, compendiums across disciplines, integration of new approaches with traditional methods? New generations of drugs that affect the neuronal network; the ever expanding neural transmitters, presynaptic substance P, and others affecting specific and nonspecific receptors and effectors are updated in these chapters. New information will address complex class drug interactions. We do know that prescribed and frequently modified medication programs must be individualized and monitored. What are the advantages and risks of the Cox I and Cox II medications? New transcutaneous, oral, sublingual, and nasal aerosol delivery systems will be reviewed. Advances in both nonnarcotic and opioid therapy are discussed. How does the patient's compliance affect the treatment program if some classes of drugs are taken abusively or, conversely, below schedule? What role does psychoneuroimmunology play in etiology and intervention? How can new approaches help trigger informational transmitters that can influence peptides and emotional well-being? What is the role of over-the-counter (OTC) and herbal medications? What may be the effect on polypharmacy, herbaceuticals, and electrotherapy treatments? These questions will be discussed in expanded chapters. Caution must be exercised in prescribing new treatment and new regimes. Is there evidence from clinical trials? Do indications described have regulatory (FDA) approval? The practicing clinician is responsible for keeping current.

Advancements in our knowledge and understanding of rehabilitation have occurred in the field of muscular and skeletal disease, and new treatments are reported in this 6th edition. The authors address outcomes of treatment and evidence-based medicine, while retaining an understanding for evaluating meaningful individual responses. Outcome studies are tools that can be used to improve care, but they can be subject to manipulation for restricting access to certain treatment. Thus, it is particularly important to understand today's political environment and to analyze treatment and the opinions expressed by health professionals concerning policy matters for important decisions, in order to comment upon the milieu of practice. The important role of the health professional is to provide both relevant specialized information and to relate the impact of such information for each patient. Treatment and social decisions depend upon fair and comprehensive assessments. When should disability be reevaluated, especially if improvement occurs or if leisurely recreational personal activities are perceived not to cause significant functional impairment? How do you re-evaluate a progressive, worsening condition?

Long-term care has at times been called "palliative care." Where a management treatment program is available to stabilize or improve quality of life, treatment has been ruled reimbursable by some courts despite the fact that a cure is not possible. On the other hand, reimbursement for palliative care programs has also been denied by many third-party reimbursement programs. It should be noted that certain classes of diseases are resistant to complete cure, for example, arthritis, cardiovascular disease, certain metabolic diseases, and certain cancer syndromes, in spite of a multidisciplinary approach and may for some be at best only managed. Chronic complex regional pain syndromes associated with ongoing functional impairment such as failed back syndrome and reflex sympathetic dystrophy (RSD) or sympathetically maintained pain (SMP) also fall into this category. Intractable pain can be managed so that the patient can be brought to the highest level of personal activities of daily living and be potentially gainfully employed through rehabilitation. Suffering from "psychological pain impairment," so well defined as "perceived nociception" by Dr. John Loeser, may be difficult to evaluate, but can often be ameliorated with an individualized, humanistic, behavioral treatment program. These issues and others will be reviewed. When are stress, anxiety, and depression (SAD) misinterpreted as malingering? An exceedingly important question. New therapies are available, based on sound psychological counseling and psychiatric experience. Home care counseling, peer counseling, and cost-effective packaged audio and visual programs are now available for selected patients. These subjects will be addressed by experienced authors.

New treatment programs combing electromodulation continue to be developed in a dynamic process as technology changes and evidence is monitored by our continuing use of outcome studies. Integrating new approaches, new routes of delivery, new roles for team members, and even new roles for the patient/client and his or her significant others is addressed in this new edition. These modalities can be adjunctive to other treatments or prescribed alone. There is preliminary evidence that a home care program can significantly reduce costs when supported with good patient education. Electrotherapy treatment modalities that combine both psychological stress, somatic pain management therapy and clarification to help patients search to rediscover meaning in life, are catapulting us to a new frontier in wellness and recovery.

Bioengineering principles that benefit and affect pathophysiogical processes, while not harming normal physiology, are the continuing quest for such modality treatment. The technology that results is controlled by regulators and agencies and may be mandated by statutory legislation. A relatively new field that I refer to as "energetics" is emerging in which psychoneuroimmunology is being studied for its ability to modulate response through noninvasive means of therapy.

New chapters which review molecular-specific neurophysiological–electrochemical events altered by receptor-specific inducement have been added to this compendium. Concurrently, one notices a move away from ablative surgery in the modulation of intractable, desultory pain syndromes.

Some of these chapters critically review newer methods of differentiating algorithmic pathways, clinically quantifying perceptual thresholds of alpha, beta, and C-fibers to wavelength-specific neural pathways of identified subsets of pain sensation. Treatments by electromodulation of spinal and cranial selective stimulation, present significant advances in pain management reported by specialists in neuromodulation of pain. New chapters in alternative medicine borrowed from European and Asian fields of healing have been added and updated. The role of spirituality is better understood in these therapies. Why do some tolerate pain better than others? These subjects will be addressed. Regulatory agencies separate experimental from investigative from approved categories of devices and further sub-classify them into three categories according to the Medical Device Act of 1976. Clinical pain associations network and have liaisons with these institutions. Clinicians are held responsible for using technology that is safe and approved for specific conditions. Scientific associations act as an important liaison between regulatory agencies. Associations help provide for testing of devices and develop guidelines and standards for protocols. The prescribing clinician, however, must be cautious and use only those devices approved for use with human subjects and understand the legal ramifications for using devices and substances for nonapproved indications. Care must be further exercised in not prescribing copied or "me, too" devices with exaggerated claims provided by the marketing department. The clinician must look for devices with established consensus by experienced investigative clinicians incorporating evidence from controlled trials and anecdotal case descriptions. This information will discussed in revised chapters.

The all important changes affecting pain management in regard to the medical–legal community are addressed in view of the changing dynamic role of the many important court discussions and new precedents. This area of inquiry assists medical, research, regulatory, legal, judicial, and legislative bodies by updating relevant new information for their respective responsibilities in decision making.

As we move forward into the 21st century with improved relations and technologies borrowed from many disciplines, we are closing the gaps in the lack of understanding conferred upon us by scientific ignorance. At the same time we are more cognizant of the need for understanding human relationships, habitats, and social policies.

History shows us that the schism of Descartes' mind–body dualism is being narrowed as we move from Aristotelian understanding of the natural order of things to Bacon's view of interrelated orders. However, we should recall an observation from Albert Einstein that "All important things cannot be measured and all things that can be measured are not necessarily important." Clinical judgment based on experience remains, therefore, paramount.

As we move into the 21st century, the emerging field of "energetics" will help modify genetics or acquired impaired neural networks that influence perceptual pain, will provide great optimism for improving the future of our ecosystem, and will improve our understanding of simple and complex syndromes. The 21st century will move us out of Descartes' "cave of ignorance" and beyond physical Newtonian concepts. We still do not understand how an anatomic neural network can also have consciousness, although general systems theory and complex theory aid our understanding. This will provide for treatments not yet imagined. The broad question whether pain perception is peripheral or centrally mediated is still debated. Is it a combination of both? What are the roles of aging, culture, and genetic predisposition? Can we not do more to understand the yin–yang and context of the psychoneural biology of acute, chronic, cancer, and psychogenic pain syndromes, each with its different mechanisms? While learning to view individuals as part of a whole, we continue to learn pattern and structure, environment and heredity, and we improve the credibility of our knowledge. The 6th edition of *Pain Management* will provide the reader with an expanding horizon as we advance, to paraphrase Delaware's former governor, Russell Peterson, into a better world by applying integrated approaches to pain management as our contribution to a meaningful legacy. According to Hippocrates, "The future is bright but fraught with difficulty." Some day we may have a dolometer or pain meter. In conclusion, according to Helen Keller, "Alone we can do little, together we do a lot."

This text is dedicated to all those who participate in these initiatives.

Pierre L. LeRoy, M.D., F.A.C.S.

Editor's Note

PAIN MANAGEMENT: A NEW APPROACH TO PAIN AND SUFFERING

We have entered a new millennium and indications are that we shall continue the odyssey and quest for affordable, quality pain management. We are witness to new emerging historic events. In 2001, the Joint Commission on Accreditation of Healthcare Organizations (JCAHO) published new Pain Management Standards. Hospitals, skilled nursing facilities, and other similar programs in the United States desiring JCAHO accreditation must comply with the new Pain Management Standards. The University of Integrated Studies became the first American University to provide distance education and degree granting (M.A. and Ph.D.) in Pain Management, and today more clinicians practice multidisciplinary pain management than ever. As a result of these trends, many people in pain can find improved care and there is renewed hope for further reduction of pain and suffering.

HISTORICAL TREATMENT OF PAIN

Throughout the millennia, problems associated with pain and attempts to control pain have historically been one of the principal reasons why individuals have sought health care. Alleviating pain is not a recent concern. Relief of suffering has been the helping profession's primary objective throughout time. However, the way we view pain and the treatments available have been altered considerably.

Individuals in prescientific cultures felt less control over their environment than is common in contemporary society. Consequently, people sought explanations and meaning for their lives in mystical, supernatural, or God-like concepts. The common thread was a feeling of very limited control over events. Attribution theory has been offered by social psychologists to explain coping mechanisms by which people ascribe a cause to an unpleasant event in the hope of establishing a difference between themselves and the "inflicted one." Such a process could comfort one into a belief of invulnerability. Thus, early men and women attributed pain to evil, at times vengeful, spirits who invaded the body of an unworthy host. However, these spirits were amenable to negotiation. Culturally differentiated rituals were used to exorcize the pain. That ancient communities paid great attention to the treatment of pain is suggested by one of the earliest vocational specialties developed by humanity: the medicine man or witch doctor. Throughout recorded history, the healer or reliever of pain was given a special status in his or her community.

Ancient healers or shamans practiced a sacred art and were viewed as catalysts who could negotiate with an angry God or who could, by ritual, restore balance with nature. In this orientation, intervention was possible, but the final outcome was not within the control of mortals. The context of the illness and pain represented more of a wholeness than presently exists in disease of the body, disease of the mind, or disease of the spirit. An illness affected the total person, who consisted of an integration of these components.

Philosophically, this concept changed when Descartes conceptually separated the body from the soul and described pain as a signal of mechanical dysfunctioning. As a result, narrow specialties, often fragmented and with little common language, developed. Although such an epistemological approach has resulted in great scientific breakthroughs in many areas of acute health care, it has often created a barrier in our understanding of intractable pain.

THE PROFESSIONAL ENVIRONMENT OF PAIN MANAGEMENT

Great strides have been made in our ability to help individuals who suffer from pain. We have gone beyond the historical method of providing treatment in which a sole practitioner works with a chronic pain patient. Interdisciplinary and multidisciplinary pain clinic facilities have demonstrated a new service delivery approach to pain management. There has been a phenomenal growth in the number and variety of inpatient and outpatient clinics. Professionals from several disciplines who work together have reintroduced an awareness that pain patients experience physical, emotional, interpersonal, financial, and spiritual problems. This reintegrated blend of art and science within the team concept helps establish the pain practitioner as a renaissance healer.

In 1988, the American Academy of Pain Management (AAPM) was incorporated so that clinical pain practitioners from all disciplines could work together for the purpose of developing standards for practice and codes of ethical conduct, and for the purpose of establishing a credentialing process for clinical pain practitioners.

CONTINUING EDUCATION

Many current pain management professionals entered the field without the benefit of specific formal graduate training in pain management. Clinicians completed a terminal degree — be that medicine, mental health, pharmacy, or one of the other therapies — and began practice. In recent years, in the United States, a select few physicians, primarily anesthesiologists, could avail themselves of a Fellowship in Pain Management.

In 2000, the AAPM developed a graduate curriculum that combined useful and practical information with the distance learning education format. A graduate committee composed of multidisciplinary clinicians and academicians developed a graduate program in Pain Studies. Graduate degrees (M.A. and Ph.D.) became available. As with the new JCAHO Pain Management Standards, the University of Integrated Studies presents evidence that the field of pain management has crossed a watershed.

EMERGING DISCIPLINE

The 6th edition of *Pain Management: A Practical Guide for Clinicians* represents a continuing commitment by the AAPM in assisting pain practitioners to more fully understand the art and science of pain management. The authors whose work is presented in this text are among the leaders in pain management. They write with a vision based on experience. The collection of their wisdom, represented here, is relevant for pain management clinicians and professionals from all disciplines who wish a consultative state-of-the-art resource for their practice. *Pain Management: A Practical Guide for Clinicians* is intended to be an updatable resource. Additional chapters will be written, and as new insights are gleaned from the real world of pain management, revisions will allow expansion, both increasing the value of this project and creating a living resource that will not soon become outdated.

Each chapter has been written to allow the reader to independently read topics of interest and thus may be viewed as a self-contained study. The collection of chapters allows an authoritative self-study on many of the pressing issues faced by pain practitioners. The writing style of each author has been left intact, further highlighting the unique contribution of each chapter to the total project.

The chapters and information presented may not represent any consensus of beliefs. We do not presuppose that all readers will agree with the sentiments that they find here, and some clinicians may disagree with others; however, we hold that by presenting this information, including divergent ideas, we provide a forum for discourse. It remains the clinician's responsibility to assure that all treatment is consistent with community standards, is lawful, and is approved for the condition being treated.

Although we have come a long way in our understanding of the impact of pain and in our ability to help reduce the toll of pain on the lives of our patients/clients, we have not yet eliminated the scourge of pain. It is my hope that this 6th edition will help illuminate our present ability and encourage future analysis.

CONCLUSION

Pain is a great leveler. Those in pain and those who suffer recognize that pain perception changes according to intensity, frequency, and duration. The multidisciplinary model remains the best hope for reducing pain and suffering as we integrate information from many disciplines to understand the whole patient. As we look ahead, past and present traveling together, we can envision the spirit of integration leading the world to a better time. The AAPM salutes multidisciplinary pain management professionals as early representatives helping to improve scientific, social, and ethical change affecting health policy in pain management. To that spirit, it is my hope that this edition will help illuminate the road we all travel.

Richard S. Weiner, Ph.D.
Executive Director
American Academy of Pain Management

Editorial Advisory Board

- Christopher R. Brown, D.D.S., M.P.S.
- B. Eliot Cole, M.D., M.P.A.
- Scott Denny, D.C., Ph.D., L.Ac.
- Arnold Fox, M.D.
- Paula L. Gilchrist, L.P.T., D.P.M.
- Jacob Green, M.D., Ph.D.
- Barbara Lum, B.S.
- Carl McNeely, A.P.R.N., P.N.P.
- Thomas Romano, M.D., Ph.D.
- Kathryn A. Weiner, Ph.D.

List of Contributors

Christine L. Algren, R.N., M.S.N., Ed.D.
Vanderbilt Children's Hospital
Nashville, TN

John T. Algren, M.D., F.A.A.P.
Vanderbilt Children's Hospital
Nashville, TN

Alfred V. Anderson, M.D., D.C.
Pain Assessment and Rehabilitation Center
Edina, MN

Lori T. Andersen, Ed.D., O.T.R./L.
Florida International University
Miami, FL

Elizabeth Ansel, R.N.
Pain Net, Inc.
Columbus, OH

James H. Ballard, D.Min., C.R.T.
The Wellness Center at Hickory Grove Baptist Church
Charlotte, NC

Robert L. Barkin, M.B.A., Pharm.D., F.A.C., N.H.A., D.A.A.P.M.
Rush Pain Center
Deerfield, IL

Stacy Barkin, M.A., M.Ed., Psy.D., D.A.A.F.C.
California School of Professional Psychology
Alliant University
San Diego, CA

Samira Kanaan Beckwith, A.C.S.W., L.C.S.W.
Hope Hospice
Ft. Myers, FL

Hal S. Blatman, M.D.
Private Practice
Cincinnati, OH

Mark V. Boswell, M.D., Ph.D.
University Hospitals of Cleveland
Cleveland, OH

James P. Boyd, D.D.S.
White Memorial Medical Center
Los Angeles, CA

David E. Bresler, Ph.D., L.Ac.
Academy for Guided Imagery
Mill Valley, CA

Clark Brill, M.D.
Maryland Spine and Sports Medicine
Columbia, MD

Christopher R. Brown, D.D.S., M.P.S.
Dental Diagnostic Services
Versailles, IN

Mary Ann Buchmeier, M.S., R.D.
Columbia Medical Plan Pain Management Group

Jan M. Burte, Ph.D., D.A.A.P.M.
Private Practice
Lido Beach, NY

C. Stephen Byrum, Ph.D.
Memorial Hermann Healthcare System
Houston, TX

Roger K. Cady, M.D.
Primary Care Network
Springfield, MO

Thomas C. Chelimsky, M.D.
University Hospitals of Cleveland
Cleveland, OH

Michael E. Clark, Ph.D.
James A. Haley Veterans Hospital
Tampa, FL

William Clewell, Ph.D.
University of Baltimore
Baltimore, MD

Misha Cohen, O.M.D., L.Ac.
Quan Yin Healing Arts Center
San Francisco, CA

B. Eliot Cole, M.D., M.P.A., F.A.P.A.
University of Integrated Studies
Sonora, CA

Richard H. Cox, M.D., Ph.D., D.Min.
Forest Institute of Professional Psychology
Springfield, MO

Jeffrey R. Cram, Ph.D.
Sierra Health Institute
Nevada City, CA

Jan Dommerholt, P.T., M.P.S.
Pain and Rehabilitation Medicine
Bethesda, MD

Stuart A. Dorow, M.D., D.C., Ph.D
Dorow's Chiropractic Clinic
Oklahoma City, OK

John Robert Essman, M.A., R.E.E.G./E.P.T., R.P.S.GT.
Forest Institute of Professional Psychology
Springfield, MO

Jan Fawcett, M.D.
Rush Medical College
Chicago, IL

Thomas Ferguson, Ph.D.
Columbia Medical Plan Pain Management Group

C. Kumerlal Fernando, M.A., L.P.T.
Island Rehabilitation
Marco Island, FL

Dale A. Ferranto, M.S.
California Department of Justice
San Clemente, CA

Arnold Fox, M.D.
Private Practice
Los Angeles, CA

Barry Fox, Ph.D.
University of Integrated Studies
Sonora, CA

Deborah Fralicker, R.N., D.C.
Southeastern Neuroscience Institute
Jacksonville, FL

R. Michael Gallagher, D.O., F.A.C.O.F.P., F.A.H.S.
School of Osteopathic Medicine
University of Medicine and Dentistry of New Jersey
Moorestown, NJ

Robert D. Gerwin, M.D.
The Johns Hopkins University School of Medicine
Baltimore, MD

Paula Lizak Gilchrist, L.P.T., D.P.M.
Dr. Gilchrist and Associates
Pittsburgh, PA

James Giordano, Ph.D.
Moody Health Center
Pasadena, TX

Ronald J. Gironda, Ph.D.
James A. Haley Veterans Hospital
Tampa, FL

Robert Gordon, B.S.(Ed.), B.S.(Bio.), D.C., D.A.A.P.M.
Cornerstone Professional Education, Inc.
Salisbury, NC

Jacob Green, M.D., Ph.D.
Southeastern Neuroscience Institute
Jacksonville, FL

Constance Haber, D.C.
Alternative Medicine Pain Management Center
Monroeville, PA

Gary M. Heir, D.M.D.
University of Medicine and Dentistry of New Jersey
Newark, NJ

Nelson H. Hendler, M.D., M.S.
Mensana Clinic
Stevenson, MD

A. R. Hirsch, M.D.
The Smell & Taste Treatment and Research Foundation
Chicago, IL

Bruce Hocking, D.Ac.
Acumed Medical
Toronto, Ontario, Canada

Linda C. Hole, M.D.
Center for Healing
Spokane, WA

Earl Horowitz, D.P.M.
Diabetic Foot Wound Center
Jacksonville, FL

Michael S. Jablon, M.S.T.
Advanced Ultrasound Imaging, LLC
Phoenix, AZ

Gary W. Jay, M.D., F.A.A.P.M., D.A.A.P.M.
Headache and Neuro-Rehabilitation Center
Lake Mary, FL

Julie Jolin, M.D.
UCLA Medical Center
Los Angeles, CA

Anne Marie Kelly, B.S.N., R.N.C.
Catholic Memorial Home
Fall River, MA

Daniel L. Kirsch, Ph.D., D.A.A.P.M.
Electromedical Products International
Mineral Wells, TX

Barbara L. Kornblau, J.D., O.T.R./L., F.A.O.T.A., D.A.A.P.M.
Nova Southeastern University
Ft. Lauderdale, FL

John Claude Krusz, M.D., Ph.D.
Private Practice
Dallas, TX

James S. Lapcevic, D.O., Ph.D., J.D., F.C.L.M.
Osteopathic Family Practice and Pain Management
Las Vegas, NV

Marilyn Lauffer, M.S., R.N.
Columbia Medical Plan Pain Management Group

Stephen A. Lawson, M.S., C.R.C., C.I.R.S.
Lawson Professional Counseling, Inc.
Riverbank, CA

W. David Leak, M.D., D.A.B.P.M.
Pain Net, Inc.
Columbus, OH

Pierre L. LeRoy, M.D., F.A.C.S.
Neurological Surgery and Pain Management Consultant
Newark, DE

Felix S. Linetsky, M.D.
University of South Florida College of Medicine
Tampa, FL
and
Assistant Professor
College of Osteopathic Medicine
Nova Southeastern University
Fort Lauderdale, FL
and
Private Practice
Palm Harbor, FL

Daniel C. Lobash, Ph.D., L.Ac.
Chinese Health Institute, KHT Systems
Hemet, CA

Timothy Lucey, B.S.
Lake Erie's College of Osteopathic Medicine, Student
Erie, PA

Richard Markoll, M.D., Ph.D.
Bio-Magnetic Therapy Systems, Inc.
Boca Raton, FL

Michael F. Martelli, Ph.D.
Concussion Care Centre of Virginia
Glen Allen, VA

Richard S. Materson, M.D.
Memorial Hermann Continuing Care Corporation
Houston, TX

Robert S. Matthews, M.D.
Mathews and Associates
Lancaster, PA

V. Robert May, Rh.D.
May Physical Therapy Services
National Association of Disability Evaluating
  Professionals
Richmond, VA

Rafael Miguel, M.D.
Professor and Chief of Anesthesiology Service
H. Lee Moffit Cancer Center
and
Director of Pain Management Fellowship Program
Professor of Anesthesia
University of South Florida College of Medicine
Tampa, FL

Mathew R. Miller, P.Ac..
Penn Orthopedics of Lancaster
Lancaster, PA

Keith Nicholson, Ph.D.
Toronto Western Hospital
Toronto, Ontario, Canada

Gretajo Northrop, M.D., Ph.D.
Southwest Blvd. Family Health Care
Kansas City, KS

Linda L. Norton, Pharm.D.
University of the Pacific School of Pharmacy and Health
  Sciences
Stockton, CA

Iva Lim Peck, L.Ac., Dipl.Ac., R.N.
Acupuncture and Aesthetics
Richardson, TX

Richard A. Peck, L.Ac., M.B.A.
Acupuncture and Aesthetics
Richardson, TX

Nick J. Piazza, Ph.D.
University of Toledo
Toledo, OH

Treven C. Pickett, A.B.D. Psy.D.
Concussion Care Centre of Virginia
Glen Allen, VA

Diane Polasky, M.A., M.H., D.O.M., Dipl.Ac., D.A.A.P.M.
Heights Acupuncture Center
Albuquerque, NM

John C. Porter, M.D.
Spine Health and Rehabilitation Center
Phoenix, AZ

Juliet Scotti Post, D.C.
Columbia Medical Plan Pain Management Group

Andrea J. Rapkin, M.D.
UCLA Medical Center
Los Angeles, CA

Anthony Rogers, M.D.
Private Practice
West Palm Beach, FL

Thomas J. Romano, M.D., Ph.D., F.A.C.P., F.A.C.R.
Private Practice
Wheeling, WV

Mary A. Romelfanger, R.N., M.S.N.
U.S. Office of Congregational Health Services for the
 Sisters of Charity Nazareth
Louisville, KY

Samuel K. Rosenberg, M.D.
University Hospitals of Cleveland
Cleveland, OH

Martin Rossman, M.D.
Academy for Guided Imagery
Mill Valley, CA

Ethan B. Russo, M.D.
Montana Neurobehavioral Specialists
Missoula, MT

Lloyd Saberski, M.D.
Yale–New Haven Hospital
New Haven, CT

Arnold Sandlow, D.C.
Sports Medicine and Rehabiliation Therapy Institute
Los Angeles, CA

Gabriel E. Sella, M.D., M.P.H., M.Sc., Ph.D., (Hon.C.), F.A.A.D.E.P., S.D.A.B.D.A., F.A.C.F.E., F.A.C.F.M., D.A.A.P.M.
Ohio Valley Disability Institute
Martins Ferry, OH

Harry Shabsin, Ph.D.
Columbia Medical Plan Pain Management Group

Afshin Alan Shargani, D.C.
Private Practice
Los Angeles, CA

C. Norman Shealy, M.D., Ph.D., D.Sc.
Holos Institutes of Health, Inc.
Springfield, MO

Richard A. Sherman, Ph.D.
Madigan Army Medical Center
Tacoma, WA

William D. Skelton, D.Ac.
The Center for Pain Management
Palmetto Baptist Medical Center
Columbia, SC

Devona J. Slater, C.M.C.P.
Auditing for Compliance and Education
Leawood, KS

Robert B. Supernaw, Pharm.D.
Texas Tech University Health Sciences Center at Amarillo
Amarillo, TX

Myrna C. Tashner, Ed.D.
State of Nevada Bureau of Disability Adjudication
Social Security Administration
Carson City, NV

Blake H. Tearnan, Ph.D.
Reno Spine Center
Reno, NV

Jane Tenberg, M.A.
Columbia Medical Plan Pain Management Group

Ole Thienhaus, M.D., M.B.A., F.A.P.A.
University of Nevada School of Medicine
Reno, NV

Robin Thomas, M.S., R.N., R.D.
Columbia Medical Plan Pain Management Group

Kathryn L. Tucker, J.D.
Perkins COIE LLP
Seattle, WA

Uday S. Uthaman, M.D., F.A.C.F.P.
Private Practice
Newark, DE

Clayton A. Varga, M.D.
Pasadena Rehabilitation Institute
Pasadena, CA

Steven D. Waldman, M.D., J.D.
Clinical Professor of Anesthesiology
Kansas City School of Medicine
University of Missouri
Leawood, KS

Michael I. Weintraub, M.D., F.A.C.P., F.A.A.N.
New York Medical College
Briarcliff, NY

Daniel T. West, D.C.
East Earl Chiropractic
East Earl, PA

Kathleen Wooding, M.A.
Columbia Medical Plan Pain Management Group

Victor John Yannacone, J.D.
Yannacone and Yannacone
Patchogue, NY

Anthony T. Yeung, M.D.
Arizona Orthopedic Surgeons
Phoenix, AZ

Nathan D. Zasler, M.D., F.A.A.P.M.&R., F.A.A.D.E.P., C.I.M.E., D.A.A.P.M.
Concussion Care Centre of Virginia
Glen Allen, VA

Chapter Consultants

- A. Elizabeth Ansel, R.N.
- Peter F. Chase, D.D.S.
- Arnold Fox, M.D.
- Bob L. Gant, Ph.D.
- Karin Hilsdale, Ph.D., L.Ac.
- Gary W. Jay, M.D.
- James S. Lapcevic, D.O., Ph.D., J.D.
- Michael K. Perry, C.R.N.A., Ph.D.
- Scott Raven
- Margaret Texidor, Ph.D.
- C. David Tollison, Ph.D.
- Tom Watson, M.Ed., P.T.

Section I

Pain in Perspective

1

Pain and Its Magnitude

Barry Fox, Ph.D.

Trying to estimate the size of the crowd at a large public gathering — such as a protest at the White House — can be difficult. People pour through the streets and parks; they do not stand still, they come and go. You cannot count the number of tickets sold or seats set out because there are neither tickets nor seats. The police give one estimate of the crowd size, the event's organizers another. Some people make "guesstimates" of crowd size by tallying up how many t-shirts or bags of popcorn were sold by vendors, or how much trash remains to be cleaned up.

Determining how many people suffer pain is also a difficult proposition. Lacking firm measuring sticks, health statisticians look to several indicators in order to develop reasonably accurate estimates of the numbers of people suffering from various types of chronic pain and the associated costs.

Unfortunately, even the "best" numbers from the most prestigious sources are only estimates. It is simply impossible to develop precise numbers, for many reasons. To begin with, we do not have a national health registration system, or a comprehensive national health database to track the numbers. Instead, the millions of people in this country are treated by a patchwork quilt of HMOs, private physicians, county hospitals, student health centers, etc., and we do not yet have a system to correlate the statistics from all these disparate entities. But even if we had a national system for tracking all complaints reported to physicians, we would not be able to account for those people who do not report their pain, preferring to ignore it, to self-treat, or to seek help from alternative health providers. To complicate matters more, there are differing ways of grouping types of pain. For example, some organizations have a very broad definition of arthritis, yielding

a greater number of arthritis sufferers, while other groups use a narrower, more restrictive definition that produces a smaller tally. One estimate of the number of people suffering from chronic pain will include those with cancer pain, while another will not.

Despite the many difficulties, several organizations have developed estimates of the magnitude of the problem in this country. According to the American Pain Foundation (APF) (2000), "over 50 million Americans suffer from chronic pain …," adding that another 25 million develop acute pain following surgery or injuries. The American Pain Society (APS) presents an expanded set of numbers, stating that while 50 million Americans suffer from chronic pain, an additional "25 million suffer with moderate-to-severe pain, and another 8 million suffer with cancer pain" (Pain Legislation, 2000). These figures, impressive as they are, may understate the problem. In the 1998 edition of this volume, Tollison noted that "some 75–80 million people in the United States are estimated to suffer chronic pain," adding that "this is generally considered a conservative estimate" (Tollison, 1998).

For seniors, pain can be a constant companion. The American Geriatrics Society estimates that "25% to 50% of older persons living in the community have pain problems," with 20% of older people taking pain medicines several times weekly (National Institutes of Health, 1998).

Let us set aside the abstract numbers for a moment to listen to some of the ways people describe their suffering: Aching, agonizing, beating, biting, burning, constant, cramping, crushing, cutting, darting, depressing, drilling, dull, excruciating, flickering, grinding, gripping, heavy, hot, intermittent, killing, light, mild, moderate, nagging, nauseating, numbing, piercing, pinching, pounding, pulsing, racking, radiating, ripping, sharp, shooting, sore,

0-8493-0926-3/02/$0.00+$1.50
© 2002 by CRC Press LLC

splitting, squeezing, stabbing, stinging, tearing, throbbing, thumping, tight, and tingling.

With such an extensive pain vocabulary, it is clear that the problem is significant. No matter whether the total number of people suffering from chronic pain is as high as 80 million or as "low" as 50 million, it is clear that the magnitude of the problem is great — and greatly troubling.

MILLIONS SUFFER FROM THE MAJOR "TYPES" OF PAIN

Chronic and intermittent pain comes in a variety of forms, most commonly joint pain, headaches, and back pain, and it may be triggered by a large number of diseases, conditions, and states, including arthritis, fibromyalgia, injuries, infection, cancer, trigemimal neuralgia, shingles, sickle cell disease, and angina. There is also the aching, burning pain of Central Pain Syndrome, which may develop after one has suffered a stroke or brain or spinal cord injury, developed multiple sclerosis, or had a limb amputated. Here are some estimates of the numbers of people suffering from some of the more common forms of pain:

- *Arthritis* — According to the National Institute of Arthritis and Musculoskeletal and Skin Diseases (1998), some 40 million Americans are afflicted by arthritis, "and many have chronic pain that limits daily activity." The total number of those suffering from arthritis is projected to reach 59 million by the year 2020. The Centers for Disease Control and Prevention (2001) give a slightly higher figure, stating "arthritis and related conditions have affected nearly 43 million Americans in 1998." The APF (2000) arrives at an even higher figure, estimating that "1 in 6 Americans suffers from arthritis." With a population of slightly over 284 million Americans as of May 2001 (U.S. Census Bureau, 2001), this means that some 47.3 million people have arthritis. Of them, 20.7 million suffer from osteoarthritis, the most common form of the disease, and 2.1 million have rheumatoid arthritis (National Institute of Arthritis, 1999).
- *Headaches* — According to the National Institute of Neurological Disorders and Stroke (NINDS, 2000b), "an estimated 45 million Americans experience chronic headaches. For at least half of these people, the problem is severe and sometimes disabling." The APF (2000) reports that more than 25 million Americans grapple with migraine headaches.
- *Back pain* — Over 25 million Americans aged 20 to 64 are hit with frequent back pain (APF, 2000). Over 5 million suffer from low back pain

so severe as to be disabling (Collacott, et al., 2000; American College of Rheumatology).* The Occupational Safety and Health Administration (1993) quotes the Bureau of Labor Statistics to report that "more than one million workers suffer back injuries each year."

- *Pelvic pain* — One out of every six women suffers from chronic pelvic pain (Adamson, 1998).
- *Cancer pain* — In 1999, the American Cancer Society estimated that "approximately 8.2 million Americans alive today have a history of cancer," and expected another 1.2 million new cases to be diagnosed that year. The Society (1998) further reports that "one out of every three being treated for cancer has related pain."
- *Jaw pain* — According to a report from The National Institute of Dental and Craniofacial Research, as many as 7.5 million Americans complain of pain in the face, or specifically in the jaw joint (Slavkin, 1996). The APF (2000) weighs in with a much higher number, stating that "20 million Americans experience jaw and lower facial pain (TMD/TMJ) each year."
- *Fibromyalgia* — Nearly 4 million Americans suffer from the pain of fibromyalgia (APF, 2000). Most of these are women.
- *Reflex Sympathetic Dystrophy Syndrome* — According to the Reflex Sympathetic Dystrophy Syndrome Association of American (2000), the severe burning pain and terrible sensitivity to touch seen with the regional pain syndrome afflict some 1.5 million people in this country. The Association describes the syndrome as being "pain-filled" and "under-treated."
- *Whiplash* — An editorial appearing in the *New England Journal of Medicine* notes that more than 1 million Americans suffer from a whiplash injury every year. Of those, 20 to 40% develop "symptoms that are sometimes debilitating and last for years (Carette, 1994)." The authors of an article in the *Archives of Neurology* offer a more conservative estimate of the lasting impact of whiplash, stating that "after 12 months, between 15% and 20% of patients remain symptomatic, and only about 5% are severely affected" (Bogduk & Teasell, 2000).
- *On the job injuries* — Reporting on work-related musculoskeletal disorders, the Occupational Safety & Health Administration ([OSHA], 1999) stated that "in 1996, more than 647,000 American workers experienced serious injuries due to overexertion or repetitive motion on the job."

---

* The American College of Rheumatology puts the number of Americans disabled at 5.4 million.

Just as we have difficulty determining the total number of people suffering from pain, we cannot pinpoint the precise number of people suffering from various "types" of pain (arthritis pain, back pain, headache pain, etc.). As you can see from the numbers above, sometimes reporting organizations are fairly close in their estimates, and other times they are far apart.

Even reasonably sound numbers put forth by advocacy organizations, such as the American Cancer Society or the Reflex Sympathetic Dystrophy Syndrome Association of American, may be attacked by those who argue that these organizations overstate the magnitude of the problem in order to draw more attention to the problem and/or to raise more money. In the same vein, critics can argue that government organizations such as the National Institute of Neurological Disorders and Stroke exaggerate the scope of a problem because it is the nature of government bureaucracies to view problems as being larger than they really are. Nevertheless, the problem is clearly dramatic, afflicting people from all walks of life.

THE DOLLAR COST OF PAIN

No one can put a price tag on a person's suffering, but we can make some estimates of the dollar cost of pain to the nation as a whole. As with the numbers of people in pain, the estimates vary.

- *Total Costs* — The APF (2000) reports that "pain costs an estimated $100 billion each year," and that over 50 million work days per year are lost to pain. The National Institute of Dental and Craniofacial Research weighs in with a lower figure, specifically for chronic pain, stating that "estimated annual costs — including direct medical expenses, lost income, lost productivity, compensation payments and legal fees — are close to $50 billion" (Slavkin, 1996).
- *Arthritis* — According to the Centers for Disease Control (2001), arthritis costs the nation "nearly $65 billion annually" and is the second leading cause of work disability. The Centers (1999) also report that "persons with arthritis and other rheumatic conditions accounted for 2.4% (approximately 744,000) of all hospital discharges and 2.4% (approximately 4 million) of days of care in 1997."
- *Back pain* — "Back pain is the leading cause of disability in Americans under 45 years old" (APF, 2000). Low back pain is responsible for more than 93 million lost workdays per year and "costs more than $5 billion in health care each year" (Slavkin, 1996). The American College of Rheumatology puts the costs of low

back pain at $16 billion a year. In an article appearing in the *Journal of the American Medical Association*, Collacott, et al. (2000) state that "the direct cost of treating low back pain is estimated at $15 billion, with indirect costs as high as $100 billion annually." The Bureau of Labor Statistics reports that back injuries are involved in 25% of all claims for workers compensation, "costing industry billions of dollars" (OSHA, 1993).
- *Headaches* — Headaches send people to their doctors for 8 million visits each year, and migraine headaches force people to lose more than 157 million workdays annually (NINDS, 2000). Some $4 billion goes to pay for headache medications every year (Slavkin, 1996).
- *Work-related musculoskeletal disorders* — The repetitive motion injuries, back pain, and other musculoskeletal problems suffered on the job are estimated to cost us between $13 billion and $20 billion annually in the form of compensation claims and lost work days (Steering Committee, 1999).

THE PERSONAL COST OF PAIN

We are all familiar with the *"watch out!"* pain that warns us, for example, that we've rested a hand on a hot stove or pushed the sewing needle just a little too far through the material and into a finger. We welcome this pain, which spurs us into taking immediately protective action. We have also experienced the *"next time you'll pay more attention"* pain that reminds us, for instance, not to leave our fingers between a rapidly closing door and the door jamb. We do not like either of these types of pain, but we understand their meaning and applaud their purpose.

Chronic pain, however, seems to have neither meaning nor purpose. Sometimes the cause of chronic pain is clear: cancer of the pancreas, for example, which has spread to the back. But oftentimes doctors and patients are baffled because the original condition has healed and the pain should have vanished. And, quite often, no one can determine why the pain developed in the first place.

Ultimately, there is no meaning to chronic pain. It is not a *"watch out!"* warning or a *"next time you'll pay more attention"* reminder. It may be telling us that tissue is being damaged, but it keeps telling us, long after we have received the message. Sometimes there is no damage for the chronic pain to be speaking about.

Long-lasting and lacking meaning, chronic pain can bring on the "'terrible triad' of suffering, sleeplessness and sadness" (NINDS, 2000a). When the "terrible triad" sets in, victims find it hard, sometimes impossible, to work. Certain movements may be difficult, even basic ones such as getting up out of bed or reaching for a glass.

Sleep may be disturbed, leading to constant fatigue and weariness. Irritability and depression may soon follow. The appetite may suffer, or the person may turn to food in an attempt to assuage distress. Hit by a pain that seems to strike without rhyme or reason, unable to find relief, perhaps told that "it's all in your head," chronic pain patients may lose hope.

Arnold Fox, M.D. (personal communication, September 12, 2000), Past President of the American Academy of Pain Management, speaks of the "Eight Ds" of chronic pain, the eight "side effects" he has seen in chronic pain patients. They are

1. *Depression* — Patients wind up feeling that there is no point in trying to get on with their lives.
2. *Distraction* — Victims focus on their pain so much that they may have difficulty handling other aspects of their lives.
3. *"Doctor Dancing"* — Patients go from one doctor to the next in their desperate search for relief.
4. *Disability* — People in pain may be unable to work or take care of themselves because of their physical or emotional symptoms. Compounding the problems, their muscles may weaken because of disuse.
5. *Disease* — Pain depresses the immune system, rendering us less able to fight off other illnesses.
6–7. *Drinking and Drugs* — Sufferers may go to great lengths in their attempts to block chronic pain.
8. *Death* — In some cases, suicide may appear to be the only way to end the suffering.

The Eight Ds may appear singly or in combination. They may attack when pain is new or after it has "settled in." In any case, they are devastating.

PROFILE OF PEOPLE IN PAIN

Everyone responds to pain uniquely, but it is possible to sketch pictures of some "typical" pain patients by looking at the results of a survey of 805 adult pain patients whose pain had lasted at least six months and was rated at "5" or more on a scale of 1 to 10, and who were not suffering from pain due to cancer (APS, 2000).

Over 50% of pain patients have been in pain for 5 years or more. Some 40% feel their pain is out of control. Just about all of them have gone to doctors looking for relief. Almost half have switched physicians at least once, primarily because they still hurt, and also because they do not feel their doctors know enough about pain and do not give the problem as much attention as it deserves. More than 20% have changed doctors three or more times for these same reasons.

Moderate to severe chronic pain takes a big bite out of quality of life. Eighty-one percent report that their pain has interfered with their ability to exercise; 79% report that it interferes with their ability to get a good night's sleep; 67% say it interferes with leisure activities and 65% with household chores; 59% report that it hampers walking; 54% report pain-related problems with sexual activity; 49% find that it hampers their ability to concentrate; and 41% say it hinders their ability to do their jobs. Emotional difficulties are triggered by uncontrolled pain. Thirty-five percent report irritability; 27% listlessness; 25% depression; 18% feelings of uselessness; 11% feeling unable to cope.

Chronic pain patients tend to feel that narcotic medications do the best job of providing relief, rating them at 7.6 on a scale of 0 to 10 (10 being total relief). Prescription NSAIDs are rated at 6.2 on the same scale, and over-the-counter medicines at 5.2. (Among those in very severe pain, the narcotics, NSAID, and OTC ratings were 7.4, 5.3, and 4.4, respectively.)

Seventy percent of the people report taking their medicines as prescribed by their physicians, but 21% say they do not follow their doctor's orders. The reasons for this include wishing to take their medicine only when they need it and wanting to decide how much they will take.

SLEEP AND PAIN

Lack of restful sleep is a common complaint among chronic pain patients. By one estimate, pain costs one third of all American adults 20 hours of sleep per month (APF, 2000). A study conducted at the University of California, San Francisco, School of Medicine utilized 24 oncology outpatients to examine the relationship between pain, sleep, and fatigue (Lamberg, 1999b). The researchers found that it took the pain patients four times longer to fall asleep, on average, than it takes healthy people. The pain patients awakened frequently. And while healthy controls had a mean sleep efficiency (time sleep compared to time in bed) of 90%, the pained subjects had a mean sleep efficiency of only 71%. In another measure of the effects of long-lasting pain on sleep, 141 patients reporting to Emory University's pain clinic were questioned: 127 of them had suffered from problems with sleep (Lamberg, 1999b). A Gallup survey conducted for the National Sleep Foundation found that one-quarter of American adults had their sleep disrupted by pain 10 nights or more every month — and headaches and back pain were the culprits cited most often. Many were able to sleep only 5 hours per night, on average, when pain struck (Lamberg, 1999a).

Arthritis patients also report difficulty in sleeping. When researchers at Texas Women's University in Denton surveyed 90 men and women with osteoarthritis or rheumatoid arthritis (Lamberg, 1999b), they found "high agreement with the statements, 'I often have trouble going to sleep' and 'Pain often awakens me.'"

Sleep studies conducted in the laboratory confirm that pain patients have sleep difficulties. Donald Bilwise, Ph.D., head of Emory University's Sleep Disorders Center, reports that "pain patients have more light sleep and less deep slow-wave sleep ... as well as more frequent brief arousals and more waking, or alpha brain activity in slow wave sleep than do healthy persons" (Lamberg, 1999a).

The disturbances in sleep patterns may be partially due to the pain itself, as well as accompanying anxiety and other emotional upset. Furthermore, many medicines used to treat pain can alter sleep patterns. For example, nonsteroidal anti-inflammatories can delay the onset of deep sleep, while steroids may decrease REM sleep (Lamberg, 1999a).

PAIN IS UNDERTREATED

Most authorities agree that a fair amount of pain is left undertreated. The National Institutes of Health report (1998) that up to "80% of nursing home residents may have substantial pain that is undertreated." The pain of cancer is "widely undertreated, even though it can be effectively controlled in up to 90 percent of all cancer patients," according to Philip Lee, M.D., Assistant Secretary for Health, Department of Health and Human Services, and Director of the Public Health Service (1994). Patients at the end of life are also at risk of suffering from inadequate pain management.

A 1999 survey released by the American Academy of Pain Medicine, the American Pain Society (APS) (1999), and Janssen Pharmaceutica found that "more than four out of every 10 people with moderate to severe chronic pain have yet to find adequate relief." Alarmingly, 56% of those with moderate to severe chronic pain have been hurting for over 5 years. Patients complain that their doctors are not able to relieve their pain, do not know enough about pain relief, and do not approach the problem aggressively or seriously enough.

Part of the problem is that we have no objective means of quantifying pain. No one can tell how your pain hurts you, or to what degree. X-rays may reveal that a bone is broken, and the presence of inflammation indicates that the body is fighting disease. But only you know if, where, and how much you hurt. It would be nice if doctors could say, for example: "Twenty sensory neurons in the patient's right little finger are signaling 18 units apiece of pressure pain; 20 times 18 equals a pain rating of 360." Unfortunately, we cannot do that because we do not know exactly how many sensory neurons each patient has in his or her body, how much stimulus is required before the nerves will begin firing off pain messages, and how patients'

emotions, psychological makeup, and past experiences affect the way their brains process pain messages.

The sensation of pain, for example, is determined to a surprising degree by a person's history of pain experience. A man who was terrified as a child after being attacked by a dog may find all dog bites extremely painful, no matter how objectively minor they may seem to a physician. Cultural attitudes or genetic makeup also may affect the way a person experiences pain. Several studies, for instance, have found that people of Nordic origin tend to be more stoic about expressing pain than are people of Jewish or Italian stock. Studies also point to differences in the way that northern and southern Italians view and respond to pain.

Soldiers fighting for a cause they hold dear are often able to shrug off pain that might force others who are less motivated to give in. But even soldiers fighting for the same cause may react differently to pain. After Allied troops stormed the Italian beach at Anzio in 1944, doctors noted that some soldiers with minor injuries reported severe pain, while others who were seriously injured registered few complaints. Likewise, athletes determined to win have shown a remarkable tolerance for bearing pain. A football player with a broken foot may run 90 yards for the touchdown without feeling any pain.

Factoring into the pain equation a person's attitudes toward pain, his fears, experiences, religious and cultural background, motivation, and other emotional and psychological factors is not yet possible. In the near future we will undoubtedly develop scanners that can count the number of sensory neurons in any part of the body, but we do not even know how to begin to measure the emotional and psychological influences on the brain's interpretation of pain. And, if we cannot agree on how acute pain should be measured, despite knowing exactly what causes the problem, how can we come to any consensus on measuring chronic pain that appears to have no objective cause, let alone set universal standards for treatment?

In the absence of objective means to measure pain, as well as generally accepted treatment guidelines, some doctors are worried that pain patients will become addicted should they be given "too much" of certain medications. Other physicians, along with some psychiatrists and psychologists, surmise that people whose pain will not respond to their ministrations are using the pain for "secondary gain," to gain sympathy or attention, for example. Or, they conclude, such people are not motivated to recover, are exaggerating their pain to get out of work or avoid responsibility, are addicted to pain-killing medications, or suffer from mental or emotional conditions.

Some patients undoubtedly invent or exaggerate pain symptoms for various reasons. But the overwhelming majority of pain patients suffer from real pain. And they want to be cured.

REFERENCES

Adamson, G.D. (1998). Chronic pelvic pain: Evaluation and management, and Chronic pelvic pain: An integrated approach (book review). *New England Journal of Medicine, 339*(17). http://www.nejm.org/content/1998/0339/0017/1252.asp

The American Cancer Society. (2001, August 2). ACS news today: Managing pain, http://www2.cancer.org/zine/Index.cfm?fn=004_12101998-0

The American Cancer Society. (1999). 1999 facts and figures: Cancer: Basic facts. http://www.cancer.org/statistics/cff99/basicfacts.html, viewed September 9, 2000.

American College of Rheumatology. Fact sheet: Back pain. http://www.rheumatology.org/patients/factsheet/backpain.html

American Pain Foundation. (2000). Fast facts about pain. http://www.painfoundation.org/medres/medresfacts.tmpl

American Pain Society. (2000, February 17). Chronic pain in America: Roadblocks to relief: Survey highlights. http://www.ampainsoc.org/whatsnew/summary030499.htm

American Pain Society. (1999, February 17). New survey of people with chronic pain reveals out-of-control symptoms, impaired daily lives. http://www.ampainsoc.org/whatsnew/release030499.htm

Bogduk, N., & Teasell, R. (2000, April). Whiplash: The evidence for an organic etiology. *Archives of Neurology, 57*, 590.

Carette, S. (1994, April 14). Whiplash injury and chronic neck pain [Editorial]. *New England Journal of Medicine, 330*(15), 1083–1084.

Centers for Disease Control and Prevention. (1999, May 7). Morbidity and mortality weekly report, *48*(17). Atlanta, GA: Centers for Disease Control and Prevention.

Centers for Disease Control and Prevention. (2001). Arthritis: The nation's leading cause of disability. http://www.cdc.gov/nccdphp/arthritis/index.htm

Collacott, E., et al. (2000). Bipolar permanent magnets for the treatment of chronic low back pain. *Journal of the American Medical Association, 283*(10), 1322.

Lamberg, L. (1999a). Chronic pain linked with poor sleep: Exploration of causes and treatment. *Journal of the American Medical Association, 281*(8), 691–692.

Lamberg, L. (1999b). Patients in pain need round-the-clock care. *Journal of the American Medical Association, 281*(8), 689–690.

National Institute of Arthritis and Musculoskeletal and Skin Diseases. (1998, January). Questions and answers about arthritis pain. http://www.nih.gov/niams/healthinfo/arthpain.htm

National Institute of Neurological Disorders and Stroke. (2000a, June 23) Chronic pain — Hope through research. http://www.ninds.nih.gov/health_and_medical/pubs/chronic_pain_htr.htm

National Institute of Neurological Disorders and Stroke. (2000b, July 27). Headache — Hope through research. http://accessible.ninds.nih.gov/health_and_medical/pubs/headache_htr.htm

National Institutes of Health. (1998, April). Gender and pain: Future directions. http://www1.od.nih.gov/painresearch/genderandpain/future.htm

Occupational Safety and Health Administration. (1999, February). Preventing work-related musculoskeletal disorders. http://www.osha-slc.gov/SLTC/ergonomics/ergofactnew.html

Occupational Safety and Health Administration. (1993, January 1). OSHA fact sheets: 01/01/1993 – Back injuries – Nation's number one workplace safety problem. http://www.osha-slc.gov/OshDoc/Fact_data/FSNO93-09.html

Pain Legislation S. 941/H.R. 2188 and H.R. 2260/S. 1272. Office of Legislative Policy and Analysis. Bethesda, MD.

Public Health Service (1994, March 2). AHCPR releases cancer pain treatment guidelines.

Reflex Sympathetic Dystrophy Syndrome Association of America. (2000, March 17). RSDSA Publishers Objective Evidence of RSD/CRPS. http://www.rsds.org/objective_evidence.htm

Slavkin, H. (1996). Insights on human health: What we know about pain. National Institute of Dental Research. http://www.nidr.nih.gov/slavkin/pain.htm

Steering Committee for the Workshop on Work-Related Musculoskeletal Injuries: The Research Base, National Research Council. Commission on Behavioral and Social Sciences and Education. (1999). *Work-related musculoskeletal disorders: Report, workshop summary, and workshop papers.* Washington, D.C.: National Academy Press.

Tollison, C.D. (1998). Pain and its magnitude. In R.S. Weiner (Ed.), *Pain management: A practical guide for clinicians* (5th ed., pp. 3–6). Boca Raton, FL: St. Lucie Press.

U.S. Census Bureau. (2001). Population clocks, 15:39 EDT May 23, 2001. http://www.census.gov.

2

Historical Perspective of Pain Management

C. Norman Shealy, M.D., Ph.D., D.Sc. and Roger K. Cady, M.D.

Most people fear death less than they fear continuing pain. Indeed, many individuals who commit suicide during terminal or potentially fatal illnesses do so to avoid pain themselves and philosophically to spare their families psychological suffering. Bonica (1990, p. 2) has estimated that 15 to 20% of the population has acute pain and 25 to 30% has some form of chronic pain. The Nuprin Pain Report (1986) suggests that pain affects a huge majority of Americans each year. Obviously, any consideration of pain has to begin with an understanding that pain is a natural part of life and has been a major factor in human development throughout time. Prehistorical evidence through archeological findings suggests that the most primitive of populations suffered from diseases which would be expected to involve pain, and in the history of every civilization of the world, there are numerous references to the plague of pain. The concept of counter-stimulation through rubbing, massaging, or pressure on painful points or around painful areas probably has been used throughout history. Theory and management have indeed evolved together.

At least 4500 years ago, the Chinese already had a well-developed system of pain management–acupuncture. Competent pain medicine clinicians today recognize that acupuncture remains one of the most powerful treatments for both acute and chronic pain. Although we are not certain of the details involved, it is clear that the Chinese used herbs and, very early in their history, opioids or narcotics.

The Egyptians chronologically stand next in line in recorded history. The Egyptians appear to have believed that pain was inflicted by either a god or a disincarnate spirit, and, as in India, the Egyptians considered the heart to be the center of sensation. The ancient Indians attached

much more significance to the emotional roots of pain. Looking forward in history, the ancient Greeks introduced the concept that the brain is the organ in which sensation becomes conscious, although that concept, introduced by Alcmaeon, was vigorously fought by Aristotle, who considered the heart the center of sensation. Hippocrates, the "father of medicine," had a concept that was very similar to the Chinese theory of five elements, except that the Chinese included only four humors: blood, phlegm, yellow bile, and black bile. An excess or deficiency of one of the humors was supposed to lead to pain. Eventually, the reality of the brain as the seat of sensation was recognized, and it was the ancient Greeks who demonstrated that the brain and the peripheral nerves were intimately connected and that there were two types of nerves: those for muscle control and those for sensation. Ancient Rome added relatively little to the concept of pain, but Galen demonstrated the central and peripheral nervous system as well as cranial and spinal nerves and sympathetic trunks. Even so, Galen continued to follow Aristotle's concept of pain as "a passion of the soul."

The center of civilization moved to Arabia approximately 1000 years ago, where Avicenna described 15 different types of pain and treatment, including exercise, heat, massage, opium, and other natural herbal remedies. Paracelsus, who died only 450 years ago, advocated the use of opium and natural herbs, but added various electrical stimulation techniques, massage, and exercise.

Remarkably, even William Harvey, who described the circulation of the blood, considered the heart to be the site where pain was felt. Descartes, who is often attacked by holistic philosophers as the individual who tore the body and mind apart, nevertheless made great contributions to the concept of pain. Unfortunately, as was true of much

0-8493-0926-3/02/$0.00+$1.50
© 2002 by CRC Press LLC

early philosophy, he was rather inaccurate. He considered that pain was a direct transfer through a tubular structure and that strong impulses were transferred directly from the periphery to the brain. He is credited with essentially creating the first "specialty" therapy for pain transmission.

Although opium and, undoubtedly, alcohol were used as analgesics from very early times, exorcism and various religious ceremonies were also an integral aspect of pain control in many cultures. Nevertheless, many early cultures used surgical trephination of the skull for headache, and acupuncture, moxibustion, massage, physical exercise, and diet have all been used for pain control in a variety of cultures. In ancient Egypt, Greece, and Rome, electric shock was used for the treatment of gout, headache, and neuralgia through the use of the electric fish.

The first major innovation in pain treatment in almost 2000 years occurred in the late 18th century when Joseph Priestley introduced nitrous oxide, and it was later found to be a significant analgesic. Throughout the 19th century, great progress was made in neurophysiology in general and pain physiology in particular. Johannes Muller introduced "The Doctrine of Specific Nerve Energies" in 1840.

Other important 19th century innovations were the isolation of morphine from crude opium; the discovery of codeine, aspirin, ether, and cocaine (especially as a local anesthetic); needles and syringes; hypnosis; the first neurological procedures for ablation of peripheral nerves of the spinal cord in the management of pain; electrotherapy, hydrotherapy, and diathermy; and the introduction of the X-ray, for both diagnostic and therapeutic purposes.

During the middle to latter portion of the 19th century, the specificity theory became the dominant concept of most scientists. Just as Galen, Avicenna, Descartes, and Muller had theorized, specificity seemed to consolidate the idea of specific pathways and specific receptors for pain. It is interesting that as early as 1858, Schiff had demonstrated analgesia by sectioning the anterior quadrants of the spinal cord of an animal, and it was over 50 years later that a clinician in Philadelphia introduced the concept of spinal cordotomy in the human being. von Frey (1894) discovered specific end organ receptors for pain and touch and expanded Muller's concept to include warmth and cold.

The origin of the pattern theory, another dominant pain theory, was introduced by Goldscheider (1894), who believed that certain patterns of nerve activation were produced by summation of sensory input from the skin in the dorsal horn. This theory was further formalized when Nafe (1934) introduced the concept that all sensation is the result of spatial and temporal patterns of nerve impulses rather than the result of specific receptors or pathways. Building upon this, Sinclair (1955) and Weddell (1955) emphasized that all fiber endings, except those innervating hair follicles, are similar and that it is only the pattern that is important in sensory discrimination. Unfortunately, both the specificity and the pattern theories were incomplete.

Hardy, Wolff, and Goodell (1952) objected to the pattern and specificity theories and insisted that there was a difference between reception of pain and reaction to pain. They, perhaps more than any others of their time, introduced the concept of major cognitive, psychological, and emotional factors as important in chronic pain management. There are numerous other minor theories related to pain, but the next major innovation and the one that sparked the most intense change in the management of pain in the past 5000 years was gate control.

Melzack and Wall (1965) introduced the theory that the information coming in over C-fibers was modulated through presynaptic inhibition from incoming beta fibers in the substantia gelatinosa. This "gating" mechanism depends upon the relative quantity of information coming in over the larger fibers versus the smaller fibers. Thus, there are two major ways in which pain "gets through" the gate: either through damage to the beta fibers, which allows spontaneous pain or sensory deprivation pain, or by activation of the C-fibers by excess stimulation through inflammation or pressure upon the C-fibers (Figure 2.1).

Later work by Shealy (1966) physiologically demonstrated that approximately 60% of C-fiber activity was crossed to the opposite side (Figure 2.1) of the spinal cord and distributed fairly diffusely in all parts of the spinal cord except the dorsal columns. That is, 60% of the total volume of central distribution of C-fiber activation goes contralaterally, not into the spinothalamic tracts but through the entire gray and white matter of the cord other than the dorsal columns, and 40% is similarly distributed ipsilaterally. Strong stimulation of beta fibers is capable of inhibiting at this initial gate the activity from the dorsal columns (Shealy & Tyner, 1966; Shealy & Taslitz, 1967).

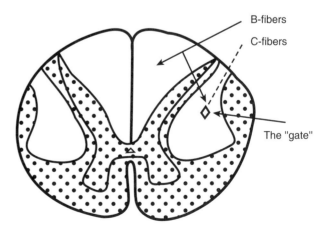

FIGURE 2.1 The dorsal columns are "pure" projections of beta fibers. The gate is closed by increased input of beta fibers and opened by excessive C-fiber activity.

It appears that the major contribution to the spino-thalamic tracts is the input from the gamma-delta fibers, which primarily bring in acute or sharp brief pain as well as touch, vibratory sensation, etc. The dominant role of the dorsal columns seems to be similar to an FM radio station, modulating input from the other sensory fibers.

Shealy (Shealy, Resnick, & Tyner, 1966; Shealy & Taslitz, 1967), after discussing the gate control theory with Wall and Melzack, reasoned that stimulation of the dorsal columns would conceivably antidromically inhibit the gate, and he demonstrated this initially in animals and later in humans. Both Melzack and Wall, in their original theory, emphasized that there were descending controls of the gates coming from the cortex and other central brain locations, as well as the peripheral control through the beta fibers. Shealy, Mortimer, and Resnick (1967) had demonstrated adequate safety of long-term stimulation of the dorsal columns, in cats and monkeys, to insert the first dorsal column stimulator in a human suffering from terminal metastatic cancer.

In 1967, Shealy resurrected an old external electrical stimulator, the Electreat™, and began encouraging the engineers at Medtronic, Inc. to make a modern solid-state electrical stimulator. Shealy, working in collaboration with Long, and each working independently, prompted Norman Hagfers (who left Medtronic to form StimTec, Inc.) and Donald Maurer (at that time still with Medtronic) to produce the first two solid-state transcutaneous electrical nerve stimulators. Shealy had already demonstrated that the two most useful types of electric current for pain relief were the spike and the square wave. Various transcutaneous electrical nerve stimulation devices were introduced in the early 1970s, using both square waves and spikes, although most devices currently use some form of modified square wave. The largest known collection of material related to the use of electrical stimulation for various purposes is at the Bakken Library of Electricity and Light (5337 Zenith Avenue, South Minneapolis, MN 55416); Earl Bakken is one of the co-founders and is the chief executive of Medtronic, Inc.

In 1969, following Shealy's presentation of the results of his first eight cases of dorsal column stimulation, a national Dorsal Column Study Group was formed. Its purpose was to have a number of neurosurgeons do the procedure and monitor the results over a 5-year period. William H. Sweet, former Chairman of the Department of Neurosurgery at Massachusetts General Hospital, declined joining the Dorsal Column Study Group, and as a result, two companies began manufacturing dorsal column stimulators, Medtronic and Avery. During the next few years, the Dorsal Column Study Group inserted approximately 480 dorsal column stimulators. In the fall of 1972, Avery began advertising dorsal column stimulators as a therapeutic technique for use by all neurosurgeons, and Medtronic followed suit in the spring of 1973.

Unfortunately, in going from a research project to a clinical application, the design of the electrodes was changed from a solid platinum plate to a tinsel wire electrode. The solid platinum plate electrodes had proven remarkably sturdy and efficacious. Numerous problems developed with the tinsel wire electrodes, which seemed to polarize and develop increased impedance or break fairly easily. The thickness of the machine-made electrodes was also greater than that of the solid platinum plate, which led to increased technical difficulties. As a result, Shealy permanently stopped doing dorsal column simulation in 1974 because he reasoned that the technology had not been adequately researched to make the procedure widely useful clinically. In his first paper on dorsal column stimulation, Shealy had emphasized the possibility of inserting dorsal column stimulators percutaneously, and it is worth noting that a variety of percutaneous dorsal column stimulators available today have less risk than the totally surgically implanted ones that require a laminectomy. Nevertheless, the long-term success rate is so poor that Shealy still considers dorsal column stimulation to be a technique that is rarely indicated and then only in extremely desperate situations.

The same year that Shealy presented his first paper on the experimental results of dorsal column stimulation, Fordyce (1966) introduced the concept of behavioral modification or operant conditioning for management of pain.

In 1970, Shealy recognized that he was selecting only 6% of the patients sent to him for dorsal column stimulation and began investigating the possibility of alternative solutions to pain management in the vast majority of such patients. In 1971, he visited Fordyce's program. Fordyce had treated approximately 100 patients with his 2-month in-patient behavioral modification program, working with up to 25 patients at a time. In 1972, Shealy organized a national meeting on the management of pain, which some 400 individuals attended. As a result of that meeting, several physicians set up similar multidisciplinary comprehensive pain clinics, modeled after the Shealy system. Over the next few years, increasing numbers of physicians established various types of pain clinics.

In 1976, *Medical World News* presented a cover article entitled "Management of Pain, Medicine's New Growth Industry." The article suggested that there were approximately 50 pain clinics in the U.S., 20 of which *Medical World News* considered "holistic," with others based upon the Bonica model. After the cover article appeared, pain clinics indeed did become one of medicine's growth industries. By 1977, Bonica reported at the Walter Reed Pain Symposium that there were some 800 pain clinics in the U.S.

Shealy and Shealy's (1976) active behavioral modification program was transformed in 1974 to place greater emphasis on biofeedback, autogenic training, and self-regulation techniques as a major modality for changing behavior. Although there have been some refinements in techniques and technology in the last two decades, there has been no further major innovation in the management of pain. Thus, as we move toward the next millennium, it is worth noting the quantum leaps in the management of pain made in the latter part of the 19th century through the introduction of transcutaneous and percutaneous electrical nerve stimulation, to some extent implanted electrical stimulators, and the use of biofeedback, autogenic training, and related techniques for behavioral modification.

The innovations in pain management sparked by the gate control theory have also led to a number of new organizations and pain-related publications. Perhaps one of the most interesting aspects of modern life is that at the end of the 20th century, the National Institutes of Health has recognized acupuncture as a useful modality in the management of pain!

Some major American-based organizations related to pain are:

- American Association for the Study of Headache
- International Association for Study of Pain
- American Pain Society (regional pain societies, e.g., Eastern, Midwestern)
- American Academy of Pain Medicine (originally American Academy of Algology)
- American Academy of Pain Management
- Some major publications related to pain are
  - *Pain*
  - *Headache*
  - *Clinical Journal of Pain*
  - *Anesthesia & Analgesia — Current Research*
  - *Pain Practitioner*
  - *The American Journal of Pain Management*

A summary of the history of development of pain treatment is provided in Table 2.1.

TABLE 2.1
The History of Pain Treatment

2600 + B.C.

Acupuncture
Massage
Exercise
Opium

TABLE 2.1 (CONTINUED)
The History of Pain Treatment

Alcohol
Herbs
Witch doctors
Medicine men
Prayer
Exorcism
Sacrifices
Religious ceremonies

18th Century

Mesmerism
Electrotherapy (crude)

19th Century

Nitrous oxide (in medical and dental field in 1863)
Hypnosis
Muller's specificity theory
Morphine
Codeine
Aspirin (introduced in 1899 by Dreser)
Diethyl ether (1846)
Needle/syringe
Cocaine (1884)
Opioid narcotics
    Opium (1806 by Serturner)
    Codeine (1832 by Robiguet)
    Papaverine (1848 by Merck)
Local anesthetics (cocaine)
Physical therapy
Hydrotherapy
Thermotherapy (diathermy)
Mechanotherapy
X-ray for diagnosis and therapy
Electrotherapy

20th Century

Procaine (introduced in 1905 by Einhorn)
Pattern theory
Cordotomy
Lobotomy
Gate control theory
Dorsal column stimulation
Transcutaneous electrical nerve stimulation
Biofeedback
Operant conditioning
Multidisciplinary pain clinics
Neurotomy/neurectomy
Modern anesthetics
Narcotic agonists/antagonists
Nonsteroidal anti-inflammatories
Steroids
Thalamic stimulation
Serotonin-altering drugs
Acupuncture approved by NIH

REFERENCES

Bonica, J. J. (1990). *The management of pain* (2nd ed., Vol. 1). Philadelphia: Lea & Febiger.

Fordyce, W. (1966). *Behavioral models for chronic pain and illness.* St. Louis: C.V. Mosby.

Goldscheider, A. (1894). *Ueber den schmerz im physiologischer und klinischer hinsicht.* Berlin: Hirschwald.

Hardy, J. D., Wolff, H. G., & Goodell, H. (1952). *Pain sensations and reactions.* Baltimore: Williams & Wilkins.

Management of chronic pain, medicine's new growth industry. (Editorial). (1976, October 18). *Medical World News, 54.*

Melzack, R., & Wall, P. D. (1965). Pain mechanisms: A new theory. *Science, 150,* 871.

Nafe, J. P. (1934). The pressure, pain, and temperature senses. In C. A. Murchison (Ed.), *Handbook of general experimental psychology.* Worcester, MA: Clark University Press.

Nuprin Pain Report (1986). A national study conducted for Nuprin by Louis Harris & Associates, New York.

Shealy, C. N. (1966). The physiological substrate of pain. *Headache, 6,* 101–108.

Shealy, M. C., & Shealy, C. N. (1976). Behavioral techniques in the control of pain: A case for health maintenance vs. disease treatment. In M. Weisenberg & B. Tursky (Eds.), *Pain: New perspectives in therapy and research* (pp. 21–33). New York: Plenum Press.

Shealy, C. N., Mortimer, J. T., & Resnick, J. B. (1967). Electrical inhibition of pain by dorsal column stimulation: Preliminary clinical report. *Anesthesia and Analgesia—Current Research, 46,* 489–491.

Shealy, C. N., Taslitz, N., Mortimer, J. T., & Becker, D. P. (1967). Electrical inhibition of pain: Experimental evaluation. *Anesthesia and Analgesia—Current Research, 46,* 299–305.

Shealy, C. N., Tyner, C. F., & Taslitz, N. (1966). Physiological evidence of bilateral spinal projections of pain fibers in cats and monkeys. *Journal of Neurosurgery, 24,* 708–713.

Sinclair, D. C. (1955). Cutaneous sensation in the doctrine of specific nerve energy. *Brain, 78,* 584.

von Frey, M. (1894). Ber. Verhandl. konig. sachs. Ges. Wiss. Leipzig. *Beitrage zur Physiologie des Schmerzsines, 46,* 185, 188.

Weddell, G. (1955). Somesthesis in chemical senses. *Annual Review of Psychology, 6,* 119.

ANNOTATED BIBLIOGRAPHY

Abbe, R. (1911). Resection of posterior roots of spinal nerves to relieve pain, pain reflex, athetosis, and spastic paralysis—Dana's operation. *Medical Records (New York), 79,* 377–381.

The first spinal rhizotomies were done by Abbe.

Anstie, F. E. (1873). Papers on electrotherapy. 1. On the relations of faradic electricity to pain. *The Practitioner: A Journal, 2351–2360.*

Francis E. Anstie published an article on the relations of faradic electricity to pain in London in 1873.

Behan, R. J. (1922). *Pain: Its origin, conduction, perception, and diagnostic significance.* New York: Appleton and Co.

This is a good early treatise.

Bonica, J. J. (1967). Management of intractable pain. In E. L. Way (Ed.), *Concepts of pain* (pp. 155–167). Philadelphia: Davis.

Bonica has emphasized the necessity for the use of a nerve block to determine if the surgical procedure would yield the desired results.

Bonica, J. J. (1976, January). Recent studies on the nature and management of acute pain. *Hospital Practice,* 6–7.

According to John Bonica, the use of narcotics as analgesics for nonsurgical pain and for surgical anesthesia goes back "2,000, 3,000 or 4,000 years." Morphine was isolated 170 years ago.

Bonica, J. J. (1990). *The management of pain* (2nd ed., Vol. 1). Philadelphia: Lea & Febiger.

"There is only one pain that is easy to bear," said the French surgeon Rene Leriche, "and that is the pain of others."

Braunwald, E., Epstein, S. E., Glick, G., Wechsler, A. S., & Braunwald, W. S. (1967). Relief of angina pectoris by electrical stimulation of the carotid-sinus nerves. *New England Journal of Medicine, 227,* 1278–1283.

Perhaps the first use of implanted stimulators for relief of pain was that of carotid sinus nerve stimulation which relieved the pain of angina.

Brockbank, W. (1954). *Ancient therapeutic arts.* London: Heinemann.

The Eber's Papyrus, written about 1500 B.C., has one of the first written records of treatment for pain. For "suffering in the abdomen," they recommended an enema of oil and honey. It is interesting to note that at the Massachusetts General Hospital, when I was a resident, milk and molasses enemas were sometimes recommended.

Cupping seems to have been practiced in primitive cultures for thousands of years, and Hippocrates mentions it as being practiced in 400 B.C. The American Indians used a buffalo horn for cupping. Leeching is mentioned at least 200 years B.C. and was an important part of medical and lay healing technique for many centuries. In fact, it is still done in some Third World countries. Blistering also seems to have been used for many years, and written accounts of the use of blistering appear in the 2nd century.

Hippocrates is quoted as having said, "Those diseases which medicines do not cure, iron cures [meaning the knife]. Those which iron cannot cure, fire cures, and those which fire cannot cure to be reckoned wholly incurable."

Fordyce, W. E. (1976). *Behavioral methods for chronic pain and illness.* St. Louis: C.V. Mosby.

Fordyce created the concept of behavioral responses of operant conditioning as the major underlying causes for pain. The Fordyce concept is that pain is a learned or conditioned response to a given stimulus or "operant" condition. "Respondents can therefore be said to be controlled by antecedent stimuli. Operants, on the other hand, in contrast, are responsive to the influence of the consequences that systematically follow their occurrence. Operants can and do occur as a direct and automatic response to antecedent stimuli, as is true of respondents." In other words, punishment vs. reward benefits from particular behaviors determine whether or not they are learned and become part of the individual.

Fordyce, W. E. (1988, April). Pain and suffering: A reappraisal. *American Psychologist*, 276–283.

Fordyce emphasizes in particular the difference between pain and suffering.

Francois-Franck, C. A. (1899). Signification physiologique de la resection du sympathique dans la maladie de basedow, l'epilepsie, l'idiotie et le glaucome. *Bulletin. Academie de Medecine (Paris), 46*, 565–594.

Sympathectomy for relief of pain was introduced by Francois-Franck.

Garrison, F. H. (1929). *History of medicine* (4th ed.). Philadelphia: Saunders.

The pattern theory has been supported by Weddell and Sinclair. A neurologist, Spiller, noted a patient with a tuberculoma of the anterior lateral quadrant of the spinal cord who lacked pain sensation on the opposite side of the body. He encouraged Frazier, a neurosurgeon, to perform a cordotomy in 1899. It was Frazier who also began sectioning roots of the fifth nerve for trigeminal neuraligia in 1901.

Hammond, B. J. (1965). A history of electric therapy: Part one. *World Medical Electronics, 3*, 44,

In 1551, Jerome Cardan differentiated between the electricity of amber and the magnetism of lodestone and introduced a "fluid therapy of electricity," which is accepted as marking the transition from supernational to physical accounts of the phenomenon.

Horsley, V., Taylor, J., & Colman, W. S. (1891). Remarks on the various surgical procedures device and the relief or cure of trigeminal neuraltic ("tic douloureux"). *British Medical Journal, 2*, 1139–1143, 1891A; 2, 1191–1193, 1891B; 2, 1249–1252, 1891C.

Victory Horsley, the great British neurosurgeon, introduced the concept of gasserian neurectomy in 1891.

Jenkner, F. L., & Schuhfried, F. (1981). Transdermal and transcutaneous electric nerve stimulation for pain: The search for an optimal wave form. *Applied Neurophysiology, 44*(5–6), 330–337.

The question of the optimal waveform for electrical stimulation has never been adequately settled. Jenkner has emphasized what he considers to be an optimal waveform.

Kellaway, P. (1946). The part played by electric fish in the early history of bioelectricity and electrotherapy. *Bulletin of Historic Medicine, 20*, 112–137.

This is a marvelous article on the role of the electric fish and was the William Osler Medal Essay. The author comments that even in the early days in the U.S., electric fish were used and often kept in tanks on plantations to be used for pain control, and these were "much favored by the Indians and the Negros."

Letievant, J. J. E. (1873). *Traite des sections nerveuses: Physiologie pathologique, indications, procedes operatoires.* Paris: Balliere.

Apparently the first book on surgery pain was written by Letievant in 1873 and was primarily concerned with neurectomies for neuralgias of the face and extremities.

Lytle, L. D., Messing, R. B., Fisher, L., & Phebus, L. (1975). Effects of long-term corn consumption on brain serotonin and the response to electric shock. *Science, 190*, 692–694.

Hyperalgesia, which appears with tryptophan deficiency (serotonin deficiency), is well discussed in this article.

Mann, F. (1971). *Acupuncture: The ancient Chinese art of healing.* London: William Heinemann.

The oldest records of acupuncture date to bone etchings of 1600 B.C., and the first book on acupuncture was written about 200 B.C.

Medtronic Neuro Division. (1983). A newsletter published by Medtronic, Inc., Minneapolis, MN,

An extensive bibliography on transcutaneous electrical nerve stimulation was published by the Medtronic Neuro Division in March 1983.

Melzack, R., & Wall, P. D. (1965). Pain mechanisms: A new theory. *Science, 150*(3699), 971–979.

It was the advent of the gate control theory by Melzack and Wall which really revolutionized modern pain therapy. Their theory incorporates both physiological specialization as well as central summation and input control. Basically, they believe that at the level of the substantia gelatinosa in the spinal cord, input over the smallest fibers, C-fibers, is presymmetrically inhibited by information coming over the larger beta fibers. Beta fiber stimulation never creates a painful sensation, whereas unopposed C-fiber sensation is perceived as very agonizing pain.

Mitchell, S. W. (1872). *Injuries of nerves and their consequences.* Philadelphia: Lippincott.

"Perhaps few persons who are not physicians can realize the influence which long continued and unendurable pain may have upon both body and mind."

Mortimer, J. T. (1968). *Pain suppression in man by dorsal column electroanalgesia.* Unpublished Ph.D. dissertation. School of Engineering, Case Western University, Cleveland, OH.

The subject of pain has been likened by Mortimer to the fable of the blind men and an elephant. Each saw and interpreted the elephant only as that particular part of the elephant with which he had come in contact. Thus, pain has been viewed throughout much of history from a noncomprehensive point of view, each person and each discipline having a rather limited view of the whole.

Reynolds, D. V., & Sjoberg, A. E. (Eds.). (1971). *Neuroelectric research: Electroneuroprosthesis, electroanesthesia and nonconvulsive electrotherapy.* Springfield, IL: Charles C Thomas.

Kratzenstein, a German physicist, was probably the first modern scientist to report therapy with "electrification" in 1744. Interestingly, he reported that it increased his pulse and allowed a better quality of sleep. He used it to treat partial paralysis as well.

Of course, we all know the work of Benjamin Franklin, who was very cautious about interpretation. He stated, "I never saw any advantage from electricity in palsies that was permanent." In the late 1800s, there was a great flurry of activity in electrotherapy. Rousell reported, "It is especially in the genital organs that electricity is truly marvelous. Impotence disappears, strength and desire of youth return, and the man, old before his time, whether by excesses or privations, with the aid of electrical fustigation, can become fifteen years younger." Machines as large as 8 feet in diameter were used to create an electrical static discharge. Out of this, of course, grew convulsive electroshock therapy. "Some treatments and instruments have been introduced as original as many as a dozen times since the early 1700s."

Schmidt, J. E. (1959). *Medical discoveries*. Springfield, IL: Charles C Thomas.

Surgeons gradually moved higher and higher in the nervous system, attempting to relieve pain with destructive procedures. Finally, in 1950 Mandel introduced the frontal lobotomy for the relief of intractable pain. It had been used, of course, over 10 years earlier for treatment of psychosis (p. 180).

Shealy, C. N. (1974). Transcutaneous electrical nerve stimulation for control of pain. *Clinical Neurosurgery, 21,* 269–277.

Shealy, C. N., & Mauer, D. (1974). Transcutaneous nerve stimulation for control of pain: A preliminary technical note. *Surgical Neurology, 2*(1), 45–47.

These are the first two scientific articles on the use of what is known as TENS or transcutaneous electrical nerve stimulation.

Smith, R. H. (1963). *Electrical anesthesia*. Springfield, IL: Charles C Thomas.

"Safe anesthesia produced by application of electrical current has been a goal for over eighty years [in 1963!]." Russian electrosleep therapy was described in 1914 by Robinovitch. "Anesthesia produced by the application of electrical current has been called electronarcosis." In 1902, Leduc published his early work with electronarcosis. He tried various frequencies of current, but mostly used 100 cycles per second of direct current square wave. Although he produced a rather cataplectic state in which patients were unable to move, they were still aware of pain. Glen Smith reported successful electronarcosis in dogs over 200 times, in rhesus monkeys 6 times, and in the chimpanzee once.

Solomon, R. A., Vierstein, M. C., & Long, D. M. (1980, February). Reduction of postoperative pain and narcotic use by transcutaneous electrical nerve stimulation. *Surgery,* 142–146.

This is another good article to quote.

Spiller, W. G., & Martin, E. (1912). Treatment of persistent pain of organic origin in the lower part of the body by division of the anterolateral column of the spinal cord. *Journal of the American Medical Association, 158,* 1489–1490.

According to Sweet and White (1955), in 1905 Spiller of Philadelphia discovered the problem with tuberculoma of pain, and Martin was the one to carry out the first successful cordotomy.

Tapio, D., & Hymes, A. C. (1987). *New frontiers in transcutaneous electrical stimulation*. Minnetonka, MN: LecTec Corporation.

Electric eels were known by ancient Egyptians and Hippocrates as potentially useful for producing an electrical shock to control pain, but it was apparently Scribonius Largus who first used the electric ray torpedic fish for treatment of both headache and gout and recorded it in 46 A.D. William Gilbert was reported to have been the first to classify and generalize the phenomenon of electricity (1544–1603). In 1756, Richard Lovett, in *The Subtil Medium*, proved dozens of cures for many diseases using electricity. John Wesley, founder of the Methodist church, was extremely enthusiastic about this treatment and also described many examples of diseases "cured" with electrotherapy, including sciatica, headache, gout, pleuritic pain, and angina pectoris. Between 1750 and 1780, 26 publications dealing with clinical electricity appeared. John Birch, an English surgeon, used electrical current to control pain in 1772. Beginning in the early 1900s, various electrical stimulators were sold to the public by door-to-door salesmen as well as in various catalogs. These instruments were very popular and came with all types of claims and cures, including curing cancer. The FDA banned the sale of such instruments in the early 1950s. In 1967, Shealy introduced the concept of dorsal column stimulation for control of pain, and that led to work with electromodulation.

Thorsteinsson, G., Stonnington, H. H., Stillwell, G. K., & Elveback, L. R. (1977). Transcutaneous electrical stimulation: A double-blind trial of its efficacy for pain. *Archives of Physical Medicine and Rehabilitation, 58,* 8–13.

A number of double-blind studies have emphasized that transcutaneous electrical nerve stimulation is not a placebo.

U.S. Department of Health, Education and Welfare. National Institutes of Health, *Pain*. (1968, September).

In 200 A.D., Galen advocated opium and mandragora as well as electrotherapy for control of pain. The first public demonstration of anesthesia on a patient was in 1846. The most important contribution to the management of pain was the development of the syringe and hypodermic needle (1845–1855). Cocaine was introduced into medical practice in 1884. Dr. William Halstead of Johns Hopkins discovered the principle of block anesthesia, which was the injection of cocaine into a nerve trunk. Spinal anesthesia was introduced in 1898. In 1967, the National Institutes of General Medicine Sciences offered the first center grant to the University of Pennsylvania and the second in 1968 to Harvard University to develop "anesthesia research and training centers where teams of scientists in many disciplines worked together in studying basic molecular research to anesthesia techniques in the operating room."

White, J. C., & Sweet, W. H. (1955). *Pain: Its mechanisms and neurosurgical control*. Springfield, IL: Charles C Thomas.

White, J. C., & Sweet, W. H. (1969). *Pain and the neurosurgeon: A forty year experience*. Springfield, IL: Charles C Thomas.

In more modern times, the classics were written by White and Sweet.

Wolff, H. G. (1963). *Headache: And other pain* (2nd ed.). New
York: Oxford University Press.

Headache, one of the most common of major pain complaints, was perhaps most well studied by Harold G. Wolff.

Section II

Elements of Multidisciplinary Pain Management

3

Implementing a Pain Management Program

Anne Marie Kelly, B.S.N., R.N.C.

The purpose of human life is to serve, to show compassion, and to help others.

Albert Schweitzer

INTRODUCTION

Relieving pain and suffering is at the heart of the healthcare profession. Despite attempts at treating pain over the decades, fear of unrelieved pain remains a major concern of patients in all healthcare settings. In 1992, the Agency for Healthcare Policy and Research (AHCPR) published guidelines on acute pain which state that the institutional responsibility for pain management begins with the affirmation that patients should have access to the best level of pain relief that may be provided safely. Regarding ethical responsibility, the guidelines stress that the ethical obligation to manage pain and relieve the patient's suffering is at the core of a healthcare professional's commitment (Acute Pain Management, 1992). Today, healthcare institutions are challenged with the responsibility and ethical obligation to develop the necessary means and resources to effectively treat pain in all patients. As the guidelines focus on improving the quality of pain relief, the need for programs that address this is becoming increasingly apparent. One of the best means to ensure optimum pain control is the availability of a pain management program that combines the expertise and commitment of a healthcare team whose members are dedicated to the prevention and treatment of pain. Formalized programs are necessary to bring pain control to its rightful place in the healthcare system. This chapter focuses on the key components and steps necessary for the successful implementation of an effective pain management program

---

TABLE 3.1
Key Components of a Successful Program

1. Institutional commitment
2. Interdisciplinary team
3. Education
4. Continuous quality improvement

IDENTIFY INSTITUTIONAL LEADERS

Well begun is half done.

Aristotle

The first step in identifying institutional leaders is the appointment of a task force to determine a plan of action. Seek out the "champions" in your institution who have a vested interest and knowledge in pain management. It is important to give those who feel a sense of commitment and ownership the opportunity to contribute to the development of the program. Peters (1987) suggests that those vested "look inward, work with colleagues and customers, work with everyone, to develop and instill a philosophy and vision that is enabling and empowering" (p. 482). Once the task force has been selected, conduct an institutional assessment to examine your organization's culture, strengths, and weaknesses related to current pain management practices. This group should address the following issues:

1. Is pain management an institutional priority?
2. Who has a knowledge base about pain management?
3. Do the policies and procedures ensure quality pain control?

0-8493-0926-3/02/$0.00+$1.50
© 2002 by CRC Press LLC

4. Who is accountable for pain management?
5. How is quality measured?

Although pain is a common problem, it remains largely an invisible one. The task force can serve as a catalyst involved in promoting increased visibility of the problem of unrelieved pain. Its focus is to collect and provide necessary data to initiate efforts to address the existing problems. The results can provide strong evidence pointing to the need to standardize pain assessment policies, make changes in institutional procedures, and develop standards of acceptable practice. Making the problem of pain visible in your institution is the initial step in developing a formalized approach to pain management.

DEVELOP A MISSION STATEMENT FOR THE PROGRAM

It is imperative that the mission statement reflect the values and purpose of the organization related to pain management practices. By articulating its purpose and what it stands for, the institution directs the work of the staff. In describing the importance of a clearly articulated purpose, Ulschak (1988) states that, "until there is agreement about purpose, an institution has no direction, no tool to measure progress, no real reason to be motivated, and no clear focus for its energy." For institutional commitment to be achieved, it must start at the top. Administration must provide leadership that can result in institutional change, encourage employee commitment, and ensure improved standards of care. Leaders in the organization will need to help staff understand why change is necessary and how it relates to the mission. Staff members must clearly see that the institution's priority and goal is to promote high standards of safe, effective pain relief to all patients within its care. Institutional commitment and administrative support are the foundation on which to build a quality program and are absolutely essential to success.

DEFINE STANDARDS OF CARE

Defining standards is a key step in developing an effective program. Pain management is arguably one of the most complex topics in medicine today. From dealing with acute, chronic, and cancer pain, to providing palliative and compassionate end-of-life care, caregivers are faced with multiple issues that extend far beyond the question of what medication to administer. Written standards are necessary to define the expectations of the caregivers and show how the care delivery system is organized and managed. The mission of the institution sets the direction for all written standards. Standards make quality a day-to-day goal.

The Joint Commission on Accreditation of Healthcare Organizations (JCAHO, 1999) set new standards for the assessment and management of pain which healthcare institutions must be prepared to meet in 2001 (Dahl, 1999). These standards call upon hospitals, home care agencies, nursing homes, behavioral healthcare facilities, outpatient clinics, and healthcare plans to:

- Recognize the right of patients to receive appropriate assessment and management of pain.
- Assess the existence and, if so, the nature and intensity of pain in all patients.
- Record the results of the assessment in a way that facilitates regular reassessment and follow up.
- Determine and assure staff competency in pain assessment and management.
- Address pain assessment and management in the orientation of all new staff.
- Establish policies and procedures which support the appropriate prescription or ordering of effective pain medications.
- Ensure that pain does not interfere with participation in rehabilitation.
- Educate patients and their families about effective pain management.
- Collect data to monitor the appropriateness and effectiveness of pain management.
- Address patient needs for symptom management in the discharge planning process.

These standards serve as guidelines in developing policies and procedures for all healthcare facilities. Clearly defined standards will positively affect the quality of patient care. The JCAHO standards establish the foundation for a system-wide initiative in pain management.

DEVELOP AN INTERDISCIPLINARY APPROACH TO PAIN MANAGEMENT

Because pain is a multidimensional experience, it requires an interdisciplinary approach. Pain profoundly affects not only the physical, but the psychological, social, cultural, and spiritual dimensions of life (Ferrell, Dean, Grant, & Coluzzi, 1995; Saunders, 1884). Successful pain control requires attention to all aspects of care and suffering, and no amount of well-prescribed analgesia will relieve the pain unless the elements that are compounding the problem are addressed. Care provided by a team of specialized healthcare professionals is required to treat the diverse aspects of pain. For modern-day pain therapy to be effective, institutions need to direct their attention to the importance of interdisciplinary teams. An interdisciplinary team is a valuable resource that serves the organization in many ways:

- It serves the organization by assisting in the development of policies and procedures, offering consultation, and providing a forum for the resolution of difficult pain management issues.
- It serves the patients by attending to the multiple dimensions of optimum pain management and integrates all aspects of care.
- It serves the families by providing support and guidance as they confront the common challenges associated with caring for a loved one coping with pain.
- It serves the community by promoting educational programs for families and the general public that focus on pain assessment, pain treatments, drug addiction, and how to communicate with healthcare professionals about pain. A holistic approach is critical to breaking down the barriers to pain management and is successful because it allows physicians, nurses, and other clinicians to learn more about the "person" than just the disease (National Institutes, 1987).

A pain management team includes professionals from various disciplines who meet regularly to discuss and develop an individualized plan of care for each patient. A typical team may include one or more physicians, nurses, pharmacists, physical therapists, occupational therapists, pastoral care counselors, social workers, dieticians, and staff educators. Depending on the setting, you may want to include a certified nursing assistant, therapeutic activity therapist, and trained volunteer. A team can address the great need for accountability in pain management and prevent further fragmentation of care (see Table 3.2). This is the best approach for responding to pain and a critical component of an effective pain management program (Gordon, Dahl, & Stevenson, 1996, pp. 10–36).

TABLE 3.2
Role of Interdisciplinary Team

1. Identify patient, family, and staff needs in pain management
2. Assure pain relief goals are met
3. Collaborate with healthcare providers to facilitate optimum pain control
4. Promote practice changes through outcome quality improvement monitoring

---

DEFINE ACCOUNTABILITY

Each team member is accountable for carrying out a specific task and plays a key role in the management of pain. Team members:

- Assess the physical, psychosocial, spiritual, functional, emotional, and cultural needs of the patient.
- Use standard tools to assess the patient.
- Discuss summary of findings with attending physician and make appropriate recommendations.
- Review treatment plan and pain relief goal with the patient and family and encourage participation in decision making.
- Include both pharmacologic and non-pharmacologic therapies.
- Attend weekly, interdisciplinary team meetings to review plan of care and problem solve.
- Communicate plan of care to appropriate staff members.
- Assess for pain relief regularly throughout the course of treatment.
- Visit the patient at least once a week to assess progress.
- Educate patient and family about pain management.
- Measure outcomes to continually improve pain management practices.

Success of the team is measured by its ability to provide pain relief in a safe and effective manner to meet the needs and expectations of the patient and family. The following case example, in which the author was part of the interdisciplinary team, illustrates these points.

CASE EXAMPLE

Mr. F. was a 79-year-old man with terminal rectal cancer who resided in a long-term care facility. He was an alert, oriented, and religious man who understood his prognosis and elected to receive comfort measures only. His pain had been fairly well controlled and his medications had been titrated up to 400 mg of Oxycontin b.i.d., Actiq 400 mg q 3 h. p.r.n. for breakthrough pain, Celebrex 100 mg b.i.d., and Nortriptyline 25 mg @ h.s. Mr. F. was able to maintain his independence and did not exhibit any major side effects from the medications. During this time, he was also referred to the pain clinic for consultation regarding pain control measures. As the rectal tumor enlarged, his pain escalated and became more difficult to manage. He was once again seen by the anesthesiologist at the pain clinic who recommended the placement of a tunneled, epidural catheter for optimum pain control. Mr. F. consented to the procedure and his attending physician agreed this was the best course to follow. However, this created a challenge for the long-term care facility for the following reasons:

1. The facility had no written policies and procedures for epidural analgesia and the nurses felt ill-prepared having little or no knowledge in this area.

2. Mr. F. wanted to come back to the facility where he felt at "home" and wished to die in a loving environment with the staff he considered his "family."

3. The facility's mission statement clearly articulated that the institution's priority was the relief of pain.

Following a discussion with administration and the interdisciplinary team, all members agreed it was the institution's responsibility and ethical obligation to provide the necessary means and resources to care for Mr. F. during his final days. With administrative support, the members of the interdisciplinary team developed the necessary policies and procedures and provided education to the clinical staff in every aspect of care. With adequate education and support from the team, the nurses felt confident and prepared for Mr. F.'s return from the hospital. The nurses knew the moment they saw Mr. F. that they had made the right decision. Upon arrival, Mr. F. looking at the nurses with a big smile on his face stated, "It's a miracle. I have no pain." His pain was controlled with 1% Bupivicaine and Fentanyl 5 mcg/cc at 6 to 14cc/h and bolus doses of Fentanyl 5 cc q 10 min via a PCA pump. His pain ratings ranged from 0 to 2 and he remained comfortable until his death, four weeks later. Although saddened by his death, the staff tempered their grief knowing that they had made a difference in his life. Mr. F. died peacefully, with dignity, and in a loving environment surrounded by dedicated staff who understood that life is a gift to be cherished up until its final moments. *His wishes had been fulfilled and the facility's goal had been met.*

During those four weeks, the interdisciplinary team invested all its skill and effort into relieving his pain and suffering. The physician monitored his condition and ordered medications for pain control; the pharmacist made certain the medications were prepared and delivered in a timely manner; the nurses assessed him regularly for pain relief and potential side effects; the nursing assistants provided physical care with a compassionate touch; the physical and occupational therapists evaluated his ability to maintain optimum independence for as long as possible and made recommendations for his comfort; the social worker listened to his expressions of fear and other emotions and offered support; the pastoral care counselor addressed his spiritual needs by praying with him daily and being present; the dietician monitored his nutritional needs and paid special attention to his food preferences and his ability to swallow; the recreational therapist provided him with musical tapes he enjoyed and taught him relaxation techniques and guided imagery

to distract him from any pain; the staff educator provided ongoing education and assessed the competency of the staff; the hospice nurse offered respite care and support to the patient, family, and staff. The interdisciplinary team, composed of dedicated professionals, was a vital force in diminishing his physical, psychosocial, and spiritual pain. When team members listen and acknowledge all aspects of pain, the patient experiences a feeling of worth, dignity, peace, and wholeness.

Although this was one of the most challenging cases for the long-term care facility, it was also the most gratifying. Everyone understood firsthand the meaning of institutional commitment and saw how a concerned and knowledgeable team is vital to successful pain management.

DEVELOP AN EDUCATION PLAN

There is no knowledge that is not power.

Ralph Waldo Emerson

Traditionally, medical and nursing schools have devoted very little, if any, time to the subject of pain management. Healthcare providers cannot be expected to practice what they do not know. Inadequacies in the education of health professionals has contributed to fears and misconceptions regarding the use of pain medications, addiction, and consequently inadequate pain management (Liebeskind & Melzack, 1998).

Education is the key step to improving pain management practices that result in institutional changes. Identifying the learning needs of your staff is vital to your educational efforts. This can be accomplished in a variety of ways:

- Administer a pretest to assess the knowledge level of your staff and to determine who has a knowledge base about pain management.
- Involve the interdisciplinary team members in conducting a survey in each of their practice areas to assess the learning needs of each discipline.
- Use the baseline data collected in your institutional assessment about current pain management practices. This is essential to planning education for the improvement of staff performance.
- Establish focus groups of about 6 to 10 people from different disciplines and ask their opinions about learning needs. Including "grass roots" input is useful for correcting inadequacies that exist.

Once you have identified the learning needs of the staff, it is important to outline an education plan including curriculum content, staff time, and programming costs. For developing a comprehensive pain management program, consider including these core content areas:

- Physiology of pain
- Pain assessment
- Types of pain
- Assessment tools and pain rating scales
- Analgesics: non-opioids, opioids, adjuvant medications
- Symptom management
- Psychosocial, spiritual, and cultural issues
- Pain management in the elderly
- Barriers to effective pain management
- Ethical issues in pain management
- Non-pharmacologic interventions

PLAN EDUCATION STRATEGIES THAT INVOLVE ALL CAREGIVERS

Organizations learn only through individuals who learn.

Peter Senge

There are a variety of formal and informal teaching strategies that can be used to enhance the learner's understanding of pain management. Healthcare educators and providers need to employ creative ways of providing education to staff, patients, families, and the community that are timely, cost-effective, and informative. Each teaching strategy is advantageous for certain outcomes and has considerations that influence its choice. Some examples of informal teaching strategies include:

Pain Management Education Week — Designate a week in your facility that is set aside just for pain management education. This time is a great opportunity to teach everyone that pain management is an institutional priority. Invite each interdisciplinary team member to set up an exhibit displaying learning materials and equipment that can help participants to understand their role in relieving pain. Team members can be available at alternating times for demonstration, skill practice, and answering questions. Communicate this event to everyone through fliers and newspaper articles. This is an excellent way for disseminating information to staff, patients, families, other healthcare providers, and the public. It stimulates interest in a dynamic way and facilitates education about the different pain control measures used in the facility. This strategy serves as a great marketing tool by conveying a strong message about

the organization's commitment to quality pain management practices.

Pain Management Poster Presentations — This is a unique and enjoyable way to involve all departments and demonstrate that pain management requires an interdisciplinary approach. Encourage creativity by inviting employees from all departments to design a poster of their choice related to pain management. Employees can work individually or as a group, and are given a deadline to complete the project. Display the posters throughout the facility. This provides valuable information to insiders and outsiders. Select different categories and ask some of your volunteers or family members to choose the winning posters. Offer prizes that can be donated by your consultants and vendors. Invite the winners to give poster presentations and offer participants continuing education credits. Ask your public relations department to take pictures of the activities and send an article to the local newspapers. This teaching method generates enthusiasm, teamwork, and publicity and clearly articulates to everyone that successful pain management is the result of interdisciplinary involvement.

Portable Educational Cart — A mobile cart displaying fact sheets and equipment is another useful way to educate staff. Keep carts in an area for a specified amount of time allowing staff members to use them when time permits. Quizzes or self-learning packets on the content can be given by the staff educator if validation is required. This is an easy way to impart information that does not require an explanation or discussion. Depending on where the cart is located, it is also a good format for providing physicians, patients, and families with updated information about pain management. This activity clearly identifies that learning about pain control is everyone's responsibility.

Pain Management Bulletin Board — Employ the use of an education bulletin board strategically placed in the facility where it is visible to everyone. The board can be used to post brochures about upcoming workshops, seminars, and programs on pain management. The facility's education calendar can be posted, indicating the times and dates of all pain management inservices. Include a spot on the bulletin board to place self-learning packets, updated articles and handouts, information on new policies and procedures, and fliers on special events related to pain management activities. This is a unique way to demonstrate to your "customers" that pain management education is considered important in the facility.

These strategies facilitate education that is system-wide and promote public awareness about the institution's efforts to provide optimum pain management. They speak loudly about the value of education to those who enter your doors.

Formal methods of education can include lectures, case studies, videotapes, audiotapes, teleconferences, CD ROMs, grand rounds, skills labs, closed circuit TV, panel discussions, seminars, and workshops. To keep educational costs at a minimum, ask members of your medical, nursing, and other professional staff who are knowledgeable about pain management to provide inservices to the staff. Videotaping the inservices is a cost-effective means of providing education to staff members who are unable to attend the presentations. Education of all healthcare providers involved in the care of the patient is crucial if you are to have an effective pain management program. Institutions need to promote education to students involved in clinical care and continuing education for practicing professionals to keep up with changing trends and maintain their skills and competency. Knowledge about pain management empowers physicians, nurses, and other clinicians to assume the most basic mission of their practice — the relief of pain and suffering.

DEVELOP A QUALITY IMPROVEMENT MONITORING PROCESS

JCAHO (1994) defines *quality of care* as "the degree to which health services for individuals and populations increase the likelihood of desired health outcomes and are consistent with current professional knowledge." Continuous quality improvement is the key component that will help to demonstrate the pain program's benefit to the institution's mission. CQI is a process that ensures optimum pain control by building excellence into every aspect of care and creating an environment that encourages all disciplines to contribute to its success (see Table 3.3). Monitoring pain management outcomes is an ongoing responsibility shared by members of the interdisciplinary team. Every organization must choose which processes and outcomes are important to monitor based on its mission and the scope of care and services provided. JCAHO (1991) has designed a 10-step quality monitoring and evaluation process for healthcare agencies (see Table 3.4). In that 10-step process, the first five steps establish the mechanism to be used for monitoring and evaluation, the sixth and seventh steps encompass collection and evaluation of relevant data, and the last

---

TABLE 3.3
Why Teamwork in Quality Improvement?

1. Instills ownership of the process
2. Involves the people who know best
3. Creates respect, cooperation, and openness
4. Breaks down barriers between departments
5. Spreads quality
6. "None of us is as smart as all of us"
   More ideas
   Better ideas

TABLE 3.4
JCAHO Ten-Step Quality Monitoring Process

1. Assign responsibility
2. Delineate scope of service
3. Identify important aspects of service
4. Identify indicators related to the important aspects of service
5. Establish thresholds for evaluation
6. Collect and organize data
7. Evaluate service when indicated by the threshold
8. Take action when opportunities for improvement or problems are identified
9. Assess the effectiveness of actions
10. Communicate relevant information to the organization-wide program for continuous quality improvement

From Joint Commission on Accreditation of Healthcare Organizations, 1991. An Introduction to Joint Commission Nursing Care Standards, Oakbrook Terrace, IL: JCAHO. With permission.

---

three steps reflect attempts to improve the provision of services rendered.

Performance monitoring and improvement are data driven. Institutions need to develop a formal plan for evaluating the quality of pain management and collect data about the needs, expectations, and satisfaction of individuals served. There are a number of ways to obtain input from these groups, including:

- Periodic satisfaction surveys of patients and families including questions about pain intensity, pain relief goals, and staff responsiveness.
- Chart audits to assess documentation of pain assessments, patients' response to treatment, and teaching outcomes.
- Chart audits to monitor analgesic drug use and treatment side effects.
- Focus groups to elicit feedback regarding pain management practices.
- Regularly scheduled meetings with family members.

The detail and frequency of data collection is determined as appropriate for monitoring ongoing performance by the organization. Whenever possible, data collection should be incorporated into day-to-day activities. High quality pain management is not a static destination to be reached, but a dynamic entity toward which we must continually strive. We must act on the basic belief…the patient is the reason we exist.

CONCLUSION

The reward of a thing well done is to have done it.

Ralph Waldo Emerson

As we look to the future, we must use our time, skills, and energy to make a defining difference in pain management. It is time for pain management programs to be incorporated into all parts of the health- care delivery system, and for physicians, nurses, and other healthcare providers to make pain control part of their routine practice. As professionals involved in a healing ministry, we must proactively promote optimum pain management by interdisciplinary teams that can enhance the quality of life and diminish pain and suffering in patients and families. As patient advocates, we must implement quality programs that increase our capabilities to serve, show compassion, and help others.

REFERENCES

Acute Pain Management Guideline Panel. (1992). *Acute Pain Management: Operative or Medical Procedures and Trauma, Clinical Practice Guideline*. AHCPR Pub. No. 920032, Rockville, MD: Agency for Health Care Policy and Research, Public Health Service, U.S. Department of Health and Human Services.

Dahl, J.L. (1999). New JCAHO standards focus on pain management. *Oncology Issues, 14*(5), 27–28.

Ferrell, B., Dean, G., Grant, M., & Coluzzi, P. (1995). An institutional commitment to pain management. *Journal of Clinical Oncology, 13*, 2158–2165.

Gordon D.B., Dahl, J.L., & Stevenson, K.K. (1996). *Building an institutional commitment to pain management*. Madison: University of Wisconsin–Madison Board of Regents.

Joint Commission on Accreditation of Healthcare Organizations (JCAHO). (1991). *An introduction to Joint Commission nursing standards*. Oakbrook Terrace, IL: JCAHO.

Joint Commission on Accreditation of Healthcare Organizations (JCAHO). (1994). *Accreditation manual for hospitals: Vol. 1. Standards*. Oakbrook Terrace, IL: JCAHO.

Joint Commission on Accreditation of Healthcare Organizations. (1999). *Joint Commission focuses on pain management*. Oakbrook Terrace, IL: JCAHO. http/www.jeaho.org/news

Liebeskind, J.C., & Melzack, R. (1998, March). The International Pain Foundation: Meeting a need for education in pain management. *Journal of Pain and Symptom Management*, 131–132.

National Institutes of Health Consensus Development Conference. (1987). The integrated approach to the management of pain. *Journal of Pain and Symptom Management, 2*, 35–44.

Peters, T. (1987). *Thriving on chaos*. New York: Harper Collins.

Saunders, C. (1884). *The management of terminal malignant disease* (2nd ed.). London: Edward Arnold.

Ulschak, F. (1988). *Creating the future of health care education*. Chicago: American Hospital Publishing.

4

The Classification of Pain

Ole Thienhaus, M.D., M.B.A., F.A.P.A. and B. Eliot Cole, M.D., M.P.A., F.A.P.A.

INTRODUCTION

The International Association for the Study of Pain (IASP) defined pain as "an unpleasant sensory and emotional experience associated with actual and potential tissue damage, or described in terms of such damage or both" (IASP, 1986). The definition emphasized the subjective and psychological nature of pain, and appropriately avoided making the authenticity of pain contingent on an externally verifiable stimulus. Pain was understood to motivate those afflicted to seek relief from it.

Price (1999) proposed an updated definition that described pain as a somatic perception containing a bodily sensation with qualities like those reported during tissue-damaging stimulation, an experienced threat associated with this sensation, and a feeling of unpleasantness or other negative emotion based on this experienced threat. By modifying the definition, there was no requirement to objectively demonstrate actual or potential tissue damage nor was there a requirement that an association be made between sensation and tissue damage. This revised pain definition was very helpful because making a linkage between sensation and tissue damage was frequently impossible to demonstrate.

In setting the stage for the 2001 implementation of pain-related standards of care, the Joint Commission on Accreditation of Healthcare Organizations (JCAHO) also linked pain to both physical and emotional responses (JCAHO, 2000). As justification for these pain-related accreditation standards, the JCAHO linked unrelieved pain to negative physiological and psychological effects, and generalized these adverse trends from the traditional acutely hospitalized patient to the majority of patients in most healthcare settings (hospitals, long-term care, surgical

centers, mental health facilities, home health services, and health system networks).

Why do we bother to classify pain? Classifying pain is necessary for research and clinical purposes. Relating a clinical database to a categorical reference system facilitates the tasks of clinical assessment, treatment planning, and formulation of an accurate prognosis. Conventionally, pain is classified according to location, underlying cause, frequency, intensity, and duration. The clinical data, thus categorized, serve as an input variable for determining the correct diagnosis and developing the optimal treatment plan. Investigators in the field of pain management work to expand the classification of pain, and to specifically tailor treatment options for each diagnostic possibility. Clinicians and researchers must attempt to know the cause of each pain problem to understand how it is to be treated. Classification improves the flow of communication between patient and clinician, ensuring that the clinician obtains a complete picture of the complaint and makes it possible for both patient and provider to speak the same language when they try to define the nature of the problem, response to treatment, and the development of secondary problems such as side effects of treatment or newly developing symptoms.

There continues to be a need for the expanded classification of pain as long as patients suffer from pains that we do not understand and that are inadequately treated. According to Wall (1989), pain classified by our ignorance about underlying mechanisms and therapy falls into three groups: (1) pains where the cause is apparent but the treatment is inadequate (deep tissue disorders, peripheral nerve disorders, root and cord disorders); (2) pains where the cause is not known but the treatment is adequate (trigeminal neuralgia, tension headaches); and (3) pains where the cause is not known and the treatment is inadequate (back pain, idiopathic pelvic and abdominal pain, migraine headache).

The classification of pain is a source of confusion for many clinicians, and as a result of this confusion pain practitioners now commonly use a number of different classification systems. Clear distinctions between pain classification systems are not always possible, but the more simplistic the classification of pain, the more omissions and overlaps occur (Pasero, Paice & McCaffery, 1999). Pain is classified according to the time course, the involved anatomy, the intensity, the type of patient, and the circumstances of the pathology. To be a successful pain practitioner one must be able to work with pain classifications encompassing all of these areas, and be capable of switching from one model to another. While the distinctions between one system and another may seem arbitrary, without some framework to categorize pain complaints, the unsophisticated clinician easily becomes lost in the pain behavior of the patient and the demand for quick solutions. Treatment options are linked to the type of pain involved, and accurate pain classification is essential for successful pain management. The pain conditions that the clinician cannot recognize and accurately diagnose cannot be satisfactorily treated.

At a more practical and human level, patients want to know if their pain will ever completely go away. Patients are frightened that their pain is attributable to unrecognized pathology and so search for the ultimate cure. Going from practitioner to practitioner serves to worsen their confusion, and patients hope that someone will be able to illuminate their difficulties. By being able to classify the pain into a recognizable and explainable syndrome, the pain practitioner, unlike the other clinicians, is able to offer some hope. Although treatment often does not yield a completely pain-free state for these patients, understanding the basis for their pain and knowing that awful diseases do not exist often provides significant relief from their suffering.

Case Example

Ms. W. was a 45-year-old woman who had seen a number of practitioners during the previous three years since her car accident. Physical therapy, massage therapy, acupuncture, and psychotherapy in isolation after thorough evaluation by neurologists, neurosurgeons, and orthopedic surgeons failed to produce lasting comfort. When she was referred to the pain clinic she was tense, angry, and argumentative. She was informed that she would never be completely pain free as a result of her well-established myofascial pain, but could eventually resume her life if she entered a pain management program. She was surprised to learn that her pain condition had a name, was recognized by the physician as a noncancer pain process, and could respond to interdisciplinary treatment. Previous clinicians had recommended that she learn to live with the pain, but did not tell her how to do this. Although no specific treatment occurred during the evaluation in a conventional sense, she was relaxed and more comfortable when she left the office.

It is not always certain that pain can be conveniently classified into some system. Some patients will present with more than one pain problem over time, and can have the pains classified simultaneously into different categories. The chronic pain patient may experience acute painful episodes unrelated to the original pain condition, the chronic non-cancer pain patient may develop cancer-related pain after years of marginal pain management, and the acute pain patient may experience a number of different aches and pains from the original pathophysiologic process, or as a consequence of the therapies to correct it.

CLASSIFICATION BY LOCATION

Pain may be classified by body location. Two overlapping schema relate the pain to the specific anatomy and/or body system thought to be involved. The anatomical classification addresses sites of pain as viewed from a regional perspective. Typical examples include lower back pain, headache, and pelvic pain. The body system pain classification focuses on classical body systems such as musculoskeletal, neurological, and vascular. Both systems of classification address only a single dimension, where or why does the patient hurt, and may ultimately fail to adequately define the underlying neurophysiology of the pain problem (Turk & Okifuji, 2001).

CLASSIFICATION BY TIME COURSE

The duration of the pain process, the temporal perspective, is the most obvious distinction that is made when classifying most pain complaints. This temporal distinction is an important consideration for understanding the neurophysiology of pain (Crue, 1983). Acute pain is limited to pain of less than 30 days, while chronic pain persists for more than six months. Subacute pain describes the interval from the end of the first month to the beginning of the seventh month for continued pain. Recurrent acute pain defines a pain pattern that persists over an extended period of time, but recurs as isolated pain episodes. Chronic pain is further divided by the underlying etiology, into non-cancer (often called "benign" pain) and cancer (often called "malignant" pain) related (Crue, 1983; Foley, 1985; Portenoy, 1988).

The primary distinction between acute and chronic pain regardless of the etiology is crucial. Acute pain is useful and serves a protective purpose. It warns of danger, limits utilization of injured or diseased body parts, and signals the departure of pathology when the limiting condition resolves. Without acute pain it is doubtful that most of us would be able to survive at all (Cousins, 1989). We would literally suffer needless burns, cuts, and other injuries. Not being able to experience pain is literally incompatible with life. Chronic pain has little protective significance, persists despite normalization after injury or disease, and ultimately interferes with productive activity. Patients with chronic pain live their lives as if they are having full-time nightmares, where pain relief is constantly sought yet rarely obtained without professional help, and the pain controls their activities of daily living. Chronic non-cancer pain occurs with or without adequate patient coping. The patients who cope with the chronic pain manage to live productive lives, while the patients who are not able to cope with their pain are disabled by chronic suffering (Crue, 1983).

ACUTE PAIN

Acute pain is almost always self-limited. When the condition that produces the pain resolves, or when the nociceptive input is blocked by a local anesthetic or altered by the use of peripheral or central analgesic medications, the pain leaves. The skin heals, the fractures mend, the inflammation subsides, and the nociceptive input stops, so the pain intensity fades away and disappears (Crue, 1983). The use of comfort measures such as applications of heat or cold, splinting, casting, or brief, time-limited analgesic medication all help to relieve this discomfort. Sentiments of concern and expected recovery from friends and family help to aid in the relief of pain for the acute pain sufferer.

Case Example
Mr. B. was a 22-year-old downhill skier who sustained a shoulder dislocation in a fall. His shoulder was relocated in the field and he was placed in a shoulder immobilizer for one week. He was assured that his injury was not significant by his physician and would not interfere with his participation in an important race later in the season. After limited physical therapy to restore his range of motion and strength, he was able to resume competitive racing with no detectable difficulties.

The pain after surgery, postoperative pain, is a specific type of acute pain. No matter how successful or how deftly conducted, operations produce tissue trauma and cause the release of potent mediators of inflammation and pain. Pain is often poorly managed because patients receive significantly less opioid analgesics than are ordered, the nursing staff are overly concerned about opioid addiction, analgesics are irration-ally selected, and many physicians have inadequate knowledge of the pharmacology of analgesics (Waldman, 1990). Although postoperative pain is experienced by millions of patients throughout the world, it is rarely recognized as producing harmful physiological or psychological effects (Cousins, 1989). The axiom, "No one ever died from pain, they just wish they could," is clearly incorrect with the modern recognition that unrelieved pain increases cardiac work, increases metabolic rate, interferes with blood clotting, leads to water retention, lowers oxygen levels, impairs wound healing, alters immune function, interferes with sleep, and creates negative emotions (Akca, et al., 1999; Dinarello, 1984; Egdahl, 1959; Kehlet, 1982; Kehlet, Brandt, & Rem, 1980; Liebeskind, 1991; Melzack, 1990). Unrelieved pain may delay the return of normal gastric and bowel function in the postoperative patient (Wattwil, 1989). Recognition of the widespread inadequacy of pain management prompted the U.S. Department of Health and Human Services to publish the *Acute Pain Management Clinical Practice Guidelines* as the first set of federal practice recommendations (AHCPR, 1992).

CHRONIC PAIN

Chronic pain confuses most sufferers because it dominates, depresses, and debilitates. If chronic pain is treated by using acute pain models only, it may become more intense and the patients may experience increased disability and suffering. Instead of comfort measures alone, chronic pain is managed by the use of rehabilitative techniques when it is primarily of a non-cancer origin, or by aggressive and supportive techniques when it is primarily due to cancer.

"Tincture of time," coupled with injury- or illness-specific therapy, may be appropriate for many acute pain conditions because most painful conditions are time limited. Acute pain is reasonably managed and usually resolves with the efforts of a single practitioner; however, chronic pain frequently requires the coordinated efforts of a broadly based treatment team bringing a number of physical, psychological, and spiritual strategies together. Chronic pain patients demand more effort and resources than a single, well-meaning practitioner can usually provide. In isolation, the solo practitioner is generally unable to address the variety of complex physical, psychosocial, and spiritual problems that chronic pain causes, and so resorts to symptom management usually by overusing a single therapeutic approach.

Case Example
Ms. D. was a 28-year-old woman referred for the management of chronic, mechanical low back pain secondary to an industrial lifting injury. Her referring neurosurgeon, who had been treating her unsuccessfully for three years, became motivated to refer her to a pain management program when his partners began to complain about her drug seeking behavior whenever they were on call for him. A full review of her medical record revealed that she had received 3900 oxycodone and acetaminophen tablets in the six months prior to referral. At the time of referral she was taking 12 to 15 of the oxycodone and acetaminophen combination tablets,

60 milligrams of diazepam, and an uncertain number of butalbital, aspirin, and caffeine-containing tablets every day to obtain marginal pain relief. She was admitted to an outpatient chronic pain management program, and over six weeks was successfully detoxified from all of her medications, while simultaneously learning many new strategies to help her deal with her chronic pain. She eventually returned to the work force in a less physically demanding position after completing the chronic pain management program.

A specialized taxonomy was introduced to facilitate the classification of chronic pain syndromes. This taxonomy turned out to be of particular utility in the area of pain research (IASP, 1986). The multiaxial approach taken in this system was hoped to be of practical use for clinicians. Using multiaxial categorization by topography, organ system, and underlying pathophysiology helped to relate the presenting complaint to the domains of traditional medical practice, and served to facilitate consultative communication with patients' primary physicians. Descriptive axes such as axis II! (pattern of occurrence) and axis IV (intensity) recognized the patients' experiential and subjective inputs. These latter two dimensions were subdivided into 10 detailed gradations by severity, reflected in numerical codes. In clinical investigations (see below), this permitted the application of parametric statistical analysis to database collections.

While acute pain usually only briefly disables patients during their initial recovery time, chronic pain often prevents patients from ever returning to any meaningful and gainful employment. Some chronic pain patients are not able to return to their former, high-paying work due to pain-related limitations, and others are unable to return to work due to the unwillingness of their employers to make reasonable accommodations because they fear losing profits (Chapman & Brena, 1989). These chronic pain patients are caught in the ridiculous position of having to maintain their disability, rather than risk returning to an entry-level position with inadequate financial compensation for their needs. Legal entanglements further cloud chronic non-cancer pain problems and contribute to the inability to resolve the suffering. The desire for the best legal settlement, often the only reward for pain problems, often prevents chronic pain patients from making full recoveries.

It is sadly said that pain problems are chronic in nature when the referral letter from one practitioner to another begins with an apology for making the referral! Chronic pain patients are so often viewed as angry, hostile, depressed, and manipulative, that they evoke feelings of anxiety, resentment, and desperation in their treating clinicians. Pain patients requesting that the results of their initial evaluations must be sent to their attorneys should alert pain practitioners to potential involvement in impending litigation. As some lawyers actually send patients for pain management assessments to strengthen their positions for claims of pain and suffering after accidents or injuries, it is necessary to understand whose interests are being served by the evaluations. Patients and lawyers stand to gain more financially from any legal action if patients do not recover from their injuries and illnesses (Chapman & Brena, 1989).

SUBACUTE PAIN AND RECURRENT ACUTE PAIN

Subacute pain is possibly the last opportunity for a full restoration and a pain-free existence, much as acute pain must be recognized before the pain becomes chronic. Subacute pain is quite similar to acute pain in its etiological and nociceptive mechanisms (Crue, 1983). Unfortunately, once the pain has been established for more than six months, the likelihood of complete pain relief is small. The first 100 days of pain appear to respond fully to therapy and return the patients to near normality. Beyond the first 100 days, most patients still may recover the majority of lost function, but do not feel fully restored or comfortable. By the time pain becomes subacute, the rehabilitative approach used for chronic pain is usually more appropriate than further acute pain management strategies.

Recurrent acute pain is the acute flare-up of peripheral tissue pathology due to an underlying chronic pathological entity and occurs with headaches, gastrointestinal motility disorders, degenerative disk and joint disease, collagen vascular disease, sickle cell disease, and similar functional processes (Crue, 1983). Unlike chronic or subacute pain, recurrent acute pain implies discrete acute episodes, which return over time. The dividing line between recurrent acute and subacute pain is often a judgment decision by the pain practitioner. Daily pain for several weeks is subacute pain, but several limited pain episodes over many months or years is typical of recurrent acute pain. The importance of recognizing recurrent acute pain is to apply a more comprehensive management approach of patient education, contingency planning, and family involvement than a single pain episode would ordinarily require.

CLASSIFICATION BY UNDERLYING PATHOLOGY

Regardless of time course of the pain, its intensity, frequency, and location, every attempt must be made to arrive at an etiologic formulation. Ideally, treating the underlying cause will bring about the definitive cure of the pain syndrome. At a minimum, etiologic clarification will tell the clinician whether causative or symptomatic treatment is possible or, commonly, whether a combination of both is necessary. Within the classificatory axis of causative factors, the differentiation between cancer pain and pain due to non-cancer causes assumes particular pertinence whenever the evaluator is confronted with pain of more than 6-months duration (chronic pain, see above).

NON-CANCER

Chronic non-cancer pain, the grist for most pain clinics, involves a number of different pathophysiologic problems that render the sufferer unable to enjoy life, but do not threaten to end life. This type of pain is often described in relationship to an anatomical site and engenders considerable anxiety. Myofascial pain, pain arising from muscle and connective tissue, accounts for a considerable amount of chronic non-cancer pain, and requires specific active therapy (stretching, trigger-point injections) and corrective actions for pain relief (Simons, Travell, & Simons, 1999; Travell & Simons, 1983).

CANCER

Chronic cancer pain is generally managed for the patient, while non-cancer pain is better managed by the patient through education, empowerment, and rehabilitation. Cancer-related pain management, like acute pain management, focuses on the comfort of the patient and involves a strategy of palliation. Palliative care involves the liberal use of medication, often opioid analgesics, with maximum comfort through symptom relief, but with toxicity from therapy kept acceptable relative to the distress produced by the symptoms being addressed.

Cancer pain is divided by the presumed pathophysiology into somatic, visceral, and deafferentation (also called neuropathic). This classification system focuses on the site of nociception (potential tissue damaging situations), being peripheral for somatic pain, intra-abdominal for visceral pain, and involving injury to afferent neural pathways for deafferentation. The pain that results from somatic processes is well localized, constant, aching, or gnawing in character. The visceral pain is poorly localized by comparison, but is constant and aching in character. It is referred to cutaneous sites. Deafferentation (neuropathic) pain is characterized by tingling, sharp paroxysmal sensations or burning dysesthesia, and is traditionally managed with adjuvant medications including antidepressants and anticonvulsants, not opioid analgesics as are visceral and somatic pains (Foley, 1985).

Bruera, Walker, and Lawlor (1999) challenged the traditional view of neuropathic pain management when they reported that more than two thirds of patients with neuropathic cancer pain achieved good analgesia with opioids alone in a prospective open study. Because the effectiveness of adjuvant medications rarely exceeded 30%, Bruera, Walker, and Lawlor recommended that opioids remain the first line of treatment for neuropathic pain patients, with adjuvants added when patients reach opioid dose-limiting toxicity.

Temporally, chronic cancer pain may worsen over time, due to the disease progression and from the various interventions (chemotherapy, radiotherapy, and surgery) used to treat the disease. The need for increasing doses of opioid analgesics is more often related to these situations, not to the rapid development of tolerance or medication abuse, as many practitioners mistakenly believe. Chronic non-cancer pain may also worsen over time, resulting in significant behavioral changes (pain behavior) and excessive use of analgesic medication.

It was recommended by Foley (1979, 1985) to classify cancer patients with pain into five groups: (1) patients with acute cancer-related pain, (2) patients with chronic cancer-related pain due to either progression or therapy, (3) patients with preexisting chronic non-cancer pain and cancer-related pain, (4) patients with a chemical dependency history and cancer-related pain, and (5) actively dying patients who must be provided comfort measures (Portenoy, 1988). This system of classifying pain according to the type of patient allowed for a rich psychosocial approach and prospective planning for the comprehensive needs of the patient, rather than too narrowly focusing on a single dimension of the pain. It also explained some of the unusual situations that developed while treating cancer pain patients, such as the following.

Case Example

Mr. P. was a 50-year-old gentleman with invasive head and neck squamous cell cancer. He had previously declined surgery but had had radiation therapy 1 year before entering the hospice program with an ulcerated, foul-smelling neck mass. His pain was initially managed by his referring physician with acetaminophen and codeine elixir, 600 mg/60 mg every 4 h, and oral lidocaine 2% viscous solution every four 4 h as needed. While not appreciated at first, it became readily obvious that he had a long-standing alcohol abuse disorder. He regularly supplemented his gastric tube feedings with liberal quantities of vodka, beer, and coffee liquor. He alleged that he only used small amounts of these beverages to cleanse the feeding tube, but was found to be intoxicated on many occasions. When his pain became more difficult to control with codeine, after 3 months of hospice involvement, he was given morphine concentrate (20 mg/ml) via the gastric tube. He quickly began to abuse the morphine, and occasionally took as much as 100 to 200 mg at a time, when only 20 to 30 mg had been prescribed. He ultimately stopped abusing the alcoholic beverages, but enjoyed the large doses of morphine at night when he wanted to sleep.

Few cancer pain patients exist in isolation, and most of these patients are cared for to some degree by concerned family members and friends. The support of the primary caregiver, with an emphasis on anticipatory bereavement, is an important element of hospice management. During the impending death of the cancer patient, the family members frequently become uncertain about their ability to provide continued care. To be able to keep the dying patient comfortable, unpleasant symptoms (nausea, vomiting, seizures, terminal restlessness) are aggressively controlled, and the caregiver is routinely provided support and respite breaks (Cole & Douglass, 1990).

CLASSIFICATION BY PAIN INTENSITY

Non-cancer-related pain is often rated along a continuum from mild to moderate to severe, but the words *incapacitating*, *overwhelming*, and *soul stealing* become necessary qualifiers for cancer pain. The intensity of the pain is perhaps the least desirable system for classifying pain, as intensity varies for most pain patients over time and is uniquely subjective. One pain patient might describe the pain experience due to some pathological condition as a 10, while another with the same pathology might feel that the intensity of pain is only a 5 (using a 0 to 10 scale where 0 signifies no pain at all and 10 represents the worse pain one could ever imagine). This has been noted under experimental conditions when identically calibrated pain stimuli, such as small electrical impulses, are administered to subjects and they rate them at widely divergent intensity levels. No clear correlation with any particular descriptor variables of the subjects could be established. Furthermore, factors lowering the cancer patient's pain threshold (the point at which a given stimulus provokes the report of pain) involve discomfort, insomnia, fatigue, anxiety, fear, anger, and depression; while restful sleep, relaxation, sympathy and understanding, elevation of mood, and diversion from the pain serve to raise the pain threshold (Twycross, 1980).

Rather than focus on a specific amount of pain, it is more useful to look at the disruption that pain causes for patients. Pain interfering with appetite, pleasurable activities, or sleep is more distressing than pain otherwise leaving an intact life, regardless of the reported intensity. Over time, most patients adapt to the pain and demonstrate either very little or markedly exaggerated pain behavior. Some patients may suffer with modest levels of pain, while others are able to function despite high levels. Suffering, an emotional response to the pain experience, is not necessarily linked to only the intensity of the pain as much as it is to the co-existence of anxiety, depression, and the failure to integrate the pain into the overall life experience. Suffering becomes an important issue when pain patients have concerns about the purpose, value, or meaning of their lives and an inability to foresee a future with function.

There is no way to know how much another person is in pain, and it is best to assume that the pain exists whenever a patient says it does and is whatever the patient says it is (McCaffery, 1999). Pain behavior is influenced and shaped by the environment, so the emphasis on function over intensity is critical for the rehabilitative approach to control chronic non-cancer pain. Family members and significant others, by altering their response to the pain behavior, are potentially involved with helping the patient to manage the chronic pain.

MENTAL HEALTH ISSUES IN PAIN CLASSIFICATION

Co-existing psychiatric disorders are not rare when pain is severe (Guggenheim, 2000). Mental health consultants are frequently asked to evaluate patients for suspected "psychogenic pain." This type of pain is included in the *Diagnostic and Statistical Manual of Mental Disorders, Fourth Edition*, where it is classified as a Pain Disorder (Table 4.1). Pain disorder is characterized by pain in one or more anatomical sites that is the predominant focus of the patient's clinical presentation and is of sufficient severity to warrant clinical attention; the pain causes clinically significant distress or impairment in social, occupational, or other important areas of functioning; psychological factors are judged to have an important role in the onset, severity, exacerbation, or maintenance of the pain; the symptom or deficit is not intentionally produced or feigned; and the pain is not better accounted for by a mood, anxiety, or psychotic disorder and does not meet criteria for dyspareunia (American Psychiatric Association, 1994). This condition further requires coding for the subtypes of pain disorder associated with psychological factors (acute or chronic), pain disorder associated with both psychological factors and a general medical condition (acute or chronic), and pain disorder associated with a general medical condition (acute or chronic).

There is little doubt that a relationship between pain and other mental disorders exists, but the exact nature of the relationship is less than clear (King, 1999). It must be emphasized that all pain is real to the patient, and little is to be accomplished by challenging the validity of the pain. Because pain is experienced in the mind and requires the interpretation of bodily sensations, there is a psychological overlay with most pain problems. It is artificial and absurd to try to partition pain into real or psychological types, especially when the distinction is too often based upon the treating practitioner's lack of ability to identify objective pathology. To fully understand the relationship between nociception and the psychological effects of acute and chronic pain, the practitioner must recognize emotional distress rather than purely nociception as a cause of pain, and understand that psychological mechanisms do intensify pain perception (Abram, 1985). An emotional reaction to pain does not mean that pain is caused only by an emotional problem (McCaffery & Pasero, 1999).

Psychosomatic pain is unfortunately synonymous with imagined pain, yet this pain may be as severe and distressing as somatogenic pain (Abram, 1985). While the threshold, the point where pain is first noted, is fairly

---

TABLE 4.1
Pain Disorder Diagnostic Features

A. Pain in one or more anatomical sites is the predominant focus of the clinical presentation and is of sufficient severity to warrant clinical attention.

B. The pain causes significant distress or impairment in social, occupational, or other important areas of functioning.

C. Psychological factors are judged to play a significant role in the onset, severity, exacerbation, or maintenance of the pain.

D. The pain is not intentionally produced or feigned as in Factitious Disorder or Malingering.

E. Pain Disorder is not diagnosed if the pain is better accounted for by a Mood, Anxiety, or Psychotic Disorder, or if the pain presentation meets criteria for Dyspareunia.

Pain Disorder is coded according to the subtype that best characterizes the factors involved in the etiology and maintenance of the pain:

307.80 Pain Disorder Associated with Psychological Factors: This subtype is used when psychological factors are judged to have the major role in the onset, severity, exacerbation, or maintenance of the pain. In this subtype, general medical conditions play either no role or a minimal role in the onset or maintenance of the pain. This subtype is not diagnosed if criteria for Somatization Disorder are also met.

Acute: This specifier is used if the duration of the pain is less than 6 months.

Chronic: This specifier is used if the duration of the pain is 6 months or longer.

307.89 Pain Disorder Associated with Both Psychological Factors and a General Medical Condition: This subtype is used when both psychological factors and a general medical condition are judged to have important roles in the onset, severity, exacerbation, or maintenance of the pain. The anatomical site of the pain or associated general medical condition is also coded.

Acute: This specifier is used if the duration of the pain is less than 6 months.

Chronic: This specifier is used if the duration of the pain is 6 months or longer.

293.83 Pain Disorder Associated with a General Medical Condition: (*Note: This subtype of Pain Disorder is not considered a mental disorder. It is included to facilitate differential diagnosis.*) The pain results from a general medical condition, and psychological factors are judged to play either no role or a minimal role in the onset or maintenance of the pain. The ICD-9-CM code for this subtype is selected based on the location of the pain or the associated general medical condition if this has been established or on the anatomical location of the pain if the underlying general medical condition is not yet clearly established—for example, low back (724.2), sciatic (724.3), pelvic (625.9), headache (784.0), facial (784.0), chest (786.50), joint (719.4), bone (733.90), abdominal (789.0), breast (611.71), renal (788.0), ear (388.70), eye (379.91), throat (784.1), tooth (525.9), and urinary (788.0).

From the American Psychiatric Association (1994). *Diagnostic and Statistical Manual of Mental Disorders* (4th ed.). Washington, D.C. American Psychiatric Press. With permission.

constant from person to person, the tolerance, what pain a person will endure, is highly variable (Bowsher, 1983). Factors such as depression, anxiety, and motivation significantly influence the tolerance for pain and may determine the amount of suffering and pain behavior generated. Secondary gain, the practical advantage resulting from the symptom of pain, is not the same as malingering or factitious disorder and does not signify that pain is purely psychological in origin (Dunajcik, 1999).

The use of placebo medication or therapy to determine the reality of pain is highly deplorable and potentially very costly (Frank-Stromborg & Christiansen, 2000). Because the ability to respond positively to a placebo has to do with the belief system of the patient, nothing about the reality of the pain will be learned from the use of sham therapies. The only accurate conclusion about a person who responds positively to a placebo is that he wants pain relief and that he trusts someone or something to help him (Edmondson, 2000). Curiously, we give placebos to patients who are the least likely to respond to them, the patients we do not like, and those who do not believe in our efforts. Rarely do we use placebos with the cooperative patients who could respond to them.

RESEARCH CLASSIFICATION

A complex pain classification system has been published by the International Association for the Study of Pain (1986), and provides the clinician with descriptive lists about pain syndromes (Table 4.2). This taxonomy defines pain syndromes, allows improved communication between clinicians and researchers, and leads to improved treatment options that are specific for each syndrome. A five axes coding scheme signifies the region of the pain (Axis I), organ system (Axis II), temporal characteristics and pattern of occurrence (Axis III), patient's statement of intensity and duration since onset of pain (Axis IV), and the presumed etiology (Axis V). Using the IASP classification of chronic pain the practitioner is able to obtain definition, site, main features, associated symptoms, laboratory findings, usual course, complications, social and physical disabilities, pathology, summary of essential features and diagnostic criteria, and differential diagnosis for most pain problems. Specific definitions with notes on usage are included, providing consistency in describing pains itself.

The IASP pain classification system is not yet proven to be reliable and valid, and has not been widely accepted since development in the 1980s. Further research is still needed to determine the psychometric properties and to facilitate modifications to the system (Turk & Okifuji, 2001). Presently, few clinicians or payment sources in the U.S. use the IASP classification system. It is the most thorough and best effort at codification available at this time. The IASP classification system allows pain syndrome diagnoses to be made with inclusion, not exclusion criteria. Pain syndromes

TABLE 4.2
International Association for the Study of Pain Coding for Chronic Pain

Axis I: Regions

Head, face, and mouth	000
Cervical region	100
Upper shoulder and upper limbs	200
Thoracic region	300
Abdominal region	400
Lower back, lumbar spine, sacrum, and coccyx	500
Lower limbs	600
Pelvic region	700
Anal, perineal, and genital region	800
More than three major sites	900

Axis II: Systems

Nervous system (central, peripheral, and autonomic) and special senses; physical disturbance or dysfunction	00
Nervous system (psychological and social)	10
Respiratory and cardiovascular systems	20
Musculoskeletal system and connective tissue	30
Cutaneous and subcutaneous and associated glands	40
Gastrointestinal system	50
Genitourinary system	60
Other organs or viscera	70
More than one system	80
Unknown	90

Axis III: Temporal characteristics of pain: pattern of occurrence

Not recorded, not applicable, or not known	0
Single episode, limited duration	1
Continuous or nearly continuous, nonfluctuating	2
Continuous or nearly continuous, fluctuating	3
Recurring irregularly	4
Recurring regularly	5
Paroxysmal	6
Sustained with superimposed paroxysms	7
Other combinations	8
None of the above	9

Axis IV: Patient's statement of intensity: time since onset of pain

Not recorded, not applicable, or not known	0.0
Mild, 1 month or less	0.1
Mild, 1–6 months	0.2
Mild, more than 6 months	0.3
Medium, 1 month or less	0.4
Medium, 1–6 months	0.5
Medium, more than 6 months	0.6
Severe, 1 month or less	0.7
Severe, 1–6 months	0.8
Severe, more than 6 months	0.9

Axis V: Etiology

Genetic or congenital disorders	0.00
Trauma, operation, burns	0.01
Infective, parasitic	0.02
Inflammatory (no known infective agent), immune reaction	0.03
Neoplasm	0.04
Toxic, metabolic, anoxia, vascular, nutritional, radiation	0.05
Degenerative, mechanical	0.06
Dysfunctional (including psychophysiologic)	0.07

TABLE 4.2 (CONTINUED)
International Association for the Study of Pain Coding for Chronic Pain

Unknown or other	0.08
Psychological origin	0.09

Examples:

Metastatic cancer (0.04) pain involving skull, shoulder, sacrum, hip, femur (900) and surrounding "soft tissue" (30); continuous in nature with fluctuations related to movement and position (3); severe intensity, more than six months in duration (0.9) is coded as 933.94.

Lower back pain (500) due to myofascial dysfunction (30); continuous and nonfluctuating (2); mild intensity for more than 6 months (0.3); exacerbated by obesity ((0.05) is coded as 532.35.

Abdominal pain (400) due to pancreatitis (50); recurring irregularly (4); severe intensity for less than 1 week per episode (0.7) associated with alcohol use (0.05) is coded as 454.75.

Note: This system establishes a five-digit code for each chronic pain diagnosis. (From International Association for the Study of Pain (1986), Classification of chronic pain: Descriptions of chronic pain syndromes and definitions of pain terms. *Pain, 3*(Suppl.), S1–S225. With permission.)

are diagnosed by what they are, not what they are not. Patients want to know what they have, not be told to live with what their clinicians cannot diagnose.

CONCLUSION

A perceptual phenomenon, like pain, is not accessible to objective validation. The subjective experience of pain is universal and one of the most common reasons that patients seek a clinician's help. An extensive armamentarium of medical, surgical, psychological, social, and rehabilitative interventions is available to address pain. In order to intervene effectively, however, the clinician must have a conceptual frame of reference. A biopsychosocial model recognizing the biological/physiological, psychological/behavioral, and environmental influences is likely the best conceptualization and the only one able to explain all patients and their pain (Robinson & Riley, 1999).

The widespread use of the Internet and the demand by healthcare payers to provide meaningful outcome data has made pain classification more than just an academic exercise. Pain practitioners from different disciplines and specialties must be able to effectively communicate with one another. Well-defined pain classification systems are necessary and must become part of the clinical record (Derasari, 2000).

Pain means suffering. It has plagued humanity as long as humans have existed. To attempt to remedy the suffering and relieve the pain, accurate assessment and diagnosis must occur. Although many pain syndromes still do not have specific therapies, by classifying pain into certain categories it is now possible to design treatment approaches to benefit most of our patients and, over time, hopefully, we will help the others.

REFERENCES

Abram, S.E. (1985). Pain pathways and mechanisms. *Seminars in Anesthesia, 4,* 267–274.

Agency for Health Care Policy and Research. (1992). *Acute Pain Management: Operative or Medical Procedures and Trauma, Clinical Practice Guideline.* (AHCPR Pub. No. 92-0032). Rockville, MD: AHCPR.

Akca, O., Melischek, M., Scheck, T., Heilwagner, K., Arkilic, C.F., Kurz, A., Kapral S., Heinz, T., Lackner, F.X., & Sessler, D.L. (1999). Postoperative pain and subcutaneous oxygen tension. *Lancet, 354,* 41–42.

American Psychiatric Association (1994). *Diagnostic and statistical manual of mental disorders* (4th ed., pp. 458–462). Washington, D.C.: American Psychiatric Press.

Bowsher, D. (1983). Pain mechanisms in man. *Resident and Staff Physician, 29,* 26–34.

Bruera, E., Walker, P., & Lawlor, P. (1999). Opioids in cancer pain. In C. Stein (Ed.), *Opioids in pain control: Basic and clinical aspects,* (pp. 309–324). Cambridge, UK: Cambridge University Press.

Chapman, S.L., & Brena, S.F. (1989). Pain and litigation. In P. D. Wall & R. Melzack (Eds.), *Textbook of pain* (2nd ed., pp. 1032–1041). Edinburgh: Churchill Livingstone.

Cole, B.E., & Douglass, M.C. (1990). Hospice, cancer pain management and symptom control. In R.S. Weiner (Ed.), *Innovations in pain management: A practical guide for clinicians,* (pp. 4–30). Orlando, FL: Paul M. Deutsch Press.

Cousins, M.J. (1989). Acute and postoperative pain. In P.D. Wall & R. Melzack (Eds.), *Textbook of pain* (2nd ed., pp. 284–305). Edinburgh: Churchill Livingstone.

Crue, B.L. (1983). The neurophysiology and taxonomy of pain. In S.F. Brena & S.L. Chapman (Eds.), *Management of patients with chronic pain,* (pp. 21–31). Jamaica, NY: Spectrum Publications.

Derasari, M.D. (2000). Taxonomy of pain syndromes: Classification of chronic pain syndromes. In P.P. Raj (Ed.), *Practical Management of Pain* (3rd ed., pp. 10–16). St. Louis, MO: Mosby.

Dinarello, C. (1984). Interleukin-I. *Reviews of Infectious Diseases, 6,* 51–95.

Dunajcik, L. (1999). Chronic nonmalignant pain. In M. McCaffery & C. Pasero (Eds.), *Pain: Clinical manual* (2nd ed., pp. 467–521). St. Louis, MO: Mosby.

Edmondson, J.C. (2000). Chronic pain and the placebo effect. In B.J. Sadock & V.A. Sadock (Eds.), *Kaplan & Sadock's comprehensive textbook of psychiatry* (7th ed., pp. 1981–2001). Philadelphia, PA: Lippincott Williams & Wilkins.

Egdahl, G. (1959). Pituitary-adrenal response following trauma to the isolated leg. *Surgery, 46,* 9–21.

Frank-Stromborg, M., & Christiansen, A. (2000). The undertreatment of pain: A liability risk for nurses. *Clinical Journal of Oncology Nursing, 4,* 41–44.

Foley, K.M. (1979). Pain syndromes in patients with cancer. In J.J. Bonica & V. Ventafridda (Eds.), *Advances in pain research and therapy* (Vol. 2, pp. 59–75). New York, NY: Raven Press.

Foley, K.M. (1985). The treatment of cancer pain. *The New England Journal of Medicine, 313,* 84–95.

Guggenheim, F.G. (2000). Somatoform disorders. In B.J. Sadock & V.A. Sadock (Eds.), *Kaplan & Sadock's comprehensive textbook of psychiatry* (7th ed., pp. 1504–1532). Philadelphia, PA: Lippincott Williams & Wilkins.

International Association for the Study of Pain. (1986). Classification of chronic pain: Descriptions of chronic pain syndromes and definitions of pain terms. *Pain, 3* (Suppl.), S1-S225.

Joint Commission on Accreditation of Healthcare Organizations. (2000). Pain management today. In *Pain assessment and management: An organizational approach,* (pp. 1–6). Oakbrook Terrace, IL: Joint Commission.

Kehlet, H. (1982). The endocrine-metabolic response to postoperative pain. *Acta Anaesthesiologica Scandinavica, 74* (Suppl.), 173–175.

Kehlet, H., Brandt, M.R., & Rem, J. (1980). Role of neurogenic stimuli in mediating the endocrine-metabolic response to surgery. *Journal of Parenteral & Enteral Nutrition, 4,* 152–156.

King, S.A. (1999). Pain disorders. In R.E. Hales, S.C. Yudofsky & J.A. Talbott (Eds.), *Textbook of psychiatry* (3rd ed., pp. 1003–1021). Washington, D.C.: American Psychiatric Press, Inc.

Liebeskind, J.C. (1991). Pain can kill. *Pain, 44,* 3–4.

McCaffery, M. (1999). Pain management: Problems and progress. In M. McCaffery & C. Pasero (Eds.), *Pain: Clinical manual* (2nd ed., pp. 1–14). St. Louis, MO: Mosby.

McCaffery, M. & Pasero, C. (1999). Assessment: Underlying complexities, misconceptions and practical tools. In M. McCaffery & C. Pasero (Eds.), *Pain: Clinical manual* (2nd ed., pp. 35–102). St. Louis, MO: Mosby.

Melzack, R. (1990). The needless tragedy of pain. *Scientific American, 262*(2): 27–33.

Pasero, C., Paice, J.A. & McCaffery, M. (1999). Basic mechanisms underlying the causes and effects of pain. In M. McCaffery & C. Pasero (Eds.), *Pain: Clinical manual* (2nd ed., pp. 15–34). St. Louis, MO: Mosby.

Portenoy, R.K. (1988). Practical aspects of pain control in the patient with cancer. *Ca–A Cancer Journal for Clinicians, 38,* 327–352.

Price, D.D. (1999). The phenomenon of pain. In *Psychological mechanisms of pain and analgesia, Progress in Pain Research and Management* (Vol. 15, pp. 3–14). Seattle, WA: IASP Press.

Robinson, M.E. & Riley, J.L. (1999). Models of pain. In A.R. Block, E.F. Kremer & E. Fernandez (Eds.), *Handbook of pain syndromes,* (pp. 23–40). Mahwah, NJ: Lawrence Erlbaum Associates, Inc.

Simons, D.G., Travell, J.G., & Simons, L.S. (1999). *Travell & Simons' myofascial pain and dysfunction: The trigger point manual* (Vol. 1, 2nd ed.). Baltimore, MD: Williams & Wilkins.

Travell, J.G. & Simons, D.G. (1983). *Myofascial pain and dysfunction: The trigger point manual.* Baltimore, MD: Williams & Wilkins.

Twycross, R.G., (1980). The relief of pain in far-advanced cancer. *Regional Anesthesia, 5*, 2–11.

Turk, D.C., & Okifuji, A. (2001). Pain terms and taxonomies of pain. In J.D. Loeser (Ed.), *Bonica's management of pain* (3rd ed., pp. 17–25). Philadelphia, PA: Lippincott Williams & Wilkins.

Waldman, S.D. (1990). Acute and postoperative pain management — An idea ripe for the times. *Pain Practitioner, 2*, 4, 9–10.

Wall, P.D., (1989). Introduction. In P.D. Wall & R. Melzack (Eds.), *Textbook of pain* (2nd ed., pp. 1–18). Edinburgh: Churchill Livingstone.

Wattwil, M. (1989). Postoperative pain relief and gastrointestinal motility. *Acta Chiurgica Scandinavica, 550* (Suppl.), 140–145.

5

Starting a Pain Clinic

Clayton A. Varga, M.D.

DEVELOPMENT CHECKLIST

1. Ask: Am I sure I want to do this?
2. Identify a leader: Am I qualified?
3. Select the clinic structure.
4. Assess the need.
5. Develop the business plan.
6. Research financial options.
7. Select the participating professionals.
8. Hire support and administrative personnel.
9. Develop the marketing plan.
10. Select the site.
11. Determine equipment needs.
12. Plan billing and collections procedures.
13. Developing a capitated contract.

ARE YOU SURE YOU WANT TO DO THIS?

The formation of any business requires a great deal of forethought and an investment of time, energy, and money to be successful. Starting a pain clinic is no exception. Individuals who wish to engage in the business of pain should ask themselves the following questions: Am I completely committed to the success of the business? Am I willing to be the effective leader of the business? If not, do I have someone to fulfill this function? Do I recognize that the financial aspects of the clinic require as much attention and expertise as the practice aspects? If the answer to any of these questions is no, then all further efforts will most likely be wasted.

IDENTIFY A LEADER

Ask yourself: Am I qualified by education and temperament to start and run a pain clinic? Do I possess the specialized clinical background necessary to develop and implement the needed structure for evaluation and treatment of patients in a multidisciplinary setting? Am I able to participate in the development of contracts and marketing plans and oversee administrative decisions? If you are unable to fulfill these requirements, then it is necessary to secure the participation of one or more individuals who can before proceeding to the next step.

SELECTION OF CLINIC STRUCTURE

Having made the decision to move forward, the desired clinic structure must be selected. Practice types and accompanying brief descriptions are as follows:

1. Single modality: A single practitioner (e.g., neurologist, acupuncturist, chiropractor) seeing and treating patients without regular input from other practitioners.
2. Multimodality: Practitioners of different specialties, treating patients in a similar location without regular, structured discussion of the patients by all practitioners.
3. Multidisciplinary: Practitioners of multiple different specialties, including a minimum of one representative from each of the following fields: physician, physical therapy, and psychology. Often present are occupational therapy,

0-8493-0926-3/02/$0.00+$1.50
© 2002 by CRC Press LLC

acupuncture, nursing, and chiropractic. The members of the clinic have made a commitment to attend regular patient conferences and to provide integrated care of the patient.

The applicability of each item discussed in this chapter will largely depend on the clinic model developed. The less complex the model, the less important certain aspects of the development process become. However, even the simplest single-modality model would benefit from following most of the steps in the development checklist.

The more complex the structure, and the greater the number of participants, the more time, energy, and money will be required to take the business from concept to a fully operational entity. The remainder of this chapter is directed toward a multidisciplinary pain clinic that has a full-time medical director and provides, as a minimum, physical therapy and psychology services and may well offer nursing, occupational therapy, and acupuncture services.

ASSESSMENT OF NEED

Once a preferred structure for the clinic has been selected, then an assessment of need must take place. The purpose of the assessment of need is to determine the demand for the product. It determines if the clinic, in the geographic area to be served, can reasonably expect to draw enough patients to pay all debt and still produce a profit. The assessment should take into account the following:

1. What is the size of the population served (i.e., what is the catchment area)?
2. What is the willingness of physicians within the catchment area to refer patients for the services you are providing?
3. Who is the competition? Are similar facilities already present?
4. What percentage of the population is served by HMOs, PPOs, or IPAs? What will be your ability to gain access to those patients?
5. Can you develop a relationship with an existing healthcare provider who will guarantee patient referrals prior to beginning operations?

The first step is to define your likely catchment area. This represents the geographic boundaries from which you can reasonably expect to draw patients.

In an urban or suburban environment, this usually represents a distance of 15 to at most 30 miles from the business. Obviously, there will be regional variation in the size of the catchment area, depending on the proximity of the clinic to major transportation arteries and traffic patterns and perceived excellence of the clinic. Once defined, the population within the catchment area should

be estimated. While no hard and fast rules exist, if the catchment area has a population of less than 100,000, its ability to support a true multidisciplinary clinic or center is questionable.

Competing service providers need to be evaluated. If one or several high-quality providers already exist in the proposed catchment area and if they have excess capacity, then concrete reasons for believing that you can capture a large enough portion of the market share to survive must be identified before business start-up. In such a situation, contracts with a PPO or IPA to be the sole provider for pain management services and verbal assurances of appropriate patient referrals from independent physicians should be obtained prior to entering the marketplace.

Talk to local HMO, PPO, and IPA administrators. Assess your ability to draw patients from these ranks. Meet with attorneys, case workers, and insurance carriers who are involved locally in the workers' compensation system and assess how many referrals are likely from these sources.

Having done the above, estimate the total number of monthly referrals you expect from all sources. If enough patients are forthcoming to support the business, then development of a detailed business plan becomes the next step. If patient referrals appear to be insufficient, then it is wise to explore other sources of patient referral before proceeding. If, after further exploration, more patients are not forthcoming, it is probably best to rethink your proposed catchment area, moving to one with a more favorable referral pattern.

THE BUSINESS PLAN

If, based on the assessment of need, it is likely that the business will be profitable in the selected catchment area, then a detailed business plan is developed. The purpose of the plan is to secure on paper a description of the components of the operation and a schedule of their implementation. This should occur prior to spending the first dollar on the program.

The business plan has two major components. The first is a narrative which contains a brief description of the business, in which the purpose and structure of the business are outlined. Included is a description of the personnel involved, the function each fulfills, an outline of the marketing plan, and a general description of the facility requirements. The narrative section should briefly address each of the following components:

1. The purpose of the business
2. The market niche served by the business
3. The personnel involved and the function of each
4. Facility requirements
5. Outline of the marketing plan
6. Plan for dissolution of the business

The second portion of the business plan is done as a spreadsheet. It can be prepared by hand using a large ledger sheet or more easily by using one of a number of commercially available electronic spreadsheets (e.g., Lotus 1-2-3).

A sample business plan for a hospital-based multidisciplinary clinic that provides primarily outpatient services is shown in Table 5.1. The business plan estimates fixed and variable costs, revenues, and the amount of start-up capital needed to begin the business and keep it running until the revenue stream produces a profit. Total cost is simply the summation of the individual cost estimates. The sample spreadsheet in Table 5.1 lists most of the individual cost estimates that are required for a multidisciplinary clinic. Each expenditure is estimated on a month-by-month basis for at least one year and entered into the spreadsheet. This produces a time estimate of how long it will take to generate a profit and estimates the revenue position of the business at any point along the time line.

The cost estimate should be as detailed as possible. It is possible to accurately predict almost all of the costs, especially fixed costs, when doing the business plan. This is in contrast to revenue estimation, which will be, at best, a rough guess. Nailing down the cost projections as accurately as possible will, in turn, allow for the greatest possible accuracy in predicting the net revenue estimate.

It is best to shift as much of the cost as possible from fixed to variable. This minimizes expenses when revenue is low. Several examples of doing this are hiring personnel on part-time or flexible-time schedules, increasing hours as patient load increases, and having billing and collection done by an outside service, with cost based on a percentage of collections.

Obtaining the revenue estimate requires developing an approximate charge per patient. If the clinic is based on one or several structured programs, in which each patient participates in a relatively uniform program for a predetermined length of time, then average charges are easy to estimate. If the clinic structure is such that revenue generation is spread over a wide range of activities, then generating an average charge per patient is more difficult. In this situation, it is necessary to develop multiple average patient charges and estimate what portion of the total predicted patient flow falls into each group.

Subtracting total cost from total revenue yields the predicted financial position of the business at any point along the time line. It is wise to do estimates using best guess, worst case, and best case revenue projection scenarios. If you are prepared to survive the worst case scenario, then the business should succeed.

FINANCING

The business plan will project the necessary capital required for business formation and development. The most common cause of a new business failure is undercapitalization. It is important to generate at least as much capital as is required based on the business plan. It is also wise to have a credit line available for emergencies. Once capitalization requirements have been determined, options for obtaining the capital must be explored. Numerous financing possibilities exist. Those most commonly employed are as follows:

1. Joint venture: This almost always consists of a limited partnership. The limited partnership consists of both limited and general partners. The general partners oversee the business formation and development and have a greater degree of legal responsibility should the enterprise fail. Limited partners invest money into the partnership but are passive in the business formation and development. Their losses are limited to their investments.

   An example of a joint venture is as follows: The director of the proposed facility develops a detailed business plan. A lawyer is hired to prepare a joint venture agreement, wherein the director is the general partner and the individuals supplying the money are limited partners. The director oversees the development and daily running of the business, for which he or she receives a portion of the profits generated by the business. The director may also receive monies generated via professional activities carried out at the business. The remaining profits are disbursed to the limited partners.

2. Borrowing of money by one or several individuals from conventional lending sources (i.e., a practice loan).

3. Utilization of personal capital to begin the business.

SELECTION OF PARTICIPATING PROFESSIONALS

The type of clinic or operating structure chosen will determine the professional components of the clinic. The quality of the professional personnel will be one of, if not the most important determinants of success. Careful thought must be given to this topic. Not only must the professionals be well trained in their own disciplines, but they must understand the fundamental difference between practicing in a unidimensional office vs. a multidisciplinary setting. They must be willing to make what are often perceived as personal sacrifices to make the system work and to regularly attend patient conference meetings and provide input in those meetings in a useful fashion. They must understand the need to promote the clinic as an entity, as

TABLE 5.1
XYZ Office Overhead First Year of Operations

Month columns are 1–12.

Item		Total Annual	1	2	3	4	5	6	7	8	9	10	11	12
Average length of stay														
Full-day nonresidential	35		20,125	20,125	20,125	20,125	20,125	20,125	20,125	20,125	20,125	20,125	20,125	20,125
Half-day nonresidential	20		7,900	7,900	7,900	7,900	7,900	7,900	7,900	7,900	7,900	7,900	7,900	7,900
Patient census														
Full-day nonresidential	56		0	0	0	3	3	4	5	7	7	8	9	10
Full-day nonresidential	33		0	0	0	1	1	2	3	4	4	5	6	7
Half-day nonresidential	23		0	0	0	2	2	2	2	3	3	3	3	3
Revenue														
Full-day nonresidential	$575	664,125	0	0	0	20,125	20,125	40,250	60,375	80,500	80,500	100,625	120,750	140,875
Half-day nonresidential	$395	181,700	0	0	0	15,800	15,800	15,800	15,800	23,700	23,700	23,700	23,700	23,700
Total revenue		845,825	0	0	0	35,925	35,925	56,050	76,175	104,200	104,200	124,325	144,450	164,575
Deductions from revenue														
80% coverage	20.00%	169,165	0	0	0	7,185	7,185	11,210	15,235	20,840	20,840	24,865	28,890	32,915
Provision for bad debt	20.00%	33,833	0	0	0	1,437	1,437	2,242	3,047	4,168	4,168	4,973	5,778	6,583
Billing expense	6.5%	10,996	0	0	0	467	467	729	990	1,355	1,355	1,616	1,878	2,139
Total deductions		213,994	0	0	0	9,089	9,089	14,181	19,272	26,363	26,363	31,454	36,546	41,637
Net revenue		631,831	0	0	0	26,836	26,836	41,869	56,903	77,837	77,837	92,871	107,904	122,938
Program personnel[a]														
Medical director[b]	90,000	90,000	7,500	7,500	7,500	7,500	7,500	7,500	7,500	7,500	7,500	7,500	7,500	7,500
Acupuncturist	35,000	45,500	3,792	3,792	3,792	3,792	3,792	3,792	3,792	3,792	3,792	3,792	3,792	3,792
Physical therapist[c]	45,000	58,500	4,875	4,875	4,875	4,875	4,875	4,875	4,875	4,875	4,875	4,875	4,875	4,875
Psychologist consultant[b]	50,000	50,000	4,167	4,167	4,167	4,167	4,167	4,167	4,167	4,167	4,167	4,167	4,167	4,167
Nurse/social worker[d]	35,000	45,500	3,792	3,792	3,792	3,792	3,792	3,792	3,792	3,792	3,792	3,792	3,792	3,792
Program personnel		289,500	24,125	24,125	24,125	24,125	24,125	24,125	24,125	24,125	24,125	24,125	24,125	24,125
Office personnel[a]														
Office manager	25,000	32,500	2,708	2,708	2,708	2,708	2,708	2,708	2,708	2,708	2,708	2,708	2,708	2,708
Receptionist	18,000	23,400	1,950	1,950	1,950	1,950	1,950	1,950	1,950	1,950	1,950	1,950	1,950	1,950
Recruitment fee	5,000	5,000	5,000											
Training	1,000	1,000	83	83	83	83	83	83	83	83	83	83	83	83
Office personnel		61,900	9,742	4,742	4,742	4,742	4,742	4,742	4,742	4,742	4,742	4,742	4,742	4,742
Administrative costs														
Accounting fees for taxes/audit		1,500	125	125	125	125	125	125	125	125	125	125	125	125
Payroll, accounting fee		480	40	40	40	40	40	40	40	40	40	40	40	40
Bank fees		150	13	13	13	13	13	13	13	13	13	13	13	13
Quality assurance		4,000	333	333	333	333	333	333	333	333	333	333	333	333
Administrative costs		6,130	511	511	511	511	511	511	511	511	511	511	511	511
Business formation														
Accounting		100	100											
Attorney corporation fee		7,500	7,500											
Business formation fees & licenses		950	950											
Reproduction/printing		500	500											
Business formation		9,050	9,050											

	Total	1	2	3	4	5	6	7	8	9	10	11	12
Capital & equipment expense													
Capital expense	53,000	53,000											
Small equipment	15,000	15,000											
Capital & equipment	68,000	68,000											
Marketing costs													
Advertising	10,000	833	833	833	833	833	833	833	833	833	833	833	833
Brochures	8,000	8,000											
Announcements	6,500	6,500											
Lectures/slides	500	167			167				167				
Marketing costs	25,000	8,833	7,333	8,833	1,000	833	833	833	1,000	833	833	833	833
Office operations													
Books	63	63	63	63	63	63	63	63	63	63	63	63	63
Business licenses/fees	800	800											
Exchange	2,700	225	225	225	225	225	225	225	225	225	225	225	225
Insurance/business overhead	1,500	1,500											
Insurance casualty	560	560											
Insurance/program liability	12,000	12,000											
Laundry/linen	1,500	125	125	125	125	125	125	125	125	125	125	125	125
Magazines	258	258											
Med supplies	24,000	2,000	2,000	2,000	2,000	2,000	2,000	2,000	2,000	2,000	2,000	2,000	2,000
Phone/6-line phone	8,430	703	703	703	703	703	703	703	703	703	703	703	703
Postage/Fed. Express	2,355	196	196	196	196	196	196	196	196	196	196	196	196
Reproduction/printing	350	29	29	29	29	29	29	29	29	29	29	29	29
Repairs/maintenance	5,700	633	633	633	633	633	633	633	633	633	633	633	633
Stationary	2,400	200	200	200	200	200	200	200	200	200	200	200	200
Supplies	5,500	458											
Taxes/IRS	[e]												
Taxes/state	800	800											
Transcription	7,836	653	653	653	653	653	653	653	653	653	653	653	653
Miscellaneous expenses	500	42											
Utilities	3,000	250											
Working capital/line of credit @ 12%	28,779	1,379	1,843	2,322	2,459	2,597	2,597	2,597	2,597	2,597	2,597	2,597	2,597
Office operations	109,718	21,441	6,036	6,515	7,286	7,424	7,424	7,424	7,424	7,424	7,424	7,424	8,224
Property, plant, equipment[f]													
Office rent (2,000 @ 2.5)	60,000	5,000	5,000	5,000	5,000	5,000	5,000	5,000	5,000	5,000	5,000	5,000	5,000
Property tax on triple net lease	750	750											
Equipment depreciation	See Capital equipment												
Amortized start-up	See Business formation												
Property, plant, equipment	60,750	5,750	5,000	5,000	5,000	5,000	5,000	5,000	5,000	5,000	5,000	5,000	5,000
Total expenses	630,048	139,618	47,747	49,726	42,497	42,635	42,801	42,635	42,635	42,801	50,236	35,036	43,435
Net operating income	1,783	(139,618)	(47,747)	(49,726)	(15,661)	(15,965)	(765)	14,268	35,203	35,036	50,236	65,270	79,503

a Employee benefits calculated at 28% (e.g., medical/dental/workers' compensation insurance/FICA/FWH labor costs will vary, depending upon urban location).

b Medical director and psychologists can be paid on a 1099 basis, assuming IRS criteria are met.

c Physical therapist's employee benefits 25%.

d This individual could function in a marketing capacity in addition to nursing/social work duties.

e Federal taxes in first year will be based on the NOI plus capitalized investment not written off in first year.

f Capital expenses and office rent could be what joint venture partners might provide for an equity interest in the clinic business. Note that both capital investment and business start-up are paid back in the first year of operation.

g Net operating income in the first year is a function of how quickly the marketing strategy/plan can tap into the clinic's catchment referral sources such HMOs, IPAs, personal injury attorneys, and workers' compensation case workers/attorneys.

well as themselves as individuals, and be willing to defer at times to other members of the team in the treatment of any particular patient. Many physicians and other professionals are not suited by character to function easily in such an environment and, despite any academic or other professional qualifications, are best excluded from the multidisciplinary setting. When selecting clinical members for the team, consideration of board certification in pain management should not be overlooked.

SUPPORT PERSONNEL

Personnel to perform all of the non-patient care activities are obviously necessary for the business to function. These areas include billing and collections, reception, ordering of supplies, scheduling, transcription, and paying bills, to name a few. These individuals should already have been taken into consideration as part of the business plan. All of these people need not be hired at the beginning of the business. It is preferable to keep start-up fixed costs as lean as possible. Even a multidisciplinary center can easily start with a single support person if time-consuming tasks, such as billing and transcription, are subcontracted to outside firms. This plan has the advantage of changing a fixed cost to a variable cost, which will be much cheaper when patient volume is low. As patient volume rises, these functions can easily be transferred in-house at such time as it becomes financially advantageous to do so.

If one individual is initially hired, then this person should be told that he or she is expected to be a jack-of-all-trades. This individual should also be someone who can become the office manager as other employees are put in place. The author believes that it is cheaper to hire one well-paid, highly motivated employee than two poorly paid, poorly motivated employees. As the business matures, additional employees can be added as need dictates.

SITE SELECTION

Having decided upon both the general geographic location and the specific structure of the clinic, it is possible to begin specific site selection. If a joint venture with a hospital has been undertaken, then the hospital may have unused space which can serve as the clinic site. This has several advantages. It serves to bind the interests of the hospital and the clinic. It provides the clinic with some instant name recognition, if the hospital name is incorporated into the clinic name, and it may help speed referrals to the clinic from members of the hospital medical staff. It also allows easy proximity between inpatient and outpatient care, if both are provided. The hospital may allow the space to be used in exchange for equity in the business, thus limiting operational costs.

If an off-hospital site is selected, then several factors need to be taken into consideration: proximity to other doctors' offices, ease of access to the likely patient base, cost per square foot, the ability of the site to be tailored to your needs, and the ability to expand into adjacent space in the future without having to relocate.

How much and what type of space will be needed will be determined by the clinic structure. Office rental cost represents one of the largest fixed expenses. The clinic structure should be well planned to maximally utilize each square foot of space. Initially, some, if not all, of the professional participants will have other practice locations. It is less expensive to time-share offices between practitioners, and it is unusual for all individuals to be seeing patients at the same time.

EQUIPMENT

Equipment used in a multidisciplinary pain clinic will depend on the clinic structure. If the clinic site is within a hospital, often all of the diagnostic, occupational, and physical therapy, and procedural (nerve block, laboratory testing, radiologic, and operating) equipment and facilities are already available. Supplying a site with the ability to see patients for medical and psychological evaluation, basic physical therapy treatment, minor office procedures (such as certain types of nerve blocks), relaxation training, biofeedback, and group as well as individual psychotherapy will require an expenditure of $50,000 to $75,000. This includes the purchase of furniture, exam and treatment tables, office and medical supplies, biofeedback equipment, fax, typewriter, photocopy equipment, and a phone system. This may or may not include computer equipment for word processing or billing. (As this is expensive, it is another reason to subcontract these services, at least during the first several years of the business.)

MARKETING

It is important to have an overall marketing plan that extends for a period of several years. This should take into consideration how much money is to be allocated to marketing efforts and what types of advertising and other promotional projects will be undertaken. It is not possible to be all things to all people. The marketing plan needs to reflect the market niche and present a consistent message.

Marketing medical services is a complicated and sometimes delicate job. Ethical standards regarding medical marketing vary regionally, and knowledge of local standards is crucial prior to beginning the marketing program. Being the first to employ a specific type of advertising in an area (e.g., radio commercials) can have a negative impact with referring physicians. However, certain techniques (discussed below) can be used in any environment.

Announcements and brochures should be sent to referring physicians, workers' compensation caseworkers, and attorneys. These should be mailed shortly after opening the practice. The announcement should be mailed first, with the brochure to follow one to two months later. This reinforces your message and is more effective than sending both at the same time.

Taking the time to personally contact and talk to local physicians, workers' compensation caseworkers, and lawyers is important in building referral patterns. PPOs, IPAs, and HMOs control a majority of the patient population in many areas. The clinic director must take the time to educate and negotiate with these groups to secure appropriate patient referral.

Lectures and community forums are useful tools for educating referring physicians as well as potential patients not only about the problem of pain, but about your business as well. Professionally prepared stationary, the development of a logo, and production of a newsletter are all effective means of advertising. The clinic's listing in the local phone directory should be easily visible. Radio, television, and print media all offer opportunities for exposure. These represent expensive and potentially sensitive areas of advertising for which local ethos should be considered and professional marketing help engaged.

A presence on the Internet by individual healthcare providers is becoming progressively more common and in the near future will become ubiquitous. A basic Web site can be developed and hosted by a good commercial Web development company relatively inexpensively. This provides an excellent avenue for continuous marketing exposure and a way for patients, providers, and third party referral sources to access information about your program at their convenience. A basic site would include information about yourself and any other service providers in your practice; your location including directions, office hours, and phone numbers; and a description of the services provided. More detailed sites can also include information about specific procedures performed by you or your colleagues including photographs or even short video segments, hot links to other complementary Web sites, and informational databases. Your Web address should be included on your business cards and all other promotional materials and activities. The author recommends dealing with an experienced Web development and hosting service. Consider starting with a basic Web page that allows for some scalability. This way you can add features or increase the complexity of the site without loosing your investment in the initial development.

Advertising and promotion make physicians and patients aware of the services the clinic provides. They do not replace the need to provide concerned, compassionate, and effective care. If the office is disorganized, the receptionist curt, or physicians and therapists chronically late, no amount of advertising can overcome the bad will spread by irate patients and referring physicians.

BILLING AND COLLECTIONS

Even the best conceived and instituted treatment program will not succeed if efficient billing/collections operations are not instituted from day one. Billing and collections can be done internally or subcontracted. This decision should be made while formulating the business plan. The billing system should be in place before the first patient is seen.

A number of local and nationwide medical billing services are available and usually charge between 6 and 10% of collections. Interview several and consider not only the cost, but also the comprehensiveness of the service rendered. Look for a company that has some expertise in billing for a similar entity or is willing to invest the start-up time to learn the peculiarities of the field. Billing externally can significantly reduce capital investment at the time of business start-up and help to reduce fixed costs at a time when cash flow will be slow.

If billing is done internally, the appropriate software, hardware, and support forms to carry out the task must be purchased. It is important to hire someone with previous billing experience to make the system work. There are numerous companies that sell medical billing systems, with a large range of capabilities. Billing, collection, scheduling, accounting, and payroll functions are all available. Software and hardware can be purchased separately or as a complete system. Prices range from $1,000 to $50,000 or more, depending on the system.

DEVELOPING A CAPITATED CONTRACT

Payment for pain management services is transitioning from a fee-for-service model to a capitated model. The extent to which this has already occurred varies dramatically from region to region. In some large metropolitan areas, the market share of managed care exceeds 80%. In other areas, total managed care penetration for 1995 was as low as 7%. Managed care will most likely continue to expand and become de facto market-driven national healthcare reform over the next 5 years, irrespective of any other national or regional political agenda. In this climate, it will be essential for the successful provider of pain management to understand the differences between fee-for-service and capitated reimbursement models and to be able to negotiate a good capitated contract.

In a capitated contract, the clinic receives a payment each month based on the number of members covered by the contract and the rate per member (the per member per month, or PMPM, rate). If the contract covers 50,000 members at a rate of $0.20 PMPM, then the payment would be $10,000 a month. This is independent of the actual number of patient visits, supplies used, or resources consumed in a particular month. If the cost of service delivery for the month was $5,000, then a $5,000 profit would be realized. Obviously, if the cost to deliver care under the contract was in excess of $10,000 for the month, then a loss would be incurred.

In order to be able to develop a price structure that makes sense, the following information should be obtained and analyzed:

1. The utilization rate for the CPT codes covered under the contract for the most recent 12-month period for the population in question.
2. Your actual reimbursement for each CPT code by insurance type. The most important, of course, is the reimbursement from the entity with which you are negotiating, if you have previous claims experience with that entity.
3. Knowledge of the range of cap rates for similar contracts in your immediate or similar geographic areas.

The above information will allow you to develop a PMPM rate that will maintain profitability. You should develop a PMPM rate based on your own analysis of prior utilization. Then check this against other contracts as a safety check. Obviously, rates can vary extensively depending on which CPT codes are covered by the contract.

It is important to build the following safeguards into the contract:

1. Input into if not direct control over utilization. If you accept the risk of fixed payments, then you must be able to control utilization to help mitigate that risk.
2. Renegotiation of the contract if actual utilization significantly exceeds projected utilization.

It is important to have in place a system to monitor utilization prior to beginning the contract. Utilization information, along with expense information, will be needed to determine the profitability of the contract. It is important to monitor this closely and move to renegotiate unprofitable contracts quickly.

BIBLIOGRAPHY

Finkler, S.A. (1992). *Finance and accounting for nonfinancial managers*. Englewood Cliffs, NJ: Prentice Hall.

Gumpert, D.E. (1992). *How to create a successful marketing plan*. Boston: Inc. Publishing.

Hammon, J.L. (1993). *Fundamentals of medical management*. Tampa, FL: ACPE.

McKeever, M. (1988). *How to write a business plan*. Berkeley, CA: Nolo Press.

Porter, M.E. (1985). *Competitive advantage*. New York: Free Press.

Sachs, L. (1987). *Marketing for the professional practice*. Englewood Cliffs, NJ: Prentice-Hall.

6

Multidisciplinary Pain Clinics

C. Norman Shealy, M.D., Ph.D., D.Sc. and Roger K. Cady, M.D.

INTRODUCTION

The management of chronic pain began to evolve from the witch doctor approach (exorcism, drugs, and ablative surgery) to the modern concept as the result of three innovations:

1. Dr. John Bonica's concept of a multidisciplinary, interdisciplinary team approach to pain management
2. The Wall-Melzack theory for gate control of pain
3. Fordyce's behavioral modification or operant conditioning concept

Bonica's concept of a multidisciplinary, interdisciplinary clinic began following World War II and evolved over a period of 10 years or so. As late as 1960, the clinic that he founded at the University of Washington was the major such clinic in the United States, but a few other university centers were beginning to follow his model. This model is called the *nerve block drug-cut psychiatry clinic* because it was originally run entirely by anesthesiologists and led to an unfortunate sequence of events. Even though a group of up to 15 to 20 different health specialists were represented in the weekly reviews of patients, the initial major approach was to look at the patient as having a reasonable physical cause of pain and as a potential anatomical specimen where one could do a peripheral or differential spinal nerve block, relieve the pain, or send the patient to the neurosurgeon for ablation of the appropriate pain pathway.

The failure of destructive neurosurgery is what led to the development of transcutaneous and dorsal column stimulation, because the only types of pain that respond to ablation successfully in the long run are cancer pain, trigeminal neuralgia, and facet joint pain. In virtually all other situations, long-term success from neurosurgical destructive procedures is roughly less than 10%. Thus, patients tend to have nerve blocks and destructive procedures, sometimes have a second set of nerve blocks and destructive procedures, try on a wide variety of drugs, and at that point are told that "it's all in their heads" and sent to see a psychiatrist.

Until at least the mid-1970s, many physicians tended to believe that if patients did not respond to surgical ablative surgery and hard drugs, then they must be "crazy" or seriously psychologically disturbed. On more than one occasion Shealy was told by a psychiatrist, "When you have taken care of the physical component of the pain, send the patient to me and I will take care of the psychological part." But Shealy never saw a patient with chronic pain helped by a psychiatrist. The major approach of psychiatrists has been to make patients feel either guilty, for being an imposition on their families or society, or angry at someone. This approach simply does not work.

On the other hand, the basic concept of a true multidisciplinary, interdisciplinary team is currently the most valid one. The model that Shealy evolved is very different from that at the University of Washington, where the primary approach has also evolved from just nerve blocks and cutting to what he would call a somewhat more comprehensive approach. At the present time in Seattle, patients have pain education, physical therapy, occupational therapy, vocational counseling, individual psychotherapy, and a modicum of relaxation therapy. The University of Washington program considers itself likely to be successful when the patient is suffering from physician-prescribed inappropriate medications, physical deactiva-

0-8493-0926-3/02/$0.00+$1.50
© 2002 by CRC Press LLC

tion, depression, superstitious behaviors and when the patient has beliefs about the body and reasonable outcome goals. The educational program at the clinic has gradually taken on many of Fordyce's concepts, as described later.

Although Bonica is responsible for the concept of a major pain clinic, Wall and Melzack's gate control theory sparked more innovation in the management of pain than any other concept in history. As a direct result of Wall and Melzack's theory, Shealy was prompted to develop dorsal column stimulation and transcutaneous electrical nerve stimulation, which by 1971 led him to start the first holistic comprehensive multimodal, multidisciplinary pain management clinic. The details of the gate control theory were covered in Chapter 2.

Fordyce's concept of pain as an operant or conditioned response also has been critically important in the development of today's pain clinics. Fordyce (1976) emphasized that the "reinforcing consequences" provided by family, friends, and acquaintances when an individual suffers from pain often reinforce pain behavior. Individuals who have been deprived of social recognition and nurturing at a subconscious level often find the tremendous attention that they receive when they suffer from chronic illness provides them a long-neglected nurturing-type environment. This reinforcement pattern must be brought to the patient's attention and often more forcefully to the attention of the spouse or other family members if the chronic cycle of an invalid pain status is to be broken.

In 1965, having been sent a copy of the gate control theory of pain prior to its publication, Shealy visited Pat Wall and then theorized that the most effective way to influence the gate was to stimulate the dorsal column of the spinal cord, because at that anatomical level the beta fibers are separated from the C-fibers, the only place in the body where that is a significant anatomical fact. This led Shealy to the development of both dorsal column stimulation (the first patient being implanted in 1967) and the concept that transcutaneous electrical nerve stimulation would be more effective in a wider variety of people than would the implanted device.

Because of the tremendous number of patients sent to Shealy for dorsal column stimulation who were not candidates for the procedure due to psychological (operant or behavioral) aspects of their illness, in 1971 Shealy opened the first nonuniversity pain clinic and the first pain clinic to offer a truly holistic approach to the concept of pain. From the beginning, the policy was that any safe modality would be included, but all the social, environmental, physical, emotional, chemical, and spiritual stresses in an individual's life would also be examined. The treatment program evolved from an inpatient treatment program to an outpatient model.

Starting in 1971, Shealy's program, with an inpatient active behavioral modification program rather than a pas-

sive behavioral modification program, lasted an average of 32 days of inpatient management, with 25 patients in a special unit where the nurses were trained to ignore pain behavior or pain complaints. The patients were advised in advance that this would be the approach. An extremely active day was planned, beginning at 7:00 A.M. following breakfast in an ambulatory dining area. During the day, patients were scheduled from morning until at least 7:00 P.M. and often until 9:00 P.M. They were assigned to walk the hall, given a number of laps which increased each day; ride a stationary bicycle for an increasing number of minutes; and do various other physical exercise activities. Five days a week they went to a swimming pool where they had 1 hour of water calisthenics. Five days a week they went to occupational therapy for 1 hour. Each patient had vigorous slapping massage of the area of pain for at least 5 min four times a day, followed by at least a 5-min rubdown of the area of pain. Patients had generalized mechanical vibratory massage for 15 minutes four times day, were in a whirlpool twice a day, and had a hands-on total body massage every other day.

Transcutaneous electrical nerve stimulation and acupuncture were intimate parts of pain management in this clinic from the beginning. For the first year, "group therapy" was handled by a psychiatrist. At the end of that time, having attended one of the group therapy sessions, Shealy believed group therapy had negative reinforcing qualities and it was discontinued. Instead, he introduced autogenic training for 30 min twice a day and began to introduce temperature, EEG, and electromyelogram (EMG) feedback.

By the end of the first year, Shealy had treated over 400 patients, of whom approximately 6% had had dorsal column stimulators inserted and 1% had had peripheral nerve implanted stimulators.

At the end of 32 days (the average hospital stay), 75% of the patients were off drugs, were markedly improved in their pain complaints and behaviors, and had a significant increase in physical activity. Over the next year and a half, reliance upon stress reduction and cognitive educational aspects increased, and during this time Shealy developed the concept of Biogenics®. The Biogenics retraining component of Shealy's pain management program (Shealy, 1978) became so prominent that the inpatient program was closed in 1974, and Shealy began to run an outpatient-only pain management program. Today, most clinicians consider it inappropriate to hospitalize chronic pain patients for anything other than drug withdrawal or severe psychiatric problems.

PAIN MANAGEMENT FOR THE 1990s

The single most important factor in managing chronic pain is evaluation of the patient. This must include the following:

Aspirin, Tylenol, etc.	up to 10 per day	10
	up to 20 per day	25
Valium, Ativan, diazepams	up to 20 mg per day	25
	up to 40 mg per day	50
	over 40 mg per day	75
Librium	up to 20 mg per day	25
	up to 40 mg per day	50
	over 40 mg per day	75
Phenothiazines, Serax, Thorazine, etc.	up to 20 mg per day	25
	up to 40 mg per day	50
	over 40 mg per day	75
Tricyclic antidepressants:	up to 4 per day	25
Elavil (10 mg), Vivactil (5 mg),	4–8 per day	30
Tofranil (10 mg), Aventyl	8–12 per day	40
	over 12 per day	50
Monoamine oxidizers	up to 4 per day	60
(antidepressants): Nardil, etc.	4–8 per day	75
Mild to moderate addicting, codeine (30–60 mg), Percodan, Talwin tablets, Darvon, Darvocet, Stadol, Nubain, barbiturates (30–60 mg)	over 8 per day	90
Demerol, injectable Talwin, morphine, Dilaudid	up to 4 doses per day	75
	up to 8 doses per day	90
	over 8 doses per day	100
Sleeping medicines	up to 1 per day	25
	2 per day	50

FIGURE 6.1 Drug usage.

1. A comprehensive history of the patient's pain problem, including:
   • Onset
   • Predisposing factor
   • Drug history (see Figure 6.1)
   • Surgical history
   • Family history
   • Social interactions
   • Symptom index
   • Pain profile (see Figure 6.2)
   • Total life stress (see Figure 6.3)
2. A review of all diagnostic tests
3. A comprehensive physical and neuromuscular examination, including particular attention to the sacrum, posture, and spinal mechanics
4. Special tests that might be needed, including:
   • Myelogram
   • CAT scan
   • MRI
   • EMG and sensory nerve conduction studies
   • Neuropsychological tests
   • Psychological tests, including:
     • California Personality Inventory (CPI)
     • Minnesota Multiphasic Personality Inventory (MMPI)
     • Myer-Briggs Type Indicator (MBTI)
   • Evaluation by a physical therapist
   • Evaluation by a psychologist
5. The minimum team needed for comprehensive pain management includes:
   • Physician (M.D. or D.O.)
   • R.N.
   • Psychologist, psychotherapist, or someone with a Master's degree in social work
   • Physical therapist

On the columns below, grade yourself (circle your choice):																					
Pain intensity (severity)	0	5	10	15	20	25	30	35	40	45	50	55	60	65	70	75	80	85	90	95	100
Decrease in physical activity	0	5	10	15	20	25	30	35	40	45	50	55	60	65	70	75	80	85	90	95	100
Percent of time pain felt	0	5	10	15	20	25	30	35	40	45	50	55	60	65	70	75	80	85	90	95	100
Effect on mood	0	5	10	15	20	25	30	35	40	45	50	55	60	65	70	75	80	85	90	95	100
Drugs consumed	0	5	10	15	20	25	30	35	40	45	50	55	60	65	70	75	80	85	90	95	100
Effect on sexual activity	0	5	10	15	20	25	30	35	40	45	50	55	60	65	70	75	80	85	90	95	100
Overall well-being	0	5	10	15	20	25	30	35	40	45	50	55	60	65	70	75	80	85	90	95	100
Overall energy	0	5	10	15	20	25	30	35	40	45	50	55	60	65	70	75	80	85	90	95	100
Pain intensity	100 = intolerable, excruciating, horrible																				
Physical activity	100% restricted = bedridden																				
	75% restricted = up and about but very little																				
	50% restricted = can't work, up and take care of myself, must rest frequently																				
	25% restricted = must rest every 4–6 hours, light work exhausts me, can't do fun activities																				
	0 = normal, I do any physical activity I choose																				
Effect on mood	0 = normal; 100 = totally withdrawn, panicked, overwhelmingly depressed																				
Drugs consumed	Doctor will do this; mark all drugs you take on reverse side of this page or separate sheet																				
Sexual function	0 = no activity; 100 = perfectly normal activity																				
Overall feeling of well-being	0 = terrible; 100 = best anybody could feel																				
Overall energy	0 = can't get up or get going; 100 = most I've ever experienced																				
Name											Date										

FIGURE 6.2 Pain profile. (©1986 C. Norman Shealy, M.D., Ph.D., Springfield, Missouri.)

Name:	Date:	

Read your stress points on the lines in the right-hand margin and indicate subtotals in the boxes at the end of each section. Then add your subtotals to determine your total score.

A.   Dietary stress

Average daily sugar consumption

Sugar added to food or drink	1 point per 5 teaspoons	_____
Sweet roll, piece of pie/cake, brownie, other dessert	1 point each	_____
Coke®, or can of pop; candy bar	2 points each	_____
Banana split, commercial milkshake, sundae, etc.	5 points each	_____
White flour (white bread, spaghetti, etc.)	5 points	_____

Average daily salt consumption

Little or no "added" salt	0 points	_____
Few salty foods (pretzels, potato chips, etc.)	0 points	_____
Moderate "added" salt and/or salty foods at least once per day	3 points	_____
Heavy salt user regularly (use of "table salt" and/or salty foods at least twice per day)	10 points	_____

Average daily caffeine consumption

Coffee	1/2 point each cup	_____
Tea	1/2 point each cup	_____
Cola drink or Mountain Dew®	1 point each cup	_____
2 Anacin® or APC tabs	1/2 point per dose	_____
Caffeine benzoate tablets (NoDoz®, Vivarin®, etc.)	2 points each	_____

Average weekly eating out

2–4 times per week	3 points	_____
5–10 times per week	6 points	_____
More than 10 times per week	10 points	_____

DIETARY SUBTOTAL [_____] A

B.   Environmental Stress

Drinking water

Chlorinated only	1 point	_____
Chlorinated and fluoridated	2 points	_____

Soil and air pollution

Live within 10 miles of city of 500,000 or more	10 points	_____
Live within 10 miles of city of 250,000 or more	5 points	_____
Live within 10 miles of city of 50,000 or more	2 points	_____
Live in the country but use pesticides, herbicides, and/or chemical fertilizer	10 points	_____

Soil and air pollution

Exposed to cigarette smoke of someone else more than 1 hour per day	5 points	

ENVIRONMENTAL SUBTOTAL [_____] B

C.   Chemical stress

Drugs (any amount of usage)

Antidepressants	1 point	_____
Tranquilizers	3 points	_____
Sleeping pills	3 points	_____
Narcotics	5 points	_____
Other pain relievers	3 points	_____

Nicotine

3–10 cigarettes per day	5 points	_____
11–20 cigarettes per day	15 points	_____
21–30 cigarettes per day	20 points	_____
31–40 cigarettes per day	35 points	_____
Over 40 cigarettes per day	40 points	_____
Cigar(s) per day	1 point each	_____
Pipeful(s) of tobacco per day	1 point each	_____
Chewing tobacco – "chews" per day	1 point each	_____

FIGURE 6.3 Personal stress assessment: total life stress test.

Average daily alcohol consumption

1 oz. whiskey, gin, vodka, etc.	2 points each	_____
8 oz. beer	2 points each	_____
4–6-oz. glass of wine	2 points each	_____
	CHEMICAL SUBTOTAL	[_____] C

D. Physical stress

Weight

Underweight more than 10 lbs.	5 points	_____
10–15 lbs. overweight	5 points	_____
16–25 lbs. overweight	10 points	_____
26–40 lbs. overweight	25 points	_____
More than 40 lbs. overweight	40 points	_____

Activity

Adequate exercise,* 3 days or more per week	0 points	_____
Some physical exercise, 1 or 2 days per week	15 points	_____
No regular exercise	40 points	_____

Work stress

Sit most of the day	3 points	_____
Industrial/factory worker	3 points	_____
Overnight travel more than once a week	5 points	_____
Work more than 50 hours per week	2 points per hour over 50	_____
Work varying shifts	10 points	_____
Work night shift	5 points	_____
	PHYSICAL SUBTOTAL	[_____] D

* Adequate means doubling heartbeat and/or sweating minimum of 30 minutes per time.

E. Holmes-Rahe Social Readjustment Rating*

(Circle the mean values that correspond with life events listed below which you have experienced during the past 12 months.)

Death of spouse	100	Change in responsibilities at work	29
Divorce	73	Son or daughter leaving home	29
Marital separation	65	Trouble with in-laws	29
Jail term	63	Outstanding personal achievement	28
Death of close family member	63	Spouse begin or stop work	26
Personal injury or illness	53	Begin or end school	25
Marriage	50	Change in living conditions	24
Fired at work	47	Revision of personal habits	23
Marital reconciliation	45	Trouble with boss	20
Retirement	45	Change in work hours or conditions	20
Change in health of family member	44	Change in residence	20
Pregnancy	40	Change in schools	19
Sexual difficulties	39	Change in recreation	19
Gain of new family member	39	Change in church activities	18
Business readjustment	39	Change in social activities	17
Change in financial state	38	Mortgage or loan less than $20,000	16
Death of close friend	37	Change in sleeping habits	15
Change to different line of work	36	Change in eating habits	15
Change in number of arguments with spouse	35	Vacation, especially if away from home	13
Mortgage over $20,000	31	Christmas or other major holiday stress	12
Foreclosure of mortgage or loan	30	Minor violations of the law	11

(Add the mean values to get the Homes-Rahe total. Then refer to the conversion table to determine your number of points.) _____

F. Emotional stress

Sleep

Less than 7 hours per night	3 points	_____
Usually 7 or 8 hours per night	0 points	_____
More than 8 hours per night	2 points	_____

FIGURE 6.3 (CONTINUED) Personal stress assessment: total life stress test.

Relaxation

Relax only during sleep	10 points	_____
Relax or meditate at least 20 minutes per day	0 points	_____

Frustration at work

Enjoy work	0 points	_____
Mildly frustrated by job	1 point	_____
Moderately frustrated by job	3 points	_____
Very frustrated by job	5 points	_____

Marital status

Married, happily	0 points	_____
Married, moderately unhappy	2 points	_____
Married, very unhappy	5 points	_____
Unmarried man over 30	5 points	_____
Unmarried woman over 30	2 points	_____

Usual mood

Happy, well adjusted	0 points	_____
Moderately angry, depressed, or frustrated	10 points	_____
Very angry, depressed, or frustrated	20 points	_____
Any other major stress not mentioned above	(10–40 points)	_____
you judge intensity (specify):		

EMOTIONAL SUBTOTAL [_____] F

Add A _____ + B _____ + C _____
+ D _____ + E _____ + F _____ = [_____]

YOUR PERSONAL STRESS ASSESSMENT SCORE

If your score exceeds 25 points, you probably will feel better if you reduce your stress; greater than 50 points, you definitely need to eliminate stress in your life.

Circle your stressor with the highest number of points and work first to eliminate it, then circle your next greatest stressor and overcome it, and so on.

Copyright ©Norman Shealy, M.D., Ph.D., 1985, Springfield, Missouri.

Conversion Table

Your Number of Points	Holmes-Rahe Less Than	Anything Over 351 = 40+	Your Number of Points	Holmes-Rahe Less Than	Anything Over 351 = 40+
0	60		16	280	
1	110		17	285	
2	160		18	290	
3	170		19	295	
4	180		20	300	
5	190		21	305	
6	200		22	310	
7	210		23	315	
8	220		24	320	
9	230		25	325	
10	240		26	330	
11	250		27	335	
12	260		28	340	
13	265		29	345	
14	270		30	350	
15	275				

HOLMES-RAHE SOCIAL READJUSTMENT RATING (CONVERTED) [_____] E

FIGURE 6.3 (CONTINUED) Personal stress assessment: total life stress test.

6. Once it is ascertained that the patient does not have a problem which needs primary surgery or medical drug management, the following modes of therapy need to be considered:
   - Educational approaches — Of critical importance to the patient are the following:
     - Understanding the anatomy and physiology of pain and appropriateness of surgical vs. drug therapy
     - Thorough understanding of stress:
       - Physical
       - Chemical
       - Emotional
       - Spiritual
     - An understanding of the concept of retraining the nervous system (Biogenics)
     - Understanding the dynamics of interpersonal relationships
   - Physical approaches
     - Acupuncture
     - Nerve blocks of:
       - Muscle trigger points
       - Facet joints
       - Sacroiliac joints
       - Caudals (rarely)
       - Intercostal blocks (rarely)
     - Miscellaneous:
       - Occipital
       - Supraorbital
       - Infraorbital
       - Mental nerves
     - Transcutaneous electrical nerve stimulation
     - Use of different types of devices:
       - Cranial electrical stimulation
       - Percutaneous electrical nerve stimulation (medium and intense)
     - Soft tissue mobilization:
       - Myofascial massage
       - Strain/counterstrain
       - Manipulative techniques
       - Vibratory massage
       - Mechanical massage
       - Heat
       - Ice
     - Exercise
       - Limbering
       - Aerobic
       - Muscle strengthening
       - Work hardening
   - Pharmacological approaches
   - Nutritional approaches
     - Special attention to vitamin C, vitamin B6, and magnesium (all deficient in a majority of patients)

   - Chemical approaches — Possible therapeutic implications include:
     - Dilantin
     - Elavil or other antidepressant drugs
     - Mexitil (especially for sensory deprivation pain)
   - Psychological and spiritual approaches
     - Pragmatic
     - Practical
     - Spiritually oriented

BIOGENICS

The backbone of Shealy's self-regulation training program is Biogenics. Biogenics incorporates the work of a number of individuals, including Dr. Elmer Green, Roberto Assagioli, Edmond Jacobson, Emil Coue, Carl Jung, and, of course, J.H. Schultz. Essentially, many of these individuals have touched on aspects that interrelate to one another. As Shealy began synthesizing the techniques of self-regulation, the following steps were most emphasized:

- Positive attitude
- A belief in self ("I can do it.") — Biofeedback proves this
- Relaxation
- Conscious control of sensation (Balancing Body Feelings) — Individuals are taught the following balancing body feelings techniques:
  - Talking to the body
  - Feeling the localizing pulsation of heartbeat
  - Imaging
  - Loving the body
  - Tensing and relaxing
  - Breathing through the body
  - Collecting and releasing
  - Circulating the electrical energy
  - Expanding the electromagnetic energy field
  - Mental induction of anesthesia
  - Balancing emotions
  - Recognizing that all distress is the result of fear of loss of:
    - Life
    - Health
    - Money
    - Love
    - Moral values
  - Logically and internally recognizing that the only solutions are:
    - Assertion to correct the problem
    - Divorcing an unacceptable problem with joy
    - Accepting and forgiving (going for sainthood)

- Programming goals (organ-specific phrases)
- Spiritual attunement

Because some 90% of individuals state that they believe in life after death, God, and living the Golden Rule, this universal belief is incorporated into teaching. Individuals are exposed to philosophical concepts to develop the transcendent will or the will of the soul, starting with the concept that all individuals have basic needs and desires in addition to those necessary for survival. The major part of cognitive understanding relates to accepting that pain, most psychologically aggravated, is the result of unfulfilled desires or failure to accept things as they are. Ultimately, individuals must learn that there are a limited number of situations that can be totally changed and that one should put effort into those that can be changed and learn total emotional–psychological detachment from those aspects of life which cannot be changed; in other words, to be at peace with the unchangeable aspects of life. At the same time, they are taught to control pain through the Biogenics techniques of Balancing Body Feelings.

Obviously, there are many models of pain clinics. Some current clinics specialize only in doing nerve blocks, especially caudal nerve blocks, whereas others primarily emphasize transcutaneous electrical nerve stimulation, and still others emphasize more physical therapy approaches. All of these techniques are valuable in managing chronic pain. The indications for specific physical approaches such as acupuncture and nerve blocks are beyond the province of this chapter. References to some of the technology can be found at the end of this chapter.

COST EFFECTIVENESS OF COMPREHENSIVE PAIN TREATMENT

No discussion of pain clinics would be adequate without attention to the catchphrase of today — cost effectiveness. Shealy's study in 1984 is one of the few that have been published.

At the Shealy Institute, over 7000 patients have been evaluated and/or treated intensely in a 13-day comprehensive program. At the present time, only 10 to 15% of patients evaluated enter the intense program. Most of the others are satisfactorily managed with one or two modalities of treatment with occasional follow-up visits. Of those who enter intense therapy, 60% have had unsuccessful back surgery, 10% have back pain without prior surgery, 10% have headaches, and the remainder have a wide variety of posttraumatic, postsurgical metabolic or degenerative pain syndromes. Sixty percent are women, and 40% are men. They range in age from 8 to 90 years, with most patients between 35 and 67 years old. Approximately 20% have had workers' compensation injuries.

Patients have been incapacitated for 1 to 7 years plus. Medical expenses have ranged from $10,000 to $450,000, with average medical expenses of over $10,000.

RESULTS FOLLOWING COMPREHENSIVE TREATMENT

In any given year, 5 to 7% of patients who enter the program fail to complete it. About 1% are sent home because of open resistance to therapy. The others who drop out do so because they "don't believe in it." Almost all of these dropouts are male smokers and are either workers' compensation or Medicaid patients.

Of the 94% who complete the program, follow-up data at 6 months and 2 to 3 years from 800 patients (600 followed up at 2 + years and 200 followed up at 6 months) consistently reveal that:

- 35% return to work.
- 90% are off all drugs except aspirin or acetaminophen.
- 70% are improved 50 to 100% (at 6 months 72% are greatly improved, and over the next 2 years this decreases to 70%).
- 30% who do not improve greatly almost invariably did not practice the techniques taught.
- 5% had a facet rhizotomy.
- 25% have continued use of transcutaneous electrical nerve stimulation for at least 6 months.
- Pain intensity is reduced an average of 70%.
- Percent of time pain is present is reduced an average of 65%.
- Mood is improved in 90% of patients.
- A majority have significant stress illness, such as hypertension, diabetes, peptic ulcer, etc.
- Less than 5% have additional surgical procedures after treatment.
- Drug expenses after therapy are reduced 85%.
- Hospitalization after therapy is reduced 90%.
- Total medical expenses are reduced after therapy 80 to 85%.
- Cost of the treatment ranges from $3,500 to $6,000 and is rarely more, depending upon need for hospitalization, drug withdrawal, etc.

In 1972, Fordyce reported that his average patient had prior expenses of $50,000. At the time, his program cost $5,000. Most pain clinics today charge from $5,000 to $35,000. Fordyce estimated that society would break even if only 10% of his patients returned to work. If one takes into account the income produced by those who return to work, even less than a 10% return-to-work success rate would produce a break even for society.

Presently, with prior medical expenses often exceeding $60,000 on average and an average cost of less than

$5,000 for the comprehensive treatment program, society breaks even if only 8% return to work. Because 35% of Shealy's patients return to work, the cost effectiveness is at least 3.4 to 1. Because total medical expenses are reduced by well over 75%, the cost of the comprehensive rehabilitation program is recouped in less than 6 months. In medical costs alone, in just a 2-year period, the cost effectiveness is 4 to 1. That is, within 2 years, society saves four times as much money as the cost of the treatment program. When the added benefit of 35% return to work is considered, the cost effectiveness is even greater than 4 to 1.

The data reported here apply only to treatment at the Shealy Institute for Comprehensive Health Care and cannot be extrapolated to other pain treatment programs or modalities (Shealy, 1976).

The advent of DRGs in 1982 began a process that is increasingly cumbersome and detrimental in all aspects of patient care. In no area has this had a greater impact than in pain management. Although the HMO, PPO, Managed Care system has continued to cover major interventional approaches such as epidurals reasonably well, almost all other aspects of pain management have been severely curtailed. In our opinion, the least effective treatment for all forms of chronic pain is epidural anesthetics. Biofeedback, transcutaneous electrical nerve stimulation, neuromuscular re-education techniques, and acupuncture, which are the hallmarks for successful pain management, are extremely poorly covered in the current situation. Thus, multidisciplinary pain clinics continue to suffer from the lack of coverage by third-party payers. Interestingly, at the Shealy Institute patients have been willing to pay out of pocket to obtain the comprehensive care that is often not covered by medical insurance.

CERTIFICATION OF PAIN CLINICS

In 1983, CARF (Commission for Accreditation of Rehabilitation of Facilities) instituted a program of accreditation for both outpatient and inpatient pain clinics. The number of pain clinics in this country is very difficult to ascertain. Fortunately, in 1996 the American Academy of Pain Management instituted its review process for certification of pain clinics and at that time certified 70 active pain clinics. These included outpatient facilities, inpatient facilities, and outpatient/inpatient facilities.

REFERENCES

Fordyce, W. (1976). *Behavioral methods for chronic pain and illness*. St. Louis: C.V. Mosby.

Shealy, C.N. (1976). *The pain game*. Millbrae, CA: Celestial Arts.

Shealy, C.N. (1978). Biofeedback training in the physician's office: Transfer of pain clinic advances to primary care. *Wisconsin Medical Journal, 77*, 41–43.

Shealy, C.N. (1984, March). Cost-effectiveness of comprehensive pain treatment. *Insurance Adjustor,* 46–47.

Shealy, C.N. (1986). *Biogenics® health maintenance*. Fair Grove, MO: Self-Health Systems.

Shealy, C.N. (1977). Biogenics: A synthesis of biofeedback and autogenic techniques for control of pain. In L.R. Pomeroy (Ed.), *New dynamics of preventative medicine* (Vol. 5, pp. 69–74).

7

Columbia Medical Plan Pain Management Group Manual

Clark Brill, M.D., Juliet Scotti Post, D.C., Thomas Ferguson, Ph.D., Harry Shabsin, Ph.D., Jane Tenberg, M.A., Kathleen Wooding, M.A., Marilyn Lauffer, M.S., R.N., Robin Thomas, M.S., R.N., R.D., and Mary Ann Buchmeier, M.S., R.D.

INTRODUCTION

All pain practitioners come to realize soon in their careers that chronic pain is a volatile mix of pathological stimuli combined with host factors of pain perception and behavioral reaction to the stimuli.

This paradigm forces us to take a more holistic approach to treatment in addressing both the organic stimulus and these host factors when necessary. Obviously, each case lies somewhere along a spectrum where some patients have a more definable pathology and fewer confounding host factors, in which case our efforts are aimed at removing the stimulus via a procedural approach. Others have either less obvious pathology or a condition that simply has no effective treatment coupled with psychological characteristics of hyperawareness or magnified response. In these patients the resources are better spent working on perception/reaction behaviors vs. pursuing multiple futile procedures.

This sounds good on paper but we all know how difficult it can be to treat these "host factors." We are also painfully aware that insurance companies seem to be willing to pay for procedural care more quickly than psychological techniques targeting these host factors.

Nonetheless, research tells us addressing these characteristics such as locus of control, depression, and coping styles is fruitful, as if our own anecdotal testimonials were not sufficient. How then do we address these host factors?

First, an analogy to other chronic diseases must be drawn. A diabetic has an incurable condition but diabetic patients can minimize the effects of the disease by making the right choices — eating properly, foot care, etc. Conversely, they can jeopardize their health and increase chances for diabetic complications by making poor choices.

Similarly, those with chronic pain can make choices to magnify their painful experience or mitigate it. To use a phrase from a family practitioner friend of mine: The pain is there — misery and suffering are optional.

This then is the mission of treating host factors — we must act as guides to help each patient live a good life despite experiencing chronic pain as opposed to living in misery with it.

A group setting is ideal for teaching these skills because it is very cost effective to bring a group of people together at one site to present this material vs. repeating oneself in an office setting ad nauseum. There is also the "group dynamic" effect where patients previously feeling isolated and hopeless are working together in a positive environment and can feed off each other's strengths.

What follows is a detailed outline of one such successful group — The Columbia Medical Plan group seminar for chronic pain patients — for those interested in starting a group of their own. This was an 8-week outpatient group experience that was intensely studied for outcomes; these were presented to the American Academy of Pain Management (AAPM) at the 1994 annual conference. Patients completing the group decreased doctor visits for pain complaints by 50%.

0-8493-0926-3/02/$0.00+$1.50
© 2002 by CRC Press LLC

The basic philosophy of the group was a simple motto — "no brain, no pain." That is, the state of mind one brings to the pain experience affects the pain itself as well as its impact on one's life.

Each group meeting consisted of a presentation and discussion of areas where patients were encouraged to make good life choices such as exercise, eating habits, and thinking patterns. These were areas they still had control over as opposed to focusing on pain levels that they may have had little control over.

Of course, the patients had to begin with a belief in this brain–pain model and this foundation was established at the initial meeting by a physician presentation on rudimentary anatomy and physiology of pain mechanisms in the human body, including Gate theory, antipain pathways, serotonin, and other neuromodulation structures.

The outline for the Columbia Medical Plan Group treatment for chronic pain follows.

PURPOSE OF MANUAL

This manual is designed to assist healthcare providers in running groups for chronic pain patients. The outlines of material to be presented are general. Providers are encouraged to add their own individual creativity and to adapt the manual to their own particular needs.

OVERALL PAIN CLINIC PROGRAM

A pain management group is an effective and cost-effective modality, and an important part of an overall pain treatment program that may include pharmaceutical management, physical therapy, injection therapy, exercise, biofeedback, and psychotherapy. An ongoing support group for chronic pain patients helps them maintain the benefits gained from the pain management group.

PAIN MANAGEMENT GROUP

   I. Objectives of Pain Management Group
     A. Educating patients in causes and treatment of pain
     B. Helping patients develop cognitive and behavioral skills for pain management
     C. Creating a support group for pain patients and those involved with them to manage pain behavior
  II. Structure of group sessions
     A. A closed 8-week group for 12 to 15 patients
     B. Group that runs for 1 h, once a week
     C. Group that is staffed by
       1. A psychotherapist who is present every week
       2. A physiatrist

       3. An exercise therapist
       4. A nutritionist
     D. Each week, the session involves
       1. Presentation on pain management
       2. Discussion time
       3. A relaxation exercise
 III. Participants
     A. Most pain patients in pain clinic recommended for the Pain Management Group
     B. Preferable that clients complete biofeedback before entering group
     C. Patients who cannot interact well in a group setting and those who have a high rate of cancellation not recommended for the group
 IV. Outline of the Pain Management Group
     A. Weekly presentations made on some aspect of pain management by a member of the treatment team covering:
       1. Anatomy and physiology of pain — physiatrist
       2. Exercise and pain management — exercise therapist
       3. Treatment of pain — physiatrist
       4. Imagery techniques in pain management — exercise therapist
       5. Cognitive treatment of pain — psychologist
       6. Behavioral treatment of pain — psychologist
       7. Nutrition and pain management — nutritionist
     B. Presentations followed by group discussion
     C. Relaxation training included in each session
     D. Homework reviewed weekly
       1. A pain management chart filled out weekly
       2. Exercise and relaxation practice charted weekly
       3. Thoughts and emotions in response to pain examined
     E. Patients referred to Chronic Pain Support Group after completing Pain Management Group

THE PROGRAM

WEEK ONE

Summary

   I. Welcome and introductions
  II. Presentation by physiatrist
     A. Anatomy and physiology of pain
     B. Discussion of presentation
 III. Homework — weekly pain management chart
     A. Explaining chart
     B. Emphasizing daily relaxation

IV. Relaxation — progressive
V. Closing

WEEK ONE

I. Welcome and introductions
   A. Group leader introducing self and welcoming group
   B. Other professionals introducing themselves
   C. Group members introducing themselves
   D. Guidelines for group
     1. Attendance
     2. Fees
     3. Outline of program
     4. Announcement of Chronic Pain Support Group (biweekly)
II. Presentation by physiatrist on anatomy and physiology of pain
   A. Definition — "Pain is a stimulus that is perceived as uncomfortable"
     1. Stimulus
       a. Torn tissue
       b. Loud noise
       c. Discomforting sight
       d. Stressful situation
     2. Perceptions
       a. Perception depends on mind set
       b. Distraction decreases perception
       c. Focusing on perception makes it stronger
     3. Being uncomfortable
       a. Not able to measure discomfort or suffering
       b. Relativity — difference among people's sensitivities and tolerances
       c. Existence of cultural differences
       d. Dependence on past history of experiences
   B. Pain pathways
     1. Stimulus site
       a. Nerve endings firing even after stimulus removed
       b. Chemicals released that enhance strength of stimulus
       c. Additive effects of stimuli
     2. Spinal cord
       a. Nerves entering at "gate" that can be open or closed
       b. Competing stimuli at this level
       c. Example of gate: rubbing skin when bump leg
     3. Brain
       a. No pain until conscious appreciation

       b. No brain — no pain!
       c. Making a conscious decision — "this is uncomfortable"
       d. Degree of discomfort depending on mind set — stress, depression
       e. If no other stimuli present, pain getting in — night pain
   C. Antipain pathways
     1. Descending pathways
       a. Nerves coming down from brain to close gates
       b. Nerves coming down from brain to release endorphins
     2. Endorphin system
       a. Body's natural pain-fighting system
       b. Responsible for placebo response
       c. Can be elevated by many means
         i. Drugs
         ii. Relaxation
         iii. Exercise
       d. Causes natural "high"
   D. Summary — pain not "all in your head" or "all in your body"
   E. Discussion of presentation
III. Homework
   A. Introducing weekly pain management chart — see Appendix 7.1
   B. Any questions/discussions arising from review of chart
IV. Relaxation
   A. Progressive relaxation — see Appendix 7.2
   B. Sharing relaxation experience
   C. Stressing importance of daily relaxation
V. Closing
   A. Thanking presenter
   B. Checking that everyone will attend next week
   C. Positive comments about today's group

WEEK TWO

Summary

I. Welcome and check-in
II. Presentation by exercise therapist
   A. Role of exercise in pain management — part I
   B. Discussion of presentation
III. Homework
   A. Recording exercise and relaxation on chart
   B. Discussing pain management section of chart
IV. Relaxation — flowing light
V. Closing

Week Two

I. Welcome and check-in
   A. Group leader and staff members reintroducing themselves
   B. Patients giving brief comments on how the week has been — especially new and good examples
   C. Group leader checking who has done relaxation and exercise
   D. Giving out Exercise Handout I*
II. Presentation by exercise therapist on role of exercise in pain management — part I
   A. Attitudes toward exercise
      1. Eliciting words from the group members that describe what comes to their minds when they think of "exercise" (writing these words on blank flip chart — both positive and negative — and discuss)
      2. Emphasizing importance of developing "positive" attitudes toward exercise
      3. "No pain, no gain"
         a. Philosophy obsolete
         b. New focus: "Train, don't strain"
   B. Benefits of exercise
      1. Physical
         a. Increases stamina, strength, flexibility, coordination
         b. Improves cardiovascular efficiency
         c. Affects medical problems
            i. Hypertension
            ii. High cholesterol levels
            iii. Diabetes
         d. Increases lung capacity
         e. Burns calories — weight control
         f. Increases pain tolerance
         g. Is associated with longevity
      2. Psychological
         a. Improves self-image/self-esteem
         b. Helps alleviate depression
         c. Enhances ability to handle stress
         d. Fosters sense of "being in control"
   C. Disadvantages of exercise
      1. Overexercise possibly causing injuries
      2. May increase pain short term
      3. Takes time
   D. Proper way to exercise — choose proper sport for your body
      1. Type
         a. Aerobic vs. anaerobic
         b. Using large muscle groups
         c. Low impact
         d. Examples
            i. Biking
            ii. Walking
            iii. Swimming
            iv. Aerobic dance
      2. Frequency
         a. 3 to 5 days per week
      3. Duration
         a. Ideal 15 to 60 min
         b. Minimum: 15 to 20 min, plus warm-up and cool-down
      4. Intensity — based on target heart rate
         a. Review of heart rate chart
         b. Level of perceived exertion
         c. Medication possibly affecting heart rate
      5. Measuring heart rate
         a. Where?
            i. Neck
            ii. Wrist
         b. How?
            i. Counting for 1 min or 15 s four times
         c. When?
            i. At rest
            ii. During exercise
            iii. After exercise
      6. Importance of practice
         a. Walking program with warm-up and cool-down
   E. Exercise precautions—be careful if the following occur:
      1. Dizziness
      2. Light headedness
      3. Chest pain or pressure
      4. Excessive fatigue
      5. Excessive shortness of breath
   F. Exercise clothing
      1. Hot weather
         a. Loose, light layered
         b. Avoiding heavy sweaters, plastic or rubberized clothing
      2. Cold weather
         a. Layered, porous clothing
         b. Avoiding overdressing
         c. Covering head, ankles, and hands
   G. Exercise shoes
      1. Choosing correct shoes for your sport
      2. Awareness of stability, cushioning
      3. Wearing absorbent socks
      4. Preventing blisters
   H. Strategies to get going
      1. Making walking a pleasure
         a. Scenery
         b. Cassettes, radio

---

* Handouts are not provided as part of this manual. It is suggested that program leaders provide material for the specific needs of their groups from materials collected and available to them.

        c. Pleasant company
     2. Linking walking with a pleasurable activity as a "reward"
     3. "Foot out the door" approach
  I. Discussion of presentation
III. Homework
  A. Commenting on weekly pain management charts by patients
  B. Stressing importance of relation — checking who did it
  C. Collecting charts and giving out new ones
  D. Giving out "Tapes and Books for Health Management" — see Appendix 7.3
IV. Relaxation
  A. Flowing light relaxation — see Appendix 7.4
  B. Sharing relaxation experience
  C. Asking how relaxation was helpful to patients this week
  V. Closing
  A. Thanking presenter
  B. Checking next week's attendance
  C. Positive comments about today's group

WEEK THREE

Summary

  I. Welcome and check-in
 II. Presentation by physiatrist
  A. Treatment of chronic pain
  B. Discussion of presentation
III. Homework — reviewing exercise and relaxation
  A. Reviewing weekly pain management charts
IV. Relaxation — breathing and beach imagery
  V. Closing

WEEK THREE

  I. Welcome and check-in
  A. Welcoming everyone back
    1. Positive comments on attendance
    2. Positive comments on adherence
  B. Checking on who has done exercise, relaxation charts
  C. Brief review of week
    1. Positive orientation encouraged
  D. Announcing Chronic Pain Support Group again
 II. Presentation by physiatrist on treatment of pain
  A. Must fight pain at all levels — cannot separate body/brain
  B. Pharmaceutical management
    1. Decreasing narcotics — interfering with natural pain-fighting systems

    2. Serotonin possibly useful — pumps up body's pain-killing system
    3. Other useful medications
     a. Anti-inflammatories
     b. Antihistamines
     c. Antivascular
     d. Antianxiety
     e. Antidepressants
  C. Physical management
    1. Exercise
     a. Increases endorphins
     b. Increases pain threshold
     c. Helps mood
     d. Reconditions body
    2. Activity gates
     a. Heat
     b. Cold
     c. Nerve stimulation
     d. Acupuncture
    3. Inactivity increasing pain by decreasing competitive stimuli
  D. Psychological management
    1. Decreasing perception using power of the mind
     a. Biofeedback
     b. Relaxation
     c. Hypnosis
     d. Imagery
    2. Addressing other cortical issues that increase pain
     a. Depression
     b. Anxiety
     c. Stress
    3. Support systems
     a. Family
     b. Pain support groups
     c. Outside activities
  E. Role of pain
    1. At first, pain may be useful — acute for protection
     a. Causes withdrawal, e.g., broken limb — not using it
    2. Later, pain can be a useless habitual signal
    3. Pain can even cause benefits at times
     a. Financial
     b. Attention
    4. Internal vs. external focus of control
     a. Making changes — flexibility
     b. Avoiding joylessness
    5. Victor vs. victim
    6. Process takes courage
  F. Discussion of presentation
III. Homework
  A. Commenting on how patients did on charts

B. Collecting old charts and giving out new ones
IV. Relaxation
  A. Breathing induction and beach imagery
  B. Sharing relaxation experience
  C. Exploring images that help patients reduce pain
V. Closing
  A. Thanking presenters
  B. Checking next week's attendance
  C. Reminding patients about charts

WEEK FOUR

Summary

I. Welcome and announcements
II. Homework — daily pain management charts
III. Relaxation — self-guided — classical music
IV. Presentation by nutritionist
  A. Nutrition and pain management
  B. Discussion of presentation
V. Closing

WEEK FOUR

I. Welcome and announcements
  A. Checking on week
  B. Checking on relaxation practice and exercise
II. Homework
  A. Introducing new daily management charts
    1. To be done for 2 weeks — see Appendix 7.4
  B. Collecting old charts and giving out new
  C. Reinforcing adherence to charts, exercise, relaxation
III. Relaxation
  A. Relaxation induction using breathing
  B. Self-guided imagery using classical music
  C. Bringing patients back to group and discussing experiences
IV. Presentation by nutritionist on nutrition and pain management
  A. Short-term/long-term effects of diet on well-being
    1. Short-term effects less obvious — therefore often neglected
      a. Affecting energy level for work, play
      b. Needed for steady supply of fuel — sugar for effective pain management
      c. Constant supply of blood sugar necessary for optimal functioning of brain, muscles, and organs
      d. Avoiding destabilizers in sugar supply (e.g., caffeine, alcohol)

      e. Considering nutrients that fight pain and depression — amino acids and B vitamins
    2. Long-term effects are preventative maintenance for the body
      a. Proper diet can help ward off
        i. Osteoporosis
        ii. Heart disease
        iii. Certain cancer types
        iv. Diabetes
        v. Gallbladder disease, etc.
      b. Need to avoid or deal with obesity to lessen certain muscle, bone, or joint pain
  B. Dietary Guidelines for Americans*
  C. NRC's dietary recommendations
    1. Eating five or more half-cup servings of vegetables and fruits every day
    2. Moderating protein intake — Recommended Daily Allowances (RDA) to twice RDA
    3. Maintaining adequate RDA calcium intake
    4. Avoiding use of dietary supplements in excess of RDA
    5. Maintaining optimal intake of fluoride
  D. Relating guidelines to balanced diet (food groups)
  E. Examining own diet (class exercise)
    1. Writing 24-hour dietary recall
    2. Comparing to dietary guidelines and food groups
    3. Determining strong and weak points of diet and prioritize any desirable changes
    4. Working on making dietary changes
  F. Diet and drug interactions
    1. Obtain a list of medications used by class participants prior to this presentation
    2. Adverse side effects with nutritional implications
      a. Drugs that may cause these side effects
      b. Dietary suggestions to alleviate or prevent side effects
  G. Arthritis (if time and relevant to class participants)
    1. No nutritional cures, though many myths abound
      a. No proof that selenium, turnips, fish oils, or vitamins help
      b. Possible that saturated fats, dairy products, chocolate, tomatoes, and citrus fruits may aggravate rheumatoid arthritic symptoms in some people

---

* Giving out nutritional handouts.

2. Achieving healthy body weight
   a. Being overweight — stress aggravating to arthritic joints
   b. Following diet low in fat, sugar, and salt and high in complex carbohydrates
   c. Increasing physical activity to burn more calories
   d. Rheumatoid arthritis — food consumption — underweight
   e. Increasing calories to offset being underweight
   f. Adjusting meal planning and food preparations to offset stiffness, pain, and fatigue
3. Reasons to eat well
   a. Boosts energy
   b. Makes you feel healthier
   c. Reduces flare-ups
   d. Helps you cope better with arthritis

H. Vitamin and other supplements
1. Reasons for taking supplements
   a. Meeting unusually high demand for nutrients
      i. Pregnancy
   b. Poor nutritional status
      i. Iron deficiency
      ii. Anemia
   c. Diet that does not meet body's nutrient needs
2. RDA vs. megadoses
   a. RDA encompassing nutrient needs of general population
   b. Megadoses usually of no benefit and often harmful to health
   c. Vitamin C only proven effective in reducing cold symptoms, yet chronic megadoses possibly cause diarrhea and kidney stones
   d. Megadoses of fat-soluble vitamins and iron are toxic
   e. Other examples
   f. Obtaining nutrients through foods safe and natural
3. Health claims on nutritional supplements
   a. How to determine legitimacy
   b. Always checking with physician before taking megadoses
   c. Asking pharmacist about potential dangers

I. Migraine headaches
1. Well-balanced diet and evenly spaced meals
2. Relatively safe foods
3. Foods to avoid list

   a. Not applicable to everyone, therefore test own reactions
   b. Most common offenders
   c. Reading food labels
4. Dietary suggestions to alleviate anorexia and nausea
J. Discussion of presentation

V. Closing
A. Thanking presenter
B. Emphasizing to patients importance of looking at their thinking patterns this week

WEEK FIVE

Summary

I. Welcome and announcements
II. Presentation by behavioral psychologist
   A. Cognitive treatment of pain
   B. Discussion of presentation
III. Discussing thought substitution chart
IV. Relaxation — progressive/imagery
V. Homework — daily pain management chart
VI. Closing

WEEK FIVE

I. Welcome and announcements
   A. Welcoming groups and positive comments regarding progress of group
   B. Checking on who has done exercise, relaxation, charts
   C. Brief check-in by patients
   D. Announcing Chronic Pain Support Group
II. Presentation by behavioral psychologist on cognitive treatment of chronic pain
   A. Henry Beecher — soldier vs. civilian story — see Appendix 7.6
      1. Meaning of story
      2. Group's reaction
   B. Pain vs. bodily sensation
      1. How we label something that will affect our experience of it
         a. Snake story — see Appendix 7.7
         b. Childbirth — the stronger the contractions, the closer the birth
         c. Difference in labeling pain as a "sensation" instead of "suffering"
      2. Control of sensory input
         a. Focusing on pain that may increase tension and therefore intensify pain
         b. Distractions such as entertainment, relaxation, and meditation decrease tension and pain

c. Some examples of controlling sensory input through altered states are dental hypnosis and fire walking

C. Meaning of patient symptoms
1. Attributing meaning to our symptoms whether we are aware of it or not
   a. e.g., religious meaning — "offer it up" — story of Job
   b. Personal identity — pain and illness possibly beginning to define who the person is
   c. Symptoms that determine the roles we play in relationships such as
      i. Victim
      ii. Martyr
      iii. Hero
   d. Spinal cord experience — paraplegics choose opposite responses story — see Appendix 7.8

D. Developing internal locus of control
1. Internal vs. external locus of control
   a. Patients with internal locus of control
   b. Relaxation and meditation ways to help develop internal locus of control
2. Man's search for meaning story — see Appendix 7.9

E. Discussion of presentation

III. Discussing thought substitution chart
A. Reviewing thought substitution chart — see Appendix 7.10
B. Having one patient describe event
C. Having other patients complete columns on chart
D. Repeating exercise for second event
E. Discussing how patients are working on their thinking/feeling patterns

IV. Relaxation
A. Progressive relaxation — Appendix 7.2
B. Imagery of place in nature

V. Homework
A. Asking patients to discuss thought substitution chart with their families
B. Collecting daily pain management charts and giving out new ones

VI. Closing
A. Reminding patients that family members are invited next week
B. Thanking presenter

Week Six

Summary

I. Welcome and introductions
II. Presentation by behavioral psychologist

A. Family interactions and pain management
B. Becoming an exceptional patient
C. Discussion of presentation

III. Small group discussion

IV. Homework — patient management chart
A. Discussing thought substitution chart with family

V. Closing

Week Six

I. Welcome and introductions
A. Welcoming and explaining why families were invited
B. Having patients introduce family members and tell why they are important
C. Any additional comments from family members
D. Checking on who did relaxation and exercise

II. Presentation by behaviorist on family interactions in management of chronic pain
A. Stranger, supportive spouse, unsupportive spouse story — see Appendix 7.11
   1. Meaning of story
   2. How others can affect pain perception
   3. How others are affected by pain
   4. Group's reaction to story
B. What others can do to help pain patients
   1. Not overreacting (not just doing something; sitting there)
      a. Letting patient care for self
      b. Not discussing/asking about symptoms
      c. Treating person in a normal fashion
   2. Attention for nonpain behavior
      a. Inappropriate attention only reminding person of symptoms
      b. Persons in pain needing to be left alone, not attended
         i. Go to their rooms
         ii. Praise for nonpain behavior
   3. Acute vs. chronic pain
   4. Other means of expressing love and concern besides attending to pain
C. Conclusion — persons with chronic pain helped best by
   1. Increasing self-reliance
   2. Increasing levels of activity
   3. Treated as well, instead of ill
D. Becoming an exceptional patient — Bernie Siegel, M.D.
   1. Defining the exceptional patient
      a. 15 to 20% of patients are
         i. Difficult
         ii. Uncooperative

iii. Assertive

iv. Demanding

v. Optimistic

vi. Rule breakers

b. Exceptional patients are the ones most likely to get well

c. Exceptional patients are willing to accept all the risks and challenges of life

2. Taking responsibility for your own health

a. Refusing to be a victim

b. Recognizing that happiness is an "inside job"

c. Asking to be educated by your doctor and becoming your own doctor

d. Refusal to hope is nothing more than a decision to die: "In the face of uncertainty, there is nothing wrong with hope" — Bernie Siegel

e. Becoming a survivor! Ignoring the statistics

f. We missed that one story — see Appendix 7.12

3. Letting go of fear

a. Exceptional patients knowing that health depends on inner peace and letting go of fear

b. Finding ways to make peace with yourself

c. Finding ways to make peace with others

d. Taking good care of yourself through relaxation (having fun), exercise, and good food

4. Helping yourself decrease or eliminate symptoms

a. Decreasing need to attend to symptoms

b. Understanding possible payoff of symptoms, e.g., avoidance of something

c. Developing positive attribution style — I am hopeful

d. Learning distraction techniques

e. Reevaluating what you can learn from your symptoms

i. Appreciating good health

ii. Having empathy with people

f. Recognizing situations that are related to the onset of symptoms

g. Avoiding onset situations such as

i. Stress

ii. Specific physical activities

iii. Anticipatory anxiety

iv. Overreacting

v. Repeated discussion of symptoms with others

5. At peace with life and death

a. Getting well not the only goal

b. Importance of learning to live without fear and to be at peace with life and death

6. How to become an exceptional patient

a. Assertiveness

b. Having information/knowledge

c. Having hope

d. Taking good care of yourself

e. Letting go of fear

f. Finding inner peace

7. Discussion of presentation

III. Small group discussion

A. Inviting group to divide up into small groups of two or three patients

B. Discussing what response from family members really helps client and what they learned from thought substitution chart

C. If appropriate, therapist intervening to confront patterns that maintain pain behavior/thinking

IV. Homework

A. Collecting daily pain management charts and giving out new weekly charts

B. Giving out another copy of thought substitution chart to work on with family member

V. Closure

A. Thanking family members for coming

B. Asking if they would like to come again in week 8

C. Thanking presenter

WEEK SEVEN

Summary

I. Welcome and announcements

II. Discussing what patients want to do in last session

III. Relaxation — healing visualization for pain management

IV. Presentation by exercise therapist

A. Exercise and pain management — part II

B. Discussion of presentation

V. Homework — weekly pain management chart

VI. Closing

WEEK SEVEN

I. Welcome and announcements

A. Discussing reactions to family coming to group

B. Reviewing charts, relaxation, exercise practice

II. Discussing what patients want to do in last session — possible options:

A. Discussing their ideas

B. Sharing and feedback

1. Patients sharing what they have learned in the group and what changes still have to be made in their lives

2. Family members sharing what changes they have seen in patient while they have been in treatment

3. Group members giving each other feedback on changes they have seen in each other and offering any suggestions for the future

C. Small group discussion

1. Patients divide into small groups based on common symptoms for discussion

a. Headaches

b. Back pain

c. Fibromyalgia, etc.

III. Healing visualization

A. Explaination of designing your own imagery — healing visualization — see Appendix 7.13

B. Patients filling out imagery sheets

C. Guiding patients through imagery

D. Patients sharing imagery in pairs

E. Discussing imagery with group

IV. Presentation by exercise therapist on role of exercise in chronic pain management — part II

A. Review

1. Targeting heart rates — discussing any problems patients may have

2. Exercise records — checking everyone is exercising regularly

B. Three parts of exercise

1. Endurance

a. Heart — increased size, decreased rate

b. Arteries — dilated

c. Muscles — increased oxygen absorption

d. Lungs — increased capacity

2. Flexibility

a. Increasing agility and mobility

b. Decreasing chances of injury

c. Improving posture

d. Relieving tension and stiffness

3. Strength

a. Cannot grow new muscles — must tone what we have

b. Muscle cells take less space than fat cells

c. Muscles burn more calories

d. Muscles contour the body

e. Firm muscles reinforce joints, reducing sprains and strains

f. Using dumbbells, circuit weights

C. Home exercise equipment

1. Exercise bikes

a. Not weather dependent

b. Transferring skills outside

c. Addition of fans, book stands, digital readouts

2. Rowing machines

a. Use of upper and lower body

b. May not be good for back problems

3. Cross-country skiing equipment

a. Uses upper and lower body

b. Can be expensive

4. Treadmills

D. Health clubs

1. Aspects to consider in a health club

a. Equipment

b. Costs — especially extras

c. Location — close by?

d. Hours — work for you?

e. Membership contracts

E. Handouts — Exercise Handout II

1. Reviewing exercise comparison

2. Reviewing cost/benefit ratios

F. Conclusion: "Adding years to your life and adding life to your years through exercise"

G. Discussion of presentation

V. Homework

A. Give out weekly pain management charts

B. Reinforce ongoing exercise and relaxation programs as lifestyle changes

VI. Closing

A. Thanking presenter

B. Reminding patients to bring family member/friend next time, but if you can't, to come anyway

C. Inviting group members to bring snacks for final session

WEEK EIGHT

Summary

I. Welcome and announcements

II. Group discussion

III. Ongoing group treatment

IV. Closing

V. Evaluation of program

VI. Refreshments

WEEK EIGHT

I. Welcoming and announcements
    A. Welcome patients and families
       1. Positive comments on progress of the group
    B. Patients reintroducing family members/friends
II. Group discussion
    A. Discuss whatever patients may have requested during last session
    B. Alternatives
       1. Patients share what they have changed in their lives as a result of being in the group
       2. Family members share positive changes they have seen
       3. Patients give each other feedback on growth they have seen in each other over the weeks
    C. Small group discussions, divided by symptoms
       1. Headaches
       2. Back pain
       3. Fibromyalgia, etc.
III. Ongoing group treatment
    A. Introducing therapist from Chronic Pain Support Group
    B. Patients committing to ongoing treatment in group
IV. Closing
V. Pain group evaluations — see Appendix 7.14
VI. Refreshments

HANDOUTS

Exercise Handout I

1. Reasons to exercise
2. Heart rate chart
3. Sample walking program
4. Information on exercise shoes
5. General stretching exercises
6. Comparisons of different forms of exercise
7. Log of exercise practice
8. Cost/benefit ratios of different forms of exercise

Exercise Handout II

1. Guidelines for working out
2. Lower-body warm-up exercises
3. Middle-body warm-up exercises
4. Upper-body warm-up exercises

Nutritional Handout

1. Nutritional guidelines
2. Foods that may increase pain — headaches
3. Nutrients that fight pain — amino acids
4. Dietary supplements/vitamins in a healthy diet
5. Caffeine content of beverages
6. Drug-nutrient information sheet

Appendices

WEEK ONE

APPENDIX 7.1   WEEKLY PAIN MANAGEMENT CHART

Name:					Date:		
Week number:							
Day (Example)	**Monday**	**Tuesday**	**Wednesday**	**Thursday**	**Friday**	**Saturday**	**Sunday**
Daily relaxation: 30 min Practice: Legs Time: Heavy Experience: Relieved Headache							
Exercise time: 40 min Type: Walking Self-talk re: Pain: This pain is terrible. When will it end? Daily medications: Aspirin							

APPENDIX 7.2   PROGRESSIVE RELAXATION

A. Using relaxation music, asking group to tense and release their muscles in the following sequence:
  1. Clenching hands and relaxing
  2. Bending hands back at wrist and relaxing
  3. Tensing biceps and relaxing
  4. Tensing forehead (raise brows) and relaxing
  5. Tensing face (squinting) and relaxing
  6. Tensing mouth and jaw and relaxing
  7. Tensing neck and upper shoulders (neck and chest) and relaxing
  8. Tensing shoulders, back, and chest (taking a large breath and pull shoulders back) and relaxing
  9. Tensing stomach and relaxing
  10. Tensing thighs (raising legs up slightly) and relaxing
  11. Tensing calves (heels off floor) and relaxing
  12. Tensing feet (curl up toes) and relaxing

B. Asking patients to bring themselves back by being aware of the room around them and of other group members

C. Asking patients to open their eyes as you count from one through five

D. Asking group members to share their relaxation experience and whether anyone had any difficulties

E. Encouraging daily relaxation practice at home

WEEK TWO

APPENDIX 7.3   TAPES AND BOOKS FOR HEALTH MANAGEMENT

Tapes

Letting Go of Stress — Emmett Miller

Images for Optimal Health — Emmett Miller

Change the Channel on Pain — Emmett Miller

Headache Relief — Emmett Miller

Healing Journey — Emmett Miller

Positive Imagery for People with Cancer — Emmett Miller

All available from: Source, P.O. Box W, Stanford, CA 94309, (415) 328–7171 or (800) 52-TAPES

Seasons for Healing — Stress and Pain Management — Jule Scotti Post (Vol. 1 — Winter-Spring; Vol. II — Summer–Fall)

Available from: Healing Imagery, 4520 Kingscup Court, Ellicott City, MD 21042

Health Journeys — Belleruth Naparstek

Cancer   Chemotherapy   Depression
Grief   General wellness

Available from: Image Paths, Inc., P.O. Box 5714, Cleveland, OH 44101

Cancer — Discovering Your Healing Power — Louis Hay

Available from: Hay House, Inc., Santa Monica, CA, (213) 394–7445

Rapid Pain Control — Carol Erickson and Thomas Condon

Self-Hypnosis for Reducing Your Stress — Carol Erickson

Available from: Changeworks, P.O. Box 4000-D, Berkeley, CA 94706

Relaxation Music

Zen Waterfall — Eliotoshu and Paul L. Warner, Global Pacific Distributions

Caverna Magica — Andreas Vollenweider, CBS Records

White Winds — Andreas Vollenweider, CBS Records

The Sky of the Mind — Andreas Vollenweider, CBS Records

Comfort Zone — Steve Halpern, Halpern Sounds

Spectrum Suite — Steve Halpern, Halpern Sounds

Winter Solstice — David Lanz and Michael Jones, Narada Productions

Pianoscapes — Michael Jones

Petals — Marcus Allen et al., Dreamwater Music

Harp and Soul — Georgia Kelly, Heru Records

Path of Joy — Daniel Kobialka, Li-Sem Enterprises

Silk Road — Kitaro, Sound Design

Silver Road — Kitaro, Sound Design

Silver Cloud — Kitaro, Sound Design

Toward the West — Kitaro, Sound Design

Silver Wings — Mike Rowland, Music Design, Inc.

Fairy Ring — Mike Rowland, Music Design, Inc.

Lovely Day — William Aura, Higher Octave

Music

Miracles — Rob Whitesides-Woo, Search for Serenity

Mountain Light — Rob Whitesides-Woo, Search for Serenity

Classical Music for Relaxation

Classic Fantasy — Anugama, Higher Octave Music

Relax with the Classics, Vol. I–IV — Lind Institute

Great Lakes Suite — Dan Gibson

The Classics — Dan Gibson

Books

Burn, David. (1981). *Feeling Good — The New Mood Therapy.* New York: Signet Penguin Books.

Catalona, Ellen Mohr. (1987). *The Chronic Pain Control Work Book.* Oakland, CA: New Harbinger Publications.

Chopra, Deepak. (1989). *Quantum Healing: Exploring the Frontiers of Mind/Body Medicine.* New York: Bantum.

Dachman, Ken and Lyons, John. (1990). *You Can Relieve Pain.* New York: Harper & Row.

Frankl, Viktor. (1984). *Man's Search for Meaning.* New York: Simon & Schuster.

Linchitz, Richard. (1987). *Life without Pain.* New York: Addison-Wesley.

Moen, Larry. (1992). *Guided Imagery,* (Vol. I–III). Naples, FL: United States Publishing.

Moyers, Bill. (1993). *Healing and the Mind.* New York: Doubleday.

Pitzele, Sefra Kobrin. (1988). *One More Day — Daily Meditations for the Chronically Ill.* Center City, MN: Hazelden.

Siegel, Bernie S. (1986). *Love, Medicine & Miracles.* New York: Harper & Row.

Sternbach, Richard. (1987). *Mastering Pain.* New York: Putnam.

APPENDIX 7.4 FLOWERING LIGHT RELAXATION — WITH RELAXATION MUSIC

A. Breathing induction — give patients the following instructions
 1. Begin by taking a few deep breaths
 2. Let go of any tension throughout your body as you breathe
 3. Notice that as you become more relaxed, your breathing becomes softer and gentler
 4. Be aware of the rising and falling of your chest while breathing in and out
B. Flowing light imagery
 1. Continue with the following instructions:
  a. In your mind's eye, picture a small ball of radiant light resting gently on top of your head; either see the light or have a sense of it being present
  b. Imagine that light is now flowing down over your head around the back of your head and around your face
  c. Let any tension in the muscles in your head and face dissolve in that flowing light; let those muscles become deeply relaxed
 2. Continue relaxation instructions, asking patients to picture a warm light flowing around the following areas:
  a. Back and front of neck
  b. Shoulders and back
  c. Arms and hands
  d. Chest and stomach
  e. Thighs and calves
  f. Feet and toes
 3. After mentioning each area, ask patients to let any tension in the muscles in that area dissolve in that warm flowing light, and let those muscles become deeply relaxed
 4. When patients have relaxed all parts of their bodies, ask them to see that warm light flowing all around them and to feel themselves floating in that light
C. Coming back
 1. Ask patients to begin bringing themselves back by having an awareness of their bodies sitting in chairs with their feet on the floor
 2. Suggest patients be aware of the sounds around them in the room and how they are currently feeling
 3. Ask patients to open their eyes as you count back from five to one
D. Sharing
 1. Ask patients to share what this relaxation was like for them
 2. Call on individuals who haven't shared much with group

WEEK FOUR

APPENDIX 7.5 DAILY PAIN MANAGEMENT CHART

Name:				
Week Number:				
Time of Symptoms	Activity	Consequences of Choices Made (Including Meds, Relaxation, etc.)	Comments	Exerciese
Daily				Daily
Change in Intensity	When Pain Level Changed	Medication	Relaxation	
Example 8:15 a.m.	Headache	Getting ready to go to work	I stayed at home	Took Demerol (amount)
I can't stand this pain.	Walking	Asprin	1/2 hour	

WEEK FIVE

APPENDIX 7.6 HENRY BEECHER — SOLDIER VS. CIVILIAN STORY — CAN HOW WE THINK AFFECT HOW WE FEEL?

Some years ago, Henry Beecher, a physician interested in human pain mechanism, designed a study to investigate the amount of tissue damage sustained in an injury and the amount of pain experienced. Dr. Beecher hypothesized that the amount of pain a person felt was directly related to the extent of an injury or the amount of damage to bone, muscle, or other tissue. To prove this theory, he studied soldiers wounded in battle. Dr. Beecher was able to ascertain the amount of injury by examining the medical record of soldiers wounded in battle. He then compared this information with the amount of morphine, a narcotic analgesic, each of the soldiers took to control pain. As he had expected, the greater the amount of bodily injury, the greater the amount of morphine used by the wounded soldiers to obtain relief from pain. From these studies, Dr. Beecher concluded that pain was solely the result of injury to tissue and did not have a higher cognitive component related to thinking or to emotional reactions to an injury.

To apply these findings to civilians, Dr. Beecher did additional research with patients who were not soldiers and who received injuries from various accidents such as falls or automobile collisions. To help make his point, Dr. Beecher even matched up the wound between soldiers and the civilians. As before, he found that the greater the injury to the civilians, the more morphine they took to control pain. However, there was one difference between the soldiers and the civilians that Dr. Beecher had trouble accounting for. For the same amount of tissue damage, civilians took almost three times as much morphine as did the soldiers to control pain. It began to appear that something else besides tissue damage was influencing the amount of pain patients were experiencing.

After further investigation, Dr. Beecher concluded that a person's reaction to injuries could affect the amount of pain experienced. When he asked the soldiers what their injuries meant to them, they told him they were primarily relieved that their wounds had not resulted in death and that they felt confident about recovering and returning home. In other words, they reacted in a positive fashion to their injuries. Civilians, on the other hand, saw their injuries from a much more negative perspective, describing their injuries and accidents as awful events resulting in their lives being disrupted. For the most part, soldiers understated their pain and felt it was minor and it was tolerable. Civilians, however, tended to describe their pain as more intense and unbearable. Since these studies, many other reports have also described how emotional or cognitive reactions to injury can affect perceptions of pain.

Based on the research of Henry Beecher and others, the response to the question, "Can how we think affect how we feel?" appears to be yes. For those of you experiencing chronic pain, this implies that by learning to react differently to your pain symptoms or by adopting different coping strategies, you can affect the amount of pain you experience. In other words, if you are willing to think more positively about your life and your symptoms, you can learn to do something to help yourself feel better.

APPENDIX 7.7   SNAKE STORY — THINKING PRECEDES FEELING

One of the contributing authors to this manual, Dr. Thomas Ferguson, described an experience he had in the following way:

> I attended graduate school at Arizona State University, and since this university is in the desert, there was an example given by one of my major professors of how thinking precedes feeling. This was a novel thought to me at that time, and I was skeptical until he gave an example that convinced me of the accuracy of this hypothesis.

The professor stated that if you went to a friend's house or apartment to water his plants while he was away on vacation and, as you opened the door, you saw what looked like a snake, you would have a thought! He said if you believed that it was a real snake, then this thought

would translate into a physiological response and then an emotion. The adrenaline would start pumping. You would then be in a "fight or flight" mode, and you would either attack the snake to kill it, if you perceived it as dangerous, or you would flee, if you were fearful. However, if you knew this friend had a great sense of humor and loved to play practical jokes, you might look at the snake a little more closely to make a determination whether it was real or not. If you decided it was not real, then you would react with calm or laughter, rather than with the adrenaline-engendered "fight or flight" syndrome.

Therefore, if you examine your emotions, you will see that how you perceive a situation makes a difference in how you respond emotionally.

APPENDIX 7.8   PARAPLEGICS CHOOSE OPPOSITE RESPONSES

In 1967, a patient at Stanford Hospital was there to have back surgery. He was struck by how differently two other patients in the ward responded to their physical conditions. Both patients had similar spinal cord injuries, leaving them paraplegic.

One patient really enjoyed listening to music, especially Aaron Copeland's "Appalachian Spring." He was very upbeat and entertaining. The other patient was con-

stantly miserable and complaining. He was obviously bitter and angry.

It was amazing to see that two people in such difficult circumstances could respond in such opposite ways. Both were paraplegic, but while one suffered constantly, the other was determined to live life as fully as he could.

We also have a choice about how we respond to our pain — to suffer constantly or make the most of the life we have.

Appendix 7.9 Man's Search for Meaning

The concept of internal vs. external locus of control is best examined by a reading of *Man's Search for Meaning* by Victor Frankl, M.D. Dr. Frankl was a Jewish psychiatrist living in Germany during the Nazi regime. At some point, he was arrested and taken to a concentration camp. During the first few nights in the concentration camp, a number of prisoners would hang themselves from the rafters out of despair. Dr. Frankl wrote that he also considered suicide as he examined his losses. The Nazis had taken his home, his profession, and his money. They had killed his family. They had even taken his bodily hair.

He felt that they had complete control over him, with the exception of one aspect of his life — they could not control how he decided to respond to this abomination. He decided that he would tell the world what happened and that he would write a book about his experiences. His heroic struggle to survive for 5 years in Nazi concentration camps is an inspirational one to read. It underlines the importance of recognizing that no one can control how you respond to your external world, no matter how traumatic that may be.

Appendix 7.10 Thought Substitution Chart

Give at least five examples of your own automatic negative thoughts in response to pain and stress, and the feelings and consequences that follow them. Think about what positive thoughts you could substitute for your automatic thoughts, and what new feelings and consequences these would bring you. See the following example.

Event	Automatic Thoughts	Feeling/Consequences Responses	Substitute Thoughts Responses	New Feeling	Consequences
e.g., Pain begins.	This is going to be terrible. I can't bear it.	I feel angry, scared, anxious. I hate the pain. The pain increases. I take my pain killer.	I become more tense.	It is time to relax through the pain. I can deal with it.	I feel calm. I am used to it. I become relaxed focused. The pain is bearable. I avoid taking pain medication.

WEEK SIX

Appendix 7.11 Supportive Spouse Story — A Sight for Sore Eyes

We have all heard the phrase "a sight for sore eyes," but what about a sight for sore backs, or heads, or arms, or stomachs, or any other part of the body? Is it possible that just the sight of another person can make us feel better or worse? The answer appears to be yes. We have all at one time or another thought about others as being a "pain in the neck." However, for most of us, this is just a way to indicate that we are experiencing stress related to another person. We usually do not mean we actually have the physical sensation of pain in our necks. However, a group of researchers reported in the journal *Pain* that just the sight of another person might actually increase or decrease the experience of painful sensations. In this study, patients in the hospital for chronic pain were observed for signs of painful discomfort under three conditions: in the presence of a supportive spouse, in the presence of a nonsupportive spouse, and in the presence of a neutral observer.

The results from this study showed that patients with chronic pain appeared to be in more pain in the presence of a supportive spouse compared with a neutral person, but seemed to experience less pain when in the company of a nonsupportive spouse compared with a neutral observer. These results may seem surprising. However, although sympathy may be appropriate for short or acute periods of pain, the researchers concluded that for patients with chronic pain, a person providing sympathy over a prolonged period of time may begin to be viewed as rewarding. Because rewards tend to increase the behavior that obtained them, the sight of a rewarding person can increase pain if that pain was the reason for obtaining the reward of sympathy in the past. The opposite also appears to be true. If a person ignores a family member's pain, that person's pain tends to decrease because there are no positive benefits for having it. If this seems far-fetched, think of the example of working for a salary. If you were paid $50,000 or $100,000 a year for going to work, the chances are good that you would continue to go to work the next day. On the other hand, if you were paid only $5,000 a year, you might soon start missing days or leave your job altogether because your salary (reward) for working was not worth the effort.

These examples illustrate how powerful the effect of rewards (or lack of rewards) can be on our behavior. Although many times we are aware of how rewards affect our behavior, we do not necessarily have to be aware of this reward–behavior relationship to be affected by it. This seems to be the case for patients with chronic pain. Even though we may not be aware of it, the way family members and friends interact with an individual with chronic pain can affect how that person feels.

APPENDIX 7.12   WE MISSED THAT ONE!

Contributing author Dr. Ferguson described another extraordinary experience in the following words:

> Dr. Bernie Siegel's quote, "In the face of uncertainty, there is nothing wrong with hope," was demonstrated to me in a courageous fashion by a 19-year-old patient that I treated during an internship at the University of Minnesota Hospital. He had been in a motorcycle accident and as a result was paraplegic. After surgery, he was sent to the rehabilitation medicine unit where I was serving as a psych intern. During our staff conferences on this patient, it was my assignment to convince him that he would never walk again, as he was in denial about the severity of his condition. He was insisting that he would overcome it. I spent the next three months working with him and after a relatively brief period of time gave up trying to convince him that he wasn't going to walk again. Instead, I supported his efforts to work hard in rehabilitation. I'll never forget the moment when he started to recover some movement in his lower extremities. By the time I finished my internship, he was walking with the aid of crutches. When I questioned the physiatrist about what had happened with the diagnosis, he shrugged his shoulders and said, "We missed that one." It taught me an important lesson: to never give up in the face of what appears to be a hopeless condition.

WEEK SEVEN

APPENDIX 7.13   HEALING VISUALIZATION: PAIN MANAGEMENT

Name: _____   Date: _____
History No: _____

1. Begining relaxation by breathing deeply
2. Imagining a warm light flowing all through your body, relaxing every muscle
3. Picturing your pain symbolically
4. Picturing the healing process symbolically
5. Seeing the healing process winning over the pain
6. Seeing your own body feeling good and relaxed and comfortable
7. Seeing yourself doing something you love to do
8. Having awareness of your body, and the room around you; when ready, opening your eyes

WEEK EIGHT

APPENDIX 7.14   PAIN GROUP EVALUATION

I. Please rate the following presentations in terms of their effectiveness for your pain management:

Very helpful	Somewhat helpful	Not helpful

Causes and treatment of chronic pain
Exercise and pain management
Changing your thinking/working with family members
Nutrition and pain management
Relaxation and imagery

II. Please use the following rating scale to answer the following questions:

1. Very much   2. Some   3. Not at all

1. How relevant were the presentations to the type of pain you experience?
2. Did you learn new information from the presentations?
3. Did the presentations change the way you think and/or feel about pain?
4. Did you feel able to speak freely in the group?
5. Overall, how much did the group experience help you?

III. Please rate the following aspects concerning pain and its effect on your life since taking this course.

Improved greatly	Somewhat improved	Not improved

1. Actual pain level experienced
2. Feelings of control over your pain
3. Feeling depressed or moody because of pain
4. Feeling good about yourself because of new skills or attitudes

IV. Please answer in your own words:
1. What did you like most about the group?
2. What would you like to see changed about the group?
3. What other comments do you have about the group?
4. Will you attend the bimonthly follow-up group?

Section III

Treatment of Commonly Occurring Pain Syndromes

8

Clinical Diagnosis of Heel Pain

Paula Lizak Gilchrist, L.P.T., D.P.M.

Heel pain (calcaneal pain) is one of the most common foot problems presenting to the clinical practitioner. In 1999, over 2 million doctor visits were involved with the treatment of heel pain. Age is not a discriminating factor. Heel pain can occur with any age group, but is most commonly found from the age of 8 to 80 years of age. Heel pain is noted in women, men, and children. It is responsible for loss of work days, loss of school days, and loss of income.

Disability from heel pain can be short term and mild to long term and fully debilitating. Problems with the heel can be associated with activity change, increase in weight, and change in shoe gear. Foot type (pronated or supinated foot) as well as atrophy of fat pads in the heel can contribute to heel pain.

In 1999 alone, a MedLine Search showed 11,849 "hits" with questions on heel pain. These questions ranged from the definition of heel pain, to causes, to treatments, to support groups.

Care for heel pain can range from the most conservative to the most radical. A myriad of treatment exists. Treatment such as rest, ice, compression, elevation, medication (oral anti-inflammatories, oral steroids, vitamin therapy), steroid injections, orthotics, physical therapy modalities, exercise for strength and flexibility, massage therapy, acupuncture, acupressure, splinting, strapping, and casts are a few of the conservative care measures. Steroid creams and anti-inflammatory creams have also been used.

Radical care, generally reserved for the most resistant cases, does include surgical measures. Plantar fasciotomy, plantar fasciectomy, exostectomy, bursectomy, calcaneal osteotomy, neurolysis and lysis of adhesions, and tendon lengthening are all within the surgical realm of possibility.

Practitioners from many arenas of traditional medicine and complementary care medicine treat heel pain. We all have our niche. Medical physicians tend to give medication for pain and inflammation. Podiatrists offer use of medication, orthotics for foot balancing, strapping, splinting, casting injections, and surgery. Osteopaths offer medication and bony adjustment (such as for a short leg). Chiropractors offer spinal alignment. Acupuncturists and acupressurists offer pain blocking care. Therapists, physical, massage, and others, offer deep tissue relief, myofascial care, scar reduction and body awareness. All have the same goal: reduction of pain, reduction of inflammation, and increase in function. There is no simple single line of treatment and no single rate of cure for those patients with heel pain.

Infectious processes as well as systemic diseases can cause heel pain. Diseases such as gout, rheumatoid arthritis, psoriatic arthritis, Reiter's syndrome, and ankylosing spondylitis can cause heel pain. However, for purposes of this discussion, the following pathologies are discussed:

1. Plantar fasciitis
2. Heel spur syndrome
3. Haglund deformity
4. Retrocalcaneal exostosis/Achilles tendon calcification
5. Achilles tendonitis
6. Tarsal tunnel syndrome
7. Flexor hallucis longus tendonitis

For an anatomical review of the foot, the reader is advised to consult a standard anatomy text for illustrations of the foot.

0-8493-0926-3/02/$0.00+$1.50
© 2002 by CRC Press LLC

There are 26 bones in the human foot. This amounts to one fourth of the bones found in the entire human body. The foot itself is divided into three bony sections.

1. Rearfoot: consisting of talus and calcaneus
2. Midfoot: consisting of navicular, cuboid, and cuneiform bones 1, 2, 3
3. Forefoot: consisting of metatarsals 1, 2, 3, 4, 5
   Five proximal phalanges
   Four middle phalanges
   Five distal phalanges

Note that the hallux (great toe) has only a proximal and a distal phalanx.

In terms of foot musculature, there are four distinct layers of plantar muscles. The layers ranging from superficial (plantar) to deep (dorsal) are

First layer: abductor digiti quinti, flexor digitorum brevis, abductor hallucis
Second layer: tendon of flexor hallucis longus, tendon flexor digitorum longus, four lumbricales, and quadratus plantae
Third layer: adductor hallucis, flexor hallucis brevis, flexor digiti minimi brevis
Fourth layer: three plantar and four dorsal interossei

Note that the tendon of the peroneus longus and tendon of the posterior tibialis muscles in the posterior half of the foot are close to this layer.

The plantar fascia, often discussed as an inflamed area in heel pain, consists of three separate compartments.

Medial fascia: encompasses abductor hallucis muscle
Central fascia: encompasses flexor digitorum brevis
Lateral fascia: encompasses abductor digiti minimi

The tarsal tunnel, located on the medial side of the ankle, is often implicated in impingement syndromes that can cause heel pain. The tarsal tunnel has four distinct canals that have the laciniate ligament (flexor retinaculum) as the roof and 2 septa that form the borders of the canals.

Canal 1: contains tibialis posterior muscle (primary function is to assist in plantar flexion and inversion of the foot)
Canal 2: contains flexor digitorum longus (assists in bending of the toes)
Canal 3: contains posterior tibial nerve (L4, L5, S1, S2, S3 nerve root) posterior tibial artery and vein
Canal 4: contains flexor hallucis longus muscle (responsible for great toe flexion and assists in push-off phase of gait; also assists in deceleration of forward motion of the tibia)

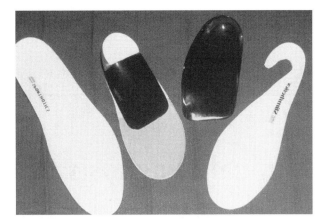

FIGURE 8.1 Different types of orthotics.

These four canal areas are prevented from bowstringing during standing and walking by the laciniate ligament (flexor retinaculum). The medial calcaneal nerve, a branch from the posterior tibial nerve, is noted to pierce through the laciniate ligament and give sensory innervation to the medial side of the heel.

PLANTAR FASCIITIS

Plantar fasciitis may perhaps be the most common heel problem presenting to the clinician. It is often associated with repetitive stress injuries and is not usually the result of direct trauma. It is a soft tissue problem that can be present for years (to some degree) before the patient seeks any type of treatment. Heel spurs can be present on radiograph without symptoms of plantar fasciitis.

Poststatic dyskinesia is often noted. Pain occurs with great intensity when the patient arises from a resting posture or from sleep. Pain is noted to diminish with activity; however, as the course of the day progresses, pain can be seen to increase. The greatest pain is noted after rest.

Inflammation can be detected at any area of the plantar fascial areas, but it is most commonly noted at the medial calcaneal tubercle attachments of the fascia onto the heel. This bony prominence serves as the point of origin of the anatomic central band of the plantar fascia, and the abductor hallucis, flexor digitorum brevis, and abductor digiti minimi muscles. Pain is generally elicited with deep palpation directly in front of the medial tubercle. Pain is also greatest at the push-off phase of gait when the already inflamed fascia is stressed and stretched as the forefoot begins to accept more body weight.

It is important to remember that the plantar fascia assists in maintaining the arch height of the foot; it connects the heel to the forefoot. With pathology present, the medial longitudinal arch of the foot can flatten. Passive toe extension with the ankle in full dorsiflexion and the knee in extension can elicit pain at the heel.

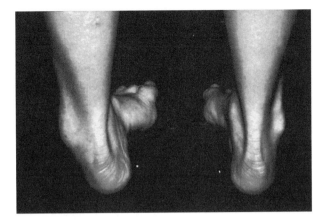

FIGURE 8.2 Cavus foot (high arch).

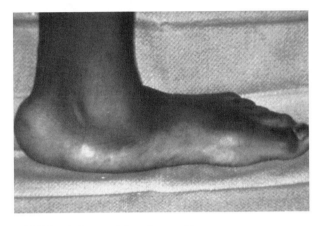

FIGURE 8.3 Pronated foot (low arch).

Pain from plantar fasciitis can be noted to increase when there is a decrease in the flexibility of the gastro-soleus (triceps surae) complex at the calf area. The triceps surae sends a slip of attachment to the plantar fascia. However, remember that when the plantar fascia is stretched, inversion of the heel occurs to a slight degree. Peroneal musculature (evertors) can be involved. Evaluation cannot always be contained to the heel itself. Musculature attachments to the heel and around the heel must be assessed.

One method to assess for calf tightness is to apply a heel lift that does not compress to less than 1/2 to 1 in. If the plantar heel pain eases, then calf tightness must be addressed in the process of eliminating heel pain. If calf tightness is noted, it is best to stretch the Achilles tendon bilaterally. The stretch should be done with the subtalar joint of the foot in neutral position. This helps maximize the stretch of the Achilles tendon. All stretches should be done as static holds, no bouncing. If heel lifts are needed, then the lifts should be worn in both shoes to reduce the risk of back pain until the flexibility of the gastro-soleus complex is restored.

Comment: When bouncing instead of static stretches is done during exercise, shortening rather than lengthening

of the muscle is apt to occur. This shortening may cause a secondary Achilles tendonitis.

Plantar fasciitis can occur in either a supinated (cavus, high-arch type of foot) or in a pronated (low-arch) type of foot. In pronation, the talus plantarflexes and adducts while the calcaneus everts. A cavus-type of foot is noted to be inherently more rigid. This foot type may require extra cushioning for relief of heel pain. A planus-type of foot is generally quite flexible. Patients with this foot type may only require a heel lift for care. Note that a hint for balance is to assess the foot with the subtalar joint in neutral position and the midtarsal joint maximally pronated. Either foot type can respond nicely with the use of a mechanically balanced custom-made orthotic to control subtalar joint motion.

In the early stages of treatment, a foot strapping to lock the first ray and transfer pressure away from the fascia and onto the tendons and toes may help relieve pain. It is not uncommon to find scar tissue formation on the medial side of the heel due to repetitive stress in an unbalanced foot. Lateral shift of the infracalcaneal fat pad and atrophy of the infracalcaneal fat pad can occur. A heel cup may eliminate lateral shift and a heel lift may assist in cushioning the foot. Scar tissue may be eradicated with deep soft tissue massage and fascial release therapy.

HEEL SPUR SYNDROME

Infracalcaneal pain (heel spur syndrome) can occur if plantar fasciitis progresses and microtears of the proximal fascia occur at the calcaneal attachments. Low-grade periostitis occurs along with thickening in the area of trauma. Edema and fibroblastic inflammatory cell infiltration can also occur. Periosteal calcification occurs near fascial and tendonous attachments. The infracalcaneal heel spur forms in this manner. A "traction" type of spur from excessive pulling of the tissue is noted.

Lateral, oblique, and calcaneal axial X-rays of the foot are helpful to assess heel pain. However, for infracalcaneal

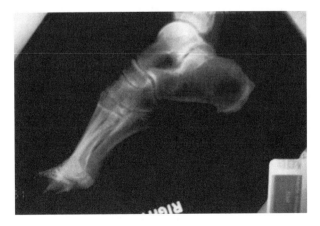

FIGURE 8.4 Infracalcaneal heel spur.

spurs, the lateral X-ray view often yields the most information as to the type and extent of spurring. Direct bony alignment of the foot can also be a contributing factor to heel spur formation.

Pain presentation is very similar to that of plantar fasciitis. Etiology can be overuse, excess weight in a pronated or supinated foot type. Conservative treatment is the same as in plantar fasciitis. The physical therapy modalities of iontophoresis and phonophoresis and electrical stimulation may be of great help to reduce inflammation.

Note that not all infracalcaneal spurs are symptomatic. Occasionally if the foot is well compensated, an infracalcaneal spur can be an incidental finding on X-ray examination.

Special attention to the thickness of the infracalcaneal fat pad is needed to assist in pain relief. Soft shoes with a long medial counter for cushioning and shock absorption may be helpful. Medial longitudinal arch support may also assist in easing inflammation.

HAGLUND DEFORMITY

Synonyms for Haglund deformity include pump bump (from female high heel shoes) and retrocalcaneal bursitis. This bony problem is often confused with Achilles tendonitis or bursitis.

This condition can occur in patients with a prominent posterosuperior aspect of the calcaneus who wear tight rigid counter shoes. It refers to the part of the shoe that "cups the heel" and gives the heel stability in the shoes. The lateral X-ray view of the foot helps to assess this problem. In this entity, the counter of the shoe rubs the heel and causes pain and further enlargement of the posterosuperior aspect of the calcaneus. Clinically, the examiner should view the posterior aspect of the heels with the patient standing. The bulge is quite evident and is seen lateral to the Achilles tendon.

Pain symptoms are generally reported as dull aching at the posterior aspect of the heel, lateral to the attachment of the tendon Achilles. The pain is greatest when the foot is dorsiflexed. A possible etiology for this pain is the pinching of the retrocalcaneal bursal sac between the Achilles tendon and the heel. An adventitious (not an anatomically correct) bursal sac can form at the superficial surface of the Achilles tendon, which can further enhance pain.

Conservative treatment for this problem includes rest, soft heel lifts, and nonsteroidal anti-inflammatory medication or drug, NSAID, occasional removal of the posterior aspect of the heel counter, or open back shoes. Heel lifts of 1/2 to 3/8 in. are used to raise the point of heel irritation just superior to the counter of the shoes. Ice massage may also help. If conservative care fails, then removal of the inflamed bursal sac and partial calcaneal exostectomy or calcaneal osteotomy may be required.

Some clinicians may advocate steroid injection into the bursal sac only; however, this must be done with great caution and skill. If steroid is inadvertently placed into the Achilles tendon, spontaneous rupture of the tendon can occur.

RETROCALCANEAL EXOSTOSIS/ACHILLES TENDON CALCIFICATION

In this malady, heel spur or calcification is noted at the insertion of the Achilles tendon onto the posterior aspect of the heel or within the tendon itself. This problem can be isolated or can be found in combination with retrocalcaneal bursitis of Achilles tendonitis. The Achilles tendon itself can become thick and wide; lateral radiographs reveal calcification in the Achilles tendon.

Pain symptoms include dull aching, especially near the insertion of the Achilles tendon onto the heel. Pain

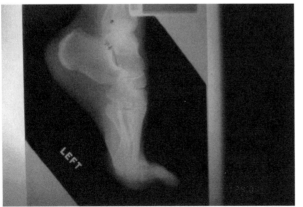

FIGURE 8.5 Haglund deformity. Note enlargement of the posterosuperior area of the calcaneus.

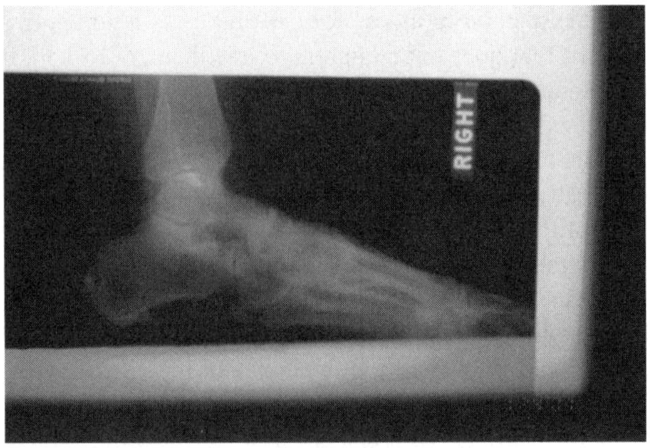

FIGURE 8.6 Retrocalcaneal and infracalcaneal spur.

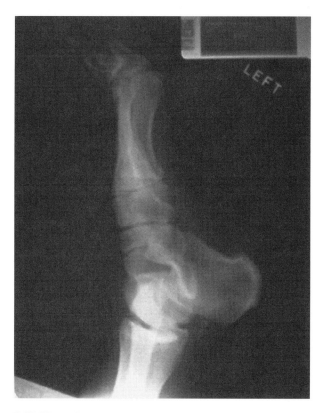

FIGURE 8.6A Note calcification in the Achilles tendon.

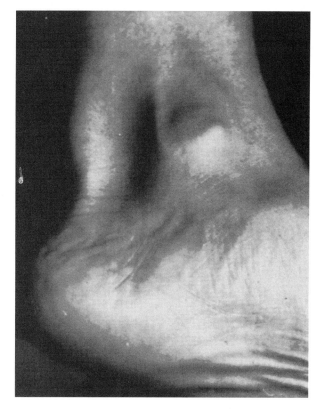

FIGURE 8.7 Achilles tendonitis.

frequently occurs in the patient who is involved in athletics or dancing activities due to the active or passive range of motion of the ankle as well as with direct palpation of the area. Slightly less dorsiflexion of the involved ankle can be noted due to bony block and crepitation of the tendon. Crepitation can occur due to chronic inflammation and fibrous deposition throughout the tendon.

Conservative care consists of rest and modality care with great emphasis placed on stretches of the triceps surae. Ice can also decrease edema and decrease post-static dyskinesia. Surgical exostectomy can require splitting of the Achilles tendon or detaching the Achilles tendon from the heel to gain exposure of the retrocalcaneal spur. The muscle does tend to lose strength with this type of radical approach.

ACHILLES TENDONITIS

Tendon disabilities can be caused by irritation around a tendon sheath (paratenosynovitis), pathology of the sheath itself (tenosynovitis), lesions between the sheath and the tendon (such as lipoma), and lesions within the tendon itself (tenosynovitis). Peritendonitis is a term used to describe inflammation of a tendon with or without a sheath. The Achilles tendon is the largest and strongest tendon in the body.

Tendonitis is an inflammation of the tendon itself generally caused from repetitive stress experienced by

athletes, dancers, and jumpers. Tendonitis crepitans can be noted due to chronic inflammation of the area.

Tendons, in general, receive blood supply from four areas: muscles, bone, paratenon, and mesotenon. The Achilles tendon has little supply from bone or muscle; much of its blood supply comes from the paratenon.

Achilles tendonitis is generally noted to be posterior on the heel with great tenderness noted approximately 3 cm proximal to the insertion of the Achilles tendon onto the heel. Pain is noted with dorsiflexion of the ankle due to tension on the heel cord itself. Tenderness can be associated with swelling, redness, and thickening of the tendon itself. In dancers, pain can be noted during landing just after a jump because the triceps surae is a decelerator of foot motion.

Treatment consists of longer warm-ups, use of heel lifts and flexibility training, cross-fiber massage, modalities, and nonsteroidal anti-inflammatories. Stretching is the key and can be done in several positions.

TARSAL TUNNEL SYNDROME

The tarsal tunnel is located on the medial side of the ankle. The roof of the tunnel is made up of the laciniate ligament. There are four distinct canals in the tarsal tunnel, which are formed by two individual septa. The contents of the canal are

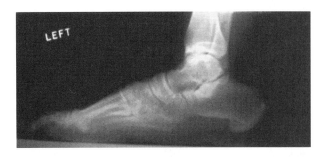

FIGURE 8.8 Radiograph of planus foot type. Note sagging of midfoot.

Canal 1: posterior tibial muscle
Canal 2: flexor digitorum longus muscle
Canal 3: posterior tibial nerve (L4 L5 S1 S2 S3) artery and vein
Canal 4: flexor hallucis longus muscle

Tarsal tunnel syndrome is generally the compression or entrapment of the posterior tibial nerve as it courses under the laciniate ligament. The posterior tibial nerve divides into the medial and lateral plantar nerves and is responsible for great areas of sensory innervation in the foot. As a result, patients may not be able to pinpoint the source of pain, but may only describe general areas of pain located at the inferior region of the medial malleolus.

Pain with this syndrome is generally of gradual onset and is described as aching, burning, and unremitting. The triad of pain, paresthesia, and numbness are not uncommon with nerve injury. Pain is noted with weight bearing and with nonweight bearing. Pain can begin in the posterior aspect of the heel and can continue forward to just below the medial malleolus and into the toes themselves. A positive Tinel (pain radiation to toes) or Vallieux sign (pain radiation to calf) can be noted with percussion and compression of the posterior tibial nerve as it courses around the medial malleolus. An electromyogram may help to clinch the diagnosis.

Causes for tarsal tunnel syndrome include pronated (flat foot) that is decompensated, hypertrophy of the abductor hallucis longus muscle (causing nerve pressure), cysts of the nerve itself, or a poorly applied cast that incorporates the foot.

Differential diagnoses are many, including plantar fasciitis, medial calcaneal neuroma, digital plantar nerve entrapment, vascular disease, and lumbosacral radiculopathy.

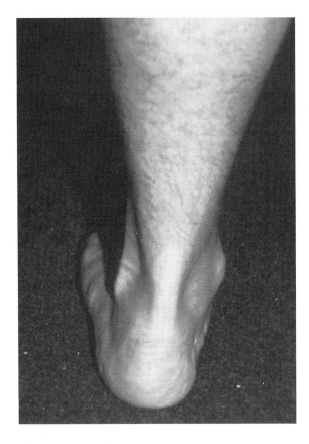

FIGURE 8.9 Low-arch foot prior to orthotic care.

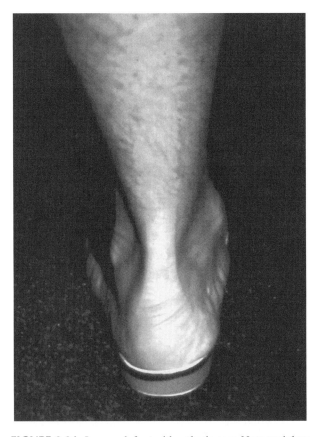

FIGURE 8.9A Low-arch foot with orthotic care. Note straighter position of Achilles tendon.

Conservative care of this lesion can include a medial longitudinal arch support, strapping, and control of the subtalar joint with a custom-made control orthotic. The goal is to control pronation. Medication and steroid injection can help in some cases when pathology is diagnosed early.

FLEXOR HALLUCIS LONGUS TENDONITIS

The flexor hallucis longus muscle assists in plantar flexion of the great toe. During the push-off phase of gait, the muscle locks the proximal phalanx of the great toe and assists in ease of weight distribution. This muscle helps decelerate the forward motion of the tibia onto a fixed foot. When tendonitis occurs here, it is generally the result of a mechanical disturbance. Overuse, other than direct trauma, is a common etiology. The patient complains of discomfort in the sole of the foot.

Tendon pain is not generally noted with passive stretch or dorsiflexion of the great toe. Pain is noted with local pressure at the point of pathology. On examination, the flexor hallucis longus tendon stands out when the toe is passively dorsiflexed. Pain can occur the length of the tendon, but is more commonly noted at the proximal

portion of the tendon. Tenderness is detected more superficial and distal to the area where heel spur tenderness is expected. The medial calcaneal tubercle is generally not tender.

Treatment for this lesion consists of soft sole shoes, modalities, and massage. A transverse archband may also help. Tendon injection with steroid medication is questionable and may cause tendon rupture.

It is hopeful that with therapeutic discussion of the prior pathologies, the practitioner may gain additional information for use in treatment of patients, or clients, with clinical heel pain.

MISCELLANEOUS

Did someone mention "heel pain?"

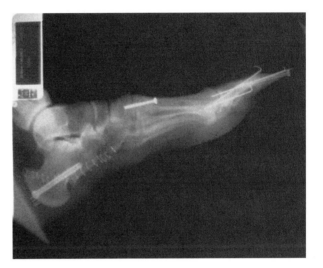

FIGURE 8.11 Did somebody mention heel pain?

REFERENCES

Anderson, J.E. (1978). *Grant's atlas of anatomy* (7th ed., pp. 4-88-4-122). A. M.r. Agur (Ed.). Baltimore: Williams & Wilkins.

Barrett, S., & O'Malley, R. (1999). Plantar fasciitis and other causes of heel pain. *American Family Physician, 59*(8), 2200-2206.

Barry, N.N., & McGuire, J.L. (1996). Overuse syndrome in adult athletes. *Musculoskeletal Medicine, 22*(3), 515-530.

Bateman, J.E. (1982). The adult heel. In M.H. Jahss (Ed.), *Disorders of the foot* (pp. 764–775). Philadelphia, PA: W.B. Saunders.

Baxter, D.E. (1994). The heel in sport. *Clinical Sports Medicine, 13*, 683–693.

Cimino, W.R. (1990). Tarsal tunnel syndrome. *Review of the Literature. Foot and Ankle, 11*, 47–52.

Cornwall, M.W., & McPoil, T.G. (1999). Plantar fasciitis: Etiology and treatment. *Journal of Orthopedic and Sports Physical Therapy, 29*(12), 756–760.

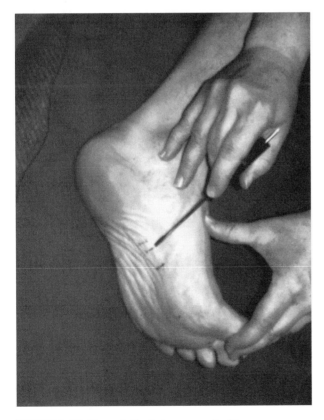

FIGURE 8.10 Flexor hallucis longus tendonitis.

Gudeman, S.D., Eisele, S.A., Heidt, R.S., Colosimo, A.J., & Stroupe, A.L. (1997). Treatment of plantar fasciitis by iontophoresis of 0.4% dexamethasone. *American Journal of Sports Medicine, 25,* 12–16.

Hoppenfeld, S. Physical examination of the foot by complaints. In M.H. Jahss (Ed.), *Disorders of the foot* (Vol. I, pp. 103–107). Philadelphia, W.B. Saunders Co.

Luther, L. (1991). Soft tissue trauma of the hindfoot. In G.J. Sammarco (Eds.), *Foot and ankle manual* (pp. 116–125). Malvern: Lea and Febiger.

Malay, D.S., & Duggar, G.E. (1992). Heel surgery. In E.D. McGlamry, A.S. Banks, & M.S. Downey (Eds.), *Comprehensive textbook of foot surgery* (Vol. 1, 2nd ed., pp. 431–455). Philadelphia: Williams & Wilkins.

Netter, F.H. (1989). *Atlas of human anatomy* (pp. 497–504). CIBA-Geigy Corporation.

Pfeffer, G.P. (1995). Plantar heel pain. In D. E. Baxter (Ed.), *The foot and ankle in sport* (pp. 195–205). St. Louis: Mosby-Yearbook.

Root, M.L., Orien, W.P., Weed, J.H., et al. (1977). Normal and abnormal function of the foot. In *Clinical biomechanics* (Vol. 2). Los Angeles: Clinical Biomechanics Corporation.

Scioli, M. (1994). Achilles tendonitis. *Orthopedic Clinics of North America, 25,* 177.

Van Wyngarden, T.M. (1997). The painful foot. Part II: Common rearfoot deformities. *American Family Physician, 55*(6), 2207–2212.

9

Cervicogenic Processes: The Results of Injury

Alfred V. Anderson, M.D., D.C.

Injuries to the cervical spine present unique problems for the health care practitioner. This fragile stem between the body and the head is extremely vulnerable. As a result of injury, the spine develops processes to accommodate the mechanical and physiological changes that inherently take place due to such injury.

This chapter is based on the author/practitioner's experience over 30 years, applying a multidisciplinary approach to chronic, intractable pain. One of the first components was an exercise regimen.

Pain is currently defined as an unpleasant sensory/emotional experience related to tissue damage or described by the patient in such terms. Chronic noncancer pain (CNCP) is generally defined as pain lasting at least 6 months, more time than expected for tissue-to-tissue healing or the resolution of the underlying disease process. It may be due to a condition where there is ongoing nociception. Chronic noncancer pain is different than acute pain in both its presentation and pathophysiology.

Progress in basic science research is gradually discovering the biochemical and structural mechanism of peripheral and central sensitization that maintains chronic pain. Over the past several decades, the author has utilized this schematic of pain. Pain becomes the center of the patient's life producing inactivity, fatigue, anger, depression, and frustration (Figure 9.1). However, the most important aspect of this patient's life is function. Function is regained with the use of appropriate modalities, exercise, and, if necessary, medication to help the patient deal with the pain associated with increased activity.

There is a wide range of pain sensitivity, even with the same "objective" findings. Variations may be dependent on several factors including the patient's early experiences with pain. Even genetics may play a role in pain perception.

CERVICAL SYNDROMES

There are numerous cervical syndromes varying from developmental and congenital disorders to degenerative processes. Also included are conditions such as strain, sprains, subluxation, and chronic conditions such as fibromylagia.

CERVICAL ACCELERATION/DECELERATION: AN EXAMPLE

Cervical acceleration/deceleration (CAD) is an ideal condition to illustrate cervicogenic processes, because this type of injury and its sequelae involve almost all of the syndromes of the cervical spine.

The CAD pain patient is sometimes misled by myths that cause as much damage to the psyche as the physical injury. **Myth:** "The injury is simple strain and sprain, it will heal in 6 to 12 weeks." **Fact:** The sudden acceleration/deceleration injuries are six to ten times more likely to develop spondylosis or degenerative changes within the joints and disks leading to prolonged recovery time (Norris and Watts, 1983).

Myth: "Permanent injuries from sudden acceleration deceleration trauma are very rare." **Fact:** Approximately 40% have some persistent recurring pain; approximately 20% have pain that alters the quality of life (Taylor and Finch, 1993).

Myth: "The client had preexisting spinal degeneration; the pain is due to this rather than the accident." **Fact:** It is the experience of the author that patients can have degenerative changes occurring down through their life without any symptoms whatsoever. However, when subjected to trauma such as a sudden accelera-

0-8493-0926-3/02/$0.00+$1.50
© 2002 by CRC Press LLC

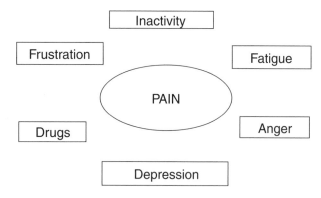

FIGURE 9.1 The results of pain.

tion/deceleration injury, these patients are predisposed to chronic pain.

ANATOMIC INJURIES

Anatomic injuries are addressed according to the intensity of the associated pain. *Facet joints* are now considered primary pain generators; they are subject to degeneration as well as capsular injury. The facets may undergo hypertrophy. They develop loss of articular cartilage, sclerosis, irregularity, and osteophytes; and these alterations take place over a number of years following trauma.

SYMPTOMS

The facet joints are supplied with proprioceptive fibers; when these are traumatized, they tend to deliver signals to the brain that can confuse the brain's perception of visual and vestibular input. This condition is referred to as *cervicogenic vertigo* and is related to symptoms of unsteadiness that patients may describe as "standing in a rocky boat." Fractures of the facets can also lead to substantial changes in the mechanical function of the joint.

Case of facet injury — A 32-year-old male, wearing a seat belt, was hit from the left at approximately 30 mi/h by a car running a stoplight. He suffered immediate pain in the cervical spine with painful range of motion. He was taken to an emergency room on a backboard; evaluations were done, including X-ray studies in which a fracture was suspected. Approximately 2 weeks later, a magnetic resonance imaging (MRI) scan was done, which did reveal a facet fracture. The patient was immobilized with a Philadelphia collar for approximately 6 weeks. A good union was obtained. However, the pain persisted in the cervical spine with radiating pain into the base of the skull as well as localized pain at the lower part of the neck. A facet nerve injection was done that substantially reduced the symptoms. As a result of this procedure, the patient elected to have a radiofrequency rhizotomy performed. This substantially reduced the pain complex. He was followed for 6 months with good results.

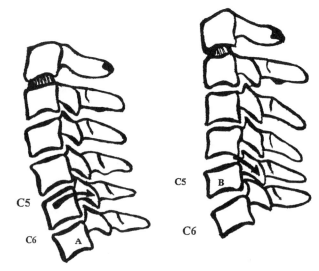

FIGURE 9.2 A, normal axis of movements of C5 on C6; B, change of axis and sudden acceleration/deceleration (SAD).

When the cervical spine incurs acceleration/deceleration injury, there is a substantial alteration of the mechanics of the spine. Studies by Ono, Daneoka, Wittek, and Kajzer (1997) and Croft (2000) have shown that there is an instantaneous change in the axis of extension of C5 on C6. The pivot point of extension normally is in the upper vertebral body of C6 (Figure 9.2). During a sudden acceleration/deceleration injury, the pivot point moves up to the lower portion of the vertebral body of C5, causing a crushing type of impact to occur with the facets of C5 onto the superior articulating surface of C6. This research shows that in a low impact accident of 6 mi/h, the spine obtains an "S" configuration with hyperflexion of the upper cervical spine and hyperextension of the lower cervical spine, particularly C5. The studies done by Ono and associates show that in *low impact accidents* the neck rarely exceeds the normal limits of range of motion; however, the substantial change in the force factors applied to the facets results in significant injury.

Bogduk and Marsland (1988) have estimated that about 60% of acceleration/deceleration injuries have their origins in the facet joints. Autopsies of persons subjected to acceleration/deceleration trauma who subsequently died of unrelated causes showed that significant trauma had occurred around the facet joints, which may not have been detectable by MRI scans. New diagnostic and treatment procedures such as facet nerve injections and radiofrequency rhizotomies have been shown to be effective in reducing the pain complex originating from facet joint injuries. Unfortunately, the hypertrophy occurring after trauma to the facet joints also adds to the possibility of stenosis in which the intervertebral foramina become narrowed, compressing the nerve root.

In chronic cases where bleeding or trauma occurs around the nerve root, fibrosis can develop following this hemorrhage, producing adhesions between the nerve and the spinal ligaments. MRI scans can detect this as perineuronal fibrosis (Seletz, 1958).

Invertebral Disk

Just opposite the nerve root is the *intervertebral disk*. In a sudden acceleration/deceleration injury the intervertebral disk at C5 to C6 is subjected to a significant shear force, causing disruption and tearing of the annular fibers. These fibers support one vertebra to the next and also retain the normal configuration of the nucleus pulposus.

There are, however, many cases in which the findings of the examination do not specifically correlate with the MRI studies. Schellhas, Smith, Gundry, and Pollei (1996) published a study relative to prospective correlation of MRI and discography in asymptomatic subjects as well as pain sufferers. Their conclusion showed that significant cervical disk annular tears often escape MRI detection and that MRI cannot reliably identify the sources of cervical discogenic pain. Clinical indications for cervical discography includes cases of chronic neck pain, head pain, or radicular pain. Discography should also be considered where normal, equivocal, or contradictory lateralizing pain complaints exist.

Freeman (1997) showed that damage to intervertebral disk results in infiltration of pain fibers into the inner third of the anulus fibrosus and into the nucleus pulposus. These findings tend to further validate the disk as a pain generator in chronic spine pain.

Although Freeman's (1997) studies were done primarily on low back pain patients, it certainly would seem feasible that this information could be extrapolated to the cervical spine as well. His findings of isolated nerve fibers that express substance P (an excitatory amino acid) deep within deceased intervertebral disks and their association with pain suggests that nerve growth into the intervertebral disk may play a role in the pathogenesis of low back pain.

Ligaments

Ligamentous injury is another result of sudden acceleration/deceleration. In a 15-mi/h collision, the head would accelerate with a force of 10 g (Macnab, 1964).

A 24-year-old female was seatbelted when hit from behind at approximately 15 mi/h. She was looking up and to the right. Following the accident she had severe neck pain with headaches. She was taken to the emergency room; X-rays were taken and she was released. Two weeks later an examination showed a normal neurological function with the exception of dizziness on range of motion testing. She had substantial loss of flexion with point

tenderness at T1 through T3. A MRI scan of the cervical spine showed interspinous tearing at C7 to T1 and T1 to T2. A later study of the 24-year-old female showed a herniated disk at the C5 to C6 and C6 to C7 level.

When disk injury occurs in the upper three to four segments of the spine, it is not unusual for headaches to arise from these areas. However, many patients who have had successful disk surgery at the C4-5 and C5-6 levels report significant relief from cervicogenic headaches.

Headaches are common to persons suffering from sudden acceleration/deceleration injuries. The headaches can result from injury to the facet structures as well as the other pain generators of the cervical spine disks. Some authorities have suggested that muscle-contracture headache diagnoses be replaced with cervicogenic headache diagnoses in the posttrauma victims. A cervicogenic headache diagnosis seems feasible considering the pain associations relating to facets and disks. Persons with prior headaches are going to be predisposed to exacerbated pain following a sudden acceleration/deceleration injury.

Muscles

Various *muscles* have been implicated in headaches. Hack, Koritzer, Robinson, Hallgren, and Greenman (1995) described the rectus capitis posterior minor muscle, in which there is a connective bridge between this muscle and the dorsal spinal dura at the atlano-occipital junction. This was observed in every muscle specimen examined. Other muscles involved in cervicogenic headaches include all the suboccipital muscles as well as the upper trapezius and levator scapulae. After significant trauma, trigger points found in these muscle structures typically refer pain to the head. Patients respond well to trigger point injections, massage therapy, and stretching exercises. Acupuncture, manipulation, and other modalities have also been useful in controlling the pain of cervicogenic headaches.

A common sequel to the process of tissue repair is the development of inflammation of the muscle and its *fascia*, commonly referred to as myofaciitis. Characteristic of myofaciitis is the presence of small sensitive nodes (trigger points), which are in the fascial sheath. Trigger points are painful hypersensitive areas within the muscle or its associative supportive tissue (fascia). Normal muscles do not contain trigger points, they do not have taut bands of muscle fibers, they are not tender to firm palpation, they do not exhibit local twitch responses, and they do not refer pain in response to applied pressure (Travell and Simons, 1992).

If the head and neck were subjected to impacts exceeding 10 to 15 mi/h, it would seem logical that muscle and ligaments would be injured, thereby generating the conditions described by Travell and Simons (1992). She describes the fibrous bands, containing trigger points, which again are considered pain generators. Pain management specialists have treated these conditions for years with good results.

Spinal Cord

Other research currently underway shows that physiological changes within the *spinal cord*, particularly the dorsal horn of the spine are associated with pain. Excitatory amino acids such as substance P, glutamate, gamma aminobutyric acid (GABA), *N*-methyl-*D*-asparte (NMDA), and other factors that sensitize the dorsal horn, are implicated in pain. Much of current research emphasizes medication that modifies the activities of these substances. An ongoing study at the University of Minnesota has demonstrated that labeled substance P normally affects the tip of the dorsal horn. However, in the study of rats subjected to lengthy periods of pain, substance P was found to migrate deeper into the dorsal horn. At the time of this publication, it is postulated that if this phenomenon continues over a period of time that a permanent alteration in the physiology of the dorsal horn may occur. Many more studies are being done concerning the hypersensitivity of the dorsal horn.

FACTORS INFLUENCING PROGNOSIS OF INJURIES

Factors influencing the prognosis of an individual include symptoms that have lasted over 6 months. As pointed out by Loeser (2000), chronic pain is different from acute pain in that measures that provide only transient pain relief do not lead to resolution of the underlying pathological process. Loeser goes on to point out that injuries to the nervous system, either because of direct trauma or because of alterations related to massive input, may lead to chronic pain. Noxious stimuli can lead to changes within the peripheral and central nervous system that alter the spinal cord, particularly the dorsal horn.

If disk injury, nerve trauma, or specific joint injury are involved, the chances of total resolution of the pain complex are significantly reduced. In this respect, older individuals, who have progressive degeneration, typically have a more difficult time in recovery due to changes within the structure of the spine, which predisposes them to additional injury when they are subjected to further trauma (Ameis, 1986).

Some elements of the trauma incident contribute to the type and severity of injury. If an individual is in a small car, hit by a large car, the impact and the forces involved probably cause more damage to the individuals occupying the smaller car.

Other risk factors involved that increase a person's chances of substantial damage would include having the head turned to one side or the chin elevated slightly such as an individual looking in the rearview mirror at the time of impact (Havsy, 1994).

How a person sits in the car is also a decisive factor in the amount of damage resulting from a collision. If a person slouches with the head tilted somewhat forward, increasing the distance between the head and the headrest, a greater stress on the cervical vertebral would occur with a rear-end collision.

Shoulder harnesses, although proven to be life-saving devices, have contributed to increased numbers of neck injuries. The shoulder belt holds the torso in place, allowing the head and neck to move forward in a much smaller arc than is allowed without the shoulder belt. A shorter radius and the chin colliding with the chest produce more damage to the structures of the neck and temporomandibular joint.

TREATMENTS

Treatments for the various conditions that are described earlier were derived from the basic premise of exercise. Exercise, however, is sometimes intolerable to patients with moderate to severe pain. Therefore, the judicious use of adjunctive medication is recommended to help the patient through the initial phases of an exercise program. Medication gives the patient confidence to proceed with exercise as well as control of the increased pain brought on by stressing the various anatomic structures.

BIOFEEDBACK

Biofeedback has been helpful in controlling stress factors involved with pain. This technique also offers the patient a method of relaxing neck muscles when they are tending toward stages of spasm. Biofeedback is especially useful in the treatment of headaches resulting from the sequelae of cervical spine injuries. Patients learn to focus on the suboccipital muscles, the muscles of the temporomandibular joints, and as has been recently discovered, the rectus capitis posterior minor muscles.

CHIROPRACTIC MANIPULATION

Chiropractic manipulation has long been effective in treating neck injuries. Manipulation of traumatized joint structures increases range of motion for damaged facet structures. Kirkaldy-Willis, et al. (1985) studied the phenomenon of manipulation and found that therapeutic effects of manipulation involved breaking interarticular adhesions, freeing the fixated joint, and stretching the supporting muscles. It is his opinion that manipulation also tends to widen and improve the opening of the foramina, thereby reducing irritation to a potentially entrapped nerve. He is also of the opinion that stimulating the joint mechanoreceptors relieves pain. The stimulation of joint mechanoreceptors tends to override the pain impulses at the dorsal horn. For example, if one hits a thumb with a hammer, the first impulse is to shake the hand and fingers. It is postulated that this tends to stimulate the joint mechanoreceptors, thereby overriding the pain impulses at the dorsal horn. This is, of course, also the concept in mobilizing the joints with exercise. Vernon, et al. (1986) also postulated that there is an increase in endorphins released after spinal manipulation.

TRIGGER POINT INJECTIONS

Trigger point injections as advocated by Travell, have been used for years by this author; the techniques and results are well documented in other chapters of this text.

OTHERS

Currently, other treatments, modalities, and systems that are implemented, include facet nerve injections, facet nerve rhizotomies, occipital nerve rhizotomies, and inter-discal electrothermy (IDET). Many of these treatments are reviewed in other chapters.

Future pain management will probably include new medications affecting the physiology of dorsal horn, medications such as COX 2 inhibitors to assist in reducing inflammatory processes, and other pharmaceuticals to modify the transmission of pain. The use of light and sound brain entrainment formerly known as evoked potentials may also prove helpful.

The author advocates the use of any treatment helpful in the care of an individual patient. After 30 years of practice it has become obvious that treatment plans must be individualized. Treatment must be geared toward increased function as well as decreased pain. When utilizing medication, the World Health Organization (WHO) criteria are appropriate and should be followed as closely as possible. This protocol starts the patients on adjunctive medication that might include antidepressants, anti-inflammatories, as well as dietary modifications and vitamin therapy. Cessation of tobacco use should be encouraged.

The next step is the prescribing of a narcotic, as well as exercise instruction to enhance overall function of the patient. The practitioner should not be fearful of including the more potent narcotics when necessary. Responses vary from patient to patient and each patient may respond differently to variations in dosages and/or types of drugs. Although one patient may respond very well to one type of narcotic, another patient may not. There is no formulary or predictive element involved in the selection of a specific narcotic for a particular patient. Judicious use of narcotics should be maintained; but the practitioner must keep in mind the variations in tolerance from one patient to the next. When chronic opioid analgesic therapy (COAT) is employed, both the patient and the doctor

must sign an informed consent narcotic agreement. Examples of these narcotic agreements are available in other chapters of this text.

Prior to starting advanced medication, priorities must be placed on increasing the patient's overall capacity for exercise, emphasizing increased function as the primary goal. Medication cannot be justified on a long-term basis if the patient is not showing some indication of increasing function. In severe cases, this may only mean regaining and maintaining the ability to perform the activities of daily living or sustaining the will to live it.

Many authors have defined pain down through the years. It is this author's opinion that Dr. Janet Travell defines pain in the most accurate terms. "*Pain is what the patient says it is.*"

REFERENCES

Ameis, A. (1986). Cervical whiplash: Considerations in the rehabilitation of cervical myofascial injury, *Canadian Family Physician*, *32*, 1871–1876.

Bogduk, N., & Marsland, A. (1988). Cervical zygapophysial joints as a source of neck pain. *Spine*, *13*, 610–617.

Freeman, A. (1997). Nerve ingrowth into disease intervertebral discs and chronic pack pain. *Lancet*, *350*, 178–181.

Hack, G.D., Koritzer, R.T., Robinson, W L., Hallgren, R.C., & Greenman, P.E. (1995). Anatomic relation between the rectus capitis posterior minor muscle and the dura mater. *Spine*, *20*(23), 2484–2486.

Havsy, A.F. (1994, January). Whiplash injuries of the cervical spine and their clinical sequelae. *American Journal of Pain Management*, 803–821.

Kirkaldy-Willis, W.H., et al. (1985). Spinal manipulation in the treatment of low back pain. *Canadian Family Physician*, *31*, 535–540.

Loeser, J.D. (2000). Pain and suffering. *Clinical Journal of Pain*, *16 Supplement*, S2–S6.

Macnab, I. (1964). Acceleration extension injuries of the cervical spine. *Journal of Bone, Joint Surgery*, *46A*(8), 1797–1799.

Norris, S.H., & Watts, I. (1983). The prognoses of neck injuries resulting from rear-end vehicle collisons. *Journal of Bone, Joint Surgery*, *65B*(5), 608–611.

Ono, K., Daneoka, D., Wittek, A., & Kajzer, J. (1997). Cervical injury mechanism based on the analysis of human cervical vertebral motion and head-neck-torso kinematics during low speed velocity rear end impacts. 41st Stapp Car Crash Conference Proceeding. SAE paper 975540, 556–559).

Schellhas, K.P., Smith, M.D., Gundry, C.R., & Pollei, S.R. (1996). Cervical discogenic pain. *Spine*, *21*(3), 300–312.

Seletz, E. (1958). Whiplash injuries: Neurophysiological basis for pain and methods used for rehabilitation, *Journal of the American Medical Association*, *168*(13) 1750–1755.

Taylor, J.R., & Finch, P. (1993). Acute injury of the neck: Anatomical and pathological basis of pain. *Annals Academy of Medicine*, *22*(2), 187–192.

Travell, J.G., & Simons, D.G. (1992). Myofascial pain and dysfunction. In J.P. Butler (Ed.), *The trigger point manual: The lower extremities* (Vol. 2). Baltimore, MD: Williams & Wilkins.

Vernon, H.T., et al. (1986). Spinal manipulation and beta endorphin: A controlled study of the spinal maniupulation on plasma beta endorphin level in normal males. *Journal of Manipulation and Physiological Therapeutics.*

ADDITIONAL READING

Allen, B.J., Li, J., Menning, P.M., Rogers, S.D., Guilardi, J., Mantyh, P.W., & Simone, D.A. (1999). Primary afferent fibers that contribute to increased supstance P receptor internalization in the spinal cord after injury. *Journal of Neurophysiology, 81*(3), 1379–1390.

Cailliet, R. (1991). *Neck and arm pain* (3rd ed.). Philadelphia: F.A. Davis.

Croft, A.C. (2000, July). Whiplash. *Journal of the American Chiropractic Association*, 32–42.

Croft, A.C. (1995). Biomechanics. In S.M. Foreman & A.C. Croft (Eds.), *Whiplash injuries: The cervical acceleration/deceleration syndrome* (2nd ed., pp. 66–71). Baltimore: Williams & Wilkins.

David, A.G. (1945). Injuries of the cervical spine. *Journal of the American Medical Association, 127*(3), 149-156.

Foreman, S.M., & Croft, A.C. (1988). Whiplash injuries: *The cervical acceleration/deceleration syndrome.* Baltimore: Williams & Wilkins.

Hohl, M. (1974). Soft tissue injuries of the neck in automobile accidents: Factors influencing prognosis. *Journal of Bone and Joint Surgery, 56A*(8), 1675–1682.

Jackson, R. (1977). *The cervical syndrome* (4th ed.). Springfield, IL: Charles C Thomas.

Kenna, C.J. (1984). The whiplash syndrome: A general practitioner's viewpoint, *Australian Family Physician, 13*(4), 256–58.

Macnab, I. (1971). The "whiplash syndrome." *Orthopedic Clinics of North America, 2*(2), 389–403.

Murphy, D.J. (1995, April). Whiplash distortions, cervical zygapophysial joint injury and chronic posttraumatic neck pain. *Journal of Clinical Chiropractic, 31.*

Nordhoff, L. (1994). *Motor vehicle collision injury for the 1990's doctor/attorney.* Automotive Injury Research Institute.

Olney, D.B., & Marsden A.K. (1986). The effect of head restraints and seat belts on the incidence of neck injury in car accidents. *Injury, 17*, 365–367.

Porter, K.M. (1989, April). Neck sprains after car accidents. *British Medical Journal, 298*, 6679, 973–974.

Quebec Task Force on Whiplash-Associated Disorders (1995). White paper. *Spine, 20*(8S).

Quintner, J.L. (1989). A study of upper limb pain and parasthesiae following neck injury in motor vehicle accidents. *British Journal of Rheumatology, 28*, 528–533.

Robinson, D.D., & Cassar-Pullicino, V.N. (1993). Acute neck sprain after road traffic accident: A long term clinical and radiological review. *Injury, 24*(2), 79–82.

Salmi, R.L. (1989). The effect of the 1979 French seat-belt law on the nature and severity of injuries to front-seat occupants: *Accident Analysis and Prevention, 21*, 589.

10

Thyroid and Parathyroid Diseases and Pain

Stuart A. Dorow, M.D., D.C., Ph.D. and Gretajo Northrop, M.D., Ph.D.

INTRODUCTION

In the current medical arena, pain is often the most important indicator of the nature and seat of disease. It frequently signals an interruption of the harmony of the bodily organs; and many physicians insist most strenuously that the distinctive characteristics of the various kinds of pain be described as accurately as possible by the patient. Pain presenting as a throbbing sensation synchronous with the heart's action is called pulsating pain. Pain described as a feeling of tightness is referred to as tensive and when combined with heat, it is called burning. On the other hand, nervous pain may be recognized by its disposition to follow a certain course, without being rigidly limited to one particular part; by its subjection to perfect intermissions; and by the suddenness with which it comes and goes. Spasmodic pain is mitigated by pressure, by frictions, and by applications of heat; it presents suddenly with greater or lesser severity, terminating abruptly. Pain that is deemed inflammatory is constant, is attended by heat and quickened pulse, is increased by movement of the affected part, by touch, or pressure, and is usually relieved by rest. Frequently, pain occurs not in the diseased part but in a distant one and this manifestation is well known as referred pain. This is all very tidy and lends itself well by extrapolation to the Fox equation, which holds that "Germ X = disease X, germ Y = disease Y" (Fox & Fox, 1992). However, as that educator and countless others have discovered, this model fails in regard to that all-too-frequently illusive pain. A pain that defies labeling by any of the preceding definitions is, in every way, equally as debilitating. Is it merely psycogenic or some supratentorial phenomenon? Thus, some rethinking of the concepts involving pain may be required, particularly the pain resulting from thyroid and parathyroid diseases.

THYROID AND PARATHYROIDS IN HEALTH

The thyroid located just below the larynx is composed of left and right lateral lobes that lie on either side of the trachea. Both lobes are connected in the midline by a mass of tissue known as an isthmus and the entire structure is in front of the trachea just inferior to cricoid cartilage. When present, there is an additional projection, which extends cephalad from its attachment at the isthmus and is known as the pyramidal lobe. This endocrine gland weighs approximately 25 g and is profused by approximately 80 to 120 ml of blood per minute. The thyroid gland has a unique configuration histologically. It is composed of spherical sacks known as thyroid follicles with the walls of each sack consisting of cells that project into the lumen of the follicle and another layer of cells that does not. Cells in contact with the lumen area are called follicular cells whereas those not in contact are called C cells or parafollicular cells. When actively secreting hormones, the cells take on a columnar appearance and when not in an active state, they appear cuboidal in shape.

Follicular cells synthesize and liberate the substance known as thyroxine, or T4, by a process known as iodination, and the coupling of two tyrosine molecules while attached to a complex protein called thyroglobulin. T4 signifies that thyroxine contains four atoms of iodine. Triiodothyronine, or T3, is synthesized as well in the colloid and contains three iodine atoms. Collectively, these two hormones comprise the thyroid hormones. Thyroxine is present in greater quantity, whereas T3 is several times more potent and is formed in peripheral tissues such as the liver and kidneys as well as in most other cells by the deiodination of T4. Reverse T3 is biologically inactive and

0-8493-0926-3/02/$0.00+$1.50
© 2002 by CRC Press LLC

is the metabolized form of T4. It is, however, the active form of T3 that binds to receptor sites and thus triggers end-organ effects. Functionally, both T3 and T4 are similar because they regulate metabolism, growth, and development, as well as the activity of the nervous system. Parafollicular C cells are not without their own manufacturing plant where they synthesize and secrete calcitonin, a compound that serves to lower the blood levels of calcium by its action on bones to increase absorption.

Clearly, thyroid cells can be seen to have three actions: the collection and transport of iodine, the synthesis of thyroglobulin for its secretion into the colloid, and the removal of the thyroid hormones from thyroglobulin for secretion into circulation (Ganong, 1989).

The parathyroid glands, four in number, are embedded in the four poles of the thyroid gland. There are two superior and two inferior glands located on the thyroid gland. These measure about the size of the tip of a small child's little finger. From the perspective of histology, two types of cells are represented, and are epithelial in nature. The chief cells, or principal cells, synthesize parathyroid hormone (PTH) and are the most numerous. PTH is released in response to a fall in extracellular ionized calcium. PTH is carried by the blood to the kidney where it causes calcium reabsorption and conversion of 25-hydroxy-vitamin D_3 to 1,25-dihydroxy vitamin D_3. This metabolite increases intestinal absorption of calcium and with PTH causes bone reabsorption of calcium. These are only a few of the actions of PTH. At different concentrations of PTH, action on target tissues may differ. Low levels of PTH result in skeletal anabolic action, whereas high levels of PTH may result in bone lysis. The remaining cells are called oxyphils and are believed to manufacture a reserve supply of PTH.

HORMONAL REGULATION

The thyroid and parathyroid glands never sleep because their role in active metabolism prohibits it. Thyroid hormones are essential for the normal maturation and metabolism of all bodily tissues. The effects of thyroid hormones on metabolism are, needless to say, diverse. Thyroid hormonal effects can be seen in their calorigenic action where T3 and T4 increase the oxygen consumption of almost all metabolically active tissues with the exception of the adult brain, testis, uterus, lymph nodes, spleen, and anterior pituitary. Nervous system effects can be seen centrally as well as in the peripheral nervous system. The effects on skeletal muscle become apparent in the patient with hyperthyroidism (thyrotoxic myopathy). Most of these patients demonstrate marked muscle weakness. Beta-adrenergic receptors on the heart are increased in number and affinity due to thyroid hormones. The increase in the number of receptors and affinity on the heart resembles the action of beta-adrenergic stimulation.

It is a well-known fact that thyroid hormones increase the rate of absorption of carbohydrate from the gastrointestinal tract, albeit most likely independently of any calorigenic action. In hyperthyroid patients, the blood glucose level can be seen to rapidly rise after a carbohydrate meal, often exceeding the renal threshold and subsequently fall just as rapidly. A topic that takes a prominent place in conversations today is cholesterol levels. The thyroid hormones are not without their effect on cholesterol levels because they have been shown to lower circulating cholesterol. The level of plasma cholesterol decreases prior to the metabolic rate rising and this action indicates that it may be independent of stimulation of oxygen consumption as well. Normal growth, development, and skeletal maturation are, in large measure, dependent on the thyroid hormones. Nowhere is this more evident than in a child who is hypothyroid and in whom bone growth is retarded and epiphyseal closure is delayed. The list of effects of the thyroid hormones on bodily tissues appears to be endless and those discussed here represent only a few of them.

The regulation of secretion of thyroid hormones can be seen in the hypothalamic–pituitary–thyroid axis where the tripeptide thyroid-releasing hormone (TRH) is secreted by the hypothalamus and triggers synthesis of a glycoprotein hormone, thyroid-stimulating hormone (TSH), from the anterior pituitary. TSH secretion sets in motion the synthesis of thyroid hormones T3 and T4. In turn, TSH production is regulated by feedback from circulating, unbound thyroid hormones (free T3 and T4). In the investigation of patients with thyroid disease, an understanding of these basics is essential for accurate interpretation of test results.

THYROID AND PARATHYROIDS IN DISEASE

Hyperthyroidism and hypothyroidism are fairly well-known disease entities, with the former being exposure of the tissues to exorbitant amounts of thyroid hormones, and the latter a paucity of those hormones. In the purest sense, for one to be hyperthyroid, there must be an overactivity of the thyroid gland itself, but thyrotoxicosis can manifest itself with ingestion of excess T4. In some cases, overstimulation of the thyroid by pituitary TSH can occur, although this is considered rare. Many factors enter into the differential diagnosis of hyperthyroidism, including overingestion of T4 as previously mentioned. Drugs frequently can be ingested and classified as goitrogens (goiter-producing agents), such as the antithyroid agents propylthiouracil (PTU), carbimazole, and methimazol (Adler, et al., 1988). Amiodarone drops have been shown to precipitate hyperthyroidism (Gaw, et al., 1995, p. 84). In addition, p-aminosalicylic acid (PAS), sulfonamides, amphenone, phenylbutazone, iodides, lithium carbonate, and cobalt have been indicated in diffuse goiter formation (Murphy, 1988, p. 107). An often-overlooked common source of iodine ingestion, which may be seasonal, but nevertheless can be taken in excess is expectorants (Hope, et al., 1996, p. 542). Among the more innocuous appearing agents in goiter formation are soy milk/flour, turnips, cabbage, brussels sprouts, and rutabagas, to mention a few. Causative agents identified here should not, by any means, be construed as all-inclusive. Multinodular goiters can be of the nodular hyperplastic type or adenomas, which are multiple. Benign adenomas, colloid nodules, thyroglossal duct cyst, granulomatous disease, lobulations of the thyroid, and hematomas comprise a miscellaneous group of solitary nodules. Malignancies such as lymphoma, anaplastic carcinoma, follicular carcinoma, medullary carcinoma (or a combination of follicular/papillary, papillary carcinoma, and metastatic disease) may also fall under the solitary classification (Burrow, 1987, p. 474).

According to Ingbar and Braverman (1986, p. 809), thyrotoxicosis or hyperthyroidism may manifest with either elevated or normal blood levels of T3 or T4. Euthyroid Graves' disease is diagnosed when blood levels of T4 and T3 are normal yet the patient has the thickened extraocular muscles associated with Graves' disease. Graves' disease is an autoimmune disease in which antibodies stimulate thyroid release from the gland. In addition, human chorionic gonadotropin (HCG) secreting tumors such as choriocarcinoma, hydatidiform moles, and testicular embryonal cell carcinomas can stimulate the thyroid gland abnormally. In cases of thyrotoxicosis without hyperthyroidism, as evidenced by a suppressed TSH in the TRH test, extrathyroidal sources of hormone such as iatrogenic or factitious ingestion may be suspect. Jod–Basedow disease is an iodine-induced source of thyrotoxicosis demonstrating reduced radioactive iodine uptake (RAIU).

Thyroiditis is considered a group of inflammatory thyroid disorders that may present as thyrotoxicosis without hyperthyroidism. This group is composed of subacute thyroiditis in either its "silent" (nonpainful) form, known as subacute lymphocytic thyroiditis, or its alternative "painful" form, known as giant cell thyroiditis (collectively referred to as simply subacute thyroiditis). However, the granulomatous form appears to be the most common cause of thyroid gland pain. Postpartum thyroiditis may evolve as hyper-, hypo-, or euthyroidism. Present thoughts are that pregnancy decreases immunologic responses whereas during the postpartum there is a "rebound effect" usually resulting in hyperthyroidism. Granulomatous thyroiditis has been known to follow upper respiratory infections of adenovirus, Epstein-Barr virus, echovirus, mumps virus, and coxsackie virus (Farwell & Brauerman, 1996). According to Bonica (1990, pp. 864–865), symptoms usually follow those of a respiratory infection as stated and include pronounced malaise and asthenia, as well as symptoms referable to stretching of the thyroid capsule, principally pain over the thyroid or pain referred to the lower jaw, ear, or occiput. Local or referred pain can predominate. Less commonly, the onset is acute, with severe pain over the thyroid accompanied by fever and occasionally by symptoms of thyrotoxicosis. Cardinal physical findings include exquisite tenderness and pain on palpation of the nodular thyroid.

Other types of thyroiditis include chronic lymphocytic thyroiditis (typically referred to as Hashimoto's thyroiditis). This disease has also been referred to as struma lymphomatosa and was first described by the Japanese surgeon H. Hashimoto who wrote his M.D. thesis on struma lymphomatosa (Firkin & Whitworth, 1990, p. 444). In the United States, it is the most common cause of goiter production, as well as the most common inflammatory thyroid gland condition (Hay, 1985; Hamburger, 1986). Dayan and Daniels (1996) indicate that lymphoma of the thyroid can be a complication of this disease but fortunately does not occur with great frequency. Several Type III autoimmune hypersensitivity reactions such as Sjogren's syndrome, rheumatoid arthritis, and systemic lupus erythematosus (SLE) have been associated with chronic lymphocytic thyroiditis. Diabetes mellitus and pernicious anemia have also been associated with chronic lymphocytic thyroiditis (Dayan & Daniels, 1996).

Acute supportive thyroiditis is an inflammatory condition resulting from invasion of the thyroid gland by *Staphylococcus aureus* or other Gram-positive organisms. It is reported that *S. aureus* is the most common invader (Dayan & Daniels, 1996). Patients may present with neck pain and/or tenderness, which appears localized to the thyroid gland. Pain associated with supportive thyroiditis does not appear in the posterior cervical region, assisting in differentiating it from that of musculoskeletal pain. The gland may also manifest rubor and calor, and cause dysphagia, which can be seen in association with pharyngitis and not surprisingly, tachycardia (Levine, 1983). Fortunately, the disease process is usually self-limiting and can be treated conservatively with microbial-sensitive antibiotics, corticosteroids, aspirin, localized heat, and restricted activity. Should an abscess develop, incision and drainage are indicated; if resolution is not obtained, surgical drainage may become a necessity.

Riedel's thyroiditis/struma (invasive fibrous thyroiditis) has the distinction of being the least common of the group of inflammatory thyroid diseases. It is a chronic thyroiditis of unknown etiology marked by localized areas of stony hard fibromas (Firkin & Whitworth, 1990). Riedel's thyroiditis is characterized by intense fibrosis of the thyroid gland and of the surrounding structures that lead to induration of the tissues of the neck, associated with some pain in the region of the neck. The condition can also be associated with mediastinal and retroperitoneal fibrosis. It is unfortunate that this slowly enlarging, or in some cases suddenly expanding, hard mass in the anterior neck is often mistaken for thyroid cancer. Hypothyroidism occurs when the insidious fibrous infiltration finally invades the entire thyroid gland (Ferri, 1998, pp. 352–353). Multifocal fibrosclerosis can be expected, as well as involvement of various sites distant to the neck. The location of the involved structures determines the manifest symptoms, which can include dysphagia, stridor, and dyspnea (Malotte, et al., 1991). This disease is frequently self-limited but on occasion, may require surgical resection (Levine, 1983; Malotte, et al., 1991). Uncommonly, the diseases classified as thyrotoxicosis may be caused by pituitary adenomas, struma ovarii, metastatic thyroid cancer, embryonal carcinoma of the testes, chorio-carcinoma, hyperemesis gravidarum, and isolated pituitary resistance to thyroid hormone (Ferri, 1994, p. 47).

GRAVES' DISEASE (TOXIC DIFFUSE GOITER)

Thyrotoxicosis is one of the most common endocrine disorders. Its incidence is highest in women 20 to 40 years of age. Thyrotoxicosis, when associated with ocular signs (ophthalmopathy) and related disturbances as well as a diffuse goiter, is given the name of Graves' disease and is the most common cause of hyperthyroidism (Graber, et al., 1994, p. 214). In European and Latin American countries, this disease may be referred to as Basedow's disease and is reported as such in their literature. This disease is interesting and often a clinical puzzle because instead of a diffuse goiter being present, a nodular toxic goiter (Hashitoxicosis) may demonstrate all the metabolic features of thyrotoxicosis and may occasionally be present without any visible or palpable enlargement of the thyroid gland. Hyperthyroidism is a condition caused by the oversecretion of hormones by the thyroid gland that ultimately influences the metabolism of cells throughout the body. Graves' disease is an autoimmune disease associated with a TSH-like immunoglobulin that binds to the TSH receptor sites of the thyroid gland, and in so doing stimulates the thyroid gland to increase production and release of thyroid hormone. The signs and symptoms of hyperthyroidism apply and are listed in Table 10.1.

Two signs that appear to be restricted to thyroid disease are pretibial nonpitting edema (infiltrative dermophathy) of myxedema and exophthalmos (proptosis). In a small number of patients with Graves' disease (less than 5%), pretibial myxedema presents as a violaceous nonpitting thickening of the skin in the pretibial region, ankles, and/or feet and is the result of mucopolysaccharide infiltration of the dermal tissue (DeBello, 1992, p. 219). Exophthalmos is considered diagnostic of Graves'

TABLE 10.1
Signs and Symptoms of Hyperthyroidism

Sign	Symptom
Restlessness	Increased bowel elimination/frequency
Nervousness	Weight loss despite increased appetite
Overactivity	Onycholysis separation at distal tuft
Tremor	Menstrual dysfunction, oligo/amenorrhea
Heat intolerance	Diffuse goiter with/without detectable bruit
Sweating	Velvet skin with moist warm hands
Hyperreflexia	Pulse pressure increases
Insomnia	Increased lacrimation
Exophthalmos[a]	Pretibial myxedema[a]
Tachycardia	Panic attacks
Lid lag	Fixed gaze stare
Photophobia	Emotional lability
Diplopia	Atrial fibrillation
Systolic flow murmur	Blurring of vision

[a] Restricted to Graves' disease.

disease when present; however, it may not be present at all or may be very minor in its presentation, and it may present at virtually any stage of the disease process. The protrusion of the globe from its orbital rim is believed to be the result of mucopolysaccharide deposition and fat accumulation behind the globe accompanied by edema of the extraocular muscles. Of interest is the fact that the cause of Graves' disease has not been elucidated. Familial predisposition to the disease has led researchers to strongly suspect genetic etiology. The classic manifestations of the disease such as goiter, ophthalmopathy, and dermopathy may well be based on thyrotoxicosis and are often present independent of each other, possibly exhibiting cyclic periods of exacerbation and remission throughout the course of the disease. The manifestations with which the patient presents, increased serum T3 and/or T4, and suppression of TSH levels found by radioimmunoassay, can confirm the increased activity of the thyroid gland. Elevated levels of antithyroid immunoglobulins evidenced on blood tests may lend credence to a diagnosis of Graves' disease. Graves' disease and its prognosis vary on a case-by-case basis. Should symptom remission and eradication of disease-associated immunoglobulins result from appropriate treatment, recovery remains while immunoglobulins are reduced. With a resurgence of thyroid-stimulating immunoglobulins (TSI), the patient again becomes hyperthyroid. A potentially fatal Graves' disease complication known as "thyroid storm," presents as a severe episode of thyrotoxicosis with rapid onset of delirium, tachycardia, sweating, fever, pulmonary edema, and congestive heart failure requiring immediate emergency medical intervention (Bulens, 1981, pp. 669–670).

HYPOTHYROIDISM (CRETINISM)

Hypothyroidism refers to a condition in which a paucity of thyroid hormones is manufactured in, or secreted by, the thyroid gland. In adults, severe thyroid deficiency is referred to as myxedema. *In utero* and in the newborn, undiagnosed and untreated hypothyroidism leads to cretinism (Fisher, 1981). Cretinism can usually be diagnosed clinically without difficulty, but at times it must be distinguished from mongolism and other genetic disturbances. Immunochemisty is important in making the diagnosis. Fortunately, cretinism is appearing with less frequency today than in the past, in part, due to more aggressive detection efforts (Fisher, 1987). Congenital hypothyroidism in the neonate is usually detected early by statewide screening programs. Since their inception in the 1970s, the incidence and complications of untreated cases of primary congenital hypothyroidism have dramatically decreased. In light of the severity of long-term effects of hypothyroidism on brain tissue maturation (mental retardation), the mandated newborn TSH, free T3, T4 testing has brought some welcome relief.

Congenital hypothyroidism results from glandular absence (athyreosis), ectopic thyroid, lingual thyroid gland, or dyshormonogenesis (Burg, 1990, pp. 134–135). Most often, infants with congenital hypothyroidism appear normal at birth but can appear placid and frequently require arousal to feed. Typically, the infant presents 6 to 12 weeks after birth with a common finding of prolonged jaundice and prolonged indirect hyperbilirubinemia. The cry of the infant sounds harsh or hoarse and the infant may also be constipated. Additionally, macroglossia similar to that seen in Down's syndrome may be apparent along with an umbilical hernia, muscle hypotonia, and bradycardia. Infants with hypothyroidism may have a history of full-term or even post-term birth.

A second category of acquired hypothyroidism may appear and in this category, an autoimmune phenomenon with lymphocytic infiltration of the thyroid gland is most common. Hypothyroidism is often insidious in onset. Complaints of a neck mass or dysphagia along with weight gain, dry skin, constipation, and intolerance to cold may be reported by a parent. A goiter is characteristic of the acquired form of hypothyroidism and is usually small and firm, having a "bosselated" texture typical of that seen with thyroiditis (Mahoney, 1987). If the disease appears during the growing years, there may be obvious failure on the part of the child to grow normally with delayed puberty manifested as well. Of interest is the often-reported observation of excellent school performance owing to the relative indistractibility of the child with hypothyroidism. Accurate diagnosis of hypothyroidism in children frequently requires the physician to painstakingly collect and synthesize a host of vague complaints on history as well as sort out nonspecific physical exam findings coupled with misinterpreted and often misleading laboratory findings. In all cases of suspected hypothyroidism in children, therapy is essential to preserve mental function in the neonate and to preserve normal growth patterns in the child. Anhalt, et al. (1956, p. 153) warn, "Despite the fact that screening for congenital hypothyroidism is now almost universal in the United States, there are certain methodologic flaws with the testing; thus, when encountering a child with suspicious signs and/or symptoms, the physician must always keep this diagnosis in mind."

HYPOTHYROIDISM (MYXEDEMA)

The thyroid gland is a uniquely regulated metabolic powerhouse and maintains its uniqueness among other glands of the body in that it can synthesize and store immense quantities of hormones and then slowly and deliberately release these hormones in response to bodily demands (Tilkian, 1993). The causes of hypothyroidism in the adult can be of primary, secondary, or tertiary origin. Primary hypothyroidism refers to thyroid hormone deficiency as a result of thyroid gland disease or dysfunction and constitutes greater than 90% of the cases of hypothyroidism. Among the etiologies comprising the primary category is Hashimoto's thyroiditis (chronic lymphocytic thyroiditis). According to Nagataki (1993, pp. 539–545), Hashimoto's thyroiditis may well be the most common producer of hypothyroidism in America with some 5% of euthyroid, Hashimoto thyroiditis-afflicted persons advancing to the hypothyroid state with each passing year. Idiopathic myxedema, which may be a nongoiterous form of Hashimoto's thyroiditis, is also included in the primary category. The category is further expanded by the inclusion of those persons who have been treated for hyperthyroidism with iodine 131 therapy or have had subtotal thyroidectomy or radiation therapy of the neck for malignant disease. Subacute thyroiditis and iodine deficiency or excess along with drugs such as lithium, *p*-aminosalicylic acid (PAS), sulfonamides, phenylbutazone, amiodarone, and thiourea or prolonged treatment with iodides add to the list. Congenital cases constituting approximately 1:4000 live births are also included. Secondary causes result from TSH deficiency in the pituitary gland and can be due to any pituitary dysfunction such as postpartum necrosis, neoplasm, and TSH deficiency secondary to infiltrative disease. Hypothalamic disease due to neoplasms, granulomas, or irradiation contributes to the tertiary category of hypothyroidism and results in a deficiency of TRH from the hypothalamus. As expected, the prevalence (number of cases of a disorder that exist) varies with location and by study. Graber, et al. (1994) indicate that hypothyroidism is present in 1 to 6% of the population. Signs and symptoms related to hypothyroidism are listed in Table 10.2.

TABLE 10.2
Signs and Symptoms of Hypothyroidism

Sign	Symptom
Fatigue	Muscle weakness
Lethargy	Weight gain
Constipation	Slowed speech & deepened voice
Arthralgias	Vocal hoarseness
Bradycardia	Reduced memory
Retarded cerebration	Loss of memory
Paresthesias	Intolerance to cold
Blunted effect	Cerebellar ataxia
Muscular stiffness	Carpal tunnel syndrom
Pericardial effusion	Distant heart sounds
Hearing impairment	DTR delayed relaxation
Dry, cool, doughy skin	Slow moving lips
Brittle, coarse hair & loss	Thickened tongue
Vitiligo	Nonpitting edema eyelids and hands
Ascites	Loss of temporal one third of eyebrows

HYPOTHYROIDISM (MYXEDEMA COMA)

Myxedema crisis or coma fortunately is rare, developing in only 1% of hypothyroid patients, but nevertheless it is a life-threatening complication of hypothyroidism (Myers, 1991). Bodily stresses such as cold, trauma, surgery, infection, and medications including iodides, narcotics, and sedatives have been identified as precipitating factors. Hypothyroid decompensation in the form of severe respiratory failure (CO_2 narcosis), hypothermia, or sluggish cerebral perfusion all contribute to the development of coma. The diagnosis is based upon the clinical presentation and therapy must be instituted before the clinical suspicions are substantiated by laboratory tests, because delay may lead to a fatal outcome in this medical emergency (Cecil, 1993). Clinical awareness of the wide spectrum of presentation and a high index of suspicion of hypothyroidism will generally serve to identify most cases. However, a number of clinical conditions such as nephritic syndrome and cirrhosis, including an associated reduction in serum TBG (thyroid binding globulin) and consequent low serum total T4 values can mimic hypothyroidism.

Patients with hypothyroidism may live for years but with some dysfunction of many organs are less able to tolerate the stress of additional illness, i.e, infection, surgery, seizures, congestive failure, stroke, drug toxicity, or exposure to extremes in heat or cold. T4 replacement is indicated. Expert modern medical management is essential. The mortality rate is still 50% and survival depends on early recognition and treatment of the hypothyroidism and any other factors contributing to the extremely serious medical condition including an altered level of consciousness. With prolonged, severe myxedema, overt psychosis may develop. Attempted suicide has also been reported with some patients never regaining sanity; "myxedema madness" has been applied to these conditions (Christy, 1975). With substitution therapy, the psychosis usually clears but on occasion, patients may develop overt psychosis with the advent of the therapy regimen.

HYPERPARATHYROIDISM, PRIMARY, SECONDARY, TERTIARY

Primary hyperparathyroidism refers to the condition in which the parathyroid glands liberate an excess of PTH (parathyroid hormone). The excess may result from one or more of the glands in spite of the fact that plasma ionizeded calcium is elevated. The normal adaptive response for the release of PTH involves parathyroid hyperplasia in reaction to lowered serum calcium levels. When prolonged for extended periods, these glands can and will hypertrophy, becoming a cause for secondary hyperparathyroidism. The majority of patients suffering with hyperparathyroidism appear to be women. The condition appears to be much less common in children. In primary hyperparathyroidism the pathogenesis appears to be unrestrained liberation of PTH but the etiology is unknown. In about 80% of patients a solitary benign parathyroid adenoma is responsible. A low percentage of hyperparathyroidism cases are due to parathyroid cancer. The small size of the gland can create a dilemma for the surgeon. Fortunately, the hormone secreted by this gland (parathyroid hormone) can be stained in paraffin sections and be used for the identification of normal parathyroid tissue or that ravaged by an invading carcinoma, particularly when the carcinoma occurs as a metastasis. This procedure takes about 30 minutes (Sherrod, 1986). An equally small percentage of hyperpathyroidism appears to be familial, with a portion of this category being associated with the syndromes of multiple endocrine neoplasia (MEN I, MEN IIa, IIb). The condition becomes suspect when routine blood chemistry reveals high calcium levels (total serum calcium > 10.5 mg/100 ml). Other conditions included in the differential may be hypercalcemia due primarily to increased bone resorption as a consequence of prolonged immobilization, hyperthyroidism, or malignancy involving bone such as metastic carcinoma to bone, leukemia, lymphoma, or multiple myeloma. Addison's disease, sarcoidosis, hypervitaminosa A or D can result in hypercalcemia. Renal calcium reabsorption increases secondary to thiazide diuretic use. Addison's disease or familial hypocalciuric hypercalcemia can also raise serum calcium levels as can ectopic hyperparathyroidism. Bronchogenic carcinoma has been known to cause hypercalcemia by enhanced absorption of calcium from the GI tract, kidney reabsorption, and resorption of calcium from bone. The ingestion of large quantities of calcium carbonate and milk (milk-alkali syndrome) also elevate serum calcium levels. The signs and symptoms of hypercalcemia are listed in Table 10.3. Symptoms are usually due to bone pain/fracture, renal stones, nonspecific abdominal pain, constipation, duodenal ulcer, pancreatitis, or depression. Ask a medical student for the symptoms of hyperparathyroidism associated with hypercalcemia and after a short moment, his or her head will begin to nod and sway rhythmically as they mentally recite the poetic mnemonic: "Bones stones, abdominal groans and psychic moans." Unfortunately, no rhythmic mnemonc exists for the additional presentations of joint stiffness, gait disturbances, hypertension, myopathy, dehydration, confusion, thirst, nocturia, and anorexia due to increased calcium levels. Approximately 25% of patients with hyperparathyroidism have prominent psychitric symptoms that may resemble mania, schizophrenia, or acute confusional states while an additional 50% may display symptoms suggesting depression (Cogan, 1987).

In hypercalcemic cases ectopic hyperparathyroidism as well as malignancy of lung, kidney, or pancreas may well come to mind. Granulomatous conditions, for example, sarcodiosis, tubercolisis, and others that may convert $25\text{-}(OH)_2D_3$ to $1,25\text{-}(OH)_2D_3$ in an unregulated fashion may lead to increased calcium adsorption from the gut as well as increased bone resorption. Routine radiographic findings may reveal osteoporosis wtih vertebral compression fractures on even more telltale subperiosteal resorption of the phlanges. Cyst-like lesions may be found in any part of the skeleton, even the skull (osteitis fibrosa cystica ostodystrophy).

These bone cysts are frequently seen and are accompanied by pain, especially when there is involvement of surrounding periosteum. Calcification of soft tissue such as lungs, tendon attachments, pancreas, or kidneys

revealing stones may serve as a clue to the hyperparathyroid condition. When there is hypocalcemia, the parathyroid glands sense the calcium reduction and begin the process of hyperplasia and initiate the secretion of PTH in an adaptive effort to restore the body's mineral balance. If or when the patient suffers from renal failure, malabsorption syndrome, vitamin D deficiency, or renal tubular defects which lead to excess loss of calcium, hypocalcemia ensues and secondary hyperparathyroidism prevails. Drugs such as phenobarbital and phenytoin actively interfere wtih metabolism of vitamin D and in so doing diminish the ability of the gastrointestinal tract to absorb calcium. Renal tubular acidosis also contributes to calcium loss.

For osteomalacia in adults and rickets in children to occur defective mineralization of bone must precede it. Multiple types of osteomalacia exist depending upon the pathophysiology of the disease or malfunctioning diseased organ. Chronic renal failure results in phosphate retention with a reciprocal decrease in calcium leading to secondary hyperparathyroidism. Because of the effects of markedly elevated PTH levels upon metabolism, osteosclerosis, osteoporosis, and "von Recklinghausens's disease of bone" (osteitis fibrosa cystica) may manifest as renal osteodystrophy (Price, 1986). Another form of oseodystrophy may develop because of the severity of the renal disease. The kidneys may no longer be capable of completing the conversion of $25\text{-}(OH)_2D_3$ into the active form 1,25-dihydroxycholecalciferol ($1,25\text{-}(OH)_2D_3$ vitamin D) resulting in the most common bone disorder, osteomalacia (adult rickets). The disease can be identified radiologically by translucent bands (Loeser's lines) that are pseudofractures involving part of the cortex perpendicular to the periostal margin of the bone. These lesion (infarctions) in the bone represent infarctions in the bone caused by compressive stresses that produce small cracks in the cortex

---

TABLE 10.3

Signs and Symptoms of Hypercalcemia (Hyperparathyroidism)

Neuromuscular	Gastrointestinal	Kidney
Myopathy	Vomiting	Renal stones
Hypotonia	Constipation	**Skin**
Muscular weakness	Ileus	Pruritus
CNS	**Pancreatitis**	**Cardiovascular**
Emotional labiality	Nausea	Hypertension
Mental confusion	Anorexia	QT interval shortened
Lethargy		Bradycardia
Stupor		Digitalis toxicity, increased potential
Coma		
Delirium		
Headache		

Azotemia (caused by effects of calcium precipitation in the renal parenchyma)

Polyuria (ADH prohibited by calcium from binding to receptor sites in the distal convoluted tubule)

and are pathognomonic of osteomalacia (Albright, 1946). Pseudofractures are frequently bilateral and symmetrical and are commonly seen in the axillary border of the scapula, the ribs, pubic and ischial rami, medial aspect of the neck of the femur, iliac bones, radii, and ulna (Aronoff, 1985). They were first described by Milkman (1930, 1934) and later became known as "Milkman's syndrome." For many years, it has been known that vitamin D (as above) is necessary for proper assimilation of calcium through the gastrointestinal tract (Hannon, 1934). Previously there was a siege of childhood rickets due to decreased vitamin D in the diet or from lack of exposure to ultraviolet rays. This siege was eventually eradicated with the fortification of many foods and food additives with vitamin D. Cases of vitamin D-resistant or persitent rickets, an X-linked autosomal dominant disease, have also occurred (Nora, 1994). Most cases of vitamin-D resistant or persistent rickets (rachitis tarda) probably represent osteomalacia caused by renal tubular insufficiency (Fanconi syndrome), a primary defect in renal tubular phosphate resorption. With the decreased active form of vitamin D, absorption of calcium from the gut is grossly impaired. Osteomalacia is seen in nearly 60% of all pateints with chronic renal failure. Defective dimineralization of the bone occurs when there is a low serum calcium level and ineffective vitamin D leading to the replacement of normal bone with osteoid tissue. Bone with wide osteoid seams is structurally inferior to normal bone and easily deforms under stress and is prone to fractures.

Osteodystrophy may be detected using plain film radiographs that show bone with decreased density, most commonly in the fingers, skull, spine, and ribs. Osteitis fibrosa cystica occurs in more than 30% of patients with hyperparathyroidism and is characterized by osteolytic resorption of bone and its replacement by fibrous tissue. The lesions of demineralization may appear to be localized and cystic, hence its name, osteitis fibroa cystica. Radiographically, the lesions may show a generalized decrease in bone density. Classically, the lesion associated with this disease is the subperiosteal resorption of bone at the phalanges with or without scattered areas of demineralization in the skull that resemble a moth-eaten appearance. Osteosclerosis is the least common bone disorder and on radiographs demonstrates a characteristic "Rugger jersy spine" appearance which gives vertebra alternating dark and light bands respresenting bone density variations. These lesions may appear solo or in any combination with other radiographic signs.

HYPOPARATHYROIDISM

Hypoparathyroidism is defined as a decrease in the production of parathormone or parathyroid hormone by the parathyroid glands. As a consequence, concentrations of circulating calcium are reduced and hypocalcemia ensues with all its ramifications. This condition is relatively rare and most commonly occurs following inadvertent removal of all four parathyroid glands during thyroid cancer surgery. Fortunately, congenital, genetic, idiopathic, and autoimmune causes are extremely rare but do exist (Damjanov, 1996, p. 423). Irradiation to the neck rarely may result in hypoparathyroidism, as can massive radioactive iodine administration for cancer of the thyroid gland. Candidiasis endocrinopathy syndrome is an inherited disease of functionally defective T cells. It is characterized by susceptibility to candidal infection with a strong predilection for parathyroid and adrenal glands. Autoimmune destruction of these glands may be due to an autoimmune disorder called multiple endrocrine deficiency, autoimmune candidiasis (MEDAC) syndrome (Camargo, 1987, p. 708). Glandular destruction regardless of the cause results in hypoparathyroidism and/or Addison's disease (Rubin & Farber, 1995, p. 84).

A severe form of deficient T-cell immunity is DiGeorge syndrome. This syndrome is caused by defective embryological development of the third and fourth pharyngeal pouches that become the thymus and parathyroid glands. In the absence of a thymus, T-cell maturation is interrupted at the pre-T-cell stage, and in the absence of parathyroid glands, hypoparathyroidism is inevitable (Sadler, 1990, p. 310). In the alcoholic patient, hypomagnesemia is a common concern; and when not replaced, it can lead to hypoparathyroidism and ultimately hypocalcemia by either impairing the secretion of PTH or interfering with end-organ responsivenss to the hormone. With an insidious onset of hypocalcemia, signs and symptoms may be negligible or absent altogether. Patients can be asymptomatic and have total serum calcium as low as 5 to 6 mg/100ml. The signs and symptoms of hypoparathyroidism are those of hypocalcemia (Dambro & Griffith, 1997) and are listed in Table 10.4.

When there is significant hypocalcemia, tetany may well be most striking in clinical presentations. Facial spasms can be so debilitating that the patient is unable to speak. Spasms affecting the hands and feet are frequently seen. When spasms become of such a magnitude that prevents the patient from talking, the clinician as well as family members must be diligent in looking for signs of laryngeal spasm requiring breathing assistance should respiration become significantly compromised. Trousseau's sign (carpal spasm in the hand) can be demonstrated by producing ischemia with a blood pressure cuff placed on the arm and inflated above the systolic blood pressure and held for 3 min. The hand will draw toward the ear and the fingers flex. The resultant carpal spasm is seen in the hand. Chvostek's sign is a facial twitch that may be induced by gently tapping the skin of the face over the area of the facial nerve slightly in front of the tragus of the ear. Numbness or tingling sensations of the face, hands, lips,

TABLE 10.4
Signs and Symptoms of Hypocalcemia (Hypoparathyroidism)

Diarrhea	Neuromuscular irritability	Fatigue
Weakness	Abdominal cramping	Alkalosis
Weight loss, dry skin	Bone pain	Tetany
Paresthesias	Carpal pedal spasm	Myalgia
Headache	Depression	Dementia
Seizures	Chvostek's sign	Trousseau's sign

and tongue are common findings in hypocalcemia, as are dryness of the skin, coarse dry hair with some hair loss, and fingernails with ridges that run longitudinally to the nail. Should extrapyramidal signs that resemble parkinsonism be exhibited, calcification of the basal ganglia may be the culprit and the plain skull film showing basal ganglia calcification can be confirmatory. Psychic disturbances (see Table 10.4) can be seen when hypocalcemia becomes chronic and the patients may exhibit signs of increased intracranial pressure with resultant papilledema. Hypotension, malabsorption syndrome, cataracts, and prolongation of the Q wave to T wave (QT) interval are all consequences of hypocalcemia. In cases of acidosis, circulating calcium is liberated from albumin and ionized calcium levels rise sharply. Conversely, alkalosis causes ionized calcium to bind to albumin binding sites that would be otherwise occupied by hydrogen ions; therefore, the manifestations of hypocalcemia become exaggerated in either respiratory alkalosis or metabolic alkalosis.

An interesting biochemical phenomenon occurs in the normocalcemic patient whereby hyperventilation can blow off CO_2, creating a respiratory alkalosis; this, in turn, reduces the amount of circulating ionized calcium, and results in low calcium tetany if prolonged. An excellent study was conducted that reviewed the metabolic and respiratory changes in 21 patients who had suffered heat stroke reported that the predominant change was that of metabolic acidosis secondary to an increased lactate content, and/or a respiratory alkalosis. The study further reported that many of the patients also had hypo-calcemia. The researchers postulated that the lactic acidosis was most likely due to increased metabolic requirements resulting from hyperthermia compounded by hypotension and hypoxemia and an impairment in liver function that decreased the capacity to dispose of the lactate once it formed. They reported that the cause of the hypocalcemia was unclear (Appenzeller, 1986, p. 70). The authors of this chapter suggest that the reason for hypocalcemia in these and heat stroke patients is hypoxemia and hyperthermia shifting the oxygen disassociation curve to the right, which resulted in additional oxygen given off to the tissues as well as increased respiratory effort to meet the

loss from blood to the tissues. In addition, increased lactic acid itself increases the respiratory effort. Thus, hypoxemia and hyperthermia plus respiratory alkalosis that lead to increased binding of ionized calcium to albumin lower the blood calcium in these patients. If tenany develops due to low calcium, additional lactate accumulates. Impairment in liver function makes lactate metabolism more difficult so a continuous cycle is established.

According to Herman and Sullivan (1959), biopsies taken from the livers of gold miners after suffering heat stroke revealed histological evidence of liver damage in the form of centrolobular necrosis and extensive cholestasis. It has been stated that the signs and symptoms of hypoparathyroidism are those of hypocalcemia. In light of the previous discussion and with continued research, heat stroke might in future literature be a viable candidate for addition to the list of etiologies in hypocalcemia.

Pseudohypoparathyroidism is an autosomal recessive disorder in which PTH target cells fail to respond to appropriate hormonal stimulation. Characteristically, the patient may be obese with short stature and round face, may be mentally retarded, and may demonstrate shortened metacarpals and metatarsals on radiographic examination (Ferri, 1998, p. 364). Resistance to multiple hormones in addition to PTH may also occur in patients with Albright's hereditary osteodystrophy. This is reported as pseudohypoparathyroidism Type I (Hope, et al., 1996, p. 542).

SUMMARY

In this chapter an attempt was made to discuss the major features of the thyroid and parathyroid glands, in health and disease and their relationship to pain. The authors now have a greater appreciation of, and renewed empathy for, the individual who sets out to go fishing with a large bucket filled with water and a cooler full of ice to safely store the catch of the day, only to look into the bucket and cooler at the end of the expedition and find a lot of water and a lot of ice. However, if you ask the fisherman how the day went, the reply might be something like, "I did not catch much, but I had a wonderful time and I learned a lot about fishing." The authors of this chapter would like to echo the sentiment by saying we didn't catch much, but we had a wonderful time and we learned a lot about thyroid and parathyroid glands during this fishing expedition. Other than the specific relationships mentioned about these glands and pain, there is paucity in the vast sea of literature concerning this relationship. Quite possibly (and more likely, probably) other researchers have embarked on this same fishing expedition and in utter exasperation simply poured out the water and the ice at the end of the day and put away the boat only to fish in more fertile waters on the next expedition. A wealth of knowledge that far exceeds the scope and intentions of

TOURO COLLEGE LIBRARY

this chapter is available on the endocrine scene concerning the thyroid and parathyroid glands; therefore, it is left for some future expedition. Our commitment was to seek out research that addresses a relationship between these two glands and pain and to report them. To this degree our expedition was a success.

Furthermore, when one reads in every book dealing with pain that it is a subjective finding encompassing a lifetime of emotions and feelings, there is small wonder why so little is written pertaining to the subject. We conclude that there may be much more to the subject of thyroid and parathyroid diseases and pain, but the difficulty may not be so much the manifestation of the pain but instead the verbal expression of it. Additionally, the pain associated with diseases of the thyroid and parathyroid glands may, in actuality, not be attributable to direct pain. Instead, pain associated with these glands may be due to the diverse effects on the body, and its cells and systems. Duress of disease influences man's ability not only to deal with the pain but also to express it.

REFERENCES

Adler, S.N., et al, (1988). *A pocket manual of differential diagnosis* (2nd ed, pp. 87–113). Boston: Little, Brown.

Albright, F., et al. (1946). Osteomalacia and late rickets: The various etiologies met in the United States, with emphasis on that resulting from a specific form of renal acidosis, the therapeutic indications for each etiological subgroup, and the relationship between osteomalacia and Milkman's syndrome. *Medicine, 25,* 399.

Anhalt, H., et al. (1996). Outpatient endocrinology and disorders of growth. In D. Bernstein & S. P. Shelov (Eds.), *Pediatrics* (p. 133). Baltimore: Williams & Wilkins.

Aronoff, G.M. (1986). *Evaluation and treatment of chronic pain.* Baltimore: Urban & Schwarzenberg. 371.

Appenzeller, O. (1986). *Clinical autonomic failure.* Amsterdam: Elsevier Science.

Bonica, J.J. (1990). *Management of pain* (Vol. 1, 2nd ed.). Philadelphia: Lea & Febiger.

Bulens, C. (1981). Neurologic complications of hyperthyroidism. *Archives of Neurology, 38,* 669–670.

Burg, F.D., et al. (1990). Treatment of infants, children and adolescents. Philadelphia: W.B. Saunders.

Burrow, G.N. (1987). The thyroid: Nodules and neoplasms. In P. Felig, et al. (Eds.), *Endocrinology and metabolism* (2nd ed., pp. 473–507). New York: McGraw-Hill.

Camargo, C.A. (1987). Endocrine disorders. In M.A. Krupp, et al. (Eds.), *Current medical diagnosis and treatment* (p. 708). Old Tappan, NJ: Appleton & Lange.

Christy, N.P. (1975). Diseases of the endocrine system: Hypothyroidism and myxedema. In P.B. Beeson & W. McDermott (Eds.), *Textbook of medicine* (Vol., II, 14th ed., p. 1722). Philadelphia: W.B. Saunders.

Cogan, M.G. (1987). Central nervous system manifestations of hyperparathyroidism. *American Journal of Medicine, 65,* 563–630.

Dambro, M.E., & Griffith, J.A. (1997). *Griffith's 5 minute clinical consult.* Baltimore: Williams & Wilkins.

Damjanov, I. (1996). *Pathology for the health-related professions.* Philadelphia: W.B. Saunders.

Dayan, D.M., & Daniels, G.H. (1996). Chronic autoimmune thyroiditis. *New England Journal of Medicine, 335,* 99–107.

DeBello, P. (1992). *Pocket clinical & drug guide* (3rd ed.). Henderson, NV: Tortoise Books.

Farwell, A.P., & Braverman, L.E. (1996). Inflammatory thyroid disorders. *Otolaryngologic Clinics of North America, 29,* 541–556.

Ferri, F.F. (1994). *The internal medicine companion.* St. Louis, MO: Mosby-Year Book.

Ferri, F.F. (1998). *The care of the medical patient* (4th ed.). St. Louis, MO: Mosby-Year Book.

Firkin, B.G., & Whitworth, J.A. (1990). *Dictionary of medical eponyms.* Park Ridge, NJ: The Parthenon Publishing Group.

Fisher, D.A., et al. (1981). Thyroid development and disorders of thyroid function in the newborn. *New England Journal of Medicine, 304,* 702–712.

Fisher, D.A. (1987). Effectiveness of newborn screening programs for congenital hypothyroidism. *Pediatric Clinics of North America, 34,* 879–888.

Fox, A., & Fox, B. (1992). Sleep and weight problems associated with pain. *Innovations in Pain Management: A Practical Guide for Clinicians, 35,* 1–24.

Ganong, W.F. (1989). The thyroid gland. *Review of Medical Physiology, 18,* 267–279.

Gaw, A., et al. (1995). *Clinical biochemistry.* New York: Churchill Livingstone.

Graber, M.A., et al. (1994). *The family practice handbook.* St. Louis, MO: Mosby-Year Book.

Hamburger, J. L. (1986). The various presentations of thyroiditis. Diagnostic considerations. *Annals of Internal Medicine, 104,* 219–224.

Hannon, R.R., et al. (1934). Calcium and phosphorus metabolism in osteomalacia, the effect of vitamin D and its apparent duration. *Chinese Medical Journal, 48,* 623.

Hay, I.D. (1985). Thyroiditis: A clinical update. *Mayo Clinic Proceedings, 60,* 836–843.

Herman, R.H., & Sullivan, B.H. (1959). Heat stroke and jaundice. *American Journal of Medicine, 27,* 154–166.

Hope, R.A., et al. (1996). *Oxford handbook of clinical medicine* (3rd ed.). New York: Oxford University Press.

Ingbar, S.H., & Braverman, L.E. (Eds.). (1986). Classification of the causes of thyrotoxicosis. In S.C. Werner (Ed.), *Werner's the thyroid: A fundamental and clinical text* (pp. 809–810). Philadelphia: Lippincott.

Levine, S.N. (1983). Current concepts of thyroiditis. *Archives of Internal Medicine, 143,* 1952–1956.

Mahoney, C.P. (1987). Differential diagnosis of goiter. *Pediatric Clinics of North America, 34,* 889–904.

Malotte, M.S., et al. (1991). Riedel's thyroiditis. *Archives of Otolaryngology Head and Neck Surgery, 117,* 214–217.

Milkman, L.A. (1934). Multiple spontaneous idiopathic symmetrical fractures. *American Journal of Roentgenology, 32,* 622–634.

TOURO COLLEGE LIBRARY

Murphy, T.A. (1988). Endocrine/metabolic system: Goiter. In S.N. Adler, et al. (Eds.), *A pocket manual of differential diagnosis* (2nd ed., p. 107). Boston: Little, Brown.

Myers, L., et al. (1991). Myxedema coma. *Critical Care Clinics, 7,* 43–56.

Nagataki, S., et al. (1993). *Eighty years of Hashimoto disease.* Amsterdam: Elsevier Science.

Nora, J.J. (1994). *Medical genetics principles and practice* (4th ed., p. 211). Philadelphia: Lea & Fabiger.

Price, S.A., & Wilson, L.M. (1986). *Pathophysiology clinical concepts of disease processes* (3rd ed). New York: McGraw-Hill.

Rubin, E., & Farber, J.L. (1995). *Essential pathology.* New York: J.B. Lippincott.

Sadler, T.W. (1990). Head and neck. In J. Langman (Ed.), *Medical embryology* (6th ed., p. 310). Baltimore: Williams & Wilkins.

Sherrod, A.E., & Taylor, C.R. (1986). Nonlymphocyte tumor markets in tissues. In N.R. Rose, et al. (Eds.), *Manual of clinical laboratory immunology* (3rd ed., pp. 938–947). Washington, D.C.: American Society for Microbiology.

Tilkian, S., et al. (1993). *Clinical implications of laboratory tests* (3rd ed). St. Louis, MO: C.V. Mosby.

11

Posttraumatic Headache: Pathophysiology, Diagnosis, and Treatment

Gary W. Jay, M.D., F.A.A.P.M., D.A.A.P.M.

INTRODUCTION

Posttraumatic headache (PTHA), as the name indicates, is a general, descriptive term for headache that occurs posttrauma. The types of trauma do not necessarily need to include an actual blow to the head, or even loss of consciousness. The majority of patients who experience PTHA do not have an associated minor traumatic brain injury (MTBI); however, PTHA is one of the most common sequelae of MTBI, but not moderate or severe traumatic brain injury.

Some have argued that PTHA is no different than nontraumatic headache in etiology or treatment. In many cases this may be true, although the assessment and diagnosis can be complex. Still, some researchers and clinicians are adamant about their feelings: PTHA is a sham; PTHA almost always has its etiology in the neck; the pathophysiology of PTHA is very different from other, primary forms of headache; and so on. This author believes that there is a spectrum of primary headache disorders, with PTHA a form of a primary headache disorder with possibly enhanced pathophysiological difficulties. Ockham's razor may be useful, but the clinical reality appears to necessitate a greater breadth of knowledge by the clinician.

On the other hand, there are pitfalls in the current classification systems, which seem to ensure difficulties in diagnosis, and not just nosologically. The ICD-10 classification system is based on criteria that primarily are concerned with the temporal relationship as well as pathogenicity between the relationship of PTHA to trauma, and ignore the clinical features of the PTHA (World Health Organization, 1997). This criterion states that the headache onset must occur within 2 weeks of the traumatic event or the patient's return to consciousness. However, posttraumatic cluster headache, for example, typically does not fit this time course. Furthermore, their criteria for acute or chronic PTHA require one of the following: loss of consciousness, a period of antrograde amnesia of at least 10 min, or abnormal neurological examination/neurodiagnostic testing. The ICD-10 criteria find that acute PTHA resolves in 8 weeks, whereas chronic PTHA lasts longer than 8 weeks. This is in counterdistinction to the IHS criteria (Headache Classification Committee [HCC], 1988).

These criteria are contrary to the most commonly accepted criteria, those of the brain injury special interest group of the American Congress of Rehabilitation Medicine (Kay & Harrington, 1993), which states that MTBI is a "traumatically induced physiological disruption of brain function" associated with at least one of the following: any period of loss of consciousness; any memory loss for events just before or after the accident; any alteration in mental state at the time of the accident, such as feeling dazed, disoriented, or confused; and focal neurological deficits that may or may not be transient. Most importantly, there is no necessity of direct head trauma to meet the diagnosis.

Another nosological problem is the synonymous use of various terminology: concussion, MTBI, postconcussion syndrome/disorder, and posttrauma syndrome. For a number of specific reasons, this author believes the postconcussion syndrome, which affects multiple organ systems, should be differentiated from MTBI (Jay, 2000). Patients with PTHA do not, by definition and clinical analysis, have to have an MTBI.

Very briefly, the basic elements found in an MTBI may include axonal shearing; marked increases in the excitotoxic neurotransmitters including acetylcholine and glutamate; a lack of the cohesiveness of the blood–brain barrier, which become "porous" for 8 to 24 h or more; and possible changes in the hemodynamics of the brain. (Please see textbook for details [Jay, 2000].) The most important aspect to keep in mind is that the "type" of PTHA must be accurately diagnosed so that appropriate treatment can be prescribed.

Typically, PTHA is noted after acceleration/deceleration injuries (whiplash) in up to 90% of patients who experience MTBI (Keidel & Diener, 1997). These headaches can be determined to be posttraumatic tension-type, migraine, cluster, or possibly cervicogenic headache. PTHAs may be secondary to work-related injuries, slip and fall injuries, and violent altercations, aside from motor vehicle injuries. These headaches are frequently part of the postconcussive syndrome, which refers to a large number of signs and symptoms that may follow a blow to the head or an acceleration/deceleration injury, which may or may not induce an MTBI.

Acute posttraumatic tension type of headache, the most frequently diagnosed PTHA, (defined as 15 headache days or less a month) may last up to 3 to 6 months; after that it becomes, nosologically, chronic. The IHS has determined that 15 headache days or more a month defines chronic headache (HCC). General pain management principles place pain as chronic after 3 to 6 months, after physiological healing has occurred. Up to 80% of PTHA patients have their pain remit within 6 months, leaving an estimated 20% of patients with chronic PTHA, which may last years in many cases.

A simple concussion may also be associated with PTHA, as well as, in the extremes, vegetative and even psychotic difficulties (Kojadinovic, Momcilovic, Popovic, et al., 1998; Muller, 1974). PTHA may also be associated with dizziness, irritability, and decreased concentration, even without the additional finding of an MTBI. (Again, for the differentiation between the postconcussive syndrome and MTBI, please see the MTBI chapter in this textbook.)

The chronic PTHA patient frequently engenders significant difficulties for the typical general practitioner, as well as the neurological specialist. This may be especially true if there is evidence of *de novo* migraine or cluster headache.

Medico-legally, PTHA is a common problem, because the patient does not "look" ill and may have few if any abnormalities on examination. In depositions, or in court, a physician is frequently asked to explain why such a significant problem was found after a relatively minor "rear-end" automobile accident or slip and fall. Why, it is asked, do professional football players, for instance, not have a high incidence of PTHA and/or MTBI. The answer is simple and is based on two circumstances: physical conditioning and the fact that when they play, these people are always very prepared and always anticipate the possibility of physical contact or trauma. This differentiates them from the vast majority of people who are not even close to being in optimal physical condition, who are injured unexpectedly, before they are even aware of the impending trauma and are therefore unable to physically prepare themselves for a trauma, for example, by bracing themselves against the headrest before their car is struck from behind.

A great deal of research has shown that when the head is free instead of confined, it is more susceptible to the effects of an acceleration/deceleration injury. Six decades ago, it was shown in cats that less force was required to produce concussion when the head was free to move, as compared with when it was fixed or confined in place (Denny-Brown & Russell, 1941). The concept of whiplash, essentially a legal term, medically known as acceleration/deceleration, is very important because it involves a multitude of medical aspects. When an acceleration/deceleration injury occurs (most frequently from a rear-end automobile accident), the physical or gravitational forces of a massive object such as a car striking another automobile are passed onto the most fragile and movable object not firmly secured in the automobile that was struck: the passenger. Even when the passenger is wearing a seat belt, the head — the ball at the end of a tether (the neck) — is first thrown forward, and then backward, when the tether can reach no farther and snaps back. If the head is turned at the moment of impact, the rotational forces are also very important, particularly when an MTBI is found.

Posttraumatic headache encompasses a number of different diagnostic entities. Specific diagnosis is needed for appropriate treatment. These diagnoses include

- Posttraumatic tension-type headache
- Posttraumatic migraine headache
- Posttraumatic cluster headache
- Cervicogenic headache
- Temporomandibular joint (TMJ)-related headache
- Neuropathic pain syndromes

POSTTRAUMATIC TENSION-TYPE HEADACHE

PTTHA (with or without secondary analgesic rebound headache) is probably the most common primary headache disorder found after trauma. Diagnostically, and clinically, this entity appears to be similar to acute and chronic tension-type headache without a traumatic etiology.

The diagnostic criteria of tension-type headache, according to the IHS (HCC, 1998), states that episodic tension-type headache is a recurrent headache occurring fewer than 15 days a month, lasting from 30 min to 7 days. The pain characteristics include two of four of the following: pain that has a pressing/tightening (nonpulsating) quality; pain that is mild to moderate in intensity and may inhibit, but not prohibit activities; pain that is always bilateral; and pain that is not aggravated by walking stairs or doing other routine physical activity. These criteria also state that both the following are true: no nausea or vomiting, but anorexia may occur, and photophobia and phonophobia are absent, or one but not the other is present. All other organic diagnoses must be ruled out first, as well as other primary headache diagnoses, including migraine and cluster headache.

In PTTHA, like non-posttraumatic tension-type headache, the pain is typically described as aching or pressure-like. The pain has also been described as feeling like a tight band, or a vice around the head. The pain is typically bilateral, although it may be unilateral. It may include various areas, some or all the occipito-nuchal, bifrontal, bitemporal, and suboccipital regions at the vertex (crown) of the head, as well as extend into the neck and shoulders.

The pain intensity may wax and wane depending on a number of factors including movement, activity level, stress, and others. Even in PTTHA, emotional/psychological aspects may increase pain. There is a female preponderance.

Unlike migraine headache patients, PTTHA patients may carry on with their activities. Most take some form of analgesic, frequently on a daily basis. Without question, PTTHA patients may also have migraine, posttraumatic or otherwise.

The chronic PTTHA patient has headache 15 or more days a month. This is also a diagnostic exercise, because most frequently, nosologically, PTTHA may be one of several headache diagnoses. All these are part of a chronic daily headache differential, which would include analgesic rebound headache, at a minimum.

PTTHA patients frequently have a headache daily or every other day. The headache is typically there when they awaken, and remains until they go to sleep. The intensity of the pain varies, decreasing for several hours after analgesics are taken. The majority of PTTHA patients, if seen early on, have associated pericranial muscle spasm or pain, whereas others do not, yet still complain of pain.

Patients with PTTHA also endure elements of depression and anxiety. There is a "chicken and egg" aspect to this, in terms of which problem comes first. In many cases, central neurochemical changes begin concurrent to the injury and manifest as both pain and affective disturbances (see later).

Nosologically, PTHA is incident to trauma. Some of the problems in making this diagnosis: the patient may not experience direct trauma to the head, but have an acceleration/deceleration injury (whiplash); there may not be significant physical findings on examination (conversely, there may be physical findings that are missed unless a good musculoskeletal examination is done); secondary to the lack of profound physical findings, the patient may be labeled with a psychogenic diagnosis, or worse, with the term malingering.

When one understands the pathophysiology of the problem, specifically PTTHA, it should be understood that the history and physical examination must be done quite specifically, not "one size fits all diagnoses." Knowing what questions to ask and what, on occasion, can be fairly subtle physical findings to look for on examination is obviously important.

PATHOPHYSIOLOGY OF POSTTRAUMATIC TENSION TYPE OF HEADACHE

The typical PTTHA begins postacceleration/deceleration injury, which most frequently occurs during a motor vehicle accident. A slip and fall accident as well as a sports-related injury or more obviously, a postviolent altercation can be the initiating event.

As described previously, the head and the neck, likened to a ball on a chain, is flung forward and backward from acceleration/deceleration forces, frequently without direct trauma to the head, or following direct trauma to the head. However it occurs, the physical forces involved cause the cervical and shoulder musculature, at a minimum, to be suddenly stretched and sustain both microtears and strain/trauma as well as endure a reflex muscle contraction after the sudden stretching. All this being said, it is obviously important to understand the myofascial pain syndrome (MPS).

Pathological changes in the musculoskeletal system may initiate, modulate, or perpetuate PTTHA. Episodic and chronic PTTHA are, at least at first, secondary to a muscle-induced pain syndrome that is typically associated with the previously mentioned MPS.

The central nervous system (CNS) controls muscle tone via systems that influence the gamma efferent neurons in the anterior horn cells of the spinal cord, which act on the alpha motor neurons supplying muscle spindles. The Renshaw cells, apparently via the inhibitory neurotransmitter gamma aminobutyric acid (GABA) influence this synaptic system. There is also supraspinal control from cortical, subcortical, and limbic afferent and efferent systems. Physiological and emotional inputs interact in the maintenance or flux of muscle tone. Adverse influences from both localized or regional myofascial nociception, with or without limbic (affective) stimulation, may produce significant muscle spasm; if prolonged, this spasm becomes tonic with the additional aspects of increased anxiety or a maintained muscle contraction–pain cycle (Diamond & Dalessio, 1980; Speed, 1983). This helps to differentiate acute vs. chronic PTTHA, to a degree.

Tonic or continued posttraumatic muscle contraction may induce hypoxia via compression of small blood vessels. Ischemia, the accumulation of pain-producing metabolites (bradykinin, lactic acid, serotonin, prostoglandins, etc.) may increase and potentiate muscle pain and reactive spasm. These nociception-enhancing or algetic chemicals may stimulate central mechanisms that, through continued stimulation, may induce continued reactive muscle spasm/contraction and maintenance of the myogenic nociceptive cycle (Dorpat & Holmes, 1955; Hong, Kniffki, & Schmidt, 1978; Perl, Markle, & Katz, 1934).

As discussed later, the myofascial aspects of tension-type headache are clinically identical to those of PTTHA; the significant difference in diagnoses is the etiology, posttraumatic or otherwise.

The MPS was, for a long while, ignored in the pathophysiology of headache of any type. Some researchers found a causal relationship between muscle spasm and headache (Martin & Mathews, 1978; Rodbard, 1970; Sakuta, 1990) whereas others have felt that muscle spasm associated with headache is an epiphenomenon, not the etiology of headache (Haynes, Cuevas, & Gannon, 1982; Philips, 1978; Philips & Hunter, 1982; Riley, 1983; Robinson, 1980; Simons, Day, Goodell, & Wolff, 1943), but a reflexive response. Other authors have indicated that muscle activity/spasm or increased tone may be more pronounced in migraine than in tension-type headaches (Bakal & Kaganov, 1977; Cohen, 1978).

Unfortunately, this research, which was obtained via electromyographic (EMG) studies, appears to be problematic, because the various authors evaluated different groups of muscles in different types of patients, many of whom had poorly defined diagnoses (Anderson & Franks, 1981; Bakal & Kaganov, 1977; Martin & Matthews, 1978; Pozniak-Patewicz, 1976). Other authors defined chronic tension-type headache (CTTHA) as an entity with or without associated pericranial muscle disorder. The concept of muscle fatigue was not taken into consideration; metabolically spent muscles that may become relatively flaccid, lose aspects of increased tonus or spasm.

Also of interest is the fact that the vast majority of research deals with tension-type headache, not PTTHA, in spite of identical physical/clinical findings as well as historical findings, all are essentially the same, except for the presence of initiating trauma.

One study found a positive correlation between pericranial muscle tenderness and headache intensity, with the former felt to be a source of nociception (Langemark & Olesen, 1987). Another study (Langmark, Jensen, Jensen, & Olesen, 1989) found that pressure pain thresholds in patients with CTTHA were highly dependent on myofascial factors. This study indicated that the generally lower pain thresholds in the chronic tension-type headache patients suggested a dysmodulation of central nociception. A lower pain threshold in chronic tension-type headache patients, when compared with normal volunteers, was also noted (Borgeat, Hade, Elie, & Larouche, 1984).

Scalp muscle tenderness and sensitivity to pain in both migraine and tension-type headache patients was measured in another study, and the author indicated that the pathophysiology of tension-type headache may involve a diffuse disruption of central pain-modulating mechanism (Drummond, 1987). Lower pain thresholds were also found in patients diagnosed with MPSs, including lower back pain (Yang, Richlin, Brand, Wagner, & Clark, 1985; Malow, Grimm, & Olsen, 1980). It should be noted that the diagnoses in the majority of research papers include tension-type headache (TTHA), but whether they were associated with trauma is not indicated.

Both PTTHA and TTHA patients frequently have a stereotypic posture, with their shoulders raised and their heads flexed forward. This tightly held posture, or muscular splinting, is effective in preventing unconscious head movement that may induce pain. The continued splinting, by maintaining tonic muscle contraction, also works to increase myogenic nociception and perpetuate this cycle.

The pericranial muscles are innervated by sensory fibers in nerves from the second or third cervical roots and in the trigeminal nerve (Langemark & Jensen, 1988). The functions of these muscles contribute to the maintenance of posture and the stabilization of the head, as well as withdrawal and protection of the head. These factors contribute to the myofascial aspects of both TTHA and PTTHA.

Muscle fatigue occurs, both metabolic and neurochemical in nature, and typically follows prolonged or tonic muscle spasm. It may be secondary to "sympatheticopenia" or the depletion of epinephrine and norepinephrine (NEP), the peripheral sympathetic transmitters (Cailliet, 1993). The muscle spindle is directly affected by the sympathetic nervous system via these neurotransmitters, particularly NEP. Prolonged and sustained peripheral sympathetic activity may lead to depletion of NEP at the synaptic receptors. Continued afferent sympathetic input from myogenic nociception, at least in part from buildup though ischemia of nociceptive metabolites, may result in sympatheticopenia (Cailliet, 1993; Jay, 1996). There are also significant sympathetic aspects of myofascial pain, which are not dealt with in this chapter (Jay, 1995).

Tenderness of the cervical, thoracic, and lumbar paravertebral muscles is also positively correlated with pericranial muscle tenderness (Langemark, Olesen,

Poulsen, & Bech, 1988). It has also been noted that the contraction of shoulder and cervical muscles as well as emotional arousal contribute to TTHA (Murphy & Lehrer, 1990). These issues also are significant factors in PTTHA.

Three mechanisms of muscle pain are thought to be relevant to acute, but more often CTTHA, which has the same physiological stigmata of PTTHA, in that myogenic nociception may be induced by (1) low-grade inflammation associated with the release of algetic, or pain-inducing substances, instead of signs of acute inflammation; (2) short- or long-lasting relative ischemia; and (3) tearing of ligaments and tendons secondary to abnormal sustained muscle tension (Langemark & Jensen, 1988). These factors do not take into consideration the possibly more significant initial trauma from acceleration/deceleration injuries, slip and fall accidents, and other reasons for direct or indirect head trauma that induces muscle trauma, primarily or secondarily.

MYOFASCIAL PAIN SYNDROME

Travell and Rinzler identified the contribution of musculoskeletal factors in the etiology of acute and CTTHA (Travell & Rinzler, 1952). They demonstrated that there are consistent patterns of referred pain from trigger points within specific muscle and defined perpetuating factors that convert acute myofascial pain into a chronic pain syndrome (Travell & Simons, 1983).

The MPS is a localized or regional pain problem associated with small zones of hypersensitivity within skeletal muscle called trigger points. With palpation of these points, pain is referred to adjacent or even distant sites. Trigger points in the head, neck, and upper back may elicit headache, as well as tinnitus, vertigo, and lacrimation, all features noted in patients with PTTHA as well as CTTHA (Jay, 1995). (Figures 11.1 to 11.8).

Trigger points may be active, with consistently reproducible pain on palpation, or latent, with no clinically associated complaints of pain but with associated muscle dysfunction. Trigger points may shift between active and latent states. Clinically, continuous myogenic nociception from active trigger points appears to be a prime instigator of the central neurochemical nociceptive dysmodulation found in patients with chronic tension-type headache as well as PTTHA.

Increased stiffness, weakness, and fatigue as well as a decreased range of motion are typically found in muscles in which trigger points are identified. These muscles may be shortened, with increased pain perceived on stretching. Patients may protect these muscles by adapting poor posture with sustained contraction, as noted previously (Fricton, 1990; Langemark & Jensen, 1988). The resulting muscular restrictions may perpetuate existing trigger points and aid in the development of others.

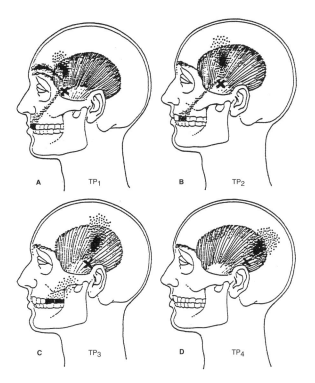

FIGURE 11.1 Referred pain patterns from trigger points (×) in the left temporalis muscle. Dark areas show essential zones; spillover zones are stippled. (A) Anterior "spokes" of pain arising form the anterior fibers — trigger point 1 region. (B) and (C) Middle spokes — trigger point 2 and 3 regions. (D) Posterior supra-auricular spoke — trigger point 4 region. (From Jay, G.W., in *Treating the Headache Patient*, Cady, R.K. and Fox, A.W. (Eds.) Marcel Dekker, New York, 1995, pp. 211–233. With permission.)

Other authors (Fricton, Kroening, Haley, & Siegart, 1985) found that a large percentage of patients suffering from an MPS of the head and neck were found to have significant postural problems, with forward head tilt and rounded shoulders, as well as poor standing and sitting posture, all findings frequently seen in both CTTHA patients as well as those with PTTHA.

An MPS of the head and neck, via myofascial trigger point referred pain, may mimic other conditions, including migraine headache, TMJ dysfunction, sinusitis, and cervical neuralgias, as well as various otological problems including tinnitus, ear pain, and dizziness (Fricton, 1990).

The onset of an acute, single muscle MPS may be associated with trauma, such as an acceleration/deceleration injury, a slip and fall, or even a direct blow. It may also come on insidiously, for example, in patients who work multiple hours at a typewriter or at the computer.

The MPS may show a spontaneous regression to a latent status, with continued muscular dysfunction, but with significant diminution of the initial pain complaints. In other patients, the MPS may "metastasize" and involve associated musculature, becoming regional, or even involving multiple muscular regions.

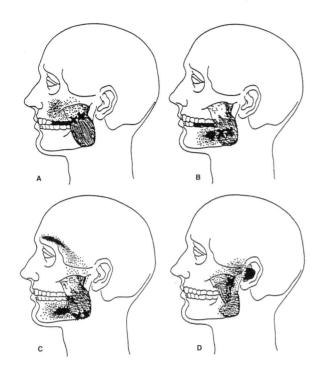

FIGURE 11.2 Each × indicates a trigger point in various parts of the masseter muscle. Dark areas show essential zones; spillover zones are stippled. (A) Superficial layer, upper portion. (B) Superficial layer, mid-belly. (C) Superficial layer, lower portion. (D) Deep layer, upper part — just below the temporomandibular joint. (From Jay, G.W., in *Treating the Headache Patient*, Cady, R.K. and Fox, A.W. (Eds.) Marcel Dekker, New York, 1995, pp. 211–233. With permission.)

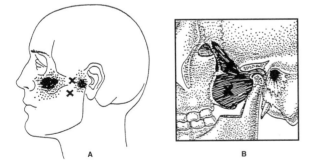

FIGURE 11.3 Referred pain pattern (A) of trigger points (×) in the left lateral pterygoid muscle (B). Note the similarity to temporomandibular disorder. (From Jay, G.W., in *Treating the Headache Patient*, Cady, R.K. and Fox, A.W. (Eds.) Marcel Dekker, New York, 1995, pp. 211–233. With permission.)

OTHER CLINICAL ASPECTS

After the onset of chronic posttraumatic tension type of headache (CPTTHA), emotional/psychological factors including stress, anxiety, and depression may become important in the maintenance or perpetuation of the

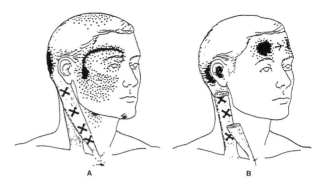

FIGURE 11.4 Referred pain patterns with location of corresponding trigger points (×) in the right sternocleidomastoid muscle. Dark areas show essential zones; spillover zones are stippled. (A) The sternal (superficial) division. (B) The clavicular (deep) dividion. (From Jay, G.W., in *Treating the Headache Patient*, Cady, R.K. and Fox, A.W. (Eds.) Marcel Dekker, New York, 1995, pp. 211–233. With permission.)

headache. This is frequently seen in the patients with the postconcussive syndrome. Patients with MTBI have other significant emotional stigmata that contribute to this headache diathesis.

A major difficulty in the literature is the fact that determinations of depression, anxiety, and other affective components to the PTTHA are found to occur in patients with CPTTHA. Without premorbid psychological analyses, it is very difficult to state with any certainty whether these patients were depressed or anxious prior to the onset of their headache problems. It is therefore possible that the neurochemical changes associated with CPTTHA, such as probable central serotonergic dysfunction, initiate depression as a response to these pain-induced neurochemical changes (see later).

Some authors have noted that the "conversion V" found in the hypochondriasis, depression, and hysteria scales of the Minnesota Multiphasic Personality Inventory (MMPI) is a marker for CTTHA as well as PTTHA, however, similar responses are found in chronic nonheadache pain patients (Jay, Grove, & Grove, 1987; Kudrow, 1986; Martin & Rome, 1967).

ASSOCIATED SLEEP DISORDERS

There appears to be an important relationship between sleep, headache, and muscle–pain syndromes. Central biogenic amines, particularly serotonin and norepinephrine, are important to sleep physiology as well as to the central pain-modulating systems. Both human and animal research indicates that central serotonin metabolism plays a role in pain modulation, affective states, and regulation of non-rapid eye movement REM sleep (Goldenberg, 1990).

A high incidence of sleep difficulties has been found in CTTHA (Matthew, Glaze, & Frost, 1958). Different

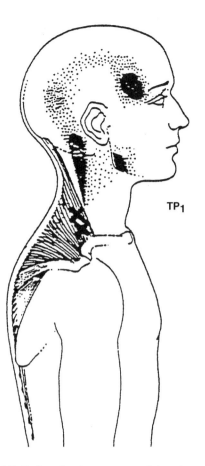

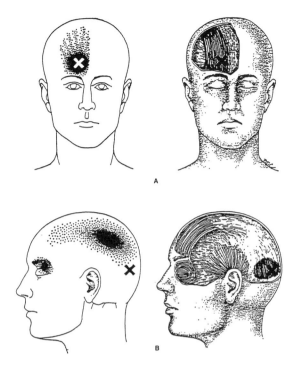

FIGURE 11.5 Referred pain pattern and location of trigger point (×) in the upper trapezius muscle. Dark areas show essential zones; spillover zones are stippled. (From Jay, G.W., in *Treating the Headache Patient*, Cady, R.K. and Fox, A.W. (Eds.) Marcel Dekker, New York, 1995, pp. 211–233. With permission.)

FIGURE 11.6 Pain patterns (shaded areas) referred from trigger points (×) in the occipitofrontalis muscle, commonly associated with unilateral, supraorbital, or ocular headache. 9a) right frontalis belly. (B) Left occipitalis belly. (From Jay, G.W., in *Treating the Headache Patient*, Cady, R.K. and Fox, A.W. (Eds.) Marcel Dekker, New York, 1995, pp. 211–233. With permission.)

sleep disorders appear to be associated with different headache entities. CTTHA and CPTTHA appear to be similar if not identical. Migraine has been found to occur in association with REM sleep, and to have an association with excessive stages 3 and 4 and REM sleep (Shahota & Dexter, 1990). Chronic TTHA has been found to be associated with frequent awakenings and decreased slow wave sleep, as well as an alpha-wave intrusion into stage 4 sleep (Drake, Pakalnis, Andrews, & Bogner, 1990).

Moldofsky et al. (1975) noted a disturbance in stage 4 sleep to be the first laboratory-based abnormality found in fibromyalgia. They induced a similar alpha-non-REM pattern of alpha-wave intrusion in delta (stage 4) sleep in normal subjects by stage 4 sleep deprivation. These subjects developed musculoskeletal pain and affective changes comparable with those seen in fibromyalgia patients. Small doses of serotonergic tricyclic antidepressant medications, which reduced the alpha intrusions into stage 4 sleep, were utilized to ameliorate the symptoms.

Alpha-wave intrusions into deep sleep have also been found in patients with other chronic pain syndromes,

including rheumatoid arthritis (Goldenberg, 1989). The alpha-non-REM disturbance has also been seen in asymptomatic people as well as in those who experience severe emotional stress, such as combat veterans (Goldenberg, 1990). In the latter group, the veterans with this sleep disorder also complained of chronic headaches, diffuse pain, and emotional distress.

Sleep disturbance is also associated with increased pain severity. As noted earlier, chronic headache patients seem to have a higher incidence of sleep abnormalities than do normal, pain-free subjects. Etiologic aspects of chronic headache may be linked to sleep abnormalities as an initiating event or as the result of the underlying pathologically dysmodulated neurochemical factors inducing a sleep disorder.

OTHER POSSIBLE ASSOCIATED FACTORS

There are several possible mechanical etiologies of chronic PTTHA. First is cervical spondylosis, which is defined as a degenerative disease affecting intervertebral disks and apophyseal joints of the cervical spine. Although several authors indicate a possible correlation between cervical spondylosis and TTHA and PTTHA (Diamond

& Dalessio, 1980; Simons, Day, Goodell, & Wolff, 1943; Speed, 1983), others conclude the contrary (Iansek, Heywood, Karnaghan, & Nalla, 1987), suggesting that the basis of existing headache is secondary to muscle contraction and/or central neurochemical dysmodulation. Cervicogenic headache, which is discussed in detail later, is a second suggestive diagnosis.

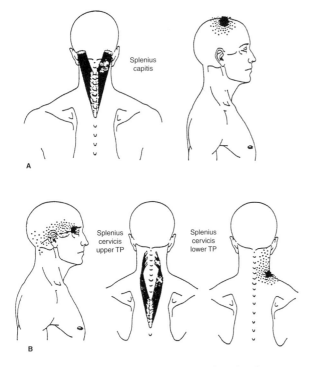

FIGURE 11.7 Trigger points (×) and referred pain patterns (shaded areas) for the right splenius capitis and splenius cervicis muscles. (A) the splenius capitis trigger point, which overlies the occipital traiangle. (B) (Left) The upper splenius cervicis trigger point (TP) refers pain to the orbit. The dashed arrow represents the pain shooting from the inside of the head to the back of the eye. (Right) Another site of pain referral. (From Jay, G.W., in *Treating the Headache Patient*, Cady, R.K. and Fox, A.W. (Eds.) Marcel Dekker, New York, 1995, pp. 211–233. With permission.)

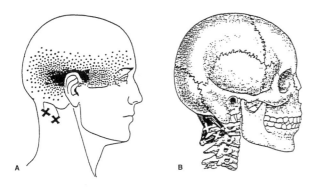

FIGURE 11.8 (A) Referred pain pattern (shaded area) of trigger points (×) in the right suboccipital muscles (B). (From Jay, G.W., in *Treating the Headache Patient*, Cady, R.K. and Fox, A.W. (Eds.) Marcel Dekker, New York, 1995, pp. 211–233. With permission.)

Finally, the dental literature has been most active in reporting a possible correlation between TMJ dysfunction and TTHA, including PTTHA (Forsell, 1985; Mikail & Rosen, 1980). The relationship appears to be dependent mainly on tenderness of the masticatory muscles, which may have other etiologies and induce TMJ dysfunction, when it exists, on a secondary basis (Langemark, Olesen, Poulsen, & Bech, 1988; Magnusson & Carlsson, 1978a, 1978b). Clinically, in the presence of direct trauma to the TMJ, the incidence of anatomic dysfunction is increased.

NEUROPHYSIOLOGICAL CHANGES

Fewer than 50% of PTTHA patients complain of mild associated autonomic symptoms such as lack of appetite, hyperirritability, dizziness, and increased light sensitivity (photophobia) (Olesen, 1988). Notably, some of these symptoms may be secondary to autonomic changes associated with active myofascial trigger points located in the head and neck.

Although muscle contraction and tenderness may be interpreted as primary symptoms of PTTHA, EMG activity and muscle tenderness increase, in some studies more often during migraine than in TTHA (Cohen, 1978; Olesen, 1978; Tfelt-Hansen, Lous, & Olesen, 1981).

In research comparing TTHA with common migraine patients exposed to auditory stimulation, TTHA patients showed a lower heart rate reactivity than migraine patients experience (Ellertsen, Norby, & Sjaastad, 1987). It was shown that TTHA patients exhibited the greatest cardiovascular arousal during headache (Haynes, 1981). In another study (Bakal & Kaganov, 1977), both migraine and TTHA patients decreased pulse velocity. In a psychophysiological comparison of migraine and tension-type headache, it was found that migraine patients are vasodilated and TTHA patients are vasoconstricted both during and between headache episodes (Cohen, 1978). During another study, administration of ergotamine tartrate, a vasoconstrictor, increased the pain of TTHA, whereas amyl nitrate, a vasodilator, yielded only transient pain relief (Tunis & Wolff, 1954).

Greater sympathetic arousal was found in TTHA patients as compared with controls (Murphy & Lehrer, 1990). Another study reported both TTHA and migraine patients demonstrated cardiovascular sympathetic hypofunction, indicated by low basal levels of norepinephrine (NEP), as well as orthostatic hypotension (Mikamo, Takeshima, & Takahashi, 1989). It has been suggested that TTHA patients have phasic hypersympathetic activity, whereas migraineurs do not differ from controls during psychogalvanic response testing (Covelli & Ferrannini, 1987).

Evidence of pupillary sympathetic hypofunction and subtle anisocoria has been found in both TTHA and migraine patients (Takeshima, Takao, & Takahashi, 1987).

It was suggested that this may have reflected a central bioaminergic system dysfunction. Another study suggested a pupillary sympathetic system imbalance in CTTHA patients, who showed asymmetrical mydriasis after tyramine instillation and in the physiological pupillary tests (Shimomura & Takahashi, 1986). Oculomotor dysfunction in the amplitude and number of corrective saccades during testing of TTHA patients has also been found (Rosenhall, Johansson, & Orndahl, 1987).

Drummond (1986) has reported increased photophobia in TTHA patients as compared with controls. He hypothesized that changes in central neurotransmitter modulation may induce increased sensitivity or hyperexcitability-induced photophobia.

Episodic platelet abnormalities with associated serotonergic dysfunction has been well documented in migraine (D'Andrea, Toldedo, Cortelazzo, & Milone, 1982; Hanington, Jones, Amess, & Wachowicz, 1981). Nonepisodic decreased platelet serotonin in CTTHA patients has also been documented (Rolf, Wiele, & Brune, 1981).

Again, it must be reiterated that the single differentiating aspect between CTTHA and CPTTHA patients is the historical factor of some form of trauma. Findings on examination, treatment techniques, and methodology are the same, with the same outcomes in both entities, if done appropriately. The research noted earlier does not differentiate the TTHA patients from those with PTTHA. Clinically and diagnostically there are few, if any, differences.

NEUROANATOMY AND NEUROCHEMISTRY

The central modulation of pain appears to originate in the brain stem and involves at least two systems. The "descending" inhibitory analgesia system appears to regulate the "gating" mechanisms of the spinal cord. This system includes the midbrain periaquaductal gray region, the medial medullary raphe nuclei, and the adjacent reticular formation, as well as dorsal horn neurons in the spinal cord (Basbaum & Fields, 1984). The "ascending" pain modulation system originates in the midbrain and is projected to the thalamus (Andersen & Dafny, 1983). Both systems utilize biogenic amines, opiod peptides and nonopiod peptides (Anderson & Dafny, 1983; Basbaum & Fields, 1984; Raskin, 1988b).

The ascending system appears to show more relevance to headache disorders. This system has projections from the brain stem to the medial thalamus, which include large numbers of serotonergic and opiate receptors. The midbrain dorsal raphe nucleus, a serotonergic nucleus, projects to the medial thalamus and is associated with pain perception. Serotonergic projections to the forebrain are implicated in the regulation of the sleep cycle, mood changes, pain perception, and hypothalamic regulation of hormone release (Raskin, 1988a).

The endogenous opiate system (EOS) within the central nervous system may act as a nociceptive "rheostat" or "algostat," setting pain modulation to a specific level. As this level changes, an individual's pain tolerance may also change. Fluctuations in pain intensity may be interpreted as being secondary to fluctuations in the function of antinociceptive pathways (Fields, 1988; Wall, 1988). Headache, along with other "nonorganic" central pain problems are thought to be the most common expression of impairment of the antinociceptive systems (Sicuteri, 1982).

The EOS modulates the neurovegetative triad of pain, depression, and autonomic disturbances that are found in only two conditions — CTTH (posttraumatic or otherwise) and acute morphine abstinence (Sicuteri, 1982). The EOS is also implicated as primary protagonists in idiopathic headache (Sicuteri, 1982; Sicuteri, Spillantini, & Fanciullacci, 1985). Reduced plasma concentrations of beta-endorphin have been found in idiopathic headache patients, including those with chronic (and posttraumatic) tension-type headache (Facchinetti & Genazzani, 1988; Genazzani et al., 1984; Mosnaim et al., 1989; Nappi et al., 1982).

A primary relationship also exists between the EOS and the biogenic amine systems that are intrinsic to both the pathophysiology of pain modulation and its treatment. Clinical and neuropharmacological information indicates that dysmodulated serotonergic neurotransmission probably generates chronic headache and head pain. It has also been noted that the ordinary, acute or periodic headache may be the "noise" of serotonergic neurotransmission (Raskin, 1988b).

Decreased levels of serotonin (Giacovazzo, Bernoni, Di Sabato, & Martelletti, 1990; Rolf, Wiele, & Brune, 1981; Shimomura & Takahashi, 1990) (with good indications of an impairment of serotonergic metabolism in patients with CTTHA), substance P, an excitatory neuropeptide (Almay et al., 1988; Pernow, 1983) and plasma norepinephrine (Takeshima et al., 1989) are found in CTTHA patients. The latter is also indicative of peripheral sympathetic hypofunction, which may also participate in the etiology or maintenance of central opiod dysfunction (Nappi et al., 1982). Platelet GABA levels are significantly increased in CTTHA patients. This may also act as a balance mechanism to deal with neuronal hyperexcitability and may also be associated with depression (Kowa, Shimomura, & Takahashi, 1992).

The opiod receptor mechanisms appear to be very susceptible to desensitization, or the development of tolerance. In CTTHA patients, opiod receptor hypersensitivity is marked, secondary to the chronically diminished secretion of neurotransmitters. This "empty neuron syndrome" may involve both autonomic and nociceptive afferent systems, as well as latent, subpathological or pathological characteristics with spontaneous manifestations (Sicuteri, Nicolodi, & Fusco, 1988).

The EOS modulates the activity of monoaminergic neurons. A chronic EOS deficiency can provoke transmitter leakage, of both opiod and bioaminergic neurotransmitters, and lead to neuronal exhaustion and "emptying," as well as compensatory effector cell hypersensitivity. The poor release of neurotransmitter along with cell/receptor hypersensitivity appears to be the most important phenomenon of the hypoendorphin syndromes. It has also been concluded that CTTHA (and, clinically, PTTHA) may result from dysmodulation of nociceptive impulses, with associated sensitized receptors (Langemark, Jensen, Jensen, & Olesen, 1989).

CTTHA, including the CPTTHA may be, along with other chronic idiopathic headaches, a "pain disease" directly linked to central dysmodulation of the nociceptive and antinociceptive systems, either latent or pathological in nature. Research indicates that at least two arms of the main endogenous antinociceptive systems, the EOS and the serotonergic systems, are involved in the pathogenesis of CTTHA. Clinical diagnosis and treatment of PTTHA demonstrates identical findings. This problem appears to be progressive, and the dysfunctions may result from neuronal exhaustion secondary to continuous activation of these systems (Facchinetti & Genazzani, 1988; Sicuteri, Nicolodi, & Fusco, 1988).

PATHOPHYSIOLOGY

By looking at the upper portion of Figure 11.9, most of the basics have been mentioned: Continuous peripheral stimulation from myofascial nociceptive input from a MPS, with or without trigger points, may effectively trigger a change in the central pain "rheostat" associated with nociceptive input, secondary to the continuous need for pain-modulating antinociceptive neurotransmitters. The affective aspects of pain — including depression, anxiety, and fear — are secondary to changes in neurotransmitters such as serotonin and NEP, directly influence myofascial nociception, and further reinforce central neurochemical changes.

After 4 to 6 and 12 weeks or so, changes in the CNS central modulation of nociception can occur. Secondary to continuous peripheral nociceptive stimulation, in association with affective changes, the central modulating mechanisms assume a primary instead of a secondary or reactive role in pain perception, as well as antinociception, shifting the initiating aspects of pain perception from the peripheral regions to the CNS.

This intrinsic shift may make innocuous stimuli more aggravating to the pain-modulating systems, the "irritable everything syndrome." The already dysmodulated internal

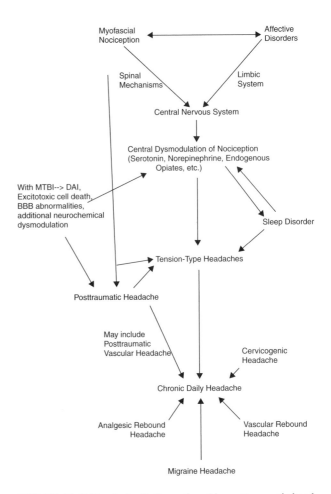

FIGURE 11.9 Headache diatheses found in posttraumatic headache patients.

feedback mechanisms may react until central neurochemical mechanisms dominate, secondary to neurotransmitter exhaustion, and receptor hypersensitivity and abnormal biogenic amine metabolism/exhaustion occurs. These neurochemical changes may induce and/or exacerbate a sleep disorder (serotonergic in nature, from the nucleus raphe magnus); by itself this disorder can perpetuate the central neurochemical dysmodulation, which is primarily responsible for CTTHA.

CPTTHA, whether or not it is associated with a MTBI, has the same pathophysiological mechanisms. In the presence of an MTBI, other significant pathophysiological changes occur that can potentiate or exacerbate the mechanisms described earlier.

In the face of dysmodulated neurochemical systems found in CTTHA, add direct myofascial trauma as an initiating event. The effects of diffuse axonal injury from MTBI, which also affects the neurochemistry of the brain as neuronal degeneration and death occurs, can exacerbate the neurotransmitter pathophysiology. This may also explain the initiation of *de novo* migraine, because brain stem trigeminovascular mechanisms may obviously be affected. Finally, excitotoxic injury that leads to cell death from the overexuberant production of acetylcholine and glutamate also may induce significant neuropathological "holes" in the primary neurotransmitter systems and exacerbate the headache pathophysiology.

Affective changes follow, with the additional problem of possible cognitive changes resulting from MTBI. The latter may make treatment of PTTHA more difficult.

PTTHA is the most common sequelae of an MTBI. It may also be associated with iatrogenic analgesic abuse. Before treatment or even diagnosis of cognitive deficits is attempted, inappropriate medications must be stopped and the headache ameliorated. Most commonly, for this to be done, the patient must be treated using an interdisciplinary headache treatment protocol. Please see *The Headache Handbook: Diagnosis and Treatment* for the details of this protocol (Jay, 1999).

The neurochemical factors leading to the perpetuation of PTTHAs appear to be further and more complexly involved than in CTTHA without associated MTBI. Treatment is most appropriately and cost-effectively performed in an interdisciplinary headache rehabilitation program. Tricyclic medications, GABAnergic medications, and nonsteriodal anti-inflammatory drugs (NSAIDs) are appropriate, whereas narcotics, Dilantin, barbiturates, and early generation benzodiazepines are not.

It is worth noting that patients with MTBI who complain of headache do not appear to perceive their headache pain the same way a headache patient without an MTBI does. These patients know that they have headaches. On a scale of 0 (no pain) to 10 (worst pain imaginable — you could not tolerate it for a moment or two), individual patients, when first seen, give you high numbers (e.g., 7 to 10). These numbers are correlated to pathophysiological myofascial findings, including decreased cervical range of motion, muscle spasm, active trigger points, and more. As they go through treatment, you see the patients regain appropriate physical functioning: normal cervical range of motion, amelioration of spasm and trigger points, etc., with a marked associated improvement of function. The patients' appear brighter; they smile, have fewer if any pain behaviors, and resume doing the physical things they enjoy.

Yet, when asked, they continue to state that their headache pain is at the same level of 7 to 10 as when they were first seen. Whether they are perseverating or are just unable to give an accurate subjective pain level (frontal lobe involvement?), their stated pain levels may not change very much at all. Therefore, you must evaluate them on improvements in function, not by self-reported subjective decrements in headache pain levels.

Evaluation and Treatment of Posttraumatic Tension-Type Headache

The neurological examination of migraine patients is, in the absence of complicated aura, negative. The examination of the cluster headache patient may yield signs of a partial Horner's syndrome. The examination of the patient with PTTHA may yield a great deal of information.

Typically, the neurological examination is negative. The musculoskeletal evaluation gives you the facts. Begin by observing the patient's shoulders. In the vast majority of cases, there is an asymmetry of the acromioclavicular joints, with one being higher than the other secondary to greater ipsilateral muscle spasm. The large muscles should be carefully palpated both for general tenderness and the presence of trigger points. These include the trapezius muscles, the deltoids, the scalenes, the rhomboids, the levaeter scapulae, and all associated muscles (including the pericranial musculature). Pay careful attention to the sternocleidomastoid muscles, particularly in patients complaining of dizziness and tinnitus. Palpate the bioccipital and bitemporal insertions. Look for true pericranial muscle tenderness, as well as masseter pain or tenderness. Observe the patient open their mouth: look for the amount of space between the teeth and see if the jaw deviates.

Perform the passive as well as the active cervical range of motion. Observe the patient's head: is it flexed forward? Is it tilted to one side? What about the shoulders: are they rounded or rolled forward? Evaluate the presence and degree of muscle spasm found in the paravertebral muscles over the entire length of the spine. If the patient is a CTTHA sufferer, posttraumatic or otherwise, or if there is a complaint of upper extremity or hand numbness, perform an axillary stretch maneuver as well as the Adson's maneuver to evaluate for a myogenic thoracic outlet syndrome. These are just the basics.

Until you know what you are dealing with physiologically, it is impossible to determine an appropriate treatment plan. Once you know, and are positive about your diagnosis reached by the history and physical/neurological examination, you can begin to formulate a treatment plan.

Treatment of Acute Posttraumatic Tension-Type Headache

The medical management of acute, or episodic PTTHA is relatively simple. Remember that the older nomenclature titled these headaches as "acute muscle contraction headache" or "tension headache." This form of headache is the most common, as previously indicated, accounting for up to 80% of all nonorganic types of headache. It has been estimated that over 90% of Americans experience an acute TTHA, with or without predisposing trauma, at some time. The majority of these headaches are self-treated with over-the-counter medications and therefore never come to the attention of a physician. This indicates that the statistics are probably low, in that a fairly large number go unnoticed by physicians.

The greatest problem in the treatment of acute PTTHA is the avoidance of the development of analgesic rebound headache, which can easily occur if a patient is overmedicated. This is one step into the development of CPTTHA or daily PTTHA. Physicians should be particularly familiar with the various types of medications that can be utilized for patients complaining of acute PTTHA.

The old adage, that less is better, certainly applies here. Many patients deal with the pain and discomfort by taking two aspirin and relaxing. Exercise is useful, as is a simple glass of wine, on an occasional basis. Any type of relaxation that distracts patients from their headache is useful.

In dealing with the medication management, physicians have a more than ample supply to chose from. It may be therefore tempting to overtreat a minor headache with medications that have a significant risk of dependency.

The simple analgesics are easily chosen by the patient, if not the physician. They are inexpensive and easy to get. They include aspirin and acetaminophen. Like the NSAIDs, aspirin appears to work by inhibiting the synthesis of prostaglandin by blocking the action of cyclooxygenase, an enzyme that enables the conversion of arachidonic acid to prostaglandin to occur. Remember that prostoglandins are synthesized from cellular membrane phospholipids after activation or injury, and sensitize pain receptors.

Aspirin, the prototypical NSAID, has anti-inflammatory and antipyretic properties, along with its pain-relieving properties. The recommended adult dose for treatment of acute PTTHA is 650 mg every 6 h. Taking the aspirin with milk or food may decrease gastric irritation. Aspirin can also double bleeding time for 4 to 7 days after taking 0.65 g. Peak blood levels are found after 45 min. The plasma half-life is 2 to 3 h.

Acetaminophen usage is common. It provides about the same amount of analgesia as aspirin, but does not have the gastrointestinal (GI) side effects. It has been suggested that acetaminophen may work by inhibiting prostaglandin synthesis in the CNS has been suggested. It has much weaker anti-inflammatory activity than that of aspirin. Peak plasma levels occur between 30 and 60 min. The plasma half-life of acetaminophen is 2 to 4 h.

Ibuprofen, an NSAID, is also available over the counter in doses of 200 mg per tablet. It can cause significant GI distress. It has a half-life of 2 to 4 h, with peak plasma levels attained in 1 to 2 h. The adult dosage is 200 to 400 mg every 4 to 6 h, with a maximum of 1200 mg/day.

These medications are frequently sold in combination with other drugs such as caffeine, which exerts no specific analgesic effects, but may potentiate the analgesic effects of aspirin and acetaminophen. There are aspirin–caffeine combination drugs (Anacin), and aspirin, acetaminophen, and caffeine combinations (Excedrin extra-strength, Excedrin migraine, and Vanquish). The recommended dosage is two tablets every 6 h as needed.

The biggest problem is that taking aspirin, acetaminophen, or combination tablets daily or even every other day for a week or more (possibly less) can induce the problem of analgesic rebound headache (which is discussed later).

As with birth control pills, when you ask patients what medications they are taking, they may forget that the birth control pill, aspirin, or acetaminophen are medications; they may forget to tell you, or even be too embarrassed to tell you, because they are taking a large number of pills each day, so you must be certain to ask specifically.

There are a number of NSAIDs that are prescribed. Because of the variability in their efficacy, pharmacokinetics, and side effects, patients may need to be tried on more than one, sequentially, not in combination, to determine the best one for them.

The NSAIDs work, as noted before, by interfering with the action of cyclooxygenase in the synthesis of prostaglandins. GI side effects are common, in up to 15 to 20% of patients; and may include epigastric pain, nausea, heartburn, and abdominal discomfort. A history of GI bleeding or ulcerations should indicate that great caution must be used, if these medications are used at all.

Most Frequently Prescribed Medications

Naproxen sodium (Anaprox) reaches peak plasma levels in 1 to 2 h, and has a mean half-life of 13 h. It can be taken at 275 or 550 mg every 6 to 8 h, with a top dosage of 1375 mg/day. Remember that this NSAID is useful in treating hormonally related migraine.

Ibuprofen (Motrin) is prescribed in dosages of 600 and 800 mg per tablet. The suggested dosage for mild to moderate pain is 400 mg every 4 to 6 h as needed.

Ketoprofen (Orudis) is a cyclooxygenase inhibitor, but also stabilizes lysosomal membranes and possibly antagonizes the actions of bradykinin. Its peak plasma level is reached in 1 to 2 h and has a 2-h plasma half-life. It is now over the counter (12.5-mg tablets), but is best used as 50 to 75 mg capsules. The recommended daily dosage is 150 to 300 mg a day in three or four divided doses. GI side effects are generally mild. Care should be taken when given to a patient with impaired renal function.

Keterolac tromethamine (Toradol) can be given orally or parentally for moderate to severe acute headache pain. Peak plasma levels occur after intramuscular (IM) injection in about 50 min. Its analgesic effect is considered to be roughly equivalent to a 10 mg dose of IM morphine. The typical injectable dose is 60 mg. Because of its potentially significant hepatic/renal side effects, the Food and Drug Administration (FDA) has stated that Toradol should be given orally, after an IM injection of 60 mg, at 10 mg, every 8 h, for a maximum of 5 days.

The cyclooxygenase-2 (COX-2) inhibitors (celecoxib and rofecoxib) are nonsteroidal anti-inflammatory agents that also have analgesic properties without, for most patients, the typical GI problems associated with NSAIDS. They appear to work by inhibiting prostaglandin synthesis, via inhibition of COX-2, which corresponds to its improved GI side effect profile, while not affecting the COX-1 isozyme, responsible for its anti-inflammatory functions. Celecoxib may be taken twice a day, 100 to 200 mg twice a day, whereas rofecoxib is taken once a day, at dosages ranging from 12.5 to 50 mg.

Muscle relaxants are given for acute TTHA by some clinicians. They are probably best utilized during the first 3 weeks of post-injury-related headache. They are useful in patients with significant muscle spasm and pain, which may be seen in acute PTTHA, but are not usually seen with an episodic TTHA. They are used appropriately after the development of muscle spasm after injury such as a slip and fall, motor vehicle accident, work and athletic injuries, or overstretching.

These medications work via the development of a therapeutic plasma level. Their exact mechanism of action is unknown, but they do not directly affect striated muscle, the myoneural junction, or motor nerves. They produce relaxation by depressing the central nerve pathways, possibly through their effects on higher CNS centers, which modifies the central perception of pain without effecting the peripheral pain reflexes or motor activity.

Carisoprodol (Soma) is a CNS depressant that metabolizes into a barbiturate, which makes it both addictive and particularly inappropriate to use for patients with pain from muscle spasm in addition to MTBI. It acts as a sedative and it is thought to depress polysynaptic transmission in interneuronal pools at the supraspinal level in the brain stem reticular formation. It is short lived, with peak plasma levels in 1 to 2 h and a 4 to 6 h half-life. Dosage is 350 mg every 6 to 8 h. It should not be mixed with other CNS depressants. It is also marketed in two other combined forms (with aspirin as Soma Compound and with codeine) for additional analgesic effects.

Chlorzoxazone (Parafon Forte DSC) is a centrally acting muscle relaxant with fewer sedative properties. It inhibits the reflex arcs involved in producing and maintaining muscle spasm at the level of the spinal cord and subcortical areas of the brain. It reaches peak plasma level in 3 to 4 h, and duration of action is 3 to 4 h. It is well tolerated, and side effects are uncommon. Dosage is 500 mg three times a day.

Metaxalone (Skelaxin) is a centrally acting skeletal muscle relaxant that is chemically related to mephenaxalone, a mild tranquilizer. It is thought to induce muscle relaxation via CNS depression. Onset of action is about 1 h, with peak blood levels in 2 h; and duration of action

is 4 to 6 h. The recommended dose is 2400 to 3200 mg a day in divided doses (tablets are 400 mg each). It should be used carefully in patients with impaired liver function, and should not be used at all in patients with significant renal or liver disease as well as a history of drug-induced anemias. Side effects include nausea, vomiting, GI upset, drowsiness, dizziness, headache, nervousness, and irritability as well as rash or pruritis. Jaundice and hemolytic anemia are rare.

Methocarbamol (Robaxin) is a centrally acting skeletal muscle relaxant. It may inhibit nerve transmission in the internuncial neurons of the spinal cord. It has a 30-min onset of action. Peak levels are found in about 2 h, and its duration of action is 4 to 6 h. It comes as 500 and 750 mg tablets. Tablets containing methocarbamol and aspirin (Robaxisal) are also available. The recommended dose of Robaxin is 750 mg three times a day. As with all these medications, it should be taken for 7 to 10 days. It is well tolerated, with initial side effects that resolve over time, including lightheadedness, dizziness, vertigo, headache, rash, GI upset, nasal congestion, fever, blurred vision, urticaria, and mild muscular incoordination. In situations of severe, seemingly intractable muscle spasm, Robaxin may be given intravenously in doses of about a gram every 8 to 12 h.

Orphenedrine citrate (Norflex, Norgesic) is a centrally acting skeletal muscle relaxant with anticholinergic properties thought to work by blocking neuronal circuits, the hyperactivity of which may be implicated in hypertonia and spasm. It is available in injectable and oral formulations. The IM dose of Norflex is 2 mg, whereas the intravenous dosage is 60 mg in aqueous solution. The oral formulation (Norflex) is given in 100 mg tablets — one tablet every 12 h. Norgesic is a combination form, including caffeine and aspirin and should be given 1 or 2 tablets every 6 to 8 h. Norgesic Forte, a stronger combination, is given one half to one tablet every 6 to 8 h. Because of its anticholinergic effects, it should be contraindicated in patients with glaucoma, prostatic enlargement, or bladder outlet obstruction. Its major side effects are also secondary to its anticholinergic properties, and include tachycardia, palpitations, urinary retention, nausea, vomiting, dizziness, constipation, and drowsiness. It may also cause confusion, excitation, hallucinations, and syncope.

Many of these medications are given in combination with other drugs, including barbiturates (butalbatal and meprobamate) and narcotics (codeine, oxycodone, propoxyphene, etc.) This is probably not a good idea, because the barbiturates and narcotics can easily help develop patient dependence.

A good combination utilized by the author is methocarbamol 750 mg three times a day for 10 days in patients with significant spasm, accompanied by ketoprofen, 75 mg every 6 to 8 h as needed, with food as needed. For the acute PTTHA, one tablet of each taken together every 6 to 8 h for two to three doses works very well. Again, narcotic medications should not be used for the patient with acute PTTHA, because the risk of dependence is too great.

Remember, too, that simple acute PTTHA is a problem that the headache specialists are rarely called to see. The patient's family physician or chiropractor most frequently sees this problem.

MEDICATION MANAGEMENT OF CHRONIC POSTTRAUMATIC TENSION-TYPE HEADACHE

The medication treatment of choice is the tricyclic antidepressants (TCAs), or the specific serotonergic reuptake inhibitors (SSRIs).

The TCA medication of choice is amitriptyline, a sedating tricyclic antidepressant. Like all the tricyclics, it works in the synapse to decrease reuptake of serotonin and (depending on the individual medication) NEP. Amitriptyline, unlike the other TCAs, also works to repair the damage in stage 4 sleep architecture. It is the most sedating tricyclic. The typical dosage is between 10 and 50 mg at night. The author has found it rare to need more than 20 or 30 mg at night.

Doxepin is also a very good tricyclic. Anticholinergic side effects such as sedation are reduced (but not by much) when compared with amitriptyline. It does *not* work on the sleep architecture. It is used at the same dosage levels of amitriptyline.

Notice that the tricyclics are not used in their antidepressant dosages, anywhere from 100 to 350 mg a day. Even though the doses are low, their effectiveness in the treatment of chronic PTTHA is there.

The SSRIs include Prozac, Paxil, and Zoloft. These medications are not typically sedating (although for some patients they may be) and with the exclusion of those patients, they are energizing. They should be given in the morning. Prozac and Paxil should start at 10 to 20 mg a day, and they can be increased to 60 to 80 mg. Zoloft should be given at 25 to 50 mg in the morning, up to 150 mg in divided doses. You should divide the doses, giving one when the patient gets up in the morning (around 7:00 A.M.) and one at noon. Explain to the patients that taking these medications later than noon can, in many cases, give them problems sleeping.

You can also safely combine 10 to 40 mg of Prozac or Paxil, or 50 mg of Zoloft with a small dose of amitriptyline or doxepin (10 to 30 mg) at night. Inappropriate dosages of these two forms of medications can, rarely, induce the serotonin syndrome.

There are other excellent antidepressants such as Wellbuterin, Serzone, and Effexor. These should be considered as needed. Do not combine these medications with the monoamine oxidase (MAO) inhibitors. It is just not a great idea.

Another excellent medication is Clonazepam, a fifth generation form of benzodiazepine. It is GABAnergic in effect. It works at the level of the internuncial neurons of the spinal cord to enhance muscle relaxation. It helps, a bit, with anxiolysis. It has a side effect of sedation. In doses of 4 to 12 mg a day, it works as an anticonvulsant. At smaller doses, 0.5 to 1 mg given at night, it is very useful in the treatment of patients with CTTHA. The sedation lasts for a shorter time than the sedation from tricyclics, and this itself is useful.

If the acute use of muscle relaxant medications is not enough to end the problem, Tizanidine is a good choice of medication after the first 3 weeks or so has gone by and the patient is still exhibiting painful neuromuscular spasm. Tizanidine is an alpha-2-noradrenergic agonist (Coward, Davies, Herrling, & Rudeberg, 1984; Sayers, Burki, & Eichenberger, 1980). It has supraspinal effects by inhibiting the facilitation of spinal reflex transmission by the descending noradrenergic pathways, as it decreases firing of the noradrenergic locus ceruleus (Palmeri & Wiesendanger, 1990). It acts presynaptically in the spinal cord inducing a polysynaptic reduction in released excitatory transmitters (Davies, Johnson, & Lovering, 1983). It also decreases hyperexcitability of the muscle without acting on the neuromuscular junctions or muscle fibers (Wagstaff & Bryson, 1997). Short acting, its maximum plasma concentrations are reached within 1 to 2 h (Wagstaff & Bryson, 1997). It has a large first pass metabolism, with a half-life of 2.1 to 4.2 h (Koch, Hirst, & von Wartburg, 1989). Dosages should be slowly increased, starting at 1 to 2 mg at night and slowly increasing to 20 to 24 mg. Maximum dosage is 36 mg in divided dosages, typically found in patients who need an antimyotonic. Interestingly, this medication appears to decrease muscle pain while providing its antimyotonic effects.

Finally, treating patients with CPTTHA with tricyclics, physical therapy, psychotherapy, etc., Will Not Work if the patient is taking daily or four times a week analgesic medications of any type! In the presence of analgesic rebound headache, nothing shows long-lasting effectiveness until the chronic analgesics are stopped.

COST-EFFECTIVE TREATMENT OF CHRONIC POSTTRAUMATIC TENSION-TYPE HEADACHE

Treatment of CPTTHA is best accomplished via an interdisciplinary rehabilitation approach, the main purpose of which is *not* to "teach the patient to live with the headache," but to properly diagnose and effectively ameliorate or stop it.

Drug detoxification is the necessary first step, whether the patient is overutilizing simple, over-the-counter analgesics, narcotics, or barbiturates. Chronic daily analgesics appear to prevent appropriate functioning of the EOS (via negative neurochemical feedback loops) and other associated antinociceptive systems, inducing analgesic rebound headaches, which are secondary problems from the medications that induce headache secondary to purely neurochemical/neurophysiological changes. Vascular rebound headaches from overutilization of vasoconstrictors may also occur and must be stopped before other treatment is applied. Clinically, an effective way to detoxify CTTHA patients is with the repetitive DHE-45 protocol described by Raskin (Raskin, 1988a). Concurrently, prophylactic medications should be started. The use of prophylactic medications, as well as physical therapy and other treatments given while a patient is enduring analgesic rebound headaches, is an ineffectual waste of time and money.

After detoxification, an outpatient interdisciplinary headache rehabilitation program utilizing neuropharmacological therapy (to restore neurochemical homeostasis), physical therapy (Jay, Brunson, & Brunson, 1989), psychotherapy, and stress management (including biofeedback-enhanced neuromuscular reeducation and muscle relaxation) is the most time and cost-effective treatment. Optimal psychotherapy or physical therapy regimes by themselves do not resolve myofascial difficulties or depression if the affective sleep and CNS neurochemical dysmodulation affecting them are not concurrently and appropriately treated. The interdisciplinary treatment paradigm also enables fine-tuning of diagnosis and possible determination of a secondary or "hidden" etiology for a patient's headaches.

Failure to treat the CPTTHA patient with an interdisciplinary, whole-person approach (see Figure 11.9) is responsible for multiple treatment failures as well as monetary waste, because long-term response — headache remediation — is most often not achieved.

POSTTRAUMATIC MIGRAINE

Posttraumatic migraine, which may begin *de novo* — without a previous personal or family history of migraine — may have neurochemical similarities with MTBI, although they are not always found together. These may include increased extracellular potassium and intracellular sodium, calcium, and chloride; serotonergic changes; decreases in magnesium; excessive release of excitatory amino acids; changes in catecholamine and endogenous opiod tonus; decreased glucose utilization; changes in neuropeptides and abnormalities in nitric oxide formation and function (Jay, 1999, pp. 17–32; Packard & Ham, 1997).

Migraine, including posttraumatic migraine, may be associated with a number of neurological symptoms or phenomena. This may include transient global amnesia (TGA), vestibular dysfunction, visual and auditory changes, and possibly increased incidence of seizures (Buchholz & Reich, 1996; Jay, 1999; Leisman, 1990).

The trigeminovascular system is of great importance in migraine (Jay, 1999). In some children who develop posttraumatic neurological deterioration without focal lesions after minor head trauma, there may be an association with an "unstable trigeminovascular reflex," which induces the release of perivascular vasodilatory peptides that can contribute to cerebral hyperemia (Sakas, Whittaker, Whitwall, & Singounas, 1997).

TGA was initially attributed to bilateral temporal lobe seizure phenomena, but more recently attributed to migraine by some (Jay, 1999), and thought to be a totally separate disorder by others, possibly due to a different form of paroxysmal disorder in the brain stem (Schmidtke & Ehmsen, 1998). TGA in the pediatric population is still felt to be secondary to ischemia of the temporo-basal structures induced by an MTBI and associated with a migrainous diathesis (Vohanka & Zouhar, 1988).

Migraine equivalents, transient neurological symptomatology not associated with headache, are not uncommon: proper diagnosis is more difficult to the generalist, as well as the neurologist. In some, possibly more susceptible individuals, minor, even trivial, head trauma can induce a migraine equivalent known as "footballer's migraine" as well as "posttraumatic cortical blindness." This particular migraine equivalent is certainly rare, but transient, total blindness may certainly be cause to call out a total, "full court press" workup (Harrison & Walls, 1990).

Another more common form of transient neurological disturbances associated with migraine are brain stem symptoms including vestibular difficulties such as dizziness, disequilibrium, vertigo, and motion intolerance. These symptoms may also present as a migraine equivalent, between migraine headache episodes or instead of the cephalic pain. Vertigo as a migraine equivalent may occur in about 25% of migraine patients, with the diagnosis made typically by history of familial migraine, because all testing is typically negative. Migraine can also mimic Meniere's disease, with vestibular Meniere's disease being more frequently but still not commonly associated with migraine (Baloh, 1997; Harker & Rassekh, 1988). Also, one should not forget the cervical causes of vertigo and dizziness, secondary to posttraumatic cervical and/or myofascial pathophysiology.

There is also a question of the possible relationship between posttraumatic migraine and posttraumatic benign encephalopathy. The latter, in children, may be associated with cortical blindness, brain stem disturbances, and seizure, lasting from 5 min to 48 h (Vohanka & Zouhar, 1990).

A significant question then arises. Posttraumatic vertigo or dizziness is a very frequent accompaniment to MTBI. It may be secondary to peripheral, labyrinthine disturbance, or brain stem disturbance secondary to trauma; or it may be a migraine equivalent. The importance of this differential is most significant, possibly, when treatment is attempted. Clinically, this would be an important avenue of treatment to explore.

As noted, trauma may induce the first migraine attack in a possibly susceptible patient or increase the frequency and possibly the severity of preexisting migraine. The etiology of these changes may be secondary to neuronal and/or axonal abnormalities secondary to trauma.

Prophylactic treatment is typically with valproic acid, an anticonvulsant medication. The use of beta-blockers such as propranolol may also be useful, but it may have significant side effects. The same is true for verapamil. The use of a triptan for abortive care is well tolerated, if used appropriately.

Cluster headache has also been seen secondary to head trauma, again possibly secondary to neuronal and/or axonal injury. The incidence ranges from 6 to 10% (Duckro, et al., 1992; Packard & Ham, 1997). Many times, this is seen as a primary chronic, instead of episodic form of cluster, or clusterlike headache. Clinically, this is one of the rarest forms of PTHA seen. Treatment, abortive or prophylactic, has been dealt with elsewhere (Jay, 1999).

OTHER ASPECTS OF POSTTRAUMATIC HEADACHE

An initial trauma may involve soft tissue injury to the scalp or face, which may be followed by an entrapment of a sensory nerve, or the sensory nerve may have been cut during the trauma via laceration. The entrapment may also occur during suturing of a laceration. Such entrapments may induce nerve, or neuropathic pain. This is easily differentiated from other primary headache types. The pain is constant, burning, and relegated to the sensory distribution of the affected nerve. Anticonvulsant medications such as carbamazepine are best for the first-line treatment. Neuronton has been used, but it has different, possibly more significant side effects in some patients, particularly in those with a concurrent MTBI. In some cases, neurolytic procedures such as radiofrequency coagulation or cryoablation may be necessary. Both are good procedures, but have varying durations of benefit, most typically between 6 and 12 months.

Without question, injuries to the cervical spine, the superficial and deep structures of the neck (muscles, ligaments, bone, disks, or nerve roots) may occur. Cervical pain from trigger points in spasmed musculature as well as from cervical joint dysfunction may be referred to the head.

If the posttraumatic pain is suboccipital with lancinating, electrical-like shooting pain attributes, secondary to involvement of the occipital neurovascular bundle (the occipital nerve, artery, and vein), or secondary to prolonged muscle spasm/contraction or excessive vascular dilatation impinging on the greater occipital nerve of Arnold, this pain is known as occipital neuralgia. It is always in the C2 distribution at the back of the head. Indomethacin may be an effective treatment for this problem. Steroidal injections may also be utilized. Neuroablative procedures should be performed only when all other treatment has failed.

Preexisting arthritis or discogenic disease may also be exacerbated by the initial trauma. An appropriate neurological evaluation helps with these entities.

The dysautonomic cephalalgia of Vijayan (1977) is associated with injury to the anterior aspect of the carotid sheath. The headache is severe and unilateral, in the frontotemporal area and associated with ipsilateral hyperhidrosis and dilatation of the ipsilateral pupil. The role of sympathetic nervous system dysfunction, although it may remain controversial, is shown in many studies, as noted earlier. Also, the signs and symptoms are, of course, similar to cluster headache.

CERVICOGENIC HEADACHE

Just as the community of headache specialty physicians were rather hesitant to accept the fact that the musculature had any role in TTHA, posttraumatic or otherwise, the idea that headache can arise from the structures of the neck still has many detractors.

Dwyer, Aprill, and Bogduk (1990) utilized fluoroscopic control to stimulate joints at segments C2–C3 to C6–C7 by distending the joint capsule with injections of contrast medium. They were able to show that each joint produced a clinically distinguishable, characteristic pattern of referred pain that enabled the construction of pain charts to be used in determining the segmental location of symptomatic joints in patients presenting with cervical zygapophyseal pain.

The diagnostic criteria for cervicogenic headache (CGHA) have been noted by several authors to differ a bit. Bogduk, et al. (1985) defined CGHA as referred pain perceived in any region of the head that was referred by a primary nociceptive source in the musculoskeletal tissues innervated by cervical nerves. Clinical features included pain that was not lancinating, and was dull or aching but could be throbbing — located in the occipital, parietal, temporal, frontal, or orbital regions, unilaterally or bilaterally. There was some indication of cervical spine abnormality such as neck pain, tenderness, impaired cervical motion, aggravation of the headache by neck movements, or history of cervical trauma.

Bogduk's diagnostic criteria included (Bogduk, et al., 1985) identification by clinical examination or by imaging of a cervical source of the pain that is found by valid antecedent studies to be reliably associated with the head pain, or complete relief of the head pain that is seen after controlled local anesthetic blockade of one or more cervical nerves or structures innervated by cervical nerves.

Sjaastad, Fredriksen, and Pfaffenrath (1990) also weighed in with specific criteria. They noted that cervicogenic headaches were one sided, but could also be bilateral "unilaterally on two sides." The duration of a headache or exacerbation ranged from several hours to several weeks. Initially the headache may be episodic, but can later chronically fluctuate. Symptoms and signs were referable to the neck, and included decreased range of cervical motion and mechanical precipitation of attacks, with autonomic symptoms such as nausea and photophobia not marked, if at all present. A positive response to appropriate anesthetic blockade is considered essential.

Sjaastad, Fredriksen, and Pfaffenrath (1990) noted several major criteria:

1. Symptoms and signs of cervical involvement
   a. Provocation of an irradiating head pain similar to the spontaneously occurring one
      i. By neck movement and/or sustained awkward head positioning
      ii. By external pressure over the upper neck or head on the side ipsilateral to the pain
   b. Restriction of cervical range of motion
   c. Ipsilateral neck, shoulder, or arm pain of a vague, nonradicular nature, or, on occasion, sharp arm pain in a radicular region
   (Symptoms and signs 1a to 1c are listed in "order of importance." One or more of these must be present for the term cervicogenic headache to be used. Point 1a is itself sufficient criteria, but 1b and 1c are not. Point 2 is a necessary additional point.)
2. Confirmation by diagnostic anesthetic blocks — necessary point
3. Unilateral pain not shifting from side to side
4. Pain characteristics
   a. Nonthrobbing pain, usually beginning in the neck
   b. Episodes of varying duration
   c. Fluctuating, continuous pain
5. Other characteristics of some importance
   a. Marginal or no effect from treatment with indomethacin
   b. Marginal or no effect from treatment with triptans or ergots
   c. Female preponderance
   d. History of head or neck trauma
   (None of the single points under 4 or 5 are essential.)
6. Other descriptions of less importance (various headache-related phenomena that are rarely present, and of only mild to moderate severity when present)
   a. Nausea
   b. Photo- and phonophobia

c. Dizziness
d. Blurred vision ipsilateral to the pain
e. Difficulty with swallowing
f. Fluid around the eye on the same side as the pain

The anatomic basis of CGHA is thought to be secondary to convergence in the trigeminocervical nucleus between nociceptive afferents from the field of the trigeminal nerve and the receptive fields of the first three cervical nerves. Headache appears to be secondary to structural problems in regions innervated by C1 to C3. These regions include the muscles, joints, and ligaments of the upper three cervical segments, as well as the dura mater of the spinal cord and the posterior cranial fossa and the vertebral artery (Bogduk, 1992).

Other anatomic causation has been identified and includes (Blume, 1997):

1. Disrupted and/or ruptured cervical disks with irritation of the sympathetic sinu-vertebral nerves (in the disk) and nerve roots by mechanical and chemical means at single or multiple levels
2. Irritation of the articular branches to the cervical zygapophyseal joints derived from the medial branches of the cervical dorsal rami
3. Irritation of the peripheral branches and unmyelinated nerve structures to the muscle attachments at the spinous process of C2 supplied by the C2 and C3 nerve roots, including the rectus capitis posterior, major obliquus capitis inferior major, semispinalis cervicis multifidus, semispinalis capitis major and rectus capitis posterior minor and interspinal, muscles at C1 to C2 and C2 to C3
4. Pain from the end fibers of the greater tertiary occipital and sympathetic nerve structures with its C fibers including the periosteum and suboccipital musculature (semispinalis capitis, rectus capitis posterior minor and major, trapezius, and occipitalis)

The treatment of CGHA begins with diagnostic anesthetic blocks that are typically mixed with long-acting steroids such as hydrocortisone. This should temporarily relieve the CGHA for hours to days. If pain relief lasts for weeks to months, blocks should be repeated.

Once a specific targeted joint or disk is identified, the latter with discography if needed, a number of procedures have been utilized for treatment of CGHA. These include

1. Neurolysis of the C2 nerve root via decompressive surgery (Poletti, 1983) as well as partial

denervation of the suboccipital and paraspinal musculature (Pikus & Phillips, 1995)

2. Radiofrequency lesions to the muscle attachments of the spinous process at C2 (Blume, Kakolewski, Richardson, & Rojas, 1982; Rogel, 1995)

3. Radiofrequency neurotomy of the sinuvertebral nerves to the upper cervical disk, as well as to the outer layer of the C3 or C4 nerve root (Sluijter, 1990)

4. Radiofrequency denaturation of the occipital nerve (Blume, 1976; Blume, Kakolewski, Richardson, & Rojas, 1981; Blume & Ungar-Sargon, 1986)

5. Radiofrequency denaturation of the C2 medial rami (Rogal, 1986)

6. Cervical discectomy and fusion

7. C2 ganglionectomy (Jansen & Spoerri, 1985)

The latter procedure is not often performed, although there remain proponents of radiofrequency lesioning vs. the "old" cervical discectomy and fusion.

It is imperative to differentiate CGHA from both migraine headache and PTTHA, because the treatments are completely different. Unfortunately, the literature in general argues the question of cervicogenic headache, although not the idea that headache may be associated with cervical pathology. It should be noted that the International Association for the Study of Pain (IASP) has recognized cervicogenic headache as a pain syndrome (Zwart, 1997). This criteria uses neck mobility as the major indicator of this diagnosis, but both TTHA and migraine have associated decrements in cervical mobility.

The different criteria for the diagnosis of CGHA make other previously recognized primary headache sufferers fall into a diagnostic hole. There appears to be too much overlap in the varying diagnoses. Likewise, patients with the diagnosis of CGHA may also fall into other diagnostic categories, or even multiple diagnostic categories (Leone, 1998; Pfaffenrath & Kaube, 1990; Treleaven, Jull, & Atkinson, 1994).

Not to be forgotten is the fact that the diagnosis specifically may follow an acceleration/deceleration injury or other cervical trauma (Obelieniene, et al., 1998; Treleaven, Jull, & Atkinson, 1994). This makes it imperative to consider the diagnosis of CGHA in patients with PTHA who do not show improvement following appropriate treatment for other diagnosed headache diatheses. On the other hand, clinically, CGHA appears to be found in less than 3 to 5% of the PTTHA population. If a PTHA patient also has an MTBI, the level of difficulty in making the diagnosis and treating that patient increases dramatically.

Psychological factors are there — the neurochemical aspects of depression and anxiety, for instance, are well known. In the presence of an MTBI they become more difficult to tease out and deal with, because the patients may be dealing with pain as well as changes in cognition and behavior, including frontal lobe difficulties such as increased irritability and labile emotionality.

CONCLUSION

Other major problems facing patients and their treating physician(s) are the questions of medico-legal disability secondary to the PTHA syndrome, with or without the question of MTBI. Patients whose injuries involved a skull fracture, subdural hematoma, or severe lacerations and whose gray matter is leaking out of their ears *may* not have a problem in regard to disability. Unfortunately for patients and their physicians, insurance problems do exist, beginning with getting approval to treat a PTHA syndrome.

Some insurance companies deny that there is such a thing as an MTBI, or PTHAs. They have a number of paid consultants to assure the legal system that this is so. They try to prevent clinicians from even getting involved with treating these patients by refusing to pay them for treatment. *It does not matter* how devastating a patient's symptoms are; the patient still faces a difficult and totally unjustified legal battle just to get treatment approved, never minding the question of disability compensation.

It is interesting that the vast majority of patients with PTHAs, particularly those with headaches as part of a postconcussion syndrome, present the same way. Maybe they all spoke together on the Internet and planned it out. They are for real and are expressing the same symptomatology from the same causation (head trauma or acceleration/deceleration injuries). This is just like patients with chicken pox who initially present, clinically, in the same way.

Then there is the M word — malingering. This is associated with the idea that settlement of litigation is all that is needed to put a stop to the PTHA syndrome. This is also a favorite theme of the insurance companies. True malingering is almost as rare as hens' teeth. There are published studies that demonstrate that legal settlement has nothing to do with the patients' symptoms ending or encouraging them to return to work (Cicerone, 1992; Elkind, 1989; Evans, 1992; Merskey & Woodford, 1972).

CPTTHAs, with or without the other aspects of the post-concussion syndrome, are extremely common after head trauma and acceleration/deceleration injury. These patients are very consistent in their presentations in their descriptions of their symptoms and sequelae. This consistency is strong evidence that their problems are organic in nature and produced by the trauma.

Most patients with PTHAs have their headaches resolve if they are given appropriate medical treatment.

About 15 to 20% have prolonged difficulties. Correct diagnosis and treatment in the majority of cases should decrease this percentage.

REFERENCES

Almay, B.G.L., Johansson, F., von Knorring, L., et al. (1988). Substance P in CSF of patients with chronic pain syndromes. *Pain, 33,* 3.

Andersen, E., & Dafny, N. (1983). An ascending serotonergic pain modulation pathway from the dorsal raphe nucleus to the parafascicularis nucleus of the thalamus. *Brain Research, 269,* 57.

Anderson, C.D., & Franks, R.D. (1981). Migraine and tension headache: Is there a physiological difference? *Headache, 21,* 63.

Bakal, D.A., & Kaganov, J.A. (1977). Muscle contraction and migraine headache: Psychophysiologic comparison. *Headache, 17,* 208.

Baloh, R.W. (1997). Neurotology of migraine. *Headache, 37,* 615–621.

Basbaum, A.I., & Fields, H.L. (1984). Endogenous pain control systems: Brainstem spinal pathways and endorphin circuitry. *Annual Review of Neuroscience, 7,* 309.

Blume, H.G. (1976). Radiofrequency denaturation in occipital pain: A new approach in 114 cases. *Advanced Brain Research Therapy, 1,* 691–698.

Blume, H.G. (1997). Diagnosis and treatment modalities of cervicogenic headaches. *Head and Neck Pain, Newsletter of the Cervicogenic Headache International Study Group, 4,* 1–2.

Blume, H.G., Kakolewski, J.W., Richardson, R.R., & Rojas, C.H. (1981). Selective percutaneous radiofrequency thermodenervation of pain fibers in the treatment of occipital neuralgia: Results in 450 cases. *Journal of Neurologic Orthopedic Surgery, 2,* 261–268.

Blume, H.G., Kakolewski, J.W., Richardson, R.R., & Rojas, C.H. (1982). Radiofrequency denaturation in occipital pain: results in 450 cases. *Applied Neurophysiology, 45,* 543–548.

Blume, H.G., & Ungar-Sargon, J. (1986). Neurosurgical treatment of persistent occipital myalgia-neuralgia syndrome. *Journal of Craniomandibular Practice, 4,* 65–73.

Bogduk, N., Corrigan, B., Kelly, R., et al. (1985). Cervical headache. *Medical Journal of Australia, 143,* 202–207.

Bogduk, N. (1992). The anatomical basis for cervicogenic headache. *Journal of Manipulative Physiology and Therapy, 15,* 67–70.

Borgeat, F., Hade, B., Elie, R., & Larouche, L.M. (1984). Effects of voluntary muscle tension increases in tension headache. *Headache, 24,* 199.

Buchholz, D.W., & Reich, S.G. (1996). The menagerie of migraine. *Seminars in Neurology, 16,* 83–93.

Cailliet, R. (1993). *Pain: Mechanisms and management* (p. 83). Philadelphia: F. A. Davis.

Cicerone, K.D. (1992). Psychological management of post-concussive disorders. *Physical Medicine and Rehabilitation: State of the Art Review, 6,* 129–141.

Cohen, M.J. (1978). Psychological studies of headache: Is there a similarity between migraine and muscle contraction headaches? *Headache, 18,* 189.

Covelli, V., & Ferrannini, E. (1987). Neurophysiologic findings in headache patients. Psychogalvanic reflex investigation in migraineurs and tension headache patients. *Acta Neurologica, 9,* 354.

Coward, D.M., Davies, J., Herrling, P., & Rudeberg, C. (1984). *Pharmacological properties of tizanidine (DS 103-282)* (pp. 61–71). New York: Springer-Verlag.

D'Andrea, G., Toledo, M., Cortelazzo, S., & Milone, F. F. (1982). Platelet activity in migraine. *Headache, 22,* 207.

Davies, J., Johnson, S.E., & Lovering, R. (1983). Inhibition by DS 103-282 of D-(^{3}H)aspartate release from spinal cord slices. *British Journal of Pharmacology, 78,* 2P.

Denny-Brown, D., & Russell, W. R. (1941). Experimental cerebral concussion. *Brain, 64,* 93.

Diamond, S., & Dalessio, D.J. (1980). *The practicing physician's approach to headache* (3rd ed.). Baltimore: Williams & Wilkins.

Dorpat, T.L., & Holmes, T.H. (1955). Mechanisms of skeletal muscle pain and fatigue. *Archives of Neurologic Psychiatry, 74,* 628.

Drake, M.E., Pakalnis, A., Andrews, J.M., & Bogner, J.F. (1990). Nocturnal sleep recording with cassette EEG in chronic headaches. *Headache, 30,* 600.

Drummond, P.D. (1986). A quantitative assessment of photophobia in migraine and tension headache. *Headache, 26,* 465.

Drummond, P.D. (1987). Scalp tenderness and sensitivity to pain in migraine and tension headache. *Headache, 27,* 45.

Duckro, P.N., Greenberg, M., Schultz, K.T., et al. (1992). Clinical features of chronic post-traumatic headache. *Headache Quarterly, 3,* 295–308.

Dwyer, A., Aprill, C., & Bogduk, N. (1990). Cervical zygapophyseal joint pain patterns. I: A study in normal volunteers. *Spine, 15,* 453–457.

Elkind, A.H. (1989). Headache and facial pain associated with head injury. *Otolaryngology Clinics of North America, 22,* 1251–1271.

Ellertsen, B., Norby, H., & Sjaastad, O. (1987). Psychophysiological response patterns in tension headache: Effects of tricyclic antidepressants. *Cephalalgia, 7,* 55.

Evans, R.W. (1992). The postconcussion syndrome and the sequelae of mild head injury. *Neurology Clinic, 10,* 815–847.

Facchinetti, F., & Genazzani, A.R. (1988). Opiods in cerebrospinal fluid and blood of headache sufferers. In J. Olesen & L. Edvinsson (Eds.), *Basic mechanisms of headache.* (p. 261). Amsterdam: Elsevier Science.

Fields, H.L. (1988). Sources of variability in the sensation of pain. *Pain, 33,* 195.

Forsell, H. (1985). Mandibular dysfunction and headache. *Proceedings of the Finnish Dental Society, 81*(Suppl. 2), 591.

Fricton, J.R., Kroening, R., Haley, D., & Siegart, R. (1985). Myofascial pain syndrome of the head and neck: A review of clinical characteristics of 164 patients. *Oral Surgery, 60*, 615.

Fricton, J.R. (1990). Myofascial pain syndrome. In J. R. Fricton & E. Awad (Eds.), *Advances in pain research and therapy* (Vol. 17, p. 107). New York: Raven Press.

Genazzani, A.R., Nappi, G., Gacchinetti, F., et al. (1984). Progressive impairment of CSF B-EP levels in migraine sufferers. *Pain, 18*, 127.

Giacovazzo, M., Bernoni, R.M., Di Sabato, F., & Martelletti, P. (1990). Impairment of 5HT binding to lymphocytes and monocytes from tension-type headache patients. *Headache, 30*, 20.

Goldenberg, D.L. (1989). Diagnostic and therapeutic challenges of fibromyalgia. *Hospital Practice, 9*, 39.

Goldenberg, D.L. (1990). Fibromyalgia and chronic fatigue syndrome: Are they the same? *Journal of Musculoskeletal Medicine, 7*, 19.

Hanington, E., Jones, R.J., Amess, J.A.L., & Wachowicz, B. (1981). Migraine: A platelet disorder. *Lancet, ii*, 720.

Harker, L.A., & Rassekh, C. (1988). Migraine equivalent as a cause of episodic vertigo. *Laryngoscope, 98*, 160–164.

Harrison, D.W., & Walls, R.M. (1990). Blindness following minor head trauma in children: A report of two cases with a review of the literature. *Journal of Emergency Medicine, 8*, 21–24.

Haynes, S.N., Cuevas, J., & Gannon, L.R. (1982). The psychophysiological etiology of muscle-contraction headache. *Headache, 22*, 122.

Haynes, S.N. (1981). Muscle contraction headache — Psychophysiological perspective. In S.N. Haynes & L.R. Gannon (Eds.), *Psychosomatic disorders: A psychophysiologyical approach to etiology and treatment*. New York, Praeger Press.

Headache Classification Committee of the International Headache Society. (1988). Classification and diagnostic criteria for headache disorders, cranial neuralgias and facial pain. *Cephalalgia, 8*(7).

Hong, S., Kniffki, K., & Schmidt, R. (1978). Pain abstracts. *Second World Congress on Pain, 1*, 58.

Iansek, R., Heywood, J., Karnaghan, J., & Nalla, J.I. (1987). Cervical spondylosis and headaches. *Clinical Experimental Neurology, 23e*, 175.

Jansen, J., & Spoerri, O. (1985). Atypical retro-orbital pain and headache due to compression of upper cervical roots. In V. Pfaffenrath, P.O. Lundberg, & O. Sjaastad (Eds.), *Updating in headache* (pp. 14–16). Berlin: Springer-Verlag, 1985.

Jay, G.W., Brunson, J., & Branson, S. J. (1989). The effectiveness of physical therapy in the treatment of chronic daily headaches. *Headache, 29*, 156.

Jay, G.W., Grove, R.N., & Grove, K.S. (1987). Differentiation of chronic headache from non-headache pain patients using the Millon Clinical Multiaxial Inventory (MCMI). *Headache, 27*, 124.

Jay, G.W. (1996). The autonomic nervous system: Anatomy and pharmacology. In P. Raj (Ed.), *Pain medicine — A comprehensive review* (pp. 461–465). St. Louis: Mosby.

Jay, G.W. (1995). Chronic daily headache and myofascial pain syndromes: Pathophysiology and treatment. In R.K. Cady & A.W. Fox (Eds.), *Treating the headache patient* (pp. 211–233). New York, Marcel Dekker.

Jay, G.W. (1995). Sympathetic aspects of myofascial pain. *Pain Digest, 5*, 192–194.

Jay, G.W. (1999). *The headache handbook: Diagnosis and treatment.* Boca Raton, FL: CRC Press.

Jay, G.W. (2000). *Minor traumatic brain injury handbook: Diagnosis and treatment.* Boca Raton, FL: CRC Press.

Kay, T., Harrington, D.E., et al. (1993). Definition of mild traumatic brain injury. *Journal of Head Trauma Rehabilitation, 8*(3), 86.

Keidel, M., & Diener, H.C. (1997). Post-traumatic headache. *Nervenarzt, 68*, 769–777.

Koch, P., Hirst, D.R., & von Wartburg, B.R. (1989). Biological fate of sirdalud in animals and man. *Xenobiotica, 19*, 1255–1265.

Kojadinovic, Z., Momcilovic, A., Popovic, L., et al. (1998). Brain concussion—A minor craniocerebral injury. *Med. Pregl., 51*, 165–168.

Kowa, H., Shimomura, T., & Takahashi, K. (1992). Platelet gamma-amino butyric acid levels in migraine and tension-type headache. *Headache, 32*, 229.

Kudrow, L. (1986). Muscle contraction headaches. In F.C. Rose (Ed.), *Handbook of clinical neurology* (Vol. 48, pp. 343). Amsterdam: Elsevier Science.

Langemark, M., & Jensen, K. (1988). Myofascial mechanisms of pain. In J. Olesen & L. Edvinsson (Eds.), *Basic mechanisms of headache* (p. 321). Amsterdam: Elsevier Science.

Langemark. M., Jensen, K., Jensen, T.S., & Olesen, J. (1989). Pressure pain thresholds and thermal nociceptive thresholds in chronic tension-type headache. *Pain, 38*, 203

Langemark, M., & Olesen, J. (1987). Pericranial tenderness in tension headache. A blind controlled study. *Cephalalgia, 7*, 249.

Langemark, M., Olesen, J., Poulsen, D.P., & Bech, P. (1988). Clinical characterization of patients with chronic tension headache. *Headache, 28*, 590.

Leisman, G. (1990). Lateralized effects of migraine and ANS seizures after closed head injury. *International Journal of Neuroscience, 54*, 63–82.

Leone, M., D'Amico, D., Grazzi, L., et al. (1998). Cervicogenic headache: A critical review of the current diagnostic criteria. *Pain, 78*, 1–5.

Magnusson, T., & Carlsson, G.E. (1978a). Comparison between two groups of patients in respect to headache and mandibular dysfunction. *Swedish Dental Journal, 2*, 85.

Magnusson, T., & Carlsson, G.E. (1978b). Recurrent headaches in relation to temporomandibular joint pain-dysfunction. *Acta Odontologia Scandinavia, 36*, 333.

Malow, R.M., Grimm, L., & Olsen, R.E. (1980). Differences in pain perception between myofascial pain dysfunction and normal subjects: A signal detection analysis. *Journal of Psychosomatic Research, 24*, 303.

Martin, M.J., & Rome, H.P. (1967). Muscle contraction headache: Therapeutic aspects. *Research in Clinical Studies of Headache, 1*, 205.

Martin, P.R., & Mathews, A.M. (1978). Tension headaches: Psychophysiological investigation and treatment. *Journal of Psychosomatic Research, 22,* 389.

Mathew, N.T., Glaze, D., & Frost, J. (1985). Sleep apnea and other sleep abnormalities in primary headache disorders. In C. Rose (Ed.), *Migraine. Proceedings of the 5th International Migraine Symposium, 1984* (p. 40). London: Basel, Karger.

Merskey, H., & Woodford, J.M. (1972). Psychiatric sequelae after minor head injury. *Brain, 95,* 521–528.

Mikail, M., & Rosen, H. (1980). History and etiology of myofascial pain-dysfunction syndrome. *Journal of Prosthetic Dentistry, 44,* 438.

Mikamo, K., Takeshima, T., & Takahashi, K. (1989). Cardiovascular sympathetic hypofunction in muscle contraction headache and migraine. *Headache, 29,* 86.

Moldofsky, H., Scariabrick, P., England, R., et. al. (1975). Musculoskeletal symptoms and non-REM sleep disturbances in patients with fibrositis syndrome and healthy subjects. *Psychosomatic Medicine, 37,* 341.

Mosnaim, A.D., Diamond, S., Wolf, M.E., et al. (1989). Endogenous opiod-like peptides in headache: An overview. *Headache, 29,* 368.

Muller, G.E. (1974). Atypical early posttraumatic syndromes. *Acta Neurologica Belgica, 74,* 163–181.

Murphy, A.I., & Lehrer, P.M. (1990). Headache versus nonheadache state: A study of electrophysiological and affective changes during muscle contraction headache. *Behavioral Medicine, 16,* 23.

Nappi, G., Gacchinetti, G., Legnante, G., et al. (1982). *Impairment of the central and peripheral opiod system in headache.* Paper presented at the Fourth International Migraine Trust Symposium, London.

Obelieniene, D., Bovim, G., Schrader, H., et al. (1998). Headache after whiplash: A historical cohort study outside the medico-legal context. *Cephalalgia, 18,* 559–564.

Olesen, J. (1978). Some clinical features of the acute migraine attack. An analysis of 750 patients. *Headache, 18,* 268.

Olesen, J. (1988). Clinical characterization of tension headache. In J. Olesen & L. Edvinsson (Eds.), *Basic mechanisms of headache* (p. 9). Amsterdam: Elsevier Science.

Packard, R.C., & Ham, L.P. (1997). Pathogenesis of posttraumatic headaches and migraine: A common headache pathway? *Headache, 37,* 142–152.

Palmeri, A., & Wiesendanger, M. (1990). Concomitant depression of locus coeruleus neurons and of flexor reflexes by an alpha$_2$-adrenergic agonist in rats: A possible mechanism for an alpha$_2$-mediated muscle relaxation. *Neuroscience, 34,* 177–187.

Perl, S., Markle, P., & Katz, L. N. (1934). Factors involved in the production of skeletal muscle pain. *Archives of Internal Medicine, 53,* 814.

Pernow, B. (1983). Substance P. *Pharmacology Review, 35,* 85.

Pfaffenrath, V., & Kaube, H. (1990). Diagnostics of cervicogenic headache. *Functional Neurology, 5,* 159–164.

Philips, C. (1978). Tension headache: Theoretical problems. *Behavior Research Therapy, 16,* 249.

Philips, C., & Hunter, M.S. (1982). A psychophysiological investigation of tension headache. *Headache, 22,* 173.

Pikus, H., & Phillips, J. (1995). Characteristics of patients successfully treated for cervicogenic headache by surgical decompression of the second cervical nerve root. *Headache, 35,* 621–629.

Poletti, C.E. (1983). Proposed operation for occipital neuralgia: C2 and C3 root decompression. *Neurosurgery, 12,* 221–224.

Pozniak-Patewicz, E. (1976). Cephalgic spasm of head and neck muscles. *Headache, 15,* 261.

Raskin, N.H. (1988a). *Headache* (2nd ed.). New York: Churchill Livingstone.

Raskin, N.H. (1988b). On the origin of head pain. *Headache, 28,* 254.

Riley, T.L. (1983). Muscle-contraction headache. *Neurology Clinic, 1,* 489.

Robinson, C.A. (1980). Cervical spondylosis and muscle contraction headaches. In D.J. Dalessio (Ed.), *Wolff's headache and other head pain* (4th ed., p. 362). New York: Oxford University Press.

Rodbard, S. (1970). Pain associated with muscle contraction. *Headache, 10,* 105.

Rogal, O.J. (1986). Successful treatment for head, facial and neck pain. *The TMJ Dental Trauma Center, 1,* 3–10.

Rogal, O.J. (1995, September). *Rhizotomy procedures about the face and neck for headaches.* Paper presented at the North American Cervicogenic Headache Conference, Toronto.

Rolf, L.H., Wiele, G., & Brune, G.G. (1981). 5-Hydroxytryptamine in platelets of patients with muscle contraction headache. *Headache, 21,* 10.

Rosenhall, U., Johansson, G., & Orndahl, G. (1987). Eye motility dysfunction in patients with chronic muscular pain and dysesthesia. *Scandanavian Journal of Rehabilitative Medicine, 19,* 139.

Sakas, D.E., Whittaker, K.W., Whitwell, H.L., & Singounas, E.G. (1997). Syndromes of posttraumatic neurological deterioration in children with no focal lesions revealed by cerebral imaging: evidence of a trigeminovascular pathophysiology. *Neurosurgery, 41,* 661–667.

Sakuta, M. (1990). Significance of flexed posture and neck instability as a cause of chronic muscle contraction headache. *Rinsho Shinkeigato, 30,* 254.

Sayers, A.C., Burki, H.R., & Eichenberger, E. (1980). The pharmacology of 5-chloro-4-(2-imidazolin-2-gamma-1-amino)-2,1,3-benzothiadiazole (DS 103 282), a novel myotonic agent. *Arzneimittelforschung, 30,* 793–803.

Schmidtke, K., & Ehmsen, L. (1998). Transient global amnesia and migraine. A case control study. *European Neurology, 40,* 9–14.

Shahota, P.K., & Dexter, J.D.S. (1990). Sleep and headache syndromes: A clinical review. *Headache, 30,* 80.

Shimomura, T., & Takahashi, K. (1986). Pupillary functional asymmetry in patients with muscle contraction headache. *Cephalalgia, 6,* 141.

Shimomura, T., & Takahashi, K. (1990). Alteration of platelet serotonin in patients with chronic tension-type headache during cold pressor test. *Headache, 30,* 581.

Shoenen, J., Pasqua, V.D., & Sianard-Gainko, J. (1991). Multiple clinical and paraclinical analyses of chronic tension-type headache associated or unassociated with disorder of the pericranial muscles. *Cephalalgia, 11,* 135.

Sicuteri, F. (1982). Natural opiods in migraine. In M. Critchley, A.P. Friedman, & S. Gorini, et al. (Eds.), *Advances in neurology* (Vol. 33, p. 65). New York: Raven Press.

Sicuteri, F., Nicolodi, M., & Fusco, B.M. (1988). Abnormal sensitivity to neurotransmitter agonists, antagonists and neurotransmitter releasers. In J. Olesen & L. Edvinsson (Eds.), *Basic mechanisms of headache* (p. 275). Amsterdam: Elsevier Science.

Sicuteri, F., Spillantini, M.G., & Fanciullacci, M. (1985). "Enkephalinase" in migraine and opiate addiction. In C. Rose (Ed.), *Migraine: Proceedings of the Fifth International Migraine Symposium* (p. 86). London: Basel, Karger.

Simons, D.J., Day, E., Goodell, H., & Wolff, H.G. (1943). Experimental studies on headache: Muscles of the scalp and neck as sources of pain. *Associated Research on Nervous and Mental Disorders Proceedings, 23,* 228.

Sjaastad, O., Bovim, G., & Stovner, L.J. (1992). Laterality of pain and other migraine criteria in common migraine. A comparison with cervicogenic headache. *Functional Neurology, 7,* 289–294.

Sjaastad, O., Fredriksen, T.A., & Pfaffenrath, V. (1990). Cervicogenic headache diagnostic criterion. *Headache, 30,* 725–26.

Sluijter, M.E. (1990). *Radiofrequency lesions in the treatment of cervical pain syndromes.* Procedure Technique Series (pp. 2–19). Holland: Radionics.

Speed, W.G. (1983). Muscle contraction headaches. In J. R. Saper (Ed.), *Headache disorders* (p. 115). Boston: John Wright.

Takeshima, T., Takao, Y., & Takahashi, K. (1987). Pupillary sympathetic hypofunction and asymmetry in muscle contraction headache. *Cephalalgia, 7,* 257.

Takeshima, T., Takao, Y.U., Urakami, K., et al. (1989). Muscle contraction headache and migraine. Platelet activation and plasma norepinephrine during the cold pressor test. *Cephalalgia, 9,* 7.

Tfelt-Hansen, P., Lous, I., & Olesen, J. (1981). Prevalence and significance of muscle tenderness during common migraine attack. *Headache, 21,* 49.

Travell, J., & Rinzler, S.H. (1952). The myofascial genesis of pain. *Postgraduate Medicine, 11,* 425–434.

Travell, J.G., & Simons, D.G. (1983). *Myofascial pain and dysfunction: The trigger point manual.* Baltimore: Williams & Wilkins.

Treleaven, J., Jull, G., & Atkinson, L. (1994). Cervical musculoskeletal dysfunction in post-concussional headache. *Cephalalgia, 14,* 273–279.

Tunis, M.M., & Wolff, H.G. (1954). Studies on headache: Cranial artery vasoconstriction and muscle contraction headache. *Archives of Neurologic Psychiatry, 71,* 425.

Vijayan, N. (1977). A new post-traumatic headache syndrome. *Headache, 17,* 19–22.

Vohanka, S., & Zouhar, A. (1988). Transient global amnesia after mild head injury in childhood. *Act. Nerv. Super. (Praha.), 30,* 68–74.

Vohanka, S., & Zouhar, A. (1990). Benign posttraumatic encephalopathy. *Act. Nerv. Super. (Praha.), 32,* 179–183.

Wagstaff, A.J., & Bryson, H. (1997). Tizanidine: A review of its pharmacology, clinical efficacy and tolerability in the management of spasticity associated with cerebral and spinal disorders. *Drugs, 53,* 435–452.

Wall, P.D. (1988). Stability and instability of central pain mechanisms. In R. Dubner & M. R. Bond (Eds.), *Proceedings of the Fifth World Conference on Pain* (p. 13). Amsterdam: Elsevier Science.

World Health Organization (1997). ICD-10 Guide for Headaches. *Cephalalgia, 17*(S19).

Yang, J.C., Richlin, D., Brand, L., Wagner, J., & Clark, W.C. (1985). Thermal sensory decision theory indices and pain threshold in chronic pain patients and healthy volunteers. *Psychologic Medicine, 47,* 461.

Zwart, J.A. (1997). Neck mobility in different headache disorders. *Headache, 37,* 6–11.

12

Posttraumatic Headache: Practical Interdisciplinary Approaches to Diagnosis and Treatment

Nathan D. Zasler, M.D., F.A.A.P.M.&R., F.A.A.D.E.P., C.I.M.E., D.A.A.P.M.
and Michael F. Martelli, Ph.D., D.A.A.P.M.

INTRODUCTION

The literature on posttraumatic headache (PTHA) appears to be replete with much confusion concerning nomenclature. Oftentimes, clinicians incorrectly assume that because someone has complaints of PTHA, they have sustained some type of insult to their brain. Individuals may develop PTHA and related disability due to a variety of causes including brain injury, cranial or cranial adnexal injury, and/or cervical acceleration/deceleration injury (Zasler, 1999).

Some individuals consider the diagnosis of PTHA to be a so-called "garbage can" diagnosis. The phrase PTHA does not tell patients, family, or other health care practitioners what they did not already know, that is, that they were involved in a trauma and subsequently have suffered from a headache condition. More importantly, many practitioners believe that it is important to specifically identify the pain generators in the context of providing diagnostic labels that may better guide clinical treatment (Zasler, 1996).

Appenzeller (1993) has been noted to have said, "No where is scientific medicine less evident than in the treatment and management of post-traumatic headaches." As practitioners in the field of brain injury care, we could not agree more. There is much confusion in the field across both medical and nonmedical disciplines as to the exact nature of the beast with regard to the diagnostic entity of

PTHA. We hope that this chapter provides some edification on the need to assess these patients in a more global manner instead of using what seems to be the traditional Ockham's razor approach. Significant deficiencies in our understanding of PTHA clearly remain which can be seen in the lack of good epidemiological, treatment, and outcomes research. These limitations must be acknowledged in the context of clinical care (Zasler, 1999).

CLASSIFICATION OF POSTTRAUMATIC HEADACHE

Current classification systems for PTHA have much to be desired given their general nature, as well as the empirical basis for the definitional criteria. If one examines the Headache Classification Committee of the International Headache Society's (IHS) (1988) classification for PTHA or the International Classification of Diseases and Related Health Problems, 10th edition (ICD-10) (World Health Organization, 1997) system, it is readily apparent that there are at least some problems with the current taxonomy for PTHA. Refer to Table 12.1 for a conversion chart between ICD-10 and IHS classification systems for PTHA.

The ICD-10 classification system uses criteria that are primarily concerned with the temporal onset and pathogenetic relationship of the headache to the trauma and not with the clinical features of the headache condition. ICD-

0-8493-0926-3/02/$0.00+$1.50
© 2002 by CRC Press LLC

TABLE 12.1
Conversion Table: IHS and ICD-10 Classification Codes

	IHS Code	ICD-10 Code	
		Etiologic Code	Headache Code
5.	Headache associated with head trauma		G44.88
5.1	Acute posttraumatic headache		G44.880
	5.1.1 With significant head trauma and/or confirmatory signs	S06	G44.880
	5.1.2 With minor head trauma and no confirmatory signs	S09.9	G44.880
5.2	Chronic post-traumatic headache		G44.3
	5.2.1 With significant head trauma and/or confirmatory signs	S06	G44.30
	5.2.2 With minor head trauma and no confirmatory signs	S09.9	

10 criteria for PTHA require that headache onset occur within 2 weeks of the traumatic event or regaining consciousness. This temporal onset criterion appears to have been determined only on the basis of empiricism. Clearly, although it tends to be the exception instead of the rule, there are patients who develop headache that is fully apportionable to their original injury beyond the 2-week rule. Another problem with the time designation of 2 weeks is that often patients may have significant multi-trauma with other more painful conditions (e.g., neck injury) than their headache, causing them to focus their attention on the more painful body part. Additionally, some may also argue that in more severe brain injury, patients' cognitive status may limit their ability to identify and/or appreciate head pain.

Also of concern is the fact that the ICD-10 criteria for either acute or chronic PTHA require one of the following: a loss of consciousness, a period of antegrade amnesia of at least 10 min, or abnormal neurodiagnostic/neurological exam. Certainly, such inclusion criteria exclude patients with various forms of PTHA including referred pain from cervical injury, as well as direct cranial and/or cranial adnexal injury, among other "posttraumatic" etiologies. Although there are classifications for other types of headache that may be applicable to these patients, they would not by definition fall under the rubric of PTHA by ICD-10 criteria. Of some import is the fact that a separate codification identifies patients with "minor head trauma and no confirmatory signs" under this classification. Acute PTHA by ICD-10 definition resolves within 8 weeks with chronic PTHA being defined temporally as any PTHA lasting longer than 8 weeks (HCCIHS, 1988); this definition is not consistent with common parlance of how chronic pain is typically defined (Zasler, 1999).

The IHS criteria were published (HCCIHS, 1988) to address the lack of operational rules and nonuniformity of nomenclature in the headache field. The classification system defines 13 major categories of headache with two broad categories (primary vs. secondary headaches). The IHS classification system has been endorsed by the World Health Organization (WHO) and the principles of the system have been incorporated into the ICD-10. The IHS criteria use both clinical features and laboratory testing to provide inclusion criteria. As with ICD-10, headache associated with "head trauma" is divided into acute and chronic PTHA. A second edition of the IHS Classification was published in 1999. There is fairly good correspondence between the ICD-10 and IHS headache classification systems.

EPIDEMIOLOGY AND OUTCOME

PTHA is clearly the most common symptom following mild brain injury and/or concussion, as well as cervical whiplash (acceleration/deceleration type injuries). Because of the lack of accurate registries and the fact that many persons with these types of injuries are never seen in acute care settings, the true incidence of this disorder in our society at large is unknown.

Surveys examining the number of individuals who develop PTHA as a result of minor head injury range anywhere from 30 to 50% (Evans, 1992; Alves et al., 1986). Additionally, there seems to be a clear, albeit to some extent controversial, correlation between severity of brain injury and incidence of PTHA. The majority of studies, as well as extensive clinical experience by professionals who have seen thousands of persons with cerebral, cranial, and cervical injuries, support the conclusion that persons with milder injury seem to have a higher frequency of headache complaints. To most, this would seem paradoxical based on the anticipated pathoetiology of PTHA. One of the classic studies examining this phenomenon was performed by Yamaguchi (1972) and published in 1992. He found that 72% of persons with mild injury vs. 33% of those with severe injury developed headache. He noted that abnormal findings on cervical radiographs including degenerative changes positively correlated with complaints of more severe headache. Just as interestingly, he noted that abnormalities on mental status testing and static brain imaging were negatively correlated with headache complaints and incidence (Yamaguchi, 1992). In a rather extensive review conducted by Appenzeller (1993), he concluded that PTHA incidence was much higher in patients with less severe brain injury.

The whole issue of correlating brain injury severity with extent of subsequent headache complaints seems, in our view, to be "missing the boat," given that there is a significant absence of literature exploring the incidence and severity of associated injury to the cranium and/or cervical spine in PTHA. Both the neck and head may be the source of pain generators in PTHA, either directly or indirectly as a result of referred pain. At the same time, however, one would expect worse cranial and cervical injuries in patients with more severe brain injury, given the magnitude of forces applied to the neural axis and therefore the skull and cervical spine. Thus, one would expect more, not less, headache in patients subjected to more significant forces across the neural and musculoskeletal axes.

Theoretically, the previously mentioned paradox may be explainable by speculating that patients with severe brain injury and/or multitrauma are commonly treated with paralytic agents, as well as prolonged bed rest, as part of their acute neurosurgical care. If one accepts that cervicogenic headache is the most frequent etiologic explanation for PTHA, although this remains controversial, one might also conclude that typically rendered treatment via muscle paralysis or prolonged immobilization may coincidentally be therapeutic for concomitant cervical musculoligamentous injury sustained by patients with more severe brain injury. In fact, this explanation, to a great extent, supports the position that the *majority* of PTHA may have nothing to do with brain injury per se.

Most studies have been unable to delineate the specific demographic factors related to the incidence of PTHA. The preponderance of data indicate that most individuals who sustain this type of posttraumatic impairment are injured in the context of motor vehicle accidents and most of these individuals are male. In order of frequency, other types of injuries that are associated with head trauma and brain injury include falls, assaults, and sports-related injuries. A rather high incidence of concurrent use of alcohol has been noted in a number of studies examining comorbidities of these types of injuries (Packard, 1999).

There has been very little methodologically sound research looking at preexisting and/or injury-related factors that may predispose to perpetuation of headache symptomatology following concussion. Aside from some literature examining the role of ongoing litigation as a factor in subjective headache complaints, there is no significant body of literature looking at musculoskeletal (including posture), neurological, and/or individual/family history issues plus their potential role in postconcussive headache symptom maintenance. A prime example of a prognostic factor associated with PTHA that is accepted as "gospel" by many physicians is that persons with preinjury headache are more prone to develop

PTHA and have a greater risk for chronic PTHA (CPTHA). However, a study by Jensen and Nielsen (1990) found that patients suffering from headache pre-injury were no more likely to suffer PTHA than patients without a preinjury headache history.

There is excellent literature with regard to cervical spine acceleration/deceleration injury and chronic pain, although not necessarily involving headache, that must be appreciated by any clinician involved with PTHA management (Freeman & Croft, 1997; Radanov et al., 1993). If one agrees with the experiential data and some research data indicating that cervicogenic referred pain is the primary etiology of PTHA, then it is not surprising to note that the observed higher incidence of PTHA in women instead of men (Jensen & Nielsen, 1990) may in fact have a pathoanatomic basis. Research has shown greater accelerative forces in whiplash injuries in women than in men, deemed to be due to differences in cervical muscle bulk and/or neck length (Siegmund, King, Lawrence, Wheeler, Brault, & Smith, 1997).

PATHOETIOLOGY

The exact pathoetiology of nontraumatic headache continues to be debated. The pain generators and pathoetiology of PTHA are even less well understood. When one considers the anatomic correlates of recurring benign head pain, one can make some general statements that are likely just as applicable for nontraumatic headache as they are for traumatic headache (Packard, 1992).

There are multiple pain-sensitive structures in the head, both intra- and extracranially, that may be pain generators. There are also pain generators more caudally in the neck that may refer pain into the head, either by direct or by indirect means. Pain, in general, is transmitted from the periphery by small myelinated fibers and unmyelinated C fibers that terminate in the dorsal horn of the spinal cord. These fibers also have end terminals in the trigeminal nucleus caudalis. Secondary neurons from the dorsal horn reach the thalamus by the spinothalamic pathways. The upper cervical spine contains pain fiber systems for the entire head/neck region. The trigeminal cervical nucleus is the anatomic structure critical to the concept of cervical headache, as well as head/neck referred pain. Sensory afferents from the trigeminal nerve, as well as the upper three cervical spinal nerves, have been theorized to relay sensory information through the trigeminal cervical nucleus (May & Goadsby, 1999). Bogduk (1982) has proposed that there are overlapping and convergent second-order neurons that serve as the pathoetiologic basis, as well as pathoanatomic basis, for referred pain. Cervical pain can, therefore, be perceived in the territory of the trigeminal nerve, particularly in the ophthalmic division due to epaptic transmission through the proximal portion of the C-2 root. This second-order neuron phenomenon is also the basis for frequent observation of referred orbital and frontal pain emanating from cervical pain generators.

The exact role that central modulation of trigeminovascular pain plays in headache, in general, and posttraumatic headache, specifically, is yet to be determined, as is the role of so-called central sensitization. This latter phenomenon, which is a well-described event in the animal literature, remains somewhat controversial in the context of various neurological and psychiatric disorders in the human population. It is manifested by increased spontaneous impulse discharges, increased responsiveness to noxious and nonnoxious peripheral stimuli, and expanded receptive fields of nociceptive neurons. So-called "windup" is a short-lasting phenomenon and therefore cannot explain central sensitization that is of longer duration and may involve changes in neuronal plasticity. Windup may, however, be the trigger to longer lasting neuronal sensitization and therefore potentially to chronic headache pain, posttraumatic or otherwise (Sessle, 1999).

In the context of assessment of a patient with PTHA, one must assess pain generators from the face, cranium (including cranial adnexal structures), cerebrum, and neck. There are multiple structures in the neck that have been hypothesized to produce head pain, including zygapophyseal joints of the second and third vertebra, musculoligamentous attachments of the atlantoaxial joints, and upper paravertebral muscles, as well as the muscles innervated by the eleventh cranial nerve (e.g., trapezius and sternocleidomastoid), the spinal dura mater (see later), the vertebral artery, and the C2–C3 intervertebral disks (Horn, 1992). There has been some manual medicine literature suggesting that attachments of the ligamentum nuchae exist to the posterior cervical spinal dura and the lateral part of the occipital bone (Mitchell, Humphreys, & O'Sullivan, 1998). This anatomic discovery may be of significance in terms of understanding the biomechanics and symptomatic sequela of cervical acceleration/deceleration (whiplash) injury, particularly in relation to rotational movements of the head in the sagittal and transverse planes, as related to cervicogenic headache following trauma.

CLINICAL ASSESSMENT

It is important for the examining clinician to keep the different mechanisms of PTHA in mind. Additionally, the mechanism of injury responsible for the initial insult should also be investigated; specifically, inquiry concerning history pertaining to three main phenomena: cerebral, cranial/cranial adnexal, and/or cervical injury.

One of the major clues for the examiner relative to the origin of the headache should come from establishing the symptom profile for that particular headache, as well as the patient's preinjury history of headache. Just because an individual had headache preinjury does not mean that he or she could not develop a different type of headache or a worsening of the preinjury condition following trauma. The major questions relative to the headache profile that need to be asked are expressed in the pneumonic COLDER: character, onset, location, duration, exacerbation, and relief. Additional questions concerning the frequency and severity of headache, time of day of headache, and associated symptomatology (including aura, pain referral patterns, and familial headache history) should be inquired about, among multiple other possibilities. Less common causes of PTHA should always be considered when the obvious ones do not pan out based on the history provided by the examinee. Some of the less commonly seen variants of PTHA include posttraumatic sinus problems, posttraumatic epilepsy, tension pneumocephalus, extraaxial collections such as subdurals and epidurals, cluster headache, paroxysmal hemicrania, dysautonomic or sympathetic headache (anterior and posterior forms), and basilar artery migraine (BAM). Drug use history, whether prescription or recreational, should also be assessed including the potential for drug-induced and/or rebound headache, the latter which is commonly iatrogenic. With the appropriate history and descriptive clues, the clinician is then armed to conduct a clinical examination to allow a more specific conclusion as to the origin of the headache condition (Zafonte & Horn, 1999).

The physical examination of the patient who presents with PTHA should be comprehensive but focused based on a good clinical history. At a minimum, the exam should include a screening neurological and musculoskeletal assessment. The basics of physical examination should be conducted with a focus to the suspected pain generators. The exam should include inspection, palpation, and, as appropriate, percussion and auscultation. Inspection should focus on posture and body asymmetries, among other areas assessed. Musculoskeletal assessment should include an adequate examination of the cranium, cranial adnexal structures, and cervicothoracic spine as deemed relevant to the patient's headache complaints. Palpatory exam might include checking for neuromatous or neuritic pain generators, myofascial trigger points, vertebral somatic dysfunction, sinus tenderness, and/or temporomandibular joint (TMJ) dysfunction (Horn, 1992; Zafonte & Horn, 1999).

MANAGEMENT

MYOFASCIAL PAIN

Myofascial pain is one of the more common etiologies of PTHA, although to some extent the diagnosis of myofascial pain remains somewhat controversial across medical specialties. Myofascial pain typically presents as a regional pain disorder characterized by localized muscle tenderness in association with discomfort/pain.

It is quite common following cervical acceleration/deceleration injuries, whether of a flexion/extension nature or lateral impulse type of force. Research has shown that referred pain, as well as so-called local twitch response, which are both characteristics of myofascial trigger points, is related to spinal cord mechanisms (Bisbee & Hartsell, 1993). It has been theorized that the taut band of skeletal muscle fibers that contain the myofascial trigger point is produced by an excessive amount of acetylcholine in the abnormal end plate (Hong & Simons, 1998).

A trigger point is defined as a localized deep tenderness in the taut band of skeletal muscles that is responsible for the pain in the zone of reference. Clinicians must differentiate between latent and active trigger points. The zone of reference is defined as the area of perceived pain referred by the irritable trigger point and is usually located over the trigger point or spreads out from the trigger point to a distant site (Travell & Simons, 1983).

Treatment for myofascial pain should be holistic. Muscle exercises should include stretching and strengthening, as well as postural. Trigger point therapy is clearly an important part of the overall armamentarium and may include such techniques as ultrasound, ischemic pressure, accupressure, and massage, among others. Counterstimulation techniques involving Fluori-Methane, diathermy, and heat and/or ice can also be used. Direct current stimulation via such techniques as electroacupuncture, transcutaneous electrical nerve stimulation, and direct current stimulation can also be considered. Acupuncture may serve as an adjutant therapy; however, its role in myofascial pain has not been well studied. Trigger point injections with local anesthetic and/or steroid and dry needling are the most common techniques used to treat this problem. Trigger point injections not only reduce pain and increase range of motion in a muscle that is typically shortened but also improve circulation to the muscle. It is not critical to inject anything into the trigger point for the needling to have a therapeutic effect, because the latter appears to be due to mechanical disruption of the trigger point by the needle, instead of the substance injected per se. Trigger point injections with local anesthetic are generally more effective and comfortable than dry needling or injecting other substances. Some clinicians have reported success modulating myofascial pain symptoms with botulinum toxin injections (Chesire, Abashian, & Mann, 1994). Spray and stretch techniques, as well as other manual strategies including strain–counterstrain, soft tissue mobilization, and myofascial release techniques, have also been found to be quite effective in ameliorating myofascial pain (Travell & Simons, 1983).

Perpetuating factors must be addressed in the treatment of myofascial pain including psychoemotional status, metabolic and hormonal factors, and, most importantly, body asymmetries and postural issues. Additionally, ergonomic issues should be examined in the workplace, as well as at home; included in the latter should be assessment of sleep habits such as use and type of head supports and bed (Travell & Simons, 1983). Therapeutic exercise is a critical component of maintaining pain relief and should include both flexibility and strengthening components. Education concerning the need for compliance with any treatment intervention should be part and parcel of any treatment regimen.

NEURALGIC AND NEURITIC PAIN

It is not uncommon after cervical whiplash to find patients with signs of occipital neuralgia, involving either the lesser or greater occipital nerves. This type of problem generally responds well to local anesthetic blockade (sometimes in conjunction with steroids) (Waldman, 1991). Unless associated myofascial dysfunction is also addressed in the context of the overall treatment, occipital nerve irritation may return fairly quickly.

Surgical decompression of the occipital nerve should be considered when entrapment is felt to be the pathoetiologic mechanism responsible for continued pain, although the procedure may not produce complete pain relief. In more intractable cases, consideration can be given for injection of neurolytic agents and/or more aggressive techniques such as destruction of the involved nerve via such procedures as cryoablation and/or open surgical neurectomy (Horowitz & Yonas, 1993). Surgical excision may result in deafferentation pain and/or neuroma formation. Of note, however, is that some experienced clinicians do not recommend the treatment due to the fact that the procedural efficacy remains poorly studied (Bogduk & Marsland, 1986).

Following more significant cranial injuries, it is not uncommon to develop neuromas in the scalp particularly after craniotomies. For more diffuse neuritic scalp irritation, topical capsaicin can be considered. When there is a question of a more focal neuromatous lesion, local anesthetic blockade can be helpful. Enteral medications traditionally used in the treatment of neuropathic pain can also be used for neuritic and neuromatous pain. These medications include nonsteroidal antiinflammatories, tricyclic antidepressants, and anticonvulsants (such as gabapentin, carbamazepine, and phenytoin), among others.

Less commonly, neuralgic problems can be encountered secondary to facial trauma. The nerves that are most commonly involved are the supraorbital and infraorbital nerves. These nerves can be injected locally with good resolution of facial pain and/or dysesthetic symptoms (Waldman, 1991). Sometimes, as with other injections, serial procedures are required.

MIGRAINE

Posttraumatic migraine accounts for up to 20% of CPTHA. It is generally treated similarly to nontraumatic migraine. There are some atypical variants of posttraumatic migraine, such as BAM, that are known to occur more frequently in young females, particularly following whiplash injury (Jacome, 1986). The exact reason for this is unknown. BAM is generally treated with atypical migraine medications such as carbamazepine or valproic acid.

Migraine treatment should include looking at all associated factors that may influence this headache picture including reduction of so-called trigger factors (this may include certain food groups as well as external and internal stressors). Treatment should be directed at minimizing the functional disability associated with the headache through other interventions including appropriate medication prescription that may be abortive, symptomatic, and/or prophylactic. A small percentage of women who take birth control pills may be exacerbating their migraines and this should be considered in the overall holistic treatment of patients with posttraumatic migraine. Other interventions such as relaxation training and biofeedback may also be used (Bell, Kraus, & Zasler, 1999).

TEMPOROMANDIBULAR JOINT DISORDERS

Although true intra-articular pathology is not frequently seen following whiplash-induced temporomandibular joint disorders (TMJD), myofascial dysfunction in the muscles of mastication is frequently noted. Appropriate workup is necessary, however, to rule out intra-articular pathology and, if present, to address it accordingly. In most cases, a referral to an oromaxillofacial surgeon would be warranted. Local treatment, as per the discussion of myofascial pain for trigger points involving the muscles of mastication (temporalis, masseter, medial pterygoid, lateral pterygoid) should be aggressively pursued. As indicated, interventions for bruxing should be suggested, for example, intraoral appliances such as occlusal splints (Fricton, 1995). Appropriate education concerning minimizing foods that require significant chewing is generally beneficial during the more acute and subacute treatment phase for myofascial pain involving the muscles of mastication. The patient should be instructed in the use of simple jaw exercises including passive jaw opening with the thumb and forefinger and a gentle scissorlike action to a position just short of pain onset. Nonsurgical treatment continues to be considered the most effective way of managing over 80% of all patients who present with symptoms of TMJD in the absence of intra-articular pathology (Dimitroulis, Gremillion, Dolwick, & Walter, 1995).

If and when it is suspected clinically and/or proven by diagnostic testing, such as magnetic resonance imaging (MRI), that there is significant intra-articular pathology, arthroscopic intervention is generally indicated. Rarely, one finds the necessity to proceed to open arthrotomy for disk repositioning and/or arthroplasty. Generally, experience has shown that surgical outcome from the latter type of procedure tends to be guarded. In extreme cases of intracapsular damage, caused by the initial injury, or by failed surgery, condylectomy and costochondral reconstruction of the articulation may be required. When there is significant meniscal injury, an artificial meniscus can be considered.

CERVICAL ZYGAPOPHYSEAL JOINT PAIN

Cervical zygapophyseal joint pain can cause both neck pain and referred head pain. Pain from the C2–C3 joint is perceived posteriorly in the upper neck extending into the occipital region, whereas pain from the C3–C4 joint and any cervical joint caudal to that does not refer into the head. Treatment considerations can include intra-articular injections of local anesthetic at the joint level for blocks of the medial branches of the dorsal rami that supply the joint. Joint blocks should be ideally performed under fluoroscopic control through either a posterior or a lateral approach. Cervical medial branch blocks are a more expedient way to block a cervical zygapophyseal joint in that they are not only easier but also less painful to the patient and provide the same diagnostic information (Lord, Barnsley, & Bogduk, 1993). Other more aggressive modalities for treatment of this type of pain include percutaneous radiofrequency neurotomy via medial branches, although this remains a controversial treatment strategy on several levels (Lord, Barnsley, & Bogduk, 1995).

SOMATIC DYSFUNCTION

Manual medicine techniques for the treatment of cervical pain remains somewhat controversial. We are quite convinced that craniocervical and cervicothoracic somatic dysfunction following traumatic neck injuries has the potential to generate head pain. There have been numerous studies involving the benefits of mobilization of the cervical spine in chronic headaches, posttraumatic and otherwise, which have shown that cervical mobilization/manipulation can be beneficial in these types of clinical conditions (Jensen, Nielsen, & Vosman, 1990). These procedures are utilized by not only chiropractors but also physical therapists, as well as appropriately trained physicians (both M.D.s and D.O.s). Mobilization with impulse (also referred to as high-velocity, low-amplitude thrust) is based on the principle of overcoming the resistive barrier in the direction of loss of range of motion. Reduction of hypertonicity in segmentally related paraspinal muscles results through a hypothesized effect on mechanoreceptors and stimulation of the afferent loop of the applicable reflex arc. There are many other techniques in the manual medicine armamentarium. Some of the direct (resistive barrier is engaged) interventions include soft tissue and articulatory muscle energy and myofascial release, as well as craniosacral manipulation. Some of the indirect (resistive barrier is not engaged) interventions include balance and hold, as well as strain–counterstrain (Greenman, 1989). Treatment contraindications, both relative and absolute, must be appreciated by any clinician using these techniques as complications have been reported (Dvorak & Orelli, 1985).

DYSAUTONOMIC HEADACHE

Certain nerve fibers in the neck, anteriorly as well as posteriorly, may be damaged from excessive flexion or extension of the neck associated with cervical acceleration/deceleration insult. These types of injuries may produce an uncommon PTHA variant known as dysautonomic cephalalgia. There may be partial or total insult to these nerves that impacts on how the condition is treated relative to medication choices (Vihayan, 1977). Involvement of posterior cervical sympathetic dysfunction (also known as Barre-Lieou syndrome) may produce symptoms of pain in the back of the head, tinnitus (buzzing in the ears), blurry vision, and vertigo (Barre, 1926).

RARE CAUSES OF POSTTRAUMATIC HEADACHE

There are multiple rare causes of headache that should also be considered in the posttrauma population. Appropriate neurodiagnostic tests such as computerized tomography (CT) or magnetic resonance imaging (MRI) scanning of the brain, plain X-rays, electrodiagnostic and vascular studies, and laboratory tests should be conducted as deemed appropriate by the treating clinician (Zafonte & Horn, 1999). These tests should not be ordered unless it is felt that the results will alter clinical treatment planning.

PSYCHOLOGICAL FACTORS

Chronic pain or pain that persists 6 months or longer after injury: (1) reflects ambiguous pathways between injury sites and the central nervous system, (2) communicates useless information that perpetuates physiological protective responses long after removal of possibility of injury extension and/or despite lack of underlying tissue damage, and (3) poses a liability to postinjury adaptation. Importantly, chronic pain is typically associated with response patterns involving decreases in, and avoidance of, activity. Decreased activity, in response, can prevent

normal restoration of function and perpetuate painful experience; and in a cyclic fashion, it reinforces avoidance, inactivity, and increased pain. Finally, the longer pain persists, the more recalcitrant it becomes and the more treatment goals move toward management of pain and coping vs. cure (Penzien, Jeanetta, & Holroyd, 1993).

According to Miller (1993) chronic pain often represents the "weak link" in the cycle of "postconcussion invalidism." Given that PTHA is the most common postconcussive symptom (Packard, 1994; Goldstein, 1991) and hence the most frequent type of posttraumatic pain associated with mild traumatic brain injury (MTBI), it follows that resolution of the postconcussion syndrome, and successful posttraumatic adaptation, may frequently rely on success in coping with PTHA symptomatology. The introduction of biopsychosocial models represents alternative theoretical approaches to dualistic and reductionistic biomedical conceptualizations that explain disease and health primarily in terms of measurable biological variables. A derived stress and coping formulation of postinjury recovery conceptualizes adaptation to injury as a series of stressful demands that require coping. Coping represents an interaction between existing coping resources and injury-related demands. Bolstering of coping resources presumably allows for improved adaptation to stressful life events. PTHA does not occur in a vacuum. Instead, it occurs in a biological system within specific psychological and social contexts. It reflects an interaction of organic and emotional factors.

Although similar to natural headaches in clinical presentation of subtypes and biochemical mechanisms, PTHA is oftentimes resistant to traditional headache treatment. Medication management alone may lead to unwanted side effects (e.g., adverse effects on sleep, mental alertness, sexual functioning, work performance) and certainly does not address adaptation to chronic pain through development of new coping skills (Martelli, Zasler, & MacMillan, 1998). Conversely, PTHA patients have been reported to exhibit minimal response to nondrug (i.e., psychological) treatments alone (Jensen, Nielsen, & Vosmar, 1990). Treatments that are holistic in nature, targeting not only the pain directly but also the patient's reaction to pain within his or her daily life, typically fare better than treatments with a more narrow focus (e.g., medication management or nondrug therapies alone). Understanding vulnerability issues as predictors of poor chronic pain adaptation is also critical in this context (Bennett, 1988) (Table 12.2). Currently, multicomponent treatment packages are the preferred treatment choice for PTHA (Packard & Ham, 1997).

The assessment phase is the starting point of any psychological treatment protocol. Detailed individual assessment is necessary to consider specific treatment issues (e.g., personality variables, social support) and facilitate the patient–therapist relationship. A thorough

TABLE 12.2
Vulnerability to Disability Rating Scale

Increased Complaint Duration	Complaint Inconsistency/ Vagueness	Previous Treatment Failure	Collateral Injury/Impairment	Pre/Comorbid Medical History	Medication Reliance
0 = < 6 Months	0 = Little	0 = Insignificant	0 = Insignificant	0 = Insignificant	0 = Little
1 = < 12 Months	1 = Mixed	1 = Mixed	1 = Mild/moderate	1 = Mild/moderate	1 = Moderate
2 = > 12 Months	2 = Mostly inconsistent	2 = Mostly or all failures	2 = Significant	2 = Significant	2 = Significant
Especially with expectation of chronicity, poor understanding of symptoms	Multiple, vague, variable sites; anatomically inconsistent; sudden onset without accident or cause; not affected by weather; performing no work or chores, or avoiding easy tasks but performing most hobbies, enjoyments; pain only occasional	Especially with complaint of treatments worsening pain or causing injury, and expectation that future treatments will fail	Especially if silent and involving adaptation reducing impairments	Seizure disorder; diabetes; hypertension; brain injury, stroke or other neurological insult or vulnerability (esp. if undiagnosed); preinjury medication reliance	> 4X/week narcotic, hypnotic or benzo-diazepine tranqulizer; perceived inability to cope without medication

Severity of Current Psychosocial Stress	Psychological Coping Liabilities	Victimization Perception	Social Vulnerability	Illness Reinforcement	Vulnerability Score
0 = Nonsignificant	0 = Few	0 = Little	0 = Little	0 = Little	
1 = Mild/moderate	1 = Mild/moderate	1 = Mild/moderate	1 = Mild/moderate	1 = Mild/moderate	
2 = Significant	2 = Significant	2 = Significant	2 = Significant	2 = Significant	_____ Total points (Max: 22)
Sum of peronal, social, financial, emotional, identity, activity stresses, life disruption, premorbid coping style disruption, etc. and including injury/ impairment X coping style incongruence; persistent premorbid psychosocial stress levels	Premorbid, comorbid: depression; posttraumatic anxiety; somatization (and repressive) defenses; emotional immaturity/ inadequacy with poor coping skills; hypochondriacal traits (e.g., postinjury MMPI-3 > 85; preinjury > 70); passive coping style; childhood trauma (esp. death of parent; child or sex abuse); anger/resentment; posttraumatic adjustment problems (see "Vulnerability to Disability" tables — psychological impediments); alcohol, substance use/abuse; limited premorbid intellect, education, skills; preinjury psychiatic treatment; poor premorbid work history	Externalized "blame" for accident, disability, etc.; perceived mistreatment; anger, fear, resentment, distrust concerning accident, treatment, understanding (family, employer, doctors, etc. — esp. given characterologic tendencies concerning victimization, resentment, suspiciousness, distrust, etc.)	Lack of family support, resources, romantic support (esp. if recent conflict, divorce); lack of community support/resources/ involvement; lack of employer, co-worker, insurance manager support; etc.	Secondary gain: attention, support in a dependency-prone person; avoidance of stressful or displeasing life or job responsibilities or demands (esp. with recent or imminent job/job duty changes or reorganization); financial compensation (esp. if litigation; or current income = preinjury/ preimpairment)	Preliminary interpretive guidlines Scores of 13 or above suggest high vulnerability to chronic disability

Vulnerability to Disability Rating Scale (VDRS) — General Version: *M.F. Martelli, Ph.D.* © 1996.

behavioral assessment may include a detailed clinical interview and other assessment instruments such as pain diaries and various standard pain and headache questionnaires. Psychophysiological assessment is an additional option, if feasible, and typically involves examination of muscle tension or electromyogram (EMG) for different muscle groups in the head (forehead, masseter, temporal, occipital) and neck (trapezius, cervical paraspinal) areas. The assessment phase concludes when the results of evaluation have produced a specific case conceptualization that identifies a specifically tailored treatment plan. Feedback to the patient using assessment results provides a framework for the treatment intervention, defines goals and patient/therapist expectations and sequences, and provides the forum for presenting general information concerning PTHA and rationale for treatment and enlisting participation.

Although there is an abundance of headache treatment outcome studies available, there are relatively few studies specifically examining the psychological treatment of PTHA as a distinct subgroup of headaches in general. The literature suggests that PTHA and natural headaches may share common pathways, and clinical presentations are generally very similar if not identical (Haas, 1993). Consequently, standard psychological treatments for headache are presumed to share common mechanisms of action. Although PTHA treatment outcome studies suggest that combined psychological treatments are generally efficacious, evidence suggests that PTHA is often more recalcitrant to standard psychological treatment compared with natural headaches. However, the severity and frequency of pain attacks and chronic pain-related sequelae such as coping abilities, depression, and anxiety may be significantly improved by combined psychological treatment protocols (Miller, 1993; Packard & Ham, 1997; Parker, 1995). Supportive counseling that begins early after trauma and is continuous results in better patient response (Ham & Packard, 1996).

Patient Education

Packard directly asked, "What does the headache patient want?" and detailed the stated treatment priorities of headache patients (Packard, 1979). Education concerning the causes of headaches was listed as a top priority. Information can be individualized for the patient and ideally presented while providing feedback after the behavioral assessment phase. It is especially important as pain professionals to emphasize to patients that their pain is real. Some patients, when told by physicians that medical tests are inconclusive or that their headache pain is due to stress, may interpret this information as "it's all in my head." Anecdotally, many patients are confused or angry when referred to a psychologist for pain treatment. Explaining the cycle of stress and pain

and validating their pain may help to gain client trust and commitment.

Biofeedback

Although an abundance of research reports the success of biofeedback for the treatment of tension-type migraine, mixed migraine, and tension-type headaches, many studies listed PTHA among the exclusionary criteria. As a result, few studies have examined the efficacy of biofeedback for PTHA specifically. A number of studies used EMG biofeedback (forehead and neck sites) in combination with other treatment modalities (e.g., cognitive–behavioral treatment, medication) and reported significant improvement in PTHA (Duckro, Tait, Margolis, & Silversintz, 1985; Medina, 1992). Ham and Packard (1996) reported that combined EMG and thermal biofeedback resulted in at least moderate improvement for 53% of 40 chronic PTHA patients, most of whom had previously received medication, physical therapy, chiropractic treatment, and/or trigger point injections without significant success. However, it is difficult to make firm conclusions concerning the efficacy of biofeedback alone for PTHA given the small sample size and the use of other simultaneous treatments in these studies. Although empirical research examining the utility of biofeedback specifically for PTHA is sparse, many clinical researchers feel that biofeedback, when combined with medical treatment and/or psychotherapy, augments the treatment response for many persons with PTHA.

Relaxation Training

Various forms of relaxation training have been used for the treatment of chronic headache (e.g., autogenics, meditation); however, progressive muscle relaxation (PMR) has been most widely studied (Blanchard, 1994). PMR involves the systematic tensing and relaxing of various muscle groups to elicit a relaxation response. Diaphragmatic breathing is generally taught in combination with relaxation exercises. Meta-analytic reviews generally conclude that relaxation training and biofeedback training are equally effective for headache reduction, producing improvement rates between 44.6 and 59.2% for tension-type headaches and migraines (Martin, 1993).

Operant Treatment

Fordyce (1976) pioneered the behavioral approach to psychological assessment and treatment of chronic pain. Although not specifically developed for use with PTHA, the concept follows the operant model to reduce general chronic pain behaviors. That is, the operant model hypothesizes that pain-related behaviors may be positively reinforced by desirable consequences (e.g., sympathy, nurturance), while simultaneously negatively reinforced by avoidance of aversive consequences (e.g., undesirable work or social obligations). Treatment based on the operant model requires altering environmental contingencies to eliminate pain behaviors (e.g., verbal complaints, inactivity) and reward "well" behaviors (e.g., exercise, increased activity level).

Cognitive–Behavioral Treatments

Cognitive approaches for headache treatment are derived from several cognitive theorists and typically train the headache patient to identify and refute maladaptive beliefs concerning pain. Specific cognitive strategies and skills are taught to replace inappropriate negative expectations and beliefs. Holroyd and Andrasik (1978) have generally led the field in cognitive therapy for chronic headache. Cognitive stress-coping therapy has been successfully applied to tension-type headache patients in group, minimal-therapist-contact, and home-based formats (Tobin, Holroyd, Baker, Reynolds, & Holm, 1988). Cognitive stress-coping therapy proposes that maladaptive cognitive responses are present that contribute to keeping the headache patient stressed/tense by keeping the sympathetic nervous system activated. Pain protocols based on this approach alter the maladaptive beliefs that mediate the stress reaction to presumably alter the stress reaction (muscle tension) leading to increased pain. In essence, the patient with PTHA is trained to shift attention from one aspect of the environment (e.g., internal pain) to another (internal or external).

Social and Assertiveness Skills Training

Miller (1993) recommended social skills training in a group format as an adjunct to standard psychotherapeutic interventions for chronic pain. Assertiveness training, in particular, may help some patients to communicate needs more effectively. This, in turn, increases the likelihood of need fulfillment and more desirable situational outcomes. Subsequent reduction of stressful events, anger, and other distressful emotional states associated with need frustration can reduce associated physiological arousal that contributes to headache pain.

Imagery and Hypnosis

Several studies have reported success with imagery-based treatments for headache in general (Martin, 1993). Procedures vary by study, but training generally includes autohypnosis and suggestions of relaxation and visual imagery. Generally, the patient is instructed to visualize the pain (i.e., give it form) and focus on altering the image to reduce the pain. Imagery-based treatment is recommended following establishment of a good therapeutic alliance to facilitate patient compliance. At least one study docu-mented the application of imagery for PTHA, in particular (Daly & Wulff, 1987).

Biofeedback-Assisted Cognitive–Behavioral Therapy

The efficacy of EMG biofeedback and cognitive–behavioral therapy (CBT), singularly and in combination in multicomponent treatment packages, has been demonstrated for the treatment of various pain disorders (e.g., headache, facial pain). The majority of multicomponent treatment packages in the literature to date utilize distinct techniques for biofeedback and CBT. Grayson (1997) presented a promising single-case research design outlining a multicomponent treatment protocol (biofeedback-assisted CBT; B-CBT) that synthesizes the two in the treatment of chronic posttraumatic pain. The B-CBT protocol combines cognitive, emotional, and physiological (e.g., muscle tension) elements to heighten awareness of self-control. It provides immediate physiological feedback during the cognitive behavior therapy process to heighten awareness of psychophysiological reactions and to facilitate change. Through the process of shaping, patients learn to monitor and control their physiological reactions in conjunction with reviewing and modifying cognitive and emotional aspects of activating stressful events. In addition, a cognitive exposure method can be utilized by having the patient repeatedly relate the activating event, while attempting to maintain physiological responding below a gradually reducing threshold level. Relaxation techniques such as deep breathing and progressive relaxation training may be also used. Initial findings for this procedure have been very encouraging and further research is warranted.

Habit Reversal

In a promising new approach to managing facial pain and tension headaches, Gramling, Neblett, Grayson, and Townsend (1996) used a habit reversal treatment approach. They taught patients with facial pain to detect, interrupt, and reverse maladaptive habits (e.g., suboptimal head/jaw posture, jaw tension, and negative cognitions). The main premise of this program is that participants can learn specific skills to reverse habits as well as reverse stressful thoughts and feelings that precipitate these habits. The treatment program begins by teaching exercises that increase awareness of the habit. Awareness training is facilitated by relaxation training exercises that are taught in conjunction with deep breathing exercises. As pain patients become more aware of maladaptive habits and the situations in which they occur, they are taught to use specific exercises (e.g., facial exercises) and deep breathing as competing responses. A similar process is used to help pain patients become more aware of habitual stress-inducing thoughts and beliefs.

IMPAIRMENT AND DISABILITY IN POSTTRAUMATIC HEADACHE

Currently, we have poor tools for gauging impairment associated with headache. For example, the American Medical Association (AMA) (1993) does not provide a *specific* methodology for calculation of impairment related to any type of headache but instead allows the rater to "estimate" the impairment. Pain is therefore rated in qualitative terms relative to frequency and intensity. One must understand, however, that the rating is based purely on patient report and therefore is totally subjective, as opposed to most of the AMA's guidelines for impairment determination that are based on objective clinical exam findings. It is also important for readers to understand that the AMA guides were established through an empirical consensus process and would not stand up to current methodologies used in the development of evidence-based standards or guidelines.

The AMA guidelines state, "An individual who complains of constant pain but who has no objectively validated limitations in daily activities has no impairment" (AMA, 1993, p. 309). This statement confuses issues germane to differentiation of impairment from functional disability. That is, impairment should not be gauged by functional ability or disability but by objective examination findings on physical and/or psychiatric examination. It is of utmost importance for clinicians, as well as lawyers, to keep the distinction between impairment (what one finds on examination) and disability (how the impairment impacts on functional abilities) clear and not intermingle and/or analogize these terms.

The AMA guidelines also state, "The vast majority of patients with headache will not have permanent impairments" (AMA, p. 312). First, this statement discusses headache in only a very general sense, and there are clearly differences in headache conditions that affect prognosis, as well as anticipated impairment and disability that are lost when making such a generalization. This statement also has the potential to bias less experienced evaluators and lead to their dismissal of chronic PTHA complaints as "nonorganic," litigious, or attention-seeking behaviors.

Finally, impairment ratings are considered appropriate only after an individual has reached maximum medical improvement (MMI); specifically, this implies that there is no more than a 3% change in whole body impairment rating expected over the ensuing year (AMA, 1993). An individual who has not been adequately assessed (e.g., there is no more specific a diagnosis than PTHA) and/or treated should not be labeled, as a rule, as MMI.

Packard and Ham (1993) proposed a reasonable alternative to the AMA impairment rating system using the acronym IMPAIRMENT and a 0 to 2 rating scale. The acronym stands for intensity, medication use, physical signs/symptoms, adjustment, incapacitation, recreation, miscellaneous activity of daily living, employment, number (frequency), and time (duration of attacks). Additionally, there are three physician modifiers scored from 0 to −4 points for motivation for treatment, overexaggeration or overconcern, and degree of legal interest. Although this paradigm for ascertaining an impairment level in PTHA is more cumbersome than the AMA Guides, the Packard and Ham methodology is one viable option that provides a more multidimensional and logical approach to rating impairment in PTHA.

CONCLUSIONS AND RECOMMENDATIONS

There is much to be learned about PTHA conditions. There must be a greater effort at bringing together the multiple disciplines involved with PTHA assessment and treatment to address many of the issues discussed in this chapter, as well as others not discussed because of space limitations. Education concerning PTHA for "frontline" clinicians in the disciplines of emergency medicine, neurology, and family practice is essential if these individuals are to receive appropriate treatment. There must be development of multidisciplinary consensus opinion concerning issues dealing with nomenclature, screening examination, classification, and accepted algorithms for treatment. PTHA classification must be more in depth and specific than that currently provided by ICD-10 or IHS. Better and more objective impairment and disability assessment techniques need to be developed for PTHA, preferably ones that have face validity and good inter-rater reliability with internal "checks" for symptom magnification, as well as response bias. Research efforts should be directed at examining PTHA subtypes in primary not tertiary PTHA patient populations that have been identified relative to historical factors and specific subpopulations (e.g., cerebral, cranial, cranial adnexal, cervical, posttraumatic psychological, or mixed impairments).

Ultimately, there is still much that is not understood about PTHA. Misinformation, lack of information, and incomplete understanding of pathoetiology, as well as natural history of the condition, continue to be problematic issues. We must commit to addressing these deficits in knowledge through multicenter, multidisciplinary, prospective research.

REFERENCES

Alves, W.M., Colohan A., O'Leary T.J., et al. (1986). Understanding post-traumatic symptoms after minor head injury. *Journal of Head Trauma Rehabilitation, 1,*1–12.

American Medical Association. (1993). *Guides to the Evaluation of Permanent Impairment* (4th ed.) Chicago: AMA.

Appenzeller, O. (1993). Post-traumatic headache. In D.J. Dalesio & S.D. Silberstein (Eds.), *Wolff's headache and other head pain* (6th ed., pp. 365–383). New York: Oxford University Press).

Barre, J.A. (1926). The posterior cervical sympathetic syndrome and its frequent cause: Cervical arthritis. *Review of Neurology, 53,* 12-46.

Bell, K.R., Kraus, E.E., & Zasler, N.D. (1999). Medical management of post-traumatic headaches: Pharmacological and physical treatment. *Journal of Head Trauma Rehabilitation, 14*(1), 34–38.

Bennett, T. (1988). Post-traumatic headaches: Subtypes and behavioral treatments. *Cognitive Rehabilitation. 6*(2), 34-39.

Bisbee L.A., & Hartsell, H.D. (1993). Physiotherapy management of whiplash injuries. In R.W. Teasell & A.P. Shapiro (Eds.), *Cervical flexion-extension/whiplash injuries* (pp. 501–516). Phildelphia: Hanley & Belfus.

Blanchard, E.B. (1994). Behavioral medicine and health psychology. In A.E. Bergin & Z.H. Garfield (Eds.), *Handbook of psychotherapy and behavior change*. New York: John Wiley & Sons.

Bogduk, N., & Marsland, A. (1986). On the concept of the third occipital headache. *Journal of Neurology, Neurosurgery, and Psychology. 49,* 775–780.

Bogduk, N. (1982). The clinical anatomy of the cervical dorsal rami. *Spine, 7,* 319–330.

Cheshire, W.P., Abashian, S.W., & Mann, J.D. (1994). Botulinum toxin in the treatment of myofascial pain syndrome. *Pain, 59*(1), 65–69.

Daly, E., &Wulff, J. (1987). Treatment of a post-traumatic headache. *British Journal of Medical Psychology, 60*(Pt 1), 85–88.

Dimitroulis, G., Gremillion, H.A., Dolwick, M.F., & Walter, J.H. (1995). Temporomandibular disorder. 2. Non-surgical treatment. *Australian Dental Journal 40*(6), 372–376.

Duckro, P.N., Tait, R., Margolis, R.B., & Silversintz, S. (1985). Behavioral treatment of headache following occupational trauma. *Headache, 25,* 180–183.

Dvorak, J., & Orelli, F.V. (1985). How dangerous is manipulation to the cervical spine? Case report and results of a survey. *Man and Medicine, 1,* 1–14.

Evans, R.W. (1992). The post-concussion syndrome and the sequelae of mild head injury. *Neurologic Clinics, 10,* 815–847.

Fordyce, W.E. (1976). *Behavioral methods for chronic pain and illness*. St. Louis: Mosby.

Freeman, M.D., & Croft, A.C. (1997). The controversy over late whiplash: Are chronic symptoms after whiplash real? In M. Szpalsk & R. Gunzburg (Eds.) *Whiplash injuries*. New York: Lippincott-Raven.

Fricton, J.R. (1995). Management of masticatory myofascial pain. *Seminars in Orthodontics, 1*(4), 229–243.

Goldstein, J. (1991). Post-traumatic headache and the post-concussion syndrome. *Medical Clinics of North American. 75,* 641–651.

Gramling, S.E., Neblett, J., Grayson, R.L., & Townsend, D. (1996). Temporomandibular disorder: Efficacy of an oral habit reversal treatment program. *Journal of Behavioral Therapy and Experimental Psychiatry, 27,* 212–218.

Grayson, R.L. (1997, November). EMG biofeedback as a therapeutic tool in the process of cognitive behavioral therapy: Preliminary single case results. Poster presented at the Association for Advancement of Behavior Therapy (AABT), 31st annual convention, Miami, Florida.

Greenman, P.E. (1989). *Principles of manual medicine*. Baltimore: Williams & Wilkins.

Haas, D.C. (1993). Chronic post-traumatic headache. In J. Olesen, P. Tfelt-Hanson, & K.M.A. Welch (Eds.), *The headaches* (pp. 629–637). New York: Raven Press.

Ham, L.P., & Packard, R.C. (1996). A retrospective, follow-up study of biofeedback-assisted relaxation therapy in patients with post-traumatic headache. *Biofeedback Self Regulation, 21*(2), 93–104.

Headache Classification Committee of the International Headache Society. (1988). Classification and diagnostic criteria for headache disorders, cranial neuralgias and facial pain. *Cephalalgia. 8*(7).

Holroyd, K.A., & Andrasik, F. (1978). Coping and the self-control of chronic tension headache. *Journal of Consulting and Clinical Psychology. 5,*1036–1045.

Hong, C.Z., & Simons, D.G. (1998). Pathophysiologic and electrophysiologic mechanisms of myofascial trigger points. *Archives of Physical Medicine and Rehabilitation, 79,* 863–872.

Horn, L.J. (1992). Post-concussive headache. In I.J. Horn & N.D. Zasler, N.D. (Eds.), *Rehabilitation of post-concussive disorders* (pp. 69–88). Philadelphia: Hanley & Belfus.

Horowitz, M.B., & Yonas, H. (1993). Occipital neuralgia treated by intra-dural dorsal nerve root sectioning. *Cephalalgia. 13,* 354–360.

Jacome, D. (1986). Basilar artery migraine after uncomplicated whiplash injuries. *Headache, 26,* 515–516.

Jensen, O.K., Nielsen, F.F., & Vosmar, L. (1990). An open study comparing manual therapy with the use of cold packs in the treatment of post-traumatic headache. *Cephalalgia, 10,* 241–250.

Jensen, O.K., & Nielsen, F.F. (1990). The influence of sex and pre-traumatic headache on the incidence and severity of headache after head injury. *Cephalalgia, 10*(6), 285–293.

Lord, S.M., Barnsley, L., & Bogduk, N. (1993). Cervical zygapophseal joint pain in whiplash. In R.W. Teasell & A.P. Shapiro (Eds.), *Cervical flexion-extension/whiplash injuries* (pp. 355–372). Philadelphia: Hanley & Belfus.

Lord, S.M., Barnsley, L., & Bogduk, N. (1995). Percutaneous radiofrequency neurotomy in the treatment of cervical zygapophyseal joint pain: Aa caution. *Neurosurgery. 36*(4), 732–739.

Martelli, M.F,, Zasler, N.D., & MacMillan, P. (1998). Mediating the relationship between injury, impairment and disability: A vulnerability, stress and coping model of adaptation following brain injury. *NeuroRehabilitation: An interdisciplinary journal, 11*(1), 51–68.

Martin, P.R. (1993). *Psychological management of chronic headaches*. New York: The Guilford Press.

May, A., & Goadsby, P.J. (1999). The trigeminovascular system in humans: Pathophysiologic implications for primary headache syndromes of the neural influences on the cerebral circulation. *Journal of Cerebral Blood Flow and Metabolism, 19*(2), 115–127.

Medina, J.L. (1992). Efficacy of an individualized outpatient program in the treatment of chronic post-traumatic headache. *Headache. 32*(4):180–183.

Miller, L. (1993). *Psychotherapy of the brain injured patient*. New York: W.W. Norton.

Mitchell, B.S., Humphreys, B.K., & O'Sullivan, E. (1998). Attachments of the ligamentum nuchae to cervical posterior spinal dura and the lateral part of the occipital bone. *Journal of Manipulative Physiology and Therapy, 21*(3), 145–148, .

Packard, R. (1979). What does the headache patient want? *Headache, 19*, 370–374.

Packard, R.C., & Ham, L.P. (1993). Impairment rating for post-traumatic headache. *Headache, 33*, 359–364.

Packard, R.C., & Ham, L.P. (1997). Pathogenesis of post-traumatic headache and migraine: a common headache pathway? *Headache, 37*(3), 142–152.

Packard, R.C. (1999). Epidemiology and pathogenesis of post-traumatic headache. *Journal of Head Trauma Rehabilitation. 14*(1):9–21.

Packard, R.C. (1994). Post-traumatic headache. *Seminars in Neurology, 14*, 40–45.

Packard, R.C. (1992). Post-traumatic headache: permanency and relationship to legal settlement. *Headache, (10)*, 496–500.

Parker, R.S. (1995). The distracting effects of pain, headaches, and hyper-arousal upon employment after minor head injury. *Journal of Cognitive Rehabilitation. 13*(3), 14–23.

Penzien, D.B., Jeanetta, C.R., & Holroyd, K.A. (1993). Psychological assessment of the recurrent headache sufferer. In C.D. Tollison & R.S. Kunkel (Eds.), *Headache: Diagnosis and treatment*. Baltimore: Williams and Wilkins.

Radanov, B.P., Di Stefano, G., Schnidrig, A., et al. (1993). Factors influencing recovery from headache after common whiplash. *British Journal of Medicine, 307*,652–655.

Sessle, B.J. (1999) Neural mechanisms and pathways in craniofacial pain. *Canadian Journal of Neurological Science, 3*:S7–11.

Siegmund, G.P., King, D.J., Lawrence, J.M., Wheeler, J.P., Brault, J.R., & Smith, T.A. (1997). Head/neck kinematic response of human subjects in low-speed rear-end collisions (pp. 357–385). SAE paper 973341.

Tobin, D.L., Holroyd, K.A., Baker, A., Reynolds, R.V.C., & Holm, J.E. (1988). Development in clinical trial of a minimal contact, cognitive-behavioral treatment for tension headache. *Cognitive Therapy and Research, 12*, 325–339.

Travell, J.G., & Simons, D.G. (1983). *Myofascial pain and dysfunction: The trigger point manual*. Baltimore: Williams & Wilkins.

Vihayan, N. (1977). A new post-traumatic headache syndrome; clinical and therapeutic observations. *Headache, 17*, 19–22.

Waldman, S.D. (1991). The role of neural blockade in the evaluation and treatment of common headache and facial pain syndromes. *Headache Quarterly Current Treatment Research, 2*(4), 286–291.

World Health Organization. (1997). ICD-10 guide for headaches. *Cephalalgia. 17*(S19).

Yamaguchi, M. (1992). Incidence of headache and severity of head injury. *Headache, 32*(9), 427–431.

Zafonte, R.D., & Horn, L.J. (1999). Clinical assessment of post-traumatic headache. *Journal of Head Trauma Rehabilitation, 14*(1), 22–33.

Zasler, N.D. (1996). Post-traumatic headache: A pain in the brain? *i.e. Magazine. 3*(3), 8–23.

Zasler, N.D. (1999). Post-traumatic headache: Caveats and controversies. *Journal of Head Trauma Rehabilitation. 14*(1):1–8.

13

Orofacial Pain and Temporomandibular Disorders

Gary M. Heir, D.M.D.

HISTORICAL PERSPECTIVE

Head and facial pain has plagued mankind throughout recorded history. In ancient times it was believed that the victim's suffering was due to evil spirits and humors that invaded the cranium. Prayers of exorcism and the application of magic potions were often performed to drive away these demons and end the victim's misery.

The search for valid etiologies over those more mystical may have begun with Hippocrates who suggested that noxious vapors from the liver and other poorly understood maladies were the cause of head pain. The release of these vapors was accomplished by the use of leeches, bleeding, and in extreme cases trephination; however, at least according to Hippocrates, these were the remedies of choice. The term *hemicrania* is attributed to the ancient Roman physician Galen, and the origins of the term *migraine* may also be traced back to this period (Kiester, 1989).

During the ensuing centuries there was slow but steady progress in the understanding of head and facial pain. The use of analgesics began in the 13th century and evolved to the use of cocaine and the discovery of other analgesic preparations, but these efforts to relieve pain did not explain its mechanism.

Thomas Willis offered a "vascular hypothesis" in the 17th century (Frank, 1990). He suggested that head pain was due to swelling of blood vessels in the cranium, a theory that was generally accepted within the medical community and became the basis for much of the 20th century pharmacotherapies. In fact, by the 19th century

the physician's approach to managing headache and facial pain was almost exclusively pharmacological, and medications were selected based on their efficacy with little understanding of their pharmacodynamics. In modern times it was the work of Wolff (1948) and his contemporaries who continued this pursuit.

While the debate as to the etiology and treatment of migraine headache continued, little effort was made to understand other forms of head and facial pain. Facial pain was thought to be mostly due to dental causes or, in some cases, thought to be of psychogenic origin. Attention was first drawn to facial pain of nonheadache and nonodontogenic origin in 1934 when Costen published his treatise on a syndrome of ear and sinus symptoms dependent on disturbed function of the temporomandibular joint (TMJ).

Now we are in a new era. Science is beginning to understand the mechanisms of pain transduction, transmission, modulation, and perception. With a more clear understanding of pain mechanisms, the healthcare sciences have been able to identify more specific etiologic factors and conditions for our patient's complaints.

For the purpose of this discussion, orofacial pain is categorized by the systems from which it may seem to arise (Merrill, 1997). This discussion reviews head and facial pain of odontogenic, vascular, musculoskeletal, neurogenous, and psychogenic origin. By evaluating symptoms on this basis, the source of the patient's suffering may be identified and appropriate therapeutic measure may be instituted.

0-8493-0926-3/02/$0.00+$1.50
© 2002 by CRC Press LLC

OROFACIAL PAIN

Orofacial pain can be acute and related to trauma, dental injuries, dental pathologies, and acute dysfunction of the masticatory system. Acute orofacial pain may include dental pathology, dysfunction of the masticatory musculature, and temporomandibular disorders (TMD). Acute pain is more readily diagnosed and treated, and often there is an identifiable precipitating event associated with the onset of acute symptoms that leads the clinician to the source of the problem.

Chronic orofacial pain is more difficult to diagnose, and the source of the patient's complaint is frequently elusive. The clinician must have the knowledge and clinical expertise to accurately pursue the assessment, diagnosis, and treatment of complex chronic orofacial pain and dysfunction disorders, including oromotor and jaw behavior disorders, chronic head, neck, and facial pain, and have knowledge of the underlying pathophysiology and mechanisms of these disorders (American Academy of Orofacial Pain [AAOP], 1998).

Chronic, complex orofacial pain may be of musculoskeletal, vascular, neurogenous, and infrequently psychological origin. There is a clear distinction between complex chronic orofacial pain and acute pain.

ACUTE PAIN

Acute pain is biologically useful. It occurs as a result of a noxious mechanical, thermal, or chemical stimulus. The symptoms and history of the onset of pain help in assessing the problem. A diagnosis for the cause of acute pain is facilitated by an assessment of the location, the duration, and the intensity of the patient's pain. Treatment efforts vary depending on the diagnosis; however, the diagnostic process is usually not difficult.

The acute pain of an infected tooth or an acute dislocation of the TMJ does not present as a significant diagnostic problem. The onset of pain symptoms presents in such a way that the diagnostic process is fairly clear.

The emotional reaction to acute pain is also somewhat predictable. The reaction to the sudden onset of acute pain is anxiety. There is fear that the sudden onset of spontaneous pain represents a life-threatening illness or that pain after trauma is due to a serious injury. However, once the patient understands the source of pain and the clinician acts to alleviate the cause and symptoms, the patient's anxiety dissipates.

CHRONIC PAIN

Unlike acute pain, chronic pain has no biological utility. Chronic pain may not be due to nociception or central neural input. The location of pain does not aid in the diagnosis. The patient may feel as though something is wrong in his or her life. Chronic pain has biological ramifications as well as sociocultural and psychological effects (Grzesiak, 1991).

Chronic pain is both a cognitive and emotional experience and can be destructive. Management may be difficult. Patients develop chronic pain syndromes that rule their lives. Chronic pain patients regularly abuse the healthcare system, overuse medications, and have difficulty with interpersonal relationships. Chronic pain is inevitably depressing, but may be synchronous with depression and not caused by it. The longer pain continues, the deeper the depression may be. Chronic pain monopolizes the patient's attention, compromising behavior and thinking. Expectations for recovery are poor (Wall, 1999).

In practice, the chronic pain patient with psychological affect may be identified by a variety of factors. The duration of their pain is longer than would be expected and, if associated with illness or injury, extends beyond the time required for normal healing or recovery. Chronic pain patients tend to dramatize their complaints. They may exaggerate symptoms verbally or demonstrate compromised functional ability beyond what would be expected. Chronic pain patients provide a history of a variety of diagnostic failures and present as a diagnostic dilemma. There may be a history of excessive use of medications both by prescription or over-the-counter preparations. Chronic pain patients demonstrate dependence on family and friends, become withdrawn, and avoid painful or potentially painful activities. Depression is evident; decision making, antisocial behavior, and rejection by friends and family may also become evident with a carefully elicited history (Rosch, 2000).

Although a psychological diagnosis may be inappropriate if made by a healthcare practitioner not trained in psychology, recognition of the emotional components of chronic pain should prompt an appropriate referral for additional assessment.

ODONTOGENIC PAIN

It is not the purpose of this chapter to discuss odontogenic pain. However, inasmuch as dental pain is the primary etiologic factor in the production of facial pain, a brief discussion is required.

Consider the tooth as a specialized primary afferent nociceptor. A tooth is a hard container composed of enamel, dentin, and cementum. It is firmly attached to the supporting bone by the periodontal ligament. This "hard case" contains the dental pulp. The dental pulp is the principal source of pain within the mouth. This pink, coherent, soft tissue is dependent on the hard tissues of the tooth for its for protection. Once exposed, it is extremely sensitive to all stimuli (Ogilvie, 1969).

Although the dental pulp is often referred to as the nerve, it is not just a mass of raw nociceptive neural tissue. The pulpal tissue of the tooth resembles other loose connective tissues of the body more than it differs from them. There are connective tissue cells of various types, as well as intercellular components made up of ground substance and fibers. Among this lies a complex network of blood vessels, lymphatics, and nerve tissue (Seltzer, 1988). Stimulation of the dental pulp elicits a painful response.

Not all dental pain is a consequence of direct stimulation of the pulpal tissue. Inasmuch as this complex structure has great similarities to other tissues in the body, it responds in a like fashion to injury or trauma. The response is inflammation and/or necrosis.

The classic signs of inflammation — heat, swelling, and, of course, pain — may all be manifest as a result of pulpal pathology or injury (Byers & Narhi, 1999). The endodontist may also bear witness to the fourth sign of inflammation, redness. Erythema is a classic characteristic of an inflamed pulp, which may be observed upon its removal during endodontic therapy. Unlike an injury to any other part of the body, once inflammation of the dental pulp begins, the swelling tissue is trapped in the hard container and, in effect, has no place to go.

An injured or diseased dental pulp may go through several stages, all of which produce pain. These stages of pulpal involvement respond differently to diagnostic testing. The clinically normal pulp is vital to testing procedures, responsive to a variety of excitations, but free of spontaneous symptoms. Histologically, it is free of any inflammatory changes.

Mild irritation of the pulpal tissue, such as caused by thermal, mechanical, or chemical irritants, may cause a dental pulp to become hyperreactive to stimulation. Of these, dental caries or tooth decay is the most familiar. In the case of stronger irritants or more advanced decay, a transitory hyperemia or reversible inflammation may occur (Scimone, 1976). An acute reversible pulpitis may become chronic and lead to pulpal necrosis and pain.

Orofacial pain of dentigerous origin may be referred throughout the face by such inflamed or diseased teeth. Various stages of dental caries may provide adequate etiology for these pulpalgias. Therefore, the patient who presents to the physician or dental office with facial pain must have a complete examination of the dentition.

The periodontal membrane, otherwise known as the periodontal ligament, responds to stimulation in the same manner as any other ligament. In fact the teeth are attached to the supporting bone by the periodontal ligament, forming a synarthrodial joint. Irritation of this generously innervated tissue results in the classic musculoskeletal symptoms of dull, aching pain. This pain is localizable to a general area and may be provoked by percussing the suspected teeth. Increased pressure on a tooth with a peri-

odontal inflammation or infection within the periodontal space produces or increases pain.

The mechanisms of periodontal injuries are either mechanical or chemical (infection). One of the most common sources of periodontal irritation is trauma from occlusion often caused by premature dental contacts or bruxism.

Bruxism may produce pain in the masticatory system, as has been documented experimentally (Christensen, 1971). The pain may arise from muscles, periodontium, and TMJ. Pain produces unbalanced, sustained, abnormal muscle activity, increasing the risk of injury (Arima, Svensson, & Arendt-Nielsen, 1999).

As stated, pain from the periodontal ligament space is musculoskeletal in character. Chronic pain arising from the periodontal ligament has the ability to refer pain to other structures. The pattern of tooth reference pain is well documented in the literature (Simons, Travell, & Simons, 1998).

From the preceding discussion of dental pain, it may be noted that an attempt is made to categorize the various symptoms as arising from vascular, neurogenous, or musculoskeletal origin. This technique is also suggested when considering head and facial pain of nondental causes.

HEADACHE

"Headache has been called the most common medical complaint of civilized man" (Dalessio, 1987). If dental structures are not the primary source of facial pain, vascular head, and facial pain, which includes such entities as migraine and cluster headaches, must be considered next. Familiarity with these entities is important because their region of onset often overlaps dental and masticatory structures.

The evaluation and management of headache disorders are adequately discussed in another section of this text. However, a basic review of various headache disorders that may present as orofacial pain is provided.

The mechanism of headache of vascular origin is currently best explained as a sterile inflammation of the trigeminovascular system (Buzzi & Moskowitz, 1993; Moskowitz, 1993). Pharmacological management of these patients is often possible. Although, it is incumbent on the dental practitioner to have the ability to recognize migraine, as well as other head or facial pains of vascular origin, the responsibility for final diagnosis and treatment of these disorders should be with our medical colleagues.

It should also be remembered that there are a number of painful vascular conditions of the face that either produce pain referred to the teeth or may on occasion affect oral vasculature, thus producing a perception of toothaches or TMD. These include facial migraine, cluster headache, angina pectoris, and temporal arteritis. These conditions must be recognized and treated (Buxbaum, Myslinski, & Myers, 1989).

MIGRAINE

Included in the classification of vascular disorders that are often confused with masticatory pain are migraine headaches. Migraine is an idiopathic, recurring headache disorder that occurs in attacks that may typically last from 4 hours to as many as 3 days. This headache is usually unilateral, moderately severe, and pulsating in quality. Migraine is generally aggravated by routine physical activity and may be associated with nausea, photophobia, and phonophobia. It is not uncommon for the migraineur to seek a dental consultation for relief from what is perceived to be dental or masticatory musculature pain.

Migraine with aura has similar characteristics, as does migraine without aura. The difference in this case is that the headache is normally preceded by a preheadache neurosensorial disturbance. This may be a series of idiopathic, recurring neurological symptoms, which usually develops over a 5- to 20-min period and may last less than 1 hour. "Nausea is the complaint of the vast majority of patients; vomiting, in addition to nausea, occurs in just over one half of the patients. These gastrointestinal disturbances usually start sometime after the onset of the pain but occasionally precede the headache" (Raskin, 1988, p. 44).

A typical aura may consist of visual disturbances, hemisensory symptoms, hemiparesis, dysphasia, or combinations of these phenomena. Gradual development, duration of less than 1 h, and complete reversibility characterized the aura, which is associated with this form of headache. Differential diagnosis of migraine headache includes myalgia, myositis or myofascial pain of the masticatory musculature, TMDs, and tooth pain.

CLUSTER HEADACHE

The presentation of cluster headache is classic. Cluster headache consists of attacks of severe, strictly unilateral pain in and around the eye and/or temporal region. This temporal, periorbital pain is frequently confused with a masticatory or dental pain. The attacks may last from a few minutes to as much as 3 h. The attacks occur from once every other day up to eight times per day. They are associated with one or more of the following: conjunctival injection, lacrimation, nasal congestion, rhinorrhea, forehead and facial sweating, miosis, ptosis, and eyelid edema. Attacks occur in series lasting for weeks or months. These are the so-called cluster periods. These periods are separated by periods of remission, which may last months or years. Cluster headache predominately affects men in a ratio of 5:1 to women. This is in contrast to migraine, which predominately affects women in a similar ratio. Differential diagnosis of cluster headache includes dental infection and acute pain of the masticatory musculature.

CHRONIC PAROXYSMAL HEMICRANIA

Another benign headache disorder known as chronic paroxysmal hemicrania has characteristics similar to cluster. Whereas cluster headache occurs more commonly in men, chronic paroxysmal hemicrania is more common in women. The attacks are more frequent and of shorter duration but distributed in similar areas as symptoms associated with cluster headache. Between attacks, there may be a continuous, sore feeling in the usually painful areas: the ocular–periocular regions, the forehead and temporal area, neck, and shoulders (Sjaastad, 1987). One diagnostic criterion of this form of headache is that it is invariably relieved by indomethacin. Differential diagnosis of chronic paroxysmal hemicrania is the same as for cluster headache.

LOWER-HALF MIGRAINE

Other forms of facial pain of vascular origin may include migraine of the midfacial region sometimes called lower-half migraine. Patients with this form of vascular pain report pain in the jaw and neck periorbitally and in the maxilla. There may be tenderness of the carotid artery (Raskin, 1988, Chapter 11); therefore, this disorder is known as carotidynia (Fay, 1932). As with migraine, this condition predominately affects women. The symptoms are of a dull pain with superimposed throbbing that may occur once or several times weekly. Exacerbations may last minutes to hours. Differential diagnosis includes TMD, pain of the myofascial pain, and masticatory musculature and dental pain.

TENSION-TYPE HEADACHE

Tension-type headache is described as recurrent episodes of headache lasting minutes to days. The pain is typically pressing or tightening in quality. Discomfort extends into the face and masticatory musculature. Many individuals describe this sensation as similar to wearing a tight hat. It is of mild or moderate intensity, is bilateral in location, and does not usually worsen with routine physical activity. Nausea is absent, but photophobia and phonophobia may be present.

The patient with tension-type headache may seek the advice of a dentist on the referral of a physician. Chronic, muscle tensionlike headaches such as these may have the capacity to refer pain to the masticatory structures (Simons, Travell, & Simons, 1998). Again, care should be taken to ensure that the patient's complaint is truly a result of masticatory function and not simply referred to the face and jaw from other areas. Differential diagnosis includes myofascial pain and dental pain.

GIANT CELL (TEMPORAL) ARTERITIS

A discussion of cephalgic and facial pain is not complete without some mention of temporal, or giant cell, arteritis. This condition is usually attended by the onset of a new headache in an individual of at least 50 years of age. One or both of the temporal regions are involved. Moderate to severe headache, polymyalgia, and claudication of the masticatory muscles may be present. The occurrence of this symptom is significant, because claudication of the masticatory musculature may be diagnosed as a TMD. There may be a swollen and tender scalp artery, usually the superficial temporal artery, which unless carefully palpated may mimic tenderness of the temporalis muscle. The patient with giant cell arteritis may have an elevated red blood cell count (RBC) sedimentation rate. A temporal artery biopsy is more definitive for giant cell arteritis (Headache Classification Committee of International Headache Society, 1998). This form of headache must not be overlooked because it has a potential for dire consequences. Untreated, temporal arteritis may cause blindness, stroke, or death.

If a patient of 50 years or older presents with a complaint of dull temporal pain, fatigue of the masticatory muscles, and joint pain and reports headache of recent onset, which is chronic, and possibly worsening, temporal arteritis must be ruled out. Differential diagnosis includes myofascial pain and dental pain.

MUSCULOSKELETAL PAIN

As stated, the dentition and supporting structures of the teeth are the primary source of facial pain. If a thorough dental evaluation eliminates the possibility of odontogenic pain, and facial pain of vascular origin has been eliminated as a possibility, pain of musculoskeletal origin should be considered next. Acute muscle pain is easily diagnosed and managed; however, the management of chronic muscle pain can be difficult. Masticatory pain of musculoskeletal origin can arise from the TMJs, the masticatory musculature, or both (Delcanho, 1995).

TEMPOROMANDIBULAR DISORDERS

TMD is defined as clinical problems that involve the masticatory musculature, the TMJs and associated structures, or both. TMDs are considered the most common musculoskeletal disorder causing orofacial pain. Pain may be of muscular origin arising from the muscles of mastication or referred to the masticatory musculature from cervical and/or shoulder structures. Myogenous pain occurs more frequently than articular disorders.

Articular disorders of the TMJs often coexist with masticatory muscle pain. Articular disorders of the TMJs include disk displacement disorders, arthritic and degenerative changes, and neoplasm (AAOP, 1996).

Myogenous pain disorders affecting the masticatory musculature are no different from those that affect other musculoskeletal structures. They include, myofascial pain, fibromyalgia, myositis, myospasm, and local myalgia.

The quality of musculoskeletal pain is deep, constant, dull, and occasionally sharp. The most important features of musculoskeletal orofacial pain are that it is made worse with movement of the jaws and that the pain is provocable. Movement of the affected joint or muscle can reproduce musculoskeletal pain. The intensity of pain is true to the degree of provocation.

In addition to the increase of pain with physical activity, chronic pain of the masticatory musculature can refer to other areas. Referred pain is the phenomenon of perception of pain at a site that is not the source of pain. Referred pain is diffuse and poorly localized. Referred pain is characteristic of myofascial pain.

MYOFASCIAL PAIN

Myofascial pain is a regional muscle disorder that is the most common cause of persistent pain in the head, face, and neck. It is characterized by one or more hyperirritable sites within the muscle called myofascial trigger points.

A myofascial trigger point is a tender point of localized deep tenderness located in a taut band of skeletal muscle, tendon, or ligament. Myofascial trigger points are approximately 2 to 5 mm in diameter and when provoked can refer pain to another region known as a zone of reference. The zone of reference is distant from the involved muscle and may not be in the same dermatome. The pattern of pain referral is reproducible and consistent, and serves as a guide to locate the source of the myofascial pain.

Myofascial pain is also characterized by increased muscle fatigue and stiffness. The patient may exhibit a mildly restricted range of motion. Pain may be elicited when the muscle is stretched. The patient may also report a sense of subjective weakness in the affected muscle or muscles. Myofascial pain can be localized involving one or two myofascial trigger points or generalized due to muscle injury. It may coexist with other conditions such as cervical or facet joint injuries.

There are two types of myofascial trigger points. A latent myofascial trigger point is painful at the site of palpation but is not associated with referred pain. An active myofascial trigger point is painful at the site of palpation and also causes spontaneous referred pain during palpation and muscle use. Myofascial trigger points cycle between an active and a latent state.

TEMPOROMANDIBULAR JOINT

Intracapsular disorders of the TMJs result from abnormal biomechanics. To appreciate the complexity of intracapsular disorders of the TMJ, a fundamental understanding of normal anatomy and biomechanics is required.

The TMJ is a synovial joint. That is, it is encapsulated and stress bearing. It is possibly the most complex joint in the body. The articulating surfaces are covered with fibrocartilage. It is a compound joint with four separate articulating surfaces; the superior aspect of the mandibular condyle functions on the inferior surface of the interarticular disk. The superior surface of the disk functions on the posterior slope of the articular eminence of the temporal bone. The disk is unique to this joint. It separates the intracapsular space into an inferior and a superior joint compartment. These are separate and isolated from one another by the disk and anterior and posterior attachment tissue. The retrodiscal tissue, a mass of loosely packed, highly innervated and vascularized connective tissue, occupies the posterior aspect of the joint space. The uppermost layer of this posterior discal tissue is composed of elastic fibers. This elastic layer composes what is called the superior retrodiscal lamina.

The interarticular disk is held tightly to the mandibular condyle by a medial and lateral colateral ligament. These ligaments are intimately incorporated within the capsular ligament. An injury to the capsule is painful.

The position of the disk should be between the condyle and the articular eminence during all mandibular movements. A displacement of the disk, typically anterior to the condyle, is the cause of most of joint sounds perceived during joint function.

ARTICULAR DISK DISORDERS

Intracapsular disorders of the TMJs involve partial or total displacement of the articular disk, inflammation of the retrodiscal tissues, and degenerative changes of the articular surfaces.

NORMAL BIOMECHANICS

The TMJ is a ginglymoid arthrodial joint. It has a rotational as well as translatory movement. The mandibular condyle is ovoid in shape, although the shape of the condyle varies from patient to patient and there may be asymmetrical condyles in the same patient.

The ovoid- or football-shaped condyle functions with the glenoid fossa of the temporal bone. The fossa is a depressed area at the base of the skull that is delineated by the TMJ capsular ligaments. The anterior aspect of the fossa includes the articular eminence, a raised ramplike structure anterior to the depressed area of the fossa. The posterior wall of the glenoid fossa is bounded by thin bone that separates the fossa from the external auditory meatus. The lateral aspect of the joints is enclosed within the capsular ligament and the medial aspect of the joint is osseous.

Interposed between the condyle and fossa is a fibrocartilagenous interarticular disk. This disk is attached to the mandibular condyle by medial and lateral collateral ligaments. This allows the disk to move anteriorly and posteriorly on the condylar head, but does not allow the disk to move away from an intimate contact with the articular surface of the condyle. Attached anteriorly to the superior lateral pterygoid muscle and posteriorly to the fossa, the disk separates the synovial space of the joint into superior and inferior compartments.

During normal function, the mandibular condyle starts its movement from a closed mouth position with the articular disk seated on the posterior slope of the mandibular condyle. Movement begins with a rotation of the condyle against the inferior articular surface of the disk. Translation combined with rotation allows the condyle–disk assembly to slide down the articular eminence to a more forward and downward position. Translation and rotation allow for full maximum opening.

ABNORMAL BIOMECHANICS

TMDs consist of three basic components: limitation of function, joint pain, and joints sounds. Limited function may result from muscle guarding or contraction following overuse or injury. Contracture, splinting, or spasm of the mandibular elevator muscles result in limited mandibular range of motion. Pain is not always present. Limitation of mandibular range of motion due to disk displacement may also occur in the absence of pain.

NEUROGENOUS PAIN

The face is the most richly innervated structure of the body and represents the majority of input to the somatosensory cortex of the brain. Facial pain is mediated by the trigeminal nerve. Specifically, nociception is transmitted to the central nervous system via two types of nerves or primary afferent nociceptors. These are the thinly myelinated A-delta fibers and the unmyelinated C fibers (Sessle, 1999).

Under normal conditions, primary afferent nociceptors are not responsive to nonnoxious stimuli. To stimulate or transduce an action potential, the primary afferent nociceptive receptor must be activated to threshold by a tissue damaging, or potentially tissue-damaging, stimulus. Such stimuli can be via mechanical deformation of tissue, noxious temperature, or chemical injury.

When an adequate noxious stimulus is encountered, a cascade of events occurs that sensitizes the nociceptive nerve ending, thereby making it receptive to further stimulation and allowing transmission information to the central nervous system. This information is modulated in the dorsal horn of the spinal chord where it is then transmitted to a second-order neuron. The peripheral sensitization is the result of the release of a variety of excitatory mediators, neuropeptides associated with inflammation, and the endogenous release of additional inflammatory mediators such as substance P. The presence of these neuropeptides in the area of the injury results in the perception of pain for the injured area until healing occurs. Once the tissue damage has resolved or the noxious stimulus has abated, peripheral sensitization ends and pain abates.

NEUROPATHIC PAIN

The mechanisms underlying neuropathic pain differ from those involved in "normal" pain. Neuropathic pain results from a dysfunction of the transmission system that carries nociception from the periphery. Neuropathic pain does not require a noxious stimulus, but may be self-propagating. It is maintained by injury or functional abnormalities of the pain transmission system (Pertes & Heir, 1991). Pain may be severe, have a delayed onset after injury, and persist for years or even decades after noxious stimulation has ceased and the damaged tissue has healed (Benoliel & Sharav, 1998).

Severity and chronicity of neuropathic pain are not clearly related to a specific etiology and may result from a variety of causes. Possible mechanisms for neuropathic pain include continued sensitization of peripheral nociceptive receptors and central neuroplasticity (Sessle, 2000). This suggests the development or activation of aberrant inputs to central, second-order pain transmission neurons. There can be a loss of afferent inhibition known as deafferentation syndrome. In deafferentation syndrome, nociceptive inputs produce an exaggerated response such as seen in postherpetic neuralgia. Neuropathic pain may also include activation of the sympathetic nervous system. In the case of sympathetically maintained pain, dysfunctional pain transmission cells are sensitized to the activity of the sympathetic system and respond with nociception (Sessle, 2000).

Neuropathic pain may be characterized by sensory deficit in the affected region or by pain, which may be bright, burning, and stimulating. Neuropathic pain may also present as dysesthesia or a mild, uncomfortable but nonpainful sensation, paresthesia, and numbness. Care must be taken in evaluating the patient with possible neuropathic pain, because differential diagnosis requires the elimination of myofascial and dental pain as the source of the patient's symptoms.

ATYPICAL ODONTALGIA

Atypical odontalgia (AO) is a poorly understood chronic pain disorder that presents as a persistent pain in apparently normal teeth and adjacent oral tissues. It is generally agreed that the term *atypical odontalgia* does not adequately describe this entity. At the time of the writing of this chapter, a taxonomy committee is hard at work to better define this

condition and provide a more descriptive and diagnostic nomenclature. It is postulated that AO is a neuropathic pain disorder (Graff-Radford & Solberg, 1992). Pain, often described as burning and spreading, may occur at the site of tooth extraction. Other concomitant factors may include traumatic injury, various routine dental procedures, endodontic therapy, endodontic surgery on teeth (apicoectomy), periodontal surgery, and dental implants (Vickers, Cousins, Walker, & Chisholm, 1998).

AO can also follow seemingly innocuous dental procedures such as crown preparation, cavity preparation, and periodontal scaling. It is more likely to develop in a tooth that was painful prior to dental intervention.

Most patients are 40- to 50-year-old females. AO is rare in younger age groups. These patients are usually examined and treated by a number of clinicians before being properly diagnosed. They often have a history of many failed dental treatments that serves to perpetuate the pain instead of relieving it. It is not uncommon for a patient with AO to have received multiple endodontic therapies and surgery, as well as multiple extractions.

Clinical characteristics of AO are continuous or almost continuous pain in a tooth or tooth site, with constant, dull, aching pain of moderate to severe intensity. There may be an associated hyperesthesia (tooth is tender to finger pressure). The clinical findings, chief complaints, and fact that pain has been present for more than 4 months with no obvious local dental cause lead to this diagnosis. The patient must have a negative clinical examination, normal radiograph, and no history or evidence of significant psychopathology. Somatic nerve block or local anesthesia does not entirely relieve the discomfort.

There are several theories for the etiology of this condition that include neurovascular, psychological, and neuropathic diagnoses. It is unlikely that AO is related to migraine, because AO is a continuous pain and migraine is episodic.

Scientific support for a psychological basis for AO is lacking. There is no increase in Minnesota Mulitphasic Personality Inventory (MMPI) scales when compared with other chronic pain patients.

Deafferentation is the most likely mechanism. Deafferentation is the partial or total loss of an afferent nerve supply from a particular area. Trauma to a nerve commonly follows dental procedures involving the dentin, pulp, or periodontal tissues. Although this type of injury may be reversible within a short time, in a small percentage of patients (less than 3%) who have undergone a dental procedure, pain persists even after healing has apparently occurred. Pain may not appear for weeks, months, or even a year after the procedure.

There may also be involvement of the sympathetic nervous system. Sympathetically maintained pain (SMP) involves a neuropathology process where the activity of the sympathetic system activates injured primary afferent nociceptors. Blockade of the sympathetic symptom may provide relief. Diagnosis of AO requires the elimination any odontogenic causes. If a dental source of the pain is not found, no dental treatment should be initiated. Differential diagnosis includes trigeminal neuralgia, facial or midface migraine, myofascial referred tooth pain, maxillary sinusitis, and TMDs.

BURNING MOUTH SYNDROME (BMS)

A review of the medical and dental literature suggests that over 40% of postmenopausal women suffer from symptoms of burning tongue or mouth. On examination, these patients have negative clinical findings for abnormalities or pathology of the oral cavity or mucogingival structures. The only common feature is the history of the onset of their symptoms after menopause.

It has been postulated that the etiology for BMS is a result of changes in estradiol levels that may have a detrimental effect on the function of the special sensory component of CN VII (chorda tympani) (Grushka, Epstein, & Kawale, 2000).

Symptoms of intraoral burning are considered idiopathic. However, a growing body of evidence indicates that BMS it is a neuropathic disorder resulting from disinhibition of nociception regulated by interactions between taste centers in the brain and CN-VII, V, and IX. BMS has also been associated with hormonal imbalance, trauma, nutritional disorders, and positive psychological findings. Conditions that may mimic BMS include denture irritation, infection, oral lesions, xerostomia, and mouth breathing, as well as gastric, rheumatologic, and other disorders. Treatment strategies depend on an accurate diagnosis (Nasri et al., 2000).

SUMMARY

Complex chronic orofacial pain syndromes have multiple etiologies and treatment possibilities. When examining and managing orofacial pain patients, it is important to set goals to achieve an acceptable degree of success. The first goal is to establish a specific diagnosis. This goal can only be achieved if the clinician has a basic understanding of, and familiarity with, those conditions that can lead to orofacial pain. Without knowledge of musculoskeletal and other systemic disorders that may cause orofacial pain, a differential diagnosis cannot be made. Having missed the first goal, diagnosis, the treating doctor cannot logically establish the second goal, management of the disorder. When an accurate diagnosis is made, the correct treatment often becomes apparent (Bell, 1980).

In some cases, despite all our best efforts and scientific knowledge, there are times when we are at a loss to help our patients. Where our skills and knowledge fail us is where our humanity must begin.

"I think that the lives of all people are linked to each other. We are always helping and have been helped by others. We can always do something to help. It is not difficult. Many times it is enough just to say something good, give a little attention, listen a little or just smile" (C. Nasri, personal communication, June 1999).

REFERENCES

American Academy of Orofacial Pain. (1998). J.P. Okeson (Ed.), *Orofacial pain, guidelines for assessment, diagnosis, and management*. Carol Stream, IL: Quintessence Books.

Arima, T., Svensson, P., & Arendt-Nielsen, L. (1999). Experimental grinding in healthy subjects: A model for post-exercise jaw muscle soreness. *Journal of Orofacial Pain, 13*(2), 104–114.

Bell, W. (1980). Lecture notes on Differential diagnosis of facial pain.

Benoliel, R., & Sharav, Y. (1998, November). Neuropathic orofacial pain. *Compendium of Continuing Education in Dentistry, 19*(11), 1099–1104.

Buxbaum, J., Myslinski, D., & Myers, D.E. (1989). Dental management of orofacial pain. In C.D. Tollison (Ed.), *Handbook of chronic pain management* (pp. 297–319). Baltimore: Williams & Wilkins.

Buzzi, M.G. & Moskowitz, M.A. (1993). The trigemino-vascular system and migraine. *Cerebrovascular and Brain Metabolism Reviews, 5*(3), 159–177.

Byers, M.R., & Narhi, M.V. (1999). Dental injury models: Experimental tools for understanding neuroinflammatory interactions and polymodal nociceptor functions, *Critical Reviews in Oral Biology and Medicine, 10*(1), 4–39.

Christensen, V. (1971). Facial pain and internal pressure of the masseter muscle in experimental bruxism in man. *Archives of Oral Biology, 16,* 102.

Costen, J.B. (1934). A syndrome of ear and sinus symptoms dependent upon disturbed function of the temporomandibular joint. *Annals of Otology, Rhinology, and Laryngology, 43,* 1–15.

Dalessio, D.J. (Ed.). (1987). *Wolff's headache and other head pain* (5th ed.). New York: Oxford University Press.

Delcanho, R.E. (1995). Masticatory muscle pain: A review of clinical features, research findings and possible mechanisms. *Australian Prosthodontic Journal, 9,* 49–59.

Fay, T. (1932). Atypical facial neuralgia, A syndrome of vascular pain. *Annals of Otolaryngology, Rhinology, and Laryngology, 41,* 1030–1062.

Frank, R.G., Jr. (1990). Thomas Willis and his circle: Brain and mind in seventeenth-century medicine. In G.S. Rousseau (Ed.), *The languages of Psyche: Mind and body in enlightenment thought*. Berkeley: University of California Press.

Graff-Radford, S.B., & Solberg, W.K. (1992). Atypical odontalgia. *Journal of Craniomandibular Disorders, 6*(4), 260–265.

Grushka, M., Epstein, J., & Kawalc, J. (2001). Burning mouth syndrome. In S. Silverman, Jr., L.R. Eversole, & E. Truelove (Eds.), *Essentials of oral medicine* (pp. 354–358). Hamilton, Ontario: B.C. Decker.

Grzesiak, R.C. (1991). Psychologic considerations in temporomandibular dysfunction. A biopsychosocial view of symptom formation. *Dental Clinics of North America, 35*(1), 209–226.

Headache Classification Committee of the International Headache Society (1998). Classification and diagnostic criteria for headache disorders, cranial neuralgias and facial pain. *Cephalalgia, 8* (Suppl. 7).

Kiester, E., Jr. (1987, December). Doctors close in on the mechanisms behind headache. *The Smithsonian Magazine*, 175–190.

Merrill, R.L. (1997). Orofacial pain mechanisms and their clinical application. *Dental Clinics of North America, 41*(2), 167–188.

Moskowitz, M.A. (1993). Neurogenic inflammation in the pathophysiology and treatment of migraine. *Neurology, 43*(6, Suppl. 3), S16-20.

Nasri, C., Okada, M., Oliveira, M.F., Formigoni, G., Teixeira, M.J., Siqueira, J.T.T., & Heir, G.M. (2000, May). *Burning mouth: A multi-disciplinary assessment*. Orofacial Pain Team, Division of Dentistry, Hospital das Clínicas, Medical School of the University of São Paulo, Brazil. Paper presented at the International Congress on Orofacial Pain, Seoul, Korea.

Ogilvie, A.L. (1969). Histology of the dental pulp. In J.L. Ingle (Ed.), *Endodontics*. Philadelphia: Lea & Febiger.

Pertes, R.A., & Heir, G.M. (1991). Chronic orofacial pain. A practical approach to differential diagnosis. *Dental Clinics of North America, 35*(1), 123–140.

Raskin, N.H. (1988). Facial pain, *Headache* (2nd ed.). New York: Churchill & Livingstone.

Rosch, P. (2000, September). The eight D's of chronic pain. Presented at the American Pain Management Society, Las Vegas.

Scimone, F.S. (1976). Bruxism, pulpal pain and restorative material. *Dental Survey, 52,* 62–63.

Seltzer, S. (1988). *Endodontology: Biologic considerations in endodontic procedures* (2nd ed.). Philadelphia: Lea & Febiger.

Sessle, B.J. (1999). Neural mechanisms and pathways in craniofacial pain. *Canadian Journal of Neurological Sciences, 26* (Suppl. 3), S7–11.

Sessle, B.J. (2000). Acute and chronic craniofacial pain: Brainstem mechanisms of nociceptive transmission and neuroplasticity, and their clinical correlates. *Critical Reviews in Oral Biology and Medicine, 11*(1), 57–91.

Simons, D.G., Travell, J.G., & Simons, L. (1998). *Myofascial pain and dysfunction: The trigger point manual* (2nd ed., Vol. 1). Baltimore: Lippincott, Williams & Wilkins.

Sjaastad, O. (1987). Chronic paroxysmal hemicrania and similar headaches. In D.J. Dalessio (Ed.), *Wolff's headache and other head pain*, (5th ed., pp. 131–135). New York: Oxford University Press.

Vickers, E.R., Cousins, M.J., Walker, S., & Chisholm, K. (1998). Analysis of 50 patients with atypical odontalgia. A preliminary report on pharmacological procedures for diagnosis and treatment. *Oral Surgery, Oral Medicine, Oral Pathology, Oral Radiology and Endodontics, 85*(1), 24–32.

Wall, P.D. (1999). *Pain: The science of suffering*. London: Weidenfelf & Nicolson.

Wolff, H.G. (1948). *Wolff's headache and other head pain*. New York: Oxford University Press.

————————14————————

Chinese Medicine and Acupuncture for Pain Management in HIV/AIDS

Misha R. Cohen, O.M.D., L.Ac.

CHINESE TRADITIONAL MEDICINE IN PAIN MANAGEMENT

Acupuncture and other forms of Chinese traditional medicine have been used for centuries to treat acute pain due to trauma, chronic pain due to injuries, and pain from organic illnesses.

In Chinese traditional medicine, pain is often associated with imbalances within the body that lead to a slowing down or blockage of the body's energy (Qi). This is known as Stagnant or Stuck Qi or with the blockage of Blood (Xue) due to an acute trauma or a worsening of the Stagnant Qi.

Pain can also be related to Damp accumulating in the Channels, to deficient Qi and Xue, to Stagnation of Cold, or to association with Heat or Damp Heat.

For example, peripheral neuropathy can be associated in the early stages with Damp in the Channels (associated with numbness), later with Heat or Cold, and — as it gets worse — Qi and Xue Deficiency-type numbness.

The most commonly used treatment in Chinese traditional medicine and acupuncture is to unblock the Qi or Xue to relieve the pain. However, removing Dampness, clearing Heat, and resolving Damp Heat may also be treatment principles for pain management.

Western science has documented some ways in which acupuncture relieves pain — there are several mechanisms. The most notable is through stimulation of endorphins. Another mechanism is through stimulation of serotonin levels within the brain, which leads to a sense of well-being as well as pain relief.

ISSUES IN HIV/AIDS PAIN MANAGEMENT

In my experience, for the last 17 years of working with people with AIDS, the assembly of a comprehensive care team is central to the treatment of people with HIV/AIDS who are dealing with various pain syndromes. The person in charge is the person with HIV/AIDS, who is the captain of the healing team.

In conjunction with the captain, there is the need to develop a whole and unified team, which may include a number of practitioners as well as caregivers. In pain management in HIV/AIDS, it is important that there be an integrated approach because pain syndromes are often difficult to manage successfully and there is a relationship to the overall treatment plan for HIV/AIDS. If a person with AIDS is in pain, it is difficult to manage other aspects of care, and vice versa.

Therefore, the pain management team would include the person with HIV/AIDS as the captain; at least one Western physician; and then other members would be included such as a licensed acupuncturist and herbalist, a massage therapist, a physical therapist, an occupational therapist, a chiropractor, an osteopathic physician, and a psychologist.

In HIV/AIDS, it is important to always have a Western baseline for ongoing care and treatment. Some pain may be resolved through changes in medications (sometimes added, sometimes subtracted). Often the pain can be associated with opportunistic infections that need to be treated with pharmaceuticals or herbal medicine. Neurological pain, for example, may be mitigated through medication,

0-8493-0926-3/02/$0.00+$1.50
© 2002 by CRC Press LLC

herbs, acupuncture, other modalities, or a combination of several modalities.

CHINESE TRADITIONAL MEDICINE (CTM) EVALUATION AND TREATMENTS

When using Chinese traditional medicine as a main form of treatment in HIV/AIDS related pain syndromes, some or all of the following comprehensive protocols could be adopted:

- Evaluation/diagnosis
- Acupuncture
- Moxibustion
- Chinese herbal medicine
- Qi Gong/other exercises
- Professional massage
- Meditation
- Food therapy

Chinese medicine is a complete medical system with its own forms of diagnosis, treatment, prognosis, and therapies. Chinese medicine treatments address disharmonies using acupuncture, moxibustion, food therapy/diet, herbal remedies, Chinese exercise, and meditation along with Western therapies.

Acupuncture is the art of inserting fine sterile metal needles into certain body or ear points to control the body's energy flow. Acupuncture is relatively painless, often accompanied with a sensation of heaviness, warmth, or movement of energy at the point of insertion or along the energy channels. Acupuncture helps to relieve pain as well as rebalance energy and heal symptoms. Electrostimulation may also be used with acupuncture for pain.

Moxibustion is the burning of the common herb mugwort over areas of the body for stimulation or warmth. Heat packs may also be used during treatment.

Chinese herbal medicine can be used for all types of disease. There are thousands of Chinese herbs. Usually they are put together into formulas to have the most effect.

Exercise includes martial arts as well as more subtle movement such as Tai Ji, Qi Gong, and Yoga. Gym workouts or aerobic exercise are also suggested.

Meditation may include traditional Asian forms as well as relaxation exercises, hypnotherapy, and biofeedback. *Massage* includes meridian pressure such as Shiatsu, Qi Gong, or Thai massage or muscle massage. *Food* therapy focuses on improving digestion, increasing energy, and balancing body energy. Food therapy often increases the effect of other treatments.

ACUPUNCTURE IN HIV PAIN MANAGEMENT

Acupuncture is often used in HIV/AIDS for various kinds of pain management.

- Abdominal pain (which may be associated with diarrhea or opportunistic infections)
- Sinus pain/headaches (which may occur as part of chronic sinusitis)
- Peripheral neuropathy (which can include pain and numbness)
- Joint pain (which may be associated both with various viral coinfections or are a result of drug side effects)

HIV ASSOCIATED PERIPHERAL NEUROPATHY

Acupuncture is used in the clinic in conjunction with other therapies for treatment of peripheral neuropathy in people with HIV/AIDS. There have been varying studies on its use. Unfortunately, none have been well designed and undertaken long enough to show conclusive results.

However, our clinical observations give us the direction for further study.

The following studies are examples of some research to date.

RESEARCH

A PILOT STUDY OF ACUPUNCTURE FOR THE SYMPTOMATIC TREATMENT OF HIV ASSOCIATED PERIPHERAL NEUROPATHY[*]

- The objective is to study the outcome of patients receiving acupuncture treatment for the symptomatic treatment of HIV-related peripheral neuropathy, not due to drug toxicity. We evaluated objective and subjective nerve function and quality of life measurements.
- Methods include 39 patients receiving acupuncture twice weekly for 6 months in a nonrandomized observational study. No particular prescription was used, with the treatment choice left to the practitioner's discretion. Neurological and QOL assessments were completed at entry, months 2 and 6.
- In summary, 26 patients returned for the first follow-up at 2 months. The 13 lost to follow-up had more severe neuropathy and lower QOL scores than those who completed the treatment.
- Significant improvement was found for QST of the toe ($p = 0.05$). No trends were found in a subjective symptom list. Five of seven QOL scales showed improved (none were significant).
- In discussion, this study suggests that there may be a role for acupuncture as a treatment

---

[*] Jonathan Ammen, AMFAR study 1991–1992, reported at HIV/AIDS and Chinese Medicine Conference 1994.

for peripheral neuropathy...future controlled studies may help further define the efficacy of this method.

This 1994 pilot study shows potential to study peripheral neuropathy using traditional Chinese medicine diagnosis and treatment. However, the pilot was too short and uncontrolled to lead to any real conclusion. It is likely that in neuropathy, 8 weeks is too short a time to really see statistically significant differences. However, the conclusion appears to be consistent with this observation.

CHINESE MEDICINE IN THE TREATMENT OF PERIPHERAL NEUROPATHY*

- The issue is that peripheral neuropathy in the HIV/AIDS population is a serious and debilitating problem that requires an effective treatment protocol.
- The project at Quan Yin Healing Arts Center — a nonprofit community-based complementary medicine clinic that has delivered Chinese medicine for over 16 years in San Francisco — involved 533 HIV/AIDS clients treated in 1996, which included 66% of its client base. Over 75% of the people with HIV/AIDS at Quan Yin Healing Arts Center presented with peripheral neuropathy, from mild to severely debilitating. All women and men with neuropathy received a combination of treatments including one or more of the following interventions: acupuncture, electroacupuncture, massage therapy, moxibustion (an herbal heat therapy), and herbal medicine. Clients received treatment in time intervals from twice a month to three times a week.
- Results were chart reviews and surveys conducted by the executive director, revealing that over 75% of HIV + clients who were reviewed had reduced symptoms including decreased pain, reduced numbness, and increased mobility (including walking/running when unable to do so previously). Variations in response were related to total number of treatments, number of weeks of treatment, compliance with self-care (such as self-moxibustion), and combination of medications that caused neuropathy. Some patients were able to discontinue treatments for neuropathy after several sessions because they no longer had neuropathy-related complaints. Others needed ongoing care for

neuropathy, especially those who continued on drug combinations that are highly likely to cause neuropathy.
- Lessons learned include a combination of Chinese medicine therapies that appears to have a high effect rate in decreasing symptoms in HIV+ people with the serious debilitating problem of peripheral neuropathy. With the apparent rate of clinical success in a large number of clients, a controlled pilot study is recommended as a follow-up to this chart review and collection of surveys.

BODY ACUPUNCTURE IN HIV-RELATED PAIN SYNDROMES BY CONDITION

- General pain: Liver 3, Large Intestine 4 (Four Gates)
- Abdominal pain: Ren 12, Stomach 25, Liver 5, Zigong, Ren 4, Ren 6
- Epigastric pain: Ren 14, Ren 12, Stomach 34, Spleen 4, Spleen 6
- Sinus pain: Bitong, Yintang, Large Intestine 4, Large Intestine 20, Gallbladder 20, Du 23, Urinary Bladder 2, Stomach 3
- Hand neuropathy: Large Intestine 4, Zhongwan, Bafeng, San Jiao 5
- Foot neuropathy: Liver 3, Stomach 41, Spleen 6, Baxie
- Muscle pain whole body: Spleen 21
- Liver/costal pain: Liver 14, Gallbladder 24, Liver 13, Japanese Mu Points
- *Herpes Zoster*/Shingles: Liver 2, Liver 5, Surround the Dragon in the local area

BODY ACUPUNCTURE IN HIV-RELATED PERIPHERAL NEUROPATHY BY CTM SYNDROMES

- Four Gates for Pain: Liver 3, Large Intestine 4
- Damp in the Channels: Spleen 6, Spleen 9
- Deficient Qi and Xue: Stomach 36, Spleen 6, Kidney 3, Spleen 4
- Stagnant Xue: Spleen 10, Large Intestine 11, Spleen 6
- Stagnant Cold: Ren 6, Kidney 7
- Heat and Damp Heat: Liver 2, Liver 5, Large Intestine 11

BODY ACUPUNCTURE IN HIV-RELATED PAIN SYNDROMES

- Four Gates for Pain: Liver 3, Large Intestine 4
- Damp in the Channels: Spleen 6, Spleen 9

*Carla Wilson, Executive Director, Quan Yin Healing Arts Center, Poster Session, 12th International AIDS Conference, Geneva, 1998.

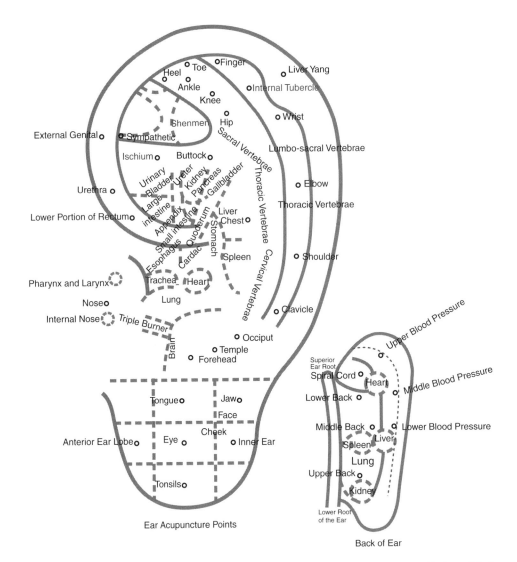

FIGURE 14.1 Ear acupuncture points. (From Cohen, M. (1996). *The Chinese Way to Healing: Many Paths to Wholeness*. New York: Perigree. With permission.)

- Deficient Qi and Xue: Stomach 36, Spleen 6, Kidney 3, Spleen 4
- Stagnant Xue: Spleen 10, Large Intestine 11, Spleen 6
- Stagnant Cold: Ren 6, Kidney 7
- Heat and Damp Heat: Liver 2, Liver 5, Large Intestine 11

EAR ACUPUNCTURE IN HIV/AIDS-RELATED PAIN SYNDROMES

- Overall pain: Ear-Shen-Men, Ear-Sympathetic, Ear-Brain
- Choice of other points according to the area in the ear associated with the organ or body part (Figure 14.1)

Moxibustion (Figure 14.2) can be used in the following ways:

- We can use it over areas of pain.
- We can use moxa on the same points as in acupuncture.
- For abdominal pain, we often use cones of moxa on salt and the herb aconite or ginger over the navel on the point Ren 8. For details, see *The Chinese Way to Healing* (Perigee, 1996) or *The HIV Wellness Sourcebook* (Henry Holt, 1998)
- Moxibustion is generally contraindicated with heat or damp heat syndromes, although there are exceptions such as abdominal cramping related to damp heat type of chronic diarrhea because there is always an underlying spleen deficiency (Figure 14.3)

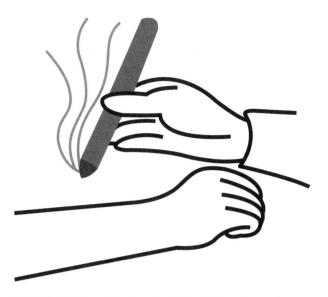

FIGURE 14.2 Moxibustion in HIV-related pain syndromes. (From Cohen, M. (1996). *The Chinese Way to Healing*: *Many Paths to Wholeness*. New York: Perigree. With permission.)

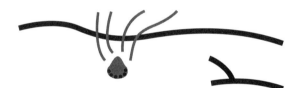

FIGURE 14.3 Abdominal treatment with navel. (From Cohen, M. (1996). *The Chinese Way to Healing*: *Many Paths to Wholeness*. New York: Perigree. With permission.)

CHINESE HERBAL MEDICINE FOR HIV/AIDS

The following formulas are examples that we use in the Chinese traditional medicine clinic on a regular basis for regulating the immune system and for differential diagnosis.

IMMUNE MODULATION

- *Enhancement* — tonifies Qi, Xue, Jing; strengthens Marrow and Spleen/Stomach/Kidney; clears Heat and toxins
- *Tremella American Ginseng* — tones Yin, Qi, Xue, Jing; strengthens Marrow and Spleen/Stomach; clears Heat and toxins
- *Cordyseng* — strengthens Qi, tones Yin and Yang, and strengthens the Spleen, Stomach, Kidney, and Lung

HERBS FOR PAIN SYNDROMES IN HIV/AIDS

ABDOMINAL PAIN

- *Channel flow* — Qi and Xue Stagnation with Cold
- *Source Qi* — for diarrhea accompanied by bloating and abdominal pain; used for the Chinese diagnosis of Spleen Qi and Yang Deficiency diarrhea with Cold

HERPES ZOSTER/SHINGLES

In this case we treat the underlying condition of Damp Heat or Liver Heat of Heat in the Xue (Blood) with formulas such as:

- Long Dan Xie Gan Tang
- Coptis Purge Fire
- Clear Heat

Peripheral Neuropathy

Cold: Mobility 3 with Channel Flow

Heat: Mobility 2 with Channel Flow

Damp in Channels: Shu Gan Wan

Damp Heat: Long Dan Xie Gan Tan or Coptis Purge Fire

Qi and Xue Stagnation with Cold: Channel Flow

Qi and Xue Deficiency: Eight Precious Pills

MASSAGE/ACUPRESSURE FOR HIV/AIDS PAIN

EAR ACUPRESSURE

- Stimulates the specific points that correspond to the areas of the body where there is pain
- Also uses Ear-Sympathetic and Ear-ShenMen

(See Figure 14.1)

BODY ACUPRESSURE

- For upper back and shoulder problems — Pericardium 6, Small Intestine 11
- For tendons, muscle pain, and tightness — Gallbladder 34
- For pain in the head and abdomen — Large Intestine 4
- To relieve Liver Qi stagnation — Liver 3
- Chest and abdomen pain — Pericardium 6

PATIENT SELF-CARE TREATMENT FOR ACHES, PAINS, AND FIBROMYALGIA

STEP ONE: STRETCHING OUT

- With chronic pain, aerobic or weight-bearing exercise can be overstimulating or aggravating to sore joints and muscles. However, gentle Qi Gong exercises can dispel tension and help you relax.
- It may also help to do mild stretching exercises, head rolls, hamstring stretches, or perhaps the Yoga routine called Bow to the Sun that gently massages each part of the body.
- A mild full-body massage is also a terrific way to relax and extend tense muscles and joints, but be careful not to overstimulate or irritate the nerves and muscles. Avoid intense Shiatsu-style massage.
- If your diagnosis indicates Dampness, Cold, and Deficiency, massage with warming and stimulating oils infused with cinnamon essential oil.
- Meditation and the practice of mindfulness — being in the moment and quieting the mind — keeps the mind from amplifying or fixating on pain.

STEP TWO: FEEL THE WARMTH

If you have not been diagnosed with a Heat disorder, and do not have a skin rash or fever, you may find hot herbal compresses are very soothing. They come premade at health supply stores and herbal outlets, but you can make them at home.

- Combine one cup fresh rosemary, thyme, and mint.
- Wrap in a double ply piece of cheesecloth. Secure the ends.
- Immerse the cheesecloth package in a pot of boiling water.
- Remove from water and wrap in thick towel.
- Place on your sore joints or muscles until the towel cools.

STEP THREE: GETTING TO THE POINT

Acupressure and moxibustion to ease pain can be done by your practitioner or at home. If you cannot reach these points yourself, use a partner to lend a hand.

Acupressure points follow:

- For upper back and shoulder problems — Pericardium 6; Small Intestine 11
- For tendons, muscle pain, and tightness — Gallbladder 34
- For pain in the head and abdomen — Large Intestine 4
- To relieve Liver Qi Stagnation — Liver 3

For ear acupuncture, stimulate the specific points that correspond to the areas of the body where there is pain. Also use Ear-Sympathetic and Ear-ShenMen. (See Figure 14.1.) Moxibustion can be applied on any area where there is pain without inflammation or redness.

ACUPUNCTURE GUIDE FOR PRACTITIONERS

For all pain, especially Stagnant Qi —
    Four Gates: Liver 3, Large Intestine 4
For pain related to Damp in the Channels —
    Spleen 6, Spleen 9
For pain related to deficient Qi and Xue —
    Stomach 36, Spleen 6, Kidney 3, Spleen 4
For pain related to stagnant Xue — Spleen 10,
    Large Intestine 11, Spleen 6
For pain related to stagnant Cold — Ren 6, Kidney 7
For pain related to Heat or Damp Heat — Liver 2,
    Liver 5, Large Intestine 11

MOXIBUSTION IN THE CLINIC AND FOR SELF-CARE

Moxibustion is especially good over areas of pain as well as appropriate points. Moxa on the same points as listed in the preceding acupuncture guide — unless diagnosis is Heat or Damp Heat. Then moxa is not recommended.

REFERENCES

Cohen, M. (1996). *The Chinese way to healing: Many paths to wellness.* New York: Perigee.

Cohen, M. (1998). *The HIV wellness sourcebook.* New York: Henry Holt.

15

Mild Traumatic Brain Injury and Pain

Gary W. Jay, M.D., F.A.A.P.M., D.A.A.P.M.

There are a number of factors that must be considered when one clinically evaluates and treats a patient with a mild or minor traumatic brain injury (MTBI) and pain. The literature is rife with overbroad terminology that when dissected makes little sense. Words are used synonymously when they most probably should not be. Most specifically, in many papers, MTBI is felt to be the same as the postconcussive syndrome. When looking at the etiology of specific problems encountered by these patients, it appears to this author that "lumping," instead of looking more specifically at both nomenclature and what each term entails, and *why* is extremely important. Therefore, prior to looking at MTBI, specifically its pathophysiology and how that affects "pain," we look at the postconcussion syndrome (PCS).

POSTCONCUSSION SYNDROME

The PCS appears to include multiple signs and symptoms consisting of neuropathological, neurophysiological, and neuropsychological as well as physical and psychological or emotional aspects secondary to MTBI (Binder, 1986).

The most common medical problems found in the patient with PCS (and MTBI) include

- Posttraumatic headache
- Posttraumatic musculoskeletal pain syndromes
- Vestibular disturbance
- Visual disturbance
- Fatigue
- Posttraumatic seizure disorder

The most common cognitive, emotional, and behavioral deficits include

- Memory impairment
- Lack of initiative
- Depression
- Problems finding work
- Irritability
- Decreased ability to concentrate
- Anxiety
- Poor impulse control
- Loss of self-esteem
- Slowed behavioral processing
- Job loss/disruption
- Behavioral/personality changes
- Denial
- Perseveration
- Difficulties with social interactions and family relationships

The PCS can be both chronic and disabling, or short lived and benign. A possible explanation for this may be the interaction between organic and psychological factors (Bohnen & Jolles, 1992). It is very difficult to differentiate between the effects of primary neurological, neurophysiological, and neuropathological injury and secondary psychosocial factors. It is thought by some that the typical PCS symptoms, including headache, dizziness, and irritability, result from emotional stress associated with diminished cognitive performance secondary to minor acquired traumatic brain injury (MATBI) (Bohnen, Twijnstra, & Jolles, 1992).

0-8493-0926-3/02/$0.00+$1.50
© 2002 by CRC Press LLC

The influence of accident mechanisms associated with more severe symptoms was studied and it was found that patients with more severe deficits at the time of a motor vehicle accident had been an unprepared occupant, had been in a rear-end collision, with or without subsequent frontal impact; and had a rotated or inclined head position at the moment of impact (Sturzenegger, DiStefano, Radanov, & Schnidrig, 1994).

The postconcussional disorder (PCD) has been accepted into and is found in an appendix of the DSM-IV. A major criterion is loss of consciousness (Anderson, 1996), and it is believed that it would be better to use the Brain Injury Special Interest Group (BISIG) definition from the American Congress of Rehabilitation Medicine (Kay, et al., 1993). This definition states: A patient with mild traumatic brain injury is a person who has had a traumatically induced physiological disruption of brain function, as manifested by at least one of the following (Kay, et al., 1993):

1. Any period of loss of consciousness
2. Any loss of memory of events immediately before or after the accident
3. Any alteration in mental state at the time of the accident (e.g., feeling dazed, disoriented, or confused)
4. Focal neurological deficit(s) that may or may not be transient

The severity of the injury does not exceed:

1. Loss of consciousness of approximately 30 min or less
2. After 30 min, an initial Glasgow Coma Scale of 13 to 15 was found
3. Posttraumatic amnesia of not greater than 24 h

Note that the definition includes patients who experience direct head trauma *as well as* those who suffer an acceleration/deceleration injury (whiplash) without specific direct head trauma. Loss of consciousness is *not* a clinical requisite for a classification of MTBI. It is also noted that the symptoms of MTBI (or MATBI) may last varying lengths of time and can consist of persistent physical, emotional, cognitive, and behavioral symptoms that may produce a behavioral disability (Kay, et al., 1993). This is our operational definition of MTBI.

Many researchers have looked for a primary psychological/emotional etiology for the PCS (Karzmark, Hall, & Englander, 1995). Gasquoine (1997) felt that symptom persistence was associated with increased emotional distress. He does note that this fact is also true in patients with severe head injury as well as back injury, and that it relates more to the patient's interpretation of the effect of the trauma than to objective "indicators of brain injury severity."

Landy (1998) looked at the more objective symptoms of headache and cervical pain and found that 70% of patients "get better" within a few weeks post-MVA, whereas about 30% continued to complain of headaches and/or cervical pain. He felt that prolonged management and slow court settlement lead to extensive introspection by the patient and thus prolongation of symptoms. His results also repeat the long-held knowledge that patients with more severe head or neck injury have a lessor incidence of chronic posttraumatic headaches or cervical symptoms.

Barrett, Ward, Boughey, et al. (1994) compared two groups of PCS patients, one of which was hospitalized for observation following a brief loss of consciousness, while the others went to the emergency department, and then home. It was found during follow-up at 2 and 12 weeks that the type and frequency of complaints were similar in both groups. However, at 12 weeks, the number of complaints/symptoms was significantly less in the group of hospitalized patients.

Several groups noted that the PCS was more frequently found after blunt head trauma and other trauma, than would have been predicted (Chambers, Cohen, Hemminger, et al., 1996; Szymanski & Linn, 1992).

By using a questionnaire, Bohnen, Van Zutphen, Twijnstra, et al. (1994) evaluated the longevity of long-term PCS complaints. Their results indicated that MTBI might not, in a percentage of patients, ever resolve.

In an attempt to evaluate the importance of psychological factors in the outcome of whiplash injuries, Mayou and Bryant (1997) utilized interviews at 3 and 12 months postinjury. The majority of the patients in their study continued to complain of persistent cervical symptoms, whereas a "sizable minority" reported specific posttraumatic psychological symptoms, such as intrusive memories and phobic travel anxiety; and this was belived to be "similar to those described by patients suffering multiple injuries." They concluded that travel, social, and psychological morbidity were more prevalent than previously recognized. They did not deal with the issue of the recognized posttraumatic stress disorder (PTSD).

Cicerone and Kalmar (1997) urged clinicians to use a great deal of caution before attributing PCS symptoms or neuropsychological deficits to a preexisting affective disorder. Leininger, Gramling, Farrell, et al. (1990) looked into the idea that MTBI patients do not develop persistent neuropsychological deficits. They found that patients with the PCS/MTBI had measurable neuropsychological deficits and the severity of these deficits was independent of gross neurological status immediately postinjury.

Looking at symptomatic patients 2 years post-whiplash injury, DiStefano and Radanov (1995) evaluated complaints of memory and attentional difficulties with neuropsychological testing. They found that memory problems were minimal, whereas problems in selective aspects of attentional functioning after whiplash were present, and these could explain the patients' cognitive complaints and induce adaptational problems in daily life.

An interesting study was performed by Parker and Rosenblum (1996) who looked at intelligence and personality difficulties after whiplash or MTBI in adults, an average of 20 months post-motor vehicle accident (MVA). They found a mean loss of 14 points of full-scale IQ from the estimated preinjury baseline (using WAIS-R) with no evidence of recovery. They also found a number of personality dysfunctions including organic or cerebral personality disorder. Of 33 patients, 30 had psychiatric diagnoses including PTSD, psychodynamic reactions to impairment, and persistent altered consciousness. They concluded that cognitive loss was induced by the interaction of brain injury with "distractions" including pain and emotional distress. This report also repeated the fact that the presence of MTBI after MVAs was probably consistently underestimated.

Although the PCS has been thought of as a reflection of the psychological response to injury, there is considerable evidence suggesting that the PCS is primarily a physiological disturbance (Szymanski & Linn, 1992). Reaction time testing, for example, has been used to support a structural, organic etiology for the PCS (Jacobson, Gaadsgaard, Thomsen, & Henriksen, 1987).

It has been found that cervical injury likely contributes to the symptomatology post-PCS/MTBI and vice versa (Barrett, Buxton, Redmond, et al., 1995). Testing has shown that cervical injuries secondary to whiplash can induce a distortion of the posture control system as a result of disorganized cervical proprioceptive activity (Gimse, Tjell, Bjorgen, & Saunte, 1996). Others note that restricted cervical movements and changes in the quality of proprioceptive information from the cervical spine region affect voluntary eye movements. Acceleration/deceleration (flexion/extension) injury to the neck secondary to whiplash may result in a dysfunction of the proprioceptive system. Oculomotor dysfunction after cervical trauma may therefore be related to disturbances in cervical afferent input (Heikkila & Wenngren, 1998). Patients who have sustained head or cervical trauma appear to exhibit an increased reliance on accurate visual input and are unable to utilize vestibular orienting information to resolve conflicting information from the visual and somatosensory systems (Rubin, Woolley, Dailey, & Goebel, 1995).

Soustiel, Hafner, Chistyakov, et al. (1995) evaluated 40 patients post-mild head trauma using brain stem trigeminal and brain stem auditory evoked potentials (BTEP, BAEP) and middle-latency auditory evoked potentials (MLAEP) within 48 h of injury and again at 3 months. They defined PCS as the presence of at least four of the following: failure to resume previous professional activity, memory deficits, headache, dizziness and vertigo, behavioral and emotional disturbances, and other neurological symptoms. Initially, all three evoked potentials were abnormal, showing prolonged latencies, indicative of disseminated axonal damage. Only the MLEAPs correlated to outcome at 3 months, particularly in its psychocognitive aspects, suggesting that organic diencephalic–paraventricular primary damage may account for the presence of the PCS.

Positron emission tomography (PET), single photon emission computed tomography (SPECT), and magnetic resonance imaging (MRI) studies have been done to attempt to correlate cerebral dysfunction to PCS symptoms. PET looks at glucose metabolism (in these studies), while SPECT looks at cerebral perfusion.

Six patients with PCS and 12 normal controls were tested. The patient group had significant hypometabolism and hypoperfusion in the bilateral parietooccipital regions, as compared with the controls. In some patients there was also hypometabolism found in other regions. It was hypothesized that parietooccipital hypometabolism can be caused by activation of nociceptive afferent nerves from the upper cervical spine (Otte, Ettlin, Nitzsche, et al., 1997).

Another study examined 13 patients with late whiplash syndrome, using PET and SPECT. The authors did not find hypometabolism in the parietotemporooccipital regions. They did find hypometabolism in the frontopolar and lateral temporal cortex and in the putamen. They did not recommend that PET or SPECT be used as a diagnostic tool for routine examination of patients with late whiplash syndrome (Bicik, Radonov, Schafer, et al., 1998).

SPECT was compared with MRI/computerized axial tomography (CAT) scans in 43 patients. The SPECT was found to be abnormal in 53% of patients, MRI was abnormal in 9%, and CAT scan was abnormal in 4.6% of patients post-MTBI/PCS. The SPECT scan appeared to be more sensitive to post-MTBI changes, especially in patients with the persistent PCS (see later) than MRI or CAT scan. No statistical relationships were found between the SPECT scan results and age, previous psychiatric history, history of substance abuse, history of multiple MTBI, or concurrent neuropsychological symptoms (Kant, Smith-Seemiller, Isaac, & Duffy, 1997).

"The truth is out there," but we do not seem to have determined the best method of identifying it. The tests noted earlier were given to patients with the PCS, by author statement. The relationship between the PCS and MTBI is discussed later, and the situation may not be that simple.

Nosologically, it is difficult to determine exactly what constitutes the PCS. Evans (1992) states that the PCS refers to the large number of signs and symptoms found alone or in combination following MATBI, including headache, memory problems, dizziness, fatigue, irritability, anxiety, insomnia, and sensitivity to light and sound.

He further indicates that studies have substantiated the existence of the PCS and that it is common, with resolution in 3 to 6 months, but with persistent symptoms and cognitive deficits persisting for months or years.

Headache, dizziness, and memory deficits are the most common combination of PCS symptoms (Young, 1985). There is no specific symptom complex found in the majority of patients with acute or chronic PCS (Alves & Jane, 1990). The multiplicity of signs and symptoms of the PCS have been well documented (Bohnen & Jolles, 1992; Brenner, Friedman, Merritt, & Denny-Brown, 1944; Brenner & Gillingham, 1974; Hoganson, Sachs, Desai, & Whitman, 1984; Jones, 1974; Oddy, Humphrey, & Uttley, 1978; Rimel & Jane, 1985; Ritchie, 1974; Rutherford, Merrett, & McDonald, 1977; Symonds, 1965; Young, 1985).

One group has suggested that the PCS should include all the consequences of head injury, regardless of its severity and the nature of the injury (Rutherford, Merrett, & McDonald, 1978–1979).

Berrol (1992) states that the term *mild traumatic brain injury* (MTBI) is preferable, because it identifies the etiology of the injury, its degree, and the pathological substrate much better than other past terms: *minor head injury, traumatic head syndrome, postconcussive syndrome, posttraumatic syndrome, postbrain-injury syndrome*, and *traumatic cephalgia*.

The term *postconcussive syndrome* (PCS) continues to be frequently used in the literature. The important nosological question is whether the PCS is secondary to the MTBI, or the cognitive/neurological deficits found after MTBI are a separate entity.

The term *PCS* would then encompass the nonneurological, neurocognitive, and neurophysiological deficits, leaving PCS to be used specifically for the other organ (noncerebral) systems that display posttraumatic signs and symptoms.

Teleologically, it appears to make more sense to separate the etiologies of the problems encountered post-MATBI. A patient with physical findings such as posttraumatic headache may indeed, posttrauma, have a PCS. Patients with neurocognitive deficits and other neurological difficulties have direct evidence of an MTBI. The author believes it is more appropriate to differentiate between the two disorders. This would mean that a patient may indeed have an MTBI as well as a PCS. Both entities must be treated, and, as discussed later, the PCS should be treated first.

Soon after injury, patients have complaints referable to several different organ systems. Alexander (1995) identifies this as the PCS. He notes that the MTBI, which can lead to brain injury, can also cause injury to the head, neck (whiplash and soft tissue damage), vestibular system, and psychological functioning. The initial complaints of deficits in cognition and sleep disorder, Alex-

ander believes, are secondary to neuronal injury, whereas the headache may be secondary to cervical injury, neuronal injury, or a combination; cervical pain secondary to soft tissue problems; dizziness secondary to peripheral vestibular dysfunction or cervical injury; and anxiety, moodiness, and irritability secondary to neurological injury, pain, and/or psychological factors.

The term *PCS*, in the author's opinion, should not include central nervous system (CNS) deficits. Vestibular dysfunction secondary to brain stem injury should be included in the MTBI, whereas peripheral dysfunction would be a part of the PCS. These differences are most important when planning and executing an appropriate treatment plan/paradigm. This appears to be more important when one encounters the difficulties obtaining insurance approval to treat an ailment (MATBI) that some insurers do not even believe exists.

To the extent plasticity allows, neuronal recovery is certainly taking place at 1 month after injury (Dikmen, McLean, Temkin, et al., 1986; Elson & Ward, 1994; Gentilini, Michelli, & Shoenhuber, 1985; McLean, Dikmen, Temkin, et al., 1984; Stuss, Stethem, Hugenholtz, et al., 1989). Neurological recovery is thought to be "substantial," by some, at 3 months (Levin, Mattis, Ruff, et al., 1987). At this point postinjury, 30 to 50% of patients have continued complaints (Dikemen, Temkin, & Armsden, 1989). Over the next 6 to 12 months (longer than a year postinjury) most patients show continued improvement and "recovery" (McFlynn, Montgomery, Feuton, & Rutherford, 1984).

It has been found that even "well-recovered" patients are still susceptible to periodic impairments secondary to physiological or psychological stress (Ewing, McCarthy, Gronwall, et al., 1980; Gronwall & Wrightson, 1974), which indicates that recovery is most likely the wrong term. That these patients have "compensated" for their injury may be more nearly correct. To say that patients may have a permanent sense of decreased mental or cognitive efficiency (Stuss, Ely, Hugenholtz, et al., 1985) would also be a function of incorrect terminology (i.e., recovered vs. compensated).

PERSISTENCE OF SYMPTOMS

At 1 year, 85 to 90% of patients are felt to be "recovered" but are still symptomatic (Rutherford et al., 1978–1979; McLean, Temkin, Dikmen, et al., 1983), leaving 10 to 15% of patients who are not only "not recovered," but also "not compensated" and still very symptomatic. The literature is replete with studies showing persistence of symptoms after the magic, if not mythical, 3-month period. This literature indicates the symptoms and deficits following MTBI and PCS may last for 6 to 12 months and even longer (Berrol, 1992; Boll & Barth, 1983; Jones, Viola, LaBan, et al., 1992; Katz & DeLuca, 1992; Leininger et al., 1990; McSherry, 1989; Stuss, et al., 1985; Wrightson & Gronwall, 1989).

Much of the literature equates MTBI and PCS, essentially using the terminology interchangeably. The majority of the literature includes cognitive and other neurological deficits in the PCS. This statement is cautionary, as one must read the literature with great care to see what exactly is being done to exactly what problem or problems.

A survey of rehabilitation specialists who followed patients with MTBI for 6 to 18 months found that 21% of the patients experienced symptoms of the PCS 2 to 6 months after their initial injury, and that 20% of these patients had the "post-MTBI syndrome" (Harrington, Malec, Cicerone, & Katz, 1993). In another survey of 51 patients, where 23 responded, 25% of the respondents reported continued sequelae from their injury. The patients with sequelae after 1 year were found to have reported more symptoms 1 week after injury (Middelboe, Anderson, Birket-Smith, & Friss, 1992).

Cicerone (1992) indicated that there was considerable evidence to show that PCS symptoms persisted in a significant proportion of patients after MTBI, and such symptoms were particularly prevalent in patients who indicated that they needed clinical attention.

Symptoms with organic etiologies, it has been noted, can mimic functional disorders (Russell, 1974). Alves (1992) indicated that as recovery occurred, persistent symptoms could be secondary to an interaction between organic and psychosocial factors. These persistent symptoms are more than would be expected from the initial organic damage alone. Alves further stated that a significant percentage of patients would exhibit persistent problems with symptoms 12 months postinjury. He felt that recovery from MTBI should also be considered in the social context in which it occurred. By recognizing the complexity of the recovery process, we should extend the concept of morbidity to include the specific socioeconomic and emotional sequelae that the patient experienced.

Mateer (1992) found that patients post-MTBI were more acutely aware of their cognitive deficits and difficulties with functional abilities. These patients would go to a physician and be found to have a negative neurological examination. They would be told that there was no organic reason for their problems. They also would be told that they should wait longer for recovery, learn to live with their problems, or seek psychiatric help.

These iatrogenically induced problems (cause and effect) most likely lengthen the patients' symptomatic period, as they begin to feel an ever increasing loss of control, fear of the unknown, and concern that they must be "going crazy."

It doesn't matter what the medical problem is, particularly when, like most patients with MTBI, they look "normal." Physicians with little or no background in the diagnosis of MTBI or PCS, or consultants who are bought

and paid for, do a great disservice to MTBI patients. Constant repetition by even well-meaning physicians of the mantra, "There is nothing wrong with you. You look fine. There's no problem here," demonstrably disrupt patients' sense of self, their life, and their feelings that there are indeed people (specifically doctors and insurance companies) "out to get them." This induces iatrogenic exacerbation of their symptoms, as the patients strive, consciously or unconsciously, to prove to *someone* that they *do* have a problem. Then, to add insult to injury, this iatrogenically induced problem is used against them both by other physicians and the legal "warriors" who are bound and determined, in the court case after a motor vehicle accident, to prove that there is nothing wrong with them, thus saving their insurance company clients money.

PERSISTENT POSTCONCUSSIVE SYNDROME

Alexander (1992, 1995) has written extensively about the "persistent postconcussive syndrome" (PPCS). These patients, after 1 year, continue to have symptoms commonly seen in acute PCS, such as headache, sleep disorder, balance problems, dizziness, sensory hyperesthesias, and cognitive symptoms including deficits in attention, memory, and executive functioning. They are also frequently noted to have prominent emotional symptoms including irritability, depression, nervousness, discouragement, and anger.

Alexander (1995) identifies some "predictors" of the development of PPCS, including the female sex, litigation, low socioeconomic status, prior MTBI, headache, and serious associated systemic injury. Although these factors may be implicated, he states that none accounts for more than a small percentage of cases of PPCS.

Other authors identify pain severity postinjury as a predictor of the development of the PPCS post-MTBI (Ettlin, Kischka, Reichmann, et al., 1993; Radanov, Di Stefano, Schnidrig, et al., 1991). Additional data suggests a greater frequency of anxiety and depression months after initial injury (Schoenhuber & Gentilini, 1988).

Dizziness is a frequent symptom of the PCS. It is noted that peripheral vestibular injury with dizziness also has a close relationship with psychiatric disorders, particularly with affective disease and anxiety. Unfortunately, the significant aspects of dizziness secondary to myofascial problems are often ignored. Zasler (1992) discusses cervicogenic dizziness. Dizziness secondary to myofascial trigger points in the sternocleidomastoid muscles is also frequently overlooked. In contradistinction, Alexander (1995) does not appear to anticipate the psychological aspects secondary to this problem, making it seem to be more of a primary psychological problem than one secondary to a true organic problem.

Chronic pain and headache are fairly universal accompaniments of the PPCS. It is also known that patients who experience chronic headache not associated with a PCS have many of the same complaints, including fatigue, sleep disorder, depression, and occasionally dizziness, as well as difficulties with concentration and memory. Psychological factors may aggravate these headaches.

It is recognized that anxiety may decrease concentration and complex mental processes (Binder, 1986; Krapnick & Horowitz, 1981). Depression can cause decreased cognitive functioning, particularly in concentration, memory and executive functions (Cicerone, 1992; Leininger & Kreutzer, 1992; Weingartner, Cohen, Murphy, et al., 1981). The latter problem has also been called "depressive pseudodementia" (Wells, 1979).

Therefore, one cannot assume that if everyone with a PCS/MTBI has impaired concentration, then everyone with impaired concentration after PCS/MTBI has a neurological etiology. The problem is that patients with PCS/MTBI associated with pain and affective difficulties may have impaired concentration for multiple reasons, including post-MTBI neuropathological changes.

Alexander (1995) asks the question: When does the physiogenesis of a clinical problem become psychogenesis? This may be difficult to determine and may have an iatrogenic component. Alexander does indicate that the major issue is physiogenesis transforming to psychogenesis, but he notes that physiogenesis can be very underestimated. He also indicates that there is no single psychological, physiological, or demographic factor leading to the PPCS.

Fenton (1996) attempted to reappraise the PCS. He reviewed data from two U.K. prospective studies of the initial aspects and course of postconcussive symptomatology using parallel psychosocial, neuropsychiatric, quantitative electroencephalogram (EEG or QEEG), and brain stem evoked potentials. Abnormal, prolonged brain stem evoked potentials were seen in between 27 and 46% of patients. Prolonged symptomatology was noted in 13% of patients and was associated with a high percentage of brain stem dysfunction. The degree of QEEG recovery is related to the intensity of early symptom reaction to trauma. Fenton believed that levels of perceived stress at the time of the injury or afterward were not related to symptom formation; however, chronic social difficulties were seen in 21% of patients who initially showed improvement but later, between 6 weeks and 6 months posttrauma, experienced an exacerbation of symptomatology.

Thus, are the PCS and MTBI absolutely two separate entities? I believe that the answer to this question is yes, with an important corollary. Because both problems begin together, after a motor vehicle accident, for instance, the presence of both problems affects each other. The physical problems found in the PCS are affected by the cognitive problems brought on by an MTBI. The affective/emotional problems found in MTBI would also affect the patient with physical problems from a PCS. However, acute and chronic pain engenders affective changes by their presence, on a neurochemical basis as well as secondary to sleep disorders (also a neurochemical problem) and learned behaviors from each patient's past.

This means that there is a lot to dissect or tease out in a patient with the PCS as well as an MTBI. Only by determining and differentiating between the physical/peripheral problems and those from the CNS resulting from an MTBI can a proper treatment plan be created and performed. For example, the author has found that it is best to treat depression and posttraumatic headache first, before endeavoring to treat the MTBI. The patient outcomes, over two decades, appear far superior to those seen when one tries to treat everything at once. Knowing a bit about what happens in the CNS to patients with a MTBI is also important, particularly when attempting to treat these patients.

MINOR TRAUMATIC BRAIN INJURY

Because we are dealing in this chapter with MTBI — the effects of direct trauma-induced focal lesions — contusions, hematomas, edema, hydrocephalus, and so on — are not covered. For those who are interested, they have been well described by Jay (2000).

Diffuse injury to the brain is seen with MTBI and is dealt with here, along with the neurochemical pathophysiology, which is of equal or possibly more importance in the entity called MTBI.

The two categories of diffuse injury important to this discussion are mild concussion and "classical" cerebral concussions (Jay, 2000).

Mild Concussion

- There is no loss of consciousness, but transient neurological disturbance may be seen.
- The patient may be confused, disoriented, and may or may not have amnesia.
- Posttraumatic headache is frequently seen.

"Classical" Cerebral Concussion

- The patient may show temporary, reversible neurological deficits secondary to trauma, associated with a brief loss of consciousness (less than 1 h) with some degree of posttraumatic amnesia.
- A mild or moderate degree of microscopic neuronal abnormalities can be found.

- There may be an associated focal brain injury (contusion).
- Posttraumatic headache, tinnitus, and subtle changes in memory or psychological functioning may be seen.

Caveats — Very Important

- Physiological and (neuro) psychological dysfunction may occur in the absence of anatomic (macroscopic) lesions.
- Functional disruption, which precedes anatomic disruption, is always the greater.
- Clinically, patients with mild concussion syndromes and "classical" cerebral concussion may have physiological dysfunction as well as microscopic anatomic disruptions that may be in contradistinction to the apparent severity of the injury.
- Traumatic brain injury (TBI) deficits are additive.

The neuropathology of TBI is, as with most aspects of the disorder, replete with knowns, unknowns, and variables. Research has established many of the basic facts, but the exact how, when, why, and where are still subject to debate.

Clinical practice indicates that a CAT scan should be performed on patients post-TBI. However, as noted earlier, the timing of the test is important. It is important to repeat a CAT scan on a patient who begins to decompensate neurologically. An acute subdural hematoma or subarachnoid hemorrhage may occur in patients with normal Glasgow Coma Scale (GCS) scores (GCS = 15) typically within 24 h. Other authors believe that when the first CAT scan is performed within 3 h of injury, another should be done within 12 h (Servadei, Nanni, Nasi, et al., 1995).

Quantitative MRI analyses have shown significant differences in TBI patients with unimodal gray matter–white matter histograms, as compared with normals, who demonstrate bimodal gray matter–white matter histograms (Thatcher, Camacho, Salazar, et al., 1997). The MRI is also better than the CAT scan at determining other postinjury pathology including diffuse axonal injury (DAI) and glial scarring. The MRI scan is also useful in morphometric analysis of the brain, showing diffuse neuronal degeneration after TBI with more severe injury. This may include larger ventricle to brain ratios and temporal horn volumes, which may relate to neuropsychological outcome (Gale, Johnson, Bigler, & Blatter, 1995).

DAI is one of the most prevalent and well-acknowledged primary and secondary postinjury pathophysiological phenomenon. The brain tissue, or parenchyma, can be severely injured secondary to axonal shearing forces during acceleration/deceleration and rotational injuries in a closed head injury. The most common locations of DAI include cerebral hemispheric gray–white matter interfaces and subcortical white matter, the body and the splenium of the corpus collosum, the basal ganglia, dorsolateral aspects of the brain stem, and the cerebellum. MRI technology is continually evolving. Nonhemorrhagic lesions can be seen via MRI using fluid attenuated inversion recovery (FLAIR) techniques, proton-density, and T2 weighted images. Old hemorrhagic lesions are best seen with the use of gradient echo sequences (Parizel, Ozsarla, Van Goethem, et al., 1998).

A good tool utilized in the investigation of DAI is beta-amyloid precursor protein (beta-APP). In one series, DAI was seen in 65 to 100% of all cases of closed head injury, fatal cerebral ischemia/hypoxia, and brain death with a survival time of greater than 3 h. Cases with a posttraumatic interval of less than 180 min did not express beta-APP (Oehmichen, Meissner, Schmidt, et al., 1998). The extent and severity of DAI cannot be predicted from biomechanical data alone, such as the height of a fall; total axonal injury in a given patient is a variable mixture of DAI and focal axonal injury from secondary mechanisms. Beta-APP immuno-staining is not able to distinguish between primary and secondary axonal injury (Abou-Hamden, Blumbergs, Scott, et al., 1997). Still another study found beta-APP immunostaining demonstrations of positive axonal swelling 1.75 h postinjury in both mild and severe TBI groups, and demonstrated a spectrum of axonal injury in TBI. The study found that axons were more vulnerable than blood vessels and those axons in the corpus callosum and fornices were the most vulnerable of all (Blumbergs, Scott, Manavis, et al., 1995).

Findings from another study express that neurofilamentous disruption is a pivotal event in axonal injury. The authors studied the progression of TBI-induced axonal change at the ultrastructural level using two antibodies (NR4, to target light neurofilament subunits, and SMI32, to target the heavy neurofilament subunit). Changes noted at 6 h postinjury entailed focally enlarged immunoreactive axons with axolemmal infolding or disordered neurofilaments. By 12 h, some axons showed continued neurofilamentous misalignment, pronounced immunoreactivity, vacuolization, and — on occasion — disconnection. Between 30 and 60 h, further accumulations of neurofilaments and organelles induced further expansion of the axis cylinder and disconnected reactive swellings were recognized. During later times, focally enlarged disconnected axons were observed in relation to axons showing less advanced reactive changes (Christman, Grady, Walker, et al., 1994).

Axonal injury including DAI was noted by several authors in the brains of patients who were victims of blunt head trauma/assault (Crooks, Scholtz, Vowles, et al., 1992; Imajo, 1996; Ramsay & Shkrum, 1995).

Other studies reinforce the fact that neuronal loss after head injury is secondary to both primary and secondary mechanisms. One study also found that microglial activation was a delayed result of TBI (Engel, Wehner, & Meyermann, 1996). Another study that evaluated Purkinje cell vulnerability in mild TBI, found that there was a close anatomic association between activated microglial cells and Purkinje cells, which suggests that Purkinje cell injury is the cause of microglial cell activation (Fukuda, Aihara, Sagar, et al., 1996).

Povlishock's (1992) and Povlishock and Jenkins' (1995) work comes to some of the same conclusions, but by a different road. They believe that the TBI itself does not cause axonal disruption. Instead, focal, subtle axonal changes that occur over time lead to impaired axoplasmic transport, continued axonal swelling, and finally disconnection. Povlishock attributes the trauma to altering the axolemmal permeability, direct cytoskeletal damage or disruption, or more overt metabolic and functional disturbances. Trauma may induce axonal change, Wallerian degeneration, and finally deafferentation. Povlishock also thinks that traumatically induced DIA leads to diffuse deafferentation and notes that posttraumatically, the cerebral parenchyma is involved with increased neuronal sensitivity to secondary ischemia. Furthermore, he believes that this increased sensitivity is secondary to the neurotransmitter storm that follows a TBI, which can induce sublethal neuroexcitation. Most importantly, Povlishock (1992) and Povlishock and Jenkins (1995) indicate that the damage noted does not take place immediately posttrauma, but takes place over days or even weeks.

NEUROCHEMICAL ASPECTS OF TRAUMATIC BRAIN INJURY

Abnormal agonist–receptor interactions related to excitotoxic processes may contribute to the pathophysiology of TBI. Activation of the muscarinic cholinergic or N-methyl-D-aspartate (NMDA) glutamate receptors appear to contribute to TBI pathophysiology.

TBI-induced membrane depolarization causes a massive release of excitatory neurotransmitters, particularly acetylcholine (ACH) and glutamate. The posttraumatic overproduction/release of these chemicals may induce abnormal activation of receptors that can produce changes in intracellular signal transduction pathways and thereby induce short-term, long-lasting, or irreversible changes in cell function. Such deficits can occur with sublethal cell disruption or cell death.

Experimental TBI is known to produce widespread neuronal depolarization, which is demonstrated by large increases in extracellular potassium (K+) resulting from neuronal discharges and not neurotransmitter release.

Increased neurotransmitter release is recruited to increase depolarization as injury severity increases. The release of these excitatory amino acids (EAAs) significantly contributes to the high levels of K+ release following TBI.

After moderate and most probably mild TBI, tissue deformation may open ion channels resulting in an influx of K+ large enough to induce abnormal levels of excitatory neurotransmitter release and therefore further depolarization.

Mild–moderate TBI induces increases in glutamate and ACH. Increased ACH release and increased cholinergic neuronal activity in some regions of the brain (such as the hippocampus) may persist for hours or longer after injury.

Posttraumatic changes in the blood–brain barrier (BBB) may also contribute to posttraumatic receptor dysfunction by allowing the abnormal passage of blood-borne excitatory exogenous neurotransmitters and neuromodulators into the brain. These additional excitatory neurochemicals may act synergistically with endogenously increased excitatory neurotransmitters (ENTs). Moderate experimental TBI without contusion in the rat leads to acute BBB dysfunction in the hippocampus and the cortex that may last more than 12 h. Other research suggests that dysfunction of the BBB secondary to TBI may allow blood plasma constituents such as ACH (at levels 7 times greater than in the cerebral spinal fluid [CSF]) to gain access to the brain and influence injury processes.

Moderate TBI can induce significant reductions in muscarinic cholinergic receptor binding. Decreased binding by glutaminergic receptors, specifically the NMDA receptors, also occurs following moderate TBI.

The predominant changes seen only in the NMDA receptors suggest that the ENT agonist–receptor interaction secondary to moderate TBI occurs predominately at this receptor subtype. This is supported by the protection given by administration of NMDA antagonists.

Reduced motor and memory deficits can be seen with pharmacological antagonism of NMDA receptors using phencyclidine, MK-801, dextrorphan, and others. This appears to be secondary to their ability to restore MG^{2+} (magnesium) levels postinjury.

Receptor activation by ENTs may contribute to cellular metabolic alterations after TBI. Further results indicate that EAA neurotransmitters may be involved in injury-induced disruption of ionic homeostasis and ion-induced cytotoxic cerebral edema.

TBI produces widespread neuronal excitation causing prolonged, usually sublethal, pathological changes in neuronal activity that disrupt many functions, including memory. Inhibitory neurotransmitters such as gamma-aminobutyric acid (GABA) and the opiods may also be released with TBI to try to decrease the excitatory state.

Oxygen free radicals (OFRs) may also be important mediators of TBI and cerebral edema. Sources for oxygen free radicals include catecholamines, amine oxidases, and peroxidases among others. Pharmacological agents being considered to decrease OFR damage include vitamin E, dimethyl sulfoxide (DMSO), and lipid peroxidation inhibitors (lazaroids).

Some conclusions that can be drawn follow.

- Excitotoxic phenomena may render neurons dysfunctional but not necessarily kill them (although that also occurs).
- TBI results in widespread depolarization and nonspecific release of many excitatory and inhibitory neurotransmitters.
- Significant changes in the BBB are found that may last for hours or more.
- The resultant sublethal toxicity appears to be mediated via increases in intracellular calcium levels.
- These processes, including DAI, may begin at the time of an accident, but take days or even weeks until they end.
- There are three subtypes of glutamate receptors: NMDA, quisqualate, and kainate.
- The NMDA receptors may protect against TBI secondary to trauma and cerebral ischemia.
- Cholinergic systems have roles in mediation of TBI and neuronal recovery, including behavioral suppression. Long-term motor deficits may be decreased by the ACH medications blocking release of excitotoxins.
- Catecholamines (especially norepinephrine) appear to help in TBI recovery.
- Alpha-noradrenergic agonists and probably dopaminergic agonists accelerated motor recovery after experimental injury to the sensorimotor cortex. Their antagonists retarded recovery.
- Early postinjury use of benzodiazipines may slow neural recovery and possible restoration of neural recovery.
- Most likely, "therapeutic cocktails" of more than one agent are necessary for appropriate treatment of TBI.

BIOGENIC AMINES AND THE ENDOGENOUS OPIATE SYSTEM

Acute traumatic injury of any type engenders the production of beta-endorphin (BE) as well as other endogenous opiates. One group looked at BE levels in the blood after trauma and found, to little surprise, that there was no correlation between serum BE and pain severity (Bernstein, Garzone, Rudy, et al., 1995). When looking at CSF BE levels, it was found that significant changes in CSF BE levels are found in patients with the full range of TBI,

mild to severe. Interestingly, the patients with mild TBI had significantly higher levels of BE than those patients with severe head trauma. The BE levels did not correlate with early prognosis (Pasaoglu, Inci Karakucuk, Kurtsoy, & Pasaoglu, 1996).

Another group of patients had lumbar punctures done on days 1, 4, and 7, head following injury; and the levels of leucine or leu-enkephalin (LENK) and methianine or met-enkephalin (MENK) were determined in the CSF. It was found that MENK levels were constantly elevated, whereas LENK levels decreased in patients with GCS scores of 8 or less, and might provide a poor prognostic factor. It was indicated that LENK and MENK appeared to be linked to different pathophysiological functions (Stachura, Kowalski, Obuchowicz, et al., 1997).

Although endogenous opiates are found in the human gut, BE is produced in the hypothalamus. It is broken down to the smaller forms of endogenous opiates, LENK and MENK. It would therefore be more likely to be found in the CSF, along with enkephalins and dynorphins, which together help mediate the central perception of pain.

Primary metabolites of norepinephrine (methoxyhydroxyphenylglycol [MHPG]), serotonin (5-hydroxyindole-acetic acid [5HIAA]) and dopamine (homovanillic acid [HVA]) were assayed in CSF taken from comatose patients after severe head injury. Samples were taken within days of the injury and again after clinical improvement (13/20 patients) or deterioration (7/20 patients) was seen. Clinical improvement was associated with significant decreases in HVA and 5HIAA. The levels of all three metabolites remained high in patients who deteriorated. These results appeared to indicate that increased turnover of CNS neurotransmitters in severe head injury normalized during recovery (Markianos, Seretis, Kotsou, & Christopoulous, 1996).

In another study, CSF levels of serotonin (5-HT), substance P (SP), and lipid peroxidation (LPx) products were measured in patients with TBI and compared with controls. The levels of SP and 5-HT in patients with head trauma were lower than those found in controls. The CSF LPx products were significantly increased in the TBI patients. There was no correlation between the CSF levels and the GCS at admission (Karakucuk, Pasaoglu, Pasaoglu, & Oktem, 1997).

The loss or decrement of cholinergic neurotransmission has been implicated in both cognitive dysfunction and memory impairment after TBI. One group looked at presynaptic markers related to cholinergic neurotransmission via choline acetyltransferase activity as well as high-affinity nicotinic receptor binding sites in the inferior temporal gyrus, cingulate gyrus, and superior parietal cortex in postmortem brains. They found that the correlation of choline acetyltransferase activity with synaptophysin immunoreactivity revealed a deficit of cholinergic presynaptic terminals in postmortem human brain after TBI (Murdoch, Perry, Court, et al., 1998).

An inverse relationship between plasma norepinephrine and thyroid hormones is found in patients with hyper- or hypothyroidism or severe stress. Head injured patients were found to have low thyroxine (T4), low triiodothyronine (T3), and high reverse T3. When phenytoin was used for seizure control, T3 and T4 were lowered, but thyroid-stimulating hormone was increased. In these patients there was no correlation between NE and T3 (Ziegler, Morrissey, & Marshall, 1990).

A great deal of evidence indicates that dopamine neurotransmission dysfunction after mild to moderate TBI is involved in the induction of posttraumatic memory deficits. By using anesthetized animals that were given MTBIs, it was found that mice were impaired in task performance. They had prolonged latencies for finding and drinking in a retention test and retest. If these animals were injected with haloperidol 15 min posttrauma, they had a shortened latency in both of the tests, which appeared to show that the use of dopamine receptor antagonists was beneficial for recovery of posttraumatic memory dysfunction. For looking closer at the receptor sites, researchers used a D1 receptor antagonist, SCH-23390, and sulpiride, a D2 receptor antagonist, in the same experimental protocol. The use of sulpiride, but not SCH-23390, improved the deficits in task performance, indicating that the D2 receptors were the major site of action. A positive interaction was noted when both D1 and D2 receptor antagonists were given together at individually subtherapeutic levels, indicating that interaction between the two receptors was involved. The dopaminergic mechanisms do appear to contribute to memory dysfunction after TBI (Tang, Node, & Nabeshima, 1997).

MINOR TRAUMATIC BRAIN INJURY AND PAIN: SOME CONCLUSIONS

The various pathophysiological aspects of MTBI and pain therefore appear to encompass several important etiologies:

- At the time of trauma, there may typically be soft tissue injuries, at a minimum. Those patients who experience significant TBI may need to be sedated, and even paralyzed; and therefore may have their perception of pain dealt with on a secondary basis.
- Moderate to severe TBI may make the patient unable to cognitively deal with pain.
- Patients with MTBI may be so overcome with pain immediately postinjury that cognitive changes and problems may not be either relevant or even looked for at that time.

- There are significant neurochemical and neurophysiological abnormalities that occur in MTBI and affect some of the same neurotransmitter systems needed by the nociceptive and antinociceptive systems; these abnormalities can lead to perturbations in the experience, perception, and appropriate recognition of pain and/or pain relief.
- The affective/emotional changes that accompany both chronic pain and MTBI are subserved by the same neurochemical systems, many of which are affected by pain as well as, pathophysiologically, trauma (from both primary and secondary effects).
- The MTBI patient with pain must therefore be dealt with on multiple levels: the soft tissue/musculoskeletal pain problems from the injury; the neuropathological changes, secondary to DAI, excitotoxic cell injury, BBB changes, and the effects of possible neurotransmitter system damage secondary to these factors; and the neurotransmitter system changes that are known to accompany chronic pain, which may be exacerbated or changed secondary to the CNS effects of the MTBI. These factors make treatment more challenging, because medication management, for example, may be more difficult as well as different when looking at a patient with only chronic benign pain.

The pathophysiological changes that occur after an MTBI may last for days or weeks. The resultant deficits may therefore not become manifested for more weeks or months. This leads to an important consideration. What if the patient complains of cognitive or emotional problems within days or several weeks of the initial insult? First, is the patient experiencing all the problems that are going to arise from the injury, or only those that have been detected at that time? Second, can you see a good reason for considering serial neurological examinations?

Somehow it has become an "urban medical legend" that all patients with an MTBI will miraculously be healed within 3 months. This may be true for a simple majority of patients who are not experiencing a significant MTBI. However, as documented earlier, anywhere from 5 to 20% of these patients do not get "all better" in 3, 6, or even 12 months.

As clinicians take the patient's history of cognitive problems, they may also find frequent complaints of posttraumatic myofascial or soft tissue pain problems, including posttraumatic headache, cervical pain, and low back pain, as well as sleep disorder.

If the patient who complains of pain is seen soon after the injury, physical therapy may be all that is needed to stop these problems before the onset of chronicity, with its attendant affective and neurochemical alterations. The use of narcotic analgesics should be strongly discouraged, because they may further enhance cognitive difficulties. If after 6 to 12 weeks there is no significant diminution of the pain and/or headache, along with depression, consideration of a specialty pain program should be given, as long as the pain practitioner understands the effects of TBI on pain.

There is an interesting dichotomy in the majority of patients with pain and MTBI. Patients in an interdisciplinary pain program are typically taught to rate their pain, on a momentary basis on a 0 (no pain) to 10 or 100 scale. When they begin treatment, the numbers are typically high and correspond with physical findings of muscle spasm, trigger points, and loss of specific function such as decreased range of motion or weakness. As treatment progresses, typically during 4 to 6 weeks, the patients' pain complaints may not change. That is, their identification of their pain level (such as 7 over 10) may not change or change only minimally, whereas functional evaluation reveals a return to a normal range of motion, for example, or absent palpable muscle spasm or trigger points.

It is extremely important to realize that this dichotomy is *not* a manifestation of malingering, but appears to be more of a learned or even perseverative response. On observation, pain behaviors are diminished and the patients' affect is improved, but they may still claim to endure what appears to be an artificially high pain level. Evaluation *must* be functional in nature, not subjective.

Even more importantly, in the presence of severe pain, a neuropsychological evaluation or cognitive evaluation is not accurate and should not be performed. This means, *MTBI patients with pain should have their pain ameliorated and their depression lifted as much as possible prior to any formal cognitive evaluation and/or treatment.*

The PCSs as well as the PPCSs are not symptoms or syndromes looking for patients. As indicated earlier, the author believes that the PCS is different from an MTBI. Still, patients from around the country, around the globe, complain of the same symptoms after an acceleration/deceleration injury. There are tests and many studies that show the presence of abnormalities. Again, we do not yet seem to know the best tests, the best window to perform them, or the best way to interpret them.

As clinicians, we also know that we have to listen to our patients. If something they say does not make sense, it is the clinician's medical responsibility to actively investigate what the patient is trying to say.

To be antagonistic to a diagnosis, to not accept the presence of a diagnosis because of preconceived notions or initial thoughts of patient malingering or because your opinion depends on who pays you, puts us back into the era of the Inquisition. That is not our job; "to do no harm" is our responsibility.

REFERENCES

Abou-Hamden, A., Blumbergs, P. C., Scott, G., et al. (1997). Axonal injury in falls. *Journal of Neurotrauma, 14,* 699–713.

Alexander, M.P. (1992). Neuropsychiatric correlates of persistent postconcussive syndrome. *Journal of Head Trauma Rehabilitation, 7*(2), 60–69.

Alexander, M.P. (1995). Mild traumatic brain injury. Pathophysiology, natural history and clinical management. *Neurology, 45,* 1253–1260.

Alves, W.M. (1992). Natural history of post-concussive signs and symptoms. *Physical Medicine and Rehabilitation: State of the Art Reviews, 6*(1), 21–32.

Alves, W.M., & Jane, J.A. (1990). Post-traumatic syndrome. In J.R. Youmans (Ed.), *Neurological Surgery* (3rd ed., pp. 2230–2240). Philadelphia: W. B. Saunders.

Anderson, S.D. (1996). Postconcussional disorder and loss of consciousness. *Bulletin of American Academy of Psychiatric Law, 24,* 493–504.

Barrett, K., Buxton, N., Redmond, A.D., et al. (1995). A comparison of symptoms experienced following minor head injury and acute neck strain (whiplash injury). *Journal of Accident and Emergency Medicine, 12,* 173–176.

Barrett, K., Ward, A.B., Boughey, A., et al. (1994). Sequelae of minor head injury: The natural history of post-concussive symptoms and their relationship to loss of consciousness and follow-up. *Journal of Accident and Emergency Medicine, 11,* 79–84, 1994.

Bernstein, L., Garzone, P.D., & Rudy, T., et al. (1995). Pain perception and serum beta-endorphin in trauma patients. *Psychosomatics, 36,* 276–284.

Berrol, S. (1992). Terminology of post-concussive syndrome. *Physical Medicine and Rehabilitation: State of the Art Reviews, 6*(1), 1–8.

Bicik, I., Radanov, B.P., Schafer, N., et al. (1998). PET with 18fluorodeoxyglucose and hexamethylpropylene amine oxime SPECT in late whiplash syndrome. *Neurology, 51,* 345–50.

Binder, L.M. (1986). Persisting symptoms after mild head injury: A review of the postconcussive syndrome. *Journal of Clinical Experiment, 8*(4), 323–346.

Blumbergs, P.C., Scott, G., Manavis, J., et al. (1995). Topography of axonal injury as defined by amyloid precursor protein and the sector scoring method in mild and severe closed head injury. *Journal of Neurotrauma, 12,* 55–72.

Bohnen, N., & Jolles, J. (1992). Neurobehavioral aspects of postconcussive symptoms after mild head injury. *Journal of Nervous and Mental Disease, 180*(11), 683–692.

Bohnen, N., Twijnstra, A., & Jolles, J. (1992) Post-traumatic and emotional symptoms in different subgroups of patients with mild head injury. *Brain Injury, 6*(6), 481–487.

Bohnen, N., Van Zutphen, W., Twijnstra, A., et al. (1994). Late outcome of mild head injury: Results from a controlled postal survey. *Brain Injury, 8,* 701–708.

Boll, T.J., & Barth, J. (1983). Mild head injury. *Psychiatric Development, 28*(5), 509–513.

Brenner, C., Friedman, A.P., Merritt, H.H., & Denny-Brown, D.E. (1944). Post-traumatic headache. *Journal of Neurosurgery, 1,* 379–391.

Brenner, D.N., & Gillingham, J.F. (1974). Patterns of convalescence after minor head injury. *Journal Royal College Surgery, Edinburgh, 19,* 94–97.

Chambers, J., Cohen, S.S., Hemminger, L., et al. (1996). Mild traumatic brain injuries in low-risk patients. *Journal of Trauma, 41,* 976–980.

Christman, C.W., Grady, M.S., Walker, S.A., et al. (1994). Ultrastructural studies of diffuse axonal injury in humans. *Journal of Neurotrauma, 11,* 173–186.

Cicerone, K.D. (1992). Psychological management of post-concussive disorders. *Physical Medicine and Rehabilitation: State of the Art Reviews, 6*(1), 129–141.

Cicerone, K.D., & Kalmar, K. (1997). Does premorbid depression influence post-concussive symptoms and neuropsychological functioning? *Brain Injury, 11,* 643–648.

Crooks, D.A., Scholtz, C.L., Vowles, G., et al. (1992). Axonal injury in closed head injury by assault: A quantitative study. *Medical Science Law, 32*(2), 109–117.

Dikmen, S.S., McLean, A., Temkin, N., et al. (1986). Neuropsychological outcome at one month post injury. *Archives of Physical and Medical Rehabilitation, 67,* 507–513,.

Dikmen, S.S., Temkin, N., & Armsden, G. (1989). Neuropsychological recovery: Relationship to psychosocial functioning and postconcussional complaints. In H.S. Levin, H.M. Eisenberg, & A.L. Benton (Eds.), *Mild head injury* (pp. 2241–2290). New York: Oxford University Press.

DiStefano, G., & Radanov, B.P. (1995). Course of attention and memory after common whiplash: A two year prospective study with age, education and gender pair-matched patients. *Acta Neurologica Scandanavica, 91,* 346–352.

Elson, L.M., & Ward, C.C. (1994). Mechanisms and pathophysiology of mild head injury. *Seminars in Neurology, 14,* 8–18.

Engel, S., Wehner, H.D., & Meyermann, R. (1996). Expression of microglial markers in the human CNS after closed head injury. *Acta Neurochirugica Suppl. (Wien), 66,* 89–95.

Ettlin, T.M., Kischka, U., Reichmann, S., et al. (1993). Cerebral symptoms after whiplash injury of the neck: A prospective clinical and neuropsychological study of whiplash injury. *Journal of Neurology, Neurosurgery, and Psychiatry, 55,* 943–948.

Evans, R.W. (1992). The postconcussion syndrome and the sequelae of mild head injury. *Neurology Clinical, 10*(4), 815–847.

Ewing, R., McCarthy, D., Gronwall, D., et al. (1980). Persisting effects of minor head injury observable during hypoxic stress. *Journal of Clinical Neuropsychology, 2,* 147–155.

Fenton, G.W. (1996). The postconcussional syndrome reappraised. *Clinical Electroencephalography, 27,* 174–82.

Fukuda, K., Aihara, N., Sagar, S.M., et al. (1996). Purkinje cell vulnerability too mild traumatic brain injury. *Journal of Neurotrauma, 13,* 255–266.

Gale, S.D., Johnson, S.C., Bigler, E.D., & Blatter, D.D. (1995). Nonspecific white matter degeneration following traumatic brain injury. *Journal of International Neuropsychology Society, 1,* 17–28.

Gasquoine, P.G. (1997). Postconcussion symptoms. *Neuropsychology Review, 7,* 77–85.

Gentilini, M., Michelli, P., Shoenhuber, R., et al. (1985). Neuropsychological evaluation ofr mild head injury. *Journal of Neurology, Neurosurgery, and Psychiatry, 48,* 137–140.

Gimse, R., Tjell, C., Bjorgen, I.A., & Saunte, C. (1996). Disturbed eye movements after whiplash due to injuries to the posture control system. *Journal of Clinical and Experimental Neuropsychology, 18,* 178–186.

Gronwall, D., & Wrightson, P. (1974). Cumulative effects of concussion. *Lancet, 1,* 995.

Harrington, D.E., Malec, J., Cicerone, K., & Katz, H. . (1993). Current perceptions of rehabilitation professionals toward mild traumatic brain injury. *Archives of Physical Medicine and Rehabilitation, 74*(6), 579–586.

Heikkila, H.V., & Wenngren, B.I. (1998). Cervicocephalic kinesthetic sensibility, active range of cervical motion, and oculomotor function in patients with whiplash injury. *Archives of Physical Medicine and Rehabilitation, 79,* 1089–1094.

Hoganson, R.C., Sachs, N., Desai, B.T., & Whitman, S. (1984). Sequelae associated with head injuries in patients who were not hospitalized: A follow-up survey. *Neurosurgery, 14,* 315–317.

Imajo, T. (1996). Diffuse axonal injury: Its mechanism in an assault case. *American Journal of Forensic Medical Pathology, 17,* 324–326.

Jacobson, J., Gaadsgaard, S. E., Thomsen, S., & Henriksen, P. B. (1987). Prediction of post-concussional sequelae by reaction time test. *Acta Neurologica Scandanavica, 75*(5), 341–345.

Jay, G.W. (2000). *Mild traumatic brain injury handbook: Diagnosis and treatment.* Boca Raton, FL: CRC Press.

Jones, J.H., Viola, S.L., LaBan, M.M., et al. (1992). The incidence of post minor traumatic brain injury syndrome: A retrospective survey of treating physicians. *Archives of Physical and Medical Rehabilitation, 73*(2), 145–146.

Jones, R.K. (1974). Assessment of minimal head injuries: Indications for in-hospital care. *Surgical Neurology, 2,* 101–104.

Kant, R., Smith-Seemiller, L., Isaac, G., & Duffy, J. (1997). Tc-HMPAO SPECT in persistent post-concussion syndrome after mild head injury: Comparison with MRI/CT. *Brain Injury, 11,* 115–124.

Karakucuk, E., Pasaoglu, H., Pasaoglu, A., & Oktem, S. (1997). Endogenous neuropeptides in patients with acute traumatic head injury. II: Changes in the levels of cerebral spinal fluid substance P, serotonin and lipid peroxidation products in patients with head trauma. *Neuropeptides, 31,* 259–263.

Karzmark, P., Hall, K., & Englander, J. (1995). Late-onset postconcussional symptoms after mild brain injury: The role of premorbid, injury-related, environmental, and personality factors. *Brain Injury, 9,* 21–26.

Katz, R.T., & DeLuca, J. (1992). Sequelae of minor traumatic brain injury. *American Family Physician, 46*(5), 1491–1498.

Kay, T., et. al. (1993). Definition of mild traumatic brain injury. *Journal of Head Trauma Rehabilitation, 8*(3), 86–87.

Krapnick, J.L., & Horowitz, M.J. (1981). Stress response syndromes. *Archives of General Psychiatry, 38,* 428–435.

Landy, P.J. (1998). Neurological sequelae of minor head and neck injuries. *Injury, 29,* 199–206.

Leininger, B.E., Gramling, S.E, Farrell, A.D., et al. (1990). Neuropsychological deficits in symptomatic minor head injury patients after concussion and mild concussion. *Journal of Neurology, Neurosurgery, and Psychiatry, 53,* 293–296.

Leininger, B.E., & Kreutzer, J.S. (1992). Neuropsychological outcome of adults with mild traumatic brain injury: Implications for clinical practice and research. *Physical Medicine and Rehabilitation: State of the Art Reviews* 6(1), 169–182.

Levin, H., Mattis, S., Ruff, R., et al. (1987). Neurobehavioral outcome following minor head injury: A three center study. *Journal of Neurosurgery, 66,* 234–243.

Markianos, M., Seretis, A., Kotsou, A., & Christopoulos, M. (1996). CSF neurotransmitter metabolites in their clinical state. *Acta Neurochirugica (Wien), 138,* 57–59.

Mateer, C.A. (1992). Systems of care for post-concussive syndrome. *Physical Medicine and Rehabilitation: State of the Art Reviews* 6(1), 143–160.

Mayou, R., & Bryant, B. (1997). Outcome of "whiplash" neck injury. *Injury, 27,* 617–623.

McFlynn, G., Montgomery, F., Fenton, G.W., & Rutherford, W. (1984). Measurement of reaction time following minor head injury. *Journal of Neurology, Neurosurgery, and Psychiatry, 48,* 137–140.

McLean, A., Dikmen, S.S., Temkin, N., et al. (1984). Psychosocial functioning at one month after head injury. *Neurosurgery 14,* 393–399.

McLean, A., Temkin, N.R., Dikmen, S.S., et al. (1983).The behavioral sequelae of head injury. *Journal of Clinical Neuropsychology, 5,* 361–376.

McSherry, J.A. (1989). Cognitive impairment after head injury. *American Family Physician 40*(4), 186–190.

Middelboe, T., Anderson, H.S., Birket-Smith, M., & Friss, M.L. (1992). Minor head injury: Impact on general health after one year. A prospective follow-up study. *Acta Neurologica Scandanavica 85*(1), 5–9.

Murdoch, I., Perry, E.K., Court, J.A., et al. (1998). Cortical cholinergic dysfunction after human head injury. *Journal of Neurotrauma, 15,* 295–305.

Oddy, M., Humphrey, M., & Uttley, D. (1978). Subjective impairment and social recovery after closed head injury. *Journal of Neurology, Neurosurgery, and Psychiatry, 41,* 611–616.

Oehmichen, M., Meissner, C., Schmidt, V., et al. (1998). Axonal injury—A diagnostic tool in forensic neuropathology? A review. *Forensic Science International, 95,* 67–83.

Otte, A., Ettlin, T.M., Nitzsche, E.U., et al. (1997). PET and SPECT in whiplash syndrome: A new approach to a forgotten brain? *Journal of Neurology, Neurosurgery, and Psychiatry, 63,* 368–372.

Parizel, P.M., Ozsarla, K., Van Goethem, J.W., et al. (1998). Imaging findings in diffuse axonal injury after closed head trauma. *European Radiology, 8,* 960–965.

Parker, R.S., & Rosenblum, A. (1996). IQ loss and emotional dysfunctions after mild head injury incurred in a motor vehicle accident. *Journal of Clinical Psychology, 52,* 32–43.

Pasaoglu, H., Inci Karakucuk, E., Kurtsoy, A., & Pasaoglu, A. (1996). Endogenous neuropeptides in patients with acute traumatic head injury, I: Cerebrospinal fluid beta-endorphin levels are increased within 24 hours following the trauma. *Neuropeptides, 30,* 47–51.

Povlishock, J.T. (1992). Traumatically induced axonal injury: Pathogenesis and pathobiological implications. *Brain Pathology, 2,* 1–12.

Povlishock, J.T., & Jenkins, L.W. (1995). Are the pathobiological changes evoked by traumatic brain injury immediate and irreversible? *Brain Pathology, 5,* 415–426.

Radanov, B.P., DiStefano, G., Schnidrig, A., et al. (1991). Role of psychosocial stress in recovery from common whiplash. *Lancet, 338,* 712–715.

Ramsay, D.A., & Shkrum, M.J. (1995). Homicidal blunt head trauma, diffuse axonal injury, alcoholic intoxication and cardiorespiratory arrest: A case report of a forensic syndrome of acute brainstem dysfunction. *American Journal of Forensic Medicine and Pathology, 16,* 107–114.

Rimel, R.W., & Jane, J.A. (1985). Minor head injury: Management and outcome. In R.H. Williams & S.S. Rengachary (Eds.), *Neurosurgery* (pp. 1608–1611). New York: McGraw-Hill.

Ritchie, W.R. (1974). Recovery after minor head injury [Letter to the Editor]. *Lancet, 2,* 1315.

Rubin, A.M., Woolley, S.M., Dailey, V.M., & Goebel, J.A. (1995). Postural stability following mild head or whiplash injuries. *American Journal of Otology, 16,* 216–221.

Russell, W.R. (1974). Recovery after minor head injury [Letter to the Editor]. *Lancet, ii,* 1315.

Rutherford, W.H., Merrett, J.D., & McDonald, J.R. (1977). Sequelae of concussion caused by minor head injuries. *Lancet, 1,* 1–4.

Rutherford, W.H., Merrett, J.D., & McDonald, J.R. (1978–1979). Symptoms at one year following concussion from minor head injuries. *Injury, 10,* 225–230.

Schoenhuber, R., & Gentilini, M. (1988). Anxiety and depression after mild head injury: A case control study. *Journal of Neurology, Neurosurgery, and Psychiatry, 51,* 722–724.

Servadei, F., Nanni, A., Nasi, M.T., et al. (1995). Evolving brain lesions in the first 12 hours after head injury: Analysis of 37 comatose patients. *Neurosurgery, 37,* 899–906.

Soustiel, J.F., Hafner,H., Chistyakov, A.V., et al. (1995). Trigeminal and auditory evoked responses in minor head injuries and post-concussion syndrome. *Brain Injury, 9,* 805–813.

Stachura, Z., Kowalski, J., Obuchowicz, E., et al. (1997). Concentration of enkephalins in cerebrospinal fluid of patients after severe head injury. *Neuropeptides, 31,* 78–81.

Sturzenegger, M., DiStefano, G., Radanov, B.P., & Schnidrig, A. (1994). Presenting symptoms and signs after whiplash injury: The influence of accident mechanisms. *Neurology, 44,* 688–693.

Stuss, D.T., Ely, P., Hugenholtz, H., et al. (1985). Subtle neuropsychological deficits in patients with good recovery after closed head injury. *Neurosurgery, 17,* 41–47.

Stuss, D.T., Stethem, L.L., Hugenholtz, H., et al. (1989). Reaction time after traumatic brain injury. Fatigue, divided and focused attention and consistency of performance. *Journal of Neurology, Neurosurgery, and Psychiatry, 52,* 742–48.

Symonds, D. (1965). Concussion and its sequelae. *Lancet, 1,* 1–5.

Szymanski, H.V., & Linn, R. (1992). A review of the postconcussion syndrome. *International Journal of Psychiatry in Medicine, 22,* 357–375.

Tang, Y.P., Noda, Y., & Nabeshima, T. (1997). Involvement of activation of dopaminergic neuronal system in learning and memory deficits associated with experimental mild traumatic brain injury. *European Journal of Neuroscience, 9,* 1720–1727.

Thatcher, R.W., Camacho, M., Salazar, A., et al. (1997). Quantitative MRI of the gray-white matter distribution in traumatic brain injury. *Journal of Neurotrauma, 14,* 1–14.

Weingartner, H., Cohen, R.M., Murphy, D.L., et al. (1981). Cognitive processes in depression. *Archives of General Psychiatry, 38,* 42–44.

Wells, C.E. (1979). Pseudodementia. *American Journal of Psychiatry, 136,* 895–900.

Wrightson, P., & Gronwall, D. (1989). Time off work and symptoms after minor head injury. *Injury, 12*(6), 445–454.

Young, B. (1985). Sequelae of head injury. In R. H. Williams & S. S. Rengachary (Eds.), *Neurosurgery* (pp. 1691–1693). New York: McGraw-Hill.

Zasler, N.D. (1992). Neuromedical diagnosis and management of post-concussive disorders. *Physical Medicine and Rehabilitation: State of the Art Reviews, 6*(1), 33–67.

Ziegler, M.G., Morrissey, E.C., & Marshall, L.F. (1990). Catecholamine and thyroid hormones in traumatic injury. *Critical Care Medicine, 18,* 253–258.

16

Trauma and Soft Tissue Injuries: Clinic and Courtroom

Thomas J. Romano, M.D., Ph.D., F.A.C.P., F.A.C.R.

Astute clinicians have long known that physical trauma, sometimes seemingly trivial, can result in medical conditions characterized by persistent pain (Ashburn & Fine, 1989; Romano, 1990), fatigue (Romano, 1990), frustration, and psychological distress (Aaron, et al., 1997). It is certainly true that most patients who have sustained injuries from motor vehicle accidents, physical assaults, and falls recover fully. At the other end of the spectrum, some individuals die of their traumatically induced injuries. Typically, the clinicians who specialize in pain management do not have the opportunity to treat patients who fall into any of the preceding two categories. It is our responsibility to treat those patients who have neither died as a result of their injuries nor fully recovered. Our patient populations tend not to be composed of cross sections of society but by their very nature are skewed. We treat the patients who have not recovered and probably will not fully recover. Most have already been treated by emergency room physicians, primary care doctors, physical therapists, and other healthcare providers with less than satisfactory results. Our patients complain of chronic pain, headaches, fatigue, and neurological problems, and are often frustrated and angry. This is understandable because many have been injured in either an accident or a physical assault and are often involved in litigation at some level. Although it has been known for many years that numerous individuals suffer persistent pain following trauma (Ashburn & Fine, 1989; Romano, 1990), it is the purpose of this chapter to explain why.

Why do some patients involved in whiplash motor vehicle accident recover fully, while others do not? Why do some patients develop chronic posttraumatic headaches whereas others involved in similar traumas do not? Why do some patients develop fibromyalgia after traumatic events and others do not? The list goes on and on.

Although the answers to these questions will probably never be totally forthcoming, it is useful to think of the problem in the following way. We human beings are highly complex biological systems. We are certainly no less complex than bacteria, goldfish, or zebras. Thus, principles of biodiversity certainly should apply to how each of our individual complex biological systems (i.e., our own bodies) reacts to certain physical stressors such as physical trauma.

I often visit the American Museum of Natural History in New York City. Several years ago a new exhibit hall, the "Hall of Biodiversity," was dedicated. It celebrates the amazing and wondrous variety of plant and animal life on this planet. Not only interspecies variability but also intraspecies diversity is described and catalogued. Certainly all zebras are not exactly the same; neither are all salamanders nor all butterflies. Each individual within a species has its own unique physical and behavioral characteristics, but, of course, there are many characteristics it shares with the remainder of the members of its species.

Dr. Stephen Jay Gould — a frequent contributor to *Natural History Magazine* (a publication of the American Museum of Natural History) and a famed geologist and biologist as well as a prolific author — celebrates biodiversity in his work *Full House* (Gould, 1996). He makes a claim with which I heartily agree. He maintains that if one wishes to describe a complex biological system using measures of central tendency such as averages or means, he or she will be wrong. It is interesting to me that he uses the word *will* as opposed to *might*.

We are all distinct individuals. A mere average cannot describe our experiences or predict our future behavior. However, is that not exactly what insurance companies, managed care organizations, and even some members of the legal profession wish for us to do? How often have a patient's medical benefits following an injury been terminated because the insurance adjustor or the physician working for the insurance company has determined that the patient should have recovered?

Although it may be true that most patients with soft tissue injuries totally recover within 4 to 6 weeks, it is unscientific and, dare I say, dishonest to maintain that all soft tissue injury patients do so. Is it then fair to expect that every patient must recover in 4 to 6 weeks or in some other arbitrary length of time and that benefits will be cut off at the end of that predetermined time period regardless of whether the patient and the treating physician maintain otherwise? How frustrating it must be for the clinician and the patient to be told that the injury in question should have healed within a certain period of time, yet knowing that there is still much more to be done to get the patient back on his or her feet. Is the doctor incompetent? Is the patient malingering? Why has the patient not recovered within the specified interval of time? This chapter seeks to answer such questions and perhaps to outline a strategy for the clinician to practice to the best of his or her ability without interference and for the patient to receive whatever damages he or she is entitled to as a result of someone else's negligence.

CERVICAL SPRAIN: AND BEYOND

The scenario of a patient complaining of intense neck pain after a trauma, such as a motor vehicle accident, despite a normal cervical spine X-ray is a common occurrence in our society. What is causing the pain? There is no fracture; the speed of the respective motor vehicles was not great; the physical damage to the vehicles was negligible. Why is the patient still in pain? The answers to these questions probably lie in the ability to more fully appreciate the mechanisms of cervical injuries and the potential for such injuries to evolve into a chronic pain state that for far too long may have been underestimated.

For example, it might seem logical that the greater the impact of two vehicles in a collision and/or the greater the property damage sustained by these vehicles, the more serious and intense is the chronic pain suffered by those injured. However, the conventional wisdom identified by the previous statement seems to be incorrect. A study by Croft (1996) showed that there was no scientifically or empirically sound basis for judging injury potential from the speed of the involved vehicles or from vehicle property

damage. This actually does make sense if one remembers there is a large degree of biological variability among accident victims (Radanov & Sturzenegger, 1996). This could help explain why some high-speed impacts may leave some drivers relatively unscathed, whereas some low-impact collisions can be devastating to others.

What about the cervical spine X-ray? The cervical spine X-ray typically taken in the emergency room to rule out a fracture/dislocation of the cervical vertebral bodies probably is not a good predictor of how much chronic pain the patient will have months, and even years, after a particular trauma. One must remember that the emergency room physician is worried about acute spinal cord transection, acute cervical fractures, etc. Having worked in many emergency rooms including Bellevue Hospital in New York City and St. Louis City Hospital, I can assure you that the emergency room doctor's duty is not to concern himself or herself with chronic conditions. The duty is to keep the patient alive, diagnose any acute injuries, and refer to the appropriate follow-up physician.

An Australian study (Taylor & Taylor, 1996) revealed that even though cervical spine X-rays had been read as normal, there was a great deal of damage done to cervical spine structures. Of the 109 cases, 102 or 94% had injuries more often to the intervertebral joints than to the vertebrae. Spinal cord injuries were seen in 25% of cases, and nerve root injuries in 14 to 33% of cases. This is consistent with the findings of an earlier study (Jonssan, Bring, Rauschning, & Sahlstedt, 1991). Is it any wonder that a patient with an occult cervical spine fracture without dislocation would be in intense pain and perhaps not be given sufficient medication … or sufficient respect? After all, the cervical spine X-ray was normal. Would such a sequence of events not make the ground fertile for the development of such chrohnic problems as dizziness (Mallison, Longridge, & Peacok, 1996), headache (Lord & Bogduk, 1996), widespread musculoskeletal pain, or even fibromyalgia (Buskila, 1997a)?

Persistent symptoms after whiplash injuries have been the subject of several review articles (Curtis, Spanos, & Reid, 1995; Havsy, 1994a; Havsy, 1994b) and books (Foreman & Croft, 1988; Swerdlow, 1998; Tollison & Satterthwaite, 1992). Various factors have been demonstrated to influence long-term outcome. A statistically significant positive correlation has been shown to exist between poor prognosis (i.e., chronic pain and impairment) and the following findings shortly after the trauma: numbness and/or pain in either arm, sharp reversal of the cervical lordosis as demonstrated on cervical spine X-ray, need for a cervical collar for more than 12 weeks, need for home traction, or need to resume physical therapy more than once because of a recurrence of symptoms (Hohl, 1974). This early study also showed that recovery occurred in only 57% of patients after 5 to 6 years. Degenerative changes developed after the injury in 39%.

A later study (Gargon & Bannister, 1990) with a longer follow-up period (mean 10.8 years) revealed that only 12% of patients who had sustained soft tissue injuries of the neck recovered completely. The authors reported that residual symptoms were "intrusive" in 28% and "severe" in 12%. They further noted that after 2 years from the date of the trauma, symptoms did not tend to alter with the further passage of time. Persistent symptoms posttrauma are not limited to neck pain, stiffness, headaches, etc. Cognitive deficits have been noted in patients with cervical spine injuries (Radanov, Dvorak, & Valach, 1992). These included dizziness, poor concentration, irritability, sleep disturbances, forgetfulness, loss of control, and many others — including, most commonly, headaches.

POSTTRAUMATIC HEADACHES

Many patients complain of rather severe headaches after being involved in traumatic events such as a motor vehicle accident or a fall. The cause of posttraumatic headaches has been known for many years. Often it is a mixed headache disorder developing because of muscle tension and vascular type of headache phenomena. In fact, many patients with cervical spine trauma also have mild traumatic brain injuries (MTBIs) that can result in the patient suffering from chronic headaches resembling migraines in their intensity, characteristics, and frequency. Some neurologists have called such headaches *posttraumatic migraines*. I prefer the term *posttraumatic headaches* or *posttraumatic vascular headaches* because these terms tend not to be confused with common migraine headaches, typically idiopathic in nature. Often patients who complain of headaches after an injury are treated symptomatically but little is done to look into the mechanism of the headaches or to validate the patient's complaints with objective testing. Perhaps it is because such patients are not believed or are thought to be exaggerating their pain. Many such patients are involved in litigation, making their motives suspect to the inadequately trained clinician. It must be stressed that there is no medical evidence that faking such symptoms is common.

A study (Packard, 1992) written to put this question to rest consisted of a large series of patients diagnosed with posttraumatic headaches. These patients continued to seek treatment and had persistent symptoms, often severe, despite the resolution of their litigation. That being the case and knowing that certain medications such as calcium channel blockers, beta-blockers, and tricyclic agents can be used prophylactically to prevent vascular headache symptoms (*vis a vis* migraine), then the need to indentify those patients whose posttraumatic headaches have a vascular component becomes obvious.

A method to detect vascular instability in the cerebral circulation (often a harbinger of intense vascular-type headaches) is available. Brain Single Photon Emission Computerized Tomography (SPECT) scanning is a useful, relatively noninvasive (i.e., one intranvenous injection of a radioactive isotope), fairly safe, and sensitive test (Holman & Devous, 1992; Nedd, et al., 1993; Newton, et al., 1992; Wyper, 1993). Although the SPECT scan does not make the diagnosis (the clinician needs to correlate the results with all other aspects of the patient's problem), it can be a very useful tool in making an accurate diagnosis and in directing therapy. If a patient has an imbalance in brain circulation as measured by a brain SPECT scan, the rationale for the use of such prophylactic agents mentioned earlier is obvious and compelling. On the other hand, if the posttraumatic headaches have their origin in muscle tension or intervertebral joint pathology with little, if any, contribution from abnormalities in cerebral circulation, then the treatment plan would weigh more heavily in favor of trigger point therapy, anti-inflammatory/anti-arthritic medication, or physical modalities such as manipulation/adjustment, etc.

Patients with cervical spine injuries who complain of headaches may also have a MTBI that should be evaluated thoroughly. One must not assume that the chronic headache is cervicogenic, although there may be a cervicogenic component. Brain SPECT scanning is a relatively noninvasive and potentially very helpful test and is much more sensitive than magnetic resonance imaging (MRI) or computed tomography (CT) (Tikofsky, 1994) and twice as sensitive as computerized electroencepholography (Romano, 1995) for detecting chronic traumatic brain injury. I must stress that in the initial evaluation of patients suspected of having an acute brain injury, MRI and/or CT can be invaluable. Such problems as subdural hematomas and intracerebral hemorrhage can be promptly identified with the preceding techniques and emergency measures can be taken. Brain SPECT scanning in the context of posttraumatic headaches should be utilized if the patient has persistent headaches and/or cognitive dysfunction months, or even years, after the trauma. At that point intracerebral pathology either had been ruled out or was no longer a realistic consideration.

Many patients who have suffered whiplash injuries also complain of a veritable litany of symptoms including light-headedness, dizziness, vertigo, double vision, blurred vision, ringing of the ears, being hard of hearing, memory problems, trouble concentrating, being easily distracted, fatigue, anxiety, excessive sweating, sadness, trouble sleeping, moodiness, irritability, changes in menstrual periods, impaired vaginal lubrication, impotence, and lack of interest in sex. Do these patients have sufficient injuries to their brains to be considered as suffering postconcussional problems?

Such conditions can arise even if there is only a momentary change in the level of consciousness — and even if no change in consciousness — at the time of the trauma. Closed head injuries have been associated with depression, anxiety, personality changes, cognitive deficits, and other such symptoms (Kant, 1996). This neurobehavioral morbidity is more common than once believed (Brown, Fann, & Grant, 1994) and, if not treated, can cause severe impairment, resulting in a marked deterioration in the quality of life. This often manifests itself as the loss of one's job, marital difficulties, and the loss of friendships. Economic hardship often accompanies these other problems.

MYOFASCIAL PAIN SYNDROME

The definition and characteristics of myofascial pain syndrome (MPS) have been amply covered in this textbook (Margoles, 1998; Gerwin & Dommerholt, 1998) and other texts (Travell & Simons, 1983; Rachlin, 1994). The diagnosis of MPS is based on the detection of objective abnormalities on careful physical examination. These include the findings of trigger points, taut myofascial bands, local twitch responses of the taut bands (Simons, 1987), and even characteristic electrical activity of trigger points measured by the electromyogram (Hubbard & Berkoff, 1993; Romano & Stiller, 1997).

The role of trauma in the generation and perpetuation of trigger points, long known to be the hallmark physical findings of MPS, was perhaps most succinctly stated by Rachlin (1994): "Injuries and surgical procedures may lead to the formation of trigger points causing repeated episodes of pain."

The worst cases of MPS seem to be the result of traumatic events such as an automobile accident or fall. Simons (1987) noted that such patients "suffer greatly and are difficult to help." He went on to write, "They exhibit a posttraumatic hyperirritability of their nervous system and of their trigger points." The trauma in question, according to Simons, is "severe enough to damage the sensory pathways of the central nervous system." In a study of Israeli trauma victims (Buskila, Neumann, Vaisberg, Alkalay, & Wolfe, 1997a), the authors suggested that the reason fibromyalgia syndrome (FS) followed neck injury 13 times more often than lower extremity injury was because of this very mechanism. The involvement of the nervous system probably is very important in the perpetuation and prolongation of the pain, thus preventing full recovery. Simons (1987) opined that damage to the nervous system " … apparently acts as an endogenous perpetuating factor susceptible to augmentation by severe pain, additional trauma, vibration, loud noises, prolonged physical activity, and emotional stress." In describing the patients who developed such severe MPS, Simons noted, "From the date of the trauma, coping with pain typically becomes the focus of life for these patients who previously paid little attention to pain. They are unable to increase their activity substantially without increasing their pain

level." Once the nervous system exhibits "posttraumatic hyperirritability" or other perpetuating factors exist and are left untreated, "an acute myofascial pain syndrome characteristically becomes chronic."

When I first read the preceding description, I immediately knew that Dr. Simons and I had something in common. We both saw numerous chronic pain patients and we both took the time to analyze their situations. He could have easily been describing patients I see and treat every day. He and I know these patients are suffering and in trouble. They did not choose to be injured; they need our help.

The concept of perpetuating factors has been known for many years (Travell & Simons, 1983), yet many patients who have severe, chronic MPS (often posttrauma) are met with skepticism and even disbelief. Bayer (1999, p. 171) wrote, "It is amazing if not amusing that insurers and their attorneys cannot believe that a patient who has suffered an injury can continue to experience symptoms of pain months or years after the injury."

However, the reality of the situation can be summed up as follows: (1) some patients develop severe, chronic MPS and even FS as the result of an injury; (2) some of these patients are treated unfairly and are not evaluated thoroughly because they may not be believed, especially when personal injury litigation is pending; and (3) the pain management specialist must rely on medical knowledge and scientific validity in formulating diagnoses and prognoses — not on bias or innuendo.

Stress plays a role in the severity of illness — any illness, not just musculoskeletal or neurological. What sane physician would encourage a patient with high blood pressure, heart disease, or ulcers to continue a stressful and unhealthy lifestyle? Thus, in treating the patient with chronic MPS, the clinician needs to help minimize stress — not contribute to it. The evaluation and treatment must be done honestly and professionally, realizing that the vast majority of patients diagnosed with posttraumatic MPS (PTMPS) are in a great deal of pain; they also are probably anxious, depressed, and frustrated due to the severity and longevity of their pain as well as probably having previously been given "short shrift" by a system that is supposed to help them. If patients with PTMPS are not treated promptly or if their pain cannot be controlled, they may even develop FS.

POSTTRAUMATIC FIBROMYALGIA SYNDROME

FS is a soft tissue rheumatic disorder characterized by widespread musculoskeletal pain associated with a deficiency of deep (i.e., stage 4, non-rapid eye movement, delta wave) sleep, headaches, fatigue, decreased stamina, and other symptoms (Romano, 1990). A committee appointed by the American College of Rheumatology (ACR) published FS criteria (Wolfe, et al., 1990) that are still in use today not only in the United States but also throughout the world.

The concept of posttraumatic fibromyalgia syndrome (PTFS) has been discussed in another chapter in this book (Romano, 1998a). However, additional remarks concerning the validity of a PTFS diagnosis need to be stressed. There have been numerous reports and book chapters in which the authors link trauma and FS (Bennett, 1989; Greenfield, Fitzcharles, & Esdaile, 1992; Moldofsky, Wong, & Lue, 1993; Rice, 1987; Saskin, Moldofsky, & Lue, 1986; Smythe, 1989). Despite this wealth of information, most doctors at a conference in Vancouver, British Columbia, in 1994 could not link trauma to FS in a cause–effect relationship. They concluded that at the time "…data from the literature are insufficient to indicate whether a causal relationship exists between trauma and FM (fibromyalgia)" (Wolfe, 1996). Many of the conference attendees opined that based on only four studies published up to that time (Greenfield, Fitzcharles, & Esdaile, 1992; Moldofsky, Wong, & Lue, 1994; Romano, 1990; Saskin, et al., 1986) they did not have enough evidence to conclude that trauma could cause FM. The committee chairman, Dr. Wolfe, was quick to add that the absence of evidence "…however, does not mean that causality does not exist, rather that appropriate studies have not been performed." Since the Vancouver conference, subsequent articles have been published (Aaron, et al., 1997; Alexander et al., 1998; Waylonis & Perkins, 1994) linking trauma and FM including a case report (Wolfe, 1994) and a controlled study of 161 cases of traumatic injury (Buskila, et al., 1997a) — both authored by Wolfe. In the latter study, Wolfe and the other authors conclude that FM was 13 times more frequent following neck injury than following lower extremity injury. Furthermore, the article ends with the following two sentences: "Thus, trauma may cause FMS (fibromyalgia syndrome), but it does not necessarily cause work disability. These findings have important implications for many industrialized countries."

Despite these new data, the Vancouver conference proceedings continue to be quoted out of context and sections of the text have been unfairly used to discredit patients who have developed PTFS. As an attendee of the Vancouver FS Conference and a participant in the discussions, I did not initially appreciate that this academic endeavor would be used for purposes unintended by most, if not all, participants. When I returned from the conference, I witnessed firsthand how attorneys and even medical evaluators have incorrectly stated the findings of the Vancouver conference to gain an advanatge in such medico-legal proceedings as depositions and even trials.

Such misrepresentations, often blatant, of what happened at that meeting motivated some attendees to publish a report to correct any misconceptions about the Vancouver conference (Yunus, Bennett, Romano, Russell, et al.,

1997). These authors correctly state that the Vancouver Consensus Report is likely to be used in the legal setting and further aptly remark that in such a setting "…causality entails only 51% certainty, usually stated in terms of reasonable medical probability." They go on to state that "…it seems more than 51% likely that trauma does play a causative role in some FMS (fibromyalgia) patients…". They cite articles on clinical patterns (Bennett, 1993; Moldofsky, et al., 1993; Pellegrino, 1996; Romano, 1990; Wolfe, 1994), other case studies (Bengtssom, et al., 1986; Buskila, et al., 1997a; Greenfield, et al., 1992; Yunus & Alday, 1993), and biological plausability concerning central nervous system plasticity (Coderre, Katz, Vaccarino, & Melzack, 1993; Dubner & Ruda, 1992; Yunus, 1992) as the basis of that statement.

FS does not develop after all, or even most, traumatic events but it can evolve after such traumas as physical assaults, motor vehicle accidents, and/or falls. FS takes at least 3 months to evolve according to ACR criteria (Wolfe, 1990). Thus, FS does not occur at the exact time of the trauma, but instead can develop weeks to months later as a direct consequence of the trauma. The real question confronting the clinician and about which he or she may need to offer legal testimony is whether a specific trauma caused a specific FS in a specific patient at a specific time. To determine that, a careful record review, a thorough medical history, and a physical examination must be obtained so that a conclusion can be reached based on the facts as opposed to prejudice or bias.

Infections can also trigger or precipitate the development of FS. An association between infections and FS has been known for a long time (Beetham, 1979). There have been numerous case reports of patients developing FS as a result of certain infections. For example, FS has been reported to have been caused by hepatitis virus (Buskila, et al., 1997b), human immunodeficiency virus (HIV) (Simms, et al., 1992), *Borrelia burgdorferi* (Lyme disease) (Dinerman & Steere, 1992), and coxsackie virus and parvovirus (Leventhal, Naides, & Freundlich, 1991). Goldenberg (1993) attempted to explain how infections trigger FS by theorizing that such infections may "promote a maladaptive behavior pattern which secondarily leads to fibromyalgia." Other explanations, including a disruption of normal sleep pattern and/or endocrine abnormalities, may be equally valid.

Regardless of how infections trigger FS, they can and do cause FS in some patients. Considering that the presence of FS diminishes the quality of life (Burckhardt, Clark, & Bennett, 1993; Martinez, Ferraz, Sato, & Atra, 1995; Turk, Okifuji, Sinclair, & Starz, 1996), the development of FS as a result of an infection is an important component of the patient's medical history. If the infection comes about as the result of negligence or even malice, the clinician may be called on to render an expert opinion concerning causation, severity, and prognosis.

If asked to testify in court concerning soft tissue injuries, the healthcare professional must remember that the court needs to know (1) what the patient is suffering from, (2) whether the medical problem (e.g., FS or MPS) could have been precipitated or caused by trauma, (3) whether the problem was indeed precipitated or caused by the accident/incident in question (i.e., if the trauma had not occurred, would the patient have this problem), (4) whether the problem is temporary or permanent, and (5) what the cost of future care will be for the patient for the injuries sustained in the accident/incident. The court needs to know these facts to a reasonable degree of medical probability or certainty. The physician's education, training, and experience, as well as his or her knowledge of the particular patient in question, should be the basis for giving such opinions.

There is no cure for FS and it does not decrease longevity. Therefore, the use of standard actuarial/mortality tables such as those provided by government agencies (Vital Statistics of the United States, 1992) is a reasonable way to determine the number of additional years a given patient is expected to live.

With that information and the knowledge of what the individual PTFS patient would need for his or her future care, the practitioner would be in a good position to render an opinion as to the cost of future medical care for the treatment of the injuries in question. Typically this treatment would include office visits, oral medications (e.g., muscle relaxants, analgesics), topical preparations (liniments), local injections, physical modalities (e.g., massage therapy, manipulation, or adjustment), and blood tests to determine whether the oral medications were causing side effects, etc.

The treatment of FS can result in diminution of symptoms with resultant clinical improvement, albeit temporary. A cure, thus far, has not been forthcoming (Kennedy & Felson, 1996; Wolfe, et al., 1997a; Wolfe, et al., 1997b). It has been reported that cost of treatment of FS patients is substantial (White, Speechley, Harth, & Ostbye, 1999; Wolfe, 1995), in part due to the chronicity of this syndrome. Often the cost of future treatment for the remainder of a patient's life is in six figures, especially if the patient is under the age of 40, and therefore is likely to live another 30 to 40 years (Vital Statistics, 1992), or if the patient in question requires a large number of medications or procedures. Of course, these projections must be tailor-made for each individual patient.

An even greater challenge to the pain practitioner is the task of estimating the relative contribution of each of several traumas to the patients' chronic pain state. Although the clinician must call on his or her years of education, training, and experience to perform such an apportionment, a method to help do this using mathematical formulas has been published (Romano, 1998b). This method can be applied to patients with either PTFS, PTMPS, or both. However, the author notes that there is no substitute for clinical acumen and that these formulas must not be used as a substitute for sound clinical judgment.

DISABILITY

The assessment of impairment and disability can be a difficult task, especially when the patient in question has chronic pain (Teasell & Merskey, 1997) with little or no skeletal deformity as is the case with soft tissue rheumatic syndromes such as FS and MPS (Bennett, 1996; Crook, Moldofsky, & Shannon, 1998; Monsein, 1994; Reilly, 1998). Because the issues are varied and complex, only clinicians with sufficient knowledge and experience in the evaluation and treatment of such patients should render opinions concerning disability (Bennett, 1996).

The majority of patients who suffer from painful soft tissue problems remain in the workforce. However, some are so impaired that they need to seek disability benefits. For example, patients with FS caused by trauma or illness are more disabled than other FS patients (Greenfield, et al., 1992). FS is as disabling as rheumatoid arthritis (Bombardier, et al., 1986; Cathey, Wolfe, & Kleinheksel, 1988; Russell, Fletcher, Tsui, & Michalek, 1989). The FS patient can be disabled because of not only pain but also inability to perform repetitive muscular tasks (Bennett, 1993); the disability is probably because of fatigue, abnormal hormone production, and other factors including lesions in muscle that result in low levels of high-energy phosphates and altered microcirculation. Some FS patients can remain employed only if there are significant workplace modifications. These include reverting to part-time status, freelancing if possible, and alteration of the patient's workstation itself including the provision of special ergonomically suitable aids. When these fail or are impractical, FS patients often enlist the aid of their doctors in obtaining disability benefits.

What is meant by the term *disability*? The Social Security Administration (1998) defines *disability* as, "An inability to perform any substantial gainful activity because of a medically determinable physical or mental impairment which can be expected to last for a continuous period of not less than 12 months." Of course, there are numerous other sources of potential disability benefits ranging from private insurance disability policies to benefits offered by companies and state agencies. The definition of disability by these other entities must be ascertained by reading the individual policies. Consequently, a discussion of this topic must of necessity be limited to the Social Security system's definitions and procedures. To that agency, "substantial gainful activity" means work that "(a) involves doing significant and productive physical or mental duties; and (b) is done (or intended) for pay or profit."

There are several reasons why a person would not be eligible for Social Security disability benefits. If a person is working (except in a "sheltered" setting) even if chronically ill or if he or she has recovered within 12 months of the onset of a potentially disabling illness, benefits are not granted. Furthermore, benefits are denied if the claimant is judged not to have a medically determinable impairment. That is where the patient's treating physician becomes a part of the disability process.

The role of the physician in the disability process is a crucial but often frustrating one. Often the patient does not understand that the determination of partial or total disability does not rest in the hands of the doctor. In truth, the physician may be able to rate impairment but disability is usually determined by a board that not only takes into account the patient's impairment but also considers other factors such as the individual's age and education, job opportunities, and local economy. Although the doctor may be convinced that the patient is disabled, he or she often is put in the unenviable position of having to explain the vagaries and intricacies of this system to the patient who has just been denied disability benefits.

This turn of events is especially likely for the patient with FS. The reasons for this are numerous. Despite the establishment of FS criteria by the ACR in 1990 and in subsequent studies showing that FS patients have numerous objectively measurable abnormalities (e.g., low magnesium levels (Romano and Stiller, 1994); decreased growth hormone levels (Bennett, Clark, Campbell, & Burkhardt, 1992)), the very existence of FS is doubted by those who have not kept up with the medical literature. Furthermore, the physician may have a difficult time in rating impairment and justifying that rating to disability boards because the American Medial Association Guide to the Evaluation of Permanent Impairment does not address FS. In fact, this publication needs revision for a number of different reasons (Cocchiarella, Turk, & Anderson, 2000; Speiler, Barth, Burton, Himmelstein, & Rudolph, 2000). Finally, the FS patient typically does not look ill.

However, despite all these apparent disadvantages, the FS patient who cannot work should apply for disability benefits with the expectation that fairness and reason will prevail. For this to happen, a collaborative effort between patient, physician, and — in most instances — attorney is necesary (Potter, 1992).

The treating physician's medical report is essential for the awarding of disability benefits, but the doctor must take care to provide detailed and clear (and, of course, honest) statements concerning the patients' impairments. Terse opinions that the patient cannot work or is disabled are insufficient. The narrative report should follow a familiar forensic format with a detailed history, a thorough physical examination, an enumeration and explanation of relevant test results, and a discussion that directly addresses itself to the patient's pain and the credibility of the patient. Where applicable the physician should also indicate that he or she has expertise in FS and has treated many such patients. Because of the nature of FS and unfounded bias against this diagnosis, it is worthwhile for the doctor to state emphatically that the patient is not exhibiting secondary gain or is not a malingerer. It is essential to state that the patient's symptoms are consistent with the findings and diagnosis of FS.

The Social Security system tends to be slow and somewhat reluctant in granting disability benefits in general. Therefore, if the initial application is rejected, the truly disabled FS patient needs to follow an orderly and logical process to obtain disability benefits. There are several steps ranging from a request for reconsideration to a hearing before an administrative law judge to an appeal through the U.S. District Court. An attorney, of course, is necessary for these latter two steps in the disability process. Paradoxically, even the denials can be helpful to the applicant, because they usually contain suggestions for alternative work possibilities (practical or not) and may suggest changes in strategy.

For example, because there is no specific listing for FS (as is also the case with newly described diseases and syndromes) and if the patient is denied disability benefits on the basis of FS, the physician may be able to find "acceptable" disease entities (i.e., those that are listed) that could explain the patient's symptoms. Many FS patients exhibit, in addition to musculoskeletal pain and fatigue, many psychiatric symptoms such as anxiety, and/or depression (listing 12) or may be considered to have a somatoform disorder (listing 12.07). This is not to suggest that FS is a psychiatric disease but the ravages of FS with its concomitant chronic pain, sense of loss, and ecnomic hardship certainly can predispose one to psychological problems. Another tactic is to attempt to get disability benefits based on organic brain dysfunction (i.e., diffuse impairment of cerebral tissue function), which is listed as 12.02. Many FS patients have significant cognitive problems that have been correlated with brain abnormalities detected by cranial SPECT imaging (Romano & Govindan, 1996), an objective neurodiagnostic test. Although this may not be the most ideal way to obtain benefits, it may be the only recourse for some FS patients, especially under the present circumstances.

The FS patients who are denied disability benefits frequently ask me to explain why they were not granted what they felt they deserved. I cannot answer this question fully because I am not privy to the machinations and workings of the disability boards. However, I have a good idea why FS patients frequently run into problems. It stems from how the FS patient is perceived. There are many different ways the FS patient may be viewed depending on the nature and/or bias of the observers. For example, managed care and health maintenance organizations claim that healthcare costs must be curbed. That translates into the very real possibility that doctors are to be limited in what they can do for their patients — FS and MPS sufferers included. If chronic soft tissue problems such as FS and MPS are perceived to be less important than other disorders, these patients may go undiagnosed, untreated, or undertreated. It certainly seems that it is in the best interest of the health insurance industry to withhold or delay issuing funds for care. Anyone who doubts this statement has only to read articles that appeared in *American Medical News* (Jacob, 1998; Mitka, 1996) describing the high salaries of managed care executives. Governmental agencies, moreover, experience budgetary constraints. This has been especially true as the national debt has risen. Thus, patients whose problems are not immediately life-threatening make handy scapegoats for the healthcare providers who treat them.

What is the answer? How is the FS patient to proceed? If the FS patient is truly unable to work, he or she must become thoroughly familiar with the disability determination process and proceed accordingly. The treating physician's report is a very important part of this process. The FS patient, however, must not be unduly discouraged by a system that is less that ideal. It is only through dogged determination and persistance that justice is truly served not only for the individual FS patient presently seeking disability benefits but also for all FS patients who ultimately need respect and understanding from our society in addition to medical treatment.

Even more frustrating and challenging is the task of rendering an opinion as to the extent of partial disability or impairment. How does one give such an opinion for FS patients, for example, whose symptoms wax and wane depending on such variables as weather changes, stress, and severity of concomitant illnesses? One way to perform such an analysis is to do so by having the patient fill out pain and activity questionnaires (Callahan, Smith, & Pincus, 1989; Meenan & Pincus, 1987; Pincus, Summey, Soraci, Hummon, & Wallston, 1983; Wolfe, 1995) on multiple occasions or keep a daily diary of symptoms and activities. If, for example, half the time a particular patient is totally incapacitated (even bed-bound) due to severe FS pain, fatigue, or excrutiating headaches, but the remainder of the time, normal activities can be pursued, then it is reasonable to assign that particular patient a 50% impairment of the "whole person." There is no easy formula to estimate impairment and/or disability for the patient with FS or other forms of painful soft tissue rheumatic problems. That is where the skill and experience of the clinician truly comes into play.

Bennett (1996) noted that for FS patients a biopsychosocial model of disease must be used in their disability evaluations and that opinions need to be expressed in terms of reasonable probability. He further states that some physicians feel "uncomfortable" in the assessment of chronic pain and "others will not have acquired the broad knowledge base necessary for understanding the biopsychosocial concept of disease." I heartily agree with his opinion that it is "preferable that both (those) groups exempt themselves, from the disability evaluation process." One can but hope … and dream.

THE CLINICIAN IN THE COURTROOM

The pain management clinician should take an active role in the legal process. First, as a member of the community he or she should get involved in community matters, especially those that affect his or her patients. Obviously this may include the medical/legal arena. If the clinician has knowledge concerning a patient's medical condition that would benefit the court, the practitioner has a duty to present that knowledge at the proper time whether it be in the form of a deposition or as an expert witness giving testimony in a courtroom. I am not alone in this opinion. As a member of the American Medical Association (AMA) and as a Fellow of the American College of Physicians, I have reviewed the ethics manuals for each group (American College of Physicians, 1998; American Medical Association Council on Ethical and Judicial Affairs, 1996–1997). Both publications clearly state that if the physician has knowledge that can be useful to the court, it is his or her duty to present such knowledge when asked.

I have participated in hundreds of trials and depositions mostly as a witness giving expert medical testimony concerning patients that I am actively treating. Some attorneys have wrongly intimated that because of this, I cannot be objective, that I have an interest in the outcome of the case, and/or that I am being less than truthful in my responses because the plaintiff in question is my patient. These are common tactics used to undermine the credibility of expert witnesses. However, despite the innuendo I willingly testify at trials because I believe it is the right thing to do, especially considering my unique perspective as a pain management specialist. This is even more so if the patient in question is being treated by me and I have examined him or her on numerous occasions. When I perform a medical evaluation for the purpose of rendering an opinion only, I strive to be objective, relying on established criteria for FS and MPS as well as testing with a dolorimeter and a tissue compliance meter (Smiley, Cram, Margoles, Romano, & Stiller, 1992).

The court is not interested in "may be" or "could be." The court wants to know whether a patient has a particular condition as a result of a particular trauma "to a reasonable degree of medical probability." That means is it more likely than not that the trauma in question caused the patient to develop a medical problem for which he or she is being treated. For example, did the motor vehicle accident of 3 years ago cause the patient to develop FM? One does not need to know with 100% certainty that a given trauma caused a patient's medical problem in question;

however, based on the clinician's education, training, and experience he or she often can given an opinion "to a reasonable degree of medical probability" whether the trauma in question caused a patient's injuries. This is an important concept and one that is often lost on academicians and scientists who are used to expressing their thoughts to a degree of certainty approaching 95 to 100%.

The court is especially interested in the objective findings that help form the bases for the opinions rendered. After performing a range of motion and/or a trigger point examinations, the clinician in the role of expert witness must stress that such findings on physical examination are objective. Other objective findings include muscle spasm, jump signs, swelling, discoloration, especially reticular skin changes, taut myofascial bands, muscle atrophy, asymmetry of muscle size or strength, and deep tendon reflex abnormalities. The greater the skill of the examiner, the more likely such abnormalities will be observed and recorded. Most neurologists and orthopedists do not have the required expertise to perform an FS tender point count or an MPS trigger point exam. According to Simons (1987), the diagnosis of FS and/or MPS "…would probably be missed on routine conventional examination. The examiner must know precisely what to look for, how to look for it, and then must actually be looking for it." Is it any wonder that patients who have been diagnosed with either FS and/or MPS are sent by insurance companies to doctors with little or no experience in the diagnosis of these disorders? Is it not in the best economic interest of such corporations to muddy the waters, so that the true extent of the patients' injuries are not appreciated?

However, absence of proof is not proof of absence. It is beyond the control of the pain practitioner to alter the view of the insurance industry that invididuals who claim not to have recovered from an injury and therefore suffer resultant chronic painful conditions are exaggerating their pain, malingering, or suffering from mental problems.

However, it is within the expertise of the knowledgeable clinician to be diligent in taking a medical history, circumspect in reviewing pertinent medical records, and thorough in performing a physical examination so that he or she can make an accurate diagnosis in the office and explain the salient findings in legal proceedings. What is wrong with the best trained and most skilled examiners testifying in court? It appears to be in the best interest of the insurance companies to place blame on the patient and to ignore important facts about MPS and/or FS as well as other important details about those individuals suffering from disorders stemming from a traumatic event.

The clinician as an expert witness must not take sides in a personal injury lawsuit. He or she must be honest, truthful, and professional at all times. However, having sworn to tell the whole truth, he or she must point out to the court if and how insurance company adverse medical evaluations were either inadequate, inappropriately performed, or lacking in scientific/medical validity. Doing so does not make the clinician an advocate in court, but instead it helps the court make a decision based on sound medical principles as opposed to ignorance and/or misrepresentations.

It should be remembered that medicine is an art that uses scientific principles, but an art, nonetheless. Some medical experts are more skilled than others. The clinician who specializes in pain and has particular expertise in evaluating individuals claiming chronic painful problems posttrauma deserves to have his or her opinions regarded carefully and with respect. So, too, do our patients deserve our respect and that of the courts.

REFERENCES

Aaron, L.A., Bradley, L.A., Alarcon, G.D., Triana-Alexander, M., Alexander, R.W., Martin, M.Y., & Alberts, K.R. (1997). Perceived physical and emotional trauma as precipitating events in fibromyalgia. *Arthritis and Rheumatism, 40,* 453–460.

Alexander, R.W., Bradley, L.A., & Alarcon, G.S., Trina-Alexander, M., Aaron, L.A., Alberts, K.R., Martin, M.Y., & Stewart, K.E. (1998). Sexual and physical abuse in women with fibromyalgia: Association with out-patient health care utilization and pain medication usage. *Arthritis Care and Research, 11,* 102–115.

American College of Physicians. (1998). Ethics manual (4th ed.). *Annals of Internal Medicine, 128,* 576–592.

American Medical Association. (1993). *Guide to the evaluation of permanent impairment.* Chicago: American Medical Association.

American Medical Association Council on Ethical and Judicial Affairs (1996–1997 edition). Code of medical ethics. Current opinions with annotations. Section 9.07 (pp. 148–149). Chicago: American Medical Association.

Ashburn, M. A., & Fine, P. G. (1989). Persistent pain following trauma. *Military Medicine, 154,* 86–89.

Bayer, J.D. (1999). Defense of a trigger point patient: Trigger points are myogenic, not psychogenic. In M. Margoles & R. Weiner (Eds.), *Chronic pain assessments, diagnosis and management* (pp. 171–178). Boca Raton, FL: CRC Press.

Beetham, W.P. (1979). Diagnosis and management of fibrositis syndrome and psychogenic rheumatism. *Medical Clinics of North America, 63,* 433–439.

Bengtsson, A., Henrikson, K.C., Jorfeldt, L. Kagedal, B., Lennmarker, C., & Lindstron, F. (1986). Primary fibromyalgia. A clinical and laboratory study of 55 patients. *Scandinavian Journal of Rheumatology, 15,* 340–347.

Bennett, R.M. (1989). Fibrositis. In W.N. Kelley, E.D. Harris, S. Ruddy, & C.B. Sledge (Eds.), *Textbook of rheumatology* (3rd ed., pp. 541–553). Philadelphia: W. B. Saunders.

Bennett, R.M. (1993). Disabling fibromyalgia: Appearance versus reality [Editorial]. *Journal of Rheumatology, 11,* 1821–1824.

Bennett, R.M. (1996). Fibromyalgia and the disability dilemma. *Arthritis and Rheumatism, 39,* 1627–1634.

Bennett, R.M., Clark, S.R., Campbell, S.M., & Burkhardt, C.S. (1992). Somatomedin C levels in patients with the fibromyalgia syndrome: A possible link between sleep and muscle pain. *Arthritis and Rheumatism, 35,* 1113–1116.

Bombardier, C., Ware, J., Russell, I.J., Larson, M., Chalmers, A., & Read, J.L. (1986). Auranofin therapy and quality of life in patients with rheumatoid arthritis — results of a multicenter trial. *American Journal of Medicine, 81,* 565.

Brown, S.J., Fann, J.R., & Grant, I. (1994). Post concussional disorder. Time to acknowledge a common source of neurobehavioral morbidity. *Journal of Neuropsychiatry, 6,* 15–22.

Burckhardt, C.S., Clark, S.R., & Bennett, R.M. (1993). Fibromyalgia and quality of life. A comparative analysis. *Journal of Rheumatology, 20,* 475–479.

Buskila, D., Neumann, L., Vaisberg, G., Alkalay, D., & Wolfe, F. (1997a). Increased rates of fibromyalgia following cervical spine injury. *Arthritis and Rheumatism, 40,* 446–452.

Buskila, D., Shnaider, A., Neumann, L. Zilberman, D., HilBuskila, D., Shnaider, A., Neumann, L. Zilberman, D., Hilzenrat, N., & Sikuler, E. (1997b). Fibromyalgia in hepatitis C infection. *Archives of Internal Medicine, 157,* 2497–2500.

Callahan, L.F., Smith, W.J., & Pincus, T. (1989). Self-report questionnaires in five rheumatic diseases. *Arthritis Care Research, 2,* 122–131.

Cathey, M.A., Wolfe, F., & Kleinheksel, S.M. *Arthritis Care Research, 1,* 85.

Cocchiarella, L., Turk, M.A., & Anderson, G. (2000). Improving the evaluation of permanent impairment. *Journal of the American Medical Association, 283,* 532–533.

Coderre, T.J., Katz, J., Vaccarino, A.L., & Melzack, R. (1993) Contribution of central neuroplasticity to pathological pain. Review of clinical and experimental evidence. *Pain, 52,* 259–285.

Croft, A.C. (1996). Low speed rear impact collision: In search of an injury threshold. *Journal of Musculoskeletal Pain, 4,* 39–46.

Crook, J., Moldofsky, H., & Shannon, H. (1998). Determinants of disability after a work related musculoskeletal injury. *Journal of Rheumatology, 25,* 1570–1577.

Curtis, P., Spanos, A., & Reid A. (1995). Persistent symptoms after whiplash injuries. Implications for prognosis and management. *Journal of Clinical Rheumatology, 1,* 149–157.

Dinerman, H., & Steere, A. (1992). Lyme disease associated with fibromyalgia. *Annals of Internal Medicine, 117,* 281–285.

Dubner, R., & Ruda, M.A. (1992) Activity-dependent neuronal plasticity following tissue injury and inflammation. *Trends in Neurosciences, 15,* 96–103.

Foreman, S.M., & Croft, A.C. (1988). *Whiplash injuries. The cervical acceleration/deceleration syndrome.* Baltimore: Williams & Wilkins.

Gargon, M.F., & Bannister, G.C. (1990). Long-term prognosis of soft-tissue injuries of the neck. *Journal of Bone and Joint Surgery, 72-B,* 904–906.

Gerwin, R.D., & Dommerholt, J. (1998). Treatment of myofascial pain syndromes. In R. S. Weiner (Ed.), *Pain management: A practical guide for clinicians* (5th ed., pp. 217–230). Boca Raton, FL: St. Lucie Press.

Goldenberg, D.L. (1993). Do infections trigger fibromyalgia? *Arthritis and Rheumatism, 36,* 1489–1492.

Gould, S.J. (1996). *Full house.* New York: Harmony Books.

Greenfield, S., Fitzcharles M.A., & Esdaile, J.M. (1992) Reactive fibromyalgia syndrome. *Arthritis and Rheumatism, 35,* 678–681.

Havsy, S.L. (1994a). Whiplash injuries of the cervical spine and their clinical sequellae. Part I. *American Journal of Pain Management, 4,* 23–31.

Havsy, S.L. (1994b). Whiplash injuries of the cervical spine and their clinical sequellae. Part II. *American Journal of Pain Management, 4,* 73–82.

Hohl, M. (1974). Soft-tissue injuries of the neck in automobile accidents. Factors influencing prognosis. *Journal of Bone and Joint Surgery, 56-A,* 1675–1682.

Holman, B.L., & Devous, M.D., Sr. (1992). Functional brain SPECT: The emergence of a powerful clinical method. *Journal of Nuclear Medicine, 33,* 1888–1904.

Hubbard, D.R., & Berkoff, G.M. (1993). Myofascial trigger points studied by needle EMG. *Spine, 18,* 1803–1807.

Jacob, J. (1998, October 5). HMO top salaries average $2 million in 1997. *American Medical News,* 28.

Jonssan, H., Jr., Bring, G., Rauschning, W., & Sahlstedt, B. (1991). Hidden cervical spine injuries in traffic accident victims. *Journal of Spinal Disorders, 4,* 251–263.

Kant, R. (1996). Post concussion syndrome — A neuropsychiatric perspective. *St. Francis Journal of Medicine, 2,* 111–114.

Kennedy, M., & Felson, D.T. (1996). A prospective study of fibromyalgia syndrome. *Arthritis and Rheumatism, 39,* 682–682.

Leventhal, L J., Naides, S.J., & Freundlich, B. (1991). Fibromyalgia and parvovirus infection. *Arthritis and Rheumatism, 34,* 1319–1324.

Lord, S.M., & Bogduk, N. (1996). The cervical synovial joints, as sources of post traumatic headache. *Journal of Musculoskeletal Pain, 4,* 81–94.

Mallison, A.J., Longridge, N.S., & Peacok, C. (1996). Dizziness, imbalance and whiplash. *Journal of Musculoskeletal Pain, 4,* 105–112.

Margoles, M.S. (1998). Myofascial pain syndrome: Clinical examinaton and management of patients. In R. S. Weiner (Ed.), *Pain management: A practical guide for clinicians* (5th ed, pp. 191–216). Boca Raton, FL: St. Lucie Press.

Martinez, J.E., Ferraz, M.B., Sato, E.I., & Atra, E. (1995). Fibromyalgia versus rheumatoid arthritis: A longitudinal comparison of the quality of life. *Journal of Rheumatology, 22,* 270–274.

Meenan, R.F., & Pincus, T. (1987). The status of patient status measures. (Editorial). *Journal of Rheumatology, 14,* 411–414.

Mitka, M. (1996, February 5). HMO executives claim fat paychecks. *American Medical News,* 3.

Moldofsky, H., Wong, M.T.H., & Lue, F.A. (1993). Litigation sleep symptoms and disabilities in post accident pain (fibromyalgia). *Journal of Rheumatology, 20,* 1935–1940.

Monsein, M. (1994). Disability evaluation and management of myofascial pain. In E.S. Rachlin (Ed.), *Myofascial pain and fibromyalgia* (pp. 91–119). St. Lous: Mosby.

Nedd, K., Sfakianakis, G., Ganz, W., Uricchio, B., Vernberg, D., Villanveva, P., Jabir, A.M., Bartlett, J., & Kena, J. (1993). $^{99m}T_c$-HMPAO SPECT of the brain in mild to moderate traumatic brain injury patients: Compared with CI — A prospective study. *Brain Injury, 7,* 469–479.

Newton, M.R., Greenwood, R.J., Britton, K.E., Charlesworth, M., Nimmon, C.C., Carroll, M.J., & Dolke, G. (1992). A study comparing SPECT with CT and MRI after closed head injury. *Journal of Neurology and Psychiatry, 55,* 92–94.

Packard, R.C., (1992). Posttraumatic headache: Permanency and relationship to legal settlement. *Headache, 32,* 496–500.

Pellegrino, M.J. (1996). *Understanding post-traumatic fibromyalgia.* Columbus, OH: Anadem Publishing.

Pincus, T., Summey, J.A., Soraci, S.A., Jr., Hummon, N.P., & Wallston, K.A. (1983). Assessment of patient satisfaction in activities of daily living using a modified Stanford health assessment questionnaire. *Arthtritis and Rheumatism, 26,* 1346–1353.

Potter, J.W. (1992). Helping fibromyalgia patients obtain Social Security benefits. *Journal of Musculoskeletal Medicine, 9,* 65–74.

Rachlin, E.S. (1994). Trigger points. In E.S. Rachlin (Ed.), *Myofascial pain and fibromyalgia* (pp. 146–147). St. Louis: Mosby.

Radanov, B.P., Dvorak, J., & Valach, L. (1992). Cognitive deficits in patients after soft tissue injury of the cervical spine. *Spine, 17,* 127–131.

Radanov, B.P., & Sturzenegger, M. (1996). The effect of accident mechanism and initial findings on the long-term outcome of whiplash injury. *Journal of Musculoskeletal Pain, 4,* 47–59.

Reilly, P.A. (1998). Work disability and soft tissue rheumatism. *Journal of Rheumatology, 25,* 1454–1456.

Rice, J.R. (1987). Fibromyalgia. A disorder for all clinicians. In J.I. Walker, J.T. Brown, & R.A. Gallis (Eds.), *The complicated medical patient* (pp. 58–70). New York: Human Sciences Press, Inc.

Romano, T J. (1990). Clinical experiences with post-traumatic fibromyalgia syndrome. *West Virginia Medical Journal, 86,* 198–202.

Romano, T.J. (1995). Abnormal central nervous system neurodiagnostic testing in post traumatic fibromyalgia (Abstr). *Journal of Musculoskeletal Pain, 3* (Suppl. 1), 106.

Romano, T.J. (1998a). A rheumatologist's perspective on pain management. In R.S. Weiner (Ed.), *Pain management: A practical guide for clinicians* (5th ed., pp. 355–371). Boca Raton, FL: St. Lucie Press.

Romano, T.J. (1998b). Proposed formula for the estimation of pain caused by each of several traumas involving soft tissue. *American Journal of Pain Management, 8,* 118–123.

Romano, T.J. (1999). Fibromyalgia. In M. S. Margoles & R. Weiner (Eds.), *Chronic pain, assessment, diagnosis, and management* (pp. 95–103). Boca Raton, FL: CRC Press.

Romano, T.J., & Govindan, S. (1996). Abnormal cranial SPECT scanning in fibromyalgia patients with headaches. *American Journal of Pain Management, 6,* 118–122.

Romano, T.J., & Stiller, J.W. (1994). Magnesium deficiency in fibromyalgia syndrome. *Journal of Nutrition and Medicine, 40,* 165–167.

Romano, T.J., & Stiller, J.W. (1997). Needle EMG in myofascial pain patients, correlation with physical findings in general rheumatology practice. *American Journal of Pain Management, 7,* 19–21.

Russell, I.S., Fletcher, E.M., Tsui, J., & Michalek, J.E. (1989). Comparisons of rheumatoid arthritis and fibrositis/fibromyalgia syndrome using functional and psychological outcome measures. *Arthritis and Rheumatology, 32,* 570, B121.

Saskin, P., Modolfsky, H., & Lue, F.A. (1986). Sleep and posttraumatic rheumatic pain disorder (fibrositis syndrome). *Psychosomatic Medicine, 48,* 319–323.

Simms, R.W., Zerbini, C.A.F., Ferrante, N., Anthony, J., Felson, D.T., Crager, D.E., & the Boston City Hospital AIDS Team (1992). Fibromyalgia syndrome in patients infected with human immuno deficiency virus. *Annals of Internal Medicine, 92,* 368–374.

Simons, D.C. (1987). Myofascial pain syndromes due to triger points. In M. Osterweis, A. Kleinman, & D. Mechanic (Eds.), *Pain and disability* (pp. 285–292). Washington, D.C.: National Academy Press.

Smiley, W.M., Cram, J.R., Margoles, M.S., Romano, T.J., & Stiller, J. (1992). Innovations in soft tissue jurisprudence. *Trial Diplomacy Journal, 15,* 199–208.

Smythe, H. A. (1989). Nonarticular rheumatism and psychogenic musculoskeletal syndromes in arthritis and allied conditions. D.J. McCarthy (Ed.), *A textbook of rheumatology* (11th ed., pp. 1241–1254). Philadelphia: Lea & Febiger.

Social Security Administration (1998, January). Disability evaluation under Social Security, Office of Disability.

Spieler, E.A., Barth, P.S., Burton, J.F., Jr., Himmelstein, J., & Rudolph, L. (2000). Recommendations to guide revision of the guides to the evaluation of permanent impairment. *Journal of the American Medical Association, 283,* 519–523.

Swerdlow, B. (1998). *Whiplash and related headache.* Boca Raton, FL: CRC Press.

Taylor, J.R., & Taylor, M.M. (1996). Cervical spine injuries: An autopsy study of 109 blunt injuries. *Journal of Musculoskeletal Pain, 4,* 61–79.

Teasell, R.W., & Merskey, H. (1997). Chronic pain disability in the workplace. *Pain Research Management, 2,* 197–225.

Tikofsky, R.S. (1994). Evaluating traumatic brain injury: Correlating perfusion patterns and function. *Journal of Nuclear Medicine, 35,* 227.

Tollison, C.D., & Satterthwaite, J.R. (Eds.). (1992). *Painful cervical trauma.* Baltimore: Williams & Wilkins.

Travell, J.G., & Simons, D.G. (1983). *Myofascial pain and dysfunction: The trigger point manual.* Baltimore: Williams & Wilkins.

Turk, D.C., Okifuji, A., Sinclair, J.D., & Starz, T.W. (1996). Pain, disability, and physical findings in subgroups of patients with fibromyalgia. *Journal of Rheumatology, 23,* 1255–1262.

Vital Statistics of the United States (1992). Life tables, Volume II, Section 6 (p. 12). U.S. Dept. Health and Human Services. Public Health Service.

Waylonis, G.W., & Perkins, R.H. (1994). Post-traumatic fibromyalgia, a long-term follow-up. *American Journal of Physical Medicine and Rehabilitation, 73,* 403–412.

White, K.P., Speechley, M., Harth, M., & Ostbye, T. (1999). The London fibromyalgia epidemiology study: Direct health care costs of fibromyalgia syndrome in London. *Canadian Journal of Rheumatology, 26,* 885–889.

Wolfe, F. (1994). Post-traumatic fibromyalgia: A case report narrated by the patient. *Arthritis Care and Research, 7,* 161–165.

Wolfe, F. (1995). Health status questionnaire. *Rheumatism Clinics of North America, 21,* 445–464.

Wolfe, F. (1996). The fibromyalgia syndrome: A consensus report on fibromyalgia and disability. *Journal of Rheumatology, 23,* 534–539.

Wolfe, F., Anderson, J., Harness, D., Bennett, R.M., Caro, X.J., Goldenberg, D.L., Russell, I.J., & Yunus, M.B. (1997a). Health status and disease severity in fibromyalgia. Results of a six-center longitudinal study. *Arthritis and Rheumatism, 40,* 1571–1579.

Wolfe, F., Anderson, J., Harkness, D., Bennett, R.M., Caro, X. J., Goldenberg, D.L., Russell, I.J., & Yunus, M.B. (1997b). Work and disability status of persons with fibromyalgia. *Journal of Rheumatism, 24,* 1171–1178.

Wolfe, F., Smythe, H.A., Yunus, M.B., Bennett, R.B., Bombardier, C., Goldenberg, D.L., Tugwell, P., Campbell, S.M., Abeles, M., Clark, P., Fam, A.G., Farber, S J., Fiechtner, J J., Franklin, C.M., Gatter, R.A., Hamaty, D., Lessard, J., Lichtbroun, A.S., Masi, A.T., McCain, G.A., Reynolds, W.J., Romano, T.J., Russell, I J., & Sheon, R.P. (1990). The American College of Rheumatology criteria for the classification of fibromyalgia. *Arthritis and Rheumatism, 33,* 160–172.

Wyper, D.J. (1993). Functional neuroimaging with single photon emission computerized tomography (SPECT). *Cerebrovascular and Brain Metabolism Reviews, 5,* 199–217.

Yunus, M.B. (1992). Towards a model of pathophysiology of fibromyalgia: Aberrant central pain mechanisms with peripheral modulation. *Journal of Rheumatology, 19,* 846–850.

Yunus, M.B., & Alday, J.C. (1993). Clinical and psychological features of regional fibromyalgia: Comparison with fibromyalgia syndrome. *Arthritis and Rheumatism, 36,* S221.

Yunus, M.B., Bennett, R.M., Romano, T.J., Russell, I.J., & other members of the Fibromyalgia Consensus Report Additional Comments Group (1997). Fibromyalgia consensus report, additional comments. *Journal of Clinical Rheumatology, 3,* 324–327.

17

Neuropathic Pain: Mechanisms and Management

Mark V. Boswell, M.D., Ph.D., Samuel K. Rosenberg, M.D., and Thomas C. Chelimsky, M.D.

INTRODUCTION

Neuropathic pain is a common cause of chronic pain. Neuropathic pain is a challenge to clinicians because it is difficult to diagnose and often is resistant to analgesics, such as opioids (Arner & Meyerson, 1988; Dellemijn, 1999; Portenoy, Foley, & Inturrisi, 1990). Classic examples of neuropathic pain include trigeminal neuralgia, postherpetic neuralgia, diabetic neuropathy, phantom limb pain, and pain associated with plexopathy and radiculopathy (see Table 17.1). Neuropathic pain often complicates the treatment of cancer pain. For example, brachial plexopathy occurs in approximately 15% of patients with cancer and pain is the most common complaint associated with brachial plexopathy (Foley, 1987). Thus, successful management of cancer pain frequently requires management of neuropathic pain.

From a theoretical standpoint, neuropathic pain is relatively simple to define. It is an abnormal pain state that arises from a damaged peripheral nervous system (PNS) or central nervous system (CNS) (Merskey & Bogduk, 1994). Indeed, peripheral neuropathies, particularly those associated with diabetes, are a frequent cause of neuropathic pain (Galer, 1995). However, from a clinical perspective, neuropathic pain may be difficult to diagnose with certainty, because its clinical characteristics are rather nonspecific. Neuropathic pain may be hard for some patients to describe, but frequently is characterized as burning or stabbing, descriptors that are not unique to neuropathic pain. Indeed, neuropathic pain may be similar to the pain ascribed to common injuries not considered neuropathic in nature, such as burns and sprains. This ambiguity in character may simply reflect the relatively limited number of ways that pain can be encoded by the nervous system.

A peculiar property of the nervous system is its plasticity. Damage to nerves often results in alteration or amplification of the signal encoded by the nerve. For example, peripheral nerve ablation, performed with good therapeutic intentions, may result in a pain syndrome that is worse than the one originally being treated. When dealing with the nervous system, "shooting the messenger" (the nerve) often intensifies and distorts the message. The new pain syndrome may be more severe, and associated with allodynia, hyperalgesia, and spontaneous and paroxysmal pain, all in the presence of mild to moderate cutaneous numbness. This complex of signs and symptoms is paradoxical to the patient and confusing to the clinician, but quite typical of neuropathic pain.

The ambiguity notwithstanding, it is important to consider neuropathic pain in the differential diagnosis of chronic pain, because neuropathic pain may be treated with some success using adjuvant analgesics, medications not traditionally considered to be pain relievers (Hegarty & Portenoy, 1994). Adjuvant analgesics, such as tricyclic antidepressants and anticonvulsants, do not have strong antinociceptive analgesic properties in experimental or clinical studies, but have been shown to be helpful in neuropathic pain states (McQuay, et al., 1996; Swerdlow, 1984). Indeed, the mainstay of treatment of neuropathic,

0-8493-0926-3/02/$0.00+$1.50
© 2002 by CRC Press LLC

TABLE 17.1
Common Causes of Neuropathic Pain

Polyneuropathy
    Diabetes (insulin-dependent and non-insulin-dependent)
    Alcoholism
    Human immunodeficiency virus
    Hypothyroidism
    Renal failure
    Chemotherapy (vincristine, cisplatinum, paclitaxel, metronidazole)
    Anti-HIV drugs
    B-12 and folate deficiencies
Mononeuropathy
    Entrapment syndromes
    Traumatic injury
    Diabetes
    Vasculitis
Plexopathy
    Diabetes
    Avulsion
    Tumor
Root Syndromes and Radiculopathy
    Compressive lesions
    Inflammatory
    Diabetes
Postherpetic neuralgia
Trigeminal neuralgia
Phantom limb pain
RSD/Causalgia/CRPS

Modified from B.S. Galer, 1995. *Neurology, 45*(Suppl. 9), 517–525.

pain is pharmacologic, and effective regimens often require multiple medications. In addition, the possible effectiveness of opioids for neuropathic pain should not be overlooked, although doses may be considerably higher than typical antinociceptive doses. The clinician should also keep in mind that successful management of chronic pain often requires treating neuropathic pain as well as pain associated with tissue injury, because both conditions may coexist and interact to maintain the painful condition.

MECHANISMS OF NEUROPATHIC PAIN

Neuropathic pain may result from a pathological process occurring at any level of the nervous system, from the nociceptor, the distal nerve, the plexus level, the dorsal root ganglion, the root entry zone, the dorsal horn of the spinal cord, and higher levels in the CNS, particularly the medulla and thalamus. It has become popular to contrast neuropathic pain with typical postinjury, nociceptive pain. Nociceptive pain, typically thought to indicate a properly functioning nervous system, is considered physiological because it results from activation of nociceptors, specialized nerve endings that respond to high threshold noxious stimuli and generally serve a protective function.

In contrast, neuropathic pain may be thought of as pathophysiological, because it arises from a damaged PNS or CNS and provides no obvious protective benefit (Bennett, 1994; Tanelian, & Victory, 1995). However, from a clinical perspective, this distinction is seldom straightforward, because physiological pain often is associated with early clinical findings generally considered neuropathic in nature, such as allodynia and paresthesias (tingling sensations). Moreover, chronic neuropathic-like pain occasionally may follow an injury that did not appear to involve nerve damage, such as a simple soft tissue injury. On the other hand, pain associated with peripheral neuropathy may be maintained by sustained peripheral nociceptive input (Gracely, Lynch, & Bennett, 1992). Strong nociceptive input often produces central sensitization, an abnormal pain amplification process in the CNS. Therefore, the definitional borders of neuropathic pain are becoming more diffuse, not more distinct, as we gain a better understanding of the remarkable plasticity of the nervous system and its close association with the various tissues that it innervates.

Neuropathic pain may be classified as stimulus-evoked or stimulus-independent pain. Stimulus-evoked pain can result from stimulation of nervi nervorum present in connective tissue surrounding otherwise intact nerves. Painful stimuli that activate nociceptors around nerves include inflammation and tissue injury from tumor or trauma (Woolf & Mannion, 1999). Stimulus-independent neuropathic pain may result from damage to afferent sensory fibers in the PNS or CNS. In this case, ongoing inflammation is usually absent. Days to months after peripheral nerve injury, persistent abnormal primary afferent activity from the periphery may arise from hypersensitive nerve terminals or nerves (Price, Mao, Mayer, 1994).

There is substantial pharmacological evidence that abnormal nerve activity is an important mechanism underlying the spontaneous pain typical of neuropathic pain states (Devor, 1994, 1995; Tanelian & Victory, 1995). It is hypothesized that sites of ectopic foci develop on injured or regenerating nerves in the periphery, at the level of the nociceptor, neuromas, or segments of injured nerves; at the dorsal root ganglion; and in the dorsal horn of the spinal cord. Indeed, after nerve transection, increased sensitivity occurs, followed in a few days by spontaneous activity. These abnormal ectopic foci may be thought of as spontaneous pain generators, resulting in paroxysmal and spontaneous pain. Precise pathophysiology is unclear, but pharmacological evidence suggests that ectopic activity is due to an increased number of sodium channels, or more likely an abnormal subtype of sodium channel, resulting in unstable sodium channel activity (Chaplan, 2000). Pharmacological evidence supporting this hypothesis is the effectiveness of local anesthetics and some anticonvulsants (sodium channel-blocking drugs) in neuropathic pain. These drugs presumably produce frequency and voltage-dependent blockade of sodium channels on damaged neurons (Devor, 1995). The abnormal sodium channel involved in neuropathic pain states may be a tetrodotoxin-insensitive subtype, found only in neural tissue (Novakovic, et al., 1998). Accumulation of atypical as well as tetrodotoxin-sensitive sodium channels (responsible for normal nerve conduction) may explain the often inadequate therapeutic benefit of current sodium channel-blocking drugs.

Work in animal models demonstrates that voltage-dependent calcium channels may also be important in modulating neuropathic transmission. Unfortunately, the currently available calcium channel blockers are cardio-selective, and are not particularly effective in neuropathic pain. There appear to be at least six calcium channel subtypes, and studies with novel N-type calcium channel blockers are promising in animals (Chaplan, 2000). Preliminary studies with conotoxin (SNX-111) are positive, although the drug must be administered spinally.

Gabapentin, a novel anticonvulsant, appears to bind to the $\alpha2\delta$ subunit of a voltage-dependent calcium channel. Work by Chaplan (2000) and colleagues demonstrates that messenger RNA and protein for the $\alpha2\delta$ subunit are increased more than 10-fold in dorsal root ganglia following nerve injury, but are not changed after tissue injury. Blockade of a retrograde signal from the injury site (which may involve nerve growth factor) prevents upregulation of the $\alpha2\delta$ subunit. Chaplan points out that the $\alpha2\delta$ subunit does not seem to play a role in normal channel kinetics but may effect calcium channel assembly and insertion into the neuronal membrane. Thus, the subunit may act as a drug-binding site and secondarily modify channel kinetics.

Following peripheral nerve injury, concomitant alternations may be evident in dorsal root ganglia, including transmitter changes and increased density of sympathetic nerve terminals (McLachlan, Janig, Devor, & Michaelis, 1993). Tyrosine hydroxylase positive cell terminals that produce norepinephrine, migrate from vessels supplying the dorsal root ganglion to nerve ganglion cells following sciatic nerve injury. The dorsal root ganglia then expresses α-adrenergic receptors. This may be a putative link between peripheral tissue injury, nerve injury, and sympathetically maintained pain states, such as reflex sympathetic dystrophy and causalgia (complex regional pain syndromes Type 1 and 2, respectively). In the periphery, sprouting nerve terminals may exhibit sensitivity to prostaglandins, cytokines, and catecholamines. These kinds of changes further increase the complexity of the neuropathic pain picture and blur the distinctions between nociceptive and neuropathic pain.

It should be noted that not all stimulus-independent pain is mediated by spontaneous activity in primary sensory neurons. Loss of normal inhibitory mechanisms,

whether segmental, supraspinal, or both, may also cause neuropathic pain (Woolf & Mannion, 1999). After deafferentation injury, particularly following loss of C fibers, arborization of Aβ fibers into the substantia gelatinosa of the dorsal horn may result in central sensitization and allodynia (Woolf, Shortland, & Coggeshall, 1992). Available evidence supports the contention that tactile allodynia is mediated by large myelinated Aβ afferents with input that is modulated at supraspinal sites in the dorsal columns (Ossipov, Lai, Malan, & Porreca, 2000). This may explain why transcutaneous electrical nerve stimulation (TENS) and spinal cord stimulation, which produce a low threshold, tingling sensation, characteristic of large fiber afferent activation, may be effective in chronic pain states, particularly neuropathic pain. Tactile allodynia should be differentiated from thermal allodynia, which appears to be mediated by nonmyelinated C fibers and amplified by pathological spinal dynorphin (discussed later).

Various studies suggest that stimulus-evoked neuropathic pain is more sensitive to opioids than stimulus-independent pain (Dellemijn, 1999). Opioid responsiveness may be maintained in some forms of stimulus-evoked pain, because opioid receptors in the substantia gelatinosa are preserved. On the other hand, segmental loss of presynaptic central opioid receptors occurs following injury or loss of C fibers, typically seen after deafferentation injury. However, the magnitude of receptor loss is minimal and largely segmental, and only partly explains the diminished opioid-responsiveness characteristic of neuropathic pain (Ossipov, et al., 2000).

Supraspinal facilitative mechanisms may also be involved in maintenance of neuropathic pain and opioid resistance. Evidence suggests that sustained afferent drive induces *facilitation* of spinal cord pain transmission involving a descending pathway from the rostroventral medial medulla (RVM) (Ossipov, et al., 2000). Tonic facilitation may involve supraspinal cholecystokinin (CCK), traditionally thought of as a visceral hormone that regulates emptying of the gallbladder. CCK antagonists injected into the RVM in animals reverse tactile and thermal allodynia produced by spinal nerve ligation (Kovelowski, Ossipov, Sun, Malan, & Proecca, 2000). Mechanistically, these antiopioid and pronociceptive actions may occur at spinal and supraspinal sites. Spinal CCK may antagonize opioid effects at the level of the primary afferent terminal in the spinal cord. Both CCK and opioids colocalize on primary nociceptive afferent neurons in the dorsal horn. In addition, CCK may act on supraspinal opioid-dependent pathways in the RVM to reduce opioid responsiveness, and thus impair descending inhibition, an important mechanism involved in opioid pain relief. Ultimately, CCK antagonists may prove useful for treating neuropathic pain states.

The phenomenon of reduced opioid responsiveness in neuropathic pain has prompted extensive studies in animals, particularly the effects of intrathecal opioids on pain associated with thermal and tactile stimulation. The similarities between opioid tolerance and neuropathic pain are also an area of active study (Vanderah, et al., 2000). It is well known that N-methyl-D-aspartate (NMDA) antagonists appear to minimize the development of opioid tolerance. Spinal dynorphin may be a common link between NMDA, central sensitization, and reduced opioid responsiveness. Following spinal nerve ligation, dynorphin levels in the spinal cord increase, suggesting that dynorphin may act as a pronociception mediator (Ossipov, et al., 2000). Although, under certain circumstances, dynorphin appears to have analgesic properties, it is becoming increasingly clear that dynorphin also has nonopioid, antianalgesic properties. Antiserum to dynorphin blocks thermal hyperalgesia after nerve injury in rats. Moreover, antiserum to dynorphin or MK801, an NMDA antagonist, restores normal spinal morphine analgesia following spinal nerve ligation. Furthermore, both agents restore morphine synergy between the brain and spinal cord (Ossipov, et al., 2000), which is required for the full clinical analgesic effects of morphine. Therefore, current evidence suggests that the pain-promoting effect of dynorphin is mediated by the NMDA receptor. Although the full clinical ramifications of dynorphin are far from understood, it is clear that sustained nociceptive drive from the periphery maintains elevated levels of spinal dynorphin, which in turn, may have toxic effects on the spinal cord. Thus, reducing sustained peripheral nociceptive input into the spinal (i.e., pain relief) may be an important way to reduce the incidence of neuropathic pain (Caudle & Mannes, 2000).

Currently, NMDA antagonists, such as ketamine, have only limited indications because of significant side effects. Ultimately, however, medications such as NMDA antagonists may become available that can reduce the effects of pathological spinal dynorphin.

MANAGEMENT OF NEUROPATHIC PAIN: GENERAL CONSIDERATIONS

Management of neuropathic pain is a complicated endeavor and often is frustrating to patient and physician alike. This stems from our relatively poor understanding of mechanisms and the limited efficacy of currently available analgesics. Therapeutic approaches vary greatly among physicians, which reflects the paucity of randomized clinical trials, particularly those comparing different drug regimens. Given our current level of understanding of neuropathic pain mechanisms and the limitations of available drugs, nonpharmacological methods may be as effective as pharmacological approaches. Recalcitrant chronic pain syndromes warrant an interdisciplinary approach, which may include attempts to treat the underlying disease (e.g., causes of the peripheral neuropathy)

as well as formulation of a rational approach to medications, interventions such as nerve blocks, and psychological and physical therapies.

The nature, duration, and severity of pain should be evaluated in detail, including appropriate physical and neurological examinations. For example, performing a neurological examination looking specifically for evidence of nerve injury, such as the presence of hypoesthesias or reflex changes, may suggest neuropathy or radiculopathy, and help guide treatment. It is crucial that psychosocial and emotional factors be explored, because there is a high comorbidity of depression and anxiety disorders in patients with chronic pain. Moreover, given the similarities between the pharmacology of mood and depression and pain transmission (e.g., serotonin and norepinephrine), patients with concomitant systemic illness and stress may be at risk for depression and development of an abnormal chronic pain state. Pharmacological management of depression may improve neuropathic pain by addressing overlapping, but distinct mechanisms.

After multiple medication trials in which there has been minimal therapeutic benefit and perhaps significant drug-related side effects, patients may believe that they have little recourse but to undergo invasive, ablative procedures in attempts to relieve their pain. Specific treatment modalities aimed at the underlying pathophysiology are usually not possible in most neuropathies, particularly with chronic sensory polyneuropathies. In general, ablative procedures are not warranted, because of the high probability of long-term worsening of pain. Except for patients with advanced cancer-related pain, nerve ablation is likely to provide only temporary benefit, leaving the patient with sensory and perhaps motor deficits. Exceptions to this phenomenon appear to be ablation of sympathetic fibers, visceral plexi, and medial branch nerve blocks, which denervate painful facet joints in the spine. In cases of nerve entrapment, where ongoing nerve compression is likely to be responsible for pain, neurolysis or transposition of the nerve may provide benefit, as long as pain is not due to irreversible underlying nerve damage. In all cases of neuropathic pain, even when neuropathy is evident, it is appropriate from time to time to reevaluate the presumed etiology of the neurological problem.

When a medication trial proves to be ineffective, a multidimensional or interdisciplinary approach should be considered. Again, this includes an attempt to treat the underlying disease, as well as specific pharmacological, psychological, and physical therapy interventions. The outcome measure for successful treatment should include increased activity as well as decreased subjective pain ratings and improved patient satisfaction. The treatment goal in chronic neuropathic pain is different from that in acute pain. In the usual acute pain setting, the goal is nearly complete relief of pain, to allow recovery of normal function during the healing process. With chronic neuropathic pain, limitations of current analgesics usually make complete pain relief a very unrealistic goal. Therefore, attention to increasing function and comfort and treating associated problems, such as depression, become paramount. Reducing dependence on opioid medications may or may not be an important goal. The objectives to consider with chronic opioid therapy include determining whether nonopioid approaches have been tried, whether the pain syndrome is opioid responsive, and whether the patient demonstrates appropriate improvement in function, without undo side effects or evidence of abuse of medications.

Nonpharmacological approaches to treating neuropathic pain include the use of a TENS unit, although relief may be poor when burning pain is a prominent complaint. This may be explained by the fact that burning pain is a C-fiber-mediated sensation, whereas TENS units probably modulate large fiber input into the dorsal horn.

Spinal cord stimulation may be efficacious for chronic pain, including neuropathic pain (North, Kidd, Zahurak, James, & Long, 1993) and reflex sympathetic dystrophy (Kemle,r et al., 2000). Mechanisms involved are poorly understood, which reflects current understanding of neuropathic pain states in general. However, central effects may include alteration in dorsal horn processing and transmission in the tract of Lissauer (Iacono, Guthkelch, & Boswell, 1992) and suppression of sympathetic outflow from the intermediolateral gray column of the spinal cord. The latter effect may explain improved peripheral blood flow in patients with chronic peripheral vascular insufficiency. The CraigPENS technique, a novel application of electroacupuncture (percutaneous neural stimulation [PNS]) has been shown effective in herpes zoster, diabetic peripheral neuropathy, and sciatica (Ahmed, et al., 1998; Ghoname, et al., 1999; Hamza, et al., 2000).

Available evidence indicates that nonpharmacological approaches such as TENS and CraigPENS can provide an initial rational therapeutic strategy, and may obviate the need for potentially toxic medications, improve the effectiveness of current analgesic regimens, or reduce the amount of medications required. Spinal cord stimulation still tends to be a treatment of last resort, although judicious use earlier in the course of treatment is probably warranted in carefully selected patients. Considering the current high cost of medication, alternative approaches, if efficacious, may prove to be cost effective.

PHARMACOLOGY OF NEUROPATHIC PAIN

From a practical standpoint, medications remain the pillar of pain management strategies, despite their limitations. From a conceptual standpoint, adjuvant analgesic drugs may be categorized into two broad classes, membrane stabilizing agents and medications that enhance inhibitory mechanisms in the dorsal horn. This classification system may provide a simple framework with which to approach therapy; however, it should be kept in mind that most of these drugs have multiple mechanisms of action, and their effects often may overlap. Given the limitations of our current drugs, pain management often becomes an exercise in polypharmacy, where the clinician uses multiple medications to target different symptoms. This strategy may optimize the chances for success, but complicates management issues when side effects develop.

Membrane stabilizing agents include local anesthetics such as lidocaine and some anticonvulsant drugs, including carbamazepine, phenytoin, and valproic acid (Tanelian & Victory, 1995). Their molecular mechanism of action involves blockade of frequency and voltage-dependent sodium channels on damaged or regenerating neuronal membranes (Devor, 1994, 1995). It appears that minimal doses of suppressive drugs may inhibit ectopic discharges without interfering with normal neuronal function. It is also possible that the sodium channel targets are atypical and not involved in normal neuronal conduction. Although the evidence is less substantial, corticosteroids also appear to have effects on membrane conductance (Castillo, et al., 1996; Devor, Govrin-Lippmann, & Raber, 1985). In addition, tricyclic antidepressants, such as amitriptyline, have effects on sodium channels (Pancrazio, Kamatchi, Roscoe, & Lynch, 1998), an action that is distinct from their effects on the reuptake of serotonin and norepinephrine. The latter are traditionally thought to be responsible for their effects on depression and pain.

Conventional wisdom maintains that the adjuvant analgesics, particularly the tricyclic antidepressants, and clonazepam and baclofen, modulate inhibitory mechanisms in the spinal cord and brain. Inhibitory pathways descend from the periaqueductal gray, reticular formation, and nucleus raphe magnus in the dorsolateral funiculus to the dorsal horn. These pathways mediate antinociception by adrenergic, serotonergic, GABAergic (γ-amino butyric acid), and opioid mechanisms (Yaksh, 1979). Although the putative mechanisms are complex and poorly understood, serotonergic effects are mediated in part by action on GABAergic interneurons (Alhaider, Lei, & Wilcox, 1991). For example, facilitory effects of large myelinated afferent fibers may be suppressed by tonic GABAergic activity, removal of which results in allodynia (Yaksh & Malmberg, 1994).

As noted earlier, tricyclic antidepressants alter monoamine transmitter activity at neuronal synapses by blocking presynaptic reuptake of norepinephrine and serotonin, thereby modulating descending inhibitory spinal pathways. However, additional mechanisms include effects on membranes, interaction with NMDA activity (Eisenach & Gebhart, 1995), and sodium channel blockade (Pancrazio, et al., 1998).

TABLE 17.2
Adjuvant Analgesics for Neuropathic Pain

Drug Class	Mechanism of Drug Action
Anticonvulsants	
Carbamazepine	Sodium channel blockade
Phenytoin	Sodium channel blockade
Valproic acid	Sodium channel blockade
Gabapentin	Calcium channel binding
Clonazepam	GABAegic mechanism
Antidepressants	
Amitriptyline	As a group Norepinephrine and serotonin
Nortriptyline	reuptake effects, possible NMDA effects,
Imipramine	and sodium channel blockade
Desipramine	
Fluoxetine	Serotonin selective effects
Paroxetine	Serotonin selective effects
Venlafaxine	Adrenergic and opioid receptor binding effects
Antiarrhythmics	
Lidocaine	As a group sodium channel-blocking effects
Mexiletine	
EMLA cream	
Miscellaneous	
Corticosteroids	Antiinflammatory and membrane stabilizing effects
Baclofen	GABA-B agonist
Capsaicin	Vanilloid agonist and C-fiber neurotoxin

From a practical standpoint, it helpful to consider the various medications useful for neuropathic pain in terms of their traditional pharmacological indications (eg, anticonvulsants and antidepressants). However, it is necessary to keep in mind that all these drugs have incompletely understood mechanisms of action, and the drug categories are more conventional than mechanistic (Table 17.2).

ANTICONVULSANTS

Anticonvulsants are useful for trigeminal neuralgia, postherpetic neuralgia, diabetic neuropathy, and central pain (Hegarty & Porteny, 1994; Swerdlow, 1984). Although anticonvulsants have traditionally been thought of as most useful for lancinating pain, they may also relieve burning dysesthesias. Chemically, anticonvulsants are a diverse group of drugs, are typically highly protein bound, and undergo extensive hepatic metabolism. At present it is uncertain whether anticonvulsants or antidepressants are better for neuropathic pain, because similar results have been obtained with both types of drugs (McQuay, et al., 1996). Indeed, the choice of a particular drug, whether anticonvulsant or antidepressant, may be based more on a clinician's experience with the drug, the expected time to therapeutic benefit, or a drug side effect profile, instead of theoretical mechanisms of action.

Carbamazepine has a long history of use for neuropathic pain, particularly trigeminal neuralgia. Trigeminal neuralgia is an FDA-approved indication for the drug. Carbamazepine is chemically related to the tricyclic antidepressant imipramine, has a slow and erratic absorption, and may produce numerous side effects, including sedation, nausea, vomiting, and hepatic enzyme induction. In 10% of patients, transient leukopenia and thrombocytopenia may occur, and in 2% of patients hematologic changes can be persistent, requiring stopping the drug (Hart & Easton, 1982; Sobotka, Alexander, & Cook, 1990; Tohen, Castillo, Baldessarini, Zarate, & Kando, 1995). Aplastic anemia is the most severe complication associated with carbamazepine, which may occur in 1:200,000 patients. Although requirements for hematologic monitoring remain debatable, a complete blood cell count, hepatic enzymes, blood urea nitrogen (BUN), and creatinine are recommended at baseline; and these are checked again at 2, 4, and 6 weeks, and every 6 months thereafter. Carbamazepine levels should be drawn every 6 months and after changing the dose to monitor for toxic levels and verify that the drug is within the therapeutic range (4 to 12 μg/cc). Patients with low pretreatment white blood cell counts are at increased risk of developing leukopenia (WBC < 3000/mm^3). Because toxicity is entirely unpredictable, it is important to instruct patients to recognize clinical signs and symptoms of hematologic toxicity, such as infections, fatigue, ecchymosis, and abnormal bleeding, and to notify the physician if they develop. To improve compliance, carbamazepine should be started at a low dose (e.g., 50 mg twice daily) and increased over several weeks to a therapeutic level (200 to 300 mg four times a day).

Phenytoin also has well-known sodium channel-blocking effects and is useful for neuropathic pain (Swerdlow, 1984). However, carbamazepine is more effective than phenytoin for trigeminal neuralgia (Blom, 1962). Phenytoin has a slow and variable oral absorption. Toxicity includes CNS effects and cardiac conduction abnormalities. Side effects are common and include hirsuitism, gastrointestinal and hematologic effects, and gingival hyperplasia (Brodie & Dichter, 1996). Allergies to phenytoin are common, and may involve skin, liver, and bone marrow. Phenytoin doses in the range of 100 mg twice or three times a day may be helpful for neuropathic pain; therapeutic blood levels are in the range of 10 to 20 μg/ml. There are numerous potential drug interactions, including induction of cytochrome P450 enzymes, which may accelerate the metabolism of other drugs. Because of side effects and toxicity, phenytoin is not a first-line drug for neuropathic pain.

Valproic acid appears to interact with sodium channels but may also alter GABA metabolism. The principle use of valproic acid for neuropathic pain is for the prophylaxis of migraine headache (Matthew, et al., 1995). Potential toxicity includes hepatic injury and thrombocytopenia, particularly in children on multiple antiepileptic medications, although valproic acid is generally considered safe for adults.

Divalproex sodium is better tolerated than valproic acid. The recommended starting dose is 250 mg twice daily, although some patients may benefit from doses up to 1000 mg/day. As a prophylactic drug, valproic acid can reduce the frequency of migraine attacks by about 50% (Matthew, et al., 1995). Although there is little published information on the efficacy of valproic acid for other neuropathic pain syndromes, based on its mechanism of action it may be useful alone or in combination with other adjuvant drugs.

Clonazepam may be useful for radiculopathic pain and neuropathic pain of a lancinating character. Clonazepam enhances dorsal horn inhibition by a GABAergic mechanism. The drug has a long half-life (18 to 50 h), which reduces the risk of inducing an abstinence syndrome on abrupt withdrawal. The major side effects of clonazepam include sedation and cognitive dysfunction, especially in the elderly. Although the risk of organ toxicity is minimal, some clinicians recommend periodic complete blood count (CBC) and liver function tests for monitoring. Starting doses of 0.5 to 1.0 mg at bedtime are appropriate to reduce the incidence of daytime sedation.

Gabapentin is a popular anticonvulsant for neuropathic pain. Gabapentin was released for use in the United States in 1994, for the treatment of adults with partial epilepsy. Almost immediately after its release, physicians began to use gabapentin for various neuropathic pain disorders, such as diabetic peripheral neuropathy and postherpetic neuralgia. The structural similarity of gabapentin to GABA suggested that the drug might be useful for neuropathic pain. Although tricyclic antidepressants have been proven clinically effective for neuropathic pain for years, they often fail to provide adequate pain relief or cause unacceptable side effects. Therefore, when gabapentin became available, its benign side effect profile quickly made it very popular among physicians. Although initial enthusiasm for the drug was based largely on word of mouth, anecdotal published reports, and discussions at clinical meetings, animal studies have substantiated the efficacy of gabapentin in various types of neuropathic pain. Over time, a growing consensus concerning the usefulness of gabapentin has emerged.

It is clear that gabapentin is not a direct GABA agonist, although indirect effects on GABA metabolism or action may occur. A leading hypothesis suggests that gabapentin interacts with a novel receptor on a voltage-activated calcium channel (Chaplan, 2000; Taylor, et al., 1998). Inhibition of voltage-gated sodium channel activity (such as occurs with classical anticonvulsants, e.g., phenytoin and carbamazepine) and amino acid transport, which alters neurotransmitter synthesis, may also occur.

Although gabapentin is not an NMDA antagonist, there is evidence that gabapentin interacts with the glycine site on the NMDA receptor (Jun & Yaksh, 1998).

Ligation of rat spinal nerves L5 and L6 (the Chung model) produces characteristic pain behaviors, including allodynia, which are typical of neuropathic pain. Chapman, Suzuki, Chamarette, Rygh, and Dickenson (1998) demonstrated that gabapentin reduces pain in the Chung model. Gabapentin appears to act primarily in the CNS, in contrast to amitriptyline, which seems to act centrally and peripherally (Abdi, Lee, & Chung, 1998). Gabapentin also is effective in reducing pain behavior in phase 2 of the formalin test, a model of central sensitization and neuropathic pain (Shimoyama, Shimoyama, Davis, Inturrisi, & Elliott, 1997). Gabapentin reduces spinally mediated hyperalgesia seen after sustained nociceptive afferent input caused by peripheral tissue injury. Gabapentin also enhances spinal morphine analgesia in the rat tail-flick test, a laboratory model of nociceptive pain (Shimoyama, Shimoyama, Inturrisi, & Elliott, 1997).

Gabapentin is effective in reducing painful dysesthesias and improving quality of life scores in patients with painful diabetic peripheral neuropathy (Backonja, et al., 1998). Of patients randomized to receive gabapentin, 56% achieved a daily dosage of 3600 mg divided into three doses per day. The average magnitude of the analgesic response was modest, with a 24% reduction in intensity at the completion of the study compared with controls. Side effects were common. Dizziness and somnolence occurred in about 25% of patients, and confusion occurred in 8% of patients.

Morello, Leckband, Stoner, Moorhouse, and Sahagian (1999) compared gabapentin with amitriptyline for diabetic neuropathy and found both equally effective. Although gabapentin probably has fewer contraindications than tricyclic antidepressants, it is considerably more expensive.

Postherpetic neuralgia (PHN) is another difficult neuropathic syndrome. PHN affects approximately 10 to 15% of patients who develop herpes zoster, and is a particularly painful syndrome associated with lancinating pain and burning dysesthesias. The incidence of PHN is age-related, with up to 50% of patients older than 60 years of age developing persistent pain after a bout of herpes zoster. Pain relief usually requires pharmacological therapy. Unfortunately, most medications are not very effective. For example, only about one half of patients obtain adequate relief with antidepressants.

Rowbotham, Harden, Stacey, Bernstein, and Magnus-Miller (1998) evaluated the efficacy of gabapentin for the treatment of PHN. Of patients taking gabapentin, 65% achieved a daily dosage of 3600 mg. Although the average magnitude of pain reduction with gabapentin was modest, with approximately a 30% reduction in pain compared with controls, statistically pain reduction was highly significant. In addition, gabapentin improved sleep parameters and quality of life scores. Adverse effects that occurred more commonly in the gabapentin group included somnolence (27%), dizziness (24%), ataxia, peripheral edema, and infection (7 to 10%). Based on the data of Rowbotham and colleagues, it is reasonable to consider gabapentin as first-line therapy for postherpetic neuralgia. Gabapentin probably is at least as effective as antidepressants, with fewer contraindications. Gabapentin may be used as monotherapy or add-on treatment.

Although gabapentin can be started at 300 mg three times a day with most patients, giving the drug three times a day with meals and again at bedtime may be more effective. Use of a bedtime dose may assist with sleep and prevent pain from developing at night. With some patients, a more gradual titration may be better tolerated. In addition, this reduces the risk of patients stopping the drug because of side effects, before a therapeutic dose is achieved (David Longmire, personal communication, 2000). For example, start with a bedtime dose of 100 mg and then increase the daily dose to 100 mg twice a day with meals and at bedtime, for 2 days. Thereafter, the dose can be increased to three times a day with meals and at bedtime. Further titration every 3 to 7 days can be continued until pain relief, side effects, or a maximum daily dose in the range of 2400 to 3600 mg/day is reached. An instruction sheet for the patients is helpful in clarifying the dosage schedule and explaining possible side effects.

Gabapentin is generally well tolerated, even in the geriatric population, and has a safer side effect profile than tricyclic antidepressants. In the PNH study, the majority of patients were titrated to 3600 mg/day, and the median patient age was 73 years. The kidneys excrete gabapentin, and the dosage must be reduced for patients with renal insufficiency (Beydoun, Uthman, & Sackellares, 1995).

ANTIDEPRESSANTS

Tricyclic antidepressants have been used for years for the management of neuropathic pain syndromes, including diabetic neuropathy, postherpetic neuralgia, and migraine headache (Max, 1994; McQuay, et al., 1996; Onghena & van Houdenhove, 1992). However, pain relief is often modest and accompanied by side effects. Controlled studies indicate that approximately one third of patients will obtain more than 50% pain relief, one third will have minor adverse reactions, and 4% will discontinue the antidepressant because of major side effects (McQuay, et al., 1996). Fortunately, some patients obtain excellent pain relief.

Because comparisons between tricyclic antidepressants have not shown great differences in efficacy (Max, 1994; McQuay, et al., 1996), the choice of which antidepressant to use often depends on the side effect profile of a given drug. For example, when a patient is having difficulty sleeping because of pain, a more sedating drug, such as amitriptyline, may be indicated. On the other hand, desipramine, which is less sedating, may be better tolerated in elderly patients.

The tricyclic antidepressants are generally highly protein bound with large volumes of distribution and long elimination half-lives. They undergo extensive hepatic first-pass metabolism and typically have active metabolites. Although effective doses may be lower than typically used for depression, this is often not the case. Patients must be warned of potential side effects including sedation, cognitive changes, and orthostatic hypotension from α-adrenergic blockade. Anticholinergic side effects are common and include constipation, urinary retention, and exacerbation of glaucoma. Antihistaminic effects may cause sedation. Because of their long half-lives, these drugs may be given as a single bedtime dose. To minimize side effects, small doses (e.g., 10 to 25 mg) are used initially and increased over several weeks to a therapeutic dose, generally in the range of 50 to 150 mg/day. An electrocardiogram (ECG) is recommended if there is a history of cardiac disease. ECG changes such as QRS widening, PR and QT prolongation, and T wave flattening can be induced by these agents. Tricyclic antidepressants may have quinidine-like actions, consistent with their sodium channel-blocking effects, particularly in patients with underlying ischemic cardiac disease or arrhythmias (Glassman, Roose, & Bigger, 1993). Because abrupt discontinuation of antidepressants may precipitate withdrawal symptoms, such as insomnia, restlessness, and vivid dreams, a gradual taper over 5 to 10 days is recommended. Occasional blood levels are recommended, as well as CBC and hepatic studies to monitor for organ toxicity.

Amitriptyline is a tertiary amine that inhibits norepinephrine and serotonin reuptake equally (*American Medical Association Drug Evaluations Annual*, 1993). Amitriptyline is probably the most commonly used tricyclic agent for neuropathic pain. Amitriptyline also is the most sedating of the tricyclic antidepressants and has the most potent anticholinergic effects. A starting dose of 25 mg at bedtime is recommended.

Amitriptyline is metabolized into nortriptyline, a secondary amine with twice as much inhibition of norepinephrine reuptake, compared with serotonin. Nortriptyline is less sedating than amitriptyline with less anticholinergic side effects. A starting dose of 10 mg at bedtime is generally well tolerated.

Imipramine is a tertiary amine with equal inhibition of norepinephrine and serotonin uptake. This drug is moderately sedating and has average anticholinergic effects. The suggested starting dose is 25 mg at bedtime. Because of unpredictable metabolism, occasional blood levels are suggested. Imipramine is metabolized to a secondary amine, desipramine, which is a much more selective inhibitor of norepinephrine uptake. Desipramine is less sedating and has fewer anticholinergic effects than imipramine or amitriptyline, is at least as effective for pain control, and is better tolerated by elderly patients.

Compared with tricyclic agents, serotonin selective reuptake inhibitors (SSRIs) for neuropathic pain have been relatively disappointing. In addition, they are more expensive than the older generic agents. Nonetheless, at relatively high doses, (e.g., 60 mg) paroxetine is effective for diabetic neuropathy (Sindrup, Gram, Brosen, Eshj, & Morgensen, 1990). Fluoxetine may also be useful in the treatment of rheumatic pain conditions, many of which have neuropathic components (Rani, Naidu, Prasad, Rao, & Shobhar, 1996). SSRIs are better tolerated than tricyclic antidepressants and should be considered as first-line drugs in patients with concomitant depression. In this group they may serve double duty.

Venlafaxine is a novel phentylethylamine antidepressant that is chemically distinct from the older tricyclic antidepressants and the serotonin selective uptake inhibitors. Although venlafaxine blocks serotonin and norepinephrine reuptake, its analgesic actions may be mediated by both an opioid mechanism and adrenergic effects (Shreiber, Backer, & Pick, 1999). The drug may be at least as well tolerated as tricyclic agents and more effective for pain than standard doses of serotonin-selective drugs. Indeed, an initial report suggests that venlafaxine is effective for neuropathic pain (Galer, 1995). Venlafaxine should be started at one half of a 37.5 mg tablet twice daily and titrated weekly to a maximum of 75 mg, taken twice a day. Nausea appears to be the most common side effect.

ANTIARRHYTHMICS

Antiarrhythmics block ectopic neuronal activity at central and peripheral sites (Chabal, Jacobson, Mariano, Chaney, & Britell, 1992). Lidocaine, mexiletine, and phenytoin — type I antiarrhythmics — stabilize neural membranes by sodium channel blockade. Lidocaine suppresses spontaneous impulse generation on injured nerve segments, dorsal root ganglia, and dorsal horn wide dynamic range neurons (Abram & Yaksh, 1994; Sotgiu, Lacerenza, & Marchettini, 1992). Lidocaine infusions have been used to predict the response of a given neuropathic pain disorder to antiarrhythmic therapy (Burchiel & Chabal, 1995). Lidocaine may be effective at subanesthetic doses, and following nerve blocks analgesia may outlast conduction block for days or weeks (Burchiel & Chabal, 1995; Chaplan, Flemming, Shafer, & Yaksh, 1995; Jaffe & Rowe, 1995). It has been reported that patients with PNS injury experience better pain relief than those with central pain syndromes (Galer, Miller, & Rowbotham, 1993). If a trial

infusion of lidocaine is effective, a trial of oral mexiletine is worth considering.

Prior to starting mexiletine, a baseline ECG is recommended if the patient has underlying ischemic heart disease. Dosages may be increased from 150 to 250 mg three times a day over several days. Taking the medication with food may minimize gastric side effects, which are common and a major reason for discontinuing the drug. Other side effects of mexiletine are nervous system effects such as tremor and diplopia. Once on a stable dose, a serum level should be obtained (the therapeutic range is between 0.5 and 2.0 µg/ml).

Topical preparations of local anesthetics may be effective for neuropathic pain when there is localized allodynia or hypersensitivity. Topical blockade of small- and large-fiber nerve endings should reduce mechanical and thermal allodynia. A topical lidocaine patch (Lidoderm 5% lidocaine) has become available, which can be applied to painful areas in shingles (herpes zoster). Up to three patches may be applied at one time to the painful area. The patches can be worn for up to 12 h a day. A topical cream, eutectic mixture of local anesthetic (EMLA cream), a mixture of lidocaine and prilocaine, may also be useful for cutaneous pain. The cream may be applied three or four times a day to the painful area.

CORTICOSTEROIDS

Corticosteroids are clearly useful for neuropathic pain, particularly in stimulus-evoked pain such as lumbar radiculopathy. The anti-inflammatory effects of corticosteroids are well known, which may partly explain their efficacy for pain. When administered epidurally for treatment of discogenic radiculopathy, corticosteroids inhibit phospholipase A2 activity and suppress the perineural inflammatory response caused by leakage of disk material around the painful nerve root (Saal, et al., 1990). However, corticosteroids also act as membrane stabilizers by suppressing ectopic neural discharges (Castillo, et al., 1996; Devor, Govrin-Lippmann, & Raber, 1985). Therefore, some of the pain-relieving action of corticosteroids may be due to a lidocaine-like effect.

Depot forms of corticosteroids injected around injured nerves provide pain relief and reduce pain associated with entrapment syndromes. Corticosteroids are also effective if given orally or systemically. In cancer pain syndromes, steroids such as dexamethasone may be first-line therapy for neuropathic pain. The potential side effects of corticosteroids are well known and may be seen whether given orally, systemically, or epidurally.

BACLOFEN

Baclofen is useful for trigeminal neuralgia and other types of neuropathic pain (Fromm, Terrence, & Chattha, 1984), particularly as an add-on drug. Baclofen is a GABA-B agonist and is presumed to hyperpolarize inhibitory neurons in the spinal cord (Yaksh & Malmberg, 1994), thereby reducing pain. This GABA effect appears to be similar to benzodiazepines, such as clonazepam. Side effects of baclofen can be significant and include sedation, confusion, nausea, vomiting, and weakness, especially in the elderly. A typical starting dose is 5 mg three times a day. Thereafter, the drug can be increased slowly to 20 mg four times a day. Abrupt cessation may precipitate withdrawal with hallucinations, anxiety, and tachycardia. The drug is excreted by the kidneys and the dosage must be reduced in renal insufficiency.

CAPSAICIN

Capsaicin is a C-fiber-specific neurotoxin and is one of the components of hot peppers that produces a burning sensation on contact with mucous membranes. Topical preparations are available over the counter and are widely used for chronic pain syndromes. Capsaicin is a vanilloid receptor agonist and activates ion channels on C fibers that are thermotransducers of noxious heat (> 43°C) (Caternia, et al., 1997). With repeated application in sufficient quantities, capsaicin can inactivate primary afferent nociceptors. For patients with pain due to sensitized nociceptors, capsaicin may be effective, if they can tolerate the pain induced by the medication. The drug causes intense burning, which may abate with repeated applications and gradual inactivation of the nociceptors. However, in patients with tactile allodynia, which is probably mediated by large fibers, capsaicin may not be as effective. Capsaicin extracts are available commercially as topical preparations, containing 0.025 and 0.075% and should be applied to the painful area three to five times a day. The preparation may be better tolerated if it is used after application of a topical local anesthetic cream.

SUMMARY AND RECOMMENDATIONS

Neuropathic pain is a common cause of chronic pain and tends to be resistant to usual doses of traditional analgesic medications. Classic examples of neuropathic pain include trigeminal neuralgia, postherpetic neuralgia, and diabetic neuropathy. Neuropathic pain is often described as lancinating or burning in nature. Both types of pain may be present at the same time, often accompanied by allodynia.

Neuropathic pain may be manageable with one or more adjuvant analgesic drugs, often prescribed as part of a comprehensive treatment plan. From a theoretical point of view, it may be helpful to categorize adjuvant analgesics into two broad classes of drugs, agents that act as membrane-stabilizing agents and drugs that enhance dorsal horn inhibition. Membrane-stabilizing drugs may act by blocking sodium and calcium channels on damaged neural membranes. Medications that enhance dorsal horn inhibition appear to act by augmenting spinal biogenic amine and GABAergic mechanisms. From a clinical standpoint, given the paucity of our understanding of neuropathic pain mechanisms and how the medications actually work, it is probably more useful to classify adjuvant drugs according to their traditional therapeutic indications (e.g., antidepressants and anticonvulsants). This point of view is strengthened by the fact that most drugs appear to have multiple mechanisms and sites of action, making further subclassification arbitrary and probably inaccurate.

Anticonvulsants, particularly carbamazepine (and more recently gabapentin), are useful for neuropathic pain. Although conventional wisdom suggests that anticonvulsants may be most effective for lancinating pain, anticonvulsants also are useful for burning dysesthesias. The mechanism of action of gabapentin is poorly understood, but the drug has been demonstrated to bind to a novel voltage-dependent calcium channel receptor. Gabapentin reduces the pain due to diabetic peripheral neuropathy and postherpetic neuralgia; and the overall safety record with gabapentin is good, making it an attractive alternative to carbamazepine and tricyclic antidepressants, particularly for elderly patients.

Clonazepam is another option and also poses minimal risk from the standpoint of organ toxicity. Clonazepam may be useful for radicular pain and pain associated with tumors, such as plexopathy. In addition, clonazepam may be used to supplement other adjuvant drugs. When given at bedtime, the mild sedating effect of clonazepam can be helpful for patients who have difficulty sleeping because of pain.

Antidepressants have been used effectively for years in the management of multiple pain syndromes, including diabetic neuropathy, postherpetic neuralgia, rheumatoid arthritis, osteoarthritis, migraine headache, low back pain, and fibromyalgia. However, pain relief is often modest and accompanied by side effects. Studies indicate that only one third of patients obtain more than 50% pain reduction. However, some patients obtain dramatic pain relief.

The choice of which antidepressant to use for neuropathic pain often depends on the particular side effect profile of a given drug, because comparisons of individual tricyclic antidepressants have not shown great differences in efficacy. When a patient is having difficulty sleeping because of pain, a more sedating drug, such as amitriptyline is appropriate. On the other hand, desipramine, which is considerably less sedating and has fewer anticholinergic effects, may be much better tolerated in elderly patients.

Serotonin-selective reuptake inhibitors for neuropathic pain have been disappointing, although paroxetine at relatively high doses is useful for diabetic neuropathy. Fluoxetine may be useful in the treatment of rheumatic pain conditions, many of which have neuropathic components. As with the tricyclic agents, the SSRIs are probably interchangeable. However, SSRIs are better tolerated than tricyclics and may be extremely effective in treating patients with chronic pain and concomitant depression.

It remains unclear whether anticonvulsants or antidepressants should be first-line therapy for neuropathic pain. Similar results have been obtained with both, and current evidence concerning drug efficacy does not support the use of one drug over another. In many cases, selection of a particular drug may depend more on expected side effects (e.g., sedation) or the clinician's experience with the drug, than theoretical considerations about mechanisms of drug action. It must be remembered that treatment of neuropathic pain remains largely empirical. In addition, for maximum analgesic benefit, more than one drug may be necessary. Until more effective medications become available, polypharmacy will remain the rule instead of the exception. This is probably understandable, given the multiple mechanisms involved in the pathophysiology of neuropathic pain.

In general, for neuropathic pain either gabapentin or amitriptyline (or a similar tricyclic antidepressant) should be first-line therapy. When considering issues such as time to effective analgesic action and toxicity, gabapentin is more attractive. In our clinic, gabapentin often is our first choice, followed by a tricyclic antidepressant, such as nortriptyline. Both drugs must be started slowly and titrated to effect, perhaps to rather high levels, for full benefit. However, tricyclics have many potential side effects that must be considered, particularly anticholinergic and cardiac interactions and organ toxicity. Clearly, gabapentin is a safer drug, but may cause sedation or dysphoria in some patients. Occasionally, patients complain of weight gain and nonpitting edema. Other disadvantages of gabapentin include its cost (approximately ten times the cost of a generic tricyclic antidepressant at usual starting doses) and the need to take the drug three or four times a day. Keep in mind that the dosage of gabapentin must be reduced appropriately for patients with renal insufficiency. A comparison of gabapentin with tricyclic antidepressants is provided in Table 17.3.

When an appropriate medication trial has been ineffective, an interdisciplinary approach should be considered. With chronic neuropathic pain, limitations of current analgesics usually make complete pain relief a very unrealistic goal. Therefore, improving function and comfort and treating associated problems, such as depression, become important goals. Reducing dependence on opioid medications may or may not be a primary goal, depending

---

TABLE 17.3

Comparison of Gabapentin and Generic Tricyclic Antidepressants: Dosages, Side Effects, and Cost

Drug	Dosage	Side effects	Approximate Cost to Patient
Gabapentin (Neurontin)	Starting dose: 300 mg b.i.d. to t.i.d. (patient may start with bedtime dose) Elderly patients: 100 mg twice a day Effective dose: 1800 to 2400 mg/day (25 mg/kg/day); e.g., 600 mg with meals and at bedtime) Note: studies used doses as high as 3600 mg/day Titrate by increasing daily dose every 3 to 7 days, patient instruction sheet helpful	Somnolence, dizziness, ataxia, and peripheral edema. Reduce dosage in renal insufficiency	300 mg capsules t.i.d.: $106/month ($118/100 capsules) No laboratory studies needed to monitor therapy.
Amitriptyline	Starting dose: 25 mg at bedtime; elderly patients: 10 mg at HS Effective dose: 25 to 150 mg/day Titrate by increasing daily dose every 7 days; patient instruction sheet helpful	Sedation, cognitive problems, anticholinergic side effects, weight gain, orthostatic hypotension, arrhythmias; rare hepatic injury	25 mg tablets at bedtime: $7.80/month ($26/100 tablets) Laboratory studies needed to monitor therapy; consider baseline ECG
Nortriptyline	Starting dose: 10 mg at HS; effective dose: 10 to 100 mg/day Titrate by increasing daily dose every 7 days; patient instruction sheet helpful	Less sedation, fewer anticholinergic effects than amitriptyline; otherwise same effects as amitriptyline	10 mg tablets at bedtime: $12/month ($40/100 tablets) 25 mg tablets at bedtime: $24/month ($80/100 tablets) Lab studies, ECG
Desipramine	Starting dose: 25 mg at bedtime; elderly patients: 10 mg HS Effective dose: 25 to 150 mg/day Titrate by increasing daily dose every 7 days, patient instruction sheet helpful	Less sedation, less anticholinergic effects, otherwise same effects as amitriptyline	25 mg tablets at bedtime: $9/month ($30/100 tablets) Lab studies, ECG

on whether the pain syndrome is opioid responsive, the patient is demonstrating appropriate improvements in function, and there are not undo side effects or evidence of drug abuse.

Current evidence indicates that nonpharmacological approaches may be reasonable, obviate or reduce the need for potentially toxic medications, and improve the effectiveness of analgesic regimens. Spinal cord stimulation may reduce pain in selected patients. Less invasive techniques, including TENS units and percutaneous nerve stimulation, are also beneficial.

Effective management of neuropathic pain requires patience on the part of the clinician and the patient, and the willingness to evaluate different treatment approaches, including trials of various medications. This may be a time-consuming process. Insofar as possible, it is helpful to target specific symptoms, for example, burning pain with tricyclic antidepressants and lancinating pain with anticonvulsants. However, from a practical standpoint, pharmacological choices are often based on physician comfort with a given drug and expected side effects. Moreover, the high cost of newer drugs may make the older tricyclic antidepressants, such as amitriptyline, the only cost-effective alternative for some patients. Until more effective drugs become available, the pharmacological approach remains largely one of trial and error. In the meantime, nonpharmacological strategies may assume a larger role in clinical practice.

REFERENCES

Abdi, S., Lee, D.H., & Chung, J.M. (1998). The anti-allodynic effects of amitriptyline, gabapentin, and lidocaine in a rat model of neuropathic pain. *Anesthesia and Analgesia, 87,* 1360–1366.

Abram, S.E., & Yaksh, T.L. (1994). Systemic lidocaine blocks nerve injury-induced hyperalgesia and nociceptor-driven spinal sensitization in the rat. *Anesthesiology, 80,* 383–391.

Ahmed, H.E., Craig, W.F., White, P.F., et al. (1998). Percutaneous electrical nerve stimulation: an alternative to antiviral drugs for acute herpes zoster. *Anesthesia and Analgesia, 87,* 1–4.

Alhaider, A.A., Lei, S.Z., & Wilcox, G.L. (1991). Spinal 5-HT3 receptor-mediated antinociception: Possible release of GABA. *Journal of Neuroscience, 11,* 1881–1888.

Arner, S., & Meyerson, B.A. (1988). Lack of analgesic effect of opioids on neuropathic and idiopathic forms of pain. *Pain, 33,* 11–23.

American Medical Association (1993). Drugs used in mood disorders. *AMA Drug Evaluations Annual* (pp. 277–306). Chicago: American Medical Association.

Backonja, M., Beydoun, A., Edwards, K.R., Schwartz, S.J., Fonseca, V., Hes, M., LaMoreaux, L., & Garafalo, E. (1998). Gabapentin for the symptomatic treatment of painful neuropathy in patients with diabetes mellitus. A randomized controlled trial. *Journal of the American Medical Association, 280,* 1831–1836.

Bennett, G.J. (1994). Neuropathic pain. In P.D. Wall & R. Melzack (Eds.), *Textbook of pain* (3rd ed., pp. 201–224). Edinburgh: Churchill Livingstone.

Beydoun, A., Uthman, B.M., & Sackellares, J.C. (1995). Gabapentin: Pharmacokinetics, efficacy, and safety. *Clinical Neuropharmacology, 18,* 469–481.

Blom, S. (1962). Trigeminal neuralgia: Its treatment with a new anticonvulsant drug (G-32883). *Lancet, 1,* 839–840.

Brodie, M.J., & Dichter, MA. (1996). Antiepileptic drugs. *New England Journal of Medicine, 334,* 168–175.

Burchiel K.J., & Chabal C. (1995). A role for systemic lidocaine challenge in the classification of neuropathic pains. *Pain Forum, 4,* 81–82.

Castillo, J., Curley, J., Hotz, J., Uezono, M., Tigner, J., Chasin, M., Wilder, R., et al. (1996). Glucocorticoids prolong rat sciatic nerve blockade *in vivo* from bupivacaine microspheres. *Anesthesiology, 85,* 1157–1166.

Caternia, M.J., Schumacher, M.A., Tominga, M., et al. (1997). The capsaicin receptor: A heat-activated ion channel in the pain pathway. *Nature, 389,* 816–824.

Caudle, R.M., & Mannes, A J. (2000). Dynorphin, friend or foe? *Pain, 87,* 235–239.

Chabal, C., Jacobson, L., Mariano, A., Chaney, E., & Britell, C.W. (1992). The use of oral mexiletine for the treatment of pain after peripheral nerve injury. *Anesthesiology, 76,* 513–517.

Chaplan, S.R. (2000). Neuropathic pain: Role of voltage-dependent calcium channels. *Regional Anesthesia and Pain Medicine, 25,* 283–285.

Chaplan, S.R., Flemming, B.W., Shafer, S.L., & Yaksh, T.L. (1995). Prolonged alleviation of tactile allodynia by *intravenous* lidocaine in neuropathic rats. *Anesthesiology, 83,* 775–785.

Chapman, V., Suzuki, R., Chamarette, H.L.C., Rygh, L.J., & Dickenson, A.H. (1998). Effects of systemic carbamazepine and gabapentin on spinal neuronal responses in spinal nerve ligated rats. *Pain, 75,* 261–272.

Dellemijn, P. (1999). Are opioids effective in relieving neuropathic pain? *Pain, 80,* 453–462.

Devor, M. (1994). The pathophysiology of damaged peripheral nerves. In P.D. Wall & R. Melzack (Eds.), *Textbook of pain* (3rd ed., pp. 79–100). Edinburgh: Churchill Livingstone.

Devor, M. (1995). Neurobiological basis for selectivity of sodium channel blockers in neuropathic pain. *Pain Forum, 4,* 83–86.

Devor, M., Govrin-Lippmann, R., & Raber, P. (1985). Corticosteroids suppress ectopic neural discharge originating in experimental neuromas. *Pain, 22,* 127–137.

Eisenach, J.C., & Gebhart, G.F. (1995). Intrathecal amitriptyline acts as an *N*-methyl-D-aspartate receptor antagonist in the presence of inflammatory hyperalgesia in rats. *Anesthesiology, 83,* 1046–1054.

Foley, K.M. (1987). Pain syndromes in patients with cancer. *Medical Clinics of North America, 71,* 169–184.

Fromm, G.H., Terrence, C.F., & Chattha, A.S. (1984). Baclofen in the treatment of trigeminal neuralgia: Double-blind study and long-term follow-up. *Annals of Neurology, 15,* 240–244.

Galer, B.S. (1995). Neuropathic pain of peripheral origin: Advances in pharmacologic treatment. *Neurology, 45* (Suppl. 9), S17–S25.

Galer, B.S., Miller, K.V., & Rowbotham, M.C. (1993). Response to intravenous lidocaine infusion differs based on clinical diagnosis and site of nervous system injury. *Neurology, 43,* 1233–1235.

Ghoname, E.A., White, P.F., Ahmed, H.E., Hamza, A., Craig, W.F., & Noe, C.E. (1999). Percutaneous electrical nerve stimulation: An alternative to TENS in the management of sciatica. *Pain, 83,* 193–199.

Glassman, A., Roose, S., & Bigger, J. (1993). The safety of tricyclic antidepressants in cardiac patients. Risk-benefit reconsidered. *Journal of the American Medical Association, 269,* 2673–2677.

Gracely, R.H., Lynch, S.A., & Bennett, G.J. (1992). Painful neuropathy: Altered central processing, maintained dynamically by peripheral input. *Pain, 51,* 175–194.

Hamza, M.A., White, P.F., Craig, W.F., Ghoname, E.S., et al. (2000). Percutaneous electrical nerve stimulation: A novel analgesic therapy for diabetic neuropathic pain. *Diabetes Care, 23,* 365–370.

Hart, R.G., & Easton, J.D. (1982). Carbamazepine and hematological monitoring. *Annals of Neurology, 11,* 309–312.

Hegarty, A., & Portenoy, R.K. (1994). Pharmacotherapy of neuropathic pain. *Seminars in Neurology, 14,* 213–224.

Iacono, R.P., Guthkelch, A.N., & Boswell, M.V. (1992). Dorsal root entry zone stimulation for deafferentation pain. *Stereotactic and Functional Neurosurgery, 59,* 56–61.

Jaffe, R.A., & Rowe, M.A. (1995). Subanesthetic concentrations of lidocaine selectively inhibit a nociceptive response in the isolated rat spinal cord. *Pain, 60,* 167–174.

Jun, J.H., & Yaksh, T.L. (1998). The effect of intrathecal gabapentin and 3-isobutyl gamma-aminobutyric acid on the hyperalgesia observed after thermal injury in the rat. *Anesthesia and Analgesia, 86,* 348–354.

Kemler, M.A., Barendse, G.A.M, van Kleef, M., de Vet, H.C.W., Rijks, C.P.M., Furnee, C.A., & van den Wildernber, F.A.J.M. (2000). Spinal cord stimulation in patients with chronic reflex sympathetic dystrophy. *New England Journal of Medicine, 343,* 618–624.

Kovelowski, C.J., Ossipov, M.H., Sun, H., Malan, T.P., & Porecca, F. (2000). Supraspinal cholecystokinin may drive tonic descending facilitation mechanisms to maintain neuropathic pain in the rat. *Pain, 87,* 265–273.

Matthew, N.T., Saper, J.R., Silberstein, S.D., Rankin, L., Markley, H G., Solomon, S., et al. (1995). Migraine prophylaxis with divalproex. *Archives of Neurology, 52,* 281–286.

Max, M. (1994). Antidepressants as analgesics. In H.L. Fields & J.C. Liebskind (Eds.), *Pharmacological approaches to the treatment of chronic pain: New concepts and critical issues. Progress in pain research and management* (Vol. 1, pp. 229–246). Seattle: IASP Press.

McLachlan, E.M., Janig, W., Devor, M., & Michaelis, M. (1993). Peripheral nerve injury triggers noradrenergic sprouting within dorsal root ganglia. *Nature, 363,* 543–546.

McQuay, H.J., Tramer, M., Nye, B.A., Carroll, D., Wiffen, P.J., & Moore, R.A. (1996). A systematic review of antidepressants in neuropathic pain. *Pain, 68,* 217–227.

Merskey, H., & Bogduk, N. (Eds.). (1994). *Classification of chronic pain. Descriptions of chronic pain syndromes and definitions of pain terms* (2nd ed.). Seattle: IASP Press.

Morello, C.M., Leckband, S.G., Stoner, C.P., Moorhouse, D.F., & Sahagian, G.A. (1999). Randomized double-blind study comparing the efficacy of gabapentin with amitriptyline on diabetic peripheral neuropathy. *Archives of Internal Medicine, 159,* 1931–1937.

North, R.B., Kidd, D.H., Zahurak, M., James, C.S., & Long, D.M. (1993). Spinal cord stimulation for chronic, intractable pain: Experience over two decades. *Neurosurgery, 32,* 383–394.

Novakovic, S.D., Tzoumaka, E., McGivern, J.G., et al. (1998). Distribution of the tetrodotoxin-resistant sodium channel PN3 in rat sensory neurons in normal and neuropathic conditions. *Journal of Neuroscience, 18,* 2174–2187.

Onghena, P., & van Houdenhove, B. (1992). Antidepressant-induced analgesia in chronic non-malignant pain: A meta-analysis of 39 placebo controlled studies. *Pain, 49,* 205–220.

Ossipov, M. H., Lai, J., Malan, T. P., & Porreca, F. (2000). Spinal and supraspinal mechanisms of neuropathic pain. *Annals. New York Academy of Sciences, 909,* 12–24.

Pancrazio, J J., Kamatchi, G.L., Roscoe, A.K., & Lynch, C., III. (1998). Inhibition of neuronal Na^+ channels by antidepressant drugs. *Journal of Pharmacology and Experimental Therapeutics, 284,* 208–214.

Portenoy, R.K., Foley, K.M., & Inturrisi, C.E. (1990). The nature of opioid responsiveness and its implications for neuropathic pain: New hypotheses derived from studies of opioid infusions. *Pain, 43,* 272–286.

Price, D.D., Mao, J., & Mayer, D.J. (1994). Central neural mechanisms of normal and abnormal pain states. In H.L. Fields & J.C. Liebskind (Eds.), *Pharmacological approaches to the treatment of chronic pain: New concepts and critical issues. Progress in pain research and management* (Vol. 1, pp. 61–84). Seattle: IASP Press.

Rani, P.U., Naidu, M.U.R., Prasad, V.B.N., Rao, T.R.K., & Shobha, J.C. (1996). An evaluation of antidepressants in rheumatic pain conditions. *Anesthesia and Analgesia, 83,* 371–375.

Rowbotham, M., Harden, N., Stacey, B., Bernstein, P., & Magnus-Miller, L. (1998). Gabapentin for the treatment of postherpetic neuralgia. A randomized controlled trial. *Journal of the American Medical Association, 280,* 1837–1842.

Saal, J.S., Franson, R.C., Dobrow, R., Saal, J.A., White, A.H., & Goldthwaite, N. (1990). High levels of inflammatory phospholipase A2 activity in lumbar disc herniations. *Spine, 15,* 674–678.

Schreiber, S., Backer, M.M., & Pick, C.G. (1999). The antinociceptive effect of venlafaxine in mice is mediated through opioid and adrenergic mechanisms. *Neuroscience Letters, 273,* 85–88.

Shimoyama, N., Shimoyama, M., Davis, A.M., Inturrisi, C.E., & Elliott, K.J. (1997). Spinal gabapentin is antinociceptive in the rat formalin test. *Neuroscience Letters, 222,* 65–67.

Shimoyama, M., Shimoyama, N., Inturrisi, C.E., & Elliott, K.J. (1997a). Gabapentin enhances the antinociceptive effects of spinal morphine in the rat tail-flick test. *Pain, 72*, 375–382.

Sindrup, S.H., Gram, L.F., Brosen, K., Eshj, O., & Morgensen, E.F. (1990). The selective serotonin reuptake inhibitor paroxetine is effective in the treatment of diabetic neuropathy symptoms. *Pain, 42*, 135–144.

Sobotka, J.L., Alexander, B., & Cook, B.L. (1990). A review of carbamazepine's hematologic reactions and monitoring recommendations. *DICP, Annals of Pharmacotherapy, 24*, 1214–1219.

Sotgiu, M.L., Lacerenza, M., & Marchettini, P. (1992). Effect of systemic lidocaine on dorsal horn neuron hyperactivity following chronic peripheral nerve injury in rats. *Somatosensory and Motor Research, 9*, 227–233.

Swerdlow, M. (1984). Anticonvulsant drugs and chronic pain. *Clinical Neuropharmacology, 7*, 51–82.

Tanelian, D.L., & Victory, R.A. (1995). Sodium channel-blocking agents. Their use in neuropathic pain conditions. *Pain Forum, 4*, 75–80.

Taylor, C.P., Gee, N.S., Su, T.Z., Kocsis, J.D., Welty, D.F., Brown, J.P., Dooley, D.J., Boden, P., & Singh, L. (1998). A summary of mechanistic hypotheses of gabapentin pharmacology. *Epilepsy Research, 29*, 233–249.

Tohen, M., Castillo, J., Baldessarin, R.J., Zarate, C., & Kando, J.C. (1995). Blood dyscrasias with carbamazepine and valproate: A pharmacoepidemiological study of 2,228 patients at risk. *American Journal of Psychiatry, 152*, 413–418.

Vanderah, T.W., Gardell, L.R., Burgess, S.H., et al. (2000). Dynorphin promotes abnormal pain and spinal opioid antinociceptive tolerance. *Journal of Neuroscience, 20*, 7074–7079.

Woolf, C.J., & Mannion, R.J. (1999). Neuropathic pain: Aetiology, symptoms, mechanisms, and management. *Lancet, 353*, 1959–1964.

Woolf, C.J., Shortland P., & Coggeshall, R.E. (1992). Peripheral nerve injury triggers central sprouting of myelinated afferents. *Nature, 355*, 75–77.

Yaksh, T.L. (1979). Direct evidence that spinal serotonin and noradrenaline terminals mediate the spinal antinociceptive effects of morphine in the periaqueductal gray. *Brain Research, 160*, 180–185.

Yaksh, T.L, & Malmberg, A.B. (1994). Central pharmacology of nociceptive transmission. In P.D. Wall & R. Melzack (Eds.), *Textbook of pain* (3rd ed., pp. 165–200). Edinburgh: Churchill Livingstone.

18

Primary Headache Disorders

R. Michael Gallagher, D.O., F.A.C.O.F.P., F.A.H.S.

MANAGEMENT OF PRIMARY HEADACHE DISORDERS

INTRODUCTION

Headache disorders are an exceedingly common patient complaint that have been described throughout recorded medical history. Symptoms of head pain were noted as early as 7000 B.C. (Lyons & Petrucelli, 1978), and Neolithic trepanned skulls suggest the extreme measures once taken to relieve head pain that was attributed to evil spirits (Venzmer, 1972, p. 19). Currently, the National Headache Foundation (2000) reports that more than 45 million Americans have chronic, recurring headaches. Each year, U.S. businesses lose approximately $50 billion to absenteeism and medical expenses caused by headache, and headache sufferers spend in excess of $4 billion on nonprescription analgesics (NHF, 2000). Headache is responsible for approximately 10 million physician consultations per year (Linet & Stewart, 1987), and it is the fourth most common reason for emergency room visits in the United States.

Although the last two decades of the 20th century produced significant advances in our understanding of headache, the precise pathophysiology of the primary headache disorders remains unknown. For many years, primary headaches were classified symptomatically, as eithervascular headaches (migraine and cluster) or nonvascular headaches (tension type). Technological advances in the 1980s allowed researchers to see for the first time that changes in cerebral blood flow during headache episodes, particularly in migraine, did not occur exclusively in areas defined by vascular boundaries.

The Headache Classification Committee of the International Headache Society (IHS) ([ACCIHS], 1988) published a classification system for headache disorders. Although they were designed to help diagnose patients for clinical trials, the IHS criteria reflect international expert consensus and, unlike earlier headache diagnostic criteria (Friedman, Finley, & Graham, 1962), they outline the specific characteristics necessary to confirm and to exclude a broad range of headache disorders. According to the IHS, most chronic or recurring head pain can be classified as one of the "primary headache disorders": tension type, migraine, or cluster. Each of these headache types, as the descriptor suggests, can occur without the presence of an underlying disorder. The IHS system classifies all other types of headache as "secondary headache disorders," because they can always be attributed to one of hundreds of indirect causes of head pain (e.g., fever, trauma, subarachnoid hemorrhage, medication). This chapter reviews the diagnosis and treatment of the three primary headache disorders.

OVERALL APPROACH

The vast majority of headache patients can be successfully treated. When therapy is successful, the management of headache can be extremely rewarding for the patient and for the physician. Therapy can be time consuming and difficult in some cases, however. When it does not succeed, or it succeeds only partially, the challenge can quickly become frustrating. Help for headache sufferers rests with the empathetic, knowledgeable medical professional who is willing to establish an honest partnership that aims at relieving symptoms, restoring function, and reducing disability, not toward "curing" their "problem." In many cases, a clinician's ability to educate patients is key; all headache patients should clearly understand the goals of their treatment plan. Unfortunately, many headache

0-8493-0926-3/02/$0.00+$1.50
© 2002 by CRC Press LLC

patients seek medical attention during severe attacks, which demand immediate attention and prevent the evaluation necessary to making an accurate diagnosis. The most productive time for assessment is when the patient is headache free or not so debilitated as to interfere with a complete history taking and examination. After the diagnosis is made, the clinician and patient can develop a realistic, achievable treatment plan.

There are two main elements of headache treatment. *Abortive treatment* aims at relief once a headache attack has begun, and *prophylactic treatment* is used to prevent or reduce the likelihood of headache episodes before they occur. Abortive treatment is used for patients whose headaches are infrequent and for those headaches that break through in spite of prophylactic therapy. When headaches are frequent or unresponsive to abortive medication, prophylactic measures should be taken. Many clinicians begin prophylaxis when a patient has more than three severe headache attacks per month.

Whether preventive or abortive therapy is indicated, management should follow a definite plan incorporating the physician and the patient into a team that works actively to reduce the frequency and/or severity of headaches. The physician's impressions and physical findings should be completely explained to the patient no matter what level and pace are required to ensure complete understanding. The headache condition should also be explained, emphasizing the fact that the disorder is real, not imagined, and that it is controllable, not curable. Once a plan is developed, follow-up and continuing care are important elements in a successful outcome.

TENSION-TYPE HEADACHE

In the 1988, IHS classification of headache, a headache type once known as "muscle contraction headache" was renamed "tension-type headache" (TTH) (HCCIHS, 1988). Traditionally, it was believed that TTH was caused by sustained muscle contraction of the neck, jaw, scalp, and facial muscles. It has since been learned, however, that the sustained contraction of pericranial muscles associated with TTH may occur as an epiphenomenon to possible central disturbances, not as a primary process. Alterations in the levels of serotonin (5-HT), substance P (SP), and neuropeptide Y in the serum or platelets have been shown in patients affected by TTH, leading to speculation that these neurotransmitters are involved in the genesis and modulation of pain in the condition (Ferrari, 1993; Gallai, et al., 1994; Nakano, Shimomura, Takahashi, & Ikawa, 1993; Rolf, Wiele, & Brune, 1981; Schoenen, 1990; Shukla, Shanker, Nag, Verma, & Bhargava, 1987; Takeshima, Shimomura, & Takahashi, 1987). Without concrete evidence of central activity, however, the cause of TTH remains unknown.

TTH is the most common type of headache and is considered to have episodic (ETTH) and chronic (CTTH) variants. One-year period prevalence estimates using the IHS criteria indicate that as many as 93% of the general population have at least one tension-type headache per year (Rasmussen, Jensen, Schroll, & Olesen, 1991), although some investigators have found ETTH rates as low as 14.3% (Lavados & Tenhanun, 1997). CTTH sufferers (more than 180 headache attacks per year) are far less common than ETTH sufferers; the highest 1-year period prevalence ever recorded for CTTH was 8.1% (Tekle Haimanot, Seraw, Forsgren, Ekborn, & Ekstedt, 1995).

Both ETTH and CTTH are characterized by intermittent or persisting bilateral pain, often described as a squeezing pressure or a tight band around the head. Some patients experience pain in the temporal or occipital regions, the forehead, or the vertex. The location of symptoms can vary from attack to attack, and associated tightness of the neck and shoulders is common. Unlike migraine, TTH is not preceded by prodromal symptoms, and TTH are not episodes typically associated with nausea or vomiting. The intensity of pain in TTH varies widely, but it is not usually incapacitating. TTH can last from hours to days and, in some cases, persist for months. The IHS diagnostic criteria for ETTH and CTTH are listed in Table 18.1 (HCCIHS, 1988).

PRECIPITATING FACTORS

TTH frequently occurs during periods of stress or emotional upset. Some CTTH patients may display evidence of anxiousness, as well as poor coping and adaptation skills. If headaches are frequent or near daily, depression may be involved and should be considered, even in the absence of obvious signs, such as mood changes, crying spells, or loss of appetite. Organic processes may also be involved in the precipitation of TTH. When the cause is organic instead of psychogenic, the pain may also be resistant to usual treatment modalities. Organic causes can be numerous, but the more commonly encountered in clinical practice include degenerative joint disease of the cervical spine, head or neck trauma, temporomandibular joint dysfunction, or ankylosing spondylitis.

TREATMENT

ETTH can be resolved with nonpharmacological measures, analgesic medications, or some combination of these modalities. Nonpharmacological options for TTH include manipulation, massage, exercise, cold or warm compresses, stress avoidance, and relaxation techniques (Table 18.2) (Stevens, 1993). When these approaches do not provide adequate relief, simple analgesics, such as acetaminophen (APAP), aspirin (ASA), or ibuprofen (IB), often relieve the symptoms of ETTH. If simple analgesics

TABLE 18.1
IHS Diagnostic Criteria for Episodic Tension-Type Headache

A. At least 10 previous headache episodes fulfilling criteria B to D listed next; number of days with such headache < 180/year (< 15/month)

B. Headache lasting from 30 min to 7 days

C. At least two of the following pain characteristics:

Pressing/tightening (nonpulsating) quality

Mild or moderate intensity (may inhibit, but does not prohibit activities)

Bilateral location

No aggravation by walking stairs or similar routine physical activity

D. Both of the following:

No nausea or vomiting (anorexia possibly occurring)

Photophobia and phonophobia are absent, or one but not the other is present

E. At least one of the following:

History, physical, and neurological examinations not suggesting one of the disorders listed in groups 5 to 11

History and/or physical and/or neurological examinations suggesting such disorder, but ruled out by appropriate investigations

Such disorder present, but tension-type headache not occurring for the first time in close temporal relation to the disorder

From HCCIHS (1988). *Cephalalgia, 8*(Suppl. 7), 1–96. With permission.

fail, caffeinated combination analgesics often provide effective relief. In TTH studies, it has been shown that it takes about 40% more of a simple analgesic to equal the analgesic potency of the simple analgesic plus caffeine (Laska, et al., 1984; Migliardi, Armellino, Friedman, Gillings, & Beaver, 1994). If a prescription is required to provide adequate relief, some patients with ETTH benefit

TABLE 18.2
Nonpharmacological Management of Headache

Topical heat or cold packs

Topical analgesic balms

Respite from stressors (rest, sleep)

Stress-reduction techniques (e.g., exercise, sexual activity, relaxation modalities)

Regular exercise

Physical therapy

Relaxation techniques (including biofeedback, hypnotherapy, vacation)

Manipulative therapy

From Stevens, M.B. (1993). *American Family Physician, 47,* 799–805. With permission.

from the combination of isometheptene, acetaminophen, and dichloralphenazone. Other options include the alpha-agonist tizanidine, ASA combined with the muscle relaxants orphenadrine or carisoprodol, or APAP added to chlorzoxazone. In some patients, the symptoms of TTH can be extremely severe and require potentially addictive analgesic combination drugs containing butalbital, meprobromate, or an opioid. These drugs provide analgesia and reduce the anxiety often associated with pain (Table 18.3). As with any potentially addicting drug, however, limit the amounts prescribed and make sure that patients understand that they should contact you about a change in prescription instead of beginning daily or near-daily use of a medication with a high risk of addiction.

Patients with CTTH require a different approach. Prescribing the stronger medications in this patient subset greatly enhances the risk of abuse. Prophylactic treatment may be needed for CTTH patients or for those whose attacks are caused by organic abnormalities. Pharmacological treatment of CTTH can include the judicious use

TABLE 18.3
Selected Prescription Medications for Tension-Type Headache

Drug	Brand Name	Dose — Prn
Aspirin	Bayer	650 mg every 4–6 h
Acetaminophen	Tylenol	500–1000 mg every 4–6 h
Aspirin/acetaminophen/caffeine	Excedrin	2 tablets every 4–6 h
Ibuprofen	Advil/Motrin	400 mg every 4–6 h
Naproxen	Aleve	275–550 mg every 6–8 h
Orphenadrine/aspirin/caffeine	Norgesic	2 tablets every 4 h
Isometheptene/dichloralphenazone/acetaminophen	Midrin	2 tablets at onset followed by 1 tablet hourly (up to 5 tablets)
Carisoprodol/aspirin	Soma compound	2 tablets every 4 h
Chlorzoxazone	Parafon Forte	1 tablet every 4–6 h
Butalbital/aspirin/caffeine	Fiorinal	1 tablet every 4 h
Butalbital/acetaminophen/caffeine	Fioricet/Esgic	1 tablet every 4 h
Tizanidine	Zanaflex	2–4 mg every 4 h

of sedatives or muscle relaxants, but most patients who respond do so only temporarily, and the risk of habituation is significant.

The nonsteroidal anti-inflammatory drugs (NSAIDs) and antidepressants appear to be the most useful in preventing TTH (Gallagher & Freitag, 1987b). Most CTTH patients who improve with NSAID treatment do so in 2 to 3 weeks. Side effects of the NSAIDs include fluid retention, nausea, diarrhea, dizziness, and gastric and duodenal irritation. Renal function monitoring must be done periodically to avoid renal injury in patients who take NSAIDs regularly. Antidepressants, in a single bedtime dose, may also be effective in reducing the frequency of CTTH pain. Therapeutic response can take as long as 4 weeks. The regimen should begin with a low dose and gradually be titrated to the individual patient's needs. Side effects vary depending on the agent and the patient, but they most frequently include drowsiness, postural hypotension, weight gain, constipation, and dry mouth.

Nonpharmacological options for CTTH include manipulation and soft tissue massage techniques to the scalp, cervical, or thoracic areas, reduction of stress and muscle tension, and biofeedback. Consider psychotherapeutic interventions for patients whose headaches are related to significant emotional conflict or are treatment refractory. Choices can range from supportive to long term and may involve the family physician, psychiatrist, or psychologist.

MIGRAINE

An estimated 28 million Americans, about 18% of women and 6% of men, suffer from migraine (Stewart, Lipton, Celentano, & Reed, 2000). This chronic, neurologic disorder is characterized by periodically recurring attacks of head pain that are accompanied by gastrointestinal, visual, and auditory disturbances (HCCIHS, 1988). Although the intensity and severity of attacks tend to vary throughout the migraine population, as well as within the same migraineur over a series of episodes, estimates suggest that pain and disability are mild in approximately 5 to 15% of attacks, moderate to severe in 60 to 70% of attacks, and incapacitating in 25 to 35% of attacks (Stewart, Schecter, & Lipton, 1994). The disorder occurs most frequently among persons aged 25 to 55 (Stewart, Lipton, Celentano, & Reed, 1992), concentrating its burden on those who are typically in their most productive years. Migraine patients consistently report lower mental, physical, and social well-being than do unaffected controls (Terwindt, et al., 2000; Lipton, et al., 2000).

According to the IHS, migraine is "an idiopathic, recurring headache disorder manifesting in attacks lasting 4–72 hours. Typical characteristics of headache are unilateral location, pulsating quality, moderate to severe

intensity, aggravation by routine physical activity, and association with nausea, photo-, and phonophobia" (HCCIHS, 1988). Migraine does not occur on a daily basis; typical frequency is one to four per month. In some patients, the migraine may occur once yearly or as often as 15 to 20 times per month.

Migraine pain typically affects one side of the head, and may switch sides. The headache can become generalized. Many patients report that their pain localizes around or behind the eye, or in the frontotemporal area. The pain may radiate toward the occiput or upper neck during an attack. The shoulder and lower portion of the neck may also be involved. In some cases, the pain radiates to the face.

A number of associated symptoms can accompany the pain of an acute attack. Nausea or vomiting, in addition to either photophobia or phonophobia, are required for the diagnosis of migraine (HCCIHS, 1988). However, dizziness, lightheadedness, blurred or double vision, anorexia, constipation, diarrhea, chills, tremors, cold extremities, ataxia, and dysarthria may also be present. Some patients may experience lethargy and fatigue for several days following an attack.

A prodrome or aura often precedes migraine attacks. Aura symptoms are usually visual, typically start just before the acute headache, and continue for less than 1 h. Prodromal symptoms include scotomata, teichopsia, fortification spectra, photopsia, paresthesias, visual and auditory hallucinations, hemianopsia, and metamorphopsia (Diamond, 1997). Despite the absence of visual and other prodromal characteristics, migraine without aura sufferers have also described premonitions of impending migraine attacks. These symptoms are usually vague and can occur from 2 to 72 h before an attack. The list of painless warnings includes hunger, anorexia, drowsiness, depression, irritability, tension, restlessness, talkativeness, excess energy, and euphoria. Table 18.4 lists the complete IHS criteria for migraine with aura and migraine without aura (HCCIHS, 1988).

PRECIPITATING FACTORS

Certain factors, known as "triggers," can play a precipitating role in the onset of migraine attacks. Migraine triggers can be categorized as physiological, psychological, or external stimuli. Although they are highly individualized, some of the most common migraine triggers appear in Table 18.5.

Physiological

Migraine sufferers can be particularly sensitive to changes in eating and sleeping patterns. Fasting or missing a meal is a known headache trigger. All migraine patients should be encouraged to maintain a regular meal schedule. Over- or undersleeping can also precipitate a migraine. Migraine attacks that occur on weekends, on

TABLE 18.4
IHS Diagnostic Criteria for Migraine without Aura and Migraine with Aura

Migraine without Aura

A. At least five attacks fulfilling B–D
B. Attack lasts 4–72 h (untreated or unsuccessfully treated)
C. Attack with at least two of the following characteristics:
   Unilateral location
   Pulsating quality
   Moderate or severe intensity (inhibits or prohibits daily activities)
   Aggravation by walking stairs or similar routine physical activity
D. During attack at least one of the following:
   Nausea and/or vomiting
   Photophobia and phonophobia
E. At least one of the following:
   History, physical, and neurological examinations not suggesting a secondary disorder
   History, physical, and/or neurological examinations suggesting such disorder, but ruled out by appropriate investigations
   Such disorder present, but migraine attacks not occurring for the first time in close temporal relation to the disorder

Migraine with Aura

A. At least two attacks fulfilling B
B. At least three of the following four characteristics:
   One or more fully reversible aura symptoms indicating focal cerebral cortical and/or brain stem dysfunction
   At least one aura symptom developing gradually over more than 4 min or, 2 or more symptoms occuring in succession
   No aura symptom lasting more than 60 min, if more than one aura symptom present, accepted duration is proportionally increased
   Headache following aura with a free interval of less than 60 min (may also begin before or simultaneously with the aura)
C. At least one of the following:
   History, physical, and neurological examinations not suggesting a secondary disorder
   History, physical, and/or neurological examinations suggesting such disorder, but ruled out by appropriate investigations
   Such disorder present, but migraine attacks not occurring for the first time in close temporal relation to the disorder

TABLE 18.5
Recognized Migraine Triggers

Physiological	Psychological	External
Fasting, missing a meal, or other changes in eating patterns	Stress (external or unconsciously created by patient)	Bright or flickering lights
Over- or undersleeping	Repressed hostility	Loud noises
Oral contraceptives in migraine patients	Depression	Strong odors
Cyclical hormonal changes; hormone replacement therapy in postmenopausal women	Fear	Rapid changes in barometric pressure; travel to areas with different altitudes
Food triggers including:	Anger	Airline flights
Alcoholic drinks		
Coffee, tea, and cola		
Aged cheese		
Chocolate		
Cured meats		
Chinese food		
Smoked fish, nuts, and pickled or marinated foods		
Drugs	Anxiety	Allergens
Atenolol		
Caffeine (and caffeine withdrawal)		
Danazol		
Diclofenac		
H2 receptor blockers		
Hydralazine		
Indomethacin		
Nifedipine		
Nitrofurantoin		
Nitroglycerin		
Oral contraceptives		
Reserpine		

holidays, or during vacations have been linked to oversleeping (Wilkinson, 1986). To avoid "weekend" headaches, patients should be instructed to go to bed only when they are tired and to arise at the same time each day. Lack of sleep and fatigue may also provoke an acute migraine attack.

A relationship between the menstrual cycle and migraine attacks is well documented and partially accounts for the higher prevalence of migraine in women. Among female migraineurs, 60 to 70% note a menstrual link to their migraine attacks, with severe attacks occurring immediately before, during, or after their period (Dia-

mond, 1997). Many report a remission of migraine after the first trimester of pregnancy. Many female patients see a reduction in frequency or complete remission of their headaches after menopause (Honkasalo, Kaprio, Heikkilä, Sillanpää, & Koskenvuo, 1993). Oral contraceptives should be used judiciously in migraine patients, because these drugs have long been known to increase the frequency, severity, duration, and complications of migraine (Whitty, Hockaday, & Whitty, 1966). Also, hormone replacement therapy (HRT) should be avoided in postmenopausal migraineurs, because these hormones can exacerbate or restart migraine attacks. However, side effects have been reduced with the patch delivery system and lower doses of estrogen, as well as with progesterones.

The link between diet and migraine depends on the individual patient. The amines, including tyramine and phenylethylamine, nitrates, monosodium glutamate (MSG), and alcohol, have all been implicated as triggers. Tyramine is found in aged cheese, pickled foods, fresh-baked yeast breads, and marinated foods. Another amine, phenylethylamine, is contained in chocolate. The nitrates, which promote vasodilation, are found in cured meats. Many food additives and Chinese foods contain MSG, which has been associated with headache. Alcohol has both central and direct vasodilating properties, and, in some patients, migraine attacks can be precipitated, especially with wine. Other possible triggers for migraine include caffeine, nicotine, ergotamine, hypoglycemia, allergy, ingestion of ice cream, and monoamine oxidase inhibitors (MAOIs). Migraineurs who are sensitive to dietary triggers should be instructed to avoid the substances to which they are susceptible whenever possible.

Psychological

Stress is probably the most readily identified psychological trigger of an acute migraine attack. However, many migraine patients remain headache free during a stressful period only to experience a severe headache when the stress has resolved. Depression, fear, anger, anxiety, and repressed hostility may also be associated with migraine. Although avoiding stress is difficult, reducing stress is not, and instruction on coping methods may be beneficial for "overloaded" patients. Other psychological triggers may require additional counseling, concomitant treatment, or both.

External Stimuli

Some migraine patients describe a relationship between their headaches and weather. Rapid changes in barometric pressure as well as extreme variations in weather have been shown to provoke a migraine attack in certain patients (Diamond, Nursal, Freitag, & Gallagher, 1989). During or subsequent to travel to an area with an altitude substantially different from the patient's norm (i.e., the mountains for those who live at sea level and vice versa), a patient may report an increase in headache frequency. A diuretic, such as acetazolamide, used on the day of a flight may help to prevent these headaches. Other external migraine triggers include bright or flashing lights, loud noises, and strong odors (such as smoke, perfume, or cleaning fluids).

TREATMENT

With a confirmed diagnosis of migraine, the clinician and patient should begin to devise a treatment plan that accounts for the practical realities of the patient's lifestyle. Migraine treatment plans usually involve some combination of behavioral change (avoiding triggers, increasing exercise, and relaxation) and pharmaceutical

and nonpharmaceutical pain management approaches (prophylactic or abortive medications, manipulation and massage, cold compresses, or warm baths). Determining the relative value of these strategies for each patient shapes the course of both acute and long-term therapy.

Behavioral changes and nonmedicinal treatments can be valuable, particularly in patients with frequent or severe migraine attacks. Most treatment plans incorporate behavioral modification in the form of avoiding foods, beverages, or situations that trigger attacks; each patient is unique in this regard. Similarly, the use of cold compresses, warm baths, or massage for migraine should be governed by the nature of the individual's disorder.

If medication is a part of the treatment plan, the selection can be tailored to the migraine patient's needs. Before recommending or prescribing any medication for migraine, however, it is crucial to determine all remedies the patient may have already tried before consulting, because detailed information in this area may reveal important therapeutic limitations and opportunities. Familiarity with the wide range of options for migraine pharmacotherapy can increase the likelihood of meeting an individual patient's needs.

Standard Migraine Medications

Pharmacological therapy is often the main component in migraine therapy. There are three broad categories of pharmacological treatment of migraine: prophylactic, abortive, and symptomatic. If migraine attacks occur four or more times per month, or if attacks are incapacitating, many clinicians consider prophylactic therapy. If a patient has three or fewer migraine attacks per month, abortive treatment may be indicated. When acute pain does not respond to abortive measures, symptomatic therapy can be employed as a backup.

Prophylactic Treatment

Prophylactic medications are used to prevent the onset of migraine attacks and to reduce their frequency and severity. The decision about which class to use generally depends on comorbidities and interactions with concomitant medications. Beta-blockers, for example, could be used in patients with hypertension but are contraindicated in those with asthma (Rapoport & Adelman, 1998); a depressed patient taking a selective serotonin reuptake inhibitor (SSRI) should not take an MAOI for migraine because of dangerous interactions. Drugs currently approved for long-term use in migraine prophylaxis include propanolol, timolol, divalproex sodium, and methysergide (Diamond, 1997).

Propanolol, an adrenergic blocker, one of the most frequently used drugs in the prophylactic therapy of migraine, must be given carefully in patients with coronary heart disease and thyrotoxicosis. It may exacerbate coronary ischemia and can produce unstable angina or myocardial infarction (Diamond, 1997). Propanolol is contraindicated in patients with asthma, chronic obstructive lung disease, congestive heart failure, or arterioventricular conduction disturbances. In some patients, administration may cause depression, nightmares, lethargy, fatigue, sexual dysfunction, and weight gain (Rapoport & Adelman, 1998). Patients being treated with insulin, oral hypoglycemia drugs, or MAOIs should not be treated with propanolol. Propanolol is administered from 60 to 240 mg/day in a simple, long-acting dosage or in divided doses. If propanolol is not tolerated, timolol, another beta-blocker, can be used in doses of 5 to 30 mg/day. Other beta-blockers, such as nadolol, atenolol, and metoprolol, have been used with varying degrees of success.

The alpha agonist, clonidine, may be useful for migraineurs who are sensitive to cheeses and other foods containing tyramine (Diamond, 1997). Side effects are usually mild and include drowsiness, dry mouth, constipation, and occasional disturbance of ejaculation. Mild orthostatic hypertension and depression may also occur.

Divalproex sodium is FDA approved for migraine prevention and is particularly indicated for migraineurs with epileptic seizures, bipolar disorder, and possibly head trauma (Rapoport & Adelman, 1998). An extended-release formulation of divalproex, which produces less fluctuation in plasma concentrations than the standard therapy, is also available. The recommended starting dose for the extended-release formulation is 500 mg daily and can be increased to 1000 mg daily. Divalproex sodium should be avoided in any patient with a history of hepatitis or abnormal liver function; it is contraindicated in pregnancy, because it is associated with neural tube defects. Divalproex sodium can be effectively combined with tricyclic antidepressants in patients with chronic recurrent migraine.

Closely related (and similar in some long-term effects) to ergotamine and its derivatives, methysergide promotes serotonin inhibition and mild vasoconstriction. This agent is usually prescribed in doses of 2 mg three times a day (t.i.d.) and should not be used for more than 4 consecutive months, after which a minimum 1-month hiatus is required before resuming therapy. Approved by the FDA for migraine prophylaxis, the drug's sustained use is contraindicated because of the potential for cardiopulmonary and retroperitoneal fibrosis (Diamond, 1997). During the treatment period, the patient should be examined at regular intervals to detect the development of fibrotic conditions, murmurs, or pulse deficits.

Topiramate, a polysaccharide anticonvulsant with several mechanisms of action, has also been assessed in an open label study of migraine. With an average daily dose of 325 mg/day in two divided doses, investigators noted an average decrease in attack frequency of 72% and an average decrease in the severity of attacks of 55% (Kruzs

& Scott, 1999). Among migraine prevention medications, a unique side effect of topiramate is that it may cause some patients to lose weight during a course of therapy. With a positive efficacy and safety profile, topiramate appears to be a promising treatment option for patients with refractory migraine.

Abortive Treatment

Abortive medications used in the treatment of migraine include the nonprescription agents, IB and APAP/ASA/CAF, as well as a range of prescription-only medication (including isometheptene mucate, ergotamine preparations, prescription-strength NSAIDs, dihydroergotamine mesylate (DHE) and DHE nasal spray), and the 5-HT_{1D} receptor agonists (including sumatriptan, naratriptan, rizatriptan, and zolmitriptan). Selected abortive agents are reviewed next.

APAP/ASA/CAF — Lipton, Stewart, Ryan, Saper, Silberstein, and Sheftell (1998) published the results of three studies comparing the nonprescription combination of APAP 250 mg, ASA 250 mg, and CAF 65 mg with placebo. A single two-tablet dose of this nonprescription compound was highly effective in relieving both migraine pain and associated symptoms. There were no serious side effects.

Ergotamine preparations — The utility of these medications in arresting migraine attacks is due to their ability to counteract the dilation of some arteries and arterioles, primarily the branches of the external carotid artery. Nausea is a common side effect of ergotamine-treated patients. Once used, ergotamine should not be repeated for 4 days to avoid the possibility of ergotamine rebound headache, a relatively prevalent side effect characterized by a self-sustaining cycle of daily or almost daily migraine headaches coupled with the irresistible use of ergotamine tartrate to alleviate them (Gallagher, 1983). Ergotamine and its derivatives should be avoided in elderly and, because of their ability to induce labor, in pregnant patients. Dihydroergotamine, which was developed as an improvement over ergotamine tartrate, has a better safety profile. It is available in parenteral and nasal formulations. A 2-mg dose of the nasal spray formulation of this agent has a rapid onset of action, a low recurrence rate, and completely resolves a migraine attack in up to 70% of patients within 4 h (Gallagher, 1996).

NSAIDs — In prescription doses, NSAIDs have been shown to be superior to placebo and equivalent to other reference drugs in the abortive treatment of migraine (Pradalier, Clapin, & Dry, 1988). Two nonprescription formulations of IB have also been approved for the treatment of acute migraine. Although fewer side effects are reported with NSAIDs than with ergotamine preparations, the gastrointestinal, renal, and hepatic risks linked with NSAID use are well documented (Rapoport & Adelman, 1998).

Isometheptene — This sympathomimetic with vasoconstrictive effects is found in combination with acetaminophen 325 mg, and dichloralphenazone 100 mg. The combination can be effective in migraine without aura. It is taken orally, two capsules at onset and one each hour thereafter, to a maximum of five capsules in 1 day. Side effects include drowsiness and nausea, and it is contraindicated in patients with hypertension and renal disease, as well as those taking MAOIs.

Selective serotonin reuptake inhibitors — Sumatriptan, an SSRI, is a mainstay in migraine therapy. A single subcutaneous dose of 6 mg relieves the majority of migraine attacks successfully (Subcutaneous Sumatriptan Study Group, 1991); oral and nasal preparations are also available. However, because of sumatriptan's low oral bioavailability, significant headache recurrence (Goldstein, 1996), and contraindication in large subgroups of patients, newer agents have been developed and introduced.

The migraine drugs being marketed as "next generation" agents are similar to sumatriptan, 5-HT$_{1B/1D}$ receptor agonists. As of this writing, there are six new compounds, only three of which have been approved for marketing by the FDA: naratriptan, rizatriptan, and zolmitriptan. Three others, almotriptan, eletriptan, and frovatriptan, should be available in the near future.

Reports of clinical experience with the approved medications suggest that, although they are effective, response to them is highly individualized. For instance, Freitag, Diamond, Diamond, Urban, & Pepper (2000), in a retrospective study of clinical experience with naratriptan, rizatriptan, and zolmitriptan, found that all the newer acute treatments for migraine were highly effective, but they observed no clear differences between the 5-HT medications that might distinguish one agent as the "best." However, one trial comparing zolmitriptan with sumatriptan found that zolmitriptan (2.5 mg) was significantly more effective than sumatriptan (50 mg) in terms of headache response at 2 and 4 h posttreatment (Gallagher, Dennish, Spierings, & Chitra, 2000). In other work, investigators compared rizatriptan 10 mg with zolmitriptan 2.5 mg and reported that patients treated with rizatriptan were 31% more likely to be pain free and 23% more likely to have pain relief sooner than patients who were treated with zolmitriptan (Diener, Pascual, & Vega, 2000).

It has been suggested that naratriptan may have the lowest rate of headache recurrence of the 5-HT oral agents (Ryan, 1998), but headache recurrence remains a problem for all the triptans. Up to one third of patients taking almotriptan (Pascual, et al., 2000), 40% of patients taking sumatriptan, 28% taking naratriptan, 40 to 47% taking rizatriptan, about 30% taking zolmitriptan have experienced recurrence of their migraine symptoms within 24 h (Goldstein, Keywood, & Hutchinson, 1999). Preclinical data indicate, however, that frovatriptan may have a prolonged duration of action, and pharmacokinetic studies show that the elimination half-life is the longest in the class (Buchan, 1998). This characteristic may be responsible for the low rate of headache recurrence seen in frovatriptan-treated patients (Goldstein, Keywood, & Hutchinson, 1999). Eletriptan effectively relieves the symptoms of an acute migraine attack at both the 40 and 80 mg doses. In clinical trials, therapeutic response to eletriptan is generally superior to sumatriptan, and the rate of headache recurrence among eletriptan-treated subjects is low (19%) (Pryse-Phillips, 1999). More investigations and additional clinical experience with the 5-HT$_{1B/1D}$ class are needed to determine how the use of these medications can be optimized across the wide range of migraine patients.

Symptomatic Treatment

When first-line nonprescription and second-line prescription abortive agents fail, symptomatic treatment is indicated. Symptomatic agents are sometimes referred to as rescue medications. Transnasal butorphanol, a nasal preparation, is one of the more useful drugs in patients with infrequent attacks. Pain relief has been demonstrated within 15 min (Goldstein, Marek, & Winner, 1998), and the nasal formulation is particularly convenient for patients who are suffering from severe nausea or vomiting. Other options for rescue therapy include injectable NSAIDs and butalbital combinations, opioids, and opioid-like combinations. Because of their abuse potential and the possibility of rebound effects, precautions must be observed when using symptomatic medications.

Intractable Migraine

Episodic migraine may become incessant and refractory to standard care (Mathew, Reuveni, & Perez, 1987). For many of these patients, drug dependence is a factor; for others, disabling headaches continue, unabated, seemingly indefinitely. In such cases, clinicians should be aware of several approaches to the management of intractable migraine. DHE, administered in a protocol developed by Raskin, can produce a headache-free state in 90% of intractable migraine patients within 2 days (Raskin, 1986). Metoclopramide is used adjunctively with DHE to suppress withdrawal symptoms (Ramaswamy & Bapna, 1987). Alternative treatments for intractable migraine include dexamethasone (4 mg intravenously) (Gallagher, 1986), ketorolac (30 to 60 mg intramuscularly or intravenously), chlorpromazine (0.1 mg/kg intravenously every 6 to 8 h) (Newman, 2000).

CLUSTER HEADACHE

Cluster headache is a devastatingly severe type of recurrent vascular headache. It also sometimes is referred to as histaminic cephalalgia, histaminic headache, Horton's cephalalgia, Horton's headache, Horton's syndrome, or migrainous neuralgia. Its clinical constellation of symptoms with the characteristic patient behavioral tendencies during attacks should make it easy to recognize and distinguish from migraine or TTH. Of the recurrent headache syndromes, it is probably the most distressing and brutal to the afflicted.

A cluster attack is characterized by severe unilateral pain, often described as a burning, boring, or stabbing sensation in the area of the eye, temple, or forehead with radiating to the jaw, ear, or neck. During attacks, sufferers often pace or become extremely active, similar to patients experiencing renal colic. Frequently associated with the pain are ipsilateral lacrimation, eye injection, rhinorrhea, congestion, facial droop, or sweating. The pain usually builds quickly over several minutes and lasts approximately 30 to 90 min.

Cluster headache attacks can occur numerous times daily, sometimes at the same hour each day. Early morning awakening with headache 2 to 3 hours after retiring is common. In its typical form, episodic cluster, the headaches cluster or group for periods of weeks to months and mysteriously disappear for months to years; thus the name "cluster headache." In its chronic form, which affects approximately 10 to 15% of sufferers (Ekbom & Olivarius, 1971), the headaches continue to occur indefinitely, affording the patients few headache-free days. The IHS criteria for cluster headache are shown in Table 18.6 (HCCIHS, 1988).

The typical onset of cluster headache is in the third or fourth decade of life although cluster attacks have been reported from as early as 1 to 3 years to the late 60s (Lance, 1993). Unlike migraine, cluster is more prevalent in men; its gender ratio favors men by 5:1. The

---

TABLE 18.6
IHS Diagnostic Criteria for Cluster Headache

A. At least five attacks fulfilling B–D
B. Severe unilateral orbital, supraorbital, and/or temporal pain
    lasting 15 to 180 min untreated
C. Headache associated with at least one of the following signs that
    have to be present on the pain side:
    1. Conjunctival injection
    2. Lacrimation
    3. Nasal congestion
    4. Rhinorrhea
    5. Forehead and facial sweating
    6. Miosis
    7. Ptosis
    8. Eyelid edema
D. Frequency of attacks: from one every other day to eight per day
E. At least one of the following:
    History, physical, and neurological examinations not
        suggesting a secondary disorder
    History, physical, and/or neurological examinations suggesting
        such disorder, but ruled out by appropriate investigations
    Such disorder present, but cluster headache not occurring for
        the first time in close temporal relation to the disorder

---

etiology remains poorly understood. However, it has been proposed that vasomotor, hypothalamic, or neurohormonal disturbances may be involved (Moskowitz, 1984; Saper, 1983; Kudrow, 1983).

Unlike migraine, diet does not seem to precipitate cluster, although an occasional patient reports that chocolate can be a factor. The one exception, however, is the consumption of alcohol during cluster periods. Most, but not all, cluster patients are heavy smokers and drinkers. During remission periods when patients are not on preventive medications, alcohol appears to have no provoking effect.

TREATMENT

The preferred approach to the treatment of cluster headache patients is prophylactic. The tremendous pain and relatively short but frequent attacks makes symptomatic treatment less practical and often ineffective. Appropriate pharmacological prophylactic regimens can reduce the frequency and severity of attacks in most patients. When treating cluster patients, the benefits of therapy should be weighed against the hazards of taking medication. Patients should be monitored closely, because some of the medication prescribed in treatment can potentially cause problems. Ergotamine and DHE preparations, methysergide, calcium channel blockers, corticosteroids, and lithium are commonly used. Other agents, such as cyproheptadine, indomethacin, chlorpromazine, antidepressants, and ergonovine have been used with limited success.

For cluster patients, ergotamine tartrate is administered orally in divided doses throughout the day and often limits the severity and frequency of cluster attacks. The daily dose should be kept as low as possible (1 to 2 mg daily), and additional ergotamine for breakthrough headaches should not be permitted. Individual tolerance and sensitivity varies greatly, and patients should be followed closely for untoward reactions and complications.

Methysergide, an ergotamine derivative, may also be used to treat cluster headache patients. It is administered orally in divided doses not to exceed 8 mg/day. On initiation of therapy, some patients experience transient mental confusion, nausea, vomiting, muscle cramps or takes, and insomnia. If the symptoms persist for more than 3 days or the patient develops evidence of peripheral vasoconstriction, claudication, or angina, the medication should be stopped. Methysergide is contraindicated in patients who have peripheral vascular or cardiovascular disease, hypertension, active ulcer, cardiac vascular disease, and hepatic or renal dysfunction; or who are pregnant.

Corticosteroids, alone or in combination with methysergide, are frequently effective for difficult patients. Their mechanism of action is not completely understood, but it is thought to involve suppression of hormonal mechanisms. This treatment is more suited for patients with episodic cluster headache, because its long-term use could be hazardous. However, because of the extreme distress and suffering of some chronic cluster patients, corticosteroids can provide temporary relief whereas other drugs are being introduced.

Prednisone or triamcinolone are commonly prescribed, although others are effective. The steroids are given in divided doses that must be titrated to the individual. The average daily starting dose is 60 mg of prednisone or 16 mg of triamcinolone. The medication is then tapered over 2 to 4 weeks with adherence to usual steroid precautions. Side effects include fluid retention, weight gain, gastrointestinal disturbances, lethargy, and Cushing's syndrome. Contraindications are hypertension, diabetes, peptic ulcer disease, infection, active immunization, or pregnancy.

Calcium channel-blocking drugs have been helpful to many patients, especially those with the chronic form of cluster. It is believed that they alter smooth muscle tone of cerebral arteries by interfering with calcium ion function (Gallagher & Freitag, 1987a). Verapamil is generally well tolerated and more frequently utilized. It has been suggested as a first-line pharmacological treatment for the prevention of cluster headache, although weeks of therapy may be required before control of the condition is established (Saper, 2000, pp. 76–77). It is given in divided doses with an average daily dosage of 360 mg/day. The most frequent side effects with verapamil are constipation and fluid retention. Verapamil is contraindicated in hypotension, cardiac conduction disease, and significant renal or hepatic disease. Other calcium channel blockers sometimes used are nifedipine (40 to 280 mg/day) and nimodipine (30 to 60 mg/day).

Lithium carbonate is reported to be affected in reducing frequency and severity of attacks in the treatment of patients suffering with chronic form of cluster headache. Its mechanism of action has been debated, but it may involve its effect on cyclic changes in serotonin and histamine (Gallagher & Freitag, 1987a) or electrical conductivity in the central nervous system (Diamond & Dalessio, 1980). It is administered orally in divided doses with a daily dosage of 600 to 1200 mg. Serum lithium level monitoring is necessary to avoid toxicity. Effective therapeutic ranges vary greatly, but generally should not exceed 1.2 meq/l. Nonsteroidal anti-inflammatory drugs and thiazide derivatives should be used with caution; when used concomitantly, these agents raise the potential risks of toxicity. Side effects include fatigue, tremor, sleep disturbance, diarrhea, decreased thyroid function, goiter, and fluid retention. Lithium is contraindicated in the presence of significant renal or cardiovascular disease.

Abortive therapy for cluster patients is a limited effectiveness because of the relatively brief headaches and the time necessary for medication absorption. Few nonpharmacological measures are helpful to cluster patients. However, the complete abstinence from alcohol during cluster periods is imperative. Drinking alcohol, without question, interfere with prophylactic therapy. Reducing cigarette smoking and caffeine consumption (Gallagher & Freitag, 1987a), as well as avoidance of daytime napping (Stensrud & Sjaastad, 1980), may benefit some patients. The inhalation of oxygen during a cluster attack is a relatively safe and effective treatment. In the majority of sufferers, oxygen aborts attacks within 12 min (Kudrow, 1981). Oxygen is administered at a rate of 7 l/min by facial mask at the onset of attack continued for up to 15 min. The main drawback to the use of oxygen is cumbersome equipment, which makes it difficult to transport for patients whose attacks are unpredictable.

For patients who experienced longer headaches and those who are not sufficiently controlled by preventive medication, abortive medication may be needed. This is generally limited to ergotamine or analgesic/sedatives. Ergotamine and its derivatives can be administered early in a cluster attack, sublingually, intramuscularly, or by inhalation. This may give relief to some, whereas simply delaying the completion of the headache in others. The usual ergotamine limitations must be observed, which limit the amount that can be taken and the number of headaches that can be treated. Analgesics and sedatives are a limited help, but they aid certain patients psychologically and reduce the anxiety associated with cluster attacks. Unmonitored use of these medications should be avoided, because potential habituation or toxicity can develop.

MIXED HEADACHE SYNDROME

Most headache patients experience one or possibly two distinct headache types, with pain-free periods between attacks. However, there is a group of patients who experience intermittent migraine attacks superimposed on a daily or near daily, less intense headache similar to that of the tension type. This pattern is characteristic of the mixed headache syndrome. The mixed headache syndrome is one of the most difficult headache patients to manage.

The typical mixed headache patient, in many cases, has a long history of evaluations and failed therapeutic attempts. Their constant fear of the daily or near-daily headaches worsening sometimes leads to self-treatment and excessive medication use. The frequent use of any immediate-relief medication for head pain can cause rebound headache, which perpetuates the problem and often renders other treatments ineffective until all medications are stopped. Psychogenic factors, such as chronic stress, anxiety, burnout, or depression, are often present and further contribute to the ongoing problem.

The patient–doctor relationship is critical in the management of mixed headache patients. A definitive, comprehensive treatment plan that addresses each element of the patient's problem must be developed and supervised by a single physician. The patient must be educated as to the nature of his or her headaches and how each aspect of treatment is expected to contribute to the control of the headaches. Once a plan is begun, continuity of care with regular follow-up visits is vital.

The treatment of the mixed headache syndrome usually requires prophylactic medications in addition to non-pharmacological measures, such as diet, exercise, stress reduction, biofeedback, social adjustments, and counseling. Because these patients, in effect, experience coexisting tension-type and migraine headache, each individual component requires its own appropriate therapy. The management of tension-type and migraine headache has been described earlier in this chapter. Patients who do not respond to outpatient therapy or who are unable to withdraw from frequent analgesic or ergotamine use may benefit from hospitalization at dedicated in-patient, tertiary care facilities (Diamond, Freitag, & Maliszewski, 1986).

REFERENCES

Buchan, P. (1998). Pharmacokinetics of frovatriptan (VML 251/SB 209509) in male and female subjects. *Functional Neurology, 13,* BC3(abstr.), 177.

Diamond, S. (1997). Recommendations for primary care providers: Diagnosis and treatment of migraine. *Headache Quarterly, 8*(Suppl.), 6–14.

Diamond, S., & Dalessio, D. (1980). *Practicing physician's approach to headache* (2nd ed.). Baltimore: Williams & Wilkins.

Diamond, S., Freitag, F., & Maliszewski, M. (1986). In-patient treatment of headache: Long-term results. *Headache, 26,* 189–197.

Diamond, S., Nursal, A., Freitag, F.G., & Gallagher, R.M. (1989). The effects of weather on migraine frequency. *Headache, 29,* 322.

Diener, H.C., Pascual, J., & Vega, P. (2000). Comparison of rizatriptan 10 mg versus zolmitriptan 2.5 in migraine (Poster). *Headache Quarterly, 11,* 51–52.

Ekbom, K., & Olivarius, B. (1971). Chronic migrainous neuralgia: Diagnosis and therapeutic agents. *Headache, 11,* 97–101.

Ferrari, M.D. (1993). Biochemistry of tension-type headache. In J. Olesen & J. Schoenen (Eds.), *Tension-type headache: Classification, mechanisms, and treatment* (pp. 115–126). New York: Raven Press.

Freitag, F.G., Diamond, S., Diamond, M., Urban, G.J., & Pepper, B.J. (2000). The new treatments in migraine: First year clinical experience. *Headache Quarterly, 11,* 33–36.

Friedman, A.P., Finley, K.H., & Graham, J.R. (1962). Classification of headache. *Archives of Neurology, 6,* 173–176.

Gallagher, R.M. (1983). Ergotamine withdrawal causing rebound headache. *Journal American Osteopathic Association, 82*(9), 677.

Gallagher, R.M. (1986). Emergency treatment of intractable migraine headache. *Headache, 26,* 74–75.

Gallagher, R.M. (1996). Acute treatment of migraine with dihydroergotamine nasal spray. *Archives of Neurology, 53,* 1285–1291.

Gallagher, R.M., Dennish, G., Spierings, E.L.H., & Chitra, R. (2000). A comparative trial of zolmitriptan and sumatriptan for the acute oral treatment of migraine. *Headache, 40,* 119–128.

Gallagher, R.M., & Freitag, F. (1987a). Cluster headache: Diagnosis and treatment. *Journal of Osteopathic Medicine, 1,* 10–18.

Gallagher, R.M., & Freitag, F. (1987b). Muscle contraction headache: Diagnosis and treatment. *Journal of Osteopathic Medicine, 1*(6), 8–17.

Gallai, V., Sarchielli, P., Trequattrini, A., Paciaroni, M., Usai, F., & Palumbo, R. (1994). Neuropeptide Y in juvenile migraine and tension-type headache. *Headache, 34,* 35–40.

Goldstein, J. (1996). Current developments in 5-HT$_{1D}$ receptor agonists. *Headache Quarterly, 7*(Suppl. 2), 17–20.

Goldstein, J., Keywood, C., & Hutchison, J. (1999, June 22–26). *Low 24-hour recurrence during treatment with frovatriptan.* Poster session presented at 9th Congress of the International Headache Society, Barcelona, Spain.

Goldstein, J., Marek, J.G., & Winner, P. (1998). Comparison of butorphanol nasal spray and Fiorinal with codeine in the treatment of migraine. *Headache, 38,* 516–522.

Headache Classification Committee of the International Headache Society. (1988). Classification of the diagnostic criteria for headache disorders, cranial neuralgias, and facial pain. *Cephalalgia, 8*(Suppl. 7), 1–96.

Honkasalo, M L., Kaprio, J.A., Heikkilä, K., Sillanpää, M., & Koskenvuo, M. (1993). A population-based survey of headache and migraine in 22,809 adults. *Headache, 33,* 403–412.

Kruzs, J.C., & Scott, V. (1999). Topiramate in the treatment of chronic migraine and other headaches. *Headache, 39,* 363.

Kudrow, L. (1981). Response of cluster headache to oxygen inhalation. *Headache, 21,* 1–4.

Kudrow, L. (1983). Cluster headache. *Neurologic Clinic, 1,* 370.

Lance, J.W. (1993). Cluster headache. In J.W. Lance (Ed.), *Mechanisms and management of headache* (5th ed., pp. 163–187). Oxford: Butterworth Heinemann.

Laska, E.M., Sunshine, A., Mueller, F., et al. (1984). Caffeine as an analgesic adjuvant. *Journal of the American Medical Association, 251,* 1711–1718.

Lavados, P.M., & Tenhamm, E. (1997). Epidemiology of migraine headache in Santiago, Chile: A prevalence study. *Cephalalgia, 17,* 770–777.

Linet, M.S., & Stewart, W.F. (1987). The epidemiology of migraine headache. In J. N. Blau (Ed.), *Migraine: Clinical and research aspects* (pp. 451–477). Baltimore: The Johns Hopkins University Press.

Lipton, R.B., Hamelsky, S.W., Kolodner, K.B., et al. (2000). Migraine, quality of life, and depression: A population-based case-control study. *Neurology, 55,* 629–635.

Lipton, R.B., Stewart, W.F., Ryan, R.E., Saper, J., Silberstein, S., & Sheftell, F. (1998). Efficacy and safety of the nonprescription combination of acetaminophen, aspirin, and caffeine in alleviating headache pain of an acute migraine attack: Three double-blind, randomized, placebo-controlled trials. *Archives of Neurology, 55,* 210–217.

Lyons, A.S., & Petrucelli, R.J. (1978). *Medicine: An illustrated history.* New York: Harry N. Abrams.

Mathew, N.T., Reuveni, U., & Perez, F. (1987). Transformed or evolutive migraine. *Headache, 27,* 102–106.

Migliardi, J.R., Armellino, J.J., Friedman, M., Gillings, D.B., & Beaver, W.T. (1994). Caffeine as an analgesic adjuvant in tension headache. *Clinical Pharmacology and Therapeutics, 56,* 576–586.

Moskowitz, M. (1984). The neurobiology of vascular head pain. *Annals of Neurology, 16,* 157–168.

Nakano, T., Shimomura, T., Takahashi, K., & Ikawa, S. (1993). Platelet substance P and 5-hydroxytryptamine in migraine and tension-type headache. *Headache, 33,* 528–532.

National Headache Foundation (2000, October). *NHF headache facts.* http://www.headaches.org/factsheet.html

Newman, L.C. (2000, November 3). *Inpatient treatment strategies for intractable headache* [Abstract]. Scottsdale Headache Symposium, American Headache Society, Scottsdale, AZ.

Pascual, J., Falk, R.M., Piessens, F., Prusinski, A., Docekal, P., Robert, M., Ferrer, P., Luria, X., Segarra, R., & Zayas, J.M. (2000). Consistent efficacy and tolerability of oral almotriptan in the acute treatment of multiple migraine attacks: Results of a large, randomized, double-blind, placebo-controlled study. *Cephalalgia, 20*(6), 588–596.

Pradalier, A., Clapin, A., & Dry, J. (1988). Treatment review: Nonsteroidal anti-inflammatory drugs in treatment and long-term prevention of migraine attacks. *Headache, 28,* 550–557.

Pryse-Phillips, W. (1999, June 22–26). *A randomised, placebo-controlled study of eletriptan vs. sumatriptan for the treatment of acute migraine attack.* Poster session presented at 9th Congress of the International Headache Society, Barcelona, Spain.

Ramaswamy, S., & Bapna, J. S. (1987). Antagonism of morphine tolerance and dependence by metoclopramide. *Life Sciences, 40,* 807–810.

Rapoport, A., & Adelman, J. (1998). Cost of migraine management: A pharmacologic overview. *Americal Journal of Managed Care, 4*(4), 531–545.

Raskin, N.H. (1986). Repetitive intravenous dihydroergotamine as therapy for intractable migraine. *Neurology, 36,* 995–997.

Rasmussen, B.K., Jensen, R., Schroll, M., & Olesen, J. (1991). Epidemiology of headache in a general population — A prevalence study. *Journal of Clinical Epidemiology, 44,* 1147–1157.

Rolf, L.H., Wiele, G., & Brune, G.G. (1981). 5-Hydroxytryptamine in platelets of patients with muscle contraction headache. *Headache, 21,* 10–11.

Ryan, R.E. (1998). *Newer modalities for migraine.* Presentation to the Diamond Headache Clinic, Orlando, FL.

Saper, J. (1983). *Headache disorders: Current concepts and treatment strategies.* Boston: John Wright-PSG.

Saper, J. (2000, November 4). *Cluster headache* [Abstract]. Scottsdale Headache Symposium, American Headache Society, Scottsdale, AZ.

Schoenen, J. (1990). Tension-type headache: Pathophysiologic evidence for a disturbance of "limbic" pathways to the brain stem [Abstract]. *Headache, 30,* 314–315.

Shukla, R., Shanker, K., Nag, D., Verma, M., & Bhargava, K.P. (1987). Serotonin in tension headache. *Journal of Neurology, Neurosurgery, and Psychiatry, 50,* 1682–1684.

Stensrud, P., & Sjaastad, O. (1980). Comparative trial of tenormin (atenolol) and inderal (propanolol) in migraine. *Headache, 20,* 204.

Stevens, M.B. (1993). Tension-type headaches. *American Family Physician, 47,* 799–805.

Stewart, W.F., Lipton, R.B., Celentano, D.D., & Reed, M.L. (1992). Prevalence of migraine in the United States: Relation to age, income, race, and other sociodemographic factors. *Journal of the American Medical Association, 287,* 64–69.

Stewart, W.F., Lipton, R.B., Celentano, D.D., & Reed, M.L. (2000, February). *American Migraine Study II.* Paper presented at the Diamond Headache Clinic Research and Education Foundation, Palm Springs, CA.

Stewart, W.F., Schecter, A., & Lipton, R.B. (1994). Migraine heterogeneity: Disability, pain intensity, and attack frequency and duration. *Neurology, 44,* S24–S29.

Subcutaneous Sumatriptan Study Group. (1991). Treatment of migraine attacks with sumatriptan. *New England Journal of Medicine, 325,* 316–321.

Takeshima, T., Shimomura, T., & Takahashi, K. (1987). Platelet activation in muscle contraction headache and migraine. *Cephalalgia, 7,* 239–243.

Tekle Haimanot, R., Seraw, B., Forsgren, L., Ekborn, K., & Ekstedt, J. (1995). Migraine, chronic tension-type headache, and cluster headache in an Ethiopian rural community. *Cephalalgia, 15,* 482–488.

Terwindt, G.M., Ferrari, M.D., Tijhuis, M., et al. (2000). The impact of migraine on quality of life in the general population: The GEM study. *Neurology, 55,* 624–629.

Venzmer, G. (1972). *Five thousand years of medicine.* New York: Taplinger Publishing.

Whitty, C.M.W., Hockaday, J.M, & Whitty, M.M. (1966). The effect of oral contraceptives on migraine. *Lancet, 1,* 856.

Wilkinson, M. (1986). Clinical features of migraine. In P.J. Vinken, G.W. Bruyn, H.L. Klawans, & F.C. Rose (Eds.), *Headache* (Vol. 48, *Handbook of clinical neurology,* pp. 117–133). New York: Elsevier.

19

Muscular Parafunction of the Masticatory System: Headache, Face, Jaw, and Sinus Pain (Temporomandibular Disorders)

James P. Boyd, D.D.S.

Some of the most difficult diagnoses to make are those that are without objective signs, that is, conditions that present with subjective symptoms only. Some of the most common pain complaints: headache, face, jaw, and sinus pain, usually present with no objective signs, and treatment is based on the patient's subjective report. The diagnosis of parafunction of the masticatory musculature falls into this category (Figure 19.1).

Before parafunction of any muscle can be addressed, one must become familiarized with the function of that muscle. As with all skeletal muscles, the form of the muscle dictates its function, and the function of the muscle follows its form. This chapter specifically addresses only two of the muscles of mastication: the *temporalis* and the *lateral pterygoid*.

TEMPORALIS

The temporalis origin covers the entire side of the skull and resides within the temporal fossa. With the anterior portion of the temporal fossa being deepest, the anterior portion of the temporalis is thickest, and therefore the strongest portion of the muscle. With the insertion of this muscle as the coronoid process of the mandible, the sole function of the temporalis is to elevate the mandible. Anthropologically speaking, the temporalis functions closely with the canine teeth. Carnivores who typically have prominent canine teeth also have well-developed temporalis muscles. Following the opening of the mouth (to capture prey), the role of the temporalis is to forcibly attempt to elevate the mandible (close the mouth) through the objects that are engaged with the canine teeth. Conversely, the herbivores have much less developed *temporalis* muscles and canine teeth, instead having better well-developed masseters, which work together with flattened occlusal patterns of the teeth, to facilitate mastication.

LATERAL PTERYGOID

In 90° opposition to the orientation of the temporalis (i.e., the alignment is horizontal instead of vertical) is the lateral pterygoid muscle. The name is derived from its origin, which is the lateral side of the pterygoid (winglike) plate of the sphenoid bone (which houses the maxillary sinuses). The insertion (of its inferior belly) is at the neck of the condyle (the superior belly attaches to the articular disc, which rides on top of the condyle). During unilateral contraction, the lateral pterygoid pulls the condyle in the anterior-medial direction of its fibers (form dictates function), with the overall effect of the mandible shifting laterally. For example, when the right lateral pterygoid contracts, the mandible moves to the left, and vice versa. When both lateral pterygoids contract simultaneously, the mandible is advanced and the mouth opens as the condyles ride down the articular eminence of the temporal bone.

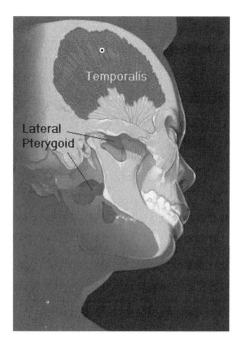

FIGURE 19.1   Masticatory musculature.

FUNCTION VS. PARAFUNCTION

In humans, these two pairs of muscles work together to bite and tear food, and to position the mandible while chewing. Once the jaws have come together and the teeth have occluded, the particular arrangement of the teeth is referred to as the *occlusion*, or occlusal scheme. It is important to make the distinction between the occlu*ding* of the teeth (a muscular act) and the scheme of occlu*sion* (the relationship of the teeth following their occluding). During mastication, there is no purpose in having the teeth in occlusion (food is supposed to be in between the upper and lower teeth) for anything more than a fraction of second. In fact, the instant the teeth occlude with each other, an opening stroke is initiated. Other than chewing and swallowing, *any muscular act that occludes the teeth (provided by the temporalis) is considered parafunctional.* Symptoms and signs that may develop depend on the intensity, frequency, and duration of the parafunctional muscular contraction.

ETIOLOGY

The field of dentistry has obviously been assigned to treat conditions of the masticatory system. Dentistry typically acknowledges that the activity synonymous with muscular parafunction is *bruxism*, which had traditionally been defined as "teeth grinding." However, although the current standard treatment for bruxism (an intraoral splint or "nightguard") may prevent against the signs of teeth grinding (worn and loose teeth), it may not be entirely effective at resolving the *symptoms*. The problem lies not in dentistry's

mistreatment, but in its misconception of the diagnosis and definition of bruxism. This lack of understanding of the true nature of bruxism has resulted in the current standard of care for chronic temporomandibular disorder (TMD): management of symptoms (McNeil, 1990; Okeson, 1989, p. 160). By using a traditional interocclusal splint, the practitioner has succumbed to the patient's intensity of occluding, which plays the largest etiologic role in his or her symptoms (regardless of the patient's occlusal scheme). Unfortunately, dentistry has stipulated that treatment with an interocclusal splint results in one of three scenarios: the patient may improve (the intensity of parafunction is disrupted and decreases), remain unchanged (intensity is unaffected), *or get worse.* (Clark & Solberg, 1987, p. 130; Dao, et al., 1994; Hansson, 1991) (muscle contraction activity intensifies). Without a full understanding of the nature of bruxism's destructive forces, the practitioner cannot inform the patient of the outcome potential when using a traditional interocclusal nightguard/splint (Figure 19.2).

One of the problems with treating muscular parafunction has been where to start. Due to the unpredictability of the outcome of a traditional intraoral splint (which is *intended* to reduce muscular parafunction, but may not), varying opinions of TMD treatment have developed within dentistry. Two basic philosophies have evolved: the patient's jaw orientation is inappropriate and therefore must be altered, or the patient's occlusal scheme is inappropriated and therefore must be altered. However, an individual with an ideal jaw relationship (the way the condyle of the mandible seats into the temporal fossa) and/or ideal occlusal scheme may suffer from chronic debilitating headaches and/or face and jaw pain (TMD), whereas another with a less-than-ideal jaw relationship and/or "improper" occlusal scheme may be completely asymptomatic. (Okeson, 1989, p. 160). When it comes to

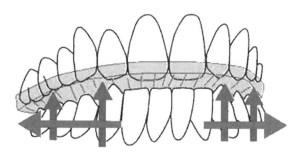

FIGURE 19.2   A flat and smooth surface reduces the efforts of the lateral pterygoids (green arrows). Eliminating the resistance of occluding cusps reduces the strain on the origins of the lateral pterygoid (the pterygoid plate of the sphenoid bone resulting in a reduction of facial symptoms) and insertions (the neck of the condyle resulting in a reduction of TMJ strain and symptoms). However, the same surface provides a more efficient resistance to the effort of the temporalis at clenching, therefore increasing the clenching intensity (red arrows).

TMD, etiologic research continues to show that, essentially, it does not matter what a person *has* or where it is (the occlusal scheme and jaw relationship) (Kahn, et al., 1999; McNamara, Seligman, & Okeson, 1995; Rodrigues-Garcia et al, 1998). What matters is what one *does* with what one has (the nature of the muscular activity—the occlu*ding*) (Israel, 1999; Ito, et al., 1986).

UNDERSTANDING BRUXISM

To gain an upper hand on bruxism, a new understanding of the term, and therefore the condition itself, is necessary. Bruxism is not a condition of the teeth. Teeth do not cause an activity, they are merely being affected by an activity. (Okeson, 1989, p. 160). Dentistry is essentially the art and science of how healthy teeth occlude with each other. Therefore, dentistry has been reflexively treating a condition by addressing the health of the teeth and their occlusal scheme. (Wilkinson, 1991). However, signs and symptoms of bruxism do not result simply from the creation of an occlusal scheme; they result from the intensity of the occluding of the teeth. The resulting scheme of occlusion may modify and direct the forces generated during the occlusion, but it may not alter the intensity of the occluding.

Bruxism is best described as a function of clenching. The intensity of clenching dictates the severity of grinding. There is no teeth grinding unless the jaws are first clenched together to some degree. The jaws must be clenched together intensely enough to provide adequate resistance to alternating lateral pterygoid activity, which then grinds the teeth in excursive movements. As the intensity of temporalis contraction (clenching) increases, resistance to lateral mandibular movement increases. The required increased efforts of the lateral pterygoids to translate the condyles (pull them down the articular eminence of the temporal bone) provide the strain on the temporomandibular joints (TMJs), which is a major source of joint pathology (Israel, 1999).

As the intensity of clenching approaches maximum, the lateral pterygoids ability to move the mandible laterally (i.e., translate the condyles) decreases or is prevented entirely. Ultimately, the most intense clenching would prevent any movement of the jaw or grinding of the teeth. Clenching in a centered position, with a balanced occlusal scheme, would provide the most stable and protected environment for the TMJs. With this observation, the appropriate definition of bruxism becomes apparent: "Jaw-clenching, with or without forcible excursive movements." The patient who presents with severely worn teeth, obviously a result of vigorous grinding, may have no symptoms to report because he or she never exerts adequate clenching intensity to become symptomatic (but enough to vigorously rub the teeth together). Another patient with no indication of occlusal wear, but who complains of severe headaches and neck pain and has no facial

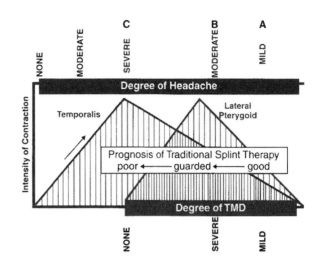

FIGURE 19.3 As temporalis contraction increases to maximum, lateral pterygoid ability to translate the condyle for potential joint strain is eliminated. As temporalis contraction intensity reduces, the opportunity for the lateral pterygoid to translate the condyle increases, thereby increasing signs and symptoms of TMD. A: In this example, minimal lateral pterygoid intensity produces mild TMD, and minimal temporalis intensity produces mild headache. Traditional splint therapy has a good prognosis. B: Intense lateral pterygoid contractions resulting from significant occlusal resistance, provided by moderate to severe temporalis intensity, allow for severe TMD. C: Intense temporalis clenching (nonexcursive) stabilizes the condyles, which presents with tension-type headache without typical signs or symptoms of TMD.

or TMD signs or symptoms, may be clenching intensely in centric position. Only by recognizing bruxism as a function of clenching can these patients be accurately diagnosed and treated (Figure 19.3).

In a study of chronic tension-type headache patients without signs or symptoms of TMD, clenching during sleep was shown to be, on average, 14 times more intense than in asymptomatic control subjects (Clark, 1997). Clenching in centric and balanced position maintains a stabilized TMJ environment. However, the typical patient with chronic TMD (headaches, face and jaw pain, tooth wear) forcibly grinds his or her teeth to an excursive position, and then clenches in that position ("grinding to a clench"), placing severe and often damaging strain on the TMJs (Hannam, 1991). If both lateral pterygoids were to maintain an isometric contraction during a centric clench, or even more significantly, with the jaw slightly advanced, a strain is placed on the pterygoid plates of the sphenoid bone (the origins of the lateral pterygoids), thereby generating sinus symptoms (in the absence of objective disease). There exists a dynamic relationship between the temporalis and lateral pterygoids, from which signs and/or symptoms may result. The intensity of the temporalis activity combined with the degree of lateral

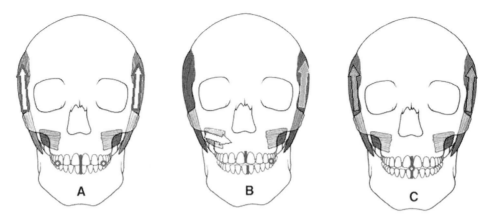

FIGURE 19.4 The relationship between occlusal scheme, joint strain, and muscle contraction intensity. A: Bilateral, posterior equal contact (red dots) allows for maximal clenching (and headache) without joint strain. B: A unilateral posterior contact (maintained by the same side temporalis) provides the opposite lateral pterygoid with resistance to its contraction in a medial direction, thereby straining the joint. Even with a well-adjusted splint, the contortion of the mandible in excursive movement can create this scenario. C: With anterior midline point contact, there is minimal temporalis contraction intensity. Resistance to lateral pterygoid contraction is minimal (therefore minimal contraction intensity) and in an anterior/superior direction, thereby seating the condyle into its optimal orientation.

pterygoid activity (if possible), dictates the presentation of headache, TMD, or tooth wear (Figure 19.4).

TREATING AND PREVENTING BRUXISM

Ultimately, to treat and prevent bruxism, clenching intensity must be suppressed. Unfortunately, the traditional interocclusal splint, while decreasing resistance to lateral movement (thereby relieving lateral pterygoid contraction and TMJ strain), provides ideal (or in some cases, enhanced) resistance to the temporalis, allowing clenching to persist or intensify (Clark, Beemserboer, & Rugh, 1981).

The success or failure of the traditional interocclusal splint is a function of the intensity of clenching. If clenching intensity persists or increases after using a splint, bruxism/TMD treatment becomes bruxism/TMD management. Therefore, to treat and prevent bruxism/TMD, clenching suppression must be addressed. This is achieved by exploiting the nociceptive trigeminal inhibition (NTI), reflex also known as the jaw-opening reflex (Okesan, 1989, p. 160; Stohler & Ash, 1986), and by creating an occlusal scheme for the least efficient muscular contraction (i.e., least intense). NTI is created by direct pressure stimulation of the mandibular incisor periodontal ligament (PDL), activating a reflex loop, which suppresses the contraction intensity of the temporalis (conversely, anesthetization of the mandibular incisor PDL allows clenching intensity to increase) (Hannam, 1991).

Historically, an anterior deprogrammer (such as a Lucia jig) or an anterior point stop (Clark, Beemsterboer, & Rugh, 1981) has been advocated to establish and record optimal condylar position (CR) and to suppress acute muscular symptoms on a short-term basis. These are effective for clenching suppression in a jaw-centered position, but

are contraindicated for therapeutic use because of the complications caused by excursive (protrusive, retrusive, lateral) movements of the mandible. During an excursive movement of the mandible, deprogramming jigs can allow a mandibular canine to contact the device, resulting in ipsilateral near-maximal clenching (Stohler & Ash, 1986) and joint strain. Protrusive movement of the mandible with the simple anterior point stop allows for occluding of the posterior teeth, again allowing for high-intensity clenching. All mandibular excursive positions, not just centric, must be considered when attempting to suppress temporalis clenching in a dynamic environment (Figure 19.5).

To accommodate for parafunctional, protrusive, and retrusive movements, an anterior midline point stop can be extended anteriorly and distally, providing clenching suppression in all mandibular movements (a prefabricated, retrofitted device is available commercially through NTI-TSS).* Used primarily during sleep, a modified anterior midline point stop (AMPS) reduces voluntary clenching intensity to one third of maximum (Becker, et al., 1999). A modified AMPS design allows for the best "musculoskeletally stable" (CR) position of the condyles, while suppressing hyperactive musculature. In addition, by providing for no unilateral canine or posterior contacts (as can happen with a full-coverage splint when the mandible contorts during excursive movement [Clark & Solberg, 1987, p. 130]), the modified AMPS allows for the least

Two misconceptions of a modified AMPS are not uncommon: posterior teeth may supraerupt, and mandibular

---

* *NTI Tension Suppression System. FDA marketing allowance, July 1998: "For the prevention of chronic tension and temporal mandibular joint syndrome that is caused by chronic clenching of the posterior mandibular and maxillary teeth by the temporalis muscle. The device is custom made for the individual." NTI-TSS, Inc., Mishawaka, IN.

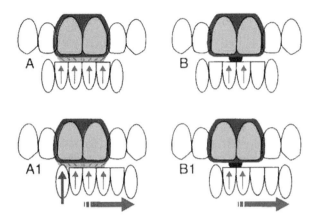

FIGURE 19.5 Both the anterior deprogrammer (A) and a modified AMPS (B) allow for minimal muscular contraction intensity and optimal seating of the condyle. An excursive movement (A1) allows an opposing canine to contact the deprogrammer, thereby providing an opportunity for intense temporalis contraction on the same side as the translated condyle, resulting in significant joint strain. The same excursive movement with a modified AMPS (B1) reduces the possibility of canine contact, thereby allowing the modified AMPS to be used therapeutically.

incisors may intrude. However, for a posterior tooth amount of potential joint strain in any excursive or protrusive movements, thereby allowing for optimal joint healing and remodeling (Schames, Boyd, Schames, & King, 2000).

To supraerupt, it must go unopposed without any contact for at least 8 days (Kinoshita, et al., 1982). With a modified AMPS in place, mastication is impossible because of the trauma experienced by the incisors opposing the device. Therefore, because an AMPS must be removed whenever the patient eats, the daily masticatory stimulation of the molars prevents their supraeruption (Kinoshita, et al., 1982).

As for incisor intrusion, there is no opportunity without a constant apical force, which is required to intrude teeth (clenching efforts last minutes, and are suppressed). Even in the case of a clinician's oversight, where the discluding element of the modified AMPS (which provides the point stop) is not perpendicular to the long axis of the mandibular incisor, the patient reports a tenderness to the tooth immediately after the first night of use. The patient resists wearing the device until the dentist addresses the problem, long before there is any orthodontic tipping movement.

Although the modified AMPS device itself does not cause any orthodontic movement, it does allow for optimal (re)positioning of the condyle, thereby potentially changing the occlusal scheme. By providing for the most musculoskeletally stable condylar position, a change in occlusal scheme is most noticeable in patients whose condyles seat more posteriorly and superiorly in the fossa

as symptoms resolve. For example, as chronic tension of the lateral pterygoids resolves, the condyles may seat more posteriorly and superiorly (a tensed lateral pterygoid may have maintained the condyles in a position anterior and inferior to the optimum). Therefore, the mandible may rotate at the last molars, with the anterior mandible rotating inferiorly and posteriorly, possibly resulting in a degree of anterior open bite (depending on the original degree of incisal overlap). After any repositioning of the condyles, some degree of occlusal equilibration or restoration may be necessary.

A modified AMPS requires less fabrication and adjustment time than the traditional methods of splint fabrication and delivery (which typically requires impressions, models, laboratory fees, and potential for several adjustment appointments). The commercially available prefabricated devices require one simple chairside procedure where the device can be retrofitted and delivered (in most cases by a supervised auxiliary) in a 20-min appointment and one follow-up appointment. Compared with the bulky and often irritating traditional splint and the unpredictable outcome, the relatively smaller size of a modified AMPS and secure fit make for excellent patient compliance. The clinical efficacy of a modified AMPS makes it a viable treatment alternative for the treatment and prevention of occlusal trauma, bruxism, and TMD.

REFERENCES

Becker, I., Tarantola, G., Zambrano, J., et al. (1999). Effect of a prefabricated anterior bite stop on electromyographic activity of masticatory muscles. *Journal of Prosthetic Dentistry, 82*(1), 22–26.

Clark, G.T. (1997). Waking and sleeping temporalis EMG levels in tension-type headache patients. *Journal of Orofacial Pain, 11*(4), 298–306.

Clark, G.T., Beemsterboer, P.L., & Rugh, J.D. (1981). Nocturnal masseter muscle activity and the symptoms of masticatory dysfunction. *Journal of Oral Rehabilitation, 8*(3), 279–286.

Clark, G.T., & Solberg, V.V.K. (1987). *Perspectives in temporomandibular disorders.* Chicago: Quintessence.

Dao, T.T., Lavigne, G.J., Charbonneau, A., et al. (1994). The efficacy of oral splints in the treatment of myofascial pain of the jaw muscles: A controlled clinical trial. *Pain, 56*(1), 85–94.

Hannam, A.G. (1991). Musculoskeletal biomechanics in the mandible. In C. McNeil (Ed.), *Current controversies in temporomandibular disorders* (pp. 72–80) Chicago: Quintessence.

Hansson, T.L. (1991). Orthopedic appliances. In C. McNeil (Ed.), *Current controversies in temporomandibular disorders* (pp. 159–161). Chicago: Quintessence.

Israel, H. (1999). The relationship between parafunctional masticatory activity and arthroscopically diagnosed temporomandibular joint pathology. *Journal of Oral Maxillofacial Surgery, 57*(9), 1034–1039.

Ito, T., Gibb, C.H., Marguelles-Bonnet, R., et al. (1986). Loading on the temporomandibular joints with five occlusal conditions. *Journal of Prosthetic Dentistry, 56*(4), 478–484.

Kahn, J., Tallents, R.H., Katzberg, R.W., et al. (1999). Prevalence of dental occlusal variables and intraarticular temporomandibular disorders: Molar relationship, lateral guidance, and nonworking side contacts. *Journal of Prosthetic Dentistry, 82*(4), 410–415.

Kinoshita, Y., Tonooka, K., Chiba, M., et al. (1982). The effect of hypofunction on the mechanical properties of the periodontium in the rat mandibular first molar. *Archives of Oral Biology, 27*(10), 881–885.

McNamara, J.A. Jr, Seligman, D.A., & Okeson, J.P. (1995). Occlusion, orthodontic treatment, and temporomandibular disorders: A review. *Journal of Orofacial Pain, 9*(1), 73–90.

McNeil, C. (1990). *Temporomandibular disorders: Guidelines for classification, assessment, and management.* Chicago: Quintessence.

Okeson, J.P. (1989). *Management of temporomandibular disorders and occlusion* (2nd ed.). St Louis: Mosby.

Rodrigues-Garcia, R.C., Sakai, S., Rugh, J.D., et al. (1998). Effects of major Class II occlusal corrections on temporomandibular signs and symptoms. *Journal of Orofacial Pain, 12*(3), 185–192.

Schames, J., Boyd, J., Schames, M., & King, E. (2000). Therapeutic motion of the joint. Manuscript submitted for publication.

Stohler, C.S., & Ash, M.M. (1986). Excitatory response of jaw elevators associated with sudden discomfort during chewing. *Journal of Oral Rehabilitation, 13*(3), 225–233.

Wilkinson, T.M. (1991). The lack of correlation between occlusal factors and TMD. In C. McNeil (Ed.), *Current controversies in temporomandibular disorders* (pp. 90–93). Chicago: Quintessence.

20

Complex Regional Pain Syndrome, Types I and II

Nelson H. Hendler, M.D., M.S.

CLINICAL SIGNS AND SYMPTOMS

Complex regional pain syndrome, type I (CRPS I) (formerly known as reflex sympathetic dystrophy [RSD]) and complex regional pain syndrome, type II (CRPS II) (formerly known as causalgia) are symptom complexes that evoke a great deal of confusion. Very often, physicians do not recognize that these are separate and distinct entities, and commonly assume that they are disorders of the same etiology, as well as responsive to the same treatment. Clinically, this has not proven accurate. CRPS, type I is a group of symptoms and clinical signs that usually follows a minor injury to a limb. In contradistinction, CRPS, type II is usually associated with peripheral nerve injury, classically from a bullet wound or some other partial nerve damage. Throughout this chapter, for the sake of consistency, earlier references that used the terms of reflex sympathetic dystrophy (RSD) are referenced or quoted as CRPS, type I, despite the original nomenclature. This same approach is used for references using the term causalgia, which are changed for the sake of continuity, to CRPS, type II. In a very fine review article, Payne (1986) clearly defined the distinction between CRPS, type I and CRPS, type II, although at the time he called them RSD and causalgia, respectively. This has been further expanded by the International Association for the Study of Pain in a supplement edited by Merskey (1986) (Table 20.1). A further expansion of this comparison is offered by Baron, Blumberg, and Janig (1996) (Table 20.1A).

Clinically, one can make the distinction between the two disorders on the basis of signs and symptoms. This is a more important set of criteria than results of laboratory tests or response to treatment, because test results for this disorder are highly variable, and the accuracy of diagnosis of this disorder is low. If a disorder is misdiagnosed, then how can a physician rely on the response to treatment as a way of establishing a diagnosis? However, sometimes physicians establish a diagnosis based on a response to treatment. This circular logic predicts that all disorders respond equally well to a given treatment, and those who do not are the fault of the patient. This ego-protective trap is a convenient one into which an unsuspecting physician might easily fall. However, there is valuable information that can be derived from a patient's response to treatment, from both a retrospective and a prospective research position. Obviously, the variables in clinical research are legion, and include the variable responses patients have to a single pathological etiology; the similar manifestations patients have to diseases of multiple etiologies; the variability of accurate diagnosis; the variability of the skill of the physician performing a procedure; and the variable response to a single, well-performed procedure. Without much trouble, five variables have already been mentioned, giving rise to a 5-factorial analysis, or 120 possible combinations of factors. Therefore, in analyzing the results of clinical research in humans, one has to be very circumspect. This is certainly true for CRPS, type I and CRPS, type II.

0-8493-0926-3/02/$0.00+$1.50
© 2002 by CRC Press LLC

TABLE 20.1
Comparison between CRPS Type I and Type II

	Complex Regional Pain Syndrome Type II (Causalgia)
Definition	Burning pain, allodynia, and hyperpathia, usually in the hand or foot, after a partial injury to a nerve or one of its major branches
Site	In the region of the limb innervated by the damaged nerve, not around the entire limb
Main features	Onset usually immediately after partial nerve injury or, may be delayed for months; CRPS, type II of the radial nerve very rare; the nerves most commonly involved are the median, the sciatic and tibial, and the ulnar; spontaneous pain; pain described as constant, burning, exacerbated by light touch, stress, temperature change or movement of involved limb, visual and auditory stimuli (e.g., a sudden sound or bright light, emotional disturbances)
Associated symptoms	Atrophy of skin appendages, secondary atrophic changes in bones, joints and muscles
	Cool, reddish, clammy skin with excessive sweating; sensory and motor loss in structure innervated by damaged portion of nerve
Signs	Cool, reddish, clammy, sweaty skin with atrophy of skin appendages and deep structures in painful area
Laboratory findings	Galvanic skin responses and plethysmography revealing signs of sympathetic nervous system hyperactivity, roentgenograms possibly showing atrophy of bone
Usual course	If untreated, the majority of patients having symptoms that persist indefinitely; spontaneous remission occurring
Relief	In early stages of CRPS, type II (first few months) sympathetic blockade plus vigorous physical therapy usually providing transient relief; repeated blocks usually leading to long-term relief; when a series of sympathetic blocks not providing long-term relief, sympathectomy indicated; long-term persistence of symptoms reducing the likelihood of successful therapy
Social and physical disabilities	Disuse atrophy of involved limb; complete disruption of normal daily activities by severe pain; risk of suicide, drug abuse if untreated
Pathology	Partial injury to major peripheral nerve; actual cause of pain unknown; peripheral central and sympathetic mechanisms involved in an unexplained way
Essential features	Burning pain and cutaneous hypersensitivity with signs of sympathetic hyperactivity in portion of limb innervated by partially injured nerve
	Complex Regional Pain Syndrome Type I (Reflex Sympathetic Dystrophy)
Definition	Continuous pain in a portion of an extremity after trauma that may include fracture but does not involve a major nerve, associated with sympathetic hyperactivity
Site	Usually the distal extremity adjacent to a traumatized area; all around the limb
System	Peripheral nervous system; possibly the central nervous system
Main features	The pain follows trauma (usually mild), not associated with significant nerve injury; the pain described as burning, continuous, exacerbated by movement, cutaneous stimulation, or stress; onset usually weeks after injury

TABLE 20.1 (CONTINUED)
Comparison between CRPS Type I and Type II

Associated symptoms	Initially there is vasodilatation with increasing temperature, hyperhidrosis, edema, and reduced sympathetic activity also occurring; atrophy of skin, vasoconstriction and appendages, cool, red, clammy skin variably present; disuse atrophy of deep structures possibly progressing to Sudeck's atrophy of bone; aggravated by use of body part, relieved by immobilization; sometimes follows a herniated intervertebral disc, spinal anesthesia, poliomyelitis, severe iliofemoral thrombosis or cardiac infarction; may appear as the shoulder–hand syndrome; later vasospastic symptoms becoming prominent with persistent coldness of the affected extremity, pallor or cyanosis, Raynaud's phenomenon, atrophy of the skin and nails, and loss of hair, atrophy of soft tissues and stiffness of joints; without therapy these symptoms possibly persisting; not necessary for one patient to exhibit all symptoms together; an additional limb or limbs possibly affected as well
Signs	Variable; may be florid sympathetic hyperactivity
Laboratory findings	In advanced cases, X-rays possibly showing atrophy of bone, and bone scan changes over time
Usual course	Persists indefinitely if untreated; small incidence of spontaneous remission
Relief	Sympathetic block and physical therapy; sympathectomy if long-term results not achieved with repeated blocks; may respond in early phases to high doses of corticosteroids (e.g., Prednisone, 50 mg daily)
Complications	Disuse atrophy of involved limb; suicide and drug abuse if untreated; sometimes spreads to countralateral limb
Social and physical disabilities	Depression, inability to perform daily activities

	CRPS I	CRPS II
Pathology	Unknown	Partial nerve lesion
Essential features	Burning pain in distal extremity usually after minor injury without nerve damage	Nerve damage
Differential diagnosis	Unrecognized local pathology (fracture, strain, sprain)	Posttraumatic vasospasm, nerve entrapment syndromes radiculopathies, or thrombosis

TABLE 20.1A
Criteria for Differential Diagnosis of Complex Regional Pain Syndromes (CRPS) Types I and II

	CRPS I	CRPS II
Etiology	Any kind of lesion	Partial nerve lesion
Localization	Distal part of extremity, or entire limb; independent from site of lesion	Any peripheral site of body; mostly confined to territory of affected nerve
Spreading of symptoms	Obligatory	Rare
Spontaneous pain	Common, mostly deep and superficial orthostatic component	Obligatory, predominately superficial, no orthostatic component
Mechanical allodynia	Most of patients with spreading tendency	Obligatory in nerve territory
Autonomic symptoms	Distally generalized with spreading tendency	Related to nerve lesion
Motor symptoms	Distally generalized	Related to nerve lesion
Sensory symptoms	Distally generalized	Related to nerve lesion

Note: From Merskey, H. (Ed.). (1986). *Pain,* 3 Suppl., pp. 28–29. Reprinted with permission.

COMPLEX REGIONAL PAIN SYNDROME TYPE I (CRPS I) (REFLEX SYMPATHETIC DYSTROPHY)

Following the distinction drawn by Payne (1986), one considers CRPS, type I as the result of minor trauma; inflammation following surgery, infection, or lacerations resulting in some degree of swelling in the affected limb; infarctions; degenerative joint disease; frostbite; and burns. One should add to this list the possibility of any compression, such as casting or swelling due to injury, that may cause prolonged pressure on peripheral nerves. As an example of this, we have seen at least two or three cases per year of CRPS, type I brought about from arthroscopy. The probable etiology is not injury to the nerve from the use of the arthroscope, but instead from using the tourniquet for a long period of time to create a bloodless operating field. A differential diagnosis between nerve entrapments and CRPS I is critical and based on the distribution of the pain, which follows nerve pathways for nerve entrapments, and is circumferencial for CRPS I.

According to Schwartzman and McKellan (1987), there seem to be three phases to CRPS, type I. Additionally, physicians should recognize that CRPS, type I is a symptom complex that is a cluster of symptoms and signs, and that patients do not present with all signs and symptoms during the course of their disease. In fact, very often they may have only one or two of the signs and symptoms of the disorder.

As described by Payne (1986) and by Schwartzman and McKellan (1987), the acute stage of CRPS, type I is characterized by spontaneous pain, usually aching or burning, that follows the distribution of blood vessels or peripheral nerves. The acute stage may manifest as "hyperpathia" (this is described as a painful syndrome of overreaction to a stimulus or after-sensation following a stimulus) and may include hypesthesia or hyperesthesia (described as a decreased or an increased sensation to pain stimulation, respectively), or dysesthesia (described as an unpleasant abnormal sensation). Associated with these tactile sensations are usually a warm, dry, red skin, or cold, blue, sweaty skin, with some swelling; and, surprisingly, increased hair and nail growth. A number of authors have interjected the notion of allodynia, or a painful response to a normally nonpainful stimulus. (Chaplan, Bach, Pogrel, Chung, & Yaksh, 1994; Kim & Chung, 1995; Lee, Kayer, Desmeules, & Guilbaud, 1994). Additionally, the patient has dependent redness and reduced motion in the damaged extremity. This summarizes the acute stage of this disorder, which may last several weeks, and may begin immediately or several days after the onset of the injury. However, it is possible for CRPS I to remain in this stage, and never progress to stage II or stage III. This is a highly individualized response.

The second stage of CRPS, type I, which usually begins about 3 to 6 months after the injury, is called the dystrophic stage by Payne (1986). During this stage, the patient experiences a burning type of pain, which radiates either above or below the site of the injury, and increased hypersensitivity or hyperalgesia (an exquisite sensitivity to touch or temperature—in counterdistinction to allodynia, a painful response to a normally nonpainful stimulus—a most important distinction that is discussed later in the chapter). The patient has changes in the nails on occasion, as well as decreased hair growth. This seems to be a variable finding, and certainly is not a *sine qua non* of the diagnosis of CRPS, type I. Joints may become stiff, with decreased range of motion, and possible thickening, associated with some degree of muscle wasting. Edema may be present, as well as bullous skin lesions, that are not related to an autoimmune disease (Baron, et al., 1996). Osteoporosis may be noted, with proper testing (Payne, 1986). Movement disorders may begin at this stage, with either dystonias, or contractures noted (Schwartzman & Kerrigan, 1990; Webster, Schwartzman, Jacoby, Knobler, & Uitto, 1991). Symptoms may vary, and fluctuate from individual to individual.

The third stage described by Payne is the atropic stage, which usually occurs 6 months or longer after the injury. According to Payne, the patient experiences pain, decreased skin temperature, trophic changes in the skin associated with a smooth glossy skin, stiff fixed joints associated with contractures, increased or decreased sweating in the affected extremity, and demineralization of the bone associated with wasted muscles and reduced strength (Payne, 1986). Again, the progression to this stage is highly variable, and may progress, in a rapidly fulminating case, in less than 2 to 3 months. As always, in medicine, there are only guidelines, but no hard and fast rules. (A summary of many of the clinical symptoms is shown later in Table 20.2.)

COMPLEX REGIONAL PAIN SYNDROME, TYPE II (CRPS, TYPE II)(CAUSALGIA)

CRPS type II, is usually associated with peripheral nerve injury and severe pain. According to Payne (1986), pain occurring in CRPS, type II follows an injury to a nerve trunk, usually a major proximal nerve branch, and is described as a persistent burning pain, but does not necessarily have to be burning in quality. It is unrelated to associated damage from surrounding tissue, and seems to be worsened by emotional or environmental stimuli. Most importantly, the pain seems to persist more than 5 to 6 weeks, which seems to be the length of time needed for surrounding tissue to recover from injury. Typically, the injury is due to damage by a bullet, a knife, sharpened rocks or parts propelled by a

TABLE 20.2
Clinical Symptoms Associated with CRPS, Type II and CRPS, Type I

Clinical Symptoms	Mechanism	Diagnostic Studies	Treatment
CRPS, Type II			
a. Burning pain[a,b]	a. Unmyelinated C fibers[c]	a. Rarely have cold hyperalgesia (2/7) or heat hyperalgesia (0/9)[b]; do have mechanical hypersensitivity[b]; use a drop of acetone and Von Frey hairs to test	a. Phenoxybenzamine DREZ[a] sympathectomy 12% to 97% effective[a], clonazepam[e], gabapentin[f]
b. Paroxysms of pain[a]	b. Nerve stretch and axon disruption[a]	b. Clinical reports	b. None
c. Partial motor paralysis (70%)[d]	c. Peripheral nerve injury, proximal nerve trunk[a,b]	c. EMG/nerve conduction velocity studies	c. No relief with sympathetic blocks[b]; no success with beta-blockers[d]
d. Worse with stress[a]	d. Lots of theory, no proof	d. Clinical reports	d. Clonidine
e. Vasomotor changes, but rare trophic change[d]	e. Unknown	e. Clinical observation	e. Sympathetic blocks
CRPS, Type I			
Hyperalgesia and Allodynia			
a. Mechanical-hypersensitivity to light touch[c]	a. Ectopic alpha-adrenergic chemosensitivity[g]; sensitization of WDR neurons in the spinal cord[i]; central nervous system mediated[k]; intact low-threshold mechanoreceptor with A-delta afferents[c]	a. All patients have mechanical hypersensitivity use Von Frey hairs to test[b]	a. Sympathectomy possibly relieving it[c] sympathectomy not relieving it[j]; low-dose naltrexone possibly working[l] nifedipine[m]? gabapentin[f]?
b. Thermal-hypersensitivity	b. No mechanism delineated	b. Patients having either cold either heat or cold[b,c,k] hyperalgesia (3/4), and/or heat hyperalgesia (4/5); use a drop of acetone to test[b]	b. 6/6 receiving relief with sympathetic blocks or sympahtectomy[b], nifedipine?
Dystrophy Phase			
a. Osteoporosis[n]	a. No mechanism delineated	a & b. X-ray did not correlate well with clinical symptoms, but bone scan did[r] (abnormal flow images, 83% abnormal static images)[r] (also true for clinical features c. and e.[a]); if clinically had CRPS, Type I, 22/23 had positive delay image bone scan[s]	a. & b. Maybe calcitonin[n,o,p]
b. Diffuse or patchy, bony[n,o,p] demineralization[r]	b. No mechanism delineated	b. X-ray and bone scan[s]	b. Calcitonin[n,o,p,r]
c. Molted skin[a,b,r]	c. No mechanism delineated	c. Themography[t,u]	c. Prednisone 60 to 80 mg, tapering[r]
d. Hair loss[b,n]	d. No mechanism delineated	d. Clinical observation[r]	d. Steroids[n,r]
e. Vasomotor instability[r]	e. No mechanism delineated	e. History or longitudinal observation[r]	e. Sympathetic blocks,[n] steroids[r]
f. Nail brittleness[a,n]	f. No mechanism delineated	f. Clinical observation	f. Sympathetic blocks,[n] steroids[r]
g. Muscle spasm[n,v,w]	g. No mechanism delineated	g. EMG biofeedback used as test[u]	g. Trigger point injections[a] baclofen[l]

continued

TABLE 20.2 (CONTINUED)
Clinical Symptoms Associated with CRPS, Type II and CRPS, Type I

Clinical Symptoms	Mechanism	Diagnostic Studies	Treatment
h. Contractures[a,n]	h. May be attributed to disuse, may be central dystonia[x]	h. Longitudinal observation[n]	h. Physical therapy[n] sympathectomy
i. Contralateral involvement[n,w]	i. Cross-communication between sympathetic chain in 80% of cadavers[w]	i. Effective countralateral block[w]	i. Contralateral sympathectomy[w]
j. Edema[a,n]	j. No mechanism delineated[y]	j. History and clinical observation	j. Nifedipine,[m] spironolactone, acetazolamide, epidural, spinal cord stimulation[aa]
k. Lower skin temperature[u]	k. Not vasospasm, but maybe an afferent and efferent reflex arc[bb]	k. Thermography[t,u]	k. Phentolamine,[a,b,t,u] Bier block with reserpine[bb] guanethidine i.v.,[n] sympathetic blocks[b,n]
l. Joint stiffness[a,s] and tenderness[r]	l. No mechanism delineated	l. Proximal interphalangeal joint 12.9 mm greater (average) n affected hand; negative rheumatoid and connective tissue blood studies[r]	l. Maybe calcitonin[p]
m. Pathological fractures	m. May be related to osteoporosis or patchy demineralization	m. 72 hours after a break 95% of bone scans are positive[cc]	m. Maybe calcitonin,[n,o] maybe Fosamax
n. Pins and needles[u] and dysesthesias[a]	n. No mechanism delineated	n. History	n. Sympathectomy[u]
o. Skin lesions[q,y,z,dd]	o. Disruption of basement membrane and destruction of colagenous anchoring fibrils,[y] circulating immune complexes[q]	o. Observation and electron microscopy[y]	o. Prednisone not working,[y] maybe tetracycline[y]
p. Dystonia[x,z] myoclonus[z]	p. Spinal cord mediated?	p. Observation	p. Epidural bupivicaine, epidural baclofen, epidural clonidine, sympathetic blocks[ee]

[a] Payne (1986); [b] Raja, et al. (1996); [c] Ochoa, et al. (1985); [d] Ghostine, et al. (1984); [e] Bouckoms & Litman (1985); [f] Mellick and Mellick (1995); [g] Devor (1983); [h] Allen & Morety (1982); [i] Roberts (1986); [j] Hoffert, et al. (1984); [k] Meyer, et al. (1985); [l] Gillman & Lichtigfeld (1985); [m] Prough, et al. (1985); [n] Schott (1986); [o] Gobelet, Waldburger, & Meier (1992); [p] Webster, Iozza, Schwartzman, Tahmoush, Knobler, & Jacoby (1993); [q] Van der Laan, Veldman, & Goris, (1998); [r] Kozin, et al. (1981); [s] Holder & MacKinnon (1984); [t] Uematsu, et al. (1981); [u] Hendler, et al. (1982); [v] Long (1982); [w] Kleinman (1954); [x] Schwartzman & Kerrigan (1990); [y] Baron, et al. (1996); [z] Greipp & Thomas (1994); [aa] Peuschl, et al. (1991); [bb] Janoff, et al. (1985); [cc] Matin (1979); [dd] Hamamcu, Dursun, Ural, & Cakci (1996); [ee] Webster, et al. (1991).

machine, or other such objects. When the injury is associated with a high-velocity missile, one must consider not only actual damage to the tissue itself, but also hydrostatic effects caused by shock waves. When one takes into account the fact that the body is made up largely of water, it is easy to see how a high-velocity missile can cause damage not only to the actual tissue that has been penetrated by the missile but also to surrounding tissue as a result of hydrostatically transmitted shock waves. If the reader desires additional information concerning the hydrostatic effects of high-velocity missiles, he or she is referred to a most amazing book titled *Split Seconds* (Dalton, 1984). Photographs in the book

clearly illustrate the hydraulic effect in soft tissue caused by a bullet.

Typically, patients with CRPS, type II report an onset of pain within several hours to a week after the injury, and describe the pain using words such as stinging, aching, burning, or tingling. Superimposed on the regular pain, patients may experience paroxysms of deep pain (Payne, 1986).

Long (1982) clearly made the distinction between CRPS, type II and CRPS, type I. CRPS, type II is secondary to partial injury to major mixed nerves, caused by low- or high-velocity missiles; and manifests as trophic changes in the distribution of the nerve associated with extreme hypersensitivity. The pain is diffuse and burning, and true CRPS, type II almost always responds to sympathectomy. Long suggested performing three or more sympathetic blocks, sometimes every day for up to a week or longer, with the expectation that longer relief should follow each subsequent block. With positive responses to sympathetic blocks, Long would suggest a sympathectomy; on the other hand, CRPS, type I usually follows a minor injury and does not involve a major nerve root. Frequently, the site of injury is the knee, ankles, or wrist; and the pain seems to get worse with cold but not with emotional upset, unlike CRPS, type II. Demineralization of the bone occurs, with fibrosis of tendons and sheaths and spasm of the muscle. Dysesthesia suggests that there will be less success with sympathectomy.

SYMPATHETICALLY MAINTAINED PAIN

This term has come into use in an effort to further define diagnostic accuracy, which would then allow better selection of treatment methods, and have some predictive value in terms of outcome. Raja and Hendler (1990) report clinical features of sympathetically maintained pain to be (1) spontaneous pain, (2) hyperalgesia to both mechanical and cooling stimuli, (3) soft tissue swelling, (4) vasomotor disturbances, (5) trophic skin changes, (6) diminished motor function, and (7) pain relief after sympathetic blockade. By using these criteria, one can have sympathetically maintained pain that could have features of either CRPS, type I or CRPS, type II because either of these conditions could have features of sympathetically maintained pain.

Hendler (1982) originally described the use of oral phentolamine to treat CRPS, type I using the rationale that this drug was a postsynaptic alpha-1-blocker. Raja and his co-workers (1991) later described the use of intravenous phentolamine as a diagnostic test to confirm whether or not the pain a patient had was sympathetic in origin, that is, "sympathetically maintained." There is evidence that the mechanism of sympathetically maintained pain is present not only in CRPS, type I but also in some cases of CRPS, type II, however, because various authors have reported the benefit of sympathetic blocks in both disorders (Long, 1982; Ghostine, et al., 1984; Hannington-Kiff, 1979). Perhaps the best conceptual framework to use is one that takes into account both neurophysiologically (i.e., the presence or absence of major peripheral nerve injury documented by electromyography [EMG], nerve conduction velocities [NCV] studies, and the somatosensory-evoked potential [SSEP]) and response to pharmacological intervention (i.e., response to IV phentolamine testing, or sympathetic blocks). A physician might consider six separate types of disorders, as shown in Table 20.3.

USING THE CLINICAL HISTORY AND SENSORY EXAMINATION FOR DIFFERENTIAL DIAGNOSIS

A number of authors have advanced the notion that there are other types of sensory mechanism, other than hyperalgesia evident in CRPS I and II (Chaplan, et al., 1994; Kim & Chung, 1995; Lee, et al., 1994; Lee & Yatsh, 1996). Unfortunately, the vast majority of the research reports are in animal models, using animals fairly low on the philogenetic scale. There is always a danger in extrapolating from animal models to clinical work in humans, because there are species-specific differences, and some of the sensory values assigned to a rat reveal more about the creativity of the researcher than they do about the sensory experience of the rat. However, bearing these caveats in mind, clinicians should be aware of the research observations that may have significant value for their patients. A sensation called allodynia has been described, which is a painful response to a *normally nonpainful* stimulus. It is important to make a distinction between this sensation and hyperalgesia, which is a more intense response to a *normally painful* stimulus. This distinction bears reemphasis, for this is the most commonly confused terminology in the hands of inexperienced clinicians. Clinically, hyperalgesia, a more intense response to a *normally painful* stimulus, is seen in the early phases of nerve entrapments, and radiculopathies. In counterdistinction, allodynia, a painful response to a *normally nonpainful* stimulus, is seen in CRPS, types I and II.

Also, it is important to make a distinction between cold hyperalgesia, heat hyperalgesia, and mechanical hyperalgesia. Both cold and heat hyperalgesia are rarely seen in CRPS II (Meyer, Campbell, & Raja, 1985; Raja, et al., 1986). Moreover, it is important to make a distinction between cold allodynia, and mechanical allodynia. Cold thermal allodynia is most often seen in CRPS, types I and II, whereas mechanical allodynia is seen commonly in CRPS, types I and II; nerve entrapment syndromes; and radiculopathies (Hendler & Raja, 1994). This clinical distinction has led to the use of the Hendler alcohol drop and swipe test to make a distinction between CRPS, types I and II, with cold allodynia (which has a painful response to an alcohol dropped on an affected limb [allodynia]); and CRPS, types I and II, nerve entrapment syndromes, and radiculopathies, with mechanical allodynia, demonstrated by lightly stroking the affected limb with the used swab (Hendler, 1995). Concisely stated, mechanical allodynia is of less use diagnostically, because it may be present in CRPS, types I and II, nerve entrapment syndromes, and radiculopathies; whereas thermal allodynia is a more useful clinical feature, usually being limited mostly to CRPS, type I and occasionally to CRPS II (Meyer et al, 1985; Raja, et al., 1986).

TABLE 20.3
Diagnostic Considerations

Response to IV	Positive Response to Phentolamine IV	No Response to Phentolamine IV	Partial Response to Phentolamine IV
EMG/nerve conduction velocity/somatosensory-evoked potential: all negative	CRPS, type I sympathetically maintained pain (SMP)	Microvascular damage with swelling and mechanical hyperalgesia; sympathetically independent pain (SIP)	Mixed injury
EMG/nerve conduction velocity/somatosensory-evoked potential: at least one positive	CRPS, type II	Neuroma or nerve entrapment at site of injury; SIP	Mixed injury
Positive response to alcohol drop test	CRPS, type I, SMP	Too low a dose phentolamine	Too low a dose phentolamine
Positive response nerve to a local nerve block (radial, ulnar, median, peroneal, saphenous, tibial) with 100% relief of all symptoms	Nerve entrapment syndrome with sympathetic component	Nerve entrapment syndrome without any sympathetic component	Nerve entrapment syndrome with sympathetic component
Positive response to sympathetic block or (a warm limb and 100% relief of all symptoms)	CRPS, type I, SMP	Too low a dose of phentolamine, or too slow an infusion	Too low a dose of phentolamine; too slow an infusion
Partial relief of pain with local nerve block	Mixed injury	Poor nerve block	Mixed injury

Additionally, a cool limb is not diagnostic of CRPS I and II, despite many reports in the literature to that effect (Hannngton-Kiff, 1979; Prough, et al., 1985). First and foremost, for a clinician to hold an affected limb in one hand, and a normal limb in another, and pronounce that the temperatures are either equal or different is a demonstration of arrogance, more than clinical skills. The ability to detect temperature differences varies due to the ambient temperature of the clinical setting, and the "physiological zero" of the organism sensing the temperature change, which lowers the "threshold of detection for thermal sensation of the opposite quality" (Geldard, 1962, p. 137). In an extensive report, by Uematsu, Hendler, Hungerford, Ono, and Long (1981), reviewing 803 cases at Johns Hopkins Hospital, the authors found that (as expected) patients with CRPS I and II had cold limbs most of the time, with ranges of 0.5°C to more than 3.0°C coldness being reported for over 79% of the cases diagnosed with CRPS I. However, in 89% of the cases in which there were abnormal EMG or nerve conduction velocity studies, the affected limb was also cold, although not to the same severity as the patients with CRPS I. These figures included cases of CRPS II, as well as patients with radiculopathies, and nerve entrapment syndromes.

The anatomic distribution of the pain is another important feature to consider. Sympathetic fibers travel with the sensory nerves, so an injured sensory nerve may have a component of sympathetic damage reported, such as coldness, or hyperalgesia. However, the actual location of the pain is a critical factor. If the pain is in the distribution of a peripheral nerve, even if all the sensations for CRPS, type I are present, then the clinical syndrome is really a nerve entrapment, with the sympathetic sensory components of it coming from the sympathetic fibers traveling with the sensory nerve. CRPS, type I has a circumfrencial pain distribution (i.e., it is all around the limb, in the pattern of the blood flow, not in a discrete nerve distribution or in a radicular distribution). Failure to recognize this distinction has lead to the misdiagnosis of a number of nerve entrapment syndromes, which get mistakenly called CPRS, type I (Hendler & Kozikowsku, 1993; Hendler, Bergson, & Morrison, 1996). In an article in preparation, Hendler and colleagues will report that 70% of the patients sent to Mensana Clinic with the diagnosis of CRPS, type I actually have nerve entrapment syndromes.

TREATMENTS

Appropriate treatments for CRPS, type I and type II have been described in Consensus Report, sponsored by the International Association for the Study of Pain (IASP) (Stanton-Hicks, et al., 1998). In this report, the participants emphasized the need for functional restoration, and psychological counseling, as well as medical intervention. Not only is there disuse as the result of a painful limb, creating multiple disabilities and atrophy but there is also evidence that once the disorder of CRPS, type I spreads, that there may be a centrally mediated muscle disorder, resembling dystonia (Schwartzman & Kerrigan, 1990). Therefore, the problem of a painful limb in CRPS, type I and type II is compounded by a real motor disorder.

The psychological problems associated with both CRPS, type I and type II have been well described for chronic pain patients in general. Hendler (1982, 1984) has long reported that patients with both chronic pain and depression really have become depressed as the result of their chronic pain. The earlier psychiatric "wisdom" of feeling that depression manifests as chronic pain has not been supported by more care observations (Hendler & Talo, 1989). Therefore, the use of group therapy seems to be the most efficient and productive way of providing support for patients with all types of chronic pain problems, and certainly is applicable to patients with CRPS, type I and type II (Hendler, Vierstein, Shallenberger, & Long, 1981). Family counseling and patient education is also of great use, when available.

The pharmacological management of CRPS, type I and type II is complicated (Hendler, 2000). The treatments shown in Table 20.2 are meant to deal with the specific symptoms associated with CRPS, type I and type II. However, there is a role for a more generalized pharmacological approach, especially dealing with the issue of depression and pain relief. Antidepressants, in and of themselves, provide relief of many of the symptoms by (1) reducing depression, (2) reducing anxiety, and (3) promoting natural sleep; and actually have some limited pain-relieving properties (Max, et al., 1991; Watson, et al., 1991; Watson, et al., 1981). For symptomatic relief in CRPS, type I and type II, narcotics are problematic. A number of authors have reported reduced efficacy, or variable effects, of narcotics in the palliative treatment of pain in patients with CRPS, type I and type II (Arner & Meyerson, 1988; Lee, Chaplan, & Yaksh, 1995; Portenoy, Foley, & Inturrisi, 1990). The variability and usual lack of efficacy of narcotics for CRPS, type I and type II may be explained by recent elegant research, which shows only a kappa-2 opioid agonist blocks the pain of hyperalgesia and allodynia, seen with peripheral neuritis and neuropathy, by inhibiting the activity of the N-methyl-D-aspartate (NMDA) receptor in the spine (Eliav, Herzberg, & Caudle, 1999). Although this research is in animals, with all the attendant problems of translating to human use, this avenue seems to hold a great deal of promise, because the formulation of a kappa-2 opioid agonist is a feasible endeavor for major drug companies. However, as of the date of writing this material, there is no practical kappa-2 agonist available for human use; thus the use of narcotics in CRPS, type I and type II for allodynia and hyperalgesia is of limited usefulness. Opioids may help pain caused by other symptoms of CRPS, type I and type II, such as muscle spasm and pathological fractures. A review of other pharmacological approaches for the management of pain can be found in several chapters by the author (Hendler, 1997, 2000).

Sympathetic blocks have always been the mainstay of diagnosis and treatment. The important feature of these blocks is to be certain of the efficacy of the block, before interpreting the result. The clinical criterion that best correlates with an efficacious block is the report of total limb warming. This tells the clinician that the sympathetic block did what it was supposed to do (i.e., blocked the sympathetic input to a limb, thereby producing warming of the limb). At this point, the next question to ask the patient is, "What do you feel?" If the patient has a warm limb, and 100% total absolute relief of all pain, then one may consider that the block was (1) effective and (2) appropriate for pain relief. From this, a clinician may conclude that the pain is sympathetic in origin. If, however, the block did not warm the limb, then the clinician must conclude that the block was not effective; and no information of any value can be determined from this type of block, except that another block, at a later date, is needed. If the block produces a warm limb, but only partial relief of the symptoms, then the question is, "Where do you still have pain?" If the remaining pain is reported in a nerve distribution, then the patient has both CRPS, type I and a nerve entrapment syndrome, which coexist, or a nerve entrapment syndrome, with a sympathetic component. If the limb is warm, and the patient has no relief, then the chances are the patient has a pure nerve entrapment syndrome (see Table 20.3).

After a clinician determines a block is effective, then the patient should have a series of six to ten blocks. After this series of blocks, several results are possible: (1) the CRPS, type I or II may go away, (2) the CRPS, type I or II may temporarily go away for weeks or months, only to return; or (3) the CRPS, type I or II may temporarily go away for hours or days, after the blocks, only to return. If scenario (1) occurs, the diagnostic blocks have also provided the cure. If scenario (2) or (3) occurs, then the patient is a candidate for sympathectomy. This author favors the surgical sympathectomy, because direct visualization of the sympathetic chain, and pathology reports on the tissue are more reassuring than a blind ablation techniques. Moreover, the author has seen disastrous results in patients, in which phenol was used for a neuroablative procedure. Despite the obvious benefit of direct visualization for sympathectomy, there are still some physicians, mostly anesthesiologists, who continue to use blind chemoablative techniques, with neurolytic agents, such as phenol, or radiofrequency lesions (Stanton-Hicks, et al., 1998).

In extreme cases, the use of epidural stimulation has been reported efficacious, although there are only a small number of cases in the literature (Barolat, Schwartzman, & Woo, 1989; Peuschl, Blumber, & Lucking, 1991; Robaina, Dominguez, & Diaz, 1989). The epidural infusion of SNX-111 has been suggested as a possible treatment for CRPS, type I or II, as has the infusion of baclofen. SNX-111 is a conotoxin that works on specific calcium channels to block the message of pain, whereas baclofen is a gabaminergic muscle relaxer. Epidural opioid infusion has been reported (Broseta, Roldan, & Gonzales-Darder, 1982), but the absence of a kappa-2 agonist may have reduced the potential results (Eliav, et al., 1999). Clonidine actually seems more effective than morphine in humans, for deafferentation pain, after spinal cord injury (Hassenbusch, Stanton-Hicks, & Covington, 1995). Other researchers have explained this difference, based on the independence of the opioid and noradrenergic pathways of the spinal cord (Glynn, Dawson, & Sanders, 1988). Opioid receptors exist in only a small group of neurons in the dorsal horn, and have various subsets, of which only the kappa-2 subset seems to be effective in reducing the allodynia of CRPS, type I (Eliav, et al., 1999). On the other hand, clonidine has multiple sites of action, such as inhibiting pain transmission in the dorsal horn of the spinal cord, and inhibiting norepinephrine release, due to its alpha-2 partial agonist effect, which inhibits the release of norepinephrine.

THEORY

With the clinical descriptions from Table 20.3 in mind, one can then make an effort to define the various anatomic, neuroanatomic, and physiological bases for these two disorders. Ghostine and colleagues (1984) have suggested multiple etiologies for CRPS, type II. Various considerations include ephapse, in which there seems to be an erosion of the insulation between nerve fibers, allowing for short-circuiting between somatic afferent fibers and sympathetic efferent fibers; and experimentally produced neuromas, with resultant ephapses occurring both acutely and chronically between myelinated fibers. Because of the delay in developing the ephapses, which does not correspond to the clinical observations of a relatively rapid onset of CRPS, type I and type II, however, the theory of ephapses as the etiology of CRPS, type II has fallen from favor. To replace this theory, the concept of nerve sprouts or free nerve endings that are sparsely myelinated seems feasible. Axonal sprouting has been noted to occur early after an injury, with a high frequency and without total axonal disruption. The possibility that causalgia is produced by these sparsely myelinated fibers is supported by evidence that the blood–nerve barrier, which is similar to the blood–brain barrier, has been destroyed in the injured nerve.

Perhaps the most comprehensive review of the neurophysiological basis of CRPS, type I and type II has been advanced by Roberts (1986). In his extensive review article, Roberts dealt with the neural mechanisms associated with pain of CRPS, types II and I. He called these disorders SMP. His hypothesis concerning SMP is based on two assumptions: "(1) that a high rate of firing in spinal wide dynamic range (WDR) or multireceptive neurons results in painful sensation and (2) that a nociceptor response is associated with trauma which can produce long-term sensitization of the WDR neurons." Furthermore, his theory postulates that SMP is mediated by low-threshold, myelinated mechanoreceptors, and that these impulses, which carry messages to the brain, are the result of sympathetic fibers carrying messages from the spine and brain to act on the receptors, or to act on the fibers carrying messages to the brain. The most important part of this hypothesis is the fact that Roberts does not postulate the need for nerve injury or for dystrophic tissue. Before one can more fully appreciate Roberts' theories, however, one has to explore the basic anatomy of the sympathetic chains.

Bennett (1991) at the National Institute of Health has advanced a brilliant theory that integrates clinical observations with basic neurophysiology. Bennett synthesizes three theories that show that damaged nerves, when they regenerate, have sprouts that are sensitive to norepinephrine; they will discharge on exposure to norepinephrine; there is enough norepinephrine produced by sympathetic fibers to trigger firing of damaged nerves; damaged nerves actually produce norepinephrine receptors at the damaged end; and nociceptors (pain receptors) in intact nerves fire more in response to norepinephrine. "All of these mechanisms may be operating in the case of patient nerve damage due to physical trauma," he says; and "these events are likely to sensitize surviving afferent terminals, perhaps to the point of inducing an ongoing discharge …". Bennett further differentiates between the type of injury: constriction or entrapment vs. partial destruction of a major peripheral nerve. The former injury (constriction) does not seem to respond to sympathetic blocks 1 to 2 weeks after the injury, and this is attributed to the loss of noradrenergic vasomotor innervation, which takes several weeks to develop. The latter injury (partial nerve destruction) becomes painful within hours of the injury, remains painful for months, and responds to sympathetic blocks even months after the injury. Other researchers have expanded on a purely neuron-mediated mechanism, and have suggested that autoimmune factors may be involved. The Schwartzman group, at Thomas Jefferson University School of Medicine, Philadelphia, found inflammatory skin lesions in the late stages of CRPS, type I, and attribute these lesions to a deposition of immune complexes in the skin. They believe the skin lesion supports the concept that cytokines and lymphokines such as interleukin-2 (IL-2) are produced as the result of the activation of complement; this in turn is excited by the progression of events beginning with local injury causing nerve growth factor release, thus activating sympathetic neurons and causing recruitment of neutrophils and monocytes, which in turn activate complement (Webster, et al, 1991). Interestingly, IL-2 has been found to selectively stimulate sympathetic neurons, whereas nerve growth factor (NGF) is produced in high concentrations after injury, which stimulates inflammation and in turn activates complement. Knobler (1996) has expanded on this, and advanced the notion of aberrant immunologic mechanism, as a cause for CRPS, type I. He traces trauma, as the cause for the release of NGF, which then stimulates inflammation and activates the complement components of the immune response, "promoting the expansion of antibody-producing B cells of the immune system." He reports that substance P and the lymphokine IL-2 are released in response to NGF, with both of these factors acting on the sympathetic nerves to activate it. As research progresses, the various factors described earlier need to be explored, with rigorous controls for (1) the type of lesion (crush vs. cut), (2) the stage of the disease, correlating with anatomic and neurohumoral changes over time, and (3) the attempt to correlate the clinical symptoms with response to various treatments.

In a discovery that led to her Nobel Prize, Rita Levi-Montalcini described the effect of NGF on sympathetic nerve (Levi-Montalcini, Skaper, Toso, Petrelli, & Leon 1996). In response to an injury or lack of innervation, the end organ, sensory receptor, releases NGF, which chemotaxically stimulates a nerve to grow toward the newly denervated receptor. This chemotaxic agent was found to be NGF. Clearly, sympathetic ganglion grow profusely in response to the addition of NGF to their growth medium. This is not limited to just sympathetic nerves. Skin and sensory nerves also have sprouted after injury (Inball, Rousso, Ashur, Wall, & Devor, 1987).

A study by Ro, Chen, Tang, & Jacobs (1999) shows that this process can be reversed, in rats, by the administration of anti-nerve growth factor antibodies. Previous work shows that anti-NGF antibodies prevented collateral sprouting of dorsal root ganglion in rats (Mearow & Kril, 1995). Ro and others (1999) studied the specific sensory response to anti-NGF, which showed that, in a dosage and time-dependent fashion, heat and cold hyperalgesia can be reduced, as well as collateral sprouting.

Finally, one of the most seminal concepts to emerge from animals studies is the idea of plasticity of the central nervous system (i.e., its ability to change in response to stimuli). Nowhere is this more important than for the understanding of CRPS, types I and II. In response to a chronically painful stimulus, the cells of the dorsal horn of the spinal cord actually alter their cytoarchitecture (the structure of the chemistry of the cell). Hyperalgesia and allodynia are largely created by the enhancement of NMDA receptor activity in the spinal cord, and treated by blocking the NMDA receptor (Ren & Dubner, 1993). The central role of NMDA receptor activity in the creation of allodynia must be emphasized. Unfortunately, there is not a practical way to modify the NMDA receptor in man, so the treatment of hyperalgesia and allodynia

remains elusive. Therefore, mechanisms other than NMDA inhibition need to be explored.

To briefly summarize the material presented earlier, three sensations are associated with CRPS, types I and II: (1) pain, which is a sensation usually experienced when tissue damage occurs; (2) hyperalgesia, which is an increased response to a normally painful stimulus; and (3) allodynia, which is a painful response to a normally nonpainful stimulus. This can be hot, cold, mechanical, or even chemical. The message of pain is initiated at two receptor sites: (1) a nosioceptor, which is usually a free nerve ending, or unmyelinated C fiber, which detects tissue damage such as temperature or chemical changes; (2) a mechanoreceptor, which is sensitive to pressure, like a Pachinian corpusle. When tissue is damaged, it produces a primary hyperalgesia, which is a sensitivity to pain, at the site of the pain; and a secondary hyperalgesia, surrounding the zone of primary hyperalgesia, in the absence of tissue damage. A sensitized nosioceptor has a lower threshold to pain, and produces hyperalgesia, whereas a sensitized mechanoreceptor transmits a message of pain, to a normally nonpainful stimulus (i.e., allodynia). Both hyperalgesia, and allodynia are the result of spinal dorsal horn body sensitization. The afferent fibers carry the sensory message to the brain, and the efferent fibers modify the sensory input from the brain back to the periphery. They have their origins in the brain stem, medulla, and periaquaductal gray; and are called descending afferent pathways. These pathways modify sensation. At the spinal cord level, increased sensory input from the peripheral nosioceptor actually changes cell functioning in the spinal cord, by altering chemical mediators, and receptor activity. The persistent sensory stimuli activates NMDA at certain cells of the dorsal horn of the spinal cord, called WDR neurons or NS. Phosphorylation of the NMDA receptor is the result of constant sensory input, which then activates the NMDA receptor, and this creates central sensitization of the receptor ion channel. Mg^{2+} is removed, so Ca^{2+} enters the channel, which causes cell sensitization. This spinal cord change produces allodynia in the peripheral nerves. Therefore, tissue damage produces damage to the nosioceptor in the periphery, causing sensitization, or hyperalgesia; and the result of this chronic increase in activity at the spinal cord level produces central sensitization. Likewise, damage to the nerve causes growth hormone to produce nerve sprouts; these are very sensitive, which cause continued input the spinal cord, producing central sensitization. This increased sensory input, which produces central sensitization, actually changes the cells in the dorsal horn of the spinal cord, which results in allodynia. The damaged nerve produces sprouts, as the result of NGF stimulation. These sprouts have alpha-2 adreno-receptors on them, which are sensitive to norepinephrine circulating in the bloodstream.

GROSS ANATOMY

The most startling finding, and one that flies in the face of commonly held beliefs, is a report by Kleinman (1954) in which sympathetic chains were found to have communication between them, in up to 80% of cases. This is an important finding, because this anatomic consideration is rarely, if ever, discussed in surgical textbooks or clinical papers. This finding also explains why some cases of CRPS, type I do not respond to sympathetic denervation, and why, paradoxical as it may seem, some cases do respond to countralateral blocks (i.e., if a patient has pain in the left leg, blocking the right lumbar sympathetic chain may produce relief).

Additional anatomy has been described by Allen and Morety (1982). When one traces the pathway of the sympathetic nerves, cell bodies are located in the lateral columns of the cervical, thoracic, and lumbar spinal cord. Cell bodies then give off axons, which form the preganglionic fibers of the sympathetic nervous system. From C7 to L2, these fibers are associated with the anterior spinal nerve roots, and leave the spinal cord in this pathway. They then separate from the nerve root and become the white rami communicantes, which then continue on to the paravertebral ganglia, forming a chain running from the skull to the coccyx. From the ganglia themselves postganglionic fibers run back to nerve roots, or become separate nerves supplying various organs.

It is important to note that some ganglion cells are found in the anterior roots, as well as the white and gray rami. By the same token, some pre- and post-ganglionic fibers do not pass through sympathetic trunks, which again indicates that there is residual sympathetic innervation due to either normal variants or aberrant fibers that bypass the sympathetic trunk. This anatomic finding explains the failure of some ganglionectomies, and suggests that one might need to do anterior nerve root sections and preganglionic rami sectioning (Smithwick procedure) in patients in whom ganglionectomy has failed.

Cervical outflow, coming from the upper portion of the cervical chain, sends fibers to the pupils and the eyelids. These fibers radiate from the upper stellate ganglion, which also supplies various fibers in the head and face. The upper thoracic sympathetic chain receives preganglionic input from upper thoracic roots, and supplies the upper extremity through postganglionic fibers that pass through the brachial plexus. The lower extremities receive input from the T11 to L3 nerve roots, forming ganglia; and from the lower two lumbar and upper sacral nerve roots, with gray rami (postganglionic) to the lumbosacral plexus.

MICROANATOMY

As described earlier in the gross anatomy portion, there are various sites along the sympathetic chain where

damage can occur to a nerve. Additionally, there are several sites where chemical intervention is possible, notably at the synapses that occur along the sympathetic pathways. Additionally, the various fibers that carry sympathetic messages are important. It has been widely held that C fibers, which are small unmyelinated fibers carrying sensory messages, are responsible for the transmission of pain. Some theories consider that SMP is mediated by activity in A fibers, however, because C-fiber blockade fails to eliminate pain in patients with SMP (Roberts, 1986). Therefore, one must start at the very beginning of the onset of pain (i.e., the receptor itself) to fully understand SMP and CRPS, types I and II. Originally, it was thought that nociceptor afferents (nerves that carry the message of pain from the periphery to the cord and the brain) were responsible for the continuous pain of SMP and CRPS, type I and CRPS, type II (Bonica, 1970; Devo & Janig, 1981; Roberts, 1986). In Roberts' (1986) article, however, he adheres to a theory first advanced by Loh and Nathan (1978) that indicates low-threshold mechanoreceptors are responsible for SMP. Roberts takes this position because nociceptor afferents, which are typically considered unmyelinated C fibers, do not have appropriate responses to sympathetic activity; therefore, both practically and conceptually cannot be included as the receptors that mediate SMP. Roberts (1986) reported that mechanoreceptors do respond appropriately to both touch and sympathetic activity, however. For CRPS, type II, others have proposed a neuroma formation as the cause of pain. Roberts believes that the sympathetic action of a neuroma is not capable of explaining why treatments that occur distal to the injury (in the form of either a nerve block or guanethidine infusion) are able to ameliorate CRPS, type II, however; even so, Roberts (1986) used the summation theory, or convergence theory, to say that both the peripheral receptors (in this case, mechanoreceptors) that arise in the neuroma and those that arise in the skin itself are transmitting painful messages to the cord, and that distal blocks eliminate only the mechanoreceptors from the skin, which is not enough to trigger responses in the WDR neurons in the spinal cord. Additionally, the concept of a neuroma causing prolongation of CRPS, type II-type pain does not fit the clinical observation that SMP may occur even in cases in which the nerve is not injured.

Ochoa, et al. (1985) advanced the theory that mechanical A-delta nociceptor endings become sensitized to multiple sensory inputs. This gives rise to the thermal hyperalgesia that is seen in CRPS, type I. On the other hand, Ochoa believes that there are abnormalities in distal nociceptor fibers that seem to have a low threshold. These low-threshold mechanoreceptors reside within large myelinated fibers, and are nonsympathetic dependent, because they transfer their information to nociceptor pathways proximal to the site of injury. These fibers may account for the mechanical hyperalgesia, manifesting as sensitivity to light touch. The previously mentioned receptors, which are the source of the hyperalgesia seen in CRPS, type I, are different than the burning pain receptors seen in CRPS, type II. Ochoa and colleagues (1985) believe that the burning pain of CRPS, type II is mediated by unmyelinated C fibers, whereas Payne (1986) believes that this pain is due to nerve stretch and axon disruptions. Another consideration is the fact that such pain may be mediated by nerve fascicles where all three types of C fibers exit (Ochoa, et al., 1985). Therefore, in summary, the current thinking seems to suggest that sparsely myelinated C fibers carry the message of burning pain found in CRPS, type II, whereas sparsely myelinated afferent fibers or the A-delta nociceptors may be responsible for pain in CRPS, type I.

SYNAPSES

Both synaptic considerations and axonal considerations have been raised as possible factors controlling both CRPS, types I and II. Ephapses, or artificial synapses, have been demonstrated in normal peripheral nerves. The concept of synaptic factors in CRPS, types I and II pain was first advanced by Granit, Leksell, & Skoglund (1944) when they found that stimulating the motor root of a damaged mixed motor sensory nerve also produced recordable electrical events in the sensory root. According to the review by Payne (1986), the formation of ephapses after nerve injury may allow a short circuiting or shunting of current from sympathetic fibers coming from the cord to the peripheral nerve into somatic fibers arising at the site of injury, carrying the message of pain back to the cord. Unfortunately, these cross-connections between fibers coming from the cord to the periphery, and conversely coming from the periphery to the cord, have been demonstrated in animal models, but not in humans (Payne 1986). Another consideration is the possibility of an ectopic impulse resulting from alterations in calcium, sodium, and potassium channels (Payne, 1986). In effect, the damaged nerve becomes "epileptic," and the spontaneous discharges from the sensory nerve may give rise to the episodic pain noted in some individuals. This could be due to lowered threshold or heightened mechanical sensitivity.

Neurosynaptic mediation of CRPS, types II and I, holds great promise for the future. When reviewing the synapses that are present within the sympathetic chain, it is apparent that these provide a potential site of mediation for sensory input. To understand synaptic mediation, one must review the anatomy of a synapse per se. By borrowing heavily from Roberts (1986), one can define the functional neuroanatomy, and delineate the location of various synapses. First, the trauma occurs, with receptors in the skin detecting various components of the trauma. Initially,

the C-fiber nociceptors carry the message to the dorsal root ganglion, and then back to the spinal cord neuron, where they synapse. After synapsing with the neuron in the spinal cord, these multiple neurons transmit information to the WDR neurons, which then send messages, via their axons, to the central nervous system or higher levels of the spinal cord. With use of Roberts' model, additional light touch activates the mechanoreceptors, which travel in the A fibers instead of the C fibers. Because the WDR neurons are already sensitized by the C fibers nociceptors, they respond to what is usually subthreshold stimuli to the A fiber mechanoreceptors. These mechanoreceptors travel in the A fiber, reaching a neuron within the spinal cord, which again impinges on the WDR neuron; this, in turn, again sends messages up the spinal cord to the brain. Sympathetic fibers exist within the lateral portions of the thoracic cord, sending efferent messages to the sensory receptor. These efferent messages (i.e., messages traveling from the cord to the periphery, mainly to the sensory receptors) may occur in the absence of cutaneous stimulation. According to Roberts' theory, however, the sympathetic efferent activity requires no cutaneous stimulation, and is the cause of the SMP. In response to this efferent activity, the WDR neurons fire, again sending messages to the spinal cord and brain. The key to Roberts' theory is the fact that the WDR neurons in the spinal cord remain sensitized, and they give a vigorous response to mechanical stimulation of A-fiber mechanoreceptors even after healing has occurred. In this schema, multiple synapses occur within the spinal cord, at the WDR neuron, and in the sympathetic ganglion. Therefore, synaptic regulation can occur at the spinal cord level or at the sympathetic ganglion level. When reviewing the actual synapse, one must conceptualize a presynaptic area wherein various chemicals are formulated, becoming neurosynaptic transmitters. The two synaptic transmitters that are of most interest to the study of CRPS, types I and II are the indolamines, of which serotonin is an example; and the catecholamines, of which norepinephrine, epinephrine, dopa, and dopamine are examples. In the presynaptic area of the nerve, precursor substances are manufactured into neurosynaptic transmitters, which confer a degree of specificity on nerve transmission. L-Tryptophan becomes 5-hydroxytryptophan, which becomes 5-hydroxytryptamine (serotonin); dopa becomes dopamine, which can be converted to norepinephrine and epinephrine.

The specific type of the neurosynaptic transmitter determines whether it will occupy a specific postsynaptic receptor site. Biogenic amines, such as the indolamines and catecholamines, are constantly being formulated and broken down by monoamine oxidase (MAO). Thus, chemically, the presynaptic area may be described as an area of high flux, with formulation and degradation of the same chemical occurring in the relatively steady state. As electrical impulses travel down the axon, pore diameter changes, altering the permeability of the membrane and causing the release of neurosynaptic transmitters. These synaptic transmitters flow across a minute gap between nerves and occupy postsynaptic receptor sites. The gap, of course, is called the synapse. The postsynaptic receptor sites determine the strength and duration of the electrical impulse that the synapse propagates. This is done by the degree of specificity that the neurosynaptic transmitters have for a particular receptor site. It also depends on the affinity that a specific neurosynaptic transmitter has for a particular receptor site, and whether it is easily displaced or forms a tight bond. Almost all neurosynaptic transmitters have their activity ended by presynaptic reuptake; that is, the chemical that occupies the postsynaptic receptor site is then taken back into the presynaptic area. Acetylcholine is an exception, being degraded on the postsynaptic receptor site by acetylcholinesterase. Additionally, some small amount of degradation of biogenic amines occurs in the synapse itself by catechol-O-methyltransferase (COMT). It is thought that less than 5% of the chemical degradation of synaptic transmitters occurs in the synapse by COMT, and 95% of the degradation occurs presynaptically, by MAO. Of course, there is constant rebuilding of the neurosynaptic transmitter presynaptically, creating the steady state mentioned earlier.

Obviously, there are multiple ways to modify the synapse. One can inhibit MAO, thereby enhancing the buildup of a monoamine neurosynaptic transmitter, such as the indolamines or the catecholamines. In fact, a class of drugs called MAO inhibitors do exactly that. By the same token, certain drugs can function as MAO exciters, which facilitate the degradation of biogenic amine neurosynaptic transmitters, such as the indolamines (serotonin) and the catecholamines (epinephrine, norepinephrine, dopamine, and dopa). Because the majority of the neurosynaptic transmitters have their activity ended by presynaptic reuptake, one can enhance the synaptic transmission by blocking presynaptic reuptake. This is how tricyclic antidepressants work. Conversely, one can diminish synaptic transmission by facilitation of presynaptic reuptake. Finally, one can work at the receptor end by using drugs that mimic the action of the presynaptic transmitters and occupy receptor sites, thereby triggering them as if the actual chemical had been released. By the same token, other drugs can be used that occupy the receptor sites but have no pharmacological activity other than to inhibit the presynaptic transmitter from occupying the receptor site. For example, curate effects a total blockade of the acetylcholine receptor. In this sense, these drugs become inhibitors of neurosynaptic transmission. Receptor sites are found not only postsynaptically but also presynaptically, very often for the same presynaptic neurosynaptic transmitter. As the number and sensitivity of these receptors change, so does the response to the neurosynaptic transmitter itself.

DIAGNOSIS OF COMPLEX REGIONAL PAIN SYNDROME, TYPE II

With the foregoing theoretical information, the clinical components of CRPS, types I and II should be more readily differentiated by appropriate diagnostic studies. According to both Raja, et al. (1986) and Payne (1986), CRPS, type II manifests as a burning pain, which is not a consistent finding of CRPS, type I. Additionally, CRPS, type II patients may experience paroxysms of pain, especially after stress, whether it be emotional or environmental. In an elegant study, Raja, et al. (1986) found that patients with CRPS, type II rarely have cold hyperalgesia (two of nine), and they do not have heat hyperalgesia (none of nine). Additionally, these patients obtain no relief from sympathetic blocks. Raja, et al. (1986) differentiated various types of hyperalgesia using sensory testing with either Von Frey hairs for touch, a drop of acetone for cold, or laser thermal stimulation for heat. Ochoa, et al. (1985) believe that CRPS, type II is not always sympathetically mediated, and instead is mediated by unmyelinated C fibers. Stretch injuries to the nerve or axon disruption of a major nerve branch is one explanation favored by Payne (1986). Usually, the CRPS, type II patient has a history of a nerve injury to a peripheral nerve, or surgery, that has damaged the proximal portion of the nerve trunk (Payne, 1986; Raja, et al., 1986). The CRPS, type II may be related to damage of nerve fascicles where all three types of C fibers exist (Ochoa, et al., 1985).

TREATMENT OF COMPLEX REGIONAL PAIN SYNDROME, TYPE II

Various authors have reported that sympathetic blocks are or are not effective, with efficacy for sympathectomy being reported to be between 12 and 97% (Payne, 1986). No relief with sympathetic blocks was reported by Raja, et al. (1986; 1991). Payne has suggested that a dorsal root entry zone (DREZ) procedure may prove effective. Ghostine, et al. (1984) have suggested the use of phenoxybenzamine. They reported 40 consecutive cases of CRPS, type II, all of which involved nerve injuries from bullet or shrapnel wounds. The Ghostine group noted partial motor paralysis in the distribution of the damaged nerve in 70% of the cases. Over time these deficits resolved in many of the cases, however. They also noted vasomotor changes, usually severe vasodilatation and sweating and less often vasoconstriction (Dalton, 1984). Rarely were trophic changes noted. The majority of the cases involved the sciatic nerve, median nerve, brachial Plexus, cauda equina, and occipital nerve, in descending order. The treatment that Ghostine, et al. (1984) used was phenoxybenzamine, which is a postsynaptic alpha-1-blocker and a presynaptic alpha-2-blocker. As mentioned earlier under the etiology of CRPS, type II, nerve sprouts, which are one of the theoretical origins of this disorder, seem to be highly excitable on the administration of norepinephrine; these can be reversed with alpha-blocking agents such as phentolamine but which are unaffected by beta-blocking agents. The dosage of the drug used by Ghostine, et al. initially was 10 mg three times a day, although this varied from patient to patient. Eventually maximum dosages of 40 to 120 mg/day were reached, with treatment lasting 6 to 8 weeks. Common side effects were orthostatic hypotension in about 45% of the patients and reduced ejaculatory ability in about 8% of the patients. In some instances, treatment lasted as long as 16 weeks. It is important to note that the patients were all treated within 2 to 70 days after the onset of their injury, however.

For this treatment to be effective, it is most important that rapid diagnosis and institution of treatment occur. Another possibility for the pharmacological treatment of CRPS, type II would be the use of clonazepam, which has been reported by Bouckoms and Litman (1985) to be effective for "burning" pains.

Surgical sympathectomy has been recommended as a treatment for CRPS, type II, after repetitive sympathetic blocks. Additionally, guanethidine, which is a ganglionic blocking agent, has proved effective in treating some forms of CRPS, type II. Guanethidine must be used with caution, however, because it causes the release of norepinephrine prior to occupying the receptor sites itself; and the time course of the cessation of activity is variable. The fact that one may occlude an affected limb below the site of the CRPS, type II and still achieve effective blocks with guanethidine suggests that its activity is not at the ganglion but instead on the peripheral sensory nerves, which produces its effect on CRPS, type II (Hannington-Kiff, 1979). Surgical intervention, in the form of surgical sympathectomy, has been used to treat CRPS, type II with variable cure rates, ranging from 12 to 97%. The variability may be ascribed to lack of precision and diagnosis, with an overlap of CRPS, type I with CRPS, type II, or CRPS, type I mistakenly diagnosed as CRPS, type II; varying skills in performing blocks; collateral reinnervation of postganglionic sympathetic fibers; and delay in performing a sympathectomy (Payne, 1986). For CRPS, type II that is not responding to sympathectomy, the possibility of a contralateral sympathectomy has been raised (Kleinman, 1954).

DIAGNOSIS OF COMPLEX REGIONAL PAIN SYNDROME, TYPE I

The clinical diagnosis of CRPS, type I is more complicated than that of CRPS, type II. Some authors believe that there is a very definite set of criteria to establish the diagnosis, whereas other authors think that only several symptoms from a whole list of symptom complexes need

be present to establish the diagnosis of CRPS, type I. Kozin, et al. (1981) have established the criteria for CRPS, type I as a patient presenting with pain and tenderness in an extremity associated with vasomotor instability (particular temperature or color changes) and generalized swelling in the same extremity. The second group of patients they consider are those with pain and tenderness associated with a vasomotor instability or swelling in an extremity; they call this group "probable CRPS, type I." This system lacks precision, however, because it does not take into account the particular type of pain that patients with CRPS, type I experience.

Raja, et al. (1986) define patients as having CRPS, type I if they have pain associated with signs of sympathetic hyperactivity (i.e., lower skin temperature, skin discoloration, increased sweating, and some trophic changes) and symptomatic relief after sympathetic blocks; they found that those with CRPS, type I also had thermal hyperalgesia either to cold or to heat. In contrast, their patients with CRPS, type II did not experience thermal hyperalgesia to heat, and only two out of seven experienced hyperalgesia to cold. Both the CRPS, type II and CRPS, type I patients experienced hyperalgesia to mechanical stimulation (Raja, et al., 1986). On the other hand, Ochoa, et al. (1985) found mechanical hyperalgesia, which they called allodynia, in their patients with CRPS, type I. Additionally, hypersensitivity to temperature was also found in patients with CRPS, type I, whether it be to heat or to cold (Meyer, Campbell, & Raja, 1985; Ochoa, 1985; Raja, et al., 1986).

One proposed mechanism for mechanical hypersensitivity is ectopic alpha-adrenergic chemosensitivity (Devor, 1983). Another consideration is a secondary abnormality in distal nociceptor fibers that escaped injury, or intact low-threshold mechanoreceptors with large myelinated fibers that are not sympathetic dependent because of transfer of information to nociceptor pathways proximal to the site of injury (Ochoa, 1985). Additionally, Ochoa, et al. (1985) advanced the concept of alpha-receptor sensitization, whereas others believe that the hypersensitivity of the mechanoreceptors could possibly be a central nervous system event (Meyer, Campbell, & Raja, 1985).

TREATMENT OF COMPLEX REGIONAL PAIN SYNDROME, TYPE I

Treatments for the mechanical hypersensitivity or hyperalgesia of CRPS, type I have been advanced by several authors, without clear-cut definition. One group of authors believes that sympathectomy may relieve mechanical hyperalgesia, whereas another group of authors reports that sympathectomy does not (Meyer, Campbell, & Raja, 1985; Hoffert, et al., 1984). Another group has advanced the notion that nifedipine, a calcium channel-blocking agent, may prove effective (Prough, et al., 1985). Finally, a group from South Africa suggested that low-dose naloxone, and possibly longer acting naltrexone, may prove effective for reducing mechanical hyperalgesia, because of the existence of a hypergesic kappa system of opiate receptors (Gillman and Lichtigfeld, 1985). Again, the area of mechanical hyperalgesia is quite muddy, because all the patients with either CRPS, type II or CRPS, type I had mechanical hypersensitivity (Raja, et al., 1986).

Thermal hypersensitivity to either heat or cold (hyperalgesia) has been reported by several groups (Meyer, Campbell, & Raja, 1985; Ochoa, et al., 1985; Raja, et al., 1986). The mechanism behind the thermal hypersensitivity is not well elucidated, but one can clinically differentiate mechanical from thermal hypersensitivity by the use of a drop of acetone. Patients with CRPS, type I in the series studied by Raja, et al. (1986) had hyperalgesia to cold (three of four, as tested by acetone drop) or to heat (four of five, as tested using a laser thermal stimulator). Some patients had hypersensitivity and hyperalgesia to both heat and cold; however, these patients did not have CRPS, type II, but instead CRPS, type I. Of the group of patients with hyperalgesia to temperature change, six of six got relief with sympathetic blocks or sympathectomy (Raja, et al., 1986). Other authors have reported that nifedipine is effective for treating hyperalgesia (Prough, et al., 1985). Specifically, in 13 patients with pain having a burning character, dysesthesia, and cold intolerance, nifedipine beginning at 10 mg three times a day, and increasing to 30 mg three times a day, proved effective in 7 of 13 patients. Nifedipine is a calcium channel-blocking agent, and as such may work by dilating blood vessels and antagonizing the effects of norepinephrine on arterial and venous muscle (Payne, 1986). Also, nifedipine may interfere with ectopic impulse formation that occurs in regenerating nerves, by blocking calcium channel protein.

The dystrophic component of CRPS, type I is more difficult to delineate. Some authors have reported a diffuse or patchy bony demineralization (Kozin, et al., 1981), whereas others have reported frank osteoporosis late in the disorder (Schott, 1986). A number of authors have reported molted skin, again late in the disorder (Kozin, et al., 1981; Payne, 1986; Raja, et al., 1986). Some authors have reported hair loss, yet again late in the disorder (Raja, et al., 1986; Schott, 1986). Vague terms such as vasomotor instability have also been reported, as well as trophic skin changes (Kozin, et al., 1981). The etiology for these components is not well defined, but the consensus seems to be reduced blood flow to the various involved organs.

A more precise diagnostic assessment was advanced by Holder and MacKinnon (1984). They evaluated patients with CRPS, type I, which they defined as diffuse hand pain, diminished hand function, joint stiffness, and skin and soft tissue trophic changes with or without vaso-

motor instability. They also used three other control groups, including patients with diffuse pain, focal pain, or vascular disease. Holder and MacKinnon (1984) found that 22 of the 23 patients who met their criteria for diagnosing CRPS, type I had positive delayed image bone scans, 12 of the 23 patients had positive blood pool images, and 10 of the 23 patients had positive radionucleotide angiograms. Approximately half the patients with CRPS, type I had positive early phase bone scans, whereas almost all patients with CRPS, type I had positive delayed image bone scans.

This study compared favorably with work done by Kozin, et al. (1981), who found that radiography is not a useful tool for diagnosing CRPS, type I (Bonica, 1970). Kozin, et al. (1981) did find that 83% of the patients with CRPS, type I had positive static (delayed) bone scans, however, whereas 69% of the patients had positive flow studies. Therefore, it is apparent that between 50 and 60% of patients with CRPS, type I will have positive early phase bone scans, but between 83 and 96% of patients will have positive delayed image bone scans (Holder & Mackinnon, 1984; Kozin, et al., 1981). Treatment for this component of CRPS, type I is difficult to assess. Kozin, et al. (1981) reported that 90% of patients with a positive bone scan had good to excellent steroid response, beginning with steroids at the level of 60 to 80 mg/day and tapering the dosages.

Schott (1986) has reported a variety of therapeutic modalities, including steroids, nonsteroidal anti-inflammatory drugs, alpha- and beta-blocking agents, griseofulvin, calcitonin, transcutaneous electrical nerve stimulation, physical therapy, sympathetic blocks, and intravenous guanethidine. None of these treatments has been studied in a systematized fashion, however.

Nail brittleness has been reported by Schott (1986) and Payne (1986) late in the disorder. The etiology of this is not clear and there is not any clear-cut treatment. Muscle spasm has been reported by a number of authors (Kleinman, 1954; Long, 1982; Schott, 1986), again without a clear-cut mechanism describing the etiology (Payne, 1986). Interestingly, electromyography (EMG) nerve conduction velocity studies seem to be relatively negative in CRPS, type I (Uematsu, et al., 1981). The treatments that seemed most effective for muscle spasm were trigger point injections (Payne, 1986) and the use of baclofen. Baclofen is a gamma aminobutyric acid (GABA)-minergic drug that centrally reduces muscle spasm. The inhibition of substance P may be implicated as part of its mechanism for reducing spasm and the pain associated with spasm (Gillman & Lichtigfeld, 1985). Soma and quinine have also been tried, with only limited success (Hendler, unpublished observations). Contractures, usually in the hand, have also been reported (Payne, 1986; Schott, 1986). The etiology of this is unclear, but is probably related to disuse.

Again, there is an absence of positive EMG-nerve conduction velocity studies (Uematsu, et al., 1981), and the only treatment seems to be preventative, by the use of passive range-of-motion exercises and physical therapy.

Contralateral involvement has been reported by several authors (Kleinman, 1954; Schott, 1986). The etiology for this may be quite direct. In approximately 80% of examined cadavers there is cross-communication between the sympathetic fibers and the sympathetic chains (Kleinman, 1954). Countralateral blocks and denervation have been recommended (Kleinman, 1954). Edema of the affected limb (Payne, 1986; Schott, 1986), as well as swelling of a specific joint (Kozin, et al., 1981), has been reported. Again, the etiology is unclear. The diagnosis is established by measuring the proximal interphalangeal joint, which averages 12.9 mm larger in the affected hand than in the control hand (Kozin, et al., 1981). No treatment has been advanced for this, although nifedipine is suggested to be effective (Prough, et al., 1985). At Mensana Clinic, Stevenson, MD, we have observed some benefit from the use of spironolactone, or carbonic anhydrase inhibitors, but not on a consistent basis.

Lower skin temperature has been reported by a variety of authors (Hendler, Uematsu, & Long, 1982; Payne, 1986; Raja, et al. 1996), but it does not seem to be due to vasospasm (Janof, Phinney, & Porter, 1985). Reflex contraction due to altered activity within the afferent and efferent nerves is proposed as the etiology (Janoff, et al., 1985). Thermography is an excellent diagnostic tool to document the reduced skin temperature (Hendler, et al., 1982; Uematsu, et al., 1981). In fact, very often patients with CRPS, type I are diagnosed as having psychosomatic disorders, and thermography can be a most convincing diagnostic tool to confirm the otherwise subjective complaint (Hendler, et al., 1982). However, nerve entrapments and radiculopathies can also lower limb temperature (Uematsu, et al., 1981).

Treatment for lower skin temperature associated with pain is best effected using regional sympathetic blocks employing reserpine. It is important to note that these reserpine blocks, or Bier blocks, are not effective for vasospasm, but specifically seem to function best for treating CRPS, type I. Therefore, vasospasm does not seem to be the etiologic mechanism for the coldness noted in the limb in CRPS, type I (Janoff, et al., 1985). Stiffness (Holder & MacKinnon, 1984; Payne, 1986) and tenderness (Kozin, et al., 1981) of the joints have been reported; again, the etiology is not clear (Payne, 1986). Very often, the involvement of the joint leads to misdiagnosis and confusion with other diseases that can affect the joint, notably infective arthritis, rheumatoid arthritis, Reiter's syndrome, systemic lupus erythematosus, and arthritides (Kozin, et al., 1981). In one series, 71% of the patients with joint tenderness and stiffness had a poor response to stellate ganglion blocks. Steroids, notably prednisone (60

to 80 mg) for 2 to 4 days, then 40 to 60 mg for 2 to 4 days, and then 30 to 40 mg for 2 to 4 days, in four equally divided doses, were the initial therapy. Subsequently, the dose was rapidly tapered using a single morning dose of 40 mg, then 30 mg, 20 mg, 10 mg, and 5 mg over 2 or 3 days at each dose. By using this regimen, 82% of the patients with joint stiffness and tenderness obtained good or excellent relief.

An unusual complication of CRPS, type I is the appearance of pathological fractures subsequent to minor trauma. In patients complaining of persistent pain in the limb that seems to be bony in origin, instead of part of the CRPS, type I, it would be imperative to obtain bone scanning to confirm the presence or absence of an undetected break. In our experience, one patient with long-standing CRPS, type I received a minor trauma (i.e., bumping her ankle while walking in a train) that resulted in a chronic intense worsening of pain in the heel. Radiographs of this area were within normal limits, but the pain persisted for several days after the event, and a bone scan was obtained. Only on bone scan did the break in the calcaneus appear, which had been totally missed by routine radiograph. Of any breaks present, 95% will have a positive bone scan after 72 h (Matin, 1979). Interestingly, after the fracture is healed, 90% of the bone scans have returned to normal 2 years from the date of the injury. Therefore, in patients with CRPS, type I who have minor injuries and complain of bony pain, it would be prudent to obtain a bone scan, and not rely on radiographs.

Payne (1986) has enumerated many attempted treatments for CRPS, type I. Unfortunately, there seems to be a lack of systematic investigation for these treatments, and most are based on clinical reports instead of systematized trials. Reported pharmacological interventions that may work for CRPS, type II are the use of propranolol, a beta-blocking agent; prazosin, an alpha-1-adrenergic-blocking agent; phenoxybenzamine, both an alpha-1- and an alpha-2-blocker; and guanethidine, a drug that produces a chemical "sympathectomy." Physical therapy has been advanced for the treatment of CRPS, type I, specifically to minimize muscle contractures and joint stiffness. It is never a definitive treatment, however, and should not be considered such. Electrical stimulation of the central nervous system, using either electrodes centrally implanted into the periaqueductal or periventricular gray or epidural stimulators, may prove effective, as might transcutaneous electrical nerve stimulation. Tricyclic antidepressants, nonsteroidal anti-inflammatory drugs, narcotics, and anticonvulsants have all been reported as treating some components of CRPS, type I, with varying degrees of success.

Surgical intervention is a treatment that is reserved until all other modalities of treatment have been attempted. In all cases, the criterion for surgical intervention would

TABLE 20.4
Recommended Treatment Flow Sheet

Treatment	Dosage	Time Course	If Ineffective, Next Step
1. Prednisone	80 mg to start and taper by 10 mg q.i.	8 days	Go to 2
2. Physical therapy	3 times a week	2 weeks	Go to 3
3. Transcutaneous electrical stimulation	Wear constantly	1 week	Go to 4
4. Sympathetic blocks	3 times a week	2 weeks	If lasting relief, stop; if 100% pain relief but temporary, go to 5
5. Sympathectomy	——	1-week recovery	If lasting relief, stop; if no relief, go to 6
6. Contralateral blocks	3 times a week	2 weeks	If lasting relief, stop; if 100% pain relief but temporary, go to 7, if no relief, go to 8
7. Contralateral sympathectomy	—	1-week recovery	If relief, stop; if no relief, go to 8
8. Epidural spinal cord stimulator	—	1-week recovery	If relief, stop; if no relief, go to 9
9. Epidural pump	Start with clonidine (Rauck, et al., 1993)	1-week recovery	If relief, stop; if no relief, try other meds in combination or alone, go to 10
10. Psychotherapy (supportive)	Use antidepressants	6 months to 2 years	Maintenance

be repetitive successes with repeat sympathetic blocks. The most commonly employed surgical interventions are resection of the lower third of the stellate ganglion and resection of the upper two thoracic ganglia; however, some surgeons resect the second through fifth thoracic ganglia in an attempt to treat upper-extremity difficulties. There are four surgical approaches to upper extremity sympathectomies (Allen & Morety, 1982):

1. Above the clavicle (anterior cervical approach)
2. Posterior resection of the transverse processes of ribs 2 and 3, and proximal section of ribs 2 and 3
3. Anterior transpleural entry through the pectoralis muscle to the third intercostal space, pressing the lung, to reach the operative area
4. The axillary approach, which is through a transaxillary incision over the second intercostal space

Also, a lumbar approach can be made through the external and internal obliques, and then the transversalis muscle, below the twelfth rib, behind the kidney; others have suggested a thoracolumbar presacral neurectomy. Side effects of surgical approaches are postsympathectomy neuralgia, beginning 7 to 10 days after surgery, and postsympathectomy dysesthesia that may last 2 to 14 weeks, and is described as continuous, severe, and worse at night. Anticonvulsants, such as diphenylhydantoin or carbamazepine, may be used to treat this (Allen & Morety, 1982). Medication, such as valproic acid and gabapentin may be useful (Mellick & Mellick, 1995). Dorsal root entry zone procedures, which produce

lesions in the dorsal root interrupting the nociceptive pathways in the tract of Lissauer and in laminae I-V of the dorsal horn of the spinal cord, may prove to be an effective modality for treating CRPS, type II for stretch injuries (Payne, 1986). A treatment guideline is shown in Table 20.4.

CONCLUSIONS

In summary, it is quite apparent that a great deal of confusion has arisen concerning the diagnosis of CRPS, type I and CRPS, type II. This is evidenced by the lack of uniformity in clinical criteria for establishing the diagnosis. Because of this lack of uniformity, assessment of various articles detailing treatment of CRPS, type I and/or CRPS, type II is difficult. What some clinicians take as symptoms of CRPS, type I are not always present in their entirety. Unfortunately, if one adheres rigorously to these criteria, proper diagnosis, and more importantly proper treatment, may be withheld. The various clinical symptoms that have been reported as associated with CRPS, type I and CRPS, type II are shown in Table 20.2. A patient should be considered to have CRPS, type I if he or she has at least one type of hyperalgesia (either mechanical or thermal), lower skin temperature, and the sensation of pins and needles. However, the presence of allodynia is a more consistent finding. At a minimum, diagnostic studies that would facilitate the diagnosis of CRPS, type I would be thermography, sympathetic blocks, and bone scan. Clinical diagnostic studies that would prove important would be testing with a drop of acetone for cold hyperalgesia and allodynia, and testing using Von Frey hairs for mechanical hyperalgesia and allodynia. All patients suspected of having CRPS, type I should have at least three sympathetic blocks. After that, one should use various diagnostic and treatment techniques, including pharmacological intervention, depending on the patient's type of complaints.

To make the diagnosis of CRPS, type II, one certainly should establish that the symptoms of burning pain are constantly present, in association with a partial peripheral nerve injury. Electromyographic and nerve conduction velocity studies should be conducted to detect whether there is an associated nerve injury. Certainly, patients should receive a peripheral nerve block; sympathetic blocks; and a trial with phenoxybenzamine, valproic acid, and gabapentin.

Regardless of whether a patient has CRPS, type I or CRPS type II, one must be aware of the need to make a distinction between the two diagnoses, because the treatments vary. More importantly, if the patient has even a single symptom of CRPS, type I, a diagnostic assessment involving the previously recommended modalities would be warranted, and further diagnostic studies should be pursued if the diagnosis of CRPS type I is not confirmed. Kozin, et al. (1981) clearly defined a number of overlapping conditions that may originally be misdiagnosed as CRPS, type I. Of the patients who were found not to have CRPS, type I, 25% had peripheral neuropathy or trapped peripheral nerves, and half the patients misdiagnosed as having CRPS, type I had inflammatory arthritis (Kozin, et al., 1981). Therefore, laboratory studies, including erythrocyte sedimentation rate, antinuclear antibody, rheumatoid factor, Lyme disease, HIV, and the like, should be conducted in patients thought to have CRPS, type I but in whom the diagnosis is not complete. In any event, CRPS, types II and I require clinical acumen to establish the diagnosis, and persistence to effect appropriate treatment. Aggressively pursuing all the diagnostic studies available, as well as relying on clinical judgment, provides better care for these patients.

REFERENCES

Allen, M.B., Jr., & Morety, W.H. (1982). Sympathectomy. In J. Youmans (Ed.), *Neurological surgery* (2nd ed., Vol. 6, pp. 3717–3726). Philadelphia: W. B. Saunders.

Arner, S., & Meyerson, B.A. (1988). Lack of analgesic effect of opioids on neuropathic and idiopathic forms of pain. *Pain, 33,* 11–23.

Barolat, G., Schwartzman, R J., & Woo, R. (1989). Epidural spinal cord stimulation in the management of reflex sympathetic dystrophy. *Stereotactic and Functional Neurosurgery, 53,* 29–39.

Baron, R., Blumberg, H., & Janig, W. (1996). Clinical characteristics of patients with complex regional pain syndrome in Germany, with special emphasis on vasomotor function, in reflex sympathetic dystrophy: A reappraisal. In W. Janig & M. Stanton-Hicks (Eds.). *Progress in pain research and management* (Vol. 6, pp. 25–48). Seattle: IASP Press.

Bennett, G.J. (1991). The role of the sympathetic nervous system in painful peripheral neuropathy. *Pain, 45,* 221–223.

Bonica, J.J. (1970). Causalgia and other reflex sympathetic dystrophies. In J.J. Bonica (Ed.), *Advances in pain research and therapy* (Vol. 3, pp. 141–166). New York: Raven Press.

Bouckoms, A.L., & Litman R.E. (1985). Clonazepam in the treatment of neuralgic pain syndrome. *Psychosomatics, 26,* 933–936.

Broseta, J., Roldan, P., & Gonzales-Darder, J. (1982). Chronic epidural dorsal column stimulation in the treatment of causalgic pain. *Applications in Neurophysiology, 45,* 190–194.

Chaplan, S.R., Bach, F.W., Pogrel, J.W., Chung, J.M., & Yaksh, T.L. (1994). Quantitative assessment of tactile allodynia in the rat paw. *Journal of Neuroscience Methods, 53,* 55–63.

Dalton, S. (1984). *Split seconds — The world of high speed photography* (pp. 21, 28, 30, 31, 32, 34, 36). Salem, NH: Salem House.

Devor, M. (1983). Nerve pathophysiology and mechanisms of pain in causalgia. *Journal of the Autonomic Nervous System, 7,* 371–384.

Devor, M., & Janig, W. (1981). Activation of myelinated afferents ending in a neuroma by stimulation of the sympathetic supply in a rat. *Neuroscience Letters, 24,* 43–47.

Eliav, E., Herzberg, U., & Caudle, R. M. (1999). The kappa opioid agonist GR89 696 blocks hyperalgesia and allodynia in rat models of peripheral neuritis and neuropathy. *Pain, 79,* 255–264.

Ganit, R., Leksell, L., & Skoglund, C.R. (1944). Fiber interaction in injured or compressed region of the nerve. *Brain, 67,* 125–140.

Geldard, F.A. (1962). *Fundamentals of psychology.* New York: John Wiley & Sons.

Ghostine, S.Y., Comair, Y.G., Turner, D.M., et al. (1984). Phenoxybenzamine in the treatment of causalgia (report of 40 cases). *Journal of Neurosurgery, 6,* 1263–1268.

Gillman, M.A., & Lichtigfeld, R.J. (1985). A pharmacological overview of opioid mechanisms mediating analgesia and hyperalgesia. *Neural Research, 7,* 106–119.

Glynn, C.J., Dawson, D., & Sanders, R. (1988). A double-blind comparison between epidural morphine and epidural clonidine in patients with chronic non-cancer pain. *Pain, 34,* 123–128.

Gobelet, C., Waldburger, M., & Meier, J.L. (1992). The effect of adding calcitonin to physical treatment on reflex sympathetic dystrophy. *Pain, 48,* 171–175.

Greipp, M.E., & Thomas, A.F. (1994). Skin lesions occurring in clients with reflex sympathetic dystrophy syndrome. *Journal of Neuroscience Nursing, 26*(6), 342–346.

Hamamci, N., Dursun, E., Ural, C., & Cakci, A. (1996). Calcitonin treatment in reflex sympathetic dystrophy. A preliminary study. *British Journal of Clinical Practice, 50*(7), 373–375.

Hannington-Kiff, J.G. (1979). Relief of causalgia in limbs by regional intravenous guanethidine. *British Medical Journal, 12,* 367–368.

Hassenbusch, S., Stanton-Hicks, M., & Covington, E.C. (1995). Long term intraspinal infusion of opioids in the treatment of neurpathic pain. *Journal of Pain and Symptom Management, 10,* 527–543.

Hendler, N. (1982). The four stages of pain. In N. Hendler, D. Long, & T. Wise (Eds.), *Diagnosis and treatment of chronic pain* (pp. 1–8). Boston: John Wright-PSG.

Hendler, N. (1984). Depression caused by chronic pain. *Journal of Clinical Psychiatry, 45*(3, Sec. 2), 30–36.

Hendler, N. (1995). Reflex sympathetic dystrophy: Clearing up the misconceptions, *Journal of Workers Compensation, 5,*(1), 9–20.

Hendler, N. (1997). Pharmacology of chronic pain. In R. North & R. Levy (Eds.), *Neurosurgical management of pain* (pp. 117–129). Amsterdam: Springer-Verlag.

Hendler, N. (2000). Pharmacotherapy of chronic pain. In P. P. Raj (Ed.), *Practical management of pain* (3rd ed., pp. 145–155). Philadelphia: C.V. Mosby.

Hendler, N., Bergson, C., & Morrison, C. (1996). Overlooked physical diagnoses in chronic pain patients involved in litigation: Part 2. *Psychosomatics, 37*(6), 509–517.

Hendler, N., & Kozikowski, J. (1993). Overlooked physical diagnoses in chronic pain patients involved in litigation. *Psychosomatics, 34*(6), 494–501.

Hendler, N., & Raja, S. (1994). Reflex sympathetic dystrophy and causalgia. In C. D. Tollison (Ed), *Handbook of pain management* (2nd ed., pp. 484–496). Baltimore: Williams & Wilkins.

Hendler, N., & Talo, S. (1989). Chronic pain patients versus the malingering patient. In K. Foley & R. Payne (Eds.), *Current therapy of pain* (pp. 14–22). Philadelphia: B.C. Decker.

Hendler, N., Uematsu, S., & Long, D. (1982). Thermographic validating of physical complaints in "psychogenic pain" patients. *Psychosomatics, 23,* 282–287.

Hendler, N., Vierstein, M., Shallenberger, C., & Long, D. (1981). Group therapy with chronic pain patients. *Psychosomatics, 22*(4), 333–340.

Hoffert, M.I., Greenburg, P.P., Wolskee, P.J., et al. (1984). Abnormal and collateral innervation of sympathetic and peripheral sensory fields associated with a case of causalgia. *Pain, 20,* 1–12.

Holder, L.E., & MacKinnon, S.E. (1984). Reflex sympathetic dystrophy in the hands: Clinical and scintigraphic criteria. *Radiology, 152,* 517–522.

Inball, R., Rousso, N., Ashur, H., Wall, P.D., & Devor, M. (1987). Collateral sprouting in skin and sensory recovery after nerve injury in man. *Pain, 39,* 141–154.

Janoff, K.H., Phinney, E.S., & Porter, I.M. (1985). Lumbar sympathectomy for lower extremity vasospasm. *American Journal of Surgery, 150,* 147–152.

Kim, S.H., & Chung, J.M. (1995). Sympathectomy alleviates mechanical allodynia in an experimental animal model for neuropathy in the rat. *Neuroscience Letters, 134,* 131–134.

Kleinman, A. (1954). Causalgia: Evidence of the existence of crossed sensory sympathetic fibers. *American Journal of Surgery, 87,* 839–841.

Knobler, R. (1996). The pathogenesis of reflex sympathetic dystrophy: Immune and viral mechanisms. *American Journal of Pain Management, 6*(3), 83–85.

Kozin, F., Ryan, L.M., Carerra, G.E., et al. (1981). The reflex sympathetic dystrophy (RSDS). *American Journal of Medicine, 70,* 23–30.

Lee, Y.W., Chaplan, S.R., & Yaksh, T.L. (1995). Systemic and supraspinal, but not spinal opiates supress allodynia in a rat neuropathic pain model. *Neuroscience Letters, 199,* 111–114.

Lee, Y.W., Kayer, V., Desmeules, J., & Guilbaud, G. (1994). Differential action of morphine and various opioid agonist on thermal allodynia and hyperalgesia in mononeuropathic rats. *Pain, 57,* 233–240.

Lee, Y.W., & Yatsh, T.L. (1996). Pharmacology of the spinal adenosine receptor which mediates the anti-allodynic action of intra-thecal adenosine agonists. *Journal of Pharmacology and Experimental Therapeutics, 277,* 1642–1648

Levi-Montalcini, R. Skaper, S.D., Toso, R.D., Petrelli, L, & Leon, A. (1996). Nerve growth factor: From neurotrophin to neurokine. *Trends in Neuroscience, 19,* 514–520.

Loh, I., & Nathan P.W. (1978). Painful peripheral states and sympathetic blocks. *Journal of Neurology, Neurosurgery, and Psychiatry, 41,* 664–671.

Long, D.M. (1982). Pain of peripheral nerve injury. In J. Youmans (Ed.), *Neurological surgery* (2nd ed, Vol. 6, pp. 3634–3643). Philadelphia: W. B. Saunders.

Matin, P. (1979). The appearance of bone scans following fractures, including immediate and long-term studies. *Journal of Nuclear Medicine, 20,* 1227–1231.

Max, M. B., Kishmore-Kumar, R., Schafer, S. C., et. al. (1991). Efficacy of desipramine in diabetic peripheral neuropathy: A placebo controlled trial. *Pain, 45,* 69–73.

Mearow, K.M., & Kril, Y. (1995). Anti-NGF treatment blocks the upregulation of NGF receptor mRNA expression associated with collateral sprouting of rat dorsal ganglion neurons. *Neuroscience Letters, 184,* 55–58.

Mellick, G.A., & Mellick, L.B. (1995). Gabapentin in the management of reflex sympathetic dystrophy. *Journal of Pain Symptoms and Management, 10,* 265–266.

Merskey, H. (ed) and the Subcommittee on Taxonomy. (1986). Classification of chronic pain. *Pain, 3*(Suppl.), 28–29.

Meyer, R.A., Campbell, J.N., & Raja, S.N. (1985). Peripheral neural mechanism of cutaneous hyperalgesia. In H.L. Fields, R. Dubner, & F. Cevero (Eds.), *Advances in pain research and therapy* (Vol. 9, pp. 53–71). New York: Raven Press.

Ochoa, J., Torebjorte, E., Marchetti, H., et al. (1985). Mechanisms of neuropathic pain: Cumulative observations, new experiments and further speculation. In H. L. Fields, R. Dubner, & F. Cevero (Eds.), *Advances in pain research and therapy* (Vol. 9, pp. 431–450). New York: Raven Press.

Payne, R. (1986). Neuropathic pain syndromes, with special reference to causalgia and reflex sympathetic dystrophy. *Clinical Journal of Pain, 2,* 59–73.

Peuschl, G., Blumber, H., & Lucking, C.H. (1991). Tremor in reflex sympathetic dystrophy. *Archives of Neurology, 48,* 1247–1252.

Portenoy, R.K., Foley, K.M., & Inturrisi, C.E. (1990). The nature of opioid responsiveness and its implications for neuropathic pain: A new hypothesis derived from the study of opioid infusions. *Pain, 43,* 273–286.

Prough, D.S., McLeskey, C.H., Poehling, G.G., et al. (1985). Efficacy of oral nifedipine in the treatment of reflex sympathetic dystrophy. *Anesthesiology, 2,* 796–799.

Raja, S.N., Campbell J.N., Meyer R.A., et al. (1986, November 6–9). *Sensory testing in patients with causalgia or reflex sympathetic dystrophy.* Abstract presented at 6th Annual Meeting of American Pain Society, Washington, D.C.

Raja, S.N., & Hendler N. (1990). Sympathetically maintained pain. In M. Rogers (Ed.), *Current practices in anesthesiology* (pp. 421–425). New York: C. V. Mosby Year Book.

Raja, S.N., Treede R.D., Davis R.D., et al. (1991). Systemic alpha-adrenergic blockade with phentolarrine: A diagnostic test for sympathetically maintained pain. *Anesthesiology, 74,* 691–698.

Rauck, R.I., Eisenach, J.C., & Jackson, K. (1993). Epidural clonidine treatment for refractory reflex sympathetic dystrophy. *Anesthesiology, 79,* 1163–1169.

Ren, K., & Dubner, R. (1993). NMDA receptor antagonists attenuate mechanical hyperalgesia in rats with unilateral inflammation of the hindpaw. *Neuroscience Letters, 163,* 22–26.

Ro, L.S., Chen, S.-T., Tang, L.-M., & Jacobs, J.M. (1999). Effect of NGF and anti-NGF on neuropathic pain in rats following chronic constriction injury of the sciatic nerve. *Pain, 79,* 265–274.

Robaina, F., Dominguez, M., & Diaz, M. (1989). Spinal cord stimulation for relief of chronic pain in vasoplastic disorders of the upper limbs. *Neurosurgery, 24,* 63–67.

Roberts, M.A. (1986). Hypothesis on the physiological basis for causalgia and related pain. *Pain, 24,* 297–311.

Schott, G.D. (1986). Neurologic manifestation of bone and joint disease. In A. K. Ashbury, G. M. McKham, W. C. McDonald, et al. (Eds.), *Diseases of the nervous system* (pp. 1523–1537). Philadelphia: W. B. Saunders.

Schwartzman, R.J., & Kerrigan, J. (1990). The movement disorder of reflex sympathetic dystrophy. *Neurology, 40,* 57–61.

Schwartzman, R.J., & McKellan, T.L. (1987). Reflex sympathetic dystrophy: A review. *Archives of Neurology, 44,* 555–561.

Stanton-Hicks, M., Baron, R., Boas, R., Gordh, T., Harden, N., Hendler, N., Koltzenberg, M., Raj., P., & Wilder, R. (1998). Complex regional pain syndrome: guidelines for therapy. *The Clinical Journal of Pain, 14*(2), 155–166.

Uematsu, S., Hendler, N., Hugerford, D., Ono, S., & Long, D.M. (1981). Thermography and electromyography in the differential diagnosis of chronic pain syndromes and reflex sympathetic dystrophy. *Electromyography and Clinical Neurophysiology, 21,* 165–182.

Van der Laan, L., Veldman, P.H.J.M., & Goris, R.J.A. (1998). Severe complications of reflex sympathetic dystrophy: Infection, ulcers, chronic edema, dystonia, and myoclonus. *Archives of Physical Medicine and Rehabilitation, 79,* 424–429.

Watson, C.P., Chipman, M., Reed, K., et. al. (1991). Amitriptyline vs. maprotiline in post herpetic neuralgia: A randomized, double blind, cross-over trial. *Pain, 48,* 29–36.

Watson, C.P., Evans, R.J., Reed, K., et. al. (1981). Amitriptyline vs. placebo in post herpetic neuralgia. *Neurology, 32,* 671–673.

Webster, G.F., Iozzo, R.V., Schwartzman, R.J., Tahmoush, A. J., Knobler, R.L., & Jacoby, R.A. (1993). Reflex sympathetic dystrophy: Occurrence of chronic edema and non-immune bulious skin lesions. *Journal of the American Academy of Dermatology, 28*(1), 29–32.

Webster, G.F., Schwartzman, R.J., Jacoby, R.A., Knobler, R.L., & Uitto, J.J. (1991). Reflex sympathetic dystrophy: Occurrence of inflammatory skin lesions in patients with stages II and III disease. *Archives of Dermatology, 127,* 1541–1544.

21

Treatment of Myofascial Pain Syndromes

Robert D. Gerwin, M.D. and Jan Dommerholt, P.T., M.P.S.

INTRODUCTION

The treatment of persons with myofascial pain syndrome (MPS) follows the general principles that apply to all medical disorders. The nature of the pain problem first must be understood through developing an appropriate differential diagnosis and evaluating the contributions of coexisting disorders, until a single working diagnosis emerges. Following the initial assessment and formulation of diagnostic hypotheses, new data are collected. A regular review at each encounter and modification of the hypotheses facilitate a more efficient and effective management of patients with MPS and dictate the actual program components (Higgs & Jones, 1995; Jones, 1994). After addressing the issue of diagnosis, the practitioner must determine the structural or biomechanical functioning of the patient and the contribution that any dysfunction may have to the individual's pain. Medical and psychological disorders that may alter the presentation of MPS or that may predispose to its becoming chronic are assessed. Treatment of persons with MPS addresses each of these issues specifically (Figure 21.1). There must be relief of pain by the direct inactivation of the myofascial trigger point (MTrP) itself. The mechanical and structural factors that affect or overload the muscle and aggravate the pain must be resolved or alleviated. The medical and psychological problems that affect muscle function, including those that alter and impair intracellular metabolism, must be identified and corrected where possible. Inactivation of the MTrP may occur with direct intervention at the MTrP itself, through correction of the mechanical factors that produced it or through improvement in the underlying medical disorders that predispose to the development or maintenance of the MTrP.

DIAGNOSIS

The diagnosis of MPS should be suspected when there is a nonneuropathic pain complaint almost anywhere in the body, including headache. At first glance, such a statement may seem to be so nonspecific as to be meaningless, but it emphasizes the need to be aware of the role of soft tissue or muscle in all types of pain. Indeed, MPS has been reported as the most common diagnosis responsible for chronic pain and disability (Fricton, 1990; Masi, 1993; Rosomoff, et al., 1989; Skootsky, Jaeger, & Oye, 1989). MPS is often thought of as a regional pain syndrome in contrast to fibromyalgia as a widespread syndrome; however, as many as 45% of patients with chronic MPS have generalized pain in three or four quadrants (Gerwin, 1995b). Patients with widespread MTrPs should be diagnosed with MPS and not with fibromyalgia, even though the classification criteria for fibromyalgia suggested making the diagnosis of fibromyalgia "irrespective of other diagnoses" (Wolfe, et al., 1990). In clinical practice the diagnosis of fibromyalgia should not be made without considering all differential diagnoses (Dommerholt, 2001; Gerwin, 1999). A survey of members of the American Pain Society showed general agreement with the concept that MPS exists as an entity distinct from fibromyalgia (Harden, et al., 2000).

Muscle pain tends to be dull, poorly localized, and deep, in contrast to the precise location of cutaneous pain. The diagnosis of MPS is confirmed when the MTrP is identified by palpation. Systematic palpation differentiates between myofascial taut bands and general muscle spasms (Janda, 1991). An active MTrP is defined as a focus of hyperirritability in a muscle or its fascia that causes the patient pain (Simons & Travell, 1984). The key features

0-8493-0926-3/02/$0.00+$1.50
© 2002 by CRC Press LLC

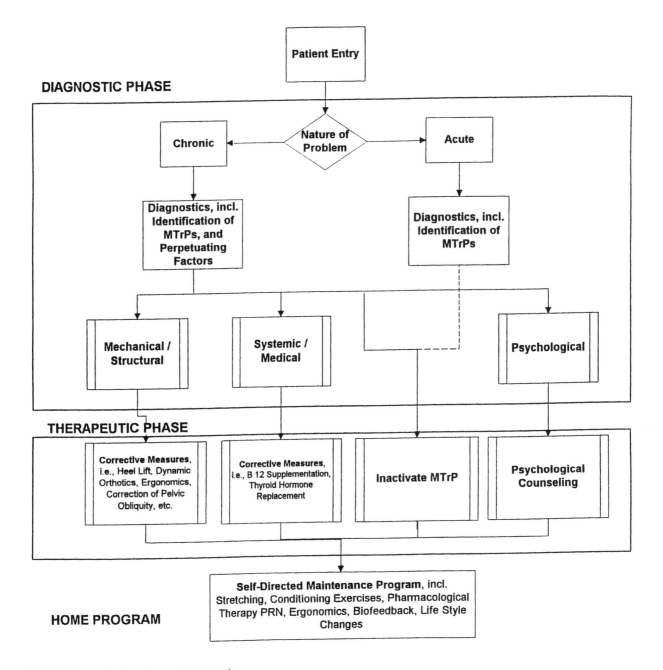

FIGURE 21.1   Treatment program example.

of the trigger point have been established by Simons, Travell, and Simons (1999) and are listed in Table 21.1. The interrater reliability of the clinical examination has been established by Gerwin, et al. (1997) for the five major features of the trigger point. Individual features of the trigger point are differentially represented in different muscles. For example, the local twitch response is easier to obtain and therefore more commonly found in the extensor digitorum communis than in the infraspinatus muscle. One should not expect to find each feature of the trigger point in every muscle by physical examination. The minimum criteria that must be satisfied in order to

distinguish an MTrP from any other tender area in muscle are a taut band and a tender point in that taut band. The presence of a local twitch response, referred pain, or reproduction of the person's symptomatic pain increases the certainty and specificity of the diagnosis.

Making a diagnosis of MPS may be therapeutic in itself and may constitute the first step in treatment, because many patients may not have been given a correct diagnosis previously. Patients are often depressed, confused, or frustrated, as they may not have been given an appropriate explanation of their pain in previous evaluations. They often appear relieved when the practitioner can literally

---

TABLE 21.1
Myofascial Trigger Point Characteristics

1. Focal exquisite tenderness in a taut band of muscle
2. Referral of pain to a distant site upon activation of the trigger point
3. Contraction of the taut band (local twitch response) upon mechanical activation of the trigger point
4. Reproduction of the person's pain by mechanical activation of trigger point
5. Restriction of range of motion
6. Weakness without muscle atrophy
7. Autonomic phenomenon such as piloerection or changes in loca circulation (regional blood flow and limb temperature) in response to trigger point activation

---

put the finger on the source of the pain, which usually results in instant rapport between patient and clinician.

The introduction of pressure algometers has improved the assessment of sensitivity significantly (Fischer, 1986c; Keele, 1954); however, only recently have pressure algometers been applied to the assessment of MTrPs (Fischer, 1984, 1986a,b). Several studies have confirmed the reliability of pressure measurement for the assessment of pain sensitivity (Jensen, et al., 1986; Merskey & Spear, 1964), for pressure sensitivity of MTrPs, and for the detection of their location (Delaney & McKee, 1993; Jaeger & Reeves, 1986; Ohrbach & Gale, 1989; Reeves, Jaeger, & Graff-Radford, 1986). Tenderness and the presence of a taut band in muscle may be quantified by pain pressure algometry and tissue compliance measurements (Fischer, 1986a,c, 1993). Fischer (1997) discussed the role of algometry and tissue compliance testing in the diagnosis of MPSs. He incorporated the two main criteria for the diagnosis of MTrPs, local point tenderness (as quantified by algometry) and recognition of patient's symptoms, into his concept of segmental sensitization, radiculopathy, and paraspinal spasm.

Hubbard and Berkoff (1993) identified a characteristic electrical discharge emanating from the trigger point and unique to it. Simons, Hong, and Simons (1995) have further studied this activity, whereas Chu (1995) has reported finding it in the trigger points of persons with lumbosacral radiculopathy. Phentolamine infusion reduced the average integrated signal of the spontaneous electrical activity by about one third in the experimental animal model. This result shows that there is a modulating effect of the sympathetic nervous system on the motor activity of the trigger point (Chen, et al., 1998). Thus, an objective electromyographic (EMG) signature of the trigger point is now available for diagnostic and research purposes.

PRINCIPLES OF TREATMENT

The ultimate goal of treatment of persons with MPS is restoration of function through inactivation of the trigger

point, restoration of normal tissue mobility, and elimination of pain (Dommerholt, 2001; Miller, 1994). The patient and the clinician need to identify appropriate goals and develop the means to implement them through therapy. Inactivation of the trigger point is a means to achieve relief of pain, to improve biomechanical function, and thus to improve the ability of the patient to better perform whatever desired tasks have been selected as goals. Relief of pain or increased range of motion, both of which can be the result of trigger point inactivation, are not in themselves the final goals of treatment. For some individuals, an initial goal may be to simply sleep through the night. For another patient, it may be eating out of bed at a table, or fastening a bra behind the back. For yet another, it may be regaining sexual ability, or returning to work or to a recreational activity. Reasonable goals that can be achieved and measured as being reached or not, are more important to focus on than simply the inactivation of a tender point or an increase in the range of a particular movement (Gerwin, 2000).

Inactivation of the MTrP can be achieved manually, by correcting structural mechanical stressors, by direct injection of a local anesthetic into the muscle, or by dry needle intramuscular stimulation of the MTrP. Treatment of the patient with MPS can be very effective when used in the context of a comprehensive diagnostic and treatment spectrum (Yue, 1995). After establishing an accurate medical diagnosis with identification of systemic, mechanical, and psychological perpetuating factors, the patient with chronic MPS is best treated through an interdisciplinary team approach (Turk & Okifuji, 1999). The term *interdisciplinary* is preferred to *multidisciplinary* because it reflects the coordinated working relationship between members of the treatment team (Melvin, 1980; Turk & Rudy, 1994). Essential members of the interdisciplinary team include the patient, physicians, psychologists, clinical social workers, occupational therapists, physical therapists, ergonomists, massage therapists, and others actively involved in patient care (Ghia, 1992; Khalil, et al., 1993). Not every MPS patient necessarily requires such an extensive collaboration. For example, patients with acute MPS may only require treatment by physicians and physical therapists. The treatment plan can be divided into a pain control phase and a training or conditioning phase (Saal & Saal, 1991). During the pain control phase, the most essential components are manual therapy, trigger point injection, dry needling, and elimination of mechanical perpetuating factors. Throughout the treatment process, much attention should be paid to educating the patient concerning the etiology, perpetuating factors, and self-management. Patients must learn to modify their behaviors and avoid overloading the muscles without resorting to total inactivity (Simons & Simons, 1994). Following the pain control phase, patients should be introduced to therapeutic exercises, movement reeducation, and overall conditioning. Too often, patients with chronic myofascial pain dysfunction are introduced too soon to isotonic training and conditioning, causing further aggravation of active trigger points and increase of pain and dysfunction. Likewise, work hardening programs should never be conducted during this phase of treatment. This can lead to further discouragement and depression, as well as an increase in pain. On the other hand, the pain control phase must be time limited, and patients must understand that progressing to the conditioning phase is imperative. If they do not move beyond the pain control phase, patients can be restricted in their functional abilities and be at greater risk of reinjury (Saal & Saal, 1991). In daily practice, the various aspects of the rehabilitation process are addressed simultaneously and not treated as separate entities.

MANUAL THERAPY

Manual therapy is one of the basic treatment options for MPS. In conjunction with manual therapy approaches, Simons, Travell, and Simons (1999) advocate the stretch and spray technique, which combines use of a vapocoolant spray with passive stretching of the muscle. Application of vapocoolant spray stimulates thermal and tactile A-beta skin receptors, thereby inhibiting C-fiber and A-delta fiber afferent nociceptive pathways and muscle spasms, MTrPs, and pain when stretching. Prior to applying the stretch and spray method, the patient is positioned comfortably. The muscle involved is sprayed with a few sweeps of a vapocoolant spray, after which the muscle is stretched passively. With the muscle in the stretched position, the spray is applied again over the skin overlying the entire muscle, starting at the trigger zone and proceeding in the direction of, and including, the referred pain zone. Following the stretch and spray, the area is heated with a moist heat pack for 5 to 10 min. The patient is encouraged to move the body part several times through the full range of motion. The stretch and spray technique can be used in physical therapy as a separate modality or following MTrP injections. In the United States, Fluori-Methane (Gebauer Chemical Co., 9410 St. Catherine Avenue, Cleveland, OH 44104) has been used, whereas in Europe the use of liquid nitrogen or ethyl chloride is the norm (Dejung, 1988a). Fluori-methane is being replaced due to its potentially damaging effects on the ozone layer. An environmentally safe substitute is being prepared.

Lewit (1991) suggests using the stretch technique for short or taut muscles and fascia, while promoting postisometric relaxation for treatment of trigger points. Postisometric relaxation is also known as muscle energy technique (Mitchell, 1993) or hold–relax technique (Knott & Voss, 1968) and can easily be combined with stretch and spray techniques either in the clinic or as part of the patient's home program. The muscle is gently lengthened,

taking up the slack until a barrier is reached. The patient is then asked to contract the muscle isometrically against resistance for about 10 s at approximately 10% of maximal effort. Because it is difficult for patients to gauge a level of effort, the clinician presents a force against which the patient pushes. The patient is instructed, "Meet my force, but do not exceed it." Thus, the clinician is in complete control of the effort exerted by the patient, and an appropriately slight contraction of muscle is achieved. Then the patient relaxes the muscle. Once total relaxation is achieved, the slack is taken up again and the process is repeated for three to five times (Lewit, 1991; Lewit & Simons, 1984; Simons & Simons, 1994). Respiratory facilitation of muscle relaxation utilizes the contraction of nonrespiratory muscles that occurs with inspiration and the relaxation of the same muscles during expiration. During the relaxation phase, the patient is asked to exhale and look down to facilitate muscular relaxation (Lewit, 1988). A variation on Lewit's approach combines isometric contractions, reciprocal inhibition, and stretch (Fischer, 1995).

Soft tissue mobilization is an essential component of the treatment. Soft tissue biomechanics including stress–strain patterns; the normal inflammatory, repair, and remodeling stages following soft tissue injury (Carlstedt & Nordin, 1989; Nolan & Nordhoff, 1996; Soderberg, 1992); the reactivity of the tissues; and tolerance level and comfort of the patient are considered (Ellis & Johnson, 1996). The intratissue (muscle tone) and intertissue mobility (muscle play) of the structures involved and of the adjacent muscles, fascia, and joints must be evaluated and treated as well. Myofascial adhesions may develop with secondary or "satellite" trigger points in nearby muscles. MTrPs appearing in muscles that are part of a functional unit must be treated together. Muscles that work together as agonists, or that work in opposition to each other as antagonists, constitute a functional muscle unit. The same muscles can be related to each other both as agonists and antagonists, depending on the action being performed. For example, the muscles that move or stabilize the shoulder form a functional unit. The trapezius and levator scapula muscles display this relationship well. These two muscles work together as agonists in elevation of the shoulder, but are antagonists in rotation of the scapula, the trapezius rotating the glenoid fossa upward and the levator scapula rotating it downward. When one of these two muscles contracts to rotate the scapula, the other must relax. If these or some other shoulder muscles become dysfunctional, because of the presence of MTrPs that weaken or shorten them and restrict their range of motion, excessive loading on other muscles in the shoulder functional unit may occur. Trigger points in the levator scapula limit upward rotation of the lateral border of the scapula, thereby placing a greater load on the trapezius, which is unable to accomplish the movement with usual effort, or perhaps is not able to accomplish the movement at all, causing a compensatory lifting of the entire shoulder to raise the arm.

The functional relationships of muscles may differ at each end of the muscle, because the agonists and antagonists for each muscle may be different at the proximal and distal ends of the muscle. MTrPs may spread from one region to another because of these relationships. Bilateral axial muscles like the trapezius, sternocleidomastoid, quadratus lumborum, and iliopsoas act as both agonists and antagonists to each other, facilitating the spread of MTrPs across the midline. Muscles that bridge regions, like the latissimus dorsi, and those that influence posture, like the effect of the iliopsoas or quadratus lumborum muscles on scoliosis, also facilitate the spread of MTrPs. Thus, MPS can involve a single region of the body or it can spread to involve all four quadrants of the body. Effective treatment should address all the affected areas. Otherwise, remaining dysfunctional muscle units may lead to the recurrence of active or spontaneously painful MTrPs.

Myofascial release techniques and gentle, sustained pressure may soften or elongate shortened or hardened muscles. The principle of the least possible force is applied, instead of applying high stress to the muscle. Effective myofascial release techniques include strumming, perpendicular and oscillating mobilizations, tissue rolling, and connective tissue massage, among others (Cantu & Grodin, 2001; Ellis & Johnson, 1996). Deep muscle massage consisting of effleurage (stroking massage technique) and pétrissage (kneading massage technique) is also recommended (Lehn, 1990; Vis, Raats, & Van der Voort, 1987). After the introductory superficial approach over the entire muscle and adjacent muscles, massage therapy can be applied directly to the taut band and trigger points. Massage and exercise were found to be effective in reducing the number and intensity of trigger points, but the addition of therapeutic ultrasound did not improve the outcome (Gam, et al., 1998).

Soft tissue mobilizations may result in improved local circulation, normalization of muscle tone and muscle play, and reduction of reflex activity and pain (Vis et al., 1987; Wells, 1994). By combining gentle approaches with more aggressive techniques, the Swiss physician and psychologist Dejung (1988a) has developed a seven-step treatment approach to myofascial dysfunction. Dejung's approach combines sustained compression, stretch and spray techniques, myofascial release, restoration of muscle play, active and passive movements, and dry needling (Dejung, 1987a, 1988b; Grosjean & Dejung, 1990). As part of Dejung's protocol, the patient actively moves the involved muscle, while the physician or therapist maintains constant pressure over the trigger point (Dejung, 1987b, 1994).

Simons, et al. (1999) also describe direct manual compression of the trigger point to inactivate trigger points.

Although it previously has been described as *ischemic compression*, it is now termed *trigger point pressure release* or *trigger point compression*. The patient can apply direct compression for self-treatment using a Thera Cane® (Thera Cane Co., P.O. Box 9220, Denver, CO 80209; Phone 800–947–1470) or a similar device. Acupressure may be another form of direct compression of trigger points (Kodratoff & Gaebler, 1993). Following the Simons et al. protocol or using acupressure guidelines, compression of trigger points is moderately painful. In contrast with these relatively gentle compression techniques, Tsujii (1993) suggests using at least 10 to 20 kg of force over the trigger point and 50 to 60 kg in chronic cases with a strong elbow pressure technique. He presumes that successful treatment of chronic muscle pain is dependent on opioid-induced analgesia and that only intermittent painful stimuli for more than 30 min produce such analgesia. Because Tsujii's approach results in tissue damage, treatments are scheduled with at least 10 days in between appointments to allow the tissues involved to heal prior to the next application.

Trigger points may also be directly related to underlying articular dysfunction (Ellis & Johnson, 1996). In the treatment of myofascial pain, the practitioner must evaluate and, when indicated, treat both soft tissue and joint dysfunction. Muscular and joint dysfunction are closely related and should be considered as a single functional unit (Janda, 1994). Restrictions in joint capsules inhibit muscle function for those muscles overlying the particular joint. Conversely, muscle dysfunction results in joint capsule restrictions (Dvořák & Dvořák, 1990; Warmerdam, 1992). Zygopophyseal joints may have referred pain patterns similar to MTrPs (Bogduk & Simons, 1993; Dwyer, Aprill, & Bogduk, 1990; McCall, Park, & O'Brien, 1979). In addition, Butler (2000) suggests that impaired mechanics and physiology of the nervous system may be another contributing factor in the overall etiology of various pain problems, including myofascial pain. Somatic dysfunction affecting muscle and joint may result in restricted range of motion and weakness that can be rather quickly reversed by manual therapy.

INVASIVE INACTIVATION OF THE MYOFASCIAL TRIGGER POINT

Inactivation of the MTrP by injection appears to be the result of the mechanical action of the needle in the trigger point itself, because it can be successfully accomplished by dry needling without the use of local anesthetics or other materials (Chu, 1995; Gunn, Milbrandt, Little, & Mason, 1980; Hong, 1994b). When using injection needles, the use of a local anesthetic is more comfortable for many patients and results in a longer lasting reduction in trigger point pain (Hong, 1994b; Travell, 1976). The use of solid acupuncture needles vs. injection needles has not been examined at this time. After identifying and manually stabilizing the tender area in the taut band with the fingers, the needle is quickly passed through the skin and then into the trigger zone. A local twitch response or a report of referred pain indicates that the trigger zone has been entered. A small amount, usually 0.1 or 0.2 ml, of local anesthetic may be injected into the trigger zone. The needle is withdrawn to just below the skin, the angle of the needle is changed, and the needle is again passed through the muscle to another trigger zone. A conical volume of muscle can thus be examined for active trigger points without withdrawing the needle through the skin. The trigger zone is explored in this manner until no further local twitch responses are obtained. At this point, the taut band is usually gone, and the spontaneous pain of the trigger point has subsided. Patients who have previously undergone treatment can tell when trigger points remain, and when they have been sufficiently inactivated. A knowledgeable patient urges the clinician to continue in an area until a key trigger point is inactivated, at which time there is a noticeable decrease in pain. The process is repeated until the symptomatic MTrPs are treated throughout the functional muscle unit (Hendler, Fink, & Long, 1983; Hong, 1993, 1994a).

Trigger point injections can be performed without anesthetic, so-called dry needling, or with a local anesthetic (Hong, 1994b). Historically, procaine has been used for this purpose, although lidocaine is also commonly used today. Procaine, in a dilute solution of 0.5%, has a short half-life, which is an advantage if the anesthetic solution spreads between tissue planes and produces a nerve block. Other local anesthetics, such as bupivicaine and etidocaine, are also used, but no study has been conducted to determine whether the longer duration of action of these latter drugs offers any therapeutic advantage. Glucocorticosteroids and ketorolac have also been used in MTrP injections, but they too have not been the subject of controlled studies comparing their effectiveness against either local anesthetic or dry needling. Steroids have the disadvantage that they are locally myotoxic and that repeated administration of steroids can produce all the unwanted side effects associated with them. Saline or dry needling can be performed on persons allergic to local anesthetics. Botulinum toxin has been tried successfully in MTrP inactivation, although it can cause a flulike myalgia lasting days to a week, and occasionally weakness beyond the area of injection (Cheshire, Abashian, & Mann, 1994; Childers, 1999; Childers, et al., 1998; Yue, 1995).

There is no limit to the number of MTrP that can be needled. Common sense and patient comfort dictate restraint. Nevertheless, when treating a regional MPS, a sufficient number of muscles in the region must be treated to resolve the problem and allow effective postneedling stretching. All the muscles in a functional muscle unit

must be released and returned to full length, if possible, either by needling or by trigger point compression and stretching. Inadequate treatment that leaves critical trigger points within a functional muscle unit usually results in the recurrence of trigger points throughout the muscles of the functional unit. Five to ten different MTrP sites can readily be treated per session, and some physicians skilled in MPS management treat considerably more in one session. Repeat injections or dry needling into the same area are best done after an interval of 1 week to allow the muscle to recover. Muscles of the affected functional unit must always be stretched, to their full length if possible, after MTrP needling. Moist heat is applied to the muscle to improve the local circulation and to reduce postinjection soreness. Otherwise, MTrPs recur because of residual significant muscle dysfunction. Local anesthetic patches can be applied to reduce the superficial or cutaneous soreness from needling. Complications of MTrP injections are listed in Table 21.2.

Trigger point injections or dry needling are a highly effective way to reduce the local pain and contraction of the taut band. This does not, however, constitute the whole treatment of MPS. The causes that led to the condition must be corrected, when possible. Mechanical, medical, and psychological perpetuating factors must also be eliminated or alleviated to reduce the chance of recurrence. Inadequate attention to these aspects of treatment leads to failure to relieve the pain (Table 21.3).

TABLE 21.2
Complications of Trigger Point Injections

1. Local hemorrhage into muscle
2. Local edema
3. Painful contraction of a taut band from inadequate MTrP inactivation (missing the MTrP)
4. Infection
5. Perforation of a viscus, most commonly the lung
6. Nerve injury from direct trauma by the needle
7. Transient nerve block
8. Syncope
9. Allergic reaction from the anesthetic

TABLE 21.3
Causes of Trigger Point Injection Failure

1. Missing the trigger point
2. Injecting the secondary or satellite trigger point and not the primary trigger point
3. Inadequate stretching of the muscle following the injection in the clinic
4. Inadequate stretching of the muscle by the patient at home
5. Failure to correct perpetuating factors

Acupuncture is used to treat many different types of pain, including myofascial pain (Baldry, 1993). Acupuncture can be performed by the traditional method of using predetermined acupuncture points along set meridians or by the more recently developed method of placing the needle close to the point of pain (Liao, Lee, & Ng, 1994). Japanese acupuncture (shallow needling) reduced the pain of chronic myofascial neck pain in one study (Birch & Jamison, 1998). Baldry (1993) has developed a technique of subdermal needling over the trigger point, while Gunn, Milbrandt, Little, and Mason (1980) and Gunn, Sola, Loeser, and Chapman (1990) use a method of dry needling called intramuscular stimulation (IMS). IMS involves the insertion of the needle into the taut band without necessarily considering the actual trigger point. It may be combined with electrical stimulation delivered through the needle (percutaneous electroneural stimulation).

MECHANICAL PERPETUATING FACTORS

Biomechanical perpetuating factors have long been known to cause persistent musculoskeletal pain (Simons et al., 1999; Travell & Simons, 1992). Major mechanical factors to be considered in the management of MPS include anatomic variations, poor posture, and work-related stress (Simons & Simons, 1994).

CORRECTION OF ANATOMIC VARIATIONS

According to Simons et al. (1999), the most common anatomic variations are leg length discrepancy and small hemipelvis, the short upper arm syndrome, and the long second metatarsal syndrome.

The leg length inequality syndrome produces a pelvic tilt that results in a chronic shortening and activation of a chain of muscles in an effort to straighten the head and level the eyes. Any asymmetrical position of the pelvis or spine requires a regulatory adjustment of the neck muscles to maintain equilibrium and an appropriate head position (Janda, 1994). The quadratus lumborum and paraspinal muscles contract to correct the deviation of the spine caused by the pelvic tilt. This correction in turn causes a tilt of the shoulder in the direction opposite to that of the pelvic tilt when a simple C-shaped scoliosis occurs. The shoulder and neck muscles then chronically contract and shorten to correct the subsequent neck tilt. Excessive loading perpetuates MTrPs and may result in low back, head, neck, and shoulder pain (Gerwin, 1995a). Trigger points in these chronically shortened and constantly contracted muscles are not readily inactivated until the muscles are unloaded. The combination of trunk muscles that undergo shortening as they constantly pull the spine toward one side or the other is more complex in an S-shaped scoliosis, but the problem is the same. A similar loading of trunk, shoulder, and neck muscles occurs when one hemipelvis

has a diminished height relative to the other or in the presence of pelvic obliquity. According to Grieve (1994), the quadratus lumborum may be less likely to develop trigger points during the teenage years, and typically, unilateral low back pain is located on the side of the shorter leg, because of early attenuation of the annulus fibrosis on that side. In adults, it occurs on the side of the longer leg, due to later arthrotic and spondylotic changes and shortening of the quadratus lumborum. A true leg length discrepancy is corrected by placing a heel lift on the shorter leg. The asymmetry caused by a small hemipelvis is corrected by placing an ischial or "butt" lift under the ischial tuberosity.

A distinction must be made between a true and an apparent leg length discrepancy. An apparent leg length discrepancy or functional shortening may be caused by a pseudo-scoliosis where the legs are actually of equal or nearly equal length, by hip adductor contractures, by hip capsule tightness, or by posterior innominate rotation, because the acetabulum is anterior to the iliosacral rotation axis (LeVeau, 1994; Mitchell, 1993; Reid, 1992). The cause must be identified and then corrected where possible. If the problem is an ilial rotation, the rotation should be corrected. If it is combined with a sacroiliac joint dysfunction, that should be corrected as well. Quadratus lumborum or iliopsoas muscles shortened by trigger points, a cause of pseudo-scoliosis, must be inactivated by stretching or by other means, such as MTrP injections. Placing a heel lift under an apparent shorter leg may increase the leg length discrepancy. Functional shortening, pseudo-scoliosis, and pelvic obliquity can be corrected via osteopathic mobilizations and muscle energy techniques (Fowler, 1994; Greenman, 1991).

When clinical determination by physical examination is uncertain, a radiographic study of the pelvis and lumbar spine utilizing a plumb line can be useful (Travell & Simons, 1992). A functional scoliosis can be corrected or reduced by a heel lift, even if it has been present for years. A fixed skeletal cause of scoliosis does not correct with a heel or butt lift. Functional scoliosis must be distinguished from those asymmetries that cannot be corrected before attempting to use a heel or butt lift. Relief of pain in the neck, shoulder, low back, and legs can result from the complete or partial correction of leg length inequality and scoliosis.

Saggini, et al. (1996) describe the incomplete resolution of pain in persons with peroneus longus MTrPs and leg length inequality corrected only by a heel lift. The peroneus longus has an increased shear force in the medial-lateral plane when loading, which increases eccentric muscle involvement, leading to muscle injury. Correcting abnormal loading associated with leg length discrepancy with a dynamic insole eliminated both the pain and the trigger points.

Short upper arms result in forward shoulder roll, pectoral muscle shortening, and abnormal loading of neck and trunk muscles, as the individual attempts to find a comfortable position when seated. Another cause of biomechanical stress on muscles that can lead to the persistence of MTrPs is a long second metatarsal bone. In this situation, the normal, stable tripod support of the foot created by the first and second metatarsal bones anteriorly and the heel posteriorly may not be present. Instead, in some individuals with this foot configuration, weight is carried on a knife edge from the second metatarsal head to the heel, overloading the peroneus longus that attaches to the first metatarsal bone. Diagnostic callus formation occurs in these individuals in the areas of abnormal loading, under the second metatarsal head, and on the medial aspect of the foot at the great toe and first metatarsal head. Correction is accomplished with support under the head of the first metatarsal, restoring the normal tripod support of the foot (Travell & Simons, 1992).

POSTURE CORRECTION

In addition to postural deviations due to anatomic variations, muscle imbalances and altered movement patterns play an extremely important role in the etiology and management of poor posture. The clinician should become familiar with Vladimir Janda's extensive research in posture and muscle dysfunction. Janda distinguished "tonic or postural" muscles from "phasic or dynamic" muscles. Postural and phasic muscles are physiologically different in their oxidative ability and their ability to contract over a specified time period. Tonic muscles are slow twitch (Type I) muscles. Phasic muscles are fast twitch (Type II) muscles. MTrPs can develop in both tonic and phasic muscles. Tonic muscles include the hamstrings muscles, rectus femoris, iliopsoas, quadratus lumborum, erector spinae muscles, pectorals, sternocleidomastoids, descending trapezius muscles, and levator scapulae. Phasic muscles include the rectus abdominus, serratus anterior, rhomboids, ascending and transverse trapezius, deep neck flexors, suprahyoid, and mylohyoid (Cantu & Grodin, 2001; Carriere, 1996; Janda, 1983, 1993, 1994). Tonic muscles have a tendency to tighten in response to abnormal stress or dysfunction, whereas phasic muscles have a tendency to become weak. These typical response patterns result in the "upper and lower crossed syndromes" (Janda, 1993, 1994). The upper crossed syndrome or forward head posture is the most common postural deviation in patients with MPS (Fricton, et al., 1985; Janda, 1994; Mannheimer, 1994).

In the forward head posture, total body alignment is severely affected. There is posterior cervical rotation with hypomobility of the upper cervical and subcranial motion segments and hypermobility of the mid and lower cervical spine. Muscle imbalances occur between the anterior and posterior cervical muscles and between the anterior and posterior shoulder muscles. The shoulder girdle protracts, and there is an increase in thoracic kyphosis, a loss of lumbar lordosis, and an increase in posterior pelvic rotation. Muscular imbalances may lead to abnormal afferent input and MTrPs (Cantu & Grodin, 2001). There is a statistically significant relation between the degree of forward head posture, posterior cervical rotation, and pain (Haughie, Fiebert, & Roach, 1995). Poor body alignment, forward head posture, and muscle imbalances predispose and perpetuate chronic pain problems including MPS.

Correcting poor body posture and alignment is an important component of treating patients with MPS, even when posture seemingly may not be directly related to the region of musculoskeletal pain. Core (trunk) stabilization as part of a closed kinetic chain rehabilitation allows optimal control of the lumbopelvic complex and improves the recovery of persons with a kinetic chain dysfunction manifest as a postural stress syndrome (Clark, Fater, & Reuteman, 2000). Good posture minimizes stress and improves efficiency in the use of muscles (Sahrmann, 1988). The physical therapist needs to determine on an individual basis whether manual therapy procedures should precede postural corrections or vice versa. In some instances, joint and myofascial restrictions must be removed prior to any postural corrections. Without the mobilizations, shortened muscles may restrict movement so much that treatment to correct postural abnormalities may not succeed. In other cases, patients may be able to alter their posture prior to or even without any manual therapy (Dommerholt & Norris, 1996).

Correction and prevention of abnormal postures requires a comprehensive program that includes exercises to restore normal dynamic pelvic and vertebral stabilization and mobility, motor control, muscle balances, strength, endurance, and breathing patterns. Certain activities of daily living may predispose a patient to chronic musculoskeletal overload, increasing the risk of myofascial dysfunction. A dynamically stable trunk in neutral position is essential, as is normal pelvic mobility (Carriere, 1996). Paradoxical breathing should be corrected with functional abdominal breathing. Paradoxical breathing is a common cause of overload of the auxiliary breathing muscles, most notably the scalene muscles (Travell & Simons, 1983; Carriere, 1996). To improve posture, the individual components must be integrated into total motor patterns (Walpin, 1994). Both the Alexander technique (Barlow, 1973; Jones, 1992; Knebelman, et al., 1994) and the Feldenkrais method (Feldenkrais, 1977; Rywerant, 1983) aim to restore function to body awareness and movement retraining and can be used in combination with physical therapy (Dommerholt, 2000).

Although posture is usually described in terms of relative alignment of body parts, it is important to realize that a person's posture reflects more than just biomechanical principles. Buytendijk (1964) states that "posture is an individual's innermost means of expression." People express their emotions, feelings, and overall well-being through their posture. Therefore, posture must be viewed as a physiological, biomechanical, and psychological phenomenon. Addressing biomechanical issues without consideration of a more phenomenological approach to posture reduces the treatment approach to strict mechanistic intervention.

WORK-RELATED STRESS

Certain jobs and work-related activities are associated with an increased risk of developing cumulative trauma disorders or work-related musculoskeletal disorders (Kuorinka & Forcier, 1995). In certain instances, MPS may be associated with work exposures (Grosshandler & Burney, 1979). In the ergonomics literature, the term *tension neck syndrome* is preferred over MPS (Viikari-Juntura, 1983). Ergonomics is a broad profession and incorporates knowledge from anatomy, physiology, and psychology. More specifically, ergonomics includes anthropometry and biomechanics, work and environmental physiology, and skill and occupational psychology (Singleton, 1972). Thompson (1991) defines ergonomics as "the application of the human physical and behavioral sciences together with the engineering sciences in the study of humans working with machines and tools." Ergonomics is based on the so-called human-machine system. In designing the ideal human-machine system, ergonomics recognizes four strategies, namely, stress reduction, machine and task design, match between the job demands and human abilities, and education and training (Ayoub, 1994; Khalil, et al., 1993). Pheasant (1991) summarizes the field as "the science of matching the job to the worker and the product to the user."

Awareness of generic risk factors in work-related musculoskeletal disorders is important. They include awkward postures, musculoskeletal loading, task invariability, cognitive demands, and organizational and psychosocial work characteristics (Kuorinka & Forcier, 1995). Prolonged static postures, awkward postures, excessive force, and repetitiveness are the most likely specific risk factors for MPS (Armstrong, 1986a). Several studies have confirmed that occupational groups with repetitive arm movements and constrained work postures have high rates of MPS (Amano, et al., 1988; Bjelle, Hagberg, & Michaelsson, 1979; Hünting, Läubli, & Grandjean, 1981). Awkward postures include wrist flexion and extension, ulnar and radial abduction, forearm supination and pronation, extended reaches beyond the shoulder-reach envelope, and pinch grips that are either too wide or too narrow (Armstrong, 1986b; Feuerstein & Hickey, 1992). For example, the intramuscular pressure in the supraspinatus muscle exceeds 30 mmHg at 30 degrees flexion or abduction,

resulting in impairment of blood circulation, mechanical overload of the muscles and adjacent muscles, and increased risk for myofascial pain (Järvholm, et al., 1988). Particular occupational groups at increased risk include data entry operators, typists (Hünting, et al., 1981), musicians (Norris & Dommerholt, 1996), teachers and nurses (Onishi, et al., 1976), and industrial and assembly line workers (Amano, et al., 1988; Silverstein, 1985).

Considering work-related aspects of myofascial pain enhances treatment outcomes. Modifying the workplace or the patient's work habits is critical. If a patient continues to be exposed to certain workplace stress factors without modification of the conditions, the potential cause of myofascial dysfunction may not be addressed adequately. Physical therapists and occupational therapists can contribute significantly to integrating basic ergonomic principles into therapeutic practice, although specific training in ergonomics is indicated (Berg Rice, 1995). More complicated ergonomic problems require the assistance of ergonomists (Ayoub, 1994; Khalil, et al., 1994).

SYSTEMIC MEDICAL FACTORS

The problem of unresolved or persistent MTrPs can be the result of systemic medical factors that affect muscle metabolism primarily or affect muscle function secondarily. These factors can be categorized broadly as nutritional, hormonal, metabolic, infectious, autoimmune, etc. An important principle that Janet Travell often emphasized in her lectures is that insufficiency states impair the ability of stressed or overloaded muscle to respond adequately to therapy. Levine and Hartzell (1987) have applied this concept to vitamin C insufficiency. They propose that the optimum concentration of an enzyme cofactor (vitamin or mineral) is that which allows each enzymatic reaction to proceed maximally (not rate limited) when required. For example, many vitamin or mineral enzyme cofactors, such as ascorbic acid (vitamin C) or iron, participate in a number of different enzymatic reactions that are not all equally active at any one time. However, if a limited concentration of an enzyme cofactor becomes rate limiting, then the products of the associated reaction may be insufficient, like the underproduction of high-energy organic phosphates for certain iron-dependent enzymes or the underproduction of serotonin or norepinephrine for certain vitamin-C-dependent enzymes. It is postulated that the needs of the body under physical stress are different than when unstressed and what may be an adequate concentration of enzyme cofactor under normal conditions may be insufficient at times of physical stress. Hence, the concept of nutritional insufficiency states is distinguished from that of disease-producing deficiency states like scurvy, the disease associated with vitamin C deficiency. Vitamin C taken in the amount of

10 mg/day prevents scurvy, but 250 mg/day is considered the optimum daily intake for good health.

Four nutritional or hormonal factors have repeatedly been found to be low or in the lower quartile of the normal range in persons studied in our clinic who have persistent myofascial pain, namely, iron insufficiency, folic acid insufficiency, vitamin B12 insufficiency, and thyroid hormone insufficiency. Of women with a chronic sense of coldness and chronic myofascial pain, 65% have a low normal or below normal serum level of ferritin, largely from an iron intake insufficient to replace menstrual iron loss. Other causes of low serum ferritin include blood loss associated with chronic intake of mixed cyclooxygenase (COX)-1 and -2 nonsteroidal anti-inflammatory drugs, and gastrointestinal blood loss associated with parasitic disease. Ferritin represents the tissue-bound nonessential iron stores in the body that supply the essential iron for oxygen transport and iron-dependent enzymes. Serum levels of 15 to 20 ng/ml mean that muscle and other storage sites for iron (liver and bone marrow) are depleted of ferritin. Anemia is common at levels of 10 ng/ml or less. The disease of iron deficiency is anemia. Symptoms of iron insufficiency are fatigue, muscle cramps, and coldness. The association between iron insufficiency and chronic myofascial pain suggests that iron-requiring enzymatic reactions like reduced nicotinamide adenine dinucleotide (NADH) dehydrogenases and the cytochrome oxidase reaction may be limited in such persons. This may in turn produce an energy crisis in muscle when it is overloaded and thereby produce metabolic stress. MTrPs may not easily resolve in such circumstances. Iron supplementation in persons with chronic MPSs and serum ferritin levels below 30 ng/ml prevents or corrects these symptoms.

Vitamin B12 and folic acid metabolism are closely related. They function not only in erythropoiesis but also in central and peripheral nerve formation. Studies have shown that in a subset of patients, serum levels of vitamin B12 as high as 350 pg/ml may be associated with a metabolic deficiency manifested by elevated serum or urine methylmalonic acid or homocysteine and may be clinically symptomatic (Pruthi & Tefferi, 1994). Preliminary studies show that 16% of patients with chronic MPS either were deficient in vitamin B12 or had insufficient levels of vitamin B12, and that 10% had low serum folate levels (Gerwin, 1995b). Replacement of vitamin B12 is lifelong, either orally, transmucosally, or intramuscularly.

Hypothyroidism is suspected clinically in chronic MPS when there is a complaint of coldness, dry skin or dry hair, constipation, and fatigue. Hypothyroidism occurred in 10% of chronic MPS subjects in one study (Gerwin, 1995b). The MTrPs tend to be widespread in hypothyroid persons. The thyroid-stimulating hormone (TSH) level may only be in the upper range of normal, but, as shown by thyroid-releasing hormone (TRH) stimulation tests, may still be abnormal for a given individual.

Thyroid hormone supplementation to restore the thyroid state may resolve many myofascial complaints and allow resolution of the problem by the usual means of physical therapy and trigger point inactivation. Thyroxine (levothyroxine) is generally used to treat hypothyroidism. However, not all tissues are equally able to convert thyroxine to triiodothyronine, the active form of thyroid hormone. The addition of triiodothyronine to thyroxine has been shown to result in an improved sense of well-being; an improvement in cognitive function and mood; and an increase in serum levels of sex-hormone-binding globulins, a sensitive marker of thyroid hormone function (Bunevicius, et al., 1999; Toft, 1999).

Other less commonly associated medical problems that are found in patients with chronic MPS and that act as perpetuating factors include recurrent candida yeast infections, particularly in women who have been given courses of antibiotic therapy for recurrent urinary tract infections. Persons with myofascial pain dysfunction syndromes affecting the temporal mandibular joint often complain of sore throat or earache and may be given antibiotics, thereby predisposing them to candida overgrowth. Women who present with widespread MTrPs resistant to usual treatment should be investigated for candida infection. If the history is very suggestive, treatment is indicated even if the organism cannot be implicated by hanging drop examination or culture. Men and postmenopausal women who have elevated uric acid levels may also have persistent MTrPs. Parasitic infections can also be associated with widespread MTrPs, often complicated by fatigue and an often nonspecific sense of discomfort, and occasionally gastrointestinal distress. Amoebiasis is the most common parasite encountered in MPS in the United States, but giardia, trematode, and nematode infection have also been found. Treatment of these infections results in an overall improvement, and often in a diminution of the extent of trigger point involvement of muscle. Of course, persons with osteoarthritis, rheumatoid arthritis, Sjögren's syndrome, carpal tunnel syndrome, or peripheral neuropathy caused by diabetes mellitus are more prone to develop MTrP. The postlaminectomy syndrome is frequently caused by MTrP. Treatment is always directed toward the underlying condition, as well as the trigger point where possible.

Sleep disturbance can be a major factor in the perpetuation of musculoskeletal pain. Pain is magnified in the presence of insomnia, whether the insomnia is caused by pain or by other factors. There is the rare case in which chronic musculoskeletal pain is eliminated by the restoration of normal sleep when caffeine was reduced or eliminated from the diet. More often, however, sleep must be addressed directly, noting that sleep disturbance is increased in persons with chronic pain. Attention is paid to pain control at night, to sleep apnea, and to mood disorders like depression or anxiety. Management is both pharmacological and nonpharmacological. Pharmacological treatment utilizes drugs that promote a normal sleep architecture, induce and maintain sleep through the night, and do not cause daytime sedation. Nonpharmacological treatment emphasizes sleep hygiene, such as using the bed only for sleep and sex, and not for reading, television viewing, and eating (Menefee, et al., 2000).

Psychological stress may aggravate MPS and activate MTrP (Lewis, et al.,1994; McNulty, et al., 1994). Trigger point EMG activity has been shown to increase dramatically in response to mental and emotional stress, whereas adjacent nontrigger point muscle EMG activity remained normal. Thus, the effect of stress on the trigger point can be highly selective, instead of generalized throughout the muscle. MPS may be the major symptomatic expression of psychological distress. In addition, pain-related fear and avoidance can lead to the development of a chronic musculoskeletal pain problem (Vlaeyen & Linton, 2000). Treatment directed toward reducing stress has been shown to diminish MPS symptoms (Banks, et al., 1998). The clinician must be sensitive to this possibility and refer the patient for psychological counseling when appropriate.

SUMMARY

In summary, treatment of MPS begins with the identification of the MTrP as a source of the pain or as a contributing factor, and a delineation of the extent of the problem. The problem may be confined to a few muscles or may be more widespread, regional, or generalized. Direct inactivation of the MTrP is accompanied by correction of mechanical and systemic medical factors that contribute to the development of the syndrome. Exercise to restore physical conditioning reduces the chances of recurrence. Persons with chronic MPS who have not responded as expected to appropriate therapy must be evaluated for further mechanical, medical, or psychological problems that have been associated with persistent MPS. Attention to the postural and physical stresses of work and awareness of the effect that psychological stress has on muscle pain identify those areas that need to be addressed. These problems must be corrected or alleviated to effectively treat the MPS. Effective treatment can be provided through the application of a variety of manual techniques, by invasive inactivation of the trigger point, and by carefully identifying and correcting the factors that interfered with recovery.

REFERENCES

Amano, M., et al. (1988). Characteristics of work actions of shoe manufacturing assembly line workers and a cross sectional factor control study on occupational cervicobrachial disorders. *Japanese Journal of Industrial Health, 30*(1), 3–12.

Armstrong, T.J. (1986a). Ergonomics and cumulative trauma disorders: Symposium on occupational injuries. *Hand Clinics of North America, 2*(3), 553–565.

Armstrong, T.J. (1986b). Upper extremity posture: Definition, measurement and control. In N. Corlett, J. Wilson, & I. Manenica (Eds.), *The ergonomics of working postures: Models, methods, and cases.* Proceedings of the First International Occupational Ergonomics Symposium, Zadar, Yugoslavia, 1985. London: Taylor & Francis.

Ayoub, M.A. (1994). Ergonomic considerations in the workplace. In C.D. Tollison, J.R. Satterthwaite, & J.W. Tollison (Eds.), *Handbook of pain management* (pp. 640–666). Baltimore: Williams & Wilkins.

Baldry, P.E. (1993). *Acupuncture, trigger points and musculoskeletal pain.* Edinburgh: Churchill Livingstone.

Banks, S.L., et al. (1998). Effects of autogenic relaxation training on electromyographic activity in active myofascial trigger points. *Journal of Musculoskeletal Pain 6*(4), 23–32.

Barlow, W. (1973). The Alexander technique. New York: Alfred A. Knopf.

Berg Rice, V.J. (1995). Ergonomics: An introduction. In K. Jacobs & C.M. Bettencourt (Eds.), *Ergonomics for therapists* (pp. 3–12). Boston: Butterworth-Heinemann.

Birch, S., & Jamison, R.N. (1998). Controlled trial of Japanese acupuncture for chronic myofascial neck pain: Assessment of specific and nonspecific effects of treatment. *Clinical Journal of Pain, 14,* 248–255.

Bjelle, A., Hagberg, M., & Michaelsson, G. (1979). Clinical and ergonomic factors in prolonged shoulder pain among industrial workers. *Scandanavian Journal of Work Environment and Health, 5,* 205–210.

Bogduk, N., & Simons, D.G. (1993). Neck pain: Joint pain or trigger points. In H. Værøy & H. Merskey (Eds.), *Progress in fibromyalgia and myofascial pain* (pp. 267–273). Amsterdam: Elsevier.

Bunevicius, R., et al. (1999). Effects of thyroxine as compared with thyroxine plus triiodothyrinine in patients with hypothyroidism. *New England Journal of Medicine, 340,* 424–429.

Butler, D.S. (2000). *The sensitive nervous system.* Adelaide, Australia: Noigroup publications.

Buytendijk, F.J.J. (1964). *Algemene theorie der menselijke houding en beweging.* Utrecht, The Netherlands: Het Spectrum.

Cantu, R.I., & Grodin, A.J. (2001). *Myofascial manipulation: Theory and clinical application* (2nd ed.). Gaithersburg, MD: Aspen Publishers.

Carlstedt, C.A., & Nordin, M. (1989). Biomechanics of tendons and ligaments. In M. Nordin & V.H. Frank (Eds.), *Basic biomechanics of the musculoskeletal system* (pp. 59–74). Philadelphia: Lea & Febiger.

Carriere, B. (1996). Therapeutic exercise and self-correction programs. In T.W. Flynn (Ed.), *The thoracic spine and rib cage: Musculoskeletal evaluation and treatment* (pp. 287–307). Boston: Butterworth-Heinemann.

Chen, J.-T., et al. (1998). Phentolamine effect on the spontaneous electrical activity of active loci in a myofascial trigger spot of rabbit skeletal muscle. *Archives of Physical and Medical Rehabilitation, 79,* 790–794.

Cheshire, W.P., Abashian, S.W., & Mann, J.D. (1994). Botulinum toxin in the treatment of myofascial pain syndrome. *Pain, 59,* 65–69.

Childers, M.K., et al. (1998). Treatment of painful muscle syndromes with botulinum toxin: A review. *Journal of Back and Musculoskeletal Rehabilitation, 10,* 89–96.

Childers, M.K., Wilson, D.J. & Simison, D. (1999). *Use of botulinum toxin type A in pain management* (pp. 30–50). Columbia, MO: Academic Information Systems.

Chu, J. (1995). Dry needling (intramuscular stimulation) in myofascial pain related to lumbosacral radiculopathy. *European Journal of Physical and Medical Rehabilitation, 5*(4), 106–121

Clark, M.A., Fater, D., & Reuteman, P. (2000). Core (trunk) stabilization and its importance for closed kinetic chain rehabilitation. *Orthopaedic Physical Therapy Clinics of North America, 9*(2), 119–135.

Dejung, B. (1987a). Die Verspannung des M. iliacus als Ursache lumbosacraler Schmerzen. *Manuelle Medizin, 25,* 73–81.

Dejung, B. (1987b). Verspannungen des M. serratus anterior als Ursache interscapularer Schmerzen. *Manuelle Medizin, 25,* 97–102.

Dejung, B. (1988a). Die Behandlung "chronischer Zerrungen." *Schweizerische Zeitschrift fur Sportmedizin, 36,* 16–168.

Dejung, B. (1988b). Triggerpunkt-und Bindegewebebehandlung neue Wege in Physiotherapie und Rehabilitationsmedizin. *Physiotherapeutics, 24*(6), 3–12.

Dejung, B. (1994). Manuelle Triggerpunktbehandlung bei chronischer Lumbosakralgie. *Schweizerische Medizinische Wochenschrift, 124* (Suppl. 62), 82– 87.

Delaney, G.A., & McKee, A.C. (1993). Inter- and intra-rater reliability of the pressure threshold meter in measurement of myofascial trigger point sensitivity. *American Journal of Physical and Medical Rehabilitation, 72,* 136–139.

Dommerholt, J. (2000). Posture. In R. Tubiana & P. Amadio (Eds.), *Medical problems of the instrumentalist musician* (pp. 399–419). London: Martin Dunitz.

Dommerholt, J. (2001). Muscle pain syndromes. In R.I. Cantu and A.J. Grodin (Eds.), *Myofascial manipulation* (pp. 93–140). Gaithersburg: Aspen.

Dommerholt, J., & Norris, R.N. (1996). Physical therapy management of the injured musician. *Orthopaedic Physical Therapy Clinics of North America, 5,* 185–206.

Dvořák, J., & Dvořák, V. (1990). *Manual medicine: Diagnostics.* Stuttgart, Germany: Georg Thieme Verlag.

Dwyer, A., Aprill, C., & Bogduk, N. (1990). Cervical zygopophyseal joint pain patterns. 1. A study in normal volunteers. *Spine, 15*(6), 453–457.

Ellis, J.J., & Johnson, G.S. (1996). Myofascial considerations in somatic dysfunction of the thorax. In T.W. Flynn (Ed.), *The thoracic spine and rib cage* (pp. 211–262). Boston: Butterworth-Heinemann.

Feldenkrais, M. (1977). *Awareness through movement.* New York: Harper and Row.

Feuerstein, M., & Hickey, P.F. (1992). Ergonomic approaches in the clinical assessment of occupational musculoskeletal disorders. In D.C. Turk & R. Melzack (Eds.), *Handbook of pain assessment* (pp. 71–99). New York: The Guilford Press.

Fischer, A.A. (1984). Diagnosis and management of chronic pain in physical medicine and rehabilitation. In A.P. Ruskin (Ed.), *Current therapy in psychiatry* (pp. 123–145). Philadelphia: W. B. Saunders.

Fischer, A.A. (1986a). Pressure threshold measurement for diagnosis of myofascial pain and evaluation of treatment results. *Clinical Journal of Pain, 2*(4), 207–214.

Fischer, A.A. (1986b). Pressure threshold meter: Its use for quantification of tender spots. *Archives of Physical and Medical Rehabilitation, 67,* 836–838.

Fischer, A.A. (1986c). Pressure tolerance over muscles and bones in normal subjects. *Archives of Physical and Medical Rehabilitation, 67,* 406–409.

Fischer, A.A. (1993). *Pressure threshold and tolerance meter* (manual). Great Neck, NY: Pain Diagnostics & Thermography.

Fischer, A.A. (1995). Local injections in pain management; trigger point needling with infiltration and somatic blocks. In G.H. Kraft & S.M. Weinstein (Eds.), *Injection techniques: Principles and practice* (pp. 851–870). Philadelphia: W. B. Saunders.

Fischer, A.A. (1997). New developments in diagnosis of myofascial pain and fibromyalgia. *Physical Medicine and Rehabilitation Clinics of North America, 8*(1), 1–21.

Fowler, C. (1994). Muscle energy techniques for pelvic dysfunction. In J.D. Boyling & N. Palastanga (Eds.), *Grieve's modern manual therapy* (pp. 781–791). Edinburgh: Churchill Livingstone.

Fricton, J. R. (1990). Myofascial pain syndrome: Characteristics and epidemiology. *Advances in Pain Research and Therapy, 17,* 107–128.

Fricton, J.R., Kroening, R., Haley, D., et al. (1985). Myofascial pain syndrome of the head and neck: A review of clinical characteristics of 164 patients. *Oral Surgery, Oral Medicine, and Oral Pathology, 60*(10), 615–623.

Gam, A.N., et al. (1998). Treatment of myofascial trigger point with ultrasound combined with massage and exercise in a randomized controlled trial. *Pain, 77,* 73–79.

Gerwin, R. (1995a). Myofascial back and neck pain. In M.A. Young & R.A. Lavin (Eds.), *Physical medicine and rehabilitation state of the art reviews* (Vol. 9, pp. 657–671). Philadelphia: Hanley & Belfus.

Gerwin, R. (1995b). A study of 96 subjects examined both for fibromyalgia and myofascial pain. *Journal of Musculoskeletal Pain, 3*(Suppl. 1), 121.

Gerwin, R.D., et al. (1997). Interrater reliability in myofascial trigger point examination. *Pain, 69,* 65–73.

Gerwin R.D. (1999). Differential diagnosis of myofascial pain syndrome and fibromyalgia. *Journal of Musculoskeletal Pain 7,* 209–215.

Gerwin, R.D. (2000). Management of persons with chronic pain. In M.N. Ozer (Ed) *Management of persons with chronic neurologic illness* (pp. 265–290) Boston: Butterworth-Heinemann.

Ghia, J.N. (1992). Development and organization of pain centers. In P. P. Raj (Ed.), *Practical management of pain* (pp. 16–39). St. Louis: Mosby-Year Book.

Greenman, P.E. (1991). Osteopathic manipulation of the lumbar spine and pelvis. In A.H. White & R. Anderson (Eds.), *Conservative care of low back pain* (pp. 200–215). Baltimore: Williams & Wilkins.

Grieve, G.P. (1994). The masqueraders. In J.D. Boyling & N. Palastanga (Eds.), *Grieve's modern manual therapy* (pp. 841–856). Edinburgh: Churchill Livingstone.

Grosjean, B., & Dejung, B. (1990). Achillodynie ein unlosbäres Problem? *Schweizerische Zeitschrift für Sportmedizin, 38*, 17–24.

Grosshandler, S., & Burney, R. (1979). The myofascial pain syndrome. *North Carolina Medical Journal, 40*, 562–565.

Gunn, C.C., Milbrandt, W.E., Little, A.S., & Mason, K.E. (1980). Dry needling of muscle motor points for chronic low-back pain. *Spine, 5*, 279–291.

Gunn, C.C., Sola, A.E., Loeser, J.D., & Chapman, C.R. (1990). Dry-needling for chronic musculoskeletal pain syndromes clinical observations. *Acupuncture, 1*, 9–15. .

Harden, R.N., et al. (2000). Signs and symptoms of the myofascial pain syndrome: A national survey of pain management providers. *Clinical Journal of Pain, 16*, 64–72.

Haughie, L.J., Fiebert, I.M., & Roach, K.E. (1995). Relationship of forward head posture and cervical backward bending to neck pain. *Journal of Manual and Manipulative Therapy, 3*(3), 91–97.

Hendler, N., Fink, H., & Long, D. (1983). Myofascial syndrome: Response to trigger-point injections. *Psychosomatics, 24*, 990–999.

Higgs, J., & Jones, M. (1995). Clinical reasoning. In J. Higgs & M. Jones (Eds.), *Clinical reasoning in the health professions* (pp. 3–23). Oxford: Butterworth-Heinemann.

Hong, C.-Z. (1993). Myofascial trigger point injection. *Critical Reviews in Physical Medicine and Rehabilitation, 5*(2) 203–217.

Hong, C.-Z. (1994a). Considerations and recommendations regarding myofascial trigger point injection. *Journal of Musculoskeletal Pain, 2*, 29–59.

Hong, C.-Z. (1994b). Lidocaine injection versus dry needling to myofascial trigger point. *American Journal of Physical and Medical Rehabilitation, 73*, 256–263.

Hubbard, D.R., & Berkoff, G.M. (1993). Myofascial trigger points show spontaneous needle EMG activity. *Spine, 18*, 1803–1807.

Hünting, W., Läubli, T., & Grandjean, E. (1981). Postural and visual loads at VDT workplace. 1. Constrained postures. *Ergonomics, 24*(12), 917–931.

Jaeger, B., & Reeves, J.L. (1986). Quantification of changes in myocardial trigger point sensitivity with the pressure algometer following passive stretch. *Pain, 27*, 203–210.

Janda, V. (1983). Muscle function testing. London: Butterworths.

Janda, V. (1991). Muscle spasm: A proposed procedure for differential diagnosis. *Journal of Manual Medicine, 6*, 136–139.

Janda, V. (1993). Muscle strength in relation to muscle length, pain, and muscle imbalance. In K. Harms-Rindahl (Ed.), *Muscle strength* (pp. 83–91). New York: Churchill Livingstone.

Janda, V. (1994). Muscles and motor control in cervicogenic disorders: Assessment and management. In R. Grant (Ed.), *Physical therapy of the cervical and thoracic spine* (pp. 195–216). New York: Churchill Livingstone.

Järvholm, U., et al. (1988). Intramuscular pressure in the supraspinatus muscle. *Journal of Orthopaedic Research, 6*, 230–238.

Jensen, K., et al. (1986). Pressure pain threshold in human temporal pain. Evaluation of a new pressure algometer. *Pain, 25*, 313–323.

Jones, F.P. (1992). Body awareness in action. In M. Murphy (Ed.), *The future of the body*. Los Angeles: Jeremy P. Tarcher.

Jones, M.A. (1994). Clinical reasoning process in manipulative therapy. In J. D. Boyling & N. Palastanga (Eds.), *Grieve's modern manual therapy* (pp. 471–482). Edinburgh: Churchill Livingstone.

Keele, K.D. (1954). Pain-sensitivity tests: Pressure algometers. *Lancet, 1*, 636–639.

Khalil, T.M., et al. (1993). *Ergonomics in back pain*. New York: Van Nostrand Reinhold.

Khalil, T.M., et al. (1994). The role of ergonomics in the prevention and treatment of myofascial pain. In E. S. Rachlin (Ed.), *Myofascial pain and fibromyalgia: Trigger point management* (pp. 487–523). St. Louis: Mosby-Year Book.

Knebelman, S., Ralson Dressler, P., Mathews Brion, M., et al. (1994). The essentials of the Alexander technique. In H. Gelb (Ed.), *New concepts in craniomandibular and chronic pain management* (pp. 177–185). London: Mosby-Wolfe.

Knott, M., & Voss, D.E. (1968). *Proprioceptive neuromuscular facilitation*. New York: Hoeber.

Kodratoff, Y., & Gaebler, T. (1993). *Meridian shiatsu*. Basel: Sphinx Verlag.

Kuorinka, I., & Forcier, L. (1995). *Work related musculoskeletal disorders (WMSDs): A reference book for prevention*. Bristol: Taylor & Francis.

Lehn, C. (1990). Massage. In W.E. Prentice (Ed.), *Therapeutic modalities in sports medicine* (pp. 257–285). St. Louis: Times Mirror/Mosby.

LeVeau, B. (1994). Hip. In J.K. Richardson & Z.A. Iglarsh (Eds.), *Clinical orthopaedic physical therapy* (pp. 333–398). Philadelphia: W.B. Saunders.

Levine, M., & Hartzell, W. (1987). Ascorbic acid: The concept of optimum requirements. Third Conference on Vitamin C. *Annals of the New York Academy of Science, 498*, 424–444.

Lewis, C., et al. (1994). Needle trigger point and surface frontal EMG measurements of psychophysiological responses in tension-type headache patients. *Biofeedback and Self-Regulation, 3*, 274–275.

Lewit, K. (1988). Postisometric relaxation in combination with other methods of muscular facilitation and inhibition. *Manuelle Medizin, 2*, 101–104.

Lewit, K. (1991). *Manipulative therapy in rehabilitation of the locomotor system.* Oxford: Butterworth-Heinemann.

Lewit, K., & Simons, D.G. (1984). Myofascial pain: Relief by post-isometric relaxation. *Archives of Physical and Medical Rehabilitation, 65,* 452–456.

Liao, S.J., Lee, M.H.M., & Ng, L.K.Y. (1994). *Principles and practice of contemporary acupuncture.* New York: Marcel Dekker.

Mannheimer, J.S. (1994). Prevention and restoration of abnormal upper quarter posture. In H. Gelb (Ed.), *New concepts in craniomandibular and chronic pain management* (pp. 93–161). London: Mosby-Wolfe.

Masi, A.T. (1993). Review of the epidemiology and criteria of fibromyalgia and myofascial pain syndrome: Concepts of illness in populations as applied to dysfunctional syndromes. In S. Jacobsen, B. Danneskiold-Samsøe, & B. Lund (Eds.), *Musculoskeletal pain, myofascial pain syndrome, and the fibromyalgia syndrome* (pp. 113–136). Binghampton: Haworth Press.

McCall, I.W., Park, W.M., & O'Brien, J.P. (1979). Induced pain referral from posterior lumbar elements in normal subjects. *Spine, 4,* 441–446.

McNulty, W., et al. (1994). Needle electromyographic evaluation of trigger point response to a psychological stressor. *Psychophysiology, 31,* 313–316.

Melvin, J. (1980). Interdisciplinary and multidisciplinary activities and ACRM. *Archives of Physical Medicine, 61,* 379–380.

Menefee, L. A., et al. (2000). Sleep disturbance and nonmalignant chronic pain: A comprehensive review of the literature. *Pain Medicine, 1,* 156–172.

Merskey, H., & Spear, F.G. (1964). The reliability of the pressure algometer. *British Journal of Social and Clinical Psychology, 3,* 130–136.

Miller, B. (1994). Manual therapy treatment of myofascial pain and dysfunction. In E.S. Rachlin (Ed.), *Myofascial pain and fibromyalgia: Trigger point management* (pp. 415–454). St. Louis: Mosby-Year Book.

Mitchell, F.L. (1993). Elements of muscle energy technique. In J.V. Basmajian & R. Nyberg (Eds.), *Rational manual therapies* (pp. 285–321). Baltimore: Williams & Wilkins.

Nolan, R.A., & Nordhoff, L.S. (1996). Basic concepts of soft tissue healing and clinical methods to document recovery. Part 1. Soft tissue injury repair. In L.S. Nordhoff (Ed.), *Motor vehicle collision injuries* (pp. 131–141). Gaithersburg, MD: Aspen Publishers.

Norris, R.N., & Dommerholt, J. (1996). Applied ergonomics: Adaptive equipment and instrument modification for musicians. *Orthopaedic Physical Therapy Clinics of North America, 5,* 159–183.

Ohrbach, R., & Gale, E.N. (1989). Pressure pain thresholds in normal muscles: Reliability, measurement effects, and topographic differences. *Pain, 37,* 257–263.

Onishi, N., et al. (1976). Shoulder muscle tenderness and physical features of female industrial workers. *Journal of Human Ergology, 5,* 87–102.

Pheasant, S. (1991). *Ergonomics, work and health.* Gaithersburg, MD: Aspen Publishers.

Pruthi, R.K., & Tefferi, A. (1994). Pernicious anemia revisited. *Mayo Clinic. Proceedings, 69,* 144–150.

Reeves, J.L., Jaeger, B., & Graff-Radford, S.B. (1986). Reliability of the pressure algometer as a measure of myofascial trigger point sensitivity. *Pain, 24,* 313–321.

Reid, D.C. (1992). *Sports injury assessment and rehabilitation.* New York: Churchill Livingstone.

Rosomoff, H.L., et al. (1989). Myofascial findings with patients with "chronic intractable benign pain" of the back and neck. *Pain Management, 3,* 114–118.

Rywerant, Y. (1983). *The Feldenkrais method: Teaching by handling.* New Canaan, CT: Keats Publishing.

Saal, J.A., & Saal, J S. (1991). Rehabilitation of the patient. In A.H. White & R. Anderson (Eds.), *Conservative care of low back pain* (pp. 21–34). Baltimore: Williams & Wilkins.

Saggini, R., et al. (1996). Myofascial pain syndrome of the peroneus longus: Biomechanical approach. *The Clinical Journal of Pain, 12,* 30–37.

Sahrmann, S.A. (1988). Adult posturing. In S. Kraus (Ed.), *TMJ disorders: Management of the craniomandibular complex* (pp. 295–309). New York: Churchill Livingstone.

Silverstein, B.A. (1985). *The prevalence of upper extremity cumulative trauma disorders in industry.* Unpublished Ph.D. thesis, University of Michigan, Ann Arbor.

Simons, D.G., Hong, C.-Z., & Simons, L. (1995). Prevalence of spontaneous electrical activity at trigger spots and control sites in rabbit muscle. *Journal of Musculoskeletal Pain, 3,* 35–48.

Simons, D.G., & Simons, L.S. (1994). Chronic myofascial pain syndrome. In C.D. Tollison, J.R. Satterthwaite, & J.W. Tollison (Eds.), *Handbook of pain management* (pp. 556–577). Baltimore: Williams & Wilkins.

Simons, D. G., & Travell, J. G. (1984). Myofascial pain and dysfunction. In P. D. Wall & R. Melzack (Eds.), *Textbook of pain* (pp. 263–276). Edinburgh: Churchill Livingstone.

Simons, D.G., Travell, J.G., & Simons, L.S. (1999). *Myofascial pain and dysfunction: The trigger point manual* (Vol. 1). Baltimore: Williams & Wilkins. 2nd edition.

Singleton, W.T. (1972). *Introduction to ergonomics.* Geneva: World Health Organization.

Skootsky, S.A., Jaeger, B., & Oye, R.K. (1989). Prevalence of myofascial pain in general internal medicine practice. *Western Journal of Medicine, 151,* 157–160.

Soderberg, G.L. (1992). Skeletal muscle function. In D.P. Currier & R.M. Nelson (Eds.), *Dynamics of human biologic tissues* (pp. 74–96). Philadelphia: F. A. Davis.

Thompson, D.A. (1991). Ergonomics. In A.H. White & R. Anderson (Eds.), *Conservative care of low back pain.* Baltimore: Williams & Wilkins.

Toft, A.D. (1999). Thyroid hormone replacement-one hormone or two? (Editorial). *New England Journal of Medicine, 340,* 469–470.

Travell, J. (1976). Myofascial trigger points: Clinical view. In J. J. Bonica, et l. (Eds.), *Advances in pain research and therapy* (pp. 919–926). New York: Raven Press.

Travell, J.G., & Simons, D.G. (1992). Myofascial pain and dysfunction: The trigger point manual. Baltimore: Williams & Wilkins.

Tsujii, Y. (1993). *Myotherapy: Treatment of muscle hardenings.* Nagoya, Japan: Nagoya University College of Medical Technology.

Turk, D.C., & Rudy, T.E. (1994). A cognitive-behavioral perspective on chronic pain: Beyond the scalpel and syringe. In C. D. Tollison, J. R. Satterthwaite, & J. W. Tollison (Eds.), *Handbook of pain management* (pp. 136–151). Baltimore: Williams & Wilkins.

Turk, D.C., & Okifuji, A. (1999) Assessment of patients' reporting of pain: An integrated perspective. *Lancet, 353,* 1784–1788.

Viikari-Juntura, E. (1983). Neck and upper limb disorders among slaughterhouse workers. *Scandanavian Journal of Work Environment and Health, 9,* 283–290.

Vis, A J., Raats, G.J., & Van der Voort, E.J. (1987). *Massagetherapie: Een fysiotherapeutische handelen.* Zevenaar, The Netherlands: Van der Voort.

Vlaeyen, J.W.S. & Linton, S.J. (2000). Fear-avoidance and its consequences in chronic musculoskeletal pain: A state of the art. *Pain, 85,* 317–332.

Walpin, L.A. (1994). Posture: The process of body use; principles and determinants. In H. Gelb (Ed.), *New concepts in cranio-mandibular and chronic pain management* (pp. 13–76). London: Mosby-Wolfe.

Warmerdam, A. (1992). *Arthrokinetic therapy: Improving muscle performance through joint manipulation.* Paper presented at the Proceedings of the 5th International Conference of the International Federation of Orthopaedic Manipulative Therapists, Vail, CO.

Wells, P.E. (1994). Manipulative procedures. In P.E. Wells, V. Frampton, & D. Bowsher (Eds.), *Pain management by physical therapy* (pp. 187–212). Oxford: Butterworth-Heinemann.

Wolfe, F., et al. (1990). The American College of Rheumatology 1990 criteria for the classification of fibromyalgia. Report of the multicenter criteria committee. *Arthritis and Rheumatism, 33,*160–172.

Yue, S.K. (1995). Initial experience in the use of botulinum toxin for the treatment of myofascial related muscle dysfunctions. *Journal of Musculoskeletal Pain, 3*(Suppl. 1), 22.

22

Chronic Pelvic Pain

Andrea J. Rapkin, M.D. and Julie Jolin, M.D.

INTRODUCTION

Chronic pelvic pain is, by definition, pain that persists for more than 6 months. In its various forms, chronic pelvic pain affects an estimated 12 to 15% of women in the United States, accounting for more than $881 million spent each year on outpatient visits associated with this chronic pain (Mathias, Kupperman, Liberman, Lipschutz, & Steege, 1996). It is one of the most common but taxing problems in gynecologic practice. Even after a thorough workup, the etiology may remain obscure, and the relationship between certain types of pathology and the pain response may be inconsistent and often inexplicable. In the patient who has no obvious pathology, it may be tempting to remove pelvic structures for their physiological variations. Approximately 12% of all hysterectomies are performed for pelvic pain and 30% of patients who present to pain clinics have already had a hysterectomy (Chamberlain & La Ferla, 1987; Reiter, 1990a).

The purpose of this chapter is to outline the anatomy and physiology of pelvic pain and to explore the differential diagnosis and management of chronic pelvic pain, including the role of surgery, psychotherapy, and the multidisciplinary pain clinic.

NEUROANATOMY AND NEUROPHYSIOLOGY OF PELVIC PAIN

The pelvic viscera receive afferent (sensory) innervation by way of the autonomic nerve trunks (Kumazawa, 1986). The major neural pathways for visceral pain from the female pelvic organs travel with the sympathetic nerve bundles and have cell bodies in a thoracolumbar distribution. Sensory afferents that travel with the parasympathetic (sacral) fibers are probably of secondary importance for pain transmission from the pelvic organs. These latter nerves have their cell bodies in the sacral dorsal root ganglia (Kumazawa, 1986). The innervation of the female pelvic viscera and somatic structures is depicted in Figure 22.1.

The lower abdominal wall and anterior vulva, urethra, and clitoris are innervated by mixed (motor and sensory) somatic nerves deriving from lumbar 1 and 2 (L1 and L2) (Renaer, 1981). The dorsal rami derived from L1 and L2 innervate the lower back, often a region of referred pelvic pain. The anus, perineum, and lower vagina are innervated by somatic branches of the pudendal nerve, which is derived from the second through fourth sacral root ganglia (S2 to S4) (Renaer, 1981).

Pain impulses from the upper vagina, cervix, uterine corpus, inner one third of the fallopian tube, broad ligament, upper bladder, terminal ilium, and terminal large bowel travel with the thoracolumbar sympathetics via the vaginal, uterine, and hypogastric plexes to the hypogastric nerve, through the superior hypogastric plexus and to the lower thoracic and lumbar sympathetic chain (Kumazawa, 1986). The afferents then pass through the dorsal roots of thoracic 11, 12 and lumbar 1 (T11, T12, L1) and enter the spinal cord at this level. There is some duplication of afferent fibers in the thoracolumbar and sacral regions and there are probably some pain impulses from the upper vagina, cervix, and lower uterine segment that travel in the pelvic nerve (nerve erigentes) via pelvic parasympathetics (sacral autotomics) to spinal segments sacral 2 through 4 (S2 to S4) (Kumazawa, 1986). Urogenital sinus structures including the lower vagina, rectum, and lower bladder are innervated by both thoracolumbar and sacral afferents (Kumazawa, 1986).

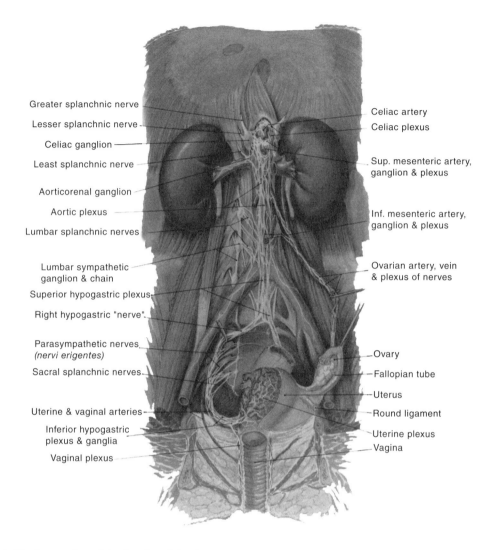

FIGURE 22.1 The innervation of the female pelvic viscera.

Afferents from the ovary, outer two thirds of the fallopian tube, and upper ureter travel along the ovarian artery entering the sympathetic nerve chain at lumbar spinal segment 4 (L4) ascending with the chain to penetrate the cord at T9 and T10 (Kumazawa, 1986). The superior hypogastric plexus carries no afferents from the ovary that accounts for the failure of presacral neurectomy (the transection of the superior hypogastric nerve) to diminish lateralizing pain or pain of adnexal origin. In sum, the transmission of painful stimuli from the pelvic organs relies on an intact sympathetic nervous system (Cervero & Tattersall, 1986). However, the parasympathetic (sacral) system is crucial for urination, defecation, and reflex regulation of the reproductive organs (Kumazawa, 1986). The role of the sacral autonomics in the genesis of pelvic pain remains to be delineated.

A large proportion of the sacral afferents from the colon and urinary bladder are usually silent. Only 5% of colon afferents and 2.5% of bladder afferents can be activated by mechanical distension. A proportion of the nonmechanosensitive unmyelinated sacral afferents are chemosensitive and can develop *de nouveau* mechano sensitivity (Janig, Haupt-Schade, & Kohler 1993). These usually "silent" fibers may be activated by and sensitized by inflammation or unusually strong mechanical stimulation and may play a role in pelvic pain of urinary tract or gastrointestinal etiology and theoretically from the internal reproductive organs as well.

The cell bodies of the afferent axons from the pelvic organs are located in the dorsal (sensory) ganglia of the spinal nerves (Fields, 1987). Before entering the spinal gray matter of the dorsal horn, branches of these afferent axons may extend for two or more segments beyond the level at which the original axons entered the cord. Much of neuronal modulation occurs in the dorsal horn. Evidence from animal studies indicates that supraspinal factors interact at the level of the dorsal horn to modulate the sensory perception of pain from the pelvic viscera (Berkley & Hubscher, 1995; De Groat, 1994).

The dorsal horn is an important site of modulation of afferent input (Cervero & Tattersall, 1986). The second-order neurons are subjected to excitatory and/or inhibitory interactions. For example, if a visceral structure and a cutaneous (somatic) structure transmitting to the same second-order neuron in the dorsal horn are stimulated simultaneously, the second-order neuron response may be greater than either the cutaneous or the visceral stimulus would evoke on its own. These viscero-somatic neurons tend to have larger receptive fields than the somatic neurons. There are also many more somatic second-order neurons than there are viscero-somatic neurons (Cervero & Tattersall, 1986). Both of these facts may account for the vague, poorly localizable quality of visceral pelvic pain.

GENERAL CONSIDERATIONS OF VISCERAL PAIN

The neurophysiology of pain transmission from the viscera (internal organs such as bowel, bladder, rectum, uterus, ovaries, and fallopian tubes) differs from that of somatic structures (cutaneous elements, fascia, muscles, parietal peritoneum, mesentery, external genitalia, anus, urethra). Nociceptors receive pain evoked at somatic nerves, whereas a plentitude of nonspecific receptors receive pain induced in the viscera (Berkley, 1994; Cervero, 1994). Visceral pain, in contrast to somatic pain, is usually deep; difficult to localize; and frequently associated with various autonomic reflexes such as restlessness, nausea, vomiting, and diaphoresis (Procacci, Zoppi, & Maresen, 1986). Early surgical studies performed under local anesthesia have shown that cutting, crushing, or burning the bowel, for example, evokes no pain, whereas distension of muscular organs or hollow viscera, stretching of the capsule of solid organs, hypoxia or necrosis of viscera, production of algesic (pain producing) substances, rapid compression of ligaments or vessels, and inflammation may cause severe pain. In contrast, cutting or crushing a somatic structure produces exquisite pain that is well localized (Procacci, et al., 1986).

PERIPHERAL CAUSES OF CHRONIC PELVIC PAIN

ADHESIONS

The differential diagnosis of the peripheral component of pelvic pain is listed in Table 22.1. Laparoscopic studies for the evaluation of chronic pelvic pain, would suggest that adhesions play a prominent role. However, when these studies were performed, nonobvious sources of pelvic pain such as abdominal wall pain, irritable bowel syndrome, and interstitial cystitis (IC) were often not excluded prior to laparoscopy. Adhesions were present in 16 to 44% of the patients undergoing laparoscopy for chronic pelvic pain (depending on the series) (Rapkin, 1986; Kresch,

---

TABLE 22.1
Peripheral Causes of Chronic Pelvic Pain

Gynecologic
    Noncyclic
        Adhesions
        Endometriosis
        Salpingo-oophoritis
         Acute
         Subacute
        Ovarian remnant syndrome
        Pelvic congestion syndrome (varicosities)
        Ovarian neoplasms
        Pelvic relaxation
    Cyclic
        Primary dysmenorrhea
        Secondary dysmenorrhea
Imperforate hymen
Transverse vaginal septum
Cervical stenosis
Uterine anomalies (congenital malformation, bicornuate uterus, blind uterine horn)
Intrauterine synechiae (Asherman's syndrome)
Endometrial polyps
Uterine leiomyoma
Adenomyosis
Pelvic congestin syndrome (varicosities)
Endometriosis
        Atypical cyclic
Endometriosis
Adenomyosis
Ovarian remnant syndrome
Chronic functional cyst formation
Gastrointestinal
    Irritable bowel syndrome
    Ulcerative colitis
    Granulomatous colitis (Crohn's disease)
    Carcinoma
    Infectious diarrhea
    Recurrent partial small bowel obstruction
    Diverticulitis
    Hernia
    Abdominal angina
    Recurrent appendiceal colic
Genitourinary
    Recurrent or relapsing cystourethritis
    Urethral syndrome
    Interstitial cystitis
    Ureteral diverticuli or polyps
    Carcinoma of the bladder
    Ureteral obstruction
    Pelvic kidney
Neurologic
    Nerve entrapment syndrome
    Neuroma
    Trigger points

(continued)

TABLE 22.1 (CONTINUED)
Peripheral Causes of Chronic Pelvic Pain

Musculoskeletal
    Low back pain syndrome
        Congenital anomalies
        Scoliosis and kyphosis
        Spondylolysis
        Spondylolisthesis
        Spinal injuries
        Inflammation
        Tumors
        Osteoporosis
        Degenerative changes
        Coccydynia
    Myofascial syndrome
    Fibromyalgia
Systemic
    Acute intermittent porphyria
    Abdominal migraine
    Systemic lupus erythematosus
    Lymphoma
    Neurofibromatosis

Seifer, Sachs, & Barrese, 1984; Lundberg, Wall, & Mathers, 1973; Liston, Bradford, Downie, & Kerr, 1972; Renaer, 1981). Do adhesions actually cause pelvic pain? Of 100 patients Kresch laparoscoped for chronic pelvic pain, 38% had adhesions and 10% had bowel adhesions. However, of 50 asymptomatic patients undergoing laparoscopy for sterilization, only 12% had adhesions and only 2% exhibited adhesions involving the bowel. These differences were highly significant (Kresch, et al., 1984). Keltz, et al. in a combined retrospective/prospective study found colon to side-wall adhesions in a higher proportion of patients (93 vs. 13%) with pelvic pain than the control group (sterilization) (Keltz, Peck, Liu, Kim, Arici, & Olive, 1995).

In comparison, Rapkin (1986) noted that many infertility patients with severe adhesions had no pain and compared the results of laparoscopies performed on two groups of patients — the first group complained of chronic pelvic pain and the second group had infertility, without complaints of pain. When evaluating both the site *and* density of adhesions, it was notable that there were no significant differences between the group with chronic pelvic pain and asymptomatic patients in the infertility group. The results of this study question the role of pelvic adhesions as a common cause of chronic pelvic pain (Rapkin, 1986). If adhesions cause pain, then lysis of adhesions should relieve pain. A prospective noncontrolled nonrandomized study of lysis of adhesions did not show significantly lower postoperative pain ratings (Steege & Scott, 1991). However, post hoc analysis consisting of separation of the subjects into those with and without psychosocial dysfunction revealed a significant improvement in pain scores in the group without psychosocial dysfunction. The only prospective randomized study of adhesiolysis in the literature revealed no differences in the pain scores between the groups (adhesiolysis vs. no adhesiolysis). Again, post hoc analysis of the data suggested there was a significant improvement (although only on two of the three methods of pain assessment) in pain scores in the subgroup of patients with dense vascular adhesions involving small bowel (Peters, Van Dorst, Jellis, VanZuuren, Hermans, & Trimbos, 1991). Advances using a 3-mm laparoscope have enabled development of "conscious pain mapping" whereby patients under local anesthesia and conscious sedation guide in determining which adhesions are those associated with pain (Palter, 1999). In an observational pain mapping study of 50 women under local anesthesia, manipulation of appendiceal and pelvic adhesions was observed to contribute significantly to pelvic pain (Almeida & Val-Gallas, 1997). Though adhesions may be prevalent in patients with chronic pelvic pain, these adhesions may or may not be the cause of pain. No prospective studies of adhesiolysis and outcome based on pain mapping have been published.

ENDOMETRIOSIS

Another "peripheral" cause of chronic pelvic pain is endometriosis. The actual incidence of endometriosis is unknown because many individuals undoubtedly have endometriosis without sufficient symptomatology to warrant surgical intervention. It seems that the incidence of endometriosis is increasing. However, this apparent increase in prevalence may be a reflection of the more liberal use of laparoscopy and of the recognition of atypical forms of endometriosis. Endometriosis is noted in patients undergoing laparoscopy for chronic pelvic pain in anywhere from 5 to 37% of the cases (Kresch, et al., 1984; Liston, et al., 1972; Lundberg, et al., 1973).

The diagnosis of endometriosis is usually made in the third or fourth decade; however, it has been noted to be a prominent diagnosis in adolescents and women in their twenties who are evaluated for chronic pelvic pain (Chatman & Ward, 1982). In fact, endometriosis has been suggested by one study to be the etiology in up to 70% of adolescents with chronic pelvic pain unresponsive to medical treatment (Probst & Laufer, 1999).

The most common symptoms of endometriosis are dysmenorrhea, dyspareunia, infertility, and abnormal uterine bleeding, usually from a secretory endometrium (Kitchen, 1985). Pelvic pain in women with endometriosis may occur at any time in the menstrual cycle, though dysmenorrhea is the most classic symptom. Dysmenorrhea may be so prolonged that the patient may complain of what seems like acyclic, continuous pain; beginning 7 to 10 days before the onset of the menstrual period and persisting until 1 week or so after the bleeding has ceased. The patient often describes pressurelike pain and aching in the lower abdomen, back, and rectum. There may be radiation of pain into the vagina, thighs, or perineum. Dyspareunia is common when the disease involves the cul-de-sac (pouch of Douglas), uterosacral ligaments, or rectovaginal septum. Pain with defecation (dyschezia) may also be present even in patients without direct bowel wall involvement. These symptoms may be due to endometrial implants near the rectum. Urinary urgency, frequency, and bladder pain may also be associated with urinary tract involvement. Because endometriosis may be present in unusual locations, the manifestations of endometriosis are protean (Kitchen, 1985). Usually the previously noted common symptoms and signs are present but, rarely, patients may complain of rectal bleeding, symptoms similar to bowel obstruction, suprapubic pain, and/or urinary symptoms (such as frequency, dysuria, or hematuria). If ureteral involvement is present, there may be flank pain, backache, or hypertension. Signs and symptoms of an acute abdomen occur infrequently and are usually related to rupture of an endometrioma.

Examination of patients with endometriosis may reveal tenderness and nodularity on the rectovaginal examination of the uterosacral ligaments and posterior cul-de-sac (Kitchen, 1985). Progressive disease results in findings of obliteration and fibrosis of the cul-de-sac, and fixed retroversion of the uterus. Enlarged ovaries (endometriomas) with decreased mobility may be noted.

Laparoscopy is necessary for definitive diagnosis of endometriosis though the diagnosis may be suggested by history and pelvic examination. A study by Ling (1999) for the Pelvic Pain Study Group reported the efficacy and safety of medical treatment with depot leuprolide before laparoscopy based on empirical, clinical diagnosis. Ultrasound is not diagnostic and cannot differentiate an endometrioma from a benign or malignant ovarian neoplasm, scattered small implants are not detectable by ultrasound. Laboratory studies are usually not specific. CA 125 and erythrocyte sedimentation rate (ESR) can be elevated in women with endometriosis.

Endometriosis can be treated hormonally using androgenic hormones (Danocrine®), progestins, or gonadotropin-releasing hormone analogs to create pseudomenopause and to atrophy ectopic endometrial implants. For those undergoing long-term therapy (12 month or greater), hormonal add-back therapy, norethindrone acetate with or without estrogen, prevents long-term hypoestrogenic side effects such as bone loss (Hornstein, Surrey, Weisberg, & Casino, 1998). Laparoscopic electro- or laser surgery or laparotomy with resection of disease often is reserved for treatment of severe endometriosis. However, in a prospective randomized double-blinded study of 63 women with minimal to moderate endometriosis, laparoscopic laser treatment was noted to benefit 90% of those women who

initially responded at 1-year follow-up (Sutton, Pooley, Ewen, & Haines, 1997). Patients who do not desire fertility may opt for radical surgery for endometriosis, which consists of a total abdominal hysterectomy with bilateral salpingo-oophorectomy as well as removal of any residual gastrointestinal (GI), genitourinary (GU), or peritoneal disease. It should be noted that patients with endometriosis, who have failed hormonal or conservative surgical therapy, may still benefit from the pain management approach (Rapkin & Kames, 1987). At least 30% of patients with recurred pain after treatment of endometriosis do not have residual disease at the time of repeat laparoscopy.

Endometriosis is a common finding in reproductive aged women, but it is clear that in many women with chronic pelvic pain and endometriosis the latter may not be the cause of the pain and may be only a contributing factor. There is no significant correlation between the amount of disease and pain severity although higher stage disease tends to be associated with a greater prevalence of and increased intensity of pain. Additionally, there is no correlation between location of pain and site of endometriotic lesions (Fukaya, Hoshiai, & Yajima, 1993) and as many as 30 to 50% of patients regardless of stage have no pain. However, deeply infiltrating lesions, particularly of the uterosacral ligaments, are strongly associated with pain (Cornillie, Oosterlynck, Lauweryns, & Koninckx, 1990). Vaginal and uterosacral endometriosis has been associated with complaints of deep dyspareunia (Vercellini, Trespedi, De Giorgi, Cortesi, Parazzini, & Crosignani, 1996).

Clinically it is possible to determine whether there is a relationship between pain and endometriosis in a specific patient because of the hormonal sensitivity of the disease and the potential to surgically cure disease. Clearly, pain that does not respond to adequate surgical and medical management of endometriosis should be reevaluated for another source, pain, or other contributing central factors.

PELVIC CONGESTION

For the last 100 years there has been waxing and waning interest in the role of pelvic congestion in the genesis of chronic pelvic pain without obvious pathology. The concept of autonomic nervous system dysfunction leading to a vascular disorder affecting the uterine and ovarian veins was outlined by Taylor (1954). Taylor suggested that emotional stress could lead to smooth muscle spasm and congestion of the veins draining the ovaries, uterus, and vulva. Taylor's series of 100 cases consisted of women in their reproductive years with the chief complaint of lower abdominal pain. Subjects also complained of secondary dysmenorrhea, low back pain, dyspareunia, infertility, and menorrhagia. Their pain was usually bilateral, lower pelvic in distribution, and was exacerbated with the menstrual period. Two thirds of the patients also complained of nervous tension, chronic fatigue, breast tenderness, and spastic colon, as well as symptoms similar to the premenstrual syndrome. Personality characteristics noted by Taylor included immaturity and decreased sexual drive.

On exam, patients manifested tenderness over the uterus. The fundus of the uterus and cervix were often bulky and the ovaries often enlarged with multiple functional cysts. The parametria, especially the uterosacral ligaments, were noted to be tender and indurated. At laparotomy, the uterus was usually soft, enlarged, and purplish or mottled. There was increased fluid in the cul-de-sac and edema of surrounding subserosal connective tissue and occasionally ovarian varicosities were prominent (Taylor, 1954).

The concept of pelvic congestion has been resurrected to explain chronic pelvic pain (Hobbs, 1976). Beard, Highman, Pearce, and Reginald (1984) performed the only blinded study of venograms in patients with chronic pelvic pain. Larger mean ovarian vein diameters, delayed disappearance of contrast medium, and ovarian plexus congestion were present in a significantly greater proportion of women with chronic pelvic pain without pathology than those with pathology or controls. Other diagnostic means include transvaginal ultrasound, which may reveal uterine enlargement, thickened endometrium, cystic ovaries, and dilated pelvic veins (Adams, Reginal, Franks, Wadsworth, & Beard, 1990; Stones, Rae, Rogers, Fry, & Beard, 1990), or more recently for more detailed visualization of structures, magnetic resonance imaging (MRI) (Gupta & McCarthy, 1994).

Because many patients were noted to have polycystic ovaries, and all were of reproductive age, hormonal suppression consisting of a hypoestrogenic environment was considered as a mode of treatment for pelvic congestion. Medroxyprogesterone acetate (MPA) given in doses of 30 mg daily for 3 months was administered in a randomized, placebo-controlled treatment trial for women with chronic pelvic pain with pelvic congestion (abnormal venograms) (Farquhar, Rogers, Franks, Pearce, Wadsworth, & Bland, 1989). A study of 84 subjects included four separate groups: MPA alone, MPA and psychotherapy, placebo plus psychotherapy, and placebo alone. MPA was significantly more effective after the 3-month treatment period than psychotherapy or placebo. Patients reported a 50% reduction in pain in the MPA group and 33% reduction in pain score after receiving placebo. However, pain returned in the MPA group after stopping treatment but did not return in the placebo group. Psychotherapy did not reduce pain in the short term, but there was a positive interaction between MPA and psychotherapy 9 months after the treatment was concluded. However, 9 months posttreatment, improvement was reported irrespective of the treatment group. This response coupled with a strong placebo response reaffirms central factors in this condition. It also suggests that hormonal suppression with MPA or gonadotropin-releasing hormone (GnRH) agonists with or without low-dose estrogen and progestin hormone addback may be therapeutic. A few small non-controlled studies have assessed the more invasive technique of transcatheter embolotherapy of the ovarian and internal iliac veins to treat pelvic congestion, with results revealing good short-term success (Capasso, Simons, Trotteur, Dongelinger, Henroteaux, & Gaspard, 1997; Sichlau, Yao & Vogelzang, 1994; Tarazov, Prozorovskij & Ryzhkov, 1997). Long-term efficacy remains to be evaluated (Venbrux & Lambert, 1999).

SALPINGO-OOPHORITIS

Salpingo-oophoritis can cause chronic pelvic pain, though patients usually present with symptoms and signs of acute or subacute infection before the pain becomes chronic. More commonly, a patient will present with frequent recurrent infections.

Sweet and Gibbs (1985) proposed criteria for making the diagnosis of salpingitis on clinical grounds. Patients should have a history of lower abdominal pain as well as lower abdominal tenderness (with or without rebound), cervical motion tenderness, and adnexal tenderness. In addition, they must have one of the following: temperature greater than 38°C, leucocytosis (greater than 10,500 white blood cells per cubic millimeter); culdocentesis fluid containing white cells and bacteria on Gram stain; presence of an inflammatory mass; elevated ESR; a Gram stain from the endocervix revealing Gram-negative intracellular diplococci; or a monoclonal smear from the endocervical secretions revealing chlamydia (Sweet & Gibbs, 1985).

Patients may complain of having had numerous episodes of pain associated with fever and may have been given the diagnosis of pelvic inflammatory disease. When these episodes become recurrent, the patient is often considered to have chronic salpingo-oophoritis, though it is not clear that a chronic inflammatory condition exists. Instead, subacute or subclinical disease with recurrent acute infections may be present. An additional possibility is that the patient may not have salpingitis at all. In all these situations, laparoscopy with peritoneal fluid cultures is diagnostic, though an experienced clinician can often make the diagnosis on the basis of clinical criteria. Broad spectrum antibiotics and anaerobic coverage represent the standard treatment of acute or recurrent salpingo-oophoritis. Only rarely is hysterectomy and salpingo-oophorectomy required.

OVARIAN REMNANT SYNDROME

Chronic pelvic pain in a patient who has had a hysterectomy and bilateral salpingo-oophorectomy for severe endometriosis or pelvic inflammatory disease may be caused by the ovarian remnant syndrome. Ovarian remnant syndrome results from residual ovarian cortical tissue that is left *in situ* after a difficult dissection in an attempt to perform an oophorectomy (Steege, 1987). Often the patient has had multiple pelvic operations with the uterus and adnexa removed sequentially.

The diagnosis is suspected on the basis of history and physical examination (Price, Edwards, & Buchsbaum, 1990). The patient usually complains of pelvic pain that is often cyclic and may be accompanied by peritoneal signs. The patient may have a history of flank pain and frequent urinary tract infections; and there is on occasion intermittent, partial bowel obstruction. The painful symptoms usually arise 2 to 5 years after surgery. Pelvic exam may reveal a tender mass in the lateral region of the pelvis and ultrasound following ovarian stimulation with 50 mg daily for 5 days of clomiphene usually confirms a mass with the sonographic characteristics of ovarian tissue. In a patient who has had bilateral salpingo-oophorectomy and is not on hormonal replacement, estradiol and follicle-stimulating hormone (FSH) assays reveal a characteristic premenopausal picture, though on occasion the remaining ovarian tissue may not be active enough to suppress FSH levels. Laparotomy and removal of residual ovarian tissue is necessary for treatment (Pettit & Lee, 1988). Importantly, it has been shown that those who have achieved pain relief with GnRH-agonist hormonal therapy prior to surgery, are usually those who also receive relief with surgical removal of the remnant (Carey & Slack, 1996).

CYCLIC PELVIC PAIN

Cyclic pelvic pain consists of primary and secondary dysmenorrhea but also includes atypical cyclic pain, such as pain beginning 1 week prior to menses and lasting for up to 1 week following the cessation of menstrual flow with occasional midcycle pain as well. Atypical cyclic pain is a variant of secondary dysmenorrhea. The diagnosis of cyclic pain often depends on the review of a daily pain diary that patients should be asked to maintain. With the availability of nonsteroidal anti-inflammatory agents and compounds that alter the female sex steroids, cyclic pelvic pain has become significantly more manageable.

Dysmenorrhea or "difficult monthly flow" is a common gynecologic disorder affecting up to 50% of menstruating women (American College of Obstetricians and Gynecologists, 1983). Primary dysmenorrhea refers to pain with menses when there is no pelvic pathology, whereas secondary dysmenorrhea is painful menses with underlying pelvic pathology. Primary dysmenorrhea usually appears within 1 to 2 years after menarche, with the establishment of ovulatory cycles. The disorder primarily affects younger women with ovulatory cycles, especially teens, but may persist into the forties. The

pain of primary dysmenorrhea begins a few hours prior to or just after the onset of menstrual flow and usually lasts for 48 to 72 hours. The pain is laborlike with suprapubic cramping that may be accompanied by lumbosacral backache, pain radiating down the anterior thighs, nausea, vomiting, and diarrhea.

Secondary dysmenorrhea, on the other hand, usually, though not always, occurs years after menarche and may occur with anovulatory cycles (ACOG, 1983). The most common cause of secondary dysmenorrhea is endometriosis. Other common causes, listed in Table 22.1, include vaginal, cervical, uterine, fallopian tube, adnexal, and peritoneal pathology. The differential diagnosis of secondary dysmenorrhea includes primary dysmenorrhea and noncyclic pelvic pain and entails ruling out primary dysmenorrhea and confirming the cyclic nature of the pain. The etiology of primary dysmenorrhea has been established to be increased uterine prostaglandin production (Filler & Hall, 1970). Prostaglandin synthetase inhibitors are effective for the treatment of primary dysmenorrhea in 70 to 80% of the cases (The Medical Letter, 1979). For the patient with primary dysmenorrhea who has no contraindications to oral contraceptive agents and desires contraception, the birth control pill is the agent of choice (Chan & Dawood, 1980). More than 90% of women with primary dysmenorrhea have relief with birth control pills.

If the patient does not respond to prostaglandin synthetase inhibitors and does not desire oral contraceptive pills for contraception, or if either of them are contraindicated, narcotic analgesics should be administered for 2 to 3 days per month. Prior to the addition of narcotic medication, psychological factors and other organic pathology should be ruled out. Other modes of hormonal menstrual suppression include high dose progestins (oral or depo intramuscular injection) continuous oral contraceptive pill administration, or GnRH agonists with or without continuous low-dose hormone (menopausal dosage) add back. Breakthrough bleeding and associated pain are potential problems with these regimens.

A patient with dysmenorrhea who does not respond to prostaglandin synthetase inhibitors and/or birth control pills and in whom organic disease has been ruled out may also respond to the pain management approach and, in particular, acupuncture or transcutaneous electrical nerve stimulation (Helms, 1987; Mannheimer & Whaler, 1985). In one study, Kaplan, et al., (1994) reported a 30% marked pain relief, 60% moderate pain relief, and 10% no pain relief in women with primary dysmenorrhea undergoing transcutaneous electrical nerve stimulations (TENS). To more fully evaluate the evidence for treating primary dysmenorrhea with TENS or acupuncture, a forthcoming study by the Cochrane Library aims to analyze all prospective randomized controlled trials comparing those modalities with medical treatment or placebo (Wilson, Farquhar, Kennedy, & Jin, 2000).

The distinction between primary and secondary dysmenorrhea requires a thorough history as to the nature and onset of the pain, the duration of pain or symptoms, and a pain diary (if on first query the pain does not appear to be cyclic). A complete physical and pelvic examination is important, with focus on the evaluation of the size, shape, and mobility of the uterus and adnexal structures and for nodularity and fibrosis of the uterosacral ligaments and rectovaginal septum. Genital cultures for gonorrhea and chlamydia and a complete blood count (CBC) with ESR are usually warranted. If no abnormalities are found, a tentative diagnosis of primary dysmenorrhea may be made and the patient started on oral contraceptive pills and/or prostaglandin synthetase inhibitors. Having made a diagnosis of primary dysmenorrhea, a 4- to 6-month trial of oral contraceptives and/or prostaglandin synthetase inhibitors is warranted before laparoscopy is performed to rule out secondary dysmenorrhea and, in particular, endometriosis. A strong family history of endometriosis and any clinical signs of endometriosis on exam may suggest that laparoscopy be performed sooner.

Surgical approaches to dysmenorrhea include laparoscopic uterine nerve ablation, presacral neurectomy, and, in selected cases of secondary dysmenorrhea, hysterectomy (Malinak, 1980). The uterosacral ligaments carry the main afferent supply from the uterus, and if complete, the uterosacral ablation should be as effective as the presacral neurectomy, though Doyle (1955) described a 70% success rate. Long-term or controlled studies of the neurectomy procedures are lacking. The management of secondary dysmenorrhea involves treatment of the underlying pathology.

GASTROENTEROLOGIC CAUSES OF CHRONIC PELVIC PAIN

Many of the patients referred to gynecologists with chronic pelvic pain actually have GI pathology (Rapkin & Mayer, 1993; Reiter, 1990b). Because the cervix, uterus, adnexa, lower ileum, sigmoid colon, and rectum share the same visceral innervation, with pain signals traveling via the sympathetic nerves to spinal cord segments T10 to L1, it is often difficult to determine whether lower abdominal pain is of gynecologic or enterocoelic origin (Hightower & Roberts, 1981). In addition, as is true with other types of visceral pain, pain sensation from the GI tract is often diffuse and poorly localized. Skillful medical history and examination are usually necessary to make the diagnosis.

Irritable bowel syndrome (IBS) is one of the more common causes of lower abdominal pain and may account for as many as 7 to 60% of referrals to a gynecologist for chronic pelvic pain (Reiter, 1990b). The predominant symptom of irritable bowel syndrome is abdominal pain (Ritchie, 1979). Other symptoms include excessive flatulence and alternating diarrhea and constipation. The pain is usually intermittent cramplike and predominantly left lower quadrant in location but, occasionally the pain is constant. Pain is often improved after a bowel movement. The pain may last for only a few minutes, but 50% of patients may have pain for hours to days, and 20% of patients may complain of pain for weeks or longer. Symptoms are usually worse during periods of stress tension, anxiety, depression, and with the premenstrual and menstrual phases of the cycle (Ritchie, 1979).

The diagnosis of the IBS is usually made on the basis of the history but cannot be made without first excluding other conditions. Sigmoidoscopy or barium enema is often necessary and is routinely negative though there may be mucosal hyperemia on sigmoidoscopy and increased haustral contractions or loss of haustration on barium enema (Hightower & Roberts, 1981). IBS is a waxing and waning disorder and treatment consists of reassurance, education, stress reduction, and antcholinergic or other antispasmodic pharmaceutical agents. Bulk-forming agents such as Metamucil® and high-fiber diet are also usually added as well (Ritchie, 1979). Low-dose tricyclic antidepressants are also useful.

Patients with chronic diarrhea must be evaluated carefully, often with a gastroenterologist in consultation. Though symptoms may have become chronic, it is possible that the patient may have contracted infectious diarrhea due to any one of a number of bacteria or parasites including *Shigella, Escherichia coli, Salmonella, Camphylobacter, or Amoeba* (Hightower & Roberts, 1981).

Though appendicitis is a common cause of abdominal pain, the abdominal pain of appendicitis is severe enough that the patient presents to the physician within 12 to 48 h after the onset of the symptoms. The practitioner treating a patient for chronic pelvic pain should be cautious when the patient suddenly has an increase in abdominal pain, especially if it is accompanied by localized right lower quadrant pain, as well as anorexia, nausea, vomiting, and peritoneal signs on exam. It is not uncommon that a patient under treatment for chronic pelvic pain develops acute appendicitis or other acute pelvic condition while in the process of evaluation for the chronic pain problem. Chronic appendicitis is a controversial entity, but in the opinion of Lee, Bell, Griffen, & Hagihara (1985), it does exist.

Another cause of chronic enterocoelic pain is diverticular disease of the colon (Young, Alpers, Norland, & Woodruff, 1976). Of the adult population over 40, 5% have been noted to have diverticulae (Painter, 1970). This percentage increases to 40% in individuals over the age of 70 although most patients never develop diverticulitis. Though diverticulosis is usually asymptomatic, diverticulitis results in severe pain. Diverticulitis results from perforation of one or more of the diverticula and usually leads to the formation of a pericolonic abscess. The principal symptom of diverticulitis is left lower quadrant abdominal pain. A tender mass may be palpable on exam. Fever and leukocytosis are usually present. Sigmoidoscopy is diagnostic. These symptoms and signs, however, are usually those of an acute pathological pain process bringing the patient to a physician early in the course of pain.

Inflammatory bowel disease such as ulcerative colitis or granulomatous disease (Crohn's disease) similarly do not usually present as chronic pelvic pain because their presentation is usually more acute with diarrhea, fever, vomiting, and anorexia (Hightower & Roberts, 1981). A sigmoidoscopy or barium enema is diagnostic.

Tumors of the GI tract can cause chronic lower abdominal pain in women (McSherry, Cornell, & Glenn, 1969). The most frequent and early symptoms of bowel carcinomas are change in bowel habits (74% of patients) and abdominal pain (65% of patients). Rectal bleeding and weight loss may be signs of advanced disease (McSherry, et al., 1969). Most rectal tumors can be palpated on rectal examination. Sigmoidoscopy and biopsy as well as barium enema are diagnostic.

Included in the differential diagnosis of lower abdominal pain is hernia though there is a relatively low incidence of hernia in females (Hightower & Roberts, 1981). Anterior and posterior perineal hernias, usually limited to cystocele, rectocele, or enterocele, may cause lower abdominal/perineal pain in women though the pain is usually not severe. This type of pain usually responds to a pessary though the management is surgical.

UROLOGIC CAUSES OF CHRONIC PELVIC PAIN

Chronic pelvic pain of urologic origin may be related to recurrent cystoureteritis, urethral syndrome, interstitial cystitis (IC), infiltrating bladder tumors, ectopic pelvic kidney, or various ureteral causes of pelvic pain such as ureteral obstructions or endometriosis (Vereecken, 1981; Summit, 1993).

The patient with cystitis presents with complaints of suprapubic pain, dysuria, frequency, urgency; has pyuria on urinalysis; and has a positive urine culture (Vereecken, 1981). The symptoms usually respond to adequate antibiotic therapy. Relapses and reinfection can be diagnosed with the aid of history, urinalysis, and culture. The antibiotic and duration of therapy may have to be adjusted and on occasion, if the patient has recurrent cystoureteritis, antibiotics may have to be administered postcoitally possibly for a prolonged period of time (Vereecken, 1981).

The urethral syndrome is a common condition in women and may present as chronic pelvic pain (Bodner, 1988). Symptoms of dysuria, urinary frequency, suprapubic pain, and dyspareunia are prominent and the diagnosis is one of exclusion. A negative urine analysis, urine culture, and urethral cultures, as well as negative evaluation for vulvovaginitis, increase the suspicion for the diagnosis of urethral syndrome. Treatment consists of a trial of antibiotics, preferably tetracycline for 2 to 3 weeks; and, if without success, urethral dilatation in reproductive aged women and vaginal estrogen for peri- and postmenopausal women (Bergman, Karram, & Bhatia, 1989). Attention should be paid to psychological factors as well.

When a patient complains of symptoms of urinary frequency, urgency, and suprapubic pain but laboratory studies are negative, the patient may actually have IC (Karram, 1993; Messing & Stamey, 1978). The evaluation of patients with the preceding symptoms should include urinalysis and culture, urethral culture for chlamydia, mycoplasma, and gonorrhea, and cystoscopy with hydrodistension and possible biopsy. The consensus criteria for the diagnosis of IC include at least two of the following: pain or bladder filling relieved by emptying; pain in suprapubic, pelvic, urethral, vaginal or perineal region, glomerulations on endoscopy; or decreased compliance on cystometrogram (Karram, 1993). Therapy consisting of intravesical distension with dimethylsulfoxide, intravesical instillation of analogs of glycosaminoglycan, TENS and biofeedback including pelvic floor muscle biofeedback training have all reduced pain in uncontrolled studies of patients with IC. Because treatment of the condition remains empiric and less than optimal, oral drugs such as anticholinergics, antihistamines, antispasmodics, nonsteroidal anti-inflammatories, tricyclic antidepressants, narcotics, and pentosan polysulfate sodium (which is Food and Drug Administration [FDA] approved for IC treatment) (Sant, 1998) have all been utilized with some success.

Very severe chronic suprapubic pain may be caused by infiltrating carcinomas of the bladder, cervix, uterus or rectum (Vereecken, 1981). These conditions should be apparent after performing the history, pelvic examination, urine analysis, and cystoscopy, though intravenous pyelogram (IVP) or CT urogram may be necessary.

NERVE ENTRAPMENT OR INJURY

Abdominal cutaneous nerve entrapment or injury should always be considered in the differential diagnosis of chronic lower abdominal pain, especially if no visceral etiology is apparent. The syndrome most commonly occurs months to years after Pfannenstiel skin or other lower abdominal and even laparoscopic incisions (Sippo, Burghardt, & Gomez, 1987) but can also follow trauma or exercise. Commonly involved nerves include ilioinguinal (T12 and L1), iliohypogastric (T12 and L1), and genitofemoral (L1 and L2).

Symptoms of nerve entrapment include pain that is typically elicited by exercise and relieved by bedrest (Hammeroff, Carlson, & Brown, 1981; Sippo, et al., 1987). The pain is described as stabbing, colicky, and sudden; and is usually judged as coming from the abdomen and not from the skin. The pain is located along the line of the lateral edge of the rectus margin and may be associated with a burning pain radiating horizontally or diagonally toward the linea alba and back to the flank or sacroiliac region. Nausea, bloating, menstruation, and full bladder may exacerbate the pain of nerve entrapment (Sippo, et al., 1987).

On exam, the pain can usually be localized with the fingertip (MacDonald, 1993). The maximal point of tenderness is the neuromuscular foramen at the rectus margin medial and inferior to the anterior iliac spine or, in the case of spontaneous nerve entrapment, at the site of exit from the aponeurosis of the other thoracic/abdominal cutaneous nerves. A maneuver that helps to make the diagnosis is to ask the patient to tense the abdominal wall by raising shoulders or raising and extending the lower limbs in a straight leg raising maneuver. The outer side of the rectal muscle is then pressed with a single finger. The pain is exacerbated if nerve entrapment syndrome is present. With the abdominal wall relaxed, the pain is relieved and becomes more diffuse. The tentative diagnosis is confirmed with a diagnostic nerve block consisting of injection of 2 to 4 ml of 1% lidocaine or 0.25% bupivocaine. Patients usually report immediate relief with symptoms after injection and many patients require no further intervention, though some patients require 2 or 3 weekly injections. Only as a last resort should patients be considered for surgical removal of the involved nerves if no other psychological factors predominate and if visceral pathology can be ruled out. Deafferentation pain is a probable sequel to surgery and there are no long-term studies of nerve excision. Medications such as low-dose tricyclic antidepressants and anticonvulsants are also useful for pain control. Physical therapy may be necessary to educate the patient concerning strengthening other muscles to prevent reinjury.

MUSCULOSKELETAL CAUSES OF CHRONIC PELVIC PAIN

Women complaining of lower back pain without complaints of pelvic pain rarely have gynecologic pathology as the cause of their pain; however, low back pain may accompany pelvic pathology. Back pain may be caused by gynecologic, vascular, neurological, psychogenic, or spondylogenic (related to the axial skeleton and its structures) pathology (Morscher, 1981). Musculoskeletal abnormalities commonly contribute to the symptoms of chronic pelvic pain (Baker, 1993).

MYOFASCIAL PAIN

Myofascial pain is defined as "pain and/or autonomic phenomena referred from active myofascial trigger points, with associated dysfunction" (Travell, 1976). Reports of the prevalence of the syndrome vary, but only two papers assessing chronic pelvic pain patients for trigger points have been published. Reiter and Gambone found myofascial syndrome in 15% of their patients with somatic pathology (Reiter, 1990b). [Patients with somatic pathology represented 47% of all patients referred to their pelvic pain clinic (Reiter, 1990b).] Slocumb (1984), in comparison, noted trigger points in most women presenting to the pain clinic with chronic pelvic pain irrespective of underlying pelvic pathology. Clinically, myofascial pain is exacerbated by activity within the muscle or muscle group and, in the case of abdominal wall trigger points and pelvic floor muscle, is exacerbated by activity in deeper visceral structures (bladder or rectal fullness, menses, and cervical motion and intercourse), which share the same dermatomal innervation (Slocumb, 1984; Slocumb, 1990; Travell, 1976). On digital exam of dermatomas of abdomen, back, or vagina, pressure on the trigger point evokes local and referred pain. Pain is exacerbated by the straight leg raising maneuver described earlier. Treatment of myofascial trigger points includes injecting the trigger points with local anesthetic, as well as treating any physical and psychological factors such as depression, anxiety, and learned behavior patterns that may accompany and exacerbate the condition (Travell, 1976; Slocumb, 1984). Medications such as tricyclic antidepressants and anticonvulsants or physical therapy may also be useful.

CENTRAL (BRAIN) FACTORS IN CHRONIC PELVIC PAIN

Descending pain modulating mechanisms, including those originating in the brain or spinal cord, probably involve various chemicals such as classical neurotransmitter, endogenous endorphin and nonendorphin analgesic systems, and excitatory amino acids. Anxiety, depression, and other psychological states may be facilitators or inhibitors of neurological transmission. Wall (1988) has suggested that it is "necessary to consider the lability of central transmission pathways as well as seeking peripheral pathology in all painful conditions." From a psychological perspective, there are various factors that may promote the chronicity of pain. Described as a "diathesis-stress" model of pain, a woman is more susceptible in certain social contexts to develop chronic pain based on her pre-existing vulnerabilities including those related to cognitive, affective, biological, and behavioral functioning (Jacobs, 1997).

Studies on women with chronic pelvic pain have documented a high level of psychological disturbance. The Minnesota Multiphasic Personality Inventory (MMPI) conversion "V" profile (elevated scores on the hypochondriasis, hysteria, and depression scales) was described by Castelnuova-Tedesco and Krout (1970) in a survey of 40 women with pelvic pain. Gross, Doerr, Caldirole, Guzinski, and Ripley (1980) reported high levels of psychopathology in women with pelvic pain, as well as a past exposure to childhood sexual abuse in 90% of their sample. Studies using the MMPI have failed to find a correspondence between psychological and physiological findings. Renaer, Vertommen, Nijs, Wagemans, and Van Hemelrijk (1979) compared MMPI profiles of women having chronic pain without obvious pathology with those of women having pain arising from endometriosis and a control group. They found the two pain groups differed from controls but not from each other. Interestingly, treatment resulting in subjective improvement in pain severity and increased activity level produces a significant improvement in personality profile (Duleba, Jubnyik, Greenfield, & Olive, 1998).

Other studies have focused on the specific diagnosis of depression and pain (Magni, Salmi, deLeo, & Ceola, 1984; Walker, Katon, & Harrop-Griffiths, 1988). Magni, (1984) examined the role of depression and found higher depression scores for women with chronic pelvic pain without pathology compared with women found to have chronic pelvic pain and pathology as established by laparoscopy. They also found a higher likelihood of depressive disorders in the family histories of women whose pain could not be attributed to organic pathology. A comparison of women with pelvic pain of unknown etiology and a pain-free control group revealed the pain group to have a significantly higher prevalence of episodes of major depression. In 12 of the 16 women with a past history of depression, the depression preceded the onset of the pain (Magni, et al., 1984; Walker, et al., 1988). It has been suggested that pain may reflect a masked depression, in view of the common neurotransmitter pathways mediating both pain and mood.

Studies have also examined the role of sexual abuse as a specific risk factor for chronic pelvic pain. Gross and associates (1980) reported a high prevalence (90%) of sexual abuse in their sample. A sample of 25 women with chronic pelvic pain of mixed etiology showed no differences in psychological functioning when divided according to presence or absence of organic findings (Harrop-Griffiths, et al., 1988). However, when compared with a control group of gynecologic patients without pain, there was a higher prevalence of prior substance abuse, functional dyspareunia, inhibited sexual desire, higher scores on the SCL-90, and greater prevalence of sexual abuse — both as youths prior to age 14 and as adults. The authors identified a history of sexual abuse as a child, along with a past history of depression, as strongly related to the subsequent persistence of pelvic pain.

The association between prior abuse and pelvic pain was studied by Rapkin, Kames, & Darke (1990). The study was designed to assess whether prior abuse is more likely in pelvic pain patients than in women with chronic pain in other sites or a painful control group, and whether the abuse was specifically sexual or extended to physical abuse as well. The prevalence of childhood sexual abuse did not differ significantly between the three groups: 19% of pelvic pain, 16% of other pain patients, and 12% of controls. There was a significant difference in the prevalence of physical abuse: highest for the pelvic pain patients (39%), compared with 18 and 9% in the other two groups. This study suggested abuse of any kind is linked to chronic pain. Walling and colleagues (1994) compared women having chronic pelvic pain with women having nonpelvic chronic pain (headache) and pain-free women, finding that women suffering pelvic pain reported a higher lifetime prevalence of major sexual abuse (56%) and physical abuse (50%). By drawing on the learned helplessness model for depression, abuse may predispose to chronicity of pain because it increases the vulnerability to depression and helplessness in the face of adversity (Abramson, Seligman, & Teasdale, 1978). Toomey reaffirmed the importance of obtaining sexual and physical abuse histories in chronic pelvic pain patients (Toomey, Hernandez, Gittelman, & Hulka, 1993).

Renaer (1980) has suggested the diagnosis "chronic pelvic pain without obvious pathology" refers to patients who lack somatic pathology. Often these patients have been considered to have psychogenic pain. As noted in the previous discussion, the majority of patients with chronic pain have abnormal psychogenic profiles, but those patients without pathology do not appear to be psychologically different from those with organic disease (Harrop-Griffiths, et al., 1988; Renaer, et al., 1979). Furthermore, the potential role of as yet unknown neurophysiological mechanisms on the brain and spinal cord in the maintenance of chronic pain cannot be ignored. Abdominal wall, lower back, and pelvic floor muscle trigger points; nerve entrapment in surgical scars; IBS; and IC represent the most common sources of nonreproductive system chronic pelvic pain (Reiter 1990a), all of which probably entail alterations of central processing. Interestingly, these patients also have a high incidence of concurrent psychopathology (somatoform pain disorder), somatization, or depression (Reiter 1990a; Wood, Weisner, & Reiter, 1990). It may be reasonable, therefore, to suggest that chronic pelvic pain without, or even with, pathology is likely to involve all levels of the neuraxis and to direct management approaches accordingly.

DIAGNOSIS AND MANAGEMENT OF CHRONIC PELVIC PAIN

Successful diagnosis and management of patients with chronic pelvic pain requires a meticulous yet compassionate, multidisciplinary approach. As with the investigation of any other physical symptom, a thorough history should be obtained, and often must be acquired in stages. The nature of the pain, location and radiation, aggravating and alleviating factors, timing, effect of menses, exercise, work, stress, intercourse, and orgasm should be queried. The context in which the pain arose should be ascertained. Did the pain begin postpartum, postabortal, or postrape? Have there been previous episodes of pain or inability to perform one's occupation. Is there pending litigation or worker's compensation? Other somatic symptoms should be noted: genital tract (abnormal vaginal bleeding, discharge, mittelschmerz, dysmenorrhea, dyspareunia, infertility); enterocoelic tract (constipation, diarrhea, flatulence, tenesmus, blood, changes in color or caliber of stool); musculoskeletal system (predominant low back distribution, radiation down posterior thigh, association with injury, fatigue, postural changes); and urologic tract (dysuria, urgency, frequency, suprapelvic pain). Historical questions specific to all the peripheral pathologies noted in Table 22.1, should be queried. Past history including medical, surgical, gynecologic, obstetric, medication intake, and prior evaluations for the pain should be documented. Operative and pathology reports are important if the patient has had surgery.

Current and past psychological history — including psychosocial factors; history of past (or current) physical, sexual, and/or emotional abuse; history of hospitalization; suicide attempts; and chemical dependency — should be asked. The attitude of the patient and her family toward the pain, resultant behavior of the patient's family with respect to the pain, and current upheavals in the patient's life should be discussed. The part of the history addressing sensitive issues may have to be reobtained after establishing rapport with the patient.

Symptoms of an acute process such as fever, anorexia, nausea, emesis, significant diarrhea or constipation, abdominal distension, uterine bleeding, pregnancy, or recent abortion should alert one as to the possibility of an acute condition requiring immediate medical or surgical intervention. This is especially called for if accompanied by orthostasis, peritoneal signs, pelvic or abdominal mass, abnormal CBC, positive genital or urinary tract cultures, or positive pregnancy test.

One should perform a complete physical examination, with particular attention to the abdominal, back vaginal, bimanual, and rectovaginal examination. The exam should include evaluation of the abdomen with muscles tensed (head raised off the table or with straight leg raising) to differentiate abdominal wall and visceral sources of pain.

Abdominal wall pain is augmented and visceral pain is diminished with the preceding maneuvers. The patient should be examined while standing for hernias, abdominal (inguinal and femoral) and pelvic (cystocele, enterocele). An attempt should be made to locate by fingertip palpation of the tissues (abdominal, pelvic, external genital, and lower back) that reproduce the patient's pain. The patient should be evaluated by, or in concert with, a gynecologist.

Laboratory studies to obtain the first visit include CBC, ESR, urine analysis and culture, cervical and urethral cultures (gonorrhea and chlamydia), wet mount of vaginal secretions, pap smear, stool guaiac, and — if diarrhea is present — stool culture. If the pelvic or abdominal exam is confusing or suggestive of a mass, ultrasound evaluation is indicated. If symptoms and signs are suggestive of other system involvement, fiberoptic or other appropriate imaging studies of other organ systems should be considered (e.g., upper and lower intestinal barium studies or computerized axial tomography [CAT] scan, intravenous pyelogram, and MRI of the spine).

The patient should be given a daily pain diary in which to note the onset and intensity of pain. Medication intake and aggravating and alleviating factors should be noted in the diary. A simple diary utilizes a visual analog scale from 1 (no pain) to 10 (most severe pain ever). The diary should be maintained for at least 2 months. Previous medical records, surgical and pathological reports or scans, should be requested at the time of, or prior to, this first visit. The second visit should be scheduled for approximately 2 weeks later.

During the second visit, one should again pursue the psychosocial and sexual history. The pain diary, laboratory results, and previous records should be reviewed with the patient. Subacute conditions should be treated (e.g., cervicitis, salpingo-oophoritis, urethritis, cystitis); and the abdominal, back, and pelvic exam should be repeated with thorough evaluation for abdominal, lumbosacral, and vaginal trigger points if not performed on the first exam. A description of the evaluation and treatment of trigger points is provided by Slocumb (1984).

At the time of the second visit the patient should be evaluated by a psychologist familiar with the evaluation and management of chronic pain. The psychologist should preferably be located within the same office or clinic suite.

Psychological referral accomplishes both evaluation, as well as opens the possibility for introducing cognitive behavioral pain management. The assessment should be designed to evaluate the pain complaint, its impact on life circumstances, and the controlling factors and coping mechanisms. Assessment in a chronic context involves a broader range of measures, reflecting social and psychological influences and sequelae, than may apply in the acute setting.

Assessment must evaluate the impact of the pain on the woman's lifestyle. Pelvic pain is likely to affect sexual functioning, which may have additional repercussions in terms of the quality of the patient's relationship and self-esteem. As with mood, a careful history is needed to establish whether the sexual problems existed before the pain or developed subsequently. Previous sexual abuse or trauma should be evaluated, as well as the impact of the pain on day to day functioning. Standardized psychological testing is helpful to determine if affective disturbance is present, as well as to establish a baseline against which to measure treatment response and guide treatment approaches.

If somatic pathology is suspected or confirmed, workup and management should proceed as per treatment of the somatic condition (see Table 22.1). Consultation with a urologist, gastroenterologist, orthopedist, or neurologist should be requested if indicated.

The third visit should be scheduled for 1 or 2 weeks later. This visit should include another review of the pain diary. Patients with cyclic or atypical cyclic pain should be evaluated for primary or secondary dysmenorrhea.

Evaluation of pelvic pain, especially cyclic pain, may require a diagnostic laparoscopy. Pelvic ultrasound or transuterine venography may be indicated if pelvic congestion is suspected, but treatment can proceed on the basis of clinical suspicion. If trigger points were injected and pain has persisted, injection should be repeated weekly or biweekly up to five injections. In addition, consideration should be given to a physical therapy consultation, especially if activity increases the pain or if low back pain is prominent.

A follow-up appointment (fourth visit) should be scheduled for 1 or 2 weeks later. Before the third and fourth visits, the "pain manager," the gynecologist (if not the pain manager), and psychologist should consult.

If pain persists, the patient should initiate cognitive behavioral pain management and various centrally acting pharmaceutical agents should be tried. Tricyclic antidepressants and anticonvulsants have been used successfully in pelvic pain patients. To date, only one randomized controlled trial assessed the effect of selective serotonin reuptake inhibitors on pelvic pain, and the short 14-week trial of 23 women failed to show significant difference in measures of pain and functional disability (Engel, Walker, Engle, Bullis, & Armstrong, 1998). The patient should continue to have scheduled visits with the gynecologist on a regular basis.

MANAGEMENT OF CHRONIC PELVIC PAIN: SURGICAL

Diagnostic Laparoscopy

Diagnostic laparoscopy has become a standard procedure in the evaluation of patients with chronic pelvic pain. Between 14 and 77% of patients have no obvious pathol-

ogy and two thirds of patients have findings of adhesions that may or not play a role in their pain. Furthermore, nonsurgical management of chronic pelvic pain (multidisciplinary pain clinics or trigger point injections) is successful in 65 to 90% of patients regardless of presence of minimal pathology (Rapkin & Kames, 1987; Reiter, Gambone, & Johnson, 1991; Slocumb, 1984). Laparoscopy should probably be reserved for patients in whom other pathology has been ruled out; and for those with signs and/or symptoms of endometriosis, cyclic pelvic pain, or infertility. Some retrospective and prospective evidence suggests that laparoscopy provides pelvic pain patients a positive psychological impact (Elcombe, Gath, & Day, 1997); however, it is costly and not without surgical and anesthetic risks.

Lysis of Adhesions

The role of pelvic adhesions in the genesis of pain is unclear. Lysis of adhesions at laparotomy is frequently undermined by a high incidence of adhesion reformation (Holtz, 1984). Laparoscopic lysis of adhesions may be less likely to result in significant reformation of adhesions; however, 20 to 90% of adhesions reform or form *de nouveau* after an adhesiolysis procedure. It is not unreasonable, therefore, to lyse adhesions at the time of diagnostic laparoscopy, but controlled studies have yet to be definitive.

Hysterectomy

Hysterectomy has long been performed to cure pelvic pain. In fact, up to 19% of hysterectomies are performed for the sole indication of chronic pelvic pain (Reiter, 1990a). However, 30% of patients presenting to pelvic pain clinics have already undergone hysterectomy without experiencing relief of pain (Chamberlain & La Ferla, 1987). Reiter and associates (1991) noted a decline in the incidence of hysterectomy for the indication of chronic pelvic pain from 16.3 to 5.8% after the initiation of a multidisciplinary approach to the diagnosis and treatment of chronic pelvic pain. A prospective cohort study, the Maine Womens Health Study, revealed 18% of women had a hysterectomy for chronic pelvic pain with significant improvement in pain and associated symptoms. Their underlying diagnoses, however, were not described (Carlson, Miller, & Fowler, 1994). Hillis, Marchbanks, and Peterson (1995) studied a prospective cohort of 308 women who underwent hysterectomy for chronic pelvic pain, thought to be of uterine origin. The outcome revealed a 74% response rate, with observed persistent pain associated with multiparity, prior history of pelvic inflammatory disease (PID), lack of pathology, and Medicaid payer status (Hillis, et al., 1995). Hysterectomy remains an option for appropriately selected patients with pain of uterine origin. In recognition of the fact that hysterectomy treats at best only some women, the American College of Obstetricians and Gynecologists (1998) established criteria to be met prior to performing such invasive surgery for pelvic pain. The criteria include that no remediable pathology is found on laparoscopic examination and that a 6-month presence of pain occurs with negative effect on the patient's quality of life.

PRESACRAL NEURECTOMY

Presacral neurectomy or sympathectomy (PSN) was first described by Cotte (1937) for the indication of dysmenorrhea. As is apparent from the discussion of the neuroanatomy of the pelvic organs, the presacral nerve, which is actually the superior hypogastric plexus, receives the major afferent supply from the cervix, uterus, and proximal fallopian tubes. Afferents traveling with the sympathetic nerve supply from the bladder and rectum also pass through the superior hypogastric plexus. Normal micturition and defecation are dependent on an intact sacral autonomic nerve supply and are relatively unaffected by resection of the superior hypogastric plexus. The nerve supply to the adnexal structures bypasses the hypogastric plexus, as the afferents from the ovary travel with sympathetic fibers accompanying the ovarian artery to the superior mesenteric plexus to enter the spinal cord at T9 and T10. These autonomic relationships constitute the rationale for Cotte's (1937) emphasis on differentiating dysmenorrhea with the maximum intensity of the pain localized to the uterus with radiation to the sacrum from lateralizing pain radiating to the lumbar region.

PSN has been studied in the management of central pelvic pain in the setting of both cyclic and noncyclic pain (Ingersoll & Meigs, 1948; Lee, Stone, Magelssen, Belts, & Benson, 1986; Polan & DeCherney, 1980). Though most studies of PSN are uncontrolled, Polan and DeCherney's (1980) study did include a control group of patients who had infertility surgery without PSN. In the latter group, only 26% experienced relief of pain as compared with 75% of patients who also underwent PSN. In another randomized controlled study by Tjaden, Schlaff, Kimball, and Rock (1992), the study was prematurely terminated due to the overwhelming response to PSN compared with resection of moderate to severe endometriosis (Tjaden, et al., 1992). However, when Candiani, Fedele, Vercellini, Bianchi, and DiNola (1992) studied PSN vs. resection of moderate or severe endometriosis, initial central pain was reduced though 6-month follow-up revealed no significant difference in pain. The value of PSN remains controversial.

MULTIDISCIPLINARY PAIN MANAGEMENT

MULTIDISCIPLINARY PAIN MANAGEMENT

Multidisciplinary pain management is an excellent approach to chronic pelvic pain. Peripheral factors are managed by the pain manager. Spinal cord and central factors related to possible abnormalities of modulation of pain impulses are addressed with trigger point injections, centrally acting medications, acupuncture, or TENS (Helms, 1987; Mannheimer & Whaler, 1985; Rapkin & Kames, 1987; Slocumb, 1984). Cognitive behavioral and other psychological factors are addressed by the psychologist.

One program was successful in reducing pain by at least 50% in 85% of the subjects (Rapkin & Kames, 1987). Other studies have suggested that similar results may be obtained with a multidisciplinary team (Milburn, Reiter, & Rhomberg, 1993; Pearce, Knight, & Beard, 1982; Peters, et al., 1991; Reiter, et al., 1991; Wood, et al., 1990). In a prospective randomized study, the multidisciplinary approach was found to be more effective than traditional gynecologic (medical and surgical) management (Peters, et al., 1991).

REFERENCES

Abramson, L.Y., Seligman, M.E.P., & Teasdale, J.D. (1978). Learned helplessness in human: Critique and reformation. *Abnormal Psychology, 87*, 49–74.

Adams, J., Reginal, P.W., Franks, S., Wadsworth, J., & Beard R.W. (1990). Uterine size and endometrial thickness and the significance of cystic ovaries in women with pelvic pain due to congestion. *British Journal of Obstetrics and Gynecology, 97*, 583–587.

Almeida, O.D, & Val-Gallas, J.M. (1997). Conscious pain mapping. *Journal of American Association of Gynecologic Laparoscopists, 4*, 587–590.

American College of Obstetricians and Gynecologists. (1983). Dysmenorrhea (Vol. 68, pp. 1–5). Washington, D.C.: American College of Obstetricians and Gynecologists.

American College of Obstetricians and Gynecologists criteria set. (1998). Hysterectomy, abdominal or vaginal for chronic pelvic pain. Number 29, November 27. Committee on Quality Assessment. American College of Obstetricians and Gynecologists. *International Journal of Gynaecology and Obstetrics, 60*, 316–317.

Baker, P.K. (1993). Musculoskeletal origins of chronic pelvic pain. In F. W. Ling (Ed.), *Obstetrics and gynecology clinics of North America: Contemporary management of chronic pain* (pp. 719–742). Philadelphia: W. B. Saunders.

Beard, R.W., Highman, J.H., Pearce, S., & Reginald, P.W. (1984). Diagnosis of pelvic varicosities in women with chronic pelvic pain. *Lancet, 2*, 946–949.

Bergman, A., Karram, M., & Bhatia, N.N. (1989). Urethral syndrome: A comparison of different treatment modalities. *Journal of Reproductive Medicine, 34*, 157–160.

Berkley, K.J. (1994). Communications from the uterus (and other tissues). In J. M. Besson (Ed.), *Pharmacological aspects of peripheral neurons involved in nociception, pain research and clinical management* (pp. 39–47). Amsterdam: Elsevier.

Berkley, K.J., & Hubscher, C.H. (1995). Visceral and somatic sensory tracks through the neuroaxis and their relation to pain: Lessons from the rat female reproductive system. In G. F. Gebhart (Ed.), *Visceral pain: Progress in pain research and management* (Vol. 5, pp. 195–216). Seattle: IASP Press.

Bodner, D.R. (1988). The urethral syndrome. *Office Urology, 15*, 699–704.

Candiani, G.B., Fedele, L., Vercellini, P., Bianchi, S., & Di Nola, G. (1992). Presacral neurectomy for the treatment of pelvic pain associated with endometriosis: A controlled study. *American Journal of Obstetrics and Gynecology, 167*, 100–103.

Capasso, P., Simons, C., Trotteur, G., Dondelinger, R.F., Henroteaux, D., & Gaspard, U. (1997). Treatment of symptomatic pelvic varices by ovarian vein embolization. *Cardiovascular Interventional Radiology, 20*, 107–111.

Carey, M.P., & Slack, M.C. (1996). GnRH analogue in assessing chronic pelvic pain in women with residual ovaries. *British Journal of Obstetrics and Gynecology, 103*, 150–153.

Carlson, K.J., Miller, B A., & Fowler, F.J., Jr. (1994). The Maine Women's Health Study: I. Outcomes of Hysterectomy. *Obstetrics and Gynecology, 83*, 557–565.

Castelnuova-Tedesco, P., & Krout, B.M. (1970). Psychosomatic aspects of chronic pelvic pain. *Psychiatry in Medicine, 1*, 109–126.

Cervero, F. (1994). Sensory innervation of the viscera: Peripheral basis of visceral pain. *Physiological Reviews, 74*, 95–138.

Cervero, F., & Tattersall, J.E.H. (1986). Somatic and visceral sensory integration in the thoracic spinal cord. In F. Cervero & J. Morrison (Eds.), *Visceral sensation* (pp. 189–205). New York: Elsevier Science Publications.

Chamberlain, A., & La Ferla, J. (1987). The gynecologist's approach to chronic pelvic pain. In J.D. Burroughs, et al. (Eds.), *Handbook of chronic pain management* (Vol. 33, pp. 371–382). Amsterdam: Elsevier.

Chan, W.Y, & Dawood, M.Y. (1980). Prostaglandin levels in menstrual fluid of non-dysmenorrheic and of dysmenorrheic subjects with and without oral contraceptive or ibuprofen therapy. *Advances in Prostaglandin and Thromboxane Research, 8*, 1443–1447.

Chatman, D.L., & Ward, A.B. (1982). Endometriosis in adolescents. *Obstetrics and Gynecology, 27*, 186–190.

Cornillie, F J., Oosterlynck, D., Lauweryns, J.M., & Koninckx, P.R. (1990). Deeply infiltrating pelvic endometriosis: Histology and clinical significance. *Fertility and Sterility, 53*, 978–983.

Cotte, G. (1937). Resection of the presacral nerves in the treatment of obstinate dysmenorrhea. *American Journal of Obstetrics and Gynecology, 33*, 1034–1040.

De Groat, W.C. (1994). Neurophysiology of the pelvic organs. In D. N. Rushton (Ed.), *Handbook of neuro-urology* (pp. 55–93). New York: Marcel Dekker.

Doyle, I.B. (1955). Paracervical uterine denervation by transection of the cervical plexus for the relief of dysmenorrhea. *American Journal of Obstetrics and Gynecology, 70*, 1–16.

Drugs for dysmenorrhea. (1979). *The Medical Letter on Drugs and Therapeutics, 21*, 81–84.

Duleba, A J., Jubnyik, K J., Greenfield, D.A., & Olive, D.L. (1998). Changes in personality profile associated with laparoscopic surgery for chronic pelvic pain. *Journal of American Association of Gynecologic Laparoscopists, 5*, 389–395.

Elcombe, S., Gath, D., & Day, A. (1997). The psychological effects of laparoscopy on women with chronic pelvic pain. *Psychological Medicine, 27*, 1041–1050.

Engel, C.C., Jr., Walker, E.A., Engel, A.L., Bullis, J., & Armstrong, A. (1998). A randomized, double-blind crossover trial of sertraline in women with chronic pelvic pain. *Journal of Psychosomatic Research, 44*, 203–207.

Farquhar, C.M., Rogers, V., Franks, S., Pearce, S., Wadsworth, J., & Bland, R.W. (1989). A randomized controlled trial of medroxyprogesterone acetate and psychotherapy for the treatment of pelvic congestion. *British Journal of Obstetrics and Gynaecology, 96*, 1153–1162.

Fields, H. (1987). *Pain* (p. 41). New York: McGraw-Hill.

Filler, W.W., & Hall, W.C. (1970). Dysmenorrhea and its therapy. *American Journal of Obstetrics and Gynecology, 106*, 104–109.

Fukaya, T., Hoshiai, H., & Yajima, A. (1993). Is pelvic endometriosis always associated with chronic pain? A retrospective study of 618 cases diagnosed by laparoscopy. *American Journal of Obstetrics and Gynecology, 169*, 719–722.

Gross, R.J., Doerr, H., Caldirola, D., Guzinski, G., & Ripley, H. (1980). Borderline syndrome and incest in chronic pelvic pain patients. *International Journal of Psychiatry and Medicine, 10*, 79–96.

Gupta, A., & McCarthy, S. (1994). Pelvic varices as a cause for pelvic pain: MRI appearance. *Magnetic Resonance Imaging, 12*, 679–681.

Hammeroff, S.R., Carlson, G.L., & Brown, B.R. (1981). Ilioinguinal pain syndrome. *Pain, 10*, 253–257.

Harrop-Griffiths, J., Katon, W., Walker, E., Helm, L., Russo, J., & Hickok, C. (1988). The association between chronic pelvic pain, psychiatric diagnoses and childhood sexual abuse. *Obstetrics and Gynecology, 71*, 589–594.

Helms, J.M. (1987). Acupuncture for the management of primary dysmenorrhea. *Obstetrics and Gynecology, 69*, 51–56.

Hightower, N.C., & Roberts, J.W. (1981). Acute and chronic lower abdominal pain of enterologic origin in chronic pelvic pain. In M.R. Renaer (Ed.), *Chronic pelvic pain in women* (pp. 110–137). New York: Springer-Verlag.

Hillis, S.D., Marchbanks, P.A., & Peterson, H.B. (1995). The effectiveness of hysterectomy for chronic pelvic pain. *Obstetrics and Gynecology, 86*, 941–945.

Hobbs, J.T. (1976). The pelvic congestion syndrome. *Practitioner, 216*, 529–540.

Holtz, G. (1984). Prevention and management of peritoneal adhesions. *Fertility and Sterility, 41,* 497–507.

Hornstein, M.D., Surrey, E.S., Weisberg, G.W., & Casino, L.A. (1998). Leuprolide acetate depot and hormonal add-back in endometriosis: A 12-month study. *Obstetrics and Gynecology, 91,* 702–708.

Ingersoll, F.M., & Meigs, J.V. (1948). Presacral neurectomy for dysmenorrhea. *New England Journal of Medicine, 238,* 357–360.

Jacob, M.C. (1997). Pain intensity, psychiatric diagnosis, and psychosocial factors. In J. Steege, D. Metzger, & B. Levy (Eds.), *Chronic pelvic pain: An integrated approach* (pp. 67–76). Philadelphia: Saunders.

Janig, W., Haupt-Schade, P., & Kohler, W. (1993). Afferent innervation of the colon: The neurophysiological basis for visceral sensation and pain. In E.A. Mayer & H.E. Raybould (Eds.), *Basic and clinical aspects of chronic abdominal pain* (pp. 71–86). Amsterdam: Elsevier.

Kaplan, B., Peled, Y., Pardo, J., Rabinerson, D., Hirsh, M., Ovadia, J., & Neri, A. (1994). Transcutaneous electrical nerve stimulation (TENS) as a relief for dysmenorrhea. *Clinical Experiments in Obstetrics and Gynecology, 21,* 87–90.

Karram, M.M. (1993). Frequency, urgency, and painful bladder syndrome. In M.D. Walters & M.M. Karram (Eds.), *Clinical urogynecology* (pp. 285–298). St. Louis, MO: Mosby.

Keltz, M.D., Peck, L., Liu, S., Kim, A.H., Arici, A., & Olive, D.L. (1995). Large bowel-to-pelvic sidewall adhesions associated with chronic pelvic pain. *Journal of the American Association Gynecologic Laparoscopists, 3,* 55–59.

Kitchen, J.D. (1985). Endometriosis. In J. Sciarra (Ed.), *Gynecology and obstetrics* (pp. 1–25). New York: Harper and Row.

Kresch, A.J., Seifer, D.B., Sachs, L.B., & Barrese, I. (1984). Laparoscopy in 100 women with chronic pelvic pain. *Obstetrics and Gynecology, 64,* 672–674.

Kumazawa, T. (1986). Sensory innervation of reproductive organs. In F. Cervero & J. Morrison (Eds.), *Visceral sensation* (pp. 115–131). New York: Elsevier Science Publications.

Lee, A.W., Bell, R.M., Griffen, W.O., Jr., & Hagihara, P. (1985). Recurrent appendiceal colic. *Surgical Gynecology and Obstetrics, 161,* 21–24.

Lee, R.B., Stone, K., Magelssen, D., Belts, R., & Benson, W. (1986). Presacral neurectomy for chronic pelvic pain. *Obstetrics and Gynecology, 68,* 517–521.

Ling, F.W., & Pelvic Pain Study Group, (1999). Randomized controlled trial of depot leuprolide in patients with chronic pelvic pain and clinically suspected endometriosis. *Obstetrics and Gynecology, 93,* 51–58.

Liston, W. A., Bradford, W. P., Downie, J., & Kerr, M.G. (1972). Laparoscopy in a general gynecologic unit. *American Journal of Obstetrics and Gynecology, 113,* 672–677.

Lundberg, W.I., Wall, J.E., & Mathers, J.E. (1973). Laparoscopy in the evaluation of pelvic pain. *Obstetrics and Gynecology, 42,* 872–876.

MacDonald, J.S. (1993). Management of chronic pain. In F. W. Ling (Ed.), *Obstetrics and gynecology clinics of North America: Contemporary management of chronic pain* (pp. 817–838). Philadelphia: W. B. Saunders.

Magni, G., Salmi, A., deLeo, D., & Ceola, A. (1984). Chronic pelvic pain and depression. *Psychopathology, 17,* 132–136.

Malinak, L.R. (1980). Operative management of pelvic pain. *Clinical Obstetrics and Gynecology, 23,* 191–199.

Mannheimer, J.S., & Whaler, E.C. (1985). The efficacy of transcutaneous electrical nerve stimulation in dysmenorrhea. *Clinical Journal of Pain, 1,* 75–83.

Mathias, S.D., Kuppermann, M., Liberman, R.F., Lipschutz, R.C., & Steege, J. F. (1996). Chronic pelvic pain: Prevalence, health-related quality of life, and economic correlates. *Obstetrics and Gynecology, 87,* 321–7.

McSherry, C.K., Cornell, G.N., & Glenn, F. (1969). Carcinoma of the colon and rectum. *Annals of Surgery, 169,* 502–509.

Messing, E.M., & Stamey, T.A. (1978). Interstitial cystitis: Early diagnosis, pathology, and treatment. *Urology, 12,* 381–392.

Milburn, A., Reiter, R.C., & Rhomberg, A.T. (1993). Multidisciplinary approach to chronic pelvic pain. In F. W. Ling (Ed), *Obstetrics and gynecology clinics of North America: Contemporary management of chronic pain* (pp. 643–661). Philadelphia: W. B. Saunders.

Morscher, E. (1981). Low back pain in women. In M.R. Renaer (Ed.), *Chronic pelvic pain in women* (pp. 137–154). New York: Springer-Verlag.

Painter, N.S. (1975). Diverticular disease of the colon, a 20th century problem. *Clinical Gastroenterology, 1,* 3–21.

Palter, S.F. (1999). Microlaparoscopy under local anesthesia and conscious pain mapping for the diagnosis and management of pelvic pain. *Current Opinion on Obstetrics and Gynecology, 11,* 387–393.

Pearce, S., Knight, C., & Beard, R.W. (1982). Pelvic pain — A common gynaecological problem. *Journal of Psychosomatic Obstetrics and Gynaecology, I(I),* 12–17.

Peters, A.A., Van Dorst, E., Jellis, B., VanZuuren, E., Hermans, J., & Trimbos, J.B. (1991). A randomized clinical trial to compare two different approaches in women with chronic pelvic pain. *Obstetrics and Gynecology, 77,* 740–744.

Pettit, P.D., & Lee, R.A. (1988). Ovarian remnant syndrome: Diagnostic dilemma and surgical challenge. *Obstetrics and Gynecology, 71,* 580–583.

Polan, M.L., & DeCherney, A. (1980). Presacral neurectomy for pelvic pain in infertility. *Fertility and Sterility, 34,* 557–560.

Price, F.V., Edwards, R., & Buchsbaum, H.J. (1990). Ovarian remnant syndrome: Difficulties in diagnosis and management. *Obstetrics and Gynecology Surgery, 45,* 151–156.

Probst, A.M., & Laufer, M.R. (1999). Endometriosis in adolescents. Incidence, diagnosis and treatment. *Journal of Reproductive Medicine, 44,* 751–758.

Procacci, P., Zoppi, M., & Maresen, M. (1986). Clinical approach to visceral sensation. In F. Cervero & J. Morrison (Eds.), *Visceral sensation* (pp. 21–36). New York: Elsevier.

Rapkin, A.J. (1986). Adhesions and pelvic pain: A retrospective study. *Obstetrics and Gynecology, 68,* 13–15.

Rapkin, A.J., & Kames, L.D. (1987). The pain management approach to chronic pelvic pain. *Journal of Reproductive Medicine, 32,* 323–327.

Rapkin, A.J., Kames, L.D., & Darke, L.L. (1990). History of physical and sexual abuse in women with chronic pelvic pain. *Obstetrics and Gynecology, 76,* 90–96.

Rapkin, A.J., & Mayer, E.A. (1993). Gastroenterologic causes of chronic pelvic pain. In F.W. Ling (Ed.), *Obstetrics and gynecology clinics of North America: Contemporary management of chronic pain* (pp. 663–683). Philadelphia: W.B. Saunders.

Reiter, R.C. (1990a). A profile of women with chronic pelvic pain. *Clinical Obstetrics and Gynecology, 33,* 130–136.

Reiter, R.C. (1990b). Occult somatic pathology in women with chronic pelvic pain. *Clinical Obstetrics and Gynecology, 33,* 154–160.

Reiter, R.C., Gambone, J.C., & Johnson, S.R. (1991). Availability of a multidisciplinary pelvic pain clinic and frequency of hysterectomy for pelvic pain. *Journal of Psychosomatic Obstetrics and Gynaecology, 12*(Suppl.), 109.

Renaer, M. (1980). Chronic pelvic pain without obvious pathology in women: Personal observation and a review of the problem. *European Journal of Obstetrics and Gynecology, 10,* 415–463.

Renaer, M. (1981). *Chronic pelvic pain in women.* New York: Springer-Verlag.

Renaer, M., Vertommen, H., Nijs, P., Wagemans, M., & Van-Hemelrijk, T. (1979). Psychosocial aspects of chronic pelvic pain in women. *American Journal of Obstetrics and Gynecology, 134,* 75–80.

Ritchie, J. (1979). Pain in IBS. *Practical Gastroenterology, 3,* 17–23.

Sant, G.R. (1998). Interstitial cystitis – a urogynecologic perspective. *Contemporary Obstetrics and Gynecology,* 119–130.

Sichlau, M.J., Yao, J.S.T., & Vogelzang, R.L. (1994). Transcatheter embolotherapy for the treatment of pelvic congestion syndrome. *Obstetrics and Gynecology, 83,* 892–896.

Sippo, W.C., Burghardt, A., & Gomez, A.C. (1987). Nerve entrapment after Pfannensteil incision. *American Journal of Obstetrics and Gynecology, 157,* 420–421.

Slocumb, J.C. (1984). Neurological factors in chronic pelvic pain: Trigger points and the abdominal pelvic pain syndrome. *American Journal of Obstetrics and Gynecology, 149,* 536–543.

Slocumb, J.C. (1990). Chronic somatic myofascial and neurogenic abdominal pelvic pain. In R.P. Porreco & R.C. Reiter (Eds), *Clinical obstetrics and gynecology* (pp. 145–153). Philadelphia: J.B. Lippincott & Co.

Steege, J.F. (1987). Ovarian remnant syndrome. *Obstetrics and Gynecology, 70,* 64–67.

Steege, J.F., & Scott, A.L. (1991). Resolution of chronic pelvic pain after laparoscopic lysis of adhesions. *American Journal of Obstetrics and Gynecology, 165,* 278–283.

Stones, R.W., Rae, T., Rogers, V., Fry, R., & Beard, R.W. (1990). Pelvic congestion in women: Evaluation with transvaginal ultrasound and observation of venous pharmacology. *British Journal of Radiology, 63,* 710–711.

Summit, R.L. (1993). Urogynecologic causes of chronic pelvic pain. In F.W. Ling (Ed.), *Obstetrics and gynecology clinics of North America: Contemporary management of chronic pain* (pp. 685–698). Philadelphia: W.B. Saunders.

Sutton, C.J., Pooley, A.S., Ewen, S.P., & Haines, P. (1997). Follow-up report on randomized controlled trial of laser laparoscopy in the treatment of pelvic pain associated with minimal to moderate endometriosis. *Fertility and Sterility, 68,* 1070–1074.

Sweet, R.L., & Gibbs, R.S. (1985). Pelvic inflammatory disease. In R.L. Sweet & R.S. Gibbs (Eds.), *Infectious diseases of the female genital tract* (Part 1, pp. 53–77). Baltimore: Williams & Wilkins.

Tarazov, P.G., Prozorovskij, K.V., & Ryzhkov, V.K. (1997). Pelvic pain caused by ovarian varices. Treatment by transcatheter embolization. *Acta Radiologica, 38,* 1023–1025.

Taylor, H.C., Jr. (1954). Pelvic pain based on a vascular and autonomic nervous system disorder. *American Journal of Obstetrics and Gynecology, 67,* 1177–1196.

Tjaden, B., Schlaff, W.D., Kimball, A., & Rock, J.A. (1992). The efficacy of presacral neurectomy for the relief of midline dysmenorrhea. *Obstetrics and Gynecology, 167,* 100–103.

Toomey, T.C., Hernandez, J.T., Gittelman, D.F., & Hulka, J.F. (1993). Relationship of sexual and physical abuse to pain and psychological assessment variables in chronic pelvic pain patients. *Pain, 53*(1), 105–109.

Travell, J. (1976). Myofascial trigger points: Clinical view. *Advances in Pain Research and Therapy, 1,* 919–926.

Venbrux, A.C., & Lambert, D.L. (1999). Embolization of the ovarian veins as a treatment for patients with chronic pelvic pain caused by pelvic venous incompetence (pelvic congestion syndrome). *Current Opinion in Obstetrics and Gynecology, 11,* 395–399.

Vercellini, P., Fedele, L., Bianchi, S., & Candiani, G.B. (1991). Pelvic denervation for chronic pain associated with endometriosis: Fact or fancy? *American Journal of Obstetrics and Gynecology, 165*(3), 745–749.

Vercelini, P., Trespedi, L., De Giorgi, O., Cortesi, I., Parazzini, F., & Crosignani, P.G. (1996). Endometriosis and pelvic pain: Relation to disease stage and localization. *Fertility and Sterility, 65,* 299–304.

Vereecken, R.L. (1981). Chronic pelvic pain of urologic origin. In M.R. Renaer (Ed.), *Chronic pelvic pain in women* (pp. 155–161). New York: Springer-Verlag.

Walker, E., Katon, W., & Harrop-Griffiths, J. (1988). Relationship of chronic pelvic pain of psychiatric diagnoses and childhood sexual abuse. *American Journal of Psychiatry, 145,* 75–80.

Wall, P.D. (1988). The John J. Bonica distinguished lecture. Stability and instability of central pain mechanisms. In R. Dubner (Ed.), *Proceedings of the fifth world congress on pain* (pp. 13–24). Amsterdam: Elsevier Science Publishers BV.

Walling, M.K., Reiter R.C., O'Hara,, M.W., Milburn, A.K., Lilly, G., & Vincent, S.D. (1994). Abuse history and chronic pain in women: I. Prevalence of sexual abuse and physical abuse. *Obstetrics and Gynecology, 84*, 193–199.

Wilson, M., Farquhar, C., Kennedy, S., & Jin, X. (2000). Transcutaneous electrical nerve stimulation and acupuncture for primary dysmenorrhea [Protocol]. Software Update. Oxford: The Cochrane Library,

Wood, D.P., Weisner, M.G., & Reiter, R.C. (1990). Psychogenic chronic pelvic pain. *Clinical Obstetrics and Gynecology, 33*, 179–195.

Young, S.J., Alpers, D.H., Norland, C.C., & Woodruff, R. (1976). Psychiatric illness and the irritable bowel syndrome: Practical implications for the primary physician. *Gastroenterology, 70*, 162–166.

Section IV

Specialty Approaches to Pain Management through Team Management

23

Pain Medicine and the Primary Care Physician

Uday S. Uthaman, M.D., F.A.C.F.P. and Pierre L. LeRoy, M.D., F.A.C.S.

Pain is a more terrible lord of mankind than even death itself.

Albert Schweitzer

This chapter is dedicated to John J. Bonica, M.D., for his outstanding contributions to pain medicine and humanity.

INTRODUCTION

The dynamics of the present health care system has forced many patients to seek managed care. This has not provided the anticipated results or satisfied the expectations of many to offer individualized care. The current system is largely a pharmacological system-based treatment program that does not address etiology or causation.

NEW STATE OF THE ART

Due to five new considerations, these and other shortcomings can be remedied:

1. New advances in the field of clinical pain medicine
2. Recent advances in diagnoses
3. New and diversified treatment programs
4. Progress in laboratory studies
5. Availability of focused integrated studies

Individually and collectively, these provide a new frontier and opportunity for primary care physicians (PCPs) to diversify their clinical practice and acquire advanced certifications and degrees.

MISSION STATEMENT FOR CLINICIANS

We offer the following ten considerations:

1. Reduce human pain and suffering
2. Individualize patient care
3. Reduce economic and psychosocial losses
4. Concurrently treat co-morbidity and social productivity
5. Reduce loss of workforce skills
6. Reduce healthcare expenditures
7. Reduce occurrence of preventable disease and injury
8. Pursue educational resources
9. Communicate with the patient with empathy
10. Never give up hope for the patient

How can these goals be accomplished?

The professional, annual continuing education of physicians is now mandated by licensing Medical Boards, but the focus on personal selection of pain medicine is elective. Some state Medical Boards are already identifying pain medicine as a subspecialty.

THE ROLE OF SPECIALTY ASSOCIATIONS

Some specialty scientific societies have long recognized the need for additional specialties in the field of pain medicine. For example, the American Association of Neurological Surgeons (AANS) has organized five divisions, of which there is a section on pain management that concentrates on both the medical and surgical treatment of pain. Anesthesiology, orthopedic, and other

0-8493-0926-3/02/$0.00+$1.50
© 2002 by CRC Press LLC

societies have also followed this trend, offering educational course material, conferences, seminars, certification, and accreditation. The world medical community, led by Dr. John J. Bonica, in the 1970s recognized the need for further research and professional interaction and founded the International Association for the Study of Pain (IASP). Dr. Bonica and several others realized at the first IASP meeting in 1975 in Florence, Italy, that there was no American Pain Society. Thus, it was quickly organized and became known as the APS. Others followed, but remained exclusive in their membership, focus, and formulated regional sections. Realizing that these organizations were primarily for specialties, the American Association of Pain Management (AAPM) was organized to be more inclusive, recognizing the need to bring together all health professionals that expressed interest in the complex field of pain medicine, a multidisciplinary approach that brings diversification, interaction, expanding education, and credentialing to the field of pain medicine.

The purpose of this chapter is to bring together a syllabus for the PCP and other interested health professionals, providing a clinical overview of the field and referring to other specific chapters for additional information.

THE DEFINITIONS OF PAIN

This subject has been a Herculean task and was assigned to Professor Mersky, on whose committee the co-author (Pierre LeRoy) was privileged to be a member. For 5 years, the Taxonomy Committee of the IASP struggled for a definition that would satisfy the somatic and psychologic criteria and be translatable into other languages to clarify the existing Babylonian confusion.

MERSKY

> Pain is an unpleasant sensory and emotional experience associated with actual or potential tissue damage or described in terms of such damage.

Since then, other concepts have emerged.

MOUNT CASTLE

> Sensory experience evoked by stimuli that injure or threaten to destroy tissue, defined introspectively by every man as that which hurts.

ARNOFF

> Operational definition of pain is that of a complex, personal, subjective and unpleasant experience which

may or may not have any correlation with bodily injury or tissue damage.

Later, other definitions evolved to show the definitive progress that has been provided by the basic scientist and technology in neuroanatomy and physiology, which act as the foundation for the improved clinical management of pain medicine.

The fundamental nociceptive stimuli for pain can provoke irritation, which is reversible, or can produce tissue damage that is not reversible and accounts for chronic spontaneous pain perception, which eventually may be interpreted by the limbic-forebrain system as "it hurts"; and becomes associated with psychological discontent and depression. If the inflammatory response, the reaction of tissue to an irritation continues, is associated with the classic, long-known, four characteristics of *Dolore, Calor, Temor*, and *Rubor* (or pain, heat, swelling, and redness). These are discussed later in this chapter and in more detail by Richard S. Materson, M.D., in *Techniques for Assessing and Diagnosing Pain.*

THE INCIDENCE OF PAIN

Actual, accurate data is not yet available but many estimates have been made that recognize an enormous human and economic burden in society. It is felt by many colleagues that the incidence of pain is underreported. Data banks have now been established to correct this. An estimate by The Information Specialists of Tampa, Florida, is that "pain costs the U.S. economy about 100 billion dollars a year, including 515 million workdays lost and about 410 million office visits to doctors." It is estimated that one in every five adult Americans experiences chronic pain and seeks relief from a doctor.

These staggering estimates are addressed in more detail in *Pain and Its Magnitude*, by Barry Fox, Ph.D.

THE CLASSIFICATION OF PAIN

Many classification systems have been proposed, but the acute, chronic, cancer, and psychogenic pain divisions appear practical for clinicians.

- Acute: From onset in time of perception, it may be variable, lasting from seconds to months.
- Chronic: A consensus is developing that after 6 months, it is considered to be chronic and frequently associated with varied emotional responses.
- Cancer: Initially, many malignancies have no symptoms and are silent. Pain perception due to tumefaction, vascular, cytochemical, and pathophysiological changes may develop insidiously

with symptoms of cancer. Special pain management is needed for this patient population.

- Psychogenic pain syndromes: These can be diagnosed when the patient complains of pain, but no physical assessment or laboratory test can corroborate the complaint. It can be considered a symptomatic response, however, that can be managed.

No classification is yet considered complete but Drs. Thienhaus and Cole address this in detail in this text.

PATHOPHYSIOLOGY FOR THE CLINICIAN

He who understands pain, knows medicine.

Sir William Osler

Basic anatomical and physiological considerations can be simplified. We will review current concepts of incoming pain signals. They are referred to as afferents or arrival sensations. We can identify four fundamental divisions that can be classified as sensory receptors, peripheral nerve networks, spinal modulation, and central brain discrimination and affective correlates.

RECEPTORS FOR PAIN

Receptors for pain are thought to be free nerve endings, but Meissner's corpuscles and bulbs of Krause, for example, have thresholds for pressure and cold temperature changes, as do many other receptor organelles. Such receptors can act like a symphony orchestra and transmit specific sensory information, but can also relay to pain networks when the stimulus becomes nociceptive. In the normal resting state, receptors are "on call," but do not "talk" unless certain thresholds are reached. This is true for neuropathic, myofascial, vascular, scleral, and visceral pain.

PERIPHERAL SENSORY NERVES

Some peripheral sensory nerves are named but the vast majority remain unnamed. These networks are more complex than previously realized because they are not only composed of somatic and autonomic afferents, but also efferent outgoing motor neurons transmitting electrochemical action potentials that regulate many forms of interactive ionic channel electrolytes such as calcium, sodium, and potassium — thus conducting a propagation action potential wave of millivolt energy similar to a small battery, but which eventually must be recharged. In addition, we now know that the ganglion cells produce neuropeptides, such as catecholamines, bradykinin, histamine, cytokines, and many other modulating substances that influence the nerve impulse. These can also be sensitized in injury area cross-talk, interact with other nerves, and produce hyperalgesia. This also explains how a light-touch stimulus can exacerbate a previously injured area that has not healed, and explains why an acute pain can become chronic and produce regional allodynia. In addition, the autonomic nervous system can produce a transmitted substance under nociceptive stimulation. This helps to explain the sensitization to allodynia in patients with reflex sympathetic dystrophy (now being called Complex Regional Pain Syndrome), in which patients avoid touch or clothing contacts that produce dysesthesias or disagreeable painful sensations.

THE SPINAL LEVEL

At the spinal level, further modulation takes place prior to sending the messages proximally as well as distally. Incoming afferent peripheral nerve impulses moving at speeds recorded in milliseconds, from low or high thresholds, neurons such as A-beta, A-delta, and C-fibers, or from sensitized receptors separating the dorsal horn of the spinal cord into zones called Rexed layers. The outermost layer is called Lissauer's tract or Substantia Gelatinosa. Here, unmyelinated C- and A-delta high-threshold nerve fibers transmit specific sensations that have burning, touch, and pressure characteristics. Other A-beta fibers go deeper into the Rexed layer five and transmit non-nociceptive sensations. These fibers integrate with marginal neurons and cross-talk when nociception occurs so that a network discriminates localizing intensity and transmits centrally, temporal-based impulses through the cord proportionate to the input stimulus. These clinical characteristics of the sensory pain signal can be identified by the patient and communicated to the physician. These deeper second-order neurons are called wide dynamic neurons (WDN). These also ascend and descend, forming the main pain tract known as the spinothalamic tract — the main pain pathway to the brain for further modulation.

THE BRAIN

The spinothalamic tract ends superiorly in the basal thalamus. This main tract carries pain and temperature sensory signals and also has a homunculus, layered localization within the thalamus itself. Non-nociceptive A-beta fibers may now trigger pain perception and help explain central sensitization. It is this tract — the main pain highway — that neurosurgeons interrupt by carefully cutting or heating with controlled radio-frequency lesions in order to relieve intractable pain. Over the years, neurosurgeons and other scientists realized that pain symptoms temporarily improved symptoms but the pain sensation returned. It was then realized that other pathways and tracts must be carrying pain sensations to perceptions not previously realized. Basic scientific research then demonstrated that other tracts, such as in the posterior section of the spinal cord, the medial and lateral tracts ending in gracilis and cuneate nucleus, not only transmit light touch, vibrations, and proprioception, but also pain. Moreover, they too cross in the sensory decussation in the brain stem. In addition, the reticular formation and spinal–spinal tracts also transmit pain sensation. Other homologous tracts transmit facial head and neck pains through the extremely complex trigeminal network.

Thereafter the thalamic afferents relay to the primary somatosensory and secondary cortical centers organized in a homunculus for localization and lateralization. An example is provided in identifying the left great toe's medial aspect as a source of pain. This tract integrates with the limbic lobe to generate the discriminatory and affective emotions components of the pain, from which the objective anatomic and physiologic basis for nociception pain and suffering is expressed as "I hurt."

In summary, we have reviewed and elucidated the basis for anatomic, discriminatory, and affective psychologic responses associated with the the nociceptive, peripheral, central, and psychological components for your consideration. The types of pain, intensity, duration, and localization due to a focal injury or disease process can have a spreading component by convergence, facilitation, inhibition, cross-talk, or sensitization responding to an inflammatory process. For example, when one has sunburn and steps into a warm shower, the pain response is exaggerated and is called hyperalgesia. These responses are compensated in addition by complex ionic and molecular neurochemical systems providing a self-adjusting, discriminatory-affective defense system. Sometimes, depending on the type of mechanical, thermal, or chemical stimulus, the intensity can not be modulated sufficiently; and when self-care fails, the patient seeks medical attention.

The pathophysiology of chronic pain perception can also shift from a relatively high threshold stimulus needed to produce pain sensation to a low mechanical, chemical, or temperature threshold stimulus of any kind to cause increased pain to be felt and lays the foundation for the sensitization and explanation of pain after injury when the stimulus has left; this has been referred to as spontaneous pain. The reader is referred to other chapters for additional information. As technology advances and clinical informational data banks develop, the progress will continue to close our gap of ignorance so that improvements in the diagnosis and treatment of pain syndromes can be achieved. This basic science provides the foundation of home care, pharmacology, physical therapy, modality, treatment, and improved rehabilitation.

DIAGNOSIS OF PAIN

The diagnosis of pain can vary from simple to complex, but is based on a thorough history, physical and basic neurologic examinations, correlation of appropriate laboratory tests, specialty consultations when needed, and the outcomes of medical, surgical, and alternative treatment programs.

In more complex pain syndromes, especially those associated with co-morbidity, the diagnosis cannot be made immediately but may require serial follow-up consultations and this should be communicated to the patient and documented in well-kept medical records. It should also be remembered that no medical information should be sent to requesting agencies without the patient's express written permission.

TREATMENT OF ACUTE, CHRONIC, AND CANCER PAIN

For successful pain management, individualization by diagnosis, personality traits, intellect, age, and outcome of prior treatments must all be seriously considered.

Based on prior educational/training experience, the PCP is in an excellent position to not only know the patient, but also the patient's family and supporting friends and groups, all of which have assistive value.

Administrative managed care and third-party reimbursement programs, however, may place barriers on a model individualized treatment plan and alternatives must be sought, but documentation for the clinical changes must be kept due to the utilization and legal considerations addressed in other chapters.

Treatment programs have at least twelve areas to consider:

1. Self-care
2. Pharmacology
3. Physical modalities
4. Surgery
5. Alternative medicine
6. Psychological/psychiatric assessment
7. Physical medicine and rehabilitation
8. Management of co-morbidity
9. Specialty consultations
10. Occupational and vocational evaluations
11. Disability evaluation
12. Medical/legal considerations

SELF-CARE

In self-care, is important to involve the patient's cooperation, compliance, and motivational initiatives to get well.

Lacking these, the treating physician is hard-pressed to achieve a successful outcome.

PHARMACOLOGIC TREATMENT

Pharmacologic treatment is usually sought when self-care fails. Pain medicine has four pillars of treatment; however, when sensitivities, untoward reactions, or complications occur in each class of drugs prescribed for the patient, caution must be exercised.

Analgesics

Analgesics are employed for symptomatic pain relief. They include (1) non-narcotic, aspirin-type salicylate compounds; and (2) opioids. Opoids are controlled substances and require special handling, based on two principles: to benefit the patient and to be in compliance with regulatory agencies. Pharmacologic drug selection and dosage schedules must be individualized.

Anti-inflammatories

Anti-inflammatories have made significant advances in becoming more receptor specific in therapy, moving from (COX) cyclooxygenases (with 14 subclasses) to the new (COXII) generation with reportedly less undesirable side effects, targeting gastrointestinal, renal, hepatic, and pulmonary organ systems. These individuals still require close monitoring because adverse effects can occur at any time in a treatment program to any patient.

Antispasmodics

Antispasmodics are prescribed when there is sufficient clinical/objective evidence of involuntary muscle spasm that itself causes pain and limitation of function. The three classes act: (1) peripherally at myoneural junctures; (2) at the spinal cord level, influencing afferent-efferent modulation; and (3) central inhibition at cortical and possibly subcortical levels.

Antidepressants

Antidepressants can play a major role in pain management because they are a class of medications that result in several synergistic effects: (1) antidepressant-serotonergic, (2) antispasmodic, and (3) analgesic. These three effects vary depending on the type of selective serotonin reuptake inhibitor (SSRI) prescribed.

These four classes of medicine can be prescribed singularly or in combination. Frequently, polypharmacy results and careful trials of various compounds must be made to produce an optimum treatment plan.

This is far from an exhaustive review, but serves as an outline for more detailed chapters in pharmacotherapeutic, psycho- and immunopharmacology.

LABORATORY TESTING FOR PAIN MEDICINE

Laboratory testing for pain medicine includes hematopoietic, serologic, imaging, and electrodiagnostic tests. Frequently, functional tests that evaluate impairment and related ergonomics that cannot be evaluated by the above are necessary and reasonable to assist in determining medical impairment and serve as a foundation for legally determined disability ratings. Functional testing comes in two categories: (1) physical or somatic, and (2) emotional or psychological. It should be noted that the latter has gained increased credibility because federal mandates direct that disability be determined by physical or mental impairment, or both.

The reader is referred to various chapters that relate more specifically to these concerns. Recall that clinical judgment is necessary because, to paraphrase Albert Einstein, "All that is important cannot be measured and all that is measured is not necessarily important." The test for clinicians is that they be able to provide a basis for their ordered tests (i.e., that the tests be reasonable and necessary) because they may be challenged or adjudicated by the legal community.

MODALITIES

Modalities are gaining increased use in medical pain management because of the lack of complete efficacy of selected chemical compounds we call pharmaceuticals. We are in no way being critical of the pharmacologic approach to pain medicine, but there are limitations of dosage schedules, intolerance reactions, and lack of efficacy that must be recognized. Some patients are averse to take medicine. Modalities offer an alternative.

Two types of modalities are recognized:

1. Mechanical
2. Electrical

Both prescribed therapies require individualization and outcome documentation.

Mechanical or physical modalities include self-care, rubbing massage, pressure, ultrasound, stretching, traction, hydrotherapy, and heat and cold techniques. These can be self-administered, or provided by trained assistants and professionally experienced physical therapists, and also manual medicine techniques performed by osteopathic and chiropractic physicians. These offer a variety of options and combinations to assist in the healing process. All, in various ways, have the potential to accelerate the normalization of the pathophysiology of disease and injury processes.

Electrical modalities are gaining wider acceptance as our basic knowledge of physics as applied by medical researchers and bio-engineering has progressed. This progress then lends itself to the clinical practitioner.

Electrical energy used as a therapy has long been recognized as beneficial. As we move from a pharmaco-logic-allopathic and homeopathic system of care, we are using more electronically based therapies. Based on the classic research of Gibert, Faraday, Nordenstrom, Becker, Avery, Sheely, Kirsch, and so many others, many clinical applications are now available to the PCP.

Transcutaneous electrical nerve stimulation (TENS) has been available by prescription since the Medical Service Act passed in 1975. There are now probably 100 types of devices on the market, but great care should be exercised in selecting the most suitable model — with special attention given to the electrode placement pattern, electrical settings of waveform, pulse width, and individual tolerance requirements — before prescribing a unit. In over 40 years of experience, we recommend a trial of four to six treatments in the office setting with physician and clinical assistant supervision before prescribing home-use units that cost between $200 and $800. A rental trial is often desirable for home care to see if the patient understands how to use the device. When effective, we found that TENS provided a substantial savings (in oral medication) when individualized frequency and pulse settings and optimal electrode pad placement were employed. Care must be taken not to prescribe TENS during first and second trimesters of pregnancy, or with cardiac pacemaker patients. Never place the electrode adhesive pad over the cervical region of the carotid sinus, due to the possibilities of affecting the cardiac rhythms.

Electromedicine has made other significant clinical advances in providing relief of physical pain by, probably, closing the spinal gate that hinders the perception of pain by stimulation of the A-beta fibers but also causing a mild vasodilation (not yet reported in the literature). This Alpha-Stim type of stimulation is different from TENS in that it provides a somatic as well as an emotional modulation pattern mediated by the serotonergic system.

Microcurrent electrical therapy (MET) reported by Kirsch and Mercola, is based on bio-electric data and provides, for the first time, a combination therapy for the modulating the perception of somatic pain and its emotional affective symptoms. It has been approved by the FDA.

Using probes or clip electrodes applied to the ear-lobes, selected patients can use the alpha-stim device for office or home care applications. Not all patients benefit from these modalities, but they do offer a variety of options for patients who do not, will not, or cannot take medication.

The reader is referred to chapters that address these subjects in more detail, permitting the PCP to enter a new field of electromedicine therapy that we call medical energetics.

PHYSICAL MEDICINE AND REHABILITATION

Physical medicine and rehabilitation are recommended for therapies of acute, chronic, and cancer pain because they provide more than modality treatment. For the PCP, it supplements the therapy program in the patient who continues to have symptoms and impairments of daily activities involving personal and work tasks. It provides a second opinion for the PCP, and it enhances the patient's probability of improving while documenting progress or lack thereof. We refer the reader to the appropriate chapters on ergonomics by Dr. Sella and others.

The psychological and psychiatric assessment and management of the pain patient presents a special field for consideration. Because the discriminatory-affective component is complex and is superimposed on a preexisting emotional character profile, diagnosis of personality characteristics can be identified as pre- and post-disease and/or injury. Attitude and behavioral components can be evaluated and managed in conjunction with the PCP's treatment of pain syndromes and co-morbidity. Special consideration is made for energizing stress, anxiety, and depression. Reflective care can be offered for lack of complaint; lifestyle and drug abuse without symptom magnification must be evaluated very carefully, with further consideration of secondary gain but also secondary losses. Munchausen's syndrome and psychogenic pain patients should be seen in conjunction with specialists in the field. The reader is referred to appropriate chapters in this text for further reference.

OCCUPATIONAL AND VOCATIONAL REHABILITATION

Occupational and vocational rehabilitation are important aspects of pain management for the PCP because they can be made part of the necessary therapy, especially for those with chronic and cancer pain symptoms. Resource services are available from both private and state-supported programs, the latter of which have no service fees. This allows the PCP to be captain of a multidisciplinary team to coordinate diagnosis, treatment, and rehabilitation plans and to assist the patient in returning to an economically productive lifestyle. Insurance programs frequently do not pay for job retraining but are ready to support job modification services in returning the patient to work, thereby reducing their monetary outlay.

The reader is referred to other chapters that address the challenges and barriers faced by patients returning to the workplace.

MEDICAL/LEGAL ASPECTS OF PAIN MEDICINE

The medical and legal aspects of pain medicine present a different sort of challenge because they are based on the adversarial approach to medical management, in which the PCP is frequently not as experienced as the clinical medicine physician. Simply stated, the PCP is in a position to provide both factual and expert witness reports, and, when needed, testimony as the treating physician who has consulted with the patient many times. PCPs are able to provide credible history, physical examination, treatment, pertinent laboratory findings, outcome, and diagnosis. They can also provide estimates for future medical care, prognosis, and disability determination by documentation or oral testimony. These are all subject to challenge by opposing counsel as well as the medical testimony of physicians retained by opposing counsel. These retained physicians often render reports that tend to minimize findings, testifying about the co-morbidity, preexisting disease or injuries, or a contributing cause of the plaintiff (patient's medical and psychological problems) from a retrospective point of view.

The treating PCP, however, can provide evidence-based opinion and testimony that the diagnosis, treatment, and related services being addressed are, in fact, reasonable and necessary. The treating physician should also charge for the medical/legal services performed, based on a usual and customary fee schedule that can be made available to requesting agencies prior to rendering these administrative services. Because the rules of testimony and evidence change and vary from state to state, the reader is referred to the medical/legal chapters of this text to update further information.

DISABILITY DETERMINATION

Disability determination is a legal concept and has become the purview of the legal community and state and federal agencies. The PCP, however, is in an eminent position to determine functional impairment. How is this determined? By clinical experience, medical literature, and consultation, an impairment rating can be determined quantitatively based on mild, moderate, and severe impairment classifications. When mild, the patient can perform home, self-care, return to usual occupational work and need not have professional treatment or see a physician, except on occasion. In the moderate category, the patient has impairment that interferes with activities of daily living (ADLs) and must modify these; professional treatments are needed and physician care is important. Return to work must be modified. In severe impairment, the patient has continued symptoms and needs continued treatment and ongoing professional medical care. He or she is not able to return to work and is considered totally and permanently disabled as determined by Social Security Disability Entitlement

Programs. Periodic reevaluation visits are performed to verify the continuing disability. The reader is referred to the chapters on disability in this text for more information.

In conclusion, we are of the opinion that:

1. PCPs are in an eminent position to become specialists in pain medicine.
2. Educational resources are available for in-office, local, regional, and national services offering continuing education credits, certification, and advanced degrees.
3. The PCP can become coordinator and captain of the ship in pain medicine, providing an individualized, humanized treatment program for the patient.
4. Specialty consultations are available to offer second opinions in complex pain syndromes available locally or at academic university centers.
5. The PCPs can concurrently manage co-morbidity while practicing pain medicine.
6. The PCP's office staff can be trained in special techniques for in-office care at substantial cost savings.
7. The PCP can provide a supportive and counseling role in the areas of pain medicine in conjunction with psychological and psychiatric consultations.
8. The PCP can refer the patient with special behavior, abuse, compliance or lifestyle impairments to specific evaluation and treatment programs and to share the care of difficult patients.
9. The PCP can provide medical testimony that is evidence-based and provide impairment ratings for further disability determination.

To paraphrase Hypocrites: The future is bright, but fraught with difficulty. We will be trained beyond our intelligences, so the real test for physician is at the bedside.

The ball is in your court. Primary care physicians should consider the following value concepts in medical decision making.

1. **Clinical:** Accumulate as much relevant medical information as possible, employing acceptable services to benefit the patient. Less than that is not acceptable.
2. **Educational:** Every patient encounter provides an accumulation of data contributing to clinical experience, but can also be shared with others through anecdotal or published peer review literature.
3. **Research:** Evaluation of unconventional approaches to unusual problems adds to the total fund of knowledge and should be shared.

4. **Administrative:** Simplify documentation; it has created a burdensome task for clinicians and staff as well as significantly escalating the cost of medical care. How can this be accomplished? The PCP's help is needed.
5. **Fiscal:** Cost constraints instituted by third-party payors have inhibited medical programs. What other options are available?
6. **Regulatory affairs:** Agencies mandated by legislative actions to maintain and control health care delivery systems often go beyond the spirit of the legislation and are dismantling the finest health care system in the world. Together, can PCPs make a difference by acting in an advisory capacity due to the significant advances that produce the gaps in agency updating?
7. **Political:** Correctness creates a trend toward mediocrity. Having served, can PCPs take a leadership position?
8. **Medical/legal:** Responsibilities have grown complex and costly, developing an adversarial system in which many health professionals and patients have lost confidence. It still is considered the best we have. How can PCPs help regain credibility?
9. **Personal:** Has this entire effort of dedicating one's life and career to the care of others been of value?

> Guerir quelquefois
> Soulager souvent
> Consoler tousjours
>
> **Anonymous**

24

The Impact of Pain on Families

James H. Ballard, D.Min., C.R.T.

INTRODUCTION: THE IMPACT OF PAIN

From the moment actor Christopher Reeve suffered his accident riding horseback, not only was his life changed, but also the lives of his wife and family. Whether one's pain is the result of an accident or an illness of spirit, soul, or body, its impact is like a rock dropped into a pond … it has a ripple effect.

Phyllis was referred to me by a local physician. The victim of a serious automobile accident, she had spent months in physical recovery. In the later phases of her physical therapy, she experienced pain in her body that could not be traced to any physical cause. She had begun to have flashbacks to a very painful and abusive past. After sessions dealing with spiritual and psychological issues, I remarked that she had not mentioned the physical pain for which she had entered counseling. Her remark was, "It's gone!" Relief of pain in spirit and soul had brought about physical healing. These sessions took place several years ago and there has been no recurrence of her pain.

After years of counseling from a Christian perspective, I am finding many whom I counsel to be in physical or psychological pain. Very often, such pain comes from deep spiritual and psychological issues that have not been faced and resolved. Rejection, abuse, and abandonment often result — not only in spiritual or psychological crises, but physical ones as well.

The victim does not stand alone. Family structures are also vitally involved and affected. Treatment of pain not only impacts the victim but all those who are part of his or her world.

A number of years ago, my wife, two children, and I lived in South Brazil where we served as missionaries. While there, I came down with extreme pain in the abdomen. The attempt to diagnose its origin led to deep depression on my part. All of that resulted in an emergency medical furlough and 6 weeks of hospitalization. At the end of that time the doctor recommended that we not return to Brazil because of the possibility of the disease returning. Needless to say, my physical and psychological pain resulted in emotional and relational pain for my wife and our two preschool-aged children. The trauma of all that took place sent shock waves through our family at the time and for several years after our return to the U.S.

I agree with Carl McNeely (2000) when he states that patients, along with family members, may frequently have adjustment difficulties because of changes in roles and limitations of the functioning of the patient. Look with me at the impact of pain on families in the following areas.

PAIN IS INTERGENERATIONAL

Karl, in his mid-fifties, has had both heart catherization and bypass surgery. He is presently separated from his wife due to repeated martial infidelities on his part. The probability of reconciliation is very slim. His family of origin gives evidence of heart trouble for several generations. Emotional, relational, and physical dysfunction has carried over into his generation and it has become clear that, with each succeeding generation, the toxicity has increased. There have been boundary violations within the family of origin structure. Karl is not the first to commit adultery. He is carrying into his generation the lifestyle of earlier generations. Such behavior ensures that familial pain from the past is carried forward. Karl has two sons. It is Karl's perspective, however, that his separation and divorce from their mother will not affect his boys because

0-8493-0926-3/02/$0.00+$1.50
© 2002 by CRC Press LLC

"they are adults." It is difficult to move beyond denial. Often, hurts go deeper in adult children of divorce than in those who experience that trauma in their earlier years. There is a probability that Karl's sons will continue his behavior for another generation or else emotionally separate themselves from their father's irresponsible actions.

I have spent more time counseling George and his fourth wife, Nora, than most of my other clients. There was deep-seated anger and personality conflicts between them. Nora has a very co-dependent personality. Her record of failed marriages closely resembles George's. They both brought a child into their marriage. These children witnessed the pain and anger that permeated their parents' relationship. Both of these children are now approaching their teenage years. I am very concerned that the past irresponsibility of their parents may wash over into their lives, thus carrying the toxicity of the past into the present and drastically affecting their futures.

After a number of sessions with George, there was a breakthrough. He admitted that much of his anger, which surfaced frequently, was the result of the sexual molestation and abuse he had experienced as a child.

Sexual molestation between the ages of birth and 18 years is affecting one out of four women and one out of five men. The trauma of these events, often many violations over a period years, has devastating effects on the victim and those around him or her. The pain of guilt and shame exacts a high price on the victim. Scars remain with them for years, whereas the perpetrator often does not remember actions toward the victim.

Traumas from past violations of one's personhood can have a devastating effect upon one's self-esteem. It can affect the victim's approach to personal intimacy. Evidence of the negative effect of such traumas can be seen in many victims of rape. Marriage bonds are strained and often broken because of this violation of one's person. Although violation of one's physical being may not be evident in many cases, it can be in other areas.

PAIN IS INTERRELATIONAL

When a family is healthy in its relationships, it allows appropriate boundaries and personal privacy. There is a clear distinction between adults and children. Children are allowed to be who they are … children. When there is dysfunction and enmeshment, children are often the major source of affirmation and affection for the adults. I frequently hear from clients that they were never allowed to have a positive, happy childhood. They had to continually replenish their parents' sense of well-being. The child in such a relationship often becomes a parent to the parent (or parents). When children grow up in such a toxic environment, they experience relational pain. The consequence of having to meet parental emotional needs can result in low self-esteem and burnout, or in a perfectionism

that is self-destructive. These traits can develop in young children as well as in older ones. Unconditional love and care within families of origin are extremely vital for healthy relationships to form. Where conditional love or absence of any type of deep, parental caring is evident, there is pain within one's personhood.

Unmet parental needs often find children going into professions of parental choosing rather than those of their own choice. Dennis was such a person. His future was laid out for him by his doctor father who wanted his son to follow in his footsteps. Dennis went to medical school and through medical residency, much to the delight of a doting dad. After Dennis completed his residency and set up a medical practice, his father died. Freed from his father's shadow, Dennis left medicine to become a musician, something he had desired to do since childhood.

Warren was the son of a woman who had risen rapidly in governmental service. She was perfectionistic and controlling in her family. Warren's father left the marriage because of the mother's dominating personality. Warren, unable to escape the power of his mother took out his anger and rage on four different wives. As of this writing, he is allowing his mother to continue to "bail him out." He does not tell his mother where to go; rather, he chooses another woman to become a victim of his dysfunctional relationship with his mother. Warren's failed marriages have caused much pain, not only for his ex-wives, but also for their immediate families.

In the procession of pain within families, whether that pain is spiritual, psychological, or physical, there are other dimensions to consider.

THE TRAUMA OF THE TEMPORARY

Whether it is a broken bone because of an accident or a broken heart that is the result of a failed relationship within teen years, there is trauma that impacts the family structure.

Our knowledge and discernment tells us that this, too, shall pass. Yet, during the disconcerting days of its happening, schedules are interrupted and the focus of attention is shifted with the victim leaving other important tasks undone. Stress often becomes the order of day, particularly if it involves the victim's hospitalization. Life often seems to be filled with times of temporary paining. One knows there will come an end to the hurts, but the journey through the valleys of pain are real while the family member is in crisis. There is often a toll on the health of the family.

THE CRISIS OF THE CHRONIC

The processing of pain within families of Alzheimer's patients can be ongoing and often debilitating. The decline of mental and physical faculties of the patient are often years in duration. Alice was a strong independent woman who, with her husband Glenn, had a good life on a farm in Piedmont, North Carolina. After Glenn's death, Alice began to show signs of early Alzheimer's and began a slide into its depths over an 8-year period. Judy, Alice's daughter, took care of Alice at home for the duration of Alice's life. During that time, Judy worked full-time as a nurse in a regional hospital and spent most of her time away from work caring for her mother. Alice's decline, slow at first, began with Alice's constant wandering around the community and progressed more rapidly with time. When living with Judy, Alice often set off the house alarm at night while attempting to leave the premises. The possibility of a normal life between Judy and her husband and children became secondary and often nonexistent because of the demands of Alice's illness. Alice was a large woman and incontinence became an increasing problem that necessitated much lifting and changing. Outside help was difficult to obtain because few people were physically able to manage Alice. The strain of years of dealing with Alzheimer's had its effect on every family member.

Cancer is another chronic disease that takes its toll on family members. The Wards were a close-knit family. Lowell and Ruth, elderly in years, were deeply distressed when their daughter Carole, with a family of her own, came down with cancer of the pancreas. For several years, Carole endured an endless series of chemotherapy treatments. With each treatment, the quality of Carole's life decreased. Lowell and Ruth spent much of their time and energy caring for her.

I recall, during one of my pastoral visits, watching Ruth massage Carole's back as the cancer spread within her body. I do not believe the touching alleviated much pain, but the tenderness of her mother's massage had a soothing effect on Carole's mind and spirit. Six weeks after that scene, Carole died. Just a couple of months later, Ruth was diagnosed with a rapidly growing cancer. Refusing any treatment, she died within weeks. The pain of a double loss so close together had its impact on Lowell, who was 80 years old. The stress of watching his daughter and wife deteriorate, and the grief following their deaths, took a fatal toll on Lowell. He experienced kidney failure and died within weeks of his diagnosis. The impact of such chronic pain exacted the ultimate price on the family.

Similar to Alzheimer's, AIDS takes it toll on family members, often not just psychologically, but physiologically. I visited John's hospital room often and every time I went, Mary was there sitting beside her son John who was critically ill with AIDS. As John deteriorated, the strain of his illness became more evident on Mary's demeanor. There were two victims of this terrible disease in that room. When John died, I conducted his funeral. Not only John's companion, but members of the gay community who had been John's friends, gave evidence of their pain from the loss of his life.

Genetics often play a tragic role in the family structure. Increasingly, bipolar disorders have a devastating effect on the family structure. With the severe mood swings of the victim, there often comes a breakdown of the family structure. Aberrant behavior often causes strains in a breakup of marriages. Trace this disease back and one often finds genetic links. The same can be true with schizophrenia. With both bipolar disorder and schizophrenia, entire families can be affected by the disease of one member. Grace and Harry have a son, Clarence, in his early twenties, who has been diagnosed with schizophrenia. When Clarence is on his medication, his behavior is stabilized; but like some, he periodically thinks he can do without his medication. When this takes place, the chronicity of this psychiatric problem takes its toll on family structure. Henry and Grace do not have to tell me when Clarence is not taking his medication because I can see the pain on their faces and in their eyes.

PAIN AND PERSONALITY

Dick is the older of two boys. William, his younger brother, is 9 years his junior. In his teen years and early twenties, Dick acted very immaturely and irresponsibly, causing his parents to spend an abnormal amount of time in rescue mode — devoting time they should have been spending with William — coping with Dick's continuing crises.

Dick got involved in the drug and alcohol scene and almost lost his life in a wreck. Seeing the actions of his brother, William withdrew into himself and became a very private person, not expressing his feelings to family or friends. Extremely brilliant, he chose to rebel in another way. He refused to attend college and he became extremely critical of societal institutions, particularly in the areas of education, politics, and religion. William chose a track opposite to that of his brother. He became fiercely independent, hardworking, and sought to free himself from causing any financial drain on his parents. The pain of the problems in the lives of these young men had a long-lasting effect on both parents. At one time, the strain was so great that the parents contemplated separation and divorce. The parents' approaches to the concerns of their children caused them to act in opposite ways. One parent became over-controlling and the other passive-aggressive.

PAIN AND PERSONHOOD

In I Thessalonians 5:23, Paul the apostle prayed that the Christians at Thessalonica would be preserved complete in spirit, soul, and body at the coming of Christ (NASV). Both the Old and New Testaments use separate words in describing these three entities of who we are.

Whenever we experience pain in one aspect of our being, it affects the other areas. There is often spiritual or psychological pain before physical pain is evident. Stresses within one's personality often cause the body to fall victim to diseases it otherwise has the capability to overcome.

We are now living in a time where the body is looked at as more than a free-standing mechanistic instrument that allopathic medicine can fix. Psycho-spiritual entities must be brought into play as well.

Emotional dysfunction that has been a pattern for several generations may ultimately express itself through physical symptoms. In a conference sponsored by The National Institute of Clinical and Behavioral Medicine, Dr. Paula Reeves (1994) presented a paper dealing with the effect of somatic belief patterns on emotional, physiological, and behavioral change. She stated that our biography is our biology, beginning with conception. Her belief is that all disease is psychosomatic, with symptoms being one-tenth instinct and nine-tenths metaphor. The majority of physical illnesses are the result of emotional and spiritual crises that occur in lives that experience a lack of love and family involvement.

Core messages that spring from family concerns result in illnesses. Dr. Reeves offers these examples:

Core Message	Illnesses
Don't feel	Phobias, depression
Don't think	Headache; ear, neck, throat problems
Don't be a child	Eating disorders, substance abuse, kidney and bowel problems
Don't exist	Respiratory/circulatory problems, sexual dysfunction, allergies
Don't be yourself	Skeletal: facial and balance problems
Don't be a bother	Muscle problems, nerve disorders (multiple sclerosis, muscular dystrophy)

All of the above involve pain. Such pain causes family concerns and pain as well. Anyone experiencing the above, according to Dr. Reeves, needs to trust that symptoms have meaning for one spiritually, emotionally, physically, and mentally.

THE ASSISTANCE OF THE FAMILY

Carl McNeely (2000) states that positive interaction between family members and the person with chronic pain is crucial. Often, when pain levels are high and the dependency of the patient is great, things can be very difficult as well as frustrating. As much as possible, clear, open communication is vital to keep at bay the mounting resentments and counterproductive emotions and reactions.

The establishment of routines and goals is vital to both the patient and family, whether the pain is physiological, psychological, or spiritual. Family help and assistance are crucial in up to 70% of patients experiencing pain.

Not only is the assistance of the family crucial for the patient, but the family itself has needs that cannot be ignored. Caregivers need to have time and energy for their other varied roles within the structure of family.

Boundaries must be visible. There must be a differentiation between caregiving (which has boundaries) and caretaking (where boundaries are nonexistent). It is crucial that goals be established concerning family involvement. Being proactive rather than reactive in this area can be of assistance in the ability of the patient to get better.

It is unwise to treat a complex, chronic pain patient separately from his family and social network. This approach could doom or, at best, retard the treatment process.

FACING THE FAITH FACTOR

In the Old Testament, Job, from the depths of pain that encompassed his whole being, states that "… I know that my Redeemer lives … even after my skin is destroyed, yet, from my flesh I shall see God." (Job 19:25–26). In the midst of traumatic testing, Job's faith was not destroyed, but refined. Several years ago, I visited a lady who was in the terminal stages of cancer. She remarked, "I am so glad I have cancer." Taken aback by that statement, I asked, "Why?" Her reply was that through the pain of cancer she had met many wonderful Christians whom she otherwise would never have known. Although her body was wasting away, due to the disease, her soul and spirit were at peace.

Allopathic medicine seeks the cure and alleviation of pain. There can be healing of soul and spirit without a cure for the body. You see, we are eternal beings in soul and spirit who live in temporal bodies.

A number of years ago, my grandmother developed pancreatic cancer. Her disease progressed slowly. My father remarked toward the end of her life that, up until that point, he had emotionally held on to her. When he was able to release her, my grandmother died within a short time.

And history repeated itself with my father. He almost died of kidney failure. At that time, my mother prayed, "Lord, whatever it takes, let Harold live." Dad lived for 6 more years. My mother, during those years, administered peritoneal dialysis every other day. As his condition worsened, mother one day remarked to me, "I am ready for your dad to go on home now." Dad died a short time later. I believe that God, in His mercy, allows loved ones to live until that time of emotional release by relatives.

STRATEGIES FOR POSITIVE ACTION

All of the illustrations set forth in this chapter have a common thread: the faith factor. Christians are not perfect;

they are pilgrims. Through painful traumas, both the victim and family members indicated that their faith was often deepened.

Andrew knew that he was losing his battle with cancer. His family had put his hospital bed in the living room so that he could see outside. On one of my visits, near the end of his life, Andrew told me that the night before had been a long and painful one. As he lay awake in the midst of his pain, he had begun thinking of how blessed he was with both his family and his faith. And in the midst of the darkness of the night, he had burst out singing. I recalled the scripture from Job 35:10b, "He (God) gives us songs in the night."

A friend of mine, Dr. Ronna Fay Jevne, has Crohn's disease. Yet in the midst of her pain, she has ministered to many cancer patients in Edmonton, Alberta, Canada. She is the author of several books centered around the theme of hope. She is also the founder of The Hope Foundation. She shares the following from her book, *The Voice of Hope, Heard across the Heart of Life* (Jevne, 1994):

"THE VOICE OF ILLNESS"

Illness is an introduction to the fragility and sacredness of life. With illness we learn we are not immune. Nor are those whom we love. We learn that our sense of invulnerability is an illusion. Illness is the great equalizer. We come to understand that life and death are intimately and ultimately connected. For everyone.

Illness comes with a formidable invitation to notice the sacredness of life. It is a wake-up call to life's preciousness. A call to notice the everyday, to be present "here" and "now." To place our lives in perspective to others, to our universe. To accept the place we have in infinity and eternity. To ask the "big" questions and enjoy the "simple" answers. To do this, we must find a rightful place for suffering. A perspective that allows room for hope. Serious illness is a journey, a hopeful journey, an unknown destination. In illness the dichotomies are vivid. Hope is the space between symptoms and diagnosis, between diagnosis and prognosis. It is the wrestling match between science and compassion, between body and spirit, between pain and relief. It is the dilemma between fearing to be alone and hungering for privacy.

Hoping is waiting: for test results, for appointments, for the organism to heal and the spirit to rekindle. Hoping is walking the line between tolerating constant probing and invasions, and declaring "no more, not now." The hope for survival is not the only hope; many days, not even the overriding hsope. The real hope is not to be "invalid."

Hoping is knowing that someone is making an effort to help. That family is never far away. That the system cares. That what happens is the best of technology and the best of humanness. Hoping is being attended by people who understand that caring makes a difference. An immeasurable difference.

Hoping is being treated, not as another case of a particular disease, but as a person. By people who understand, this could happen to them. It is knowing there are no secrets. Being a partner on the treatment team. Being encouraged to do as much as possible for one's self. Hoping is trying again. Moving against the odds. Knowing everything that can be done is being done. Knowing the caring will go on when the limits of science are reached.

Hoping is denying the statistics. Reaching beyond the traditional. Keeping open the possibility of being the exception. Hoping is listening to the unconscious. Having dreams in the world of sleep and dreams in the world of the consciousness. Wondering if there are miracles. Being fascinated with the little miracles: the words that heal, the memories that let us forget.

Hoping is having passion for life. Noticing life. Wanting life. Inching toward life. Being willing to embrace life despite the risks. Hoping is recognizing that death is not the enemy — never living is.

Suffering humbles us; hoping takes us forward. We come to understand that we are among many who are ill. Among many who hurt and fear. And who need. We come to trust the unusual experiences we cannot explain. The experiences for which we have no words. There is a knowing that accompanies suffering; a knowing that emerges from deep within us. That speaks from another dimension to life.

Pain affects not only individuals and their family structure, but impacts the human family. We, despite our many differences, are fellow pilgrims on this planet. Perhaps the one thing that is a common factor is pain.

The Apostle Paul, writing to the Corinthians, made a statement regarding not only the physical body, but the body of Christ, the Church: "… members should have the same care for one another … if one member suffers, all the members suffer with it; if one member is honored, all the members rejoice with it" (I Corinthians 12:25–26, NASV).

During my years in the ministry, my family and I have experienced periods of pain, either relational or physical. During those times, I questioned why. I now know that those times of trauma were to better equip us to understand and minister to ones trapped in prisons of pain. May it be so with you as well.

REFERENCES

Jevne, R. F. (1994). *The voice of hope, heard across the heart of life.* San Diego: Lura Media.

McNeely, C. (2000). The role of the family in the treatment of chronic pain. *The Practitioner, 10*(2), 5.

Reeves, P. (1994). Spontaneous movement: The effect of somatic belief patterns. National Institute for the Clinical Application of Behavioral Medicine Conference, Vol. A, 482, 493. Mansfield Center, CT: National Institute for the Clinical Application of Behavioral Medicine.

25

The Impact of Nursing on Pain Management

Chris L. Algren, R.N., M.S.N., Ed.D. and Mary Romelfanger, R.N., M.S.N.

INTRODUCTION

Pain is the most common reason patients seek out health-care professionals. The National Institutes of Health (NIH, 1987) published a consensus statement in 1987 that stressed the "caring" and "curing" role in pain management. Since that time, great strides have been made in the assessment and understanding of the multiple dimensions of pain. Advances have been made in both the pharmacologic and nonpharmacologic methods of treating pain. The number of multidisciplinary pain centers has grown rapidly. Comprehensive, holistic pain management using a multidisciplinary team of health professionals with an integrated approach has gained wide acceptance.

The NIH consensus statement expressed concern that the education of many professionals — including nurses, physicians, dentists, and physical therapists — did not put sufficient emphasis on contemporary pain assessment and management. The need for communication and collaborative approaches among professionals was noted (NIH, 1987).

The U.S. Congress created the Agency for Health Care Policy and Research (AHCPR) in December 1989 as the federal government's focal point for health services research. The agency's mission is to enhance the quality of patient care services by generating knowledge that can be used to meet society's healthcare needs. The AHCPR is responsible for developing and updating guidelines that will be used to manage clinical conditions. To meet these challenges and others, agency activities include database development, effectiveness and outcome research, and dissemination of research findings and guidelines to providers, policy makers, and the public (Acute Pain Management Guideline Panel, 1992).

Pain-related guidelines were among the first sets developed by interdisciplinary expert panels representing medicine, nursing, pharmacology, psychology, rehabilitation therapy, ethics, and consumers/patients. Nurse clinicians, educators, researchers, administrators, and professional nursing organization representatives provided input. The first edition of the Acute Pain Management Guidelines was published by the AHCPR in February 1992 (Acute Pain Management Guideline Panel, 1992). The American Society of Anesthesiologists promulgated guidelines for acute pain management in the perioperative setting in 1995 (Ready, 1995).

Most recently, the Joint Commission on Accreditation of Healthcare Organizations (JCAHO) published Pain Standards for 2001 (JCAHO, 2001). These new standards are effective for surveys conducted after January 1, 2001. Aspects of pain management are covered in six of the eleven chapters of functions or activities required of accredited healthcare organizations. Organizations — including ambulatory care, behavioral healthcare, home care, hospice, hospitals, and long-term care facilities — now have a mandate to address pain management.

The integration of the pain management team's knowledge and skill is enhanced through an understanding of the perspective and scope of practice of each discipline. Pain manuals specific to nursing practice are available (McCaffery & Pasero, 1999).

Because "patient" is used by pain management practitioners from many disciplines and because "patient" is used in a majority of settings where nurses practice in the world, "patient" rather than "client" is used in this chapter. The rights and responsibilities associated with the use of "client" are intended.

0-8493-0926-3/02/$0.00+$1.50
© 2002 by CRC Press LLC

THE NURSE'S ROLE IN PAIN MANAGEMENT

Nurse decision-making is performed step by step using the nursing process, including assessment, diagnosis, planning, implementation, and evaluation (Gordon, 2000). Based on the establishment of a trusting relationship and a good rapport with the patient and family, this systematic process provides a framework for nurses to provide care for patients with pain in all settings.

The move to multidisciplinary planning and plans of care is supported by accrediting bodies such as the JCAHO and the American Academy of Pain Management, Pain Program Accreditation. Current hospital and home health JCAHO standards require coordination, collaboration, and continuity of services to each patient by all disciplines through an established plan of care. Critical pathways are a means of organizing patient care that relate care and services by disciplines and time frames to costs and measurable outcomes. Critical pathways are population specific and provide a database for performance improvement, including outcome-driven, competency-based staff development. Sample diagnosis-related critical paths are available in the literature (Aspen Reference Group, 1995; Cronin & Bahrke, 1996; Ignatavicius & Hausman, 1995).

Nurses play an essential role in the assessment of a patient's pain. The information the nurse obtains from assessing the patient's pain is used to identify goals for managing that pain. The goals for the patient can be accomplished using a combination of both pharmacologic and nonpharmacologic means. Assessing the effectiveness of interventions and monitoring for adverse effects are important aspects of the nurse's role. The nurse serves as an advocate for the patient when the intervention is not effective in relieving pain. The nurse also serves as an educator to the patient and family. Teaching about pain and measures to relieve it lessens anxiety and gives the patient and family a sense of control.

NURSING MANAGEMENT OF CHRONIC NONMALIGNANT PAIN

One of the most widely accepted definitions of pain is that "pain is an unpleasant sensory and emotional experience associated with actual or potential tissue damage, or described in terms of such damage" (IASP, 1979). Pain is not determined by tissue damage alone. Patients with chronic nonmalignant pain (CNP), pain not associated with a neoplastic process, may have pain for which little or no tissue damage can be found.

Pain is subjective and personal. McCaffery's (1968) definition — "Pain is whatever an individual says it is, and it occurs whenever he says it does" — seems especially relevant for the patient with CNP. The practitioner can only observe signs and obtain information about symptoms. The pain belongs to the patient, not to the practitioner. The person with pain is the best judge of the existence, duration, and severity of the pain and the success of pain management treatments.

The patient as expert rather than the healthcare practitioner can be difficult for the practitioner to accept. Until recently, pain has been viewed as a symptom, not as a diagnosis. Pain was thought to be something the healthcare provider could cure, or at least control. Many times, the cause of chronic pain is not discovered quickly or easily. The healthcare provider as well as the patient becomes frustrated.

Many healthcare providers had and still have little training about pain, particularly chronic pain, and the relief of pain. Often times, pain management is not considered a priority.

The nurse is a key player on the chronic pain management team, regardless of the setting. Nurses who work in community settings are likely to regularly help patients and families manage chronic as well as acute pain. Table 25.1 outlines how home health standards for practice and reimbursement can be applied to a diagnosis of pain (Marrelli, 1994).

The nurse, as well as everyone caring for the patient, needs to know the meaning that pain has for the patient. No chemical or neurophysiological tests exist that can accurately measure pain. Because the question of whether

---

TABLE 25.1
Home Care Pain Management

- Documentation Guidelines
- General considerations
- Need for initial visit
- Potential diagnoses and codes (medical-surgical)
- Associated nursing diagnoses (e.g., home maintenance management, impaired)
- Skilled services (e.g., RN to implement nonpharmacological interventions, titrate medication dose to achieve outcome with acceptable level of side effects)
- Other services (e.g., home health aide to assist with activities of daily living; MSS to assess financial ability to comply with pain treatment plan; physical therapist to teach energy conservation, apply heat or cold)
- Homebound status factors
- Short-term goals by discipline (e.g., RN to daily control pain and other symptoms)
- Long-term goals by discipline (e.g., RN, patient, and/or caregiver knowledgeable about pain management measures)
- Discharge plans
- Education needs: patient/family/caregiver
- Reimbursement tips

Adapted from Marrelli, T.M. (1994), *Handbook of Home Health Standards and Documentation Guidelines for Reimbursement* (2nd ed., pp. 243–248). St. Louis: Mosby, Inc.

the patient has "real pain" cannot be answered, healthcare providers must accept the patient's report of pain. The nurse must determine what the patient thinks is needed in order to deal with chronic pain. Nurses, particularly those who are discharge planners or who work in the community, need to know what resources are available to patients in pain. Support groups established to assist individuals in pain and referral services for patients are needed. One such group in the United States, with chapters throughout the country, is the National Chronic Pain Outreach Association. Nurses and physicians often serve as advisers or as coordinators for local chapters. If the practitioners are certified in pain management by the American Academy of Pain Management, they bring valuable knowledge and expertise that might not otherwise be available to many members of the group.

Regardless of the setting, the nurse functions as patient advocate, educator, counselor, provider, and coordinator of care.

NURSING MANAGEMENT OF PAIN IN THE ELDERLY

For purposes of the discussion that follows, the term "elderly" refers to those persons 65 years of age or older. However, it is important to note that many of the physiological changes associated with the aging process have an onset as early as the fourth decade. Therefore, although this discussion focuses on an age-related cohort, individual variation is a hallmark of any investigation of the sequelae of human aging.

The axiom that "aging is not for sissies" may have found its origin in the many factors of aging that support the nursing diagnosis "alteration in comfort." Carpenito (1999) states unequivocally that pain is omnipresent in the elderly. This is a particularly startling revelation in view of Wolanin's (1976) observation that pain is primary and, until it is relieved, no person functions adequately. This discussion explores these concepts in more detail and addresses other factors that combine to make the elderly a population uniquely vulnerable to pain.

The myriad physiologic and pathophysiologic changes of human aging that result in either acute or chronic pain may manifest themselves in a variety of ways in the elderly. Some of these manifestations are obvious and accompanied by typical signs and symptoms of a specific problem, while others are subtle, atypical, or even paradoxical (Caird, Dall, & Williams, 1987). Although the mechanisms of pain have been well described (Thompson, 1984), variation in pain perception in the elderly remains an area of contradictory subjective opinion and objective data (Caird et al., 1987; Corso, 1971; Matteson, 1988). However, it is generally accepted that pain threshold increases with age (Carpenito, 1999; Charleton & Buckley, 1984; Jacox, 1977; McConnell, 1988). In addition to an increased pain threshold, other factors are known to alter pain perception in the elderly. These include peripheral and central nervous system impairments, drug therapies, cognitive impairments, co-existing pathologies, individual psychophysiological or cultural experiences, and adaptation (Caird et al., 1987; Carpenito, 1999; McConnell, 1988; McCue, 1987).

Whether a result of increased pain threshold or other factors, certain conditions are reported to be less painful in older adults than in younger persons. Conditions frequently presenting with significant pain in younger persons but with only mild discomfort in the elderly include peptic ulceration, appendicitis, pneumonia, and mesenteric infarction (Charlton & Buckley, 1984). In the elderly, these events may be heralded only by vague signs such as restlessness or confusion.

Another factor confusing the symptom pattern in the elderly is the tendency for pain to be referred to other sites in the body. Chest pain may be referred from abdominal or esophageal pathologies (Charlton & Buckley, 1984; Dymock, 1985), while abdominal pain may arise from musculoskeletal or spinal problems or abdominal wall entrapment syndromes. Back pain may be the presenting symptom of a host of pathologies, including disc degeneration, arthritis, osteoarthritis, metastatic disease, and Paget's disease. These conditions may present as lower limb pain (Charlton & Buckley, 1984). Spondylosis of the cervical vertebrae may present as pain, muscular spasticity, or paresthesia in one upper limb (Grahame, 1985; Pathy, 1985).

Perhaps the most frequently cited clinical manifestation of paradoxical pain perception in the elderly is cardiac pain. Although elderly persons experiencing angina pectoris report the same need to cease exertion and similar dyspnea and pain radiation patterns as younger persons, they also report much less severe pain. It is postulated that the modified severity of pain results from either the presence of afferent denervation of the heart or the occurrence of disease in the smaller coronary vessels which produces less pain than disease in the larger vessels (Caird et al., 1987).

In addition to modified chest pain, it is not unusual for the elderly patient with clinically severe ischemic heart disease to present totally absent of pain. One study found that 31% of the elderly patients who experienced myocardial infarction reported no pain, while 40% reported clinically atypical symptoms (Caird et al., 1987; Charlton & Buckley, 1984). This phenomenon may be the result of the presence of multiple pathologies that severely limit activity, such as arthritis, parkinsonism, blindness, or hemiplegia. The presence of other pathologies may also present the patient with other symptoms so noxious that chest pain is not noticed (Caird et al., 1987).

Clearly, determining the origin of pain in the elderly presents a challenge to the healthcare practitioner and patient alike. Pain is a subjective phenomenon. Variables such as coexisting chronic pathologies, underreporting of pain, and the increased incidence of cognitive impairment all combine to make pain evaluation much more difficult among the elderly than among other adult populations (Ferrell & Ferrell, 1987). Although practitioners observe the elderly for behavioral manifestations of pain such as facial grimacing, positional guarding, etc., such observations, or even the perceptions of the experienced practitioner, are not reliable assessments of whether pain is present and, if so, how severe that pain may be. As is the case with nonelderly patients presenting with pain, the elderly patient's report of pain must be accepted as the most reliable clinical description. This requires that the patient with pain be trusted (Wright & Gal, 1987). It has been reported that the inability of an elderly patient to walk on a broken thigh was ascribed to hysteria (Pitt, 1982).

Although this is an extreme example of failure to trust, attributing pain to psychogenic origin may occur in those circumstances where no clear-cut etiology for the pain is found. In reality, it is not always possible to discover an etiology for the discomfort experienced by patients. This reality can lead to frustration or guilt on the part of the clinical practitioner, which in turn can lead to avoidance of the patient or minimization of the patient's pain by the practitioner, neither of which benefits either party (McConnell, 1988). Compounding the difficulty of establishing trust and gathering accurate data from the patient is the fact that older persons tend to be more reluctant to report pain than younger persons (Charlton & Buckley, 1984; Matteson, 1988; McConnell, 1988). Additionally, due to increased pain tolerance and adaptation, the elderly individual also does not tend to demonstrate expected objective signs of pain as readily as a younger person (Carpenito, 1999). While this adaptive behavior by the elderly patient may be necessary for continued survival, particularly in the presence of chronic pain, it may lead to inaccurate assessment by the practitioner, ineffective pain management, reduced comfort and mobility, and increasing dependence and isolation, anger and frustration, and, in some cases, confusion on the part of the patient (Pitt, 1982).

Clearly, an individual touched by pain experiences that perception across the broad spectrum of physical, emotional, and spiritual aspects of human experience. The experience also includes the human diminishments pain evokes in the individual, both organically and spiritually. This view of the integrated wholeness of the human person experiencing life events is reaching new awareness in a healthcare environment and era that had found comfort in the high-tech-low-touch approach to problem solving. During the past decade, however, the traditional philosophies and healthcare practices of Western society have become increasingly receptive to a cultural renewal of the ancient and Eastern philosophies of holistic health. This openness is resulting in increasingly active interest in the modalities associated with those traditions. As a result, it appears that we are witnessing the emergence of sociocultural legitimacy of a holistic health paradigm, perhaps best described as a renaissance moment. A singular outcome of this ongoing trend is without doubt the consciousness-raising constellation of external and internal variables integral to the individual and personal experience of health/illness events, such as pain.

Seaward (1994) posits that the primary reason for this readiness to transition originates from the socioeconomic reality that the "American healthcare system is crumbling under its own economic weight." The burgeoning recognition that Eastern traditions and Western traditions are in fact not mutually exclusive but rather complementary is perhaps best illustrated by recent activities at the federal level of healthcare policy. The NIH is transitioning the Office of Alternative Medicine (OAM) into the mainstream by funding and staffing the office to serve as the primary agency to engage in and support research in the area of complementary and alternative medicine, or CAM (Villaire, 1995). The evolution of this new emphasis is reflected in the creation of six to eight additional research centers devoted to specific clinical problems, including, but not limited to, stroke, women's health, and pain issues.

The readiness of the healthcare community to learn and share new realities and awareness of the power of integrating East and West and high-tech and high-touch has found a common ground in the search for higher clinical efficacy and healthcare cost savings. These were also the discussion triggers for the participants in the OAM-sponsored Conference on Technology Assessment during the fall of 1995. The two specific clinical foci of that conference were treatment modalities for insomnia and chronic pain, and the outcome recommendations give new direction for plausible and efficient modalities for efficacious interventions (Chilton, 1996). By nature of the everyday adaptations these realities demand of the older adult, the outcome recommendations of this panel have benchmark implications for healthcare providers serving this population.

For example, Garner and Kinderknecht (1993) address the responsibility of healthcare workers to empower clients in pain by teaching them coping skills that will allow clients to actively engage in the process of ameliorating pain. In their discussion of the gate theory of pain perception, the authors provide an overview of pain management and coping modalities designed to insert self-control back into the equation of health status, even in the face of the reality of illness. This is a most powerful and appealing idea. The concept is a natural evolution of the psychological theory of "self-efficacy." This theory, in turn, is giving rise to the model of self-efficacy training, which is reportedly being proven as an intervention for indigenous peoples in Canada, Latinos in California, and those with chronic co-morbid conditions (Chilton, 1996).

Results of scientific investigation into the phenomenon of pain experienced by the elderly may assist the elderly in achieving the best possible quality of life. Although instruments have been developed to quantify and qualify pain experienced by the elderly and non-elderly (Kane & Kane, 1984; Wright & Gal, 1987), this remains an area of need for additional nursing research. Unfortunately, until recently, pain research in the elderly has received limited attention. This is despite the fact that the special vulnerability to pain experienced by this cohort is commonly reflected in the literature as a given. For example, the Clinical Practice Guideline for Management of Cancer Pain states: "The elderly should be considered an at-risk group for the undertreatment of cancer pain because of inappropriate beliefs about pain sensitivity, pain tolerance and ability to use opioids. Elderly patients, like other adults, require aggressive pain assessment and management" (Agency for Health Care Policy and Research, 1994).

Some of the factors that singly and in combination explain why the elderly population is at high risk for the nursing diagnosis alteration in comfort are presented in Table 25.2.

THE LOCUS OF ASSESSMENT: THE PATIENT

Gratefully, the past decade has brought important changes in both the knowledge and performance parameters of pain management across all health professions. The most cru-cial change in thinking is the clinical foci of control of pain residing with the patient, rather than the individual professional whose capacity to address subjective symptoms may be biased by a host of intellectual, cultural, professional, and personal variables which influence effective treatment interventions for the elderly.

The awareness of pain and its influence on the quality of life has garnered the attention of the graying American public. Thanks to the influences of communications media from print to the Internet, the level of healthcare consumer knowledge today is more sophisticated than in previous generations. Concurrently, the health industry, with its renewed focus on quality assurance, has found the focus of care delivery once again returning to the patient. Performance expectations, measurable behavioral outcomes of patient care, and other outcome performance tools are all examples of the shifting model of healthcare service delivery. The shift is consonant with a heightened awareness of the criticality of pain management throughout the clinical professions.

The clinical discourse on quality assurance of pain control has also translated into a new organizational awareness. Policy and standard-setting institutions such as the Agency for Healthcare Research and Quality, and the JCAHO are developing new pain management standards (Acute Pain Management Guideline Panel, 1992; JCAHO, 2001). Significantly, the JCAHO developed new standards for pain control with a radical change in thinking — that pain management is the responsibility of healthcare organizations. In introducing the new standards (effective January 2001), which include the elderly in all care delivery settings, the quality of pain management is addressed through a systematic assessment of pain using a 10-point scale. More detail regarding the specific revisions in the six standards chapters (Rights and Ethics; Assessment of Persons with Pain; Care of Persons with Pain; Education of Persons with Pain; Continuum of Care, and Improvement of Organization Performance) is available on the JCAHO Web site (http://www.jcaho.org) (Phillips, 2000).

TABLE 25.2
Risk Factors Associated with Nursing Diagnosis: Alterations of Comfort in the Elderly

- Pain threshold increases with age.
- Physiologic/pathophysiologic changes may alter perception of pain.
- Pain in the elderly may be referred from site of origin.
- Physiologic changes of aging give rise to chronic pain.
- Multiple pathologies may result in the paradoxical absence of pain.
- Severe pain and chronic discomfort in the elderly may manifest as confusion.
- Cultural/psychological expectations may diminish reporting of pain.
- Concern for overmedication may result in insufficient pain management modalities.
- Societal acceptance of pain in the elderly leads to avoidance or minimalization of pain.
- Depression is present and most frequently associated with chronic pain.
- Constellation of symptoms in chronic pain states includes behavior commonly associated with maladaptation to the aging process, including sleep disturbances, appetite disturbances, decreased libido, irritability, withdrawal of interests, weakening of relationships, and increased preoccupation with ill health.
- Underreporting of symptoms occurs frequently.
- Communication difficulties increase history-taking problems.

NURSING MANAGEMENT OF PAIN IN INFANTS AND CHILDREN

Although pain relief is a primary goal of nurses, pain management in children has often been ignored and has received limited attention in the literature. In 1977, Eland and Anderson documented the undertreatment of pain in children. Following this study, subsequent research findings supported the idea that pain in children is an ignored dimension of care (Wong & Hockenberry-Eaton, 2001). Recently, significant advances in the management of children's pain have been facilitated by the development of clinical practice guidelines for pain (Acute Pain Management Guideline Panel, 1992) management from the federal

---

TABLE 25.3
Myths Associated with the Undertreatment of Pain in Children

- Infants and children are unable to perceive and experience pain.
- Children have no memory of pain.
- Pain produces no harmful effects.
- Children become easily addicted to narcotics.
- Children are more likely to experience respiratory depression.

AHCPR and the development of acute pain services in hospitals.

Experts have proposed many explanations for undertreatment of pain in children (Table 25.3). The inability to assess children's pain, however, has presented the biggest challenge for pediatric nurses. Preverbal infants, intubated patients, and developmentally challenged children are not able to verbally describe their pain. Pediatric nurses must be able to assess pain and understand that infants and children respond to pain with reactions based on age and cognitive processes. Because of the problems associated with the measurement of pain in children, assessment requires a multifaceted approach.

Research findings indicate that infants and children do experience pain and respond to that pain both physiologically and behaviorally (Deshpande & Anand, 1996; Jorgensen, 1999). These pain cues may be more subtle than those expressed by adults. Observation of these responses provides the basis for nursing assessment. Other assessment parameters include: (1) obtaining a thorough history from the child and/or parents; (2) using a self-report tool, if appropriate; and (3) eliciting parental input about the child's pain.

Behavioral changes may indicate pain in children who are unable or unwilling to verbally report pain. Behavioral responses associated with children's pain include:

- Vocal communication, such as moaning, whimpering, or crying
- Facial expressions, such as a grimace
- Body language, such as positioning, posturing, splinting, pushing away, or kicking
- Emotional responses, such as withdrawal, depression, irritability, and unusual quietness
- Changes in daily routines, such as loss of appetite and disturbed sleep patterns

Behavioral responses modulate over time and require careful assessment throughout a child's illness. Parents are often the first to detect these subtle behaviors, and their input is essential.

Physiological parameters that demonstrate the presence of pain include changes in vital signs, skin color, sweating, and nausea and/or vomiting. Flushed skin;

increased temperature, pulse, and blood pressure; poor tissue perfusion; and dilated pupils may be associated with pain. These signs of autonomic nervous system arousal and the body's stress response are self-limiting. The body cannot continue the response. Adaptation occurs and a state of homeostasis follows, although the child is still in pain. These physiological responses, therefore, are only helpful when they are combined with other assessment data.

Assessment tools offer a systematic approach to the evaluation of pain. A valid and reliable tool reduces bias. Various tools exist, and one tool is not appropriate for all children. The selection of an assessment tool should be based on the child's age and developmental level (Wong & Hockenberry-Eaton, 2001).

A specific assessment form should be used to document assessment findings. Documentation should include the location and intensity of the pain, the type of assessment tool used, observed behavioral manifestations, physiological parameters, the pain intervention, and the response to that intervention (Lux, Algren, & Algren, 1999).

The AHCPR publication, "Clinical Practice Guideline for Acute Pain Management" (Acute Pain Management Guideline Panel, 1992), provides information for the assessment and management of pain in infants, children, and adolescents. The goal for pediatric pain management is preventing or relieving pain as much as possible using pharmacological or nonpharmacological strategies, or a combination of the two.

Pharmacological agents used to manage pain in children include both opioid and nonnarcotic analgesics. The ideal analgesic should be easy to administer, have a rapid onset, and produce the desired degrees of analgesia. Physiological parameters and respiration should be minimally altered. The discussion of specific pharmacological agents is beyond the scope of this chapter. Extensive information can be found in Chapter 39 on the "Management of Procedural and Perioperative Pain in Children."

A variety of routes of administration are now being utilized in pediatric pain management. Oral and rectal administration are less traumatizing than intramuscular injection. In fact, injections are strongly discouraged in most pediatric institutions. Topical anesthetics, regional anesthesia and analgesia, and epidural analgesia have also become commonplace in treating children's pain (Algren & Algren, 1994; Wong & Hockenberry-Eaton, 2001).

In most children's hospitals, patient-controlled analgesia (PCA) is the mainstay of pediatric pain management. Pain resulting from etiologies such as surgery, trauma, sickle cell crisis, and cancer can be successfully managed by PCA. Using an infusion pump, patients can administer a preset amount of opioid, usually morphine, by simply pressing a button. The patient, however, cannot repeat a dose before a specified period of time, usually

8 to 15 minutes. PCA gives the patient control over pain management, permits individual titration, and provides superior analgesic effect (Lux et al., 1999).

Patient-controlled analgesia was first used in adolescents, but its use has quickly spread to younger children. Children as young as 5 years of age can safely and effectively control their own analgesia (Yaster et al., 1997). A degree of safety is maintained by the patients when they no longer feel the need to "push the button" or when they become sedated. The key to successful use of PCA in children is adequate patient and parent education. The control of PCA pumps by a surrogate such as a parent or nurse is controversial because it compromises the inherent safety of PCA. If parents or nurses control the PCA system, frequent assessment and conservative dosing is desirable (Lux et al., 1999).

Nonpharmacological strategies may be very helpful in the management of mild to moderate pain and procedural pain. These techniques are noninvasive, inexpensive, and offer some control to the child and parent. Strategies such as distraction, guided imagery, and relaxation techniques decrease anxiety, reduce pain perception, and enhance the effectiveness of analgesics (Vessey & Carlson, 1996). Guided imagery, such as imagining being at the beach, can be used in children who are capable of abstract thinking. Relaxation activities such as holding, rocking, reading stories, and listening to music may reduce the stress associated with pain and thus provide pain relief.

Cutaneous stimulation can also be used as a noninvasive pain relief measure. Activities such as stroking or rubbing an injured area stimulate the large A-alpha peripheral fibers and block the transmission of noxious impulses at the spinal cord. Applications of heat and cold may also promote analgesia.

In summary, nurses play a vital role in pediatric pain assessment and management. Health professionals must create a climate that makes effective pain management a priority. Developmentally appropriate pain assessment tools must be utilized in evaluating children's pain. Clinical practice must be evaluated through research and quality improvement programs. Finally, all practitioners must be advocates for the child and the family for effective pain management.

NURSING MANAGEMENT OF CANCER PAIN

Approximately one million Americans are diagnosed with cancer each year. In the early and intermediate stages, 30 to 45% experience moderate to severe pain. In the advanced stages of cancer, 75% of patients experience pain; 25 to 30% of these patients describe their pain as severe. Good to excellent pain relief is possible in 95% of these patients if adequately treated with pharmacological therapy (Jacox et al., 1994). The majority of cancer patients in the U.S. receive inadequate pain management. The literature suggests that healthcare providers continue to have misconceptions about cancer pain (Pargeon & Hailey, 1999). Patients may hamper their own treatment due to misconceptions about pain and fears about opioids.

Cancer pain is multifaceted and is generally classified as pain from direct tumor involvement, invasive diagnostic and therapeutic procedures, infection, or toxicity of chemotherapy and radiation therapy. Because cancer most often occurs at ages when other maladies causing pain develop (e.g., arthritis and chronic back problems), the practitioner must attempt to identify the source of the pain and intervene appropriately. Cancer-related pain may be difficult for the patient to explain. Thorough and accurate nursing assessment is paramount to the diagnosis and management of cancer pain.

The Standards of Oncology Nursing Practice emphasize the systematic and continuous collection of data to plan appropriate interventions with the patient (ANA, 1996). Cancer patients may underreport pain if they think pain indicates their disease is not responding to treatment. Some patients simply do not want to complain even if analgesics are available to relieve the pain because they think it is part of the fate of the disease. Other variables such as financial concerns, anxiety, and limited family support may add to the perceived pain experienced. The absence of standardized assessment tools makes it difficult for nurses to consistently and effectively assess the extent of pain, evaluate the efficacy of the intervention, and accurately communicate this information. Lack of knowledge about the cause of cancer pain, as well as attitudes toward pain and its management, can be barriers to adequate assessment.

The Oncology Nursing Society has long recognized the need for a consistent approach to cancer pain management and barriers to that management. In a recent revision of its Position Paper on Cancer Pain Management (Oncology Nursing Society, 2000), emphasis is placed on multidisciplinary management that is collaborative and involves ongoing assessment, planning, intervention, and evaluation of pain and pain relief.

The site of the cancer and the stage of the disease factor into the incidence and prevalence of pain. As the disease progresses, patients with metastatic disease are more likely to experience pain, particularly those with bone involvement from primary infiltration or metastasis. Interference with organ function or structure or nerve invasion intensifies pain. Terminal patients report significant increases in pain. It is evident that the management of cancer pain may need to be multimodal secondary to the many dimensions of its etiology. However, the treatment of acute and chronic cancer pain continues to remain primarily within the realm of pharmacologic management.

Effective cancer pain management has been described in practice quidelines by organizations such as the AHCPR (Jacox et al., 1994). While advocating a team approach, details such as assessment, pharmacological management, adjuvant therapy, and psychological interventions are outlined in the guidelines.

Analgesics are extremely effective in most patients when used correctly. In 1986, the World Health Organization recommended a three-step "analgesic ladder" that emphasizes the use of standard drugs classified as nonopioids, weak opioids, and strong opioids. Sequential use of the drugs is advocated with the addition of a weak opioid in combination with the nonopioid, or a strong opioid should relief not be obtained. Adjuvant drugs are added if required for specific indications, and they are often needed in patients with pain secondary to nerve injury. Nonopioid drugs such as the nonsteroidal anti-inflammatory drugs interfere with peripheral receptors by inhibiting prostaglandin release, thus reducing pain from resulting inflammation. Opioid drugs (narcotics) bind to receptors that interfere with the transmission of painful stimuli. Because of the difference in action, a combination of the two types of drugs results in efficacious pain management. Adjuvant drugs are used to treat specific types of pain and to alleviate other symptoms that may occur in cancer patients. Anticonvulsants, antidepressants, and corticosteroids are used to reduce anxiety and depression, which often exacerbate cancer pain and interfere with other activities of the patient.

Other interventions may be useful, particularly for pain that is not responsive to analgesics. Nerve blocks, transcutaneous nerve stimulation, and neuroablative techniques may benefit cancer patients.

Nurses in acute and chronic pain settings can add a unique perspective to the assessment and care of each cancer patient. Changes in a patient's comfort that occurs every 24 hours can be observed and reported and interventions evaluated more closely because of the increased contact with the patient. Combining nursing therapies with behavioral therapies and pharmacotherapies offers a broader approach to pain management. Comfort measures helpful for patients with cancer pain are summarized in Table 25.4.

The Oncology Nursing Society (2000) supports nurse design of individualized physical and psychosocial interventions that are intended to achieve stated outcomes and are prioritized according to the patient's needs. The nurse also collaborates and communicates with appropriate members of the multidisciplinary team in designing the plan of care.

It is imperative that information be as complete as possible and be available to all practitioners involved in treating the patient's pain or discomfort. Outcome crite-

---

TABLE 25.4
Nursing Therapies for Cancer Pain

- Rest and sleep
- Adequate nutrition
- Daily elimination
- Activities of daily living
- Encourage movement
- Environmental control
- Encourage independence
- Medications
- Thermal therapy
- Communication
- Therapeutic touch
- Relaxation techniques
- Distraction
- Emotional support
- Availability of spiritual support

---

ria for the patient, in relation to comfort, state that the patient will:

1. Communicate alterations in comfort level
2. Identify measures to modify psychosocial, environmental, and physical factors that increase comfort and promote the continuance of valued activities and relationships
3. Describe the source of discomfort, the treatment, and the expected outcome of the proposed intervention
4. Describe appropriate interventions for potential or predictable problems such as pain

To do so requires a comprehensive approach to pain control for the cancer patient. Accountability and responsibility of the professionals involved with the care are demanded and advocated. The challenge is for the nurse to identify, assess, treat, evaluate at specific intervals, make alterations if necessary, and further evaluate. It is the professional and ethical responsibility of caregivers to assist the patient and family in identifying and managing factors that promote comfort.

SUMMARY

In conclusion, the AHCPR and other major organizations have widely disseminated pain guidelines. The absence of knowledge is no longer a factor in caring for patients with pain. Pain management as a multidisciplinary, collaborative practice is still too new for many practitioners to be competent, confident members of the team. In *Seizing the Future*, Zey (1994) addresses mentoring as an effective developmental tool routed in caring and individualized learning that provides the emotional support often missing in society's high-tech cognitive approach to solutions.

To assist patients with pain and to help them integrate its management into their life, practitioners need cognitive, affective, and psychomotor practice skills. Formal pain mentoring programs established in hospitals and other settings (Kachoyeanos, 1966) and less-formal mentoring through the American Academy of Pain Management, the American Society of Pain Management Nurses, and other pain organizations can develop practitioners to better serve patients and mentor other colleagues in the future.

Nurses are ubiquitous, just as pain and the need for pain management is ubiquitous. Nurses have more contact with patients in pain than any other practitioner. Nursing practice, research, and mentoring are vital components of pain management practice, and nurses are valuable participants who help determine how the healthcare systems in the U.S. and throughout the world deal with pain management.

REFERENCES

Acute Pain Management Guideline Panel (1992). *Acute pain management: Operative or medical procedures and trauma* (AHCPR Publ. No. 92-0032). Rockville, MD: Agency for Health Care Policy and Research, U.S. Department of Health and Human Services Public Health Service.

Agency for Health Care Policy and Research. (1994). *Management of cancer pain*. Clinical guideline number 9. (AHCPR Publication No. 94-0592). Rockville, MD: Agency for Health Care Policy and Research.

Algren, C.L., & Algren, J.T. (1994). Pain management in children. *Plastic Surgical Nursing, 14*(2), 65–70.

American Nurses Association: Oncology Nursing Society (1996). *Standards of oncology nursing practice*. Kansas City, MO: American Nurses Association.

Aspen Reference Group (1995). *Pain management: Patient education manual* (S. Neimeyer & S. N. DiLama, Eds.). Gaithersburg, MD: Aspen Publishers.

Caird, F.L., Dall, J.C., & Williams, B.O. (1987). The cardiovascular system. In J.C. Brocklehurst (Ed.), *Textbook of geriatric medicine and gerontology* (3rd ed., pp. 230–267). Edinburgh: Churchill Livingstone.

Carpenito, L.J. (1999). *Nursing diagnosis: Application to clinical practice* (8th ed.). Philadelphia: Lippincott, Williams & Wilkins.

Charlton, J.E., & Buckley, F.P. (1984). Management of chronic pain. In J.G. Evans & F.I. Caird (Eds.), *Advanced geriatric medicine* (Vol. 4, pp. 17–32). London: Pittman Press.

Chilton, M. (1996). Panel recommendations integrating behavioral and relaxation approaches into medical treatment of chronic pain, insomnia. *Alternative Therapies, 2*(1), 18–28.

Cleary, B.L. (1997). Age-related changes in the special senses. In M. A. Matteson, E.S. McConnell, & A.D. Linton (Eds.), *Gerontological nursing: Concepts and practice* (2nd ed., pp. 385–405). Philadelphia: W. B. Saunders.

Corso, J.F. (1971). Sensory processes and age effects in normal adults. *Journal of Gerontology, 26,* 90–105.

Cronin, Y., & Bahrke, L.S. (1996). An epidural clinical pathway: A new generation for clinical pathways. *ASPMN Pathways, 5*(1), 1, 3–4.

Deshpande, J.K., & Anand, K.J. (1996). Basic aspects of acute pediatric pain and sedation. In J. Deshpande & J. Tobias (Eds.), *The pediatric pain handbook* (pp. 1–48). St. Louis: Mosby.

Dymock, I.W. (1985). The gastrointestinal system-the upper gastrointestinal tract. In J.C. Brocklehurst (Ed.), *Textbook of geriatric medicine and gerontology* (3rd ed., pp. 508–519). Edinburgh: Churchill Livingstone.

Eland, J., & Anderson, J. (1977). The experience of pain in children. In A. Jacox (Ed.), *Pain: A sourcebook for nurses and other health professionals* (pp. 453–473). Boston: Little, Brown & Company.

Ferrell, B.R., & Ferrell, B.A. (1997). Care of elderly patients with pain. In *Expert pain management*. Springhouse, PA: Springhouse Corporation.

Garner, J.D., & Kinderknecht, C. (1993). Living productively with arthritis. In J.D. Garner and A. Young (Eds.), *Women and healthy aging* (pp. 61–81). Binghamton, NY: Haworth Press.

Gordon, M. (2000). *Manual of nursing diagnosis* (9th ed.). St. Louis: Mosby.

Grahame, R. (1985). The musculoskeletal systemæ disease of the joints. In J. C. Brocklehurst (Ed.), *Textbook of geriatric medicine and gerontology* (3rd ed., pp. 795–819).

Ignatavicius, D., & Hausman, K. (1995). *Clinical pathways for collaborative practice*. Philadelphia: W.B. Saunders.

International Association for the Study of Pain (IASP) Subcommittee on Taxonomy (1979). Pain terms: A list with definitions and notes on useage. *Pain, 6*(2), 249.

Jacox, A. (1977). Sociocultural and psychological aspects of pain. In A. Jacox (Ed.), *Pain: A sourcebook for nurses and other health professionals* (pp. 57–87). Boston: Little, Brown & Company.

Joint Commission on Accreditation of Healthcare Organization (2001). *2001 Accreditation manual*. Oakbrook Terrace, IL: Joint Commission on Accreditation of Healthcare Organizations. http://www.jcaho.org/standard/pm.html

Jorgensen, K. (1999). Pain assessment and management in the newborn infant. *Journal of Perianesthesia Nursing, 14*(6), 349–356.

Kachoyeanos, M.K. (1966). Establishing a pain mentoring program. *ASPMN Pathways, 5*(1), 7–8.

Kane, R., & Kane, R. (1984). *Assessing the elderly: A practical guide to measurement*. Lexington, MA: Lexington Books.

Lux, M., Algren, C., & Algren, J. (1999). Management strategies for ensuring adequate analgesia in children. *Disease Management and Health Outcomes, 6*(1), 37–47.

Marrelli, T.M. (1994). *Handbook of home health standards and documentation guidelines for reimbursement* (2nd ed.). St. Louis: Mosby.

McCaffery, M. (1968). *Nursing practice theories related to cognition, body pain, and man-environment interaction*. Los Angeles: University of California, Students' Store.

McCaffery, M., & Pasero, C. (1999). *Pain: Clinical manual.* St. Louis: C.V. Mosby.

McConnell, E.S. (1988). Nursing diagnoses related to physiological alterations. In M.A. Matteson & E.S. McConnell (Ed.), *Gerontological nursing concepts and practice* (pp. 331–428). Philadelphia: W. B. Saunders.

McCue, J.D. (1987). Medical screening of the relatively asymptomatic elderly patient. In C. S. Rogers & J. D. McCue (Eds.), *Managing chronic disease* (pp. 391–399). Oradell, NJ: Medical Economics Books.

National Institutes of Health Consensus Development Conference. (1987). The integrated approach to the management of pain: Consensus development conference statement. *Journal of Pain and Symptom Management, 2*(1), 35–44.

Oncology Nursing Society. (2000). *Position paper on cancer pain.* Pittsburgh: Oncology Nursing Society.

Pargeon, K, & Hailey, B. (1999). Barriers to effective cancer pain management: A review of the literature. *Journal of Pain and Symptom Management, 18*(5), 358–368.

Pathy, M.J. (1985). The central nervous system. Clinical presentation and management of neurological disorders in old age. In J. C. Brocklehurst (Ed.), *Textbook of geriatric medicine and gerontology* (3rd ed., pp. 795–819). Edinburgh: Churchill Livingstone.

Phillips, D. (2000). JCAHO pain management standards are unveiled. *Journal of the American Medical Association, 284*(4), 428–429.

Pitt, B. (1982). *Psychogeriatrics: An introduction to the psychiatry of old age* (2nd ed., pp. 2–14, 31–38). Edinburgh: Churchill Livingstone.

Ready, L.B. (1995). Practice guidelines for acute pain management in the perioperative setting: A report by the American Society of Anesthesiologists Task Force on Pain Management, Acute Pain Section. *Anesthesiology, 82,* 1071.

Seaward, B.L. (1994, September). Alternative medicine complements standard. *Health Progress,* 52–57.

Thompson, J.W. (1984). Pain: Mechanisms and principles of management. In J. G. Evans & F. I. Caird (Eds.), *Advanced geriatric medicine* (Vol. 4, pp. 3–16). London: Pittman Press.

Vessey, J.A., & Carlson, K. (1996). Nonpharmacological interventions to use with children in pain. *Issues in Comprehensive Pediatric Nursing, 19,* 169–182.

Villaire, M. (1995). A fresh start: OAM charts its course for the future. *Alternative Therapies, 1*(5), 18–20.

Wolanin, M.O. (1976). Nursing assessment. In L.M. Burnside (Ed.), *Nursing and the aged* (pp. 398–420). New York: McGraw-Hill.

Wong, D., & Hockenberry-Eaton, M. (2001). *Wong's essentials of pediatric nursing* (6th ed.). St. Louis: Mosby.

World Health Organization. (1986). *Cancer pain relief.* Geneva, Switzerland: World Health Organization.

Wright, A.B., & Gal, P. (1987). Assessment and treatment of pain. In C.S. Rogers & J.D. McCue (Eds.), *Managing chronic disease* (pp. 28–34). Oradell, NJ: Medical Economics Books.

Yaster, M., et al. (1997). *Pediatric pain management and sedation handbook.* St. Louis: Mosby.

Zey, M.G. (1994). *Seizing the future.* New York: Simon & Schuster.

26

The Psychiatrist's Role in Pain Diagnosis and Management

Nelson H. Hendler, M.D., M.S.

INTRODUCTION

The role of a psychiatrist in chronic pain management is multiple. He or she must be a diagnostician, a pharmacologist, a sociologist, a psychotherapist, and even, on occasion, patient advocate. Therefore, by definition, the psychiatrist must have an eclectic orientation, and be broadly schooled in all forms of diagnostic and therapeutic interventions.

There are at least three approaches to chronic pain that a psychiatrist can use. Each has its own advantages and disadvantages.

The medical model. Using this paradigm, pain is defined as a manifestation of a disease. This approac lends clarity to the problems of pain, and offers predictive capabilities for outcome. It may offer a cure where none existed before. As an example, "pain in the back and the leg" is a description, but "a herniated disc with radiculopathy" is a diagnosis. Surgery on the disc may cure the pain. However, should the surgery not work, or should there be psychological problems or social problems compounding the recovery, response to surgery may not be as predicted.

The psychiatric model. Using this approach, a psychiatrist tries to establish a psychiatric diagnosis to explain the behavior of a pain patient who is troublesome or not responding in the predicted fashion. Using this tack, personality disorders, affective disorders, or anxiety traits that might be the source of a patient's complaints are identified and treated. Unfortunately, the use of psychiatric intervention in this fashion very often leads to an "either-or" type of thinking, with psychiatric diagnosis being established to the exclusion of medical diagnosis. A person with a histrionic personality disorder, who has surgical excision of a disc and does not get well, may run afoul of the system. His or her lack of recovery is ascribed to "secondary gain" or "dependency needs," but not to retained disc material missed by the first surgery

The integrated response model. Using this model, the psychiatrist tries to establish both medical and psychiatric diagnoses, not only from the point in time at which a patient is seen, but also based on the historical perspective of the patient, that is, the "pre-morbid" or "pre-pain" personality. In this fashion, one can determine the appropriateness of response to pain, and to treatment. This approach is time-consuming and involves a multidisciplinary approach, with multilevel diagnoses and integration of material. In this model, both medical and psychiatric diagnoses can exist.

MEDICAL MODEL

Adherence to the medical model is often found within pain treatment centers or in clinical practices that utilize only medical evaluation of the patient. The absence of a psychiatric or psychological professional to assist in evaluation and diagnosis limits the evaluation of the chronic pain patient to only medical assessment. It disregards the possibility that a patient may have psychiatric problems, the result of chronic pain, which can lead to diagnostic oversight. Indeed, some authors believe that the incidence of depression, in dissociation with chronic pain, is remarkably high (Hendler, 1984b; Krishnan, et al., 1985; Pilowsky & Bassett, 1982). Other authors have advanced the theory that chronic pain may be a manifestation of an underlying

0-8493-0926-3/02/$0.00+$1.50
© 2002 by CRC Press LLC

depression (Engel, 1959; Maruta, Swanson, & Swanson, 1976). Therefore, the medical assessment of chronic pain without psychiatric assessment (to determine the preexisting personality characteristics and motivations that may lead to an exaggerated response to chronic pain, or may, in fact, lead to the expression of psychiatric disease as a chronic pain process) would compromise any medical diagnostic endeavor. By the same token, severe and chronic illness certainly produces depression, and perhaps other psychiatric disorders, which would benefit from therapeutic intervention. The use of a purely medical model cannot be endorsed.

Likewise, the purely psychiatric model suffers from many of the same problems. In a most thorough review of the problem, Dr. Charles Ford (1986) discusses what has been called "somatizing disorders." In this article, Ford discusses the concept of the sick role, which allows the ill person to be released from regular duties and obligations. He further differentiates illness from disease, describing the latter as objectively measured, while illness discusses the change in functioning of an individual. He further clarifies the point, indicating that disease can occur in the absence of illness, while conversely, illness can occur in the absence of disease. Dr. Ford further describes somatization as "the process by which an individual uses the body, or bodily symptom, for psychological purpose or personal gain." However, Ford does concede that somatization can occur in the presence of' demonstrable physical disease, with amplification of the response to a real physical disorder. Ford then lists nine reasons why people somatize:

1. To avoid unpleasant tasks, or to achieve primary or secondary gains, in the form of payment
2. To solve family problems
3. To allow an individual to focus on physical symptoms rather than psychological problems
4. As a form of communication of displeasure
5. As a way of expressing oneself when they are not capable of expressing themselves otherwise
6. A culturally determined response
7. Using a physical symptom because is it more culturally acceptable than a psychiatric one
8. Focusing on physical problems that are manifestations of underlying stress
9. Utilizing the fashionable diagnosis to explain underlying/psychiatric disease, such as hypoglycemia

Ford further feels that patients may utilize somatic symptoms instead of expressing depression, and further indicates that these depressions are unrecognized. Anxiety may also manifest as a somatic complaint, which he also believed could go undiagnosed. According to Ford, "chronic pain syndromes are one of the more common forms of somatization." He also includes disability syndromes under the description of somitizing disorders. He describes hard-working individuals who have an accident, and then fall apart. This inability to function allows the individual to have support and secondary gains, and allows an underlying dependency to manifest itself.

PSYCHIATRIC MODEL

In a superb review article, Drs. Turk and Flor (1984) reviewed the psychological models contributing to chronic back pain. In this article, they discuss theoretical constructs, which explain the transition from acute to chronic back pain, with the exception of the psychoanalytic approach. In this approach, unexplained back pain is considered a conversion neurosis, a manifestation of underlying tension, and manifess as increased muscle activity and spasm. Using this model, various authors have suggested that pain of unexplained origin should be treated as depression with the use of antidepressant drugs. Another explanation for unexplained back pain advances the family system theory. In this approach, the basic idea is that "symptoms of the patient fulfill the emotional needs of other family members." They suggest that the sick role is used for conflict avoidance. Another theory that is advanced is the observational learning theory based on cognitive behavioral assumptions. In this model, the patient expresses feelings of helplessness aand hopelessness, and loss of control over his or her environment. Another theory, originally advanced by Flor, discusses the diathesis-stress model of chronic back pain. In this model, interactions lead to the development of chronic back pain. This is an attempt to integrate the physical, psychological, and social factors that lead to the development of illness. In this diathesis-stress model, hyperactivity of the back muscles may be due to (1) the existence of a response stereotypy (diathesis) involving the back muscles, (2) recurrent or very intense adverse situations perceived as stressful, and/or (3) inadequate coping abilities of the individual.

Another attempt to explain pain of unknown etiology utilizes the diagnostic manual of the American Psychiatric Association (1994). Reich, Rosenblatt, and Tupin (1983) have attempted to explain the use of this diagnostic system for chronic pain patients. They indicate that attempts to categorize chronic pain patients "merely in terms of the prime physical complaints has obvious shortcomings." They describe the prime physical complaints as having five categories, or axes, in the *Diagnostic and Statistical Manual of Mental Disorders* (DSM-III), that correspond to five major areas of concern:

Axis I: used to describe thought disorders, such as schizophrenia and manic depressive disease, and drug abuse;

Axis II: used to describe personality characteristics

Axis III: used to describe medical diagnoses, or physical complaints;

Axis IV: used to describe the severity of' psychosocial distress

Axis V: used to describe the highest level of functioning during the past year

Reich and colleagues (1983) feel that an entire category of diagnoses, "the somatoform disorders," can be used to categorize chronic pain patients, in whom there is a strong psychological component that could explain a pain unexplained by physical diagnosis. The major diagnosis within this group is "psychogenic pain disorder." The criteria for utilizing this diagnosis are (1) the absence of appropriate physical findings, and (2) the presence of psychological factors that may explain the etiology of the complaint. Attendant to this diagnosis are a variety of subjective assessments, such as the severity of the pain, the inability of the pain to conform with anatomical distribution, and, perhaps the most subjective assessment of all, that the severity of the pain be out of proportion to what one might anticipate. Further diagnostic categories under the somatic disorders include hypochondriasis and conversion disorder. In the former, the patient is concerned with the development of a severe, debilitating illness, despite the lack of objective findings. In this instance, the patient's concerns are considered inordinate because the organic condition was not substantiated. In conversion disorders, the physical condition suggests an underlying organic disease, but the basis of the illness is purely psychological. The authors then offer several examples of DSM-III diagnoses, in which the predominate features are highly subjective, and the use of words "inconsistent with physical findings" or "pain, etiology unknown," and prior surgeries with residual pain. The authors advocate the use of DSM-III taxonomy because it has achieved better reliability than previous psychiatric diagnostic systems.

With the advent of the Diagnostic and Statistical Manual of Mental Disorders, fourth edition, which was published in 1994, there have been some modifications to the approach to pain, with a wide range of options. At one extreme, there is a group of patients who actually fabricate symptoms for subconscious psychological, but not financial gain. These patients have factious disorders, with predominantly physical signs and symptoms (DSM-IV code 300.19) or with combined psychological and physical signs and symptoms (DSM-IV code 300.19). An entire chapter is devoted to "Somatoform Disorders," and contains a wide-ranging list. Included are Hypochondriasis (DSM-IV code 300.7), Somatization Disorder (DSM-IV code 300.81), Undifferentiated Somatoform Disorder (DSM-IV code 300.81), Conversion Disorder (DSM-IV code 300.11), Pain Disorder with several subtypes: Pain Disorder Associated with Psychological Factors (DSM-IV code 307.80), or Pain Disorder Associated with both Psychological Factors and General Medical Conditions (DSM-IV code 307.89). Most noteworthy is the addition of a concept of Pain Disorder Associated with a General Medical Condition, divided into acute (less than 6 months) or chronic (greater than 6 months). This category is not considered a mental disorder and is coded under Axis III to facilitate differential diagnosis, and then uses the ICD-9 codes of the medical disorder to classify the diagnosis. This is a major advance in psychiatric thinking; it advances the notion that chronic pain can produce psychiatric disorders, rather than the reverse. (APA,1994).

INTEGRATED RESPONSE MODEL

The third approach to diagnosing chronic pain patients, utilizing an integrated response model, avoids the diagnostic dualism of the previous two models. In this model, an attempt is made to study the normal response to chronic pain in a previously well-adjusted individual, and then using these responses as a benchmark against which other responses can be measured. Only by thoroughly understanding the normal patterns of response can one determine what is abnormal. It is for this reason that a medical student studies anatomy before he or she studies pathology, physiology, or pathophysiology. This approach also attempts to integrate responses, taking into account physical, psychological, and environmental factors, including sociological and legal considerations. One such attempt at integration has been advanced by Richard Black, M.D. (1982). Black asserts that a patient with a chronic pain syndrome must be assessed simultaneously for physical, mental, and environmental factors. He believes that sociological and economic factors rarely get considered, except when litigation is involved.

In an effort to further clarify this issue, Hendler and Talo (1989a) offer a diagnostic system that takes into consideration (1) the pre-morbid (pre-pain) adjustment of the individual (pathological or well-adjusted), (2) the response to the pain (pathological or appropriate), and (3) the actual physical diagnosis (the presence or absence of objective findings). Central to this formulation are two basic concepts:

1. Chronic pain can create psychological problems in a previously well-adjusted individual
2. Regardless of the pre-morbid (pre-pain) personality characteristics, if a person has a normal response to chronic pain, then the chances of a valid organic basis for the complaint of pain are quite high. This would be true even in the absence of objective laboratory studies or physical finding. Restated for emphasis, if a patient's response to pain is appropriate but there are no objective physical findings, it is incumbent upon the physician to keep looking for the organic basis of the patient's complaints.

Hendler (1981) has divided chronic pain patients into four groups, based on the three factors mentioned previously; that is: (1) pre-morbid adjustment, (2) response to pain, and (3) the presence or absence of objective upon physical findings in laboratory studies or physical examination. These four categories are:

1. Objective pain patient, defined as an individual with:
   a. Good pre-morbid adjustment,
   b. Normal response to chronic pain
   c. A definable organic lesion
2. Exaggerating pain patient, defined as an individual with:
   a. Pathology as part of a pre-morbid adjustment
   b. An unusual response to pain, in that there might be an absence of anxiety, or depression
   c. Minimal organic findings
3. An undetermined pain patient, defined as an individual with:
   a. Good pre-morbid adjustment
   b. A normal response to pain
   c. An absence of objective physical findings or physical examination (it is this individual who warrants further investigation)
4. Affective or associative pain patient, defined as an individual with:
   a. A poor pre-morbid adjustment
   b. An unusual response to chronic pain
   c. A total absence of objective physical findings or positive laboratory studies

By studying the normal response to chronic pain, one can then compare any patient against a known standard. In this case, the objective pain patient serves as the "normal" model against which all other responses to chronic pain should be judged. The objective pain patient has a good pre-morbid adjustment, which can be defined (Hendler, 1982a) as:

1. A good work record
2. A stable family background
3. A negative psychiatric history, with no previous suicide attempts or depression
4. The absence of alcohol or drug abuse
5. A good marital history
6. Lack of financial difficulties prior to the pain
7. A good sexual adjustment
8. No sleep difficulties
9. No radical changes in weight, other than conscious attempts to change it
10. The absence of any anti-social or sociopathic behavior

Hendler (1982b) further expands upon the objective pain patient, indicating that this individual goes through four stages in response to the chronic pain:

1. The acute stage, anywhere from 0 to 2 months, is when the individual expects to get well and has no psychological problems. Psychological testing administered during this time is within normal limits.
2. The subacute stage, which occurs anywhere from 2 to 6 months, is when the individual begins to experience somatic concerns and may have elevated Scales 1 and 3 on the Minnestoa Multiphasic Personality Inventory (MMPI).
3. The chronic stage of chronic pain occurs anywhere from 6 months to 8 years after the acquisition of the pain. The previously well-adjusted individual then develops depression and has elevated scales 1, 2, and 3 on the MMPI, with Scale 2 depression being higher than Scales 1 and 3 (hypochondriasis and hysteria).
4. The subchronic stage of chronic pain occurs anywhere from 3 to 12 years after the acquisition of the pain, during which time the depression resolves, but hypochondriacal and hysterical Scales of the MMPI remain elevated as one might expect, because the patient still has somatic concerns.

If all of the above occurs in an individual with a definable organic lesion and with positive objective testing, then one categorizes this type of patient as an objective pain patient. If all of the above psychological features are present, but no objective testing is positive, then one considers this individual an undetermined pain patient who still needs further medical investigation (Hendler, 1981).

To facilitate diagnosis using the four categories described previously, Hendler and co-workers (1985b) have devised the Mensana Clinic Back Pain Test. Using a simple, 15-question screening test, chronic pain patients can be divided into the four diagnostic categories, as described by Hendler. The screening test had good predictive values because *women* scoring in the objective pain patient category (17 points or less) had positive findings on electromyogram (EMG), nerve conduction velocity studies, thermography, CT scan, myelogram, or X-ray 77% of the time. If women scored in the exaggerating pain patient category (21 points or greater), none of the 53 women studied had objective physical findings, which is in counter-distinction to the MMPI, which had a great deal of scatter, with only the Depression Scale correlating with all with the absence or presence of physical findings. Hendler, et al., (1985a) also published results for the predictive volume of the test for *men*, showing that in 31 men there was a 91% chance of organic pathology if the patient scored in the objective pain patient range. Overall, the predictive value of the test was 85% (Hendler, Mollett, Talo, & Levin (1988). The usefulness of the four diagnostic categories for chronic pain patients is highlighted by the ability to predict the presence or absence of objective physical findings, based on the pre-morbid adjustment to the response to chronic pain and the description of the pain itself. The fact that the MMPI, which measures personality traits, was not a useful predictor of organic pathology lends support to the belief that personality characteristics and physical abnormalities are independent events, which reduces the accuracy of the DSM-III diagnostic manual, for validating the complaints of pain (Hendler and Talo, 1989a).

Patients with chronic pain are often misdiagnosed. This is neither a local nor regional phenomenon. Data from research reports from the Mensana Clinic, in Stevenson, Maryland, reflect a national picture because 75% of the referrals to the Clinic are from 42 states and 8 foreign countries. Hendler and Kozokowski (1993) and Hendler, Bergson, and Morrison (1996) found that 40 to 67% of the patients referred to Mensana Clinic arrived with overlooked physical diagnoses, which were later diagnosed and treated at Mensana Clinic. Failure to have a diagnosis for medical conditions, and even worse, having a psychiatric diagnosis assigned to a patient to explain the symptoms, leads to frustration, resentment, and certainly a well-justified psychological response in a previously well-adjusted individual. In these instances, chronic pain certainly leads to depression, as described previously. Moreover, after the proper diagnoses are found at Mensana Clinic, 50 to 55% of the patients are referred for surgery. Finally, once proper diagnosis and treatment are obtained, the patients get better. This is amply demonstrated by objective measures, such as return to work rates. Liberty Mutual, one of the largest workers' compensation insurance carriers in the U.S., reports that when a claimant is out of work for 2 years or more on a workers' compensation claim, the return-to-work rate is less than 1%. At Mensana Clinic, for the same group of patients, the return-to-work rate is 19.5% for workers compensation patients and 62.5% for auto accident cases (Hendler, 1989). This is in stark contrast to the results of the more psychologically and behaviorally oriented pain treatment centers, very few of which have any published statistics on these outcome measures.

The preceding lengthy preamble regarding the psychiatric diagnosis is critical in defining the role of a psychiatrist in treating chronic pain patients. It is essential to have a diagnosis of an individual *before* instituting the therapy. By offering a clinician a variety of diagnostic systems from which to choose, the selection of appropriate therapy becomes a less formidable task. Whether one strictly adheres to DSM-IV diagnoses or less conventional diagnostic systems is a matter of which system gives the best results in the hands of a particular practitioner. This should facilitate selection of an appropriate therapy. Although many types of psychotherapy are available, treatment results are not well documented for any of the forms of therapy. This chapter deals with the more conventional modalities, such as

1. Individual psychotherapy
2. Biofeedback
3. Family therapy
4. Group psychotherapy
5. Pharmacotherapy
6. Narco-synthesis
7. Hypnosis.

PSYCHOTHERAPY

Very few reports in the psychiatric and medical literature support the contention that individual psychotherapy is a useful treatment for chronic back problems, or pain of any sort. For the purpose of definition, one should consider psychotherapy as an individual session, conducted between a patient and a therapist without the use of specialized techniques, such as hypnosis, biofeedback, or narcosynthesis. Likewise, group psychotherapy (or conditioning therapy) is separate and distinct from individual, insight-oriented, dynamic psychotherapy. When one imposes these parameters on the definition of psychotherapy, reports on its efficacy are sparse indeed. However, some components of individual psychotherapy have therapeutic benefits, although it is difficult to substantiate their efficacy. Rutrick (1981) reports that psychotherapy can be effective if the therapist directs his or her activity toward understanding the "psychosomatic" personality, which is described as those individuals who (1) have difficulty with psychological thinking, (2) have difficulty expressing emotion, and (3) are impulsive.

Very often, psychotherapy is administered in conjunction with other modalities of therapy. As such, eclectic studies employing numbers of interventions provide some evidence for the usefulness of comprehensive treatment programs. However, the lack of control groups, the lack of a comprehensive pain assessment, and the uncertainty about the effective component do not allow definite conclusions to be drawn. Here too, a wide variety of patients have been treated with a lack of or widely divergent sample descriptions. It needs to be determined which patients profit from what treatment. Component analysis of eclectic and cognitive behavioral treatments are needed to determine the effective interventions and thus reduce cost and treatment time and enhance the effectiveness of the treatment (Turk & Flor, 1984).

One element of psychotherapy, which is present whether an individual therapist recognizes it or not, is the component of modeling. This process occurs when patients observe another person with chronic pain who is functioning despite their physical damage. This other individual serves as a model for the patient's behavior and straddles the bridge between individual psychotherapy, and behavioral therapy. Some therapists have used videotapes of patients in pain coping with their problem, while others have used a directive approach, actually instructing a patient about which behaviors are acceptable and which are not (Webb, 1983).

BIOFEEDBACK

The use of biofeedback as a modality for assisting patients with chronic pain has created much controversy. Some authors feel that biofeedback does not offer any advantage over relaxation techniques, and attributed its efficacy to its placebo effect (Webb, 1983). Other authors have conducted a more comprehensive review and concluded that EMG biofeedback may be a promising treatment modality for chronic back pain (Turk & Flor, 1984). In their most evenhanded review of biofeedback techniques, Turk and Flor report only the results of EMG biofeedback. This modality seems to have the most usefulness for patients with muscle tension-type pain. Turk and Flor found that there were three types of reports in the literature: (1) anecdotal or systematic case studies, (2) group outcome or comparison studies, and (3) controlled group studies. The efficacy of EMG biofeedback was further complicated by the fact that in a review of over 20 articles, all researches — save one — utilized concomitant medication, and not biofeedback exclusively. In the two controlled studies reviewed by Turk and Flor, both showed strong effects of EMG biofeedback on reducing pain and tension levels. In one study, a decrease of 60% in pain intensity and duration, as suffered by the patients, was noted. As expected, as muscle tension levels drop, pain intensity also drops. However, interestingly, at 3-month follow-up, although muscle tension increased, pain reduction was maintained. In the other study reviewed, EMG biofeedback was compared to medical treatment and "psychotherapy." In this study, conducted by Flor and co-workers, they found that EMG biofeedback was more efficacious than psychotherapy and control groups receiving just medical treatment alone. They noted that EMG readings decreased and the patients sought less medical attention when utilizing EMG biofeedback. Turk and Flor concluded that muscle relaxation alone does not necessarily contribute to the beneficial effects of EMG biofeedback, but rather that a cognitive process is important. Hendler, et al. (1977) attributed EMG biofeedback effectiveness to other factors. In their study, they found two groups of patients: (1) those who responded to biofeedback and (2) those who did not respond to biofeedback. In this study, 13 patients were evaluated using EMG biofeedback. Six of the 13 reported that they had less pain

on at least 4 out of 5 days of EMG biofeedback training, but 11 of the 13 were unable to alter EMG biofeedback in the affected muscle group. EMG relaxation consisted of reduction of muscle tension in the forehead. Therefore, one might conclude that specific muscle relaxation was not the therapeutic component of the EMG biofeedback. There were no significant differences between either the starting EMG muscle tension levels or the final levels between the two groups. However, the response rate (i.e., 6 out of 13) was double what one might expect from a placebo response alone on a consistent basis (Hendler & Fernandez, 1980). The difference between the two groups was thought to be due the stage at which the patient was in his or her chronic pain process; that is, whether they were in the acute stage, subacute stage, chronic stage, or subchronic stage. The difference between the patients who responded and those who did not respond was the presence of depression in the responders. Those who did not respond did not have elevated depression scales, using the SCL-90.

Another component that might contribute to the efficacy of biofeedback therapy is the issue of the patient's motivation or preparedness for change (Large, 1985). Large utilized a measure for "illness attitudes" in an effort to determine which patients might respond to therapeutic interventions. He used an illness behavior questionnaire, developed by Pilowsky and Spence, and expanded upon this by using a repertory grid technique, which has been described by Bannister and co-workers. Seven of the 18 patients did not experience overall relief of symptoms, while 11 did. In this report by Large (1985), 48 ratings were analyzed to determine the discrepancy between how patients perceived themselves, and how patient wished they would be. Correlating these findings with response to biofeedback showed that people who were dissatisfied with their condition (i.e., chronic and persistent pain) were more likely to respond well to biofeedback.

FAMILY THERAPY

The role of the family in the maintenance of chronic pain behavior may be one factor to consider when dealing with treatment failures. The poorest outcome among patients with chronic pain was found in families with the greatest degree of agreement when rating the severity of the patient's pain (Webb, 1983) Webb interprets this as "tertiary gain," indicating that the pain is maintained because of the psychological importance to other family members. A more likely explanation is the fact that a person with severe debilitating disease would have difficulty concealing the deficit from the family members and that they would be in agreement with his assessment of the pain. Webb describes family studies in which it is clear that the spouse and children of patients with chronic pain experience distress, as might be expected. This is particularly true in families where the patient is unemployed, while less so in families where the patient is retired. Webb (1983) feels that families can reinforce the pain and worsen the prognosis.

A more empathetic study involved that of the spouse of chronic pain patients. Two nurses (Rowat & Knafl, 1985) studied the impact of pain on 40 spouses of chronic pain sufferers (21 males and 19 females). They found that 60% of the spouses were uncertain as to the cause or persistence of the pain in their partners. Additionally, 83% of the spouses reported experiencing emotional, physical, or social disturbances that they directly attributed to the pain in their spouses. And 69% of the spouses felt that they were experiencing emotional difficulties as a result of their partners' pain. The most frequent forms of emotional disturbance were sadness or depression, fear, irritability, and nervousness; 40% ofthe spouses reported that there was a sense of helplessness because they were unable to effect any change in their partner's pain, and they were uncertain about how to proceed in doing so. They expressed feelings of loss of control. Some 75% of the spouses felt that they could delineate which factors influenced their mate's pain, such as increased activity that reduced or increased the pain, and medications reducing the pain.

In a very fine review article, Payne and Norfleet (1986) examined the factors influencing family relationships and believe that certain family characteristics and behaviors contribute to the problem of chronic pain, as well as influencing outcome. In their review, Payne and Norfleet found that some authors believe that there might be a relationship between the maintenance of pain and large family size. The rationale for this is obvious. In a large family, one of the only ways to get attention and reduce tension would be the expression of disability or invalidism. Some authors have reported that the majority of their patients come from families with four or more children. Birth order was also considered as a factor influencing the complaint of pain. One author found that the youngest or the oldest child complained, while another author found that the complaint of pain might even effectively reduce tension for younger children in large families. These findings have not been supported by other authors.

Socioeconomic status may also influence the expression of pain. The fact that a majority of pain patients are blue-collar workers has been interpreted as the inability of working-class people to express emotional conflict, thereby using somatizing terms. Of course, one must take into account that there are probably more blue collar workers than there are professionals, and it is the blue-collar workers who have the physically strenuous jobs that put them at higher risk. Other equivocally substantiated theories have been offered, such as the quality of relationships with parents, early loss of a family member, maintenance

of pain or illness in the family, and location of the pain corresponding to that of the family member. Depression in the family member has also been explained in psychodynamic terms, which are equally as difficult to substantiate. No doubt, patients with chronic pain have reduced sexual activity and poor sexual adjustment, which may contribute to poor marital relationships. Unfortunately, the majority of studies in this area discuss only the patient, and they appear at the time that they are seen by the physician, without an adequate historical perspective. One questions whether or not marital difficulties develop as the result of the chronic pain, or if marital difficulties predated the chronic pain and if the chronic pain became a convenient excuse to avoid further sexual contact. When chronic pain patients with depression were compared to patients with just depression, the former group had a more disturbed marital relationship than the latter. In another study, pain patients with no documented organic lesion were found to have more frequent "upsets, blows, conflicting interests, or separation" than those patients with definable organic lesion. Payne and Norfleet (1986) further report that 91% of couples interviewed at the Chronic Pain Treatment Center reported sexual problems and a decline in their social lives since the onset of their pain problems. This was confirmed by other researchers. The authors conclude that studies on marital relationships involving chronic pain patients consistently indicate high rates of sexual and marital maladjustment, even in previously stable relationships. However, they also advance the notion that the family can maintain the pain of an individual patient. Based on Payne and Norfleet's review of the literature, they feel there are four factors that contribute to the persistence of chronic pain in a patient:

1. The patient's pain is an expression of dysfunction within the family system, and it is easier to utilize the complaint of pain rather than say there are difficulties with the relationships.
2. The family acts as a reinforcer for pain behavior by nurturing and caring for the injured member.
3. The patient may use the symptom of pain to control his or her family members and is reinforced when this works.
4. The stresses of family life may produce physiological effects that predispose an individual to stress and disease.

The review article considers the three approaches to family therapy: (1) behavioral, (2) transactional, and (3) systems approach of structural family therapy. The behavioral approach has been discussed in previous chapters in this volume. The transactional approach tries to make family members aware of the ways a patient can use pain for psychological "payoffs" and how they might foil these attempts. The systems approach deals with the family as an organization and tries to change the structure so that no one family member has to be in the sick role. Most articles report that family therapy is a combination of behavioral, transactional, and systems approaches. Unfortunately, it is quite difficult to assess the efficacy of family therapy. However, follow-up studies designed to reassess the recurrence of symptoms are the best way to determine efficacy. One study, conducted at the Northwest Pain Center, compared 25 successful patients with 25 patients who did not maintain gains made at the pain treatment center. Interestingly, they found that there were more divorced or separated people in this success group, while the failure group had done little to change the patterns of behavior in their environment. They concluded that the role of the family in maintaining pain behavior contributed to the failures. Payne and Norfleet (1986) concluded that family members contribute to treatment outcome by reinforcing or not reinforcing pain behavior. They suggested that if a patient has a family that is appropriately supportive, and has learned not to reinforce pain behavior, the chance of success with pain treatment is greatly improved. If family members have not participated in the program, or resist change to their own behavior, then the family member with pain will probably persist. When compared to these resistant family groups, a single (unmarried) pain patient will probably have a better chance at success although they do not have family support.

GROUP PSYCHOTHERAPY

Group psychotherapy has been an adjunctive treatment for patients with terminal disease, rheumatoid arthritis, and chronic, intractable benign pain. These three groups of patients share four common features (Hendler, Viernstein, Shallanberger, & Long, 1981):

1. They have not had success with conventional therapy.
2. They feel isolated and burdensome to their family and friends.
3. They are angry at physicians and disappointed about treatment failure.
4. They have reactive depressions, frustration, and reduced physical activity.

Group therapy can be utilized on both an inpatient and outpatient basis, although the structure and format for these two groups is somewhat different (Hendler, 1981). In the inpatient setting, the patient is involved in group therapy for a relatively short period of time, usually 8 to 12 sessions. In this context, the group psychotherapy format more closely resembles a mixture of educational and free-interaction group psychotherapy, with more of a focus on the depressive components of the chronic pain process. The most common themes of inpatient groups

deal with depression and frustration including (Hendler, et al., 1981):

1. The feeling that treatment in a pain treatment center is a last resort
2. Expression of displeasure and anger toward physicians for not helping
3. A willingness to do anything to get rid of the pain
4. A feeling of helplessness and guilt, compounded by feelings of inadequacy and frustration because of an inability to function with the pain
5. Indications about the relationship between the patient and his or her family that clearly indicate whether the family is supportive of the patient behavior, or in conflict with it
6. A questioning of religious faith and the selection process (why me?)
7. Explorations regarding feelings of dependency,
8. Resentment towards the disbelief of family members, physicians, and associates
9. A fear about the origin of the pain and its progression

These same authors then described outpatient group therapy that was more protracted and allowed exploration of different themes including:

1. Feelings of physical inability or handicaps
2. Resentment toward vocational rehabilitation
3. Difficulty in readjusting life goals
4. Concern about other group members
5. Frustration regarding the slowness of the process of rehabilitation
6. Fear regarding the loss of a spouse because of the chronic pain

As with all forms of psychotherapy, it is difficult to access the efficacy of group treatment. However, Ford (1984) utilized an objective measure of efficacy (i.e., the amount of medical care sought by patients prior to and after group psychotherapy) and reviewed the literature on this topic. Ford offers a cogent argument for psychotherapy — if it able to reduce the number of medical visits, on a cost-effective basis, if for no other reason. Various authors have reported between a 50 and 75% reduction in medical clinic visits while patients with somatic illness were undergoing group psychotherapy concomitantly. Ford's own experience was not quite as dramatic, but he attributes this to patients belonging to a low socioeconomic group, and underscores the need for very long-term group treatment before any benefit was noted. The most important patient benefit appeared to be in the area of gaining control over his or her life. Other authors have advanced the notion that "peer modeling" and "interaction with other group members" allow patients to more freely express their emotions, to learn new coping methods, and to be more verbal when soliciting help (Gamsa, Braha, & Catchlove, 1985). Although these authors conclude that group psychotherapy is a useful adjunct to their chronic pain treatment program, they do not offer any objective evidence. Hendler, et al. (1981) studied patients assigned to group therapy or individual therapy. In their study, 8 of the 11 patients assigned to group therapy had remained in therapy, and 7 of the 8 had abstained from narcotic and hypnotic use. This was contrasted with a group of 12 patients, 7 of whom continued to use hypnotics, narcotics, or benzodiazepines prescribed by other physicians. At the end of 3 months, 6 of the 12 had discontinued sessions. A much more comprehensive report (Hall, Hall, & Gardner, 1979) compared the efficacy of combined group therapy and tricyclic antidepressants vs. supportive individual therapy, analytically oriented therapy, and management by surgical specialists, using narcotics or antidepressants. Using the Zung Rating Scales as an indication of the severity of depression, Hall's group found that group psychotherapy combined with tricyclic antidepressants was the most efficacious modality of therapy, while individual psychotherapy and surgical management, using narcotics or antidepressants, were least effective.

Although it is difficult to accurately assess the efficacy of group therapy, and many reports do not have objective measures of outcome, the technique is cost-effective and provides a degree of modeling and social reinforcement that is not available from other forms of therapy. The effectiveness of other self-help groups, such as Alcoholics Anonymous, would lend credence to the contention that group therapy is an effective modality for treating chronic pain patients.

NARCOSYNTHESIS

Several recent articles in the psychiatric literature, as well as in the chronic pain literature, suggest that many undiagnosed chronic pain problems are really conversion reactions or hysterical conversion disorders. Most of these articles are unsubstantiated, or deal with single cases or a few cases, after which the authors attempt to apply their limited experience to the broad range of chronic pain patients. In reality, the number of conversion disorders presenting as chronic pain problems is probably very small. In this author's experience (more than 25 years), after treating over 7000 chronic pain patients at the Chronic Pain Treatment Center of Johns Hopkins Hospital, while under the direction of the Department of Neurosurgery, and at the Mensana Clinic, the incidence of hysterical conversion disorders was three cases. Of course, these cases are quite memorable and represented enormous therapeutic challenges.

One must be quite careful in making the diagnosis of hysterical conversion reaction. In one of the classic stud-

ies, Slater (1965) did a 9-year, follow-up study on 85 people originally diagnosed as having hysterical conversion reaction, who had been seen at the Queens Square Hospital in London. At the time of follow-up, only 19 of the 85 patients were free of symptoms. Of these 85 patients, 7 were found to have recurrent endogenous depression, 2 were schizophrenic, 3 had undetected neoplasms, and of the 4 who committed suicide, 2 had atypical myopathy and disseminated sclerosis. Each died of natural causes. Two of the patients were found to have trigeminal neuralgia and one woman was finally diagnosed as having thoracic outlet syndrome. Three people were finally diagnosed as having early, previously undetected, dementia, while one woman, who had pain in the right shoulder and arm, was later diagnosed as having Takayasu's syndrome. The remainder had a multiplicity of organic diseases, including epilepsy, vestibular lesions, and total block of the spinal cord. Of the 85 patients with the original diagnosis of "hysteria" meaning conversion reaction, only 7 were really found to have an acute psychogenic reaction resulting in formation of a conversion symptom, while 14 were diagnosed as having Briquet's syndrome, which is a polysomatic hysterical neurosis more compatible with hypochondriasis, or somatizing disorders.

In a most thorough review of the literature, encompassing nearly a 50-year period of time, Stephens and Kamp (1962) found that the incidence of hysterical conversion reaction at a psychiatric hospital (Phipps Clinic of Johns Hopkins Hospital) was approximately 2% of all psychiatric admissions. Therefore, one must be quite cautious in assigning the diagnosis of conversion neurosis, or hysterical conversion disorder. Additionally, many clinicians have difficulty differentiating between histrionic personality disorders, and a hysterical personality disorder resulting in many somatic complaints, which has been called Briquet's syndrome. These two disorders are different from a hysterical conversion reaction because the last of these three disorders can occur in a previously well-adjusted individual subjected to extreme stress (Hendler, 1981). A review of histrionic personality disorders vs. hysterical, polysomatic Briquet syndrome vs. hysterical conversion reactions vs. malingering can be found in Hendler's book (Hendler, 1981). Also, Hendler and Talo (1989a) published a chapter in which the differential diagnosis of these disorders is summarized.

If hysterical conversion reaction is suspected in the differential diagnosis, amobarbital narcosynthesis can be quite useful in assisting in the diagnosis. One of the leading proponents of this technique, Dr. Walters (1973), of the University of California School of Medicine, has recommended dosages between 200 and 500 mg, taking a patient through the surgical pains of anesthesia, including loss of corneal reflex which produces full relaxation of "psychogenic tissue pain." Indeed, using too small a dose of amobarbital may contribute to many of the failures associated with the lack of effectiveness of this technique (Hendler, Filtzer, Talo, Panzetta, & Long, 1987). In fact, Hendler and co-workers specifically found that a diagnostic failure, using amobarbital narcosynthesis, was directly related to an inadequate dosage of amytal (dosage range 200 to 250 mg). When the dosage was increased to between 450 and 600 mg, effective narcosynthesis was obtained.

HYPNOSIS

When considering hypnosis for the patient in pain one must make a distinction between acute pain and chronic pain. There is no question that hypnosis is an effective treatment for acute pain problems. Scott (1974) has discussed the usefulness of hypnotic techniques for treating badly burned patients and for surgical candidates. However, even Scott admits that the effectiveness of this technique is variable and unreliable. In theory, hypnosis can be used to treat the patient with acute pain, by altering his or her perception of the amount of time the pain is experienced. In this fashion, Teitelbaum (1965) has proposed that hypnosis can be used for hypnoanalgesia and calls this phenomenon "time distortion."

For chronic pain states, generalized relaxation therapy, as described by Jacobson (1964) seems to be quite useful. As with biofeedback, hypnotic relaxation techniques seem to work best with chronic pain patients who have myofascial pain or chronic muscle tension. Unfortunately, it is difficult to assess the efficacy of hypnosis, especially in chronic pain states, and the technique does not lend itself to controlled studies. The question of the efficacy of hypnosis with chronic back pain awaits controlled empirical research (Turk & Flor, 1984). The major objection to hypnosis lies in the fact that it might provide temporary relief for the patient with chronic pain, but long-term relief has not been adequately documented. However, hypnosis may be a useful diagnostic tool for uncovering underlying hysterical conversion reactions, although it may be less than narcosynthesis, as previously discussed.

DIAGNOSIS AND TREATMENT OF DEPRESSION

No discussion about the psychotherapy of chronic pain patient would be complete without a thorough understanding of the depression associated with chronic pain. One of the major difficulties one encounters in diagnosing chronic pain patients with depression pertains to the etiology of the depression. France and Krishnan (1985) make a distinction between despondency, or grief reaction in response to serious physical disease, and depression, stating that despondency is similar to grief reaction and must be differentiated from depression in chronic pain states

(Krishnan, et al., 1985). France and co-workers believe that one can differentiate various subtypes of depression in chronic low-back pain patient, and distinguish between (1) major depression, (2) minor depression, (3) intermittent depression, (4) chronic low back pain patients without depression. One way of making this distinction is the use of the dexamethasone suppression test. The former chairman of the Department of Psychiatry at Duke University, Bernard Carroll, first advanced the notion of elevated plasma cortisol, resistant to suppression by dexamethasone, in severe depressive illness (Carroll, Martin, & Davies, 1968). Subsequent to this original article in 1968, Carroll and co-workers published extensively about the use of the dexamethasone suppression test. Randall France, formerly of Duke University, and later the University of Utah, studied a group of 80 chronic back pain patients, with and without depression, using the dexamethasone suppression test (DST) (France & Krishnan, 1985). France and co-workers selected a uniform group of chronic low-back pain patients, that is, those with chronic low-back pain associated with organic pathology, and divided them into two groups based on the presence or absence of major depression, using DSM-III criteria. They then examined the cortisol response to dexamethasone in each group. Of this group of 80 patients, 35 patients were diagnosed as having major depression, while 45 patients did not satisfy the criteria for major depression. However, of the 45 patients who did not have major depression, 10 satisfied the criteria for dysthymic disorder. In the group of patients with the diagnosis of major depression, 14 of the 35 had a positive dexamethasone suppression test, while none of the 45 patients who did not have major affective disorder had a positive dexamethasone suppression test. Again, of this group of 45 patients, 10 were diagnosed as having a dysthymic disorder, which might be more appropriately described as reactive depression. France very appropriately concluded that the abnormal dexamethasone suppression test is in response to a major depressive disorder, and not to chronic pain itself. Additionally, France noted that the incidence of anormal cortisol response to dexamethasone is higher in depressed patients without organic findings. As a conclusion, France and co-workers stated that the "difference in the rate of non-suppression in chronic back pain patients with and without depression suggests that the notion of conceptualizing chronic back pain as a variant of depression or as a marked (sic) (masked) depression might be an oversimplification" (France & Krishnan, 1985).

In another study of 63 patients, conducted at the University of Washington Pain Clinic, 49% of the sample met the DSM-III criteria for major depression (Haley, et al., 1985). In this study, depressed patients did not differ significantly from nondepressed patients in the ratio of male vs. female, use of narcotics, use of sedative-hypnotics or antidepressant medication, number of years in chronic pain, age, or number of surgeries. However, for women, depression was more closely related to subjective reports of pain; while in men, depression was more closely related to impairment of activity. In a review of 454 chronic pain patients at Columbia-Presbyterian Medical Center, Department of Anesthesiology Pain Treatment Service, New York, 100 patients were selected at random, and eventually 82 patients were contacted by telephone for long-term follow-up of a sub-sample of the original number of patients (Dworkin, Richlin, Handlin, & Brand, 1986). In evaluating the original 454 chronic pain patients, 79 of these patients were found to be depressed, while 375 were not considered depressed. Between the two groups, there was no significant difference in the percentage of males, females, age, marital status, education, or compensation. The only significant differences existed between the percentage of patients undergoing litigation or being employed. The depressed patients had a higher percentage of litigation and a lower percentage of employment when compared with nondepressed chronic pain patients. When compared with pain-related characteristics, chronic pain patients with depression more often had constant pain, and a higher self-reported scale of pain than the non-depressed patients. In non-depressed patients, significant variables contributing to the ability to predict treatment outcome were number of treatment visits, compensation, number of previous therapies, and the location of pain. In depressed patients, the predictors of treatment outcome were employment and duration of pain.

Atkinson and his group in San Diego have defined three subgroups of chronic pain patients based on MMPI scores and the type of depression they experience (Atkinson, Ingrani, Kremer & Saccuzzo, 1986). Using Research Diagnostic Criteria, Atkinson, et al. found that 44% of the 52 patients examined had major depression, 19% had minor depression, 13% had other psychiatric disorders, and 22% had no mental disorder. Patients with a major depression were found to have a discrete MMPI profile, with Scales F, Hs, D, Hy, Pd, Pa, Pt, Sc, Ma, and Si being significantly higher, and Scale K being significantly lower than the other three groups. The best predictors were Scales Sc, Pt, and D. When the patients were divided by clinical characteristics of somatization, depression, or hypochondriasis, patients with major depression fell into three depression MMPI profile groups (2, 1, 3, for rank order elevation of MMPI scales, or D, Hs, Hy). Despite these distinctions, there was "an even distribution of objective evidence for pain across all MMPI subgroups." This supports the contention that Hendler, et al. (1985a,b) have long maintained, that is, the MMPI cannot predict the validity of the complaint of pain, and patients with psychiatric problems can also have real physical problems at the same time.

By using a psychiatric diagnostic system for delineating the various types of depression in chronic pain patients and adhering rigorously to DSM-IV diagnostic criteria, one can identify a group of chronic pain patients who will respond to interventions for depression. There is no doubt that the use of antidepressant medication in the chronic pain patients with major depression will prove the most efficacious modality of therapy. To appropriately prescribe medication, physicians should understand the pharmacological contributions to normal sleep, pain perception, anxiety, and depression. In a review of the literature, Hendler (1982a) describes the common pharmacological substrate of normal sleep, pain perception, and antidepressant activity within the central nervous system as being elevation of serotonin levels. Therefore, drugs that enhance serotonin activity within the central nervous system are beneficial, and these include tricyclic antidepressants as well as the newer bicyclic and tetracyclic antidepressants. Thus, an antidepressant given at bedtime may promote natural sleep, reduce the perception of pain, and reduce anxiety and depression. Unfortunately, the selective serotonin reuptake inhibitors (SSRIs), which would be thought to be ideal for augmenting the treatment of pain, have not been as effective as the tricyclic antidepressants (Hendler, 2000). Moreover, there seems to be a paradoxical worsening, or even creation of anxiety with the use of certain SSRIs, in certain sensitive individuals (Hendler, 2000).

Antidepressant dosage should be individually tailored to suit the patient's age and tolerance for medication, but as a starting dose, one might recommend 50 to 100 mg amitriptyline, or doxepin, in patients who are both anxious and depressed, while one might consider using nortriptyline or desipramine at dosages between 25 and 75 mg in patients who are depressed and report lack of energy or a feeling of sluggishness. Dosage can be escalated in 25- to 50-mg increments, depending on the patient's response to the medication. It should be noted that the anti-anxiety effects of medication usually occur within the first 2 days, as does enhancement of sleep. However, it usually take 2 to 4 weeks before the antidepressant effect of these medications are fully appreciated. This seems to correlate well with the amount of time it takes for the down-regulation of the post-synaptic serotonin receptors (Hendler, 2000). If the use of antidepressants does not prove productive by the end of 4 weeks, therapeutic monitoring, using serum levels, will allow adjustment of the dosage into the proper range.

The use of specialized treatments for depression, such as monoamine oxidase inhibitors or electroconvulsive therapy, is best left in the hand of psychiatrists, and the selection of patients for these types of therapies should be done only after psychiatric consultation has been obtained.

RESULTS

Describing a pain patient can be likened to the famous fable of the five blind men describing an elephant for their king.

Each clinic, each physician, and each hospital sees a different type of patient. Therefore, to assess results properly, the demographics of the chronic pain patient population under study must be defined. On this point, the literature is in shambles. Even more chaotic is the reporting of results.

Few, if any, individual psychiatrists have published any results documenting the efficacy of their intervention. Reporting is hampered by the absence of objective criteria for improvement. What parameters should be measured to determine if a patient has benefited from the intervention of a psychiatrist? How do you measure pain? Is pain relief or improved activity the desired goal? Can they exist independently? How long has the patient had pain? Is litigation involved?

Hendler and Talo (1989) reviewed the literature of chronic pain clinics that had published results of treating their pain patient population. Most clinics were either multidisciplinary or behavior modification clinics. Of note, 1 year after discharge from the clinic, most clinics reported that only 25% of their patients had maintained the improved level of activity they had experienced at discharge from the clinic. Pain relief ranged from slight to great in only 33 to 63% of the patients. That is, only about half the patients experienced any relief, even slight relief, and only 25% maintained any improvement in their level of activity (Hendler & Talo, 1989a). Using a more objective set of criteria, Hendler (1989) reviewed 60 patients who had been diagnosed and treated at the Mensana Clinic. All 60 patients were involved in litigation and had been out of work an average of 4.9 years. By all accounts, this group of patients was considered to be difficult to treat because of the involvement of litigation and the chronicity of their problem. Although 90% of the patients had no difficulty discontinuing narcotics, hypnotics, and/or tranquilizers, only 50% had pain relief, but 91% improved their sleep and levels of activity. However, the most startling statistic was the number of undiagnosed surgical problems; 50% of the patients were referred on for further surgery (one to four additional operations) because they had not been properly diagnosed before referral (Hendler, 1989). Subsequent reports by Hendler and colleagues show that 40 to 67% of the patients are misdiagnosed, and the referral to surgery rate is 50 to 55% (Hendler & Kozokowski, 1993; Hendler, et al., 1996). Referral diagnosis was very often a vague or descriptive one in 41% of the cases (25/60), with such terms as "psychogenic pain," "pain neurosis," "low-back pain," "chronic muscle strain," etc. being used instead of any attempt at diagnosis. Because 96% of the referrals came from orthopedic or neurosurgeons, internists, rheumatologists, and physical medicine and rehabilitation medicine physicians, the failure to diagnose surgically correctable lesions is especially troubling. This was not a local or regional phenomenon because 75% of Mensana Clinic patients came from around the country (43 states)

and eight foreign countries, as of the year 2000. Therefore, the need to accurately diagnose patients, both medically and psychiatrically is of paramount concern for the psychiatrist. The psychiatrist cannot rely on the medical diagnosis of nonpsychiatric physicians. If he or she feels the patient merits further diagnostic evaluations, it is incumbent upon the psychiatrist to order additional diagnostic studies and to obtain consultation with top-quality surgical colleagues.

THE PSYCHIATRIST AS EDUCATOR

Patients with chronic pain are frightened because, very often, they do not know or understand what is wrong with them. Once an accurate diagnosis has been established, the psychiatrist should explain — in simple and concise terms — the anatomic origin of the pain problem, the options for treatment, the expected treatment outcome, and alternatives to treatment. Chronic pain is a devastating problem; but once a patient is fully informed about his or her options, anxiety is reduced and the patient has been given an active role in the decision-making process. Patients appreciate this involvement and respond in a positive fashion. Little has been written about the educator role for a psychiatrist; but in the author's opinion, it is one of the most beneficial interventions that he or she performs.

PSYCHOLOGICAL TESTS

Simply put, if a psychiatrist wants to measure personality traits, then he or she should use the MMPI or the Millon. If one wishes to measure psychological states, then the SCL-90, Beck Depression Test, Stress Vector Analysis, and Holmes-Rahe Life Events tests should be used. To measure the validity of the compliant of pain, only the Mensana Clinic Back Pain Test is designed to do so, independent of preexisting personality traits or psychological states (Hendler, et al., 1979, 1985a, b, 1988). The fact that not one single scale of the MMPI ever correlates with the presence or absence of organic pathology clearly illustrates the need to use the proper test to measure the pathology of interest.

SUMMARY

Psychotherapy of chronic pain patients is a difficult task at best. In part, the process is complicated by the lack of precision of diagnosis within the realm of psychiatry, but also within the realm of medicine. For this reason, chronic pain patients engender controversy. Improved treatment can be achieved by improved precision of diagnosis, both in the medical and psychiatric realms. Unfortunately, the efficacy of psychotherapy is difficult to establish, but improved levels of functioning, less depression, better family relationships, and improvements in sleep and pain levels can all be achieved with appropriate interventions. Most important, the psychiatrist should serve as an objective observer and recorder of patient complaints and be a diagnostician. Without accurate diagnosis, all treatments are doomed to fail.

REFERENCES

American Psychiatric Association (APA). (1994). *Diagnostic and statistical manual of mental disorders* (4th ed.). Washington, D.C.: APA.

Atkinson, J.H., Ingram, R., Kremer, E., & Sacctizzo, D. (1986). MMPI subgroup: Affective disorders in chronic pain patients. *Journal of Nervous and Mental Disease, 174*(7), 408–413.

Black, R.G. (1982). *The clinical managment of chronic pain.* In N. Hendler, D. Long, & T. Wise (Eds.), *Diagnosis and treatment of chronic pain* (pp. 211–224). Littleton, MA: John Wright–PSG.

Carroll, E.J., Martin, F.R., & Davies, B. (1968) Resistance to suppression by dexamethasone of plasma II–OHCS in severe depressive illness. *British Medical Journal, 3,* 285–287.

Dworkin, R., Richlin, D., Handlin, D., & Brand, I. (1986). Predicting treatment response in depressed and non-depressed chronic pain patients. *Pain, 24*(3), 343–353.

Engel, G. (1959). Psychogenic pain in the pain prone patient. *American Journal of Medicine, 26,* 899–918.

Ford, C.V (1984). Somatizing disorders. In H. Roback (Ed.), *Helping patients and their families cope with medical problems* (pp. 39–59). San Francisco: Jossey-Bass.

Ford, C.V. (1986). Somatizing disorders. *Psychosomatics, 27*(5), 327–337.

France, R., & Krishnan, K.R.R. (1985). The dexamethasone suppression and a biological marker of depression and chronic pain. *Pain, 21*(1), 49–55.

Gamsa, A., Braha, R., & Catchlove, R. (1985). The use of structure group therapy sessions in the treatment of chronic pain patients. *Pain 22*(1), 91–96.

Haley, W., Turner, J., & Romano, J. (1985). Depression in chronic pain patients: Relation to pain, activity, and sex differences. *Pain, 24*(3), 343–353.

Hall, R.C., Hall, A.K., & Gardner, E.R. (1979). *Comparison of tricyclic antidepressants and analgesic: The management of chronic post-operative surgical pain.* Paper presented at the Annual Meeting of the Academy of Psychosomatic Medicine, San Francisco.

Hendler, N. (1981). *Diagnosis and nonsurgical management of chronic pain.* New York: Raven Press.

Hendler, N. (1982a). The anatomy and psycho-pharmacology of chronic pain. *Journal of Clinical Psychiatry, 43,* 15–20.

Hendler, N. (1982b). *The four stages of pain.* In N. Hendler, D. Long, & T. Wise (Eds.), *Diagnosis and treatment of chronic pain* (pp. 1–8). Littleton, MA: John Wright–PSG.

Hendler, N. (1984a). Chronic pain. In H. Roback (Ed.), *Helping patients and their families cope with medical problems* (pp. 79–106). San Francisco: Jossey-Bass.

Hendler, N. (1984b). Depression caused by chronic pain. *Clinical Journal of Psychiatry, 43*(3), 30–36.

Hendler, N. (1989). Validating the complaint of pain: The Mensana clinic approach. *Clinical neurosurgery, 35,* 385–397.

Hendler, N. (2000). Pharmacological management of pain. In P. Prithvi Raj (Ed.), *Practical management of pain* (3rd ed., pp. 145–155). Philadelphia: Mosby.

Hendler, N., Bergson, C., & Morrison, C. (1996). Overlooked physical diagnoses in chronic pain patients involved in litigation, Part 2. *Psychosomatics, 37*(6), 509–517.

Hendler, N., Derogatis, L., Avella, J., & Long, D. (1977). EMG biofeedback in patients with chronic pain. *Diseases of the Nervous System, 38,* 505–509.

Hendler, N., & Fernandez, P. (1980) Alternative treatments for patients with chronic pain. *Psychiatric Annals, 10*(12), 25–33.

Hendler, N., Filtzer, D., Talo, S., Panzetta, M., & Long, D. (1987). Hysterical scoliosis treated with amobarbital narcosynthesis. *The Clinical Journal of Pain, 2*(3), 179–182.

Hendler, N., & Kozokowski, J. (1993). Overlooked physical diagnoses in chronic pain patients involved in litigation. *Psychosomatics, 34*(5), 494–501,

Hendler, N., Mollett, A., Viernstein, M., Schroeder, D., Rybock, J., Campbell, J., Levin, S., & Long, D. (1985a). A comparison between the MMPI unit the "Hendler back pain test" for validating the complaint of chronic back pain in *men.* The Journal of Neurological & Orthopaedic Medicine & Surgery, 6*(4), 333–337.

Hendler, N., Mollett, A., Viernstein, M., Schroeder, D., Rybock, J., Campbell, J., Levin, S., & Long, D. (1985b). A comparison between the MMPI and the "Mensana Clinic back pain test" for validating the complaint of chronic back pain in *women.* Pain, 23*(3), 243–252.

Hendler, N., Mollett, A., Talo, S., & Levin, S. (1988). A comparison between the Minnesota multiphasic personality inventory and the "Mensana Clinic back pain test" for validating the complaint of chronic back pain. *Journal of Occupational Medicine, 30*(2), 98–102.

Hendler, N., & Talo, S. (1989a). Chronic pain patients versus the malingering patient. In K. Foley & R. Payne (Eds.), *Current therapy of pain* (pp. 14–22). Toronto: B. C. Decker.

Hendler, N., & Talo, S. (1989b). Role of the pain clinic. In K. Foley & R. Payne (Eds.), *Current therapy of pain* (pp. 23–32). Toronto: B. C. Decker.

Hendler, N., Viernstein, M., Gucer, P., & Long, D. M., (1979). A pre-operative screening test for chronic back pain patients. *Psychosomatics, 20* (12) 801–808.

Hendler, N., Viernstein, M., Shallanberger, C., & Long, D. (1981). Group psychotherapy with chronic pain patients. *Psychosomatics, 22*(4), 332–340.

Jacobson, E. (1964). *Anxiety and tension control* (pp. 108–111). Philadelphia: J. B. Lippincott.

Krishnan, K.R.R., France, R.D., Belton, S., McCann, U.D., Davidson, J., & Urban, B.J. (1985). Chronic pain and depression 1, Classification of depression and chronic lower back pain patients. *Pain, 22*(3), 279–287.

Large, R. (1985). Prediction of treatment response in pain patients: The illness self-concept repertory grid and EMG biofeedback. *Pain, 21*(3), 279–287.

Maruta, E., Swanson, D., & Swanson, W. (1976). Pain as a psychiatric symptom: Comparison between low back pain and depression. *Psychosomatics, 17*, 123–127.

Payne, B., & Norfleet, M. (1986). Chronic pain and the family: A review. *Pain, 26*(1), 1–22.

Pilowsky, I., & Bassett, D. L. (1982). Pain and depression. *British Journal of Psychiatry, 141*, 30–36.

Reich, J., Rosenblatt, R., & Tupin, J. (1983). DSM-III: A new nomenclature for classifying patients with chronic pain. *Pain, 16*(2), 201–206.

Rowat, K.M., & Knafl, K.A. (1985). Living with chronic pain: The spouse's perspective. *Pain, 23*(3), 259–271.

Rutrick, D. (1981). Psychotherapy with chronic intractable benign pain patients. *Pain, Suppl. 1*(331), S271.

Scott, D.L. (1974). *Modern hospital hypnosis.* Chicago: Yearbook Medical Publishers.

Slater, E. (1965). Diagnosis of "hysteria." *British Medical Journal, 1*, 1395–1399.

Stephens, J. & Kamp, M. (1962). On some aspects of hysteria: A clinical study, *Journal of Nervous and Mental Disease, 134*, 305–315.

Teitelbaum, M. (1965). *Hypnosis induction techniques* (pp. 22–24). Springfield, IL: Charles C Thomas.

Turk, D., & Flor, H, (1984). Ideological theories and treatments for chronic back pain, II: Psychological models and interventions. *Pain, 19*(3), 209–233

Walters, A. (1973). Psychiatric consideration of pain. In J. Youmans (Ed.), *Neurological surgery* (1st ed., Vol. 3, pp. 1516–1645). Philadelphia: W. B. Saunders.

Webb, W., Jr. (1983). Chronic pain. *Psychosomatics, 24*(2), 1053–1063.

27

A Rheumatologist's Perspective on Pain Management

Thomas J. Romano, M.D., Ph.D., F.A.C.P., F.A.C.R.

INTRODUCTION

Pain can be defined as an unpleasant sensation that is thought to originate from a particular body part and which is usually associated with processes that are capable of causing damage to body tissue. Pain can be acute, such as one might experience in the case of a fractured bone. If pain persists beyond the customary time it takes the affected part to heal or recuperate, the pain is termed "chronic." Acute pain typically occurs when a noxious stimulus activates sensitive peripheral endings of primary afferent nociceptors. The noxious stimulus is then turned into a form of electrochemical energy by a process called transduction, whereupon the message is then transmitted via peripheral nerves to the spinal cord and then on to the brain, where the inputs are modulated and pain is consciously perceived (reviewed in great detail by Fields, 1987). It is clear that pain is more than just a sensation. It has two components: sensory and affective. Regardless of the cause of the pain, both components must be considered.

No greater interplay between the sensory and affective aspects of pain can be found than in the rheumatic diseases. Not only is the central nervous system of a patient suffering from arthritis bombarded by afferent signals from inflamed swollen tissue, but the conscious (or unconscious) interpretation of the significance of the painful stimuli (perhaps the harbinger of crippling, loss of independence, etc.) may influence pain perception, as can other factors such as the development of a secondary fibromyalgia syndrome or psychiatric/psychological problems that may complicate the course of a

patient with chronic (i.e., incurable and probably progressive) disease.

Rheumatologists are concerned with many problems and/or potential problems that affect the clinical course of the patients under their care. Patients need to be kept ambulatory, if possible, or at least their ability to care for themselves must be maximized to prevent progressive joint and spine deformity. Physicians want to minimize or eliminate the chance that the patient's underlying disease (e.g., systemic lupus erythematosus, rheumatoid arthritis) will affect their internal organs (e.g., nephritis in systemic lupus erythematosus, Felty's syndrome [splenomegaly and neutropenia] in RA), and optimize the length and quality of the patient's life.

When the vast majority of patients first present for consultation and treatment, it is the complaint of pain, above all other symptoms, that dominates the initial patient-physician encounter. Certainly, the fear of having a potentially crippling disease or of not being able to perform certain tasks because of weakness, stiffness, or loss of dexterity comes to the forefront after the impact of the illness is explored. However, it is the worsening of pain or the fear of increased pain that has brought the patient for treatment at that particular time, although other symptoms may have been present for months or even years.

To better appreciate how the rheumatologist approaches the problem of pain, and to gain an understanding of the role of pain control in the rheumatic diseases, one must first know what a rheumatologist is, how he/she was trained, and what concerns him/her when con-

0-8493-0926-3/02/$0.00+$1.50
© 2002 by CRC Press LLC

fronted with a patient who is in pain and who often has other symptoms/problems. Frequently, the rheumatologist's patient is confused as to the diagnosis and prognosis, often having seen numerous other health professionals before contacting the rheumatologist.

A rheumatologist typically treats many types of musculoskeletal diseases. The spectrum of rheumatologic disease is vast, and classifications are constantly being updated. The most recent classification can be found in the latest *Primer on Rheumatic Diseases* (Schumacher, 1997). In his/her day-to-day practice, the rheumatologist typically encounters patients with inflammatory conditions such as rheumatoid arthritis (RA), systemic lupus erythematosus, and the like, or degenerative joint disease such as osteoarthritis and myofascial pain syndromes of both the regional and generalized (i.e., fibrositis/fibromyalgia) forms. Quite frequently, he/she is also confronted with musculoskeletal problems that arise out of or complicate other diseases. Infectious diseases (e.g., AIDS, tuberculosis, rheumatic fever), endocrine abnormalities (e.g., diabetes mellitus, thyroid disease, hyperparathyroidism), malignancy, and other pathologic conditions may first manifest themselves as neuromuscular or musculoskeletal problems. Therefore, the rheumatologist must use his/her acumen as an internist to understand and treat patients thus afflicted.

It would be easier to understand the treatment of rheumatologic diseases if general categories were established and analyzed separately. For purposes of clarity and trying to follow general pathophysiologic guidelines, I propose dividing rheumatologic diseases into four main groups:

1. Degenerative diseases
2. Inflammatory conditions
3. Myofascial pain syndromes
4. Other (e.g., infectious, neoplastic, endocrine, congenital) conditions

Naturally, there may be considerable overlap, and any one patient may have several of the above conditions, but these distinctions should prove useful in systematically analyzing and treating patients with either simple or complex problems. Conspicuous in its absence in the above format is the impact of psychological forces that may play a part in the suffering of rheumatologic disease patients. Although rheumatologists do not primarily treat psychological disease, its presence is recognized in some patients. Therefore, problems such as depression and anxiety will be discussed in terms of their impact on specific diseases, as opposed to creating a separate category.

DEGENERATIVE DISEASES

The category of degenerative diseases contains, but is not limited to, degenerative joint disease; degradation of joint,

TABLE 27.1
Possible Causes of Secondary Osteoarthritis

A.	Joint damage due to:
	• Infectious (septic arthritis)
	• Hemophilia
	• Neuropathy (Charcot joint)
	• Gout and other crystal-induced arthritis
	• Rheumatoid or other inflammatory arthritis
B.	Multiple epiphyseal dysplasia
C.	Congenital dislocation of the hip
	• Slipped capital epiphysis
D.	Inherited metabolic disorders
	• Wilson's disease
	• Hemochromatosis
	• Alkaptonuria
	• Morquio's disease
E.	Paget's disease of bone
F.	Acromegaly
G.	Other processes that damage articular cartilage

bone, and other connective tissue by repeated trauma or inflammation; and low back pain that usually arises from a combination of factors.

Degenerative arthritis or osteoarthritis (OA) (osteoarthrosis in Great Britain and The Commonwealth) is probably the most common rheumatic disease affecting bones and joints (Creamer & Hochbery, 1997). It may be primary (idiopathic) or secondary to other diseases (Table 27.1). It is characterized by the narrowing of joint space by progressive loss of articular cartilage, usually accompanied by reactive changes at the joint margins and underlying subchondral bones. Many patients describe a "bone-on-bone" sensation in weight-bearing joints, such as the knees and/or hips, especially during exercise or simply upon ambulation. It must be remembered that OA is a disease of the joints and it has no systemic component (Bergstrom, 1985; Forman, Malamet, & Kaplan, 1983).

The prevalence of OA increases with age and some form of OA is present in almost all patients 65 or older. Many times, the patient experiences transient and/or mild to moderate discomfort and does not see a rheumatologist. Often, over-the-counter analgesics, combined with resting of the affected area, tend to provide sufficient relief. Other patients have more prolonged symptoms or have more severe pain than they can control themselves, so they initially seek relief from their family doctor. Many such patients obtain relief with the chronic use of nonsteroidal anti-inflammatory drugs (NSAIDs) such as prescription-strength aspirin preparations (Zorprin, Easprin), nonsalicylate medications such as ibuprofen (Motrin, Rufen), diclofenac (Voltaren), naproxen (Naprosyn), flurbiprofen (Ansaid), ketoprofen (Orudis), piroxicam (Feldene), indomethacin (Indocin, Indocin SR), and many others. These have been amply reviewed (Fowler and Arnold,

1983) and their effectiveness has been established. A word of caution: if a patient with OA on an NSAID obtains objective improvement (e.g., decreased swelling, redness, warmth) but still complains of pain, a secondary myofascial pain or fibromyalgia syndrome should be considered (Romano, 1996). Many OA patients also suffer from regional (e.g., anserine bursitis) or generalized (e.g., fibromyalgia) soft tissue myofascial pain syndromes. Unless these are addressed separately and treatment initiated, the patient will continue to complain of pain — which is the primary reason he/she sought medical attention in the first place — despite a good response to OA treatment. These are the types of patients whom the rheumatologist is apt to see. These OA sufferers who do well with NSAIDs or other therapy prescribed by their family doctor have no reason to visit a rheumatologist's office. While NSAIDs are excellent medications, they should not be used in a cavalier fashion, due to potentially severe and even life-threatening side effects. The potential gastrointestinal toxicity of these medications is very well-known (Huskisson, Woolf, Balme, Scott, & Franklin, 1976), as are the effects of these drugs on renal plasma flow (Brezin, Katz, Schwartz, & Chintz, 1979) and platelet aggregation (Roth & Majerus, 1975). These effects are the result of prostaglandin inhibition and seem to affect patients in a direct proportion to their age and the presence of other disease (e.g., peptic ulcer disease, liver disease, kidney disease).

One way to prevent the untoward effects of prostaglandin inhibitors is the use of anti-inflammatory medications that are selective prostaglandin inhibitors, such as salsalate (Disalcid, Salflex, Monogesic) or choline magnesium trisalicylate (Trilsate). Misoprostol (Cytotec) can be introduced to prevent NSAID gastropathy (Graham, Agranval, & Roth, 1988) because it is a synthetic prostaglandin E analog that allows the stomach to proceed with its endogenous cytoprotective mechanisms even in the presence of NSAID-induced prostaglandin inhibition. It is generally prescribed for patients who are elderly or who have had upper gastrointestinal problems in the past. Patients using nonacetylated salicylates do not need to use misoprostol. Recently, a new class of NSAIDs has been approved for use for arthritis sufferers (Osiris & Moreland, 1999). Celecoxib (Celebrex®) (Simon, et al., 1999) and rofecoxib (Vioxx®) (Langman, et al., 1999) selectively inhibit cyclooxygenase-2 (COX-2), thus minimizing potential adverse effects on the gastrointestinal tract. Furthermore, topical capsaicin (McCarthy, & McCarthy, 1992) and topical preparations of NSAIDs (Russell, 1991) (Ginsberg & Famaey, 1991) have been shown to be effective in relieving symptoms in OA patients.

Often, topical and NSAID therapy is not enough to relieve the pain in a particular joint. In such cases, the use of intra-articular injections of a local anesthetic-corticosteroid mixture can provide prompt, dramatic relief (Hollander, 1972). While the relief is usually temporary, lasting

from weeks to months, it can aid the patient in taking advantage of exercise or physical therapy that previously may have been difficult to endure. More recently, viscous/elastic intra-articular preparations composed of mixtures of hyaluronic acid and saline such as sodium hyaluronate (Hyalgan®) (Altman & Moskowitz, 1998) have been employed to treat painful knee OA. While these visco-supplementation medications are superior to oral NSAID treatment alone, their role in the long-term management of OA remains to be determined. Other regimens to help reduce pain and relieve mechanical stress on affected (especially weight-bearing) joints are weight loss, muscle strengthening, use of orthotics (e.g., cane, walker, crutches), and local heat/massage.

A word of warning: NSAIDs should be given with great caution in patients taking oral anticoagulants, sulphonylurea anti-diabetes medication, or other highly protein-bound drugs because NSAIDs compete with such medication for plasma protein binding sites and often displace a sufficient amount of the drug in question to cause untoward effects (e.g., a further prolongation of the prothrombin time or an exaggerated hypoglycemic response). In addition, NSAIDs can interfere with diuretic therapy, and adjustments in type or dosage of these medications may need to be made (Day, Graham, Champion, & Lee, 1984).

When the pain or deformity of OA become overwhelming, consideration should be given to orthopedic consultation, especially if the patient has symptoms involving a weight-bearing joint like the hip or knee. The technology for the replacement of these joints is superior than for other joints, and orthopedists generally have more experience with this type of replacement. However, not every patient with recalcitrant knee OA needs total knee replacement. High tibial osteotomy and other corrective procedures may be more appropriate in selected patients.

Often, patients with OA develop associated painful conditions, such as carpal tunnel syndrome, fibromyalgia, or a local myofascial pain syndrome, all of which need to be identified and treated.

Joints under increased mechanical stress would seem to be likely candidates for the development of OA, although the medical literature is far from clear on this issue, as illustrated in recent papers regarding runners (Lane, et al., 1986; Panush, et al., 1986).

Some studies have found that there is a relationship between prolonged stress and OA (e.g., spine OA in coal miners [Schlomka, Schroter, & Ocherwal, 1955] and shoulder OA in bus drivers [Lawrence, 1969]), while other studies have not found this to be the case (Burkle, Fear, & Wright, 1977; Puranen, Ala-Ketola, Peltokallio, & Saarela, 1975).

Each patient's problem must be evaluated individually, and aggravating factors minimized or removed if and when they are identified. This is particularly true for patients with back problems.

Back pain may come from a single problem or a combination of pathologic processes. Spinal OA is a disease of the apophyseal joints. It is frequently associated with disc disease and the terms *degenerative disc* and *joint disease, or spondylosis,* are often used. While anatomic changes may be well-defined by an X-ray or CT scan showing osteophytic lipping and sclerosis, often these correlate poorly with the clinical picture. The development of spondylosis is probably inevitable in most patients with microtrauma where everyday activities contribute to the symptoms. However, preventive measures, such as the maintenance of ideal weight, good posture, moderate exercise, and proper methods of lifting and carrying, can do much to ease symptoms. The use of NSAIDs, as well as adequate rest and the use of heat or cold applications to the affected areas, may be helpful. In some patients, traction and/or bracing may be needed (Lee, et al., 1989). If the cervical spine is involved, the use of a cervical pillow (preferably a four-in-one cervical pillow or Wal-Pil-O [Roloke Co., 8919 Sunset Blvd., Los Angeles, CA 90069]), which prevents neck flexion and hyperextension, is helpful in relieving night pain. Using chairs with a headrest and avoidance of reading or watching television while recumbent can also help. Posterior neck muscles can be strengthened by isometric exercises (Thiske, 1969). The patient tightens the muscles in the back of the neck and makes a double chin (military posture) to the count of five; this is repeated 10 times. Patients are encouraged to do this four or five times per day.

As far as the lumbar area is concerned, pain in the buttocks, thighs, and legs is caused by a combination of entrapment of nerve roots by discs, apophyseal joints, and adjacent soft tissue. There is often a long-standing history of recurrent low back pain related to a congenital narrowing of the neural canal. Aging and degenerative changes bring on further narrowing and the clinical syndrome of spinal stenosis.

Spinal stenosis, especially of the lumbar spine, most commonly occurs in elderly patients with spondylosis with encroachment of osteophytes into the spinal canal or exit foramina. This causes a phenomenon known as neurogenic claudication in which the patient experiences calf and/or thigh/buttock pain while walking. Relief typically occurs when the patient sits down, which helps to differentiate the problem from vascular claudication. The symptoms of vascular claudication are often alleviated when ambulation ceases, but sitting down is not usually necessary for relief. The presence of the above history in an elderly patient (or one who suffers from Paget's disease) with strong distal pulses, should make the clinician very suspicious. A CT scan of the spine should be taken and, if stenosis is present, orthopedic or neurosurgical consultation should be obtained. Corrective surgery often gives

dramatic relief. Age alone should not be a deterrent in cases of spinal stenosis, especially since medical management of this condition is far from ideal and the quality of life can be greatly enhanced by a relatively safe and effective procedure.

INFLAMMATORY CONDITIONS

Unlike degenerative diseases such as OA, inflammatory conditions, such as systemic lupus erythematosus (SLE), rheumatoid arthritis (RA), and vasculitis (e.g., polyarteritis nodosa, giant cell arteritis, or cryoglobulinemia), are not only painful conditions, but can be life-threatening. The musculoskeletal manifestations of these systemic diseases can be quite severe, and can affect the nervous system directly through the deposition and activity of immune complexes.

Rheumatoid arthritis (RA) is a chronic inflammatory connective tissue disease that can be potentially crippling and even life-threatening (Harris, 1990). It typically affects diarthrodial joints, but can also cause such extra-articular manifestations as scleritis, pericarditis, lymphadenopathy, arteritis, nodulosis, splenomegaly, neutropenia, anemia, and pleural effusions/pleuritis. The systemic nature of RA is reflected by the presence of an increased erythrocyte sedimentation rate, the presence of rheumatoid factor, antinuclear antibody, other autoantibodies, anemia (usually chronic disease, but iron deficiency anemia may also be present), or low plasma albumin in some, but not necessarily all patients.

Rheumatoid arthritis is found worldwide and is extremely common (approximately 1% of the U.S. population is believed to be affected) with a female to male ratio of 3:1. Peak incidence is between the ages of 40 and 60. Mild cases are usually treated symptomatically by patients using over-the-counter preparations, while more seriously afflicted individuals seek the services of their primary care doctor. Rheumatologists usually see more severe cases, especially when disease-modifying antirheumatic drugs (DMARDs) or remittive agents are needed in addition to NSAIDs and/or oral glucocorticosteroids. DMARDs are slow-acting agents whose function is to prevent RA from crippling and are also helpful in controlling systemic problems (Furst, 1990). Gold salts (injectable or oral), d-penicillamine, and hydroxychlorogorine have been used in the past, over a decade ago, with some success; but recently, immunosuppressive agents such as methotrexate, azathioprine, and cyclosporin have been successful in halting the ravages of RA. However, even the immunosuppressive agents were less than ideal, either due to unacceptable side effects (e.g., bone marrow failure, hepatotoxicity, nephrotoxicity, etc.) or the lack of efficacy. More recently, leflunomide (Arava®), etanercept (Enbrel®), and infliximab (Remicade®), have been introduced. Each works differently but all have been shown to be effective in treating many RA patients already on methotrexate (Smolen, et al., 1999; Weinblatt, Kremer, & Bankhurst, 1999; Maini, Breedveld, & Kalder, 1998). Leflunomide inhibits pyrimidine synthesis while etanercept blocks the action of tumor necrosis factor (TNF), a substance necessary for the autoimmune inflammatory synovitis in RA. Infliximab, a monoclonal antibody, neutralizes the activity of TNF, thus reducing disease activity.

For patients with particularly severe RA that is unresponsive to various combinations of one NSAID and a single DMARD, combinations of DMARDs have been used with success (McCarty, Harman, Grassanovich, Qian, & Klein, 1995b). The treatment pyramid for RA is shown in Figure 27.1.

Lately, many rheumatologists have chosen to treat RA much more aggressively, initiating treatment with NSAIDs plus DMARDs earlier rather than later (Wiske & Healey, 1990). Suffice it to say, the rationale regarding RA therapy has undergone some changes recently (Mikuls & O'Dell, 2000). Each patient is unique and, given the variety of medications and techniques now at our disposal, it is more likely than ever that a safe, individualized treatment can be designed to fit each patient.

A word of caution: DMARDs with NSAIDs tend to have potentially more serious side effects than NSAIDs used alone. Alopecia, lowering of blood count (red blood count and/or white blood count and/or platelet count), hepatotoxicity, gastrointestinal upset, and oral ulceration are common to all DMARDs. Gold salts can cause renal problems and rashes, as can d-penicillamine, which can also cause such bizarre problems as polymyositis (a myasthenia gravis-type syndrome) and obliterative bronchiolitis. Cyclosporin use can cause renal failure.

Leflonamide can cause hepatotoxicity and other side effects such as rash, diarrhea, and reversible alopecia. Etanercept must not be given to patients at risk for serious infection because it is immunosuppressive and may exacerbate infectious processes. One disadvantage in using etanercept is that it needs to be injected subcutaneously (25 mg) twice a week. Another is cost — the wholesale price for 6 months of treatment would be $6000 to $7000. For severe refractory RA, intravenous infliximab has been given in multiple administrations. The cost of three doses for a 70-kg patient would easily cost several thousand dollars. This cost must be weighed against the potential benefit and, of course, potential life-threatening side effects.

Like OA, RA can involve weight-bearing joints in addition to its capacity to involve the small joints of the hands, wrists, feet, ankles, and elbows in a symmetrical manner. Often when knees are involved, large effusions result and aspiration and injection can be dramatically effective (McCarty, Harman, Grassanovich, & Quin, 1995). Analysis of synovial fluid generally shows an elevated white cell count (usually 10,000 to 50,000 per microliter) with a predominance of polymorphonuclear

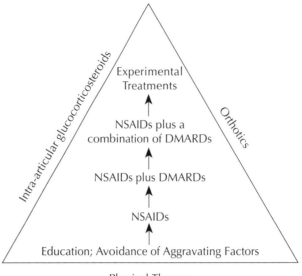

FIGURE 27.1 Treatment pyramid for RA.

leukocytes. Complement levels in RA synovial fluid are generally low and rheumatoid factors are often found; however, this testing tends to be of only limited benefit as it usually does not affect the course of treatment. A more dramatic, convenient, and inexpensive test is the observation that RA synovial fluid is watery compared to the more viscous fluid found in joint fluid from OA patients and normal controls. This is because the hyaluronic acid and other macromolecular synovial fluid components have been degraded by the inflammatory mediators (e.g., superoxides, enzymes, lymphokines) present in the affected joint.

If an inflamed RA knee develops a large effusion that becomes chronic, a popliteal or Baker's cyst may develop. Most of the time, the communication between the joint space and the cyst is one-way and this valve effect can cause high pressures in the popliteal space. Because fluid is incompressible, a rupture of the cyst can occur. The release of a large volume of fluid that contains inflammatory mediators posteriorly between the medial head of the gastrocnemious muscle and the tendinous insertion of the biceps muscle can cause the affected calf to become swollen, red, and intensely painful. The patient thus involved can present to the physician with a problem that resembles acute thrombophlebitis. The Homan's sign is frequently positive, thus causing some confusion. A positive arthrogram (with or without a negative venogram, depending on the circumstances) can confirm the presence of a Baker's cyst. Treatment with intra-articular steroids, rest, elevation, and attention to the underlying rheumatological conditions should be effective in the vast majority of cases. Surgical synovectomy may occasionally be necessary. A word of caution: treating a patient with a Baker's cyst using an intravenous anticoagulant, such as heparin (the preferred treatment for acute thrombophlebitis), is not only ineffective, but may be counterproductive, causing painful ecchymoses in the calf tissues that have become hyperemic from the inflammation.

Although many reports of improved and "unorthodox" treatments for RA are sprinkled throughout the lay press and touted by some health care professionals, it is important to remember that testimonials and endorsements are not a substitute for sound scientific research. However, one must keep an open mind regarding new RA therapies. Three recent studies offer examples of the utility of treatments not ordinarily thought of as antirheumatic but have been shown to be effective in treating RA: fish oil (Kremer, et al., 1995) and the antibiotic minocycline (Kloppenburg, Breedveld, Terwiel, Mallee, & Dijkmans, 1994; Tilley, et al., 1995). The clinician must weigh what he/she feels is the potential benefit vs. the possible risks/toxicities of each therapeutic intervention and prescribe accordingly. RA may be unpredictable and often periodic reassessments of the patients' conditions need to be made with attendant adjustments in therapeutic regimen changes in therapy.

Other painful problems that can occur in RA are the development of fibromyalgia, severe metatarsalgia (often helped by wearing 3/8-in. metatarsal bars on the outside of the shoes), carpal tunnel syndrome (median nerve compression neuropathy), chest pain due to either pleuritis or pericarditis, and Sjogren's syndrome (a chronic autoimmune/inflammatory disorder that results in keratoconjunctivity sicca and xerostomia). The dry eyes associated with the latter condition are painful and annoying, and other mucous membranes can also become affected. The lack of vaginal secretions can make sexual intercourse painful. If food is not chewed well and eaten with frequent sips of water, it may become lodged in the throat. The paucity of saliva (with its attendant antibacterial activity) can lead to painful dental caries and frequently loss of teeth. Other complications of RA are legion but their enumeration and description fall outside the scope of this chapter.

MYOFASCIAL PAIN SYNDROME

It is important for the rheumatologist to realize that, in terms of the general population, the majority of patients with musculoskeletal complaints do not have arthritis. The pain usually results from problems (i.e., disease or injury) in structures near or around the joint, such as nerves, muscles, tendons, fascia, ligaments, bursae, or bones (Simons, 1990). This section focuses on pain caused by these non-articular areas. The problem may be localized or generalized (reviewed in Fricton & Awad, 1990). Localized myofascial pain syndromes have plagued man since the beginning of time. These syndromes are characterized by complaints of regional pain (e.g., neck, shoulder, hip) that can be reproduced by palpation of specific trigger points that may be

present at a site distant from the painful area and often possess taut myofascial bands which may even restrict movement. These are amply illustrated (Travell & Simons, 1983; Sheon, Moskowitz, & Goldenberg, 1982) (see Figure 27.2). The trigger point has been shown to have a characteristic pattern on needle electromyographic testing (Hubbard & Berkoff, 1993; Romano & Stiller, 1997). Furthermore, some patients with myofascial pain syndrome have been shown to have magnesium deficiency (Romano, 1994). Trauma, especially sustained repetitive trauma, can bring on these syndromes, and part of therapy is to avoid aggravating conditions.

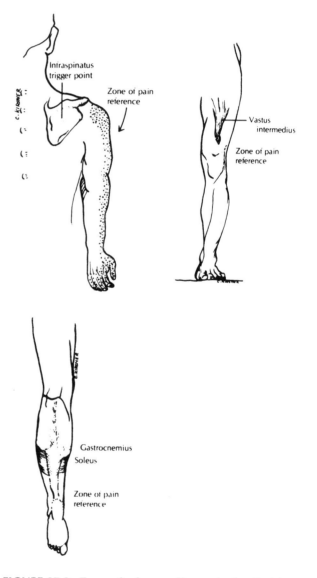

FIGURE 27.2 Zones of reference: Upon palpating the trigger point, pain is produced at some distant point. This zone is quite characteristic for each trigger point. (From Shoen, R.P., Markowitz, R.W., & Goldberg, V.M. (Eds.) (1987). *Soft tissue rheumatic pain: Recognition, management and prevention* (p. 224). Philadelphia: Lea & Febiger. Copyright ©1987. Reprinted by permission.)

Men and women appear to be affected equally. Treatment usually consists of local trigger point injections with a local anesthetic — long-acting corticosteroid preparation followed by massage of the affected area. This can cause a dramatic response with prompt relief and better range of motion. The use of a moist heating pad several times a day for 5 to 15 minutes is encouraged as is trying to get family members involved in the treatment scheme, because recurrences may be preempted with easily learned acupressure techniques (Prudden, 1980) before the pain becomes unbearable. Education and reassurance are extremely helpful and usually result in fewer visits and a diminished requirement for trigger point injections.

For the patient with chronic myofascial pain that is recalcitrant or recurrent (and for the generalized myofascial pain patient), a counselor/psychologist trained in biofeedback, relaxation techniques, and a cognitive-behavioral approach to pain may prove invaluable. Often, such patients benefit from treatment by a physical therapist with interest and training in myofascial release techniques or spray and by a chiropractor who is able to manipulate certain muscle groups that are in spasm or very taut. In so doing, pain can be relieved and postural problems corrected.

FIBROMYALGIA SYNDROME

The epitome of a widespread soft tissue pain syndrome is fibromyalgia (previously termed *fibrositis*) syndrome (FS). Intense research efforts over the past decade have provided good evidence that FS is a distinct rheumatological disorder, and widely accepted definitive criteria for its diagnosis were published in early 1990 (Wolfe, et al., 1990). The 1990 criteria are given in Table 27.2. FS occurs predominantly (80 to 90%) in women from their teens to mid-thirties, but in the Upper Ohio Valley area, the female:male ratio is 3:1 (Romano, 1988b). Children have also been diagnosed as having FS (Yunus & Masi, 1985; Romano, 1991a).

FS is a very common problem, and it confronts rheumatologists on a daily basis (Bohan, 1981; Mazenac, 1982). FS patients usually complain of musculoskeletal pain, stiffness, and easy fatigability, often linked to non-restful sleep. Generalized achiness and diffuse musculoskeletal pain are very common and, although joint swelling cannot be documented, it is often a complaint. Feelings of weakness cannot be documented, but are commonly encountered. They cannot be correlated with the usual tests of muscle strength and routinely available tests (e.g., blood muscle enzyme levels, routine muscle biopsies, and electromyographic studies) are normal. However, more sophisticated testing has demonstrated abnormalities in histochemical (Awad, 1990), immunological (Caro, 1986; Romano, 1991b), and neurological

---

TABLE 27.2

The American College of Rheumatology 1990 Criteria for the Classification of Fibromyalgia

1. **History of widespread pain**
   Definition: Pain is considered widespread when all of the following are present: pain in the left side of the body, pain in the right side of the body, pain above the waist, and pain below the waist. In addition, axial skeletal pain (cervical spine, anterior chest, thoracic spine, or low back) must be present. In this definition, shoulder and buttock pain is considered as pain for each involved side. "low back" pain is considered lower segment pain.

2. **Pain in 11 of 18 tender point sites on digital palpation.**
   Definition: Pain, on digital palpation, must be present in at least 11 of the following 18 tender point sites:
   - *Occiput:* Bilateral, at the suboccipital muscle insertions
   - *Low cervical:* Bilateral, at the anterior aspects of the intertransverse spaces at C5-C7
   - *Trapezius:* Bilateral, at the midpoint of the upper border
   - *Supraspinatus:* Bilateral, at origins, above the scapula spine near the medial border
   - *Second rib:* Bilateral, at the second costochondral junctions, just lateral to the junctions on upper surfaces
   - *Lateral epicondyle:* Bilateral, 2 cm distal to the epicondyle
   - *Gluteal:* Bilateral, in the upper outer quadrants of buttocks in anterior fold of muscle
   - *Greater trochanter:* Bilateral, posterior to the trochanteric prominence
   - *Knee:* Bilateral, at the medial fat pad proximal to the joint line Digital palpation should be performed with an approximate force of 4 kg. For a tender point to be considered "positive," the subject must state that the palpation was painful. "Tender" is not to be considered "painful."

Adapted from Wolfe, et al., 1990, *Arthritis and Rheumatism, 33,* 160–172.

(Romano & Stiller, 1988; Cohen, Arroyo, & Champion, 1990; Romano & Govindan, 1996) testing. This may help explain the presence of such neuritic complaints as paresthesias, lancinating pains, and headache that affect over 50% of FS sufferers (Wolfe, et al., 1990). Fatigue is an extremely common symptom in FS patients and many have been shown to have FS and chronic fatigue syndrome (Goldenberg, Simms, Geiger, & Komaroff, 1990). Fatigue may be the major reason why some FS patients are impaired. A defect in stage 4, non-REM, delta-wave sleep is often present (see Figure 27.3) leading to a nonrestorative sleep after which the FS patient feels as tired, or more tired, upon arising than when he or she retired. Nocturnal myoclonus has been found to be very common in FS patients (Romano, 1999). This disturbing symptom often responds to clonazepam (Klonopin®) taken at bedtime.

Patients with FS are reported to have a poor quality of life (Burkhardt, Clark & Bennett, 1993; Bernard, Price, Edsoll, 2000) and may become so impaired that

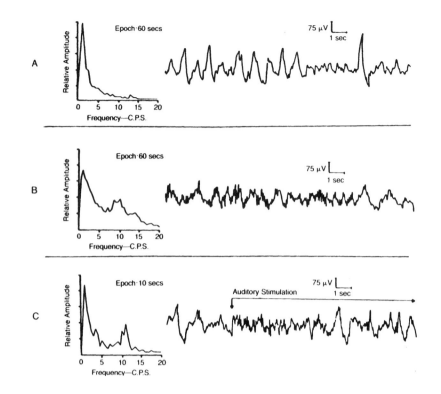

FIGURE 27.3 (A) Frequency spectra and raw EEG from non-REM (stage 4) sleep in a healthy 25-year-old subject. The spectrum shows that most amplitude is concentrated at 1 cps (delta). (B) Non-REM sleep in a 42-year-old "fibrositis" patient. The spectrum shows amplitude at both 1 cps (delta) and 8–10 cps (alpha). (C) Non-REM sleep of a healthy 21-year-old during stage 4 sleep deprivations. In the EEG, there is a clear association between the external arousal (auditory stimulation) and alpha onset. Again, the frequency spectrum (obtained by 10-second analysis from stimulus onset) shows amplitude concentrated in the delta and alpha bands. (From *Primer on the rheumatic diseases* (9th ed.). Copyright ©1988. Used by permission of the Arthritis Foundation.)

they are disabled from gainful employment (Bennett, 1993). This may be because the central nervous system is affected. Yunus (1992) postulated a pathophysiological model of FS that described aberrant central pain mechanisms with peripheral modulation. Recent studies lend support to this hypothesis. Abnormalities of regional cerebral blood flow have been demonstrated in FS patients (Mountz, et al., 1995; Romano & Govindan, 1996). Cognitive difficulties have also been demonstrated in patients with FS (Clauw, Morris, Starbuck, Blank, & Gary, 1994), as has abnormal central processing of nociceptive stimuli (Bradley, et al., 1995).

Many modulating factors affect the FS sufferer. Most FS patients report worsening symptoms due to cold damp weather, loud noises, emotional stress, anxiety, and/or overexertion. Patients seem to report improvement in symptoms in warmer, dryer months, and after hot baths, mild to moderate activity, and/or vacations. Often, numerous medications (e.g., NSAIDs, analgesics) have been tried without success. Many patients report that chiropractic help gives relief, albeit temporary. A complete history should help the clinician in making diagnosis of FS in that the physical examination would definitely include a tender point count, as well as good general examination. The hallmark of the FS patient's examina-

tion is the presence of typical tender points at characteristic locations (Wolfe, et al., 1990). A dolorimeter examination is not necessary for diagnosis, but helps in achieving more objectivity in the analysis of tender points (Campbell, Clark, Forehand, Tindall, & Bennett 1983; Fischer, 1987). Not all FS patients are aware of the presence of many of these discrete points of tenderness and often express surprise when the trained physician seems to locate these points with relative ease. The examination of the primary FS patient often does not reveal any other abnormalities. There is no synovitis or joint swelling. Range of motion of all appendicular joints is usually normal, and edema is absent. Neurological examination reveals no abnormalities in gait or station (although poor posture may be present). There is normal sensation to pinprick and vibratory sense, and reflexes are normal. If a localized myofascial pain syndrome also afflicts the FS patient, then a trigger point or constellation of trigger points is usually present. As opposed to a tender point that causes local pain when palpated, pressure on a trigger point causes pain to be referred to nearby regional sites. The rheumatologist needs to be aware that many conditions may present with FS-like symptoms. These include, but are not limited to, early SLE or RA, polymyalgia rheumatica, polymyositis, Sjogren's syndrome, metabolic myopathies, regional myofascial pain syndromes, hypothyroidism, hyperparathyroidism, and widespread generalized OA.

Before initiating treatment, the physician needs to stress that patients must be actively involved in their treatment and not just a passive recipient of health care (Bennett, 1986; Romano, 1988a). Patients need to understand that FS does not kill or cripple; it can nonetheless be very painful, and they must minimize stress in their lives and be compliant with the treatment plan.

The treatment of FS consists of prompt symptomatic relief, along with a plan for long-term management. NSAIDs are not very useful, except as analgesics. Because of a paucity of potential adverse reaction (especially important in those FS sufferers who also have irritable bowel syndrome, irritable bladder, tension headaches, temporomandibular joint syndrome, migraine, and dysmenorrhea), use of one of the nonacetylated salicylates (salsalate: Disalcid, Monogesic, Salfex; choline magnesium trisalicylate: Trilisate) prescribing up to 3 g/day in divided doses is preferred. FS patients may get temporary benefit from heat therapy, massage, acupuncture, spray-and-stretch techniques, injection of tender points with local anesthetic (such as 1% procaine or 1% xylocaine with or without a corticosteroid preparation), transcutaneous nerve stimulation, physical therapy, and/or postural correction. Medications that help restore normal sleep patterns, such as amitriptyline, nortriptyline, chlorpromazine, doxepin, trazodone, or cyclobenzaprine, can be very useful if taken in the evening. The dosages may need to be individualized to each particular patient, but typical starting doses are: amitriptyline (Elavil), 10–50 mg; nortriptyline (Pamelor), 10–25 mg; chlorpromazine (Thorazine), 25–100 mg; doxepin (Sinequan), 10–50 mg; trazodone (Desyrel), 50–150 mg; and cyclobenzaprine (Flexeril), 10–20 mg. Gabapentin (Neurontin®) (Neville, 2000) at 100 to 3600 mg/day in divided doses helps many FS patients who have prominent neuritic symptoms. Tramatol (Ultram®) 50 mg q 4–6h prn) has been reported by many FS researchers to be helpful as a safe and effective analgesic. Other strategies, including the use of narcotic analgesics and growth hormones have been reviewed by Bennett (1999). Brand-name medications instead of generic drug preparations are preferred, despite the cost savings. Too many questions have been posed concerning the quality control and bioavailability of generic drugs to have confidence in them, and therefore, their use is discouraged. Narcotic preparations that provide moderate analgesic effect may be helpful in some patients, but the need for their use should diminish with time. Recent studies have demonstrated a deficiency of magnesium in some FS patients (Clauw, Blank, Hewitt-Moulman, & Katz, 1993; Romano & Stiller, 1994) and dietary supplementation has been suggested (Abraham & Flechas, 1992)

as an important treatment for these patients. As FS is still incompletely understood and treatment far from ideal, successful management of FS patients requires a good physician-patient relationship, with the realization that progress can be made through mutual trust and effort. As is the case with other rheumatic diseases, a "cookbook" approach has little chance of success and shortchanges both the physician and the patient.

TRAUMA AND SOFT TISSUE RHEUMATISM CONDITIONS

It is important to realize that there are three types of FS. The first is idiopathic FS or FS that occurs for a reason but one that cannot be readily identified. Another form of FS is called secondary or concomitant FS, where the FS comes as a direct consequence of a chronic medical condition, such as rheumatoid arthritis, chronic lung disease, chronic heart disease, etc. The third type of FS, known as post-traumatic FS, comes as a result of an accident, such as a motor vehicle accident or fall. In terms of severity, a recent study has shown that reactive FS (either post-traumatic FS or secondary/concomitant FS) is more severe and more disabling than the idiopathic variety (Greenfield, Fitzcharles, Esdaile, 1992). There is no doubt that fibromyalgia (also known as fibrositis) can be caused by trauma (Bennett, 1989; Smythe, 1989). The question is whether a specific trauma caused a specific FS in a specific patient at a specific time. To determine that, a careful history and physical examination must be obtained so that a conclusion based on the facts as opposed to prejudice or bias can be reached. However, because many physicians are unfamiliar with FS and/or myofascial pain syndromes, their relationship to a traumatic event can be overlooked. Dr. David Simons (1987) wrote, "Myofascial trigger points are one of three musculoskeletal dysfunctions that are commonly overlooked and deserve particular attention. The other two are fibrositis/fibromyalgia and articular dysfunction. None has a diagnostic laboratory imaging test at this time. All three conditions presently require diagnosis by history and physical examination alone. In each case, the diagnosis would probably be missed on routine conventional examination. The examiner must know precisely what to look for, how to look for it, and then must carefully be looking for it." Since this was written, techniques such as dolorimetry, tissue compliance testing, etc., have aided the pain practitioner, but it is ultimately the "hands-on" examination by an experienced examiner that can correctly diagnose a given situation. This is incredibly important in dealing with patients who suffer from these nonarticular or soft tissue rheumatism conditions especially when such patients and their advocates are criticized for maintaining that these patients are in a great deal of pain when diagnostic studies such as MRI, CT, etc., are negative or normal. An article in a law journal (Smiley, Cram, Margoles, Romano, Stiller, 1992) underscores the importance of obtaining a good history, performing a methodical and accurate physical examination, and obtaining the appropriate tests to allow the pain practitioner to determine the presence or absence of one or another soft tissue pain syndrome. The jury can then determine the extent of compensation based on the manner in which these tools are used to describe the patient's injuries (or lack of them). Once a patient is diagnosed as having post-traumatic FS, he/she is likely to return for treatment even when litigation is over (Romano, 1990), a phenomenon that has also recently been observed in patients with post-traumatic headache disorder (Packard, 1992).

To understand how a local injury can cause FS, one needs to understand that most patients with soft tissue trauma, and even with fractures, recover uneventfully after a reasonable period of time, usually several months. However, some patients do not recover and have widespread pain that seems to get worse with time. Several noted rheumatologists have described the connection between trauma and FS. Smythe (1989) wrote, "Trauma may initiate a chronic fibrositis syndrome with a frequency of 25% in one study of 92 patients." In addition; "injury to the neck was described in 40% before the onset of symptoms and in the low back in 31%." More recently, several rheumatologists described an increased incidence of FS after cervical spine injury as opposed to injuries to the lower extremity (Buskila, Neumann, Vaisberg, Alkalag, & Wolfe, 1997). Bennett (1989) described how a sequence of events can take place to generate a widespread FS from a local myofascial pain syndrome.

FS can be as painful and disabling as rheumatoid arthritis (Russell, 1990). It can adversely affect lifestyle (Burkhart, Clark and Bennett, 1993), so much so that FS patients consistently scored among the lowest in all domains measured compared with patients with RA, OA, permanent ostomies, chronic obstructive pulmonary disease, insulin-dependent diabetes, and health controls. This may be a surprising finding for the uninitiated, but this is absolutely true and is something that is seen on an almost-daily basis.

Because traumatically induced FS usually starts as a local myofascial pain syndrome (Bennett, 1989) or "regional fibromyalgia" (Yunus, 1993), and then spreads to involve other areas of the body, possibly as the result of expanded receptive fields (Dubner, 1992) and neuroplasticity of the nervous system (Mense, 1994), it is no surprise that the resultant FS is intensely painful and difficult to treat. These "persistent pain syndromes can dramatically affect the patient's life, leading to long-term disability and a significant decrease in quality of life." (Ashburn & Fine, 1989).

If asked to testify in court regarding soft tissue injuries, the physician must remember that the court needs to know (1) what the patient is suffering from; (2) if the soft tissue problem (e.g., FS, myofascial pain syndrome, etc.) could be precipitated or caused by trauma; (3) if the problem was precipitated or caused by the accident/incident in question (i.e., if the trauma would not have occurred, would the patient have this problem); (4) if the problem is permanent; and (5) the cost of future care for the patient for the injuries sustained in the accident/incident. The court needs to know these things to a reasonable degree of medical probability or certainty. How this standard applies to testimony given by a rheumatologist was outlined in a paper authored by several prominent FS researchers (Yunus, et al., 1997). A method to assess the contribution of several different traumas regarding patients' painful medical problems has been determined (Romano, 1998). Ultimately, however, the physician's education, training, and experience, as well as his knowledge of the particular patient in question, should be the basis for giving such opinions.

MISCELLANEOUS CONDITIONS

Perhaps in no other area is the skill of the rheumatologist (vis-à-vis internist) put to more of a test than in the realm of such miscellaneous conditions as endocrine, metabolic, infectious, or neoplastic diseases that present with musculoskeletal signs and symptoms. The patient with a disease that fits into one of the above categories has more than a muscle, joint, bone, or soft tissue problem, but this may not be obvious early in the course of the disease, less so if the condition behaves in an atypical manner. One must remember, however, that FS can coexist with any of these disorders (Hudson, Goldenberg, Pope, Keck, & Schlesinger, 1992). In fact, FS has even been described in patients infected with human immunodeficiency virus (Simms, et al., 1992).

The musculoskeletal problems attendant to certain endocrine diseases may be the first clue that an endocrinopathy is present. The rheumatological signs and symptoms are often eminently treatable and even curable if the underlying endocrine abnormality is rectified (Bland, Frymoyer, Newberry, Revers, & Norman, 1979). If the patient presents with myofascial pain (especially fibromyalgia), carpal tunnel syndrome, shoulder capsulitis (i.e., periarthritis), crystal deposition disease (e.g., pseudogout due to calcium pyrophosphate deposition disease), proximal myopathy, or osteopenia (osteoporosis and/or osteomalacia), the presence of an underlying endocrine disorder should be strongly considered. Endocrine problems including, but not limited to, parathyroid disease (both hypo- and hyperparathyroidism), adrenal disorders, and diabetes mellitus can be causative or contributing to the development of the above rheumatologic problems.

The patient suffering from hyperparathyroidism often presents with back pain and even vertebral fractures that mimic osteoporosis senilis (Dauphine, Riggs, & Schlotz, 1975). Generalized muscular aching and stiffness, joint laxity (and accompanying arthralgia from hypermobility), erosive OA (Resnick, 1974), spontaneous tender avulsion/rupture, and neuromyopathy (Patten, et al., 1974) can also raise the suspicion of the presence of hyperthyroidism, especially if serum calcium determinations are elevated. Some 35% of hyperparathyroidism patients have chondracalcinosis (Pritchard & Jessop, 1977). Acute arthritis in the setting of an acute myocardial infarction or postoperatively may be due to gout or pseudogout. A synovial fluid analysis, which includes a crystal examination, helps establish this diagnosis.

At the opposite end of the spectrum, the patient with hypoparathyroidism may present with signs and symptoms (typically back pain) of ankylosing spondylitis (Chaykin, Frame, & Sigler, 1969), carpopedal spasm with tingling due to the low serum calcium, as well as muscle cramps.

Musculoskeletal complaints seem to be associated with adrenal overactivity and adrenal underactivity, the latter condition (Addison's disease) frequently manifesting itself as severe muscle cramping.

Cortisol excess (Cushing's syndrome) can be idiopathic or due to treatment with glucocorticosteroids, and in severe osteoporosis may ensue with compression fractures of the spine and ribs, proximal muscle wasting, and possible aseptic necrosis of bone (especially the femoral head). When exogenous corticosteroids are withdrawn, pseudorheumatism (diffuse muscle, joint, and bony aching) may occur. It is imperative to be aware of this, as such a problem can have the same symptoms as a flare of certain types of arthritis for which the medication may have been prescribed. When and if such symptoms occur, their interpretation in light of the patient's clinical course is crucial for optimal management, because pseudorheumatism usually abates gradually with a slowing down of the steroid tapering schedule and the administration of mild non-narcotic analgesics. However, a flare of RA, for example, could entail a much more thorough reassessment and revision of the treatment plan.

Thyroid disease often affects the musculoskeletal system and its manifestations are protean. Hypothyroidism often presents with a myopathy, with profound muscle weakness and elevated serum muscle enzymes. It can be confused with inflammatory disorders of muscles, such as polymyositis or dermatomyositis. The peripheral joints of hypothyroid patients with myxedema may be swollen in a symmetrical fashion much like the joints in rheumatoid arthritis (Dorwart & Schumacher, 1975).

In contrast to the joint fluid from RA patients, the synovial fluid aspirated from the joints of hypothyroid patients is definitely not inflammatory (i.e., it is thick and highly viscous, with white cell counts of 1000 cells/mm³ or less). Thyroid replacement often results in dramatic resolution of the above rheumatic problems.

If a patient has an overactive thyroid, rheumatic problems often manifest. Diffusely swollen and painful hands and feet associated with periositis (thyroid acropachy) can be seen in Graves' disease, as can thyrotoxic myopathy, bone pain caused by osteopenia, shoulder periarthritis, and shoulder-hand syndrome complicating adhesive capsulitis (Wohlgethan, 1987). Musculoskeletal pain may also occur with Hashimoto's thyroiditis. This disorder has been seen with increased frequency in association with RA and possibly other connective tissue disease (Smiley, Husain, & Indenbaum, 1980; Gordon, Klein, Dekker, Rodnan, & Medsger, 1981). Ironically, one of the treatments of hyperthyroidism, the administration of propylthiouracil, has been reported to cause such rheumatic diseases as SLE (Amrheim, Kenney, & Ross, 1970) and vasculitis (Houston, Crouch, Brick, & DiBartolomeo, 1979).

Diabetes mellitus, probably the most common endocrine disease, also has numerous rheumatologic manifestations (Gray & Gottlieb, 1976). Painful neuropathy may first bring the diabetic patient to the attention of the pain specialist. Other problems, such as Charcot joints (Sinha, Munichoodappa, & Kozak, 1972) (often not completely painless and confused with osteomyelitis, another condition to which diabetic patients are susceptible), shoulder periarthritis (Bridgman, 1972), carpal tunnel syndrome and palmar flexor tendinitis (Jung, et al., 1971), and a scleroderma-like digital sclerosis (Seibold, 1982), can plague the diabetic patient. The rheumatologist often encounters patients with both adult and juvenile onset diabetes who have painless contractures of the proximal and distal interphalangeal joints; recognition of these conditions is important because such microvascular complications as nephropathy and retinopathy may parallel the development and progression of these contractures (Fitzcharles, Duby, Waddell, Banks, & Karsh, 1984).

Excess pituitary secretion of growth hormone, which causes acromegaly, can result in a characteristic arthropathy that mirrors the enhanced action of this hormone on bone, cartilage, and periarticular soft tissue. With regard to the diarthrodral joints, early cartilage hypertrophy causes the joint space to be abnormally wide, as seen on X-ray. This cartilage tends to break down more easily than normal cartilage and such patients develop OA at a relatively early age. Carpal tunnel syndrome is also common. The spinal pain and polyarthritis have been reported to respond dramatically when the underlying pituitary disorder is treated successfully (Lachs & Jacobs, 1986). This principle (i.e., the importance of the identification and treatment of the underlying endocrine problem) is crucial in alleviating the pain and suffering of patients with endocrine disease in whom musculoskeletal manifestations may be severe.

TABLE 27.3
Differential Diagnosis of Generalized Osteopenia in Adults

Osteoporosis	Parallel loss of mineral and matrix Predisposing factors include aging, menopause, female sex, white or Asian race, immobilization, low physical activity, inadequate dietary calcium, smoking, alcohol, corticosteroid therapy, family history
Osteomalacia	Inadequate mineralization of bones, matrix Differential diagnosis includes: • Vitamin D deficiency: Inadequate intake, low sunlight exposure, drug-induced catabolism of vitamin D, intestinal malabsorption • Phosphate-wasting syndrome: Acquired renal tubular defects, with isolated phosphate loss, combined tubular defects (Fanconi's syndrome), renal tubular acidosis, antacid abuse
Osteitis fibrosa	PTH-induced increase in mineral and matrix reabsorption Differential diagnosis includes: • Primary hyperparathyroidism • Secondary hyperparathyroidism: Vitamin D deficiency states, primary decrease in intestinal calcium absorption with age, reduced renal mass (chronic renal insufficiency)
Glucocorticoid-induced osteopenia	Differential diagnosis includes: • Iatrogenic • Adrenal corticosteroid overproduction: Indiopathi (Cushing's syndrome)
Other disorders	• Hyperparathyroidism • Diffuse osteolytic malignancies (e.g., multiple myeloma) • Congenital disorders: Osteogenesis imperfecta tarda, vitamin D–resistant rickets

From *Seminars in Arthritis and Rheumatism.*

It should be noted that FS often coexists with endocrine problems (Crofford, 1996; Griep, Buersmat, & de Kloet, 1993), necessitating even more vigilance and circumspection on the part of the clinician. Clearly, the most common metabolic disease that causes musculoskeletal pain in the general population is osteopenia. The scope of this problem is enormous and the differential diagnosis lengthy (see Table 27.3). Acute bone fracture can result from osteopenia, and thousands of patients suffer from hip fractures annually, making it a major public health problem with high morbidity and mortality. Metabolic bone disease can also cause muscular pain and weakness, symptoms of which are often confused with other musculosk-

eletal conditions. Osteopenia can also occur in patients who have other rheumatic diseases, especially those receiving long-term glucocorticosteroid treatment (Hahn & Hahn, 1976). The scope of the problem is so vast that a chapter devoted to it could not even begin to outline the problem and discuss therapy. However, some major factors need to be considered. The patient with osteopenia usually has osteoporosis (loss of bone mineral and matrix in parallel), osteomalacia (accumulation of unmineralized matrix after loss of bone mineral), hyperparathyroidism with osteitis fibrosa (replacement of bone by fibrous tissue), or cortisteroid-induced osteopenia. The last problem is often unavoidable due to the patients' need for such medication, but the ability of steroids to interfere with calcium absorption from the intestine may be partially overcome by the administration of calcium and vitamin D supplementation (Hahn, Halstead, Teitelbaum, & Hahn 1979). The use of these medications is recommended for patients with osteoporosis senilis, as is estrogen, fluoride, calcitonin, or a combination of these agents based on the individual patient's needs. The best method of treating osteoporosis is prevention, if feasible. Patients at risk (typically sedentary, small-framed women approaching menopause who smoke and drink alcohol and who have low calcium and vitamin D intake) should use preventative measures such as regular exercise, adequate intake of calcium and vitamin D (Matkovic, et al., 1979; NIH Consensus Conference, 1984), and consultation with a physician who may feel that other measures, such as estrogen therapy, are necessary.

The most common causes of osteomalacia in adults are decreased absorption of vitamin D due to intestinal or biliary tract disease, accelerated catabolism of vitamin D due to drug-induced increases in hepatic oxidase activity, and acquired renal tubular defects with phosphate wasting. Correcting the cause of the metabolic problem is necessary for reversal of the osteomalacia.

While not as common as osteopenia, Paget's disease of bone is a frequent cause of bony pain, and is estimated to affect 1 to 3% of people over the age of 45 in the U.S. It is usually polyostotic, and men tend to predominate. While the cause of Paget's disease (osteitis deformans) is unknown (late manifestation of viral infection has been suggested), it is characterized by excessive bone resorption followed by excessive bone formation, culminating in a bizarre mosaic pattern of lamellar bone associated with increased local vascularity and increased fibrous tissue in adjacent marrow (Smiger, et al., 1977). The disease is a focal disorder as normal bone exists even in patients severely affected. The sites most commonly involved are the pelvis, skull, femur, tibia, and spine. In addition to pain, gross deformity, compression of neural structures, fracture of involved bone, and alteration of joint structure/function, often result. Increased serum alkaline phosphatase and urinary hydroxproline reflect the increased bone turnover in this disease. An infrequent (<1%), but dreaded, complication of Paget's disease is osteosarcoma; other associated neoplasms include non-neoplastic granulomas and giant cell tumors. Paget's disease can be asymptomatic with little clinical disability and, therefore, no therapy may be necessary (Altman & Singer, 1980). However, specific therapy is available for patients who are suffering. While NSAIDs help control pain, they do not affect the biochemical abnormalities. Disodium etidronate, a diphosphonate compound (Krane, 1982), decreases bone resorption, but this oral agent should be given for no longer than 6 months at a time. Bone pain usually responds to this medication, but a temporary paradoxical increase in bone pain may occur in some patients. Subcutaneous injections of synthetic salmon calcitonin are also used to provide pain relief and help prevent deformity. Clinical improvement usually occurs within a month or two. Some patients may become refractory to this medication if they produce neutralizing antibodies to this salmon protein.

Joint pain can be caused by a variety of pathophysiological mechanisms. While disorders such as RA, OA, and SLE are chronic and incurable causes of arthritis and arthralgia, infectious agents can cause an acute arthritis which, with early detection and proper management, can be cured with little or no permanent sequellae.

While any infectious agent can cause septic arthritis, pyogenic bacterial arthritis causes the most rapidly destructive form of infectious arthritis. Bacterial arthritis is usually divided into two groups, that caused by *Neisseria gonorrhea* and that caused by other bacteria (e.g., staphylococci, enteric organisms, etc.). Most cases of bacterial arthritis are the result of hematogenous spread to the affected joint(s). Other causes include direct infection from a puncture wound or skin infection. Once inside the joint space, the infectious agent multiplies rapidly, and the inflammatory response can become very severe, causing so much joint swelling and intense pain that the patient can neither actively extend nor flex the affected joint. Usually, such patients are febrile with high peripheral white blood cell counts. If untreated, the infection can cause destruction of cartilage and bone, as a result of a direct toxic effect of the bacteria and enzymatic destruction from purulent inflammatory exudates (Goldenberg & Reed, 1985). *Staphylococcus aureus* and Gram-negative bacilli often destroy joints rapidly, whereas other organisms, such as *Streptococcus pneumoniae* and *Neisseria gonorrhea*, cause damage much more slowly. To make a correct diagnosis, an aspiration of the affected joint needs to be performed under aseptic conditions and the fluid sent for cell count, differential, and culture. A septic joint typically has a white cell count in excess of 50,000 cells/mm³, with a predominance (often 90%) of polymorphonuclear leukocytes. It may take several days for the offending organism to grow in culture, and therapy should not be delayed. The prompt initiation of intravenous antibiotics

(the exact nature of which depends on the likelihood of having a particular organism under certain clinical conditions) may be critical. Periodic joint aspiration and reassessment need to be performed while the patient is hospitalized. Depending on the organism, intravenous antibiotics need to be administered for 2 to 6 weeks. Some patients can be managed with home intravenous therapy at the discretion of the physician. Patients at risk for the development of septic arthritis include patients taking systemic or locally injected corticosteroids, immunocompromised patients, and patients with hemarthroses. Among otherwise young, healthy patients, disseminated gonococcal infection is the most common cause of septic arthritis in the urban population. Increasing in prevalence (Veasy, et al., 1987), although still considered uncommon, is acute rheumatic fever, an inflammatory disease induced by an antecedent group A beta-hemolytic streptococcal pharynigitis. The most common features are carditis and polyarthritis. The Jones criteria enable the physician to establish the diagnosis (Stollerman, Markowitz, Toronta, Wannamaker, & Whittemore, 1965) and act as a guide in the evaluation of patients with polyarthritis of unknown etiology.

Patients with neoplastic diseases often are seen by a rheumatologist for musculoskeletal symptoms. Primary neoplasms of bursae, joints, and tendon sheaths are uncommon (Jaffe, 1958). Most arise from the synovium and are benign. Tumor-like swelling in and around a joint most likely is the result of inflammatory and traumatic lesions and which hence should not be considered true neoplasms. However, tumors can occur (see Table 27.4).

TABLE 27.4

Types of Tumors of Joint, Tendon Sheaths, and Bursae

Benign

Neoplasms and tumoral conditions
- Pigmented villonodular synovitis
- Synovial chondromatosis (osteochondromatosis)
- Other benign tumors: lipoma including lipoma arborescens, chondroma, hemangioma, fibroma

Tumor-like lesions
- Ganglion, bursitis, synovial cyst, parameniscal cyst, nodules

Malignant

Primary
- Synovial sarcoma (malignant synovioma); biphasic and monophasic
- Clear cell sarcoma
- Epithelioid sarcoma
- Synovial chondrosarcoma

Secondary
- Metastatic carcinomatous arthritis
- Joint invasion by leukemia, lymphoma, myeloma
- Continuous spread of malignant bone tumors

More often, secondary neoplastic involvement of joints occurs as a complication of contiguous spread of primary bone sarcomas, invasion by hematologic malignancies (e.g., leukemia, lymphoma, myeloma), or carcinomatous metastases (Schajowica, 1982).

Most subtle involvement of the musculoskeletal system with malignancy manifests itself as the group of disorders termed *paraneoplastic syndromes*. True paraneoplastic syndromes include myopathies, arthropathies, and other conditions such as hypertrophic pulmonary osteoarthropathy, amyloidosis, and secondary gout. Polyarthritis resembling RA may be the presenting sign of malignancy (Calabro, 1967). The cause is unknown, but the action of circulating immune complexes and alterations in cellular immunity have been offered as explanations (Robins & Baldwin, 1978; Awerbuch & Brooks, 1981). In addition, a syndrome similar to SLE has been reported in association with underlying malignancies (Wallack, 1977; Pierce, Stern, Jaffe, Fullman, & Talan, 1979). Unfortunately, other rheumatic conditions, such as polymyalgia rheumatica, scleroderma, necrotizing vasculitis, cryoglobulimenia with Raynaud's Phenomenon (seen most commonly with metastatic malignancy), and reflex sympathetic dystrophy have also been associated with various malignancies. This confusing picture often requires much in the way of energy and expertise to understand and properly treat the specific condition(s).

ROLE OF THE RHEUMATOLOGIST IN THE MULTIDISCIPLINARY APPROACH TO THE TREATMENT OF THE PAIN PATIENT: THE RHEUMATOLOGIST AS "TEAM PLAYER"

To paraphrase the eminent poet John Donne: no physician is an island, especially when it comes to the treatment of the pain patient. Often, the physician needs to coordinate the efforts of several health care professionals (e.g., orthopedists, neurologists, anesthesiologists, counselors, psychologists, physical therapists) and educate his/her colleagues regarding the special requirements of such patients. Physical therapy, for example, is an extremely useful adjunct in the treatment of many patients who require specialty (e.g., rheumatological) care. However, the approach of the physical therapist needs to be individualized to each and every patient he or she sees. Most physical therapists see patients with such varied disorders as strokes, arthritis, post-surgical states, sports injuries, and myofascial pain syndromes. The stroke victim has a different pathology and hence different needs than the patient with RA or adhesive capsulitis of the shoulder. While general principles of physical therapy usually are the same for all patients, the practical application of these principles can vary greatly from patient to patient, depending on the problem. The patient with arthritis of the knees, for example, who requires quadriceps muscle strengthening therapy to combat atrophy of the thigh muscles due to disuse requires different management if a concomitant myofascial pain syndrome (MPS) is also present. The same is true for work-hardening programs. If the deconditioned patient with a regional MPS enrolls in a standard program, he/she will be unable to tolerate the strengthening exercises because they will exacerbate the condition (Janet Travell, personal communication). It is only when the rheumatologist or other pain specialist treats the MPS successfully that work-hardening can proceed. The physical therapist can play a pivotal role in treating MPS with spray-and-stretch techniques, massage, acupressure, local heat, or ultrasound. In fact, the therapist often can alert the referring physician to the possibility that the patient may have a regional MPS if the patient in question has a paradoxical response to correctly applied physical therapy modalities. As mentioned above, if work-hardening causes increased pain, one should suspect a regional MPS. The same principle holds true for cervical traction, a very useful treatment for chronic cervical radiculopathy(ies). If, in addition, the patient has a regional MPS in the vicinity of the occiput or cervical musculature or trapezius/rhomboid areas, the force of the correctly applied traction applied to taut muscles usually results in more pain rather than less. Such a scenario should alert the therapist to the possibility of a regional MPS, and this information should be shared with the referring physician. If the MPS persists, rheumatologic consultation should be obtained.

Often, FS patients with bothersome neuritic symptoms need the expertise of a neurologist to help determine if peripheral neuropathy, nerve entrapment, or another neurological problem exists. Tests such as electromyograms (EMGs), nerve conduction studies, and radiographic studies (e.g., CT scans, MRI scans) may need to be done to complement the neurological examination and more precisely define (or rule out) a particular problem. FS sufferers tend to have an exacerbation of their symptoms after EMGs, probably due to their abnormal perception of pain and aberrant central processing. In fact, the first clue that a patient may have FS is often the observation that the patient in question, who is being treated or evaluated by a neurologist for numbness, tingling, or lancinating pain, behaves quite differently than other patients with similar symptoms. The patient may report that the EMG was very painful and may, in fact, terminate his/her participation in the study before it is completed due to unbearable pain. The neurologist can be of great help to the patient referred for neuritic symptoms but for whom no definable neurological abnormality can be found. As mentioned earlier, gabapentin may be helpful in the management of neuropathic pain. These patients may be suffering from FS and should be referred to a rheumatologist for further evaluation.

The orthopedist is frequently called upon to help the rheumatologist when medical management of rheumatologic conditions fails. As mentioned, patients with end-stage osteoarthritic or rheumatoid arthritic changes in knee or hip joints often require total joint replacement. It is up to the rheumatologist to help select suitable candidates for such procedures. The ideal surgical candidate not only has failed conservative measures but is not overweight (the heavier the patient, the more likely the prosthesis may loosen or dislodge), is motivated and intelligent (so as not to take undue risks after the procedure is performed [i.e., avoid activities that put increased mechanical stress on the prosthetic joint]), and is sufficiently advanced in years such that, statistically speaking, the life span of the prosthesis should exceed that of the patient. Conversely, many practicing orthopedists evaluate patients with joint pain who, inspired by media hype, self-refer themselves for total joint replacement. Some need the procedure, but many others do not. Their arthritis can be managed quite well with a program of anti-inflammatory drug therapy, weight reduction, physical therapy, and orthotic use (e.g., a cane, if necessary). Conservative medical management of this type can often help patients avoid premature and possibly unnecessary surgery while adequately controlling their pain.

The rheumatologist is most likely to call upon the services of his/her colleagues in anesthesiology when a patient requires a nerve block for such diverse conditions as occipital neuralgia (as the cause of some chronic headache conditions) and reflex sympathetic dystrophy (which can often complicate arthritic conditions). Many "failed back" patients benefit from lumbar nerve root blocks, which often give effective, albeit temporary, relief from severe pain. Other modalities (outlined in Chapter 23) can be extremely effective, especially if timely referrals are made.

Frequently, the orthodontist and the rheumatologist need to work together in the treatment of FS patients with temporomandibular disorders, as these two entities frequently coexist in the same patient and one can exacerbate the symptoms of the other (see Chapter 15).

A valuable ally in treating patients in pain is the psychologist or counselor. Often, patients with chronic painful states such as RA, fibromyalgia, and/or OA are anxious, depressed, or lack coping skills necessary to deal with their pain. Cognitive behavioral approaches to pain such as pain imaging, for example, may be very useful tools in helping patients take an active role in controlling their pain level and not just become a victim of their disorder. Biofeedback training may help some patients, especially those afflicted with myofascial pain states. Families whose members have painful diseases are often under a great deal of stress and become dysfunctional. Family counseling and/or marital counseling can go a long way in aiding the patient and those around him/her in coping with chronic illness. The patient suffering from chronic pain must avoid the feelings of helplessness and despair that can occur, especially when the patient feels that he/she is a victim and has no control over his/her pain. Overcoming such obstacles is essential for optimal care of the patient with chronic painful states. Insight into how certain aspects of a patient's lifestyle can aggravate the underlying painful condition can also be attained through counseling, thus further benefiting patients and conceivably lessening their need for analgesics and other medications.

While multidisciplinary pain clinics have been a great boon in the treatment and further understanding of the pain patient, they are beyond the reach of many — probably most — patients. However, that does not mean that such an approach to patients in pain cannot be attempted at the community level. Such an endeavor, however, requires that the professional caring for the patient strive to cooperate and communicate with each other in order to provide the most conducive atmosphere for encouragement and eventual improvement.

CONCLUSIONS

For the patient who comes to the rheumatologist with a complaint of pain, it is not sufficient for the physician to offer only symptomatic relief. As an internist, as well as a specialist in rheumatic diseases, the rheumatologist needs to accurately pinpoint the cause of the pain and take appropriate measures to minimize associated morbidity. Investigations necessary for the accurate and prompt identification of the scope of the patient's illness may be costly in terms of time and money, but the advantages of an accurate, early diagnosis and prompt effective treatment far outweigh these other considerations. Patients trust their physicians to care for them when they are suffering. That trust must never be betrayed; patients deserve no less.

REFERENCES

Abraham, G.E., & Flechas, J.D. (1992). Management of fibromyalgia: Rationale for the use of magnesium and malic acid. *Journal of Nutritional Medicine, 3,* 49–59.

Altman, R.D., & Moskowitz, R. (1998). Intrarticular sodium hyalovernate (hyalganr) in the treatment of patients with osteoarthritis of the knee; A randomized clinical trial. *Journal of Rheumatology, 25,* 2203–2211.

Altman, R.D., & Singer, F. (Eds.). (1980). Proceedings of the Kroc Foundation Conference on Paget's disease of bone. *Arthritis and Rheumatism, 23,* 1073–1240.

Amrheim, J.A., Kenney, F.M., & Ross, D. (1970). Granulocytopenia, lupus-like syndrome, and other complications of propylthiouracil therapy. *Journal of Pediatrics, 74,* 54–63.

Ashburn, M.A., & Fine, P.G. (1989). Persistent pain following trauma. *Military Medicine, 154*(2), 86–89.

Awad, E.A. (1990). Histopathological changes in fibrositis. In J.R. Fricton & E.A. Awad (Eds.), *Advances in pain research and therapy* (pp. 249–258) New York: Raven Press.

Awerbuch, M.S., & Brooks, P.M. (1981). Role of immune complexes in hypertrophic osteoarthropathy and nonmetastatic polyarthritis. *Annals of Rheumatic Disease, 40,* 470–472.

Bennett, R.M. (1986). Current issues concerning the management of the fibromyalgia syndrome. In R.M. Bennett (Ed.), Proceedings of symposium on the fibrositis/fibromyalgia syndrome. *American Journal of Medicine, 81*(A), 15–18.

Bennett, R.M. (1989). Fibrositis. In W. Kelley, E. Harris, S. Ruddy, & C. Sledge (Eds.), *Textbook of rheumatology* (3rd ed., pp. 541–553). Philadelphia. W. B. Saunders.

Bennett, R.M. (1993). Disabling fibromyalgia. Appearance versus reality. *Journal of Rheumatology, 20,* 1821–1823.

Bennett, R.M. (1999). Treatment strategies for fibromyalgia syndrome. *Journal of Musculoskeletal Medicine, 16* (Suppl.), S20–S25.

Bergstrom, G. (1985). *Joint impairment and disorders at ages 70, 74 and 79.* Unpublished master's thesis, University of Gothenburg, Sweden.

Bernard, A.L., Prince, A., & Edsall, P. (2000). Quality of life issues for fibromyalgia patients. *Arthritis Care and Research, 13,* 42–50.

Bland, J.H., Frymoyer, J.W., Newberry, A.H., Revers, R., & Norman, R.J. (1979). Rheumatic syndromes in endocrine disease. *Seminars in Arthritis and Rheumatism, 9,* 23–65.

Bohan, A. (1981). The private practice of rheumatology. *Arthritis and Rheumatism, 25,* 1304–1307.

Bradley, L.A., Alarcon, F.S., Alexander, R.W., Alexander, M.T., Aaron, L.A., Alberta, K.R., & Martin, M.Y. (1995). Abnormal central processing of dolorimeter stimuli in patients and community residents with fibromyalgia (FM): One year reliability. *Arthritis and Rheumatism, 38,*(9, Suppl.), 991.

Brezin, J.H., Katz, S.M., Schwartz, A.B., & Chintz, J.L. (1979). Reversible renal failure and nephrotic syndrome associated with non-steroidal anti-inflammatory drugs. *New England Journal of Medicine, 301,* 1271–1273.

Bridgman, J.F. (1972). Periarthritis of the shoulder and diabetes mellitus. *Annals of Rheumatic Disease, 31,* 9–71.

Burkhardt, C.S., Clark, S.R., & Bennett, R.M. (1993). Fibromyalgia and quality of life: A comparative analysis. *Journal of Rheumatolology, 20,* 475–479.

Burkle, M.J., Fear, E.C., & Wright, V. (1977). Bone and joint changes in pneumatic drillers. *Annals of Rheumatic Disease, 36,* 276–279.

Buskila, D., Neumann, L., Vaisberg, G., Alkalay, D., & Wolfe, F. (1997). Increased rates of fibromyalgia following cervical spine injury. *Arthritis and Rheumatism, 40,* 446–452.

Calabro, J.J. (1967). Cancer and arthritis. *Rheumatism, 10,* 553–567.

Campbell, S.M., Clark, S., Forehand, M.E., Tindall, E.A., & Bennett, R.M. (1983). Clinical characteristics of fibromyalgia: A "blinded" controlled study of symptoms and tender points. *Arthritis and Rheumatism, 26,* 817–824.

Caro, X. J. (1986). Immunofluorescent studies of skin in primary fibrositis syndrome. *American Journal of Medicine, 81* (Suppl. 3A), 43–49.

Chaykin, L.B., Frame, B., & Sigler, J.W. (1969). Spondylitis: A clue to hypoparathyroidism. *Annals of Internal Medicine, 70,* 995–1000.

Clauw, D., Blank, C., Hewitt-Moulman, J., & Katz, P. (1993). Low tissue levels of magnesium in fibromyalgia [Abstract]. *Arthritis and Rheumatism, 36,* S161.

Clauw, D.J., Morris, S., Starbuck, V., Blank, C., & Gary, G. (1994). Impairment in cognitive function in individuals with fibromyalgia. *Arthritis and Rheumatism, 37*(9, Suppl.), 1119.

Cohen, M.L., Arroyo, J.F., & Champion, G.D. (1990). Evidence for neuropathic mechanisms in diffuse musculoskeletal pain syndrome (Fibromyalgia) [Abstract]. *Arthritis and Rheumatism, 33*(9, Suppl.), 74, S22.

Creamer, P., & Hochbery, M.C. (1997). Osteoarthritis. *Lancet, 350,* 503–509.

Crofford, L. (1996). Stress-response systems in fibromyalgia. *Lyon Mediterranee Medical Tome, 32,* 2138–2142.

Dauphine, R.T., Riggs, B.L., & Schlotz, D.A. (1975). Back pain and vertebral crush fractures: An unemphasized mode of presentation for primary hyperparathyroidism. *Annals of Internal Medicine, 83,* 365–367.

Day, R.O., Graham, G.G., Champion, G.D., & Lee, E. (1984). Anti-rheumatic drug interactions. *Clinics of Rheumatic Disease, 10,* 251–275.

Dorwart, B.B., & Schumacher, H.R. (1975). Joint effusion, chondrocalcinosis and other rheumatic manifestations in hypothyroidism. *American Journal of Medicine, 59,* 780–790.

Dubner, R. (1992). Hyperanalgesic and expanded receptive fields. *Pain, 48,* 3–4.

Fields, H.L. (1987). *Pain.* New York: McGraw-Hill.

Fischer, A.A. (1987). Pressure algometry over normal muscles. Standard values validity and reproducibility of pressure threshold. *Pain, 30,* 115–126.

Fitzcharles, M. A., Duby, S., Waddell, R.W., Banks, E., & Karsh, J. (1984). Limitation of joint mobility (chiroarthropathy) in adult noninsulin-dependent diabetic patients. *Annals of Rheumatic Disease, 43,* 251–257.

Forman, M.D., Malamet, R., & Kaplan, D. (1983). A survery of osteoarthritis of the knee in the elderly. *Journal of Rheumatology, 10,* 282–287.

Fowler, R.W., & Arnold, K.G. (1983). Non-steroidal analgesic and anti-inflammatory agents. *British Medical Journal, 287,* 835.

Fricton, J., & Awad, E.A. (Eds.) (1990). *Advances in pain research and therapy* (Vol. 17). New York: Raven Press.

Furst, D.E. (1990). Rational use of disease-modifying anti-rheumatic drugs. *Drugs, 39,* 19–37.

Ginsburg, F., & Famaey, J.P. (1991). Double-blind, randomized cross over study of the percutaneous efficacy and tolerability of a topical indomethacin spray versus placebo in the treatment of tendinitis. *Journal of International Medical Research, 19*, 131–136.

Goldenberg, D.L., & Reed, J.I. (1985). Bacterial arthritis. *New England Journal of Medicine, 312*, 764–771.

Goldenberg, D.L., Simms, R.W., Geiger, A., & Komaroff, A.L. (1990). High frequency of fibromyalgia in patients with chronic fatigue seen in a primary care practice. *Arthritis and Rheumatism, 33*, 381–387.

Gordon, M.B., Klein, I., Dekker, A., Rodnan, G.P., & Medsger, T.A., Jr. (1981). Thyroid disease in progressive systemic sclerosis: Increased frequency of glandular fibroids and hypothyroidism. *Annals of Internal Medicine, 95*, 431–435.

Graham, D.J., Agranval, N.M., & Roth, S.H. (1988). Prevention of NSAID-induced gastric ulcer with misoprostol: Multicentre, double-blind, placebo-controlled trial. *Lancet, 2*, 1277–1280.

Gray, R.B., & Gottlieb, N.L. (1976). Rheumatic disorders associated with diabetes mellitus: Literature review. *Seminars in Arthritis and Rheumatism, 6*, 19–34.

Greenfield, S., Fitzcharles, M.A., & Esdaile, J.M. (1992). Reactive fibromyalgia syndrome. *Arthritis and Rheumatism, 35*, 678–681.

Griep, E.N., Boersma, J.W., & deKloet, E.R. (1993). Altered reactivity of the hypothalamic-pituitary-adrenal axis in the primary fibromyalgia syndrome. *Journal of Rheumatology, 20*, 469–474.

Hahn, T.J., & Hahn, B.H. (1976). Osteopenia in patients with rheumatic disease: Principles of diagnosis therapy. *Seminars in Arthritis and Rheumatism, 6*, 165–188.

Hahn, T.J., Halstead, L.R., Teitelbaum, S.L., & Hahn, B.H. (1979). Altered mineral metabolism in glucocorticoid-induced osteopenia: Effect of 25-hydroxyvitamin D administration. *Journal of Clinical Investigation, 64*, 655–665.

Harris, E.D. (1990). Mechanisms of disease: Rheumatoid arthritis. Pathophysiology and implications for therapy. *New England Journal of Medicine, 322*, 1277–1289.

Hollander, J.L. (1972). Intrasynovial corticosteroid therapy in arthritis. *Maryland Medical Journal, 19*, 62–66.

Houston, B.D., Crouch, M.E., Brick, J.E., & DiBartolomeo, A.G. (1979). Apparent vasculitis associated with propylthiouracil use. *Arthritis and Rheumatism, 22*, 925–928.

Hubbard, D.R., & Berkoff, G.M. (1993). Myofascial trigger points studied by needle EMG. *Spine, 18*, 1803–1807.

Hudson, J.I., Goldenberg, D.L., Pope, H.G., Keck, P.E., & Schlesinger, L. (1992). Comorbidity of fibromyalgia with medical and psychiatric disorders. *American Journal of Medicine, 92*, 363–367.

Huskisson, E.C., Woolf, D.L., Balme, H.W., Scott, J., & Franklin, S. (1976). Four new anti-inflammatory drugs: Responses and variations. *British Medical Journal, i*, 1048–1049.

Jaffe, H.L. (1958). *Tumors and tumorous conditions of the bone and joints.* Philadelphia: Lea & Febiger.

Jung, Y., Hohmann, T.C., Gerneth, J.A., Novak, J., Wasserman, R.C., D'Andrea, B.J., Newton, R.H., & Danowski, T.S. (1971). Diabetic hand syndrome. *Metabolism, 20*, 1008–1015.

Krane, S.M. (1982). Etidronate disodium in the treatment of Paget's disease of bone. *Annals of Internal Medicine, 96*, 619–625.

Kremer, J.M., Lawrence, D.A., Petrillo, G.F., Litts, L.L., Mullaly, P.M., Rynes, R.I., Stocker, R.P., Parhami, N., Greenstein, N.S., Fuchs, B.R., Mathur, A., Robinson, D.R., Sperling, R.I., & Bigaouette, J. (1995). Effects of high-dose fish oil on rheumatoid arthritis after stopping nonsteroidal antiinflammatory drugs. *Arthritis and Rheumatism, 38*(8), 1107–1114.

Kloppenburg, M., Breedveld, F.C., Terwiel, J. ., Mallee, C., & Dijkmans, B A. (1994). Minocycline in active rheumatoid arthritis. A double-blind, placebo-controlled trial. *Arthritis and Rheumatism, 37*(5), 629–636.

Lachs, S., & Jacobs, R.P. (1986). Acromeglic arthropathy: A reversible rheumatic disease. *Journal of Rheumatology, 13*, 634–636.

Lane, N.E., Bloch, D.A., Jones, H.H., Marshall, W.H., Jr., Wood, P.D., & Fries, J.F. (1986). Long-distance running, bone density, and osteoarthritis. *Journal of the American Medical Association, 255*, 1147–1151.

Langman, M.J., Jensen, D.M., Watson, D.J., Harper, S.E., Zhao, P.-L., Quan, H., Bolognese, J.A., & Simon, T.J. (1999). Adverse upper gastrointestinal effects of rofecoxib compared with NSAIDs. *Journal of the American Medical Association, 282*, 1929–2933.

Lawrence, J.S. (1969). Generalized osteoarthritis in a population sample. *American Journal of Epidemiology, 90*, 381–389.

Lee, M.H.M., Itoh, M., Yang, G.W., & Eason, A.L. (1989). Physical therapy and rehabilitation medicine. In J.J. Bonica (Eds.), *The management of pain* (2nd ed., pp. 1769–1788). Philadelphia: Lea & Febiger.

Maini, R.N., Breedveld, F.C., Kalder, J.R., et al. (1998). Therapeutic efficacy of multiple intravenous infusions of antitumor necrosis factor-alpha monoclonal antibody combined with low dose weekly methotrexate in rheumatoid arthritis. *Arthritis and Rheumatism, 41*, 1552–1563.

Matkovic, V., Kostial, K., Simonovic, I., Buzina, R., Broarec, A., & Nordin, B.E. (1979). Bone status and fracture rates in two regions in Yugoslavia. *American Journal of Clinical Nutrition, 32*, 540–549.

Mazenac, D.J. (1982). First year of a rheumatologist in private practice. *Arthritis and Rheumatism, 25*, 718–719.

McCarty, D.J., Harman, J.G., Grassanovich, J.L., & Qian, C. (1995). Treatment of rheumatoid joint inflammation with intrasynovial triamcinolone hexacetanide. *Journal of Rheumatology, 22*, 1631–1635.

McCarty, D.J., Harman, J.G., Grassanovich, J.L., Qian, C., & Klein, J.P. (1995). Combination drug therapy of seropositive rheumatoid arthritis. *Journal of Rheumatology, 22*, 1636–1645.

McCarthy, G.M., & McCarty, D.J. (1992). Effect of topical capsaicin in the therapy of painful osteoarthritis of the hands. *Journal of Rheumatology, 19*, 604–607.

Mense, S.D. (1994). Referral of muscle pain. New aspects. *APS Journal, 3,* 1–9.

Mikuls, T.T., & O'Dell, J. (2000). The changing face of rheumatoid arthritis therapy: Results of serial surverys. *Arthritis and Rheumatism, 43,* 464–465.

Mountz, J.M., Bradley, L.A., Modell, J.G., Alexander, R.W., Triana-Alexander, M., Aaron, L.A., Stewart, K.E., Alarcon, G.A., & Mountz, J.D. (1995). Fibromyalgia in women. Abnormalities of regional cerebral blood flow in the thalamus and the caudate nucleus are associated with low pain threshold levels. *Arthritis and Rheumatism, 38*(7), 926–938.

Neville, M.W. (2000). Gabapentine in the management of neuropathic pain. *American Journal of Pain Management, 10,* 6–12.

NIH Consensus Conference. (1984). Osteoporosis. *Journal of the American Medical Association, 252,* 799–802.

Osiri, M., & Moreland, L.W. (1999). Specific cyclooxygenase alpha inhibitors: A new choice of nonsteroidal anti-inflammatory drug therapy. *Arthritis Care and Research, 12,* 351–362.

Packard, R. (1992). Posttraumatic headache: Permanency and relationship to legal settlement. *Headache, 32,* 496–499.

Panush, R. S., Schmidt, C., Caldwell, J. R., Edwards, N. D., Longley, S., Yonker, R., Webster, E., Nauman, J., Stork, J., & Pettersson, H. (1986). Is running associated with degenerative joint disease? *Journal of the American Medical Association, 255,* 1152–1154.

Puranen, J., Ala-Ketola, L., Peltokallio, P., & Saarela, J. (1975). Running and primary osteoarthritis of the hip. *British Medical Journal, 2,* 424–425.

Patten, B.M., Bilezikian, J.P., Mallette, L.E., Prince, A., Engel, W.K., & Aurbach, G.D. (1974). Neuromuscular disease in primary hyperparathyroidism. *Annals of Internal Medicine, 80,* 172–183.

Pierce, D.A., Stern, R., Jaffe, R., Fullman, J., & Talan, N. (1979). Immunoblastic sarcoma with features of Sjogren's syndrome and systemic lupus erythematosus in a patient with immunoblastic lymphadenopathy. *Arthritis and Rheumatism, 22,* 911–916.

Pritchard, M.H., & Jessop, J.D. (1977). Chondrocalcinosis in primary hyperparathyroidism. *Annals of Rheumatic Disease, 36,* 146–151.

Prudden, B. (1980). *Pain erasure.* New York: Ballantine Books.

Resnick, D.L. (1974). Erosive osteoarthritis of the hand and wrist in hyperparathyroidism. *Radiology, 110,* 263–269.

Robins, R. A., & Baldwin, R. W. (1978). Immune complexes in cancer. *Cancer Immunology and Immunotherapy, 4,* 1–3.

Romano, T.J. (1988a). Fibromyalgia: It's the real thing. *Postgraduate Medicine, 83,* 231–243.

Romano, T.J. (1988b). Fibrositis in men. *West Virginia Medical Journal, 84,* 235–237.

Romano, T.J. (1990). Clinical experiences with post-traumatic fibromyalgia syndrome. *West Virginia Medical Journal, 86,* 198–202.

Romano, T.J. (1991a). Fibromyalgia in children; diagnosis and treatment. *West Virginia Medical Journal, 87,* 112–114.

Romano, T. J. (1991b). Presence of anticardiolipin antibodies in the fibromyalgia syndrome. *The Pain Clinic, 4,* 147–153.

Romano, T.J. (1994). Magnesium deficiency in patients with myofascial pain. *Journal of Myofascial Therapy, 1,* 11–12.

Romano, T.J. (1996). Fibromyalgia syndrome in other rheumatic conditions. *Lyon Mediteranee Medical Medecine Sudest, Tome, 32*(5/6), 2143–2146.

Romano, T.J. (1998). Proposed formula for the estimation of pain caused by each of several traumas involving soft tissue. *American Journal of Pain Management, 8,* 118–123.

Romano, T.J. (1999). Presence of nocturnal myoclonus in patients with fibromyalgia syndrome. *American Journal of Pain Management, 9,* 85–89.

Romano, T.J., & Govindan, S. (1996). Abnormal cranial SPECT scanning in fibromyalgia patients with headaches. *American Journal of Pain Management, 6,* 118–122.

Romano, T.J., & Stiller, J. (1994). Magnesium deficiency in fibromyalgia syndrome. *Journal of Nutritional Medicine, 4,* 165–167.

Romano, T.J., & Stiller, J. (1997). Needle EMG in myofascial pain syndrome. Correlation with physical findings in a general rheumatology practice. *American Journal of Pain Management, 7,* 19–21.

Romano, T.J., & Stiller, J.W. (1988). Abnormal current perception testing in fibromyalgia [Abstract]. *Arthritis and Rheumatism, 31*(1, Suppl.), R44.

Roth, G.J., & Majerus, P.W. (1975). The mechanism of the effect of aspirin on human platelets. *Journal of Clinical Investigations, 56,* 624–632.

Russell, A.L. (1991). Piroxicam 0.5% topical gel compared to placebo in the treatment of acute soft tissue injuries: A double-blind study comparing efficacy and safety. *Clinical and Investigative Medicine, 14,* 35–43.

Russell, I.J. (1990). Treatment of the patient with fibromyalgia syndrome. In J. R. Fricton & E. A. Awad (Eds.), *Advances in pain research and therapy* (Vol. 17, pp. 305–314). New York: Raven Press.

Schajowica, F. (1982). *Tumors and tumor-like lesions of bones and joints.* New York: Springer-Verlag.

Schlomka, G., Schroter, G., & Ocherwal, A. (1955). Uber der Bedeutung der bernflischer Belastung far die entsehring der degenerativen. *Gelenkleiden Z. Gesamte Internal Medicine, 447*(10), 993.

Schumacher, H.R. (1997). *Primer on rheumatic disease* (11th ed.). Atlanta, GA: Arthritis Foundation.

Seibold, J.R. (1982). Digital sclerosis in children with insulin-dependent diabetes mellitus. *Arthritis and Rheumatism, 25,* 1357–1361.

Sheon, R.P., Moskowitz, R.W., & Goldenberg, V.M. (1982). *Soft tissue rheumatism pain recognition management: Prevention.* Philadelphia: Lea & Febiger.

Simms, R.W., Zerbini, C.A.F., Ferrante, N., Anothony, J., Felson, D.T., Craven, D.E., & Boston City Hospital Clinical AIDS Team (1992). Fibromyalgia syndrome in patients infected with human immunodeficiency virus. *American Journal of Medicine, 92,* 368–374.

Simon, L.D., Weaver, A.L., Graham, D.Y., Kivitz, A.J., Lipsky, P.E., Hubbard, R.C., Isakson, P.C., Verburg, K.M., Yu, S.S., Zhao, W.W., & Geis, G.D. (1999). Anti-inflammatory and upper gastrointestinal effects of celecoxib in rheumatoid arthritis. *Journal of the American Medical Association, 282,* 1921–1928.

Simons, D. (1990). Muscular pain syndromes. In J.R. Fricton & E.A. Awad (Eds.). *Advances in pain research and therapy* (Vol. 17, pp. 24–27). New York: Raven Press.

Simons, D.G. (1987). Myofascial pain syndromes due to trigger points. In A. Kleinman & D. Mechanic (Eds.), *Pain and disability, clinical, behavioral and public policy perspectives* (pp. 285–292). Washington, D.C.: M. Osterweis Institute of Medicine, National Academy Press.

Sinha, S., Munichoodappa, C.S., & Kozak, G.P. (1972). Neuropathy (charcot joints) in diabetes mellitus. *Medicine, 51,* 191–210.

Smiger, F.R., Schiller, A.L., Pyle, E.B., et al. (1977). Paget's disease of bone. In L.V. Avioli & S.M. Kane (Eds.), Metabolic bone disease (pp. 490–575). New York: Academic Press.

Smiley, A.M., Husain, M., & Indenbaum, S. (1980). Eiosinophilic faciitis in association with thyroid disease: A report of three cases. *Journal of Rheumatology, 7,* 871–876.

Smiley, W.M., Cram, J.R., Margoles, M.S., Romano, T.J., & Stiller, J. (1992). Innovations in soft tissue juriprudence. *Trial Diplomacy Journal, 15,* 199–208.

Smolen, J.S., Kalden, J.R., Scott, D.L., Rozman, B., Kvien, T.K., Larsen, A., Loew-Friedrich, I., Oed, C., Rosenburg, R., & The European Leflunomid Study Group. (1999). Efficacy and safety of leflunomide compared with placebo and sulphasalazine in active rheumatoid arthritis; a double-blind, randomised, multicentre trial. *Lancet, 353,* 259–266.

Smythe, H.A. (1989). Nonarticular rheumatism and psychogenic musculoskeletal syndromes. In D.J. McCarty (Ed.), *Arthritis and allied conditions. A textbook of rheumatology* (11th ed., pp. 1241–1254). Philadelphia: Lea & Febiger.

Stollerman, G.H., Markowitz, M., Toronta, A., Wannamaker, L.W., & Whittemore, R. (1965). Jones criteria (revised) for guidance in the diagnosis of rheumatic fever. *Circulation, 32,* 664–668.

Thiske, M.G. (1969). Neck and shoulder pain: Evaluation and conservative management. *Medical Clinics of North America, 53,* 511–524.

Tilley, B.C., Alarcon, G.S., Heyse, S.P., Trentham, D.E., Neuner, R., Kaplan, D.A., Clegg, D.O., Leisen, J.C., Buckley, L., Duncan, H., Pillemer, S.R., Tuttleman, M., & Fowler, S.E. (1995). Minocycline in rheumatoid arthritis. *Annals of Internal Medicine, 122,* 81–89.

Travell, J.G., & Simons, D. (1983). *Myofascial pain and dysfunction: The trigger point manual.* Baltimore: William & Wilkins.

Veasy, L.G., Wiedmeier, S.E., Orsmond, G.S., Ruttenberg, H.D., Boucek, M.M., Roth, S.J., Tait, V.F., Thompson, J.A., Daly, J.A., Kaplan, E.L., & Hill, H.R. (1987). Resurgence of acute rheumatic fever in the intermountain area of the United States. *New England Journal of Medicine, 316,* 421–427.

Wallack, H.W. (1977). Lupus-like syndrome associated with carcinoma of the breast. *Archives of Internal Medicine, 137,* 532–535.

Weinblatt, M.E., Kremer, J.M., & Bankhurst, A.D. (1999). A trial of etanercept, a recombinant tumor necrosis factor receptor: Fc fusion protein in patients with rheumatoid arthritis receiving methotrexate. *New England Journal of Medicine, 340,* 253–259.

Wiske, K.R., & Healey, L.A. (1990). Challenging the therapeutic pyramid: A new look at treatment strategies for rheumatoid arthritis. *Journal of Rheumatology, 17* (Suppl. 25), 4–7.

Wohlgethan, J.R. (1987). Frozen shoulder in hyperthyroidism. *Arthritis and Rheumatism, 30,* 936–939.

Wolfe, F., Smythe, H.A., Yunus, M.D., Bennett, R.M., Bombardier, C., Goldenberg, D.L., Tugwell, P., Campbell, S.M., Abeles, M., Clark, P., Fam, A.G., Farber, S.J., Fiechtner, J. J., Franklin, C.M., Gatter, R.A., Hamaty, D., Lessard, J., Lichtbroun, A.S., Masi, A.T., McCain, G.A., Reynolds, W.J., Romano, T.J., Russell, I.J., & Sheon, R.P. (1990). The American College of Rheumatology 1990 criteria for the classification of fibromyalgia. *Arthritis and Rheumatism, 33,* 160–172.

Yunus, M.B. (1992). Towards a model of pathophysiology of fibromyalgia: Aberrant central pain mechanisms with peripheral modulation. *Journal of Rheumatology, 19,* 846–850.

Yunus, M.B., & Aldag, J.C. (1993). Clinical and psychological features of regional fibromyalgia: Comparison with fibromyalgia syndrome (abstr.). *Arthritis and Rhematism, 36*(9), S221.

Yunus, M.B., & Masi, A.T. (1985). Juvenile primary fibromyalgia syndrome. *Arthritis and Rheumatism, 28,* 138–144.

Yunus, M.B., Bennett, R.M., Romano, T.J., Russell, I.J., & other members of the FCRAC Group (1997). Fibromyalgia consensus report: Additional comments. *Journal of Clinical Rheumatology, 3,* 324–327.

28

The Role of the Neurologist in a Multidisciplinary Pain Clinic

Jacob Green, M.D., Ph.D.

INTRODUCTION

It has been said that many of the multidisciplinary pain clinics take on the characteristic interests of their director. True to this comment, as neurologist–director of a large multidisciplinary pain clinic, I place a significant emphasis in our institution on the *evaluation* of the nervous system. We never lose sight that pain is "an experience" and our approaches to the individual patient are always pluralistic, multidisciplinary, and multifaceted in character. We evaluate the patient as a whole and do, in fact, always use the traditional multidisciplinary approach, including those beneficial aspects of both behavioral and organic approaches to each person in our consideration of their pain problems.

This chapter is a synopsis of the various neurodiagnostic studies commonly employed in our multidisciplinary pain clinic in order to ascertain the state of function of the nervous system as used in the day-to-day approach to any patient. These diagnostic studies typically include an analysis of peripheral nerve and spinal cord functions.

Newer studies such as electronic brain imaging ("brain mapping") that ascertain the cerebral mechanisms involved in the "appreciation" of pain are now coming online. Our very preliminary research shows a potential side-to-side difference in the brain mapped somatosensory input tests in chronic unilateral pain patients. The brain map study helps us to evaluate the way the cerebrum handles nociceptive (sensory) incoming information. Technical change is certain, ongoing, and ever-present. Needless to say, we will probably be rewriting this chapter on these newer aspects of central-brain neurophysiology tests in the future. Surely, future assessments of the cerebral influences will be included in a physiologic assessment study of the appreciation of the pain experience. The study of the brain's ongoing adaptation to chronic pain states will also be included in future considerations of the clinical neurophysiology (neurology) studies of pain. Such a compilation has been accomplished by Chen (1993).

The physician can objectively evaluate the chronic pain patient with concomitant peripheral nerve and/or spinal dysfunction using various diagnostic methods that are currently available in most neurodiagnostic laboratories and affiliated pain clinics and that are truly multidisciplinary and multitasking.

More information can now be gained with motor nerve conduction studies using late responses, which provide data concerning the most proximal course of the motor nerve. Sensory nerve conductions via computer averaging techniques now make information concerning sensory complaints alone more easily understandable. Thermography (high resolution infrared imaging), using the electronic infrared technique, indicates when the autonomic nerves are dysfunctional. All of this information aids in our interpretation of dysfunctional mixed peripheral nerves. Cerebrally recorded, peripherally stimulated evoked potentials provide a method of determining the input pathways from the sensory tracts through the spinal cord into the cerebral cortex and give a measure of the cerebral processing of nociceptive information.

Often, the physician who is treating a patient suffering radicular pain must assess all the information available

0-8493-0926-3/02/$0.00+$1.50
© 2002 by CRC Press LLC

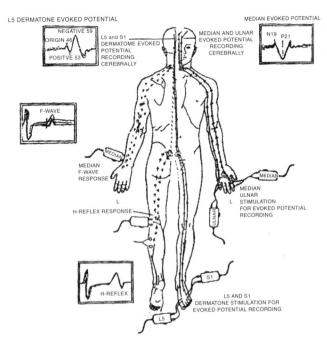

FIGURE 28.1 Schematic demonstrating recording of information obtained in neurophysiological evaluation. (From *Contemporary Orthopaedics*, Nov. 1987, Vol. 15, No. 5. Reproduced with permission.)

and obtainable by all the neurodiagnostic studies performed. Electromyography (EMG) tests only the motor component of the mixed peripheral nerve. EMG gives no information about the sensory component (nociception), which frequently is involved when the patient presents with a chronic pain complaint. Electromyography is simply a needle study to assess damage to only motor nerves or muscles. It is incumbent upon the physician to have a working knowledge of all the neurodiagnostic methods currently available for thoroughly testing the peripheral nervous system, spine, and brain when evaluating chronic pain patients.

NEUROPHYSIOLOGIC STUDIES

The term *clinical neurophysiological evaluation* involves the assessment of a patient using various available electrodiagnostic methods to detect relevant changes that may correlate with the clinical pain condition. In addition to traditional EM), these diagnostic tests include electroneurography (motor and sensory nerve conduction velocity studies), evoked potential studies, and high-resolution infrared imaging.

ELECTRONEUROGRAPHY

By definition, electroneurography is an electrical stimulation study of the peripheral nerves. In addition to studying the motor nerve from a point proximal to one more distal,

now it also is possible to evaluate "late responses." In these late responses, the neural message travels down to the electrode recording pick-up placed over a designated muscle belly, and it also travels proximally (upward) into the central (spinal cord) neuraxis and then back out (again) to the final recording site, arriving later. Computerized averaging techniques make these tiny voltage neurophysiological events (late responses) useful evaluative tools in patients suffering chronic radicular pain from proximal nerve lesions. The sensory component of the mixed peripheral nerve is also tested using direct nerve stimulation techniques.

Motor Nerve Conduction Studies

In motor nerve conduction velocity studies, a recording electrode is applied on the skin over the active belly of a selected distal muscle, with a reference electrode placed distally over a nonactive area (Figure 28.1). Stimulation of the motor fibers of the mixed peripheral nerve is then carried out, and the time it takes to create the muscle contraction is recorded.

An example of this technique is the placement of a recording electrode over the abductor pollicis brevis muscle, with a reference electrode placed distally over the thumb (Figure 28.2). The median nerve and its motor components are then stimulated in sequence at the supraclavicular region, forearm, and wrist (8 to 10 cm above the muscle). By varying these stimulation points and dividing the time elapsed at each stimulus site into the distance to the muscle stimulated, a conduction "velocity" is determined on a segmental basis for the motor nerve from the supraclavicular region point to point down to the hand (Buchthal & Rosenfalck, 1966; Hodes, Larrabee, & German, 1948; Jebsen, 1967; Melvin, Harris, & Johnson 1966).

A similar strategy is used for the ulnar nerve (Figure 28.3), proceeding sequentially from the supraclavicular

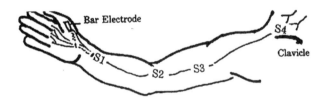

FIGURE 28.2 Placement of recording electrodes in a motor nerve conduction velocity study. Median nerve (C6, 7, 8, T1): Bar electrode over abductor pollicis brevis muscle (ABD). S1—10 cm, directly over carpel tunnel. S2—Elbow (antecubital fossa)—medial to the palpable brachial artery. S3—Axilla—groove between muscles (must be 10 cm from elbow stimulator). S4—Supraclavicular—approx. 5–6 cm from clavicular notch. F-wave—supramaximal stimulator (take shortest wave of ten trials). (From *Contemporary Orthopaedics*, Nov. 1987, Vol. 15, No. 5. Reproduced with permission.)

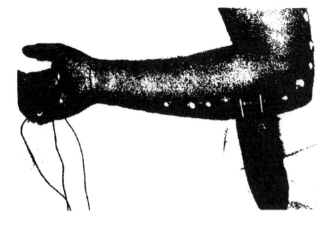

FIGURE 28.3 Use of inching technique to accurately determine the site of a nerve block (ulnar nerve). (From *Contemporary Orthopaedics*, Nov. 1987, Vol. 15, No. 5. Reproduced with permission.)

area to the axillary region, to the elbow, to a pick-up over the abductor digiti minimi muscle in the hand (Kimura, 1974).

In the lower extremity, typically a stimulus is sent from the popliteal fossa down the peroneal nerve to the lateral portion of the foot and similarly down the posterior tibial nerve to the medial portion of the foot (Figure 28.4), where recordings are made over the selected muscles.

For the peroneal nerve, these recordings are made over the extensor digitorum brevis; for the posterior tibial nerve, the recordings are made over the abductor muscles (Hodes et al., 1948; Jimenez, Easton, & Redford, 1970; Lamontagne & Buchthal, 1970). Under special circumstances, magnetic or needle stimulation of the sciatic nerve can be carried out in the lumbosacral area, with recordings obtained distally over any point of the sciatic innervated muscles (Yap & Hirota, 1967).

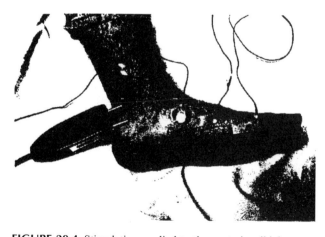

FIGURE 28.4 Stimulation applied to the posterior tibial nerve at the ankle. (From *Contemporary Orthopaedics*, Nov. 1987, Vol. 15, No. 5. Reproduced with permission.)

Late Response Studies

Late response studies (F-times) are carried out by stimulation of a motor nerve and recording the response from the muscle distally, with the averaging computer looking for a sufficiently long period of time for the stimulating neural impulse to climb up the motor nerve in retrograde antidromic fashion (Eisen, Schomer, & Melnod, 1977a, b; Kimura, 1983; Mayer & Feldman, 1967; Panayiotopoulos & Scarpalezos, 1977). There is then a synapse in the internuncial neuronal pool of the spinal cord, and a subsequently generated neural impulse, which comes back down in an orthodromic fashion to be recorded over the muscles of the hand or foot. This F-wave late response uses supramaximal current (Figure 28.5A) and shows a somewhat variable responses (Kimura, 1974).

The quickest of ten supramaximal shocks for each nerve studied is the designated F-time (latency for this activity). A significantly prolonged F-time (2 msec or more), compared to the reading for the opposite side, may well correlate with a typical proximal motor nerve deficit.

In the lower extremities, in addition to the F-time determination, posterior tibial nerve stimulation may be conducted using a submaximal current (Figure 28.5B), with a late response phenomenon recorded over the soleus muscle. This is known as the Hoffmann reflex or H-reflex (Braddom & Johnson, 1974; Cook, 1968; Magiadery, Porter, Park, & Teasdale, 1952). This action potential denotes the time taken for the stimulus at the popliteal fossa to climb in a normal orthodromic fashion, up the 1-A sensory input fibers, which usually are used by the muscle spindles to send messages into the spinal internuncial neuronal pool; then these neural impulses subsequently go down the motor component of the sciatic-posterior tibial nerve. H-reflexes are quite accurate. In an adequate study performed in a controlled setting, a 2-msec delay in a side-to-side comparison may well indicate a proximal lesion of the S1 nerve root (i.e., a herniated disc) or other proximal peripheral nerve lesion.

Magnetic Motor Nerve Stimulation

The magnetic motor system stimulating coil device can be used at the skin surface to painlessly "excite" both the central neuraxis (brain and spinal cord) and the peripheral motor nerves. Pending FDA release for cerebral study, we chose to utilize only the peripheral motor nervous system alone. All neural structures within the entire intra- and extraspinal course of the final motor component of the peripheral nerve are accessible for this magnetic (motor) study.

Several practical advantages of this new noninvasive motor nerve stimulation technique are apparent. The magnetic stimulator is placed directly over the spinal column (on the skin) in the neck and also in similar fashion over

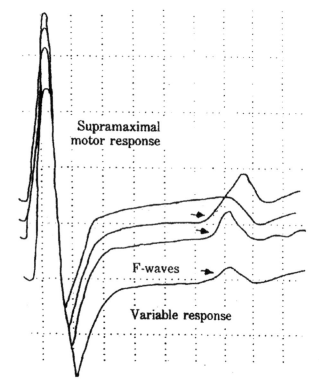

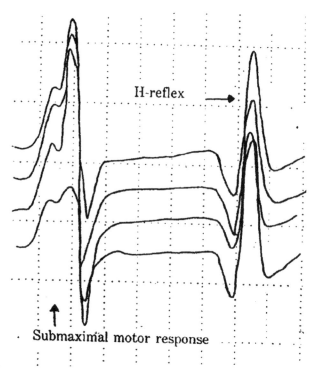

FIGURE 28.5A (Recording of supramaximal shock wave to provide F-time for comparison with opposite side. (From *Contemporary Orthopaedics*, Nov. 1987, Vol. 15, No. 5. Reproduced with permission.)

FIGURE 28.5B (Use of submaximal current for posterior nerve stimulation to record late phenomenon over the soleus muscle. (From *Contemporary Orthopaedics*, Nov. 1987, Vol. 15, No. 5. Reproduced with permission.)

the skin of the low back area (both in the midline) to symmetrically study the activity of the final motor neuron's entire pathway.

In the past, one of two methods of spinal motor nerve root exit zone evaluation was to insert deep needle electrodes within the paraspinal muscles in order for the stimulator to become juxtaposed to the emerging (cervical and lumbosacral) motor nerve roots as they exited from the spinal column. The relatively invasive (direct) motor nerve needle stimulations were done to obtain physiologic information from the motor nerve roots near their origin. The deep needle stimulation procedure was typically quite painful.

The only other previously available method utilized to obtain clinically relevant information from this important paraspinal area (i.e., the motor spinal root exit zone) was the use of "late response" nerve conduction studies previously described. This "F-time" neurophysiologic technique typically called for the "ricocheting" of an antidromic (nerve) message up the motor nerve into the spinal internuncial neuronal spinal pool. This intraspinal neuronal pool would then, in turn, respond to the generated incoming stimulus with an outward-bound elicited motor nerve response. Clinically, the F-time was obtained by the repetitive use of supramaximal (painful) electrical shocks applied to the distal peripheral nerve to

be tested. This F-time late response technique typically required the repetitive use of 10 to 20 of these supermaximum shocks delivered to each mixed peripheral nerve. This repetitive shock study was done to ascertain the quickest F-time of the motor transmission times for each of the nerves studied. This late response information was used to compare, in side-to-side (symmetry) fashion, the motor root entry and exit zone functions of each spinal-accessible nerve pair.

This new magnetic stimulation technique, utilizing a painless skin surface magnetic coil stimulation system, allows for a positive patient evaluative experience. The central neuraxis (C-spine and LS-spine) to peripheral motor system transmission information is measured by recording the motor responses at the hand muscles and similarly at the foot muscles. This information (nerve function values) is now readily derived in a painless manner from the most proximal part of the motor nerve. Central motor (CNS, brain, and spinal cord) conduction times have been recorded in this manner (Pascual-Leone, et al., 1993).

Sensory Nerve Condition Studies

Sensory nerve conduction velocity studies depend on the ability to record messages transmitted from purely sensory nerves. Sensory nerve action potentials (SNAP) are of low

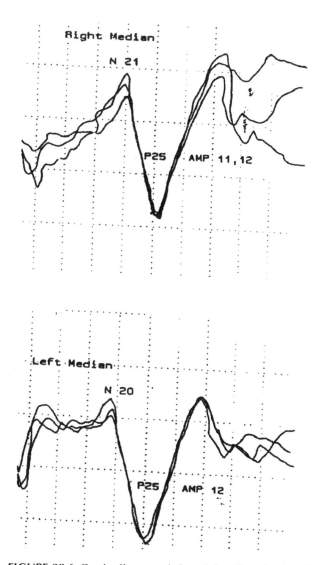

FIGURE 28.6 Cerebrally recorded peripherally stimulated median nerve potentials obtained for comparison between the affected and unaffected extremities (normal study). (From *Contemporary Orthopaedics*, Nov. 1987, Vol. 15, No. 5. Reproduced with permission.)

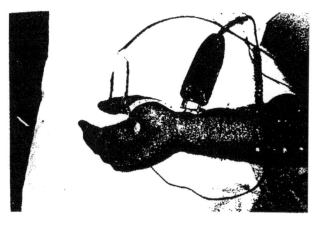

FIGURE 28.7 Radial nerve orthodromic sensory study. (From Contemporary Orthopaedics, Nov. 1987, Vol. 15, No. 5. Reproduced with permission.)

voltage (15 uV) compared to motor potentials (5 to 15 mV). SNAPs are well observed by the averaging techniques now widely used in modern-day clinical neurophysiology laboratories equipped with microprocessing computers (Behse & Buchthal, 1971; Buchthal & Rosenfalck, 1966; Ludin & Beyeler, 1977).

A sensory nerve conduction study can provide information concerning the competency of the sensory portion of the mixed peripheral nerves (Burk, Skuse, & Lethlean, 1974; Lefebvre-D'Amour et al., 1979). Testing of the sensory components of a peripheral nerve (e.g., median, ulnar) is conducted in a fashion similar to that for motor nerves. The stimulus is applied starting at the axillary region and proceeding to the elbow and wrist, while a recording of an "antidromic" sensory

conduction velocity is made from the fingers (Kimura, 1974; Lachman, Shahani, & Young 1980). Similar timing of the response from point to point can provide segmental sensory nerve conduction velocity, a study that can be used for comparison with the opposite, clinically "unaffected" side (Figure 28.6).

Noting that the fingers contain only sensory nerves, the recording can be made in an orthodromic manner, coming upward from the fingers as the impulses reach the wrist, elbow, axillary, and supraclavicular regions (Figure 28.7).

These sensory techniques can also be used to stimulate at the dorsal thumb region and a more proximal site in order to record the sensory potentials of the radial nerve.

In the lower extremities, sensory nerve conduction studies can be used to gain information concerning the integrity (or lack thereof) of the sural nerve. The sural nerve is a combination of branches from the peroneal and posterior tibial nerves that carries purely sensory impulses from the foot and lower leg up to the spinal cord. The sensory latency of the sural nerve is tested by applying stimulation in an antidromic (outward) fashion.

Specific information as to the individual components of the sensory nerve C, 1A, and 1D fibers can be obtained via neurometer testing. This test is the most sensitive measure of sensory nerve function, in my opinion (Green, et al., submitted; Katims, et al., 1991).

EVOKED POTENTIAL CEREBRAL RECORDING STUDIES

Evoked potential studies are a further offshoot of biomedical computer averaging techniques. In these painless and fully reproducible studies, stimuli are applied at the peripheral nerves, that is, the median and ulnar nerves in the hand and the posterior tibial and peroneal nerves in the foot (Bergamini, Bergamasco, & Fra, 1969; Green, Gildmeser, & Hazelwood, 1983; Hume & Cant, 1978). The dermatomes of the foot (L5, S1, etc.) can also be stimulated to send sensory messages in an orthodromic (inward) manner to the spinal cord and subsequently to the brain. These tiny electrical messages are continually conducted up the neuraxis to be recorded as the impulses arrive at the cranial vault (Magiadery & McDougal, 1950).

Dermatomal stimulation of the lumbar roots by stimulating patches of skin known to be innervated by a specific nerve root has been helpful in the diagnosis of lumbar disc disease. Examples of this include stimulation over the dorsum of the foot between the first and second interspaces to test an L5 dermatome, and stimulation of the lateral plantar surface of the foot to test an S1 dermatome. Patients having herniated lumbar discs may demonstrate significant delay or distortion of the signals from these dermatomes.

Because of the interlacing of the cervical nerve roots within the brachial plexus, less specific information is gained on a dermatomal basis in the upper extremities. However, information from anatomic areas subserved by the radial, median, and ulnar nerves occasionally can be detected by a distortion of the cerebrally recorded signal generated by dermatomal skin stimulation.

There are a number of proponents of intraoperative monitoring of evoked potentials during spinal surgery. Most operative formats suggest bilateral stimulation of specific nerves by placement of indwelling subcutaneous needle electrodes near the nerve being evaluated. Stimulation from the upper extremity is part of the paradigm for ensuring that recording apparatus is intact. Halogenic anesthetics must be avoided because of the distortion of the cerebrally recorded evoked signal. Meticulous recording techniques are typically performed throughout the operative procedure. In some cases, reversible spinal pathway abnormalities have been detected with these testing methods, preventing spinal cord damage during surgical procedures for scoliosis and other conditions.

ELECTROMYOGRAPHY

In the technique used to obtain an electromyogram, the actual EMG, a thin Teflon-coated needle is inserted into the various muscles being studied (Figure 28.8) (Buchthal, 1975).

In a pure radiculopathy, among the first EMG changes noted following injury (at approximately 10 days) often will be electrographic signs of unstable muscle cell membrane potentials in the paraspinal areas alone. Within 3 weeks or so, more peripheral changes can usually be found in the extremity muscles of the involved limb. The earliest EMG changes seen also include reduction of motor unit potential amplitudes (Petajan & Philip, 1969).

Motor nerve root irritation may also be evidenced by the finding of unstable muscle cell membrane potentials (fibrillations and positive sharp waves, previously called denervation potentials) in the various groups of extremity muscles (Figure 28.9).

Decreased recruitment of motor unit action potentials elicited during EMG testing also is a reliable sign of neuropathic dysfunction (Petajan, 1974; Sacco, Buchthal, & Rosenfalch, 1962; Wexler, 1983a).

In long-standing neuropathic changes, renervation can occur and high-voltage prolonged motor unit action potentials with many positive and negative turns can be found (Fig 28.10).

A careful study of multiple sites in multiple muscles in the back is essential in ascertaining whether a motor nerve root, individual nerve, or a group of nerves (i.e., brachial plexus, L-s plexus) is involved.

On some occasions, perplexing data can occur at the C5–6 level even in myelographically verified root lesions (Uyematsu, 1983; Wexler, 1983b). For example, positive sharp waves may be found in the deltoid and bicep muscles, both innervated by C5–6, but not in the cervical paraspinal muscles, as expected. In some nerve root abnormalities, findings of unstable muscle cell membrane potentials and decreased recruitment may be discovered. As an example, occasional abnormalities may be found in the medial gastrocnemius and soleus muscles of the leg, while other muscle groups, which are not innervated by S1, are spared.

Findings of positive sharp waves and fibrillations in the multifidus muscles alone (deep paraspinal muscles) may be a good indication of motor root nerve irritation via the motor root primary dorsal ramus. Motor abnormalities alone may not be associated with pain per se unless the sensory nerve fibers also are involved.

THERMOGRAPHY (HIGH-RESOLUTION) INFRARED IMAGING

The newest neurophysiologic examination technique is high-resolution (electronic) infrared thermography, also known as neurothermography or HRI. This technique depends on the use of a highly sensitive electronic infrared scanning camera to ascertain the autonomic sympathetic peripheral nerve output (Figure 28.11).

Normalcy is manifested by showing little or no side-to-side variations in skin surface temperatures. When the individual is equilibrated and repetitive infrared scanning photos are taken, damage to the autonomic nerve component is revealed by the persistence of abnormality. These thermographic abnormalities in the extremities and related areas of the back have been correlated with a high degree of accuracy with other neurophysiological studies (Green, Noran, Coyle, & Gildemeister, 1985). According to reports in the literature, the correlation between thermographic findings and myelography may be as high as 90%. Ochoa, a student of basic pain mechanisms, has stated that it is the best test of the autonomic peripheral system (Ochoa, 1990).

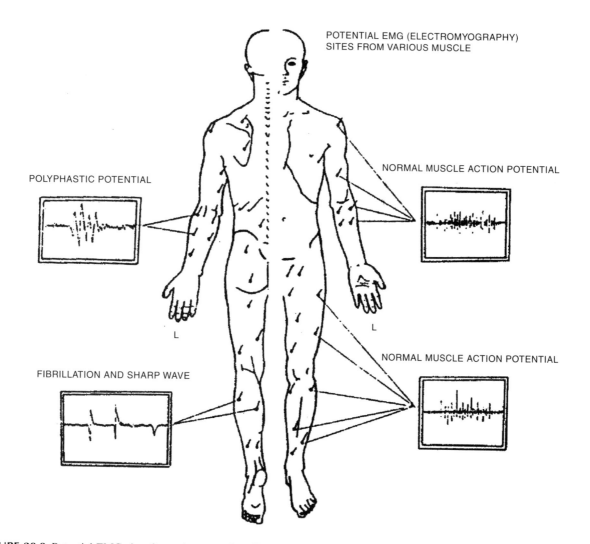

FIGURE 28.8 Potential EMG sites for various muscles. (From *Contemporary Orthopaedics*, Nov. 1987, Vol. 15, No. 5. Reproduced with permission.)

Comments

Comments concerning the use of thermography (HRI) include:

- "Thermography, a culminate temperature mapping achieved by this procedure allows delineation of the territory of the skin affected by dysfunction of peripheral nerves. The fiber types evaluated with telethermography are sympathetic C-fibers" (Pulst & Haller, 1981). "At present, thermography is the most valuable test available for evaluationg the autonomic nervous system" (Ochoa, 1990).
- "Thermography is a safe, noninvasive test which does not involve the use of ionizing radiation. It is a test of physiological function and may aid in the interpretation obtained by the other tests. Thermography can be useful in diagnosis of selective neurological or musculoskeletal conditions. "Thermography is useful in the diagnosis of reflex sympathetic dystrophy syndrome" (American Academy of Physical Medicine and Rehabilitation, 1990).
- "There is absolutely no diagnostic method more specific for cutaneous autonomic dysfunction than thermography. Thermography is the only means by which initial signs of vasomotor instability occurring in sympathetic dysfunction may be observed. The value of this in diagnosis, prognosis and treatment cannot be achieved by any other laboratory or clinical diagnostic device at present available to medicine" (Stanton-Hicks, 1990).
- "Many cases of SMP/RSD are less than obvious and may require adjunctive diagnostic tests, which may include an assessment of surface temperature, particularly by infrared

thermography" (Harden, 1990). In an editorial response to his comments, he stated that the term *SMP* should be used whenever an autonomic abnormality is detected by thermograms (Brenna, 1990).

CASE REPORTS

CASE 1

A 38-year-old male who was working as a brick mason fell 6 feet from a scaffold and landed on his buttocks. The patient initially had severe pain in the buttocks that resolved within 3 weeks. Continual pain radiated down his right leg in a sciatic distribution. Conservative therapy, including 2 weeks of bed rest, analgesics, and anti-inflammatory medication, reduced the pain by 50%. During the following 3 months, the patient worked 4 days per week.

Based on the slow clinical improvement in a patient whose neurological examination, including reflex, motor, and sensory nerve tests, was normal, a decision was needed regarding whether to proceed with myelography. Noting that the patient had experienced a reaction to IVP dye one year previously, it was decided to continue with additional conservative therapy and to perform comprehensive neurophysiological testing.

The EMG showed no paraspinal or peripheral muscle signs of denervation such as fibrillations, positive sharp waves, or decreased recruitment pattern. Cerebrally recorded, peripherally stimulated dermatomal evoked potentials showed no delay or distortion of the evoked responses. Motor and sensory nerve conduction studies were normal with the exception of the right H-reflex, which was 4 msec slower than the left. According to laboratory criteria, this is an abnormal finding. Electronic infrared thermography showed a deviation of the midline heat stripe to the right on the back, with a persistent decreased temperature on the right calf, suggestive of S1 radiculopathy.

Based on the positive thermogram and delayed H-reflex, a myelogram was performed, which showed a large S1 disc herniation. The patient experienced no adverse effects from the myelography and was referred for surgery and not included for long-term pain management services.

CASE 2

A 47-year-old female patient complained of severe pain in the back, radiating down the right leg for approximately 1 month. Four months previously, the patient had undergone a lumbar laminectomy for a myelographically demonstrated L4–5 disc protrusion on the right.

Examination showed a reduced right ankle jerk reflex compared to the left. Right Lasegue's test was positive at 30E. Physical examination revealed no other motor or sensory changes. The patient was hostile toward the orthopaedic surgeon who had performed the laminectomy and had considered obtaining legal redress.

Neurophysiological investigation showed needle EMG findings of positive sharp waves and fibrillations within 3 cm of the midline of the low back. Fibrillations, positive sharp waves, and decreased recruitment were found in the right medial gastrocnemius muscle. It should be noted that permanent changes within 3 cm of the midline of the low back can occur following laminectomy and have no clinical significance.

Dermatomal level evoked potentials showed the S1 dermatome to be delayed by 4 msec and decreased in amplitude by 40% compared to the opposite side. Motor and sensory nerve conductions were normal, and no delays in the H-reflex or F-times were noted.

Electronic infrared thermography showed an increase in the midline heat stripe at the area of the laminectomy scar. Decreased temperature was noted in the area of the right calf. This was a positive thermogram strongly suggestive of an S1 abnormality.

The patient was told that another myelogram was indicated, noting there could be a recurrence of the previous disc abnormality or that another disc could be ruptured. The patient confessed that 1 month following her previous laminectomy, she had fallen down a flight of stairs. The onset of her current symptoms had in fact appeared after her postoperative fall. A myelogram was performed, and a huge S1 right herniated disc was identified, suggestive of surgical intervention in the immediate future.

CASE 3

A 29-year-old male who had been employed as a railroad worker for 1.5 months stated that he had slipped and fallen backward on grease that had leaked from an engine. The patient had been off work for 90 days, complaining of severe back pain with numbness in his right foot and right testicle.

Neurologic examination showed no motor or reflex asymmetries and a varying sensory examination. Needle electromyography of the back and legs and a thermogram were also completely normal.

After being informed of this series of normal studies, the patient was more accepting of our psychiatrist's advice and our rehabilitation team's advice without further medical intervention that might reinforce the notion that he had been "seriously" injured on the job.

CASE 4

A 38-year-old male was seen because of pain in the back running down both legs, with some occasional numbness of the posterolateral aspect of the left leg. There was no numbness or pain in the anterior thigh or the area of the saphenous nerve. There was an occasional weak feeling and giveaway of the left leg over the right. The patient had fallen on the job. Knee jerks were diminished as were ankle jerks. An MRI-myelogram was done and was indicative of a lumbar disc. Noting the newness of the technique, the MRI-myelogram, the patient also had a lumbar Metrizamide invasive myelogram that showed, in essence, a less significant picture of the same lesion that was much better demonstrated on the MRI and myelogram alone. This indicates a new technique that is not invasive, which corroborates the patient's history and physical findings of back pain with radiation into the leg.

REFERENCES

American Academy of Physical Medicine and Rehabilitation, Subcommittee on Assessment of Diagnostic and Therapeutic Modalities (1990, December).

Behse, F., & Buchthal, F. (1971). Normal sensory conduction in the nerves of the leg in man. *Journal of Neurology, Neurosurgery, and Psychiatry, 34,* 404.

Bergamini, L., Bergamasco, B., & Fra, L. (1969). Somatosensory evoked cortical potentials in subjects with peripheral nerve lesions. *Electromyography, 5,* 121.

Braddom, R. I., & Johnson, E. W. (1974). Standardization of H-reflex and diagnostic use in S1 radiculopathy. *Archives of Physical and Medical Rehabilitation, 55,* 161.

Brenna, S. (Ed.). (1990, Fall). *Issues in Pain, 3*(1),

Buchthal, F. (1975). Electromyography (Part A). Amsterdam: Elsevier Biomedical Press.

Buchthal, F., & Rosenfalck, A. (1966). Evoked action potential and conduction velocity in human sensory nerves. *Brain Research, 3,* 1.

Burke, D., Skuse, N. F., & Lethlean A. K. (1974). Sensory conduction of the sural nerve in polyneuropathy. *Journal of Neurology, Neurosurgery, and Psychiatry, 37,* 647.

Chen, A. C. N. (1993). Human brainmeasures of clinical pain: A review. II. Tomographic recordings. *Pain, 54,* 133.

Cook, W. (1968). Effects of low frequency stimulation on the monosynaptic reflex (H-reflex) in man. *Neurology, 18,* 47.

Eisen, A., Schomer, D., & Melmod, C. (1977a). The application of F-wave measurements in the differentiation of proximal and distal upper limb entrapments. *Neurology, 27,* 662.

Eisen, A., Schomer, D., & Melmod, C. (1977b). An electrophysiological method for examining lumbosacral root compression. *Canadian Journal of Neurological Science, 4,* 117.

Green, J., Gildemeister, R., & Hazelwood, C. (1983). Dermatomally stimulated somatosensory cerebral evoked potentials in the clinical diagnosis of lumbar disc disease. *Clinical Electroncephalography, 14,* 152.

Green, J., Noran, W. H., Coyle, M. C., & Gildemeister, R. G. (1985). Infrared electronic thermography (ET): S noninvasive diagnostic neuroimaging tool. *Contemporary Orthopaedics, 11*(1), 39.

Green, J., Reilly, A., Schnitzlein, H. N., & Clewell, W. (1986). Comparison of neurothermography and contrast myelography. *Orthopedics, 9,* 1699–1704.

Green, J., et al. (submitted). An alternate method of objectively assessing subjective sensory complaints by perceptual threshold testing in a series of silicone exposed female patients complaining of dysesthesia, numbness, and/or tingling of one or more extremities. *American Journal of Pain Management.*

Harden, N. (1990, Fall). *Issues in Pain, 3*(1).

Hodes, R., Larrabee M. G., & German W. (1948). The human electromyogram in response to nerve stimulation and conduction velocity of motor axons. *Archives of Neurology and Psychiatry, 60,* 340.

Hume, A. L., & Cant, B. R. (1978). Conduction time in central somatosensory pathways in man. *Electroencephalography and Clinical Neurophysiology, 45,* 361.

Jebsen, R.H. (1967). Motor conduction velocities in the median and ulnar nerves. *Archives of Physical and Medical Rehabilitation, 48,* 185.

Jimenez, J., Easton, J. K. M., & Redford, J. B. (1970). Conduction studies of anterior and posterior tibial nerves. *Archives of Physical and Medical Rehabilitation, 51,* 164.

Katims, J., et al. (1991). Current perception threshold screening for carpal tunnel syndrome. *Archives of Environmental Health, 45*(4), 207–212.

Kimura, J. (1974). F-wave velocity in the central segment of the median and ulnar nerves: A study in normal subjects and in patients with Charcot-Marie-Tooth disease. *Neurology, 24,* 339.

Kimura, J. (1983). Electrodiagnosis in disease of nerve and muscle. Philadelphia: F. A. Davis.

Lachman, T., Shahani, B. T., & Young, R. R. (1980). Late responses as aids to diagnosis in peripheral neuropathy. *Journal of Neurology, Neurosurgery, and Psychiatry, 43,* 150.

Lamontagne, A., & Buchthal, F. (1970). Electrophysiological studies in diabetic neuropathy. *Journal of Neurology, Neurosurgery, and Psychiatry, 33,* 442.

Lefebvre-D' Amour, M., Shahani, B. T., et al. (1979). Importance of studying sural conduction and late responses in the evaluation of alcoholic subjects. *Neurology, 29,* 1600.

Ludin, H. P., & Beyeler, F. (1977). Temperature dependence on normal sensory nerve action potentials. *Journal of Neurology, 216,* 173.

Lundervold, A., Bruland, H., & Stensrud, P. (1965). Conduction velocity in peripheral nerves: A general introduction. *Acta Neurologica Scandinavica, 13,* 259.

Magiadery, J. W., Porter, W. E., Park A M., & Teasdale R. D. (1952). Electrophysiological studies of nerve and reflex activity in normal man. *Bulletin, Johns Hopkins Hospital, 88,* 449.

Magiadery, J., & McDougal, D. B. (1950). Electrophysiological studies of nerve and reflex activity in normal man. I. Identification of certain reflexes in the electromyogram and the conduction velocity of peripheral nerve fibers. *Bulletin, Johns Hopkins Hospital, 86,* 265.

Mayer, R. F., & Feldman, R. G. (1967). Observations on the nature of the F-wave in man. *Neurology, 17,* 147.

Melvin, J. L., Harris, D. H., & Johnson, E. W. (1966). Sensory and motor conduction velocities in the ulnar and median nerves. *Archives of Physical and Medical Rehabilitation, 47,* 511.

Ochoa, J. (1990). Contemporary techniques in assessing peripheral nervous system function. *American Journal of EEG Technology, 30,* 29–44.

Panayiotopoulos, C. P., & Scarpalezos, S. (1977). F-wave studies in the deep peroneal nerve: Part 1, Chronic renal failure; Part 2, Limb-girdle muscular dystrophy. *Journal of Neurological Science, 31,* 331.

Pascual-Leone, A., Houser, C. M., Rease, K., et al. (1993). Safety of rapid-rate transcranial magnetic stimulation in normal volunteers. *Electroencephalography and Clinical Neurophysiology, 84,* 120.

Petajan, J. H. (1974). Clinical electromyographic studies of the diseases of the motor unit. *Electroencephalography and Clinical Neurophysiology, 36,* 395.

Petajan, J. H., & Philip, B A. (1969). Frequency control of motor unit action potentials. *Electroencephalography and Clinical Neurophysiology, 27,* 66.

Sacco, G., Buchthal, F., & Rosenfalck, P. (1962). Motor unit potentials at different ages. *Archives of Neurology, 6,* 44.

Stanton-Hicks, M. (1990, December). Director of Pain Clinic at the Cleveland Clinic, Cleveland, OH.

Uricchio, J. V. (1983). Electronic thermography. *Journal, Florida Medical Association, 70,* 889.

Uyematsu, S. (1983). *Telethermography in the differential diagnosis of reflex sympathetic dystrophy and chronic pain syndrome.* New York: Elsevier Biomedical Press.

Wexler, C. E. (1983a). *Atlas of thermographic patterns.* Tarzana, CA: Thermographic Services, Inc.

Wexler, C. E. (1983b). *An overview of liquid crystal and electronic lumbar, thoracic, and cervical thermography.* Tarzana, CA: Thermographic Services, Inc.

Yap, C. B., & Hirota, T. (1967). Sciatic nerve motor conduction velocity study. *Journal of Neurology, Neurosurgery, and Psychiatry, 30,* 232m.

Section V

Approaches to Chronic and Acute Pain

29

Epidural Steroid Injection: A Review of Indications, Techniques, and Interpretation of Results

W. David Leak, M.D., D.A.B.P.M. and A. Elizabeth Ansel, R.N.

INTRODUCTION

This chapter is written with the specific focus as an applied clinical tool for practitioners of pain management. Acute applications for epidural injection, such as labor and delivery and elective surgical regional anesthesia, are not within the parameters of this chapter. The information imparted is directed to clinicians with a basic understanding of normal and pathologic anatomy, physiology, pharmacology, and basic physics.

The placement of chemicals for diagnostic, prognostic, and therapeutic purposes in the epidural space is widely practiced and published. More than 447 references are available from the National Library of Medicine for the search phrase *epidural injection* and 20,471 for the keyword *epidural*. The practice of medicine has become more complicated not by the nature of disease, but by the maze of authoritative yet illogical denial "rationale" by third-party payers. The use of epidural injection, although a very useful clinical tool, is also underappreciated and thus undervalued relative to associated risk. This chapter assists not only in the clinical application of epidural injection, but the administrative practice as well.

The key clinical pearl: Epidural injection is not experimental or investigational.

HISTORICAL BACKGROUND

Clinical reports of the earliest epidural anesthesia have been credited to James Corning. Corning used intraspinal cocaine on two subjects: a dog, to stop the animal from masturbating, and a human with "spinal weakness and seminal incontinence." These were classified as neurological illnesses. The results were reported in the fall of 1885 in the *New York Medical Journal*. European urologists Cathelin and Sicard of France documented epidural placement via the sacral route in the early 1900s. Epidural injection to treat sciatica was described by Viner in 1925. Edwards and Hingson reported continuous caudal epidural anesthesia in 1942 (Kafiluddi & Hahn, 2000). Interventional procedures can be partitioned into three major purposes: (1) diagnostic, (2) prognostic, and (3) therapeutic. Historically, epidural steroid injection has been viewed as therapeutic, applied in many cases to sciatica. Epidural injection with various agents may be diagnostic. Injection of epidural steroids yielding relief suggests inflammatory disease. Injection of epidural local anesthetics with lower extremity pain relief well beyond the duration of the local anesthetic suggests autonomic dysfunction. If pain does not return after diagnostic epidural injection, the procedure is therapeutic. Should pain return after a short duration of relief (hours, days, weeks), the procedure is prognostic for future interventions.

The key clinical pearl: Epidural injection and infusion are neither new nor investigational.

0-8493-0926-3/02/$0.00+$1.50
© 2002 by CRC Press LLC

ANATOMY

The epidural space is confined to the cranial and spinal canal. The most common reference is the space between the walls of the vertebral canal and the dura mater of the spinal cord (Stedman, 1999). It extends from the most cephalad aspect of the cranium surrounding the brain with compartmental interruption at the formen magnum. In the spinal canal, it extends caudally to the sacrococcygeal junction. Thus, epidural therapies and pathology may occur from the cranium to the caudal canal. Accessing the epidural space in the spinal column had been traditionally taught as a "blind technique," palpating surface anatomy and advancing the needle using proprioceptive feedback. Numerous terms have been used to describe the sensations one should appreciate during various phases of this "blind procedure." The terms include words such as give, pop, release, and loss of resistance. When taught by experts, an appreciation of these mystical sensations can be regarded as universal truths that guarantee proper procedural performance. Numerous tissue plains that are below the skin have give, and will pop, release, and lose resistance but will direct a needle far away from the epidural space. The advent of fluoroscopic guidance for spinal injection procedures has revealed that massive amounts of misinformation existed relative to the anatomy, proprioception, and behavior of infusions into the epidural space.

Leak demonstrated that board-certified anesthesiologists who routinely performed blind epidural injections could not reliably identify spinal levels when surface anatomy identification techniques were used alone. When compared to fluoroscopy, vertebral interspaces (specifically the L3–4) could not be identified using conventional anatomy surface landmarks in patients in the prone position. Clinicians and researchers have published significant prospective studies demonstrating the essential need for fluoroscopy when performing epidural blocks for painful diseases (Bogduk, Aprill, & Derby, 1995; Manchikanti & Bakhit, 1999). Derby and White published a missed target rate of over 30% using blind techniques for epidurals. The traditional teachings suggested that the spread of injection solutions in the epidural space could be calculated. Teaching that the volume of an anesthetic solution would cover predictable anatomic areas has been proven erroneous by numerous clinical reports (Bogduk, et al., 1995). Figure 29.1 demonstrates the alignment of an epidural needle in the midline of an adult male patient. Attempts to maintain anatomic symmetry are demonstrated. Equal distance of the pedicles from the spinous process in a true anterior posterior radiographic projection should yield midline needle placement. Figure 29.2 demonstrates a unilateral flow of an 8-cc water-soluble contrast injection in the thoracic epidural space. Despite midline needle placement, the contrast migrated to the right side of the patient's spinal canal. The flow is not uniform in the cephalad caudad direction either.

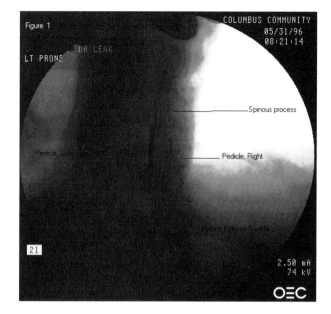

FIGURE 29.1 The alignment of an epidural needle in the midline of an adult male patient.

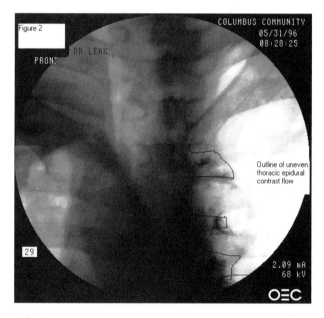

FIGURE 29.2 A male patient injected in the prone position via midline epidural needle placement with 8 cc of contrast agent.)

Figures 29.1 and 29.2 demonstrate a single aberrancy that could lead to misinterpretation of the effectiveness of an epidural injection. If the patient's multilevel neuritis was left sided the clinical conclusion might be that the patient was disingenuous with his pain complaint because the epidural failed to relieve his pain. This anatomic mishap could lead to catastrophic events for the patient, including behavioral modification in the face of unrelieved organic pain. A missed diagnosis could lead to a medical liability judgment against the physician.

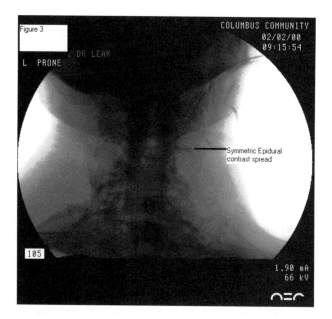

FIGURE 29.3 Normal-appearing anatomy of the cervical spine.

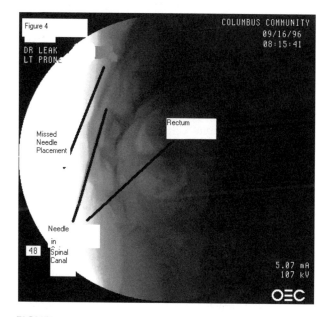

FIGURE 29.4 A needle placed in the caudal canal using direct fluoroscopic guidance.

Headaches of cervical origin have been reported as often as 50% of the time. Knowledge of cervical spinal anatomy for injection is paramount (Dwyer, Aprill, & Bogduk, 1990). Reportedly, one of the most frequently missed spinal injections is the blind caudal approach. Knowledge of anatomy is critical, but there is no substitute for direct fluoroscopic visualization. Figure 29.3 demonstrates the normal-appearing anatomy of the cervical spine. A misplaced needle in the cervical region can have rapid and irreversible aberrant results. Avoidance of the spinal cord, dome of the lung, and carotid and vertebral arteries is easier said than done using blind techniques.

Figure 29.4 shows a needle placed in the caudal canal using direct fluoroscopic guidance. The hazards are not insignificant. Interosseous injection, rectal injection, bladder injection, and simple missed blocks can have catastrophic effects.

The key clinical pearl: Knowledge of radiographic anatomy and the use of radiographic guidance is the standard of care for diagnostic, prognostic, and therapeutic spinal injection procedures.

THE WORK-UP

Although mastery of anatomy for execution of the epidural injection is required, the most important component of the procedure is performing it correctly. The right physician should do the right procedure on the right patient for the right reason. Standard requirements for epidural injections are not widely known, although they do exist from several sources. Guidelines have been written by The American Society of Anesthesiologists (ASA), the International Spinal Injection Society (ISIS), and the Pain Net, to name a few. There is variation between the "guidelines" of the various organizations.

Patient history and physical examination should generate substantial subjective and objective evidence for the procedure. The impressions and plan should be consistent with the history and physical. Avoidance of being the "itinerant surgeon" is of paramount importance. A patient may be referred for a series of epidural injections for back pain or sciatica. The performance of a transient palliative procedure that masks or delays diagnosis of cancer, discitis, or other progressive and deadly diseases is below the standard of care. Thus, a review of records, history, and physical examination, and a review of relevant laboratory and radiographic studies constitute the minimum standard prior to performance of the procedure.

WORK-UP COMPONENTS

The specific components of the work-up should cover the following general standard:

History

1. Chief complaint.
2. History of present illness (include other work-ups and treatment for the current problem).
3. Past medical and surgical history (e.g., age is an important factor in the work-up of complaints of low-back pain from a 20-year-old subject).
4. Social history (e.g., work, smoking, substance abuse, and secondary gain factors should be explored).

5. Family history (rheumatoid disease, coagulopathy, cancer, etc.).

6. Allergies and specific reactions and where the events are documented:
   a. Beware of patients who are allergic to "all nonsteroidal anti-inflammatory drugs."
   b. Supplementation of pain relief with scheduled drugs may not excuse the practitioner from contributory negligence or malpractice claims in the event of drug-related morbidity or mortality.
   c. When total classes of nondependency producing agents are reported without any healthcare professional's objective documentation, consider allergy testing.

7. Medication history (a copy of all pharmacy printouts from the previous 12 months is recommended).

8. Review of systems.

Physical Examination

1. Vital signs:
   a. They will change in association with performance of epidurals.
   b. Noxious stimulation associated with traumatic introduction of a trochar into an already hyperalgesic area may produce a potentially fatal change in a patient who is already hyperdynamic.
   c. A patient rendered "normotensive" by antihypertensive agents may be volume deficient and suffer fatal consequences from epidural infusion and associated vasodilation.

2. Cardiovascular exam:
   a. Mortality associated with epidural injection in the face of uncompensated aortic valvular stenosis is a preventable circumstance. The epidural may cause massive vasodilatation that may not be adequately compensated for in an individual with severe aortic valvular stenosis, resulting in profound and irreversible hypotension.

3. Neurologic exam:
   a. Sensory, motor, and reflex findings normal and aberrant should be documented prior to commencing a procedure with the capacity to cause neurologic damage.

4. Musculoskeletal exam:
   a. Tenderness pre- and post-procedure.
   b. Noxious range of motion.
   c. Pain-alleviating range of motion.
   d. Documentation of range of motion.

5. Integument:
   a. Infectious lesions of the skin in the path of the epidural are direct contraindications to performing the procedure.
   b. Psoriatic lesions should not be traversed if in the path of an epidural injection:
      i. Displacing keratinotic and possibly nonsterile tissue into the epidural space may be hazardous.
   c. Bruises may suggest coagulation problems:
      i. Epidural hematomas are associated with severe morbidity and mortality.

Laboratory

1. Complete blood count (CBC):
   a. Evidence of infection or, more important, absence of infection should be documented.
   b. Leukopenia that may risk serious infection.
   c. Anemia that may become clinically significant with required volume expansion.
   d. Thrombocytopenia resulting in insufficient clotting.

2. Coagulation profile:
   a. Prolonged bleeding times may result in bleeding and anemia.
   b. Prolonged coagulation times may result in paralyzing intraspinal hematomas.

3. Electrolytes plus calcium and magnesium:
   a. Sodium has been observed to drop after exposure to anesthetics.
   b. Sodium, potassium, calcium, and magnesium may be low in association with chronic painful diseases via renal elimination.
   c. Glucose may have dangerous fluxes in susceptible individuals, such as diabetics, when epidural steroids are administered.

4. Erythrocyte sedimentation rate (ESR) and C-reactive protein (CRP):
   a. Inflammatory processes, both infectious and noninfectious, may yield elevated ESR and CRP.
   b. The CRP can be followed to determine whether the inflammation is progressive because it responds very quickly to circulating pyrogens and complement complexes.

5. Urinalysis:
   a. Provides a broad snapshot of endocrine, immune, and metabolic functions.
   b. Specific gravity may indicate volume depletion or overload.
   c. Glucose level may indicate risk for undiagnosed diabetes.
   d. Infectious processes revealed in the urine are a relative contraindication to epidural injection

Radiographic Studies

1. Plain radiographs:
   a. The target region must be imaged in the anterior/posterior and lateral views to eliminate the presence of dangerous anatomic anomalies that may create complications in an otherwise uncomplicated procedure.
   b. Spina bifida presence should be known prior to needle introduction.
   c. Hypertrophic spinous processes and facets may impede successful injection.
   d. Calcification of interspinous ligaments may wreak havoc with an intraspinal approach.
2. Scintillation scans:
   a. Primary metastatic oncologic disease may be revealed.
   b. Discitis or osteomyelitis may be discovered.
3. Computerized axial tomography (CAT):
   a. Depending on the history and physical examination, a CAT scan may be indicated.
   b. With a history of cancer, a CAT scan is a must due to the potential for metastatic or recrudescent disease.
4. Magnetic resonance imaging (MRI):
   a. Prior to embarking on an invasive therapeutic trial, comprehensive information concerning soft tissue structures of the spine should be known.
   b. Discovery of damage or destruction of tissue after an invasive procedure, such as an epidural injection, subjects the procedure and the physician performing the procedure to being considered pathologic etiology.

Electrophysiologic Studies

1. Somatosensory evoked potentials (SSEP):
   a. Measures sensory (the pain) aspects of nerve function
   b. Electromyography (EMG) looks for significant motor dysfunction
2. Selective tissue conductance (STC):
   a. A direct measure of autonomic dysfunction that responds instantly to change
   b. Evaluates changes in sudomotor and vasomotor activity
3. Cold pressor:
   a. Another assessment of autonomic vasomotor function

Note that overlapping aberrancies in all three electrophysiologic studies direct the clinician to a more focused work-up. Objective data do reflect the presence or absence of nociception. The selective tissue conductance, cold pressor, and somatosensory evoked potential allow the physician to quantify physiologic change brought about through therapeutic intervention.

The work-up includes trial responses to the physical therapy, fitness conditioning, transcutaneous electrical nerve stimulation, smoke cessation, laboratory, and appropriate radiographic and electrophysiological capture of data prior to epidural injection. The radiographic data minimally consists of plain film. As the case becomes more complex and recalcitrant to conservative measures, CAT and MRI scans should be obtained.

Good outcomes go largely unnoticed except by the occasional grateful patient. A bad outcome due to poor preparation may result in alienation of colleagues and patients. The list of known complications and adverse events may appear to grow exponentially if preparation is not systematic and meticulous. The diagnosis must be specific and match the procedural plan.

The term "rule out" negates a diagnosis and leads to third-party rejection of the procedural claim. The cancellation of the work-up may be included in the denial as the impression was reduced to "rule out." The Healthcare Finance Administration (HCFA), the administrative and regulatory body for Medicare, requires that the documentation for epidural injection meet their criteria for diagnosis and treatment prior to issuing reimbursement. This is not innately evil; it is just difficult to find in the voluminous policy manual. The manual is available to all Medicare providers. It will be sent to the billing address, which may or may not be the mailing office address. If your Medicare remittances are routed to a lockbox, so is your Medicare Policy Manual. The manual can also be found on the Internet at www.hcfa.gov. The manual can be printed from the Internet and contains over 350 pages. Familiarity with the manual will improve the economic and social relationship between the patient and practitioner. The coverage policies with HCFA are dynamic. By the time this chapter is published, the policies will have changed. The HCFA Web site will be the best source for current coverage information on epidural or any other injection.

Clinical impressions that may be appropriate for epidural injection include but are not limited to:

991.1   Frostbite of hand
991.2   Frostbite of foot
53.13   Post-therapeutic polyneuropathy
722.2   Displacement of intervertebral disc, site unspecified, without myelopathy
Discogenic syndrome NOS
Herniation of nucleus pulposus NOS
Intervertebral disc NOS:
   Extrusion
   Prolapse

Protrusion

Rupture

Neuritis or radiculitis due to displacement or rupture of intervertebral disc

337.21 Reflex sympathetic dystrophy of the upper limb

337.22 Reflex sympathetic dystrophy of the lower limb

724.3 Sciatica neuralgia, or neuritis of the sciatic nerve

353.6 Phantom limb (syndrome)

577.0 Acute pancreatitis

Giving a disease a name does not necessarily mean that is what the patient has; thus, objective criteria should be used when possible. The U.S. healthcare culture may contain numerous third-party administrative encumbrances. The administrative information request for documentation can be overcome with proper radiographs, laboratory, and electrophysiology studies. Objective evidence of motor, sensory, or autonomic function allows the practitioner to practice evidence-based medicine. The known hazards of the procedure mandate the laboratory assessment.

Electrophysiologic studies were previously mentioned as instruments of objective measurement. Included in this is an explanation to the third-party payer of why such instruments are medically necessary and are indicated for epidural injections. The detailed scientific answers follow.

Somatosensory evoked potential: SSEP studies (or somatosensory evoked potentials) are the evaluation of the central nervous system via sensory tracts in the spinal cord connecting the extremities to the brain. This is the mechanism by which humans are able to perceive pain and temperature.

Selective tissue conductance: The operational definition is the relative ability of biological tissue to conduct a weak (DC) electrical signal which is applied for a selected period of time to a selected limited and restricted surface area of that tissue.

Conductance is considered to include any or all of the methodological aspects of instrumentation, measurement, assessment procedures, applications, and analysis of selective tissue conductance data.

One of the most important roles of the autonomic nervous system is to maintain a relative constancy of the internal milieu of the body. Because tissues and organs can function optimally only within a relatively small range of physical conditions, the neural and hormonal control of internal temperature, circulation, and fluid and electrolyte contents must be maintained at all times. Otherwise, the results of even brief periods of autonomic subsystem failure can result in illness, tissue dysfunction, or death.

To provide adequate control of the internal environment, the homeostatic mechanism must operate efficiently to compensate for rapid changes in the conditions outside the body. The responsive action, often exemplified by physiological change, which is caused by exposure to heat or cold, is mediated primarily through vasomotor and sudomotor divisions of the sympathetic systems.

Figures 29.5 and 29.6 demonstrate pre- and post-procedural selective tissue conductance studies that corresponded to the patient's clinical subjective complaint. The key clinical pearl: to document objective parameters prior to interventions.

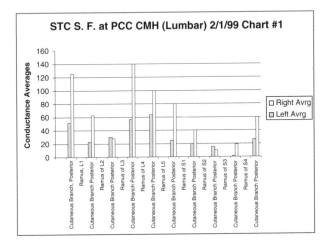

FIGURE 29.5 The asymmetry and increased activity of the nerve roots that correspond to the patient pattern of pain prior to an epidural injection and decompression of nerve roots.

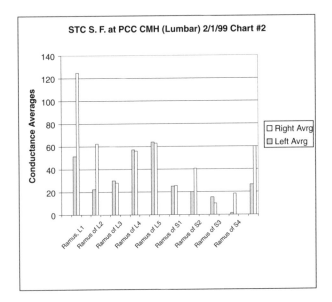

FIGURE 29.6 Substantial reduction of nerve activity of L-4, L-5, and S-1 24 hours after epidural decompression and adhesioloysis associated with elimination of the subjective complaint of pain.

PHARMACOLOGY

Numerous agents are used in the injection of the epidural space. Agents include but are not limited to:

1. Saline
2. Local anesthetics
3. Steroids
4. Alpha-2-adrenergic agonists
5. Antimicrobials
6. Neurolytics
7. N-Methyl-D-Aspartate Agonist

Below is a description of the two classes of agents most frequently injected into the epidural space — steroids and local anesthetics. The other agents are addressed elsewhere in the text. The information below is primarily from the Generex CD manufacturer's description of the drug with little modification. Note that although injection of steroids is one of the most popular applications, epidural injection is not one of the labeled uses.

STEROIDS

Methylprednisolone acetate is an "anti-inflammatory glucocorticoid, for intramuscular, intrasynovial, soft tissue, or intralesional injection. It is available in three strengths: 20 mg/ml; 40 mg/ml; 80 mg/ml. Glucocorticoids (e.g., hydrocortisone), which also have salt-retaining properties, are used in replacement therapy in adrenocortical deficiency states." Their synthetic analogs are used primarily for their potent anti-inflammatory effects in disorders of many organ systems. Glucocorticoids cause profound and varied metabolic effects. In addition, they modify the body's immune response to diverse stimuli. The product contains benzyl alcohol, which is potentially toxic when administered locally to neural tissue.

Prolonged use of corticosteroids may produce posterior subcapsular cataracts, glaucoma with possible damage to the optic nerves, and may enhance the establishment of secondary ocular infections due to fungi or viruses.

Avascular necrosis has been reported with a wide variety of doses and durations of recurrent exposures to steroids.

Average and large doses of cortisone or hydrocortisone can cause elevation of blood pressure, salt and water retention, and increased excretion of potassium. All corticosteroids increase calcium excretion. The list below is a partial compilation from numerous sources that lends some insight into the dangers of unmonitored steroid use. There will be no declaration that the maximum number of injections is three. One should follow electrolytes, cortisol, glucose, weight, complete blood counts, and manufacturer recommendations for diagnosing and management of toxicity when using these agents.

Prolonged or repeated exposure to steroids may result in:

- Fluid and electrolyte disturbances:
  - Sodium retention
  - Potassium loss
  - Fluid retention
  - Hypokalemic alkalosis
  - Congestive heart failure in susceptible patients
  - Hypertension
- Musculoskeletal disturbances:
  - Muscle weakness
  - Vertebral compression fractures
  - Steroid myopathy
  - Aseptic necrosis of femoral and humeral heads
  - Loss of muscle mass
  - Osteoporosis
  - Pathologic fracture of long bones
- Gastrointestinal disturbances:
  - Peptic ulcer with possible subsequent abdominal distention, perforation and, hemorrhage
  - Ulcerative esophagitis
  - Pancreatitis
- Dermatologic disturbances:
  - Impaired wound-healing
  - Facial erythema
  - Thin fragile skin
  - Hyperhidrosis sweating
  - Petechiae and ecchymosis
  - May suppress reactions to skin tests
- Neurological disturbances:
  - Convulsions
  - Vertigo
- Endocrine disturbances:
  - Menstrual irregularities
  - Decreased carbohydrate tolerance
  - Development of Cushinoid state
  - Manifestations of latent diabetes mellitus
  - Suppression of growth in children
  - Secondary adrenocortical and pituitary suppression
- Ophthalmic disturbances:
  - Posterior subcapsular cataracts
  - Glaucoma
  - Increased intraocular pressure
  - Exophthalmos
- Metabolic disturbance:
  - Negative nitrogen balance due to protein catabolism

Methylprednisolone is indicated for many inflammatory diseases. The specific indication for intraspinal disc disease is not specifically listed. The Food and Drug Administration Bulletin of April 12, 1982 provides information about off-label use of FDA-certified drugs.

LOCAL ANESTHETICS

Local anesthetics block the generation and conduction of nerve impulses, presumably by increasing the threshold for electrical excitation in the nerve, by slowing the propagation of the nerve impulse, and by reducing the rate rise of the action potential. The progression of anesthesia is related to the diameter, myelination, and conduction velocity of affected nerve fibers. Clinically, the order of loss of nerve function is as follows: (1) pain, (2) temperature, (3) touch, (4) proprioception, and (5) motor function.

Systemic absorption of local anesthetics can produce effects on the cardiovascular and central nervous systems. At blood concentrations achieved with therapeutic doses, changes in cardiac conduction, excitability, refractoriness, contractility, and peripheral vascular resistance are minimal. Toxic blood concentrations depress cardiac conduction and excitability, which may lead to atrioventricular block, ventricular arrhythmias, and to cardiac arrest, sometimes resulting in mortalities. Myocardial contractility is depressed and peripheral vasodilation occurs, leading to decreased cardiac output and arterial blood pressure. Incremental dosing is necessary with blind injection. Fluoroscopy with contrast reduces the incidence of adverse reactions associated with injection of local anesthetics anywhere other than the target site.

Following systemic absorption, local anesthetics can produce central nervous system stimulation, depression, or both. Apparent central nervous system stimulation is usually manifested as restlessness, tremors, and shivering, progressing to convulsions, followed by depression and coma, and progressing ultimately to respiratory arrest. Local anesthetics have a primary depressant effect on the medulla and on higher centers. In some European countries, slow infusion of lidocaine has been used to treat seizures. The depressed stage may occur without a prior excited stage.

COMPLICATIONS

Informed consent is critical as complications do occur. Patients should be asked to make decisions that a reasonable person would make if placed in a similar circumstance as the patient. Guarantees and assurances should not be promised, but failure of expectation constitutes a perceived and real breach of contract. Do not say, "This will definitely take all your pain away, and there is no risk of anything bad happening to you." The following components should be included in the informed consent and thought process for treating complications:

1. The patient should be aware of the nature (invasive vs. noninvasive) of the procedure.
2. The patient should be aware of the purpose (diagnostic, prognostic, or therapeutic) of the procedure.
3. The patient should be aware of the alternatives to the procedure (e.g., behavioral, pharmacological, physiotherapy, less-invasive procedures).
4. The patient should be aware of the course of the disease without the procedure (e.g., remain the same with unacceptable pain, get worse relative to pain and physiologic dysfunction).
5. The patient should be aware of the risk of the procedure. This is the predominant issue relative to informed consent in liability cases. The consent as a whole is important, but lack of disclosure of salient risks is often an important point of contention. The following is a brief list that should be disclosed when consenting for epidural procedures:.
   a. Bleeding (perioperative CBC and vital signs)
   b. Infection (perioperative CBC and vital signs)
   c. Adverse reactions to drugs (monitoring, perioperative CBC and vital signs)
   d. Allergic reactions to materials used (monitoring, perioperative cbc, and vital signs)
   e. Injury to any/all organs/organ systems (monitoring, perioperative CBC, and vital signs)
   f. Pain may be made worse (monitoring, pain rating scales, vital signs, SSEPs, and STCs)
   g. Pain may not be relieved (monitoring, pain rating scales, vital signs, SSEPs, and STCs)
   h. May need further procedures
   i. Paralysis (monitoring with emphasis on neurological, pain rating scales, vital signs, SSEPs, and STCs)
   j. Seizures (monitoring, pain rating scales, vital signs, CBC, electrolytes, drug levels, toxicology screen for additional agents such as cocaine, electroencephalogram, chest X-ray to follow potential seizure related aspiration, arterial blood gases)
   k. Collapsed lung (monitoring, vital signs, chest X-ray, arterial blood gas if vitals are unstable or patient is otherwise not healthy)
   l. Pulmonary embolism (monitoring, vital signs, chest X-ray, arterial blood gas if vitals are unstable or patient is otherwise not healthy)
   m. Headache (monitoring, vital signs, CBC, electrolytes, bedrest, fluid, caffeine, adrenocorticotropic hormone (ACTH), dural repair)
   n. Numbness (CBC, monitoring with emphasis on neurological, pain rating scales, vital signs, SSEPs, and STCs)

o. Weakness (CBC, monitoring with emphasis on neurological, pain rating scales, vital signs, SSEPs, and STCs)

p. Sexual dysfunction (monitoring with emphasis on neurological, pain rating scales, vital signs, SSEPs, and STCs)

q. Bowel dysfunction (monitoring with emphasis on gastrointestinal function, pain rating scales, vital signs, SSEPs, and STCs)

r. Bladder dysfunction (monitoring with emphasis on urological function, pain rating scales, vital signs, SSEPs, and STCs)

s. Death (advanced cardiopulmonary resuscitation)

SUMMARY

The clinical economic benefits of indicated epidural injection in properly selected patients are positive. Patients have experienced alleviation from the intractable side effects of painful diseases. This has facilitated completion of otherwise failed physical therapy. The agents commonly used are frequently applied in an off-label but widely published and acceptable manner.

Knowledge of radiographic anatomy, pharmacology, physiology, and medical management of perioperative co-morbid disease is critical. Equal importance must be placed on early recognition of complications by constant monitoring (physical exam as well as electronic monitors).

The procedure can be performed safely by properly trained physicians, but must always be respected for its capacity to precipitate severe and deadly consequences.

The evolution of additional agents that may be effective in long-term pain relief make epidural injection one of the most valuable current and future skills in the physician's repertoire.

REFERENCES

Bogduk, N., Aprill, C., & Derby, R. (1995). Epidural steroid injections. In *Spine care operative treatment* (Vol. 1, pp. 322–343). St. Louis: Mosby Yearbook.

Dwyer, A., Aprill, C. N., & Bogduk, N. (1990). Cervical zygapophyseal joint pain pattern:. A clinical evaluation. *Spine, 15*(6), 458–461.

Kafiluddi, R., & Hahn, M. B. (2000). Epidural neural blockade. *Practical Management of Pain 45*, 637–650.

Manchikanti, L., & Bakhit, C. E. (1999). Fluoroscopy is medically necessary for the performance of epidural steroids response. *Anesthesia and Analgesia, 89*, 1330.

Stedman's Medical Dictionary. (1999). Baltimore, MD: Williams & Wilkins.

30

Myofascial Trigger Point Injection

Hal S. Blatman, M.D.

INTRODUCTION

This chapter discusses injection of trigger points as a technique for treating the increased muscle tension and pain that is caused by trigger points. As such, trigger point injection is one of several "body work" techniques that have been shown to be effective in treating myofascial pain. Other techniques include acupressure, vapo-coolant spray with stretching, myofascial release, reflexology, acupuncture, aromatherapy and chiropractic adjustment.

Myofascial pain is defined as pain that is generated by myofascial trigger points. Trigger points form in muscle, fascia, and tendon as a tissue response to injury. Fascia is the connective tissue that intertwines through muscle and ligamentous structures. Tendons attach muscle to bone at both ends. Examples of injuries that activate or cause formation of trigger points include repetitive strain, lifting something too heavy, and sudden high-velocity stretching.

LOCATIONS OF TRIGGER POINTS

Trigger points can be located and treated in three anatomic zones in muscle tissue. These include the ligamentous/tendinous origin, the insertion of the muscle, and the muscle belly. Trigger points at the origin and insertion of the muscle may not be discretely palpable. These areas will be tender, however, and may refer pain to distant sites with palpation and needling. A trigger point in the muscle belly will create a taut band of muscle fibers extending from the origin to the insertion of the muscle. Trigger points in the muscle belly will usually be palpable as nodular densities within the taut band.

TREATMENT OF MYOFASCIAL PAIN

The successful treatment of myofascial pain involves stretching the involved muscles to their normal (healthy) resting length. Trigger point injection is a tool that "unlocks," or releases a trigger point, thereby allowing this stretch to occur. Unlocking trigger points with injection techniques may be an essential component of a treatment plan. Additionally, treatment will be more effective when all the musculature and trigger points involved in a particular pain pattern are collectively treated at the same time. Some trigger points can be treated with non-injection techniques, while other trigger points are injected. After injection, the injected muscles should be stretched with hands-on myofascial release techniques.

ACTIVE VS. LATENT TRIGGER POINTS

Optimal treatment of a myofascial pain condition requires the physician to understand that latent trigger points are usually a very important component of the patient's pain pattern. Limiting trigger point injection therapy to active, very tender, and pain-referring trigger points will severely limit the success of this treatment modality. Palpable latent trigger points that can be expected to refer pain to the area of complaint should usually be treated with injection therapy, even if they are not tender.

TRIGGER POINT INJECTION

Trigger point injection means placing a needle into a trigger point, and then injecting a liquid solution or suspension into the area. The term "dry needling" refers to placing a needle into a trigger point without injection of

0-8493-0926-3/02/$0.00+$1.50
© 2002 by CRC Press LLC

fluid, such as in acupuncture. Introducing a needle into a trigger point usually elicits a characteristic "twitch" response. With this twitch, the trigger point releases and the taut band relaxes. The twitch and subsequent relaxation are therapeutic, even without injection of fluid. Injection of fluid can have a synergistic effect by enhancing the relaxation response and/or decreasing post-needling discomfort.

Occasionally, needle insertion into a trigger point will not elicit a characteristic "twitch" response; however, the tissue may otherwise respond as expected, with concomitant relaxation and post-treatment soreness.

INDICATIONS FOR TRIGGER POINT INJECTION

Trigger point injections are indicated for the treatment of any patient with myofascial pain. Injection techniques will almost always facilitate relief of pain and restoration of function. Moreover, clinical improvement may not be possible without trigger point injection therapy. In general, the more chronic and more severe the condition, the more medically necessary injections become.

CONTRAINDICATIONS FOR TRIGGER POINT INJECTION

Contraindications for trigger point injection include infection at the injection site and allergy to injection medication. Relative contraindications for trigger point injection include patient use of anticoagulants and illness. In acutely ill patients, it may be best to limit treatment to one or two trigger point injections, administering these into the most active or important trigger point areas.

The duration of pain is not a contraindication for trigger point injection. Pain patterns of 20, 30, or more years will still respond to injection techniques.

PATIENT EVALUATION

An interim history should be obtained from every patient at the start of each office visit. It is important for the practitioner to understand how the patient's pain pattern is evolving in response to treatment. This helps determine which areas are more likely to require injection treatment at the time of the office visit.

A physical examination should also be performed on every patient prior to trigger point injection. During this examination, tenderness and activity of trigger points is evaluated. Treatment is best determined at the time of the office visit, based on the interim history, a thorough assessment of treatment results, and physical examination at the time of the office visit.

PATIENT INFORMED CONSENT

It is a good idea for patients to sign a document that represents informed consent prior to performing this invasive procedure. In addition, the American Academy of Pain Management Accreditation requires that the clinic documents informed consent for trigger point injections. The document should include the purpose of the procedure, alternative methods of treatment, common untoward effects, and risks of treatment.

CPT/BILLING CODE

The CPT/billing code for myofascial trigger point injections is 20550.

TECHNIQUE

The patient needs to be placed in a comfortable position, and the musculature to be injected should be totally relaxed. For most injections, the patient will be supine or prone. A patient will rarely be seated during injection. Some muscles are best injected with the patient lying on their side. With the muscles more relaxed, the technique is more easily performed and it is also less uncomfortable.

The muscle to be injected should be isolated as much as possible from major nerves, blood vessels, and visceral cavities. For example, when injecting the quadriceps, an effort should be made to isolate the femoral artery and nerve by palpation. When injecting the middle trapezius muscles, the needle should be kept mostly tangential to the chest wall, and the taut band should be isolated by palpation. Specific anatomical techniques are well illustrated elsewhere (Travell & Simons, 1983).

Most of the time, treatment will be effective if trigger points in the muscle belly are injected. For some conditions, it may be more important to also treat trigger points in the origin or insertion of the involved muscles. Optimal treatment of epicondylitis, for example, may require injection of both the origin and muscle belly trigger point zones.

It is usually not helpful to mark the skin over trigger points prior to injection. Palpating the taut band, eliciting a twitch response, and then marking the skin is likely to result in partial treatment of the trigger point. When a trigger point is even partially treated, the patient's pain pattern may shift to that of a more active trigger point. It is generally more time efficient if the area to be treated is identified by history and light palpation shortly before an injection is to be administered. With this in mind, however, it may be helpful for a partner to mark the painful areas they work on or find most tender.

The skin at the injection site should always be cleaned. Anything that is applied to the skin for cleaning can be absorbed — almost as if it were ingested. The best and least toxic cleaning agent may be ethyl alcohol. In diluted form it is commonly ingested in small amounts. Isopropyl alcohol is more commonly used for skin cleaning; its use is discouraged here because it is too toxic to drink.

Sterile gloves are not necessary, although gloves may be worn by the practitioner for protection from blood-borne pathogens. For practitioners who insist on not using rubber gloves, barrier creams may offer some protection. Good hand-washing techniques are also important for protecting the patient.

Needle size should be determined by the procedure. It is best to use the smallest diameter needle that is long enough to reach through the trigger point and allow adequate control by the technician. Cervical and intra-oral trigger points may be reached with a 1-in., 30-gauge needle. In larger people, a 1.5-in., 27-gauge needle may be necessary. Injecting trigger points in the gluteal muscles may require 2-in., 25-gauge needles. Some larger people require 3-in. or even 6-in. long spinal needles for buttocks trigger point injections. It takes considerable skill and practice to be able to use a 3-in., 25-gauge needle; 22-gauge needles are easier to use and are most necessary when the needle is 6-in. long.

Syringe size should be chosen so that the syringe is easy to hold and use and there is control over how much fluid is injected. Three-milliliter (3-ml) syringes may be the best choice most of the time. One-milliliter syringes are too small, and 5- and 10-cc syringes hold much more fluid than is necessary for an area of trigger points.

SOLUTIONS FOR INJECTION

For the most part, success with trigger point injection is much more related to where the needle is inserted than to which fluid is injected. This is underscored by the success of "dry needling."

SHORT-ACTING LOCAL ANESTHETIC AGENTS

Trigger point injection area soreness is generally lessened by local anesthetics. Short-acting local anesthetic agents usually work very well. Lidocaine and procaine may be the most commonly used of the local anesthetics for trigger point injections. Procaine is well tolerated and may have physiologic benefit beyond its local anesthetic effect. Allergic reactions are usually due to preservatives in the solution. Procaine can be purchased preservative-free, making allergic reactions rare.

The procaine purchased from standard medical supply companies is acidic, and infusion is accompanied by burning discomfort at the injection site. Some of this burning can be lessened by buffering the solution prior to injection. One method is to inject 3 cc of sodium bicarbonate into the typical 30-cc bottle of 1% procaine prior to using the bottle. This will neutralize the pH and injections will be

more comfortable. Preservative free procaine ordered from a compounding pharmacy can be buffered at the pharmacy with sodium hydroxide.

LONG-ACTING LOCAL ANESTHETIC AGENTS

Trigger point injection soreness may be lessened for a longer period of time by long-acting local anesthetics. Etidocaine and bupivocaine are two examples of long-acting local anesthetics that have been used for trigger point injections. The use of bupivocaine has been associated with myotoxicity, and this should be considered.

Although long-acting local anesthetics may prolong some level of anesthesia and thereby ease stretching and rehabilitation, I have not found this to be a noticeable advantage over the use of procaine.

HOMEOPATHIC AGENTS

There are various homeopathic agents that are currently used for trigger point injections. These agents may be very helpful, and they have not been shown to be harmful.

CORTICOSTEROID AGENTS

Corticosteroid agents should rarely be used for trigger point injections. There is little or no benefit in steroid injection compared with local anesthetic injection, provided the injection area is cleared of trigger points and the muscles are properly stretched afterward.

BOTULINUM TOXIN

Trigger points that are resistant to injection with local anesthetic and vapo-coolant spray-and-stretch may relax for a longer period of time after injection with botulinum toxin. Use of this agent for routine trigger point injections is discouraged.

EPINEPHRINE

Epinephrine decreases blood flow and should not be injected into a trigger point. Likewise, anesthetic agents that contain epinephrine should not be used for trigger point injection.

AMOUNT OF FLUID INJECTED

For the most part, success with trigger point injection is not related to how much fluid is injected. This is underscored by the success of "dry needling." To minimize the amount of fluid that is injected, first insert the needle through the skin and through the trigger point, eliciting a twitch response. Then withdraw the needle back through the trigger point, while maintaining gentle pressure on the plunger of the syringe. This will place a few drops of fluid into the trigger point.

When several trigger points are injected and more fluid is used during a treatment session, it is important to consider the dose-related toxicity of the injected solution.

HOW MANY INJECTIONS SHOULD BE ADMINISTERED DURING AN OFFICE VISIT?

Optimal treatment for myofascial pain is for all of the trigger points in the pain pattern to be treated at the time of each office visit. This is not likely to be possible for a patient with a total body pain pattern. An effective and more limited treatment plan is to treat the more severe trigger points causing an area-wide pain pattern. Within any area, there may be several trigger point areas that can be injected. If the pain pattern involves both sides of the body, it is important to keep the body balanced by treating both sides. Treatment, however, does not need to be totally symmetric and can be focused on one side or the other.

TIMING OF INJECTIONS

The practitioner may find that the initial office visit should include history taking, physical examination, and instructions for stretching and dietary modification. Injections during the first visit are rarely of lasting benefit for chronic and diffuse pain patterns. Most patients are ready for injections by the time of their second visit. Their nutritional status has improved and they have been stretching as instructed. This stretching starts development of a healing routine and also prepares the body for more aggressive treatment.

It is usually best to limit the first trigger point injections to two areas, the same on each side of the body. For upper body pain, it may be best to inject bilateral shoulder trapezius or infraspinatus muscles, even if pain is mostly perceived on one side of the body. Myofascial pain is sympathetically mediated, and the sympathetic nervous system is not discrete with respect to one side or the other. Additionally, if treatment is discontinued after unilateral injection of shoulder trapezius musculature, it is possible for the patient to lose balance and fall when trying to walk.

During subsequent office visits, the patient will tolerate more aggressive therapy and more injections. For upper body pain, it may be possible to address muscles in the jaw, neck, upper shoulder, and upper back at the time of a single office visit. Some patients respond best to such a more diffuse and involved treatment session. In such a situation, it is not unreasonable to inject 7 to 14, or more, separate sites during a single office visit.

SYMPATHETIC NERVOUS SYSTEM CAUTIONS

Myofascial trigger point injection by this procedure can affect the body very deeply and very quickly. Each injection into a trigger point "touches" the sympathetic nervous system. If this system is stimulated too much, it may instigate a complex, uncomfortable reaction. The patient may become cold, light-headed, nauseous, and/or start to shiver. Sometimes this will occur after as few as two injection sites.

It is very important for the patient that the health care personnel remain calm and confident. Do not suggest that "you have never seen this before," without admitting that you have read about appropriate procedures for treating the reaction.

This reaction may resolve quickly and easily, or it may require an hour of direct attention and effort from a staff member. Keep the patient warm, hydrated, and resting. Do not perform additional injections. Craniosacral therapy, massage therapy, healing touch, aromatherapy, moist heat, and hydrotherapy may be particularly helpful, and generally have a profound effect on stopping the episode and restoring balance to the nervous system.

The patient will most likely be exhausted and perhaps a little disoriented when this is over. It may be prudent for the office to arrange transportation home for the patient.

LOCAL CAUTIONS

There may be bleeding at the injection site and deep into the muscle as a result of the needle puncturing a blood vessel. Hemostasis is best accomplished with direct pressure to the area of the injection, directly after removal of the needle. The most important time for application of pressure for this purpose is in the first 45 seconds after needle removal. This will minimize bleeding and bruising.

Extra precautions to prevent bleeding and bruising are especially important in the patient that has ingested aspirin-related products. Pressure may be applied during injection by using a firmer grip on the muscle. Pressure should be applied right after injection and may need to be maintained for a few additional minutes.

Vitamin C supplementation reduces bruising and bleeding at injection sites. This effect is generally optimized with ingestion of 1000 mg twice daily. Bleeding will often be noticed at the needle entrance after one or two missed doses from the previous 24 hours.

Additionally, trigger point injections seem to "use up" the patient's vitamin C stores. This will be manifested during a treatment session by bleeding at the needle sites of later injections. In these cases, increasing daily vitamin C supplementation should be considered. Illness may also deplete vitamin C resources, and this should be taken into account when recommending a change in dose.

DISCOMFORT CAUTIONS

After trigger point injection, there is usually relaxation of the entire treated taut band of muscle. At 15 or 20 minutes after injection of trigger points with a short-acting local anesthetic, the muscle will usually begin to get sore. This soreness typically feels like the muscle had been exercised with weightlifting the day before, after not having exercised for some time. This soreness typically subsides in 24 to 48 hours, just like what can be expected with most weightlifting. Occasionally, soreness will persist for a week or longer. With relaxation of a trigger point, the patient's pain pattern is likely to lessen in severity and shift its location. This apparent shift of location represents the quieting of some trigger points and the noticing of others that are now relatively more active.

Occasionally, a pain pattern will worsen after trigger point injection. This phenomenon represents muscle tightening and increased activity with respect to trigger points that may or may not have been treated during the particular treatment session. This is more likely to occur if the patient being injected is anxious or tense during the treatment session, or if the patient undergoes too much treatment during a particular treatment session.

Once in awhile, during post-injection stretching, an injected muscle may retighten. A taut band will be palpable, trigger points will be active, and the patient will be very uncomfortable. This is likely to occur if the patient was not relaxed during the injection treatment. When this happens, the best option is usually to re-inject the muscle and re-stretch it before the patient is discharged from the office. Other options include craniosacral therapy, aromatherapy, and deep tissue massage. This extra care and time from the physician and staff may disrupt a busy schedule, but it is extremely important and will usually prevent several days of misery and an emergency appointment during the next few days. Until the patient is more stable and can easily tolerate more bodywork, the physician should consider less aggressive treatment during future office visits.

COMPLICATIONS

More serious complications are related to the location of the needle. If the needle pierces the pleural cavity, pneumothorax may result. If the needle pierces a major blood vessel in the forearm or lower leg, a compartment syndrome may result. Treatment for pneumothorax may require intubation, and treatment of compartment syndrome may require surgical decompression.

Other serious complications are related to reactions to medications. Severe allergies to the injected solution may require treatment for rash and swelling, or resuscitation.

AFTERCARE

After trigger point injections, the injected muscles and other related muscles involved in the pain pattern should be gently, firmly, and fully stretched toward their normal resting length. It is important to remember that injection is the tool that makes this level of stretch possible, and that stretch is the treatment for myofascial pain.

The body is like a rubber band — it tends to tighten after stretching. It is important to keep the treated muscles from tightening back up, and the most concerted effort should be made during the first hours and then days after treatment. Patients should be advised to stretch slowly, gently, and even briefly anytime it feels like the muscle is tightening. Sometimes, this will be only 10 minutes after previous stretching. Usually, the treated muscles are more stable after a couple of hours and then should be stretched every hour or so until sleep.

The patient should be advised to drink a lot of water, usually at least one glass every hour for several hours. Trigger point injections relax muscle spasm and tension, improving circulation and bloodflow through the muscle. Toxins of metabolism will be released into the body and the water is important for detoxification. People who do not drink enough water may experience fever, nausea, and general malaise.

BIBLIOGRAPHY

Bourne, I. H. J. (1984). Treatment of chronic back pain comparing corticosteroid-lignocaine injections with lignocaine alone. *Practitioner, 228,* 333–338.

Byrn, C., Olsson, I., Falkheded, L., et al. (1993). Subcutaneous sterile water injections for chronic neck and shoulder pain following whiplash injuries. *Lancet, 341,* 449–452.

Campbel, S. M. (1989). Regional myofascial syndromes. *Rheumatology Disease Clinics of North America, 15,* 31–43.

Carlson, C. R., Okeson, J. P., Falace, D. A., et al. (1993). Reduction of pain and EMG activity in the masseter region by trapezius trigger point injection. *Pain, 55,* 397–400.

Fischer, A. A. (1988). Documentation of myofascial trigger points. *Archives of Physical and Medical Rehabilitation, 69,* 286–291.

Fischer, A. A. (1995). Trigger point injection. In T. A. Lennard (Ed.), *Physiatric Procedures in Clinical Practice* (pp. 28–36). Philadelphia: Hanley & Belfus.

Fricton, J. R. (1993). Myofascial pain: Clinical characteristics and diagnostic criteria. *Journal of Musculoskeletal Pain 1,* 37–47.

Garvey, T. A., Marks, M. R., & Wiesel, S. W. A prospective, randomized, double-blind evaluation of trigger point injection therapy for low-back pain. *Spine, 14,* 962–964, 1989

Gerwin, R. D., Shannon, S., & Hong, C.-Z. (1995). Identification of myofascial trigger points: Interrater agreement and effect of training. *Journal of Musculoskeletal Pain 3*(Suppl. 1), 55.

Gerwin, R. D. (1995). A study of 96 subjects examined both for fibromyalgia and myofascial pain. *Journal of Musculoskeletal Pain, 3*(Suppl. 1), 121.

Gerwin, R. D. (1994). Neurobiology of the myofascial trigger point. *Balliéres Clinical Rheumatology, 8,* 747–762.

Hong, C.-Z. (1994). Consideration and recommendations regarding myofascial trigger point injections. *Journal of Musculoskeletal Pain, 2,* 29–58.

Hong, C.-Z. (1994). Lidocaine injection versus dry needling to myofascial trigger point: The importance of the local twitch response. *American Journal of Physical Medicine and Rehabilitation, 73,* 256–263.

Hubbard, D. R., & Berkoff, G. M. (1993). Myofascial trigger points show spontaneous needle EMG activity. *Spine, 18,* 1803–1807.

Lewit, K. (1979). The needle effect in the relief of myofascial pain. *Pain, 6,* 83–90.

Njoo, K. H., & Van der Does, E. (1994). The occurrence and inter-rater reliability of myofascial trigger points in the quadratus lumborum and gluteus medius: A prospective study in non-specific low back pain patients and controls in general practice. *Pain, 58,* 317–323.

Simons D. G., Hong C.-Z., & Simons L. S. (1995). Nature of myofascial trigger points, active loci. *Journal of Musculoskeletal Pain, 3*(Suppl. 1), 62.

Simons D. G., Hong C.-Z., & Simons L. S. (1995). Prevalence of spontaneous electrical activity at trigger points and at control sites in rabbit skeletal muscle. *Journal of Musculoskeletal Pain, 3,* 35–48.

Simons D. G. (1988). Myofascial pain syndromes: Where are we? Where are we going? *Archives of Physical and Medical Rehabilitation, 69,* 207–212.

Travell J. G., & Simons D. G. (1983). *Myofascial pain and dysfunction: The trigger point manual.* Baltimore: Williams & Wilkins.

The Role of Cannabis and Cannabinoids in Pain Management

Ethan B. Russo, M.D.

INTRODUCTION

The herb cannabis is derived from the Old World species *Cannabis sativa* L. *Cannabis indica* and *C. ruderalis* may also merit species status. Cannabis has a history as an analgesic agent that spans at least 4000 years, including a century of usage in mainstream Western medicine. Quality control issues, and ultimately political fiat eliminated this agent from the modern pharmacopoeia, but it is now resurgent. The reasons lie in the remarkable pharmacological properties of the herb and new scientific research that reveals the inextricable link that cannabinoids possess with our own internal biochemistry. In essence, the cannabinoids form a system in parallel with that of the endogenous opioids in modulating pain. More important, cannabis and its endogenous and synthetic counterparts may be uniquely effective in pain syndromes in which opiates and other analgesics fail.

Despite hundreds of supportive journal articles over the past decade, the news about cannabis and cannabinoids has only slowly filtered into public and even professional acknowledgment. The attendant politics remain contentious, with certain states and countries acknowledging a role for cannabis in medicine, while other governmental bodies languish in inactivity or outright opposition.

No major medical text on pain has previously covered this topic to the author's knowledge. This chapter may then represent one point of departure in what I believe will be a major renaissance of interest in this plant, its healing attributes, and what it might tell us about our own internal mechanisms of analgesia. A unique set of clinical tools may be added to an armamentarium in pain management that never seems wholly adequate to the task at hand.

This chapter examines the use of cannabis and cannabinoids historically, scientifically, and anecdotally in relation to a variety of pain syndromes. The author has previously addressed this topic with respect to migraine — in short (Russo, in press) and at great length (Russo, 2001).

CANNABIS AND PAIN TREATMENT: A HISTORICAL SURVEY

CHINA

Traditional knowledge of cannabis in China may span 5000 years, dating to the legendary emperor and "Divine Plowman," Shên-Nung. Julien (1849) wrote of the physician Hoa-tho in the early 2nd century and his use of a cannabis extract in surgical anesthesia:

> He gave to the sick person a preparation of hemp (Ma-yo), and, in a few moments, he became so insensible that it were as if he was plunged into rapture of loss of life. Then, following this instance, he practiced some overtures, incisions, amputations, and removed the cause of the malady; then he repaired the tissues with suture points, and applied liniments. (p. 197, translation EBR)

0-8493-0926-3/02/$0.00+$1.50
© 2002 by CRC Press LLC

INDIA

The *Atharva Veda* of India dates to between 1400 and 2000 BCE and mentions a sacred grass, *bhang,* which remains a modern term of usage for cannabis. Medical references to cannabis date to Susruta in the 6th to 7th centuries BCE (Chopra & Chopra, 1957). Dwarakanath (1965), described a series of Ayurvedic and Arabic tradition preparations containing the herb indicated for migraine, neuralgic, and visceral pains.

EGYPT

Previous scholars had thought cannabis to be absent from Ancient Egypt, but Nunn (1996) cited six supporting experts, indicating that it was utilized medicinally. These authors agree with the view of Dawson that the hieroglyphic *shemshemet* means cannabis. Physical proof includes discoveries of hemp remnants in the tomb of Akhenaten (Amenophis IV) around 1350 BCE, and cannabis pollen in the tomb of Rameses II, who died in 1224 BCE (Mannische, 1989). Cannabis has remained in the Egyptian pharmacopoeia since pharaonic times, administered orally, rectally, vaginally, on the skin, in the eyes, and by fumigation.

Mannische (1989) cites the following from Papyrus Ramesseum III, 1700 BCE: "A treatment for the eyes: celery; hemp; is ground and left in the dew overnight. Both eyes of the patient are to be washed with it early in the morning" (p. 82). This suggests a parallel to modern use of cannabis in glaucoma treatment.

Another passage (Ebers Papyrus 821) is reminiscent of the 19th-century use of cannabis as an aid to childbirth (Ghalioungui, 1987): "Another: *smsm-t* [shemshemet]; ground in honey; introduced into her vagina *(iwf).* This is a contraction" (p. 209). Passage E618 refers to treatment of a toenail with a bandage containing hemp resin.

SUMER/AKKAD/ASSYRIA

Thompson (1924; 1949) documented 29 citations of the use of cannabis in Assyrian medical documents, and attested to its analgesic and psychogenic effects by various methods, including fumigation. The bulk of the references date to the second millennium BCE and pertain to *A.ZAL.LA* in Sumerian and *azallû* in Akkadian. Through philological arguments, Thompson (1924) concluded that:

> The evidence thus indicates a plant prescribed in AM [Assyrian manuscripts] in very small doses, used in spinning and rope-making, and at the same time a drug used to dispel depression of spirits. Obviously, it none other than hemp, *Cannabis sativa,* L. (p. 101)

Specifically, according to Thompson (1949), hemp, or *azallû,* was employed to bind the temples (possibly for headache?). Furthermore, the Sumerian texts recommended internal use for depression and staying the menses, and "for 'poison' of all limbs, dry, pound, sift, and fumigate..." (p. 222).

ANCIENT ISRAEL/PALESTINE/JUDEA

Physical evidence of medicinal cannabis use in Israel/Palestine was recently discovered (Zias, et al., 1993) in a burial tomb in Beit Shemesh where the skeleton of a 14-year-old girl was found along with 4th century bronze coins. Contained in her pelvic area was the skeleton of a term fetus, of sufficient size to disallow a successful vaginal delivery. In her abdominal area, gray carbonized material was noted and analyzed, yielding chromatographic and nuclear magnetic resonance spectroscopy evidence of delta-6-tetrahydrocannabinol, a stable metabolite of cannabis. The authors stated: "We assume that the ashes found in the tomb were cannabis, burned in a vessel and administered to the young girl as an inhalant to facilitate the birth process" (p. 363). They further remarked that cannabis retained an indication as an aid to parturition into the 19th century.

GREEK AND ROMAN EMPIRES

In the 1st century of the Common Era, Dioscorides published his *Materia Medica* and described the analgesic role of cannabis (Dioscorides, 1968): "Cannabis is a plant of much use in this life for ye twistings of very strong ropes, ... but being juiced when it is green is good for the pains of the ears" (p. 390).

Pliny (1951) described additional indications for hemp: "The root boiled in water eases cramped joints, gout too and similar violent pains. It is applied raw to burns, ..." (Book XX, XCVII, p. 153).

THE ISLAMIC WORLD

In the 9th century, Sabur ibn Sahl in Persia cited the use of cannabis several times in his dispensatorium, *Al-Aqrabadhin Al-Saghir* (Kahl, 1994). According to the translation and interpretation of the text by Dr. Indalecio Lozano (personal communication, 2000), ibn Sahl prescribed a compound medicine containing cannabis juice that was used to treat a variety of aching pains and migraine that was instilled into the nostril of the afflicted patient.

Also in the 12th century, Al-Biruni (Biruni & Said, 1973) noted: "Galen says: 'The leaves of this plant [cannabis] cure flatus — Some people squeeze the fresh (seeds) for use in ear-aches. I believe that it is used in chronic pains'" (p. 346).

Umar ibn Yusuf ibn Rasul also suggested cannabis for ear and head pains at the end of the 13th century (Lewis, Menage, Pellat & Schacht, 1971).

Some time later, an electuary named *bars,* or *barsh,* containing a variety of ingredients, sometimes including cannabis, became popular as an analgesic treatment in the Arab world. (Lozano Camara, 1990).

At the close of the 17th century in Indonesia, Rumphius studied cannabis use, including treatment of pleuritic chest pains and hernias (Rumpf & Beekman, 1981).

WESTERN MEDICINE

Medicinal uses persisted in England. In 1640, in the *Theatrum Botanicum: The Theater of Plants* (Parkinson & Cotes, 1640) John Parkinson indicated:

> Hempe is cold and dry … the *Dutch* as one saith doe make an Emulsion out of the seede, … for it openeth the obstructions of the gall, and causeth digestion of choller therein: … the Emulsion or decoction of the seede, stayeth laskes and fluxes that are continuall, easeth the paines of the collicke: and allayeth the troublesome humours in the bowels: … The decoction, of the roote is sayd to allay inflammations in the head or any other part, the herbe it selfe, or the distilled water thereof performeth the like effect; the same decoction of the rootes, easeth the paines of the goute, the hard tumours, or knots of the joynts, the paines and shrinking of the sinewes, and other the like paines of the hippes: it is good to be used, for any place that hath beene burnt by fire, if the fresh juyce be mixed with a little oyle or butter. (p. 598)

In 1758, Marcandier published his *Traité du chanvre [Treatise on Hemp],* which was translated into English several years later (1764):

> The grain and the leaves being squeezed, while they are green, and applied, by way of cataplasm, to painful tumours, are reckoned to have a great power of relaxing and stupefying. … The root of it boiled in water, and applied in the form of a cataplasm, softens and restores the joints of fingers or toes that are dried and shrunk. It is very good against the gout, and other humours that fall upon the nervous, muscular, and tendinous parts. It abates inflammations, dissolves tumours, and hard swellings upon the joints. Beat and pounded in a mortar, with butter, when it is still fresh, it is applied to burns, which it relieves greatly when it is often renewed. (pp. 24, 26)

Linnaeus acknowledged the pain-reducing properties of cannabis in his list of its medical applications in his *Materia Medica* (Linné, 1772): "narcotica, phantastica, dementans, anodyna, repellens" (p. 213).

In France, Chomel (1782) noted once more the benefits of hemp seed oil on burn treatment, promoting both pain and healing.

The medical use of cannabis, or what became known as "Indian hemp," was reintroduced to the West by O'Shaughnessy in 1839. His treatise on the subject dealt with the apparent utility of a plant extract administered to patients suffering from rabies, cholera, tetanus, infantile convulsions, but also a series of painful rheumatological conditions.

Shortly after Indian hemp came to England, Clendinning (1843) described his results of treatment of 18 patients: three with headaches, one with abdominal pain secondary to tumor, one with pain secondary to a laceration, two with rheumatic joint pain, and one with gout. In each case, the tincture of Indian hemp provided relief, even in cases of morphine withdrawal symptoms. He observed:

> I have no hesitation in affirming that in my hand its exhibition has usually, and with remarkably few substantial exceptions, been followed by manifest effects as a soporific or hypnotic in conciliating sleep; as an anodyne in lulling irritation; as an antispasmodic in checking cough and cramp; and as a nervine stimulant in removing languor and anxiety, and raising the pulse and spirits; and that these effect have been observed in both acute and chronic affections, in young and old, male and female. (p. 209)

In Ireland in 1845, Donovan (1845) extensively described his own extensive trials with small doses of cannabis resin, mainly in patients with various types of neuropathic and musculoskeletal pain. Effects were fairly uniformly impressive, with few side effects. He also described the benefits of local application of hemp leaf oil on hemorrhoids and neuralgic pains.

Christison (1851) endorsed benefits of cannabis in treating tetanus, augmenting labor, and treatment of neuralgic and musculoskeletal pain.

Grigor (1852) examined to role of cannabis in facilitating childbirth. In nine cases, little was noticeable; but in seven, including rive primiparous women, "the contractions acquire great increase of strength … it is capable of bringing the labour to a happy conclusion considerably within a half of the time that would other have been required" (p. 125). No untoward effects were observed on mother or child.

Over the next decades, numerous authorities recognized cannabis as helpful for painful conditions. Sir John Russell Reynolds was eventually to become Queen Victoria's personal physician. He successfully treated her dysmenorrhea with a cannabis extract throughout her adult life. Reynolds (1868) reported on various successes with Indian hemp, theorizing that:

> This medicine appears capable of reducing over-activity of the nervous centres without interfering with any one of the functions of organic, or vegetal life. The bane of

many opiates and sedatives is this, that the relief of the moment, the hour, or the day, is purchased at the expense of tomorrow's misery. In no one case to which I have administered Indian hemp, have I witnessed any such results. (p. 160)

Silver (1870) reported five cases in detail of menorrhagia and dysmenorrhea, all relieved nicely with cannabis. He also referred to a colleague, who had never failed in over 100 cases to control pain and discomfort in these disorders within three doses.

In 1874, a popular textbook, *Practical Therapeutics* (Waring, 1874) stated of cannabis: "Of a good extract, gr. 1/4 to gr. 1/2, rarely gr. j, in the form of pill, is very effective in some forms of neuralgia" (p. 159).

In the French literature, Michel (1880) extensively reviewed and endorsed the success of cannabis in treating neuralgic afflictions.

In 1883, two letters to the *British Medical Journal* attested to the benefits of extract of *Cannabis indica* in menorrhagia, treating both pain and bleeding successfully with a few doses. (Batho, 1883; Brown, 1883)

Rennie (1886) reported from India on the therapeutic value of a cannabis tincture in curing acute and chronic dysentery and its attendant pain in some dozen patients.

Dr. Hobart Hare published an article that dealt with the indications of cannabis at length:

CANNABIS INDICA has been before the profession for many years as a remedy to be used in combating almost all forms of pain, yet, owing to the variations found to exist as to its activity, it has not received the confidence which I think it now deserves. ... I have found the efficient dose of a pure extract of hemp to be as powerful in relieving pain as the corresponding dose of the same preparation of opium. ... During the time that this remarkable drug is relieving pain a very curious psychical condition sometimes manifests itself; namely, that the diminution of the pain seems to be due to its fading away in the distance, so that the pain becomes less and less, just as the pain in a delicate ear would grow less and less as a beaten drum was carried farther and farther out of the range of hearing. (pp. 225–226)

Soon thereafter, Farlow (1889) penned a treatise on the use of rectal preparations of cannabis: "Cannabis has few equals in its power over nervous headaches such as women with pelvic troubles are subject to" (p. 508).

Aulde (1890) lauded the drug as follows: "As a remedy for the relief of *supraorbital neuralgia* no article perhaps afford better prospects than cannabis ..." (p. 118).

In the French literature, Sée (1890) submitted a detailed report on the use of cannabis in the treatment of various disorders producing gastric and intestinal pain. He

found it preferable in efficacy and side effects to other agents of the day, including opiates and bismuth that remain on the modern scene.

In the article "On the Therapeutic Value of Indian Hemp," Suckling (1891) declared: "I have met with patients who have been incapacitated for work from the frequency of the attacks [of migraine], and who have been enabled by the use of Indian hemp to resume their employment" (p. 12). This echoes modern claims of clinical cannabis users who partake lightly of the drug and return to work or study.

Mattison was effusive in his praise in 1891:

... Indian hemp is not here lauded as a specific. It will, at times, fail. So do other drugs. But the many cases in which it acts well, entitle it to a large and lasting confidence.

My experience warrants this statement: *cannabis indica* is, often, a safe and successful anodyne and hypnotic. (pp. 270–271)

Mackenzie (1894) described the utility of cannabis in treating neuralgias, headache, including chronic daily headache, tabetic (syphilitic) pain, functional gastrointestinal pain (corresponding to modern idiopathic bowel syndrome, or "spastic colon"), and pruritic disorders.

That year in India, among many other indications, the encyclopedic Indian Hemp Drugs Commission (1894) reported that a small piece of *charas* (hashish) placed in a carious tooth would relieve aching pain.

An American 1898 drug handbook stated the following quaint prose under "Actions and Uses" for cannabis (Lilly, 1898): "Not poisonous according to best authorities, though formerly so regarded. Antispasmodic, analgesic, anesthetic, narcotic, aphrodisiac. Specially recommended in spasmodic and painful affections ..." (p. 32).

Dixon (1899), a famed British pharmacologist, studied cannabis extensively and recognized its value "as a useful food accessory," supporting its current indications in the cachexia of cancer chemotherapy and HIV-positive patients. He also reintroduced the concept of smoking the drug to Western medicine:

In cases where an immediate effect is desired the drug should be smoked, the fumes being drawn through water. In fits of depression, mental fatigue, nervous headache, and exhaustion a few inhalations produce an almost immediate effect, the sense of depression, headache, feeling of fatigue disappear and the subject is enabled to continue his work, feeling refreshed and soothed. I am further convinced that its results are marvellous in giving staying power and altering the feelings of muscular fatigue which follow hard physical labour. (p. 1356)

The same year, Shoemaker (1899) reported on a large series of patients with pain conditions, including migraine, dental neuralgia, gastralgia, enteralgia, cerebral tumor, and herpes zoster, all successfully treated with *Cannabis indica*.

As late as 1915, Sir William Osler (Osler & McCrae, 1915) the acknowledged father of modern medicine stated of migraine treatment: "*Cannabis indica* is probably the most satisfactory remedy. Seguin recommends a prolonged course of the drug" (p. 1089). This statement provided support of its use for both acute and prophylactic treatment of migraine.

In 1918, *The Dispensatory of the United States of America* (Remington, et al.) stated, "Cannabis is used in medicine to relieve pain, to encourage sleep, and to soothe restlessness. … For its analgesic action it is used especially in pains of neuralgic origin, such as *migraine,* but is occasionally of service in other types" (p. 280).

In 1922, Hare still advocated the use of cannabis noting that: "For the relief of *pain,* particularly that depending on nerve disturbance, hemp is very valuable" (p. 181).

Hoechstetter, as late as 1930, noted the ability of cannabis to achieve a labor with pain burden substantially reduced or eliminated, followed by a tranquil sleep. He stated: "As far as is known, a baby born of a mother intoxicated with cannabis will not be abnormal in any way" (p. 1165).

In 1942, despite its political disenfranchisement, Morris Fishbein, the editor of the *Journal of the American Medical Association* still advocated oral preparations of cannabis in the treatment of menstrual (catamenial) migraine (Fishbein, 1942).

Cannabis remained in the British armamentarium somewhat longer, and was extolled above opiates and barbiturates in the treatment of the pain of hospitalized patients with duodenal ulcers (Douthwaite, 1947).

Modern Ethnobotany of Cannibis in Analgesia

In Tashkent in the 1930s, cannabis, or *nasha,* was employed medicinally, despite Soviet prohibition (Benet, 1975): "A mixture of lamb's fat with *nasha* is recommended for brides to use on their wedding night to reduce the pain of defloration. The same mixture works well for headache when rubbed into the skin; it may also be eaten spread on bread" (pp. 46-47).

In Southeast Asia, cannabis remains useful (Martin, 1975):

> Everywhere it is considered to be of analgesic value, comparable to the opium derivatives. Moreover, it can be added to any relaxant to reinforce its action. Cooked leaves, which have been dried in the sun, are used in quantities of several grams per bowl of water. This

decoction helps especially to combat migraines and stiffness… (p. 70).

A more recent study documents the ethnobotanical uses of cannabis by the Hmong minority in the China-Vietnam border region (Gu & Clarke, 1998): "Some older Hmong men may rarely smoke cannabis to 'relieve discomfort,' but they are not daily smokers" (p. 6).

In a book (Dastur, 1962) about medicinal plants of India, we see the following:

> Charas is the resinous exudation that collects on the leaves and flowering tops of plants [equivalent to the Arabic *hashish*]; it is the active principle of hemp; it is a valuable narcotic, especially in cases where opium cannot be administered; it is of great value in malarial and periodical headaches, migraine, acute mania, whooping cough, cough of phthisis, asthma, anaemia of brain, nervous vomiting, tetanus, convulsion, insanity, delirium, dysuria, and nervous exhaustion; it is also used as an anaesthetic in dysmenorrhea, as an appetizer and aphrodisiac, as an anodyne in itching of eczema, neuralgia, severe pains of various kinds of corns, etc. (p. 67)

In Colombia, the analgesic effects of a cannabis tincture was lauded (Partridge, 1975): "The knowledge that cannabis can be used for treatment of pain is widespread…" (p. 161).

Rubin (1976; Rubin & Comitas, 1975) documented extensive usage of cannabis in Jamaica for a variety of conditions, including headache. In Brazil, Hutchinson (1975) noted:

> Such an infusion [of marijuana leaves] is taken to relieve rheumatism, "female troubles," colic and other common complaints. For toothache, marijuana is frequently packed into and around the aching tooth and left for a period of time, during which it supposedly performs an analgesic function. (p. 180)

MODERN DATA ON CANNABIS AND ANALGESIA

Recent Theory and Clinical Data

A popular treatise (Margolis & Clorfene, 1969) on marijuana noted medicinal effects:

> You'll also discover that grass is an analgesic, and will reduce pain considerably. As a matter of fact, many women use it for dysmenorrhea or menorrhagia when they're out of Pamprin or Midol. So if you have an upset stomach, or suffer from pain of neuritis or neuralgia, smoke grass. If pains persist, smoke more grass. (p. 26)

Solomon Snyder (1971), the discoverer of opiate receptors, examined cannabis' pros and cons as an analgesic, commenting:

> For there are many conditions, such as migraine headaches or menstrual cramps, where something as mild as aspirin gives insufficient relief and opiates are too powerful, not to mention their potential for addiction. Cannabis might conceivably fulfill a useful role in such conditions. (p. 14)

Subsequent experimental studies by Noyes explored these reported analgesic effects of cannabis. One article examined pain tolerance thresholds (Milstein, MacCannell, Karr, & Clark, 1975). Both naïve (8% increase) and experienced human subjects (16% increase) noted statistically significant increases in pain threshold after smoking cannabis.

In humans, Noyes (Noyes & Baram, 1974) described case studies of five patients who voluntarily employed it to treat their painful conditions. Another study (Noyes, Brunk, Baram, & Canter, 1975) pertained to oral tetrahydro-cannabinol (THC) in cancer patients. Pain relief with escalating doses significant to the $P < 0.001$ level was observed. Peak effects occurred at 3 hours with doses of 10 and 15 mg, but were delayed until 5 hours after the 20-mg oral dose.

Noyes' research group compared the analgesic effect of THC to codeine (Noyes, Brunk, Avery, & Canter, 1975). In short, 10 mg of oral THC reduced subjective pain burdens by similar decrements to 60 mg codeine, as did 20 mg THC vs. 120 mg codeine. The 20-mg dose was sedative and not as well tolerated in some elderly, cannabis-naïve subjects.

Hollister (1986) addressed possible cannabis indications, including analgesia. He concluded that it seemed that no THC homologue would be an analgesic of choice, but that "It is too early to be sure, however" (p. 15). These were prophetic words in light of upcoming cannabinoid receptor research.

In 1991, a series of case studies on the utility of cannabis in treating chronic pain were published (Randall, 1991). One pertained to Lynn Hastings, an Idaho woman with severe juvenile rheumatoid arthritis, whose symptoms of pain, spasm, and depression were resistant to standard medicine, but were effectively treated with cannabis. A state Supreme Court finding of "medical necessity" followed her initial arrest for cultivation of cannabis. Eventually, the charges were dropped.

In 1993, the landmark book *Marihuana, The Forbidden Medicine,* was first published and has since been revised (Grinspoon & Bakalar, 1997). Although criticized in some quarters as anecdotal, the book contains numerous compelling testimonials from patients and their doctors attesting to the clinical efficacy of cannabis where con-

ventional pharmacotherapy failed. Cases of painful conditions responding to cannabis are legion: osteoarthritis, ankylosing spondylitis, pruritus from allergic dermatitis, premenstrual syndrome (PMS), menstrual cramps, labor pains, gingival pain (with local application of cannabis tincture), migraine, phantom limb pain, Crohn's disease, and "functional" gastrointestinal pain. Often, these patients improved with cannabis, worsened without it, and were improved once more upon its resumption. These accounts fulfill criteria of "N-of-1 studies" and have been accepted by epidemiologists as proof of efficacy in rare conditions or ones in which blinded controlled trials are technically difficult (Guyatt, et al., 1990; Larson, 1990).

The *American Journal of Public Health* (1996) "Access," issued a particularly strong plea for liberalization of laws pertaining to medical cannabis in 1996, citing its activity in "decreasing the suffering from chronic pain…."

Hollister (2000) has recently reviewed indications for cannabis "for exploratory purposes, any patient with pain unrelieved by conventional analgesics should have access to smoked marijuana if they so desire" (p. 5).

CANNABINOID AND ENDOCANNABINOID NEUROCHEMISTRY

In recent years, scientists (Barinaga, 1992; Devane, et al., 1992; Marx, 1990; Matsuda, Lolait, Brownstein, Young, & Bonner, 1990) have provided elucidation of the mechanisms of action of cannabis and THC (tetrahydrocannabinol, the primary psychoactive component) with the discovery of an endogenous cannabinoid (endocannabinoid) ligand, arachidonylethanolamide, nicknamed anandamide, from the Sanskrit word *ananda,* or "bliss." Anandamide inhibits cyclic AMP mediated through G-protein coupling in target cells, which cluster in nociceptive areas of the central nervous system (CNS) (Herkenham, 1993). Early testing of its pharmacological action and behavioral activity indicate similarity to THC (Fride & Mechoulam, 1993), although anandamide differs from THC in not causing dynorphin release (Strangman & Walker, 1999). Pertwee (1997) has examined the pharmacology of cannabinoid (CB) receptors in detail. CB_1 receptors are mainly confined to the CNS, while CB_2 receptors are found in the periphery, often in conjunction with immune mechanisms.

Further research has elucidated analgesic mechanisms of cannabinoids, which will be examined system by system.

Cannabinoids and Serotonergic Systems

Serotonergic mechanisms are implicated in many pain conditions, especially migraine and cluster headaches.

THC reduces serotonin release from the platelets of human migraineurs (Volfe, Dvilansky, & Nathan, 1985).

Cannabis has been observed to stimulate 5-HT synthesis, its brain content, decrease its synaptosomal uptake, while stimulating its release (Spadone, 1991).

Anandamide and other cannabinoid agonists inhibit rat serotonin type 3 ($5\text{-}HT_3$) receptors (Fan, 1995) that mediate emetic and pain responses. The recent advent of alosetron, a $5\text{-}HT_3$ blocker employed in the treatment of irritable bowel syndrome ("Alosetron," 2000), would seem to support claims of the efficacy of cannabis in that disorder on the basis of this mechanism.

Recently, Boger and his group (1998) have demonstrated an 89% relative potentiation of the $5\text{-}HT_{1A}$ receptor response, and a 36% inhibition of the $5\text{-}HT_{2A}$ receptor response by anandamide. Similar effects by THC are likely, supporting efficacy for cannabinoids in acute symptomatic migraine treatment due to agonistic activity at $5\text{-}HT_{1A}$ or $5\text{-}HT_{1D}$, and in prophylactic treatment of chronic headache due to antagonistic activity at $5\text{-}HT_{2A}$ (Peroutka, 1990a,b).

Kimura, Ohta, Watanabe, Yoshimura, and Yamamoto (1998) showed that high concentrations of anandamide decreased serotonin and ketanserin binding (a $5\text{-}HT_{2A}$ antagonist). 11-OH-delta 8-THC and 11-oxo-delta 8-THC metabolites of cannabis were also observed to modify serotonin receptor binding.

Ultimately, this author and colleagues (Russo, Macarah, Todd, Medora, & Parker, 2000) have shown that essential oil components of cannabis demonstrate potent serotonin receptor activity that supports putative synergism with THC in the modulation of analgesia.

Dopaminergic Systems

The importance of dopaminergic mechanisms in the treatment of migraine and other types of pain has received recent emphasis (Peroutka, 1997). However, existing neuroleptics are significantly sedating.

Ferri, Cavicchini, Romualdi, Speroni, and Murari (1986) were able to demonstrate that 6-hydroxydopamine, which causes degeneration of catecholamine terminals, was able to block THC antinociception.

In a more recent review article (Mechoulam, Fride, & diMarzo, 1998), a number of studies were reviewed as demonstrating that cannabimimetic drugs cause "inhibition of the dopaminergic nigrostriatal system" (p. 12).

Müller-Vahl and colleagues (Müller-Vahl, Kolbe, Schneider, & Enrich, 1998) cited Mailleux (Mailleux & Vanderhaeghen, 1992) in their discussion of cannabinoid interactions with the dopaminergic system stating that: "cannabinoid receptors were found to be co-localized both with dopamine D_1 receptors on striatonigral dynorphin/substance-P-containing neurones and with dopamine D_2 receptors on striatopallidal enkephalinergic neurones" (p. 504).

Carta, Gessa, and Nava (1999) demonstrated that antinociceptive effects of THC are mediated by CB_1 and dopamine D_2 receptors, and that combination of the agents improved analgesic effects in rats.

Inflammatory Mechanisms

Modern authors (Burstein, 1992; Evans, Formukong, & Evans, 1987; Formukong, Evans, & Evans, 1988, 1989) have examined the relationship between cannabinoids and inflammation. McPartland (2001) provides an excellent summary and analysis of the subject.

Burstein, Levin, & Varanelli (1973) demonstrated that THC and other cannabinoids inhibit prostaglandin E-2 synthesis. In 1979, experiments showed that smoked cannabis reduced platelet aggregation (Schaefer, Brackett, Gunn, & Dubowski, 1979).

In 1981, cannabichromene, often the second-most abundant cannabinoid in marijuana after THC, was demonstrated to be a more effective anti-inflammatory agent than phenylbutazone in carrageenan-induced rat paw edema and the erythrocyte membrane stabilization method (Turner & ElSohly, 1981). The authors stated: "The activity of cannabichromene through the oral route, its safety and its lack of behavioral-type (psychotomimetic) activity characteristic of THC(I) indicate its therapeutic potential for the treatment of inflammatory diseases" (pp. 288S–289S).

Evans (1991) has stated that: "Experiments involving oral administration of THC suggested that THC was 20 times more potent than aspirin and twice as potent as hydrocortisone" (p. 565). Cannabidiol (CBD) functioned as a dual cyclooxygenase and lipoxygenase inhibitor in various assays.

Klein (Klein, Friedman, & Specter, 1998) noted that THC had variable effects on tumor necrosis factor (TNF) production, depending on the cells and culture system selected.

In 1998, Jaggar and colleagues issued two reports addressing visceral and inflammatory pain in rats (Jagger, Hasnie, Sellaturay, & Rice, 1998; Jagger, Sellaturay, & Rice, 1998). The endocannabinoid anandamide, a CB_1 ligand, prevented and reduced viscero-visceral hyperreflexia (VVH) in the inflamed bladder. In contrast, palmitoylethanolamide, a presumptive endogenous CB_2 ligand that accumulates in inflamed tissues and reduces edema by down-modulating mast cells, only reversed VVH once previously established. The authors posited the possibility of development of non-sedating analgesic anti-inflammatory drugs based on CB_2 receptor agonism.

In a 1999 review (Fimiani, et al., 1999), the authors noted: "Delta-9-THC blocks the conversion of arachidonic acid into all metabolites derived by cyclooxygenase activity, whereas it stimulates lipoxygenase, resulting in an increase in lipoxygenase products" (p. 27). The COX inhibition of THC may in fact be selective for the COX-2 isozyme, as more fully discussed by McPartland (2001). Clinically, no increased incidence of gastric ulceration was reported in chronic cannabis users (New York (City), 1973; Rubin & Comitas, 1975; Stefanis, Dornbush, & Fink, 1977), thus supporting its likely selectivity for COX-2. In 1978, cannabis was believed to reduce gastric acidity in humans (Nalin, et al., 1978), while another group demonstrated THC to have anti-ulcer effects in rats (Sofia, Nalepa, Harakal, & Vassar, 1973). In fact, one essential oil sesquiterpene component of cannabis, caryophyllene, has recently been demonstrated to have a gastric cytoprotective effect (Tambe, Tsujiuchi, Honda, Ikeshiro, & Tanaka, 1996).

Fimiani and co-workers (Fimiani, et al., 1999) also observed that the morphine-cannabinoid system modulates the eicosanoid cascade and its pro-inflammatory cytokine activity through induction of nitric oxide synthesis, averting damaging effects on tissues. They stated in summary (p. 30): "Thus, we can surmise cannabinoid-morphine systems are down-regulators of inflammatory processes in an attempt to restore homeostasis."

A recent report has demonstrated the efficacy of oral cannabidiol (CBD), a minimally psychoactive cannabis component, at a dose of 5 mg/kg/d in treating mice against collagen-induced arthritis, a model for human rheumatoid arthritis (Malfait, et al., 2000). Benefits were produced through a combination of immunosuppressive effects (diminished CII-specific proliferation and IFN-gamma production) and anti-inflammatory effects (decreased release of tumor necrosis factor by synovial cells).

Cannabis seed also has dietary benefits as an anti-inflammatory agent. It yields linolenic acid, which promotes formation of anti-inflammatory metabolites, and gamma-linolenic acid, which inhibits the formation of pro-inflammatory products from arachidonate (Conrad, 1997; Russo, 2000; Wirtshafter, 1997).

Flavonoid and terpenoid essential oil components of cannabis demonstrate anti-inflammatory effects at physiologically appropriate levels (McPartland & Mediavilla, in press). Cannflavin A and B inhibited prostaglandin E-2 production in human rheumatoid synovial cells 30 times more potently than aspirin (Barrett, Scutt, & Evans, 1986).

The cannabis flavonoid apigenin has anti-inflammatory actions on interleukin, TNF, carrageenan-induced edema, and by inhibition of up-regulation of cytokine-induced genes (Gerritsen, et al., 1995).

Quercetin, another flavonoid in cannabis, serves as an antioxidant and inhibits hydrogen peroxide-mediated NF-kappa B activity (Musonda & Chipman, 1998).

Burstein and co-workers have demonstrated eugenol to be a potent prostaglandin inhibitor (Burstein, Varanelli, & Slade, 1975).

Subsequently, both the alpha-pinene and caryophyllene components of cannabis have proven to demonstrate anti-inflammatory activity in the rat hindpaw edema model (Martin, et al., 1993).

Cannabinoid Interactions with Opiates and Endogenous Opioids

THC experimentally increases beta-endorphin levels Wiegant, Sweep, & Nir, 1987). Depletion of endorphins has been measured in the CSF of migraineurs during attacks (Fettes, Gawel, Kuzniak, & Edmead, 1985), and theoretically contributes to migraine effects such as hyperalgesia and photophobia.

Early exposure to THC in rat pups boosted adult levels of beta-endorphins in specific brain areas (Kumar, et al., 1990).

Mailleux and Vanderhaeghen (1994) have also demonstrated that THC regulates substance P and enkephalin mRNA levels in the basal ganglia. Manzanares and co-workers have shown that THC is able promote increases in beta-endorphin in rats (Manzanares, et al., 1998).

Meng and colleagues demonstrated that THC is involved in an analgesic brainstem circuit in the rostral ventromedial medulla that interacts with opiate pathways (Meng, Manning, Martin, & Fields, 1998).

Cichewicz, Martin, Smith, and Welch (1999) have suggested an opiate sparing effect of THC might be employed clinically in pain patients, echoing claims of the 19th century pioneers of Indian hemp. Similarly, Welch and Eads (1999) noted that cannabinoid-induced analgesia produced antinociception through spinal dynorphin release with synergistic effects with opiates. They stated, however: "THC, in comparison to the morphine derivatives, has a greater therapeutic range" (p. 188)

Many analgesic effects of cannabinoids cannot be reproduced by opiates, however, particularly in cases of neuropathic pain (Hamann & di Vadi, 1999). Nicolodi (1998) examined opiate aggravation of migraine.

Recently, Manzanares and colleagues cited that chronic cannabinoid administration could similarly promote hypothalamic production of beta-endorphin (Manzanares, Corchero, Romero, Fernandez-Ruiz, Ramos, & Fuentes, 1999).

Strangman and Walker (1999) demonstrated that a cannabinoid antagonist was able to decrease wind-up in spinal nociceptive neurons, producing hyperalgesia and allodynia in chronic pain states. The same group showed that cannabinoids selectively affect nociceptive neurons in the spinal cord and ventroposterolateral nucleus of the thalamus in a manner that promotes antinociception without anesthesia (Walker, Hohmann, et al., 1999). In all, seven sites in the CNS involved in pain processing produced effects after microinjections of cannabinoids, effecting a circuit that mediates the descending pain suppressing effects of opiates.

Cannabinoids and the Periaqueductal Gray Area

In 1996, researchers demonstrated antinociceptive effects of delta-9-THC and other cannabinoids in the periaqueductal gray matter (PAG) in rats (Lichtman, Cook, & Martin, 1996). The PAG is a putative migraine generator area (Goadsby & Gundlach, 1991; Raskin, 1988). The PAG has received a lengthy analysis (Behbehani, 1995), citing its importance in the processes of ascending and descending pain pathways. A detailed review of effects of the PAG and cannabinoids in migraine is contained in Russo (2001).

Manzanares, Corchero, Romero, Fernandez-Ruiz, Ramos, and Fuentes suggested that cannabinoid-mediated antinociception in the PAG is produced by activation of endogenous opioids, supported by the fact that subchronic THC administration elevates proenkephalin gene expression in the area (Manzanares, et al., 1998).

Recently Walker and colleagues demonstrated that electrical stimulation of PAG in the rat stimulated anandamide release and CB_1 receptor-mediated analgesia (Walker, Hohmann, Martin, Strangman, Huang, & Tsou, 1999). The system seemed to be tonically active and cannabinoid antagonists produced hyperalgesia. The authors posited that this cannabinoid-modulated pain system would support the prospect of approaches with cannabinoids to opiate-resistant syndromes.

NMDA and Glutamate

A trigeminovascular system has long been implicated as subserving pain, inflammatory and vascular effects, again reviewed in Russo (2001).

In 1996, Shen and co-workers elucidated basic mechanism of cannabinoids in glutamatergic systems (Shen, Piser, Seybold, & Thayer, 1996). Through G-protein coupling, cannabinoid receptors inhibit voltage-gated calcium channels and activate potassium channels to produce presynaptic inhibition of glutamate release. Subsequently, it has been shown (Shen & Thayer, 1999) that THC is a partial agonist acting presynaptically via CB_1 to modulate glutamatergic transmission through a reduction without blockade.

Hampson and colleagues (Hampson, Bornheim, Scanziani, Yost, Gray, Hansen, Leonoudakis, & Bickler, 1998) demonstrated a 30 to 40% reduction in delta-calcium-NMDA responses by THC, which was eliminated by a cannabinoid antagonist. THC and CBD components of cannabis act as neuroprotective antioxidants against glutamate neurotoxicity and cell death mediated via

NMDA, AMPA and kainate receptors (Hampson, Grimaldi, Axelrod, & Wink, 1998). Effects are independent of cannabinoid receptors. The natural cannabinoids were more potent in their anti-oxidant effects than either alpha-tocopherol or ascorbate.

Italian researchers Nicolodi, Sicuteri, and colleagues have recently elucidated the role of NMDA antagonists in eliminating hyperalgesia in migraine, chronic daily headache, fibromyalgia, and possibly other mechanisms of chronic pain (Nicolodi & Sicuteri, 1995, 1998; Nicolodi, Del Bianco, & Sicuteri, 1997; Nicolodi, Volpe, & Sicuteri, 1998). Gabapentin and ketamine were suggested as tools to block this system and provide amelioration. Given the above observations and relationships, it is logical that prolonged use of THC prophylactically may exert similar benefits, as was espoused in cures of chronic daily headache claimed in the 19th century with regular use of extract of Indian hemp (Mackenzie, 1887).

This concept is bolstered by examination of another series of articles by Richardson and co-workers. One study (Richardson, Kilo, & Hargreaves, 1998) examined peripheral mechanisms, wherein cannabinoids acted on CB_1 to reduce hyperalgesia and inflammation via inhibition of neurosecretion of calcitonin gene-related peptide (CGRP) in capsaicin-activated nerve terminals.

At the spinal level, they noted an antihyperalgesic effect of cannabinoids, mediated by the CB_1 receptor (Richardson, Aanonsen, & Hargreaves, 1998a). Additionally, experimental cannabinoid receptor blockade induced a glutamate-dependent hyperalgesia, suggesting a tonic activity of cannabinoids in averting such a development. The authors suggested the clinical utilization of cannabinoids in disorders "characterized by primary afferent barrage" (p. 152). Inasmuch as an increased potency of cannabinoids was observed in hyperalgesia this "may mean that there are dosages of cannabinoids that would be effective as antihyperalgesic agents but subthreshold for the untoward psychomimetic effects." This is akin to Dixon's (1899) observations of patients able to return to work after treating their headaches with a few inhalations of cannabis.

Elaborating on these themes, Richardson noted that a decrease in lumbar cannabinoid receptor numbers correlated with hyperalgesia, and could provide an etiology for certain chronic pain states, especially those unresponsive to opiates (Richardson, Aanonsen, & Hargreaves, 1998b).

In a more recent study (Li, Daughters, Bullis, Bengiamin, Stucky, Brennan, & Simone, 1999), the synthetic cannabinoid agonist WIN 55,212-2 was employed to block capsaicin-induced hyperalgesia in rat paws, much as has been observed for THC in formalin treatment.

Ko and Woods (1999) examined local THC administration and its activity on capsaicin-induced pain in rhesus monkeys. THC effectively reduced pain, which was blocked by a CB_1 antagonist and was effective at a parenteral dose that produced no behavioral change or sedation.

Maneuf, Nash, Crossman, and Brotchie (1996) examined similar issues at higher CNS levels, and were able to show a tonic activation of the cannabinoid system serving to reduce GABA uptake in the globus pallidus.

Synergism and the Entourage Effect

Palmitylethanolamide (PEA) is another endogenous cannabinoid with analgesic effects, released with from a phospholipid in conjunction with anandamide (Calignano, La Rana, Giuffrida, & Piomelli, 1998). Ensemble, the two substances effect a 100-fold synergism on CB_1 type peripheral receptors in cutaneous tissues.

Endocannabinoids and their inactive metabolites combine to boost physiological responses (the "entourage effect") (Mechoulam & Ben-Shabat, 1999). Given the likely contributions of cannabis flavonoids and essential oils to therapeutic effects on mood, inflammation, and pain reviewed in McPartland and Pruitt (1999), one may readily accept Mechoulam's quotation: "This type of synergism may play a role in the widely held (but not experimentally based) view that in some cases plants are better drugs than the natural products isolated from them" (Mechoulam & Ben-Shabat, 1999, p. 136)

PRACTICAL APPLICATION OF CANNABINOIDS TO ANALGESIA

MARINOL® (DRONABINOL): PROS AND CONS

Marinol® is a synthetically derived THC dissolved in sesame oil, developed by Unimed Pharmaceuticals and marketed by Roxane Laboratories. It is available in capsules of 2.5, 5, and 10 mg and is marketed in the United States, Canada, Australia, and some areas in Europe (Grotenherman, in press a). Until 1999, Marinol® was a Schedule II drug in the U.S. with close scrutiny to its usage, which was restricted to indications of AIDS-associated anorexia and cancer chemotherapy. After safety studies revealed a low potential for abuse or diversion (Calhoun, Galloway, & Smith, 1998), dronabinol was "down-scheduled" to Schedule III, allowing refill prescriptions for up to 6 months, and its "off-label" administration for any indication.

Clinicians have utilized Marinol® to only a limited degree. Its bioavailability is only 25 to 30% of an equivalent smoked dose of THC (British Medical Asociation [BMA], 1997). Additional problems include the first pass effect of hepatic metabolism, which results in the production of a more psychoactive metabolite 11-hydroxy-THC, and its considerable cost, which may exceed U.S.$600 per month for the lowest dosage of 2.5 mg t.i.d. Considerable anecdotal data supports preference by patients of smoked

cannabis over dronabinol (Grinspoon & Bakalar, 1997; Russo, in press).

Reports of dronabinol use in painful clinical conditions are few, but it has had some variable success in migraine prophylaxis (Mikuriya, 1997; Russo, 1998; 2000; in press).

Maurer, Henn, Dittrich, and Hoffman (1990) demonstrated efficacy of analgesia of 5 mg p.o. THC to 50 mg codeine in treatment of pain in a young paraplegic after removal of a spinal tumor. However, THC also limited spasticity, whereas codeine and placebo did not.

Holdcroft, et al. were able to demonstrate an analgesic benefit ($p < 0.001$) of THC 50 mg per day in five split doses in a patient with relapsing familial Mediterranean fever in a double-blind placebo-controlled trial (Holdcroft, et al., 1997).

NABILONE

Nabilone is a synthetic cannabinoid said to be pharmacologically similar to THC, but more potent, less apt to produce euphoria, and possessing lower "abuse potential" (BMA, 1997). It is produced by Eli Lilly Company as Cesamet® and is available in the United Kingdom, Canada, Australia, and certain countries in Europe (Grotenhermen, in press a) as an agent for nausea in chemotherapy. Some scattered reports have noted benefit on spasticity in multiple sclerosis, and effects on dyskinesias. Lethal toxicity in dogs has been noted with chronic use (Mechoulam & Feigenbaum, 1987).

A group in the U.K. recently assessed the analgesic effects of nabilone in patients, including some with neuropathic pain (Notcutt, Price, & Chapman, 1997). Side effects of drowsiness and dysphoria were troubling. Several patients claimed improved pain relief and fewer side effects with smoked cannabis and preferred it to this legal alternative. Nabilone's cost was also estimated to be 10 times higher than cannabis, even at "black market" rates.

LEVONANTRADOL

Levonantradol is a synthetic cannabinoid developed by Pfizer. Although analgesic responses of up to 6 hours were noted in postoperative pain patients (Jain, Ryan, McMahon, & Smith, 1981), no dose-response effects were observed and side effects were a significant issue. The latter included somnolence (50 to 100%) and dysphoria (30 to 50%), according to the British Medical Association (BMA, 1997), and were labeled "unacceptable" by that formal body.

AJULEMIC ACID (CT3)

Ajulemic acid is synthetic derived from delta-8-THC that does not bind to cannabinoid receptors. CT3 is being developed by Atlantic Pharmaceuticals. It has shown analgesic and anti-inflammatory properties in animal models without COX-1 inhibition side effects, and reportedly will be soon in Phase 1 human trials (Burstein, 2000, in press).

CANNABIS PROPER

Use of cannabis for pain conditions is extensive in the United States and some European countries. A survey of patients attending the Oakland Cannabis Buyers' Club revealed (Gieringer, in press):

> By far the largest category of patients interviewed by Mikuriya use cannabis for analgesia to treat conditions including: migraines and neuralgias; arthritis and rheumatism; spinal, skeletal and back disorders due to injury, deformity, or degenerative disease; inflammatory gastrointestinal disorders, and a host of miscellaneous diseases.

Analysis of the totals revealed that at least 1133 of 2480 patients (or 46%) sought cannabis for analgesia in treatment of chronic pain conditions.

Cannabis is traditionally employed therapeutically by smoking or ingestion. Each has advantages and disadvantages. Grotenhermen (2001, in press b) has produced an excellent summary of "Practical Hints," as have Brazis and Mathre (1997).

Dosing of therapeutic cannabis must be titrated to the patient's need. In general, 5 mg represents a threshold dose for noticeable effects in the average adult. Whereas tolerance to cardiovascular effects (tachycardia) and psychoactive effects ("high") are achieved after some days to weeks of chronic usage, observed clinical and "anecdotal" reports support retention of analgesic efficacy over the long term. Occasionally, upward dose titration is necessary, as is true for any agent.

Allergies to cannabis are rare, although some may experience rhinitis symptoms, particularly when exposed to the smoke of the unrefined product.

More severe psychiatric conditions present a relative contraindication to the use of cannabis, while many milder emotional afflictions may benefit from the drug (Grinspoon & Bakalar, 1997; Russo, 2000). Although concerns have been raised about subtle neuropsychological sequelae in children born to mothers employing cannabis in pregnancy (Fried, in press), other studies have shown no significant abnormalities (Dreher, 1997). Certainly, no mutagenic or teratogenic potential has been demonstrated in humans.

Concerns about our youth employing cannabis are often well intentioned. However, there is some evidence that very young children may be relatively resistant to its psychoactive properties. A research group in Israel examined the antiemetic effects of delta-8-tetrahydrocannabinol (a natural isomer) in a series of children undergoing chemotherapy (Abrahamov & Mechoulam, 1995). Excellent efficacy and

tolerance were observed at doses that would be expected to produce significant psychoactivity in adults.

People employing cannabis therapeutically must be warned of the usual caveats assigned to any potentially sedative drug, especially due care with the operation of machinery and motor vehicles.

Acute overdosages of cannabis are self-limited and most frequently consist of panic reactions. These are uniquely sensitive to reassurance ("talking down") and are quite unusual once a patient becomes familiar with the drug. Cannabis has a unique distinction of safety over four millennia of analgesic usage: no deaths due to direct toxicity of cannabis have ever been documented in the medical literature.

Some cannabis-drug interactions are apparent, but are few in number or consequence. Additive sedative effects with other agents, including alcohol, may be observed. Similarly, however, additive or synergistic anti-emetic and analgesic benefits may accrue when combining dopamine agonist neuroleptics and cannabis (Carta, et al., 1999). Cannabis may accelerate metabolism of theophylline, while slowing that of barbiturates. Anticholinergic-induced tachycardia may be accentuated by cannabis, while this effect is countered by beta-blockers (Grotenhermen, in press b). Indomethacin appears to slightly reduce the psychoactive and tachycardic effects of cannabis (Perez-Reyes, Burstein, White, McDonald, & Hicks, 1991). As discussed, synergistic analgesic benefits may accrue with concomitant usage of cannabis and opioids (Cichewicz, et al., 1999; Hare, 1887).

Crude cannabis contains most of its THC in the form of delta-9-THC acids that must be decarboxylated by heating to be activated. This occurs automatically when cannabis is smoked, whereas cannabis that is employed orally should be heated to 200–210°C for 5 minutes prior to ingestion (Brenneisen, 1984).

Contrary to disseminated propaganda in the United States, *average* cannabis potency has varied little over the last 3 decades (ElSohly, Ross, Mehmedic, Arafat, Yi, & Banahan, 2000; Mikuriya & Aldrich, 1988). It is true that the *maximum* potency has increased through applied genetics, cultivation, and harvesting techniques. This goal is achieved through production of clonal cultivation of the preferred female plants and maximization of the yield of unsterilized flowering tops known as *sinsemilla* (Spanish for "without seed"). In this manner, a concentration of stalked trichomes where THC and therapeutic terpenoids are produced is effected. Resultant yields of THC may exceed 20% by weight. This is potentially advantageous, particularly when smoked, because a therapeutic dosage of THC is obtained with fewer inhalations, thereby decreasing lung exposure to tars and carcinogens.

A considerable concentration of THC, and other cannabinoids and terpenoids as well, may also be achieved through some simple processing of crude, dried cannabis.

Techniques for sieving or washing of cannabis to isolate the trichomes to produce hashish are well described (Clarke, 1998; Rosenthal, Gieringer, & Mikuriya, 1997) and may produce potential yields of 40 to 60% THC. Clarke (1998) demonstrates a simple method of rolling the resultant powdery material into a joint of pure hashish, termed "smoking the snake," providing a relatively pure product for inhalation.

Cultivation techniques are beyond the scope of this review, but are freely available through a variety of guidebooks (Clarke, 1981; Rosenthal, Gieringer, & Mikuriya, 1997), magazines such as *Cannabis Culture* or *High Times,* or via the Internet to those who live in jurisdictions where this endeavor is legal. Outdoor, indoor, or hydroponic techniques are possible. Emphasis should focus on potent medicinal strains, scrupulous organic cultivation of female plants, clonal selection and augmentation, and appropriate processing.

Oral Use of Cannabis

A variety of issues attend this mode of cannabis administration. The most important concerns bioavailability. Oral absorption of cannabinoids is slow and erratic at best, often requiring 30 to 120 minutes. In HIV-positive or chemotherapy patients and in acute migraine with nausea and emesis, oral usage may be precluded altogether. Additionally, oral THC is subject to the "first pass effect" of hepatic metabolism yielding 11-hydroxy-THC, considerably more psychoactive than THC itself. Thus, some patients become "too high" even on low doses of medicine, such as 2.5 mg THC as dronabinol.

Advantages of oral usage are its avoidance of lung exposure in those who are immunosuppressed or have impaired pulmonary function, and its prolonged half-life. This may be of advantage for nocturnal complaints where sedation is less of an issue.

Grotenhermen (2001, in press b) suggests dose titration beginning with 2.5 mg oral THC b.i.d. with increases as needed and tolerated. For cannabis of 5% THC content, this would represent 50 mg herb per dose. For 10% THC cannabis, only 25 mg plant material would be required. Most painful clinical conditions require t.i.d. dosing of cannabis.

THC, CBD, and terpenoids are all highly lipophilic. Gastrointestinal absorption is markedly enhanced by inclusion of lipids in the cooked preparations. Traditional Indian cannabis cookery makes good use of *ghee,* or clarified butter. When cannabis tea is employed, added cream will enhance clinical benefits. Therapeutic tincture extraction in alcohol is also possible.

SMOKED CANNABIS

Techniques of smoking cannabis are legion and include marijuana cigarettes ("joint," "reefer," etc.), pipes,

waterpipes ("hookahs"), and bongs. Pharmacodynamically, smoking would be an ideal method of application of clinical cannabis, except for the attendant pulmonary issues. Clinical effects are noted within seconds to minutes after smoking. Inhalation avoids the first pass effect that hampers oral use, and allows effective dosage titration. Doses as low as 5 mg may provide relief of clinical symptoms, while hundreds of testimonials indicate the ability to continue work or study with unimpaired effectiveness. When symptoms return, repeat dosage is achieved quickly and easily. Overdosage is effectively avoidable.

In chronic usage of smoked cannabis, it is true that isolated cases of head and neck carcinogenesis have been noted (Tashkin, in press). Precancerous cytological changes in the airways of heavy cannabis smokers have been observed via bronchoscopy, but do not seem to lead to emphysematous deterioration (Tashkin, Simmons, Sherrill, & Coulson, 1997).

The "amotivational syndrome" has been largely relegated to the dustbin of drug war propaganda (Zimmer & Morgan, 1997). In fact, the interested reader may wish to seek out three rare books of the past generation on chronic usage that are remarkable for their careful documentation of the few distinguishing features between chronic cannabis smokers and age-matched controls (Carter, Coggins, & Doughty, 1976; Rubin & Comitas, 1975; Stefanis, et al. 1977). These are rarely mentioned in current alarmist reviews of the dangers of cannabis.

Some old myths die hard. Traditional smoking techniques in the U.S. make prolonged holding of a marijuana "toke" *de rigueur.* From a dose-response standpoint, this is unnecessary. Inhaled THC is well absorbed after a very brief interval, and subjective high and serum THC levels do not increase beyond a maximum 10-second inhalation (Azorlosa, Greenwald, & Stitzer, 1995). Furthermore, prolonged breath-holding under pressure increases the potential for hypoxia or pneumothorax (Tashkin, in press).

Contamination of herbal cannabis by pesticides, herbicides, and bacterial or fungal agents is possible and may represent a threat to the smoker, especially immunosuppressed patients (McPartland & Pruitt, 1997; McPartland, in press; Tashkin, in press). Scrupulous cultivation techniques avoid some of these issues. McPartland (in press) recommends pasteurization of herbal cannabis by heating in an oven at 150°C for 5 minutes.

Waterpipes and bongs are popular techniques for cooling smoke. Although they may reduce particulate matter as well, THC content and pharmaceutical efficiency appear to be compromised (Gieringer, 1996a,b). Surprisingly, the unfiltered "joint" seems to represent the most efficient means for conventional smoking, although use of hashish in a pipe (without tobacco) was not examined.

Vaporizers for Cannabis Administration

Vaporization of herbal cannabis may allow THC and terpenoid components below the flash point of the leaf, thereby reducing exposure to smoke, tar, and carcinogens. The technology has been hampered in its development by paraphernalia laws. Initial investigations of available devices to date have had disappointing results (Gieringer, 1996a, b), but further studies are currently underway and appear very promising.

Rectal Administration

Suppository preparations of cannabis were employed in the 19th century and may be an acceptable alternative route of administration for some conditions. The first-pass effect is largely avoided, although the ability for close dose titration is lost. THC suppositories, particularly as a hemisuccinate, have proven to be twice as bioavailable as oral THC (Brenneisen, Egli, ElSohly, Henn, & Spiess 1996; ElSohly, Little, Hikal, Harland, Stanford, & Walker, 1991; Mattes, Engelman, Shaw, ElSohly, 1994). No studies have examined the use of this preparation with respect to analgesia, but one might expect comparison to dronabinol at least with regard to the spectrum of activity. Synergistic combinations of cannabis components may be more valuable.

Suppositories are not a popular method of drug delivery in the United States.

Sublingual Tincture of Cannabis

This method of administration is under investigation by GW Pharmaceuticals in the United Kingdom, employing combinations of specific strains of cannabis that are rich in THC or CBD. Terpenoids and other minor components that may be important to therapeutics effects of cannabis are retained in this fashion. Dose-metered sublingual sprays are currently in Phase 1 and Phase 2 clinical trials for a variety of indications. Initial results indicate good bioavailability, patient tolerance, and clinical effects.

Aerosol THC Preparations

Cannabis has a long history of use in asthma, even as a smoked preparation. A pure THC aerosol has been attempted numerous times in the past. Physical and delivery issues have been challenging, but more interestingly, pure THC seems to have an irritating and even bronchoconstrictive effect when employed in isolation (Tashkin, 1977). This author (Russo) believes that anti-inflammatory effects of concomitant terpenoid and flavonoid administration is necessary for full effects and tolerance in pursuit of the pulmonary route. Further research is underway by GW Pharmaceuticals, Inhale Therapeutic Systems, and possibly others.

Transdermal Administration

The American Cancer Society has received a large grant to examine the use of a THC skin patch. No pharmacokinetics data are currently available to ascertain whether transdermal THC administration is a viable option (Brenneisen, 2001, in press).

REFERENCES

Abrahamov, A., & Mechoulam, R. (1995). An efficient new cannabinoid antiemetic in pediatric oncology. *Life Sciences, 56*(23–24), 2097–2102.

Access to therapeutic marijuana/cannabis. (1996). *American Journal of Public Health, 86,* 441–442.

Alosetron (Lotronex) for the treatment of irritable bowel syndrome. (2000). *Medical Letters, 42*(1081), 53–54.

Aulde, J. (1890). Studies in therapeutics—Cannabis indica. *Therapeutic Gazette, 14,* 523–526.

Azorlosa, J.L., Greenwald, M.K., & Stitzer, M.L. (1995). Marijuana smoking: Effects of varying puff volume and breathhold duration. *Journal of Pharmacology and Experimental Therapeutics, 272*(2), 560–569.

Barinaga, M. (1992). Pot, heroin unlock new areas for neuroscience. *Science, 258,* 1882–1884.

Barrett, M.L., Scutt, A M., & Evans, F.J. (1986). Cannflavin A and B, prenylated flavones from *Cannabis sativa* L. *Experientia, 42*(4), 452–453.

Batho, R. (1883, May 26). Cannabis indica. *British Medical Journal, 1,* 1002.

Behbehani, M.M. (1995). Functional characteristics of the midbrain periaqueductal gray. *Progress in Neurobiology, 46*(6), 575–605.

Benet, S. (1975). Early diffusion and folk uses of hemp. In V. Rubin (Ed.), *Cannabis and Culture* (pp. 39–49). The Hague: Mouton Publishers.

Biruni, M.I.A., & Said, H.M. (1973). *al-Biruni's book on pharmacy and materia medica.* Karachi: Hamdard Academy.

Boger, D.L., Patterson, J.E., & Jin, Q. (1998). Structural requirements for 5-HT2A and 5-HT1A serotonin receptor potentiation by the biologically active lipid oleamide. *Proceedings, National Academy of Science (USA), 95*(8), 4102–4107.

Brazis, M.Z., & Mathre, M.L. (1997). Dosage and administration of cannabis. In M.L. Mathre (Ed.), *Cannabis in medical practice: A legal, historical and pharmacological overview of the therapeutic use of marijuana* (pp. 142–156). Jefferson, NC: McFarland.

Brenneisen, R. (1984). Psychotrope Drogen. II. Bestimmung der Cannabinoide in *Cannabis sativa* L. und in Cannabisprodukten mittels Hochdruckflüssigkeitschromatographie (HPLC) [Psychotropic drugs. II. Determination of cannabinoids in Cannabis sativa L. and in cannabis products with high pressure liquid chromatography (HPLC)]. *Pharmaceutica Acta Helvetiae, 59*(9–10), 247–59.

Brenneisen, R. (2001, in press). Pharmacokinetics. In F. Groten-hermen & E.B. Russo (Eds.), *Cannabis and cannab-inoids: Pharmacology, toxicity and therapeutic potential*. Binghamton, NY: Haworth Press.

Brenneisen, R., Egli, A., Elsohly, M.A., Henn, V., & Spiess, Y. (1996). The effect of orally and rectally administered delta 9-tetrahydrocannabinol on spasticity: A pilot study with 2 patients. *International Journal of Clinical Pharmacology and Therapeutics, 34*(10), 446–452.

British Medical Association (1997). *Therapeutic uses of cannabis*. Amsterdam: Harwood Academic Publishers.

Brown, J. (1883). Cannabis indica: A valuable remedy in men-orrhagia. *British Medical Journal, 1*(May 26), 1002.

Burstein, S. (1992). Eicosanoids as mediators of cannabinoid action. In L. Murphy & A. Bartke (Eds.), *Marijuana/can-nabinoids: Neurobiology and neurophysiology of drug abuse. I. (pp. 73–91). Boca Raton, FL: CRC Press.

Burstein, S.H. (2000). Ajulemic acid (CT3): A potent analog of the acid metabolites of THC. *Current Pharmaceutical Design, 6*(13), 1339–1345.

Burstein, S.H. (2001, in press). The therapeutic potential of ajulemic acid (CT3). In F. Grotenhermen & E.B. Russo (Eds.), *Cannabis and cannabinoids: Pharmacology, tox-icology and therapeutic potential*. Binghamton, NY: Haworth Press.

Burstein, S., Levin, E., & Varanelli, C. (1973). Prostaglandins and cannabis. II. Inhibition of biosynthesis by the nat-urally occurring cannabinoids. *Biochemical Pharmacol-ogy, 22*(22), 2905–2910.

Burstein, S., Varanelli, C., & Slade, L. . (1975). Prostaglandins and cannabis. III. Inhibition of biosynthesis by essential oil components of marihuana. *Biochemical Pharmacol-ogy, 24*(9), 1053–1054.

Calhoun, S.R., Galloway, G.P., & Smith, D.E. (1998). Abuse potential of dronabinol (Marinol). *Journal of Psychoac-tive Drugs, 30*(2), 187–196.

Calignano, A., La Rana, G., Giuffrida, A., & Piomelli, D. (1998). Control of pain initiation by endogenous cannabinoids. *Nature, 394*(6690), 277–281.

Carta, G., Gessa, G.L., & Nava, F. (1999). Dopamine D(2) recep-tor antagonists prevent delta(9)-tetrahydrocannabinol-induced antinociception in rats. *European Journal of Pharmacology, 384*(2–3), 153–156.

Carter, W.E., Coggins, W J., & Doughty, P.L. (1976). *Chronic cannabis use in Costa Rica: A report by the Center for Latin American Studies of the University of Florida to the National Institute on Drug Abuse*. Gainesville: Uni-versity of Florida Press.

Chomel, P.J.B. (1782). *Abrégé de l'histoire des plantes usuelles*. Paris: Libraires Associés.

Chopra, I.C., & Chopra, R.W. (1957). The use of cannabis drugs in India. *Bulletin on Narcotics, 9,* 4–29.

Christison, A.. (1851). On the natural history, action, and uses of Indian hemp. *Monthly Journal of Medical Science of Edinburgh, Scotland, 13,* 26–45, 117–121.

Cichewicz, D.L., Martin, Z.L., Smith, F.L., & Welch, S.P. (1999). Enhancement of mu opioid antinociception by oral delta9-tetrahydrocannabinol: Dose-response analysis and receptor identification. *Journal of Pharmacology and Experimental Therapeutics, 289*(2), 859–67.

Clarke, R.C. (1998). *Hashish!* Los Angeles, CA: Red Eye Press,

Clarke, R.C. (1981). *Marijuana botany: An advanced study: The propagation and breeding of distinctive cannabis*. Ber-keley, CA: And/Or Press.

Clendinning, J. (1843). Observation on the medicinal properties of *Cannabis sativa* of India. *Medico-Chirurgical Trans-actions, 26,* 188–210.

Conrad, C. (1997). *Hemp for health: The medicinal and nutritional uses of Cannabis sativa*. Rochester, VT: Healing Arts Press.

Dastur, J.F. (1962). *Medicinal plants of India and Pakistan*. Bombay: D.B. Taraporevala Sons.

Devane, W.A., Hanus, L., Breuer, A., Pertwee, R.G., Stevenson, L.A., Griffin, G., Gibson, D., Mandelbaum, A., Etinger, A., & Mechoulam, R. (1992). Isolation and structure of a brain constituent that binds to the cannabinoid recep-tor. *Science, 258*(5090), 1946–1949.

Dioscorides, P. (1968). *The Greek herbal of Dioscorides*. Lon-don: Hafner Publishing.

Dixon, W.E. (1899). The pharmacology of *Cannabis indica*. *British Medical Journal, 2,* 1354–1357.

Donovan, M. (1845). On the physical and medicinal qualities of Indian hemp *(Cannabis indica)*; With observations on the best mode of administration, and cases illustrative of its powers. *Dublin Journal of Medical Science, 26,* 368–402, 459–461.

Douthwaite, A.H. (1947). Choice of drugs in the treatment of duodenal ulcer. *British Medical Journal, 43,* 43–47.

Dreher, M.C. (1997). Cannabis and pregnancy. In M. L. Mathre (Ed.), *Cannabis in medical practice: A legal, historical and pharmacological overview of the therapeutic use of marijuana* (pp. 159–170). Jefferson, NC: McFarland.

Dwarakanath, C. (1965). Use of opium and cannabis in the traditional systems of medicine in India. *Bulletin on Narcotics, 17,* 15–19.

ElSohly, M.A., Little, T.L., Jr., Hikal, A., Harland, E., Stanford, D.F., & Walker, L. (1991). Rectal bioavailability of delta-9-tetrahydrocannabinol from various esters. *Phar-macology, Biochemistry, and Behavior, 40*(3), 497–502.

ElSohly, M.A., Ross, S.A., Mehmedic, Z., Arafat, R., Yi, B., & Banahan, B.F., III (2000). Potency trends of delta9-THC and other cannabinoids in confiscated marijuana from 1980–1997. *Journal of Forensic Sciences, 45*(1), 24–30.

Evans, A.T., Formukong, E.A., & Evans, F.J. (1987). Actions of cannabis constituents on enzymes of arachidonate metabolism: Anti-inflammatory potential. *Biochemical Pharmacology, 36*(12), 2035–2037.

Evans, F.J. (1991). Cannabinoids: The separation of central from peripheral effects on a structural basis. *Planta Medica, 57*(7), S60–S67.

Fan, P. (1995). Cannabinoid agonists inhibit the activation of 5-HT3 receptors in rat nodose ganglion. *Journal of Neuro-physiology, 73,* 907–910.

Farlow, J.W. (1889). On the use of belladonna and *Cannabis indica* by the rectum in gynecological practice. *Boston Medical and Surgical Journal, 120,* 507–509.

Ferri, S., Cavicchini, E., Romualdi, P., Speroni, E., & Murari, G. (1986). Possible mediation of catecholaminergic path-ways in the antinociceptive effect of an extract of *Can-nabis sativa* L. *Psychopharmacology, 89*(2), 244–247.

Fettes, I., Gawel, M., Kuzniak, S., & Edmeads, J. (1985). Endorphin levels in headache syndromes. *Headache, 25*(1), 37–39.

Fimiani, C., Liberty, T., Aquirre, A.J., Amin, I., Ali, N., & Stefano, G.B. (1999). Opiate, cannabinoid, and eicosanoid signaling converges on common intracellular pathways nitric oxide coupling. *Prostaglandins and Other Lipid Mediators, 57*(1), 23–34.

Fishbein, M. (1942). Migraine associated with menstruation. *Journal of the American Medical Association, 237*, 326.

Formukong, E.A., Evans, A.T., & Evans, F.J. (1988). Analgesic and antiinflammatory activity of constituents of *Cannabis sativa* L. *Inflammation, 12*(4), 361–371.

Formukong, E.A., Evans, A.T., & Evans, F.J. (1989). The inhibitory effects of cannabinoids, the active constituents of *Cannabis sativa* L. on human and rabbit platelet aggregation. *Journal of Pharmacy and Pharmacology, 41*(10), 705–709.

Fride, E., & Mechoulam, R. (1993). Pharmacological activity of the cannabinoid receptor agonist, anandamide, a brain constituent. *European Journal of Pharmacology, 231*(2), 313–314.

Fried, P.A. (in press). Pregnancy. In F. Grotenhermen & E. Russo (Eds.), *Cannabis and cannabinoids: Pharmacology, toxicology and therapeutic potential*. Binghamton, NY: Haworth Press.

Gerritsen, M.E., Carley, W.W., Ranges, G.E., Shen, C.P., Phan, S.A., Ligon, G.F., & Perry, C.A. (1995). Flavonoids inhibit cytokine-induced endothelial cell adhesion protein gene expression. *American Journal of Pathology, 147*(2), 278–292.

Ghalioungui, P. (1987). *The Ebers papyrus: A new English translation, commentaries and glossaries*. Cairo: Academy of Scientific Research and Technology.

Gieringer, D. (1996a). Waterpipe study. *Bulletin of the Multidisciplinary Association for Psychedelic Studies, 6*, 59–63.

Gieringer, D. (1996b). Why marijuana smoke harm reduction? *Bulletin of the Multidisciplinary Association for Psychedelic Studies, 6*, 64–66.

Gieringer, D. (in press). Medical use of cannabis: Experience in California. In F. Grotenhermen & E. Russo (Eds.), *Cannabis and cannabinoids: Pharmacology, toxicology, & therapeutic potential*. Binghamton, NY: Haworth Press.

Goadsby, P.J., & Gundlach, A.L. (1991). Localization of ^{3}H-dihydroergotamine-binding sites in the cat central nervous system: Relevance to migraine. *Annals of Neurology, 29*(1), 91–94.

Grigor, J. (1852). Indian hemp as an oxytocic. *Monthly Journal of Medical Sciences, 14*, 124.

Grinspoon, L., & Bakalar, J.B. (1997). *Marihuana, the forbidden medicine* (Rev. & exp. ed). New Haven, CT: Yale University Press.

Grotenhermen, F. (in press a). Definitions and explanations. In F. Grotenhermen & E. Russo (Eds.), *Cannabis and cannabinoids: Pharmacology, toxicology, & therapeutic potential*. Binghamton, NY: Haworth Press.

Grotenhermen, F. (in press b). Practical hints. In F. Grotenhermen & E. Russo (Eds.), *Cannabis and Cannabinoids: Pharmacology, toxicology, & therapeutic potential*. Binghamton, NY: Haworth Press.

Gu, W., & Clarke, R.C. (1998). A survey of hemp (*Cannabis sativa* L.) use by the Hmong (Miao) of the China/Vietnam border region. *Journal of the International Hemp Association, 5*(1), 4–9.

Guyatt, G.H., Keller, J.L., Jaeschke, R., Rosenbloom, D., Adachi, J.D., & Newhouse, M.T. (1990). The n-of-1 randomized controlled trial: Clinical usefulness. Our three-year experience. *Annals of Internal Medicine, 112*(4), 293–299.

Hamann, W., & di Vadi, P.P. (1999). Analgesic effect of the cannabinoid analogue nabilone is not mediated by opioid receptors. *Lancet, 353*(9152), 560.

Hampson, A.J., Bornheim, L.M., Scanziani, M., Yost, C.S., Gray, A.T., Hansen, B.M., Leonoudakis, D.J., & Bickler, P.E. (1998). Dual effects of anandamide on NMDA receptor-mediated responses and neurotransmission. *Journal of Neurochemistry, 70*(2), 671–676.

Hampson, A.J., Grimaldi, M., Axelrod, J., & Wink, D. (1998). Cannabidiol and (-)Delta9-tetrahydrocannabinol are neuroprotective antioxidants. *Proceedings, National Academy of Science (USA), 95*(14), 8268–8273.

Hare, H.A. (1887). Clinical and physiological notes on the action of *Cannabis indica. Therapeutic Gazette, 2*, 225–228.

Hare, H.A. (1922). *A text-book of practical therapeutics, with especial reference to the application of remedial measures to disease and their employment upon a rational basis* (18th ed.). Philadelphia: Lea & Febiger.

Herkenham, M.A. (1993). Localization of cannabinoid receptors in brain: Relationship to motor and reward systems. In S. G. Korman & J. D. Barchas (Eds.), *Biological basis of substance abuse* (pp. 187–200). London: Oxford University.

Hoechstetter, S.S. (1930). Effects of alcohol and cannabis during labor. *Journal of the American Medical Association, 94*(15), 1165.

Holdcroft, A., Smith, M., Jacklin, A., Hodgson, H., Smith, B., Newton, M., & Evans, F. (1997). Pain relief with oral cannabinoids in familial Mediterranean fever. *Anaesthesia, 52*(5), 483–486.

Hollister, L.E. (1986). Health aspects of cannabis. *Pharmacological Reviews, 38*(1), 1–20.

Hollister, L.E. (2000). An approach to the medical marijuana controversy. *Drug and Alcohol Dependency, 58*(1–2), 3–7.

Hutchinson, H.W. (1975). Patterns of marihuana use in Brazil. In V. Rubin (Ed.), *Cannabis and culture* (pp. 173–183). The Hague: Mouton.

Indian Hemp Drugs Commission (1894). *Report of the Indian Hemp Drugs Commission, 1893–94*. Simla, India: Govt. Central Print. Office.

Jaggar, S.I., Hasnie, F.S., Sellaturay, S., & Rice, A.S. (1998). The anti-hyperalgesic actions of the cannabinoid anandamide and the putative CB_2 receptor agonist palmitoylethanolamide in visceral and somatic inflammatory pain. *Pain, 76*(1–2), 189–199.

Jaggar, S.I., Sellaturay, S., & Rice, A.S. (1998). The endogenous cannabinoid anandamide, but not the CB2 ligand palmitoylethanolamide, prevents the viscero-visceral hyper-reflexia associated with inflammation of the rat urinary bladder. *Neuroscience Letters, 253*(2), 123–126.

Jain, A.K., Ryan, J.R., McMahon, F.G., & Smith, G. (1981). Evaluation of intramuscular levonantradol and placebo in acute postoperative pain. *Journal of Clinical Pharmacology, 21*(8–9 Suppl.), 320S–326S.

Julien, M.S. (1849). Chirugie chinoise—Substance anesthétique employée en Chine, dans le commencement du III-ième siecle de notre ère, pour paralyser momentanement la sensibilité. *Comptes Rendus Hebdomadaires de l'Académie des Sciences, 28,* 223–229.

Kahl, O. (1994). *Sabur ibn Sahl: Dispensatorium parvum (al-Aarabadhin al-Saghir).* Leiden, The Netherlands: E.J. Brill.

Kimura, T., Ohta, T., Watanabe, K., Yoshimura, H., & Yamamoto, I. (1998). Anandamide, an endogenous cannabinoid receptor ligand, also interacts with 5-hydroxytryptamine (5-HT) receptor. *Biological and Pharmaceutical Bulletin, 21*(3), 224–226.

Klein, T.W., Friedman, H., & Specter, S. (1998). Marijuana, immunity and infection. *Journal of Neuroimmunology, 83*(1–2), 102–115.

Ko, M.C., & Woods, J. H. (1999). Local administration of delta9-tetrahydrocannabinol attenuates capsaicin-induced thermal nociception in rhesus monkeys: A peripheral cannabinoid action. *Psychopharmacology (Berlin), 143*(3), 322–326.

Kumar, A.M., Haney, M., Becker, T., Thompson, M L., Kream, R.M., & Miczek, K. (1990). Effect of early exposure to delta-9-tetrahydrocannabinol on the levels of opioid peptides, gonadotropin-releasing hormone and substance P in the adult male rat brain. *Brain Research, 525*(1), 78–83.

Larson, E.B. (1990). N-of-1 clinical trials. A technique for improving medical therapeutics. *West Journal of Medicine, 152*(1), 52–56.

Lewis, B., Menage, V.L., Pellat, C.H., & Schacht, J. (1971). *The encyclopedia of Islam.* Leiden, The Netherlands: E.J. Brill.

Li, J., Daughters, R.S., Bullis, C., Bengiamin, R., Stucky, M.W., Brennan, J., & Simone, D.A. (1999). The cannabinoid receptor agonist WIN 55,212-2 mesylate blocks the development of hyperalgesia produced by capsaicin in rats. *Pain, 81*(1–2), 25–33.

Lichtman, A.H., Cook, S.A., & Martin, B.R. (1996). Investigation of brain sites mediating cannabinoid-induced antinociception in rats: Evidence supporting periaqueductal gray involvement. *Journal of Pharmacology and Experimental Therapeutics, 276*(2), 585–593.

Lilly (1898). *Lilly's Handbook of Pharmacy and Therapeutics.* Indianapolis: Lilly and Company.

Linné, C.A. (1772). *Materia medica per regna tria naturae.* Lipsiae et Erlangae: Wolfgang Waltherum.

Lozano Camara, I. (1990). *Tres tratados arabes sobre el Cannabis indica: Textos para la historia del hachis en las sociedades islamicas, S. XIII–XVI.* Madrid: Agencia Española de Cooperacion Internacional Instituto de Cooperación con el Mundo Arabe.

Mackenzie, S. (1887). Remarks on the value of Indian hemp in the treatment of a certain type of headache. *British Medical Journal, 1,* 97–98.

Mackenzie, S. (1894). Therapeutique médicale: De la valeur therapeutique speciale du chanvre indien dans certains états morbides. *Semaine Médicale, 14,* 399–400.

Mailleux, P., & Vanderhaeghen, J.J. (1992). Localization of cannabinoid receptor in the human developing and adult basal ganglia. Higher levels in the striatonigral neurons. *Neuroscience Letters, 148*(1–2), 173–176.

Mailleux, P., & Vanderhaeghen, J.J. (1994). Delta-9-tetrahydrocannabinol regulates substance P and enkephalin mRNAs levels in the caudate-putamen. *European Journal of Pharmacology, 267*(1), R1–3.

Malfait, A.M., Gallily, R., Sumariwalla, P.F., Malik, A.S., Andreakos, E., Mechoulam, R., & Feldmann, M. (2000). The nonpsychoactive cannabis constituent cannabidiol is an oral anti-arthritic therapeutic in murine collagen-induced arthritis. *Proceedings, National Academy of Science (USA), 97*(17), 9561–9566.

Maneuf, Y.P., Nash, J.E., Crossman, A.R., & Brotchie, J.M. (1996). Activation of the cannabinoid receptor by delta 9-tetrahydrocannabinol reduces gamma-aminobutyric acid uptake in the globus pallidus. *European Journal of Pharmacology, 308*(2), 161–164.

Mannische, L. (1989). *An ancient Egyptian herbal.* Austin: University of Texas.

Manzanares, J., Corchero, J., Romero, J., Fernandez-Ruiz, J.J., Ramos, J.A., & Fuentes, J.A. (1998). Chronic administration of cannabinoids regulates proenkephalin mRNA levels in selected regions of the rat brain. *Brain Research, Molecular Brain Research, 55*(1), 126–132.

Manzanares, J., Corchero, J., Romero, J., Fernandez-Ruiz, J.J., Ramos, J.A., & Fuentes, J.A. (1999). Pharmacological and biochemical interactions between opioids and cannabinoids. *Trends in Pharmacological Sciences, 20*(7), 287–294.

Marcandier, M. (1758). *Traité du chanvre.* Paris: Chez Nyon.

Marcandier, M. (1764). *Treatise on hemp.* London: T. Becket and P. A. de Hondt.

Margolis, J.S., & Clorfene, R. (1969). *A child's garden of grass (The official handbook for marijuana users).* North Hollywood, CA: Contact Books.

Martin, M.A. (1975). Ethnobotanical aspects of cannabis in Southeast Asia. In V. Rubin (Ed.), *Cannabis and Culture* (pp. 63–75). The Hague: Mouton Publishers.

Martin, S., Padilla, E., Ocete, M.A., Galvez, J., Jimenez, J., & Zarzuelo, A. (1993). Anti-inflammatory activity of the essential oil of *Bupleurum fruticescens. Planta Medica, 59*(6), 533–536.

Marx, J. (1990). Marijuana receptor gene cloned. *Science, 249*(4969), 624–626.

Matsuda, L.A., Lolait, S.J., Brownstein, M.J., Young, A.C., & Bonner, T.I. (1990). Structure of a cannabinoid receptor and functional expression of the cloned cDNA. *Nature, 346*(6284), 561–564.

Mattes, R.D., Engelman, K., Shaw, L.M., & Elsohly, M.A. (1994). Cannabinoids and appetite stimulation. *Pharmacology, Biochemistry, and Behavior, 49*(1), 187–195.

Mattison, J.B. (1891). *Cannabis indica* as an anodyne and hypnotic. *St. Louis Medical and Surgical Journal, 61,* 265–271.

Maurer, M., Henn, V., Dittrich, A., & Hofmann, A. (1990). Delta-9-tetrahydrocannabinol shows antispastic and analgesic effects in a single case double-blind trial. *European Archives of Psychiatry and Clinical Neuroscience, 240*(1), 1–4.

McPartland, J. (2001). Cannabis and eicosanoids: A review of molecular pharmacology. *Journal of Cannabis Therapeutics, 1*(1), 71–83

McPartland, J.M. (in press). Contaminants and adulterants in herbal cannabis. In F. Grotenhermen & E.B. Russo (Eds.), *Cannabis and cannabinoids: Pharmacology, toxicology, & therapeutic potential.* Binghamton, NY: Haworth Press.

McPartland, J M., & Mediavilla, V. (in press). Non-cannabinoids in cannabis. In F. Grotenhermen & E. B. Russo (Eds.), *Cannabis and cannabinoids.* Binghamton, NY: Haworth Press.

McPartland, J.M., & Pruitt, P.L. (1997). Medical marijuana and its use by the immunocompromised. *Alternative Therapies in Health and Medicine, 3*(3), 39–45.

McPartland, J.M., & Pruitt, P.L. (1999). Side effects of pharmaceuticals not elicited by comparable herbal medicines: The case of tetrahydrocannabinol and marijuana. *Alternative Therapies in Health and Medicine, 5*(4), 57–62.

Mechoulam, R., & Ben-Shabat, S. (1999). From gan-zi-gun-nu to anandamide and 2-arachidonoylglycerol: The ongoing story of cannabis. *Natural Product Reports, 16*(2), 131–143.

Mechoulam, R., & Feigenbaum, J.J. (1987). Toward cannabinoid drugs. In G. Ellis & G. West (Eds.), *Progress in medicinal chemistry* (pp. 159–207). Amsterdam: Elsevier Science.

Mechoulam, R., Fride, E., & Di Marzo, V. (1998). Endocannabinoids. *European Journal of Pharmacology, 359*, 1–18.

Meng, I.D., Manning, B.H., Martin, W.J., & Fields, H.L. (1998). An analgesia circuit activated by cannabinoids. *Nature, 395*(6700), 381–383.

Michel, L. (1880). Propriétés médicinales de l'Indian hemp ou du *Cannabis indica. Montpellier Medical, 45,* 103–116.

Mikuriya, T.H. (1997). Chronic migraine headache: Five cases successfully treated with marinol and/or illiciit cannabis. http://206.61.184.43/schaffer/hemp/migrn1.htm

Mikuriya, T.H., & Aldrich, M.R. (1988). Cannabis 1988. Old drug, new dangers. The potency question. *Journal of Psychoactive Drugs, 20*(1), 47–55.

Milstein, S.L., MacCannell, K., Karr, G., & Clark, S. (1975). Marijuana-produced changes in pain tolerance. Experienced and non-experienced subjects. *International Pharmacopsychiatry, 10*(3), 177–182.

Müller-Vahl, K.R., Kolbe, H., Schneider, U., & Emrich, H.M. (1998). Cannabinoids: Possible role in patho-physiology and therapy of Gilles de la Tourette syndrome. *Acta Psychiatrica Scandinavica, 98*(6), 502–506.

Musonda, C.A., & Chipman, J.K. (1998). Quercetin inhibits hydrogen peroxide (H_2O_2)-induced NF-kappaB DNA binding activity and DNA damage in HepG2 cells. *Carcinogenesis, 19*(9), 1583–1589.

Nalin, D.R., Levine, M.M., Rhead, J., Bergquist, E., Rennels, M., Hughes, T., O'Donnel, S., & Hornick, R.B. (1978). Cannabis, hypochlorhydria, & cholera. *Lancet, 2*(8095), 859–862.

New York (City). Mayor's Committee on Marihuana, Wallace, G. B., & Cunningham, E. V. (1973). *The marihuana problem in the city of New York.* Metuchen, NJ: Scarecrow Reprint Corp.

Nicolodi, M. (1998). Painful and non-painful effects of low doses of morphine in migraine sufferers partly depend on excitatory amino acids and gamma-aminobutyric acid. *International Journal of Clinical Pharmacology Research, 18*(2), 79–85.

Nicolodi, M., Del Bianco, P.L., & Sicuteri, F. (1997). Modulation of excitatory amino acids pathway: A possible therapeutic approach to chronic daily headache associated with analgesic drug abuse. *International Journal of Clinical Pharmacology Research, 17*(2–3), 97–100.

Nicolodi, M., & Sicuteri, F. (1995). Exploration of NMDA receptors in migraine: Therapeutic and theoretic implications. *International Journal of Clinical Pharmacology Research, 15*(5–6), 181–189.

Nicolodi, M., & Sicuteri, F. (1998). Negative modultors [sic] of excitatory amino acids in episodic and chronic migraine: Preventing and reverting chronic migraine. *International Journal of Clinical Pharmacology Research, 18*(2), 93–100.

Nicolodi, M., Volpe, A.R., & Sicuteri, F. (1998). Fibromyalgia and headache. Failure of serotonergic analgesia and N-methyl-D-aspartate-mediated neuronal plasticity: Their common clues. *Cephalalgia, 18*(Suppl. 21), 41–44.

Notcutt, W., Price, M., & Chapman, G. (1997). Clinical experience with nabilone for chronic pain. *Pharmaceutical Sciences, 3,* 551–555.

Noyes, R., Jr., & Baram, D.A. (1974). Cannabis analgesia. *Comprehensive Psychiatry, 15*(6), 531–535.

Noyes, R., Jr., Brunk, S.F., Avery, D.A.H., & Canter, A.C. (1975). The analgesic properties of delta-9-tetrahydrocannabinol and codeine. *Clinical Pharmacology and Therapeutics, 18*(1), 84–9.

Noyes, R., Jr., Brunk, S.F., Baram, D.A., & Canter, A. (1975). Analgesic effect of delta-9-tetrahydrocannabinol. *Journal of Clinical Pharmacology, 15*(2–3), 139–43.

Nunn, J. F. (1996). *Ancient Egyptian medicine.* Norman: University of Oklahoma Press.

O'Shaughnessy, W.B. (1838–1840). On the preparations of the Indian hemp, or gunjah *(Cannabis indica)*; Their effects on the animal system in health, and their utility in the treatment of tetanus and other convulsive diseases. *Transactions of the Medical and Physical Society of Bengal,* 71–102, 421–461.

Osler, W., & McCrae, T. (1915). *The principles and practice of medicine.* New York: Appleton and Company.

Parkinson, J., & Cotes, T. (1640). *Theatrum botanicum: The theater of plants.* London: Tho. Cotes.

Partridge, W.L. (1975). Cannabis and cultural groups in a Colombian *municipio.* In V. Rubin (Ed.), *Cannabis and culture* (pp. 147–172). The Hague: Mouton Publishers.

Perez-Reyes, M., Burstein, S.H., White, W.R., McDonald, S. A., & Hicks, R.E. (1991). Antagonism of marihuana effects by indomethacin in humans. *Life Sciences, 48*(6), 507–515.

Peroutka, S.J. (1990a). Developments in 5-hydroxytryptamine receptor pharmacology in migraine. *Neurologic Clinics, 8*(4), 829–839.

Peroutka, S.J. (1990b). The pharmacology of current antimigraine drugs. *Headache, 30*(1 Suppl.), 5–11; discussion, 24–28.

Peroutka, S.J. (1997). Dopamine and migraine. *Neurology, 49*(3), 650–656.

Pertwee, R.G. (1997). Cannabis and cannabinoids: Pharmacology and rationale for clinical use. *Pharmacetical Science, 3,* 539–545.

Pliny (1951). *Pliny: Natural history.* Cambridge, MA: Harvard University.

Randall, R.C. (1991). *Muscle spasm, pain & marijuana therapy.* Washington, D.C.: Galen Press.

Raskin, N.H. (1988). *Headache* (2nd ed.). New York: Churchill Livingstone.

Remington, J.P., Wood, H.C., Sadtler, S.P., LaWall, C.H., Kraemer, H., & Anderson, J.F. (1918). *The dispensatory of the United States of America* (20th ed.). Philadelphia: J. B. Lippincott.

Rennie, S.J. (1886). On the therapeutic value of *tinctura Cannabis indica* in the treatment of dysentery, more particularly in its sub-acute and chronic forms. *Indian Medical Gazette, 21,* 353–354.

Reynolds, J.R. (1868). On some of the therapeutical uses of Indian hemp. *Archives of Medicine, 2,* 154–160.

Richardson, J.D., Aanonsen, L., & Hargreaves, K.M. (1998a). Antihyperalgesic effects of spinal cannabinoids. *European Journal of Pharmacology, 345*(2), 145–153.

Richardson, J.D., Aanonsen, L., & Hargreaves, K.M. (1998b). Hypoactivity of the spinal cannabinoid system results in NMDA-dependent hyperalgesia. *Journal of Neuroscience, 18*(1), 451–457.

Richardson, J.D., Kilo, S., & Hargreaves, K.M. (1998). Cannabinoids reduce hyperalgesia and inflammation via interaction with peripheral CB₁ receptors. *Pain, 75*(1), 111–119.

Rosenthal, E., Gieringer, D., & Mikuriya, T. (1997). *Marijuana medical handbook: A guide to therapeutic use.* Oakland, CA: Quick American Archives.

Rubin, V. (1976). Cross-cultural perspectives on therapeutic uses of cannabis. In S. Cohen & R. Stillman (Eds.), *The therapeutic potential of marihuana* (pp. 1–17). New York: Plenum Medical.

Rubin, V.D., & Comitas, L. (1975). *Ganja in Jamaica: A medical anthropological study of chronic marihuana use.* The Hague: Mouton.

Rumpf, G.E., & Beekman, E.M. (1981). *The poison tree: Selected writings of Rumphius on the natural history of the Indies.* Amherst: University of Massachusetts Press.

Russo, E.B. (1998). Cannabis for migraine treatment: The once and future prescription? An historical and scientific review. *Pain, 76,*(1–2), 3–8.

Russo, E.B., Macarah, C.M., Todd, C.L., Medora, R.S., & Parker, K.K. (2000). Pharmacology of the essential oil of hemp at 5HT₁ₐ and 5HT₂ₐ receptors. Poster, 41st Annual Meeting of the American Society of Pharmacognosy, Seattle, WA. *Journal of Natural Products.*

Russo, E.B. (2000). *Handbook of psychotropic herbs: A scientific analysis of herbal remedies for psychiatric conditions.* Binghamton, NY: Haworth Press.

Russo, E.B. (2001). Hemp for headache: An in-depth historical and scientific review of cannabis in migraine treatment. *Journal of Cannabis Therapeutics, 1*(2), 21–92.

Russo, E.B. (in press). Migraine: Indications for cannabis and THC. In F. Grotenhermen & E. B. Russo, E. B. *Cannabis and cannabinoids.* Binghamton, NY: Haworth Press.

Schaefer, C.F., Brackett, D.J., Gunn, C.G., & Dubowski, K.M. (1979). Decreased platelet aggregation following marihuana smoking in man. *Journal, Oklahoma State Medical Association, 72*(12), 435–436.

Sée, M.G. (1890). Usages du *Cannabis indica* dans le traitement des névroses et dyspepsies gastriques. *Bulletin de l'Academie Nationale de Medecine, 3,* 158–193.

Shen, M., Piser, T.M., Seybold, V.S., & Thayer, S.A. (1996). Cannabinoid receptor agonists inhibit glutamatergic synaptic transmission in rat hippocampal cultures. *Journal of Neuroscience, 16*(14), 4322–4334,.

Shen, M., & Thayer, S.A. (1999). Delta-9-tetrahydrocannabinol acts as a partial agonist to modulate glutamatergic synaptic transmission between rat hippocampal neurons in culture. *Molecular Pharmacology, 55*(1), 8–13.

Shoemaker, J.V. (1899). The therapeutic value of *Cannabis indica. Texas Medical News, 8*(10), 477–488.

Silver, A. (1870). On the value of Indian hemp in menorrhagia and dysmenorrhoea. *Medical Times and Gazette, 2,* 59–61.

Snyder, S.H. (1971). *Uses of marijuana.* New York: Oxford University Press.

Sofia, R.D., Nalepa, S.D., Harakal, J.J., & Vassar, H.B. (1973). Anti-edema and analgesic properties of delta9-tetrahydrocannabinol (THC). *Journal of Pharmacology and Experimental Therapeutics, 186*(3), 646–655.

Spadone, C. (1991). Neurophysiologie du cannabis [Neurophysiology of cannabis]. *Encephale, 17*(1), 17–22.

Stefanis, C.N., Dornbush, R.L., & Fink, M. (1977). *Hashish: Studies of long-term use.* New York: Raven Press.

Strangman, N.M., & Walker, J.M. (1999). Cannabinoid WIN 55,212-2 inhibits the activity-dependent facilitation of spinal nociceptive responses. *Journal of Neurophysiology, 82*(1), 472–477.

Suckling, C. (1891). On the therapeutic value of Indian hemp. *British Medical Journal, 2,* 12.

Tambe, Y., Tsujiuchi, H., Honda, G., Ikeshiro, Y., & Tanaka, S. (1996). Gastric cytoprotection of the non-steroidal antiinflammatory sesquiterpene, beta-caryophyllene. *Planta Meicad, 62*(5), 469–470.

Tashkin, D.P. (2001, in press). Respiratory risks from marijuana smoking. In F. Grotenhermen & E. B. Russo (Eds.), *Cannabis and cannabinoids: Pharmacology, toxicology and therapeutic potential.* Binghamton, NY: Haworth Press.

Tashkin, D.P., Reiss, S., Shapiro, B.J., Calvarese, B., Olsen, J.L., & Lodge, J.W. (1977). Bronchial effects of aerosolized delta 9-tetrahydrocannabinol in healthy and asthmatic subjects. *American Review of Respiratory Disease, 115*(1), 57–65.

Tashkin, D.P., Simmons, M.S., Sherrill, D.L., & Coulson, A.H. (1997). Heavy habitual marijuana smoking does not cause an accelerated decline in FEV1 with age. *American Journal of Respiratory and Critical Care Medicine, 155*(1), 141–148.

Thompson, R.C. (1924). *The Assyrian herbal.* London: Luzac and Co.

Thompson, R.C. (1949). *A dictionary of Assyrian botany.* London: British Academy.

Turner, C.E., & Elsohly, M.A. (1981). Biological activity of cannabichromene, its homologs and isomers. *Journal of Clinical Pharmacology, 21,* 283S–291S.

Volfe, Z., Dvilansky, A., & Nathan, I. (1985). Cannabinoids block release of serotonin from platelets induced by plasma from migraine patients. *International Journal of Clinical Pharmacology Research, 5*(4), 243–246.

Walker, J.M., Hohmann, A.G., Martin, W.J., Strangman, N.M., Huang, S.M., & Tsou, K. (1999). The neurobiology of cannabinoid analgesia. *Life Sciences, 65*(6–7), 665–673.

Walker, J.M., Huang, S.M., Strangman, N.M., Tsou, K., & Sañudo-Peña, M.C. (1999). Pain modulation by the release of the endogenous cannabinoid anandamide. *Proceedings, National Academy of Science (USA), 96*(21), 12198–12203.

Waring, E. (1874). *Practical Therapeutics.* Philadelphia: Lindsay and Blackiston.

Welch, S.P., & Eads, M. (1999). Synergistic interactions of endogenous opioids and cannabinoid systems. *Brain Research, 848*(1–2), 183–190.

Wiegant, V.M., Sweep, C.G., & Nir, I. (1987). Effect of acute administration of delta 1-tetrahydrocannabinol on beta-endorphin levels in plasma and brain tissue of the rat. *Experientia, 43*(4), 413–415.

Wirtshafter, D. (1997). Nutritional value of hemp seed and hemp seed oil. In M. L. Mathre (Ed.), *Cannabis in medical practice* (pp. 181–191). Jefferson, NC: McFarland and Company.

Zias, J., Stark, H., Sellgman, J., Levy, R., Werker, E., Breuer, A., & Mechoulam, R. (1993). Early medical use of cannabis. *Nature, 363*(6426), 215.

Zimmer, L.E., & Morgan, J.P. (1997). *Marijuana myths, marijuana facts: A review of the scientific evidence.* New York: Lindesmith Center.

32

Nutrition for Pain Management

Hal S. Blatman, M.D.

The human body has built-in mechanisms for the purpose of healing. Some of these are more visible, such as callous formation after a bone fracture or scab formation after an injury to the skin. Other mechanisms of healing, such as the repair of oxidative damage, work at the level and size of molecules.

Nutrition affects pain and healing at three basic levels. One level is that food has to provide the basic raw materials for the body to build or manufacture parts for repair and development of body tissues. Another level of nutrition is that dietary supplements can enhance particular biochemical pathways, altering inflammation and affecting healing. A third level is that poisons can be ingested that negatively affect the body's ability to heal.

There is a mathematical formula that describes the basics of the relationship of nutrition to pain, healing, and wellness.

$$G - B + R \rightarrow P$$

In this equation, G represents the good things that can be done for or to the body, as well as good things that can be put into the body. B represents the bad things that can be done for or to the body, as well as bad things that can be put into the body. R represents the reserve that the body has left. This is an abstract measure of the life force that has been provided at birth and then partly used up with aging. These three categories (G, B, and R) imply the number P, which represents the degree of pain or problems (conversely, wellness) that a person experiences.

Patients seek medical attention because they are not happy with "P," the degree of pain and problems that they might be having. People pray to negotiate for how much "R" reserve their body has left. "G" and "B" are under more direct control by each person. By modifying the ratio of "G" good and "B" bad exposures to the body, the degree of "P" pain and problems will change. In other words, the body will create a level of function and healing that is directly related to nutrition.

To explain the impact of diet and nutrition on successful pain treatment and management, I have simplified the concepts into three rules.

RULE NO. 1: THOU SHALT NOT PUT "POISON" INTO THY BODY.

A poison is an ingested substance that adversely affects basic body functions. Two prevalent nutritional "poisons" should not be put into the body. These are aspartame and hydrogenated oil. Aspartame converts in the human body to methanol and formaldehyde. Formaldehyde is used in embalming fluid and has toxic effects on the body. Methanol is toxic to the nervous system and has been related to increased incidence of brain cancer. It is slowly excreted and accumulates in the body with frequent exposure. Additionally, aspartame outside the body is converted to methanol when it is heated to 85°F.

Sugar-free drinks and diet yogurt are examples of foods that contain aspartame. Recently, the food industry has been given permission by the FDA to add small amounts of aspartame to food without including it in the labeled list of ingredients.

Many people ingest aspartame without any noticeable adverse health effects. Other people will experience diffuse and body-wide pain symptoms. In some people, one diet soda every other day is enough exposure to cause this widespread pain. Pain symptoms will progressively lessen during the first 2 months after exposure is discontinued.

0-8493-0926-3/02/$0.00+$1.50
© 2002 by CRC Press LLC

Hydrogenated oil is the other commonly ingested poison. Approximately 100 years ago, a scientist bubbled hydrogen gas into vegetable oil, forming margarine. In the United States, this discovery became important during World War II when there was a shortage of butter. Production of margarine quickly became an industry. Then it was discovered that bugs would not eat it, mold would not grow on it, and it would not sustain or support life.

At that time in the United States, the retail food industry needed product shelf-life to be extended. It was discovered that the shelf-life of food could be greatly increased if essential fatty acids were replaced by hydrogenated oil.

These processed oils have several effects on the human body. They increase cholesterol risk factors and contribute to atherosclerotic heart disease. In addition, they alter prostaglandin synthesis pathways, increasing inflammation. Most profoundly, however, they affect cell membrane synthesis and repair.

Every cell in the body has a cell membrane that separates the contents of the cell from the material outside. This membrane is composed primarily of two layers of fat. The basic functions of the cell membrane include bringing nutrients into the cell, sending waste products out of the cell, and maintaining flexibility. Cell membrane composition determines the quality of these processes.

Ingested fatty acids are raw materials that are incorporated into cell membranes in approximately the same ratio as what is in the food. The most important of these are the omega-3 and the omega-6 fatty acids. These raw materials are called "essential" fatty acids because the human body cannot synthesize them. Historically, fat in the unaltered or unprocessed human food supply was approximately four parts omega-6 fatty acids to one part omega-3 fatty acids. Indeed, cell membranes function best when their omega-6:omega-3 ratio approximates 4:1. For people who cannot get quality fatty acids from fruits, vegetables, fish, and nuts, the diet can be supplemented with oils such as borage oil, flax seed oil, evening primrose oil, and fish oil. Borage oil and evening primrose oil are primarily omega-6 oils; fish oil is composed of omega-3 oils; and flax seed oil is composed of mostly omega-3 and partly omega-6 oils.

Hydrogenation alters the shape and function of fatty acids and hydrogenated oils are foreign to the natural biology of life. When hydrogenated oils are eaten, they are incorporated into cell membranes throughout the body in the same ratio as the foods that supplied them. Cell membranes that contain hydrogenated fats do not function as well as cell membranes that are composed of omega-6 and omega-3 fatty acids in a 4:1 ratio. These cell membranes then do not transmit nutrients and waste as effectively, and they lose their flexibility. With these changes, the basic body parts become less able to respond and heal

from injury. In other words, the body becomes "like a genuine GM truck that has been fixed with plastic parts."

In addition, when cells become injured, they release parts of their cell membranes into the general circulation. These cell membrane parts are integral components of biochemical inflammation processes. Some of these released cell membrane parts are pro-inflammatory and others are anti-inflammatory. Indeed, cellular membrane composition directly affects the biochemical process of inflammation and healing in this way also.

Many foods contain (partially) hydrogenated vegetable oil. These include margarine, peanut butter that does not require refrigeration after opening, donuts, cakes, crackers, potato chips, and pretzels. If a jar of peanut butter can be kept in the pantry for many months without growing mold, then it must have "poison" in it to keep the mold from growing. Restaurants are likely to cook egg dishes in margarine. Most important, virtually all foods cooked in a deep fat fryer have been bathed in this "poison" oil.

Patients should be advised to cook with olive oil, sesame oil, and butter. They should dispose of margarine and they should not eat foods that include hydrogenated or partially hydrogenated oil as an ingredient. Foods that have been cooked in deep fat should also not be eaten. These recommendations are not only very important for patients with pain, but also for patients with heart disease and high cholesterol.

RULE NO. 2: WHEN YOU ARE TRYING TO RUN A RACE CAR, USE 100-OCTANE FUEL.

The human body is a high-performance, biochemical "Ferrari." A brief look at children will show that they accelerate quickly, corner well, and wear out their tires. It makes sense that the energy level (octane) of food will affect the ability of the body to generate energy and heal. The lowest octane fuels that most people eat include sugar, wheat, and potatoes (white and red). Sugar drains the body of its energy, weakens the immune system, and affects personality. A typical serving of soda contains approximately 10 teaspoons of sugar. Moreover, to keep this much sugar in solution, phosphates are added to the mix. Processing these phosphates results in a loss of calcium. This loss of calcium has been associated with osteoporosis and childhood bone fractures. Soda should therefore be eliminated from the diet. Most store-bought fruit juices (including orange juice) also have very high sugar contents and are low-octane fuels. Food made from wheat (bread, pasta) is also of lower octane, and many people will do better if they avoid it. When there is a choice of bread to be made, wheat, multi-grain, and rye breads are higher on the octane list than white bread. Some breads, crackers, and pasta also do not contain wheat grain. Some patients are sensitive enough to wheat food octane that eating a dinner roll will cause significant fatigue the following day. Finally, a medium-sized potato can be likened to half a cup of sugar. Patients with pain and fatigue should be especially counseled to avoid wheat and potatoes. Rice is generally a much better choice and can often be substituted for potatoes and pasta. Brown rice is higher up the octane scale than white rice (long grain and not instant). Sweet potatoes and yams are usually well tolerated.

RULE NO. 3: THE RULE OF CRITTERS.

Inside the human intestine are approximately seven or eight pounds of microorganisms. These organisms make up the intestinal flora, which can be loosely categorized as symbiotic or dysbiotic. A symbiotic relationship is mutually beneficial, helping both the microorganisms and the human body. Symbiotic organisms include acidophilus and lactobacillus. These bacteria are important for digestion of food, production of B vitamins, and regulation of the immune system. A dysbiotic relationship is not mutually beneficial, helping the microorganisms while harming the human body. Yeast is a dysbiotic organism. Dysbiotic organisms contribute to injury and destruction of intestinal endothelium, the cells that line the digestive tract.

The health of this endothelial lining is of major importance for the entire human organism, affecting the immune, nervous, and digestive systems. For the immune system, endothelial cells produce immunoglobulin A (IgA). IgA provides the front-line defense for the body. When the body is deficient with respect to production of IgA, white blood cells must work harder to "pick up the slack." When body energy is diverted to production of white blood cells, there is less energy left to "run the engines." The result of this decreased IgA is fatigue.

Intestinal endothelial cells also produce 95% of the seratonin in the human body. Seratonin is an important neurotransmitter for the brain and for the digestive system. If these cells do not produce enough seratonin, the person is likely to become constipated and depressed.

The endothelial lining also functions as a barrier to the toxins and waste that are always present in the large intestine. When endothelial injury causes this barrier to become incompetent, the colon leaks foreign proteins, pathogenic organisms, and other toxins into the body. This toxic exposure causes what is called leaky gut syndrome. It can be likened to the process of a toxic waste dump leaking "poison" into the body's water supply. This phenomenon occurs especially in patients with irritable bowel syndrome (IBS) and Crohn's disease.

To improve health, the endothelial lining needs to be restored and symbiotic flora need to flourish. L-glutamine is a safe nutritional supplement that can be prescribed for healing the endothelium. Nutrition is provided to symbiotic flora by eating green leafy vegetables. These organisms must be fed like pet fish in a fish tank. Dysbiotic flora eat sugar, wheat, and potatoes. To change the balance of flora and promote the health of the gut, diet must be adjusted accordingly. The cleaner a patient becomes with respect to these food choices, the more likely it is that healing will occur.

Finally, it is important to remember that the human body needs water. In addition to basic hydration needs, water helps the body to detoxify. Massage and body work increase this requirement for water, as the toxins released from muscle will cause flu-like symptoms if they are not flushed from the body. The estimated daily need for water is up to one quart for every 50 pounds of body weight.

Motivating patients to make better food choices can be extremely challenging. The healthcare professional must be confident that following these recommendations will lead to noticeable clinical improvement. Most chronic pain and fatigue patients will experience a dramatic change in their levels of pain and energy after following the guidelines and recommendations presented in this chapter. Many will notice improvement within the first 2 weeks. It is also important that the healthcare provider show a good example. Patients are much less likely to pay attention to these recommendations when they see their doctors drink a diet soda and eat french fries.

BIBLIOGRAPHY

Gianotti, L., et al. (1995). Oral glutamine decreases bacterial translocation and improves survival in experimental gut-origin sepsis. *Journal of Parental and Enteral Nutrition, 14*, 69–74.

Kaminski, M., & Boal, R. (1992). An effect of ascorbic acid on delayed-onset muscle soreness. *Pain, 50*, 317–321.

Krause, W., Matheis, H., & Wulf, K. (1969). Fungaemia and funguria after oral administration of Candida albicans. *Lancet, 1*, 598.

Lee, L. (1998). Good dietary fat is beneficial for health. *Women's Health Connection 5*, 1–5.

Meisenberg, G., & Simmons, W. (1998). *Principles of medical biochemistry.* St. Louis: Mosby.

Percival, M. (1997). Nutritional support for connective tissue repair and wound healing. *Clinical Nutrition Insights*, 1–5.

Salisbury, A. (1997). Is NutraSweet safe, or sweet poison? *International Congress for Medical Professionals Journal, 7*, 2.

Travell, J., & Simons, D. (1983). *Myofascial pain and dysfunction: The trigger point manual.* Baltimore: Williams & Wilkins.

Werbach, M. (2000). Nutritional strategies for treating chronic fatigue syndrome. *Alternative Medicine Review, 5*(2), 93–108.

33

Pain Management with Regenerative Injection Therapy (RIT)

Felix S. Linetsky, M.D., Rafael Miguel, M.D., and Lloyd Saberski, M.D.

The whole of science is nothing more than a refinement
of everyday thinking.

Albert Einstein

INTRODUCTION

The purpose of this chapter is to provide pain management
clinicians with a review of the pertinent literature, and clinical
and anatomic considerations in relation to an interventional
regenerative treatment for chronic musculoskeletal pain.

There is an omnipresence of the connective tissue
throughout the body. Structurally and biomechanically, they
represent a heterogenous group with variations in collagen
orientation, cross linking, shape, cell properties, and presence of synovial lining in various locations. Without connective tissue, the "musculoskeletal system" will cease to
exist. A large variety of functions depend on the proper
homeostasis of connective tissue. For example, without the
storage and release of energy in connective tissue during
locomotion, much higher energy requirements would be
encountered (Dorman, 1992; Gray, 1995). On the other
hand, many dysfunctional and painful syndromes may arise
from pathologic conditions of the connective tissue.

The injury occurs when the internal or external forces
exceed the threshold of failure for the specific connective
tissue. This may be in the form of a ruptured or strained
ligament, tendon, fascia, or bone fracture, or a prolapsed disc.

Pain arising from connective tissue pathology, such as
degenerative and posttraumatic changes in the intervertebral
disc, ligaments, tendons, aponeuroses, fasciae, and sacroiliac
and facet joint capsular ligaments, is often difficult to differentiate based solely on clinical presentation. Individual variations in innervation further complicate the differential diagnosis. Left untreated, posttraumatic and overuse injuries of
ligaments and tendons can linger indefinitely, leading to the
progression of degenerative changes, loss of function, deconditioning, and perpetuation of disability and chronic pain
(Bogduk, et al., 1991; Dreyfuss, 1997; Hackett, 1958; 1991;
Merskey, et al., 1994; Shuman, 1958; Steindler, et al., 1938).

Interventional regenerative modalities for painful
musculoskeletal pathologies have been described for more
than two millenniums. For example, the technique of collagen thermomodulation, now known as *thermocapsulo-
graphy,* was originally described by Hippocrates, who had
created thermocoagulation of the anteroinferior capsule
for treatment of recurrent shoulder dislocations "with red
hot slender irons" (Dorman, et al., 1991; Shuman, 1958).
It is currently recognized that sufficient thermomodulation
of collagen can be achieved with lower temperatures to
stimulate a proliferative and regenerative/reparative
response. This concept has led to the development of
intradiscal electrothermal (IDET) procedures, currently
utilized with the intent to achieve nuclear shrinkage, seal
annular fissures, and thermocoagulate nociceptors (Darby,
et al., 1998; Saal, et al., 1998a, 1998b).

The coexistence of physical and chemical methods is
well demonstrated in the contemporary practice of dermatology and plastic surgery, where chemical (carbolic acid/
phenol) and laser-induced facial peels are utilized for
regeneration and rejuvenation by chemo- and thermomodulation of the skin collagen.

0-8493-0926-3/02/$0.00+$1.50
© 2002 by CRC Press LLC

A less-known but long-practiced method of interventional regenerative modalities is regenerative injection therapy (RIT), also known as prolotherapy or sclerotherapy (Linetsky, 1999a; Linetsky, et al., 2000). It was originally described by Celsus for treatment of hydroceles, with injections of saltpeter (Hoch, 1939; Linetsky, 1999b). The current technique combines addressing the affected connective tissues with diagnostic local anesthetic blocks, followed by injection of solutions that, by virtue of their chemical properties, are able to stimulate a regenerative, reparative process in the injured tissues.

Application of RIT for low back pain has been described in numerous textbooks and articles; comparatively adequate applications for cervical and thoracic pain are lacking. We choose to emphasize cervicothoracic pain problems treated with RIT in this chapter (Cyriax, 1969; 1982; Dorman, et al., 1991, 1993; Hackett, 1991; Ombregt, et al., 1995).

ETYMOLOGY OF SOME TERMINOLOGY

Biegelesen (1984) first used the term "sclerotherapy" in 1936. 'Sclero': derived from the word *skleros* (Greek, hard). Hackett (1958) felt that sclerotherapy implied scar formation; therefore, he coined the term "prolotherapy" and defined it as: "the rehabilitation of an incompetent structure by the generation of new cellular tissue" (derived from the word *proli* (Latin, offspring)). "Proliferate": to produce new cells in rapid succession. The former, however, is an integral attribute of a malignant, unsuppressed growth. Moreover, with advances in basic science and the contemporary understanding of the healing process, these authors prefer RIT because it is recognizes that regeneration extends beyond the proliferative stage. On a cellular level, RIT induces chemomodulation of collagen through repetitive stimulation of the inflammatory and proliferative phases in a sophisticated process of tissue regeneration and repair, mediated by numerous growth factors leading to the restoration of tensile strength, elasticity, increased mass, and load-bearing capacity of the affected connective tissue (Klein, et al., 1989; Liu, et al., 1983; Maynard, et al., 1985; Ongley, et al., 1987). These capabilities make RIT a specific treatment for degenerative, chronic, painful conditions such as enthesopathy, tendinosis, and ligament laxity, versus commonly utilized steroid injections and denervation procedures (Klein, et al., 1997; Reeves, 1995).

LOCAL ANESTHETICS IN DIAGNOSIS OF MUSCULOSKELETAL PATHOLOGY: BRIEF HISTORY

In 1930, Leriche introduced the application of procaine for differential diagnosis and treatment of ligament and tendon injuries of the ankle and other joints at their fibroosseous insertions. In 1934, Soto-Hall and Haldeman reported on the benefits of procaine injections in the diagnosis and treatment of painful shoulders. Subsequently in 1938, they published a study on diagnosis and treatment of painful sacroiliac dysfunctions with procaine injections. After infiltration of posterior sacroiliac ligaments, interspinous ligaments at L4–5 and L5-S1 levels, and zygapophyseal joint capsules with procaine, they observed a marked relaxation of spastic musculature and added the routine use of sacroiliac joint manipulations, establishing manipulation of axial joints under local anesthesia (Haldeman, et al., 1938).

In 1938, Steindler and Luck made a significant contribution to currently validated approaches in the diagnosis and treatment of low-back pain based on procaine injections. The authors pointed out that posterior divisions of the spinal nerves provide the sensory supply to the musculature; tendons; supraspinous, interspinous, iliolumbar, sacroiliac, sacrotuberous, and sacrospinous ligaments; and origins and insertions of aponeurosis of tensor fascia lata, gluteal muscles, and thoracolumbar fascia. They emphasized that, based on clinical presentation alone, no definite diagnosis could be made and postulated that five criteria must be met to prove that a causal relationship exists between the structure and pain symptoms (see Table 33.1).

Subsequently, in 1948, Hirsch demonstrated relief from sciatica following intradiscal injection of procaine (Hirsch, 1948).

Local anesthetic diagnostic blocks are currently the most reliable and objective confirmation of the precise tissue source of pain and clinical diagnosis (Bonica, et al., 1990; Cousins, et al., 1988; Merskey, et al., 1994; Wilkinson, 1992).

HISTORY AND EVOLUTION OF RIT

The scientific rationale for implementing RIT regenerative injection therapy in chronic painful pathology of ligaments and tendons evolved from clinical and histologic research performed for injection treatment of hernias, hydroceles and varicose veins. The therapeutic action of the newly formed connective tissue was different in each

---

TABLE 33.1
Radiating/Referral Pain Postulates

1. Contact with the needle must aggravate the local pain.
2. Contact with the needle must aggravate or elicit the radiation of pain.
3. Procaine infiltration must suppress local tenderness.
4. Procaine infiltration must suppress radiation of pain.
5. Positive leg signs must disappear.

From Steindler, et al., 1938. *Journal of the American Medical Association, 110,* 106–113. With permission.

condition. In hernias, the proliferation and subsequent regenerative/reparative response led to fibrotic closure of the defect (Riddle, 1940; Warren, 1881; Watson, 1938). In hydroceles, hypertrophied subserous connective tissue reinforced the capillary walls of serous membrane and prevented further exudate formation (Hoch, 1939; Linetsky, 1999b). The latter mode of action was employed in the treatment of chronic olecranon and pre-patellar bursitis by Poritt in 1931. He drained the fluid from the sac and injected 5% sodium morrhuate. In cases of persistence, he injected a 5% phenol solution into the bursae (Poritt, 1931).

In 1935, Schultz, while searching for a better way to treat painful subluxations of TMJs, conceived the idea that strengthening of the joint capsule by induced ligament fibrosis would lead to capsular contraction and prevent subluxations. Animal experiments were conducted with several solutions, among those, Sylnasol provided the best outcomes and therefore was chosen for the clinical trials. (*Note:* Sylnasol-sodium psyllate was an extract of psyllium seed oil produced by Searle Pharmaceutical and discontinued in 1960s.) A clinical study of 30 human subjects after biweekly injections of 0.25 to 0.5 ml Sylnasol demonstrated "entire patient satisfaction." Schultz (1937) concluded that the principle of induced hypertrophy of the articular capsule by injecting a fibrosing agent might be applied to other joints capable of subluxations or recurrent dislocations. He also concluded that Sylnasol was a dependable agent. Injections restored normal joint function and the method was within the scope of treatment of a general practitioner. Twenty years later, Schultz presented the positive results of Sylnasol injections on several hundred patients, successfully cured of painful hypermobility of TMJs (Schultz, 1956).

Also in 1937, Gedney reported some details of collateral ligament injections for painful unstable hypermobile knees and posterior sacroiliac ligaments of unstable painful sacroiliac articulations. Small amounts of sclerosant solutions were injected along the entire affected structures. Six months later, he extended this treatment to recurrent shoulder dislocations, acromioclavicular separations and sternoclavicular subluxations (Gedney, 1937; 1938).

In 1939, Kellgren injected volunteers with hypertonic saline and implicated interspinous ligaments as a significant source of local and referred pain. He published maps of referred pain from deep somatic structures, including interspinous ligaments (Kellgren, 1939).

In 1940, Riddle included a chapter on "The Injection Treatment of Joints" in his text and described the injection treatment of TMJs and shoulders in great detail, giving Schultz the appropriate credit for initiation of this treatment.

Shuman described injection treatment of recurrent shoulder dislocations via strengthening of the inferior capsular ligaments with Sylnasol in 1941. Subsequently, in 1949, he adopted the term "sclerotherapy" for this injection modality, modifying it later that year to "joint sclerotherapy" (Shuman, 1949a, 1949b).

In 1945, Bahme published the first retrospective study of 100 patients who improved after injection of Sylnasol to the sacroiliac ligaments. Patients were under his care for an average of 4 months. The average number of injection treatments was five; 80% reported complete resolution of symptoms. He also found these injections to be very helpful in the treatment of unstable ribs, and reported improvement in 12 patients. He described a significant coexistence of painful hypermobile ribs with hypermobile sacroiliac joints, explaining the phenomenon by concomitant functional scoliosis.

By 1944, Lindblom demonstrated radial annular fissures during cadaveric disc injections and later described nucleographic patterns of 15 discs in 13 patients. Thereafter, in 1948, Hirsch relieved sciatic pain with intradiscal injection of procaine. These two articles prompted Gedney, and subsequently Shuman, to explore therapeutic applications of sclerosants for pain related to intervertebral disc (IVD) pathology.

By 1951, Gedney had extended treatment with sclerosant injections to painful degenerative lumbar disc syndromes and described the detailed technique of Sylnasol injections into the lateral annulus of the lumbar disc without fluoroscopic guidance. He reported L4 disc involvement in 95% of cases and a 50% clinical improvement after treatment of this disc alone (Gedney, 1952a). In the treatment of hypermobile sacroiliac joints, he emphasized that the amount of solution and quantity of treatments were highly individual and depended on the patient's response (Gedney, 1952b). In a retrospective study, Gedney (1954a) emphasized the significant statistical coexistence of sacroiliac pathology with disc pathology at L3, L4, and L5 levels. By 1954, he had completed a prospective study of 100 patients; 65 were initially treated with the injections into the disc, and 35 were initially treated with injections into the posterior sacroiliac ligaments. The latter group required fewer intradiscal injections. Thus he concluded that, in the presence of sacroiliac pain and hypermobility, adequate stabilization of the sacroiliac joint should be achieved in all cases prior to addressing discogenic pain (Gedney, 1954a). He emphasized the importance of interspinous and iliolumbar ligament injections in the treatment of lumbar spondylolisthesis (Gedney, 1954b).

In 1954, Shuman evaluated the effectiveness of sclerosant injections to the sacroiliac joints, intervertebral discs, spondylolisthesis, zygapophyseal joint capsules, knees, and shoulders in 93 respondents in a retrospective survey. Improvements ranged from 75 to 98%. Only those patients who were able to perform their usual occupations were considered to have positive results. Subsequently, he detailed many aspects of treatment with integration of manipulative techniques, including manipulation under local anesthesia (introduced 20 years earlier by Haldeman and Soto-Hall). Shuman stated that zygapophyseal joint pathology (emphasized by Hackett in 1956) and disc pathology were the more common causes of lower back pain than sacroiliac joint pathology (Shuman, 1958).

Hackett, the inventor of prolotherapy, postulated in 1939 that ligaments were responsible for the majority of back pain (Hackett, 1953). By 1958, he came to the conclusion that tendons at the fibroosseous junctions were another significant source of chronic pain syndromes (Hackett, 1958). In a retrospective study, he reported on 84 patients with sacroiliac pain treated by sclerosant injections of Sylnasol, five to seven times to each affected area. In this study, 82% reported themselves entirely symptom-free for a duration of 6 to 14 years (Hackett & Henderson, 1955). In the initial animal experiments, he demonstrated a 30 to 40% increase in tendon size after injections of Sylnasol (Hackett, 1956) (Figures 33.1 and 33.2). Not satisfied with the term "sclerotherapy," because it implied hardening of the tissue and scar formation, Hackett introduced the term "prolotherapy" in 1956. He did this because the results of his experimental study did not support scarring but rather hypertrophy induced by proliferation of connective tissue in a linear fashion (Hackett, 1956). Hackett employed and emphasized the importance of the earlier referenced postulates of Steindler. He confirmed ligament or tendon involvement as pain generators reproducing local and referred pain by "needling" and abolishing the pain by infiltration of local anesthetic prior to injecting the proliferants (Hackett, 1956). He published maps of referred pain from ligaments and tendons, initially of the lumbopelvic region. These were derived from 7000 injections in over 1000 patients treated over 17 years. He subsequently developed maps of the cervicothoracic region (Hackett, 1958) (Figure 33.3). Later, he pointed out that loose-jointed individuals had a lesser ability to recuperate from sprains, because of the congenital laxity of their ligaments, and have a predisposition to chronic lingering pain for decades. He emphasized their positive response to prolotherapy (Hackett, 1959).

In several subsequent publications, Hackett emphasized the common pathogenesis of impaired local circulation in chronic conditions such as neuritis, headaches, whiplash, osteoporosis, bone dystrophy, bronchospasm, and arteriosclerosis. Excess antidromic, sympathetic, and axon reflex stimulation caused local vasodilatation and edema, with a perpetuating vicious cycle, of "tendon relaxation," the condition now understood as degenerative changes, enthesopathy, tendinosis, and laxity (Hackett 1959a, 1959b, 1960a, 1960b, 1961, 1966a, 1966b, 1966c, 1966d, 1967; Hackett et al., 1961, 1962).

Extended subsequent animal experiments with multiple solutions conducted by Hackett revealed that the strongest fibroosseous proliferations were achieved with Sylnasol, zinc sulfate solutions, and silica oxide suspensions. The strongest acute inflammatory reaction was obtained

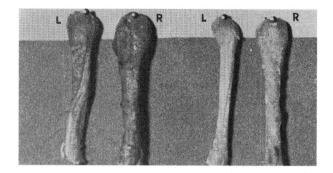

FIGURE 33.1 Hypertophied rabbit tendons 9 and 12 months after injection with proliferant; controls (L), treated (R). (From Hackett, G. (1958) *Ligament and tendon relaxation (skeletal disability)-treated by prolotherapy (fibro-osseous proliferation)*, 3rd ed., Springfield, IL: Charles C Thomas. With permission.)

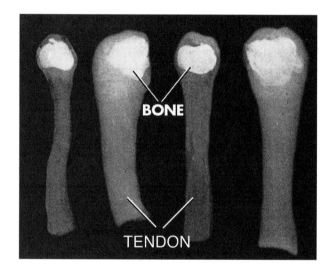

1 month   3 months

FIGURE 33.2 Paired radiograph of hypertrophied rabbit tendons, fibro-osseous attachment 1 and 3 months after injection of proliferant. Treated tendons are on the right side of each pair, controls on the left. (From Hackett, G. (1958) *Ligament and tendon relaxation (skeletal disability)-treated by prolotherapy (fibro-osseous proliferation)*, 3rd ed., Springfield, IL: Charles C Thomas. With permission.)

with Sylnasol and zinc sulfate, followed by silica oxide the whole blood moderately stimulated fibroosseous proliferation. Hydrocortisone used alone or in combination with proliferants inhibited proliferation for 3 to 4 weeks. At the fracture sites, proliferants increased callus formation in 3 weeks; whereas, used in combination with steroids the callus formation was markedly inhibited (Hackett, et al., 1961).

Hackett's positive results were initially corroborated by others (Compere, et al., 1958; Green, 1956, 1958; Myers, 1961; Neff, 1959). In fact, Myers reported improvement in 82% of patients.

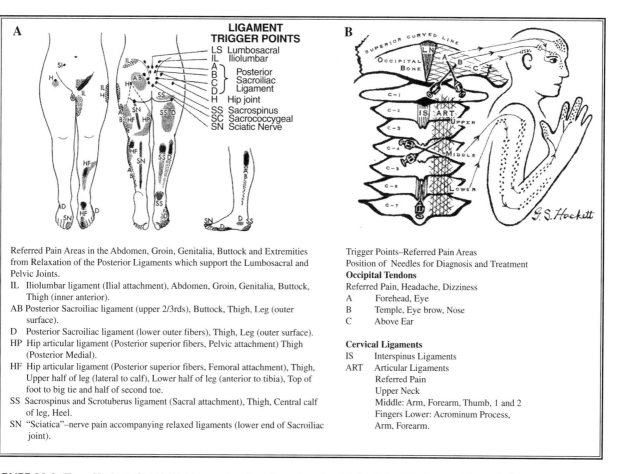

FIGURE 33.3 (From Hackett, G. (1958) *Ligament and tendon relaxation (skeletal disability)-treated by prolotherapy (fibro-osseous proliferation)*, 3rd ed., Springfield, IL: Charles C Thomas. With permission.)

In 1961, Blaschke reported the first prospective study of 42 patients treated with prolotherapy for lower back pain. Thirty-two were workers' compensation cases, notoriously the most difficult cases to treat, and ten were private insurance cases. Complete recovery was achieved in 20 patients observed for 3 years. Thirteen patients reported no change in their condition and nine underwent surgery. Four patients with clinical presentation of acute herniated disc, in whom prolotherapy was utilized without hope of success, had better results than any other patients in this study. In three instances of surgical intervention, specimens were obtained from the sites of injections and were reported as "normal fibrous tissue."

A multicenter study conducted by Kayfetz, et al. was published in 1963. Of 264 patients treated by prolotherapy for headaches, 78% had headaches of traumatic origin, 58% had non-traumatic headaches, and 56% had symptoms of Barre–Lieou syndrome. In addition, 86% had symptoms longer than 1 month and 46% had symptoms longer than 1 year. The traumatic group reported satisfactory results in 79%, with excellent results in 60%. The non-traumatic group reported satisfactory results in 47% and excellent results in 29%. Of 264 cases, 60% of patients

were followed for over 1 year and 27% were followed for 3 to 5 years. There were no infections or other complications following prolotherapy.

Also in 1963, Kayfetz reported a 5-year follow-up study of 189 cases with whiplash injuries treated by prolotherapy. Of these, 149 cases (79%) were due to automobile accidents; 153 (81%) had associated injuries to the thoracic and lumbar areas; 98 (52%) had an associated Barre–Lieou syndrome; and 55% had symptoms longer than 1 month's duration and 21% longer than 1-year duration. The majority of patients received 6 to 30 injections in one setting and were treated on one to ten occasions. Duration of treatment was from 1 to 6 months. Excellent results, in terms of pain, were obtained by 113 (60%), good results by 15 (8%) and fair results by 34 (18%). Some 75% of patients considered themselves cured of pain.

In response to adverse effects published after alleged incidental intrathecal injections of zinc sulfate, experiments were conducted with intrathecal injections of this solution in rabbits (Schneider, 1959; Keplinger, 1960; Hunt, 1961). Clinical doses (4 to 5 drops) did not produce any noticeable effect. Those animals receiving increased doses that produced spinal anesthesia, completely recovered after the anesthetic wore off. "It was necessary to use much greater than clinical dosage to induce paraplegia for a few weeks duration, which also cleared up" (Hackett, et al., 1961).

In 1967, Coleman brought medicolegal aspects of prolotherapy to the attention of the medical community. He pointed out that Hackett's technique was accepted as a standard of care. It was declared by a California court that a physician treating a patient had deviated from the method as described by Hackett. Conclusion was made that one did not have to follow the method of treatment followed by the majority of the physicians in the community. A physician is permitted to follow a method or a form of treatment followed by a minority of physicians if they are reputable and in good standing. But if he or she varies from the minority method of treatment he or she does so in violation, just as if he or she deviated from the generally accepted method of treatment.

The court concluded: " ... as a matter of law that prolotherapy as a method of treatment cannot be said to be inappropriate or to be malpractice even though it has not been accepted as a common method of treatment by the medical profession generally" (Coleman, 1968).

Abroad, positive results with Hackett's method were obtained by Ongley, Cyriax (1969, 1982), Barbor (1964), and Coplans (1972). Barbor presented a study of 153 patients with back pain for up to 20 years duration. Of 153, 111 (74%) of them reported relief to their satisfaction; 17 (11%) failed to improve; 25 (16%) were lost for follow-up; and 31 (23%) required periodic booster injection for relief. The solution utilized was dextrose phenol-glycerine (DPG) mixed in proportions of 2 cc DPG to 3 cc local anesthetic.

Cyriax (1969, 1982, 1993) included detailed descriptions of "sclerosant injections" to interspinous and facet joint capsular ligaments of the cervical, thoracic, and lumbar regions in his texts. Further, he described "a clinical blind study of 'sclerosant therapy' presented by Sanford in 1972. Of 100 patients, only 3 were lost for follow-up." The following three solutions were compared: (1) 2 ml DPG sclerosant mixed with 8 ml saline; (2) 10 ml of 0.5% procaine; and (3) 10 ml normal saline. The diluted sclerosant and procaine solutions were almost equally effective, by relieving pain in more than 50% of cases. Procaine and normal saline were equally ineffective by not helping in 50% of cases. Saline solution helped less than a third of patients. The dilution of DPG sclerosant down to 20% of the original strength significantly impaired its proliferant action.

In 1974, Blumenthal reported two cases of migraine headache and one case of cluster headache successfully cured by prolotherapy and a minor modification of Hackett's technique in the treatment of cervicodorsal pain.

By 1976, Leedy had reported a 70% improvement in the condition of 50 low-back pain patients treated with sclerosant injections and followed for 6 years. He also published several descriptive articles of the method (Leedy, 1977; Leedy, et al., 1976).

Also in 1976, Vanderschot compared prolotherapy with acupuncture in the treatment of chronic musculoskeletal pain and concluded that prolotherapy has a faster onset of action and longer-lasting pain relief (Vanderschot, 1976a,b).

In 1978, Chase reported up to 70% or better improvement in long-standing cases of painful head, neck/shoulder, and low-back syndromes.

Also in 1978, Koudele reported findings of Haws and Willman on histologic changes in human tissue treated up to five times with sclerosant injections for low-back pain. The following changes were observed and documented on slides. DPG solution produced early coagulation necrosis, followed by early collagen formation. By 6 months, a small zone of residual inflammatory cells were documented in an area of very dense collagen. In two other specimens treated with DPG, a dense collagen with fibrosis, occluded blood vessels, and a dense whirl of scar were observed.

After injection of a pumice suspension, an area of dense collagen and fibrosis surrounding a "lake" of pumice was documented, without foreign body reaction but with a capsule formation (Koudele, 1978).

In 1982, Hirschberg, et al. reported a prospective study of 16 patients with the iliolumbar syndrome. Nine were treated with infiltration of lidocaine at the insertion of the posterior iliolumbar ligament to the iliac crest, and seven were injected with a mixture containing equal amounts of 50% dextrose and 2% xylocaine (a total of 5 cc). Significant recovery was reported by ten patients. Six out of the seven treated with dextrose/xylocaine recovered, whereas only four out of the nine treated with xylocaine recovered.

Liu, et al., in a 1983 double-blind study, injected rabbit medial collateral ligaments (MCLs) and demonstrated that repeated injections of 5% sodium morrhuate at the fibroosseous attachments (enthesis) significantly increased its bone–ligament–bone junction strength by 28%, ligament mass by 44%, and thickness by 27%, when compared with saline controls. Morphometric analysis of electron micrographs demonstrated a highly significant increase in the diameter of collagen fibrils in the experimental ligaments vs. controls. These findings confirmed that sodium morrhuate had a significant regenerative influence on dense connective tissue at the insertion sites.

Maynard and co-workers reported a decrease in collagen fibrils and hydroxyproline content and an overall increase in the mass of tendons in experimental animals injected with sodium morrhuate. The average tendon circumference increased up to 25%.

Ongley, et al. (1987) in a double-blind, randomized study of chronic low-back pain in 81 subjects, statistically demonstrated a significant improvement greater than 50% in patients injected with a DPG solution vs. saline. In terms of disability scores, the experimental groups demonstrated a greater improvement than the control group: (p < 0.001), (p < 0.004), and (p < 0.001), respectively (Ongley, 1987). Subsequently, Ongley demonstrated a significant statistical improvement in five patients treated for painful instability of the knees with prolotherapy. Ligament stability data was obtained via three-dimensional computerized goniometry, integrated with force measurements (Ongley, et al., 1988).

Bourdeau (1988) published a 5-year retrospective survey of patients with low back pain treated with prolotherapy. Seventeen patients (70%) reported excellent to very good results.

Klein, et al. (1989) histologically documented proliferation and regeneration of ligaments in human subjects in response to injections of DPG solution, accompanied by decreased pain and increased range of motion, as documented by computerized inclinometry.

Roosth (1991) described gluteal tendinosis as a distinct clinical entity and Klein (1991) described the treatment of gluteus medius tendinosis with proliferant injections.

Also in 1991, Schwartz et al. reported a retrospective study of 43 patients with chronic sacroiliac strain who received three series of proliferant injections at biweekly intervals. Improvement was reported by all but three patients, and ranged from 95% reported by 20 patients to 66% reported by four patients; ten patients reported recurrence. Schwartz concluded that induced proliferation of collagen and dense connective tissue of the ligament is associated with a reduction of painful subluxations.

Hirschberg, et al. (1992) reported positive results in treating iliocostal friction syndrome in the elderly with proliferant injections and a soft brace.

Klein, et al. (1993) reported a double-blind clinical trial of 79 patients with chronic low-back pain who had failed to respond to previous conservative therapy. Subjects were randomly assigned to receive a series of six injections in a double-blind fashion at weekly intervals of either lidocaine/saline or lidocaine/DPG solution into the posterior sacroiliac and interspinous ligaments, fascia, and facet capsules of the low back from L-4 to the sacrum. All patients underwent pretreatment MRI or CT scans. Patients were evaluated with a visual analog, disability, and pain grid scores, and with objective computerized triaxial tests of lumbar function 6 months following the conclusion of injections. Thirty of the 39 patients randomly assigned to the proliferant group achieved a 50% or greater decrease in pain or disability scores at 6 months compared to 21 of 40 in the group that received lidocaine (p = 0.042). Improvements in visual analog (p = 0.056), disability (p = 0.068), and pain grid scores (p = 0.025) were greater in the proliferant group.

Massie, et al. (1993) reported that it was possible to stimulate fibroplasia in the intervertebral discs with proliferant injections. Also in 1993, Mooney advocated proliferant injections for chronic painful recurrent sacroiliac sprains if the clinician was skilled (Mooney, 1993a, b).

Grayson (1994) reported a case of sterile meningitis after injection of lumbosacral ligaments with proliferating solutions. Matthews (1995) found significant improvement in painful osteoarthritic knees after injection of the ipsilateral sacroiliac ligaments with proliferant solutions. Also in 1995, Reeves pointed out that degenerative changes of enthesopathy may be painful, and prolotherapy with a less aggressive solution such as 12% dextrose with xylocaine is the only type of specific treatment for these pathologic changes of ligaments and tendons.

Eek (1996) reported on the benefit of proliferating injections for intradiscal pain. Klein and Eek have described proliferant injections for low-back pain in detail (Klein, 1997).

The clinical anatomy in relation to RIT/prolotherapy for low-back pain was reviewed by Linetsky & Willard (1999). The presence of the connective tissue stocking surrounding various lumbar structures, dictating their function as a single unit in a normal state and the necessity to include multiple segmental and extrasegmental structures in differential diagnosis of low-back pain, was emphasized (Linetsky, 1999).

Subsequently, in March of 2000, Reeves demonstrated in a randomized, double-blind, placebo-controlled study the beneficial effects of 10% dextrose with lidocaine in knee osteoarthritis with anterior cruciate ligament laxity. Goniometric measurements of knee flexion improved by 12.8% (p = 0.005) and anterior displacement difference improved by 57% (p = 0.025). By 12 months (six injections), the dextrose-treated knees improved in pain (44% decrease), swelling complaints (63% decrease), knee buckling frequency (85% decrease), and flexion range (14° increase). He concluded that proliferant injection with 10% dextrose stimulated growth factors and regeneration, and resulted in a statistically significant clinical improvements in knee osteoarthritis (Reeves, et al., 2000). The history of RIT/prolotherapy from the 1930s through the 1980s was recently reviewed (Linetsky, et al., 2000, 2001).

To understand the essence of RIT/prolotherapy, it is important to review the basic science related to the healing process, as well as some anatomical and biomechanical properties of connective tissue and clinical anatomy.

INFLAMMATORY-REGENERATIVE/ REPARATIVE RESPONSE AND DEGENERATIVE PATHWAYS

The inflammatory response is intertwined with the regenerative, reparative process. A complex inflammatory reaction induced in vascularized connective tissue by endogenous or exogenous stimuli may lead to two distinct repair pathways. The first is regeneration, which replaces injured cells by the same type of cells; and the second is fibrosis, or the replacement of injured cells by fibrous connective tissue. Often, a combination of both processes contributes to the repair. Initially in both processes a similar pathway takes place with migration of fibroblasts, proliferation, differentiation, and cell-matrix interaction. The latter, together with the basement membrane provides a scaffold for regeneration of pre-existing structures (Cotran, et al., 1999). " … modulation of these cell matrix responses regardless of the method, provides an intriguing challenge" (Leadbetter, 1992). Cell replication is controlled by chemical and growth factors. Chemical factors may inhibit or stimulate proliferation, whereas growth factors such as cytokines/chemokines, TGF-β1 (transforming growth factor β1), PDGF (platelet derived growth factor), FGF (fibroblast growth factor), VEGF (vascular endothelial growth factor), IGF (insulin-like growth factor), CTF (connective tissue growth factor), and NGF (nerve growth factor) stimulate proliferation. The regenerative potential depends on cell type, genetic information, and the size of the defect. In the presence of a large connective tissue defect, fibrotic healing takes place (Cotran, et al., 1999; Reeves, 2000).

Under the best circumstances, natural healing restores connective tissue to its pre-injury length but only 50 to 75% of its pre-injury tensile strength (Leadbetter, 1992; Reeves, 1995). Connective tissues are bradytropic (their reparative capability is slower than that of muscle or bone). In the presence of repetitive microtrauma, unjudicious use of nonsteroidal anti-inflammatory drugs (NSAIDs) and steroid medications, tissue hypoxia, metabolic abnormalities, and other less-defined causes, connective tissue may divert toward a degenerative pathway (Leadbetter, 1992, 1994, 1995; Reeves, 1995, 2000). "A judicious utilization of anti-inflammatory therapy remains useful, albeit adjunctive therapy …" (Leadbetter, 1995). Biopsies of these tissues demonstrate disorganized collagen, excessive matrix, insufficient elastin, disorganized mesenchymal cells, vascular buds with incomplete lumen, few or absent white blood cells, neovasculogenesis, and neoneurogenesis (Jozsa, 1997; Leadbetter, 1994). Degenerative changes in tendons may be hypoxic, mucoid, mixoid, hyaline, calcific, fibrinoid, fatty, fibrocartilaginous and osseous metaplasia, and any combination of the above (Jozsa, 1997).

Similar degenerative changes were found in fibromyalgia syndrome with dense foci of rough, frequently hyalinized fibrillar connective tissue. Vascularization occurred at the periphery of these foci, only where thin nervous fibrils and sometimes small paraganglions were seen with severe degenerative changes of the collagen fibers, and marked decrease of fibroblasts. Inflammatory markers were absent (Tuzlukov, et al., 1993).

Repeated eccentric contractions diminish muscle function and increase intramuscular pressure. For example, the intramuscular pressure in the supraspinatus and infraspinatus is four to five times higher than that in the deltoid or trapezius at the same relative load (Ranney, 1997). Edema arising in one muscle compartment secondary to overuse does not spread to adjacent compartments. Prolonged static muscular efforts predispose to edema, which leads to a decrease in perfusion pressure and a subsequent reduction of blood flow with granulocyte plugging of the capillaries and further metabolite accumulation and vasodilatation (Jozsa, 1997; Leadbetter, 1994; Ranney, 1997).

Further repeated eccentric contractions are notorious for microtraumas with microruptures either at the fibroosseous junctions, in the mid substance of the ligaments and tendons, or at the myotendinous interface. Repetitive microtrauma with insufficient time for recovery leads to an inadequate regenerative process that turns to a degenerative pathway in tendons, muscles, discs, joint ligaments, and cartilage. Improper posture, in combination with eccentric contractions (such as driving with both hands on a steering wheel or typing on a computer with improperly positioned keyboard and monitor), are the most common examples of eccentric contraction (Jozsa, 1997; Leadbetter, 1992, 1994, 1995; Ranney, 1997; Reeves, 2000).

Impaired circulation at the fibromuscular and fibroosseous interface eventually leads to impaired intraosseous circulation with diminished venous outflow and increased intraosseous pressure. This, in turn, stimulates intraosseous baroreceptors and contributes to nociception transmitted through fine myelinated and nonmyelinated fibers that accompany nutrient vessels into bone and located in perivascular spaces of Haversian canals. Decreased circulation leads to hypoxia, affects calcium metabolism, and contributes to the progression of osteoarthritis (Gray, 1995; Hackett, 1959, 1960a, 1960b, 1961, 1966a, 1966c, 1966d, 1967; Hackett, et al., 1961, 1962; Shevelev, et al., 2000; Sokov, et al., 2000; Zoppi, et al., 2000).

SOME ANATOMICAL AND BIOMECHANICAL PROPERTIES OF LIGAMENTS AND TENDONS

Ligaments are dull white, dense connective tissue structures that connect adjacent bones. They may be intraarticular, extraarticular, or capsular. Collagen fibers in ligaments may be parallel, oblique, or spiral. These orientations represent adaptation to specific directions in restriction of joint displacements.

Tendons are glistening white collagenous bands interposed between muscle and bone that transmit tensile forces during muscle contraction. There are considerable variations in shape of fibroosseous attachments from cylindrical, fan shaped to wide, flat, and ribbon shaped. The myotendinous junctions have significant structural variations from end to end, to oblique and singular intermuscular fibers. The collagen content of tendons is approximately 30% wet weight, or 70% dry weight (Butler, et al., 1978; Gray, 1995).

Under the light microscope, ligaments and tendons have a crimped, wave-form appearance. This crimp is a planar zigzag pattern that unfolds during initial loading of collagen (Butler, et al., 1978; Gray, 1995). Elongated below 4% of original length, ligaments and tendons return to their original crimped wave appearance; beyond 4% elongation, they lose the elasticity and become permanently laxed. However, in degenerative ligaments, subfailure was reported as early as 1.5% elongation. Laxity of ligaments obviously leads to joint hypermobility. Experimental studies have confirmed that the medial collateral ligament (MCL) failed more abruptly than either the capsular ligaments or the anterior cruciate ligament (ACL). This happens because the MCL has more parallel fibers with uniformity in length and, therefore, they fail together. The capsular fibers are less organized than the MCL or ACL, and their lengths and orientations vary. Because these fibers are loaded and fail at different times a large joint displacement is needed before capsular failure is complete.

Three principal failure modes exist. The first and most common is ligament failure. The second is a bone avulsion fracture; and the third, the least common, is a shear or cleavage failure at the fibroosseous interface.

Collagenous tissues are deleteriously affected by inactivity and are favorably influenced by physical activity of an endurance nature. They are also deleteriously affected by NSAIDs and steroid administrations.

In fact, "Administration of even a single dose of corticosteroids directly into ligaments or tendons can have debilitating effects upon their strength. Intraarticular injections of methyl-prednisolone acetate given either once or at intervals of several months may be less detrimental to ligament or tendon mechanical properties" (Butler, et al., 1978).

Tendons are strongly attached to the bones by decussating and perforating Sharpey's fibers. Current understanding of OTJ (osseo tendinous junction, a.k.a. enthesis, fibroosseous junction) is such that the fibers insert to the bone via four zones: tendon zone, fibrocartilage zone, mineralized fibrocartilage zone, and lamellar bone. However, it does not shed much light on the mechanism of tendon avulsion and overuse-induced pathology, as was emphasized by Hackett, et al. (1991) and Jozsa (1997). The tensile strength of tendons is similar to that of bone and is about half that of steel. A tendon with a cross section of 10 mm in diameter can support a load of 600 to 1000 kg (Butler, et al., 1978; Gray, 1995; Jozsa, 1997).

Three types of nerve endings in posterior ligamentous structures of the spine were confirmed microscopically. They are free nerve endings, and Pacini and Ruffini corpuscles. The free nerve endings were found in superficial layers of all ligaments, including supraspinous and interspinous, with a sharp increase in their quantity at the spinous processes attachments (enthesis). Paciniform corpuscles are located in adipose tissue between supraspinous ligaments and lumbosacral fascia and in the deep layers of supraspinous and interspinous ligaments acting as nociceptors in all locations and as mechanoceptors with a low threshold, and are stimulated by stretch of the ligaments and muscle actions. Ruffini receptors are located in the interspinous and flaval ligaments; they respond to stretch; and they control the reflex inhibitory mechanism (Yahia, et al., 1989).

Neoneurogenesis and neovasculogenesis have been documented in chronic connective tissue pathology. The nerve and vascular tissue ingrowth into diseased intervertebral discs, posterior spinal ligaments, hard niduses of fibromyalgia, together with neuropeptides in the facet joint capsules, have been observed (Ashton, et al., 1992; El-Bohy, et al., 1988; Freemont, et al., 1997; Tuzlukov, et al., 1993).

During postnatal development, tendons enlarge by interstitial growth, particularly at the myotendinous junction (a.k.a. fibromuscular interface) where there is a high concentration of fibroblasts. The nerve supplies are largely sensory (Best, 1994; Butler, et al., 1978; Gray, 1995; Jozsa, 1997).

Insertion pathology of the trunk muscles (enthesopathy at the fibroosseous junctions) most commonly affects the following sites: occipital and scapular insertions; the spinous processes, especially at the cervicodorsal and thoracolumbar regions; iliac crest; sternum; and symphysis pubis (Figures 33.4 and 33.5). Histopathologically, the following findings were observed: calcium deposits and mineralization of the fibrocartilaginous zone (Jozsa, 1977). A large study examined traumatically ruptured tendons from 891 patients in comparison with 445 tendon specimens obtained from similar local sites in similar age and gender groups of "healthy" individuals who died accidentally. Degenerative changes were well-documented in 865 ruptured tendons (97%) and only in 149 control tendons (27%). Similar statistical differences were observed comparing tendons of individuals who died 3 years after quadriplegia and those who died accidentally. Irreversible lipoid degenerations at the muscle tendon junctions were documented as early as 3 months after onset of quadriplegia (Jozsa, 1977).

The cervical zygapophyseal joint (z-joint) is responsible for 54% of chronic neck pain after "whiplash" injury. The prevalence may be as high as 65% (Barnsley, et al., 1994). In populations presenting with headaches after whiplash, over 50% of the headaches stem from the C2–3

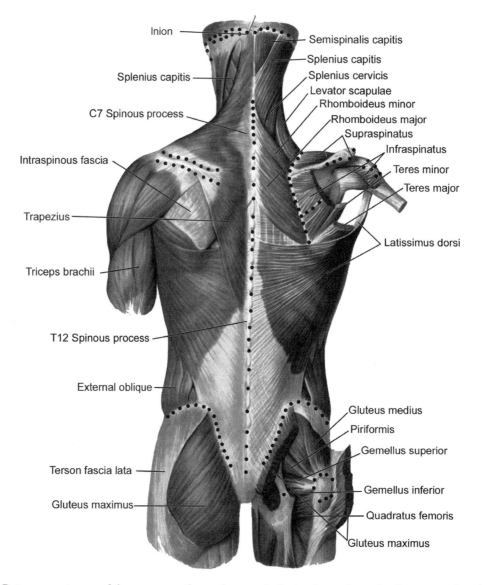

FIGURE 33.4 Dots represent some of the common enthesopathy areas in the trunk muscles at the fibroosseous insertions (enthesis), at the occipital, scapular, humeral, trochanteric, iliac crests, and spinous processes. Dots also represent the most common locations of needle tips during RIT droplet infiltrations. (Please note: not all of the locations must be treated in each patient.) (From *Sinelnikov Atlas of Anatomy*, (1972) Vol. I, Moscow: Meditsina. Modified by Tracey Slaughter.)

z-joint (Bogduk, 1986, 1996; Bogduk, et al., 1996; Lord, 1986). Intraarticular corticosteroid injections are ineffective in relieving chronic cervical z-joint pain (Barnsley, et al., 1994). These data strongly suggest that there is a presence of nociceptors other than z-joints and intervertebral discs. Pain patterns from synovial joints at the cranio-cervical junction overlap with the pain patterns from the lower z-joints and suboccipital soft tissues (Aprill, et al., 1990; Dreyfuss, et al., 1994a; Hackett, 1958, 1960a; Hackett, et al., 1962, 1991; Travell, et al., 1983). Their contribution to nociception requires confirmation with intraarticular blocks under fluoroscopic guidance by a practitioner with a significant amount of experience (Bogduk, 1988; Dreyfuss, et al., 1994a).

CLINICAL ANATOMY OF CERVICOCRANIAL, CERVICAL, AND CERVICODORSAL REGIONS IN RELATION TO RIT

It is important to realize that various ligaments, tendons, and fasciae of the cervical, thoracic, and lumbar regions form a continuous connective tissue stocking which incorporates and interconnects various soft tissue, muscular, vascular, and osseous structures. Although each of the connective tissues has a slightly different biochemical content, they blend at their boundaries and function as a single unit. The innervation is generally segmental and posteriorly provided by

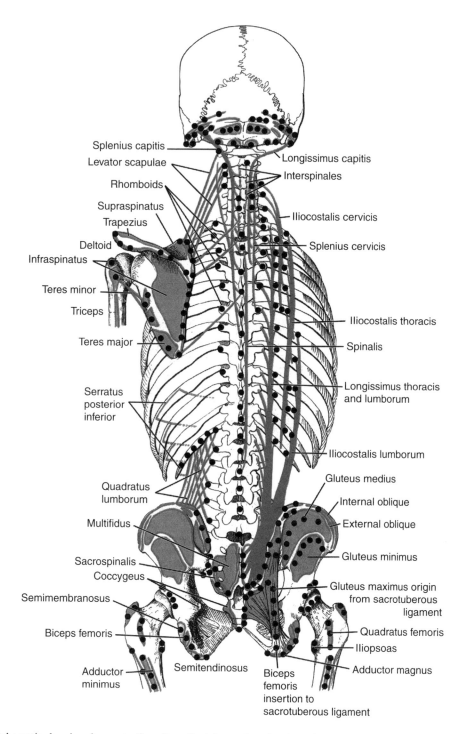

FIGURE 33.5 Schematic drawing demonstrating sites of origins and tendon insertions (enthesis) of the vertebral, paravertebral and peripheral musculature in the cervical, thoracic, and lumbar regions and partly upper and lower extremities. Clinically significant painful enthesopathies are common at these locations defined by dots. Dots also represent most common locations of needle insertions and infiltration during RIT (Please note: not all of the locations must be treated in each patient.) (From *Sinelnikov Atlas of Anatomy*, (1972) Vol. I, Moscow: Meditsina. Modified by Tracey Slaughter.)

the respective medial and lateral branches of the dorsal rami (Agur, et al., 1991; Gray, 1995; Linetsky, 1999; Willard, 1995).

Differential diagnosis is based on a thorough understanding of the regional and segmental anatomy and pathology. Currently prevailing trends in diagnostic efforts are addressing discogenic, facetogenic, and neurocompressive components of spinal pain. Consequently, therapy is directed toward neuromodulation or neuro-ablation with radiofrequency generators. Also, surgical ablations and fusions correct the mass effects in neurocompressive models, or discogenic pain.

In the mid-cervical area, blocking the putative medial branches of the dorsal rami at the waist of the articular pillars, as the initial step in differential diagnosis, is considered diagnostic and prognostic for z-joint pain (Bogduk, 1988; Lord, 1996). However, such an approach as an initial step in differential diagnosis may be misleading for two reasons. First, it interrupts orthodromic and antidromic transmission at the proximal segment of the medial branch of the dorsal rami (MBDR), excluding other putative nociceptors located distally on its course from the differential diagnosis. Second, there is significant individual variation in the location of the dorsal rami bifurcations into the medial and lateral branches (Willard, personal communication, October 9, 2000).

All cervical spinal nerves divide into ventral and dorsal rami. The dorsal rami in turn divide into the medial and lateral branches, except for the first dorsal ramus, which is also called the suboccipital nerve. The first dorsal ramus supplies the muscles of the suboccipital region — rectus capitis posterior minor and major, inferior and superior oblique, and semispinalis capitis — and has an ascending cutaneous branch that connects with the greater and lesser occipital nerves and may contribute to the occipital and suboccipital headaches (Bogduk, 1986, 1988; Gray, 1995). The second cervical dorsal ramus also supplies the inferior oblique, connects with the first one, and divides into lateral and medial branches (MBDR). Its medial branch (the greater occipital nerve) pierces the semispinalis capitis and trapezius at their insertion to the occipital bone on its ascending course. Thereafter, it connects with the branches from the third occipital nerve along the course of the occipital artery supplying the skin of the skull up to the vertex (Bogduk, 1986, 1988; Gray, 1995).

Anatomical texts (Agur, et al., Gray, 1995) indicate that the dorsal ramus proper of the lower five cervical nerves is located laterally at the waist of the articular pillars (Figures 33.6 and 33.7). On the other hand, current trends in therapeutic and diagnostic blocks are based on the assumption that the anatomy and course of the MBDR is constant, and that it arises from the intertransverse space and wraps around the waist of the respective articular pillars (Aprill, et al., 1990; Bodguk, 1988). However, the clinical observations supported by ongoing research and microdissections of Willard (personal communication, October 9, 2000) indicate that bifurcations into medial and lateral branches are not consistent in their location and may originate in the intertransverse space or in the projections of the lateral and posterior aspects of articular pillars (Figures 33.6 and 33.7). Quite often, the course of the medial (MB) and lateral branches (LB) is parallel at the waists of the

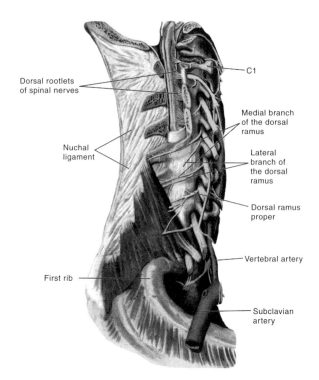

FIGURE 33.6 The course of the medial, lateral branches and the dorsal ramus proper, represented semi-schematically. (From *Sinelnikov Atlas of Anatomy*, Vol. I, Meditsina Moskow, 1972. Modified by Tracey Slaughter.)

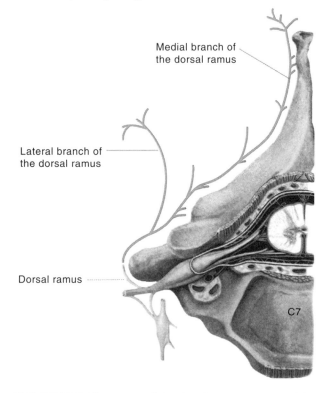

FIGURE 33.7 The course of the dorsal ramus proper and its medial and lateral branches, represented semi-schematically. (From *Sinelnikov Atlas of Anatomy*, Vol. I, Meditsina Moskow, 1972. Modified by Tracey Slaughter.)

articular pillars with the MB being proximal to the osseous structure. Thereafter, the MB of the dorsal ramus (MBDR) furnishes twigs to zygapophyseal joint capsules and continues along the lamina and spinous process toward its apex, innervating structures inserting or originating at the lamina and the spinous process on its course (Agur, et al., 1991; Gray, 1995; Willard, personal communication, October 9, 2000). For example, the fourth and fifth cervical MBDRs supply the semispinalis cervices and capitis, multifidi, interspinalis, splenius and trapezius, supraspinous ligaments, and end in the skin. The lowest three MBDRs have a similar course (Figures 33.6 and 33.7).

Lateral branches supply the iliocostalis, longissimus cervices, and longissimus capitis. Similar anatomic relationships are observed in the thoracic region where medial branches of the upper six thoracic dorsal rami supply the zygapophyseal joints, semispinalis thoracis, multifidi, piercing trapezius, and rhomboid, and reach the skin most proximal and lateral to the spinous processes (Agur, et al., 1991; Gray, 1995).

RIT/PROLOTHERAPY MECHANISM OF ACTION

The RIT mechanism of action is complex and multifaceted.

1. The first is the mechanical transection of cells and matrix by the needle, causing cellular damage and stimulating inflammatory cascade.
2. The second is compression of cells by the extracellular volume of the injected solution, stimulating intracellular growth factors (Reeves, 2000).
3. The third step is chemomodulation of collagen through inflammatory proliferative, regenerative/reparative response induced by the chemical properties of the proliferants and mediated by cytokines and multiple growth factors (Cook, 2000; DesRosiers, et al., 1996; Kang, et al., 1999; Lee, et al., 1998; Harui, et al., 1997; Nakamura, et al., 1998; Reeves, 1995, 2000; Rudkin, et al., 1996; Spindler, et al., 1996).
4. The fourth is chemoneuromodulation of peripheral nociceptors and antidromic, orthodromic, sympathetic, and axon reflex transmissions (Hackett, 1958, 1960b, 1961, 1966a, 1966b, 1966c, 1966d; Hackett, et al., 1961, 1962).
5. The fifth is modulation of local hemodynamics with changes in intraosseous pressure leading to a reduction of in pain. Empirical observations suggest that a dextrose/lidocaine combination has a much more prolonged action than lidocaine alone (Hackett, 19598, 1960b, 1961, 1966a, 1966b, 1966c, 1966d; Hackett, et al., 1961, 1962; Shevelev, et al., 2000; Sokov, et al., 2000; Zoppi, et al., 2000).
6. The sixth is a temporary repetitive stabilization of the painful hypermobile joints induced by inflammatory response to the proliferants, providing a better environment for regeneration and repair of the affected ligaments and tendons (Bahme, 1945; Gedney, 1952a, 1952b, 1954a, 1954b; Hackett, 1958; Hackett, et al., 1991; Shuman, 1958).

PUTATIVE PAIN-GENERATING STRUCTURES ADDRESSED BY RIT/PROLOTHERAPY

1. Ligaments: Intraarticular, periarticular, capsular
2. Tendons
3. Fascia
4. Enthesis: The zone of insertion of ligament, tendon, or articular capsule to bone (Dorland, 1985; Jozsa, 1997; Klein, et al., 1997; Mirman, 1989) (a.k.a. fibroosseous junctions of ligaments and tendons). In the orthopedic literature, this is referred to as OTJ (osseo/tendinous junction) (Jozsa, 1997; Leadbetter, 1992, 1994, 1995; Reeves, 2000). For the purpose of this chapter, enthesis and fibroosseous junction are interchangeable.
5. Intervertebral discs

TISSUE PATHOLOGY TREATED WITH RIT/PROLOTHERAPY

1. Sprain: Ligamentous injury at the fibroosseous junction or intersubstance disruption. A sudden or severe twisting of a joint with stretching or tearing of ligaments; also, a sprained condition (Leadbetter, 1994; Merriam-Webster, 1995; Reeves, 1995; Simon, et al., 1987).
2. Strain: Muscle/tendon injury at the fibromuscular or fibroosseous interface. When concerned with the peripheral muscles and tendons sprains and strains are identified as separate injuries and in three-stage gradations: first-, second-, and third-degree sprain, and similarly for strain. With regard to vertebral and paravertebral ligaments and tendons, no consensus exists among authors and the definitions are quite vague (Dorland, 1985; Leadbetter, 1994; Mirman, 1989).

3. Enthesopathy: A painful degenerative pathological process that results in the deposition of poorly organized tissue, degeneration and tendinosis at the fibroosseous interface and transition toward loss of function (Jozsa, 1997; Klein, et al., 1997; Leadbetter, 1994; Linetsky, 1999a; Reeves, 1995).

4. Tendinosis/ligamentosis: A focal area of degenerative changes due to a failure of cell matrix adaptation to excessive load and tissue hypoxia, with a strong tendency toward chronic recurrent pain and dysfunction (Best, 1994; Jozsa, 1997; Klein, et al., 1997; Leadbetter, 1994; Reeves, 1995; Roosth, 1991).

5. Pathologic ligament laxity: A post-traumatic or congenital condition leading to painful hypermobility of the axial and peripheral joints (Dorland, 1985; Dorman, et al., 1991; Hackett, 1958; Leedy, 1977; Reeves, 1995, 2000; Reeves, et al., 2000; Simon, et al., 1987).

INDICATIONS FOR RIT/PROLOTHERAPY

1. Chronic pain from ligaments or tendons secondary to sprains or strains

2. Pain from overuse or occupational conditions known as repetitive motion disorders (i.e., neck and wrist pain in typists and computer operators, "tennis" and "golfer's" elbows, chronic supraspinatus tendinosis).

3. Painful chronic postural neck and cervicodorsal junction problems

4. Painful recurrent somatic dysfunctions secondary to ligament laxity that improve temporarily with manipulation. Hypermobility and subluxation at a given peripheral or spinal articulation or mobile segment(s), accompanied by a restricted range of motion at reciprocal segment(s).

5. Thoracic vertebral compression fractures with a wedge deformity that exerts additional stress on the posterior ligamento-tendinous complex.

6. Recurrent painful subluxations of ribs at the costotransverse, costovertebral, and/or costosternal articulations.

7. Spondylolysis and spondylolisthesis

8. Intolerance to NSAIDs, steroids, or opiates. RIT may be the treatment of choice if the following modalities are contraindicated. Or failure to improve after physical therapy, chiropractic, or osteopathic manipulations, steroid injections or radiofrequency denervation, or surgical interventions in aforementioned conditions.

SYNDROMES AND DIAGNOSTIC ENTITIES CAUSED BY LIGAMENT AND TENDON PATHOLOGY THAT HAVE BEEN SUCCESSFULLY TREATED WITH RIT/PROLOTHERAPY

1. Cervicocranial syndrome (cervicogenic headaches, alar ligaments sprain, atlanto-axial and atlanto-occipital joint sprains)
2. Temporomandibular pain and dysfunction syndrome
3. Barre–Lieou syndrome
4. Spasmodic torticollis
5. Cervical segmental dysfunctions
6. Cervical and cervicothoracic spinal pain of "unknown" origin
7. Cervicobrachial syndrome (shoulder/neck pain)
8. Hyperextension/hyperflexion injury syndromes
9. Cervical, thoracic, and lumbar facet syndromes
10. Cervical, thoracic, and lumbar sprain/strain syndromes
11. Costo-transverse joint pain
12. Costovertebral arthrosis/dysfunction
13. Slipping rib syndrome
14. Sternoclavicular arthrosis and repetitive sprain
15. Thoracic segmental dysfunction
16. Tietze's syndrome/costochondritis/chondrosis
17. Costosternal arthrosis
18. Intercostal arthrosis
19. Xiphoidalgia syndrome
20. Acromioclavicular sprain/arthrosis
21. Shoulder–hand syndrome
22. Recurrent shoulder dislocations
23. Scapulothoracic crepitus
24. Myofacial pain syndromes
25. Ehlers–Danlos syndrome
26. Osgood-Schlatter disease
27. Marie–Strumpell disease
28. Failed back syndrome

CONTRAINDICATIONS TO RIT/PROLOTHERAPY

1. Allergy to anesthetic or proliferant solutions or their ingredients, such as dextrose, sodium morrhuate, or phenol
2. Acute nonreduced subluxations or dislocations.
3. Acute sprains or strains of axial and peripheral joints
4. Acute arthritis (septic or posttraumatic with hemarthrosis)
5. Acute bursitis or tendinitis

6. Capsular pattern shoulder and hip designating acute arthritis accompanied by tendinitis

7. Acute gout or rheumatoid arthritis

8. Recent onset of a progressive neurologic deficit, including but not limited to severe intractable cephalgia, unilaterally dilated pupil, bladder dysfunction, and bowel incontinence

9. Requests for a large quantity of sedation and/or narcotics before and after treatment

10. Paraspinal neoplastic lesions involving the musculature and osseous structures

11. Severe exacerbation of pain or lack of improvement after local anesthetic blocks

12. Relative contraindications: central spinal canal, lateral recess and neural foraminal stenosis

CLINICAL PRESENTATIONS

Patients may present with a variety of complaints ranging from one area of localized pain and tenderness to any combination of referred pain patterns known with cervical disc, cervicocranial, and cervicobrachial or cervical and thoracic facet syndromes. Headaches accompanied by cervical muscle spasms are a common complaint. Other compaints include: (1) exacerbation of pain while standing or sitting in the same position for a given period of time, and increased pain after exertion or physical activity are typical; (2) a feeling of weakness in the neck, back, or extremities and extreme fatigability; (3) pseudoradicular patterns of change in sensation, such as burning, numbness, and tingling; (4) difficulties in maintaining balance, ringing in the ears, and blurred vision; (5) feeling the need for repetitive self-manipulations, or chiropractic or osteopathic manipulations; (6) painful clicking, popping, or locking of axial or peripheral joints; (7) dropping of objects, weakness of the hands, and "heaviness of the head" (Dorman, et al., 1991; Hackett, et al., 1991; Kayfetz, 1963; Kayfetz et al., 1963; Reeves, 1995, 2000).

Physical Examination

Tenderness is the most common finding over the chronically strained or sprained ligaments or tendons. Provoked tenderness rarely reproduces radiating or referral pain; it is a local phenomenon. However, intensity of such tenderness may be changed or abolished completely after manipulation. Patients are able to point out such pain with their finger in the posterior cervicodorsal region.

Such local tenderness, as well as referred and radiating pain, can often be abolished by infiltration of nociceptors in the involved tissue with local anesthetic. Tenderness is an objective finding, especially when elicited at posterior structures (Borenstein, et al., 1996; Broadhurst, et al., 1996; Hackett, 1958; Hackett, et al., 1991; Linetsky, 1999).

RADIOLOGIC EVALUATION PRIOR TO RIT/PROLOTHERAPY

1. Plain radiographs are of limited diagnostic value in painful pathology of the connective tissue; however, they may detect:

   a. Structural or positional osseous abnormalities

   b. Anterior or posterior listhesis on lateral views (flexion, extension)

   c. Degenerative changes in general and deformity of zygapophyseal articulation (Browner, et al., 1998; Harris, et al., 1981; Resnick, 1995; Watkins, 1996).

2. Videofluoroscopy or digital motion radiography is currently a valuable diagnostic method in evaluating painful hypermobility and instability due to posttraumatic and degenerative pathology of capsular and axial ligaments. Evaluation of certain axial and peripheral joints in motion affords a noninvasive opportunity to identify specific segments responsible for nociception. At the upper cervical levels, this technology is capable of identifying excessive motions at atlanto occipital, lateral and median atlanto axial joints, and, indirectly, pathology of their respective fibrous articular capsules and periarticular ligaments (Figures 33.8, 33.9, and 33.10). Capsule-related pathology with hypo- and hypermobility can be identified and documented in caudally situated cervical zygapophyseal articulations. The integrity of the posterior ligamentous complex con-

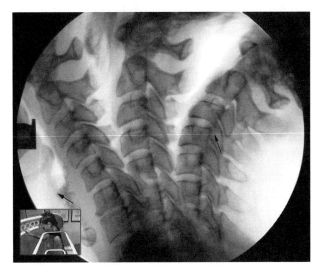

FIGURE 33.8 Posterior listhesis of C3 on C4 during extension identified with digital motion radiography. This was not identified with plain flexion, extension radiography. (Images acquired utilizing Visualizer 2000 from VF-Works, Inc. Modified by Tracey Slaughter.)

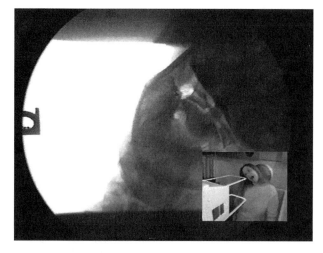

FIGURE 33.9 Listhesis of C1 on C2 during lateral flexion. Identified by digital motion radiography. This was not identified by plain film radiography. (Images acquired utilizing Visualizer 2000 from VF-Works, Inc. Modified by Tracey Slaughter.)

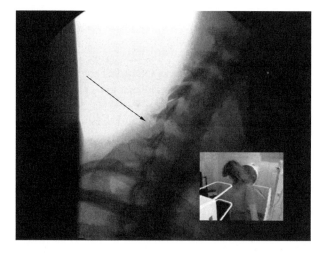

FIGURE 33.10 Flexion oblique view demonstrating widening of the facet joint suggestive of capsular ligament tear identified by digital motion radiography. This was not well visualized by plain film radiography. (Images acquired utilizing Visualizer 2000 from VF-Works, Inc. Modified by Tracey Slaughter.)

tributing to listhesis-related pathology can be documented. Small avulsion fractures of articular pillars as well as vertebral bodies or spinous processes can be identified. The pathology of TMJs is visualized and correlated with audio/video captioning. Painful instability of peripheral joints such as shoulder, elbows, wrists, knees, and ankles has also been identified and documented (Antos, et al., 1990; Buonocore, et al., 1996; Fielding, 1957, 1963; Jones, 1967; Tacharski, et al., 1981). Such studies must be performed with high-quality digitized equipment by well-trained technologists to produce film quality contrast resolution and to be of diagnostic value, as

currently available from VF Works, Inc. Combined with computerized range of motion studies, this technology may afford the opportunity to objectively document progress after RIT/prolotherapy, or other procedures directed toward the stabilization of axial and peripheral articulations such as facets, shoulders, knees and TMJs.

3. MRI may detect intervertebral disc pathology, enthesopathy, ligamentous injury, interspinous bursitis, zygapophyseal joint disease and sacroiliac joint pathology, evaluation of the neural foraminal pathology, bone contusion, neoplasia infection or fracture, as well as exclude or confirm spinal cord disease and pathology related to intradural, extramedullary, and epidural space (Resnick, 1995; Stark, et al., 1999).

4. CT scan may detect small avulsion fractures of the facets, laminar fracture, fracture of vertebral bodies and pedicles, or degenerative changes (Resnick, 1995).

5. Bone scan is useful in the assessment of the entire skeleton, ruling out metabolically active disease processes (Resnick, 1995).

SAFE INJECTION SITES

Common sites for injections are the enthesis of the structures that insert or originate at the spinous processes and are innervated by the medial branches of the dorsal rami. At the cervicodorsal junction, from superficial to deep, these include the supraspinous ligament, superficial layers of the cervicodorsal fascia, and multiple tendons. The apex of the spinous process may be considered a "spinous rotator cuff" (Figures 33.11 and 33.12). At the cervicocranial junction, these are fibroosseous insertions at the superior and inferior nuchal lines, lateral aspects of the apex at the C2 spinous process and C2-3 posterior z-joint capsule.

The following step-by-step approach to a differential diagnosis is based on knowledge of anatomy and pathology, to investigate all potential nociceptors in the distribution of the medial and lateral branches extending it beyond z-joints, as is currently accepted (Aprill, et al., 1990; Barnsley, et al., 1994; Bogduk, 1986, 1988, 1996; Bogduk, et al., 1996; Dreyfuss, et al., 1994b, 1995; Dussault, et al., 1994; Dwyer, et al., 1990; Lord, 1996).

Accordingly, in the presence of significant midline tenderness, the most painful medial structures innervated by terminal filaments of the MBDRs are blocked initially. If after local anesthetic block, the paramedian pain persists, laminar enthesis of structures are blocked. If pain still persists, the posterior cervical or thoracic facet joint capsules are blocked, because the facet joints are the most proximal structures innervated by MBDRs on their emerging course from the dorsal ramus. Pathology of the

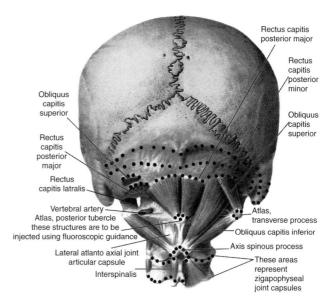

FIGURE 33.12 Sites of tendon origins and insertions (enthesis) of the vertebral and paravertebral musculaturein the upper cervical and occipital region. Clinically significant painful enthesopathies are common at these locations defined by dots. Dots also represent the most common locations of needle tips during RIT droplet infiltrations. (*Please note*: not all of the locations must be treated in each patient.) (From *Sinelnikov Atlas of Anatomy*, Vol. I, Meditsina Moskow, 1972. Modified by Tracey Slaughter.)

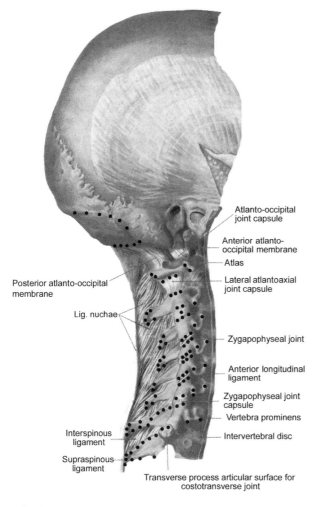

FIGURE 33.11 Cervical ligaments and joint capsules at their enthesis. Clinically significant painful enthesopathies are common at the locations defined by dots. Dots also represent most common locations of needletips during RIT droplet infiltrations. (Please note: not all of the locations must be treated in each patient.) (From *Sinelnikov Atlas of Anatomy*, Vol. I, Meditsina Moskow, 1972. Modified by Tracey Slaughter.)

capsular ligaments and periarticular tendons is an integral part of the facet joint syndrome.

Laterally positioned structures are innervated by the lateral branches of the dorsal rami. If laterally arising pain persists, enthesis at posterior tubercles of the cervical transverse processes and in the thoracic area capsules of costotransverse articulations are injected. If the pain persists, the iliocostalis cervices and thoracis tendons, at their respective fibroosseous rib insertions, are blocked.

Regarding z-joints, the intention is to inject the joint capsule posteriorly, initially with lidocaine utilizing the posterior approach, and thereafter with a mixture of bupivacaine and proliferating solution. Patients usually experience slight unsteadiness after injection of the C2-3 or C3-4 z-joint capsules, indicating a disturbance of postural tonic reflexes and indirectly successful blocks of the medial branches.

SOLUTIONS UTILIZED

The most common solution is 12.5% dextrose. Dilution is made with local anesthetic in 1:3 proportion, (i.e., 1 ml of 50% dextrose mixed with 3 ml of 1% lidocaine (Hackett, et al., 1991; Reeves, 1995, 2000).

For intra-articular injection of the knee, Hemwall has recommended a 25% dextrose solution (Hackett, et al., 1991). Reeves, et al. (2000) have pointed out that a 10% dextrose solution may be equally effective. If this proves ineffective, gradual progression to sodium morrhuate full strength has been described (Dorman, et al., 1991; Hackett, et al., 1991).

Sodium morrhuate (5%) is a mixture of sodium salts of saturated and unsaturated fatty acids of cod liver oil and 2% benzyl alcohol, which acts as a local anesthetic and a preservative. Note that benzyl alcohol is chemically very similar to phenol.

Dextrose/phenol/glycerine solution, originally produced in England by Boots Company Ltd. of Nottingham for treatment of varicose veins, was introduced to pain management by Ongley, et al. (1988). The solution consists of 25% dextrose, 2.5% phenol, and 25% glycerine and is referred to as DPG (a.k.a. P2G). Prior to injection it is diluted in concentrations of 1:2; 1:1, or 2:3 with a local anesthetic of the practitioner's choice. Some authors exclusively use this solution in 1:1 dilution (Dorman, et al., 1991). Others modified it, reducing the percentage of glycerine to 12.5%

The 6% phenol in glycerine solution was utilized by Poritt in 1931 and reintroduced in the late 1950s by Maher (1957) of England for intrathecal injections in the treatment of spasticity. Subsequently, after gaining sufficient experience with intrathecal use of this solution, Wilkinson (1992), a neurosurgeon trained at Massachusetts General Hospital, began injecting it at the donor harvest sites of the iliac crests for neurolytic and proliferative responses.

CONCLUSIONS

1. RIT/prolotherapy is a valuable method of treatment for correctly diagnosed, chronic painful conditions of the locomotive systems.
2. Thorough familiarity of the physician with normal, pathologic, cross-sectional, and clinical anatomy, as well as anatomical variations and function is necessary.
3. Current literature supports manipulation under local joint anesthesia.
4. The use of RIT in an ambulatory setting is an acceptable standard of care in the community.
5. The current literature suggests that NSAIDs and steroid preparations have limited utility in chronic painful overuse conditions and in degenerative painful conditions of ligaments and tendons. Microinterventional regenerative techniques and proper rehabilitation up to 6 months or a year, supported with mild opioid analgesics, are more appropriate.

The future is such that, instead of indirect stimulation of growth factors through inflammatory cascade, specific growth factors will become available. The challenge will remain as to what specific growth factors to utilize. Most probably, a combination of several growth factors will be utilized, together with specific genes responsible for production of these growth factors. It appears that the delivery mode will be injections for deep structures; however, superficial structures will probably be addressed through transdermal delivery systems (Cook, 2000; DesRosiers, et al., 1996; Kang, et al., 1999; Lee, et al., 1998; Marui, et al., 1997; Nakamura, et al., 1998; Reeves, 1995, 2000; Rudkin, et al., 1996; Spindler, et al., 1996).

A physician who is versatile in manipulation as well as diagnostic and therapeutic injection techniques as described previously may have ample opportunity for RIT use in the practice of pain management.

BIBLIOGRAPHY

Readers interested in incorporating RIT/prolotherapy in their pain management practice are referred to the following textbooks containing the bulk of information about this subject. These books were published in the 1980s and 1990s but remain reliable sources of basic principles and information.

The *Illustrated Manual of Orthopaedic Medicine* by Cyriax (1993) is available from Butterworth & Heinemann.

Diagnosis and Injection Techniques in Orthopedic Medicine and *Prolotherapy in the Lumbar Spine and Pelvis* (Dorman, 1995) is available from T. Dorman, M.D. at 2505 South 320th St., #100, Federal Way, WA 98003.

Hackett, et al.'s (1991) text is available from the Institute in Basic Life Principles (IBLP), Box 1, Oak Brook, IL 60522–3001.

Lennard's text, *Pain Procedures in Clinical Practice* (see Reeves, 2000) is available from Hanley & Belfus.

A System of Orthopaedic Medicine (see Ombregt, et al., 1995) by Ombregt, is available from W.B. Saunders.

Movement, Stability and Low Back Pain: The Essential Role of the Pelvis, by Vlemming, et al. (1997) is available from Churchill Livingstone.

The Failed Back Syndrome Etiology and Therapy, by Wilkinson (1992) is available from Springer-Verlag.

ACKNOWLEDGMENTS

The authors would like to extend special thanks to Pamela Ward and Dianne Zalewski for their invaluable help in the preparation of this manuscript, and to Tracey Slaughter for preparing the illustrations for publication.

REFERENCES

Agur, A., et al. (1991). *Grant's atlas of anatomy* (9th ed.). Baltimore: Williams & Wilkins.

Anderson, D.M. (1985). *Dorland's illustrated medical dictionary* (26th ed.). Philadelphia: W. B. Saunders.

Antos, J., et al. (1990). Interrated reliability of fluoroscopic detection of fixation in the mid-cervical spine. *Chiropractic Technique, 2*(2), 53–55.

Aprill, C., et al. (1990). Cervical zygapophyseal joint pain patterns II: A clinical evaluation. *Spine, 15,* 6.

Ashton, I., et al. (1992). Morphological basis for back pain: The demonstration of nerve fibers and neuropeptides in the lumbar facet joint capsule but not in the ligamentum flavum. *Journal of Orthopaedic Research, 10,* 72–78.

Bahme, B. (1945). Observations on the treatment of hypermobile joints by injections. *Journal of the American Osteopathic Association, 45*(3), 101–109.

Bannister, L.H., Berry, M.M., Collins, P., & Dussek, L.E. (Eds.) (1995). *Gray's anatomy* (38th British ed.). New York: Churchill Livingston, Pearson Professional Limited.

Barbor, R. (1964). A treatment for chronic low back pain. Proceedings from the IV International Congress of Physical Medicine, Paris, September 6–11, pp. 661–663.

Barnsley, L, et al. (1994). Lack of effect of intraarticular corticosteroids for chronic pain in the cervical zygapophyseal joints. *New England Journal of Medicine, 330*(15), 1047–1050.

Bell, G. (1990, September). Skeletal applications of videofluroscopy. *Journal of Manipulative and Psychological Therapeutics, 13,* 7.

Best, T. (1994). Basic science of soft tissue. In J.C. Delee & D. Drez, Jr. (Eds.). *Orthopedic Sports Medicine Principles and Practice* (Vol. 1, pp. 7–35). Philadelphia: W.B. Saunders.

Biegeleisen, H.I. (1984). *Varicose veins, related diseases and sclerotherapy: A guide for practitioners.* Montreal: Eden Press.

Blaschke, J. (1961, September). Conservative management of intervertebral disk injuries. *Journal of Oklahoma State Medical Association, 54,* 9.

Blumenthal, L. (1974, September). Injury to the cervical spine as a cause of headache. *Postgraduate Medicine, 56,* 3.

Bogduk, N. (1986). On the concept of third occipital headache. *Journal of Neurology, Neurosurgery and Psychiatry, 49,* 775–780.

Bogduk, N. (1988). Back pain: Zygapophysial blocks and epidural steroids. In M. Cousins, et al. (Eds.), *Neural blockage in clinical anesthesia and management of pain* (pp. 935–954). Philadelphia: J.B. Lippincott.

Bogduk, N. (1996). Post-traumatic cervical and lumbar spine zygapophyseal joint pain. In R.W. Evans (Ed.), *Neurology and trauma* (pp. 363–375). Philadelphia: W.B. Saunders.

Bogduk, N. (1997). *Clinical anatomy of the lumbar spine and sacrum* (3rd ed.). New York: Churchill Livingstone.

Bogduk, N., et al. (1991). *Clinical anatomy of the lumbar spine* (2nd ed.). Melbourne: Churchill Livingstone.

Bogduk, N., et al. (1996). Precision diagnosis of spinal pain. In T.S. Jensen (Ed.), *Pain 1996—An updated review refresher course syllabus* (pp. 507–525). IASP Refresher Courses on Pain Management, held in conjunction with the 8th World Congress on Pain, Vancouver, BC, August 17–22.

Bonica, J., et al. (1990). *The management of pain* (Vol, 1, 2nd ed., pp. 7, 136–139). Philadelphia: Lea & Febiger.

Borenstein, D., et al. (1996). *Neck pain medical diagnosis and comprehensive management.* Philadelphia: W. B. Saunders.

Bourdeau, Y. (1988). Five-year follow-up on sclerotherapy/prolotherapy for low back pain. *Manual Medicine, 3,*155–157.

Broadhurst, N., et al. (1996). Vertebral mid-line pain: Pain arising from the interspinous spaces. *Journal of Orthopaedic Medicine, 18*(1), 2–4.

Browner, B., et al. (1998). *Skeletal trauma* (Vol. 1, 2nd ed.). Philadelphia: W. B. Saunders.

Buonocore, E., et al. (1996). Cineradograms of cervical spine in diagnosis of soft tissue injuries. *Journal of the Americal Medical Association, 198*(1), 143–147.

Butler, D., et al. (1978). Biomechanics of ligaments and tendons. *Exercises and Sport Sciences Reviews, 6,* 125–182.

Chase, R. (1978, December). Basic sclerotherapy. *Osteopathic Annals, 6,* 514–517.

Coleman, A. (1968). Physician electing to treat by prolotherapy alters the method at his peril. *Journal of the National Medical Association, 60*(4), 346–348.

Compere, E., et al. (1958). Persistent backache. *Medical Clinics of North America, 42,* 299–307.

Cook, P. (2000, August/September). Wound repair system assists body in regenerating tissue. *Outpatient Care Technology, 1.*

Coplans, C. (1972). The use of sclerosant injections in ligamentous pain. In A. Heflet, L. Grueble, & M. David (eds.), *Disorders of the lumbar spine* (pp. 165–169). Philadelphia: Lippincott.

Cotran, R.S., et al. (1999). *Robbins pathologic basis of disease.* Philadelphia: W. B. Saunders.

Cousins, M., et al. (1988). *Neural blockage in clinical anesthesia and management of pain.* Philadelphia: J. B. Lippincott.

Cyriax, J. (1969). *Textbook of orthopaedic medicine. Vol. 1, Diagnosis of soft tissue lesion* (5th ed.). Baltimore: Williams & Wilkins.

Cyriax, J. (1982). *Textbook of orthopaedic medicine. Volume 1: Diagnosis of soft tissue lesion* (8th ed.). London: Bailliere Tindall.

Cyriax, J. (1993). *Illustrated manual of orthopaedic medicine* (2nd ed.). Oxford: Butterworth Heinemann.

Darby, R., et al. (1998). *Intradiscal electro-thermal annuloplasty.* Presentation at IITS 11th Annual Meeting, San Antonio, TX, May.

DesRosiers, E., et al. (1996). Proliferative and matrix synthesis response of canine anterior cruciate ligament fibroblasts submitted to combined growth factors. *Journal of Orthopaedic Research, 14,* 200–208.

Dorman, T. (1992). Storage and release of elastic energy in the pelvis: Dysfunction, diagnosis and treatment. In A. Vleeming, V. Mooney, C. Snijders, & T. Dorman (Eds.), *Low back pain and its relation to the sacroiliac joint* (pp. 585–600). San Diego, CA: E.C.O.

Dorman, T. (1995). *Prolotherapy in the lumbar spine and pelvis.* Philadelphia: Hanley & Belfus.

Dorman, T., et al. (1991). *Diagnosis and injection techniques in orthopedic medicine.* Baltimore: Williams & Wilkins.

Dreyfuss, P. (1997, December). Differential diagnosis of thoracic pain and diagnostic/therapeutic injection techniques. *ISIS newsletter,* 10–29.

Dreyfuss, P., et al. (1994a). Atlanto-occipital and lateral atlanto-axial joint pain patterns. *Spine, 19*(10), 1125–1131.

Dreyfuss, P., et al. (1994b). Thoracic zygapophyseal joint pain patterns: A study in normal volunteers. *Spine, 19*(7), 807–811.

Dreyfuss, P., et al. (1995). MUJA: Manipulation under joint anesthesia/analgesia: A treatment approach for recalcitrant low back pain of synovial joint origin. *Journal of Manipulative & Physiological Therapeutics, 18*(8), 537–546.

Dussault, R., et al. (1994, June). Facet joint injection: Diagnosis and therapy. *Applied Radiology*, 35–39.

Dwyer, A., et al. (1990). Cervical zygapophyseal joint pain patterns. I: A study in normal volunteers. *Spine, 15*, 6.

Eek, B. (1996). New directions in the treatment of disc pain. In *Diagnosis and treatment of discogenic pain. International Spinal Injection Society 4th annual meeting syllabus* (pp. 47–48), Vancouver, BC, August 16.

El-Bohy, A., et al. (1988). Localization of substance P and Neurofilament immunoreactive fibers in the lumbar facet joint capsule and supraspinous ligament of the rabbit. *Brain Research, 460*, 379–382.

Fielding, J. (1963). Cineradiography. *Journal of Bone and Joint Surgery (American Volume), 45*, 1543.

Fielding, J. (1957). Cineroentgenography of the normal cervical spine *Journal of Bone and Joint Surgery (American Volume), 57*, 1280–1288

Freemont, A., et al. (1997). Nerve ingrowth into diseased intervertebral disc in chronic back pain. *Lancet, 22*, 178–181.

Gedney, E. (1937, June). Special technic hypermobile joint: a preliminary report. *The Osteopathic Profession*, 30–31.

Gedney, E. (1938). *The hypermobile joint — further reports on injection method.* Paper presented at Osteopathic Clinical Society of Pennsylvania, February 13.

Gedney, E. (1951, September). Disc syndrome. *The Osteopathic Profession*, pp. 11–13, 34, 38, 40.

Gedney, E. (1952a, April). Use of sclerosing solution may change therapy in vertebral disk problem. *The Osteopathic Profession*, 34, 38 & 39. 1113.

Gedney, E. (1952b, August). Technique for sclerotherapy in the management of hypermobile sacroiliac. *The Osteopathic Profession*, 16–19, 37–38.

Gedney, E. (1954a, August). Progress report on use of sclerosing solutions in low back syndromes. *The Osteopathic Profession*, 18–21, 40–44.

Gedney, E. (1954b, September). The application of sclerotherapy in spondylolisthesis and spondylolysis. *The Osteopathic Profession*, 66–69, 102–105.

Grayson, M. (1994). Sterile meningitis after lumbosacral ligament sclerosing injections. *The Journal of Orthopaedic Medicine, 16*, 3.

Green, S. (1956, April). Hypermobility of joints: Causes, treatment and technic of sclerotherapy. *The Osteopathic Profession*, 26–27, 42–47.

Green, S. (1958, January). The study of ligamentous tissue is regarded as key to sclerotherapy. *The Osteopathic Profession*, 26–29.

Hackett, G. (1953). Joint stabilization through induced ligament sclerosis. *Ohio State Medical Journal, 49*, 877–884.

Hackett, G. (1956). *Joint ligament relaxation treated by fibro-osseous proliferation.* Springfield, IL: Charles C Thomas.

Hackett, G. (1958). *Ligament & tendon relaxation (skeletal disability)—Treated by prolotherapy, (fibro-osseous proliferation)* (3rd ed.). Springfield, IL: Charles C Thomas.

Hackett, G. (1959). Ligament relaxation and osteoarthritis, loose jointed vs. closed jointed. *Rheumatism* (London), *15*(2), 28–33.

Hackett, G. (1959, September). Low back pain. *Industrial Medicine and Surgery, 28*, 416–419.

Hackett, G. (1960a). Prolotherapy in low back pain from ligament relaxation and bone dystrophy. *Clinical Medicine, 7*(12), 2551–2561.

Hackett, G. (1960b). Prolotherapy in whiplash and low back pain. *Postgraduate Medicine, 27*, 214–219

Hackett, G. (1961). Prolotherapy for sciatic from weak pelvic ligament and bone dystrophy. *Clinical Medicine, 8*, 2301–2316.

Hackett, G. (1966b, February). Uninhibited reversible antidromic vasodilation in pathophysiologic diseases: Arteriosclerosis, carcinogenesis, neuritis and osteoporosis. *Angiology, 17*(2), 109–118.

Hackett, G. (1966c, July). Cause & mechanism of headache, pain and neuritis. *Headache, 6*, 88–92.

Hackett, G. (1966d, August). Uninhibited reversible antidromic vasodilatation in bronchiogenic pathophysiologic diseases. *Lancet, 86*, 398–404.

Hackett, G. (1967, September). Prevention of cancer, heart, lung and other diseases. *Clinical Medicine, 74*, 19.

Hackett, G., & Henderson, D. (1955, May). Joint stabilization: An experimental, histologic study with comments on the clinical application in ligament proliferation. *American Journal of Surgery, 89*, 968–973.

Hackett, G., et al. (1961, July). Back pain following trauma and disease prolotherapy. *Military Medicine*, 517–525.

Hackett, G., et al. (1962, April). Prolotherapy for headache: Pain in the head and neck, and neuritis. *Headache, 2*, 20–28.

Hackett, G., et al. (1991). *Ligament and tendon relaxation—Treated by prolotherapy* (5th ed.). Oak Park, IL: Gustav Hemwall, M.D.

Haldeman, K., et al. (1938). The diagnosis and treatment of sacroiliac conditions by the injection of procaine (novocain). *Journal of Bone and Joint Surgery, 20*(3), 675–685.

Harris, J., et al. (1981). *The radiology of emergency medicine* (2nd ed.). Baltimore: Williams & Wilkins.

Hirsch, C. (1948). An attempt to diagnose the level of a disc lesion clinically by disc puncture. *Acta Orthopaedia Scandinavica, 18*, 131–140.

Hirschberg, G., et al. (1982). Treatment of the chronic iliolumbar syndrome by infiltration of the iliolumbar ligament. *Western Journal of Medicine, 136*, 372–374.

Hirschberg, G., et al. (1992). Diagnosis and treatment of iliocostal friction syndromes. *Journal of Orthopedic Medicine, 14*(2), 35–39.

Hoch, G. (1939). Injection treatment of hydrocele. In F. Yeoman (Ed.), *Sclerosing therapy, the injection treatment of hernia, hydrocele, varicose veins and hemorrhoids* (pp. 141–156). London: Bailliere, Tindall & Cox.

Hunt, W. (1961). Complications following injections of sclerosing agent to precipitate fibro-osseous proliferation. *Journal of Neurosurgery, 18*, 461–465.

Jones M. (1967). Cineradiographic studies of abnormalities of the high cervical spine. *Archives of Surgery, 94*, 206–213.

Jozsa, L., & Kannus, P. (1997). *Human tendons, anatomy, physiology and pathology*, Champaign, IL: Human Kinetics.

Kang, H., et al. (1999). Ideal concentration of growth factors in rabbit's flexor tendon culture. *Yonsei Medical Journal, 40*(1), 26–29.

Kayfetz, D. (1963, June). Occipito-cervical (whiplash) injuries treated by prolotherapy. *Medical Trial Technique Quarterly*, 109–112, 147–167.

Kayfetz, D., et al. (1963). Whiplash injury and other ligamentous headache. Its management with prolotherapy. *Headache*, 3(1), pp??.

Kellgren, J. H. (1939). On the distribution of pain arising from deep somatic structures with charts of segmental pain areas. *Clinical Science, 4*, 35–46.

Keplinger, J. (1960). Paraplegia from treatment with sclerosing agents—Report of a case. *Journal of the American Medical Association, 73*, 1333–1336.

Klein, R. (1991). Diagnosis and treatment of gluteus medius syndrome *Journal of Orthopaedic Medicine, 13*, 1373–1376.

Klein, R. (1997, May). Prolotherapy: An alternative approach to managing low back pain. *Journal of Musculoskeletal Medicine*, 45–59.

Klein, R., et al. (1989). Proliferation injections for low back pain: Histologic changes of injected ligaments and objective measurements of lumbar spine mobility before and after treatment. *Journal of Neurological and Orthopaedic Medicine and Surgery, 10*(2), 123–126.

Klein, R., et al. (1993). A randomized double-blind trial of dextrose-glycerine-phenol injections for chronic, low back pain. *Journal of Spinal Disorders, 6*(1), 23–33.

Koudele, C. (1978). Treatment of joint pain. *Osteopathic Annals, 6*(12), 42–45.

Leadbetter, W. (1992). Cell-matrix response in tendon injury. *Clinical Sports Medicine, 11*, 533–578.

Leadbetter, W. (1994). *Soft tissue athletic injuries: Sports injuries: Mechanisms, prevention, treatment.* Baltimore: Williams & Wilkins.

Leadbetter, W. (1995). Anti-inflammatory therapy and sport injury: The role of non-steroidal drugs and corticosteroid injections. *Clinical Sports Medicine, 14*, 353–410

Lee, J., et al. (1998). Growth factor expression in healing rabbit medial collateral and anterior cruciate ligaments. *Iowa Orthopaedic Journal, 18*, 19–25.

Leedy, R. (1977, August). Applications of sclerotherapy to specific problems. *Osteopathic Medicine*, 79–81, 85, 86, 89–91, 94–96.

Leedy, R., et al. (1976). Analysis of 50 low back cases 6 years after treatment by joint ligament sclerotherapy. *Osteopathic Medicine, 6*, 15–22.

Leriche, R. (1930). Effets de l'anesthesia a la novocaine des ligaments et des insertion tenineuses periarticulares dans certanes maladies articulares et dans les vices de positions foncitionnells des articulations. *Gazette des Hopitaux Civils et Militaires, 103*, 1294.

Lindblom, K. (1944). Protrusions of the discs and nerve compression in the lumbar region. *Acta Radiologica Scandanavica, 25*, 192–212.

Linetsky, F.S. (1999a). Regenerative injection therapy for low back pain. *The Pain Clinic, 1*(1), 27–31.

Linetsky, F. S. (1999b). History of sclerotherapy in urology. *The Pain Clinic, 5*(2), 30–32.

Linetsky, F.S. et al. (2001). A history of the applications of regenerative injection therapy in pain management, Part II 1960s–1980s. *The Pain Clinic, 3*(2), 32–36.

Liu, Y., et al. (1983). An in situ study of the influence of a sclerosing solution in rabbit medial collateral ligaments and its junction strength. *Connective Tissue Research, 11*, 95–102.

Lord, S. (1996). Chronic cervical zygapophyseal joint pain after whiplash: A placebo-controlled prevalence study. *Spine*, 21(15), 1737–1745.

Maher, R. (1957, January). Neuron selection in relief of pain. Further experiences with intrathecal injections. *Lancet*, 16–19.

Marui, T., et al. (1997). Effect of growth factors on matrix synthesis by ligament fibroblasts. *Journal of Orthopaedic Research, 15*, 18–23.

Massie, J., et al. (1993). Is it possible to stimulate fibroplasia within the intervertebral disc? *Journal or Orthopaedic Medicine, 15*(3), 83.

Matthews, J. (1995). A new approach to the treatment of osteoarthritis of the knee: Prolotherapy of the ipsilateral sacroiliac ligaments. *American Journal of Pain Management, 5*(3), 91–93.

Maynard, J., et al. (1985). Morphological and biochemical effects of sodium morrhuate on tendons. *Journal or Orthopaedic Research, 3*, 234–248.

Merriam Webster's Desk Dictionary. (1995). Springfield, MA: Merriam-Webster.

Merskey, H., et al. (1994). *Classification of chronic pain, descriptions of chronic pain syndromes and definitions of pain terms* (2nd ed.). Seattle: IASP Press.

Mirman, M. (1989). *Sclerotherapy* (4th ed.). Springfield, PA: Merrill Jay Mirman.

Mooney, V. (1993a, January). Sclerotherapy in back pain? Yes, if clinician is skilled. *Journal of Musculoskeletal Medicine*, 13.

Mooney, V. (1993b, July). Understanding, examining for, and treating sacroiliac pain. *Journal of Musculoskeletal Medicine*, 37–49.

Myers, A. (1961). Prolotherapy treatment of low back pain and sciatica. *Bulletin, Hospital for Joint Diseases, 22*, 48–55.

Nakamura, N., et al. (1998). Early biological effect of in vivo gene transfer of platelet-derived growth factor (PDGF)-B into healing patellar ligament. *Gene Therapy, 5*, 1165–1170.

Neff, F. (1959, March). A new approach in the treatment of chronic back disabilities. *Family Physician, 9*, 3.

Neff, F. (1960). Low back pain and disability. *Western Medicine, 1*, 12.

Ombregt, L., et al. (1995). *A system of orthopaedic medicine.* Philadelphia: W. B. Saunders.

Ongley, M., et al. (1987, July 18). A new approach to the treatment of chronic low back pain. *Lancet*, 143–146.

Ongley, M., et al. (1988). Ligament instability of knees: A new approach to treatment *Manual Medicine, 3*, 152–154.

Poritt, A. (1931). The injection treatment of hydrocele, varicocele, bursae and nevi. *Proceedings, Royal Society of Medicine, 24*, 81.

Ranney, D. (1997). *Chronic musculoskeletal injuries in the workplace.* Philadelphia: W. B. Saunders.

Reeves, D. (1995). Prolotherapy: Present and future applications in soft-tissue pain and disability. *Physical Medicine and Rehabilitation Clinics of North America, 6*(4), 917–926.

Reeves, D. (2000). Prolotherapy: Basic science clinical studies and technique. In T.A. Lennard (Ed.), *Pain procedures in clinical practice* (pp. 172–189). Philadelphia: Hanley & Belfus.

Reeves, K, et al. (2000). Randomized prospective double-blind placebo-controlled study of dextrose prolotherapy for knee osteoarthritis with or without ACL laxity. *Alternative Therapy, 6*(2), 68–74, 77–80.

Resnick, D. (1995). *Diagnosis of bone and joint disorders* (Vol. 1–6, 3rd ed.). Philadelphia: W. B. Saunders Co.

Riddle, P. (1940). *Injection treatment*. Philadelphia: W. B. Saunders.

Roosth, H. (1991, November). Low back and leg pain attributed to gluteal tendinosis. *Orthopedics Today,* 10 et seq.

Rudkin, G., et al. (1996). Growth factors in surgery. *Plastic and Reconstructive Surgery, 97*(2), 469–476.

Saal, J., et al. (1998a). A novel approach to painful internal disk derangement: Collagen modulation with a thermal percutaneous navigable intradiscal catheter: A prospective trial presented at the *NASS-APS first joint meeting* Charleston, SC, April.

Saal, J., et al. (1998b). Percutaneous treatment of painful lumbar disc derangement with a navigable intradiscal thermal catheter: A pilot study presented at the *NASS-APS first joint meeting* Charleston, SC, April.

Schneider, R. (1959). Fatality after injecting of sclerosing agent to precipitate fibro-osseous proliferation. *Journal of the American Medical Association, 170,* 1768–1772.

Schultz, L. (1937, September). A treatment for subluxation of the temporomandibular joint. *Journal of the American Medical Association, 256.*

Schultz, L. (1956, December). Twenty years' experience in treating hypermobility of the temporomandibular joints. *American Journal of Surgery, 92.*

Schwartz, R., et al. (1991). Prolotherapy: A literature review and retrospective study. *Journal of Neurologic and Orthopaedic Medicine and Surgery, 12,* 220–223.

Shevelev, A., et al. (2000). Interosseous receptor system as the modulator of trigeminal afferent reactions. *Worldwide Pain Conference: July 15–21, Abstract* p. 34.

Shuman, D. (1941). Luxation recurring in shoulder. *The Osteopathic Profession, 8*(6), 11–13.

Shuman, D. (1949a, March). Sclerotherapy—Injections may be best way to restrengthen ligaments in case of slipped knee cartilage. *The Osteopathic Profession* (preprint).

Shuman, D. (1949b, October). The place of joint sclerotherapy in today's practice. *Bulletin of the New Jersey Association of Osteopathic Physicians and Surgeons* (preprint).

Shuman, D. (1954, July). Sclerotherapy: Statistics on its effectiveness for unstable joint conditions. *The Osteopathic Profession,* 11–15, 37–38.

Shuman, D. (1958). *Low back pain.* Philadelphia: David Shuman.

Simon, R., et al. (1987). *Emergency orthopedics: The extremities* (2nd ed.). Norwalk, CT: Appleton & Lange.

Sokov. E., et al. (2000). Are herniated disks the main cause of low back pain. In abstract book of *Worldwide Pain Conference,* p. 74.

Spindler, K., et al. (1996). Patellar tendon and anterior cruciate ligament have different mitogenic responses to platelet-derived growth factor and transforming growth factor b. *Journal of Orthopaedic Research, 14,* 542–546

Stark, D., et al. (1999). *Magnetic resonance imaging* (Vol. 1 & 2, 3rd ed.). St. Louis, MO: Mosby.

Steindler, A., et al. (1938). Differential diagnosis of pain low in the back allocation of the source of pain by the procaine hydrochloride method. *Journal of the American Medical Association, 110,* 106–113.

Tacharski, C. C., et al. (1981). Dynamic atlanto-axial aberrations: A case study and cinefluorographic approach to diagnosis. *Journal of Manipulative and Psychological Therapeutics, 4*(2), 65–68.

Travell, J., et al. (1983). *Myofacial pain and dysfunction-trigger point manual—The upper extremities* (Vol. 1). Baltimore: Williams & Wilkins.

Tuzlukov, P., et al. (1993). The morphological characteristics of fibromyalgia syndrome. *Arkhiva Patelogie, 4*(2), 47–50.

Vanderschot, L. (1976a). The American version of acupuncture. Prolotherapy: Coming to an understanding. *American Journal of Acupuncture, 4,* 309–316.

Vanderschot, L. (1976b).Trigger points vs. acupuncture points, *American Journal of Acupuncture, 4,* 233–238.

Vleeming, A., et al. (1997). *Movement, stability and low back pain: the essential role of the pelvis.* New York: Churchill Livingstone.

Warren, J. (1881). *Hernia-strangulated and reducible with cure by subcutaneous injection.* Boston: Charles C Thomas.

Watkins, R. (1996). *The spine in sports.* St. Louis: Mosby.

Watson, L. (1938). *Hernia* (2nd ed.). St. Louis: C.V. Mosby.

Wilkinson, H. A. (1992). *The failed back syndrome etiology and therapy* (2nd ed.). Berlin: Springer-Verlag.

Willard, F. (1995). The lumbosacral connection: The ligamentous structure of the low back and its relation to back pain. In A. Vleeming, U. Mooney, C. Snijders, & T. Dorman (Eds.), *Proceedings of the Second Interdisciplinary World Congress on Low Back Pain, the Integrated Function of the Lumbar Spine and Sacroiliac Joints, Part I* (pp. 29–58), San Diego, CA, November 9–11.

Yahia, H., et al. (1989). A light and electron microscopic study of spinal ligament innervation. *Zeitschrift fuer Mikroskopische-Anatomische, 103,* 664–674.

Zoppi, M., et al. (2000). From "intraosseous pain syndrome" to osteoarthritis. In abstract book of *Worldwide Pain Conference,* p. 412.

34

Prescription NSAIDs: Choices in Therapy

Linda L. Norton, Pharm.D.

GOALS

The goal of this chapter is to help clinicians select appropriate nonsteroidal anti-inflammatory drugs (NSAIDs) for patients with specific risk factors by:

Providing an overview of these agents
Increasing the understanding of NSAID pharmacology
Increasing the awareness of characteristics of NSAIDs that make individual NSAIDs better or worse choices in specific patients

This information is presented in the hope and belief that selection of the most appropriate pharmacologic agent will improve patient outcomes by decreasing side effects and improving compliance and tolerability.

INTRODUCTION

Nonsteroidal anti-inflammatory drugs (NSAIDs) have been in use since the 1900s. They have been developed from a variety of sources, including natural products and as the result of developments and advances in our understanding of medicinal chemistry and pharmacology. Not all NSAIDs that have been developed, used medicinally, and marketed in the United States. have stood the test of time and prospective and retrospective investigation. For example, an NSAID approved by the Food and Drug Administration (FDA) in July 1997 for short-term use in acute pain (i.e., less than or equal to 10 days) was released to the U.S. market and then voluntarily withdrawn in June 1998 following reports of liver failure when the drug was used for extended periods of time (FDA, 1998). However, several products discovered early in the NSAID timeline

have stood the test of time and extensive use, and are still available and in use today. For example, willow bark, a natural product with an active ingredient called salicin, was first isolated in 1829 and still appears in some natural products listings and texts (Insel, 1996). Similarly, the use of sodium salicylate to treat rheumatic fever was reported in 1875, and products containing sodium salicylate are still marketed today. Interestingly, one of the most commonly used NSAIDs, aspirin, was developed and later marketed by Dresser in 1899, based on work from the 1850s by the chemist Gerhardt. Later Hoffman, a chemist at Bayer, prepared acetylsalicylic acid (ASA); and, as mentioned, ASA was marketed in 1899 as aspirin. Numerous other NSAIDs have been developed and marketed, mostly in the latter half of the 20th century, with most being marketed in the past 20 to 30 years. Cyclooxygenase (COX)-2 inhibitors are the latest class of NSAID to be marketed in the U.S., with the first of the class approved by the FDA in December 1998 and actually reaching the market in 1999 (Kaplan-Machlis & Klostermeyer, 1999). Peer-reviewed publications on the long-term safety and efficacy of COX-2 inhibitors are currently in progress with one containing the results of the CLASS study published in September of 2000 (Silverstein, et al., 2000).

NSAIDs and related products are used to reduce pain, stiffness, inflammation, platelet aggregation, and temperature, and are among the most frequent products prescribed by physicians or selected for self-care. ASA is the most commonly used household analgesic and one of the most widely prescribed analgesic, antipyretic, and anti-inflammatory agents in the United States. (APhA, 1999; Insel, 1996). Some estimates place the number of NSAID prescriptions in the U.St. at 50 to 100 million annually (APhA, 1999; Fung & Kirschenbaum, 1999). Furthermore, each

0-8493-0926-3/02/$0.00+$1.50
© 2002 by CRC Press LLC

day, more than 13 million Americans use NSAIDs (Kaplan-Machlis & Klostermeyer, 1999). In the U.S., the cost of these products is greater than $1 billion annually, with some estimates ranging as high as $2.2 billion per year (Boyce & Takiya, 2000; Kaplan-Machlis & Klostermeyer, 1999). The range in costs is based, in part, on the large number of factors that affect cost, including which cost is being discussed (i.e., consumer cost, medical center acquisition cost, or third-party payer cost), and it is largely artificial. These numbers are presented only to demonstrate the magnitude of use of these medications. The 1995 estimates of worldwide sales listed sales at greater than $5.7 billion (Kaplan-Machlis & Klostermeyer, 1999). And, as much as 10,000 to 20,000 tons of ASA may be used in the U.S. annually (Insel, 1996). It is difficult to visualize 20,000 tons of aspirin; but picture a line of pick-up trucks, each with a half-ton of ASA in the back. If the trucks were parked end to end, the line would stretch from New York City to Hartford, Connecticut. By any estimate, ASA and other NSAIDs are widely used and widely prescribed.

PRIMARY ACTIONS/MECHANISMS OF ACTIONS

When considered in its simplest form, inflammation is a series of physiologic reactions that result in erythema, edema, tenderness, or pain (Insel, 1996). Inflammation can be caused by a variety of factors that may be as easily identified as an injury, infection, or ischemia, or as difficult to trace as a previously unidentified antigen-antibody reaction. Inflammation occurs in three phases. The first phase is what patients often report. In this phase, the events are usually easily noticed and are usually reported as swelling and redness. The swelling and redness result from local vasodilation that leads to increased capillary permeability. Next, a delayed phase results in the migration of leukocytes and phagocytic cells. Finally, a chronic phase can occur in which tissue degeneration and fibrosis are seen. These are the events that anti-inflammatory medications are intended to block. In most cases, the anti-inflammatory agent of choice is an NSAID. A large part of this choice is due to the fact that although NSAIDs can have significant, even lethal adverse effects, they are associated with fewer problems than the other large category of anti-inflammatory drugs, the steroids.

Acetaminophen (APAP) is often not considered a non-steroidal anti-inflammatory drug because it has no anti-inflammatory activity at recommended doses, and unlike many NSAIDS, APAP has no anti-platelet effect (Insel, 1996). It is included in this chapter, however, because of the tight connection between APAP and NSAIDs in clinical use and because APAP is often the drug of choice in noninflammatory pain in patients for whom NSAIDs should not be used or in patients who cannot tolerate NSAIDs (Kastrup, 2000; McEvoy, 1999). Additionally, it is included because clinicians may not provide adequate information to patients/consumers on the differences between APAP and NSAIDs, and although APAP is generally well tolerated, it, too, is associated with significant risk, especially risk of hepatoxicity. APAP is effective in decreasing mild to moderate pain and for decreasing temperature, but it may not be the best choice of agents to treat pain associated with inflammation and should not be used to decrease platelet aggregation. The importance of this general lack of efficacy as an anti-inflammatory agent and also as an anti-platelet agent should be explained to patients, because many patients have used recommended doses of APAP successfully to relieve aches and pains with very few, if any, side effects. Due, in part, to its low side-effect profile and low cost, APAP appears to patients/consumers to be an attractive alternative to NSAIDs. Unfortunately, in the absence of adequate information, patients may substitute APAP for an NSAID when an anti-inflammatory or anti-platelet effect is needed. Patient/consumer education by clinicians may be the key to avoiding this confusion.

APAP's antipyretic activity is at the hypothalamic heat-regulating center (Kastrup, 2000; McEvoy, 1999). This action increases vasodilation and sweating and allows heat loss. Additionally, the action of endogenous pyrogens on the heat-regulating centers is inhibited, and central, but not peripheral, inhibition of prostaglandin synthetsis occurs. APAP's mechanism for reducing pain is not fully known. The question of APAP and anti-inflammatory action is complex. Although under some circumstances weak anti-inflammatory effects may be seen, these actions are rarely seen at doses safe for clinical use. This may be because APAP is only a weak inhibitor of cyclooxygenase (COX), and this weak inhibition appears to be seen only in low concentrations of peroxide. Interestingly, areas of inflammation tend to have increased levels of peroxides produced by leukocytes (Insel, 1996).

Salicylates are organic acids that are hydrolyzed to salicylic acid (Insel, 1996; Kastrup, 2000; McEvoy, 1999). Salicylamide and diflunisal are products that are structurally similar to salicylates, but are not hydrolyzed to salicylic acid (Kastrup, 2000; McEvoy, 1999). The salicylates and related products are effective in decreasing pain, temperature, and inflammation, but have a variable impact on platelet aggregation. Aspirin, but not other salicylates, inhibits platelet aggregation for 4 to 11 days, which is the life of the platelet (Insel, 1996; Kastrup, 2000; McEvoy, 1999). In addition to aspirin, salicylamide, and diflunisal, other products considered in this category include choline salicylate, magnesium salicylate, combinations of choline and magnesium salicylate, sodium salicylate, sodium thiosalicylate, and salsalate (salicylsalicyclic acid).

Salicylates tend to accumulate at sites where inflammation is present, and can be particularly effective when it is

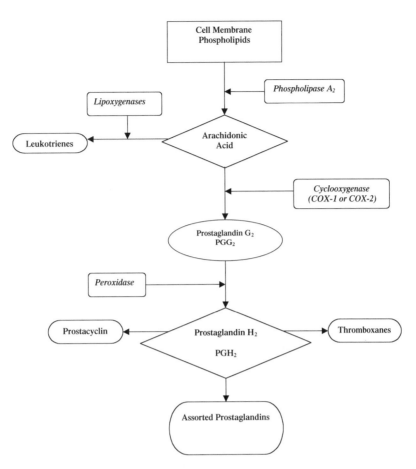

FIGURE 34.1 Arachidonic acid, prostaglandins, and COX: The role of COX-1 and COX-2. (Adapted from Campbell & Halushka, 1996; Kaplan-Machlis & Klostermeyer, 1999; McEvoy, 1999; Simon, 1999.)

their anti-inflammatory action that is needed (Insel, 1996). Reduction of pain and the anti-inflammatory action of salicylates are primarily due to inhibition of prostaglandin synthesis (Kastrup, 2000; McEvoy, 1999) (see Figure 34.1). The irreversible anti-platelet action of ASA has been attributed to the irreversible acetylation of COX, especially COX-1, resulting in decreased thromboxane A_2 synthesis and eventually decreased platelet aggregation. The duration of the effects of ASA are related to the turnover rate of COX in cells (Insel, 1996). Because platelets have little or no ability to synthesize COX or other proteins, the effect of ASA in platelets is for the life of the platelet (Insel, 1996; Kastrup, 2000; McEvoy, 1999). The antipyretic actions of the salicylates are due to inhibition of prostaglandins that have an effect in the hypothalmus and by peripheral vasodilation that increases heat loss.

Many combination products are marketed as pain relievers. Some of these include combinations of acetaminophen and salicylates or salicylate-like products, and barbiturates, caffeine, phenyltoloxamine citrate, pyrilamine maleate, pamabrom, antacids, and meprobamate. These combination products are not specifically discussed in this chapter.

NSAIDs are organic acids that also tend to accumulate at sites of inflammation (Insel, 1996). One exception to the organic acid classification is the non-organic nabumetone. However, nabumetone is converted to a form of acetic acid *in vivo*. NSAIDs are also effective in decreasing pain, temperature, and inflammation and have variable impact on platelet aggregation. They are generally considered to be effective analgesics for mild to moderate pain; but for some pain, such as certain types of postoperative pain, they may be more effective than opioid analgesics. The NSAIDs are classified chemically as acetic acids, fenamates, anthranilic acids, naphthylalkanones, pyrazolidinediones, oxicams, propionic acids, pyranocarboxylic acids, pyrrolizine carboxylic acids, or COX-2 inhibitors (Kastrup, 2000; McEvoy, 1999).

Listings of these classifications are not constant, with some listings including the naphthylalkanones in the acetic acid category along with other similarly minor changes (Boyce & Takiya, 2000; Insel, 1996; Kastrup, 2000; McEvoy, 1999). And, these differences are quite accurate. Nabumetone, mentioned above, is an inactive pro-drug that is metabolized to an active acetic acid form. It is the one product marketed in the U.S. that is listed in the naphthylalkanone class. Other single-agent classes of NSAIDs, the pyranocarboxylic acids (i.e., etodolac) and the pyrrolizine carboxylic acids (i.e., ketorolac), are sometimes also listed as subcategories of acetic acid NSAIDs. Additionally, pyrazolidinediones (phenylbutazone) have only one NSAID in the class. Other classes such as the acetic acids, fenamates, oxicams, propionic acids, and the COX-2 inhibitors have more than one product per class. Members of the acetic class are diclofenac, indomethacin, sulindac, and tolmetin. Two products, meclofenamate and mefenamic acid, are classified as fenamates; and two products are classified as oxicams (i.e., piroxicam and meloxicam). The propionic acids include fenoprofen, flurbiprofen, ibuprofen, ketoprofen, naproxen, and oxaprozin; the COX-2 inhibitors are celecoxib, a sulfonamide-like agent, and rofecoxib, a furanone.

For some of the NSAID chemical classes, such as the propionic acids, there is considerable similarity in efficacy and safety although, between products in this class, there is large variability in half-lives and duration of action (Boyce & Takiya, 2000). For many others of the NSAID chemical classes, the only consistency within the class appears to be in the chemical structure. However, for some chemical classes, these chemical and structural similarities allow clinicians to predict side-effect profiles and potentially which patients may have allergic reactions. For example, knowing that celecoxib is a COX-2 inhibitor should suggest that this product might have fewer GI side effects than products from another class. In addition, knowing that celecoxib is a sulfonamide-like COX-2 agent will help a clinician predict that patients who are allergic to sulfonamide antibiotics should avoid this product because they may also be allergic to this sulfonamide-like agent. Interestingly, this same type of logic may not hold true for ASA. In general, patients who are allergic to ASA should be instructed to avoid all NSAIDs. However, the likelihood of an ASA allergic patient having an allergic reaction is actually greater with non-salicylate NSAIDs that with nonaspirin salicylates (Insel, 1996; Lipman, 1996).

The anti-platelet activity of the NSAIDs, as well as their effects in reducing pain and inflammation, are primarily a result of inhibition of prostaglandin synthesis (Insel, 1996; Kastrup, 2000; McEvoy, 1999). The inhibition of prostaglandin synthesis occurs when the enzymatic action of cyclooxygenase (COX) is blocked, thereby preventing the conversion of arachidonic acid to prostaglandin G2 and H2 and eventually to a more diverse series of prostaglandins (see Figure 34.1). Additionally, NSAIDs may inhibit the movement of leukocytes and contribute to a reduction in superoxide radicals as well as induction of apoptosis (Kastrup, 2000; McEvoy, 1999). Decreases in nitric oxide synthetase, tumor necrosis factor-alpha, and interleukin-1, and changes in lymphocyte activity and cellular membrane function are believed to play a role in decreasing inflammatory action. Diclofenac, ibuprofen, indomethacin, and ketoprofen have been shown, in animal models, to have central analgesic activity. Antipyretic activity is due to the inhibition of prostaglandin-E2 synthesis in the central nervous system in and/or near the hypothalamic area (Kastrup, 2000; McEvoy, 1999).

As mentioned, NSAIDs inhibit COX. Depending on the NSAID used, the inhibition may be of both COX-1 and COX-2, primarily COX-1, or primarily COX-2. As shown in Figure 34.1 and described previously, inhibiting COX-1 and/or COX-2 inhibits the conversion of arachidonic acid to prostaglandins. With less prostaglandin production, there is less pain and inflammation; however, nonenzymatic pathways produce products that contribute to inflammation and are not affected by NSAIDs.

Currently, most NSAIDs used in the U.S. are nonselective inhibitors of COX-1 and COX-2 (Insel, 1996). However, some — including aspirin, ketoprofen, flurbiprofen, indomethacin, piroxicam, and sulindac — have modest selectivity for inhibiting COX-1, while ibuprofen, naproxen, and diclofenac may have less selectivity for COX-1 (Fung & Kirschenbaum, 1999; Kaplan-Machlis & Klostermeyer, 1999; Kastrup, 2000). Nabumetone and possibly etodolac are slightly selective for COX-2 inhibition (APhA, 1999; Kastrup, 2000). Meloxicam has intermediate COX-2 inhibition selectivity. Celecoxib and rofecoxib are selective for COX-2 inhibition. Thus, inhibition of COX, whether it is selective or nonselective, is the primary mechanism for NSAIDs and appears to provide the majority of the effect in decreasing pain and inflammation. Inhibition of COX also contributes to other activities of the NSAIDs and to their side-effect profile. However, when COX selectivity of the NSAIDs is discussed, some differences are listed. For example, some sources state that at low doses, aspirin is almost exclusively COX-1 selective (APhA, 1999). In addition, there is some disagreement as to the selectivity of etodolac, with some sources listing nabumetone as the only agent with some, but less than intermediate, COX-2 selectivity (Insel, 1996).

Structurally, NSAIDs that primarily inhibit the actions of the enzyme COX-2 differ from nonselective NSAIDs (i.e., inhibitors of COX-1 and/or COX-2 enzymes) by the presence of a rigid side extension on the COX-2 inhibitor molecule. The COX-2 inhibitor's side extension fits into a "pocket" on the COX-2 enzyme, preventing the activity of the COX-2 enzyme (APhA, 1999; Simon, 1999). Think of the COX-2 selective products as a hand with the fingers closed but the thumb extended. The COX nonselective products would then look like a hand with the fingers and thumbs closed. The hand with the fingers and thumb closed (nonselective NSAID) would fit easily into a mitten (COX-2 receptor) or a tube sock (COX-1 receptor). The hand with the fingers closed and the thumb extended (COX-2 selective NSAID) would fit into the mitten, but would be difficult to fit in the tube sock.

The activities of COX are many and varied. COX-1 is considered a constitutive enzyme that has a "housekeeping role" (APhA, 1999; Kaplan-Machlis & Klostermeyer, 1999; Simon, 1999). It is present in all tissues and cell types. Its major impact is on prostaglandin production and the production of thromboxane A2. Remember, thromboxane A2 has effects on increasing platelet aggregation and may affect vasoconstriction. COX-1 is also responsible for normal renal function, hemostasis, and most notably, GI mucosal integrity. Prostaglandins produced under the influence of COX-1 decrease gastric acid secretion, increase mucous secretion, increase mucosal blood flow, and aid in the maintenance of the stomach lining. Renal function is also affected by prostaglandins produced under the influence of COX-1. These prostaglandins contribute to dilation of the renal vasculature, especially under circumstances where there is reduced renal blow flow due to such problems as decreased systemic blood flow, blood volume depletion, and low cardiac output. There is also some compensation for the effects of the renin-angiotnesin-aldosterone and sympathetic activity.

COX-2 is an inducible enzyme known for its role in the inflammatory process (APhA, 1999; Kaplan-Machlis & Klostermeyer, 1999; Simon, 1999). Under normal circumstances, it is usually undetectable in most tissues. The tissues that are exceptions, where it appears to have a fairly constant role, include parts of the brain, in bones, in normal kidneys, and in the female reproductive system, especially the ovaries and uterus (Simon, 1999; Wallace, 1999). Effects in these areas that appear to be mediated by COX-2 are those involved in mitogenesis and growth, regulation of the reproductive process in females, bone formation, and renal function where it is involved in the regulation of sodium, circulatory volume, and blood pressure. However, in most tissue, pro-inflammatory products such as interleukin-1, lipopolysaccharide, tumor necrosis factor, mitogens, and others induce COX-2 activity (Kaplan-Machlis & Klostermeyer, 1999). Once COX-2 activity is induced in damaged tissue, there is an increase in the production of prostaglandins that contributes to the inflammatory process. Thus, blocking COX-2 is an effective way to decrease inflammation and pain. The problem is that COX-2 affects more than just the pain. For example, while COX-2 is almost undetectable in the GI tract in normal circumstances, when the GI tract is injured, the effects of COX-2 contribute to the healing process (Wallace, 1999). Despite this contribution, the information to date (October 2000) supports the use of selective inhibition of the COX-2 enzyme to decrease the adverse effects of NSAIDs on the GI tract. This means that, overall, the effects that occur when the COX-1 enzyme is blocked must contribute more to GI problems than

the effect that COX-2 contributes to healing an injury of the GI tract.

FACTORS AFFECTING PRODUCT SELECTION

For most types of medications, product selection is based on patient symptoms, and other patient factors and product factors. For NSAIDs, this is also the product selection process. If all these factors are equal, the choice of NSAIDs is largely empirical (Boyce & Takiya, 2000; Insel, 1996; Kastrup, 2000). When the product is selected, it should be given for 1 week or more, depending on the agent's half-life, to assess efficacy. Agents with a long half-life (e.g., piroxicam) should be given for 2 weeks or more to allow time for the effects of the drug to be seen. If an adequate therapeutic response is seen, the product should be continued for the duration of the need at the lowest effective dose, unless toxicities occur or the product is only approved for short-term use. Of note, there are large variations in the responses of individuals to individual NSAIDs, even if the NSAIDs are from the same chemical class (Insel, 1996). For example, in studies that compared the activity of some propionic acids, patients preferred naproxen for relief of pain and morning stiffness. When considering side effects, naproxen was preferred, followed by ibuprofen and fenoprofen. However, there were large interpatient variations in preference and no effective way to predict, before starting therapy, which product would work best with the fewest side effects in any given patient.

When all factors are not equal, selecting a medication becomes even more difficult. However, the factors mentioned previously can help to narrow the selection process (APhA, 1999). Patient characteristics that should be considered include the patient's age, concurrent disease states, organ function, medication allergies, and what products have worked or not worked well in the past. In addition, the patient's reproductive status and any physical limitations are important. The reproductive status of women of child-bearing age should always be considered, in part because about 50% of the pregnancies in the U.S. today are unplanned pregnancies, but also because of the potential of medications to contribute to difficulties in conception and harm to a developing fetus. The patient's vision and physical limitations, such as difficulties with opening vials and bottles, identifying tablets and capsules, measuring liquids, and even swallowing, should be considered. This is especially true when these difficulties are related to specific dosage forms (e.g., syrups, suspensions, tablets, or capsules) because many of these issues can be avoided with thoughtful prescribing. Factors to consider that are related to patient symptoms include the patient's description of the problem, along with details of the onset of symptoms and factors that increase or decrease the symptoms, and the frequency, nature, and severity of symptoms. Finally, product characteristics to consider are the efficacy of the ingredient for the particular symptom, COX selectivity, availability (i.e., from local sources as well as formulary restrictions), cost, dosage form and regimen, and the inactive ingredients in the product such as dyes and lactose content (APhA, 1999).

As mentioned, a general recommendation is to begin with the lowest dose that is expected to produce an adequate response and evaluate response and toxicities. However, as also mentioned, it is difficult to predict which medication will be the most effective in any given patient; even in clinical trials, the doses given were often too low to be effective. However, there is some good news. Recently, physicians in Australia have reported success in general practice with single-patient trials (Nikles, et al., 2000). The objective of the trials was to improve decision-making in the use of long-term medications for chronic medical conditions by piloting a single-patient trials design. Investigators in academic general practice designed the single-patient trials as a 12-week within-patient, randomized, double-blind, placebo-controlled, crossover comparison of two medications. In the design, which included 2-week treatment periods grouped into three pairs, patients with osteoarthritis were tested on ibuprofen and acetaminophen. To be included in the trials, patients must have had pain of at least 1 month's duration with the expectation that ongoing, long-term use of pain medication would probably be needed. Outcome measures were pain and stiffness, comparative measures of arthritis, preference for each product at the end of the product's 2-week period of use, use of escape medication, side effects, and changes in therapy as a result of participation in the trial. A survey of the results showed that 8 of 14 participants completed the trials with useful information that improved the decision-making process for each of the eight. Medications were changed for six of the eight completing the trial. The authors concluded that this type of trial can be used in a general-practice setting and may help identify patients who will respond to medications as well as which medication may be a better choice.

INDICATIONS AND UNLABELED USES

Acetaminophen is approved for a variety of nonvisceral analgesic and antipyretic uses such as muculoskeletal pain, headache, earache and the aches, pains, and fever of colds, flu, and other infections. In contrast, the salicylates, including aspirin, are approved for relief of various inflammatory conditions as well as the treatment of mild to moderate pain and fever (Kastrup, 2000; McEvoy, 1999). In addition to these uses, ASA has also been used to decrease the risk of stroke and heart attacks. Unlabeled uses of aspirin abound. It has been considered as a possible

prevention for cataract formation and even for possible prevention of toxemia of pregnancy. Similar to the salicylates, the NSAIDs are approved for a variety of pain and inflammatory indications. These include rheumatoid and osteoarthritis, treatment of mild to moderate pain, primary dysmenorrhea, tendintis and bursitis, as well as for gout and fever (Kastrup, 2000). Each NSAID has been used successfully for its FDA-approved (i.e., labeled) indications; but in most cases, APAP and the NSAIDs are also used for an assortment of pain-related uses that are not FDA approved (i.e., unlabeled) uses (see Table 34.1).

When the indications are viewed, reports of the trials are read, and clinicians are questioned, several interesting points emerge as being worthy of discussion. First, for many types of pain, any of the NSAIDs appear to be as effective as any other NSAID in reducing pain when given at equal analgesic dose — which is, more or less, the definition of equal analgesic doses. However, APAP is not included in this group, and an exception to this general rule of efficacy is that the salicylate NSAIDs do not seem to be as effective as the non-salicylate NSAIDs for relieving pain associated with dysmenorrhea (APhA, 1999; McEvoy, 1999). Of note, although only one of the currently available COX-2 inhibitors (rofecoxib) is indicated for primary dysmenorrhea, the COX-2 selective agents would be expected to be particularly effective for this use. This is due to the expected efficacy of the COX-2 inhibitors in preventing the increase in prostaglandins seen following ovulation when an increase in leutenizing hormone induces the COX-2 enzyme (APhA, 1999; Simon, 1999). Increased amounts of COX-2, in the presence of adequate substrate (arachidonic acid) result in increased production of prostaglandin, as is seen during the luteal and menstrual phases of the cycle and especially when dysmenorrhea is present. Blocking COX-2 should result in less prostaglandin production and a decrease in dysmenorrhea. However, NSAIDs, including COX-2 inhibitors, should be used with caution in women of childbearing age because their full effects on conception and the developing fetus are still not completely understood.

Another point suggested from trials and clinician experience is that the dosing of NSAIDs for pain is different than the dosing NSAIDs for anti-inflammatory use (Kastrup, 2000; McEvoy, 1999; Vlessides, 2000). In general, for pain, dosing of NSAIDs should be toward the lower end of the dosing range at the lowest dose that is expected to be adequate for relief of pain. This has been referred to as an osteoarthritis dose. Again, in general, for treatment of inflammation, dosing of many NSAIDs should be from about mid-range to the higher end of the dosing range. This has been referred to as a rheumatoid or anti-inflammatory dose. For NSAIDs with shorter half-lives, a significant degree of pain relief should be noticed within a day to up to a week (Insel, 1996). For longer half-life drugs, significant pain relief can take longer. The

TABLE 34.1
Selected Indications and Unlabeled Use of NSAIDs

Generic	Trade/Brand Name	Select Indications	Select Unlabeled Uses
Aspirin	Many (e.g., Bayer®, Ecotrin®, Empirin®)	Mild to moderate pain, fever, inflammation, others (see text)	(see text)
Acetaminophen	Many (e.g., Tylenol®, Feverall®, Aspirin Free Pain Relief®, Panadol®)	Analgesic, antipyretic (especially in patients who should not take aspirin), musculoskeletal pain, headache, earache, toothache, and relief of discomfort of conditions that cause fever and chills	Prophylaxis in children receiving DPT injections
Etodolac	Lodine®	Rheumatoid arthritis, osteoarthritis, pain	Tendinitis, bursitis, fever, ankylosing spondylitis
Ibuprofen	Many (e.g., Motrin®, Advil®, Nuprin®)	Rheumatoid arthritis, osteoarthritis, juvenile rheumatoid arthritis, mild to moderate pain, primary dysmenorrhea, fever in children	Migraine (abortive and prophylactic), resistant acne vulgaris, psoriatic arthritis, ankylosing spondylitis, gout, juvenile rheumatoid arthritis
Ketoprofen	Orudis®	Rheumatoid arthritis, osteoarthritis, mild to moderate pain, primary dysmenorrhea, OTC for minor aches and pains and reduction of fever	Juvenile rheumatoid arthritis, migraine (prophylactic and menstrual), ankylosing spondylitis, Reiter's syndrome, gouty arthritis
Ketorolac	Toradol®	Moderately severe acute pain	Long-term use for chronic pain
Nabumetone	Relafen®	Rheumatoid arthritis, osteoarthritis	None located
Naproxen	Many (e.g., Aleve®, Anaprox®, Naprosyn®)	Rheumatoid arthritis, osteoarthritis, ankylosing spondylitis, mild to moderate pain, primary dysmenorrhea, juvenile rheumatoid arthritis (not naproxen sodium), tendinitis, bursitis, acute gout	Migraine (abortive, prophylactic, menstrual), premenstrual syndrome, Paget's disease of bone, Bartter's syndrome, OTC as an antipyretic
Sulindac	Clinoril®	Rheumatoid arthritis, osteoarthritis, acute gouty arthritis, inflammatory conditions (ankylosing spondylitis, tendinitis, bursitis, acute painful shoulder)	Juvenile rheumatoid arthritis
Rofecoxib	Vioxx®	Osteoarthritis, mild to moderate pain, primary dysmenorrhea	None located
Celecoxib	Celebrex®	Rheumatoid arthritis, osteoarthritis, familial adenomatous polyposis (FAP)	None located

Adapted from Boyce & Takiya 2000; Kastrup, 2000; McEvoy, 1999.

full anti-inflammatory effects of the NSAIDs may take from 1 to 4 weeks to occur.

DOSING ADJUSTMENTS

Dosing adjustment is most frequently considered in children, the elderly, and in patients with organ system dysfunction. Children have very specialized dosing considerations, and these are not discussed here. For the elderly, some products, such as ketoprofen and ketorolac, have specific recommendations (Kastrup, 2000; Lipman, 1996; McEvoy, 1999). In the elderly, use caution and evaluate need but, for use of most NSAIDS, start low and monitor for toxicities including renal, hepatic, central nervous system (CNS), and gastrointestinal (GI) effects that are all of greater concern with these products in this population. Medication clearance in the elderly has not really been thoroughly studied for many NSAIDs. However, we do know that clearance is

reduced for etodolac, ketoprofen, nabumetone, rofecoxib, and sulindac; and thus these NSAIDs, as well as some salicylates, may need dosing adjustments (Boyce & Takiya, 2000; Kastrup, 2000; McEvoy, 1999). Dosing adjustment may be also necessary in naproxen products. Diclofenac, however, does not appear to show reduced clearance in the elderly.

Adjusting the doses of NSAIDs in the elderly is important because the adjustment can help compensate for the potential to have increased serum levels and decreased clearance of medication. Increased monitoring for adverse events is equally important. Unfortunately, even with decreased doses and increased monitoring, many elderly users of NSAIDs are still at greater risk of adverse drug reactions (ADRs), especially those associated with renal and GI effects (Boyce & Takiya, 2000). The elderly and individuals taking large numbers of medications are also at increased risk for drug–drug interactions.

Caution should be used in recommending or prescribing NSAIDs to any patient with suspected organ damage. This is especially true because many NSAIDs have been shown to contribute directly or indirectly to damage or dysfunction of many major organ and tissue systems, including the renal, hepatic, cardiac, and endocrine systems as well as vascular, endothelial, mucous membranes, and skin tissue. Studies support adjusting the dose of selected NSAIDs in liver or kidney disease.

When liver disease is present or suspected, use caution in the use and dosing of NSAIDs due to the risk of higher than anticipated serum levels of non-plasma-protein-bound NSAID, which can contribute to an increased incidence of ADRs. This effect can be attributed to several mechanisms. Hepatic disease can contribute to decreased plasma protein production and decreased protein binding of medications. These medications include NSAIDs as well as other medications a patient may be taking. Patients with severe hepatic disease may encounter decreased drug metabolism and decreased elimination and excretion of medications. Fortunately, for many NSAIDs, dosing adjustment is usually only required in very severe disease or failure (Boyce & Takiya, 2000; Kastrup, 2000; McEvoy, 1999). For others, such as fenoprofen, naproxen products, nabumetone, sulindac, and the COX-2 inhibitors, a dosing adjustment should be considered when liver disease/failure is present. It has been recommended that ASA and potentially diclofenac should be avoided in patients with liver disease/failure because both of these medications may be more likely to contribute to hepatic changes (Boyce & Takiya, 2000). Use of NSAIDs and decreased plasma protein is not always a critical problem as far as drug-drug interactions are concerned. For example, a patient with a history of long-term use of two medications that are known to cause problems due to drug-drug interactions and changes in plasma-protein-binding can be stable and not experiencing any problems. As long as the medications and the patient's status do not change, the potential for the drugs to create problems is reasonably low. However, problems do arise when patients are taking highly protein-bound medications with narrow therapeutic indices and have a change of status or when medications are started or stopped.

In patients with renal disease, again, use caution due to the potential for decreased clearance of NSAIDs, decreased protein binding, and increased risk of GI and renal toxicities. Dosing adjustment is recommended for many of the NSAIDs, including definite recommendations for ketoprofen, oxaprozin, ketorolac, and possibly diflunisal, fenoprofen, ibuprofen, naproxen products, nabumetone, sulindac, tolmetin, and piroxicam. Patients with renal disease should avoid mefenamic acid (Boyce & Takiya, 2000; Kastrup, 2000; McEvoy, 1999).

SELECTED SIDE EFFECTS, ADVERSE DRUG REACTIONS, AND TOXICITIES

NSAIDs and related products are associated with a large number of side effects, adverse reactions, and toxicities. Select problems are discussed here. Some of the most commonly seen problems with the NSAIDs are GI in nature and range from mild dyspepsia to life-threatening GI bleeds. The GI irritation and ulceration can be attributed to two mechanisms: local irritation and a systemic effect that includes a change in gastric acid secretion, decreased mucosal blood flow, and decreased mucous production. None of the NSAIDs marketed to date that have anti-inflammatory action have completely overcome the problem of an increased risk of GI ulceration and bleeding. Notably, APAP, which at clinical effective doses does not have anti-inflammatory actions, is not usually associated with GI complaints. And, the nonacetylated salicylates are associated with fewer GI problems (Insel, 1996). The newly marketed, moderately COX-2 selective meloxicam and the selective COX-2 inhibitors rofecoxib and celecoxib are believed to have fewer GI-related problems than the nonselective NSAIDs (Kastrup, 2000; Silverstein, et al., 2000). In contrast, indomethacin, aspirin, tolmetin, ketorolac, and piroxicam are associated with significant GI problems (Kastrup, 2000; McEvoy, 1999; Redford, 2000).

Aspirin and diclofenac have been associated with an increased risk of hepatoxicity, and probably should not be used in the presence of existing liver disease (Boyce & Takiya, 2000; Redford, 2000). However, a number of the NSAIDs have been implicated in reports of hepatic problems, and have precautions listed in their package inserts. For example, the insert from a selective COX-2 inhibiting agent suggests that patients at risk should be monitored, and if clinical signs and symptoms that indicate liver problems occur, the drug should be discontinued (Celebrex™, 1999).

Indomethacin, tolmetin, piroxicam, and ketorolac have been associated with renal problems (Redford, 2000). Clinicians should use caution when prescribing any NSAIDs in patients with renal problems or insufficiency because, in general, NSAIDs are not recommended for use in patients with advanced kidney disease. The use of NSAIDs in patients reliant on prostaglandins may contribute to renal and systemic problems because inhibition of prostaglandins can decrease renal vasculature dilation. This is of particular concern in patients at increased risk, such as those with cardiac compromise due to increased age, hypertension, congestive heart failure, renal or hepatic disease, or alterations in systemic volume. Additionally, NSAIDs may contribute to fluid retention, hypertension, and congestive heart failure. Even COX-2 selective inhibitors have been associated in at least one report with complicating therapy in two patients with chronic renal insufficiency (Perazella & Eras, 2000).

TABLE 34.2
Selected Drug–Drug Interactions

Drug	Interaction	Drug	Interaction
Aspirin	Omeprazole can increase the rate of absorption of enteric coated aspirin, leading to toxic levels.	Digoxin	Ibuprofen and indomethacin can both lead to increased digoxin levels.
Celecoxib	Fluconazole can inhibit the metabolism of celecoxib that may require reduced doses.	Phenytoin	NSAIDs may lead to increased phenytoin levels, leading to toxicity.
Midazolam	Rofecoxib can induce the enzyme CYP3A4, which can increase the dose of midazolam needed.	NSAIDs	Diuretics may increase the risk of renal failure when taken with ketoprofen and possibly other NSAIDs.
Rofecoxib	Rifampin can decrease rofecoxib concentrations, increasing the dose of rofecoxib needed.	NSAIDs	Alcohol (especially heavy use) may increase the risk of GI bleeds when taken with NSAIDs.
Salicylates	Alcohol may increase the risk of GI ulceration when taken with ASA.	NSAIDs	Cyclosporine use with NSAIDs may increase the renal toxicity of both products.
Acetaminophen	Alcohol use with APAP may increase the hepatoxicity.	NSAIDs	Probenicid may lead to increased NSAID concentrations and toxicity; probenicid should not be taken with ketorolac.
Piroxicam	Ritonivir may inhibit the metabolism of piroxicam and lead to toxicity.		

CNS effects such as dizziness, drowsiness, headache, nightmares, and/or confusion have been reported with many of the NSAIDs. Tinnitis is a well-known problem associated with excessive aspirin use (Kastrup, 2000). At least one account of celecoxib-induced auditory hallucinations has been reported (Lantz & Giambanco, 2000). Aspirin has been shown to cause hypersensitivity reactions, especially in patients with asthma and nasal polyps, or chronic urticaria. As well, ASA and the salicylates have been associated with Reyes syndrome and should be cautiously used — if at all — in children (Kastrup, 2000).

SELECTED DRUG–DRUG INTERACTIONS

Drug interactions with the NSAIDs are numerous and, although similar among many of the NSAIDs, striking differences are apparent among the NSAIDs when warfarin, methotrexate, ACE inhibitors, beta-blockers, loop and thiazide diuretics, and several other medications are considered. Many of the especially problematic interactions involve medications that are metabolized by cytochrome enzymes (Boyce & Takiya, 2000; Insel, 1996; Kastrup, 2000; Nikles, et al., 2000) (see Table 34.2). Of special note are interactions between NSAIDs and warfarin. NSAIDs that inhibit platelet aggregation, most notably aspirin, when taken with warfarin can increase the risk of bleeding. The COX-2 inhibitors should have less impact on platelets and result in a lower risk of bleeding. Although limited information is available on interactions between warfarin and the COX-2 inhibitors celecoxib and rofecoxib, reports of bleeding, especially

in the elderly, have been noted with at least one of these products (Celebrex, 1999). Additionally, both of these products inhibit enzyme systems that are required for warfarin metabolism. There have been reports on this interaction with rofecoxib; none were located for celecoxib (Boyce & Takiya, 2000; Fung, et al., 1999). Prothrombin times should be closely monitored, and patients should be counseled to monitor for signs of bleeding while taking any NSAID.

Aspirin also figures prominently with regard to concomitant use of NSAID therapy and methotrexate. It has been reported to increase low-dose, methotrexate-induced liver toxicity. Diclofenac, sulindac, and rofecoxib have also been associated with alterations is methotrexate kinetics, with rofecoxib reported to cause up to a 23% decrease in methotrexate clearance. Celecoxib has not been associated with changes in methotrexate kinetics (Boyce & Takiya, 2000; Kastrup, 2000; Celebrex, 1999). NSAIDS are reported to interact with beta-blockers and thiazide and loop diuretics to generally decrease the effectiveness of these medications. Many NSAIDs have the potential to affect blood flow through the renal arteries, decreasing renal function and increasing sodium and fluid retention, but sulindac appears to be a better choice for therapy, at least where interactions with beta-blockers are concerned (Kastrup, 2000). Decreases in renal function caused by NSAIDs is also a concern when patients on NSAIDs are also taking lithium. In this scenario, serum concentrations of lithium can reach toxic levels. Again, sulindac may be a better choice for patients who must take an NSAID and lithium (McEvoy, 1999).

COST

Prices for NSAIDs vary tremendously, with major differences existing between products, between brand and generic, and between the exact same product acquired from different sources. On the low end, acquisition costs for a 5-day supply of NSAIDs dosed for acute pain range from $1.88 for indomethacin (25 mg b.i.d.) and $2.70 for ASA (650 mg q.i.d.), to $21.82 for mefenamic acid (250 mg q.i.d.). In contrast, initial anti-inflammatory dosing costs of NSAIDs range from $20.70 for a 30-day supply of generic ibuprofen (800 mg t.i.d.) to $134.01 for a 30-day supply of diclofenac potassium (50 mg t.i.d.) (Boyce & Takiya, 2000). The cost of the medication dispensed to patients can be much higher.

Overall, acquisition costs for the NSAIDs are only one component of the full cost of drug therapy for pain patients taking NSAIDs. In select cases, providing a more expensive drug can result in decreased overall costs. This may be especially true of therapy for patients at increased risk for adverse events or drug interactions from certain NSAIDs. For example, the use of a computer program to predict costs of therapy at McDonald Army Community Hospital in Newport News, Virginia, showed that the selective use of COX-2 inhibitors could save over $12,000 annually at that facility (Vlessides, 2000). The predicted cost savings would occur if all patients (n = 112) at that facility receiving NSAIDs and a proton pump inhibitor (omeprazole) were switched to the COX-2 inhibitor celecoxib. Information in the same report showed that switching patients receiving nabumetone at that institution to celecoxib would not result in a savings and, in fact, would cost the institution several thousand dollars more per year.

As discussed in the introduction, costs of medications are relative. However, when discussing medication acquisition costs for consumers (i.e., fee for service), there is tremendous variability — not only among products, but also among pharmacies. Patients should be cautioned to select a pharmacy and pharmacist much as they would select a physician. Ask friends, family, co-workers, and others about their experiences; and ask the pharmacy staff about the services they provide. Finally, patients should compare prices between pharmacies that provide the services and convenience they need. However, comparing prices for products received through a no-service mail order, an e-mail system, or a limited service facility to those at a full-service, patient-oriented pharmacy that offers clinical services may not be productive. Whatever types of healthcare services patients select, they should be counseled to communicate with all their healthcare providers to be sure that providers know what medications the patients are taking. This communication can help to reduce adverse drug reactions, medication misadventures, and costs both to patients and the healthcare system. One way to increase this communication is for patients to have a primary physician prescribe all their medications and a single pharmacy or pharmacist provide all their medications and counseling with the medication.

CONCLUSION

All medications have the potential to improve a patient's condition or to cause adverse events. NSAIDs are no different from other medications in this regard. The goal of this chapter has been to present information on NSAIDs that will help clinicians select appropriate the NSAIDs for patients with specific risk factors and thereby improve patient outcomes by decreasing medication side effects and improving patient compliance and adherence and product tolerability.

REFERENCES

American Pharmaceutical Association. (1999, October). APhA Special Report: A continuing education program for pharmacists — Emerging therapies for inflammation and pain: the role of cyclooxygenase selectivity (pp. 1–19). Washington, D.C.: American Pharmaceutical Association.

Boyce, E.G., & Takiya, L. (2000). Nonsteroidal anti-inflammatory drugs: Review of factors guiding formulary selection. *Formulary, 35,* 142–146, 149–150, 153–156, 159–162, 167–168.

Campbell, W.B., & Halushka, P.V. (1996). Lipid-derived autacoids — Eicosanoids and platelet-activating factor. In J.G. Hardman, L.E. Limbird, P.B. Molinoff, & R.W. Ruddon (Eds.), *Goodman & Gilman's The pharmacological basis of therapeutics* (9th ed., pp. 601–616). New York: McGraw-Hill.

Celebrex (package insert). (1999). Chicago: G.D. Searle.

Food and Drug Administration. (1998, June). FDA talk papers: Wyeth-Ayerst Laboratories announces the withdrawal of Duract from the market. http://www.fda.gov/bbs/topics/ANSWERS/ANS00879.html

Fung H.B., & Kirschenbaum H.L. (1999). Selective cyclooxygenase-2 for the treatment of arthritis. *Clinical Therapeutics, 21,* 1131–1157.

Insel, P.A. (1996). Analgesic-antipyretic and anti-inflammatory agents and drugs employed in the treatment of gout. In J.G. Hardman, L.E. Limbird, P.B. Molinoff, & R.W. Ruddon (Eds.), *Goodman & Gilman's The pharmacological basis of therapeutics* (9th ed., pp. 617–657). New York: McGraw-Hill.

Kaplan-Machlis, B., & Klostermeyer, B.S. (1999). The cyclooxygenase-2 inhibitors: Safety and efficacy. *The Annals of Pharmacotherapy, 33,* 979–988.

Kastrup, E.K. (Ed.). (2000). *Drug facts and comparisons 2000.* St. Louis, MO: Facts and Comparisons.

Lantz, M.S., & Giambanco, V. (2000). Acute onset of auditory hallucinations after initiation of celecoxib therapy [Letter]. *American Journal of Psychiatry, 157,* 1022–1023.

Lipman, A.G. (1996). Internal and external analgesic and anti-pyretic products. In *Handbook of nonprescription drugs* (11th ed., pp. 45–74). Washington, D.C.: American Pharmaceutical Association.

McEvoy, G.K. (Ed.). (1999). *AHFS drug information '99.* Bethesda, MD: American Society of Health-System Pharmacists.

Nikles, C.J., Glasziou, P.P., Del Mar, C.B., et al. (2000). Preliminary experiences with a single-patient trials service in general practice. *Medical Journal of Australia, 173,*100–103.

Perazella, M.A., & Eras, J. (2000). Are selective COX-2 inhibitors nephrotoxic? *American Journal of Kidney Diseases, 35,* 937–940.

Redford, T.W. (2000). *Arthritis management: Number four of a five-course home-study program.* Lawrence, KS: Pharm-At Inc.

Silverstein, F.E, Faich, G., & Goldstein, J.L., et al. (2000). Gastrointestinal toxicity with celecoxib vs. nonsteroidal anti-inflammatory drugs for osteoarthritis and rheumatoid arthritis — The CLASS study: A randomized controlled trial. *Journal of the American Medical Association, 284,* 1247–1255.

Simon, L.S. (1999). Role and regulation of cyclooxygenase-2 during inflammation. *American Journal of Medicine, 106*(5B), 37S–42S.

Vlessides, M. (2000, January). Researchers predict saving $12,000 annually with selective use of COX-2 inhibitors. *Pharmacy Practice News,* 6.

Wallace, J.L. (1999). Distribution and expression of cyclooxygenase (COX) isoenzymes, their physiological roles, and categorization of nonsteroidal anti-inflammatory drugs (NSAIDs). *American Journal of Medicine, 107*(6A),11S–7S.

35

Chronic Pain Management with a Focus on the Role of Newer Antidepressants and Centrally Acting Agents

Robert L. Barkin, M.B.A., Pharm.D., F.A.C., N.H.A., D.A.A.P.M., Jan Fawcett, M.D., and Stacy J. Barkin, M.A., M.Ed., Psy.D., D.A.A.F.C.

INTRODUCTION

Of the range of recalled negative experiences that beset human existence, pain is among the most debilitating and the most fear and anxiety provoking. Pain, defined both as an unpleasant sensory and emotional experience associated with actual or potential tissue damage (Merskey & Bogduk, 1994), or described in terms of such damage, has the capacity to subjectively affect every aspect of life. The physiological effects of pain include diminished functional capacity, endurance, autonomic and peripheral events and, in some individuals, disorders of initiating and maintaining sleep. The psychosocial effects of pain include somatic preoccupation and perceived loss of control, coupled with increased anxiety, anger, fear, agitation, and depression. The societal impact of pain includes feelings of guilt and altered relationships (e.g., social, vocational, avocational, personal, financial, familial, and marital). Anti-depressant treatment for chronic pain has been fully described elsewhere (Barkin & Fawcett, 2000) and utilized in the preparation of this chapter.

CLASSIFICATION OF PAIN

An entirely subjective experience, pain involves a highly complex array of emotional, affective, and sensory phenomena. Pain can be categorized according to whether its etiology is organic or nonorganic (psychogenic)

(Table 35.1). In addition, pain can be classified as (1) acute; (2) disease-related (e.g., pain caused by cancer, sickle cell disease, fibromyalgia syndrome, or complex regional pain [CRP] syndrome); or (3) chronic nonmalignant (Chapman, 1993). In the true sense of the word, all pain is "malignant." Discrimination among these three pain classifications is a function of the following characteristics: duration, physical pathology association, psychological challenges, autonomic and peripheral indices of prominence, nerve conduction, prognosis for resolution, treatment focus appropriateness, and biologic purpose or value associated with the pain (Barkin, et al., 1996). See Table 35.1 for current terms used in the literature.

ACUTE PAIN

Acute pain is typically precipitated by a known noxious insult such as injury or trauma. Acute pain's physiologic purpose is protective in nature; it occurs when tissues are being or have been damaged, and causes the individual to react and remove or avoid the pain stimulus. The severity of acute pain is a function of objective autonomic and peripheral events associated secondary to tissue injury, and it generally resolves following tissue regeneration and/or repair over time and may be augmented by subjective pain indices (behaviors, i.e., suffering, guardian, grimacing, etc.) Acute pain is brief by definition — generally less than 1 to 3 months (Barkin, et al., 1996).

0-8493-0926-3/02/$0.00+$1.50
© 2002 by CRC Press LLC

TABLE 35.1
Pathophysiologic Pain Classification

Organic Etiology
- Neuropathic (deafferentation):
  - Nonnociceptive
  - May be associated with involvement of peripheral nerves
  - May benefit from treatment with antidepressants, anticonvulsants, sodium channel blockers, excitatory amino acid receptor blockers
- Nociceptive (acute: somatic, visceral):
  - From peripheral tissue injury/trauma by nerve ending damage, inflammation, hyperalgesia (i.e., mechanical, thermal, chemical, ischemic stimuli)
  - Peripheral stimulation of nociception at somatic and visceral sites
  - Benefits from opioids and nonsteroidal anti-inflammatory agents
- Mixed or undetermined, unspecified, unknown:
  - Chronic cephalalgia
  - Vascular pain
  - Benefits from multidisciplinary approach of cognitive or behavioral therapy, physical therapy, pharmacotherapy

Psychogenic Etiology
- Psychologic/psychiatric conditions with significant features of pain following complete exclusion of somatic pathology

The assessment of acute pain should include pain intensity and quality, distribution, onset, duration, circumstantial variability, and functional status, coupled with patient-specific collateral issues (anxiety, insomnia, anger, frustration, depression, etc.).

The body's autonomic reaction to acute pain is consistent with sympathetic fight and/or flight responses. Such responses are approximately proportional to the intensity of the initial noxious event or stimulus. Objective responses to acute pain stimuli involve a range of autonomic and peripheral indices, including elevation in heart rate, stroke volume, and blood pressure; pupillary dilatation; muscle tension; and a decrease in gut motility and salivary flow (xerostomia). Anxiety, which is almost universally present in acute pain, represents the subjective psychological response (Barkin, et al., 1996). Pain is therefore a subjective experience lacking the objectivity of vital signs. The disorders of initiating or maintaining sleep secondary to acute pain is a predictable consequence and additionally deserves specific treatment and management.

DISEASE-RELATED PAIN

Although the progress of disease-related pain is unpredictable, the prognosis and pathophysiology are predictable and defined. Collateral pain conditions (e.g., depression,

anxiety, insomnia, frustration, and anger) are generally predictable, thus precipitating multimodal interventions (Craig, 1994). Disease states associated with painful episodes include the following (Barkin, 1997b; Barkin & Richtsmeier, 1995; Barsky, et al., 1990; Bayer, Chadha, Farag, & Pathy, 1986; Bowsher, 1995; Casadevall, et al., 1996; DeWester, 1996; Galer, 1995; Kauver, 1993; Larue, Fontaine, & Colleau, 1997):

1. Rheumatologic (articular, osteoarthritis, rheumatoid arthritis, soft tissue: fibromyalgia syndrome [FMS])
2. Orthopedic (failed low-back surgery syndrome)
3. Cardiac (myocardial infarction, angina)
4. Neurologic (migraine, multiple sclerosis, neuropathies)
5. Sympathetically mediated pain (complex regional pain syndrome [CRPS])
6. Endocrine (endometriosis)
7. Chronic pelvic pain
8. HIV pain syndromes
9. Neoplastic
10. Sickle cell vaso-occlusive crisis pain
11. Gastrointestinal (GI) tract (pancreatitis, adhesions, biliary colic, intestinal ischemia)
12. Genitourinary (renal stones, ureteral obstruction)

CHRONIC NONMALIGNANT PAIN

Chronic nonmalignant pain may, on occasion, be associated with past injury. Again, all pain is malignant in nature. It is, however, devoid of biologic purpose or value and persists far beyond the tissue damage caused by the initial etiologic insult. It is generally considered to have a duration of 1, or 3 to 6, months or more; and, except in the case of an acute exacerbation of a chronic pain complaint, autonomic responses may develop some habituation, but may resume during acute painful exacerbations of the chronic pain. Moreover, the etiology of chronic nonmalignant pain is often difficult to determine because the pain behavior and the patient's subjective sense of the pain are perceived from an objective perspective as disproportionate to the initial insult or injury (Barkin, et al., 1996). Medical management of chronic nonmalignant pain is often particularly challenging. This category of pain, hereinafter referred to as chronic pain, is the focus of this chapter (Addison, 1984; Barkin, et al., 1996; Godfrey, 1996; Lister, 1996; Pappagallo & Heinberg, 1997).

CLINICAL PRESENTATION OF CHRONIC PAIN

Chronic pain may have its source in a physical disease state (e.g., arthritis, CRPS, FMS) or it may be secondary to learned behaviors from a resolved physical insult. It may also be related to somatization disorder, conversion disorder, depression, anxiety or other pain-related psychiatric diagnoses (Barkin, Leikin, & Barkin, 1994; Dworkin, Von Korff, & LeResche, 1990; Parmalee, Katz, & Lawton, 1991). The onset of chronic pain is usually gradual and its character may be either continuous or intermittent. Chronic pain has numerous psychosocial components, including irritability, depression, somatic preoccupation, anhedonia, withdrawal from outside interests, and diminished strength of vocational, avocational, familial, and social relationships. In addition, changes in appetite, decreased sleep, and libido are frequently noted (Barkin, et al., 1996).

Regardless of the particular anatomical site of chronic pain, other organ systems are frequently involved as well. Somatic complaints, which occur in "masked depression" presenting as chronic pain, often account for the somatization of depression and further somatic complaint may present for anxiety (Barkin, et al., 1996; Gruber, Hudson, & Pope, 1996). These masked depression complaints frequently involve the GI tract and include abdominal pain, constipation, flatulence, altered appetite, and an unpleasant taste in the mouth. Such patients complain of physical symptoms and have a paucity of overt manifested depressive symptoms, and are thus atypical in their clinical presentation. Common musculoskeletal complaints include generalized muscle aches, arthritic-type pain, backaches, and fatigue (Bigos, et al., 1994; Grube,r et al., 1996). Patients with chronic pain may also have cardiac complaints, including palpitations, weakness, diminished activity due to alleged heart disease, fatigue, noncardiac chest pain, and other expenditures (Barkin, et al., 1996; Gruber, et al., 1996; Rost, Zhang, Fortney, Smith, & Smith, 1998). Table 35.2 describes pain associated with physical pathology and psychopathology.

In addition to somatic complaints, the patient with chronic pain typically presents with a number of psychological and socioeconomic issues related to diminished capacity to function (American Psychiatric Association [APA], 1994, pp. 458–461, 317–392). Characteristic features include catastrophizing affective components of pain, which are often invoked as suffering, coupled with depression, frustration, agitation, and anxiety. Loss of gainful employment and significant inactivity exacerbate these affective components (Barkin, et al., 1996; Huff & Barkin, 1994).

Further complicating the clinical picture is the fact that previous attempts at pain relief may have led to misuse of prescription and nonprescription medications (over-the-counter, phytopharmaceuticals) and/or the use of alcohol and recreational drugs. Table 35.3 lists the chronic pain syndromes, often antidepressant responsive, that are frequently encountered in the primary care setting. Effective chronic pain management requires precise therapeutic judgment in all patients, but particularly in the elderly patient,

due to pharmacotherapeutic challenges including polypharmacy, psychosocial factors, cognitive impairment, drug interactions, multi-organ dysfunction, noncompliance, and side effects (Barkin & Barkin, 1998; Barkin, et al., 1996).

TABLE 35.2
Pain Described by Physical Pathology and Psychopathology

- Peripheral and central:
    Inflammatory pain
    Neuropathic pain
    Cutaneous, somatic visceral pain
- Psychologic pain aspects:
    Emotional and cognitive pain (see *DSM-IV*)
- Soft tissue, joints, bone:
    Acute and postoperative pain
    Osteoarthritis
    Rheumatoid arthritis
    Orthopedic pain from trauma
    Skeletal muscle pain
    Low back pain (psychological origin with spinal referral also)
    Upper extremity pain
    Fibromyalgia and myofacial pain syndrome (chronic)
    Cephalalgia
    Back pain, temporomandibular disorders
    Spinal and radicular pain syndromes of cervical, lumbar, sacral, and coccygeal origins
- Visceral and deep pain:
    Chest and vascular pain
    Eye pain
    Orofacial pain
    Abdominal pain, GI distress
    Chronic gynecologic pain
    Labor pain
    Genitourinary pain (bladder, uterus, ovaries, adnexa uteri)
    Rectal, perineum, external genitalia
- Nerve root damage:
    Post-amputation and phantom limb pain
    Peripheral neuropathies
    Complex regional pain (CRP) syndrome (Type I — reflex sympathetic dystrophy; Type II — causalgia)
    Trigeminal neuralgia and atypical facial pain
    Nerve root damage and arachnoiditis
- Carcinoma/malignancy
- Central pain (neuropathic)
- Lesions:
    Failed back
    Orthopedic surgery pain
- Parkinson's pain
- Multiple sclerosis pain

Source: Adapted from *Text Book Pain* (3rd ed.) P.D. Wall and R. Melzack, 1994, New York: Churchill Livingstone, and *Classification of Chronic Pain* (2nd ed.), H. Mersky and N. Bogduk, 1994, Seattle: IASP Press.

TABLE 35.3
Chronic Pain Syndromes Frequently Encountered in Primary Care

- Low-back pain and failed low-back surgery syndrome[a]
- Cancer pain[a]
- Neuropathic pain[a]
- Complex regional pain syndrome[a] (CRPS)
- Sickle cell pain
- Primary dysmenorrhea[a]
- Chronic pelvic pain[a]
- Herpes simplex/zoster[a]
- Postherpetic neuralgia[a]
- Trigeminal neuralgia
- Atypical facial pain[a]
- Phantom limb pain (postamputation)[a]
- Fibromyalgia syndrome (FMS)[a]
- Burn pain
- Multiple sclerosis pain[a]

[a] Responds to antidepressants.

PATHOPHYSIOLOGY OF PAIN AND PAIN SIGNAL TRANSMISSION

Pathophysiologically, pain involves at least three transmission circuits: (1) a spinal cord-thalamic frontal cortex–anterior cingulate pathway, which has a role in the subjective psychological and physiological response secondary to pain; (2) a spinal cord-thalamic somatosensory cortex pathway, which plays a role in the sensation of pain; and (3) a descending pathway involving the periaqueductal gray (PAG) region, which modulates pain signals. This system can inhibit or induce pain transmission at the level of the dorsal spinal cord, modulating the lamina on the dorsal horn where endogenous opioids are concentrated (Barkin, et al., 1996; Bonica 1990; Bonica, et al., 1990; Braverman, O'Connor, & Barkin, 1993; Guilbaud, Bernard, & Besson, 1994; LaMotte, 1986; Larue, et al., 1997; Meyer, Campbell, & Raja, 1994; Ruda, 1986; Seybold, 1986; Siddall & Cousins, 1995; Tarster, 1990; Yaksh, 1996; Yaksh & Malmberg, 1994).

Pain is transmitted from peripheral pain receptors by A-delta (δ) nerve fibers (small myelinated fibers with conduction velocities of 12 to 30 ms^{-1}) and C-fibers (small unmyelinated fibers with conduction velocities of 0.5 to 2 ms^{-1}), passing the dorsal root ganglion to lamina II on the dorsal horn of the spinal cord and synapse within the substantia gelatinosa. The primary ascending somatosensory pathway for cephalad pain impulse transmission is the spinothalamic tract. Nerve impulses proceed from the thalamus to the cortical somatosensory areas. Nociceptive input perception is multilevel, modulated in the afferent sensory pathway extending from peripheral nerves to the cerebral cortex (Bennett, 1994; Bonica, 1990; Bonica, et

al., 1990; Braverman, et al., 1993; Chakour, Gibson, Bradheer, & Helme, 1996; LaMotte, 1986; Meyer, et al., 1994; Ruda, 1986; Seybold, 1986; Siddall & Cousins, 1995; Tarster, 1990; Yaksh, 1996). Repeated C-fiber stimulation at the peripheral level progressively builds up the central nervous system (CNS) response, a temporalis with increased persistent pain and increased receptive field and hyperalgesia which is known as CNS neuroplasticity.

A conceptual model of pain transmission involves ascending afferent excitatory somatosensory pathways and descending inhibitory pain pathways (utilizing NE and 5-HT), as well as various neurotransmitters and neuromodulators, including monoamines, amino acids, and neuropeptides. Pain impulse transmission can be modulated by descending inhibitory pain pathway activation, passing from the brain down the spinal cord. This results in the release of inhibitory pain neurotransmitters, which limit pain impulse transmission from pain receptors by ascending afferent fibers. The source of pain migrates up the CNS from peripheral sites. Therefore, the peripheral noxious stimulus causes nociception, pain becomes a thalamic cessation, suffering is a cortex event, and pain behaviors are learned prefrontal cortical experiences.

The gate control theory of nociceptive mechanisms implicates the spinal cord dorsal horn in the function of a gate that controls the synaptic pain impulse transmission by the spinothalamic tract. Large afferent fiber activation (as seen with transcutaneous electrical nerve stimulator [TENS] therapy) may provide a counterirritant effect by small pain fiber inhibition (Bonica, 1990; Bonica, et al., 1990; Braverman, et al., 1993; LaMotte, 1986; Melzack, 1996; Ruda, 1986; Seybold, 1986; Tarster, 1990).

Serotonergic and noradrenergic pathways in the spinal cord modulate the lamina on the dorsal horn of the spinal cord. Tramadol, for example, exerts its binary mechanism of action in part at this spinal level, with re-uptake blockade of NE and 5-HT; additionally, it provides μ_1 opiate agonist effects supraspinally (Barkin, 1995a, 1995b; Barkin, et al., 1996; Braverman, et al., 1993; Gibson, 1996; Ruoff, 1996).

MANAGEMENT OF CHRONIC PAIN

In the majority of cases, the first step in the management of chronic pain is an attempt to document a neurologic lesion. More often than not, however, an etiologic source is either elusive or nonexistent. Therefore, the optimal treatment approach is multidisciplinary, including not only efforts at pain relief but also aggressive intervention aimed at psychosocial factors. The overall treatment goal is to improve the patient's functional status and the ability to perform necessary activities of daily living without significant pain-related interruption or dysfunction (Barkin, et al., 1996; Dworkin & Gitlin, 1991).

Treatment modalities for chronic pain include therapies provided by physical medicine and rehabilitation services; surgical interventions; cognitive and behavioral therapies; vocational, physical, and occupational therapies; anesthesiology augmentation (i.e., nerve blocks) within a multidisciplinary comprehensive pain center; and pharmacotherapy (McQuay & Moore, 1997; Philipp & Fickinger, 1993). Antidepressant pharmacotherapy is the primary focus of the remainder of this chapter, although some information is provided on opiates. An optimal treatment plan amalgamates all or most of the available therapeutic options in a coordinated, multidisciplinary manner. In general, the longer the interval between the onset of chronic pain and the commencement of appropriate treatment, the poorer the prognosis for restoration of optimal functioning (Barkin, et al., 1996).

OPIOID/OPIATE ANALGESICS

Opioid analgesics are a mainstay of pain treatment. Opiates used in the management of chronic pain have been described in a variety of chronic pain states, such as Parkinson's disease, depression, and chronic low-back pain. Opiates are agonists at stereospecific endogenous opioid receptors, which are found at both presynaptic and postsynaptic central and peripheral nervous system sites (Table 35.4) (Stein & Read, 1997). Opiate receptors are guanine protein-coupled receptors, which include muscarinic (M), adrenergic (NE),

and gamma-aminobutyric acid (GABA). Naloxone-sensitive opiate-binding sites in man are classified as μ_1, μ_2, Δ, and κ receptors (Table 35.4) (Barkin, et al., 1996; Chapman, 1993; Merskey & Bogduk, 1994).

Opioid receptor activation inhibits presynaptic release of excitatory neurotransmitters from peripheral nociceptive nerve terminals. This results in neuron hyperpolarization caused by increased potassium conduction and/or calcium channel activation. Opioid receptors and endogenous ligands function as an endogenous pain suppression system. Opioid receptors are located supraspinally in the brain-stem PAG matter and spinal cord substantia gelatinosa. These areas are involved with pain perception, impulse integration, and pain response (LaMotte, 1986; Ruda, 1986; Seybold, 1986). The proposed mechanism of action of opiates/opioids involves the activation of opiate receptors (Table 35.4), leading to an efflux of potassium and the resultant hyperpolarization, which limits calcium intracellular entry. Furthermore, coupling of the opiate receptors to G_i proteins results in a decreased formation of intracellular cyclic adenosine monophosphate (CAMP), which leads to a decrease in calcium channel phosphorylation and consequent diminished calcium entry. The opioids' action upon G proteins, which are independent of CAMP formation, directly diminishes calcium channel opening and enhances the opening of potassium channels. This blocks substance P release, an 11-amino-acid neurokinin neuropeptide with vast CNS distribution belonging to the tachykinins group of neuropeptides, resulting in blockade of nociceptive transmission (Barkin, 1996, 1997; Barkin, et al., 1996; Bonica, 1990; Bonica, et al., 1990; Braverman, et al., 1993; Popp & Portenoy, 1996; Tarster, 1990).

The opiate/opioid sites of action are the primary afferent sensory presynaptic neurons, which inhibit the release of nociceptive peptide substance P. In the brain, the initial binding of opiates in the PAG signals release of inhibitory 5-HT from the raphe nucleus. This 5-HT release inhibits dorsal horn neurons. Morphine affects the descending NE pathway; and NE release in response to opiates results in spinal analgesic effects (Barkin, Barkin, & Barkin, 1997–1998; Barkin, et al., 1996; Bonica, 1990; Bonica, et al., 1990; LaMotte, 1986; Popp & Portenoy, 1996; Ruda, 1986; Seybold, 1986; Tarster, 1990; Yaksh, 1996).

THE ROLE OF SUBSTANCE P AS A FOCUS IN ANTIDEPRESSANT ACTIVITY AND PAIN

Distribution of substance P is found in cell bodies and terminals of small-diameter (Aδ- and C-fibers) primary afferent neurons. Substance P, found in the afferent sensory neurons, in the spinal cord dorsal horn and in dorsal root ganglia, is a peptide neurotransmitter facilitating nociceptive stimuli passage from peripheral sites to the spinal cord and supraspinal structures (Yaksh, 1996).

TABLE 35.4
Opiate Receptor Classification

Receptor	Effect
μ_1	Supraspinal analgesia, miosis, nausea, vomiting, pruritus, urinary retention, endorphins endogenous agonist
μ_2	Spinal analgesia, physical dependence, sedation, euphoria, hypoventilation, bradycardia, ileus, endorphins endogenous agonist
Δ $\delta_{1,2}$	μ Receptor modulation; enkephalin endogenous agonist $\delta_{1\&2}$ – Spinal and to a lesser extent supraspinal (δ_2) analgesia
$\kappa_{1, 2, 3}$	Analgesia, sedation, miosis, dysphoria, endogenous agonist, dynorphin coupled with calcium channels (N channels), κ_3 supraspinal, κ_1 spinal

Source: Adapted from *Goodman & Gilman's The Pharmacological Basis of Therapeutics,* J. G. Hardman and L. E. Limbird, (Eds.), 1996, New York: McGraw-Hill; Update on opioid receptors, R. Atcheson and D. G. Lanbert, 1994, *British Journal of Anaesthesology, 73,* pp. 132–134; and *Appropriate Use of Opiates/Opioids in Migraine Headache Pain Management,* V. T. Loh and R. L. Barkin, September 1998, Monograph A4-X009, Bristol-Myers Squibb Company, Princeton NJ, A Continuing Pharmacy Education ACPE#316-000-98-039-401.

The substantia gelatinosa has enkephalins in interneurons of the dorsal spinal cord that have antinociceptive effects. Antinociceptive effects may be initiated by pre- and post-synaptic actions, inhibiting substance P release and decreasing the cellular activity, which projects from the spinal cord to supraspinal CNS areas (Yaksh, 1996). This dorsal horn neuropeptide neurochemical, substance P, is restricted within the laminar distribution and can act as a primary afferent transmitter. Depletion from the cord provides analgesia for thermal nociception, and possibly by chemoreception and baroreception.

A possible antidepressant mechanism of action is substance P antagonism. Substance P antagonists produce analgesia following intrathecal administration, and plasma substance P is then lower in chronic-pain (neuropathic pain, fibromyalgia, low-back pain) patients than in healthy volunteers (Yaksh, 1996).

Both 5-HT and NE are involved in the descending inhibitory mechanisms and alterations in spinal cord neurochemical (monoamines, amino acids, neuropeptides) transmission. Furthermore, the interaction with endorphin/enkephalin modulating systems occurs with spinal application of 5-HT/NE and morphine-producing analgesia (Reisine & Pasternak, 1996; Yaksh, 1996).

Studies of antidepressant effectiveness in pain management include anecdotal reports, open studies, case reports, reviews, and double-blind, controlled studies. Overall, the antidepressants have had a role in the management of pain. The use of antidepressants in the comprehensive multidisciplinary treatment plan of pain should be strongly considered despite some flaws inherent in the methodology of studies evaluating antidepressants for this indication.

The mechanisms of action of antidepressants for pain relief have been described as (1) relief of underlying depression that intensifies the suffering of the patient (suffering is the affective component of pain); (2) a common underlying biochemical substrate integral to experience of pain and depression; and (3) neuromodulatory effects of antidepressants on the endogenous opioid system (Feinmann, 1985). Antidepressants have usefulness as an integral part of comprehensive multidisciplinary treatment plans for chronic pain and alone possess analgesic activity (Raj, 1992).

A distinct mechanism for antidepressant activity by blockade of central substance P receptors has been described. Substance P preferring neurokinin-1 (NK_1) is highly expressed in brain regions critical to regulation of affective behavior and neurochemical response to stress. Additionally, this provides interactions between substance P and convergent NE/5-HT pathways through which antidepressants act, suggesting substance P antagonists might also be used in the treatment of psychiatric disorders. Some NE/5-HT containing cell bodies co-express substance P. Chronic *in vivo* antidepressant administration

down-regulates substance P biosynthesis, speculating that alterations in the neurokinin system contribute to antidepressant effects.

Antidepressants block behavioral effects of central substance P receptor stimulation. There is clinical evidence that substance P antagonism represents a distinct marker for antidepressant activity. This raises the question of whether substance P antagonism and antidepressants act by distinct molecular targets (i.e., monoamine transporters or the NK_1 receptors). The amygdala, in particular, is a potential site for antidepressant activity. An output projection from the amygdala is directed to the hypothalamus and substance P provides the monosynaptic input from medial amygdala to the hypothalamus. Furthermore, another projection from the amygdala is directed to the periaquaductal gray (PAG) matter with dense substance P activity. Additionally, stress causes release of substance P (Kramer, et al., 1998).

ANTIDEPRESSANTS: A THERAPEUTIC OPTION IN PAIN MANAGEMENT

The use of antidepressant agents in the management of chronic pain has been reported in the literature for the past 40 years (Barkin, et al., 1996; Braverman, et al., 1993; Bryson & Wilde, 1996; De Angelis, 1992; Eija, Tiina, & Pertti, 1996; Galer, 1995; Magni, 1991; Sindrup, 1993; Watson, 1994). Nevertheless, these agents are probably not prescribed for this application as frequently, nor as optimally, as they should be for their beneficial therapeutic possibilities to be realized. Ample evidence exists to support the efficacy and safety of the use of antidepressant agents as part of a comprehensive treatment program for patients with chronic pain (Barkin, et al., 1996, 1997–1998; Braverman, et al., 1993).

The literature describes a broad variety of chronic pain syndromes in which antidepressants have been used (Table 35.5). The categories of chronic pain that appear to be most responsive to antidepressant pharmacotherapy include neuropathic pain, such as nerve compression or nerve destruction; deafferentation pain; dermatome distribution of pain if peripheral; and nondermatome pain if central, including diabetic neuropathy (Eija, et al., 1996; Onghena & Van Houdenhove, 1992). HIV-related neuropathy (Lister, 1996), herpetic pain, and pain of malignancy (nerve tumor involvement, [brachial, cervical, lumbosacral, plexic] peripheral neuropathy due to tumor infiltration, radiation fibrosis, chemotherapy). Patient descriptors of neuropathic pain include burning, numbness, pins/needles, shooting, electric shock, radiating, stabbing, and searing (Atkinson & Grant, 1994; Borestein, 1995; Galer, 1994; Hunter, 1994; Rowbotham, 1994). Antidepressants have also been reported to be effective in the treatment of failed back surgery syndrome, a challenging condition to manage (Taylor & Rowbotham, 1996).

TABLE 35.5
Pain Syndromes Described in the Literature with Antidepressant Nociception

Low-back pain	Coccygeal pain
Nerve damage pain	Acute diabetic neuropathy
Rheumatic pain conditions	Somatoform pain disorders
Chronic paranasal sinus pain	Somatization of pain
Abdominal migraine	Traumatic neuralgia
Fibromyalgia syndrome (FMS)	Postoperative pain
Neuropathic pain	Nocturnal ulcer pain
Pain in HIV disease	Thalamic pain syndromes
Oral facial neuralgia	Psychogenic pain
Painful diabetic peripheral neuropathy	Atypical odontalgia
Postherpetic neuralgia	Cranial mandibular pain
Neuropathic pain	Acute sickle-cell crisis pain
Head and neck cancer pain	Rheumatoid arthritis
Neuropathic pain of peripheral pain origin	Pericardial pain
Chest pain	Phantom limb pain
Noncardiac chest pain	Chronic nonmalignant pain
Chronic pelvic pain	Fibrocystic syndrome
Breast cancer pain	Lower extremity post amputation pain
Terminal cancer pain	Polyneuropathy
Atypical facial pain	Arthralgia
Chronic fatigue syndrome	Cervical disk degeneration
Cephalalgia	Central post-stroke pain
Irritable bowel syndrome	Opiate postoperative analgesia
Premenstrual dysphoric disorder pain	Idiopathic pelvic pain
Polyneuropathy	Vulvodynia
Central pain	Thalamic pain syndrome
Chronic facial pain	Sickle cell disease or occlusive pain crisis
Herpes zoster	Chronic benign pain
Fibrositis	Acute back pain with spasm
Pudendal neuralgia	Cortical origin pain
Dysesthetic pain	Brachial plexus injury pain
Deafferentation pain	Idiopathic genital pain
Psychogenic oral facial pain	Acute low-back pain and muscle spasms
Cutaneous disorders associated with psychiatric disorders	Chronic abdominal pain

It is evident that antidepressants provide analgesia independent of their antidepressant effects (Braverman, et al., 1993; Godfrey, 1996). However, there is evidence (Loeser, 1986; McQuay, et al., 1996; Sindrup, Brosen, & Gram, 1992a, 1992b; Tacey, 1996) to suggest that the mechanism of action of antidepressants in the relief of pain may be different from their action in the relief of depression. The effectiveness of antidepressants in treating chronic pain has been described. The extent of the analgesic effect is not significantly different in the following situations: pain of organic or psychologic origins; in the presence or absence of a (masked or manifested) depression; in the presence or absence of an antidepressant effect; in doses less than those effective in depression, or in therapeutic doses; and finally, in sedating or nonsedating pharmacotherapy (Onghena & Van Houdenhove, 1992). For example, the observation that antidepressants are helpful even when no depression is present suggests that these drugs have intrinsic analgesic activity (Magni, 1991).

A central (supraspinal) mechanism of action involving the monoamine and opioid systems has been postulated by several investigators. Alterations in the CNS pain modulatory system at the spinal cord level have also been hypothesized (Gonzales, 1995). Further, CNS plasticity (neuroplasticity) results in a reorganization/alteration in receptive fields and probably changes in the modulation of sensory perceptions (Braverman, et al., 1993; Coderre, Katz, Vaccarino, & Melzack, 1993). Experimental evidence has shown cellular and gene expression changes within the CNS following peripheral nerve system injury (Yaksh & Malmberg, 1994). Pain may result directly from dysfunctional peripheral nerves or from alterations in the CNS function, which may then enhance and maintain pain perception (Braverman, et al., 1993).

Some evidence suggests an interaction between antidepressant agents and opioid receptors, and this may be the mechanism by which antidepressants provide antinociception. Specifically, opioid-dependent neurons may be secondarily activated by nonopioid neurons, and this, coupled with inhibition of the re-uptake of biogenic monoamines, may lead to antinociception (Gonzales, 1995). This latter mechanism, as noted earlier, has been demonstrated in the case of the centrally acting analgesic tramadol, which has a binary mechanism of action, with both an enantiomer leading to μ_1 opioid receptor agonism and an enantiomer that blocks the spinal reuptake of 5-HT and NE. Also, antinociception with tramadol occurs when the agent is co-administered with an opioid antagonist (Barkin, 1995a, 1995b; Barkin, et al., 1996; Braverman, et al., 1993; Gibson, 1996; Ruoff, 1996). An implication of antinociceptive influence of antidepressants over substance P has also been described (Braverman, et al., 1993).

ANTIDEPRESSANT OPTIONS FOR THE MANAGEMENT OF CHRONIC PAIN

Several classes of antidepressants are currently available, and many of them have been employed in the management of chronic pain (Table 35.6) (Barkin, et al., 1996; Braverman, et al., 1993). Substantial differences exist with respect to their antinociceptive usefulness as discussed earlier (Richardson, 1993). The tricyclic antidepressants (TCAs) have the longest history of use in general, and consequently the most extensive record in the treatment of chronic pain. The mechanism of action of TCAs in chronic pain is incompletely understood but implicates substance P (as discussed previously). However, activity within the CNS brainstem-dorsal horn nociceptive modulating systems has been described, with both 5-HT and noradrenergic projections between brainstem and spinal dorsal horn nuclei with implication in nociceptive modulation (Braverman, et al., 1993; Parmelee, et al., 1991).

The impact of the TCAs on both NE and 5-HT, the two monoamines believed to be key in the etiology of depression, is also important to their effects on chronic pain. The TCAs also block other neuroreceptors, which

TABLE 35.6
Antidepressants Used in the Management of Various Pain States

Amitriptyline	Maprotiline
Bupropion	Mianserin
Carbamazepine (TCA-like structure)	Mirtazapine
Citalopram	Nefazodone
Clomipramine	Paroxetine
Desipramine	Phenelzine (MAOI)
Dibenzapine	Sertraline
Dothiepin	Trimipramine
Doxepin	Trazodone
Femoxetine	Venlafaxine
Fluoxetine	Zimelidine
Imipramine	

mediates physiologic effects unrelated to the treatment of depression and to that of chronic pain. It is the antagonism of these unrelated neuroreceptors that produces the well-known adverse nontherapeutic effects associated with the TCAs. These side effects may jeopardize compliance, thereby negating their potential therapeutic benefit as co-analgesics in a patient's treatment plan. For example, blockade of the muscarinic receptors produces amblyopia, xerostomia, sinus tachycardia, constipation, urinary tension, and memory dysfunction; while blockade of histaminergic (H_1) receptors produces sedation, drowsiness, weight gain, and potentiation of CNS depressants. Alpha$_1$ (α_1)-adrenergic blockade (also with nefazodone, trazodone) is associated with dizziness and postural hypotension, while α_2-adrenergic blockade is associated with, but not limited to, priapism and decreased antihypertensive efficacy when co-administered with such agents as clonidine, methyldopa, guanabenz, and guanadrel. A direct membrane stabilization effect is produced. Finally, dopamine receptor blockade (as seen with amoxapine) has been associated with extrapyramidal symptoms (EPS) and movement disorders, including dystonia, akathisia, rigidity, tremor, akinesia, and tardive dyskinesia, and with neuroleptic malignant syndrome and increased prolactin secretion (Barkin, et al., 1996; Braverman, et al., 1993; Cookson, 1993; Eschalier, Ardid, & Coudore, 1992).

As a group, the selective serotonin reuptake inhibitors (SSRIs) have a plasma protein binding percentage in the range of 30% (citalopram) to 99% (sertraline); the $t_{1/2}\beta$ of the SSRI parent drug is in the range of 15 to 20 hours (fluvoxamine/paroxetine), up to 48 to 72 hours (fluvoxamine); and the half-life of active metabolites is 60 hours (sertraline), up to 168 to 340 hours (fluvoxamine). All SSRIs except sertraline have linear pharmacokinetics.

Anecdotal evidence exists to support the use of the newer antidepressants as antinociceptive agents; however, no double-blind, placebo-controlled studies have been published to date. Because they exert an effect on only one monoamine, the newer SSRIs have a far more favorable 5-HT-specific adverse effect profile than the TCAs (Sindrup, Gram, Brøsen, Eshøj, & Morgensen, 1990; Zitman, Linssen, Edelbroek, & Ven Kempen, 1992). For the same reason, however, they may be less effective than the TCAs in the management of chronic pain. Nevertheless, these agents may be useful in cases in which heterocyclic antidepressants are poorly tolerated or contraindicated (Barkin, et al., 1996; Braverman, et al., 1993). SSRIs may initially create gastrointestinal symptoms, anxiety, insomnia, agitation (e.g., fluoxetine, sertraline), overstimulation (sertraline), panic (sertraline), sexual dysfunction, and sedation (paroxetine) in treatment. Pharmacokinetic drug interactions are produced by SSRIs by CYP450 inhibition (1A2, 2D6, 2Cs, 3A4). This CYP450-inhibition (e.g., with codeine and hydrocodone) will decrease both of the pro drugs' analgesic effects to their active therapeutic metabolites morphine and hydromorphone, respectively. (See Table 35.7, CYP IID6.)

Monoamine oxidase (MAO) inhibitors act by inhibiting the MAO enzyme system and causing an increase in the concentration of endogenous epinephrine, norepinephrine, and serotonin in storage sites throughout the CNS. Because they have a wide range of clinical effects and the potential for serious drug–food and drug–drug interactions, MAO inhibitors have been reserved for patients who are resistant to other antidepressants. Use in treating chronic pain is limited. As mentioned, administration to patients receiving meperidine (a reuptake blocker of 5HT and NE) can lead to potentially fatal side effects (i.e., hypertensive crisis and serotonin syndrome).

An ideal antidepressant agent for the management of chronic pain would be characterized by modulation of both NE and 5-HT, but would lack the nontherapeutic acute synaptic effects associated with the TCAs or heterocyclic antidepressants, have a robust onset of effect, once daily dosing for compliance enhancement, mild to minimal side/adverse effects, a paucity of drug interactions and minimal overdose consequences. Among the newer antidepressants, venlafaxine and mirtazapine are unique in providing the therapeutic advantages of both serotonin and noradrenergic effects, non-SSRIs, but without the acute synaptic insults of α_1- or α_2-adrenergic, histaminergic (H_1, H_2), or anticholinergic events. These two agents offer the therapeutic benefits of the TCAs and SSRIs, but without these groups of iatrogenic insults associated with the TCAs and SSRIs (Augustin, Cold, & Jann, 1997; Barkin, et al., 1996; Braverman, et al., 1993).

VENLAFAXINE: SEROTONIN NORADRENERGIC REUPTAKE INHIBITOR

Venlafaxine has been studied in several chronic pain states, including fibromyalgia, chronic pain (primarily of cephalalgia), and neuropathic pain (Barkin, et al., 1996; Godfrey, 1996; Gonzales, 1995; Rowbotham, 1995; Tamler & Meerschaert, 1996). In addition, reports in the literature suggest the usefulness of venlafaxine in other pain states, including reflex sympathetic dystrophy, sympathetically mediated pain, intercostal neuralgia, atypical facial pain, multiple sclerosis, peripheral neuropathy, post-stroke pain, post-Zoster pain, and may improve restorative rehabilitation (Davis & Glassman, 1989; Taylor & Rowbotham, 1996). Venlafaxine appears to provide an antinociceptive effect independent of its antidepressant efficacy (Songer & Schulte, 1996; Taylor & Rowbotham, 1996). Effective doses have ranged between 37.5 mg and ≥300 mg per day, with varying degrees of patient-described pain relief (Barkin, et al., 1996; Holliday & Benfield, 1995; Taylor & Rowbotham, 1996).

In our clinical experience, venlafaxine has provided pain relief equal to or greater than that achieved with TCAs or SSRIs. We have noted particular efficacy in patients suffering from neuropathic pain, post-herpetic neuralgia, polyneuropathies, cephalalgia, failed low back surgery syndrome, fibromyalgia, and HIV-related pain syndromes (Barkin, 1997b; Barkin, et al., 1996; Dwight, Arnold, O'Brien, Metzger, & Morris-Park, 1996; Gonzales, 1995; Ruoff, 1996; Yunus, 1996). In addition, patients have found venlafaxine significantly more tolerable than the TCAs and some of the SSRIs (Barkin, 1995a, 1998; Barkin, et al., 1996; Cerruto, 1996; Rani, Naidu, Prasad, Rao, & Shobha, 1996; Songer & Schulte, 1996).

Unlike the SSRIs, venlafaxine and mirtazapine have not shown a loss in efficacy with maintenance therapy (Yunus, 1996). Venlafaxine is a phenylethylamine bicyclic antidepressant, which blocks the transporter reuptake of, in order of decreasing potency, 5-HT (low dose), NE (medium dose), and dopamine (high dose). The weak inhibition of dopamine reuptake occurs primarily at doses >225 mg (Augustin, et al., 1997; Barkin, et al., 1996; Holliday & Benfield, 1995). Venlafaxine's effect on CNS β-adrenergic receptors is of interest because it demonstrates an acute subsensitivity of the β-adrenergic cAMP-generating systems (Barkin, et al., 1996, 2000; Cohen, 1997). There may be other mechanisms by which venlafaxine produces an antidepressant or antinociceptive outcome.

It is theorized that antidepressants are associated with the down-regulation of this system, most likely in the pineal gland (murine model), and it has been suggested that venlafaxine has a more robust effect on this system, with resulting early onset of therapeutic response (Davis & Glassman, 1989; Barkin, et al., 2000; Cohen, 1997; Huff & Barkin, 1994). Two racemates, the R and S enantiomers, are present within the parent compound, each with individual pharmacologic profiles. Binding of either enantiomer to cholinergic, histaminergic, α_1-, α_2-, or β-adrenergic receptors appears to be minimal, if it occurs at all. The major metabolite is O-desmethylvenlafaxine (ODV).

The pharmacokinetics of venlafaxine have been described (Augustin, et al., 1997; Barkin, et al., 1996; Feighner, 1994; Holliday & Benfield, 1995; Montgomery, 1993). The T_{max} is approximately 1.4 to 3.0 hours; the clearance (Cl) is approximately 0.58 to 1.85 l/hr/kg; the $T_{1/2}$-β is 2.2 to 11.3 hours and is prolonged in both liver and renal dysfunction. The volume of distribution (Vd) is 2 to 22.7 l/kg and protein binding is 25 to 30%. The ODV metabolite T_{max} is 3.1 to 6 hours; the Cl is 0.2 to 0.5 l/hr/kg; the $T_{1/2}β$ is 6.5 to 16 hours; the Vd is 3 to 7.5 l/kg; and plasma protein binding is 30%. Further, extensive tissue distribution is seen and metabolism is probably first pass and saturable. Dosages greater than 75 mg every 8 hours display nonlinear (zero order) distribution kinetics seen with the conversion from the parent drug to the ODV metabolite (Barkin, 1998; Holliday & Benfield, 1995).

TABLE 35.7
Pharmacotherapeutic Inhibitors, Inducers, and Substrates of Cytochrome P450 Enzymes Used in the Management of Pain

Xenobiotic CYP Enzyme	Inhibitor	Inducer	Substrate
1A2	Anastrozole	Bupropion (possible)	Acetaminophen (APAP)
Polymorphism: Yes	Bupropion	Carbamazepine	Beta-adrenergic blocking agents
≈13% or a deficit in	Cimetidine	Charcoal-broiled foods	Bupropion (possible)
activity or poor	Ciprofloxacin	Cigarette smoke	Caffeine
metabolizers	Citalopram	Cruciferous vegetable	Chlorzoxazone
(Caucasians, Asians,	Clarithromycin	Dihydralazine	Clozapine
Blacks)	Diethyldithiocarbamate	Omeprazole	Cyclobenzaprine
	Diltiazem	Phenobarbital	(demethylation)
	Enoxacin	Phenytoin	Diazepam
	Erythromycin	Primidone	Haloperidol
	Fluoroquinolones	Rifampin	Lidocaine
	Fluvoxamine	Ritonavir	Methadone
	Grapefruit juice (6–7-dihydroxy-		Mirtazapine
	bergamontin)		Naproxen
	Grepafloxacin		Olanzapine
	Isoniazid (INH)		Ondansetron
	Ketoconazole		Phenothiazines
	Levofloxacin		Propranolol
	Mexiletine		Ropivacaine
	Mibefradil		Tacrine
	Mirtazapine (very weak)		Theophylline
	Moclobemide		TCAs (tertiary amines)
	Nalidixic acid		(demethylation)
	Nefazodone		Zolpidem
	Norfloxacin		
	Omeprazole		
	Paroxetine		
	Propranolol		
	Ritonavir		
	Sertraline		
	Tacrine		
	Zileuton		
IIA6	Diethyldithiocarbamate		Nicotine
	Ketoconazole		
	Letrozole		
	Methoxsalen		
	Miconazole		
	Pilocarpine		
	Ritonavir		
IIB6	Diethyldithiocarbamate	Bupropion (possible)	Bupropion
	Ketoconazole	Carbamazepine	Diazepam (demethylation)
	Quinidine	Phenobarbital	Halothane
	Orphenadrine	Phenytoin	Temazepam
		Primidone	
IIC8–10	Amiodarone (2C9)	Dexamethasone	Amitriptyline (2C9)
IIC9	Anastrozole (2C8/9)	Bupropion (possible)	Aspirin
Polymorphism: Yes	Cannabinol	Carbamazepine(2C9)	Barbiturates (2C9)
2%–3% Caucasians;	Chloramphenicol (2C9)	Clopidogrel (2C9)	Bupropion
15%–25% Asians	Cimetidine (2C9)	Ethanol (2C9)	Carbamazepine
	Clopidogrel (2C9)	Phenobarbital (2C9)	Celecoxib (2C9)
	Delavirdine	Phenytoin (2C9)	Diazepam (2C8/9)
	Diclofenac (2C9)	Primidone (2C8)	Diclofenac (2C8/9)

TABLE 35.7 (CONTINUED)
Pharmacotherapeutic Inhibitors, Inducers, and Substrates of Cytochrome P450 Enzymes Used in the Management of Pain

Xenobiotic CYP Enzyme	Inhibitor	Inducer	Substrate
	Diethyldithiocarbamate (2C8)	Rifampin (2C9)	Fluoxetine (2C9)
	Disulfiram (2C9)	Rifapentine (2C8/9)	Flurazepam
	Efavirenz (2C9)		Flurbiprofen (2C9)
	Felbamate (2C8)		Imipramine (2C9)
	Fluconazole (2C9)		Ibuprofen (2C9)
	Flurbiprofen (2C9)		Indomethacin (2C8/9)
	Fluvastatin (2C9)		Mefenamic acid (2C9)
	Fluoxetine (suspected) (2C9)		Mirtazepine (2C9)
	Fluvoxamine (2C9)		Nonsteroidal anti-inflammatory
	Isoniazid		drugs (NSAIDs) (2C9)
	Ketoconazole		Naproxen (2C9)
	Ketoprofen (2C9)		Phenytoin (2C9)
	Leflunomide (2C9)		Piroxicam (2C9)
	Metronidazole (2C9)		Propranolol
	Miconazole (2C9)		TCAs (tertiary amines) (2C9)
	Omeprazole (2C8/9)		Warfarin (S) (2C8/9)
	Phenylbutazone (2C9)		
	Ritonavir (2C9/10)		
	Sertraline (suspected)		
	Sulfonamides (2C9)		
	Topiramate		
	Trimethoprim/		
	Sulfamethoxazole (TMP/SMX) (2C9)		
	Troglitazone (2C9)		
	Zafirlukast (2C9)		
IIC18–19	Cimetidine (2C18)	Rifampin (2C19)	Amitriptyline (2C19)
Polymorphism: Yes	Citalopram (2C19)	Bupropion (possible)	Barbiturates (2C19)
Japanese — 18%	Delavirdine		Carisoprodol (2C19)
Blacks — 8%	Efavirenz (2C19)		Citalopram (minor) (2C19)
Caucasian — 3–5%	Felbamate (2C19)		Diazepam (2C19)
Poor metabolizers	Fluoxetine (2C19)		Imipramine (2C19)
or deficit of enzyme	Fluvoxamine (2C19)		Mephenytoin
	Ketoconazole		Moclobemide
	Letrozole		Naproxen (2C18)
	Omeprazole (2C19)		Omeprazole (2C19)
	Ritonavir (2C19)		Phenytoin
	Sertraline		Piroxicam (2C18)
	Telmisartan (2C19)		Propranolol (2C19)
	Tolbutamide (2C19)		Tiagabine
	Topiramate (2C19)		Topiramate
	Troglitazone (2C19)		TCAs (tertiary amines) (2C19)
	Tranylcypromine (2C19)		Valproic acid (2C19)
	Venlafaxine (very weak) (2C19)		
IID6	Amiodarone	No inducers shown	Antidysrhythmics (Type 1C)
Subject to genetic	Amitriptyline		Amphetamine
polymorphism: Yes	Bupropion		Beta-adrenergic blockers (some
	Celecoxib		lipophilic)
Subset of:	Cimetidine		Bupropion
5–10% Caucasian	Chloroquine		Captopril
1–10% Asian	Chlorpromazine		Citalopram (minor)

(*continued*)

TABLE 35.7 (CONTINUED)
Pharmacotherapeutic Inhibitors, Inducers, and Substrates of Cytochrome P450 Enzymes Used in the Management of Pain

Xenobiotic CYP Enzyme	Inhibitor	Inducer	Substrate
2–8% Blacks: Poor metabolizers or deficits in activity	Citalopram (weak)		Chlorpheniramine (CTM)
	Clomipramine		Chlorpromazine
	Codeine		Codeine (Pro drug for morphine)
	Delavirdine		Cyclobenzaprine (hydroxylation)
	Desipramine		Dextromethorphan (DM)
	Diltiazem		Dextropropoxyphene
	Diphenhydramine		Encainide
	Doxorubicin		Ethylmorphine
	Fenfluramine		Flecainide
	Flecainide		Fluphenazine
	Fluoxetine		Fluoxetine
	Fluphenazine		Flurazepam
	Fluvoxamine		Fluvoxamine
	Haloperidol		Haloperidol
	Imipramine		Hydrocodone (Pro drug for hydromorphone)
	Lomustine		Hydroxyamphetamine
	Methadone		Lidocaine
	Metoprolol		Maprotiline
	Mexiletine		MCPP (metabolite of trazodone and nefazodone)
	Mibefradil		
	Mirtazapine (very weak)		Meperidine
	Moclobemide		Methadone
	Nefazodone		Methamphetamine
	Nicardipine		Mexiletine
	Norfluoxetine		Mirtazapine
	Nortriptyline		Morphine
	Paroxetine		Neuroleptics
	Perphenazine		Nortriptyline
	Primaquine		Opiate analgesics
	Propafenone		Oxycodone
	Propoxyphene		Paroxetine
	Propranolol		Pentazocine
	Quinidine		Phenothiazines
	Quinine		Propafenone
	Ritonavir		Propoxyphene
	Sertraline		Propranolol (minor)
	TCAs		Quazepam
	Thioridazine		Risperidone
	Timolol		Sertraline
	Venlafaxine (very weak)		TCAs (secondary amines) (hydroxylation/high first-pass effects)
	Vinblastine		
	Vinorelbine		
	Yohimbine		Tramadol (for M1 metabolite)
	Ziprasidone		Trazodone
			Venlafaxine
			Zolpidem
IIE1 Polymorphism: No	Diethyldithiocarbamate	Ethanol	Acetaminophen (hepatotoxic metabolite)
	Disulfiram	Isoniazid	
	Ritonavir		Bupropion
			Chlorzoxazone

TABLE 35.7 (CONTINUED)
Pharmacotherapeutic Inhibitors, Inducers, and Substrates of Cytochrome P450 Enzymes Used in the Management of Pain

Xenobiotic CYP Enzyme	Inhibitor	Inducer	Substrate
			Enflurane
			Ethanol
			Halothane
			Isoflurane
			Methoxyflurane
			Mexiletine
			Mirtazapine (minor)
			Sevoflurane
IIIA3	Cimetidine		Midazolam
	Nefazodone		
	Ranitidine		
	Sertraline		
IIIA4	Acetaminophen	Barbiturates	Acetaminophen (APAP)
Polymorphism: No	Amiodarone	Carbamazepine	Alfentanil
	Anastrozole	Dexamethasone	Alprazolam
(*Note:* Significant	Antifungals	Efavirenz	Antiarrhythmics
differences in CYP	Calcium channel blockers (some)	Ethosuximide	Benzodiazepines (short-acting
IIIA4 expression	Cannabinol	Glucocorticoids	triazolo type)
among patients)	Cimetidine	Griseofulvin	Bupropion (possible)
	Citalopram	Macrolide antibiotics	Caffeine
	Clarithromycin	Nevirapine	Calcium channel blockers (most)
	Clotrimazole	Phenobarbital	Carbamazepine (CBZ)
	Danazol	Phenylbutazone	Chlorpromazine
	Delavirdine	Phenytoin	Citalopram
	Dextropropoxyphene	Prednisone	Clonazepam
	Dihydroergotamine (DHE)	Primidone	Cocaine
	Diltiazem	Quinidine	Codeine (demethylation)
	Diethyldithiocarbamate	Rifabutin	Corticosteroids
	Efavirenz	Rifampicin	Cyclobenzaprine
	Erythromycin	Rifampin	(demethylation)
	Fluconazole	Rifapentine	Cyclosporin (CSP)
	Fluoxetine	Sulfinpyrazone	Dexamethasone
	Fluvoxamine	Troglitazone	Dextromethorphan (DM)
	Gestodene	Verapamil	Diazepam (minor)
	Grapefruit juice		Dihydroergotamine (DHE)
	Indinavir		Dihydropyridine
	Interferon (gamma)		Diltiazem
	Itraconazole		Calcium channel blockers
	Ketoconazole		Erythromycin
	Lovastatin		Estazolam
	Macrolide antibiotics		Ethylmorphine
	Metronidazole		Fentanyl
	Mibefradil		Fluoxetine
	Miconazole		Hydrocortisone (cortisol)
	Mirtazapine (very weak)		Itraconazole
	Naringenin		Ketoconazole
	Nefazodone		Lidocaine
	Nelfinavir		Loratadine
	Nevirapine		Midazolam
	Nifedipine		Mirtazapine

(continued)

TABLE 35.7 (CONTINUED)
Pharmacotherapeutic Inhibitors, Inducers, and Substrates of Cytochrome P450 Enzymes Used in the Management of Pain

Xenobiotic CYP Enzyme	Inhibitor	Inducer	Substrate
	Norfloxacin		Nefazodone
	Norfluoxetine		Nifedipine
	Omeprazole		Phenytoin
	Paroxetine		Prednisone
	Propranolol		Protease inhibitors
	Propoxyphene		Quetiapine
	Protease inhibitors		Quinidine
	Quinidine		Ropivacaine
	Quinine		Sertraline
	Ranitidine		Sex hormone
	Ritonavir		Sufentanil
	Saquinavir		Tiagabine
	Sertraline		Tamoxifen
	Trazodone		Tramadol
	Troglitazone		Trazodone
	Troleandomycin		Triazolam
	Verapamil		TCAs (demethylation)
	Venlafaxine (very weak)		Amitriptyline (minor)
	Zafirlukast		Clomipramine
	Ziprasidone		Imipramine
			Venlafaxine (n-demethylation)
			Verapamil
			Zolpidem
IIIA5–7	Clotrimazole	Phenobarbital	Midazolam (3A5)
	Ketoconazole	Phenytoin (PHT)	Triazolam
	Metronidazole	Primidone	
	Miconazole	Rifampin	
	Troleandomycin		

Note: From a primary care clinician's and consultant's guide to medicating for pain and anxiety, J. Huff and R. L. Barkin, 1994, *American Journal of Therapeutics, 1*, 186–190; Loss of antidepressant efficacy during maintence therapy: Possible mechanisms and treatments, S.E. Byrne and A. J. Rothschild, 1998, *Journal of Clinical Psychiatry, 59*, 279–288; Pharmacokinetics of the newer antidepressants: Clinical relevance, C.L. DeVane, 1994, *American Journal of Medicine, 97*(Suppl. 6A), 6A-13S–6A-23S; Opiate, opioids, and centrally acting analgesics and drug interactions: The emerging role of the psychiatrist, R.L. Barkin, D.S. Barkin, S.J. Barkin, and S.A. Barkin, 1998, *Medical Update for Psychiatrists, 3*(6),172–175.

Venlafaxine substrate metabolism appears to occur via the cytochrome hepatic isoenzyme (CYP-4502D6) (DeVane, 1994).

Venlafaxine's inhibition of this isoenzyme is significantly less and weaker than that reported with SSRIs and produces negligible hepatic isoenzyme inhibition. Consequently, venlafaxine has a significantly lower potential for clinically relevant pharmacokinetic interactions, including those agents used in chronic pain management (Table 35.7) (Barkin, et al., 1998, 2000; Bazine & Benefield, 1997–1998; Cohen & DeVane, 1996; Huff & Barkin, 1994). In addition, because of its low plasma protein binding (25 to 30%), interaction with agents that are highly

protein bound is unlikely. Cytochrome P-4503A4 is the isoenzyme used for the N-demethylated metabolite (Table 35.7). Approximately 1 to 10% of the drug is excreted unchanged, 30% is excreted as the ODV metabolite, 6 to 19% as the N,O-di-desmethyl metabolite, and 1% as the N-desmethyl metabolite. The $T_{1/2}$-beta of the parent compound ranges between 3 and 4 hours, while that of the ODV metabolite is about 10 hours (Barkin, 1998; Barkin, et al., 1996, 2000; Feighner, 1994; Montgomery, 1993).

Although serotonin syndrome has not been reported with venlafaxine as of this publication, the agent should not be administered with MAOIs or within a 14-day period following MAOI discontinuation (Sternbach, 1991). A 7-day pharmacokinetic-based washout period should precede initiation of an MAOI following a gradual discontinuation of venlafaxine. Prescription and nonprescription forms of cimetidine decrease the clearance of venlafaxine and increase the area under the curve (AUC) and peak plasma concentration (Barkin & Fawcett, 2000; Byrne & Rothschild, 1998). Refer to Table 35.7 for CYP450 isoenzyme induction and inhibition of agents utilized in the management of pain.

Side effects associated with venlafaxine include 5-HT-mediated nausea and vomiting, which is self-limited and dose-related and may respond to mirtazapine. Anorexia, somnolence or sedation, dizziness, and xerostomia have also been reported, and their frequency appears to be less with the extended-release dosage form (Barkin & Fawcett, 2000).

Infrequently reported side effects include NE- and 5-HT-receptor-mediated palpitations, fatigue, headache, constipation, self-limiting insomnia/anxiety (which may be treated with zolpidem, mirtazapine, or trazodone), sexual dysfunction (erectile failure, delayed orgasm, anorgasmia, impotence, abnormal ejaculations [which may be diminished by addition of mirtazapine]), blurred vision, asthenia, and diaphoresis. Slight increases in blood pressure (≤ 5 to 8 mmHg) and heart rate may be noted at doses exceeding 200 mg per day. A slight increase in serum lipid levels (2 to 3 mg/dl) may occur. The incidence of side effects such as dyspepsia, diarrhea, and headache is comparable to that associated with placebo. Overall, venlafaxine is well tolerated. A slow decremental titration is appropriate to prevent withdrawal symptoms such as GI distress, diaphoresis, or dizziness (Barkin & Fawcett, 2000).

Notably, venlafaxine is one of the few antidepressants (in addition to bupropion) associated with loss of appetite or anorexia, with an incidence of 11%. One of the authors found that, in a limited number of patients, venlafaxine may be cautiously prescribed with bupropion when necessary for concomitant or adjunctive purposes in the nicotine-dependent and/or obese patient, without iatrogenic effects. It may be possible to exploit this therapeutic side effect to the patient's advantage, because weight reduction (in obesity) and nicotine-dependency management are critical for patients with chronic pain involving the musculoskeletal system, particularly given the severe negative impact of excessive body mass on weight-bearing joints and in patients attempting to abate habituation of smoking (Barkin, 1995a, 1998; Barkin & Fawcett, 2000; Barkin, et al., 1999, 2000; Braverman, et al., 1993; Fawcett & Barkin, 1997).

Mirtazapine (NASSA)

Mirtazapine is an atypical antidepressant described as a noradrenergic serotonin-specific antagonist. NASSA has been reviewed elsewhere. This agent produces unique therapeutic antagonism at presynaptic α_2-auto and heteroreceptors, thus facilitating rapid, robust, enhanced noradrenergic and serotonin release, respectively. There is no transporter reuptake inhibition mechanics No sexual dysfunction, a decrease in migraine headaches, and decreased anxiety, agitation, and depression are associated with $5HT_2$-, H_1-, α_2-hetero-, and α_2-autoreceptor blockade, as with mirtazapine. Further antagonism occurs at $5HT_2$ receptors (decreasing anxiety and cephalalgia, agitation) and at $5HT_3$ receptors (decreasing nausea and GI distress, augmenting antidepressant effects).

Mirtazapine is rapidly and completely absorbed following oral administration and has a mean half-life ($t_{1/2}\beta$) of about 20 to 40 hours. The mean elimination half life of mirtazapine after oral administration ranges from approximately 20 to 40 hours across age and gender subgroups, with females of all ages exhibiting significantly longer elimination half lives than males (mean half life of 37 hours for females vs. 26 hours for males).

The disposition of mirtazapine was studied in patients with varying degrees of renal function. Elimination for mirtazapine is correlated with creatinine clearance. Total body clearance of mirtazapine was reduced approximately 30% in patients with moderate (Clcr = 11 – 39 ml/min/ 1.73 m²) renal impairment when compared to normal subjects.

The oral clearance of mirtazapine was decreased by approximately 30% in hepatically impaired patients. Peak plasma concentrations are reached within about 2 hours following an oral dose. Mirtazapine is extensively metabolized. Major pathways of biotransformation are demethylation and hydroxylation, followed by glucuronide conjugation. Human liver microsomes indicate that cytochrome 2D6 and 1A2 are involved in the formation of the 8-hydroxy metabolite of mirtazapine, whereas cytochrome 3A is considered to be responsible for the formation of the N-desmethyl and N-oxide metabolite. Mirtazapine has an absolute bioavailability of about 50% It is eliminated predominantly via urine (75%) with 15% in feces. Several unconjugated metabolites possess pharmacological activity but are present in the plasma at very low levels. The (–) enantiomer has an elimination half-life that is approximately twice as long as the (+) enantiomer and therefore achieves plasma levels that are about three times as high as that of the (+) enantiomer.

Plasma levels are linearly related to dose over a dose range of 15 to 80 mg. The mean elimination half-life of mirtazapine after oral administration ranges from approximately 20 to 40 hours across age and gender subgroups, with females of all ages exhibiting significantly longer elimination half-lives than males (mean half-life of 37 hours for females vs. 26 hours for males). Steady-state plasma levels of mirtazapine are attained within 5 days, with about 50% accumulation (accumulation ratio = 1.5). Mirtazapine is approximately 85% bound to plasma proteins over a concentration range of 0.01 to 10 μg/ml.

H_1 receptor antagonism at low doses (≤ 30 mg) produces drowsiness, facilitating sleep and improving appetite. No clinically significant interactions are revealed on the CYP450 system. Mirtazapine is a useful adjuvant agent with a robust onset of action in the management of chronic pain, FMS, migraine headache, failed low-back surgery syndrome, neuropathic pain, etc. Mirtazapine $5HT_3$ antagonism decreases the nausea and of some pharmacological tramadol and venlafaxine. Beneficial effects for the initial combination of venlafaxine and mirtazapine are for many pain patients needing restful sleep. At doses of 7.5 to 22.5 mg, the benefits decreased in insomnia and agitating anxiety, and enhanced appetite, especially beneficial in cachectic patients. This agents pharmacology decreases the need for benzodiazepines. Mirtazapine will provide dose-related effects, which include xerostomia, enhanced appetite, constipation, drowsiness, and of clinical importance is the low-dose-mediated appetite. Drowsiness events are much less at 45-mg than at 22.5-mg doses and below due to less prominence of the H_1 receptor pki at higher doses (Barkin, Chor, Braun, & Schwer, 1999; Barkin & Fawcett, 2000; Barkin, Oetgen, & Barkin, 1999; Barkin, et al., 2000; Bhatia, Bhatia, & Barkin, 1997; Davis & Barkin, 1999; Fawcett & Barkin, 1998a, 1998b; Kao, Barkin, and Leikin, 1997). A soluble oral tablet dosage form is available.

TRAMADOL: CENTRALLY ACTING ANALGESIC

Tramadol is centrally acting due to an analgesic binary mechanism of action. It combines centrally acting (the enantiomer binds to μ receptor), mild opioid activity with an additional spinal mechanism of monamine transporter reuptake inhibition as seen with TCAs. With its weak affinity for μ-opioid receptors, in consort with a synergistic action with serotonin ([+] enantiomer provides 5HT transporter reuptake) and norepinephrine ([−] enantiomer NE transporter reuptake blockade, tramadol interferes with central pathways that mediate pain. The spinal analgesia is modulated by descending nonadrenergic and serotonergic pathways affecting laminae I) (A-delta fiber project and synapse) on the dorsal horn of the spinal cord. Tramadol has a lower degree of respiratory depression than opioids. A very low potential for tolerance or abuse is seen with tramadol. Indications include management of moderate or moderately severe pain. The concomitant use of tramadol and nonsteroidal anti-inflammatory drugs (NSAIDs) (i.e., rofecoxib and others) may offer the therapeutic benefits of both central and peripheral analgesia, although the requisite studies have not yet been conducted. This combination is frequently initiated in clinical practice. Tramadol is a good choice for patients who are at risk for the side effects of NSAIDs but are reluctant to use opioid analgesics. The action of tramadol is without prostaglandin-mediated effects and therefore does not

exhibit the GI and renal side effects associated with traditional NSAIDs. Dose-related side effects include dizziness, nausea, headache, and constipation.

Tramadol appears in plasma within 15 to 45 minutes of oral administration, with almost complete absorption (75% bioavailable). It achieves a peak plasma concentration in about 2 hours. Onset of action following oral routes is within 25 to 35 minutes, and analgesia duration is 3 to 11 hours. Mean elimination half-life is 6 hours after single doses and 7 hours after multiple doses. About 30% of an oral dose is excreted by the kidneys, with 60% excreted as metabolites. Both CYP-450 3A4 (M1 metabolite desmethyl tramadol) and 2D6 isoenzymes (parent) are involved as a substrate in the hepatic metabolism (see Table 35.7). Renal impairment produces both a decreased extent and rate of excretion of the parent drug and active metabolites. The low plasma proteins binding (20%) provides a benefit in hypoalbuminic patients. Tramadol exhibits linear pharmacokinetics. Dialysis removes less than 7% of a given dose, which may be a benefit in patients undergoing hemodialysis (HD). Hepatic cirrhosis results in decreased metabolism of both the parent drug and its active metabolites. Tramadol has not, in clinical experience, been shown to modulate sphincteric muscles (no urinary retention, biliary tract spasms, or ampulla of Vater in the pancreas).

Tramadol has been studied in elderly populations and for a variety of conditions. It has been well tolerated overall and has proven to be effective in fibromyalgia, osteoarthritis, back pain, and neuropathic pain. Side-effect minimization can be accomplished by titrating the dose in increments of 25 to 50 mg/day every 3 days until an effective analgesic is reached, to a maximum of 400 mg/day in the non-elderly patient with normal hepatic and renal function. Any nausea may further be diminished by co-prescribing mirtazapine. The analgesic effects of tramadol will not be totally reversed with naloxone administration. In patients with a decreased seizure threshold or in patients taking antidepressants, neuroleptics, or other drugs that decrease that threshold, a risk-benefit analysis should be made. In other countries, tramadol at 1 to 2 mg/kg every 6 hours has been used in children. Children predictably have more rapid clearance of tramadol. A combination with acetaminophen (APAP) and sustained action dosage form are to be available in the near future. These dosage forms have been effectively utilized with co-pharmacotherapy (NSAIDs, membrane stabilizers, antidepressants, anxiolytics, [e.g., venlafaxine mirtazapine] anticonvulsants [e.g., topiramate, etc.] opiates, and skeletal muscle relaxants. (Barkin, 1995a, 1995b, 1996; Barkin, Lubenow, et al., 1996; Barkin, Oetgen, & Barkin, 1999; Gaynes & Barkin, 1999). A combination dose form with acetaminophen is available, with a long-acting and liquid dosage form available in the near future.

CONCLUSION

Antidepressants have a clear role in the treatment of chronic pain, whether or not depression is involved. The best choice of a particular antidepressant class for use in this application is somewhat less clear, however. The TCAs have been shown to be effective in the management of chronic pain. However, the associated adverse effects may compromise compliance. The SSRIs have a more favorable adverse-effect profile than TCAs, but they have not been well studied in patients with chronic pain. The pharmacokinetic and pharmacodynamic profiles of both venlafaxine and mirtazapine are superior to those of the TCAs, and the agent offers significant patient-specific advantages over some of the SSRIs, including a paucity of pharmacokinetic interactions. Venlafaxine and mirtazapine are certainly worthy of pharmacotherapeutic consideration in the patient with chronic pain.

REFERENCES

Addison, R.G. (1984). Chronic pain syndrome. *The American Journal of Medicine, 10*, 77(3A), 54–58.

American Psychiatric Association (1994). Mood disorders. *Diagnostic and statistical manual of mental disorders* (4th ed., pp. 458–461) Washington, D.C.: American Psychiatric Association. *Pain Disorders*, 317–392.

Atkinson, J.H., & Grant, I. (1994). Natural history of neuropsychiatric manifestations of HIV disease. *Psychiatric Clinics of North America, 17*, 17–33.

Augustin, B.G., Cold, J.A., & Jann, M.W. (1997). Venlafaxine and nefazodone, two pharmacologically distinct antidepressants. *Pharmacotherapy; 17*, 511–530.

Barkin, R.L. (1995a). Alternative dosing for tramadol aids effectiveness. *Formulary, 30*, 542–543.

Barkin, R.L. (1995b). Focus on tramadol: A centrally acting analgesic for moderate to moderately severe pain. *Formulary, 30*, 321–325.

Barkin, R.L. (1997a). Cancer pain treatment insights. *Pharmacotherapy, 17*, 397–398.

Barkin, R.L. (1997b). *Three challenging, diverse pain patient's requirements for patient-specific treatment. Economic and therapeutic implications of analgesia in hospital pharmacy.* Poster presented at the 32nd Annual ASHP Midyear Clinical Meeting, December 8, Atlanta, GA.

Barkin, R.L. (1998). Attributes, advantages of venlafaxine overlooked [Letter to the Editor]. *Formulary, 33*(1), 74–75.

Barkin, R.L., & Barkin, D. (1998). Pharmacotherapeutic challenges in the elderly: Polypharmacy, drug interactions, compliance and side effect/adverse effect predictions. *Anesthesia Today, 9*, 12–19.

Barkin, R.L., & Barkin, D.S. (2001). Pharmacologic management of acute and chronic pain: Focus on drug interactions and patient scpecific pharmacotherapeutic selection. *Southern Medical Journal, 94*, 756–767.

Barkin, R.L., Barkin, D.S., Barkin, S.J., & Barkin, S.A.. (1998). Opiate, opioids, and centrally acting analgesics and drug interactions: The emerging role of the psychiatrist. *Medical Update for Psychiatrists, 3*(6):172–175.

Barkin, R.L., Barkin, S.J., & Barkin, S.A. (1997–1998). Opiate/opioid overdose: Challenges in the emergency room which complicate management in the treatment of opiate/opioid overdose. In J.B. Leiken (Ed.), *Poisoning and toxicology compendium* (pp. 90–91). Cleveland, OH: Lexi-comp Inc. Americomp Pharmaceutics Association.

Barkin, R.L, Chor, P.N, Braun, B.G, & Schwer, W.A. (1999). A trilogy case review highlighting the clinical and pharmacologic applications of mirtazapine in reducing polypharmacy for anxiety, agitation, insomnia, depression, and sexual dysfunction, primary care companion. *Journal of Clinical Psychiatry, 1*(5), 142–145.

Barkin, R.L, & Fawcett, J. (2000). The management challenges of chronic pain: The role of antidepressants. *American Journal of Therapeutics, 7*, 31–47.

Barkin, R.L., Leikin, J.B., & Barkin, S.J. (1994). Noncardiac chest pain: A focus upon psychogenic causes. *American Journal of Therapeutics, 1*, 321–326.

Barkin, R.L., Lubenow, T.R., et al. (1996). Management of chronic pain, Parts I and II. *Disease-a-month, 42*(7), 389–456.

Barkin, R.L, Oetgen, J., & Barkin, S.J. (1999, June). Pharmacotherapeutic management opportunities utilized in chronic nonmalignant pain, *Supplement to Drug Topics.*

Barkin, R.L., & Richtsmeier, A.Y. (1995). Alternative agents in pharmacologic management of sickle cell pain crisis complicated by acute pancreatitis. *American Journal of Therapeutics, 2*, 819–823.

Barkin, R.L, Schwer, W.A, & Barkin, S.J. (2000). Recognition and management of depression in primary care: A focus on the elderly. A pharmacotherapeutic overview of the selection process among the traditional and new antidepressants. *American Journal of Therapeutics, 7*(3), 205–226.

Barsky, A.J., Hochstrasser, B., Coles, N.A., et al. (1990). Silent myocardial ischemia: Is the person or the event silent? *Journal of the American Medical Association, 364*, 1132–1135.

Bayer, A.G., Chadha, J.S., Farag, R.R., & Pathy, M.S.J. (1986). Changing presentations of myocardial infarction with increasing old age. *Journal of American Geriatric Society, 34*, 263–266.

Bazine, S., & Benefield, W.H. (1997–1998). *Psychotropic drug directory 1997–1998.* West Orange, NJ: Quay Books & Organon, Inc. 214–216.

Bennett, G.F. (1994). Neuropathic pain. In P.D. Wall & R. Melzack (Eds.)., *Textbook of pain* (3rd ed., pp. 201–224). New York: Churchill Livingstone.

Bhatia, S., Bhatia, S., & Barkin, R.L. (1997). Mirtazapine revisited [Letter to the Editor]. *American Family Physician, 56*(9), 2190–2192.

Bigos, S., Bower, O., Braen, G., et al. (1994). Acute low back problems in adults. Clinical practice guideline No. 14. Rockland, MD: Agency for Healthcare Policy and Research, Public Health Service U.S. Department of Health and Human Services. AHCPR publication 95-0642.

Bonica, J.J. (1990). Anatomic and physiologic basis of nociception and pain. In J. J. Bonica (Ed.), *The management of pain* (2nd ed., pp. 28–94). Malvern, PA: Lea and Febiger.

Bonica, J.J., et al. (1990). Biochemistry and modulation of nociception and pain. In J.J. Bonica (Ed.), *The management of pain* (2nd ed., pp. 95–121). Malvern, PA: Lea and Febiger.

Borestein, D. (1995). Prevalence and treatment outcome of primary and secondary fibromyalgia in patients with spinal pain. *Spine, 20,* 796–800.

Bowsher, D. (1995). The management of central post-stroke pain. *Postgraduate Medical Journal, 71,* 598–604.

Braverman, B., O'Connor, C., & Barkin, R.L. (1993). Pharmacology, physiology and anesthetic implications and antidepressants. In R.C. Stoelting (Ed.), *Pharmacology and physiology in anesthetic practice* (2nd ed., pp. 1–15). Philadelphia: Lippincott.

Bryson, H.M., & Wilde, M.I. (1996). Amitripyline. A review of its pharmacological properties and therapeutic use in chronic pain states. *Drugs Aging, 8,* 459-476.

Byrne, S.E, & Rothschild, A.J. (1998). Loss of antidepressant efficacy during maintenance therapy: possible mechanisms and treatments. *Journal of Clinical Psychiatry, 59,* 279–288.

Casadevall, A., Barkin, R.L., Moreno, J.A., Carcia, A., McCutchan, J.A., Sanchez, A., & Martinez, A.J. (1996). *AIDS: Combating infection and enhancing quality of life.* Cuban Medical Convention Symposium Proceeding, Albert Einstein College of Medicine CME, Miami Beach, Fl, 1996.

Cerruto, L. (1996). Venlafaxine joins ranks of psychotropic therapies to treat fibromyalgia. *Primary Psychiatry, 1,* 62–66.

Chakour, M.C., Gibson, S.J., Bradbeer, M., & Helme, R.D. (1996). The effect of age on A-delta and C fibre thermal pain perception. *Pain, 64,* 143–152.

Chapman, C.R. (1993). The emotional aspects of pain. In C.R. Chapman & K.M. Foley (Eds.), *Current and emerging issues in cancer pain: Research and practice* (pp. 83–98). New York: Lippincott-Raven.

Coderre, T.J., Katz, J., Vaccarino, A.L., & Melzack, R. (1993). Contribution of central neuroplasticity to pathological pain: Review of clinical and experimental evidence. *Pain, 52,* 259–285.

Cohen, L.J. (1997). Rational drug use in the treatment of depression. *Pharmacotherapy, 17,* 45–61.

Cohen, L.J., & De Vane, C.L. (1996). Clinical implications of antidepressant pharmacokinetics and pharmacogenetics. *Annals of Pharmacotherapy, 30,* 1471–1480.

Cookson, J. (1993). Side effects of antidepressants. *British Journal of Pyschiatry, 163*(Suppl. 20), 20–24.

Craig, K.D. (1994). Emotional aspects of pain. In P.D. Wall & R. Melzack (Eds.), Textbook of pain (3rd ed., pp. 261–274). New York: Churchill Livingstone.

Davis, J., & Barkin, R.L. (1999). Clinical pharmacology of mirtazapine: Revisited. *American Family Physician, 60*(4), 1101.

Davis, J.M., & Glassman, A.H. (1989). Antidepressant drugs. In H.I. Kaplan & B.J. Sadock (Eds.), *Comprehensive textbook of psychiatry* (pp. 1627–1654). New York: Williams and Wilkins.

De Angelis, L. (1992). "Newer" versus "older" antidepressant drugs in the treatment of chronic pain syndromes. *Advances in Therapy, 9,* 91–97.

De Wester, J.N. (1996) Recognizing and Treating the patient with Somatic Manifestations of Depression. *Journal of Family Practice, 43* (Suppl.), S3–S15.

DeVane, C.L. (1994). Pharmacokinetics of the newer antidepressants: Clinical relevance. *American Journal of Medicine, 97*(Suppl. 6A):6A-13S–6A-23S.

Dwight, M., Arnold, L., O'Brien, H., Metzger, R., & Morris-Park, E. (1996). Venlafaxine treatment of fibromyalgia. *Psychopharmacology Bulletin, 32,* 435.

Dworkin, R.H., & Gitlin, M.J. (1991). Clinical aspects of depression in chronic pain patients. *Clinical Journal of Pain, 7,* 79–94.

Dworkin, S.F., Von Korff, M., & LeResche, L. (1990). Multiple pains and psychiatric disturbance: An epidemiologic investigation. *Archives of General Psychiatry, 47,* 239–244.

Eija, K., Tiina, T., & Pertti, N.J. (1996). Amitryptyline effectively relieves neuropathic pain following treatment of breast cancer. *Pain, 64,* 293–302.

Eschalier, A., Ardid, D., & Coudore, F. (1992). Pharmacological studies of the analgesic effect of antidepressants. *Clinical Neuropharmacology, 15*(Suppl. 1, Part A), 373A–374A.

Fawcett, J., & Barkin, R.L. (1997). Efficacy issues with antidepressants. *Journal of Clinical Psychiatry, 58*(6), 32–39.

Fawcett, J., & Barkin, R.L. (1998a). A meta-analysis of eight randomized, double blind controlled clinical trials of mirtazapine for the treatment of patients with major depression and symptoms of anxiety. *Journal of Clinical Psychiatry 59*(3), 123–127.

Fawcett, J., & Barkin, R.L. (1998b). Review of the results from clinical studies on the efficacy, safety and tolerability of mirtazapine for the treatment of patients with major depression. *Journal of Affective Disorders, 51,* 267–285.

Feighner, J.P. (1994) The role of venlafaxine in rational antidepressant therapy. *Journal of Clinical Psychiatry, 55*(9, Suppl. A), 62–68.

Feinmann, C. (1985). Pain relief by antidepressants: Possible modes of action. *Pain, 23,* 1–8.

Galer, B.S. (1994). Painful polyneuropathy: diagnosis, pathophysiology, and management. *Seminars in Neurology, 14,* 237–246.

Galer, B.S. (1995). Neuropathic pain of peripheral origin: advances in pharmacologic treatment. *Neurology, 45*(Suppl. 9), S17–S25.

Gaynes, B.L., & Barkin, R.L. (1999). Analgesicsin ophthalmic practice: A review of the oral non-narcotic agent tramadol. *Optometry and Vision Science, 76*(7), 455–461.

Gibson, T.P. (1996). Pharmacokinetics, efficacy, and safety of analgesia with a focus on tramadol HCL. *American Journal of Medicine, 101*(Suppl. 1A), 47S–53S.

Godfrey, R.G. (1996). A guide to the understanding and use of tricyclic antidepressants in the overall management of fibromyalgia and other chronic pain syndromes. *Archives of Internal Medicine, 156*, 1047–1052.

Gonzales G.R. (1995). Central pain: Diagnosis and treatment strategies. *Neurology, 45*, S11–S16.

Gruber, A.J., Hudson, J.I., & Pope, H.G., Jr. (1996). The management of treatment-resistant depression in disorders on the interface of psychiatry and medicine. Fibromyalgia, chronic fatigue syndrome, migraine, irritable bowel syndrome, atypical facial pain, and premenstrual dysphoric disorder. *Psychiatric Clinics of North America, 19*, 351–369.

Guilbaud, G., Bernard, J.F., & Besson, J.M. (1994). Brain areas involved in nociception and pain. In P.D. Wall & R. Melzack (Eds.), *Textbook of pain* (3rd ed., pp. 113–128). New York: Churchill Livingstone.

Holliday, S.M., & Benfield, P. (1995). Venlafaxine: A review of its pharmacology and therapeutic potential in depression. *Drugs, 49*, 280–294.

Huff, J., & Barkin, R.L. (1994). A primary care clinician's and consultants guide to medicating for pain and anxiety associated with outpatient procedures. *American Journal of Therapeutics, 1*, 186–190.

Hunter, S. (1994). Atypical facial pain-rewarding to treat. *Practitioner, 238*, 186–193.

Kao, L., Barkin, R.L., & Leikin, J.B. (1997). Mirtazapine overdose: A case report. *Medical Update for Psychiatrists, 2*(2), 58–59.

Kauvar, D.R. (1993). The geriatric acute abdomen. *Clinical Geriatrics Medicine, 9*, 547–558.

Kramer, C., Feighner, J., Shrivastava, R., Carman, J., et al. (1998). Distinct mechanisms for antidepressant activity by blockade of central substance P receptors. *Science, 281*(1), 1640–1644.

LaMotte, C.C. (1986). Organization of dorsal horn neurotransmitter systems. In T.L. Yaksh (Ed.), *Spinal afferent processing* (pp. 97–116). New York: Plenum Press.

Larue, F., Fontaine A., & Colleau, S.M. (1997). Underestimation and undertreatment of pain in HIV disease: Multicentre study. *British Medical Journal, 314*, 23–28.

Lister, B.J. (1996). Dilemmas in the treatment of chronic pain. *American Journal of Medicine, 101*(Suppl. 1A), 2S–5S.

Loeser, J.D. (1986). Herpes zoster and postherapeutic neuralgia. *Pain, 25*, 149–164.

Magni, G. (1991). The use of antidepressants in the treatment of chronic pain. A review of the current evidence. *Drugs, 42*, 730–748.

McQuay, H.J., & Moore, R.A. (1997). Antidepressants and chronic pain. *British Medical Journal, 314*, 763–764.

McQuay, H.J., Tramer, M., Nye, B.A., Carroll, D., Wiffen, P.J., & Moore, R.A. (1996). A systematic review of antidepressants in neuropathic pain. *Pain, 68*, 217–227.

Melzack, R. (1996). Gate control theory: on the evolution of pain concepts. *Pain Forum, 5*, 128–138.

Merskey, H., & Bogduk, N. (1994). *Pain terms. Anonymous classification of chronic pain syndromes and definition of pain terms* (2nd ed., pp. 210–213) Seattle: International Association for the Study of Pain Press.

Meyer, R.A., Campbell, J.N., & Raja, S.N. Peripheral and neural mechanisms of nociception. In P.D. Wall & R. Melzack (Eds.), *Textbook of pain* (3rd ed., pp. 13–44). New York: Churchill Livingstone.

Montgomery, S.A. (1993). Venlafaxine: A new dimension in antidepressant pharmacotherapy. *Journal of Clinical Psychiatry, 54*, 119–126.

Onghena, P., & Van Houdenhove, B. (1992). Antidepressant-induced analgesia in chronic non-malignant pain: Aa meta-analysis of 39 placebo-controlled studies. *Pain, 49*, 205–219.

Pappagallo, M., & Heinberg, L.J. (1997). Ethical issues in the management of chronic nonmalignant pain. *Seminars in Neurology, 17*, 203–211.

Parmelee, P. A., Katz, I. R., & Lawton, M.P. (1991). The relation of pain to depression among institutionalized aged. *Journal of Gerontology, 46*, 15–21.

Philipp, M., & Fickinger, M. (1993). Psychotropic drugs in the management of chronic pain syndromes. *Pharmacopsychiatry; 26*, 221–234.

Popp, B., & Portenoy, R.K. (1996). Management of chronic pain in the elderly: Pharmacology of opioids and other analgesic drugs. In B.R. Ferrell & B.A. Ferrell (Eds.), *Pain in the elderly* (pp. 21–34). Seattle: International Association of the Study of Pain.

Raj, P.P. (1992). *Practical management of pain* (2nd ed.). St. Louis: Mosby Yearbook.

Rani, P.U., Naidu, M.U.R., Prasad, V.B.N., Rao, TR.K., & Shobha, J.C. (1996). An evaluation of antidepressants in rheumatic pain conditions. *Anesthesia and Analgesia, 83*, 371–375.

Reisine, T., & Pasternak, G. (1996). Opioid analgesics and antagonists. In J.G. Hardman, L.E. Limbird, P.B. Molinoff, & R.W. Ruddon (Eds.), *Goodman & Gilman's The pharmacological basis of therapeutics* (9th ed., pp. 521–555). New York: McGraw-Hill.

Richardson, P.H. (1993). Meta-analysis of antidepressant-induced analgesia in chronic pain: comment. *Pain, 52*, 247.

Rost, K., Zhang, M., Fortney, J., Smith, J., & Smith, G.R.J. (1998). Expenditures for the treatment of major depression. *American Journal of Psychiatry, 155*, 883–888.

Rowbotham, M.C. (1994). Painful polyneuropathy. *Seminars in Neurology, 14*, 247–254.

Rowbotham, M.C. (1995). Chronic pain: From theory to practical management. *Neurology, 45*, S5–S10.

Ruda, M.A. (1986). The pattern and place of nociceptive modulation in the dorsal horn: a discussion of the anatomically characterized neural circuitry of enkephalin, serotonin, and substance P. In T. L. Yaksh (Ed.), *Spinal afferent processing*. New York: Plenum Press.

Ruoff, G.E. (1996). Depression in the patient with chronic pain. *Journal of Family Practice, 43* (Suppl. 6), S25–S34.

Seybold, V.S. (1986). Neurotransmitter receptor sites in the spinal cord. In T. L. Yaksh (Ed.), *Spinal afferent processing* (pp. 117–146). New York: Plenum Press.

Siddall, P.J., & Cousins, M.J. (1995). Pain mechanisms and management: An update. *Clinical Experiments in Pharmacology and Physiology, 22,* 679–688.

Sindrup, S.H. (1993). Antidepressants in pain treatment. *Nordic Journal of Psychiatry, 47*(Suppl.), 67–73.

Sindrup, S.H., Brosen, K., & Gram, L.F. (1992a). Antidepressants in pain treatment: antidepressant or analgesic effect. *Clinical Neuropharmacology, 15*(Suppl. 1, Part A), 636A–637A.

Sindrup, S.H., Brosen, K., & Gram, L.F. (1992b). The mechanism of action of antidepressants in pain treatment: controlled cross-over studies in diabetic neuropathy. *Clinical Neuropharmacology, 15*(Suppl. 1, Part A), 380A–381A.

Sindrup, S.H., Gram, L.F., Brøsen, K., Eshøj, O., & Mogensen, E.F. (1990). The selective Serotonin reuptake inhibitor paroxetine is effective in the treatment of diabetic neuropathy symptoms. *Pain, 42,* 135–144.

Songer, D.A., & Schulte, H. (1996). Venlafaxine for the treatment of chronic pain [Letter]. *American Journal of Psychiatry, 153,* 737.

Stein, W.M., & Read, S. (1997). Chronic pain in the setting of Parkinson's disease and depression. *Journal of Pain and Symptom Management, 14,* 255–258.

Sternbach, H. (1991). The serotonin syndrome. *American Journal of Psychiatry, 148,* 705–713.

Tacey, B.R. (1996). Effective management of chronic pain. The analgesic dilemma. *Postgraduate Medicine, 100,* 281–284, 287–293.

Tamler, M.S., & Meerschaert, J.R. (1996). Pain management of fibromyalgia and other chronic pain syndromes. *Physical Medicine and Rehabilitation Clinics of North America, 7,* 549–560.

Tarster, R.R. (1990). Pain resulting from central nervous system pathology (central pain). In J. J. Bonica (Ed.), *The management of pain* (2nd ed., pp. 264–283). Malvern, PA: Lea and Febiger.

Taylor, K., & Rowbotham, M.C. (1996). Venlafaxine hydrochloride and chronic pain. *Western Journal of Medicine, 165,* 147–148.

Watson, C.P.N. (1994). Antidepressant drugs as adjuvant analgesics. *Journal of Pain and Symptom Management, 9,* 392–405.

Yaksh, T.L. (1996). Pharmacology of the pain processing system. In S.D. Waldman, A.P. Winnie (Eds.), *Interventional pain management* (pp. 141–164), Dannemiller Memorial Educational Foundation. Philadelphia: W.B. Saunders.

Yaksh, T.L, & Malmberg, A.B. (1994). Central Pharmacology of nociceptive transmission. In P.D. Wall, & R. Melzack (Eds.), *Textbook of pain* (3rd ed., pp. 165–200). New York: Churchill Livingstone.

Yunus, M.B. (1996). Fibromyalgia syndrome: Is there any effective therapy? *Consultant, 36,* 1279–1285.

Zitman, F.G., Linssen, A.C.G., Edelbroek, P.M., & Ven Kempen, G.M. (1992). Clinical effectiveness of antidepressants and antipsychotics in chronic benign pain. *Clinical Neuropharmacology, 15*(Suppl. 1, Part A), 377A–378A.

36

Drug Management of Pain

Robert B. Supernaw, Pharm.D.

INTRODUCTION

As is the case with almost any medical problem, the best pharmacotherapeutic approach to acute and chronic pain management is no drug therapy at all. However, the option of not using drugs in managing many pain syndromes is not realistic. When the clinician has determined that the pain condition is significant and beyond the scope of being treated solely with physical medicine (e.g., ice packs, massage, physical therapy), drug therapy is indicated. To determine the best pharmacotherapeutic response to pain, the nature and severity of the pain must be assessed and considered. Whether the pain is acute or chronic must be taken into account, as well as whether the pain is malignant, benign, organic, psychogenic, vascular, or depression related. Neuropathic pain is addressed in a completely different manner than nociceptive pain. Additionally, the pain should be graded as mild, moderate, severe, or excruciating before an appropriate drug regimen and drug delivery system are formulated.

Treatment plans are formulated on the basis of the categorization of the pain syndrome. For example, mild acute respondent pain is treated differently than chronic severe aberrant pain. Because the nature or categorization of the pain is important, the interdisciplinary pain treatment model is considered state-of-the-art. Unlike the basic therapeutic approach to other commonly encountered problems (e.g., hypertension, hyperlipidemia), where drug therapy is initiated in relatively small doses and built until the therapeutic threshold or desired outcome is achieved, the therapeutic approach to pain is predicated on the basis of matching the pain category to the appropriate agent.

That is, there is no need to begin drug therapy for any pain complaint with the less potent, over-the-counter analgesics before attempting more potent drug therapy. A severe, chronic, benign cluster headache will not respond to aspirin or acetaminophen therapy; thus, there is simply no justification in trying. This treatment principle underscores the need for an accurate categorization of the pain complaint. Therefore, the clinician's familiarity with the pain scales, such as those described above, is essential. The International Association for the Study of Pain deems the role of pharmacotherapy in pain management to be of such vital importance that it established a focus group for the design of a pain curriculum for all pharmacy students.

ACUTE PAIN

When a patient presents in acute distress, often the clinician's attention is first drawn to the comfort of the patient, and alleviating the pain is attempted even before the cause of the distress is considered. For this reason, the clinician must make a quick and accurate assessment of the relative degree of the pain. In acute pain, the same classification system is used as for chronic pain (i.e., mild, moderate, severe, and excruciating).

CHRONIC PAIN

Chronic pain can be thought of as a completely different medical problem than its acute phase. Chronic pain has elements of acute pain, but it is generally more psychologically innervated, debilitating the personhood as well as the physical nature of the body being treated. For this reason, the patient suffering chronic pain should be treated just as aggressively as the patient suffering acute

0-8493-0926-3/02/$0.00+$1.50
© 2002 by CRC Press LLC

distress. Quality-of-life issues are important considerations in chronic pain, whereas simply diminishing the intensity of the pain is the primary focus in the treatment approach to acute pain. Chronic pain serves no useful purpose; acute pain can be helpful in deducing the underlying cause.

MILD PAIN

FIRST-LINE PHARMACOTHERAPY

Because, by definition, acute mild pain is limited in its duration, it need not be aggressively treated. Often, it need not be treated at all. In that chronic pain is, by definition, long-term pain, often nonpharmacologic pain-mitigating therapy is indicated. However, if a decision is made to treat the mild acute or chronic pain, first consideration should be given to aspirin. For the aspirin-allergic patient, acetaminophen is an excellent alternative, although it has insignificant anti-inflammatory activity. Internal, over-the-counter (OTC) analgesics are the mainstay for mild pain, and sales of these agents (i.e., aspirin, acetaminophen, ibuprofen, naproxen sodium, and ketoprofen) totaled $2,660,831,000 in 1995 (Information Resources, 1996).

Aspirin

Aspirin, given as a 650-mg dose (two tablets) every 4 hours, is the mainstay of first-line drug therapy in various mild pain-related problems such as minor arthritis flare-ups, mild tension-type headaches, and chronic minor low-back pain. Aspirin is absorbed very rapidly in the duodenum; there are insignificant differences in absorption between buffered and nonbuffered varieties. As with all salicylates, aspirin is metabolized in the liver and is highly albumin-bound. Therefore, caution is warranted when aspirin is given to a patient taking an oral anticoagulant (OAC) in that the OAC is approximately 97% albumin-bound. The concomitant use of aspirin will displace a significant amount of the OAC from its inactive binding sites, causing an increase in the active dose (drug level) of the OAC.

Aspirin was first introduced to the U.S. market in 1899. It has analgesic, anti-inflammatory, antiplatelet, and antipyretic activity. Its mechanism of action is by inhibition of prostaglandin synthesis, and it is effective in mild and mild-to-moderate pain. The benefits of aspirin therapy are well known. It is cheap, readily available, has a very long track record, is very effective in the relief of mild or mild-to-moderate pain, and reduces inflammation, especially at higher doses. Additional benefits include its ability to reduce fever and its antiplatelet adhesion properties.

However, the use of aspirin is not without risk. The gastrointestinal (GI)-related risks include everything from mild stomach irritation to ulceration and GI bleeding. Hearing loss has been associated with very high doses of aspirin. Generally, tinnitus will forewarn the clinician of too high an aspirin dose before problems arise. Aspirin has also been implicated in blood-related problems, including decreased white blood cell and platelet counts and hemolytic anemia.

Aspirin should not be taken if the patient is allergic to salicylates, has a bleeding disorder, has peptic ulcer disease, or during the last 3 months of pregnancy (see pregnancy category note below). Clinicians should also warn patients to throw out aspirin that has an odor of vinegar, which indicates that the aspirin has chemically degraded. Extra caution is indicated if the patient (1) is taking an anticoagulant, (2) is taking an oral antidiabetic agent, (3) has a history of peptic ulcer disease, (4) has systemic lupus erythematosus, (5) is pregnant or contemplating pregnancy, (6) is scheduled for surgery, (7) is receiving a new prescription, or (8) any time the patient is experiencing a new significant adverse effect.

Aspirin has a tentative Food and Drug Administration (FDA) Pregnancy Category of D, which means that studies in pregnant women demonstrate positive evidence of human fetal risk. Aspirin is present in breast milk. For infants and children into their teens, aspirin is contraindicated in viral infections, including flu and chicken pox, as it has been implicated in Reye's syndrome, It is suggested that complete blood cell counts be monitored in patients taking daily doses of aspirin, as well as monitoring kidney function/urine analyses along with liver function.

Dosing guidelines are very specific and are formulated on the basis of weight or age:

- Children age 2–11, 64 mg/kg/day in four to six doses or
- Children age 11, 480 mg/day
- Children age 9–10, 400 mg/day
- Children age 6–8, 325 mg/day
- Children age 4–5, 240 mg/day
- Children age 2–3, 160 mg/day
- Children younger than 2, by weight
- For adults, and children over 11, 325–650 mg every 4 hours, not to exceed 4 g/day

Acetaminophen

For patients who cannot tolerate aspirin, acetaminophen is indicated. It is given in doses similar to aspirin; however, some caution is warranted in higher dosing schedules. Acetaminophen (Tylenol®) first appeared on the OTC market in 1954. It is an analgesic and has antipyretic properties. It tends to be better tolerated than aspirin in individuals who experience GI-related complications with analgesics. Its mechanism of action is similar to the salicylates; however, it possesses only very weak anti-inflammatory activity.

Acetaminophen has been widely used largely because of its reputation for safety. Although its reputation is deserved, it is not without risks. Hepatotoxicity is a significant adverse drug reaction associated with the use of acetaminophen. Because many patients with pain tend to take medications on a routine basis, it is the clinician's responsibility to warn of possible liver damage with as little as 2.6 g acetaminophen daily, over extended periods of time. Patients should not take acetaminophen if they have experienced an allergy to it, if they have diminished liver function, if they are alcoholics, if they are fasting, or if they have significant kidney damage or loss of kidney function.

Extra caution is indicated any time a patient who is contemplating taking acetaminophen (1) requires higher chronic doses, (2) is alcoholic, (3) has compromised liver or kidney function, or (4) experiences a significant adverse drug reaction.

The specific adverse drug reactions to watch for include GI bleeding, anemias, rash, and signs and symptoms of hepato- and nephrotoxicity. Acetaminophen is classified by the FDA as Pregnancy Category B, which means that animal studies are negative for fetal abnormalities, or animal studies are positive while human studies are negative. Although acetaminophen is present in breast milk, studies have shown that only an insignificant 0.88 mg is passed on with each feeding. Laboratory monitoring should include periodic liver function tests if chronic relatively high doses are being taken.

Dosing guidelines are as follows:

- Adults, 325–650 mg every 4–6 hours, not to exceed 4 g/day for acute pain
- Children age 11, 480 mg
- Children age 9–10, 400 mg
- Children age 6–8, 320 mg
- Children age 4–5, 240 mg
- Children age 2–3, 160 mg
- Children age 1–2, 120 mg
- Children age 4–11 months, 80 mg
- Children younger than 4 months, 40 mg

SECOND-LINE PHARMACOTHERAPY

If the mild pain does not respond to aspirin or acetaminophen and the doses have been pushed to the extent deemed appropriate, consideration should be given to second-line therapy. There are now three OTC nonsteroidal anti-inflammatory drugs (NSAIDs) that are readily available – ibuprofen, naproxen sodium, and ketoprofen — and they are excellent second choices for mild pain complaints. The NSAIDs exert their pharmacologic effects by virtue of their ability to inhibit the synthesis and/or release of prostaglandins.

Ibuprofen

Ibuprofen was first introduced onto the prescription market in the United States in 1969; and in 1984, the 200-mg dosage form became an OTC item (Advil®, Nuprin®). Ibuprofen is in the class of NSAIDs, and it has analgesic, anti-inflammatory, some antipyretic, and some antiplatelet activity. It is thought to work by decreasing tissue concentrations of prostaglandins and related compounds. It is approximately 80% absorbed. Perhaps the most important concept for clinicians to remember about OTC ibuprofen is that in the OTC dose (i.e., 200 mg), the drug has little anti-inflammatory effect. At this dose, its primary effects are analgesic and antiplatelet adhesion.

Ibuprofen has been shown to be an effective OTC analgesic. However, it should be monitored for its potential adverse drug reactions. Perhaps the most common side effect is GI pain or even ulceration. GI complications are thought to be dose related; thus, the OTC dose would have the least possibility of provoking GI-related complications. Nevertheless, the practitioner would be wise to warn patients of this potential problem. Patients who are particularly sensitive to NSAID-related GI distress should be counseled to take their medication with a full glass of water and not to lie down for 30 minutes. Ibuprofen is safe to crush for patients in skilled nursing facilities. Also, ibuprofen may be taken with food to limit GI irritation.

Patients should not take ibuprofen if they are subject to asthma or nasal polyps caused by aspirin, if they have active peptic ulcer disease, if they have a bleeding disorder or blood cell disorder, or if they have significant kidney damage.

The physician should be consulted any time a patient is considering using ibuprofen on an OTC basis if the patient (1) is allergic to aspirin, (2) has a history of peptic ulcer disease, (3) has a history of a bleeding disorder, (4) has diminished liver or kidney function, (5) has high blood pressure or heart failure, (6) is taking acetaminophen chronically, or (7) experiences a significant adverse drug reaction.

In addition to GI irritation, other adverse drug reactions include altered pattern and timing of the menstrual cycle (30% of women are affected). It may also give false-positives for fecal occult blood, and it may cause drowsiness in sensitive individuals.

One study has shown an increased analgesic activity when taken with caffeine; however, the drawbacks seen with caffeine intake must be weighed against its advantages.

Ibuprofen, as well as naproxen sodium, appear to be especially helpful in menstrual cramps. It has been tentatively assigned by the FDA to Pregnancy Category B, which means that animal studies are negative for fetal abnormalities, or animal studies are positive while human studies are negative. It is not recommended for use during the last 3 months of pregnancy. It is present in very small amounts in breast milk. If a patient is taking ibuprofen for extended periods of time, monitoring of CBC as well as liver and kidney function may be warranted.

The OTC dose of ibuprofen is 200 mg every 4 to 6 hours. Ibuprofen was not recommended for children on an OTC basis until 1996. Children's Motrin® and Children's Advil® are approved for OTC use. If given by prescription, the children's dosing schedule is as follows:

- Children 11–15.9 kg (24–35 lb.), 100 mg
- Children 16–21.9 kg (36–47 lb.), 150 mg
- Children 22–26.9 kg (48–59 lb.), 200 mg
- Children 27–31.9 kg (60–71 lb.), 250 mg
- Children 32–43.9 kg (72–95 lb.), 300 mg

Naproxen Sodium

Naproxen sodium was first introduced in 1974 as a prescription NSAID and was approved for OTC use in 1994 (Aleve®). It has analgesic, anti-inflammatory, some antipyretic, and some antiplatelet activity.

Naproxen sodium is thought to work by decreasing the tissue concentrations of prostaglandins and related compounds. It is virtually 100% absorbed. Naproxen sodium has been shown to be an effective OTC analgesic; however, it, too, should be monitored for potential risks. An advantage of naproxen sodium over other NSAIDs is that it has a lower incidence of adverse effects, including less GI irritation and a lower incidence of liver and kidney complications. Nevertheless, because it is an NSAID, patients should be warned to monitor GI irritation; and for those who are particularly sensitive to NSAID-related GI distress, taking their medication with a full glass of water and not lying down for 30 minutes will be helpful. Naproxen sodium is safe to crush for patients in skilled nursing facilities. Also, it may be taken with food to limit GI irritation.

Patients should not take naproxen sodium if they are subject to asthma or nasal polyps caused by aspirin, if they have active peptic ulcer disease, if they have a bleeding disorder or blood cell disorder, or if they have significant kidney damage.

The physician should be consulted any time a patient is considering using naproxen sodium on an OTC basis if the patient (1) is allergic to aspirin, (2) has a history of peptic ulcer disease, (3) has a history of a bleeding disorder, (4) has diminished liver or kidney function, (5) has high blood pressure or heart failure, or (6) experiences a significant adverse drug reaction.

As discussed earlier, naproxen sodium has less GI-related irritation potential than other NSAIDs. Adverse drug reactions include altered pattern and timing of the menstrual cycle. It may also give false-positives for fecal occult blood and may cause drowsiness in sensitive individuals. It may also cause fluid retention.

Naproxen sodium, as well as ibuprofen, appears to be especially helpful in menstrual cramps. It has been tentatively assigned by the FDA to Pregnancy Category B, which means that animal studies are negative for fetal abnormalities, or animal studies are positive while human studies are negative. It is not recommended for use during the last 3 months of pregnancy. It is present in very small amounts in breast milk. If a patient is taking naproxen sodium for extended periods of time, monitoring of CBC as well as liver and kidney function may be warranted.

The OTC dose of naproxen sodium is 220 mg every 8 to 12 hours. It is recommended that the drug be initiated as two tablets (440 mg) immediately, then one tablet every 8 to 12 hours, not to exceed 660 mg in a 24-hour period. For patients over 65, the recommended dose is one tablet every 8 to 12 hours, not to exceed 440 mg in 24 hours. It is not recommended for children under 12 on an OTC basis; however, if absolutely necessary, the recommended prescription doses of naproxen for children are as follows:

- Children 12.5 kg (29.5 lb.), 125 mg (1 tsp. of a 125-mg/5-ml suspension in two divided doses)
- Children 25 kg (55 lb.), 250 mg (2 tsp. of a 125-mg/5-ml suspension in two divided doses)

Ketoprofen

Similar to ibuprofen and naproxen sodium, ketoprofen was first approved for use as a prescription drug. In 1995, it was approved for OTC sales by the FDA as Orudis-KT® and Actron®. Ketoprofen is a phenylpropionic acid, in the same chemical family as ibuprofen and naproxen sodium. As with ibuprofen and naproxen sodium, it possesses minimal anti-inflammatory activity at the OTC dose.

Ketoprofen is available OTC as a 12.5-mg tablet and is dosed as a second-line analgesic at 12.5 mg every 4 to 6 hours for adults. If pain is not relieved within 1 hour, a second tablet may be taken. Doses above two tablets (i.e., 25 mg) are not considered appropriate for OTC use. Additionally, without prescription, doses should not exceed six tablets (75 mg) in a 24-hour period. It is not recommended for children under 16.

At the OTC dose, ketoprofen is effective in managing pain associated with colds, minor back discomfort, toothache, menstrual cramps, muscle aches, and minor pain associated with arthritis.

Peak serum concentrations of ketoprofen are reached in 30 minutes to 2 hours, and almost 100% of the drug is absorbed. Although it has a rapid onset, its relatively short duration of action necessitates dosing three to four times daily. As with other NSAIDs, the chief adverse effects are associated with GI irritation; however, these problems can be minimized by following the procedures described below. Additionally, concomitant use with antacids does not appear to affect the absorption of ketoprofen.

Ketoprofen has been assigned by the FDA to Pregnancy Category B, which means that animal studies are negative for fetal abnormalities, or animal studies are positive while human studies are negative. Its appearance in breast milk is insignificant. It is not recommended for children under 12 on an OTC basis; however, if absolutely necessary, the recommended prescription doses for children are as follows:

- Children 3 months to 14 years of age, 0.5–1.0 mg per kilogram of weight for fever
- Children with juvenile chronic arthritis, 25–50 mg

MODERATE PAIN

THIRD-LINE PHARMACOTHERAPY

As the pain complaint reaches the moderate level, the dose of aspirin, acetaminophen, ibuprofen, naproxen sodium, or ketoprofen is increased as third-line therapy. Seldom does a tension-type headache respond to the equivalent of 650 mg aspirin. The dose will need to be increased to the equivalent of 1000 mg aspirin to expect success. Lower doses will simply diminish the level of appreciation the patient has for OTC pharmacotherapy; thus, the prudent clinician best not be too timid to begin therapy at the equivalent of 1000 mg aspirin. No specific NSAID has been shown to be more effective or less toxic than others (Brooks & Day, 1991).

With increased dosing levels of NSAIDs, the procedure moves from an OTC recommendation to a prescription drug. NSAIDs account for 3.8% of all prescriptions written ("Antiarthritic," 1992), and the clinician must be ever-mindful that these prescriptions are responsible for some 20 to 25% of all adverse drug reactions reported. The chief complaint is GI irritation. With increased dosing levels, there will be an associated increase in the likelihood of an adverse effect, particularly GI irritation. Patients should be instructed to take their NSAIDs with a full glass of water and not to lie down for 30 minutes after dosing. A small amount of food may be taken with the drug. This simple procedure will significantly decrease the incidence of GI-related distress.

Recently, a new category of NSAIDs has become available. These drugs are termed COX-2 inhibitors. This term derives from their ability to selectively inhibit just the COX-2 enzyme in preference to both the COX-1 and COX-2 enzymes. This difference inhibits the cascade that converts substrates to the prostaglandins that enhance pain transmission and provoke inflammation, while not blocking the production of the prostaglandins that cause platelets to aggregate (clump) and not blocking the production of the prostaglandins that protect the gastrointestinal mucosa. Therefore, these new drugs are superior in their adverse effect profiles in that they do not significantly provoke gastrointestinal irritation. However, they do not contribute to platelet antiadhesion, so they do not possess the beneficial cardiovascular effects of aspirin and traditional NSAIDs.

The three COX-2 inhibiting drugs most widely available in the United States are celecoxib (Celebrex®), rofecoxib (Vioxx®), and meloxicam (Mobic®). Celecoxib and rofecoxib are excellent choices for the patient who is experiencing GI irritation with other NSAIDs. These are also excellent choices for the patient for whom the NSAID dose must be pushed upward, often provoking GI irritation with traditional NSAIDs. These drugs are indicated for osteoarthritis, and rofecoxib is indicated for pain, although both should be considered for pain. Meloxicam is significantly less COX-2 selective; therefore, it should be considered a third choice.

FOURTH-LINE PHARMACOTHERAPY

If the increased doses of the first- and second-line therapies (i.e., third-line therapy) are not successful, an alternate NSAID may be substituted, and COX-2 inhibitors are suggested. It is recommended that the second NSAID be selected from a different chemical family. Chemical families are described in Table 36.1. Prescription-strength ibuprofen, ketoprofen, naproxen sodium, and naproxen are the most commonly employed selections. The drug-specific information related to effective use of the NSAIDs is summarized in Table 36.2.

As previously mentioned, when NSAIDs are used, GI irritation is a concern. Studies have shown that up to 4% of patients treated with NSAIDs on a long-term basis will develop GI complications, including ulcers, bleeding, or perforation. The elderly and patients with a history of peptic ulcer disease are at highest risk.

Hepatotoxicity and nephrotoxicity are the only major adverse drug reactions with NSAIDs (GI distress is considered a minor adverse effect). Therefore, kidney and liver function should be monitored, especially in patients taking long-term doses, very large short-term doses of NSAIDs, or concomitant doses of acetaminophen. Also, significant GI irritation is widely reported in some patients taking even small amounts of NSAIDs. In this case, it appears that an individual sensitive to one NSAID will be sensitive to all NSAIDs. It is the responsibility of the clinician to recommend discontinuation of NSAID therapy before GI-related problems lead to significant GI bleeding. Even the non-oral form of these drugs can cause significant GI irritation; therefore, GI effects appear to be not just a local effect of the drug on the GI mucosa.

Injectable NSAIDs (only two are currently available) are not indicated for moderate pain, even if the pain is acute and would appear to demand a treatment that is more

TABLE 36.1
Family and Chemical Classes of Commonly Used NSAIDs

Chemical Class	NSAID
Acetylated carboxylic acid	Aspirin
Nonacetylated carboxylic acids	Choline salicylate
	Diflunisal
	Magnesium salicylate
	Salicylamide
	Salsalate
	Sodium salicyiate
Acetic acids	Carprofen
	Fenbufen
	Fenprofen
	Flubiprofen
	Ibuprofen
	Ketoprofen
	Ketorolac
	Pirofen
	Indoprofen
	Naproxen
	Naproxen sodium
	Oxaprozin
	Suprofen
	Tiaprofenic acid
Fenamic acids	Flufenamic acid
	Mefenamic acid
	Meclofenamic acid
	Meclofenamate (fenamate)
	Niflumic acid
Enolic acids	Isoxicam
	Oxyphenbutazone
	Phenylbutazone
	Piroxicam
	Sudoxicam
	Tenoxicam
Nonacidic compounds	Bufexamac
	Nabumetone
	Proquazone
COX-2 inhibitors	Celecoxib
	Rofecoxib
	Meloxicam
Pyrole acetic acid	Indomethacin

immediate in action than the oral medications. It is important to remember that the drug is to be matched to the category, and moderate pain is not matched with the injectable NSAIDs. These dosage forms are addressed later in another pain intensity category.

FIFTH-LINE PHARMACOTHERAPY

If the clinician believes that an oral medication is appropriate and also believes that a narcotic is indicated for moderate pain, the combination of aspirin or acetaminophen with codeine is an appropriate first choice.

In a study of 100 patients, codeine sulfate (65 mg) and aspirin (650 mg) was judged by the patients to be superior in its pain-alleviating activity when compared with (1) oxycodone (9.75 mg) and aspirin (650 mg); (2) pentazocine hydrochloride (25 mg) and aspirin (650 mg); (3) propoxyphene napsylate (100 mg) and aspirin (650 mg); (4) promazine hydrochloride (25 mg) and aspirin (650 mg); (5) pentobarbital sodium (32 mg) and aspirin (650 mg); (6) caffeine (65 mg) and aspirin (650 mg); (7) ethoheptazine citrate (75 mg) and aspirin (650 mg); (8) aspirin (650 mg) alone; and (9) placebo (Moertel, et al., 1974). When codeine is added to aspirin or acetaminophen, the side effects of the opiates present themselves.

Mechanism of Action of the Opioids

Drugs in the opiate family exert their analgesic and nonanalgesic effects secondary to their binding and activation of stereospecific receptors, predominantly in the central nervous system, but also in the periphery. The three most important opiate receptors are mu, kappa, and delta (Collin, et al., 1993). The sigma (PCP receptor) should not be considered an opiate receptor in that its activation is not reversible by employment of an opiate antagonist.

Opioid drugs have a high affinity for the mu receptors, which are located principally at supraspinal sites. Mu activation produces analgesia, respiratory depression, euphoria, and physical dependence. It has been determined that the relative potency of an opiate is a function of its affinity (strength of binding) to the mu receptor (Chen, Irvine, Somogyi, & Bochner, 1991).

The opioid receptors of the kappa variety are located principally within the spinal cord. Kappa activation mediates spinal analgesia, miosis, and sedation (Sabbe & Yaksh, 1995). Delta binding sites promote analgesia, yet their ultimate utility in pain management has yet to be fully determined.

Opioid agonist drugs fully occupy and activate the opioid receptors, mimicking the natural effects of endogenous endorphins and enkephalins. Thus, the greater the quantity of agonists administered, the more significant the analgesia and the more pronounced the adverse effects. Agonists are not limited by a ceiling effect.

The most bothersome of these side effects are the GI effects. It is common for patients taking these combinations to complain of constipation and gastric distress, as well as nausea. Because constipation occurs secondary to the stimulation of the opioid receptors, bulk-forming laxatives are of little benefit. Stimulant or irritant laxatives will be necessary to promote GI motility. Patients should be warned of the possibility of constipation, and it is prudent to suggest an appropriate laxative. In the category of stimulant/irritant laxatives,

TABLE 36.2
Commonly Used NSAIDs and Their Prescription Doses

Generic Name	Trade Name	Usual Prescription Dose (mg)	Dosing Schedule (h)
Aspirin	Various	325–1000	4–6
Celecoxib	Celebrex®	100–200	12
Choline magnesium trisalicylate	Triisate®	750–1000	12–24
Diclofenac potassium	Cataflam®	50–200	8
Diclofenac sodium	Voltaren®	50	8
Diflunisal	Dolobid®	250–500	8–12
Etodolac	Lodine®	200–400	6–8
Fenoprofen	Nalfon®	400	4–6
Flubiprofen	Ansaid®	50–100	8
Ibuprofen	Motrin®, Advil®, Nuprin®	200–800	4–8
Indomethacin	Indocin®	25–50	8–12
Ketoprofen	Orudis®	25–75	6–12
Ketorolac	Toradol®	30–60 i.m. stat, then 15–30 mg every 6 hours, not to exceed 150 mg 1st day or 200 mg/day thereafter	As described
Meclofenamate	Meclomen®	50–100	4–6
Mefanamic acid	Ponstel®	250	6
Nabumetone	Relafen®	500–1000	4–6
Naproxen	Naprosyn®	250–500	12
Naproxen sodium	Anaprox®	275–550	12
Oxaprozin	Daypro®	1200–1800	24
Phenylbutazone	Butazolidin®	100	6–8
Piroxicam	Feldene®	10–20	12–24
Rofecoxib	Vioxx®	12.5–25	24
		50 (acute pain)	24
Salsalate	Disalcid®	1000–1500	8–12
Sulinac	Clinoril®	150–200	6–8
Tolmetin	Tolectin®	200–800	6–8

the most frequently recommended choices are, in order, Dulcolax®, Correctol®, Ex-Lax®, and Sennakot® ("Pharmacists' Top Choices," 1996). The popular bulk-forming laxative Metamucil® would be of little or no value in opioid-induced constipation.

Sedation can also occur; therefore, patients should be warned to take precautions in driving or operating machinery. Patients should also be cautioned about the additive central nervous system (CNS) depressant activity when alcohol is consumed.

Although codeine is an effective agonist, it has a significant limitation in its unique activity. It appears to act as an agonist/antagonist or partial agonist (see explanation under seventh-line pharmacotherapy) in that it yields added analgesia up to approximately 65 mg. Doses exceeding 65 mg appear to produce no adsded benefit yet significantly increase the complications of adverse effects, especially constipation.

SIXTH-LINE PHARMACOTHERAPY

If the outcomes of moderate pain management with codeine and codeine-like combinations are not satisfac-

tory, consideration should be given to the use of tramadol (Ultram®). Tramadol has the unique ability to activate the mu-opioid receptor as well as inhibiting norepinephrine reuptake, much like the newer antidepressants. In doses of 50 to 100 mg every 4 to 6 hours, not to exceed 400 mg/day, this drug has been quite effective in some patients. However, because it has far less affinity for opioid receptors when compared with the classic opioids, it should not be given in combination with other narcotics.

Tramadol is also given intravenously (i.v.), intramuscularly (i.m.), subcutaneously (s.c.), and rectally in 100-mg doses. It can be administered to children over the age of 1 year at a dose calculated on the basis of weight (1–2 mg/ kg).

Because of tramadol's unique pharmacologic activity, it may prove to be effective in patients who have a combination of nociceptive and neuropathic pain syndromes. As with other antineuropathic pain management regimens, the effects of tramadol may be delayed, requiring a 10-day trial before final management decisions are made.

SEVERE PAIN

SEVENTH-LINE PHARMACOTHERAPY

For pain conditions that are considered severe, more potent pharmacotherapy is necessary. Three rather obvious criteria should be considered an indication for aggressive treatment of pain with a narcotic agent such as morphine: (1) if the clinician has previously tried non-narcotics in reasonable doses and has achieved less than effective results, (2) if the pain is considered significantly more debilitating than moderate pain, and (3) if the patient has a history of pain relief when narcotics are used. If any of these criteria are met and rapid relief is required, then a narcotic is appropriate.

Of the parenteral narcotics available, morphine sulfate is clearly the standard. Although it should be remembered that oral dosage forms are preferred unless the patient is in acute distress, the clinician should not hesitate to administer morphine sulfate injection in severe acute pain situations.

Morphine is an excellent narcotic analgesic because it is a pure agonist. That is, it attaches to the narcotic receptors and activates them fully. Therefore, the greater the amount of morphine administered, the greater the number of narcotic receptors occupied, and the greater the analgesia. Agonists have no therapeutic ceiling (except for codeine) and thus are effective for long periods of time as the dose is steadily increased to achieve greater pain relief. Therefore, they are very effective in progressive diseases such as cancer (malignant pain).

Mixed agonist-antagonists fully occupy both principal receptors but activate just the kappa receptors, blocking activation of the mu component of the receptor complex. Therefore, these drugs (e.g., pentazocine, nalbuphine, butorphanol) exhibit a ceiling effect, and increased doses do not provide increased analgesia above the ceiling level. This is because no matter how much of the mixed-action drug is given, the blocked component of the occupied receptor complex cannot be activated to provoke increased analgesia.

Partial agonist narcotics (e.g., buprenorphine) act similarly to mixed agonist-antagonists in that they activate only part of the receptor complex (the mu site). They do not occupy the kappa sites; however, by partially occupying the complex, they effectively block the occupation and activation of the kappa narcotic receptor component of the receptor complex.

Because of the nature of receptor occupation, there is no justification for the use of more than one type of narcotic (i.e., agonist, agonist/antagonist, partial agonist). If an agonist were to be used in conjunction with a mixed-action or partial agonist, the results would not be favorable for (enhanced) analgesia. In fact, a diminished clinical response to the agonist could be anticipated because fewer receptor sites would be available for binding and activation. Narcotic characteristics and equivalencies are summarized in Table 36.3.

Acute Severe Pain Management

For acute severe pain, unlike other drug regimens in which the practitioner starts off at a relatively low dose and gradually ascends to higher doses or adds other drugs until the

TABLE 36.3
Commonly Used Opioids and Their Prescription Doses

Opioid	Trade Name	Opioid Type	p.o./i.m. Potency	Usual Oral Dose
Morphine		Agonist	3–6	10–100 mg every 4 h
Morphine extended release	MSCotin® RoxanoISR® Kadian®	Agonist	NA	15–100 mg every 12 h
Codeine		Agonist	NA	30–65 mg every 3–4 h
Methadone	Dolophine®	Agonist	2	5–20 mg daily
Hydromorphone	Dilaudid®	Agonist	5	4–8 mg every 4–6 h
Hydrocodone	Lorcet® Lortab® Vicodin®	Agonist	NA	30 mg every 3–4 h
Oxycodone	Roxicodone® Percocet®, Percodan® Tylox®	Agonist	NA	30 mg every 3–4 h
Oxymorphone	Numorphan®	Agonist	NA	NA (i.m. 1 mg every 3–4 h)
Pentazocine	Talwin®	Agonist/antagonist	3	50–150 mg every 3–4 h
Nalbuphine	Nubain®	Agonist/antagonist	NA	(i.m. 10 mg every 3–4 h)
Butorphanol	Stadol®	Agonist/antagonist	NA	NA (i.m. 2 mg every 3–4 h)
Buprenorphine	Buprenex	Partial agonist	NA	NA (i.m. 0.3–0.4 mg every 6–8 h)

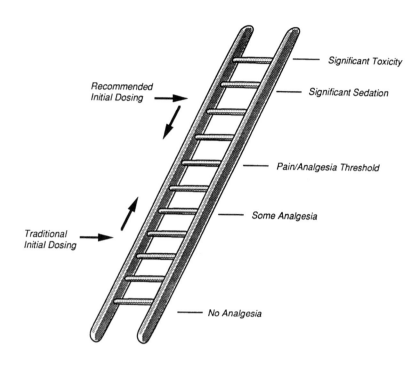

FIGURE 36.1 Analgesic dosing ladder.

condition is managed (e.g., hypertension, hyperlipidemia), the drug regimen should be equal to the task of alleviating the pain immediately. This philosophy of aggressive dosing, termed "descending the ladder," is graphically illustrated in Figure 36.1. It has gained acceptance, at least partially, because too often fears of addiction and respiratory depression have led to too timid dosing of narcotics (Marks & Sachar, 1973). Simply stated, a dose that is felt to be adequate should be administered, and the subsequent doses are slightly tapered down until the pain threshold is discovered. Then, the dose is adjusted just slightly upward to alleviate the pain on an around-the-clock basis without overdosing. This system should lead to lower maintenance doses because the patient is rapidly rather than gradually brought into the realm of comfort. Care must be taken for the opioid-naïve patient.

A usual initial dose of parenteral morphine sulfate (i.e., i.m. or s.c.) for an adult is 10 to 20 mg. If an effective oral dose of morphine is already established, then one sixth to one third of that dose should be administered parenterally. If the pain is excruciating, then a larger dose is appropriate before beginning to descend the ladder. After the initial dose, the patient will need repeated doses every 4 to 6 hours. With parenteral morphine, the patient should begin to feel relief within a few minutes. If morphine is going to be continued, it should be changed to an oral dosage form, as there is no real advantage to continuation of the parenteral form (Twycross, 1974). For long-term maintenance, consideration should be given to long-acting morphine sulfate (MSCotin®, RoxanolSR®). The long-acting dosage form appears to provide 12-hour

relief at a dosage level of approximately 75% of the immediate-release oral dosage forms (Cundiff, et al., 1988).

As with all aggressive treatment regimens, the clinician should be most diligent in monitoring side effects, especially because the opiates have CNS depressant activity. Sedation should be carefully evaluated. Significant sedation will present itself at narcotic levels above the pain threshold. The ideal dose will be achieved if sedation is not significant and pain control is maintained. Sedation later in therapy may be an indication of an accumulation toxicity effect. If this is the case, it may be difficult to cut back the dose late in therapy without causing the pain to recur. Short of reinitiating the dosing regimen, the use of amphetamines or methylphenidate (Ritalin®) may be contemplated, especially in terminal care. While the use of one drug to cover up the adverse effects of another is considered irrational polypharmacy, for patients in acute distress, intractable pain, or for the terminally ill, the use of these CNS stimulants may be indicated as long as the sedation is simple sedation and not mental confusion, symptomatic of a more serious toxicity.

Respiratory depression is also a fear of many clinicians who administer potent doses of narcotics. The fear of respiratory depression appears to be misplaced. Although respiratory depression is fairly easy to demonstrate in non-pain patients, significant respiratory depression is not common in pain patients receiving narcotics (Walsh, et al., 1981). The adverse drug effects commonly associated with chronic narcotic use, including addiction and tolerance, will be addressed in the next section on chronic severe pain management.

Epidural injection of narcotics is another method of both rapid and longer-acting narcotic administration. Epidural (or extradural) injection of morphine will result in almost immediate pain relief, and that relief will continue for approximately four times the duration expected with oral or i.m. administration (Leavans, et al., 1982). The narcotic injection must be preservative-free. The logic associated with this form of drug delivery is that the narcotic, usually morphine, can be given nearer to the CNS to work directly on the receptors. As with other parenteral routes, epidural injection of morphine eliminates the first-pass effect of hepatic degradation, thereby allowing for lower doses to be equally effective as higher oral doses. Additionally, epidural injection may allow for even slightly lower doses than required for other parenteral narcotics because of the greater general systemic absorption of i.m.- or s.c.-administered doses. Therefore, the epidural/extradural route has been shown to have significant advantages for the obstetric pain patient. However, to date, few additional benefits have been achieved with this route for other pain patients, and adverse effect profiles for these administrations appear to be no better than those for conventional injections (McQuay, 1989). Significant itching has also accompanied epidural injections of narcotics. This seems to be alleviated with the combined use of hydroxyzine (Vistaril®, Atarax®) with the narcotic.

Chronic Severe Pain Management

When a narcotic is indicated in chronic pain care, morphine sulfate is the narcotic of choice. There are no advantages to parenteral administration of morphine in chronic pain care, except in the few cases where the patient cannot take or cannot tolerate oral medications. The initial oral dose of morphine sulfate is variable, based upon the clinician's assessment of the severity and nature of the chronic pain. Doses of from 10 to 100 mg may be required. Tablet strengths customarily available are 10, 15, 30, and 100 mg. There are no established upper limits of the dose to be given to a patient suffering from severe chronic pain. Many clinicians feel that any dose that helps the patient in maintaining a relatively comfortable state, without causing mental confusion or significant respiratory depression, is justified. Because of the nature of the opioid receptors and pure agonist narcotics (e.g., morphine), raising the dose will always increase the analgesia (i.e., no therapeutic ceiling). Oral morphine will have to be redosed every 4 hours to achieve continued pain relief. Sustained-release, 12-hour oral morphine formulations (MSCotin®, RoxanolSR®) have proven to be very effective, and they have been shown to actually diminish the 24-hour total dose of morphine required. Recently, Kadian®, a sustained-release, single-daily-dose (24-hour) formulation, has been approved by the FDA.

Dosing Schedule

Some clinicians believe that when chronic pain is not manifesting itself, the patient should not be taking medication. Therefore, these practitioners feel that chronic pain medication should be administered on an as-needed (prn) basis. It has now been demonstrated that around-the-clock administration of pain medication provides superior analgesia. Not allowing the pain symptoms to recur causes less mental and physical trauma and can actually lead to less medication used with better pain control. Pain memory (when the patient begins to feel pain and anticipate continued pain distress) can be eliminated when the pain control pharmacotherapy is regularly scheduled.

Toxicity

The extended use of opioids in chronic pain management has not led to widespread toxicity in cancer patients (Kreek, 1973, 1978).

Respiratory Depression

Activation of the mu-opioid receptor will decrease the responsiveness of the respiratory centers (Mueller, et al., 1982; Martin, 1967), along with increasing analgesia. However, in chronic dosing, the clinical consequences of this are limited (Walsh, et al., 1981). It appears that if the opioid is not causing clouded thought processes, respiratory risk is minimal (Lipman, 1988).

Tolerance and Addiction

With chronic narcotic use, there persists a fear of tolerance and addiction. Clearly, these fears are overemphasized. In studies, addiction has been shown to be of minor concern in the patient with chronic pain. In one study, nearly 12,000 pain patients receiving narcotics were followed, and of these, only four patients became addicted (Porter, et al., 1980). Tolerance does not appear to be a common characteristic among pain sufferers in acute distress. Increasing doses of narcotics is likely attributable to the normal progression of the disease process rather than tolerance in acute pain cases. However, in chronic conditions, tolerance is significant. Patients on long-term narcotic therapy will require increased doses, unless therapeutic and receptor-stimulation substitution is attempted.

Drug dependence is not a significant problem in the pain patient population. In the large study of over 12,000 pain care cases, only 0.03% were inadvertently addicted to their narcotic drugs. Of course, overdependence on narcotics without a real need for them is indefensible; however, a summary of several studies indicates that toxicity and addiction are not significant problems, and efficacy is achievable in chronic nonmalignant narcotic pharmacotherapy (Portenoy, 1996).

Patient-Controlled Analgesia

Another system that has gained popularity is patient-controlled analgesia (PCA). A PCA device, about the size of a deck of playing cards, is programmed to deliver regular doses of a narcotic directly into the patient (usually i.m.), and the microprocessor is adjusted to a set dose for drug delivery around the clock. Additionally, the PCA device allows the patient to administer bolus injections of medication when the pain level increases. The device will not allow the patient to overdose, as limits are programmed into the portable device. The more sophisticated models can give the practitioner a printout of doses administered, including bolus doses administered by the patient. Studies have shown that PCA devices are very effective in controlling pain, with minimal side effects (White, 1988). A list of several commercially available PCA devices is given in Table 36.4. Most of these devices are simple microprocessors with small battery-driven motors that activate screw-driven plungers that inject predetermined amounts of medication into the muscle. Some clinicians prefer to add a steroid, such as dexamethasone (0.02 mg/ml), to the narcotic to limit needle trauma and inflammation. Also, the implant site should be rotated about every 4 days. With PCA devices, the patient has a renewed sense of being in control of his or her pain, which can be an exhilarating and liberating feeling for most chronic pain sufferers.

Pain Cocktails

The original pain cocktail is Brompton's mixture, dating back to the 1800s. It was formulated using morphine, cocaine, alcohol, and chloroform. It is now thought that the cocaine was used to numb the throat, and the chloroform was used to give the mixture a bitter taste, which was a requirement for all British medicines in those times. Because these two ingredients are not appropriate (and chloroform is not permitted in medications in the United States), contemporary pain cocktails, usually labeled as "hospice mixture," contain just morphine sulfate in solution. Some pain clinics allow their pain cocktails to include any other patient-specific medications that are physically compatible with the hydroalcoholic mixture. Frequently, antidepressant medications will be added but these are not required to justify the label "pain cocktail." The addition of other agents has been shown to have no demonstrable advantage over morphine sulfate solution alone.

OPIOID-INSENSITIVE PAIN

By definition, chronic pain that is opioid insensitive does not respond to narcotic analgesics. Usually, this pain is either aberrant or organic, with nerve compression or nerve destruction (McQuay, 1989). Nerve destruction is common in accident-related trauma, tumor-related disease, post-herpetic neuralgia, and trigeminal neuralgia. Patients that provide the greatest clinical challenge present with both opioid-sensitive (e.g., nociceptive) and opioid-insensitive (e.g., neuropathic) pain at different sites. With nerve-related chronic pain that is opioid insensitive, unconventional drug therapy is indicated. Trials with tricyclic antidepressants and anticonvulsants, such as

TABLE 36.4
Commonly Used PCA Devices

Device Name	Functions	Bolus	Prefilled Syringe	Security System	Lockout Interval Range
Abbott Lifecare Infusor 1821	PCA	Volume	Yes; 30 ml	Key	5–99 min
Abbott Lifecare Infusor 4100	PCA/continuous	mg	Yes; 30 ml	Key	5–99 min
Bard Ambulatory PCA	PCA/continuous	mg or volume	No; 100- or 250-ml reservoir	Yes	3–240 min
Baxter PCA System	PCA	Fixed volume prefilled	Use with Baxter Infusor, not mount	Optional pole	6 min fixed
Becton Dickinson PCA Infusor	PCA/continuous	mg	Yes; IMS prefilled, 30 ml, 60 ml	Key	5–99 min
Harvard PCA Pump 6464-001	PCA/continuous	Volume	Yes; 50 ml	Key	3–60 min
MiniMed PCA Device-404-S	PCA/continuous	Volume	No; 3-ml disp syringe	Case locks	0–799 min
Pancretec Provider-5000	PCA/continuous	mg or volume	No; use with 50–3,000-ml i.v. bag	Key	1 min–200 hr
Pharmacia Deltec-Model 5200 PXC	PCA/continuous	mg	No; use with medication cassette	Key	5–199 min
Stratofuse PCA PSM-9000	PCA/continuous	Volume	Yes; IMS prefilled, 30 ml	Key	5–60 min

carbamazepine (Tegretol®) and gabapentin (Neurontin®) have been shown to be effective in neuropathic and other opioid-insensitive pain syndromes.

ANTIDEPRESSANTS

While tricyclic antidepressants remain the mainstay in pharmacotherapy for neuropathic and opioid-insensitive pain, consideration must be given to the newer serotonin and norepinephrine reuptake inhibitors, of which venlafaxine (Effexor®) is the prime example. This category of antidepressant appears to mitigate neuropathic pain while presenting a minimum of side effects. It would appear that these drugs will receive significantly greater attention in pain care in the future.

Tricyclic antidepressants are rather curious analgesics. Clearly, antidepressant medications are effective in the treatment of endogenous depression. Because one of the symptoms of depression is chronic pain, usually vague in description, antidepressants exert an analgesic effect indirectly by combating the depressive illness. It has been postulated that tricyclics also have an intrinsic analgesic activity which assists in chronic pain management. This activity is secondary to the ability of tricyclics to effectively block the reuptake of serotonin. Additionally, tricyclics may also have a potentiating effect on narcotics, thereby facilitating chronic pain management. Also, tricyclics are effective for neuropathic pain. The analgesic activity of the tricyclics is most likely a combination of all three phenomena. Studies have demonstrated their effectiveness in the management of chronic pain in hundreds of patients (Tollison & Kriegel, 1988). The analgesic activity of tricyclics occurs within 5 to 7 days, rather than the 10 to 14 days required for their antidepressant effects. Usually, success is achieved at slightly lower than normal antidepressant doses.

ANTICONVULSANTS

Carbamazepine (Tegretol®) is also often effective in painful conditions not responsive to narcotics. It is dosed at 200 mg three times daily to start and then increased to as much as 800 mg daily. It is very effective in trigeminal neuralgia at higher doses.

Gabapentin (Neurontin®), another anticonvulsant, is similarly effective when dosed from 300 to 500 mg, with reports of efficacy at 900 to 1200 mg daily in divided doses (Rosner, Rubin, & Kestenbaum, 1996). Responsive patients most often describe diminished levels of pain within 48 hours.

Other Drugs

For opioid-insensitive conditions not responsive to either tricyclics or these two anticonvulsants, mexiletine (Mexitil®) should be considered. It is dosed at 450 mg daily. It

has been particularly helpful in neuropathic pain described as stabbing, burning, or warm sensations. Mexiletine should be given for a full week before pain management outcomes are evaluated.

Clonazepam (Klonopin®), dosed at 0.5 mg three times daily, is an alternative. It has been effective in combating phantom limb pain (Borg & Krijnen, 1996). It is also an agent that should be considered in combination with a tricyclic antidepressant in suspected neuropathies that are particularly nonresponsive to conventional treatments.

CHRONIC MALIGNANT PAIN

The World Health Organization (WHO) has developed a three-step approach to pain relief for the cancer patient. With malignancies that are customarily painful, the pain syndrome begins as mild pain, progresses to moderate pain, and further progresses to severe pain as the disease progresses. The three-step approach corresponds to the progressive nature of cancer. This approach is summarized in Figure 36.2 and described below.

Step 1: Aspirin, acetaminophen, or an NSAID is to be used in combination with an adjuvant for initial analgesia in malignant pain management. Analgesic adjuvants are not restricted to cases of malignant pain. These medications include tricyclic antidepressants, antihistamines, benzodiazepines, caffeine, dextroam-

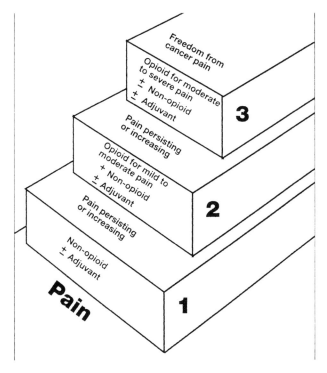

FIGURE 36.2 The WHO three-step analgesic ladder. (From World Heath Organization, 1996. Reproduced with permission.)

phetamine, steroids, laxatives, phenothiazines, and anticonvulsants. With the exception of tricyclic antidepressants and anticonvulsants (which provide direct and indirect pain relief), these analgesic adjuvants are given for their indirect benefits in pain management. The various reasons for using analgesic adjuvants include (1) direct analgesia (e.g., tricyclic antidepressants, anticonvulsants); (2) potentiation of narcotic analgesia (e.g., tricyclic antidepressants, caffeine, dextroamphetamine); (3) combating nausea (e.g., antihistamines, phenothiazines), alleviating anxiety related to pain syndromes (e.g., benzodiazepines, phenothiazines); (4) counteracting sedation (e.g., amphetamines); (5) alleviating nerve compression (e.g., steroids); (6) alleviating constipation (e.g., laxatives); and (7) alleviating itching (e.g., antihistamines).

Step 2: If the drugs used in the first step are ineffective, or become ineffective, in alleviating the pain, the initial drug should be continued in combination with an oral narcotic and adjuvant. In this step, codeine is the narcotic of choice in combination with aspirin, acetaminophen, or an NSAID. As for all persistent pain, the clinician must remember to recommend regular dosing on an around-the-clock basis. Of course, the patient need not be awakened for dosing during the night if sleeping. However, initial morning dosing should begin immediately upon awakening.

Step 3: When the patient fails to respond to second-step medications, these should be discontinued in favor of a more potent oral narcotic. Again, the preferred oral narcotic for cancer pain is morphine, in an oral dose sufficient to maintain patient comfort. This dose can be progressively increased without limit — all the while assessing the patient's respiration, mental status, and wakefulness. In cases of significant pain that requires very high morphine dosing, patients can be given stimulants (e.g., methylphenidate (Ritalin®)) to allow them to attend to personal and family-related business in the latter stages of a terminal malignancy. Theis simply no reason why terminal cancer patients should be allowed to spend their final days in pain. Physicians will surely balk at the prospect of huge doses of morphine, but the quality of life is far greater an issue than unfounded concern for the numeric value of the milligrams in a dose of analgesic medication.

MINOR CHRONIC MUSCLE PAIN

Muscle pain that is minor but bothersome can be treated topically if traditional oral analgesic and anti-inflammatory agents prove ineffective. These topical analgesic agents are classified as counterirritants, and they exhibit analgesic action by dilation of the vasculature and an increase in the blood flow to the affected muscle. The FDA advisory panel on nonprescription topical analgesics has labeled the following product ingredients as relatively more potent counterirritants, as well as safe and effective: allylisothiocyanate, ammonia water, methyl salicylate, and turpentine oil, capsaicin, capsicum, capsicum oleoresin. Many patients achieve substantial muscle pain relief with the appropriate use of these counterirritants, but patients should be warned to discontinue use of these products if excessive irritation develops.

SUMMARY

Many pain patients are undertreated because of unwarranted fears of adverse drug reactions on the part of clinicians, including respiratory depression, tolerance, and addiction. These effects would be extremely problematic; however, they do not seem to occur often enough to warrant timidity in the pain management approach. Pain is an excessively debilitating medical and psychologic problem that warrants aggressive initial treatment and diligent continued care.

REFERENCES

Anon. (1992). Antiarthritic medication usage 1991. *Statistical Bulletin, 73*, 25–34.

Anon. (1996). Pharmacists' top choices in OTCs for 1996. *Drug Topics Supplement, 140*, 17.

Bonica, J.J. (2001). History of pain concepts and therapies. In J.D. Loeser (Ed.), *The management of pain* (3rd ed., pp. 3–16). Philadelphia: Lippincott.

Bonica, J.J., & Coda, B.A.. (2001). General considerations of acute pain. In J.D. Loeser (Ed.), *The management of pain* (3rd ed., pp. 222–240). Philadelphia: Lippincott.

Borg, P.A.J., & Krijnen, H.J. (1996). Clonazepam for the treatment of lancinating phantom limb pain. *Clinical Journal of Pain, 12*(1), 59–62.

Brooks, P.M., & Day, R O. (1991). Nonsteroidal anti-inflammatory drugs—differences and similarities. *New England Journal of Medicine, 324*, 1716–1725.

Campa, J.A., & Payne, R. (1993). Pain syndromes due to cancer treatment. In R. B. Patt (Ed.), *Cancer pain* (pp. 130–143). Philadelphia: Lippincott.

Chen, Z.R., Irvine, R.J., Somogyi, A.A., & Bochner, F. (1991). Mu receptor binding of some commonly used opioids and their metabolites. *Life Sciences, 48*, 2165–2171.

Collin, E., Poulain, P., Gauvain-Piquard, A., Petit, G., et al. (1993). Is disease progression the major factor in morphine "tolerance" in cancer pain treatment? *Pain, 55,* 319–326.

Crabbe, S.J. (1990). Ketorolac: A non-narcotic analgesic. *Hospital Therapy, 15,* 755–764.

Cundiff, D., McCarthy, K., Saverese, J.J., et al. (1988). Evaluation of a cancer pain model for the testing of long-acting analgesics: The effect of MS Cotin in a double-blind, randomized crossover design. *Cancer, 63,* 2355–2359.

Giles, G.W.A., Kenny, G.N.C., Bullingham, R.E.S., et al. (1987). The morphine-sparing effect of ketorolac tromethamine. *Anesthesia, 42,* 727–731.

Information Resources. (1996). OTC sales by category—1995. *Drug Topics Supplement, 34,* 6.

Jacobson L., & Mariano, A.J. (2001). General considerations of chronic pain. In J.D. Loeser (Ed.), *The management of pain* (3rd ed., pp. 241–254). Philadelphia: Lippincott.

Kreek, M.J. (1973). Medical safety and side effects of methadone in tolerant individuals. *Journal of the American Medical Association, 223,* 665–668.

Kreek, M.J. (1978). Medical complications in methadone patients. *Annals of the New York Academy of Sciences, 311,* 110–134.

Leavans, M.E., Hill, C.S., Cech, C.A., et al. (1982). Intrathecal and intraventricular morphine for pain in cancer patients: Initial study. *Journal of Neurosurgery, 56,* 241.

Lewis, J.H. (1984). Hepatic toxicity of nonsteroidal anti-inflammatory drugs. *Clinical Pharmacy, 3,* 128.

Lipman, A.G. (1988). Pain management. In E.T. Herfindal, D.R. Gourley, & L.L. Hart (Eds.), *Clinical Pharmacy and Therapeutics* (pp. 945–962.). Baltimore: Williams & Wilkins.

Marks, R.M., & Sachar, E.J. (1973). Undertreatment of medical inpatients with narcotic analgesics. *Annals of Internal Medicine, 78,* 173.

Martin, W.R. (1967). Pharmacology of opioids. *Pharmacological Reviews, 35,* 283–323.

McQuay, H.J. (1989). Opioids in chronic pain. *British Journal of Anaesthesiology, 63,* 213–226.

Melzack, R., & Katz, J. (1994). Pain measurement in persons in pain. In P.D. Wall & R. Melzack (Eds.), *Textbook of pain* (3rd ed., pp. 337–351). New York: Churchill Livingstone.

Moertel, C.G., Ahmann, D.L., Taylor, W.F., et al. (1974). Relief of pain by oral medications. *Journal of the American Medical Association, 229,* 55.

Mueller, R.A., Lundberg, D.B., Breese, G.R., Hedner, J., Hedner, T., & Jonason, J. (1982). The neuropharmacy of respiratory control. *Pharmacological Reviews, 34,* 255–285.

O'Hara, D.A., Fragen, R.J., Kinzer, M., et al. (1987). Ketorolac tromethamine as compared with morphine sulfate for treatment of post-operative pain. *Clinical Pharmacology & Therapeutics, 41,* 556–561.

Portenoy, R.K. (1996). Opioid therapy for chronic nonmalignant pain: A review of the critical issues. *Journal of Pain and Symptom Management, 11*(4), 203–216.

Porter, J., et al. (1980). Addiction rare in patients treated with narcotics. *New England Journal of Medicine, 302,* 123.

Rosner, H., Rubin, L., & Kestenbaum, A. (1996). Gabapentin adjunctive therapy in neuropathic pain states. *Clinical Journal of Pain, 12*(1), 56–58.

Sabbe, M.B., & Yaksh, T.L. (1995). Pharmacology of spinal opioids. *Journal of Pain and Symptom Management, 5*(3), 191–203.

Seeff, L.B., et al. (1986). Acetaminophen hepatotoxicity in alcoholics—A therapeutic misadventure. *Annals of Internal Medicine, 104,* 399.

Supernaw, R.B. (1992). Alternative medical care in pain management: Selected thoughts on voodoo, science, and other things I learned in college. *American Journal of Pain Management, 2,* 52–54.

Taylor, H., & Curran, N.M. (Eds.). (1985). *The Nuprin pain report.* New York: Lou Harris and Associates.

Tollison, C.D. (1993). The magnitude of the problem. In R.S. Weiner (Ed.), *Innovations in pain management.* Orlando, FL: PMD Press.

Tollison, C.D., & Kriegel, M.L. (1988). Selected tricyclic antidepressants in the management of chronic benign pain. *Southern Medical Journal, 81*(5), 562–564.

Twycross, R.G. (1974). Clinical experiences with diamorphine in advanced malignant disease. *International Journal of Clinical Pharmacology, 9,* 184.

Walsh, T.D., Baxter, R., Bowerman, K., et al. (1981). High-dose morphine and respiratory function in chronic cancer pain. *Pain, S1,* 39.

White, P.F. (1988). Use of patient-controlled analgesia for management of acute pain. *Journal of the American Medical Association, 259,* 243–247.

World Health Organization (1986). *Cancer pain relief.* Geneva, Switzerland: WHO.

Yee, J.R., Koshiver, J.E., Allbon, C., et al. (1986). Comparison of intramuscular ketorolac tromethamine and morphine sulfate for analgesia of pain after major surgery. *Clinical Pharmacology & Therapeutics, 39,* 253–261.

Yee, J.R., Stanski, D., & Cherry, C. (1986). A comparison of analgesic efficacy of intramuscular ketorolac tromethamine and meperidine in post-operative pain. *Clinical Pharmacology & Therapeutics, 39,* 237.

37

The Role of Neural Blockade in the Management of Common Pain Syndromes

Steven D. Waldman, M.D., J.D.

INTRODUCTION

Pain is the most common medical complaint of civilized man. The Nuprin Pain Report estimates that there are over 70 million Americans with pain severe enough to require medical care (Saper, 1987). The cost of pain to society in terms of medical bills, lower productivity, and absenteeism is staggering. The purpose of this chapter is to provide the pain management specialist with an overview of the role of neural blockade in the management of common pain syndromes encountered in clinical practice. Practical suggestions to simplify the care of these sometimes-difficult patients are also included.

Neural blockade with local anesthetic can be used as a diagnostic procedure to identify specific pain pathways and to aid in the differential diagnosis as to the origin and site of pain. Neural blockade with local anesthetics can also be used in a prognostic manner to predict the effects of destruction of a given nerve. In addition to helping determine the efficacy of destruction of a given nerve, prognostic neural blockade can allow the patient an opportunity to experience the numbness, loss of function, and other side effects that may attend the destruction of a nerve. Therapeutic neural blockade with a local anesthetic, combined with steroids, or rarely a neurolytic agent, can be useful in relieving a variety of painful conditions. The addition of steroids to nerve blocks has extended the utility of this powerful pain-relieving modality. Steroids are thought to improve the efficacy of neural blockade via their ability to stabilize membranes and their salutory effect on the inflammatory process via both the prostaglandin and leukotriene cascades. Neural blockade should not be viewed as a stand-alone treatment for most pain syndromes, but should be intelligently integrated into a comprehensive treatment plan.

SYMPATHETIC NERVE BLOCKS

SPHENOPALATINE GANGLION BLOCK

Indications

Blockade of the sphenopalatine ganglion with local anesthetic is useful in the management of acute migraine, acute cluster headache, and a variety of facial neuralgias, including Sluder's, Vail's, and Gardner's syndromes (Diamond & Dalessio, 1982; Kitrelle, Grouse, & Seybold, 1985; Phero & Robbins, 1985a; Waldman, 1996a, 1998a). This technique may also be useful in status migrainous and chronic cluster headaches.

Anatomy

The sphenopalatine ganglion (pterygopalatine, nasal, or Meckel's ganglion) is located in the pterygopalatine fossa, posterior to the middle turbinate (Katz, 1994a; Waldman, 1998a). It is covered by a 1- to 5-ml layer of connective tissue and mucous membrane. The ganglion is a 5-mm triangular structure comprising the largest group of neurons in the head, outside the brain. Major branches extend from the sphenopalatine ganglion to the trigeminal nerve, carotid plexus, facial nerve, and the superior cervical ganglion.

0-8493-0926-3/02/$0.00+$1.50
© 2002 by CRC Press LLC

Technique

Sphenopalatine ganglion block is accomplished by the application of local anesthetic to the mucous membrane overlying the ganglion (Waldman, 1996a, 1998a) (see Figure 37.1). The patient is placed in the supine position. The cervical spine is then extended, and the anterior nares space is inspected for polyps, tumor, or foreign body. A small amount of 2% viscous lidocaine, 4% topical lidocaine, or 10% cocaine solution is then instilled into each nostril. The patient is asked to inhale briskly through the nose. This draws the local anesthetic into the posterior nasal pharynx, serving the double function of lubricating the nasal mucosa and providing topical anesthesia, allowing easier passage of 3½-in. cotton-tipped applicators. These applicators are saturated with the chosen local anesthetic and then advanced along the superior border of the middle turbinate until the tip comes in contact with the mucosa overlying the ganglion. Then, 1.2 ml local anesthetic is placed along the cotton-tipped applicator in each nostril. The applicator acts as a tampon, allowing the local anesthetic to remain in contact with the mucosa overlying the ganglion and then diffuse through the mucosa to the ganglion. The applicators are removed after 20 minutes. The patient's pulse, blood pressure, and respirations are monitored for untoward effects secondary to sphenopalatine ganglion block.

Practical Considerations

Clinical experience has shown that this technique can be useful in aborting the acute attack of migraine or cluster headaches (Diamond & Dalessio, 1982; Kitrelle, Grouse, & Seybold, 1985; Waldman, 1996a, 1998a). Its simplic-

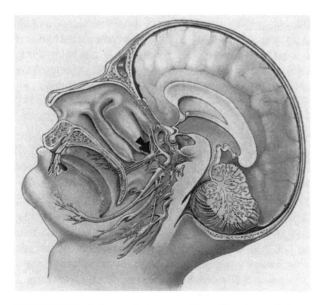

FIGURE 37.1 Sphenopalatine ganglion. (Courtesy of Astra Pharmaceutical Products, Inc. © Anazak Productions.)

ity lends itself to use at the bedside, in the emergency room, or in the headache or pain clinic. Although some experienced in this technique feel that cocaine represents a superior local anesthetic for this indication, the various political issues surrounding the use of this controlled substance make the use of other local anesthetics such as lidocaine a more practical option. For the acute headache sufferer, this technique can be combined with oxygen inhalation via mask through the mouth while the cotton-tipped applicators are in place. Experience indicates that this technique will abort approximately 80% of acute migraine or cluster headaches. This technique is utilized on a daily basis for chronic headache and facial pain conditions, with the end point being total pain relief. The author's clinical experience suggests that pain relief will generally occur within five to six daily sphenopalatine ganglion blocks.

Complications

The major complication with this technique is epistaxis. This complication occurs more frequently during the winter months when forced-air heating may cause drying of the nasal mucosa. Because of the highly vascular nature of the nasal mucosa, local anesthetic toxicity may occur if attention is not paid to the total maximum milligram dose of local anesthetic utilized to carry out sphenopalatine ganglion block. Occasionally, patients will experience significant orthostatic hypotension following sphenopalatine ganglion block. For this reason, the patient should be carefully monitored following the block, moved to a sitting position, and allowed to ambulate only with assistance.

STELLATE GANGLION BLOCK

Indications

Stellate ganglion block is indicated in the treatment of reflex sympathetic dystrophy of the face, neck, upper extremity, and upper thorax, as well as sympathetically mediated pain of malignant origin. Stellate ganglion block is also useful in the treatment of acute herpes zoster and postherpetic neuralgia (Waldman, 1998b, 2001a; Waldman & Waldman, 1987). This technique may help salvage fingers in patients suffering from vascular compromise of the upper extremity due to Raynaud's disease, frostbite, or other forms of acute and chronic vascular insufficiency (Waldman, 1998b). Clinical reports suggest that stellate ganglion blocks may also be useful in the palliation of some atypical vascular headaches and facial pain syndromes. Patients suffering from upper extremity postmastectomy pain and edema may also benefit from stellate ganglion blocks with local anesthetic and steroid.

Anatomy

The stellate ganglion is located between the anterior lateral surface of the seventh cervical vertebral body and the neck of the first rib (Katz, 1994b). The ganglion lies central to the vertebral artery and the transverse process, and is separated by the longus coli muscle. The ganglion is medial to the common carotid artery and jugular vein, and lateral to the trachea and esophagus.

Technique

The medial edge of the sternocleidomastoid muscle is identified as the level of the cricothyroid notch (C6). The sternocleidomastoid muscle is then displaced laterally with two fingers. The pulsations of the carotid artery should then be identified. The skin medial to the carotid pulsation is prepped with alcohol, and a 1½-in., 22-gauge needle is advanced until contact is made with the transverse process of C6. The needle is then withdrawn approximately 2 mm and careful aspiration is carried out; 7 ml of 0.5% preservative-free bupivicaine or 1% preservative-free lidocaine is then injected. The addition of a depot steroid preparation such as methylprednisolone to the local anesthetic solution is useful in patients suffering from reflex sympathetic dystrophy or other pain syndromes that have a significant inflammatory component (e.g., acute herpes zoster). Careful monitoring of pulse, blood pressure, and respirations is indicated following stellate ganglion block.

Practical Considerations

Daily stellate ganglion block with local anesthetic either alone or in combination with steroid is beneficial for the previously mentioned pain syndromes. Careful explanation to the patient regarding the special side effect of Horner's syndrome from blockade of the stellate ganglion should be given prior to implementation of stellate ganglion block to avoid undue patient anxiety. Local anesthetic should never be injected if the transverse process of C6 cannot be identified with the needle, as doing so will lead to an unacceptable high rate of potentially life-threatening complications.

Complications

Hematoma, hoarseness due to blockade of the laryngeal nerves, difficulty in swallowing, and pneumothorax can occur. Due to the proximity of the great vessels of the neck, intravascular injection, with almost immediate local anesthetic drug toxicity, is a distinct possibility if careful aspiration and needle placement is not carried out. Epidural, subdural, and subarachnoid anesthesia can occur if the needle is allowed to pass between the transverse process of C5 and C6 and impinge upon the cervical root.

CELIAC PLEXUS BLOCK

Indications

Celiac plexus block with local anesthetic is indicated as a diagnostic maneuver to determine if flank, retroperitoneal, or upper abdominal pain is sympathetically medicated via the celiac plexus (Portenoy & Waldman, 1991). This technique is also used in a prognostic manner to determine if celiac plexus block with neurolytic solution, such as alcohol or phenol, will provide relief of the pain of chronic pancreatitis or, more commonly, pain of upper abdominal and retroperitoneal malignancy, such as carcinoma of the pancreas, adrenal gland, etc. Daily celiac plexus block with local anesthetic and depot steroid is also used in the palliation of pain secondary to acute pancreatitis. Clinical reports suggest that early implementation of celiac plexus block with local anesthetic and/or steroid may markedly reduce the morbidity and mortality associated with acute pancreatitis (Waldman, 2001).

Anatomy

The celiac plexus is situated in the prevertebral area at the level of T12-L1 vertebral body (Raj, 1985). It is composed of the ganglia of the right and left celiac, superior mesenteric, and aorticorenal ganglia and the dense network of sympathetic nerve fibers that connect them.

Technique

Diagnostic celiac plexus block with local anesthetic can be performed without radiographic guidance. However, it is the clinical impression of many pain management specialists that neurolytic celiac plexus block can be performed most safely utilizing computed tomography (CT) guidance or, if CT guidance is unavailable, fluoroscopy. The use of radiographic guidance should improve not only the safety but also the efficacy of the following technique.

The patient is well hydrated with intravenous fluids and is placed prone on the CT scanning table. A scout film is obtained to identify the T12-L1 interspace. A CT scan is then taken through this area. The scan is reviewed for position of the aorta relative to the vertebral body, the position of intra-abdominal and retroperitoneal organs, and the distortion of normal anatomy due to tumor, previous surgery, or adenopathy. The level at which the scan was taken is then identified on the patient's skin and marked with a gentian violet marker. The skin is prepped with antiseptic solution. The skin and subcutaneous tissues at a point approximately 2½ in. from the left of the midline are then anesthetized with 1% lidocaine utilizing a 22-gauge, 1½-in. needle. A 13-cm, 22-gauge styleted Hinck needle is then placed through the anesthetized area and is advanced until the posterior wall of the aorta is encountered. The needle is then advanced into the aorta and the stylet is removed. A free flow of arterial blood should then be present. A well-lubricated, 5-cc glass syringe filled with preservative-free saline is then attached to the Hinck needle, and the needle and syringe are advanced through the anterior wall of the aorta (Feldstein, Waldman, & Allen, 1985). The glass syringe is removed, and a small amount of 0.5% lidocaine in solution with water-soluble contrast media is then injected through the needle. A CT scan at this same level is again taken. The scan is reviewed for the placement of the needle and, most importantly, for the spread of contrast. Contrast should be seen in the pre-aortic area surrounding the aorta. None of the contrast should be retrocrural. After satisfactory placement and spread of contrast is confirmed, 12 to 15 cc absolute alcohol or 6% aqueous phenol is then injected through the needle. The needle is flushed with a small amount of saline and then removed. The patient is observed carefully for hemodynamic changes, including hypotension and tachycardia secondary to the resulting profound sympathetic blockade.

Practical Considerations

CT-guided celiac plexus neurolysis utilizing the loss of resistance technique has been shown to be safe as well as efficacious for treatment of the above-mentioned pain syndromes (Liebarman & Waldman, 1990). This technique can be performed in the lateral position for patients who are unable to lie prone because of intractable abdominal pain or because of colostomy, ileostomy appliances, and the like. This technique avoids the possibility of spread of neurolytic substance onto the lumbar plexus. Posterior retrocrural spread of local anesthetic and contrast injected prior to injection of the neurolytic substance will alert the clinician to the possibility of this complication, and the needle can be repositioned. It is the author's clinical impression that the higher resolution and ease of identification of anatomic structures make the use of the CT scanner far superior to the use of fluoroscopy for this technique (Liebarman & Waldman, 1990). Celiac plexus block utilizing the anterior approach with either CT or ultrasound guidance may also be an option for patients who are unable to assume the prone position.

Complications

The most feared complication of celiac plexus neurolysis is the inadvertent injection of neurolytic substance onto the lumbar plexus, epidurally, subarachnoid, or intravascular. Inappropriate needle placement can result in damage to the kidneys. If the needle is placed too far anterior, injection into the pancreas or into the peritoneal cavity or liver can occur. As mentioned, the incidences of these complications can be markedly reduced by the use of CT guidance.

When properly performed, this technique results in profound sympathetic neural blockade. In the cancer patient who may have compromised cardiac reserve, this hypotension can be life-threatening. For this reason, the patient should be well hydrated prior to the procedure, and blood pressure should be monitored closely following the procedure. The patient should be cautioned that orthostatic hypotension may persist for a period of days, and the patient should get up only with assistance until the orthostatic hypotension has been resolved.

LUMBAR SYMPATHETIC NERVE BLOCK

Indications

Lumbar sympathetic nerve block with local anesthetic is indicated as a diagnostic maneuver to determine if lower extremity pain is sympathetically mediated via the lumbar sympathetic chain and for sympathetic dystrophy of the lower extremity. Prognostically, the lumbar sympathetic chain can be blocked with local anesthetic to determine if destruction of the lumbar sympathetic chain with neurolytic substances such as phenol and alcohol, radio-frequency neurolysis, or surgical excision of a portion of the lumbar sympathetic chain will improve blood flow and/or relief of pain of the lower extremities. This technique is used therapeutically to treat acute and chronic peripheral vascular insufficiency, ischemia secondary to frostbite, acute herpes zoster of the lower extremities, and a variety of peripheral neuropathic pains of the lower extremities (Lobstrom & Cousins, 1988). Lumbar sympathetic block has also been utilized to palliate the pain of impacted renal or ureteral calculi.

Anatomy

The lumbar sympathetic ganglion lies along the anterolateral surface of the lumbar vertebral bodies and antromedial to the psoas muscle (Raj, 1985). The anterior vena cava lies just anterior to the right sympathetic chain, and the aorta lies anterior and slightly medial to the sympathetic chain on the left. The sympathetic innervation of the lower extremity arises from preganglionic fibers that take their origin from the cell bodies located in the T10-L2 levels of the spinal cord. Nearly all postganglionic fibers to the lower extremity leave the sympathetic chain interval below L2. Anterior to the chain is the visceral peritoneum and the great vessels.

Technique

The technique of lumbar sympathetic block and neurolysis is quite similar to that described in the section on celiac plexus neurolysis. The patient is placed in the prone position on the CT scanner table with a pillow underneath the abdomen to allow flexion of the thoraco-lumbar spine. This opens up the space between adjacent transverse processes. A scout film is taken and the L2 vertebral body is identified. The skin overlying the transverse process of L2 is marked with a gentian violet marker and then prepped with antiseptic solution. Utilizing a $1^1/_2$-in., 22-gauge needle, the skin and subcutaneous tissues are anesthetized with 1% lidocaine. A 22-gauge, 13-cm styleted needle is then advanced through the previously anesthetized area until the tip rests against the vertebral body. The needle is then redirected in a trajectory to pass just lateral to the vertebral body. A well-lubricated glass syringe filled with preservative-free saline is then attached, and loss of resistance technique is utilized while the needle is advanced through the body of the psoas muscle. As soon as the needle tip passes through the fascia of the muscle, a loss of resistance is encountered. This should place the needle adjacent to the sympathetic chain. A small amount of local anesthetic and water-soluble contrast media is then injected to ensure appropriate spread of contrast material in the prevertebral region. Then 12 cc of 0.5% preservative-free lidocaine or absolute alcohol is injected via the needle. The needle is flushed with preservative-free saline and removed. The patient is then observed carefully for hypotension and tachycardia secondary to sympathetic blockade.

Practical Considerations

The use of CT guidance when performing lumbar sympathetic neurolysis can markedly decrease the risk of complications. The patient should be warned that, in all likelihood, he or she will experience some backache following the procedure due to needle trauma to the muscles of posture. The patient should also be advised that following lumbar sympathetic block, the affected lower extremity may feel hot and somewhat swollen relative to the nonaffected extremity. This side effect is normal and will go away with time. Despite the use of radiographic guidance, a small percentage of patients will suffer persistent ilioinguinal or genitofemoral neuralgia due to either direct needle trauma or from spread of the neurolytic solution onto the nerve itself.

Complications

Complications (Lobstrom & Cousins, 1988) of lumbar sympathetic block are similar to those of celiac plexus neurolysis. Because the needle tip is more medial in its trajectory, damage to lumbar nerve roots and their branches as they exit the spinal column is a distinct possibility.

Hypogastric Plexus Block

Indications

Hypogastric plexus block with local anesthetic is indicated as a diagnostic maneuver to determine if pelvic pain is sympathetically medicated via the hypogastric plexus and for sympathetic dystrophy of the pelvis. Prognostically, the hypogastric plexus can be blocked with local anesthetic to determine if destruction of the plexus with neurolytic substances such as phenol and alcohol, radio-frequency neurolysis, or surgical excision of the plexus will provide relief of pain in the previously mentioned areas. This technique is used therapeutically to treat acute and chronic pelvic pain, acute herpes zoster of the sacral roots, cancer pain of the pelvic viscera, pelvic reflex sympathetic dystrophy, and a variety of peripheral neuropathic pains of the pelvis due to trauma, endometriosis, etc. Rectal pain, including proctalgia fugax, may also respond to therapeutic hypogastric plexus block with local anesthetic and steroid (Waldman, Wilson, & Kreps, 1991).

Anatomy

The hypogastric plexus represents the caudal continuation of the lumbar sympathetic chain. The plexus lies along the anterolateral surface of the sacrum just below the L5-S1 interspace. The iliac vessels lie just anterior to the psoas muscle and just lateral to the hypogastric plexus.

Technique

The technique of hypogastric plexus block is quite similar to that described in the section on celiac plexus neurolysis. The patient is placed in the prone position on the CT scanner table with a pillow underneath the lower abdomen to allow flexion of the lower lumbar spine. This opens up the space between L5 transverse processes and the sacral alae. A scout film is taken and the L4-L5 interspace is identified. The skin overlying the interspace is marked with a gentian violet marker and then prepped with antiseptic solution. Utilizing a $1^1/_2$-in., 22-gauge needle, the skin and subcutaneous tissues are anesthetized with 1% lidocaine. A 22-gauge, 13-cm styleted needle is then advanced through the previously anesthetized area and directed approximately 30° caudad and 30° mediad toward the anterior lateral portion of the L5-S1 interspace. If the transverse process of the L5 vertebral body is encountered, the needle is withdrawn and directed slightly more caudad. If the needle impinges on the L5 vertebral body, the needle is redirected in a trajectory to pass just lateral to the vertebral body. A well-lubricated glass syringe filled with preservative-free saline is then attached, and loss of resistance technique is utilized while the needle is advanced through the body of the psoas muscle. As soon as the needle tip passes through the fascia of the muscle, a loss of resistance is encountered. This should place the needle adjacent to the hypogastric plexus. After careful aspiration, a small amount of local anesthetic and water-soluble contrast media is then injected to ensure appropriate spread of contrast material in the presacral region in the retroperitoneal space. Then, 10 cc of 0.5% preservative-free lidocaine or absolute alcohol is injected via the needle in incremental doses after repeated careful aspiration. If alcohol is utilized, the needle is flushed with preservative-free saline and removed. The patient is then observed carefully for hypotension and tachycardia secondary to sympathetic blockade or bleeding into the presacral space from the iliac vessels. Unless there is significant scarring from previous surgery or tumor mass and/or adenopathy, there will be contralateral spread of the injectate, making placement of a second needle unnecessary (Waldman, et al., 1991).

Practical Considerations

The use of CT guidance when performing hypogastric plexus neurolysis can markedly decrease the risk of complications. The patient should be warned that, in all likelihood, he or she will experience some backache following the procedure due to needle trauma to the muscles of posture. Despite the use of radiographic guidance, a small percentage of patients will suffer persistent ilioinguinal or genitofemoral neuralgia due to either direct needle trauma or from spread of the neurolytic solution onto the nerve itself. Because of the proximity of the iliac vessels to the hypogastric plexus, the potential for intravascular injection is high. The presacral space can accommodate significant amounts of blood from traumatized vessels before tamponade should occur. The use of CT guidance should help decrease the incidence of this complication as well as needle trauma to the cauda equina. The potential for bowel and bladder difficulties and sexual dysfunction is always a possibility when performing hypogastric plexus neurolysis. Furthermore, it should be remembered that many patients suffering from pelvic pain syndromes of obscure etiology may have a significant behavioral component to their pain symptomatology.

Complications

Complications following hypogastric plexus block are similar to those of celiac plexus and lumbar sympathetic neurolysis. Because the needle tip is in close proximity to the iliac vessels and cauda equina, damage to these structures is a distinct possibility. The possibility of bowel and bladder difficulties and sexual dysfunction following hypogastric plexus neurolysis makes it advisable that this technique be reserved primarily for patients suffering from pelvic pain of malignant origin, although neurolysis of the hypogastric plexus can be used in carefully selected patients suffering from intractable benign pain syndromes.

SOMATIC NERVE BLOCKS

OCCIPITAL NERVE BLOCK

Indications

Occipital nerve block with local anesthetic and steroid may be beneficial in the management of occipital neuralgia (Raj, 1989). Occipital neuralgia is characterized by suboccipital pain that is aching in nature. This pain radiates over the posterior lateral scalp. Superimposed electric-shock-like pain may also be present. With prolonged attacks of occipital neuralgia, the patient may also complain of deep retro-orbital ache. Pressure over the greater and lesser occipital nerve on the affected side may recreate the patient's pain symptomatology. In some patients, occipital neuralgia may trigger migraine headaches.

Anatomy

The greater occipital nerve perforates the semispinalis capitis and the trapezius muscles, approximately 3 cm lateral to the occipital protrubance, at the level of the linea nuchae. It is medial to the occipital artery, which can be palpated in some patients. The lesser occipital nerve is approximately $2\frac{1}{2}$ cm lateral to the greater occipital nerve and is found directly above and behind the mastoid process.

Technique

Deep palpation of the musculature overlying the greater occipital nerve will generally recreate the patient's pain symptomatology and help localize this nerve's exit from the bony skull. If the occipital artery can be palpated, this will serve as an additional guide. The skin and hair overlying the greater occipital nerve is then prepped with alcohol, and 10 ml of 0.5% bupivicaine and 80 mg methylprednisolone is injected around the greater and lesser occipital nerve. Nerve blocks are carried out on a daily or every-other-day basis.

Practical Considerations

Occipital neuralgia is greatly overdiagnosed. Many patients carrying this diagnosis actually suffer from tension-type headaches. This may explain the less than optimal long-term results that many patients who undergo occipital nerve block experience. If the patient who carries a working diagnosis of occipital neuralgia does not respond to daily blocks of long-acting local anesthetic and depot-steroid preparations, a trial of cervical epidural steroids is indicated. Because the pain of posterior fossa tumor or tumor compromising the upper cervical nerve roots may mimic the pain of occipital neuralgia, these potentially life-threatening conditions must be ruled out prior to implementation of occipital nerve block. Currently, magnetic resonance image scanning of the posterior fossa and upper cervical spine is the best way to rule out occult pathology in this anatomic region.

Complications

This block should be performed with care in patients who are anticoagulated. The needle should not be directed medially, or inadvertent subarachnoid injection with resultant total spinal anesthesia may occur.

TRIGEMINAL NERVE BLOCK

Indications

Use of trigeminal nerve block with local anesthetic and steroids serves as an excellent adjunct to drug treatment of trigeminal neuralgia (Waldman, 2000c, 2001d). The use of this technique allows rapid palliation of pain while oral medications are being titrated to effective levels (Phero & Robbins, 1985b). This technique may also be of value in patients suffering from atypical facial pain. Other indications for trigeminal nerve block include pain in maxillary neoplasm, cluster headaches uncontrolled by sphenopalatine ganglion block, and acute herpes zoster and postherpetic neuralgia in the area of trigeminal nerve not controlled by stellate ganglion block.

Anatomy

The trigeminal nerve is the largest of the cranial nerves, containing both sensory and motor fibers. The trigeminal nerve can be blocked utilizing an extra oral approach via the coronoid notch into the pterygopalatine fossa (Waldman, 1996a). The fossa is a triangular space between the pterygoid process of the sphenoid bone and maxilla of the upper part infratemporal fossa.

Technique

Palpation of the coronoid notch is facilitated by having the patient open and close the mouth. The notch should be encountered approximately 4 cm anterior to the acoustic auditory meatus (see Figure 37.2). The skin is anesthetized with antiseptic solution, and a $1\frac{1}{2}$-in., 22-gauge needle is directed through the middle of the coronoid notch. The tip of the needle may encounter the lateral lamina of the pterygoid process. If blockade of the maxillary nerve is desired, the needle is withdrawn into the subcutaneous tissue and is redirected with the tip 1 cm further anteriorly and 1 cm further superiorly from the first bony contact. Paresthesia may be elicited in the area of the maxillary nerve. If blockade of the mandibular nerve is desired, the needle is withdrawn into the subcutaneous tissue and readjusted with the tip 0 cm posteriorly and 1 cm inferiorly. Paresthesia in the distribution of the mandibular nerve may be elicited. After careful aspiration, 5

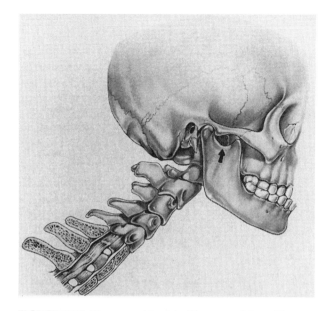

FIGURE 37.2 The coronoid notch. (Courtesy of Astra Pharmaceutical Products, Inc. © Anazak Productions.)

to 7 ml of 0.5% preservative-free bupivicaine in combination with 80 mg of methylprednisolone is injected. Subsequent daily nerve blocks are carried out in a similar manner, substituting 40 ml methylprednisolone for the initial 80-ml dose (Waldman, 2000a).

Practical Considerations

This technique represents an excellent emergency treatment for uncontrolled pain of trigeminal neuralgia. It can be utilized while carbamezepine (Tegretol), liorisal (Baclofen), phenytoin (Dilantin), or other medications are being titrated. With patients suffering from atypical facial pain secondary to temporomandibular joint dysfunction, this technique can be utilized to allow physical therapy and range of motion of the temporomandibular joint.

Complications

The major complication of trigeminal nerve block is inadvertent vascular injection. The pterygopalatine fossa is traversed with a large number of arteries and veins; and for this reason, careful and frequent aspiration should be carried out during injection of local anesthetic. Needle damage to this vasculature can result in significant hematoma formation. Although self-limited, it is recommended that patients be advised of this potential untoward effect so they will not be unduly alarmed should it occur.

EPIDURAL NERVE BLOCK

Indications

The use of epidural nerve blocks with local anesthetic and/or steroid is useful in the diagnosis and treatment of a variety of pain syndromes. The efficacy of this technique has been demonstrated for the relief of pain secondary to acute and chronic cervical, thoracic, and lumbar strain and radiculopathy, spinal stenosis, bilateral sympathetically maintained pain such as reflex sympathetic dystrophy, peripheral vascular insufficiency, or ischemic pain secondary to frostbite. Epidural neural blockade with local anesthetic and/or steroid is also useful in the management of acute herpes zoster and postherpetic neuralgia of the extremities or trunk. Epidural nerve block with local anesthetic and steroid may also be useful in the palliation of pain secondary to diabetic polyneuropathy, pain of malignant origin, phantom limb pain, peripheral neuropathies, and demyelinating diseases. Pain secondary to acute vertebral compression fractures responds to epidural nerve block with local anesthetic and steroid and allows more rapid ambulation and return to activities of daily living (Waldman, 2000a, 2000b).

Cervical epidural nerve block with local anesthetic and steroid has also been shown to be efficacious in providing long-term relief in tension-type and chronic daily cervicogenic headache. Cronen and Waldman (1988) demonstrated this finding in a prospective study in a group of patients who had failed all treatment modalities, including the optimal use of simple analgesics, nonsteroidal anti-inflammatory agents, antidepressant compounds, and biofeedback. Cervical epidural nerve blocks are also useful in the palliation of pain secondary to cervicalgia and whiplash-type injuries of the cervical spine. Clinical experience suggests that this technique is of value in patients with severe fibromyalgia of the cervical paraspinal musculature (Waldman, 2001b).

Anatomy

The epidural space extends from the foramen magnum where the periosteal and spinal layers of dura fuse together to the sacrococcygeal membrane (Bridenbaugh & Greene, 1989) (see Figure 37.3). The anterior portion of the epidural space is bound by the posterior longitudinal ligament, which covers the posterior aspect of the vertebral body and the intravertebral disc. Posteriorly, the epidural space is bound by the anterior lateral surface of the vertebral lamina and the ligamentum flavum. Laterally, the epidural space is bound by the pedicles of the vertebra and the intravertebral foramen. From a technical viewpoint, the ligamentum flavum is the key landmark for identification of the epidural space. It is composed of dense fibroelastic tissue. It is thinnest in the cervical region. In the adult male, the epidural space is narrowest in the cervical region, with an anterior/posterior diameter of 2 to 3 mm in the cervical region when the neck is flexed.

Technique

Epidural nerve block is most easily carried out if the patient is in the sitting position with the cervical spine flexed and

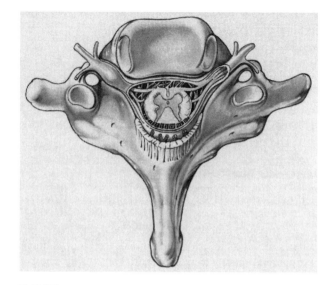

FIGURE 37.3 The epidural space. (Courtesy of Astra Pharmaceutical Products, Inc. © Anazak Productions.)

the forehead resting on a padded bedside table. The arms should rest comfortably in the patient's lap or at the patient's side. The skin overlying the appropriate vertebral interspace is prepped with antiseptic solution, and a sterile fenestrated drape is then placed. Careful palpation of the spinous process and intervertebral space is carried out. The exact midline position is then identified. The skin and subcutaneous tissues are anesthetized with 1% preservative-free lidocaine or 0.25% preservative-free bupivicaine. A 22- or 25-gauge 1.5 or 2 in. needle is then placed into the previously anesthetized area with a trajectory slightly cephalad and toward midline. A well-lubricated, 5-cc glass syringe filled with preservative-free saline or a syringe containing local anesthetic and steroid is attached to the epidural needle. With constant pressure on the plunger of the syringe, the epidural needle is carefully advanced. As the tip of the needle passes through ligamentum flavum into the epidural space, the operator will sense a sudden loss of resistance. After careful aspiration, 0.5% preservative-free lidocaine or 0.25% preservative-free bupivicaine combined with depot steroid preparations is then injected through the needle. The epidural needle is removed, a 4 × 4 gauze pad is placed on the injection site, and general pressure is applied. The patient is returned to the supine position, and careful monitoring of blood pressure, pulse, and respirations is carried out until the patient is fully recovered. Many experienced pain management specialists are utilizing these shorter and sharper 22- and 25-gauge needles for epidural blocks with a similar incidence of complications but with the advantage of less procedure-related pain (Waldman, 2000b).

Practical Considerations

Clinical experience suggests that the use of steroid epidural nerve block for the palliation of the above-mentioned pain syndromes is most efficacious when carried out in the following manner (Waldman, 1994a). The initial epidural nerve block is performed with 80 mg methylprednisolone (Depo-Medrol, Upjohn) and 7 ml of preservative-free bupivicaine (Sensorcaine, Astra) in the cervical region, 10 ml in the lower thoracic region, and 12 ml in the lumbar region. Subsequent epidural nerve blocks are administered on an every-other-day basis with 40 mg methylprednisolone and an appropriate amount of preservative-free bupivicaine in each successive nerve block. The number of blocks that can be administered in this manner varies from patient to patient. For patients with relatively acute pain problems, four or five epidural blocks carried out on a daily or every-other-day basis will often result in complete palliation of the pain symptomatology. More chronic conditions, such as postherpetic neuralgia, cancer pain, or reflex sympathetic dystrophy, may require more aggressive use of neural blockade, with eight or nine epidural blocks being necessary to achieve the desired results. The amount of methylprednisolone should be decreased in diabetics or patients who have received prior treatment with systemic glucocorticoids, as well as patients who may require more than four or five epidural blocks. It is thought that the use of large doses of methylprednisolone (i.e., greater than 120 mg in a single nerve block) significantly increases the incidence of steroid-related side effects and should probably be avoided. Epidural nerve block can be utilized early in the course of treatment for the previously mentioned pain syndromes while waiting for other treatment modalities such as antidepressants or physical therapy to become effective. The addition of preservative-free morphine may be useful in patients suffering from cancer- or trauma-related pain.

It is the author's strong belief that increasing the frequency of epidural blocks to daily or every other day will result in increased efficacy block for block when compared with weekly, every other week, or monthly regimens. This increase in frequency will generally result in a lower number of epidural blocks being required to obtain the desired level of pain relief when compared to regimens of less frequent epidural blocks. Whatever regimen is chosen, the pain management specialist should avoid "cookbook" approaches to pain management and individualize treatment to optimize pain relief. This will often require providing epidural blocks to patients suffering from acute problems such as acute herpes zoster and peripheral vascular insufficiency on weekends and holidays (Waldman, 2000b).

Complications

Because an epidural block interrupts both somatic and sympathetic nerve conduction, cardiovascular changes, including hypotension and tachycardia, may occur (Waldman, 1989a). These cardiovascular changes can produce devastating complications if not promptly identified and treated. Respiratory compromise or failure can occur if blockade of the phrenic nerve or respiratory centers of the brain stem inadvertently occurs. For this reason, epidural nerve blocks should be performed only by those trained in airway management and resuscitation. Appropriate monitoring of vital signs is imperative, and resuscitation equipment must be readily available.

Minor untoward effects and complications of epidural nerve block include pain at the injection site, inadvertent dural puncture, and vasovagal syncope. Major complications include damage to neural structures, epidural hematoma, and epidural abscess. These major complications are rare but can be life-threatening when they occur.

CAUDAL EPIDURAL NERVE BLOCK

Indications

In addition to applications for surgical and obstetrical anesthesia, caudal epidural nerve block with local anesthetics can be utilized as a diagnostic tool when performing differential neural blockade on an anatomic basis in the evaluation of pelvic, bladder, perineal, genital, rectal, anal, and lower extremity pain. If destruction of the sacral nerves is being considered, this technique is useful as a prognostic indicator of the degree of motor and sensory impairment that the patient may experience.

Caudal epidural nerve block with local anesthetics and/or steroids can be utilized to palliate acute pain emergencies in adults and children, including postoperative pain, pain secondary to pelvic and lower extremity trauma, pain of acute herpes zoster, and cancer-related pain, while waiting for pharmacologic, surgical, and/or antiblastic methods to become effective. Additionally, this technique is valuable in patients suffering from acute vascular insufficiency of the lower extremities secondary to vasospastic and vaso-occlusive disease, including frostbite and ergotamine toxicity.

Caudal nerve block is also recommended to palliate the pain of hydrenadenitis suppurativia of the groin. The administration of local anesthetics and/or steroids via the caudal approach to the epidural space is useful in the treatment of a variety of chronic benign pain syndromes, including lumbar radiculopathy, low back syndrome, spinal stenosis, postlaminectomy syndrome, vertebral compression fractures, diabetic polyneuropathy, postherpetic neuralgia, reflex sympathetic dystrophy, phantom limb pain, orchalgia, proctalgia, and pelvic pain syndromes (Waldman, 2000c).

Because of the simplicity, safety, and lack of pain associated with the caudal approach to the epidural space, this technique is replacing the lumbar epidural approach for these indications in many pain centers. The caudal approach to the epidural space is especially useful in patients who have previously undergone low-back surgery, which may make the lumbar approach to the epidural space less optimal. Because the caudal approach to the epidural space can be utilized in the presence of anticoagulation or coagulopathy, local anesthetics, opioids, and/or steroids can be administered via this route even when other regional anesthetic techniques, including the spinal and lumbar epidural approach, are contraindicated. This is advantageous in patients with vascular insufficiency who are fully anticoagulated and in cancer patients who have developed coagulopathy secondary to radiation and/or chemotherapy. The caudal epidural administration of local anesthetics, in combination with steroids and/or opioids, is useful in the palliation of cancer-related pelvic, perineal, and rectal pain. This technique has been especially successful in the relief of pain secondary to the bony metastases of prostate cancer and the palliation of chemotherapy-related peripheral neuropathy. As mentioned above, the caudal administration of local anesthetics, opioids, and/or steroids can be utilized in the presence of anticoagulation or coagulopathy.

Anatomy

The triangular-shaped sacrum consists of the five fused sacral vertebrae that are dorsally convex. The sacrum inserts in a wedge-like manner between the two iliac bones, articulating superiorly with the fifth lumbar vertebra and caudally with the coccyx. On the anterior concave surface, there are four pairs of unsealed anterior sacral foramina that allow passage of the anterior rami of the upper four sacral nerves. The posterior sacral foramina are smaller than their anterior counterparts. The vestigial remnants of the inferior articular processes project downward on each side of the sacral hiatus. These bony projections are called the sacral cornua and represent important clinical landmarks when performing caudal epidural nerve block. The triangular-shaped coccyx is made up of three to five rudimental vertebrae. Its superior surface articulates with the inferior articular surface of the sacrum. Two prominent coccygeal cornua adjoin their sacral counterparts. The tip of the coccyx is an important clinical landmark when performing caudal epidural nerve block. The sacral hiatus is formed by the incomplete midline fusion of the posterior elements of the lower portion of the S4 and the entire S5 vertebrae. This U-shaped space is covered posteriorly by the sacrococcygeal ligament, which is also an important clinical landmark when performing caudal epidural nerve block. Penetration of the sacrococcygeal ligament provides direct access to the epidural space of the sacral canal. A continuation of the lumbar spinal canal, the sacral canal continues inferiorly to terminate at the sacral hiatus (Waldman, 2000c).

Technique

The patient is placed in the prone position. The patient's head is placed on a pillow and turned away from the pain management physician. Another pillow is placed under the hips to tilt the pelvis and bring the sacral hiatus into greater prominence. The legs and heels are abducted to prevent tightening of the gluteal muscles, which can make identification of the sacral hiatus more difficult. If the lateral position is chosen because the patient is unable to lie prone, the dependent leg is slightly flexed at the hip and knee for patient comfort. The upper leg is flexed so that it lies over and above the lower leg and is also in contact with the bed. This modified Sim's position separates the buttocks, making identification of the sacral hiatus easier. Due to sagging of the buttocks in the lateral position, the gluteal fold is usually inferior to the level of the sacral hiatus and is a misleading landmark for needle placement (Waldman, 2000c).

A $1^1/_2$-in., 22-gauge needle is suitable for the vast majority of adult patients. A 1/2-in., 25-gauge needle is indicated for pediatric applications. A $1^1/_2$-in., 25-gauge needle is utilized when caudal epidural nerve block is performed in the presence of coagulopathy or anticoagulation. The use of longer needles, as advocated by some earlier investigators, will increase the incidence of complications, including intravascular injection and inadvertent dural puncture. Furthermore, the use of longer needles adds nothing to the overall success of this technique. Preparation of a wide area of skin with an antiseptic solution, such as povidone-iodine, is carried out so that all of the landmarks can be palpated aseptically. A fenestrated sterile drape is placed to avoid contamination of the palpating finger. The pain management physician's middle finger is placed over the sterile drape into the natal cleft, with the fingertip at the tip of the coccyx. This maneuver allows easy confirmation of the sacral midline and is especially important when utilizing the lateral position. After careful identification of the midline, the area under the pain management physician's proximal interphalangeal joint is located. The middle finger is moved cephalad to the area that was previously located under the proximal interphalangeal joint. This spot is palpated using a lateral rocking motion to identify the sacral cornua. The sacral hiatus will be found at this level if the pain management physician's glove size is $7^1/_2$ or 8. If the pain management physician's glove size is smaller, the location of the sacral hiatus will be just superior to the area located below the operator's proximal interphalangeal joint when the fingertip is at the tip of the coccyx. If the pain management physician's glove size is larger, the location of the sacral hiatus will be just inferior to the area located below the proximal interphalangeal joint when the fingertip is at the tip of the coccyx. Although there is normally significant anatomic variation of the sacrum and sacral hiatus, the spatial relationship between the tip of the coccyx and the location of the sacral hiatus remains amazingly constant. When the approximate position of the sacral hiatus is located by palpating the tip of the coccyx, identifying the midline, and locating the area under the proximal interphalangeal joint as described above, inability to identify and enter the sacral hiatus should occur less than 0.5% of the time.

After locating the sacral hiatus, a 22- or 25-gauge 1.5 or 2 in. needle is inserted through the anesthetized area at a 45° angle into the sacrococcygeal ligament. As the ligament is penetrated, a "pop" or "giving way" will be felt. If contact with the interior bony wall of the sacral canal occurs, the needle should be withdrawn slightly. This will disengage the needle tip from the periosteum. The needle is then advanced approximately 0.50 cm into the canal. This is to ensure that the entire needle bevel is beyond the sacrococcygeal ligament to avoid injection into the ligament. The force required for injection should not exceed that necessary to overcome the resistance of the needle. If there is initial resistance to injection, the needle should be rotated 180° in case it is incorrectly placed in the canal, but the needle bevel is occluded by the internal wall of the sacral canal. Any significant pain or sudden increase in resistance during injection suggests incorrect needle placement, and the pain management physician should stop injecting immediately and reassess the position of the needle (Waldman, 1998c).

When the needle is satisfactorily positioned, a syringe containing the drugs to be injected is attached to the needle. Gentle aspiration is carried out to identify cerebrospinal fluid or blood. Although rare, inadvertent dural puncture can occur, and careful observation for spinal fluid must be carried out. Aspiration of blood occurs more commonly. This can be due to either damage to veins during insertion of the needle into the caudal canal or, less commonly, intravenous placement of the needle. Should the aspiration test be positive for either spinal fluid or blood, the needle is repositioned and the aspiration test repeated. If negative, subsequent injections of 0.5-ml increments of local anesthetic are undertaken. Careful observation for signs of local anesthetic toxicity or subarachnoid spread of local anesthetic during the injection and following the procedure is indicated.

Local anesthetics capable of producing adequate sensory block of the sacral and lower lumbar nerve roots when administered via the caudal route include 1.0% lidocaine, 0.25% bupivicaine, 2% 2-chloroprocaine, and 1.0% mepivicaine. Current clinical practice suggests that smaller volumes of local anesthetics, i.e., 5–7 ml are as effusive as the larger volume of local anesthetics previously advocated with a decreased incidence of side effects. For diagnostic and prognostic blocks, 1.0% preservative-free lidocaine is a suitable local anesthetic. For therapeutic blocks, 0.25% preservative-free bupivicaine in combination with 80 mg depot methylprednisolone

(Depo-Medrol, Upjohn) is injected. Subsequent nerve blocks are carried out in a similar manner, substituting 40 mg methylprednisolone for the initial 80-mg dose. Daily caudal epidural nerve blocks with local anesthetic and/or steroid may be required to treat the above-mentioned acute painful conditions and sympathetically maintained pain syndromes such as reflex sympathetic dystrophy and acute herpes zoster.. Chronic conditions such as lumbar radiculopathy and diabetic polyneuropathy are treated on an every-other-day to once-a-week basis, or as the clinical situation dictates. If selective neurolytic block of an individual sacral nerve is desired, incremental 0.1-ml injections of 6.5% phenol in glycerine or alcohol to a total volume of 1.0 ml can be utilized after first confirming the level of pain relief and potential side effects with local anesthetic blocks. If the caudal epidural route is chosen for administration of opioids, 4 to 5 mg morphine sulfate formulated for epidural use is a reasonable initial dose. More lipid-soluble opioids such as fentanyl must be delivered by continuous infusion via a caudal catheter.

Practical Considerations

As with the other approaches to epidural nerve block, increased efficacy will occur if caudal epidural blocks are performed on a daily or every-other-day basis rather than weekly, biweekly, or monthly. Again, a "cookbook" approach should be avoided and the care individualized to ensure optimal pain relief. Because of the simplicity, safety, and extremely low incidence of inadvertent dural puncture, caudal epidural nerve block is preferred over the lumbar approach to the epidural space for most patients and especially in those patients who have undergone prior back surgery. The ability to utilize the caudal approach to the epidural space in the presence of anticoagulants or coagulopathy is an added advantage (Waldman, 1998c).

It is possible to insert the needle incorrectly when performing caudal epidural nerve block. The needle may be placed outside the sacral canal, resulting in the injection of air and/or drugs into the subcutaneous tissues. Palpation of crepitus and bulging of tissues overlying the sacrum during injection is indicative of this needle malposition. An increased resistance to injection accompanied by pain is also noted. A second possible needle misplacement occurs when the needle tip is placed into the periosteum of the sacral canal. This needle misplacement is suggested by considerable pain on injection, a very high resistance to injection, and the inability to inject more than a few milliliters of drug. A third possibility of needle malposition is partial placement of the needle bevel in the sacrococcygeal ligament. Again, there is significant resistance to injection, as well as significant pain as the drugs are injected into the ligament. A fourth possible needle malposition is to force the point of the needle into the marrow cavity of the sacral vertebra, resulting in very high blood levels of local anesthetic. This can occur in elderly patients with significant osteoporosis. This needle malposition is detected by the initial easy acceptance of a few milliliters of local anesthetic, followed by a rapid increase in resistance to injection as the noncompliant bony cavity fills with local anesthetic. Significant local anesthetic toxicity can occur as a result of this complication. The fifth and most serious needle malposition occurs when the needle is inserted through the sacrum or lateral to the coccyx into the pelvic cavity beyond. This can result in the needle entering both the rectum and birth canal, resulting in contamination of the needle. The repositioning of the contaminated needle into the sacral canal carries the danger of infection.

Because of the potential for hematogenous spread via Batson's plexus, local infection and sepsis represent absolute contraindications to the caudal approach to the epidural space. Pilonidal cyst and congenital abnormalities of the dural sac and its contents also represent relative contraindications to the caudal approach to the epidural space.

Complications

With the exception of the decreased incidence of inadvertent dural puncture, the complications of the caudal approach to the epidural space mirror those of the lumbar approach. Because of the proximity of the rectum, scrupulous attention to sterile technique must be observed to avoid infection, which can easily spread via Batson's plexus to the epidural space. Because of the vascular nature of the caudal epidural space, the potential for local anesthetic toxicity remains ever present. Careful aspiration and incremental dosing of local anesthetics will help avoid this potentially lethal complication. As with all procedures performed in the prone position, careful attention to the airway must be observed.

FACET NERVE BLOCK

Indications

The primary indication for injection of local anesthetic and steroid into or around the facet joint is palliation of the constellation of symptoms that has been given the rubric "facet syndrome." Facet syndrome is characterized by the following findings: (1) pain on palpation of the tissues overlying the facet joints, (2) reproduction of the patient's pain with hyperextension or rotation of extreme lateral bending of the affected spinal segments, (3) increased pain when remaining in one position for long periods of time, (4) pain localized to the affected spinal segments with no radicular symptoms or physical findings, and (5) radiographic findings of facet arthropathy. As clinicians have gained experience with facet block, it has

become apparent that the efficacy of this technique is due in large part to blockade of the medial articular branch of the posterior primary ramus rather than injection of drug into the joint itself. This explains why the efficacy of nonradiographically guided approaches to facet nerve block may be greater than radiographically guided blocks where the needle is placed directly into the facet joint itself (Waldman, 1998d).

Facet nerve block is also indicated as a diagnostic maneuver to determine if spondylolysis is the cause of the patient's back pain. The technique can also help the pain specialist determine if the pseudarthrosis that occurs between the transitional vertebra in the lumbar spine is the source of the patient's pain prior to spinal stabilization surgery.

Technique

Facet nerve block can be done in the prone or sitting position. In the prone position, a pillow is placed below the patient to rotate the patient obliquely approximately 30 to 35°. This places the facet joints and nerves in a more vertical position. After the skin is prepped with antiseptic solution, the skin and subcutaneous tissues are anesthetized with 1% lidocaine. The needle is then advanced perpendicular to the table, with a 60° trajectory from the skin at an entry point approximately 7 cm lateral to the midline. The needle is advanced until bone is encountered. The pain specialist may then attempt to walk the needle into the facet joint or, in most cases, after careful aspiration for blood and cerebrospinal fluid, simply inject 1 to 2 ml of 0.25% preservative-free bupivicaine and 10 mg methylprednisolone at each joint to block the medial branch of the facet joint nerve. Most pain specialists recommend injecting at least two levels due to the variation and overlap of innervation of the facet joints and posterior elements of the spine. Bilateral injection is usually indicated unless the degenerative process and resultant pain are limited to one side. Radiographic guidance for needle placement is generally indicated only if one needs to ascertain if a specific facet joint represents the nidus of the patient's pain or if a facet rhizotomy with phenol or radio-frequency needle is being contemplated.

Practical Considerations

Facet nerve block is gaining increasing popularity among pain specialists in the treatment of nonradicular neck and back pain. A clear understanding of the anatomy will help the pain specialist perform the procedure with less discomfort for the patient. Blockade of the medial branch is generally sufficient to provide pain relief, and actual injection into the facet joint itself is rarely required. When used as a diagnostic maneuver, radiographic guidance is useful to document needle placement, but the pain specialist should assess other behavioral factors that may impact the patient's response to facet nerve block, including chemical dependence on narcotic analgesics, and secondary gain issues.

Complications

Due to the proximity of the spinal nerve roots, direct trauma to the nerves is a distinct possibility. For this reason, intravenous sedation during facet nerve block should be avoided so the patient can warn the pain specialist of any paresthesias that occur during needle placement. Inadvertent injection of the local anesthetic into epidural, subdural, or subarachnoid space is also a possibility. Needle placement into the intervertebral disc can also occur if the initial needle placement is too far lateral and discitis has been reported.

MYOFASCIAL TRIGGER POINT INJECTION

Indications

Injection of myofascial trigger points with local anesthetic and/or steroid is indicated in the treatment of myofascial pain syndromes of the head and neck (Raj, 1989). These myofascial trigger points are discrete hypersensitive areas of muscle that in most instances result from previous trauma. Palpation of these trigger points can initiate pain, autonomic disturbance in a nonsegmental and referred distribution. Trigger points can occur essentially in any muscle of the body. They are most frequently found in the trapezius, semispinalis capitis, splenius capitis, occipitofrontalis, and the muscles of mastication and facial expression, as well as the trapezius and rhomboids.

Technique

Localization of trigger points is accomplished by deep palpation and observation of the radiation of the patient's pain (Travell, 1976). The skin overlying the area is then prepped with alcohol, and 0.25 ml of 1% preservative-free lidocaine, or 0.5% preservative-free bupivicaine alone or in combination with methylprednisolone, is injected into the trigger points.

Practical Considerations

Most patients with muscle contraction headache and atypical head and facial pain syndrome will have multiple myofascial trigger points. A more central nerve block, such as cervical epidural nerve block or trigeminal nerve block, may be more effective in treating and decreasing the number of these trigger points than actual injection into the multiple trigger points that may be present. Dis-

crete trigger points that remain after epidural or trigeminal nerve blocks can then be injected quite easily. With trigger point injection, patients should be informed that they may experience an exacerbation of pain symptomatology when the local anesthetic wears off. Recently, there has been interest in the use of botulinum toxin to inject trigger points that have failed to respond to more conservative methods (Waldman, 2001c).

Complications

Due to the highly vascular nature of the head and face, intravascular injection is a possibility. Care should be taken to avoid inadvertent subarachnoid injection with resultant total spinal anesthetic when injecting trigger points near the midline of the neck and occipital region.

INTERCOSTAL NERVE BLOCKS

Indications

Intercostal nerve block with local anesthetic and/or corticosteroid can be performed at the bedside or in the outpatient setting. This procedure may palliate pain secondary to acute traumatic or pathologic rib fractures, chest wall metastasis, postthoracotomy pain, or right upper quadrant pain secondary to hepatic metastasis (Waldman, 1998b, 1998e). Intercostal nerve blocks may also reduce pain due to percutaneous drainage devices such as chest tubes or nephrostomy tubes. Studies have demonstrated clinically significant improvement in pulmonary function in patients treated with this procedure (Waldman, 1998b).

Anatomy

The thoracic spinal nerves give off the white and gray rami communicantes of the sympathetic system which go to or come from the particular ganglion of the sympathetic chain. Distal to the rami communicantes, the nerve trunk divides into the dorsal and ventral branches. The dorsal branch innervates the skin and muscles of the back as well as the periosteum of the vertebra. The ventral branch follows the rib via the costal sulcus, into the dorsal thoracic region between the two lamina of the intercostal muscles into the lateral and ventral portion of the thorax. This intercostal nerve travels in tandem with the intercostal artery and vein (Raj, 1985).

Technique

Intercostal nerve block can be performed with the patient in the sitting, lateral decubitus, or prone position. The rib in the anatomic region to be blocked is identified by palpation, and the skin in the posterior axillary line is prepped with antiseptic solution. The intercostal nerve can be blocked more anteriorly should the clinical situation dictate. A 22-gauge, 1½-in. needle attached to a 5-ml syringe is advanced vertically until bony contact with the rib is made. The needle is withdrawn back into the subcutaneous tissues, and the needle is then walked off the inferior margin of the rib, with care being taken not to advance the needle more than 0.5 cm. After careful aspiration, 3 to 5 ml of 0.5% or 0.75% preservative-free bupivicaine is injected. The needle is then removed. This technique can be repeated at each level subserving the pain, with care being taken to carefully monitor the total milligram dosage of local anesthetic injected (Waldman, 1998e).

Practical Considerations

Therapeutic intercostal nerve block is an excellent adjunct in the armamentarium of the pain management specialist to treat a variety of acute and chronic pain syndromes. Its simplicity lends itself to performance in the emergency room or at the bedside, provided appropriate resuscitation equipment and drugs are readily available. The highly vascular nature of the intercostal region makes careful monitoring of the total milligram dosage of local anesthetic, such as 0.75% bupivicaine, important. This technique can be performed on a daily basis to provide long-lasting pain relief for trauma and acute surgical incisions.

Complications

The major complication of intercostal nerve block is inadvertent and unrecognized pneumothorax. The incidence of this complication is approximately 0.5 to 1.0%. If the patient is being maintained on ventilatory support with positive pressure ventilation, tension pneumothorax can occur. As mentioned, vascular uptake of local anesthetic with systemic toxicity is also a problem if careful dosage guidelines are not observed.

Interpleural Catheter

Indications

Recent studies have demonstrated that local anesthetic installation via interpleural catheter is effective in the management of both acute and chronic pain (Reiestad & Stomstag, 1986). This simple technique can be performed on an outpatient basis or at the bedside. Indications are essentially the same as for intercostal nerve block. In addition to these indications, several clinical reports have suggested that the intrapleural catheter technique can be used to reduce pain below the diaphragm, including pain secondary to pancreatic malignancy (Waldman, 1998f).

Technique

The patient is placed in the lateral decubitus position with the painful side upward. The eighth and ninth ribs at the posterior axillary line are identified and then prepped with antiseptic solution. Sterile drapes are placed, and skin and subcutaneous tissues are anesthetized with 1% lidocaine. After adequate analgesia is obtained, a styleted Tuohy or Hustead needle is placed through the skin and into the subcutaneous tissue. A 5-ml syringe with 0.9% preservative-free saline is attached, and the needle and syringe are walked over the superior margin of the rib to avoid damage to the neurovascular bundle. The intrapleural space is then identified utilizing either the hanging drop technique or the negative intrapleural pressure technique as described by Reiestad, et al. (1986). A catheter is then introduced through the needle and advanced approximately 10 cm through the intrapleural space, the Tuohy needle is removed, and 12 to 15 ml of local anesthetic is then injected to ensure catheter integrity and to confirm adequate pain relief from the intrapleural catheter. If long-term use is anticipated, the catheter should be tunneled to avoid the risk of subcutaneous infection (Waldman, 1989b).

Practical Considerations

This technique has proven quite useful in the acute pain management arena. Recent clinical reports have demonstrated that this technique can also be used on a long-term basis. This is accomplished by tunneling the intrapleural catheter to reduce the incidence of infection. As the pleural space is highly vascular, careful attention to the total milligram dosage of local anesthetic used is indicated. In patients with significant pleural disease or pleural effusion, this technique should be used with caution, and the total dose of local anesthetic must be decreased to avoid toxic blood levels.

Complications

The complications of this technique are similar to intercostal nerve block. In addition, if infection occurs, empyema can result.

Epidural Blood Patch

Indications

Epidural blood patch is indicated for the treatment of post-dural puncture headache following lumbar puncture, myelographic procedures, or inadvertent dural puncture that may occur during attempted epidural anesthesia (Waldman, Feldstein, & Allen, 1987). This technique can also be utilized in the treatment of spontaneous low-pressure headaches that may result from minor head or neck trauma.

Anatomy

The anatomy of the epidural space was described in the section on epidural nerve block. The epidural space is larger in the lumbar region relative to the cervical region, and clinical experience indicates that a larger volume of autologous blood will be required to relieve postdural puncture headaches in the lumbar region relative to the cervical region.

Technique

The patient is hydrated with intravenous fluids, and any co-existing nausea and vomiting is treated with antiemetics. After donning sterile surgical cap, gown, mask, and gloves, the antecubital fossa and skin overlying the area of dural puncture are prepped in a sterile manner with povidone-iodine solution. Identification of the epidural space is carried out, and autologous blood is obtained in a sterile manner from the previously prepped antecubital vein. Autologous blood (7 to 10 ml) is placed in the cervical region, with 12 to 15 ml of autologous blood required for the lumbar region.

Practical Considerations

Many patients with postdural puncture headache have severe nausea and vomiting that may lead to significant dehydration. This results in worsening of the headache and makes venous access to obtain autologous blood quite difficult. The use of preprocedure hydration is therefore indicated. The most common reason for failure of the epidural blood patch is the fact that the patient does not remain supine following the procedure. The patient and nursing staff must be instructed to closely adhere to the postepidural blood patch orders.

Complications

In addition to the complications attendant to identification of the epidural space, the most feared complication of epidural blood patch is infection. Although written about, the actual incidence of this potentially devastating complication (assuming that strict sterile technique is followed) is exceedingly rare. Occasionally, a second and rarely a third epidural blood patch may be required to palliate the above-mentioned pain syndrome.

SUMMARY

The use of neural blockade represents an excellent addition to the armamentarium of the physician caring for the patient in pain. Proper integration of these techniques into the comprehensive pharmacologic and behavioral treatment plan is essential if one is to maximize their efficacy. An understanding of the anatomic, technical, and practical considerations of each specific type of nerve block should lead to a high degree of success and minimal complications.

REFERENCES

Bridenbaugh, P., & Greene, N. (1989). Spinal neural blockade. In M. Cousins & P. Bridenbaugh (Eds.), *Neural blockade* (p. 216). Philadelphia: Lippincott.

Cronen, M., & Waldman, S. (1988). Cervical steroid epidural nerve block in the palliation of pain secondary to intractable muscle contraction headache. *Headache, 28,* 314–315.

Diamond, S., & Dalessio, D. (1982). Cluster headache. In EDITOR? *The practicing physician's approach to headache* (pp. 64–65). Baltimore: Williams & Wilkins.

Katz, J. (1994a). Sphenopalatine ganglion. In J. Katz (Ed.), *Atlas of regional anesthesia* (2nd ed., pp. 16–17). Norwalk: Appleton-Century-Crofts.

Katz, J. (1994b). Stellate ganglion. In J. Katz (Ed.), *Atlas of regional anesthesia* (pp. 50–52). Norwalk: Appleton-Century-Crofts.

Kitrelle, J., Grouse, D., & Seybold, M. (1985). Cluster headache: Local anesthetic abortive agents. *Archives of Neurology, 42,* 496–498.

Liebarman, R., & Waldman, S. (1990). Celiac plexus neurolysis. *Radiology, 175,* 874–876.

Lobstrom, J., & Cousins, M. (1988). Sympathetic neural blockade. In M. Cousins & P. Bridenbaugh (Eds.), *Neural blockade* (pp. 479–493). Philadelphia: Lippincott.

Phero, J. & Robbins, G. (1985a). Sphenopalatine ganglion block. In P. Raj (Ed.), *Handbook of regional anesthesia* (pp. 24–26). New York: Churchill Livingstone.

Phero, J., & Robbins, G. (1985b). Trigeminal nerve block. In P. Raj (Ed.), *Handbook of regional anesthesia* (pp. 18–21). New York: Churchill Livingstone.

Portenoy, R., & Waldman, S. (1991). Recent advances in cancer pain management. *Pain Management, 4,* 18–24.

Raj, P. (1985). Chronic pain. In P. Raj (Ed.), *Handbook of regional anesthesia* (pp. 102–116). New York: Churchill Livingstone.

Raj, P. (1989). Prognostic and therapeutic nerve blocks. In M. Cousins & P. Bridenbaugh (Eds.), *Neural blockade* (pp. 899–907). Philadelphia: Lippincott.

Reiestad, F., & Stomstag, K. (1986). Intrapleural catheter in the management of postoperative pain. *Regional Anesthesiology, 11,* 89–91.

Saper, J. (1987). Highlights of the Nuprin pain report. *Topics in Pain Management, 2,* 41–43.

Travell, J. (1976). Myofascial trigger points. In J. Bonica & D. Albe-Fessard (Eds.), *Advances in pain research and therapy* (pp. 919–926). New York: Raven Press.

Waldman, S.D. (1989a). Complications of cervical epidural nerve blocks. *Regional Anesthesiology, 14,* 149–151.

Waldman, S.D. (1989b). Subcutaneous tunneled intrapleural catheter in the long term relief of right upper quadrant pain of malignant origin. *Journal of Pain Symptom Management, 4*, 86–89.

Waldman, S.D. (1996a). Headache and facial pain. In P. Raj (Ed.), *Pain management: A comprehensive review of the specialty* (pp. 385–396). St. Louis: Mosby.

Waldman, S.D. (1996b). Sphenopalatine ganglion block. In M. Hahn & P. McQuillan (Eds.), *Regional anesthesia—An atlas of anatomy and techniques* (pp. 79–82). St. Louis: Mosby.

Waldman, S.D. (1998a). Caudal nerve block. In S.D. Waldman (Ed.), *Atlas of interventional pain management techniques* (pp. 337–350). Philadelphia: W.B. Saunders.

Waldman, S.D. (1998b). Intercostal nerve block. In S.D. Waldman (Ed.), *Atlas of interventional pain management techniques* (pp. 228–231). Philadelphia: W.B. Saunders.

Waldman, S.D. (1998d). Interpleural catheter. In S. D. Waldman (Ed.), *Atlas of interventional pain management techniques* (pp. 232–237). Philadelphia: W.B. Saunders.

Waldman, S.D. (1998d). Lumbar facet block: Medial branch approach. In S.D. Waldman (Ed.), *Atlas of interventional pain management techniques* (pp. 300–303). Philadelphia: W.B. Saunders.

Waldman, S.D. (1998e). Sphenopalatine ganglion block. In S. D. Waldman (Ed.), *Atlas of interventional pain management techniques* (pp. 10–12). Philadelphia: W.B. Saunders.

Waldman, S.D. (1998f). Stellate ganglion block. In S. D. Waldman (Ed.), *Atlas of interventional pain management techniques* (pp. 110–112). Philadelphia: W.B. Saunders.

Waldman, S.D. (2000a). Caudal nerve block. In S.D. Waldman (Ed.), *Interventional pain management* (2nd ed., pp. 440–454). Philadelphia: W.B. Saunders.

Waldman, S.D. (2000b). Lumbar epidural nerve block. In S.D. Waldman (Ed.), *Interventional pain management* (2nd ed., pp. 423–439). Philadelphia: W.B. Saunders.

Waldman S.D. (2000c). Neural blockade of the trigeminal nerve. In S.D. Waldman (Ed.), *Interventional pain management* (2nd ed., pp. 273–284). Philadelphia: W.B. Saunders.

Waldman S.D. (2001a). Acute Pancreatitis. In S.D. Waldman (Ed.), *Atlas of common pain syndromes* (pp. 223–227). Philadelphia: W.B. Saunders.

Waldman S.D. (2001b). Myofascial pain syndrome. In S.D. Waldman (Ed.), *Atlas of common pain syndromes* (pp. 103–106). Philadelphia: W.B. Saunders.

Waldman S.D. (2001c). Reflex sympathetic dystrophy of the face. In S.D. Waldman (Ed.), *Atlas of common pain syndromes* (pp. 123–129). Philadelphia: W.B. Saunders.

Waldman S.D. (2001d). Trigeminal neuralgia. In S.D. Waldman (Ed.), *Atlas of common pain syndromes* (pp. 89–96) Philadelphia: W.B. Saunders.

Waldman, S.D., Feldstein, G., & Allen, M. (1987). Cervical epidural blood patch for treatment of cervical dural puncture headache. *Anesthesiology Review, 23–25.*

Waldman, S.D., & Waldman, K. (1987). Reflex sympathetic dystrophy of the face and neck. *Regional Anesthesiology, 12,* 8–12.

Waldman, S.D., Wilson, W., & Kreps, R. (1991). Superior hypogastric plexus block: description of a single needle technique. *Regional Anesthesia, 16,* 286–289.

38

Myths and Misconceptions about Chronic Pain: The Problem of Mind–Body Dualism

Keith Nicholson, Ph.D., Michael F. Martelli, Ph.D., D.A.A.P.M., and Nathan D. Zasler, M.D., F.A.A.P.M.&R., F.A.A.D.E.P., C.I.M.E., D.A.A.P.M.

As with most other phenomena, there are many myths or misconceptions about chronic pain. At the risk of being mundane, pretentious, or even reinforcing existing misconceptions, this chapter explores what some of these may be. Simply, myths or misconceptions arise out of an incomplete understanding and reflect our ignorance of the material at hand. Myths or misconceptions can also arise out of apparent but possibly false dichotomies. A fundamental dichotomy permeating many domains of human activity, from at least the time of Descartes, is mind–body dualism. This can be especially problematic for the understanding of chronic pain. Much of the current chapter is devoted to one aspect or another of this dichotomy and the misconceptions or confusion that flow from a biased perspective. Although some may think that reviewing this issue is akin to "beating a dead horse," this may also represent an important misconception. Rather, it is argued that explication of what the interface between the two sides of this issue may be is a most important avenue of research. It should also be noted that many myths or misconceptions may be rooted in one's professional training or background. In this regard, it is acknowledged that the predominant perspective of the current chapter is from that of psychologists working in the field of chronic pain.

Perhaps the most elemental myth or misconception is that we know what pain is. We do not. Pain is but a four-letter word or, preferably, a construct that facilitates understanding and communication of a number of related phenomena. One touches a hot stove, experiences "pain," and pulls one's arm away or says "ouch." Certainly, there is a shared intersubjective experience of many acute pain phenomena and, in this sense, acute pain is similar to the experience of a yellow banana or red apple. There is some understanding of the underlying neurobiology of the acute pain experience traditionally associated with the specificity theory of pain and thought to involve peripheral nociception with transmission of information about pain via the lateral pain system to the brain where it is experienced (somehow) as pain. In such situations, the nociceptive stimulus is usually withdrawn or there is healing of damaged tissue and the experience of pain resolves. Although there is certainly much to be learned about this acute pain response (e.g., why one may not experience pain in the midst of battle, during hypnosis or other activity), the problem becomes more complex and mysterious when one considers the transition to chronic pain.

Unlike the situation with color perception (i.e., where specific wavelengths of light may reliably be associated with the perception of particular colors) or many other domains of experience, there is often a poor relationship between the "subjective" experience of pain and "objective" or external referents. This may be most evident in the case of chronic pain where apparently similar peripheral pathology, injury, or nociceptive input can result in markedly different presentations. Whereas patient self-report, using verbal analogue or other rating scales, is perhaps the most straightforward and appropriate means of determining pain severity (or other aspects of the pain experience), this is prone to response bias like all self-reports. In this regard, it has been suggested that less than 10% of the chronic pain

0-8493-0926-3/02/$0.00+$1.50
© 2002 by CRC Press LLC

population may consume as much as 70 to 80% of the resources (Linton, 1999), possibly due to a response bias to report pain and related problems, dependency behavior or other factors associated with the distinction between impairment and disability (Martelli, Zasler, & MacMillan, 1998; Martelli, Zasler, Mancini, & MacMillan, 1999).

A response bias to report pain may be suspected when there are extremely high severity ratings and exuberant pain behavior with high affective distress and (possibly exaggerated) suffering in the context of few, if any, clinical findings. In such cases, one might conclude that underlying emotional problems rather than pain are really the primary problem. On the other hand, many patients present with an apparent "belle indifference" and, despite giving extremely high pain severity ratings (e.g., 9/10 or even 10/10 — "the worst that pain could ever be"), they may appear entirely comfortable, in no apparent distress whatsoever, and often in much better spirits than the examiner. When challenged, such patients will typically maintain that their pain is very severe (e.g., worse than childbirth). It becomes very difficult to ascertain what the meaning of pain is in such discrepant presentations. However, it is likely that the problem of response bias, which reflects the meaning of the experience of pain, is not restricted to the unusual or extreme cases and may often confound presentation in even more "legitimate" cases.

Most clinicians have encountered patients who complain that some doctors think their pain is "all in their heads," that is, it is just psychological, has no organic basis, or is not real. Many doctors may also sometimes hold such an opinion especially if there are no signs of any relevant pathological process, the presentation is otherwise inconsistent with expectation, or the patient appears somehow quirky and with obvious psychological problems. Of course, most would readily accept that lack of a discernible pathological process does not mean that there is not one. There is obviously much to learn about the underlying biological processes involved in chronic pain as well as in many other medical conditions. It is sometimes suggested (to patients or others) that pain is always experienced in the brain and thus is actually "all in the head." However, this begs the question about whether the pain is more "psychological" or "organic" as any psychological phenomena (e.g., reading this sentence or reading the next sentence) is presumed to have a neurobiological substrate. It should be remembered that the definition of pain accepted by the International Association for the Study of Pain (IASP) states that pain is always a psychological state (Merskey & Bogduk, 1994) but this should not be misinterpreted to mean that it is only a psychological state devoid of any physical basis in reality.

Another way of expressing the question of whether pain is in the mind or body is in terms of it being either functional or organic. Organic here implies structural damage or aberration generating "real" pain, whereas functional is com-monly meant to imply that presentation is associated with (usually preexisting) psychological or psychiatric problems and that the corresponding perception or self-report of pain may be distorted or magnified. However, there is increasing realization that chronic pain problems may truly be functional but, in this sense, functional refers to the effects of distributed neural networks involved in the processing of pain in contrast with the view of pain as involving a static structural (peripheral or central) lesion generating some nociceptive or neuropathic process (Wall, 2000). This is perhaps especially true of chronic nonmalignant or idiopathic pain. Notably, distributed neural networks underlie many (or most) neuropsychological functions such as motor, vision, or language. In this regard, pain might be considered akin to vision where there is clearly a peripheral and central biological apparatus mediating function but where psychological factors are also clearly pertinent and, therefore, we tend to see what we want to see or perception is otherwise colored by experience. Much of the brain has been shown to be involved in processing of painful information in one manner or another (Besson, Guilbaud, & Ollat, 1995; Bromm & Desmedt, 1995; Chundler & Dong, 1995). There is limited understanding of how several more dedicated areas actually operate. There is also very poor understanding of how the "pain system" interacts with other systems (e.g., endocrine, immune, motor, cognitive, etc).

With regard to the functional-structural distinction, Mailis, Amani, Umana, Basur, & Roe (1997) have documented a dissociation of separable components of pain in a sample of neuropathic pain patients, i.e., a deep pain component mediated by peripheral nociceptors plus a cutaneous component (allodynia) considered to be a product of central sensitization. Several further studies by this group utilizing sodium amytal or other techniques have purported to document structural-functional dissociations in several other patient samples and that functional aspects of presentation appear to be associated with specific psychosocial factors (Cohodarevic, Mailis, & Montanera, 2000; Mailis & Nicholson, 1997). Whereas the concept of central sensitization has certainly come into vogue, most study remains at the level of the spinal cord or periphery whereas the most important effects may well be supraspinal. Of course, it is much more difficult to conduct experiments at this level. It is also important to recognize that a focus upon how the brain is processing pain does not resolve the mind–body problem, although it may take it a step closer. Caution should also be exercised about neglecting peripheral factors in favor of how the brain is processing pain. It would be unfortunate if the pendulum were to swing and one misconception about chronic pain was displaced only to be replaced by another.

There is a widespread belief that functional neuroimaging will allow us to unlock the secrets of pain or at least provide for some better "objective" indices of pain. Unfortunately, most functional neuroimaging studies of pain have involved acute pain challenges with normal controls. Results have revealed widespread patterns of activation and deactivation in multiple cortical and subcortical sites (Coghill, Sanf, Maisog, & Ladoralo, 1999; Hsieh et al., 1995; Treede, Kenshalo, Gracely, & Jones, 1999). Indeed, almost all of the brain has been shown to respond in one paradigm or another. There has been more consistent (albeit not always found) patterns of activation in the anterior cingulate, insula, somatosensory cortex (S1 and/or S2), and somatosensory thalamus, findings that might have been anticipated given what is known about the neuroanatomy of the pain system. Notably, however, the anterior cingulate is activated by almost any behavioral challenge (Cabeza & Nyberg, 1997) and the insula is activated by somatosensory stimulation whether noxious or not (Craig, Reinan, Evans, & Bushnell, 1996), although it may be that processing of pain takes place within discrete parts of these cortical areas (Davis, Taylor, Crawley, Wood, & Mikulis, 1997). Furthermore, activation may be seen in the same areas if the subject merely anticipates pain (Drevets et al., 1995; Porro, Francescato, Cettolo, & Baraldi, 1995), although one study has found that the sites of activation with actual vs. anticipated pain can be distinguished (Ploghaus et al., 1999). It remains unclear what the significance of most of these findings are, or whether this technique will fulfill the promise of providing an important inroad to the understanding of chronic pain. However, this technology by itself cannot be expected to resolve mind–body problems. Rather, such issues will only successfully be addressed with relevant psychological analysis of the phenomena of interest (e.g., fear avoidance, response bias to report pain, etc.) coupled with appropriate behavioral challenge during neuroimaging with groups of patients who have been well defined (psychologically and medically) prior to imaging.

There is a long tradition in distinguishing sensory-discriminative, motivational-affective, or cognitive-evaluative components of pain (Melzack & Casey, 1966). Such distinctions often resolve into the dichotomy between the sensory-discriminative vs. the motivational-affective, the latter subsuming the cognitive-evaluative. It seems to often be assumed, at least implicitly, that these are distinct or independent components of pain but that "real" pain necessarily involves the sensory-discriminative component, the motivational-affective or cognitive-evaluative components merely being the emotional or cognitive overlay. More recently it has been suggested that such distinctions are too simplistic or misleading, again leading into problems of Cartesian dualism (Treede et al., 1999; Wall, 2000). There has also been a tradition of distinguishing between the lateral and medial pain systems, generally corresponding to the distinction between the sensory-discriminative vs. motivational-affective and cognitive-evaluative components of pain (Vogt, Sikes, & Vogt, 1993). It remains unclear to what extent these systems are independent and

processing information in parallel or how there is interdependence of function and unification of the experience of pain (Vogt, et al., 1993; Treede et al., 1999). Notably, this same issue, integration vs. independence or differentiation of function, has also been a subject of debate with regard to the function of basal ganglia-thalamocortical loops mediating motor, visual, cognitive, affective or other functions (Alexander, DeLong, & Strick, 1986; St-Cyr, Taylor, & Nicholson, 1995).

Many instances or types of central pain occur (e.g., post-stroke central pain) when central, often supraspinal, activation of the pain system produces the experience of pain independent from any peripheral pathology (Nicholson, 2000a). Such pain can be very severe and very real. As indicated previously, chronic pain can be expressed independent from any structural lesion (central or peripheral) as a consequence of central sensitization or functional neural networks. This might account for many puzzling presentations, perhaps especially in those cases of idiopathic pain or when there is no indication of any significant peripheral pathology, but mechanisms of effect remain largely unknown.

The gate control theory initially provided great promise of an integration of peripheral and central, ascending and descending, or neurobiological and psychological factors (Melzack & Wall, 1965). Unfortunately, this paradigm has failed to generate such integration, although there has been an immense amount of work devoted to understanding the microcircuitry of the spinal cord. In the recent past, several other models with a focus on supraspinal mechanisms have been suggested (Birbaumer, Flor, Lutenberger, & Elbert, 1995; Chapman, 1995, 1996; Flor et al., 1995; Flor, Braun, Elbert, & Birbaumer, 1997; Lenz, Gracely, Zirh, Romanowski, & Dougherty, 1997; Melzack, 1999; Wood, Alpers, & Andrews, 1999). These all accept, more or less explicitly, the importance of some neuropsychobiological interface. Some have provided good detail of possible neurobiological mechanisms but there has been very poor, if any, actual integration of psychological and neurobiological factors. Rather, there has been only general suggestion of how psychological processes (e.g., emotion, memory, conditioning, stress, personality) may be related to underlying neurobiological processes. Unfortunately, the neurobiological underpinning of personality is extremely rudimentary (Grigsby & Stevens, 1999).

Gabriel (1990, 1993, 1995) has developed a model system of discriminative avoidance learning that may prove useful in providing for future integration of psychological and biological components involved in chronic pain. Gabriel distinguishes between an anterior and posterior thalamocingulate circuit. The anterior thalamocingulate circuit, centered on the medial dorsal thalamus and the anterior cingulate (area 24b), is specialized for the rapid and flexible acquisition of conditioned avoidance responses. In contrast, the posterior thalamocingulate circuit, centered upon the posterior cingulate with afferents from anterior thalamic nuclei, is specialized for the maintenance and retention of responses involved in discriminative avoidance learning. These circuits are heavily interdependent and also dependent upon inputs from several other structures (e.g., the amygdala). This model appears of interest, especially given that psychological dimensions associated with the development or expression of chronic pain problems (e.g., active-passive, motor-sensory, independent-dependent) might be mapped onto this neurobiological substrate (Nicholson, in preparation). The structure of such neuropsychobiological circuits underlying chronic pain may also be seen to be associated with aspects of social behavior and psychosocial development (i.e., maternal behavior, separation cry, etc.) (MacLean, 1986, 1993; Nelson & Panksepp, 1998). Increasing understanding of the neurobiology of attachment or other aspects of social or interpersonal behavior can be expected to facilitate understanding of chronic pain problems. It is suspected that development of animal models that explore the psychobiological substrate may be especially useful but this would require raising laboratory animals in an environment that would produce psychological vulnerability.

Whereas there has been much investigation about the possible role of psychological factors in the presentation of chronic pain patients, there is very poor understanding and even poorer empirical documentation of what this might entail. One approach to this issue is that the psychology of chronic pain is merely a matter of how people react to or cope with the ("real" or "physical") pain they have. This appears to represent what has been the dominant cognitive-behavioral perspective prevalent in at least North America. Many who adopt this approach seem to think that psychological distress, as can be measured by various brief questionnaires, is the only pertinent psychological phenomenon to be assessed. On the other hand, others consider that psychosocial factors may contribute to a vulnerability for development or expression of chronic pain problems, or that there is some "psychogenicity" in the expression of a pain problem. In such cases, a more detailed psychological analysis is usually considered. It is likely that these two approaches are often two sides of the same coin. For example, fear avoidance is a prominent problem with many chronic pain patients who may be unwilling to try to be doing things because of a fear of increasing pain, whereas other patients who do not have such fear may be coping better with pain and related problems or engaging in activity that may help to reduce the pain. Although this phenomenon is usually interpreted as a coping mechanism, it can also be considered a disposition or premorbid vulnerability.

It is likely that there are many shades of meaning to the term "psychogenic pain," some involving a weaker or stronger sense of how psychosocial factors may be causal. It is unknown to what extent any pain problem may be primarily (or even exclusively) psychogenic or independent of peripheral factors. Even in such cases as sympathetic labor pain of a man whose wife is expecting, i.e., the couvade syndrome (Bardhan, 1965), there may be associated gastrointestinal effects related to the stress and anxiety of this event and focus upon gastrointestinal sensation that might generate some peripheral nociception. However, especially if such pain is severe, one might suspect there is central magnification of any actual peripheral nociception. Again, in general, it remains very poorly understood what pertinent psychosocial factors may be or what any specific mechanisms of effect might be. There is also very poor understanding of the interaction of psychosocial factors with the pain system or other systems (i.e., motor, immune, endocrine, autonomic, etc.). Nonetheless, there has recently been increasing attention devoted to these and related issues (Block, Kremer, & Fernandez, 1999; Gatchel & Turk, 1999; Grzesiak & Ciccone, 1994; Nicholson, 2000b).

It is suspected that that there is typically an interaction of biomedical and psychological factors contributing to presentation in most cases of chronic pain. As is true for many traits, it might be expected that psychological predisposition or vulnerability is normally distributed with a minority (perhaps 5 to 15%) having marked disposition, another minority (again, perhaps 5 to 15%) being very resistant, and most of us somewhere in between. Thus, for someone with strong disposition, it may require little in the way of peripheral pathology/injury or peripherally generated nociception to activate central functional components associated with psychological factors. In others who are more resistant, it may require marked injury, perhaps under conditions of extreme stress, for a central sensitization effect associated with psychosocial factors or vulnerability to be activated. This is consistent with several recent vulnerability-diathesis-stress models of chronic pain (e.g., Dworkin & Banks, 1999). Returning to the example of fear avoidance, an individual with marked vulnerability may react with extreme fear avoidance to even little actual nociception (e.g., slight musculoskeletal strain). In an individual with little disposition, it may require much more severe injury and substantive nociception to limit activity due to fear avoidance. Notably, other vulnerability factors (e.g., genetic) should also be considered; but, again, an association or interaction with psychological factors can often be expected (e.g., gender, temperament, or other effects).

The nosological system of the American Psychiatric Association (APA, 1994) distinguishes between Pain Disorder Associated with Both Psychological Factors and a General Medical Condition versus Pain Disorder Associated with Psychological Factors. In the latter, psychological factors are considered to play the primary role in the onset, maintenance, severity, or exacerbation of chronic pain, whereas both psychological and medical factors are considered to contribute to the former. Pain Disorder Associated with a General Medical Condition is not a psychiatric diagnosis and indicates that pain is associated with medical factors alone. Whereas these distinctions are certainly heuristic and useful, it should be noted that this nosological system provides no guidance about what psychosocial factors should be considered, how these might be measured, what any specific mechanisms of effect might be, or how any interaction effects between psychological and biomedical factors might operate. Again, just because psychological factors can be associated with onset, maintenance, exacerbation or severity of pain, and although they may well be primary, it does not mean that pain is not "real" or that there is not a neurobiological substrate to this disorder. This appears to be a common misconception (Teasell & Merskey, 1997). Again, psychological states or processes (e.g., pain, fear, responsibility, reading this sentence) are not merely figments of one's imagination but are presumed to have an underlying neurobiological substrate. "Functional" pain associated with psychological factors may be quite "real" and should perhaps be considered a variant of central pain as has previously been suggested (Nicholson, 2000b). Psychiatry has grappled with similar problems of what constitutes organic, functional, and psychologic factors in the understanding of several other disorders (e.g., depression) where both psychosocial and biomedical etiological factors can be identified and both biomedical or psychosocial treatments may be indicated.

There is a widespread misconception that what constitutes psychological factors contributing to presentation in chronic pain must be gross psychopathology, psychiatric disorder, or sexual/physical abuse during childhood. Whereas there is some evidence that physical or sexual abuse may play a part in the etiology of gastrointestinal or pelvic pain problems, there is otherwise little evidence that this is a relevant etiological factor in other pain problems (Drossman, 1994; Roy, 1998), although it may be that concurrent histories of abuse plus a significant nociceptive or neuropathic pain problem can result in increased affective distress and difficulty coping. There is mixed evidence on the causal relationship between pain and depression (more generally considered negative affect and certainly not always involving premorbid clinical depression), different studies suggesting that the relationship may be causal, reactive, or recursive (Robinson & Riley, 1999). On the other hand, it has also long been noted that many chronic pain patients appear to be model citizens and, although perhaps very active, with underlying dependence-independence conflicts or other identifiable characteristics, do not have gross premorbid psychosocial problems (Blumer & Heilbronn, 1982). In some cases, there are clear indications that psychological factors are playing a major role in presentation, such as when there is complete resolution of pain

problems on administration of a placebo, when there is marked exacerbation under stress or complete resolution in a calming environment, or when there is dramatic pain behavior when attention is focused on pain but no pain behavior when distracted. In many cases, however, the markers may be much more subtle.

Another important and often very contentious issue associated with many misconceptions about chronic pain is whether patients might be malingering (Martelli, Zasler, et al., 1999; Fishbain, et al., 1999a). Although it may be cruel to suggest that (actual) pain is just in the head, suggesting that it is not real or valid, it may be a greater insult to suggest that one's (actual) pain is the product of active dissimulation or malingering, that is, that the individual is just pretending to have pain (or greatly exaggerating pain) to obtain some financial or other benefits. On the other hand, some patients may be actively malingering and this can be very costly, diverting resources from those who need them. A recent review of the literature indicates that malingering might be present in from 1.25 to 10.4% of chronic pain patients but that estimates are not considered reliable and, furthermore, that there is no reliable method for detecting malingering with chronic pain patients (Fishbain, et al., 1999a).

Some signs, often considered to be "non-organic" (i.e., non-dermatomal sensory deficits) (Mailis et al., 2001; Waddell, McCulloch, Kummel, & Venner, 1980), have been found to be associated with actual abnormalities on functional neuroimaging, that is, lack of activation or deactivation of contralateral S1 cortex and other areas on stimulation of the affected side (Mailis et al., 2000). In addition, such nondermatomal somatosensory deficits are prevalent in several pain populations and are suspected as being associated with psychosocial factors (Fishbain, Goldberg, Rosomoff, & Rosomoff, 1991; Mailis & Nicholson, 1997).

Whereas symptom validity testing has been used in other domains (i.e., assessment of memory complaints) to quite unambiguously identify conscious dissimulation. e.g., when level of performance is statistically significantly below what would be expected on the basis of random responding, this is not possible with pain because there is no objective external criteria to evaluate the subjective report. Although there appears to be a trend to use certain cut-off scores on symptom validity testing with those pain patients who concurrently complain of cognitive problems, this is considered inappropriate because such techniques have not been normed on appropriate populations (i.e., chronic pain patients with affective or other problems). Furthermore, there is a large literature documenting cognitive deficits associated with either acute pain challenges in normal volunteers or chronic pain patients (Hart, Martelli, & Zasler, 2000; Martelli, Grayson, & Zasler, 1999; Nicholson, 2000c).

Although it may be very difficult to ascertain whether there is deliberate malingering, there is much stronger evidence that compensation has the potential to influence presentation, for example, severity or duration of complaints (Cassidy et al., 2000; Loeser, Henderlite, & Conrad, 1995; Loeser & Sullivan, 1995; Nachemson, 1994; Rohling, Binder, & Langhinrichsen-Rohling, 1995). There is also consistent evidence that secondary gain, a concept that is crudely akin to social reinforcement of illness behavior, is an important factor affecting presentation (Fishbain, Rosomoff, Cutler, & Rosomoff, 1995). Again, it is often very difficult to disentangle the effect of these or other specific psychosocial factors from biomedical factors in individual cases.

Many myths and misconceptions about treatment for chronic pain also arise from our poor understanding of the phenomena or are specifically associated with a biased perspective of the mind–body problem. There appears to be a predominant misconception, on behalf of both patients and professionals, that medical science will solve the problem of pain and suffering. On the part of the patient, this may be associated with the idea that medical science is omniscient or omnipotent and can fix any and all problems. Some patients may relegate all responsibility for their pain problem(s) to their doctors. These or related attitudes can lead to persistent medical treatment seeking behavior. After repeated temporary successes (or failures) with numerous medical interventions, it might be questioned whether patients expect to be "cured" by medical science or if they really just want someone to take care of them, perhaps as their parents may once have done. Unfortunately, patients who present with much suffering and desire for treatment can usually find some physician who will provide treatment, whether or not there are good indications for any such intervention. Many interventions, especially surgical, can lead to very serious iatrogenic effects. Some patients may then end up with pain problems far worse than they previously had, wishing they had never had surgery. Iatrogenic effects are certainly not limited to medical interventions. Physiotherapy, chiropractic, or other physical therapies can also result in serious iatrogenic effects. Furthermore, psychological treatments, especially perhaps insofar as they enhance invalidism, can also greatly exacerbate problems. It should also be noted that many practitioners (whether they be plumbers, mechanics, physiotherapists, physicians, psychologists, lawyers, or others) will engage in their professional activity, applying the tools of their trade, often with little regard for the need or effectiveness of their interventions. It should not be forgotten that there are tremendous financial benefits on the part of practitioners. In this regard, it may be more pertinent to question the issue of compensation of practitioners than patients. It should also be recognized that there is a massive medical-industrial complex propagating biomedical research and treatments. Undue medicalization of a problem is not unique to the field of pain. For example, many people would rather have liposuction

for weight control than maintain a proper regimen of diet and exercise or accept a less than ideal body weight. It may be easier to administer Ritalin or other stimulants to school children rather than provide appropriate structure or stimulation for problems of activity level. Patients or their doctors may prefer to take a pill for problems of depression rather than pursue cognitive-behavioral change that may be more effective.

Although it might be demonstrated that there is an organic or biomedical substrate for a pain problem, this does not necessarily mean that there should be medical treatment. For example, there may be some mild degenerative spinal changes demonstrated on CT, or functional neuroimaging might demonstrate that there are some patterns of brain activation (or deactivation) associated with low-back pain. However, it might be that pain in this case is primarily associated with inactivity, poor posture, or poor back hygiene. The treatment of choice may be to have the person engage in an appropriate exercise regimen or other activity rather than perform back (or brain) surgery. In this context, it should be noted that a recent meta-analysis indicates that opioids provide some good effect with nociceptive pain, are less effective with neuropathic pain, and are not effective with idiopathic pain (Graven, de Vet, van Kleef, & Weber, 1999). Although no attempt will be made to review the literature, it is apparent that there are many myths or misconceptions regarding opioid treatment, ranging from the extremes of believing opioids should never be prescribed because this will lead to drug addiction, to the other extreme where no consideration is given for this possible problem and opioids are heavily prescribed whether or not there is beneficial effect.

As previously suggested, whereas it might be demonstrated that psychosocial factors are involved in the etiology, maintenance, exacerbation, or severity of pain problems, this does not mean that such pain is not "real." It also does not mean that such pain should be treated with psychological methods alone, nor that psychological interventions would necessarily be helpful at all. Indeed, pharmacological or other medical treatment might be the treatment of choice with these patients. It remains largely unknown to what extent any such pain problems would respond to psychosocial interventions or to what extent medical treatments may be required. In addition, whereas psychosocial factors may play an important or even primary role in the pain problem, with relatively little apparent peripheral pathology/nociception, it might be that alleviation of this minor peripheral component via medical intervention would be sufficient to completely resolve the problem.

Although psychosocial interventions have been shown to be effective for a wide variety of chronic pain problems, whether or not there is demonstrable peripheral pathology (Flor, Fydrich, & Turk, 1992; Holroyd & Lipchik, 1999; Morely, Eccleston, & Williams, 1999; Van Tulder, Koes, & Bouter, 1997), effect sizes are often limited and many

TABLE 38.1
Myths and Misconceptions about Chronic Pain

We know what pain is.

We know what the biological basis of pain is.

We know what the psychology of pain is.

Pain is either in the body or in the mind.

Pain has either sensory or affective and/or cognitive components.

Pain is psychogenic or pain is not psychogenic.

If there is no discernible organic basis, then pain must be "functional," that is, "only psychological."

Psychological means somehow not real or without any basis in physical reality.

If there is a psychological component, it is all in your head.

If there is a marked psychological component contributing to presentation, there is no organic substrate.

We have reliable tests that are specifically sensitive to "organic" vs. "non-organic" conditions, or we can accurately measure biomedical or psychological components contributing to presentation.

Patient self-report of pain severity or other problems is unbiased.

We know when a patient is malingering or to what extent compensation issues are affecting presentation.

Practitioners are not biased or are not influenced by compensation issues.

Medical science or biomedical treatments will solve all the problems of pain and suffering.

Psychological treatments are all that is necessary or you just need to be a better person or of better character.

If there is a major psychological component contributing to presentation, there should be psychological but not biomedical treatment.

Psychological presentation in chronic pain patients is either causal or reactive.

Psychological treatments are not helpful for real (organic) pain.

Because psychological factors may be associated with onset, maintenance, exacerbations, severity, etc., means that it is not a real.

Functional neuroimaging will allow us to unlock the secrets of pain and establish the organic vs. psychological basis of the pain.

Opioid use causes addiction or does not result in problems of addiction.

Pain does not cause cognitive problems.

All of a patient's problems are because of an accident/injury and pain.

patients do not find these helpful. It is largely unknown what specific techniques are effective for which patients. In addition, it has been suggested that any systematic treatment delivered with enthusiasm appears to be helpful, leading one to suspect placebo (or at least nonspecific) effects (Blanchard & Galovski, 1999). Indeed, placebo effects are common and prominent (Turner, Deyo, Loeser, Von Korff, & Fordyce, 1994). Again, the mechanism of effect is not well understood (Price & Fields, 1997), although it has been demonstrated that the placebo effect may be associated with a discrete neurobiological response (Benedetti, Arduino, & Aanzio, 1999; Harrington, 1997). There is clearly need for further study about how psychosocial or related interventions work.

Finally, there is a trend toward emphasizing the results of systematic reviews and meta-analyses (i.e., evidence-based medicine) to establish whether or not any specific treatment is effective. Although this is certainly laudatory and may help to weed out the "junk science" or inappropriate and possibly iatrogenic treatments, caution should be exercised about taking such reviews/analyses as "gospel." These may not always be of adequate quality, thus raising concern about conclusions (Fishbain, Cutler, Rosomoff, & Rosomoff, 1999b). Furthermore, just because a set of studies does not provide evidence for something, it does not mean that this is necessarily so. For example, although one could line up the studies indicating that there is no peripheral biological basis for fibromyalgia, this does not mean that some such process will not discovered. Following a strict set of guidelines based on the results of such reviews/analyses could prematurely limit the range of options for treatment or future research.

In conclusion, many myths or misconceptions about chronic pain exist today. These largely arise out of our poor understanding of the phenomena. This chapter focused on myths or misconceptions that are associated with the problem of mind–body dualism or the tendency to view pain problems from either an "organic" or a "psychological" perspective. In contrast, it has been repeatedly suggested that explication of the interface between these domains may be of critical importance in the understanding and treatment of chronic pain. Table 38.1 presents a summary of the primary myths and misconceptions that have been discussed in this chapter. It would be another misconception to think that many other myths and misconceptions do not exist.

REFERENCES

Alexander, G.E., DeLong M.R., & Strick, P.L. (1986). Parallel organization of functionally segregated circuits linking basal ganglia and cortex. *Annual Review of Neuroscience, 9*, 357.

American Psychiatric Association (1994). *Diagnostic and statistical manual of mental disorders* (4th ed.). Washington, D.C.: American Psychiatric Association.

Bardhan, P.N. (1965). The couvade syndrome. *British Journal of Psychiatry, 111*, 908.

Benedetti, F., Arduino, C., & Aanzio, M. (1999). Somatotopic activation of opiods systems by target-directed expectations of analgesia. *The Journal of Neuroscience, 19*, 3639–3648.

Besson, J.M., Guilbaud, G., & Ollat, H. (1995). *Forebrain areas involved in pain processing*. Paris: John Libbey Eurotext.

Birbaumer, N., Flor, H., Lutenberger, W., & Elbert, T. (1995). The corticalization of chronic pain. In B. Bromm & J.E. Desmedt (Eds.), *Pain and the brain: From nociception to cognition* (pp. 331–343). New York: Raven Press.

Blanchard, E.B., & Galovski, T. (1999). Irritable bowel syndrome. In R.J. Gatchel & D.C. Turk (Eds.), *Psychosocial factors in pain* (pp. 270–283). New York: Guilford Press.

Block, A.R., Kremer, E.F., & Fernandez, E. (Eds.). (1999). *Handbook of pain syndromes*, Mahwah, NJ: Lawrence Erlbaum Associates.

Blumer, D., & Heilbronn, M. (1982). Chronic pain as a variant of depressive disease: The pain-prone personality. *Journal of Nervous and Mental Disease, 170*, 381–486.

Bromm, B., & Desmedt, J.E. (Eds.). (1995). *Pain and the brain: From nociception to cognition.* New York: Raven Press.

Cabeza, R., & Nyberg, L. (1997). Imaging cognition: An empirical review of PET studies with normal subjects, *Journal of Cognitive Neuroscience, 9*, 1–26.

Cassidy, J.D., Carroll, L.J., Cote, P., Lemstra, M., Berglund, A., & Nygren, A. (2000). Effect of eliminating compensation for pain and suffering on the outcome of insurance claims for whiplash injury. *New England Journal of Medicine, 342*, 1179–1186.

Chapman, C.R. (1995). The affective dimension of pain: A model. In B. Bromm & J. E. Desmedt (Eds.), *Pain and the brain: From nociception to cognition* (pp. 283–301). New York: Raven Press.

Chapman, C.R. (1996). Limbic processes and the affective dimension of pain. *Progress in brain research, 10*, 63–81.

Chundler, E.H., & Dong, W.K. (1995). The role of the basal ganglia in nociception and pain, *Pain, 60*, 3–38.

Coghill, R.C., Sanf, C.N., Maisog, J.M., & Ladoralo, M.J. (1999). Pain intensity processing within the human brain: A bilateral, distributed mechanism. *Journal of Neuropsychology, 82*, 1934–1943.

Cohodarevic, T., Mailis, A., & Montanera, W. (2000). Syringomyelia: Pain, sensory abnormalities, and neuroimaging. *Journal of Pain, 1*, 54–66.

Craig, A.D, Reiman, E.M., Evans, A., & Bushnell, M.C. (1996). Functional imaging of an illusion of pain. *Nature, 384*, 258–260.

Davis, K.D, Taylor, S.J., Crawley, A.P., Wood, M.L., & Mikulis, D.J. (1997). Functional MRI of pain- and attention-related activations in the human cingulate cortex. *Journal of Neurophysiology, 77*, 3370–3380.

Drevets, W.C., Burton, H., Videen, T.O., Snyder, A.Z., Simpson, J.R., & Raichle, M.E. (1995). Blood flow changes in human somatosensory cortex during anticipated stimulation, *Nature, 373*, 249–252.

Drossman, D.A. (1994). Physical and sexual abuse and gastrointestinal illness: What is the link? *The American Journal of Medicine, 97*, 105–107.

Dworkin, R.H. & Banks, S.M. (1999). A vulnerability-diathesis-stress model of chronic pain: Herpes zoster and the development of postherpetic neuralgia. In R.J. Gatchel & D.C. Turk (Eds.), *Psychosocial factors in pain* (p. 247–271). New York: Guilford Press.

Fishbain, D.A., Cutler, R.B., Rosomoff, H.L., & Rosomoff, R.S. (1999a). *Chronic pain and disability exaggeration/malingering research and the application of submaximal effort research to this area: A review.* Poster presented at International Association of Pain 9th World Congress, Vienna, Austria.

Fishbain, D.A., Cutler, R.B., Rosomoff, H.L., & Rosomoff, R.S. (1999b). What is the quality of the implemented meta-analytic procedures in chronic pain treatment meta-anlyses? *The Clinical Journal of Pain, 16*, 73–85.

Fishbain, D.A., Goldberg, M., Rosomoff, R.S., & Rosomoff, H.L. (1991). Chronic pain patients and the nonorganic physical sign of nondermatomal sensory abnormalities (NDSA). *Psychosomatics, 32*, 294–303.

Fishbain, D.A., Rosomoff, H.L., Cutler, R.B., & Rosomoff, R.S. (1995). Secondary gain concept: A review of the scientific evidence. *The Clinical Journal of Pain, 11*, 6–21.

Flor, H., Braun, C., Elbert, T., & Birbaumer, N. (1997). Extensive reorganization of primary somatosensory cortex in chronic back pain patients. *Neuroscience Letters, 224*, 5–8.

Flor, H., Elbert, T., Wienbruch, C., Pantev, C., Knecht, S., Birbaumer, N., Larbig, W., & Taub, E. (1995). Phantom limb pain as a perceptual correlate of cortical reorganization. *Nature, 357*, 482–484.

Flor, H., Fydrich, T., & Turk, D.C. (1992). Efficacy of multidisciplinary pain treatment centers: A meta-analytic review, *Pain, 49*, 221–230.

Gabriel, M. (1990). Functions of anterior and posterior cingulate cortex during avoidance learning in rabbits. *Progress in Brain Research, 85*, 467–482.

Gabriel, M. (1993). Discriminative avoidance learning: A model system. In B.A. Vogt & M. Gabriel (Eds.), *Neurobiology of cingulate cortex and limbic thalamus: A comprehensive handbook* (pp. 478–523). Boston: Birkhauser.

Gabriel, M. (1995). The role of pain in cingulate cortical and limbic thalamic mediation of avoidance learning. In J.M. Besson, G. Guilbaud, & H. Ollat (Eds.), *Forebrain areas involved in pain processing* (pp. 197–211). Paris: John Libbey Eurotext.

Gatchel, R.J., & Turk, D.C. (Eds.). (1999). *Psychosocial Factors in Pain.* New York: Guilford Press.

Graven, S., de Vet, H., van Kleef, M., & Weber, W. (1999). *Opioids in chronic non-malignant pain: A meta-analysis of the literature.* Poster presented at International Association of Pain 9th World Congress, Vienna, Austria.

Grigsby, J., & Stevens, D. (1999). *Neurodynamics of personality.* New York: Guilford Press.

Grzesiak, R.C., & Ciccone, D.S. (Eds.). (1994). *Psychological vulnerability to chronic pain.* New York: Springer-Verlag.

Harrington, A. (Ed.). (1997). *The placebo effect: An interdisciplinary exploration.* Cambridge, MA: Harvard University Press.

Hart, R.P, Martelli, M.F., & Zasler, N.D. (2000). Chronic pain and neuropsychological functioning. *Neuropsychology Review, 10*(3), 131–149.

Holroyd, K.A., & Lipchik, G.L. (1999). Psychological management of recurrent headache disorders: Progress and prospects. In R.J. Gatchel & D.C. Turk (Eds.), *Psychosocial factors in pain* (pp. 193–212). New York: Guilford Press.

Hsieh, J.C., Stahle-Backdahl, M., Hagermark, O., Stone-Elander, S., Rosenquist, G., & Ingvar, M. (1995). Traumatic nociceptive pain activates the hypothalamus and the periaqueductal gray: A positron emission tomography study. *Pain, 64*, 303–314.

Lenz, F A., Graceley, R.H., Zirh, A.T., Romanowski, A.J., & Dougherty, P.M. (1997). The sensory-limbic model of pain memory. *Pain Forum, 6*, 22–31.

Linton, S.J. (1999). Prevention with special reference to chronic musculoskeletal disorders. In R. J. Gatchel & D.C. Turk (Eds.), *Psychosocial factors in pain* (pp. 374–389). New York: Guilford Press.

Loeser, J.D., Henderlite, S.E., & Conrad, D.A. (1995). Incentive effect of worker's compensation benefits: A literature synthesis. *Medical Care Research and Review, 52*, 34–59.

Loeser, J.D., & Sullivan, M. (1995). Disability in the chronic low back pain patient. *Pain Forum, 4*, 114–121.

MacLean, P.D. (1986). Culminating developments in the evolution of the limbic system: The thalamocingulate division. In B.K. Doane & K.E. Livingston (Eds.), *The limbic system: Functional organization and clinical disorders* (pp. 1–26). New York: Raven Press.

MacLean, P.D. (1993). Perspectives on cingulate cortex in the limbic system. In B.A. Vogt & M. Gabriel (Eds.), *Neurobiology of cingulate cortex and limbic thalamus: A comprehensive handbook* (pp. 1–15). Boston: Birkhauser.

Mailis, A., Amani, N., Umana, M., Basur, R., & Roe, S. (1997). Effect of sodium amytal on cutaneous sensory abnormalities, spontaneous pain and algometric pain pressure thresholds in neuropathic pain patients: A placebo-controlled study II. *Pain, 70*, 69–81.

Mailis, A., Downar, J., Kwan, C., Nicholson, K., Mikulis, D., & Davis, K.D. (2000). FMRI in explainable widespread somatosensory deficits (WSDs) in patients with chronic pain. Nineteenth Annual APS meeting, Atlanta, CA, *American Pain Society Abstract, 760*, 158.

Mailis, A., & Nicholson, K. (1997). Effect of normal saline controlled intravenous administration of sodium amytal in patients with pain and unexplained widespread non-anatomical sensory deficits: A preliminary report. *American Pain Society Abstract, 708*, 138.

Mailis, A., Papagapiou, M., Umana, M., Cohodarevic, T., Nowak, J., & Nicholson, K. (2001). Unexplainable widespread somatosensory deficits in patients with chronic nonmalignant pain in the context of litigation/compensation: A role for involvement of central factors. *Journal of Rheumatology, 28*, 1385–1393.

Martelli, M.F., Grayson, R., & Zasler, N.D. (1999). Post traumatic headache: Psychological and neuropsychological issues in assessment and treatment. *Journal of Head Trauma Rehabilitation, 14*(1), 49–69.

Martelli, M.F., Zasler, N.D., & MacMillan, P. (1998). Mediating the relationship between injury, impairment and disability: A vulnerability, stress & coping model of adaptation following brain injury. *NeuroRehabilitation: An Interdisciplinary Journal, 11*(1), 51.

Martelli, M.F., Zasler, N.D., Mancini, A.M., & MacMillan, P. J. (1999). Psychological assessment and applications in impairment and disability evaluations. In R.V. May & M.F. Martelli (Eds.), *Guide to functional capacity evaluation with impairment rating applications*. Richmond, VA: NADEP Publications.

Melzack, R. (1999). From the gate to the neruomatrix. *Pain Supplement, 6*, S121–S126.

Melzack, R., & Casey, K.L. (1966). Sensory, motivational and central control determinants of pain: A new conceptual model. In D. Kenshalo (Ed.), *The skin senses* (pp. 423–443). Springfield, IL: Charles C Thomas.

Melzack, R., & Wall, P.D. (1965). Pain mechanisms: A new theory. *Science, 150*, 971–979.

Merskey, H., & Bogduk, N. (Eds.). (1994). *Classification of chronic pain* (2nd ed.). Seattle: IASP Press.

Morely, S., Eccleston, C., & Williams, A. (1999). Systematic review and meta-analysis of randomized controlled trials of cognitive behaviour therapy and behaviour therapy for chronic pain in adults, excluding headache. *Pain, 80*, 1–13.

Nachemson, A. (1994). Chronic pain—The end of the welfare state? *Quality of Life Research, 3*, S11–S17.

Nelson, E.E., & Panksepp, J. (1998). Brain substrates of infant-mother attachment: Contributions of opiods, oxytocin and norepinephrine. *Neuroscience and Biobehavioral Reviews, 22*, 437–452.

Nicholson, K. (2000a). An overview of pain problems associated with lesions, disorder or dysfunction of the central nervous system. *NeuroRehabilitation, 14*, 3–13.

Nicholson, K. (2000b). At the crossroads: Pain in the 21st century. *NeuroRehabilitation, 14*, 57–67.

Nicholson, K. (2000c). Pain, cognition and traumatic brain injury. *NeuroRehabilitation, 14*, 95–103.

Nicholson, K. (in prep.) Psychogenic pain: Review of the construct, a novel taxonomy and neuropsychobiological model.

Ploghaus, A., Tracey, I., Gati, J.S., Clare, S., Menon, R.S., Matthews, P.M., & Rawlins, J.N.P. (1999). Dissociating pain from its anticipation in the human brain. *Science, 284*, 1979–1981.

Porro, C.A., Francescato, M.P., Cettolo, V., & Baraldi P. (1998). *Cortical activity during anticipation of a noxious stimulus: A fMRI study* [Abstract]. 4th International Conference on Functional Mapping of the Human Brain, Montreal, Quebec.

Price, D.L., & Fields, H.L. (1997). Where are the causes of placebo analgesia. *Pain Forum, 6*, 44–52.

Robinson, M.E., & Riley, J.L. (1999). The role of emotion in pain. In R.J. Gatchel & D.C. Turk (Eds.), *Psychosocial factors in pain* (pp. 74–88). New York: Guilford Press.

Rohling, M.L., Binder, L.M., & Langhinrichsen-Rohling, J. (1995). Money matters: A meta-analytic review of the assocaition between financial compensation and the experience and treatment of chronic pain. *Health Psychology, 14*, 537–547.

Roy, R. (1998). *Childhood abuse and chronic pain: A curious relationship?* Toronto: University of Toronto Press.

St-Cyr, J., Taylor, A., & Nicholson, K. (1995). Behavior and the basal ganglia. In W.J. Weinger & A.E. Lang (Eds.), *Behavioral neurology of the movement disorders, Advances in neurology* (Vol. 65, pp. 1–28), New York: Raven Press.

Teasell, R.W., & Merskey, H. (1997). Chronic pain disability in the workplace. *Pain Research Management, 2*, 197–205.

Treede, R., Kenshalo, D.R., Gracely, R.H., & Jones, A.K.P. (1999). The cortical representation of pain. *Pain, 79,* 105–111.

Turner, J.A., Deyo, R.A., Loeser, J.D., Von Korff, M., & Fordyce, W.E. (1994). The importance of placebo effects in pain treatment and research. *Journal of the American Medical Association, 271,* 1609–1614.

Van Tulder, M.W., Koes, B.W., & Bouter, L.M. (1997). Conservative treatment of acute and chronic nonspecific low back pain. *Spine, 22,* 2128–2156.

Vogt, B.A., Sikes, R.W., & Vogt, L.J. (1993). Anterior cingulate cortex and the medial pain system. In B.A. Vogt & M. Gabriel (Eds.), *Neurobiology of cingulate cortex and limbic thalamus: A comprehensive handbook* (pp. 313–344). Boston: Birkhauser.

Waddell, G., McCulloch, J.A., Kummel, E.G., & Venner, R.M. (1980). Non-organic physical signs in low back pain. *Spine, 5,* 117–125.

Wall, P.D. (2000). Pain in context: The intellectual roots of pain research and therapy. In M. Devor, M.C. Rowbotham, & Z. Wiesenfeld-Hallin (Eds.), *Proceedings of the 9th World Congress on Pain: Progress in pain research and management* (pp. 19–34). Seattle: IASP Press. Inclusive pages??

Wood, J.D., Alpers, D.H., & Andrews, P.L.R. (1999). Fundamentals of neurogastroenterology. *Gut, 45*(Suppl. 2), II6–II16.

Section VI

Specialty Concerns

39

Management of Procedural and Perioperative Pain in Children

John T. Algren, M.D., F.A.A.P. and Christine L. Algren, R.N., M.S.N., Ed.D.

INTRODUCTION

The relief of pain in children is a challenge to pediatric healthcare providers. Because the existence of pain in children has previously been denied and ignored (Eland & Anderson, 1977; Schechter, 1989), many children have undergone procedures and surgeries without adequate sedation, analgesia, or anesthesia. The recent interest in pediatric pain has resulted in major philosophical shifts and technical advances. Consequently, various innovative pediatric pain management strategies have evolved. This chapter addresses the care of children with acute pain associated with diagnostic and therapeutic procedures and surgery.

SEDATION AND ANALGESIA FOR PEDIATRIC PROCEDURES

Although pain is a universal experience for children, the type and intensity of pain are quite variable. Children experience brief, intermittent episodes of pain associated with cuts, bruises, and common childhood illnesses. Hospitalized children undergo painful procedures, ranging from venipunctures and intravenous catheter insertions to lumbar punctures and bone marrow aspirations. These diagnostic and therapeutic procedures can cause brief but intense pain. Children often describe these procedures as more distressing than any other aspect of their hospitalization or illness (Eland & Anderson, 1977). Unrelieved pain can have both negative physiological and emotional consequences. Effective pain prevention and treatment can

prevent these adverse effects, yielding both short- and long-term benefits.

The goals of pain management for pediatric procedures include lessening patient and parent anxiety, minimizing pain, improving patient cooperation, and facilitating the successful completion of the procedure. Appropriate preparation and adequate analgesia and sedation for painful procedures are crucial not only for minimizing pain, but also for decreasing stress and anxiety. Optimal management should take into consideration the type of procedure being performed and individual factors such as the age and physical condition. Based on a thorough pain assessment, appropriate interventions may consist of pharmacologic agents and nonpharmacological interventions. (Acute Pain Management, 1992). With appropriate nonpharmacologic intervention and sufficient sedation, analgesia, and anxiolysis, children are able to undergo procedures with little physiological or emotional stress.

MONITORING AND MANAGEMENT GUIDELINES

Recent technological and therapeutic advances have led to an increase in diagnostic and minor surgical procedures. Although anesthesiologists provide sedation or general anesthesia for many of these procedures, practical issues of cost, logistics, and availability of personnel support the practice of sedation management by other healthcare providers as well. To promote safe sedation practices, the Committee on Drugs of the American

0-8493-0926-3/02/$0.00+$1.50
© 2002 by CRC Press LLC

Academy of Pediatrics has promulgated guidelines for monitoring and managing pediatric patients undergoing conscious or deep sedation for diagnostic and therapeutic procedures (American Academy of Pediatrics, 1992). Other professional organizations have developed differing guidelines (American Academy of Pediatric Dentistry, 1993; American College of Emergency Physicians, 1993; American Society of Anesthesiologists, 1996), leading to considerable debate (Cotè, 1994; Sacchetti, et al., 1994). All have the common goal of fostering safe yet efficient sedation practices. Regardless of perspective or bias, practitioners are urged to not allow expediency to compromise patient safety.

Effective sedation management should provide anxiolysis and analgesia and facilitate patient cooperation. Patient safety and welfare, however, must remain the primary concern of practitioners and assistants because depressed consciousness increases the risk of airway obstruction, respiratory depression, and aspiration, all of which can result in serious morbidity or mortality. When selecting sedatives and analgesics, practitioners must consider the risk of serious adverse events, as well as the incidence of minor problems such as vomiting and prolonged sedation.

Sedatives and analgesics cause depression of the sensorium, ranging from minimal sedation to general anesthesia. "Conscious sedation" is commonly preferred because patients maintain protective airway reflexes and airway patency. Patients remain responsive to verbal and physical stimuli and are able to follow commands. Conscious sedation may be insufficient, however, for some patients undergoing painful procedures. Young children are likely to move and become uncooperative if they experience any discomfort or pain.

"Deep sedation" produces greater depression of consciousness, resulting in diminished responsiveness to stimuli, including pain. Unfortunately, deep sedation may also obtund protective airway reflexes and compromise the patient's ability to independently maintain a patent airway. Such a state is associated with a greater risk of adverse events (e.g., respiratory depression, airway obstruction, and aspiration) and necessitates intravenous access and close and continuous monitoring of cardiorespiratory function. Due to the variability of individual response to depressant medications, administration of sedatives and analgesics for conscious sedation can result in deep sedation, increasing the risk of adverse events. Therefore, irrespective of the planned depth of sedation, practitioners should continuously monitor all patients and be fully prepared to manage potential problems and rescue patients who develop respiratory or cardiovascular depression.

Practitioners must be knowledgeable and competent to oversee all aspects of patient sedation, including drug administration, monitoring, and management of compli-

cations. Due to the small but real risk of serious adverse events such as respiratory depression, vomiting, seizures, anaphylaxis, and cardiorespiratory arrest, resuscitation equipment and emergency drugs must be readily available. Facilities should be suitable in size and configuration to accommodate emergency equipment and personnel. Practitioners and assisting personnel must, at a minimum, be trained in basic pediatric life support (American Academy of Pediatrics, 1992).

Serious complications can best be avoided or minimized by close observation and early detection of changes in patient status. All patients must be monitored throughout the period of sedation and recovery. After recording baseline vital signs, patient assessment should include continuous oxygen saturation and heart rate monitoring, intermittent blood pressure recording, and, depending on the depth of sedation, intermittent or continuous monitoring of ventilation.

Patients should not be discharged until they have sufficient recovery of vital system functions to assure safety. This should include recovery of protective airway reflexes, stable and satisfactory cardiovascular and respiratory function, recovery of presedation neurologic function (appropriate for age or developmental level), and adequate hydration. Patients may still be somewhat sedated at discharge but should be sufficiently recovered to be able to sit in a wheelchair and, if necessary, walk with assistance.

Suitable candidates for conscious or deep sedation are American Society of Anesthesiologists Physical Status Class I or II patients (see Table 39.1). Sedation of Class III or IV patients by non-anesthesiologists should be approached with caution due to the presence of severe systemic disease, which may increase the risk of complications. In preparation for a procedure, patients as well as parents should be thoroughly informed about the procedure and receive instructions concerning preparation for the procedure and care of the child after discharge.

To minimize the risk of aspiration of gastric contents, oral intake should be suspended prior to an elective procedure (see Table 39.2) (American Society of Anesthesi-

---

TABLE 39.1
American Society of Anesthesiologists (ASA) Physical Status Classification

Class	Description
I	Healthy patient
II	Mild systemic disease; no functional limitation
III	Severe systemic disease; definite functional limitation
IV	Severe systemic disease that is a constant threat to life
V	Moribund patient not expected to survive 24 hours with or without operation

TABLE 39.2
Dietary Restrictions for Elective Sedation

Ingested Material	Minimum Fasting Period (hr)
Clear liquids	2
Breast milk	4
Infant formula	6
Nonhuman milk	6
Light meal	6

Source: From American Society of Anesthesiologists Task Force on Preoperative Fasting, *Anesthesiology*, 90, 896, 1999. With permission.

ologists Task Force, 1999). Whenever possible, unscheduled procedures should be delayed until dietary precautions are met. Urgent or emergent situations may require that sedation be provided despite recent oral intake. Under such circumstances, practitioners should proceed cautiously with sedation to avoid depression of airway reflexes and minimize the risk of aspiration. Pharmacologic treatment with drugs such as ranitidine and metaclopramide, which increase gastric pH and decrease gastric volume, may be appropriate. Airway protection provided by tracheal intubation may be advisable if deep sedation is likely to be necessary.

NONPHARMACOLOGIC APPROACHES TO PROCEDURAL PAIN MANAGEMENT

Procedural pain is often associated with stress, fears, and anxiety. Strategies that reduce fear and stress and facilitate cooperation of the child comprise a variety of nonpharmacological interventions that may be helpful in the management of procedural pain. In addition, these interventions can be utilized in the management of chronic or recurrent pain problems, as well as postoperative pain. In addition to being noninvasive and inexpensive, these interventions can give children and parents a sense of control and involvement in the management of pain.

PREPARATION

Because stress and anxiety intensify the sensation of pain, any technique that reduces fear and anxiety can alter the child's perception of pain. Age-appropriate preparation is one of the most widely used interventions for reducing stress and anxiety in children undergoing an invasive procedure. Explanations about the procedure increase the understanding of both the child and parents and reduce fear of the unknown. If possible, the child should be encouraged to express fears, and time should be allowed for questions and answers. Information about why the procedure is necessary and what will be done during the

procedure should be discussed. In addition, the explanation may include a description of how the procedure may feel. For example, a child might be told that he or she will feel a "small pinch" or prick when local anesthetic is administered. Various methods, such as tours, coloring books, dolls, puppets, and play therapy, can be used to prepare the child for the procedure.

DISTRACTION

Distraction can be a powerful coping strategy during painful procedures. Although distraction does not actually reduce the intensity of the pain, it improves pain tolerance. Preschool and older children are more easily distracted than infants.

Healthcare personnel should first identify what is of interest to the child. Distraction can then be accomplished by focusing the child's attention on something other than the procedure. Listening to music with a headset, talking about pets or school, squeezing the nurse's hand, and singing or counting are effective distraction techniques. The perception of pain is only altered, however, during the distracting activity. When the child is no longer distracted, the pain may return.

RELAXATION AND GUIDED IMAGERY

In children who are capable of abstract thinking, relaxation and guided imagery are effective adjunctive therapies for pain management during painful procedures. These techniques do not have to be complex to be effective. Muscle tension, which intensifies pain, can be alleviated by methods such as deep breathing and progressive relaxation exercises (McDonnell & Bowdem 1989). Soothing music and talking in a soft, calm voice can also produce relaxation. Both "easy listening" music and personally preferred music have been reported to significantly decrease postoperative pain (Mullooly, Levin, & Feldman, 1988). These techniques also give the child a feeling of control instead of a sense of helplessness.

Guided imagery can also be used as a means of achieving relaxation during a painful procedure. Children can be guided into imagining pleasant images such as a favorite place, playing in the sand at the beach, or floating on a cloud. Children may also use fantasy to imagine medication traveling through the body to the pain site or heroes attacking the pain.

HYPNOSIS

Hypnosis has been an effective technique for managing procedural pain in children. Zeltzer and LeBaron (1982) reported on the use of hypnosis in children with cancer who were undergoing bone marrow aspirations and lumbar punctures. Hypnotic techniques were consistently more effective than nonhypnotic techniques such as distraction and supportive counseling. Of course, the use of hypnosis requires specific training.

POSITIVE REINFORCEMENT

Positive reinforcement is a simple strategy for enhancing cooperation both during and after a procedure. For example, a child might be praised for holding still during a lumbar puncture or verbally encouraged during the procedure. After the procedure, the child might receive a tangible "reward" such as a badge of courage or sticker. A child should receive positive reinforcement for any positive behavior, even if the child cried and was distressed during the procedure. A child should not, however, be punished or ridiculed for uncooperative behavior.

PHYSICAL MODALITIES

Several physical modalities can be used to manage pain in children. Physical cutaneous stimulation as well as transcutaneous electrical nerve stimulation can be effective. These interventions are frequently used in combination with various pharmacological agents.

Cutaneous stimulation is a valuable noninvasive technique for reducing pain. Pleasant stimulation, such as stroking, patting, or massaging feet, hands, or the back, often produces muscle relaxation and reduces pain during injections, suturing, lumbar punctures, and venipunctures. Infants can frequently be soothed by allowing them to suck on a pacifier or by gently rubbing their heads. These techniques can often be performed by parents and, thus, have an emotional benefit as well.

The application of heat and cold is another cutaneous stimulation technique. Interventions such as handing an injured child an ice cube to rub above and below an injury or rubbing ice on a site prior to an injection may reduce the pain and decrease the inflammatory response. Precautions must be taken, however, to avoid skin irritation. Applying heat for approximately 15 minutes before drawing blood promotes vasodilatation and relieves the intensity of the pain.

Transcutaneous electrical nerve stimulation (TENS) delivers small amounts of electrical energy to the skin via electrodes, modulating transmission of pain impulses at the level of the spinal cord (Eland, 1991). In addition, TENS may cause endorphin release. Although little research on the use of TENS in children has been cited in the literature, Eland (1993) and Lander and Fowler-Kerry (1991) have reported its effectiveness in decreasing procedural and chronic pain in pediatric patients. Thus, TENS may be a useful adjunct in the management of chronic and recurrent pain problems.

RESTRAINTS

Papoose boards and other types of restraints have been used to restrain children for procedures. These measures are frightening and usually inappropriate. In selected situations, however, physical restraint of a child may be necessary in conjunction with appropriate use of sedatives and analgesics (Selbst, 1993). When used as an adjunct to sedation, restraint may facilitate the injection of local anesthetic or the completion of a procedure and reduce the need for deep sedation.

TOPICAL AND LOCAL ANESTHETICS

Innovations in the formulation of local anesthetics have resulted in the availability of several new compounds that provide effective local cutaneous anesthesia for minor procedures (see Table 39.3). These compounds are designed to reduce or avoid the pain associated with injection of local anesthetics. Such improvements enhance the usefulness of topical anesthetics for minor procedures and, in many instances, reduce or eliminate the need for systemic sedation or analgesia.

The eutectic mixture of prilocaine and lidocaine (EMLA cream) promotes local anesthetic penetration of intact skin, producing effective cutaneous anesthesia for minor procedures such as intravenous cannulation and percutaneous accessing of subcutaneous intravenous injection ports (Hallen, Olsson, & Uppfeldt, 1984). EMLA cream is applied in a thick layer to the skin and covered with an occlusive plastic dressing. For effective analgesia, EMLA cream should be applied at least 1 hour prior to a procedure. Analgesia increases with longer application periods of up to 4 hours (Cooper, et al., 1987). EMLA is easy to apply and can

---

TABLE 39.3
Local Anesthetics

Drug	Dosage	Route	Comments
Lidocaine 0.5–1%, with or without epinephrine 1:200,000	Maximum dose: 5 mg/kg; 7 mg/kg if with epinephrine	Subcutaneous	Buffer with 1 mEq NaHCO$_3$ per 9 ml to reduce pain with injection
TAC	Usual: 1–3 ml; Maximum: 0.09 ml/kg	Topical	Avoid mucous membranes and digits
EMLA cream	Usual: 2.5–5 g applied 1–4 hr before procedure	Topical	Apply to intact skin only

be applied by parents at home so that waiting periods are minimized. Side effects are minor and include erythema, blanching, and rash. It should be applied only to intact skin. Prior application of EMLA cream can eliminate the pain associated with infiltration of local anesthetics and may be a useful adjunct for procedures such as lumbar puncture and bone marrow aspiration. EMLA cream has also been used for neonatal circumcision (Benini, et al., 1993).

Another effective method for numbing an area of skin is an intradermal delivery system called Numby Stuff®. Using iontophoresis, a technique that uses a mild electrical current to rapidly transport a solution of 2% lidocaine hydrochloride and 1:100,000 epinephrine through intact skin, Numby Stuff® provides dermal anesthesia to a depth of 10 mm within 8 to 10 minutes. It is effective for intravenous catheter insertion of various types and for pulsed dye laser therapy (Ashburn, et al., 1997). Although this system is approved for all age patients, some young children may be frightened by the tingling sensation produced by the electrical current.

A solution of tetracaine, adrenaline, and cocaine (TAC) provides effective topical anesthesia for repair of superficial lacerations in children (Bonadio & Wagner, 1988). The solution can be prepared by the local hospital pharmacy (tetracaine 0.5%, adrenaline 1:2000, and cocaine 11.8%). Alternative formulations that have been found to be effective and have a lower risk of toxicity are tetracaine 1%, adrenaline 1:4000, and cocaine 4% (Smith & Barry, 1990) and lidocaine 4%, tetracaine 0.5%, and adrenaline 1:2000 (Ernst, et al., 1995). To avoid systemic cocaine toxicity, TAC should not be applied to mucous membranes. Also, it must not be applied to areas supplied by terminal arteries, such as the nose, penis, or fingers.

Hegenbarth, et al. (1990) found TAC anesthesia to be sufficient in 89% of patients with scalp and facial wounds; however, 57% of patients with extremity wounds required supplemental local anesthesia. The usual dose of TAC was 1 to 3 ml of solution (maximum dose 0.09 ml/kg), applied with a gauze pad held in place for 15 to 20 minutes. To avoid ischemia of the fingers, healthcare personnel should wear gloves when applying TAC.

The acid pH of local anesthetics enhances solubility and prolongs shelf life but substantially increases the pain associated with subcutaneous injection. Buffering of local anesthetic solutions reduces burning with injection and may increase efficacy. The addition of 1 mEq sodium bicarbonate to 10 ml of 1% lidocaine significantly reduces pain and stinging associated with injection, without causing precipitation of the local anesthetic (Christoph, et al., 1988).

SEDATIVE AND ANALGESICS

A variety of sedative-hypnotic drugs and opioids have been used to provide sedation and analgesia for minor procedures (see Table 39.4). Drug selection should be based on the anticipated level of sedation and analgesia required for the procedure, risk of potential side effects, and available routes of administration.

Chloral hydrate is a sedative-hypnotic agent devoid of analgesic properties. It is available for pediatric use in a liquid or suppository form and has been widely used in infants and children, primarily due to its low risk of adverse effects when administered in standard doses of 30 to 50 mg/kg. When administered in a dosage range of 35 to 75 mg/kg for computerized tomography (CT) scanning, onset ranged from 30 to 105 minutes, recovery ranged from 60 to 120 minutes, and sedation was inadequate in

---

TABLE 39.4
Sedatives and Analgesics for Procedures

Drug	Dosage	Comments
Chloral hydrate	50–100 mg/kg p.o., p.r.; maximum dose: 2 g	Higher dosage can cause respiratory depression
Pentobarbital	2–6 mg/kg i.v., i.m.	i.v. titration preferred
Midazolam	0.5–1.0 mg/kg p.o.	Onset: 10–20 min
	0.3 mg/kg intranasal	
	0.05–0.1 mg/kg i.v.; titrate to maximum of 0.2 mg/kg	Titrate to desired effect over 10-min. period
Morphine	0.1 mg/kg i.v., up to maximum of 0.2 mg/kg	Reduce dose when combining with sedatives
Meperidine	1 mg/kg i.v., up to 2 mg/kg	Reduce dose when combining with sedatives
Fentanyl	1 μg/kg i.v., titrate to maximum of 5 μg/kg	Reduce dose when combining with sedatives
Ketamine	6–10 mg/kg p.o.	
	0.5–1 mg/kg i.v.	Administer atropine or glycopyrolate
	4 mg/kg i.m.	

13% of patients (Strain, et al., 1986). Doses of 50 to 100 mg/kg (maximum of 2 g) can be used to accelerate onset and improve efficacy but may prolong recovery and increase the risk of respiratory depression (Anderson, Zeltzer, & Fanurik, 1993).

Recent concerns over possible carcinogenic effects of trichlorethanol, an active metabolite of chloral hydrate, are based on laboratory studies in rats and have no supporting clinical data. The primary disadvantages of this drug are slow onset, prolonged recovery, and a significant rate of inadequate sedation. The risk of respiratory as well as cardiac depression with higher dosages warrants continuous cardiorespiratory monitoring. Nevertheless, due to the relative ease of administration and overall safety, chloral hydrate remains a popular sedative for nonpainful procedures, such as CT scanning and magnetic resonance imaging (MRI) (Keeter, et al., 1990).

Barbiturates are also sedative-hypnotic agents devoid of analgesic properties. Short-acting barbiturates such as methohexital or thiopental have been used for induction of anesthesia and produce dose-dependent respiratory and cardiac depression. Both agents can be administered rectally to provide sedation in children. Rectal absorption, however, is somewhat variable and may result in either inadequate or deep sedation.

Pentobarbital is an intermediate-acting barbiturate that is a useful sedative for pediatric radiologic procedures. Strain, et al. (1986) studied the efficacy of intramuscular and intravenous administration of pentobarbital for CT scanning. A single intramuscular dose of 5 to 6 mg/kg produced effective sedation within 30 to 45 minutes in 86% of patients. Intravascular dosage was titrated to achieve satisfactory sedation, resulting in an average dose of 4.4 mg/kg (range, 2 to 6 mg/kg). Intravascular administration was found to be more efficacious due to more rapid onset (1 to 2 minutes), shorter recovery (55 minutes), and a low rate of failed sedation (0.5%).

Midazolam, a short-acting benzodiazepine, provides anxiolysis, sedation, and amnesia and is commonly used as a premedicant or sedative-hypnotic in children as well as adults. Due to limited oral bioavailability, doses of 0.5 to 0.75 mg/kg have been used for preoperative sedation (Feld, Negus, & White, 1990). Doses of 1 mg/kg may be required when midazolam is used as the sole sedative for procedures. Midazolam has also been administered to children by nasal and sublingual routes, which enable transmucosal absorption (Karl, et al., 1993). Transmucosal absorption increases bioavailability and shortens onset time, but children often find these routes of administration to be unpleasant.

Intravenous administration of midazolam produces rapid onset of anxiolysis and sedation and enables titration of dosage to produce the desired degree of sedation. Incremental doses of 0.05 mg/kg can be repeated every 5 to 10 minutes. Tolia, et al. (1991) found that a dose of 0.1 mg/kg

is sufficient for gastrointestinal endoscopic procedures. Up to 0.2 mg/kg may be required for oncology patients undergoing lumbar puncture and bone marrow aspiration (Sandler, et al., 1992). Because midazolam has no analgesic properties, local anesthetics or analgesics should also be administered for painful procedures.

The risk of respiratory depression increases with higher doses of midazolam, as well as with the concomitant administration of opioid analgesics. Other side effects such as nausea and vomiting or hallucinations are uncommon. Recovery from midazolam sedation usually occurs within 1 hour. Persistent sedation may be reversed with the benzodiazepine antagonist flumazenil (see Table 39.5). In addition, flumazenil antagonizes, at least partially, the respiratory depressant effects of midazolam (Gross, Weller, & Conard, 1991).

Opioids such as morphine and fentanyl provide both sedation and analgesia for painful procedures. Fentanyl, a potent synthetic opioid, is most commonly used in perioperative anesthetic management. Due to its lipid solubility, it has a rapid onset, a large volume of distribution, and a relatively short duration of action, except when administered in high doses or by continuous infusion. The dosage of fentanyl and other opioids is limited by the risk of serious dose-related side effects, such as respiratory depression and chest wall rigidity. Sandler, et al. (1992) found fentanyl, administered in incremental doses up to 4 µg/kg, to be a satisfactory agent for oncology procedures. The majority of patients in the study preferred midazolam, however, presumably due to its amnestic effect. Continuous infusion of fentanyl provides effective sedation and analgesia for ventilated patients.

Oral transmucosal fentanyl citrate (OTFC) is an innovative formulation of fentanyl in a candy matrix lozenge attached to a stick. It provides effective pre-anesthetic sedation (Friesen, et al., 1995; Steisand, et al., 1989) and analgesia and sedation for painful procedures (Schechter, et al., 1995). Sucking the lozenge causes transmucosal absorption of approximately 25% of the dose, and the remainder is swallowed, ultimately resulting in a total bioavailability of approximately 50% of the administered dose. The recommended dose is 5 to 15 µg/kg, up to a maximum of 400 µg. Children may need a higher dose (10 to 15 µg/kg) than adults (5 to 8 µg/kg).

Side effects associated with OTFC include nausea and vomiting, pruritis, and respiratory depression. Nausea and vomiting can occur in over 30% of patients and may limit the acceptability of OTFC (Schechter, et al., 1995). Continuous monitoring, including pulse oximetry, is indicated for all patients receiving OTFC (Yaster, 1995). The commercial preparation of OTFC, Fentanyl Oralet®, is approved only for use in monitored anesthesia care or as an adjunct to anesthesia.

Opioids are commonly used in conjunction with other sedative-hypnotic agents, particularly benzodiazepines. In

TABLE 39.5
Antagonists

Drug	Dosage	Comments
Naloxone	1–100 µg/kg i.v.	1–2 µg/kg for mild opioid-induced respiratory depression; 10–100 µg/kg for severe depression or apnea
Flumazenil	0.01 mg/kg i.v. up to 0.2 mg; may repeat 2 to 3 times at 1-min intervals; usual maximum adult dose is 1 mg	May not reverse benzodiazepine-induced respiratory depression; resedation may occur; may increase risk of seizure in patients with seizure disorder

a study of pediatric oncology patients, midazolam combined with morphine or fentanyl provided safe and effective sedation (Sievers, et al., 1991). Despite conservative drug dosages, however, transient oxygen desaturation occurred in 12% of patients. The potential risk of respiratory depression resulting from the combination of fentanyl and midazolam has been previously reported (Bailey, et al., 1990; Yaster, et al., 1990). Sedation with this combination of drugs requires continuous monitoring, careful titration of dosages, and full capability to manage respiratory depression or apnea. Naloxone should be available for antagonism of respiratory depression unresponsive to verbal or physical stimulation. Opioid-induced respiratory depression can usually be reversed with incremental doses of 1 µg/kg of naloxone. Larger doses of 10 to 100 µg/kg should be reserved for respiratory arrest secondary to opioid overdose (see Table 39.5).

The "lytic cocktail" (demerol, phenergan, thorazine (DPT)) is a combination of meperidine, promethazine, and chlorpromazine for intramuscular injection. It has been extensively used in children to provide sedation and analgesia for minor procedures, such as laceration repair and closed reduction of fractures. However, sedation is sometimes inadequate, recovery is often prolonged, and respiratory depression may occur (Nahata, Clotz, & Krogg, 1985). Titration of intravenous sedatives and analgesics on an individual basis produces more rapid onset, predictable depth of sedation, and faster recovery. The Committee on Drugs of the American Academy of Pediatrics has criticized the use of this drug combination (American Academy of Pediatrics, 1995).

Ketamine, a dissociative anesthetic, has been recommended as a sedative and analgesic for minor pediatric procedures (Green, Nakamura, & Johnson, 1990; Tobias, et al., 1992). Ketamine is a unique drug that produces anesthesia, analgesia, and amnesia when administered in doses of 1 to 2 mg/kg intravenously or 3 to 5 mg/kg intramuscularly. Lower doses typically produce sedation and analgesia only. Due to stimulation of sympathoadrenergic activity, cardiovascular performance is maintained or even enhanced. Airway patency, reflexes, and respiratory function are also usually well maintained. However, anesthetic doses of ketamine may alter ventilatory drive and airway reflexes, increasing the risk of aspiration,

laryngospasm, and hypoventilation. The risk of respiratory complications may be accentuated in young infants and in children with respiratory infections. Patients receiving anesthetic doses of ketamine should also receive an anticholinergic, either atropine or glycopyrolate, to prevent hypersalivation, which may complicate airway management. Ketamine increases cerebral blood flow and, consequently, may increase intracranial pressure. The prevalence of emergence delirium and hallucinations in teenagers and adults has limited the usefulness of ketamine. This problem is less severe and less frequent in children (Green, et al., 1990).

Green, et al. reported their experience with ketamine in emergency department patients. Patients received intramuscular injections of ketamine (4 mg/kg) plus atropine (0.01 mg/kg.) Only 3 of 108 were inadequately sedated. One patient developed transient laryngospasm, and another vomited during the procedure. Neither experienced any sequelae. The average time to discharge was 82 minutes. During recovery, agitation occurred in 21 patients but was considered "mild" in 18 patients. The authors concluded that intramuscular ketamine was a reliable and safe agent for minor emergency department procedures.

Oral ketamine has also been used for preoperative sedation as well as sedation for pediatric procedures. In a study of pediatric oncology patients, oral ketamine, in a dose of 10 mg/kg, produced effective sedation within 45 minutes in 87% of patients (Tobias, et al., 1992). Three of 35 patients experienced mild to moderate emergence problems, and the recovery period exceeded 2 hours.

Ketamine is a useful agent for painful procedures. However, practitioners should be mindful of the low but real risk of respiratory complications and of adverse effects such as emergence delirium and prolonged recovery. Ketamine is available only in parenteral solution.

Propofol is a sedative-hypnotic agent that is commonly used for induction as well as maintenance of general anesthesia. Its mechanism of action is unknown. Due to relatively rapid hepatic conjugation and renal excretion, propofol is useful when administered by continuous infusion for maintenance of general anesthesia or sedation. Similar to sodium thiopental, however, propofol causes dose-related loss of airway reflexes, hypoventilation, apnea, and cardiovascular depression. Although anesthesiologsits use propofol as a sedative agent, the safety of this practice by non-anesthesiologists has not been established (Litman, 1999).

MANAGEMENT OF PERIOPERATIVE PAIN IN CHILDREN

Often, children about to undergo surgery express fears regarding postoperative pain. For many of these children, their fears become a reality. Mather and Mackie (1983) studied 170 children postoperatively and found that 40% reported moderate to severe pain on the operative and first postoperative day. Using an integrated, multidisciplinary approach, however, postoperative pain can be minimized.

A comprehensive analgesia plan includes preoperative, intraoperative, and postoperative strategies for minimizing pain related to surgery (Acute Pain Management, 1992). The selection of analgesic strategies should be based on the planned surgical procedure and anesthetic techniques, the anticipated severity of postoperative pain, and the expected course of recovery (i.e., ambulation, physical therapy, dressing changes, etc.). The plan may include any or all of the following interventions for pain management: nonpharmacological approaches, regional anesthesia/analgesia, and systemic opioids and anti-inflammatory drugs. Once these interventions have been initiated, the child should be reassessed at frequent intervals. If the interventions have been ineffective, the plan should be reevaluated and modifications should be made to achieve optimal pain control.

Perioperative management begins with appropriate teaching and preparation for hospitalization and surgery. Surgery creates fear about both real and imagined events for most children and their parents. Without adequate preparation and accurate information, fantasies and fears can lead to distress and anxiety. Strategies that decrease stress and anxiety either reduce pain or enhance the patient's ability to tolerate it better. Explanations of what to expect should be simple and brief. Children should be warned that they will feel discomfort or pain following surgery, but that "medicine will help the pain go away."

PREMEDICANTS

Although preparation and teaching may allay the fears of older children, they may be less effective in toddlers and preschool children. Sedative premedications are useful in alleviating separation anxiety and facilitating induction of anesthesia. The decision to use a premedicant is based on the evaluation of the patient during preoperative assessment. Patients who are especially likely to benefit from a premedicant are young children prone to separation anxiety, uncooperative patients, children whose parents are very anxious, and children who

have had unpleasant or painful healthcare experiences. Although a variety of sedatives and anxiolytics are available, oral midazolam (0.75 mg/kg) has become popular due to its safety, efficacy, quick onset, and short duration of effect (Feld, et al., 1990).

NONPHARMACOLOGICAL INTERVENTIONS

As noted previously in this chapter, nonpharmacological interventions such as relaxation, distraction, and imagery can be very helpful in reducing pain and anxiety. These strategies can be taught preoperatively and incorporated into the postoperative analgesia plan. When used effectively, these strategies can reduce the amount of analgesics needed for pain control.

HYPERSENSITIZATION AND PREEMPTIVE ANALGESIA

Acute pain serves as a warning, alerting us to potential or actual tissue injury. Persistent pain, however, contributes to pathophysiologic processes that compromise normal mobility and function. For example, following thoracic or abdominal surgery, pain may restrict breathing and coughing, resulting in impaired ventilation, atelectasis, and pneumonia (Duggan & Drummond, 1987; Ready, 2000).

Tissue injury and pain also activate the neuroendocrine stress response, increasing sympathoadrenergic activity and releasing "stress hormones" and inflammatory mediators, including catecholamines, cortisol, growth hormone, glucagon, vasopressin, interleukin-1, substance P, and tumor necrosis factor (Fitzgerald & Anand, 1993; Kehlet, 1989). The hypermetabolic and catabolic state that follows may be complicated by impaired immune function and increased postoperative morbidity and mortality (Kehlet, 1989).

Tissue injury and inflammation accentuate peripheral nociceptor sensitivity, resulting in hypersensitivity to mechanical and chemical stimuli (Woolf & Chong, 1993). In addition, dorsal horn neurons respond to sustained afferent stimulation with neurophysiologic and morphologic changes consistent with increased excitability to afferent stimulation (Woolf & Chong, 1993). The development of peripheral and central hypersensitization accentuates pain due to noxious stimuli (hyperalgesia) and produces pain with innocuous stimuli as well (allodynia).

Administration of local anesthetics and analgesics prior to tissue injury may inhibit stimulation of nociceptive pathways and thereby prevent activation of the neuroendocrine stress response and the development of peripheral and central hypersensitivity (Woolf & Chong, 1993). General anesthesia alone is ineffective, but local anesthetics, opioids, and nonsteroidal anti-inflammatory drugs have been used with variable results. Preemptive analgesia appears to be a promising strategy for reducing postoperative pain and complications but remains a subject of some controversy and ongoing investigation (Dahl & Kehlet, 1993; Kissin, 2000).

REGIONAL ANESTHESIA/ANALGESIA

Regional blockade with local anesthetics can be used to provide postoperative analgesia as well as surgical anesthesia. Regional anesthesia techniques are commonly used in conjunction with general anesthesia in children (Dalens, 1989; Ross, Eck, & Tobias, 2000). When performed following induction of general anesthesia, regional blocks allow reduction of maintenance anesthetic requirements, enabling rapid emergence from general anesthesia. Regional analgesia usually persists for several hours, significantly reducing systemic analgesic requirements.

Peripheral and central nerve blocks are useful in infants and children. Commonly performed peripheral nerve blocks include the penile block for circumcision, ilioinguinal/iliohypogastric nerve block for inguinal hernia repair, and intercostal nerve blocks following thoracotomy. Other useful peripheral nerve blocks include brachial plexus blocks, femoral nerve blocks by various techniques, and popliteal blocks. Central blocks are useful for both intraoperative anesthesia and postoperative analgesia. They include single-shot and continuous caudal epidural blocks, and continuous lumbar and thoracic epidural blocks.

The single-shot caudal block is typically performed following induction of general anesthesia. This technique provides epidural anesthesia/analgesia for surgical procedures involving the lower abdomen, inguinal region, and lower extremities (Dalens & Hasnaoui, 1989). It is especially popular for genitourinary procedures, such as inguinal hernia repair, orchidopexy, and hypospadias repair. This block is relatively easy to perform and has a high success rate with a low risk of complications (Broadman, et al., 1987; Dalens & Hasnaoui, 1989). Injection of 0.5 to 1 ml/kg of 0.25% bupivacaine into the caudal epidural space produces effective analgesia for at least 4 to 6 hours. Caudal administration of morphine (0.03 to 0.07 mg/kg) provides analgesia for more than 12 hours but also introduces the risk of opioid-related side effects (Krane, Tyler, & Jacobson, 1989; Valley & Bailey, 1991).

Excellent postoperative analgesia can be provided by the administration of local anesthetics and/or opioids as intermittent boluses or continuous infusions through caudal, lumbar, or thoracic epidural catheters (Berde, et al. 1990; Desparmet, et al., 1987; Gunter & Eng, 1992). Epidural catheters are easily inserted via the caudal canal in infants and small children (Dalens & Hasnaoui, 1989). The tip of the catheter is commonly positioned in the lumbar region but can be advanced to the thoracic level, although this may be somewhat more difficult in children than in infants. Epidural catheters are most commonly inserted in the lumbar region in children. Insertion in the thoracic region is less common due to concern about the risk of neural injury in an uncooperative or anesthetized patient.

Epidural opioids, such as fentanyl, morphine, and hydromorphone, produce excellent analgesia but are associated with side effects that include pruritus, nausea and vomiting, urinary retention, and, rarely, respiratory depression (Taylor & Boswell, 1991). Opioid side effects can be treated with various antiemetics and antihistamines, as well as with opioid antagonists (see Tables 39.5 and 39.6). Concomitant administration of a low concentration of local anesthetic, such as 0.0625 to 0.1% bupivacaine, enables a reduction in opioid dosage, resulting in a lower incidence of opioid-related side effects and little or no motor blockade (McIlvaine, 1990). Selection of agents is usually based on the relative position of the epidural catheter tip to the surgical site. When in close proximity, a solution of fentanyl plus bupivacaine provides excellent analgesia. When the catheter tip is significantly inferior to the surgical site, an opioid that is less lipid soluble (e.g., morphine or hydromorphone) should be used to facilitate cephalad diffusion of the drug.

TABLE 39.6
Treatment of Opioid Side Effects

Side Effect	Drug	Dose	Comments
Pruritus	Diphenhydramine	0.5–1 mg/kg i.v., p.o. prn; maximum: 25 mg	Causes drowsiness
Pruritus	Naloxone	1–2 µg/kg/hr continuous i.v. (e.g., add 0.1 mg/100 ml of maintenan .iv. fluids)	Epidural patients only; antagonizes systemic opioid effects
Pruritus	Nalbuphine	0.05 mg/kg i.v. q 4–6 hr prn	Epidural patients only; partially antagonizes systemic opioid effects
Nausea and vomiting	Metoclopramide	0.1–0.2 mg/kg i.v. q 6 hr prn	Extrapyramidal reactions
Nausea and vomiting	Promethazine	0.25–0.5 mg/kg i.v., p.o., p.r. prn	Causes drowsiness
Nausea and vomiting	Ondansetron	0.1 mg/kg i.v. q 6 hr prn	Expensive

TABLE 39.7
Analgesics

Drug	Dosage	Comments
Acetaminophen	10–15 mg/kg p.o. q 4 hr	Delayed rectal absorption
	20–40 mg/kg p.r.	
Codeine	0.5–1 mg/kg p.o. q 4 hr	
Fentanyl[a]	2–4 µg/kg/hr i.v.	Continuous infusion; ventilated patients only
Ibuprofen	4–10 mg/kg p.o. q 6 hr	
Ketorolac	0.5 mg/kg i.v. q 6 hr;	Limit to 5 days; see text for side effects
	maximum dose: 30 mg	
Meperidine[a]	0.5–1 mg/kg i.v. q 2–3 hr	
Methadone[a]	0.1 mg/kg i.v. q 6–12 hr	
	0.1–0.2 mg/kg p.o. q 8–12 hr	
Morphine[a]	0.05–0.1 mg/kg i.v. q 2–3 hr	
	0.02–0.05 mg/kg/hr i.v. infusion	

[a] Continuous i.v. infusion or repeated i.v. administration of potent opioids may result in drug accumulation and respiratory depression. Periodic (usually hourly) patient assessment is advised. For infants < 3 to 6 months of age, initial dosage of potent opioids should be reduced to one third to one half of usual dose.

Routine patient assessment at many institutions includes continuous cardiorespiratory or oxygen saturation monitoring for patients receiving epidural opioids (McIlvaine, 1990). Other centers rely on close nursing observation, which includes frequent assessment of sensorium, respiratory rate, and ventilation. Continuous monitoring is reserved for patients at increased risk for respiratory depression (e.g., infants less than 6 months of age, patients with preexisting neurologic or pulmonary disorders, and patients receiving long-acting hydrophilic opioids such as morphine or hydromorphone) (Berde, et al., 1989). Complete patient assessment must also include periodic evaluation of pain status, sensorium, motor and sensory blockade, and side effects. Although somewhat complex and labor intensive, epidural delivery of anesthetics and analgesics provides excellent analgesia and is well suited for patients with severe pain problems or unique circumstances that limit the safety or efficacy of other analgesics.

OPIOID ANALGESICS

Parenteral opioids remain the mainstay of treatment for moderate to severe pain during the perioperative period. Analgesic requirements vary among individuals and over the course of a pain problem. Tolerance may develop with prolonged therapy. Therefore, dosage should be adjusted according to the severity and duration of pain. Treatment periods exceeding 7 to 10 days may result in physical dependence and require a period of weaning prior to discontinuation of opioid therapy (Shannon & Berde, 1989). Addiction rarely develops in pediatric patients receiving opioids for pain control and is not a valid reason for withholding opioid analgesics.

Common opioid side effects include nausea and vomiting, pruritus, urinary retention, and constipation. Respiratory depression can be avoided by adjusting dosage on an individual basis. For example, neonates are more sensitive to the depressant effects of morphine due to immaturity of the blood–brain barrier. Furthermore, clearance of morphine may be prolonged in infants less than 3 to 6 months of age (Shannon & Berde, 1989). Consequently, intravenous morphine should be titrated in young infants by incremental administration of lower doses (see Table 39.7). Young infants receiving intravenous opioids should receive close observation, usually supplemented by respiratory monitoring. Morphine is the gold standard for the management of severe pain. Equipotent doses of other opioids result in similar risks of side effects, (e.g., respiratory depression) (Yaster & Maxwell, 1993). Although popular, meperidine offers no significant advantage over morphine. Prolonged meperidine use, particularly in higher dosages, may result in seizures due to the accumulation of an active metabolite, normeperidine. Due to its lipid solubility, fentanyl has a relatively short duration of analgesia except when administered in high doses or by continuous infusion. Continuous infusion of fentanyl is an effective method for providing perioperative analgesia for ventilated patients. The fentanyl "patch" promotes sustained transdermal absorption of fentanyl over a 72-hour period. Onset is slow and absorption variable. Consequently, this transdermal delivery system is not suitable for management of acute pain (Gaukroger, 1993).

PATIENT-CONTROLLED ANALGESIA (PCA)

For optimum pain control, analgesics should be administered on a scheduled rather than "as-needed" (PRN) basis.

The latter approach often delays treatment and compromises pain relief. Intramuscular injection of opioids is undesirable because it is painful and less effective than other alternatives (Berde, et al., 1991). Administration of opioids by continuous infusion or by patient-controlled analgesia (PCA) pumps maintains relatively constant drug levels and provides excellent analgesia (Wilder, et al., 1992). Morphine is the most common choice for PCA, but meperidine, fentanyl, or hydromorphone can also be administered by PCA if morphine is unsuitable. With age-appropriate instruction, most school-age children can safely and effectively control opioid delivery by PCA (Berde, et al., 1991; Gaukroger, Tomkins, and van der Walt, 1989).

A routine pediatric PCA regimen for morphine includes a loading dose of 0.05 to 0.1 mg/kg, followed by interval doses of 0.015 to 0.025 mg/kg every 8 to 15 minutes as needed, with a maximum of 0.25 to 0.35 mg/kg every 4 hours. A concomitant "background" infusion, which sustains drug levels during periods of sleep, has been advocated but has not been shown to significantly improve analgesia (McNeely, Pontus, & Trentadue, 1992). Considering the potential for drug accumulation and respiratory depression, it may be prudent to limit the use of background infusions to patients with severe pain that is not likely to be controlled by interval dosing alone.

Nurse or parent control of PCA interval dosing has also been reported for children incapable of independent control of PCA (Weldon, Connor, & White, 1991). Although convenient and efficient in some settings, this approach may compromise the inherent safety of PCA. Nevertheless, Lloyd-Thomas and Howard (1994) reported safe and effective analgesia in infants and children with nurse-controlled analgesia. Their regimen included a continuous infusion of 0.01 to 0.02 mg/kg per hour, supplemented by interval doses of 0.01 to 0.02 mg/kg every 30 to 60 minutes as needed.

The authors reported effective yet safe analgesia with nurse, parent, or patient control of PCA pumps (Algren, et al., 1998). The regimen used for nurse control was similar to that described by Lloyd-Thomas and Howard (1994). In contrast, the regimen for parent control provided an interval dose of 0.02 mg/kg of morphine every 12 to 15 minutes as needed, but did not routinely include a background infusion. No serious adverse effects were observed in 206 patients managed with nurse or parent control of PCA, as well as the 240 children who managed PCA independently.

Monitto, et al. (2000) described the use of combined "parent-/nurse-controlled" analgesia (PNCA), which allowed both nurses and parents to control PCA interval dosing for 218 patients. The routine PNCA regimen included a continuous background infusion plus interval dosing as needed to administer morphine, fentanyl, or hydromorphone. For example, the usual initial morphine dose was an infusion of 0.02 mg/kg/hr plus an interval

dose of 0.02 mg/kg every 8 minutes as needed. This regimen provided effective analgesia; however, nine (4%) patients received naloxone for excessive sedation, oxygen desaturation, or apnea.

Thus, "surrogate" control of PCA interval dosing appears to be efficacious. However, the combination of a background infusion and frequent interval dosing may increase the risk of an opioid overdose. Somewhat conservative dosing regimens may be prudent, particularly with parent-controlled analgesia. Close monitoring and thorough instruction of nurses and parents regarding administration of interval doses and the risk of adverse effects are essential.

ORAL ADMINISTRATION

When gastrointestinal function permits, oral administration of opioids offers the benefits of sustained pain relief and freedom from parenteral therapy. Onset is slow, however, so oral administration is usually unsuitable during the initial management of severe acute pain. Morphine, meperidine, and methadone are available in oral as well as parenteral forms and are useful for the management of ongoing pain of moderate to severe intensity. Methadone has a prolonged elimination half-life, enabling dosing intervals of 8 to 12 hours and relatively constant analgesia (Yaster & Maxwell, 1993). However, its prolonged half-life increases the potential for drug accumulation and toxicity and may necessitate dosage adjustment. Oral methadone is useful for patients requiring prolonged treatment with opioids or weaning from opioids (Tobias, Schleien, & Haun, 1990). Oral codeine, usually in combination with acetaminophen, is an effective analgesic for moderate pain. Oxycodone and hydrocodone, alone or in combination with acetaminophen, are effective alternatives for patients who may be intolerant to oral codeine.

NON-OPIOID ANALGESICS

Nonsteroidal anti-inflammatory drugs (NSAIDs) provide effective analgesia for mild to moderate pain. In addition, they may be useful in conjunction with opioids in the management of severe pain (Watcha, et al., 1991). By inhibiting prostaglandin synthesis, NSAIDs reduce inflammation and associated pain. These drugs are particularly effective in reducing musculoskeletal pain but are relatively ineffective in treating visceral pain. Due to a "ceiling effect," increasing dosage above the recommended maximum does not significantly improve analgesia (Maunuksela, 1993).

Ketorolac is the only parenteral NSAID approved for use in the United States. Although initially approved for intramuscular administration only, intravenous administration has been shown to be safe and effective (Reinhart, et al., 1992). Intravenous ketorolac, in doses of 0.5 mg/kg (maximum dose, 30 mg) every 6 hours, is very effective in treating moderate orthopedic pain. In addition, for patients with severe pain or opioid-related side effects, ketorolac can be used to supplement intravenous or epidural opioids, thereby improving analgesia and reducing opioid requirements. Significant side effects may develop with prolonged administration of NSAIDs, particularly ketorolac. These disorders primarily result from inhibition of prostaglandin synthesis and include gastritis and gastrointestinal bleeding, platelet dysfunction, renal insufficiency, hepatocellular injury, and central nervous system stimulation. Serious side effects are uncommon for patients free of organ dysfunction. Intraoperative administration of ketorolac may increase blood loss by interfering with platelet function. Consequently, it should not be administered until hemostasis has been ensured. To avoid side effects, ketorolac administration should not exceed 5 days.

Acetaminophen, which primarily acts by interfering with prostaglandin synthesis in the central nervous system, remains popular for the management of mild pain as well as fever. Rectal administration of acetaminophen has been a common, but often inadequate, approach to the treatment of pediatric pain, such as postoperative pain following myringotomy tube insertion. Rectal administration results in slow, incomplete absorption, and dosages in excess of 35 mg/kg may be necessary to achieve therapeutic serum levels (Rusy, et al., 1995). Oral administration results in more predictable absorption. Acetaminophen can be combined with codeine, hydrocodone, or oxycodone for treatment of moderate pain.

Pediatric use of aspirin has dramatically declined since its use was linked to Reye's syndrome (Maunuksela, 1993). Ibuprofen has become very popular as both an antipyretic and analgesic in children and adults. Ibuprofen, in a dose of 6 to 10 mg/kg, is a very effective analgesic and anti-inflammatory agent. Other NSAIDs that have longer half-lives (e.g., naproxyn) are useful for chronic pain.

CONCLUSION

Contemporary pediatric management of procedural and perioperative pain strives to reduce anxiety and provide analgesia through the use of sedatives, analgesics, anesthetics, and numerous nonpharmacological strategies. Severe or recurrent pain is managed by synergistic combinations of opioids, NSAIDs, local anesthetics, and adjunctive approaches that inhibit nociceptive transmission at multiple sites along the nociceptive pathway. Such a comprehensive approach to pain management minimizes pain perception and reduces its adverse physiological and emotional consequences.

REFERENCES

Acute Pain Management Guideline Panel. (1992). *Acute Pain Management: Operative or Medical Procedures and Trauma. Clinical Practice Guideline.* AHCPR Pub. No. 92-0032, Agency for Health Care Policy and Research, Public Health Service, U.S. Department of Health and Human Services, Rockville, MD.

Algren, J T., et al. (1998). Efficacy and safety of patient-, parent, or nurse-controlled analgesia in children. *Anesthesiology, 89,* A1303.

The American Academy of Pediatric Dentistry (1993). Guidelines for the elective use of pharmacologic conscious and deep sedation in pediatric dental patients. *Pediatric Dentistry, 15,* 297.

American Academy of Pediatrics, Committee on Drugs. (1992). Guidelines for monitoring and management of pediatric patients during and after sedation for diagnostic and therapeutic procedures. *Pediatrics, 89,* 110.

American Academy of Pediatrics, Committee on Drugs. (1995). Reappraisal of lytic cocktail/demerol, phenergan, thorazine (DPT) for sedation of children. *Pediatrics, 95,* 598.

American College of Emergency Physicians Pediatric Emergency Medicine Committee. (1993). The use of pediatric sedation and analgesia—policy statement. *Annals of Emergency Medicine, 22,* 626.

American Society of Anesthesiologists. (1996). Practice guidelines for sedation and analgesia by non-anesthesiologists. *Anesthesiology, 84,* 459.

American Society of Anesthesiologists Task Force on Preoperative Fasting. (1999). Practice guidelines for preoperative fasting and the use of pharmacologic agents to reduce the risk of pulmonary aspiration: Application to healthy patients undergoing elective procedures. *Anesthesiology, 90,* 896.

Anderson, C. T., Zeltzer, L. K., & Fanurik, D. (1993). Procedural pain. In N. L. Schechter, C. B. Berde, & M. Yaster (Eds.), *Pain in infants, children and adolescents* (pp. 435–458). Baltimore: Williams & Wilkins.

Ashburn, M.A., et al. (1997). Iontopheretic administration of 2% lidocaine hydrochloride and 1:100,000 epinephrine in humans. *Clinical Journal of Pain, 13,* 22.

Bailey, P.L., et al. (1990). Frequent hypoxemia and apnea after sedation with midazolam and fentanyl. *Anesthesiology, 75,* 826.

Benini, F., et al. (1993). Topical anesthesia during circumcision in newborn infants. *Journal of the American Medical Assiciation, 270,* 850.

Berde, C.B. (1989). Pediatric postoperative pain management. *Pediatric Clinics of North America, 36,* 921.

Berde, C.B., et al. (1989). Regional analgesia on pediatric medical and surgical wards. *Intensive Care Medicine,15,* S40.

Berde, C.B., et al. (1990). Continuous epidural bupivacaine-fentanyl infusions in children following ureteral reimplantation. *Anesthesiology, 73,* A1128.

Berde, C.B., et al. (1991). Patient-controlled analgesia in children and adolescents: A randomized prospective comparison with intramuscular administration of morphine for postoperative analgesia. *Journal of Pediatrics, 118,* 460.

Bonadio, W.A., & Wagner, V. (1988). Efficacy of TAC topical anesthetic for repair of pediatric lacerations. *American Journal of Disabled Children, 15,* 203,.

Broadman, L.M., et al. (1987). "Kiddie caudals": Experience with 1,154 consecutive cases without complications. *Anesthesia & Analgesia, 66,* S18.

Christoph, R.A., et al. (1988). Pain reduction in local anesthetic administration through pH buffering, *Annals of Emergency Medicine, 17,* 117.

Cooper, C.M., et al. (1987). EMLA cream reduces the pain of venepuncture in children. *European Journal of Anaesthesia, 4,* 441.

Coté, C.J. (1994). Sedation protocols—Why so many variations? *Pediatrics, 94,* 281.

Dahl, J.B., & Kehlet, H. (1993). The value of pre-emptive analgesia in the treatment of postoperative pain. *British Journal of Anaesthesia, 70,* 434.

Dalens, B. (1989). Regional anesthesia in children. *Anesthesia & Analgesia, 68,* 654.

Dalens, B., and Hasnaoui, A. (1989). Caudal anesthesia in pediatric surgery: Success rate and adverse effects in 750 consecutive patients. *Anesthesia & Analgesia, 68,* 83.

Desparmet, J., et al. (1987). Continuous epidural infusion of bupivacaine for postoperative pain relief in children. *Anesthesiology, 67,* 108.

Duggan, J., & Drummond, G.B. (1987). Activity of lower intercostal and abdominal muscles after surgery in humans. *Anesthesia & Analgesia, 66,* 852.

Eland, J. (1991). The use of TENS with children who have cancer pain. *Journal of Pain Symptom Management, 6,* 145.

Eland, J. (1993). The use of TENS with children. In N. L. Schechter, C.B. Berde, & M. Yaster (Eds.), *Pain in infants, children and adolescents* (pp. 331–339). Baltimore: Williams & Wilkins.

Eland, J., & Anderson, J. (1977). The experience of pain in children. In S. Jacox, (Ed.), *Pain: A sourcebook for nurses and other health professionals* (pp. 453–473). Boston: Little, Brown.

Ernst, A.A., et al. (1995). Lidocaine adrenaline tetracaine gel versus tetracaine adrenaline cocaine gel for topical anesthesia in linear scalp and facial lacerations in children aged 5 to 17 years. *Pediatrics, 95,* 255.

Feld, L.H., Negus, J.B., & White, P.F. (1990). Oral midazolam preanesthetic medication in pediatric outpatients, *Anesthesiology, 73,* 831.

Fitzgerald, M., & Anand, K.J.S. (1993). Developmental neuroanatomy and neurophysiology of pain. In N.L. Schechter, C.B. Berde, & M. Yaster (Eds.), *Pain in infants, children and adolescents* (pp. 11–31). Baltimore: Williams & Wilkins.

Friesen, R.H., et al. (1995). Oral transmucosal fentanyl citrate for preanaesthetic medication of paediatric cardiac surgery patients, *Paediatric Anaesthesiology, 5,* 29.

Gaukroger, P.B. (1993). Novel techniques of analgesic delivery. In N.L. Schechter, C.B. Berde, & M. Yaster (Eds.), *Pain in infants, children and adolescents* (pp. 195–201). Baltimore: Williams & Wilkins.

Gaukroger, P.B., Tomkins, D.P., & van der Walt, J.H. (1989). Patient-controlled analgesia in children. *Anaesthetics in Intensive Care, 17,* 264.

Green, S.M., Nakamura, R., & Johnson, N.E. (1990). Ketamine sedation for pediatric procedures: Part 1, A prospective series. *Annals of Emergency Medicine, 19,* 1024.

Gross, J.B., Weller, R.S., & Conard, P. (1991). Flumazenil antagonism of midazolam-induced ventilatory depression. *Anesthesiology, 75,* 179.

Gunter, J.B., & Eng, C. (1992). Thoracic epidural anesthesia via the caudal approach in children. *Anesthesiology, 76,* 935.

Hallen, B., Olsson, G.L., & Uppfeldt, A. (1984). Pain-free venepuncture. *Anaesthesia, 39,* 969.

Hegenbarth, M.A., et al. (1990). Comparison of topical tetracaine, adrenaline, and cocaine anesthesia with lidocaine infiltration for repair of lacerations in children. *Annals of Emergency Medicine, 19,* 63.

Karl, H.W., et al. (1993). Transmucosal administration of midazolam for premedication of pediatric patients. *Anesthesiology, 78,* 885.

Keeter, S., et al. (1990). Sedation in pediatric CT: National survey of current practice. *Radiology, 175,* 745.

Kehlet, H. (1989). Surgical stress: The role of pain and analgesia. *British Journal of Anaesthetics, 63,* 189.

Kissin, I. (2000). Preemptive analgesia. *Anesthesiology, 93,* 1138.

Krane, E.J., Tyler, D.C., & Jacobson, L.E. (1989). The dose response of caudal morphine in children. *Anesthesiology, 71,* 48.

Lander, J., & Fowler-Kerry, S. (1991). Managing brief procedural pain with TENS. *Journal of Pain Symptom Management, 6,* 179,

Litman, R. (1999). Sedatives/hypnotics. In B. Kraoss & R.M. Brustowicz, *Pediatric procedural sedation and analgesia* (pp. 39–46). Philadelphia: Lippincott-Williams & Wilkins.

Lloyd-Thomas, A.R., & Howard, R.F. (1994). A pain service for children. *Paediatric Anaesthesiology, 4,* 3.

Mather, L., & Mackie, J.T. (1983). The incidence of postoperative pain in children. *Pain, 15,* 271.

Maunuksela, E. (1993). Nonsteroidal anti-inflammatory drugs in pediatric pain management. In N.L. Schechter, C.B. Berde, & M. Yaster (Eds.), *Pain in infants, children and adolescents* (pp. 135–143). Baltimore: Williams & Wilkins.

McDonnell, L., and Bowden, M.L. (1989). Breathing management: A simple stress and pain reduction strategy for use on a pediatric service. *Issues in Comprehensive Pediatric Nursing, 12,* 339.

McIlvaine, W.B. (1990). Spinal opioids for the pediatric patient. *Journal of Pain Symptom Management, 5,* 183.

McNeely, J.M., Pontus, S.P., & Trentadue, N.C. (1992). Comparison of patient controlled analgesia with and without basal morphine infusion for postoperative pain control in children. *Anesthesiology, 77,* A814.

Monitto, C. L., et al. (2000). The safety and efficacy of parent-/nurse-controlled analgesia in patients less than six years of age. *Anesthesia and Analgesia, 91,* 573.

Mullooly, V.M., Levin, R.F., & Feldman, H.R. (1988). Music for postoperative pain and anxiety, *Journal of New York State Nursing Association, 19,* 4.

Nahata, M.C., Clotz, M.A., & Krogg, E.A. (1985). Adverse effects of meperidine, promethazine, and chlorpromazine for sedation in pediatric patients. *Clinical. Pediatrics, 24*, 558.

Ready, B.L. (2000). Acute postoperative pain. In R.D. Miller (Ed.), *Anesthesia* (pp. 2323–2350). New York: Churchill Livingston.

Reinhart, D., et al. (1992). IV Ketorolac vs. sufentanil for outpatient ENT surgery, a double-blind, randomized, placebo-controlled study. *Anesthesiology, 77*, A31.

Ross, A.K., Eck, J.B., and Tobias, J.D. (2000). Pediatric regional anesthesia: Beyond the caudal. *Anesthesia and Analagesia, 91*, 16.

Rusy, L.M., et al. (1995). A double-blind evaluation of ketorolac tromethamine versus acetaminophen in pediatric tonsillectomy: Analgesia and bleeding. *Anesthesia and Analgesia, 80*, 226.

Sacchetti, A., et al. (1994). Pediatric analgesia and sedation. *Annals of Emergency Medicine, 23*, 237.

Sandler, E., et al. (1992). Midazolam versus fentanyl as premedication for painful procedures in children with cancer. *Pediatrics, 89*, 631.

Schechter, N.L. (1989). The undertreatment of pain in children: An overview. *Pediatric Clinics of North America, 36*, 781.

Schechter, N.L., et al. (1995). The use of oral transmucosal fentanyl citrate for painful procedures in children. *Pediatrics, 95*, 335.

Selbst, S.M. (1993). Pain management in the emergency department. In N.L. Schechter, C.B. Berde, & M. Yaster (Eds.), *Pain in infants, children and adolescents* (pp. 505–518). Baltimore: Williams & Wilkins.

Shannon, M., & Berde, C.B. (1989). Pharmacologic management of pain in children and adolescents. *Pediatric Clinics of North America, 36*, 855.

Sievers, T.D., et al. (1991). Midazolam for conscious sedation during pediatric oncology procedures: Safety and recovery parameters. *Pediatrics, 88*, 1172.

Smith, S.M., & Barry, R.C. (1990). A comparison of three formulations of TAC (tetracaine, adrenalin, cocaine) for anesthesia of minor lacerations in children. *Pediatric Emergency Care, 6*, 266.

Strain, J.D., et al. (1986). Intravenously administered pentobarbital sodium for sedation in pediatric CT. *Radiology, 161*, 105.

Streisand, J.B., et al. (1989). Oral transmucosal fentanyl citrate premedication in children. *Anesthesia and Analgesia, 69*, 28.

Taylor, G., & Boswell, M.V. (1991). Continuous epidural infusion of low dose morphine for postoperative analgesia in children. *Anesthesiology, 75*, A937.

Tobias, J.D., Schleien, C.L., & Haun, S.E. (1990). Methadone as treatment for iatrogenic narcotic dependency in pediatric intensive care unit patients. *Critical Care Medicine, 18*, 1292.

Tobias, J.D., et al. (1992). Oral ketamine premedication to alleviate the distress of invasive procedures in pediatric oncology patients. *Pediatrics, 90*, 537.

Tolia, V., et al. (1991). Pharmacokinetic and pharmacodynamic study of midazolam in children during esophagogastroduodenoscopy. *Journal of Pediatrics, 119*, 467.

Valley, R.D., & Bailey, A.G. (1991). Caudal morphine for postoperative analgesia in infants and children: A report of 138 cases. *Anesthesia and Analgesia, 72*, 120.

Watcha, M., et al. (1991). A comparison of ketorolac and morphine when used during pediatric surgery. *Anesthesiology, 75*, A942.

Weldon, B.C., Connor, M., & White, P.F. (1991). Nurse-controlled vs. patient-controlled analgesia following pediatric scoliosis surgery. *Anesthesiology, 75*, A935.

Wilder, R.T., et al. (1992). Patient-controlled analgesia in children and adolescents: Safety and outcome among 1,589 patients. *Anesthesiology, 77*, A1187.

Woolf, C.J., & Chong, M.S. (1993). Preemptive analgesia—Treating postoperative pain by preventing the establishment of central hypersensitization. *Anesthesia and Analgesia, 77*, 362.

Yaster, M. (1995). Pain relief. *Pediatrics, 95*, 427.

Yaster, M., et al. (1990). Midazolam-fentanyl intravenous sedation in children: Case report of respiratory arrest. *Pediatrics, 86*, 463.

Yaster, M., & Maxwell, L.G. (1993). Opioid agonists and antagonists. In N.L. Schechter, C.B. Berde, M. Yaster (Eds.), *Pain in infants, children and adolescents* (pp. 145–171), Baltimore: Williams & Wilkins.

Zeltzer, L., & LeBaron, S. (1982). Hypnosis and nonhypnotic techniques for reduction of pain and anxiety during painful procedures in children and adolescents with cancer. *Journal of Pediatrics, 101*, 1032.

40

Pain Management in Geriatrics

Samuel K. Rosenberg, M.D. and Mark V. Boswell, M.D., Ph.D.

INTRODUCTION

Elderly patients are among the fastest growing segment of the world's population and often suffer multiple medical problems, of which pain is the most common complaint that motivates patients to visit the physician (Ferrell, 1991). In 1998, the U.S. census documented over 34 million people over the age of 65, of which at least 4 million were older than 85 years (U.S. Census Bureau, 1999). Moreover, in the next three decades, the elderly population in the U.S. is expected to increase by approximately 73%.

Pain is more common in the elderly than in the young (Brattberg, Mats, & Andrews, 1989), and population-based studies have shown that 25 to 50% of community dwelling elderly suffer significant pain (Crook, Rideout, & Browne, 1984; Ferrell, 1991). It is estimated that 5% of elderly people reside in nursing homes, where the prevalence of pain is even higher, reaching 40 to 80%. Longitudinal studies suggest that 40% of people older than 65 years will spend some time in nursing homes in their lifetimes, and 20% of those older than 85 years reside in nursing homes (Ferrell, 1996).

Recent studies have shown a decrease in thermal and mechanical thresholds for pain with advancing age, while electrical thresholds for pain may not be affected by aging (Farrell, 2000). These may be due to a preferential contribution of C-fiber activation vs. A-δ fiber activation in the elderly. Studies have shown a great degree of variability in pain sensitivity in those older than 80, and some evidence even suggests a decrease in pain tolerance with advanced aging (Farrell, 2000). Zheng, Gibson, Khalil, Helm, and McMeehen (2000) demonstrated that mechanical hyperlagesia was present despite aging, and that the duration of the secondary hyperalgesia was longer in the

elderly. That may be explained by the theory that dorsal horn sensitization is dependent on a greater peripheral input, and once initiated is then less likely to resolve spontaneously. Therefore, after a stimuli exceeds a threshold, the aging nociceptive system may not respond adequately to inhibitory mechanisms, leading to more persistent levels of central sensitization, as can occur in postherpetic neuralgia.

The consequences of pain in the elderly include impaired activities of daily living and ambulation, depression, sleep disturbance, and increased healthcare costs (Ferrell, 1991). Pain may also be associated with deconditioning, gait abnormalities, falls, cognitive dysfunction, and polypharmacy.

Harkins, Kwentus, and Price (1984, 1990) described changing patterns of pain reported by the elderly visiting physicians' offices. Joint pain and fractures were more common, while back pain and headaches were relatively less frequent. In an epidemiologic study of osteoarthritis, more than 80% of elderly individuals were found to suffer some form of painful arthritis (Davis, 1988). The Nuprin pain survey (Sternbach, 1986) revealed similar findings, where headaches, back pain, dental pain and muscular pain were less frequent in those older than 65 years, but joint pain was much more prevalent. The National Health and Nutrition Survey (1987) documented an increased incidence of depression and impairment in activities of daily living in the elderly suffering pain. Cancer is more common in old age, and as many as 80% of cancer patients suffer substantial pain (Foley, 1994).

Many pain syndromes affect the elderly disproportionately, including herpes zoster and postherpetic neuralgia, temporal arteritis, polymyalgia rheumatica, and atherosclerotic peripheral vascular disease (Gordon, 1979).

0-8493-0926-3/02/$0.00+$1.50
© 2002 by CRC Press LLC

Nonetheless, care must be taken to avoid mistakenly attributing new pain symptoms to preexisting conditions.

PAIN ASSESSMENT AND THE PHYSICAL EXAMINATION

Elderly people may underreport pain because they expect pain with aging, with their disease, and in the case of cancer pain, because of the fear of cancer progression. Family members as well as caregivers are often the best source of information (Ferrell, 1991). Although cognitive impairment may be a barrier to pain assessment, it is important to recognize that most cognitively impaired patients reliably report the presence of current pain at the moment they are asked (Ferrell, Ferrell, & Rivera, 1995).

Old age may be associated with an increase in threshold but not in dynamic response of higher-frequency mechanoreceptors in the skin. However, there is little evidence that perception of pain is diminished. Moreover, there is no evidence that age per se has an impact on the unpleasantness of pain. Indeed, pain in the elderly is a major source of unnecessary suffering and limitation of activities of daily living (Harkins & Price, 1992).

Pain assessment tools that work for the young are likely to work for the elderly (Harkins & Price, 1992).

The Visual Analogue Scale is an efficient and simple way to measure pain intensity (Melzac & Katz, 1994). It consists of a 10-cm horizontal line, with two endpoints labeled "no pain" and "worst pain ever." The patient is then asked to mark on the line that corresponds to pain intensity, the line is then measured, yielding a pain score. The advantages of this tool of pain assessment include its simplicity, ease of administration, minimal intrusiveness, and proven reliability in clinical and research settings.

The McGill Pain Questionnaire provides information about the quality of the pain experienced. Its descriptors fall into four categories: sensory, affective, evaluative, and miscellaneous. This tool is reliable and discriminative, and can help in the differential diagnosis of the pain (Melzac & Katz, 1994).

A crucial aspect of pain assessment is the physical examination, particularly in the elderly. The examination should include:

- Complete history and physical examination
- Review of pain location, intensity, factors that exacerbate or alleviate the pain, and pain impact on mood and sleep
- A screen for cognitive impairment (Folstein Mini-Mental Examination) (Folstein, Folstein, & McHugh, 1975)
- A screen for depression

- A review of the patient's activities of daily living (bathing, dressing, toileting, continence, feeding) and instrumental activities of daily living (using the telephone, shopping, food preparation, housekeeping, laundry, transportation, taking medicine, managing money), and the effect of pain upon functional status
- Gait and balance assessment
- Basic visual and auditory examination to screen for sensory deprivation

An important aspect of the pain assessment is the physical examination. The examination should include not only the organ systems relevant to the patient's complaint, but also a focused neurologic evaluation. For example, a patient with a history of lung cancer, coming with severe groin pain on external rotation of the lower extremity, might suggest a pathologic proximal femur fracture. On the other hand, pain upon percussion of the spine at T12-L1 might suggest tumor metastasis to the spine, producing concomitant referred pain to the groin in a T12-L1 dermatomal pattern. The clinician should examine for evidence of a neurologic deficit, which may herald epidural spread of tumor and possible cord compression. In such cases, further diagnostic studies, such as magnetic resonance imaging (MRI) of the thoracolumbar spine, may be necessary.

Neuropathic pain conditions are common in elderly patients and can pose diagnostic and treatment challenges. Herpes zoster infection is a classic example of acute neuropathic pain that affects 1 to 2% of the elderly each year (Harkins, et al., 1990). Subsequent postherpetic neuralgia is strongly dependent on age, affecting as many as 30 to 50% elderly, vs. 5 to 10% in all age groups. A neurologic examination, specifically looking for evidence of nerve injury (such as hypoesthesias) may help confirm the diagnosis. This may be useful in the unusual case when zoster presents without a cutaneous rash. Wu, Marsh, and Dworken (2000), in a recent review of sympathetic nerve blocks, confirm their role in acute herpes zoster infections. On the other hand, there have been no randomized, double-blind studies that prove the usefulness of sympathetic blocks in postherpetic neuralgia. However, newer techniques, such as the transforaminal approach to the epidural space, which ensures the delivery of steroids and local anesthetics near or at the dorsal root ganglia, may prove to be of great value. Also, the addition of fluoroscopically guided blocks may also translate into better and longer lasting pain relief.

Low-back pain is a frequent complaint in the elderly (Ciocon, Galindo-Ciocon, Amaranth, & Galindo, 1994). The examination of the back should be done in a systematic fashion (Borenstein & Burton, 1993). Initially, the spine should be evaluated with the patient in the erect position and kyphosis, lordosis, and scoliosis should be noted. Palpation of the paravertebral muscles at each level should follow, and muscle spasms and trigger points should be noted. Palpation and percussion of the spinous processes may reveal localized tenderness, which suggests compression fracture, malignancy, or infection. Range of motion of the lumbosacral spine can reveal pain with flexion, which may suggest a herniated intervertebral disc or paraspinal muscle spasm. Pain on extension may suggest spinal stenosis, whereas pain with lateral rotation and extension can be seen with apophyseal disease, commonly known as lumbar facet pain.

Pain that radiates to the lower extremity may be due to an ipsilateral herniated intervertebral disc producing radiculopathy, particularly if the pain radiates below the knee in a dermatomal pattern. In the elderly, radiculopathy is more likely due to degenerative changes of the spine with facet and ligamentous hypertrophy and loss of disc height, than to a herniated disk (Deyo, Rainville, & Kent, 1992).

Deep tendon reflexes at the knee (L4) and ankle (S1) may be absent in the elderly, and reflexes may be significant only if asymmetric. On the other hand, hyperreflexia and a positive Babinski sign may reflect upper motor neuron disease. Motor function of the lower extremities can be tested in the supine or sitting position: knee extensors, L3-L4; knee flexors, foot evertors, hip extensors, L5-S1; dorsiflexion of the toes L4-L5; and plantar flexors, S1. The apophyseal joints (facet joints) as well as the sacroiliac joints should be palpated and tenderness ruled out, because they can be common sources of back pain (Schwarzer, April, & Bogduk, 1995). The prevalence of lumbar facet pain may be as high as 40% in the elderly (Schwarzer, Wang, McNaught, Laurent, & Bogduk, 1995).

Radiofrequency neurotomy of the lumbar median branches, an outpatient procedure, has been shown to provide at least 60 % pain relief at 1-year follow-up in 87% of those studied, and about 60% of those studied obtained at least 90% pain relief 12 months after the procedure (Dreyfuss, et al., 2000)

Patients with spinal stenosis typically have back and leg pain with standing and walking, which often resolves with sitting or lying with hips flexed. In such patients, abnormal physical findings include reproduction of the pain with back extension, wide-base gait and, in severe cases, motor weakness, particularly with ambulation. In such patients, coexisting peripheral vascular disease producing claudication must be excluded. In Amundsen, et al.'s (2000) recent, prospective 10-year follow-up in those with spinal stenosis, patients were randomized to either surgical or conservative treatment. A good result was found in 70% at 6 months, 64% at 1 year, and 57% at 4 years in those treated conservatively. The surgical group did better; that is, patients improved in 79% at 6 months, 89% at 1 year, and 84% after 4 years. The surgeries

included one level (8%), two levels (52%), three levels (28%), and four levels (11%). Interestingly, patients with multilevel operations did not have a poorer outcome than those with single-level surgeries, and the delay of surgery did not translate into a worse outcome. Also, there was no association between the degree of narrowness of the spinal canal and the results after 4 years of follow-up. The study concluded that surgery for lumbar spinal stenosis was beneficial to at least 80% of individuals, but initial conservative treatment in those with milder symptoms appeared to be appropriate, especially since delaying surgery did not worsen the final outcome.

The differential diagnosis of back pain in the elderly should include other diseases that may also cause back pain. For example, an abdominal aortic aneurysm can present with back pain in addition to the presence of a pulsatile mass, abdominal bruit, decreased peripheral pulses, and signs of cutaneous ischemia. Pancreatic cancer and perforated duodenal ulcers also can present with pain referred to the upper lumbar and thoracic spine. Metastatic tumors that commonly invade the spine include prostate, breast, and lung cancers. Indeed, a history of cancer greatly increases the probability that new-onset back pain is tumor related (Deyo, et al., 1992)

EPIDURAL ANALGESIA FOR POSTOPERATIVE PAIN

Epidural anesthesia and/or analgesia in high-risk elderly surgical patients offers substantial benefits, as demonstrated in several prospective studies. Christopherson, et al., (1993) studied 100 patients with an average age of 64 years following revascularization of the lower extremities. Cardiovascular morbidity and mortality were similar in the control and epidural groups, but there was a much lower incidence of reoperation for graft thrombosis in the epidural group. In a prospective series by Tuman, et al. (1991), elderly patients with an average age of about 70 years undergoing lower extremity revascularization with general anesthesia and postoperative epidural analgesia were compared with patients having general anesthesia and postoperative patient-controlled analgesia with intravenous opioids. The patients in the epidural group received bupivacaine and fentanyl, and had a lower incidence of thrombotic events, such as graft occlusions and coronary artery and deep venous thromboses. In addition, cardiovascular morbidity, infectious complications, and ICU days were reduced in the epidural group. Yeager, Glass, Neff, and Brinck-Johnsen (1987) conducted a prospective trial in 53 high-risk surgical patients, comparing epidural anesthesia, light general anesthesia, and postoperative epidural analgesia to general anesthesia and postoperative parenteral opioids. Patients in the epidural group had significantly less cardiovascular, respiratory, and infectious morbidity, and hospitalization costs were lower.

A review of epidural anesthesia and analgesia (Liu, Carpenter, & Neal, 1995) concluded that the benefits of epidural analgesia may transcend the immediate postoperative analgesia because perioperative coagulability is reduced, thereby decreasing the incidence of arterial and venous thromboses. In addition, there may be improved pulmonary function and gastrointestinal motility, particularly in those receiving thoracic epidural infusions with local anesthetics.

Transient postoperative reduction in cognitive function is frequently observed in the elderly and its pathogenesis is poorly understood (Berggren, et al., 1987). The nadir is seen on the second postoperative, with full recovery noted within a week (Riis, Lomholt, Haxholdt, & Kehlet, 1983). A study of postoperative patients between 50 and 80 years of age demonstrated that untreated pain — and not excessive analgesic intake — predicted decline in the first five postoperative days (Duggleby & Lander, 1994). Although prospective double-blind studies have not confirmed the beneficial effects of epidural analgesia on reducing transient cognitive dysfunction, epidural techniques may reduce the need for parenteral opioids and thereby minimize opioid-related side effects (Salomaki, Leppaluoto, Laitinen, Vuolteenaho, & Nutinen, 1993).

Epidural Steroids

Epidural steroid injections are common procedures done for patients with back pain with radiculopathy. If such injections are performed by properly trained physicians, the incidence of side effects is low (Spaccarelli, 1996).

Although there is a debate in the literature as to the efficacy of epidural steroids for back pain (Koes, Scholten, Mens, & Bouter, 1995), a recent prospective series of 30 patients with an average age of 76 years, along with radicular symptoms associated with spinal stenosis, noted significant pain relief following a course of epidural steroids. Pain relief lasted up to 10 months (Ciocon, et al., 1994). Another case report confirmed the effectiveness of epidural steroid injections for acute radiculopathy in the elderly (Ice, Dillingham, & Belandres, 1995). Lutz, Vad, and Wiseneski (1998), in an outcome prospective study of transforaminal lumbar epidural steroid injections under fluoroscopic guidance, confirmed their effectiveness in those patients with herniated discs and radiculopathy. Sixty-nine patients received one to four transforaminal epidural steroid injections under fluoroscopy, directed at the herniated disc. They were followed for an average of 80 weeks and ranged in age from 22 to 77 years. More than 75% of patients reported greater than 50% pain relief long-term, with an average of 1.8 injections.

The potential benefit of epidural steroid injections may include reduced pain, improved function, decreased analgesic medication intake, and possibly the avoidance of surgery. The use of fluoroscopic guidance may improve the accuracy of epidural injections, thus enhancing their efficacy.

PHARMACOLOGIC MANAGEMENT OF PAIN

It is important to recognize the physiologic changes that occur with aging in order to prescribe medications safely. With respect to renal function, there is a decline in creatinine clearance with aging. The decline is not linear, and clearance decreases more rapidly with advancing age. Also, renal plasma flow, tubular secretion, tubular reabsorption, hydrogen ion secretion, and water absorption and excretion are decreased with aging.

The gastrointestinal system shows less decrease in function with aging. Esophageal transit time is delayed and lower esophageal sphincter function is altered. The stomach retains relatively normal motility but there is a decrease in gastric acid production. Cytochrome P450 microsomal oxidase system efficiency declines with age. Demethylation, the process by which benzodiazepines are metabolized by the liver, is markedly decreased with aging. However, glucuronidation, a primary metabolic pathway for lorazepam, is not altered by aging. Drugs that undergo high hepatic first-pass metabolism, such as propranolol and lidocaine, may have a decreased clearance due to reduced hepatic blood flow.

From a treatment standpoint, it is clinically useful to determine whether pain is nociceptive, neuropathic, sympathetically mediated, or a combination of these types of pain. An example of this is cancer pain, which may be nociceptive due to tumor in the bone, and neuropathic pain from infiltration or compression of neural structures. Pharmacologic therapy should be directed at the mechanism of pain and based on a specific diagnosis. Neuropathic pain represents a challenge for clinicians because it is often poorly responsive to opioids and anti-inflammatory medications. Examples of neuropathic pain present in the elderly include trigeminal neuralgia, postherpetic neuralgia, diabetic neuropathy, phantom limb pain, and radiculopathy.

Neuropathic pain is commonly described as a lancinating, stabbing, at times burning pain. Allodynia, a painful reaction to a non-painful stimuli, and hyperalgesia, an exaggerated pain reaction to a painful stimuli, are hallmarks of neuropathic pain. Nociceptive pain, on the other hand, can be described as an ache, sharp and, at times, burning as well. Visceral pain, a form of nociceptive pain, can be described as a diffuse or poorly localized, crampy discomfort, which sometimes is intermittent.

Neuropathic pain can be classified as stimulus evoked or stimulus independent pain. (Orza, Boswell, & Rosenberg, 2000) Inflammation and tissue injury may be the stimulus that activates the nervi nervorum in the affected nerves, and stimulus evoked neuropathic pain may be more responsive to opioids than the stimulus independent type of neuropathic pain. Stimulus independent pain may result from an ongoing disturbance in the afferent peripheral or central nervous system, associated with physiologic and morphologic changes in the dorsal root ganglia and dorsal horn of the spinal cord. Also, loss of the normal descending inhibitory mechanisms may also be implicated in the stimulus independent neuropathic pain, and inflammation is usually absent, and opioids are usually not beneficial (Arner & Meyerson, 1988; Portenoy, Foley, & Inturrisi, 1990).

Several days to months after nerve injury, persistent small-fiber activity may be evident at peripheral sites of injury, as well as in dorsal root ganglia. In the periphery, sprouting nerve terminals may display enhanced chemical and mechanical sensitivity to prostaglandins, cytokines, and catecholamines. In addition, there is evidence for up-regulation of sodium channels in injured axons that may be a source of ongoing ectopic discharge, maintaining the painful state. Dorsal root ganglia also show morphological changes ipsilateral to the injured nerve, often with an increased density of abnormal sympathetic nerve terminals, which may contribute to hypersensitization. Recently, changes in dorsal horn have also been documented following peripheral injury, with arborization of dendrites of large-diameter afferents (Aβ fibers) into superficial lamina, such as the substantia gelatinosa (Woolf, Shortland, & Coggeshall, 1992). Thus, neuropathic pain can result from a combination of peripheral and central nervous system changes.

Adjuvant "analgesic" medications such as tricyclic antidepressants and anticonvulsants are often useful for neuropathic pain. Proposed mechanisms of action of adjuvant drugs have been recently reviewed (Tanelian & Victory, 1995; Max, 1995). Anticonvulsants such as carbamazepine and phenytoin may inhibit ectopic neuronal activity by blocking sodium channels. Other anticonvulsants, such as clonazepam and gabapentin, may activate inhibitory gabaergic mechanisms in the dorsal horn. Tricyclic antidepressants appear to enhance endogenous descending inhibitory pathways involving serotonin and norepinephrine, although N-methyl-D-aspartate (NMDA) blockade may also play a role.

ANTICONVULSANTS

Carbamazepine and phenytoin are useful for neuropathic pain, probably by action at sodium channels (Devor, 1995). Side effects can include sedation, confusion, ataxia, gastrointestinal disturbances, elevation of liver enzymes,

and bone marrow depression. Although valproic acid may cause liver toxicity and thrombocytopenia in children, the drug is remarkably safe in adults. Mexiletine, a sodium channel-blocking agent, is structurally similar to lidocaine, and was originally developed as an anticonvulsant, although currently is approved as an antiarrhythmic drug. In doses of 450 mg/day, mexiletine may be effective in reducing lancinating and burning dysesthesias (Stracke, Meyer, Schumacher, & Federlin, 1992). Side effects include nausea, vomiting, and dizziness, which can be minimized by slow titration and administration with food. Mexiletine has the potential for inducing arrhythmias, although this is more of a concern in patients with ischemic heart disease, and an electrocardiogram (ECG) may be warranted in patients with cardiac disease or a history of arrhythmia.

Clonazepam is an alternative to carbamazepine for neuropathic pain (Swerdlow, 1984; Iacono, Linford, & Sandyk, 1987) and poses minimal risk from the standpoint of organ toxicity. However, side effects in elderly patients may include sedation and memory loss. The risk of habituation appears to be small, and the potential for serious abstinence syndrome on abrupt withdrawal of clonazepam is mitigated by the drug's long half-life (18 to 50 hours). Clonazepam is generally well tolerated in the elderly if started at a low dose (e.g., 0.25 to 0.5 mg at bedtime) and it should be titrated slowly. Typical daily doses at steady state are in the range of 1.0 to 2.0 mg. A single dose given at bedtime is usually sufficient, because of the drug's long half-life, which may minimize daytime sedation. Clonazepam may also be useful in improving sleep.

Gabapentin, an analog of gamma-aminobutyric acid, is approved for partial seizures with and without generalization in adults. Gabapentin has been shown in two randomized controlled clinical trials to be effective in diabetic neuropathy and in postherpetic neuralgia (Backonja, et al., 1998; Rowbotham, Harden, Stacey, Bernstesin, & Magnus-Miller, 1998). It was shown to be as effective as tricyclic antidepressants, and may also be considered a first choice in those neuropathic pain syndromes. Gabapentin may be effective for lancinating pain and is an alternative to carbamazepine and clonazepam. The anticonvulsant mechanism of action of gabapentin is not clear (Beydoun, Ulthman, & Sackellares, 1995). Although gabapentin is presumed to enhance GABAergic activity (Honmou, Kocsis, Richerson, 1995), it does not bind to GABA receptors (Beydoun, et al., 1995), and neither GABA antagonists A or B reverse the analgesia from gabapentin (Gillin & Sorkin, 1998). Gabapentin has a high affinity for the alpha2-delta subunit of the calcium channel, but its significance remains unknown. Gabapentin has also been shown to improve pain in multiple sclerosis and cancer-related pain. It is mostly helpful in reducing spontaneous, paroxysmal pain with burning and lancinating quality, as well as allodynia to cold and tactile stimuli. It is less likely to be beneficial for the dull, aching pain, as well as for hyperalgesia. (Mao & Chen, 2000).

Gabapentin is not metabolized by the liver, nor is it an enzyme inducer, but is largely excreted unchanged by the kidneys. Therefore, the dose should be reduced in the presence of renal insufficiency. Overall, gabapentin is well tolerated, and no adverse drug interactions have been reported. Side effects, which are usually mild, include somnolence, fatigue, headache, nausea, weight gain and dizziness. In the elderly, starting doses range from 100 mg at nighttime to three times a day.

TRICYCLIC ANTIDEPRESSANTS

Antidepressants have a proven role in the treatment of neuropathic conditions such as postherpetic neuralgia and diabetic neuropathy (Max, 1995). Side effects include constipation, dry mouth, and urinary retention, attributable to the anticholinergic actions of the drugs. Cognitive side effects, including sedation, may also occur, possibly due to anticholinergic or antihistiminic effects. Adrenergic side effects include postural hypotension and tachycardia due to peripheral receptor blockade. Tricyclic antidepressants may have cardiac effects that are similar to type I antiarrhythmic agents. Electrocardiographic changes may include QRS widening, PR and QT prolongation, and T-wave flattening. Therefore, it is advisable that elderly patients with underlying ischemic cardiac disease have a baseline ECG prior to starting tricyclic antidepressants. The use of tricyclic antidepresants and paroxetine has resulted in very high doses of the former, which may result in adverse side effects. If paroxetine is to be used along with tricyclic antidepresant agents, careful monitoring of blood levels should be followed (Aranow, et al., 1989)

In the elderly, tricyclics with the least anticholinergic side effects, such as desipramine or nortryptiline, should be tried first, starting with a low dose and titrating slowly to effect. Reasonable starting doses are in the range of 10 to 25 mg at bedtime. Target doses of around 100 mg/day may be necessary to maximize analgesic effects, although such doses are often not tolerated, decreasing the clinical usefulness of antidepressants for pain management. Selective serotonin reuptake inhibitors such as fluoxetine generally do not appear to be as effective for neuropathic pain, although they are better tolerated than tricyclic antidepressants (Max, et al., 1992). However, paroxetine has been shown to be effective for diabetic neuropathy, but at doses higher than usually required for depression (Sindrup, Gram, Brosen, Eshoj, & Mogensen, 1990).

NONSTEROIDAL ANTI-INFLAMATORY DRUGS (NSAIDs)

NSAIDs are highly protein-bound organic acids that undergo extensive hepatic metabolism. Their analgesic action is mediated by inhibition of prostaglandin synthesis at sites of inflammation. In addition, NSAIDs may decrease neutrophil migration into injured tissue and inhibit the release of free radicals such as nitric oxide. Analgesic effects may also result from inhibition of prostaglandin synthesis in the dorsal horn of the spinal cord (Brooks & Day, 1991; Souter, Fredman & White, 1994).

Inhibition of prostaglandin synthesis by NSAIDs is due to a reversible inactivation of cyclooxygenase (COX), which converts arachidonic acid to prostaglandin intermediates. Two types of cyclooxygenase have been identified: COX-1 is the constitutive isoform present in blood vessels, stomach, and kidney, whereas COX-2 is inducible at sites of inflammation by cytokines and other mediators of the inflammatory process. Most NSAIDs nonselectively inhibit both forms of the enzyme, which accounts for the wide range of side effects experienced by patients, especially the elderly. Side effects include gastrointestinal bleeding, renal injury, fluid retention, platelet inhibition, constipation, and central nervous system effects such as confusion and dizziness. However, nabumetone, a selective COX-2 inhibitor, is associated with a lower incidence of ulceragenic side effects (Insel, 1996). A recent celecoxib long-term arthritis safety study (CLASS) on the gastrointestinal side effects of celecoxib at doses of 400 mg twice a day, vs. ibuprofen 800 mg three times a day or diclofenac 75 mg twice a day, demonstrated less gastrointestinal side effects, including ulcers, especially in patients not taking concomitant aspirin (Silverstein, et al., 2000). Elderly patients are at increased risk for complications from NSAIDs, having a higher incidence of gastrointestinal bleeding, renal injury, confusion, tinnitus, and hearing loss. Approximately 2 to 4% of patients taking NSAIDs on a chronic basis will develop upper intestinal bleeding, a symptomatic ulcer, or intestinal perforation per year (Fries, et al., 1989). These complications may also occur after acute administration of NSAIDs. It should be noted that abdominal pain and dyspepsia are not predictive of gastrointestinal bleeding, and up to two thirds of NSAID users have no symptoms before bleeding or perforation (Popp & Portenoy, 1996).

A randomized controlled trial of celecoxib, naproxen, or placebo in 1003 osteoarthritis patients, has confirmed the efficacy of celecoxib, especially at 100 and 200 mg twice a day doses, as well as a comparable tolerability in comparison with naproxen, but with fewer gastrointestinal side effects (Bensen, et al., 1999).

In the elderly, NSAID-related nephrotoxicity can result in acute renal failure due to renal ischemia, interstitial nephritis with nephrotic syndrome, and rarely papillary necrosis (Henrich, Agodoa, & Barrett, 1996). Patients at risk for acute renal failure have underlying volume depletion from any cause or preexisting kidney disease. There is an added risk of nephrotoxicity when NSAIDs are combined with aspirin as well as with acetaminophen (Henrich, Agodoa, & Barrett, 1996). Interestingly, misoprostol, a prostaglandin (PGE) analog used for prophylaxis against NSAIDs-induced gastrointestinal injury, has also been shown to have a protective effect against indomethacin-induced renal dysfunction in the elderly (Nesher, Sonnenblick, & Dwolatzky, 1995).

NSAIDs may also have deleterious effects to articular cartilage and bone resorption, and may be worsen osteoarthritis (Davies & Wallace, 1996).

NSAIDs can be given with food to decrease abdominal discomfort because the bioavailability of these drugs is not altered. The dose-response relationship for NSAIDs is characterized by a minimal effective dose and a ceiling dose for analgesia; therefore, doses higher than 1.5 to 2.0 times the starting dose may not offer significant added analgesia and can only increase the risk of side effects.

OPIOIDS

Morphine and other pure μ-agonist opioids are used with increasing frequency for moderate to severe pain, particularly cancer-related pain. Although pharmacokinetic data for opioids are derived mainly from young adults, several studies have demonstrated age-related differences in potency and clearance of morphine. A retrospective analysis of postoperative analgesia with morphine administered intramuscularly to cancer patients demonstrated a two-fold difference in pain relief between the extremes of adult age (Kaiko, 1980; Kaiko, Wallenstesin, Rogers, Gabrinski, & Houde, 1982). Plasma morphine levels in older patients (mean age of 71 years) were approximately twice those of the younger group (average age of 29 years), consistent with decreased

morphine clearance in the elderly patients. Although older patients experienced greater maximum pain relief, the predominant effect was a longer duration of analgesia after a given dose. Therefore, age-related increases in pain relief with parenteral morphine appear to be primarily related to increased duration of analgesia rather than peak analgesic effect.

The pharmacokinetics of intravenous and oral immediate and controlled-release morphine have been evaluated in healthy young and elderly volunteers (Baillie, Bateman, Coates, & Woodhouse, 1989). Morphine pharmacokinetic profiles were determined over a 24-hour period after administration of 10 mg morphine to young (average age, 27 years) and older subjects (mean age, 74 years). Although maximum plasma concentrations (Cmax) after intravenous administration were not significantly different between younger and older subjects, Cmax was larger in elderly subjects after both oral preparations (see Figures 40.1 and 40.2). Moreover, areas under the plasma concentration-time curves were greater in older than younger subjects for all three modes of administration, suggesting decreased systemic clearance and possibly reduced first-pass hepatic metabolism of morphine in the elderly.

When administered epidurally, morphine also appears to be more potent in elderly patients (Moore, Vilderman, Lubenskyi, McCans, & Fox, 1990). In a study comparing young (mean, 36 years) and elderly patients (mean, 77 years) following elective major abdominal surgery, the quality of analgesia after a single dose of epidural morphine (0.07 mg/kg) was consistently better in the elderly group and the duration of analgesia was longer. Plasma

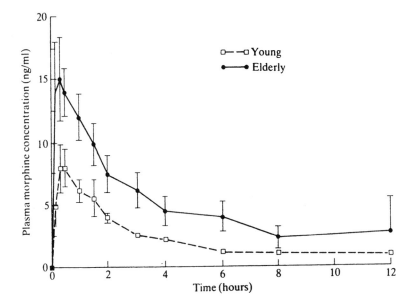

FIGURE 40.1 Plasma morphine concentrations for 12 hours after a 10-mg oral dose of immediate-release morphine solution in young and elderly healthy subjects (mean ± SEM). (From Baille, et al., *Age and Ageing*, *18*, 258, 1989. With permission.).

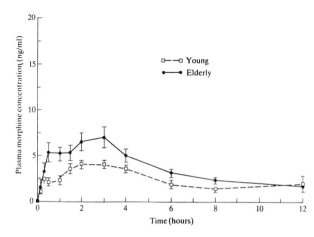

FIGURE 40.2 Plasma morphine concentrations for 12 hours after a 10-mg, oral controlled-release morphine tablet (MST Continus™) in young and elderly healthy subjects (mean + SEM). (From Baille, et al., *Age and Ageing, 18,* 258, 1989. With permission.)

morphine concentrations in both groups were not significantly different, suggesting a centrally mediated increase in sensitivity to morphine in elderly patients.

Patient-controlled analgesia (PCA) allows patients to self-administer small doses of analgesic on demand. The technology has been available for close to three decades and is safe and effective (White, 1988). In elderly patients, the use of intramuscular medication may be hazardous, particularly in frail patients. A prospective controlled trial with 83 high-risk, postoperative elderly patients compared PCA morphine to intramuscular morphine (Egbert, Parks, Short, & Burnett, 1990). Significant improvement in analgesia, without sedation, was noted in patients who received morphine by PCA. In addition, confusion and respiratory depression were less common and serum morphine concentrations showed less variability on the first postoperative day, demonstrating the advantages of PCA drug delivery for elderly patients.

Oral opioids are cost-effective, particularly for patients out of the hospital. Controlled-release preparations of opioids are convenient, minimize the number of daily doses required, and optimize patient comfort and compliance. Oxycodone, an opioid analgesic with a potency similar to morphine, has recently been recognized as an alternative to oral morphine for the management of postoperative and cancer pain (Poyhia, Vainio, & Kalso, 1993). However, in contrast to morphine, oxycodone's pharmacokinetic and pharmacodynamic parameters are not significantly different between healthy young adults and elderly subjects (Figure 40.3), and dosage reductions for healthy elderly patients in moderate to severe pain do not appear necessary (Kaiko, et al., 1996). This makes Oxycontin™, a controlled-release preparation of oxyc-

odone, an attractive alternative to controlled-release morphine for elderly patients.

Opioids are remarkably effective for nociceptive pain and remain the gold standard against which all other analgesics are measured. However, concerns about addiction and side effects, which are often overstated, may interfere with appropriate prescribing for both acute and chronic pain syndromes. The risk of addiction with opioids is probably very small, as shown in the Boston collaborative drug surveillance program, which identified only four cases of drug addiction in a follow-up of close to 40,000 patients (Porter & Jick, 1980). Opioid analgesics are the cornerstone of postoperative pain management and the incidence of addiction in this setting is virtually zero (Pasero & McCaffery, 1996). Based on a favorable experience with opioids for cancer pain, there is increasing belief that opioids may also be appropriate for some forms of chronic nonmalignant pain. For patients who have well-defined pain syndromes and no history of drug abuse, opioids may have a better therapeutic index than currently available NSAIDs. Indeed, opioids do not appear to produce organ toxicity, as shown in longitudinal studies with patients on methadone maintenance (Kreek, 1973). Issues related to opioids for chronic nonmalignant pain have been discussed in detail by Portenoy (1994). In a survey conducted by Turk, Brody, and Okifuji (1994), long-term prescribing of opioids is widespread and the legal requirements of some states for triplicate prescriptions appear to have had little impact on opioid-prescribing practices.

Recently, tramadol was released for use in the U.S., although the drug has been available in Canada and Europe since the early 1970s. Initial enthusiasm for the drug in the U.S. was probably based on the impression that tramadol was a nonopioid analgesic with a potency similar to codeine, but without the stigma of being a controlled substance. More recently, the manufacturer has addressed this issue in direct mailings to physicians, noting that the drug is a centrally acting analgesic with μ-agonist activity and therefore has the potential for abuse. In addition, a recent notification that tramadol may cause seizures at usual therapeutic doses, particularly in patients taking tricyclic antidepressants, has dampened enthusiasm for the drug. As an analgesic, tramadol may have some value for neuropathic pain because it appears to inhibit reuptake of serotonin and norepinephrine, in a manner similar to tricyclic antidepressants, which may partially account for the analgesic action of the drug. Tramadol is generally well tolerated by elderly patients, and a double-blind study evaluating 390 elderly patients with chronic pain found tramadol comparable to acetaminophen with codeine (Rauck, Ruoff, & McMillen, 1994). Side effects are similar to codeine and include nausea, constipation, dizziness, and somnolence.

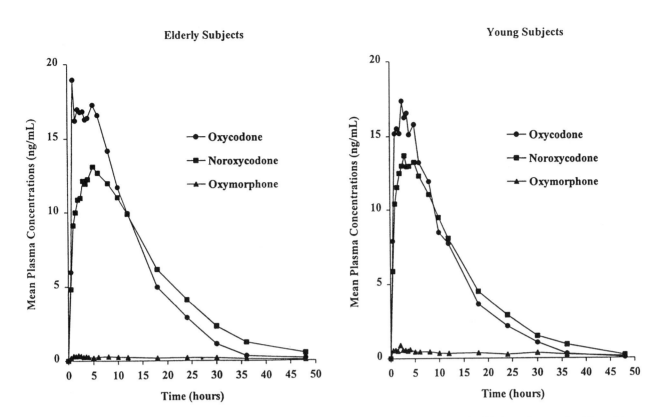

FIGURE 40.3 Mean plasma concentrations of oxycodone, noroxycodone, and oxymorphone in elderly and young healthy subjects for 48 hours after administration of a single, 20-mg, controlled-release oxycodone tablet (OxyContin™). Noroxycodone is the major metabolite in plasma and does not appear to contribute to analgesia. Although oxymorphone is more potent than oxycodone, plasma levels are not clinically significant. No differences in plasma concentrations of oxycodone or metabolites were evident between elderly and young subjects. (From The Perdue Frederick Company, Norwalk, CT, 1996. With permission.)

SUMMARY

It appears that pain perception is not altered by age. Indeed, pain is more common in the elderly. Pain assessment tools used in young adults are also useful for elderly patients. As with younger patients, other dimensions of pain should be evaluated, including cognitive, functional, and psychological status, to ensure optimum treatment and appropriate utilization of healthcare resources. The pain assessment and physical examination must be thorough, and the clinician should look for possible coexisting disease.

It is useful to determine whether pain is nociceptive or neuropathic in nature, which may help direct therapy. Although opioid analgesics are effective for nociceptive pain, adjuvant analgesics such as tricyclic antidepressants and gabapentin will be more effective for pain associated with nerve injury. Pharmacologic management should be based on a specific diagnosis if possible, and therapy directed at the mechanisms of pain. Because pharmacokinetic and pharmacodynamic parameters can vary between young adults and elderly patients, analgesic dosing regimens may need to be adjusted for older patients. To improve pain relief and minimize side effects in elderly

patients, analgesics should be started at lower doses than with younger patients and titrated more slowly to effect. Although perhaps more labor intensive than with younger patients, this approach should improve compliance and optimize patient care.

Finally, newer techniques such as radiofrequency denervation and transforaminal epidural steroid injections under fluoroscopy may help reduce the discomfort and medication use in appropriate cases.

REFERENCES

Amundsen, T., Weber, H., Nordal, H J., Magnaes, B., Abdelnoor, M., & Lilleas, F. (2000). Lumbar spinal stenosis: Conservative or surgical management. *Spine, 25*(11), 1424–1436.

Aranow, R.B., Hudson, J.I., Pope, H.G., Grady, T.A., Laage, T.A., Bell, I.R., & Cole, J.O. (1989). Elevated antidepressant plasma levels after addition of fluoxetine. *American Journal of Psychiatry, 146,* 7.

Arner, S., & Meyerson, B. A. (1988). Lack of analgesic effect of opioids on neuropathic and idiopathic forms of pain. *Pain, 33,* 11–23.

Backonja, M., Beydoun, A., Edwards, K.R., Schwartz, S.J., Fonseca, V., Hes, M., LaMoreaux, L., & Garafalo, E. (1998). Gabapentin for the symptomatic treatment of painful neuropathy in patients with diabetes mellitus. A randomized controlled trial. *Journal of the American Medical Association, 280,* 1831–1836

Baillie, S.P., Bateman, D.N., Coates, P.E., & Woodhouse, K.W. (1989). Age and the pharmacokinetics of morphine. *Age and Ageing, 18,* 258–262.

Bensen, W.G., Fiechtner, J.J., McMillen, J.I., Zhao, W.W., Yu, S.S., Woods, E.M., Hubbard, R.C., Isakson, P.C., Verburg, K.M., & Geis, G.S. (1999). Treatment of Osteoarthritis, with celecoxib, a cyclooxygenase-2 Inhibitor: A randomized control trial. *Mayo Clinic Proceedings, 74,* 1095–1105.

Berggren, D., Gustafson, Y., Eriksson, B., Bucht, G., Hanson, L. I., Reiz, S., & Weinblad, B. (1987). Postoperative confusion after anesthesia in elderly patients with femoral neck fractures. *Anesthesia and Analgesia, 66,* 497–504.

Beydoun, A., Ulthman, B.M., & Sackellares, J.C. (1995). Gabapentin: Pharmacokinetics, efficacy, and safety. *Clinical Neuropharmacology, 18,* 469–481.

Borenstein, D.G., & Burton, J.R. (1993). Lumbar spine disease in the elderly. *Journal of the American Geriatric Society, 41,* 167–175.

Brattberg, G., Mats, T., & Andrews, W. (1989).The prevalence of pain in a general population: The results of a postal survey in a county of Sweden. *Pain, 37,* 215–222.

Brooks, P.M., & Day, R.O. (1991). Nonsteroidal antiinflammatory drugs — differences and similarities. *New England Journal of Medicine, 324,* 1716–1725.

Christopherson, R., Beattie, C., Frank, S.M., Norris, E.J., Meinert, C.L., Gottlieb, S.O., Yates, H., Rock, P., Parker, S. D., & Perler, B.A. (1993). Perioperative morbidity in patients randomized to epidural or general anesthesia for lower extremity vascular surgery. Perioperative ischemia randomized anesthesia trial study group. *Anesthesiology, 79,* 422–434.

Ciocon, J.O., Galindo-Ciocon, D., Amaranth, L., & Galindo, D. (1994). Caudal epidural blocks for elderly patients with lumbar canal stenosis. *Journal of the American Geriatric Society, 42,* 593–596.

Crook, J., Rideout, E., & Browne, G. (1984). The prevalence of pain complaints among a general population. *Pain, 18,* 299–314.

Davies, N.M., & Wallace, J.L. (1996). Selective inhibitors of cyclooxygenase-2. Potential in elderly patients. *Drugs and Aging, 9*(6), 406–417.

Davis, M.A. (1988). Epidemiology of osteoarthritis. *Clinics in Geriatric Medicine, 4,* 241–255.

Devor, M. (1995). Neurobiological basis for selectivity of Na+ channel blockers in neuropathic pain. *Pain Forum, 4,* 83–86.

Deyo, R.A., Rainville, J., & Kent, D.L. (1992). What can the history and physical examination tell us about low back pain? *Journal of the American Medical Association, 268,* 760–5.

Dreyfuss, P., Halbrook, B., Pauza, K., Joshi, A., McLarty, J., & Bogduk, N. (2000). Efficacy and validity of radiofrequency neurotomy for chronic lumbar zygopophyseal joint pain. *Spine, 25*(10), 1270–1277.

Duggleby, W., & Lander, J. (1994). Cognitive status and postoperative pain: Older adults. *Journal of Pain Symptom Management, 9,* 19–27.

Egbert, A.M., Parks, L.H., Short, L.M., & Burnett, M.L. (1990). Randomized trial of postoperative patient control analgesia vs. intramuscular narcotics in frail elderly man. *Archives of Internal Medicine, 150,* 1897–1903.

Farrell, M.J. (2000). Pain and aging. *American Pain Society Bulletin, 10*(4), 1–11.

Ferrell, B.A. (1991). Pain management in elderly people. *Journal of the American Geriatric Society, 39,* 64–73.

Ferrell, B.A. (1996). Overview of aging and pain. In B.R. Ferrell & B.A. Ferrell (Eds.), *Pain in the elderly* (pp. 1–10). Seattle: IASP Press.

Ferrell, B.A., Ferrell, B.R., & Rivera, L. (1995). Pain in cognitively impaired nursing home patients. *Journal of Pain Symptom Management, 10,* 591–595

Foley K. (1994). Pain in the elderly. In W.R. Hazzard, E.L. Bierman, J.P. Blass, W.H. Ettinger, & J.P. Halter (Eds.), *Principles of geriatric medicine and gerontology* (pp. 317–331). New York: McGraw-Hill.

Folstein, M.F., Folstein, S.E., & McHugh, P.R. (1975). Mini mental state: A practical method for grading the cognitive state of patients for the clinician. *Journal of Psychiatry Research, 12,* 189–198.

Fries, J.F., Miller, S.R., Spitz, P.W., Williams, C.A., Hubert,, H.B., & Block D.A. (1989). Towards an epidemiology of gastropathy associated with nonsteroidal antiinflammatory drug use. *Gastroenterology, 96*(Suppl 2), 647–655.

Gillin, S., & Sorkin, L.S. (1998). Gabapentin reverses the allodynia produced by the administration of anti-gd-2 ganglioside, an immunotherapeutic drug. *Anesthesia and Analgesia, 86,* 111–116.

Gordon, R.S. (1979). Pain in the elderly. *Journal of the American Medical Association, 241,* 2191–2192.

Harkins, S.W., Kwentus, J., & Price, D.D. (1984). Pain and the elderly. In C. Benedetti, et al. (Eds.), *Advances in pain research and therapy* (Vol. 7, pp. 103–212). New York: Raven Press.

Harkins, S.W., Kwentus, J., & Price, D.D. (1990). Pain and suffering in the elderly. In J. J. Bonica (Ed.), *Management of pain,* (2nd ed., pp. 552–559). Philadelphia: Lea & Febiger.

Harkins, S.W., & Price, D.D. (1992). Assessment of pain in the elderly. In D.C. Turk & R. Melzack (Eds.), *Handbook of pain assessment* (pp. 315–331). New York: Guilford Press.

Henrich, W.L., Agodoa, L.E., Barrett, B., et al. (1996). National Kidney Foundation position paper. Analgesics and the kidney: Summary and recommendations to the scientific advisory board of the National Kidney Foundation from an ad hoc committee of the National Kidney Foundation. *American Journal of Kidney Disease, 27,* 162–165.

Honmou, O., Kocsis, J.D., & Richerson, G.B. (1995). Gabapentin potentiates the conductance increase induced by nipecotic acid in CA1 pyramidal neurons *in vitro*. *Epilepsy Research, 20*, 193–202.

Iacono, R.P., Boswell, M.V., & Neumann, M. (1994). Deafferentation pain exacerbated by subarachnoid lidocaine and relieved by subarachnoid morphine. *Regional Anaesthesia, 19*, 212–215.

Iacono, R.P., Linford, J., & Sandyk, R. (1987). Pain management after lower extremity amputation. *Neurosurgery, 20*, 496–500.

Ice, D.A., Dillingham, T.R., & Belandres, P.V. (1995). Epidural corticosteroid injections for acute radiculopathy in a 95-year-old woman. *Southern Medical Journal, 88*, 222–224.

Insel, P.A. (1996). Analgesic, antipyretic and antiinflammatory agents and drugs employed in the treatment of gout. In J.G. Hardman, P.B. Limbrid, et al. (Eds.), *Goodman and Gilman's: The pharmacologic basis of therapeutics*, (9th ed., pp. 617–657). New York: McGraw-Hill.

Kaiko, R.F. (1980). Age and morphine analgesia in cancer patients with postoperative pain. *Clinical Pharmacology, Therapy, and Toxicology, 28*, 823–826.

Kaiko, R.F., Benziger, D.P., Fitzmartin, R.D., Burke, B.E., Reder, R.F., & Goldenheim, P.D. (1996). Pharmacokinetic-pharmacodynamic relationships of controlled-release oxycodone. *Clinical Pharmacology, Therapy, and Toxicology, 59*, 52–61.

Kaiko, R.F., Wallenstesin, S.L., Rogers, A.G., Gabrinski, P.Y., & Houde, R.W. (1982). Narcotics in the elderly. *Medical Clinics of North America, 66*, 1079–1089.

Koes, B.W., Scholten, R.J.P.M., Mens, J.M.A., & Bouter, L.M. (1995). Efficacy of epidural steroid injections for low back pain and sciatica: A systematic review of randomized clinical trials. *Pain, 63*, 279–288.

Kreek, M.J. (1973). Medical safety and side effects of methadone in tolerant individuals. *Journal of the American Medical Association, 223*, 665–668.

Liu, S., Carpenter, R.L., & Neal, J.M. (1995). Epidural anesthesia and analgesia and their role in postoperative outcome. *Anesthesiology, 82*, 1474–1506.

Lutz, G.E., Vad, V.B., & Wiseneski, R.J. (1998). Fluoroscopic transforaminal lumbar epidural steroid: An outcome study. *Archives of Physical Medicine and Rehabilitation, 79*, 1362–1365.

Mao, J., & Chen, L.L. (2000). Gabapentin in pain management. *Anesthesia and Analgesia, 91*, 680–687

Max, M.B. (1995). Antidepressant drugs as treatments for chronic pain: Efficacy and mechanisms. In B. Bromm & D.E. Desmedt (Eds.), *Pain and the brain: From nociception to cognition. Advances in pain research and therapy* (Vol. 22, pp. 501–515). New York: Raven Press.

Max, M.B., Lynch, S.A., Muir, J., Shoaf, S.E., Smoller, B., & Dubner, R. (1992). Effects of desipramine amitriptyline, and fluoxetine on pain in diabetic neuropathy. *New England Journal of Medicine, 326*, 1250–1256.

Melzac, R., & Katz, J. (1994). Pain measurement in persons in pain. In P.D. Wall & R. Melzac (Eds.), *Textbook of pain* (3rd ed., pp. 337–351). New York: Churchill Livingston.

Moore, A.K., Vilderman, S., Lubenskyi, W., McCans, J., & Fox, G.S. (1990). Differences in epidural morphine requirements between elderly and young patients after abdominal surgery. *Anesthesia and Analgesia, 70*, 316–320.

The National Health and Nutrition Survey. (1987). Epidemiological follow-up study, 1982–1984. Vital and health statistics, Series I, No. 22, DHHS Pub. No. (PHS).

Nesher, G., Sonnenblick, M., & Dwolatzky, T. (1995). Protective effect of misoprostol on indomethacin induced renal dysfunction in the elderly. *Journal of Rheumatology, 22*, 713–716.

Orza, F., Boswell, M.V., & Rosenberg, S.K. (2000). Neuropathic pain: Review of mechanisms and pharmacologic management. *NeuroRehabilitation, 14*, 15–23.

Pasero, C., & McCaffery, M. (1996). Postoperative pain management in the elderly. In B.R. Ferrell & B.A. Ferrell (Eds.), *Pain in the elderly* (pp. 45–68). Seattle: IASP Press.

Popp, B., & Portenoy, R.K. (1996). Management of chronic pain in the elderly: Pharmacology of opioids and other analgesic drugs. In B.R. Ferrell & B.A. Ferrell (Eds.), *Pain in the elderly* (pp. 21–34). Seattle: IASP Press.

Porter, J., & Jick, H. (1980). Addiction rare in patients treated with narcotics. *New England Journal of Medicine, 302*, 123.

Portenoy, R.K. (1994). Opioid therapy for chronic nonmalignant pain: Current status. In H.L. Fields & J.C. Liebskind (Eds.), *Progress in pain research and management* (pp. 247–287). Seattle: IASP Press.

Portenoy, R.K., Foley, K.M., & Inturrisi, C.E. (1990). The nature of opioid responsiveness and its implications for neuropathic pain: New hypotheses derived from studies of opioid infusions. *Pain, 43*, 272–286.

Poyhia, R., Vainio, A., & Kalso, E. (1993). A review of oxycodone's clinical pharmacokinetics and pharmacodynamics. *Journal of Pain Symptom Management, 8*, 63–67.

Price, D.D., Mao, J., & Mayer, D.J. (1994). Central neural mechanisms of normal and abnormal pain states. In H.L. Fields & J.C. Liebskind (Eds.), *Progress in pain research and management* (pp. 61–84). Seattle: IASP Press.

Rauck, R.L., Ruoff, G.E., & McMillen, J.I. (1994). Comparison of tramadol and acetaminophen with codeine for long term pain management in elderly patients. *Current Therapeutic Research, 55*, 1417–1431.

Riis, J., Lomholt, B., Haxholdt, O., & Kehlet, H. (1983). Immediate and longterm mental recovery from general versus epidural anesthesia in elderly patients. *Acta Anaesthesiologica Scandinavica, 27*, 44–49.

Rowbotham, M., Harden, N., Stacey, B., Bernstesin, P., & Magnus-Miller, L. (1998). Gabapentin for the treatment of postherpetic neuralgia. A randomized controlled trial. *Journal of the American Medical Association, 280*, 1837–1842.

Salomaki, T.E., Leppaluoto, J., Laitinen, J.O., Vuolteenaho, O., & Nutinen, L.S. (1993). Epidural vs. intravenous fentanyl for reducing hormonal, metabolic and physiologic responses after thoracotomy. *Anesthesiology, 79*, 672–679.

Schwarzer, A.C., Aprill, C.N., & Bogduk, N. (1995). The sacroiliac joint in chronic low back pain. *Spine, 20*, 31–37.

Schwarzer, A.C., Wang, S., Bogduk, N., McNaught, P.J., & Laurent, R. (1995). Prevalence and clinical features of lumbar zygopophyseal joint pain: A study in an Australian population with chronic low back pain. *Annals of the Rheumatic Diseases, 54*,100–106.

Silverstein, F.E., et al. (2000). Gastrointestinal toxicity with celecoxib vs nonsteroidal anti-inflammatory drugs for osteoarthritis and rheumatoid arthritis. The CLASS study. A randomized controlled trial. *Journal of the Americal Medical Association, 284*, 1247–1255

Sindrup, S.H., Gram, L.F., Brosen, K., Eshoj, O., & Mogensen, E.F. (1990). The selective serotonin reuptake inhibitor paroxetine is effective in the treatment of diabetic neuropathy symptoms. *Pain, 42*, 135–144.

Souter, A.J., Fredman, B., & White, P.F. (1994). Controversies in the perioperative use of nonsteroidal antiinflammatory drugs. *Anesthesia and Analgesia, 79*, 1178–1190.

Spaccarelli, K.C. (1996). Lumbar and caudal epidural corticosteroid injections. *Mayo Clinic. Proceedings, 71*, 169–178.

Sternbach, R.A. (1986). Survey of pain in the United States: The Nuprin pain report. *Clinical Journal of Pain, 2*, 49–53.

Stracke, H., Meyer, U., Schumacher, H., & Federlin, K. (1992). Mexiletine in the treatment of diabetic neuropathy. *Diabetes Care, 15*, 1550–1555.

Swerdlow, M. (1984). Anticonvulsant drugs and chronic pain. *Clinical Neuropharmacology, 7*, 51–82.

Tanelian, D.L., & Victory, R.A. (1995). Sodium channel-blocking agents. Their use in neuropathic pain conditions. *Pain Forum, 4*, 75–80.

Tuman, K.J., McCarthy, R.J., March, R.J., DeLaria, G.A., Patel, R.V., & Ivankovich, A.D. (1991). Effects of epidural anesthesia and analgesia on coagulation and outcome after major vascular surgery. *Anesthesia and Analgesia, 73*, 696–704.

Turk, D.C., Brody, M.C., & Okifuji, E.A. (1994). Physicians' attitudes and practices regarding the long term prescribing of opioids for noncancer pain. *Pain, 59*, 201–208.

U.S. Census Bureau, Population Division, Aging Studies Branch. (1999, November 5).

White, P.F. (1988). Use of patient-controlled analgesia for management of acute pain. *Journal of the American Medical Association, 259*, 243–247.

Woolf, C.J., Shortland, P., & Coggeshall, R.E. (1992). Peripheral nerve injury triggers central sprouting of myelinated afferents. *Nature, 355*, 75–77.

Wu, C.L., Marsh, A., & Dworken, R.H. (2000). The role of sympathetic nerve blocks in herpes zoster and postherpetic neuralgia, *Pain, 87*, 121–129.

Yeager, M.P., Glass, D.D., Neff, R.K., & Brinck-Johnsen, T. (1987). Epidural anesthesia and analgesia in high risk surgical patients. *Anesthesiology, 66*, 729–736.

Zheng, Z., Gibson, S.J., Khalil, Z., Helm, R.D., & McMeeken, J.M. (2000). Age-related differences in the time course of capsaicin-induced hyperalgesia. *Pain, 85*. 51–55.

41

Sleep and Weight Problems Associated with Pain

Arnold Fox, M.D. and Barry Fox, Ph.D.

So neither ought you attempt to cure the body without the Soul, and this … is the reason why the cure of so many diseases is unknown to the physicians of Hellas, because they are ignorant of the whole which ought to be studied, also, for part can never be well unless the whole is well.

Plato

INTRODUCTION

Sleep and weight generally afflict all chronic pain patients. In addressing this topic, the authors recognize that many complex factors enter into health and disease, including stress. Pain, suffering, and disability are described as a cycle dependent, in part, on our expectations.

Problems associated with weight gain and sleep disturbance exacerbate treatment for pain and must be regarded as perpetuating factors needing resolution concomitant with pain management.

SINGLE CAUSES AND SIMPLE EQUATIONS

As a young medical student, I (Arnold Fox) was taught to look for the single cause of disease, for the specific germ, perhaps the *Mycobacterium* tuberculosis. This single cause, said the medical sages and literature, would define the disease, explain the cause, and point to the cure.

Streptococcus "explained" strep sore throat, as well as the rheumatic fever and rheumatic heart disease that struck many children and young adults. The polio virus "explained" why we had hospital floors filled with patients lying helpless in their iron lungs. Look for the germ, they told us … find the vitamin deficiency, the endocrine imbalance … the single factor that elucidates the disease process.

It was all so simple. Germ X = disease X, germ Y = disease Y. The equation was simple. Yes, the single-cause theory was exciting and enticing; it made everything so easy — cause and cure, effect and response. Unfortunately, the single-cause theory failed to consider the fact that people who are exposed to various germs and other disease-causing factors remain perfectly healthy. I spent many months in the tuberculosis ward at the Los Angeles County Hospital. I saw entire families that had been exposed to tuberculosis, who had been coughed on countless times by the patient they cared for, yet they never came down with the disease.

Clearly, disease was more than the result of being exposed to a germ. The response of the invaded body had to be considered, as well as the person's immune system, nutritional, physiologic, and psychological state, and more. Sometimes, the body's misreading of the situation leads to disease. This happens with allergies; the body labels relatively harmless pollen as a potential poison, triggering a violent reaction. The body is hit by "friendly fire," producing allergies or worse.

Obviously, the equation was more complex than we thought. And clearly, the physical factors (such as germs and vitamins) do not stand alone in the health equation. Every formula must include the psychological and spiri-

0-8493-0926-3/02/$0.00+$1.50
© 2002 by CRC Press LLC

tual factors as well as the physical factors. Indeed, we have learned that the effect of the psychological factors (stress) on the immune system are among the most powerful of all, especially those of a chronic nature (Cassel, 1986; Friedman & Glascow, 1974; Mason, et al., 1979; Syme, 1975).

IS STRESS THE SINGLE CAUSE?

"Well, just a minute," some have said. Can we consider stress to be the single cause of disease — or of many diseases? No, because we all react differently to stress. For years, those who suffered from migraine headache were characterized as suffering the effects of ongoing and severe stress. Yet it has been shown that migraine headache sufferers and individuals who do not have migraine headaches have just about the same type of life otherwise (Henry, Gutt, & Rees, 1973). Other equally interesting studies include one that measured the response to stress among women awaiting breast biopsies for presumed cancer of the breast. All the women faced the same serious, possibly deadly, disease, yet there was wide variety in their measures of cortisol (in the form of 17-hydroxycorticosteroid, which is known to be elevated with stressful situations) (Katz, et al., 1970). This and thousands of other studies have convinced most physicians and others in the health care field that there is no single cause of disease — not even stress.

A COMPLEX EQUATION

Many factors enter into the health and disease equation. The entire interaction between the person and his or her environment must be considered. This is especially true with chronic pain. All the factors must be considered, especially the psychological, for what we *think* influences how we *feel*.

Reciprocal interactions between persons/patients and their environments help determine what they think about their problems, thus influencing how they feel. One person with a history of chronic low back pain who wakes up with back pain may consider it a minor annoyance, a cost of growing older. So this person takes a hot shower, a simple analgesic (e.g., aspirin), does a few stretching exercises, then goes to work, fully expecting to be able to get through the day. Another person with similar pain may look upon the pain as a punishment, or be angry at the driver of the car that rear-ended him or her. This person expects to feel miserable and believes that he or she cannot possibly get through the day. This person may lie in bed, become angry, fight with a spouse, resent the boss for being so uncaring, go to a physician, or seek an attorney. Increasing resentment, anger, and irritability result, along with sleep disturbances. Inactivity and increased food intake (to assuage the stress) lead to weight gain — which often increase the pain and disability. Such cycles can go forever, or so it seems.

What we think, what we believe, and what we expect (cognitive factors) may have more influence on our pain than other factors. The pain equation is long and complex.

OBESITY

To complicate matters, obesity, a major problem here in the U.S., is often associated with chronic pain. All of us who care for patients have noted that those with chronic pain problems tend to gain weight. Away from work, sitting at home, not exercising, eating more to alleviate the psychic and physical pain, eating the wrong foods, and/or suffering a drop in self-esteem, pain patients tend to pack on the pounds. Gaining weight exacerbates their disability, increases joint problems, and deleteriously affects the entire pain-control process. Studies (e.g., Jamison, et al., 1990) have shown that there is a significant relationship between a chronic pain patient's weight gain and decreased physical activity, an increased tendency to have accidents, heightened emotional stress with all the associated physiologic and psychological problems, and even increased sensitivity to pain.

Such studies support the observation that obese subjects may be more sensitive to pain than non-obese subjects (McKendall & Haier, 1983). (This was felt to be related to the endogenous opiate systems, although the mechanism is far from clear.) Electrophysiologic studies measured nociceptive threshold in 30 obese women (30% or more above ideal weight) and 20 controls. The nociceptive threshold was significantly lower in the obese individuals than in the controls (Pradatier, et al., 1981). The authors' experience in raising the endogenous endorphin levels using *dl*-phenylalanine (DLPA) (Fox & Fox, 1985), plus dietary and related methods, have shown that the pain threshold can be lifted and pain decreased. This often speeds the patient's recovery.

(Authors' Note: In 1972, Dr. Candace Pert and Dr. Solomon Snyder showed that morphine [a powerful pain-killing drug] fits into certain nerve cell structures in the brain like a key fits its lock [i.e., morphine can unlock previously unknown powers of the brain]. But this was a puzzling discovery. Why do human brain cells have specific structures that interact with morphine? These two scientists, along with others, proposed a simple, yet radical, explanation: The human brain must produce its own form of morphine. Studies at major universities around the world have shown that the brain does, in fact, produce many hormone-like chemicals that bear a close functional resemblance to morphine. These morphine-like chemicals are called endorphins because they are produced by the body [they are endogenous] and are similar to morphine. Pain researchers began testing the endorphins, finding that

the endorphins are more powerful than morphine, the strongest painkiller we have. Unfortunately, the body that produces endorphins also degrades them. In fact, it was theorized that, in some pain patients, the body was keeping natural endorphin levels too low, resulting in pain. Dr. Seymour Ehrenpreis of the Chicago Medical School found that a nutritional amino acid called phenylalanine [PA] blocked the degradation of endorphins. DLPA [the dl-form of phenylalanine] protects our naturally produced endorphins, effectively extending their life in the nervous system. I (Arnold Fox) have had a great deal of success treating pain patients with DLPA. As part of the full treatment, DLPA helps in raising their threshold to pain, lifting their depression, and losing excess weight.)

PAIN, SELF-PERCEPTION, AND OBESITY

The weight gain that often accompanies chronic pain can damage the patient's self-esteem. This can lead to, among other problems, dysfunctional responses to the stress of pain and disharmony within the network of family and friends, and the medical team — the very people who should all be working together to support the patient. As patients become increasingly immobilized by their pain, weight gain, stress, and increased sensitivity to pain, they may develop feelings of helplessness and hopelessness. Convinced that they have lost control, patients wonder why they should even bother trying to get well. Manageable pains may become intolerable burdens. The pain equation is complex indeed.

OBESITY AND PAIN

I (Arnold Fox) have seen many patients whose pain was worsened by their obesity. For example, I have treated a number of obese patients with carpal tunnel syndrome who were obese and had no other predisposing factors (e.g., repetitive occupational use of wrists or hands, pregnancy myxedema, rheumatoid arthritis, acromegaly, and gout) (Swick & McQuillen, 1976). In many of these patients, significant weight loss was enough to abolish symptoms and normalize nerve velocity studies.

Osteoarthritis is characterized by a gradual loss of the joint cartilage, leading to deformities of the joints involved, plus progressive pain and loss or limitation of motion in the affected joint. Obesity may contribute to or worsen this process, especially in weight-bearing joints. Pseudogout is a form of arthritis caused by the release of calcium pyrophosphate crystals into the joint space, which, in turn, causes an inflammation of various joints. Acute exercise may trigger attacks involving one or several joints in some areas. We doctors aspirate the fluid from the joint and find the crystals in the joint fluid. We treat pseudogout with medications and rest. We help

prevent further attacks by reducing aggravating factors, including obesity.

Back pain is a major problem, the incidence of which is staggering. Approximately 80% of the population will, at some time, have back pain sufficient to interfere with their regular activities, or send them to see a doctor (Nachemson, 1976). Obesity can cause or aggravate low back (lumbar spine) pain, especially fat in the abdominal area. "Beer bellies" may cause the muscles of the abdomen to become distended, producing increased lordosis. (Picture the pregnant female in the last part of pregnancy.) The muscles of the anterior abdominal wall have a very important function: stabilizing the lumbar spine and pelvis. Obesity reduces the tonus (strength) of these muscles, increasing lordosis (curve of the lumbar spine). This produces strain of the anterior lumbar spinal ligaments, and possibly impingement of the posterior joint facets and spinous processes on occasion, adding to more back pain. There may also be disturbances of the weight-bearing duties of the feet, knees, and hips with obesity. The abnormal posture caused by obesity can lead to pain in the lower extremities and hips. In addition, with obesity there may be weakness of the pelvic floor, especially in females, that may cause referred pain to the sacrum and coccyx.

There are various pains caused by trapping of a nerve. For example, pain on the anterior (front) side of a thigh may be caused by the lateral femoral cutaneous nerve becoming entrapped beneath the inguinal ligament, producing a syndrome called neuralgia paresthestica (Kitchen & Simpson, 1972), which may often be a complication of obesity. The symptoms can include a burning, tingling pain and numbness over the anterior thigh area made worse by walking or standing. Weight loss is very effective. (This can also occur with pregnancy, or be caused by a tight girdle.)

PAIN AND SLEEP DISORDERS

Pain patients often complain about their sleep disorders, especially an inability to fall asleep. So many patients report that they are more aware of their pain in the evening and nighttime hours, and that the pain is more intense at that time. I (Arnold Fox) learned back in the 1950s that pain seems greater during the dark hours. As an intern, I was called to see patients all night long (and wound up with my own sleep problems). Patients whose chronic pain appeared to be stabilized in the daytime became unstable during the sleep hours. Why? For one thing, there was less activity at night. Various external stimuli (e.g., lights, TV, visitors) are absent. The focus of the patient's attention moves inward, settling on the pain. Patients may fear another sleepless, painful night, and their fears worsen their pain. Focus and fear are great inducers of pain.

Depression is another enemy of sleep. The link between depression and chronic pain is well-established. Many depressed chronic pain patients have difficulty in falling asleep and staying asleep. They have early-morning awakenings, fitful sleep patterns, and they wake up feeling very tired. (Some depressed people may sleep more than usual.) Antidepressants can be used to raise the person's (subjective) pain threshold, which may help restore the sleep cycle.

Patients may resist antidepressants, saying that they are not depressed, or not depressed enough to require medications. It is important to convey to these patients that the antidepressant is being used to raise their pain threshold. We must stress that we understand that their pain is real, and not imagined.

CASE HISTORY

Mr. Jones, a 35-year-old factory worker, is one of the multitude of chronic pain patients I (Arnold Fox) have seen through the years. Many of the pain factors discussed previously have played a role in his disability and recovery. He injured his low back while lifting boxes at work. The company doctor examined him, took X-rays, and prescribed medications and 4 weeks of physical therapy. The doctor's attitude, according to Mr. Jones, was negative: "He didn't believe that I was hurt."

The patient was sent back to work. His back still hurt, but he had to work to support his family, and he figured his back would improve. It did not, despite copious quantities of over-the-counter and prescribed pain medications. When I interviewed Mr. Jones, he vehemently denied depression, but did acknowledge that since the injury he had difficulty falling asleep and staying asleep, had early morning awakenings, and felt tired upon awakening. He also admitted to some other biological associates of depression, such as poor appetite, fatigue, difficulty in concentrating and focusing his thoughts, a decreased sexual interest, plus a decreased interest in formerly pleasurable activities (e.g., movies, theater, reading, family outings). His MMPI (Minnesota Multiphasic Personality Index) showed a rather significant rise in the depression scale; and although he denied depression, his voice, expression, and body language supported the impression of depression.

He stated that his sleep disturbances became notable when, 7 to 8 weeks after the injury, he realized that his pain was not going to go away as quickly as he thought it would. Eight months passed and he was still unable to work. His disability checks stopped when the company disputed the work injury. His small savings account was quickly exhausted. His wife went to work while he sat at home feeling guilty and useless. He feared that his three children would view him in a negative light. He

was careful not to complain, preferring to bear his pain and disability "like a man."

He "didn't feel like" eating. In fact, he avoided sitting down to a meal. Instead, he snacked all day. Once 5′10″ and 170 pounds, he grew to 225 pounds. His feet and knees hurt. His back pain grew worse. His blood pressure was high (for the first time). He attributed the weight gain to his lack of exercise. He saw many specialists, practicing many modalities, all of whom were helpful for a while. He took various medications, ranging from nonsteroidal anti-inflammatory drugs (NSAIDs, some of which increase weight) to narcotics. He took up smoking again, puffing his way through two packs a day, along with a six-pack of beer, to assuage his symptoms.

With each treatment failure, Mr. Jones' pain and other problems grew worse. He only slept a few hours a night, waking up tired and irritable. His morale plummeted. His physicians and other healthcare providers became more negative as his problems continued. As they became more negative, they attempted to distance themselves from him and "shuffled him over" to other specialists. (This is called the "dumping syndrome" — dump the patient on someone else.)

SKEWING THE EQUATION

Why was Mr. Jones so long in recovering? Every treatment we physicians, and others, offer to our patients carries a message. That message is there, whether or not we label it as a message, or even understand that it exists. In what we do and say, we convey to the patient an impression. It may be positive: "Yes, I am a professional. Yes, I am optimistic. Yes, we are going to lick this thing together." The message may also be negative: "There is no hope. You will have to learn to live with it. Stop complaining. If you are not getting better, it is your fault. How can I get rid of you?"

I believe that Mr. Jones received the latter message and it was reflected in continuing and even worsening symptoms, not only of his back pain but, more importantly, of his deterioration as a person — as a father, husband, son, worker, and citizen.

It is important that everyone who meets with and deals with patients — from the receptionist to all the healthcare professionals and associates — presents the most optimistic picture that can be honestly given. I was taught that there is always something that we can do to help the patient. Something. Perhaps we cannot alter the pathology, but we can offer what we know, understanding, empathy, a kind hand, and not withdraw from the patient. (The doctor for whom Barry Fox is named always offered a kind hand, and never in defeat. He sat quietly with my grandmother, holding her hand at home, as she died. He taught me that there is always something we can do.)

SOLVING THE EQUATION

In Mr. Jones's case, the interdisciplinary team was assembled. Therapy suggestions were made and considered. He was weaned from his analgesics and soporifics (sleeping pills). Antidepressants were used for a time to raise his threshold to pain, and then gradually reduced. To help him sleep, he was taught the Meditation-Relaxation Response, a technique we have used for years (Fox & Fox, 1989). The response helped him relax, setting up the mechanisms for sleep.

We also used biofeedback, demonstrating to this demoralized patient that he could control certain physiologic functions and that he had some control over his body. We also started him on the DLPA program (Fox & Fox, 1985). The DLPA program includes the use of DLPA, specific dietary instructions and nutrients, plus exercises and affirmations.

INVOLVEMENT: THE OFTEN-MISSING FACTOR

One of our main goals was to get Mr. Jones actively involved in his own treatment and recovery. We emphasized to him, and he accepted, the fact that the benefits of the various treatments were largely a result of what he did himself. The team members worked together with Mr. Jones, emphasizing that we looked upon him as a human being operating in his environment and not a low-back patient.

His family was also involved because the entire family is affected by his pain and plays a role in his recovery (or lack of). We can assume that even a well-functioning family group can become dysfunctional with time, as the chronic pain patient loses his/her family and occupational role, gradually assuming the role of "the sick one" (Roy, 1982, 1984; Maruta,1981). One must ask the question: What purpose does the pain serve for the patient or the family? It has been shown that in many family settings there may be a definite role prolonging and perpetuating the chronic pain (Swenson & Maruta, 1980).

Some 30 years ago, when I was a young, newly graduated consultant, a woman patient with severe pain was referred to me by a general practitioner. Not finding anything I could deal with or understand, I sent her to a psychiatrist. The psychiatrist promptly called me and asked, "What do you want me to do?" I replied, "Take away her pain." He said, "Arnold, don't you see that the way the family is constituted, both she and they 'need' the pain? Until this family dysfunction is resolved, there will be no resolution of the pain." I learned a valuable lesson.

We must also remember that spouses and other close family members of the chronic pain patient suffer a higher degree of depression than do members of families without chronic pain members. Furthermore, it is well-known that spouses of chronic pain patients may be even more depressed than the patients themselves. It is important to involve the entire family.

With a multidisciplinary healthcare team, with the family involved, with the patient convinced that he could recover, with the Meditation–Relaxation Response, the exercises, diet, and DLPA program, Mr. Jones began to recover. He was able to sleep at night. His self-esteem returned. He lost his excess weight, went through a special exercise program, and was eventually able to return to a full family and occupational life.

The pain equation is complex, often too difficult for one professional to solve. The factors are many: the patient; the patient's feelings and fears; the doctor's attitude; the germs; the medicines and treatments; the family; and more. There is rarely a single cause with a simple solution. It often takes a team of experts to solve the complex pain equation.

MEDITATIVE RELAXATION

The following is a "script," which may be tape-recorded, for the meditative-relaxation technique that I and others have used successfully to help chronic pain patients (and other patients) relax, sleep better, and overcome pain. Meditative relaxation may not be as glamorous or high-tech as drugs and surgery, but it worked well in many cases.

PART 1: EVERY MUSCLE NEEDS A TOTAL LOOSENING

I have found that this three-tiered program of meditative relaxation helps many chronic pain patients reduce their stress and pain, and sleep better. I suggest to patients the following:

Go into a quiet room twice a day for 10 to 15 minutes, turn off the lights, close the shades, unplug the phone, loosen all belts and ties, and tell everyone not to bother you.

Push a comfortable chair up against a wall and take a seat. Rest your feet on the floor, a little bit in front of you. Place your hands on your knees.

Tensing for Relaxation

Begin by tensing and relaxing your eyes, mouth, neck, arms, trunk, and legs. To help my patients remember the order, I tell them that *Every Muscle Needs A Total Loosening* (that is, Every = eyes, Muscle = mouth, Needs = neck, A = arms, Total = trunk, and Loosening = legs).

Every = Eyes

Begin by closing your eyes. Hold them clenched shut, as tightly as you can. Clench them still tighter. Hold those muscles taut while you count slowly: one thousand … two thousand … three thousand … four thousand … five thousand … six thousand … seven thousand … eight thousand … nine thousand … ten thousand.

Relax your eye muscles.

Now take a slow, deep breath in through your nose. Hold it. Then let it slowly out through your mouth, very slowly, taking at least 5 seconds to let it all out.

Take another slow breath. Fill your lungs. Feel your diaphragm pulling down to open the lungs wide. With your mind's eye, see your diaphragm dropping down as your lungs fill.

Now repeat. Squeeze your eyes tightly shut. Hold your eyes closed tightly while you count slowly: one thousand … two thousand … three thousand … four thousand … five thousand … six thousand … seven thousand … eight thousand … nine thousand … ten thousand.

Slowly relax your muscles, and then slowly open your eyes.

Take a deep breath in through your nose … a nice, deep breath. Feel your diaphragm pulling down to open your lungs wide. With your mind's eye, see your diaphragm dropping down as your lungs fill.

Hold your breath for a moment. Now let it out through your mouth, very slowly, taking at least five seconds to empty your lungs.

Take another big breath; fill your lungs.

Hold it for a moment. Now let it out very slowly. Take 5 seconds or more to blow it all out.

The muscles around your eyes do not feel tired anymore. They feel good.

Muscle = Mouth

Now tighten up the muscles of your mouth. Grimace. Show your teeth, and tighten up the muscles around your mouth and the front of your neck. Tilt your chin up. Now, with your teeth still bared, open your lips as wide as you can. Hold them open, teeth clenched, as you also tighten your cheek and neck muscles. Teeth clenched, cheeks and neck tight, lips pulled open. Hold these muscles tight while you count slowly: one thousand … two thousand … three thousand … four thousand … five thousand … six thousand … seven thousand … eight thousand … nine thousand … ten thousand.

Slowly relax your lips, jaw, cheek, and neck muscles.

Now take a slow, deep breath in through your nose. Hold it. Then let it slowly out through your mouth, very slowly, taking at least 5 seconds to let it all out.

Take another slow breath. Fill your lungs. Feel your diaphragm pulling down to open the lungs wide. With your mind's eye, see your diaphragm dropping down as your lungs fill.

Now repeat. Tighten the muscles of your mouth, clench your teeth, and grimace. Tilt your chin up and tighten the muscles around your mouth and in the front of your neck. Hold that for a moment, then open your lips wide as you tighten your cheek and neck muscles. Hold these muscles tight while you count slowly: one thousand … two thousand … three thousand … four thousand … five thousand-six thousand … seven thousand … eight thousand … nine thousand … ten thousand.

Slowly relax your jaw, lips, cheek, and neck muscles.

Take a deep breath in through your nose … a nice, deep breath. Feel your diaphragm pulling down to open your lungs wide. With your mind's eye, see your diaphragm dropping down as your lungs fill.

Hold the breath for a moment. Now let it out through your mouth very slowly, taking at least 5 seconds to empty your lungs.

Take another big breath; fill your lungs.

Hold it for a moment. Now let it out very slowly. Take 5 seconds or more to blow it all out.

The muscles of your mouth and the front of your neck now feel light and relaxed.

Needs = Neck

Next comes the neck: gently, but firmly, push your head against the wall behind you. This puts the muscles in the back of your neck into contraction. Hold that position while you count slowly: one thousand … two thousand … three thousand … four thousand … five thousand … six thousand … seven thousand … eight thousand … nine thousand … ten thousand.

Slowly relax, letting your head slump forward just a little.

Now take a slow, deep breath in through your nose. Hold it. Then let it slowly out through your mouth, very slowly, taking at least 5 seconds to let it all out.

Take another slow breath. Fill your lungs. Feel your diaphragm pulling down to open the lungs wide. With your mind's eye, see your diaphragm dropping down as your lungs fill.

Again. Gently, but firmly, push your head against the wall behind you. Hold that position while you count slowly: one thousand … two thousand … three thousand … four thousand … five thousand … six thousand … seven thousand … eight thousand … nine thousand … ten thousand.

Slowly relax your jaw, lips, cheek, and neck muscles.

Take a deep breath in through your nose … a nice, deep breath. Feel your diaphragm pulling down to open your lungs wide. With your mind's eye, see your diaphragm dropping down as your lungs fill. Hold the breath for a moment. Now let it out through your mouth, very slowly, taking at least 5 seconds to empty your lungs.

Take another big breath, fill your lungs.

Hold it for a moment. Now let it out very slowly. Take 5 seconds or more to blow it all out.

Now push up your shoulders so that they almost touch your ears. Tilt your chin up and your head back, so that the back of your head almost touches your raised shoulders. Push your neck down and back, into your shoulders, feeling the muscles at the base of your neck, where your neck meets your shoulders, contracting. Lift your shoulders up into your neck as high as you can. Feel the tension in the back of your neck and upper shoulders as you count slowly: one thousand … two thousand … three thousand … four thousand … five thousand … six thousand … seven thousand … eight thousand … nine thousand … ten thousand.

Slowly relax your neck and lower your shoulders.

Now take a slow, deep breath in through your nose. Hold it. Then let it slowly out through your mouth, very slowly, taking at least 5 seconds to let it all out.

Take another slow breath. Fill your lungs. Feel your diaphragm pulling down to open the lungs wide. With your mind's eye, see your diaphragm dropping down as your lungs fill.

Once more, tilt your neck back and lift your shoulders up into your neck. Hold your neck and shoulders tense as you count slowly: one thousand … two thousand … three thousand … four thousand … five thousand … six thousand … seven thousand … eight thousand-nine thousand … ten thousand.

Slowly relax your jaw, lips, cheek, and neck muscles.

Take a deep breath in through your nose … a nice, deep breath. Feel your diaphragm pulling down to open your lungs wide. With your mind's eye, see your diaphragm dropping down as your lungs fill.

Hold the breath for a moment. Now let it out through your mouth, very slowly, taking at 5 five seconds to empty your lungs.

Take another big breath, fill your lungs.

Hold it for a moment. Now let it out very slowly. Take 5 seconds or more to blow it all out.

The muscles of your shoulders and the back of your neck now feel light and tingly.

A = Arms

Put both arms straight out in front of you at about shoulder level, palms facing down. Make two very tight fists, as tight as you can make them. Bending at the wrist, push your fists down toward the floor as hard as you can. Feel the muscles in your wrists and forearms tighten, and feel the tension, especially in your forearms, up to your elbows. Hold that position while you count slowly: one thousand … two thousand … three thousand … four thousand … five thousand … six thousand … seven thousand … eight thousand … nine thousand … ten thousand.

Slowly relax. Open your fists. Rest your hands, palms down, on your knees. Feel how relaxed, refreshed, and tingly your hands, wrists, and arms feel.

Now take a slow, deep breath in through your nose. Hold it. Then let it slowly out through your mouth, very slowly, taking at least 5 seconds to let it all out.

Take another slow breath. Fill your lungs. Feel your diaphragm, pulling down to open the lungs wide. With your mind's eye, see your diaphragm dropping down as your lungs fill.

Again, put both arms straight out in front of you at about shoulder height, palms facing down. Make two very tight fists, as tight as you can make them. Bending at the wrists, push your fists down toward the floor as hard as you can. Feel the muscles in your wrists and forearms tighten, and feel the tension, especially in your forearms, up to your elbows. Hold that position and count slowly: one thousand … two thousand … three thousand … four thousand … five thousand … six thousand-seven thousand … eight thousand … nine thousand … ten thousand.

Now slowly relax your jaw, lips, cheek, and neck muscles.

Take a deep breath in through your nose … a nice, deep breath. Feel your diaphragm pulling down to open your lungs wide. With your mind's eye, see your diaphragm dropping down as your lungs fill.

Hold that breath for a moment. Now let it out through your mouth, very slowly, taking at least 5 seconds to empty your lungs.

Take another big breath; fill your lungs.

Hold it for a moment. Now let it out very slowly. Take 5 seconds or more to blow it all out.

Now hold your arms out to the sides of your body at shoulder level, palms up. Close your hands into tightly clenched fists. Bend your arms at the elbow, bringing your fists to your ears. Clench your arm and shoulder muscles, especially the biceps muscles in your upper arms. Hold tight and count slowly: one thousand … two thousand … three thousand … four thousand … five thousand … six thousand … seven thousand … eight thousand … nine thousand … ten thousand.

Slowly relax, dropping your arms to your lap as you take in a deep breath through your nose.

Take in another deep breath through your nose. Hold it for a moment. Now let it out slowly, very slowly, through your mouth, taking at least 5 seconds to empty your lungs.

Take another big breath, filling up your lungs. Hold it for a moment. Now let it out slowly, very slowly.

Again, hold your arms out to the sides of your body at shoulder level, palms up. Close your hands into tightly clenched fists. Bend your arms at the elbow, bringing your fists to your ears. Clench your arm and shoulder muscles, especially the biceps muscles in your upper arms. Hold tight and count slowly: one thousand … two thousand … three thousand … four thousand … five thousand-six thousand … seven thousand … eight thousand … nine thousand … ten thousand.

Slowly relax, dropping your arms to your lap as you take in a deep breath through your nose.

Take in another deep breath through your nose. Hold it for a moment. Now let it out slowly, very slowly, through your mouth, taking at least 5 seconds to empty your lungs.

Take another big breath, filling up your lungs. Hold it for a moment. Now let it out slowly, very slowly.

Concentrate on your arms for just a moment. Feel how light and tingly they are.

Total = Trunk

Fill your lungs with as much air as you can. Holding the air in your lungs, bear down as if you were going to have a bowel movement. While holding the air and bearing down, place your fists up by your chin. Squeeze your arms tightly against your chest. Feel the tension in your chest muscles as you count slowly: one thousand … two thousand … three thousand … four thousand … five thousand … six thousand … seven thousand … eight thousand … nine thousand … ten thousand.

Slowly relax, letting the air out of your lungs.

Now take a slow, deep breath in through your nose. Hold it. Then let it out slowly through your mouth, very slowly, taking at least 5 seconds to let it all out.

Take another slow breath. Fill your lungs. Feel your diaphragm pulling down to open the lungs wide. With your mind's eye, see your diaphragm dropping down as your lungs fill.

Fill your lungs once again, bear down, hold your fists by your chin and squeeze your arms against your chest. Hold that position, chest muscles clenched tightly, as you slowly count: one thousand … two thousand-three thousand … four thousand … five thousand … six thousand … seven thousand … eight thousand-nine thousand … ten thousand.

Slowly relax and exhale.

Take a deep breath in through your nose … a nice, deep breath. Feel your diaphragm pulling down to open your lungs wide. With your mind's eye, see your diaphragm dropping down as your lungs fill.

Hold that breath for a moment. Now let it out through your mouth, very slowly, taking at least 5 seconds to empty your lungs.

Take another big breath, fill your lungs. Hold it for a moment. Now let it out very slowly. Take 5 seconds or more to blow it all out.

Your trunk now feels relaxed.

Loosening = Legs

Straighten out your legs in front of you, lock your knees, and raise your feet off the floor. Hold them at about the level of your chair seat, toes pointing forward. Feel the tension in your calves, ankles, and in the front and outside of your thighs. Hold that position. Keep your toes pointed forward as you slowly count: one thousand … two thousand … three thousand … four thousand … five thousand … six thousand … seven thousand … eight thousand-nine thousand … ten thousand.

New slowly relax, lowering your feet to the floor. Take a slow, deep breath in through your nose. Hold it. Then let it out slowly through your mouth, very slowly, taking at least 5 seconds to let it all out.

Take another slow breath. Fill your lungs. Feel your diaphragm pulling down to open the lungs wide. With your mind's eye, see your diaphragm dropping down as your lungs fill.

Again, lift your feet off the floor, knees locked, toes pointing forward. Hold tight and count slowly: one thousand … two thousand … three thousand … four thousand … five thousand … six thousand … seven thousand … eight thousand-nine thousand … ten thousand.

Slowly relax and exhale.

Take a deep breath in through your nose … a nice, deep breath. Feel your diaphragm pulling down to open your lungs wide. With your mind's eye, see your diaphragm dropping down as your lungs fill.

Hold that breath for a moment. Now let it out through your mouth, very slowly, taking at least 5 seconds to empty your lungs.

Take another big breath; fill your lungs. Hold it for a moment. Now let it out very slowly. Take 5 seconds or more to blow it all out.

Your leg muscles feel relaxed. It feels good. You have relaxed your whole body.

Now go back to the neck and shoulders one more time: Push your neck down and slightly back. Raise your shoulders up into your neck. Hold them tight as you count slowly: one thousand … two thousand … three thousand … four thousand … five thousand … six thousand … seven thousand … eight thousand … nine thousand … ten thousand.

Relax and take a deep breath. Hold it, and then exhale slowly, taking at least 5 seconds to let it all out.

Another breath … hold it … let it out slowly.

Push your neck back down and your shoulders up one more time. Clench those muscles and count slowly: one thousand … two thousand … three thousand … four thousand … five thousand … six thousand … seven thousand … eight thousand … nine thousand … ten thousand.

The muscles in your neck feel relaxed.

PART 2: CONCENTRATION ON RELAXATION

Now your entire body is nice and relaxed. Get comfortable in your chair, keeping your feet on the floor. Close your eyes. You are going to become aware of various parts of your body. You are going to actually "feel" them. Breathe in and out slowly through your nose, concentrating on your feet. Relax and focus on your feet. See your feet with your mind's eye … both of your feet … toes … along your soles from your toes to your heels … along the top from toes to the ankles. Feel your feet relaxing. Feel all of your toes relaxing … your right and left soles..right and left heels … the tops of both your feet relaxing. Silently tell yourself that both feet are totally relaxed … your toes, soles, heels, tops and bottoms of both your feet are totally relaxed.

Now feel your ankles relaxing. Concentrate on both your left and right ankle as you continue breathing through your nose, in and out, slowly. Feel both ankles. See them, in your mind's eye, relaxing. Silently tell yourself that your ankles are relaxed.

Continue breathing in and out through your nose, slowly, as you feel relaxation spreading to your calves, on the back sides of your lower legs. See them with your mind's eye. Concentrate on the feeling as both of your calves relax. Silently tell yourself that your calves are now relaxed.

With your calves relaxed, the feeling spreads around the front of your legs to your shins. Feel your right and left shins relaxing. See your shins with your mind's eye; feel them relaxing. Silently tell yourself that your shins are relaxed.

Continue breathing slowly through your nose, eyes closed, as you feel your knees relaxing. Concentrate on your left and right knees as you tell yourself that they are relaxed. See your knees with your mind's eye. Silently tell yourself that both of your knees are now relaxed.

Eyes closed, continue to breathe slowly, in and out through your nose, as you concentrate on your upper legs. See your upper legs, left and right, in your mind's eye. Feel the front of your upper legs relaxing. Now the relaxed feeling begins to spread to the outsides of your thighs … to the bottoms of both your thighs. Concentrate on your upper legs as the relaxation moves back up the insides … around to the tops. Silently tell yourself that both of your legs, from toes to thighs, are totally relaxed. And so they are.

As you continue breathing slowly through your nose … slowly … eyes closed … feel your buttocks and genital area relaxing. Concentrate on the feeling of relaxing. Silently tell yourself that these areas are relaxed.

Continue concentrating as the relaxed feeling spreads to your lower abdomen, below your navel. Concentrate as the feeling of relaxation spreads through your lower abdomen. Eyes closed, breathing slowly through your nose, feel the relaxation. Silently tell yourself that your lower abdomen is relaxed.

Now feel your lower back relaxing, loosening up. Concentrate on the feeling of relaxation in your lower back. See your lower back in your mind's eye. Silently tell yourself that your lower back is relaxed. Feel the tension gathered in your lower back fading away.

Move your mind's eye up a little to focus on your belly, from your navel to your chest. Feel the relaxation moving up past your navel to your lower chest. Concentrate on the feeling of relaxation. Silently tell yourself that you are relaxed from your navel to your chest.

Now the relaxed feeling continues up your chest to the base of your neck. See your chest with your mind's eye. Focus on the pleasant feeling of relaxation as it covers your entire chest. Silently tell yourself that your chest is now relaxed.

Eyes still closed, breathing slowly ... in and out through your nose ... concentrate on the relaxation as it spreads over your upper back. See your upper back with your mind's eye. Concentrate on the relaxation as it covers your entire upper back. Silently tell yourself that your back, belly, and chest are now totally relaxed.

Concentrate as the great feeling of relaxation continues up into your shoulders. See your shoulders ... right and left ... in your mind's eye. Feel the tension and tightness drain from both shoulders. Eyes closed, breathing slowly in and out through your nose, concentrate as your shoulders totally relax. Silently tell yourself that your shoulders are now relaxed.

Now the feeling of relaxation spreads up through your neck, from the bottom to the top. See your neck with your mind's eye. Feel the front of your neck relax. Concentrate on the feeling as it spreads around the right side of your neck ... the back ... the left side. Silently tell yourself that your whole neck is now completely relaxed.

Eyes closed, slowly breathing in and out through your nose, concentrate on the feeling of relaxation as it moves from your shoulders down both your arms. Picture your arms in your mind's eye. From your shoulders, the feeling of relaxation moves into the left and right upper arms ... front and back ... to both elbows ... front and back ... to your forearms ... front and back. Concentrate on the relaxation as it envelops both of your arms. Now your wrists are relaxing ... both wrists are relaxing. Concentrate as your fingers relax ... the fingers on both hands ... your thumbs ... index fingers ... middle fingers ... ring fingers ... little fingers. Silently tell yourself that both of your arms ... from your shoulders to the tip of each finger ... are relaxed.

Eyes closed, breathing slowly through your nose, see your head in your mind's eye. Concentrate on your head as the relaxation spreads up from your neck to your chin ... from the sides of your neck to the sides of your head ... from the back of your neck up the back of your head. Feel the relaxation spreading over your head ... your cheeks ... mouth ... nose ... eyes ... temples ... ears ... forehead. Concentrate carefully as the relaxation spreads up your head to the very top. Silently tell yourself that your head is now relaxed.

With your whole body totally relaxed, focus on your left arm. Eyes closed, breathing slowly through your nose, silently tell yourself that your left arm is heavy, very heavy. Feel your left arm becoming heavy. See it in your mind's eye ... heavy. Concentrate on the feeling of heaviness.

Now see your right arm in your mind's eye. Concentrate on your right arm ... silently tell yourself that your right arm is heavy, very heavy. Feel your right arm becoming heavy. Concentrate on the feeling of heaviness in your right arm.

Now let the heaviness totally drain out of both arms.

Your breathing is slow and easy. Your whole body is relaxed.

Part 3: "One"

As soon as you've completed your relaxation exercise, move right into meditation.

You are totally relaxed. Keep your eyes closed. Silently, to yourself, begin saying "one" over and over. Say it slowly. If you can sense your heart beat, say "one" in time with your heart. If not, say it slowly, over and over again.

Now see the numeral "1" with your mind's eye. See it and say it silently, slowly, over and over. Do not count the numbers of times you say "one." Just keep seeing and saying it. If you get tired of the number "1" switch over to the word "one." See the three letters "o," "n," and "e" with your mind's eye.

If your mind begins to wander, if you start thinking about work or supper, gently bring your attention back to "one."

If you can, see the "one" in color. See it in soft blue with your mind's eye. See it in green, the green of trees in the woods. When you can see it in color, or against a background, you know you are doing something powerful with your mind.

Keep seeing and saying "one" until you feel it is time to stop. Do not set an alarm to go off at a certain time. You will know when the session should end. Ten or 15 minutes for the entire relaxation-meditation session should be enough, but go for no more than 20 minutes.

When you are finished, slowly open your eyes. Sit quietly for a few moments, then rise and go about your business.

LOW-FAT EATING

Weight loss is a vital part of the equation for many overweight pain patients. Dieting, difficult enough, is made more confusing by the proliferation of "light," "lean," "natural," and "heart healthy" labels. Hundreds of diet books fill the bookstore shelves, but few are effective and safe. The basic principles of the Beverly Hills Medical Diet (Fox, 1982), which was awarded four stars by Consumer Guide's Rating the Diets, are still the best: a low-fat, low-cholesterol eating regimen based on the complex carbohydrates found in fresh vegetables, fruits, and whole grains.

Watch out for the hidden fats in foods, especially processed foods. The average American takes in some 40 to 50% of his or her calories in the form of fat — way too much. Only 20% of our calories, or fewer, should come from fat. Complex carbohydrates (especially from vegetables and whole grains) should comprise the greater part of our calories.

What should you eat? The following foods are low in fat: apples, apricots, artichokes, asparagus, bananas, barley, beets, berries, black beans, broccoli, brown rice, buckwheat, buttermilk, cabbage, carrots, cauliflower, celery, cherries, chestnuts, chicken (white, no skin), cilantro, cod, corn, cranberries, cress (water and garden), cucumbers, dandelion greens, eggplant, endive, flounder, garbanzo beans, garlic, grapefruit, haddock, halibut, hoop cheese, Jerusalem artichokes, jicama, kale, kidney beans, kohlrabi, lentils, lettuce (dark green), lychee nuts, mangoes, melons, milk (skim or 1% fat), millet, mushrooms, mustard greens, nectarines, oats, okra, onions, oranges, papayas, parsley, parsnips, peaches, pears, peas, peppers, perch, pike, pineapple, pink beans, plantains, plums, popcorn, potatoes, pumpkin, radish, red beans, red snapper, rutabagas, whole grain rye, sand dabs, scallops (steamed), sea bass, sole, spinach, split peas, sprouts, sweet potatoes, tangerines, tomatoes, tuna (packed in water), turkey (white, no skin), turnips, whole grain wheat, white beans, and wild rice.

Some tips for vegetables: Vegetables are sources for many vitamins, minerals, and enzymes, as well as dietary fiber. A diet including many vegetables lowers blood fats. Cook vegetables for as short a time as possible — just until they are tender and crisp. Use more raw than cooked vegetables, as cooking destroys many vitamins and minerals.

Some tips for fruit: Fruits are packed with vitamins, minerals, and sweetness. Eat whole, fresh fruit, not cooked, canned, or frozen fruit. Eat fresh, not dried fruits.

Eat two to four fruits a day, according to your weight and sugar sensitivity.

Some tips for whole grains: Whole grains are rich sources of B vitamins, minerals, fiber, low-fat protein, and complex carbohydrates. Use whole grains as cereal and for casseroles. Use breads made of all whole grains.

Some tips for legumes: Legumes are dried beans and peas, such as black beans, garbanzo beans, Great Northern beans, kidney beans, lentils, lima beans, red beans, small white beans, and split peas. Legumes are high in vitamins B1, B6, and others. They are high in minerals, such as calcium and iron, high in fiber, low in fat, and contain up to 20% protein.

Some tips for dairy products: Drink skim or buttermilk, if desired. If you like yogurt, eat plain, low-fat yogurt. Use low-fat yogurt instead of sour cream and mayonnaise. Cheese is high in fat and salt. Use hoop cheese, up to 4 ounces a day, instead.

Nuts and seeds are high in fat. Use them sparingly, just to add flavor and crunch to your foods. Avoid processed nuts and seeds.

Finally, a note on water: Water is a terrific weight-loss helper. Not only that, we need lots of water for good health. Drink at least five 8-ounce glasses of water each day.

EATING FOR GOOD SLEEPING

The drop in blood sugar called hypoglycemia can make it difficult to fall asleep — or it may wake you up once you have fallen asleep. When your blood sugar falls, the body pumps out a slew of hormones to bring the sugar back to normal. These include epinephrine from the adrenal glands, glucagon from the pancreas, cortisol from the adrenal cortex, and growth hormone. For example, when your blood sugar drops, the adrenal medulla causes epinephrine to be secreted in order to liberate sugar from the glycogen stored in the liver. This is just one of the mechanisms by which the body maintains homeostasis — and thereby keeps the blood sugar within acceptable levels. Unfortunately, there is a "side effect." The epinephrine quickly stabilizes blood sugar, but it also raises your heart rate, causes anxiety, and wakes up your brain. How can you sleep when that is going on?

That is why it is not a bad idea to snack on a small amount of whole-grain muffin or crackers, or other complex carbohydrates before going to bed. This will help keep your blood sugar within comfortable limits. And the complex carbohydrates in the food will also help increase brain levels of serotonin, which should lead to sounder sleep.

Perhaps some people can get away with drinking caffeine-containing beverages late at night, but this is not the case for most people. The ability of the body to "deactivate" caffeine varies from person to person, but to be safe, do not drink coffee, tea, or soft drinks with caffeine, chocolate and cocoa, or even coffee-flavored candy or ice cream.

A quick note on alcohol: Many people drink alcohol late at night in order to get to sleep. The problem is that, in most people, alcohol causes the adrenal glands to secrete epinephrine, which impairs the ability to sleep. Furthermore, an essential amino acid called tryptophan, which the body can convert into the "sleep-helping" serotonin, is adversely affected by alcohol.

SUPPLEMENTS FOR SLEEP

Serotonin, which the body makes from the amino acid tryptophan, is important for getting to sleep. In the late 1980s, the Food and Drug Administration reclassified tryptophan: it was no longer available over-the-counter in health food stores, etc. Instead, it was a prescription medication. Inside the body, tryptophan is converted into 5-HTP (5-hydroxytryptophan) and then to serotonin. Because it is difficult to obtain tryptophan, we have been using 5-HTP, which is actually better, and closer than tryptophan to serotonin, the natural "sleep aid."

A number of double-blind medical studies have shown that 5-HTP decreases the number of nighttime awakenings from sleep, as well as the latent period (from the time you try to go to sleep, until you actually do). We have found that 5-HTP works even better when taken with a small amount of fruit. Additionally, 5-HTP works best when there are good body levels of magnesium and vitamins B6 and B3 because these three substances are important in the conversion of 5-HTP to serotonin in the body.

Another helpful sleep substance is melatonin, a hormone made by the pineal gland in the brain. When we close our eyes to go to sleep, the lack of light on the retina causes the pineal gland to secrete melatonin. Unfortunately, in some people melatonin levels fall low and they have trouble sleeping. We have been using melatonin for such patients for many years, and it works well in most cases. (In addition to its sleep-promoting effects, melatonin also helps stimulate the immune system.) We prefer patients to take from 0.5 mg up to 3.0 mg, sublingually, about 30 minutes before going to sleep.

Several herbs are helpful in inducing relaxation and sleep, including valerian. Clinical studies have shown that this herb has a good ability to not only help people get to sleep and stay asleep, but also to improve the quality of their sleep. (Balderer & Borbely, 1985; Lindahl & Lindwall, 1989). The standardized preparation of valerian is preferable: 300 mg at bedtime. *Note:* When you open a bottle of valerian, if it does not smell like dirty sneakers or socks, it is not valerian.

Passion flower, also called *passiflora incarnata*, has been used by civilizations as far back as the Aztecs. The active ingredient, *harmine*, appears to have the ability to slow the breakdown of serotonin; 300 mg passion flower at bedtime is a commonly recommended starting dose.

Kava, also known as *Piper methysticum*, comes from the Polynesian Islands and has been used for its calming effect. Although kava is not primarily used for sleep, it can be helpful for those who cannot sleep because they are anxious or nervous. Taking a capsule with 75 mg of kavalactones at bedtime will be effective for most people, although some may require more.

Many other substances are used to induce sleep; these are the ones we have found to be most useful.

REFERENCES

Balderer, G., & Borbely, A.A. (1985). Effect of valerian on human sleep. *Psychopharmacology, 87*, 406–409.

Cassel, J. (1986). The contribution of the social environment to host resistance. *American Journal of Epidemiology, 104*, 107–123.

Fox, A. (1982). *The Beverly Hills medical diet.* New York: Bantam Books.

Fox, A., & Fox, B. (1985). DLPA to end chronic pain and depression. New York: Long Shadow Books.

Fox, A., & Fox, B. (1989). *Immune for life.* Rocklin, CA: Prima Books.

Friedman, S.B., & Glascow, L.A. (1974). Psychosocial factors and resistance to infectious disease. In P.M. Insel & R.H. Moos (Eds.), *Health and the social environment.* Toronto: D.C. Health.

Henry, K., Gutt, R.R., & Rees, W.L. (1973). Psychosocial aspects of migraine. *Journal of Psychosomatic Research, 17*, 141–153.

Jamison, R.N., et al. (1990). Effects of significant weight gain on chronic pain patients. *Clinical Journal of Pain, 6*, 47–50.

Katz, J.J.L., et al. (1970). Stress, distress & ego defenses. *Archives of General Psychiatry, 23*, 131–142.

Kitchen, C., & Simpson, J. (1972). Neuralgiaparesthetica: A review of sixty-seven patients. *Acta Neurologica Scandinavica, 48*, 542.

Lindahl, O. & Lindwall, I. (1989). Double blind study of valerian preparation. *Pharmacology and Biochemical Behavior, 32*(4):1065–1066.

Maruta T. (1981). Chronic pain patients and spouses: Marital and sexual adjustment. *Mayo Clinic. Proceedings, 56*, 307–310.

Mason, J.W., et al. (1979). A prospective study of corticosteroid and catecholamine levels in relation to viral respiratory illness. *Journal of Human Stress, 5*, 18–27.

McKendall, J.F., & Haier, R.J. (1983). Pain sensitivity and obesity. *Psychiatry Research, 8*, 119–125.

Nachemson, A.L. (1976). The lumbar spine: An orthopaedic challenge. *Spine, 1*, 59–71.

Pradatier, A., et al. (1981). Relationship between pain and obesity: An electrophysiological study. *Psychology of Behavior, 27*, 961–964.

Roy, R. (1982). Marital and family issues in chronic pain. *Psychotherapy and Psychosomatica, 37*, 1–12.

Roy, R. (1984). Chronic pain: A family perspective. *Journal of Family Therapy, 6*, 31–43.

Swenson, D.W., & Maruta, T. (1980). The family's viewpoint of pain. *Pain, 8*, 163–166.

Swick, H.M., & McQuillen, M.P. (1976). The use of steroids in the treatment of idiopathic polyneuritis. *Neurology, 25*, 206.

Syme, S.L. (1975). Social and psychological risk factors in coronary heart disease. *Modern Concepts of Cardiovascular Disease, 14*, 17–21.

42

Hospice, Cancer Pain Management, and Symptom Control

Samira Kanaan Beckwith, A.C.S.W., L.C.S.W. and B. Eliot Cole, M.D., M.P.A., F.A.P.A.

INTRODUCTION

Death has not been conquered; we are all terminally ill to some degree. In 1900, the average life expectancy was only 50 years and infant mortality was very high. Because of sanitation efforts and immunization programs, antibiotics, better management of acute illnesses and trauma, and improved chemotherapy, Americans now live well into their late 70s or 80s (Emanuel, von Gunten, & Ferris, 1999). Due to these advances, patients now expect to have prolonged experiences of living with chronic illnesses and ultimately dying.

Some 69% of patients said they would opt for suicide if they felt their pain could not be relieved (Levin, Cleeland, & Dar, 1985). Fear of unacceptable pain was a major component of requests to physicians for assisted suicide (Helig, 1988; Emanuel, et al., 1999). The increased awareness of the public in assisted suicide, due to the activities of Dr. Jack Kevorkian during the 1990s, and the popularity of the "how to commit suicide" book *Final Exit* (Humphry, 1991) give evidence to this well-founded concern. Undertreatment of acute and chronic cancer pain persists despite decades of efforts to provide clinicians with information about analgesics (American Pain Society [APS], 1995).

When finding a cure for the patient's conditions is no longer possible, the emphasis shifts to palliation (Kaye, 1989). Palliative management, the focus of hospice care, affords relief and reduces the severity of bothersome symptoms, but does not produce toxicity or hasten the death of the patient (Johanson, 1988). Palliative care becomes necessary when the patient's disease is beyond cure, when the tumor process is the cause of symptoms, when realistic treatment goals have been established, and when clear communication exists among the professional team, the patient, and the family regarding the treatment plan (Brescia, 1987). No specific therapy is excluded from consideration. The test of palliative treatment lies in the agreement by the patient, the physician, the primary caregiver, and the hospice team that the expected outcome is relief from distressing symptoms, easing of pain, and enhancement of quality of life (National Hospice Organization [NHO], 1996). The absolute goal for palliative care is to improve the quality of the patient's life while avoiding side effects worse than the symptoms being treated (Emanuel, et al., 1999). Good palliative care focuses on pain control and symptom management to help the patient avoid a lingering and suffering death. To realize this goal, it is essential for the clinicians involved to believe and to assess the severity of each pain complaint.

Total pain management cannot be undertaken by an individual alone, but only by individuals working together as a team (Lack, 1984). This underlying principle of working together in hospice care manifests through the use of a multidisciplinary approach and a creative process of individualized patient management. This results in an empowered patient who is able to experience comfort and dignity. Hospice care integrates the best of psychological support, physical care, and spirituality for the patient directly and provides long-term bereavement assistance for the surviving loved ones.

0-8493-0926-3/02/$0.00+$1.50
© 2002 by CRC Press LLC

Hospice is based on a philosophy of caring for the terminally ill embracing a number of concepts. Death is viewed as a natural part of the life cycle. When death is inevitable, hospice will neither seek to hasten nor postpone it. Hospice exists in the hope and belief that through appropriate care and the promotion of a caring community sensitive to their needs, patients and their families may be free to attain a degree of mental and spiritual preparation for death that is optimal for them (NHO, 1996). Despite the successful growth of the hospice movement in the U.S. during the past 30 years, nearly 85% of Americans die in hospitals and long-term care facilities, making palliative care interventions relatively unused in the settings in which most of them die (Rummans, Bostwick, & Clark, 2000).

Pain relief and symptom control are appropriate clinical goals, with psychological and spiritual pain considered to be as significant as physical pain. Addressing all three simultaneously requires the skills and experience of an interdisciplinary treatment team. Such hospice teams include physicians, nurses, social workers, pharmacists, aides, chaplains, homemakers, volunteers, bereavement counselors, and other therapists as needed. Patients with their families and loved ones are the functional units of care, and this care is generally provided to them regardless of their ability to pay.

Hospice was viewed by many as unconventional at its beginning. Many thought that hospice programs actually shortened the lives of the people served through covert euthanasia practices. Nothing was farther from the truth. Hospice medicine became quite scientific and developed, with a large body of knowledge about providing care for people at the end of life (Appleton, 1996). Hospice medicine established new standards for medication dosing, medication selection, home care limitations, and the ability to provide "whole patient" care.

Hospice is now recognized as one of the standards for clinical practice. Based on these concepts of "whole patient" care, hospice is now a specialized healthcare program focusing on the provision of pain management, symptom control, emotional support, personal care, and bereavement counseling. More economical than hospital, home health, or nursing home (long-term) care, hospice provides a cost-effective choice for providing wonderful care at the end of life. Because hospice care combines the best quality and value for most terminally ill patients, it is now covered by Medicare, many insurance companies, and in most states by Medicaid programs for the medically indigent. A majority of hospice programs also look to members of their communities for additional support to assist them in providing indigent care and other unmet needs.

The primary focus of hospice care is to maintain patients in their homes for as long as possible. This is the experience of the authors; additionally, care is also provided in inpatient hospice units, long-term care nursing facilities, and contract hospitals. Electing hospice care allows patients to make choices, control their destinies, and maintain their dignity while avoiding the sense of abandonment and solitude often associated with a hospital death.

WHOLE-PATIENT ASSESSMENT AND HOSPICE CARE

Whole-patient assessment is an important skill for practitioners caring for the terminally ill. Whole-patient assessment clarifies the diagnosis and prognosis; coordinates the activities of the hospice team members; improves trust between patients, their families, and their professional caregivers; and leads to the best therapeutic effects (Emanuel, et al., 1999). Thorough assessment allows establishment of a comprehensive plan of care with the task of the multidisciplinary hospice team being to provide care that is interdisciplinary in scope.

Certain diseases can be expected to follow predictable courses. However, hospice is not about providing routine care, but instead focuses on providing an individualized hospice plan of care that is prepared uniquely for every new admission and then updated continuously. This plan of care begins the moment the patient is referred to the hospice program and evolves as the needs of the patient change. Although the initial plan of care is the collaboration of the intake nurse, attending physician, hospice medical director, and social worker, the other members of the interdisciplinary team, including chaplains, aides, volunteers, and other therapists, participate in the frequent revisions.

The whole-patient view of end-of-life care encompasses many domains simultaneously. These domains include the patient's complete illness and treatment summary, ongoing physical and psychological care requirements, decision-making capacity, communication needs, social and spiritual issues, practical day-to-day assistance, and anticipatory planning for death (Emanuel, et al., 1999). The goal of this assessment is control of bothersome symptoms, improvement in function, reduction of suffering, minimization of further laboratory testing, and bettering the overall quality of life remaining.

The referring source often has certain expectations about services for the patient, and the hospice team must consider these wishes along with the overall hospice philosophy. The orderly transition of the patient from a hospital setting to hospice necessitates a close relationship between the attending physician, discharge planners, and the hospice staff. Problems identified in the earliest stages of hospice involvement tend to reflect uncontrolled symptoms, specific equipment needs, and accessibility to the attending physician. Once the patient has settled into the program, a number of the hospice team members visit the patient to develop an appropriate plan of care.

Relocation issues are important considerations for hospice care provided in the home when either the patient or the primary caregiver has to relocate to accommodate the care demands. These changes in living arrangements often result in disruption for everyone as new routines are established. Not only must the medical aspects of care be undertaken, but in addition, the more mundane aspects of daily living must also be addressed. Who will pay the bills? Who will feed the pets? Who will do the grocery shopping? Who will get the prescription medications filled? Who will do the chore work around the house? These issues must be resolved to successfully care for any patient at home.

In a home environment there are important concerns related to the physical safety of the debilitated patient; thus, specialized adaptive equipment is often provided to improve the care of the challenged patient. Emotional support coupled with extensive and practical education provides the new caregiver with the requisite confidence to assume the challenge of providing care for the terminally ill patient. Despite all this wonderful support, it remains very difficult to prepare the new caregiver for the personal sacrifices that must be made to provide care for the very ill patient. The simplest errand often takes on monumental qualities when care for the terminally ill patient must be provided continuously. The caregiver does not have a day off unless alternate caregivers are available. This "24/7" routine often results in the exhaustion of the caregiver, physically and emotionally, and necessitates the need for respite care.

Trust issues manifest early in the care of the hospice patient. Loyalties to the attending physician and past healthcare providers must be expanded to include the hospice team members. Many attending physicians are not able to follow their patients at home and thus rely on the skills of the hospice team members to provide the day-to-day aspects of care. The reality that most hospice patients are older and seriously medically ill, yet are frequently cared for by younger family members, produces interesting reversals in generational hierarchies. The daughter, or daughter-in-law, who typically becomes the caregiver for her, or her husband's, parent, and the actual patient, must adjust to the new patterns. Long-standing, unresolved conflicts may reappear due to the stressful conditions that exist and can lead to power struggles and other dysfunctional expressions.

Hospice care embraces the idea that psychosocial, emotional, and spiritual factors all impact physical symptoms. Plato once said, "As you ought not to attempt to cure the eyes without the head or the head without the body, so neither are you to attempt to cure the body without the soul; for the part can never be well unless the whole is well; therefore, if the head and body are to be

well, you must begin by curing the soul." Later, in the 6th century, Galen wrote that melancholic women were more prone to cancer than those of sanguine temperament. In the 15th century, Lorenzo Sassoli, a physician, wrote to a patient: "To get angry and shout at times pleases me for this will keep you your natural heat; what displeases me is your being grieved and taking all matters to heart; for it is this as the whole of physics teaches which destroys our body more than any other cause."

The connections between the mind and body have continued to be the focus of attention for many researchers. Outcomes attributable to psychosocial factors range on a continuum from the readily explicable to the most controversial. These outcomes include enhanced physical comfort, increased responsiveness to medical treatment, relief from emotional anguish, extension of survival time after disease onset, and outright "psychogenic" cure. For these reasons, we believe that the psychosocial, emotional, and spiritual components of a patient's pain experience must be thoroughly addressed to understand the totality of the pain. The experience of pain, and the resulting suffering, may be greater when the pain is accompanied by anger, anxiety, depression, fear, and the meaning given to the pain by the sufferer. Because many patients report less pain when they are rested, distracted, and have other symptoms under good control, many questions are raised about what specific factors influence how an individual patient may experience pain. Factors considered involve the duration of the pain experience, the course the pain has taken during that time, the anticipation that the pain will be controlled, the expected interval before improvement will be realized, and the time anticipated until meaningful comfort will be attained. Patients must be given hope that their pain will be managed.

A comprehensive psychosocial assessment is important and must include an appropriate analysis of gender, present financial situation, family history, relationship patterns, previous coping strategies, previous losses, history of alcohol and substance abuse, past mental health problems, occupational history, and ethnic and cultural issues, as well as an exploration of religious and spiritual beliefs. The specific information regarding finances, environment, and care costs is necessary to develop a plan of care that is realistic and achievable. Many patients and their caregivers express concern about the cost of their analgesic medications and other needed services.

Fear is a major factor that adversely influences the experience of cancer pain. It is natural to be afraid of death, as death is the ultimate unknown (Ryder, 1993). Fear of pain takes at least two forms: fear of the pain itself and fear of the inability to control pain (Hill & Shirley, 1992). Most patients expect the pain from cancer to be very severe, perhaps to the point of interfering with life-prolonging treatment and causing them to die a painful death. The popular knowledge that most cancer pain is poorly controlled does not offer newly diagnosed cancer patients much reason to be hopeful about their personal pain management.

Unnecessary concerns and myths about the consequences of opioid analgesic usage, including addiction, confusion, constipation, disorientation, tolerance, and withdrawal problems, continue to prevent many patients from receiving the medications they legitimately deserve. Patients should never need to wish for death because of their physicians' reluctance to use adequate amounts of effective opioids (Reisine & Pasternak, 1996).

Fear also arises from concerns about loss of control and dignity, loss of relationships, being abandoned, becoming a burden to care for, and having bothersome symptoms poorly controlled (Emanuel, et al., 1999). Professional caregivers must explore patient fears and ultimately affirm their commitment to care for the patient. Failure to do this may lead to the patient contemplating suicide and requesting the assistance of the caregivers if unable to perform the act alone.

Untreated anxiety and depression also worsen the pain experience, resulting in interference with restful sleep, impaired cognitive processes, and altered social patterns. Depression associated with uncontrolled pain plays a significant role in suicidal ideation; and when coupled with a sense of helplessness and hopelessness, it becomes a deadly predictor of actual suicide. Pain relief clearly enhances the sense of hope and well-being for the patients. Failure to appreciate the psychological needs of the patient will render even aggressive treatment of pain with analgesics or procedures ineffective (Patt & Isaacson, 1996).

Healthcare professionals must make their treatment decisions with a focus on the whole person rather than just the specific disease state. People must be the focus of care. Caregivers need to understand that having a serious, potentially terminal condition can by itself be a reason for demoralization and loss of hope. Patients need to be reassured by their professional caregivers that care, compassion, and concern will always be available to them and that they will not be abandoned. Information about the disease, expected outcomes, and treatment options, including their effects on the quality of life, must be communicated in common terms that the patient and family can understand.

Helping the family caregiver with practical day-to-day tasks can reduce the caregiver's fatigue and potential for overload and burnout. Using the psychosocial assessment process, resources needed can be identified and provided. Giving the patient and caregiver a flowchart with the names and duties of the professional team members can clarify the roles and relationships. Done properly, the patient and caregiver can view their appropriate place in the care continuum and feel that they are valuable team participants.

Many caregivers report that much of their day is centered on the dying patient, attending to positioning, feeding, bathing, and medicating. The care needs of the patient direct the life of the caregiver. Although appropriate and encouraged during the patient's hospice care, upon the death of the patient, the routine is radically altered for the caregiver. This loss of activity and fulfillment of nurturing needs should be acknowledged as part of the emptiness experienced after death. Hospice programs provide bereavement support, maintaining continued involvement with the caregiver through the professional staff and volunteers, utilizing a variety of techniques including support groups, classes, and individual counseling. The bereavement plan of care must be based on an assessment of risk indicators (Beckwith, et al., 1990). Bereavement care demonstrates the hospice philosophy and communicates, "We still care for you, and we will help you get through this."

Bereavement, a separation or loss through death, is derived from the Old English *bereafian*, meaning "to rob," "to plunder," or "to dispossess" (Burnell & Burnell, 1989). Bereavement is the general state of being that results from having experienced a significant loss (Cook & Dworkin, 1992). It is the price paid in emotional pain for having meaningful relationships. All caregivers have loss experiences that color how they handle subsequent losses, and these losses need acknowledgment in preparation for healthy grieving after the loved one's death. Soon after the death, or often through the dying process, caregivers must look for ways to adjust their identities. Caregivers may experience an initial sense of relief and simultaneous feelings of emptiness when new coping patterns have not been developed. Confusion over identity arises with a shift in focus from the care needs of the patient to the personal needs of the caregiver.

Ultimately, the search for meaning and the exploration of spiritual issues can contribute to the alleviation of emotional distress for patients and their families. A review of things enjoyed and loved, such as people, places, events, and experiences, can bring genuine comfort and relief from suffering. Although formal psychiatric involvement may be needed for those with histories of prior psychiatric illness, supportive techniques of psychotherapy can often be helpful for most who elect to use them. This spiritual search for meaning can also impact the perception of the pain experience.

Spirituality needs require thorough exploration from the outset of hospice care. We must acknowledge that pain is not just a response to a physical problem; all facets must be addressed if we are to treat the whole person (Cosh, 1995). Almost all who connect their pain with impending death review the events of their lives and seek to determine the significance of their lives. Some return to religious values of earlier days, and others make intense demands on their faith (Lack, 1984). Rectifying previous religious traditions with present affiliations can prove problematic. When spouses are of different faith traditions or one spouse is a relative nonbeliever, the provision of spiritual care can be more complex. It is not the responisiblity of the hospice team to resolve religious matters or to "save" people, but rather to assess and attempt to provide spiritual support as desired by the patient and family. Symptom control has to precede spiritual or psychosocial support; a person cannot think about the meaning of his or her life while in pain (Kaye, 1989).

The nursing assessment focuses on the safety of the patient in the environment, the patient's chief complaint, use of medications, care needs over time, and developing the initial plan of care. In the assessment process, the nurse gathers information from the patient that allows for understanding the pain experience and its effect on the quality of life (McCaffery & Beebe, 1989; McCaffery & Pasero, 1999). It is important to avoid making assumptions about the patient's wishes. Asking the patient for ideas and opinions makes his or her wishes known (Kaye, 1989). Inquiring "How are you right now?" lets the person know that human needs will be addressed. This helps to establish trust and build the relationship that allows screening for care requirements, such as diet, appetite, bowel function, managing unpleasant side effects, sexual and intimacy issues, and successful pain management. The interdisciplinary approach to care in conjunction with trained volunteers ensures that no person has to travel the final days alone.

The hospice physician primarily attends to the management of unpleasant symptoms, serves as a supervisor for the interdisciplinary team, and acts as a liaison with the attending physician. Education of the team, support for the team members as they deal with terminal patients, and representing the hospice program are key duties for this physician. A willingness to be available, often 24 hours a day, and to work collaboratively with the interdisciplinary treatment team adds to the services provided by the traditional medical staff in the community. The house call, with care provided in the home of the patient rather than the office or the hospital, is the preferred method of management for the hospice patient. The hospice physician must be flexible, able to handle routine medical problems, and practice medicine with a minimum of complicated technology often associated with institution-based care.

CANCER PAIN MANAGEMENT

Approximately 70% of advanced cancer patients report pain as a major symptom (Bonica, 1987). For half of them, the pain is moderate to severe in intensity; while for a third, the pain is severe to excruciating (World Health Organization [WHO], 1986). It is tragic that although pain in one in ten cancer patients is difficult to control, pain in 50 to 80% of cancer patients is not satisfactorily relieved because their physicians do not aggressively treat the pain problem (Bonica, 1985). With six million newly diagnosed cancer cases in the world each year, every physician who cares for cancer patients or others at the end of life

must be able to elicit a detailed pain history and be able to bring relief to these sufferers (WHO, 1986). Cancer pain may be due to direct tumor progression and related pathology, operations and other invasive diagnostic or therapeutic procedures, toxicities of chemotherapy and radiation, infection, or from muscle aches when patients have limited physical activity (Foley, 1985).

The basic pain evaluation must begin with believing the pain complaint expressed by the patient (Foley, 1988). Pain is whatever the person experiencing it says it is, and it exists whenever the person experiencing it says it does (McCaffery & Beebe, 1989; McCaffery & Pasero, 1999). Because all pain is very real and distressing to the patient, trying to assign relative proportions to organic or functional causes is of little value. It is more useful to determine if the pain limits the activity of the patient and disturbs sleep, appetite, or the ability to engage in productive or pleasurable endeavors. Knowing what the patient can or cannot do, how medications have or have not worked, and what side effects the patient will or will not tolerate are key initial questions to be answered. It is vital that a language about the pain be developed among the patient, the caregiver, and the hospice team to allow skillful management. Descriptive words such as mild, moderate, and severe indicate the intensity of acute pain fairly well. Words such as excruciating, incapacitating, overwhelming, and soul stealing better define the pain of cancer. A number of pain scales have been developed to quantify and track the pain experience, such as the descriptive (uses words), numerical (uses numbers), visual (uses anchors of "no pain" and "worse pain") analogs.

To most thoroughly treat the pain, it is best to obtain the richest detail about the pain complaint that the patient and family can provide. A careful, comprehensive physical examination that is global in scope should be performed, because many cancer pain patients have been recently cared for by specialists who might not have provided total care for them. If necessary, the physician should order and personally review needed diagnostic studies to better elaborate the overall problems of the cancer patient (Portenoy, 1988). All of the possible methods of controlling the pain — not just pharmacological means — must be considered and blended to individualize the plan of care for the patient. Finally, the level of pain control and patient satisfaction after each intervention must be assessed. There is no point in frequently changing methods until compliance with what was previously ordered has occurred. Establishing clear and reasonable goals with the patient and the family is necessary to enssure a successful outcome. Everyone must understand that analgesics are not anesthetics; although absolute pain elimination may not be a realistic goal, improved comfort can be provided.

With a clear understanding of the pain problem, treatment can be staged from least to most complicated.

Through hospice, medical equipment and supplies that are needed to facilitate even complex care of the patient can be provided either in the home or in the hospice inpatient unit. The capacity and emotional status of non-professional caregivers should be assessed to be certain that they are not overwhelmed or at risk for burnout. A balance must be struck among the capabilities of medical science, the wishes of the patient, and the realistic abilities of the caregiver. The loss of the caregiver at home is a frequent reason for a patient needing to enter a long-term care nursing facility or an inpatient setting.

PHARMACOTHERAPY

The correct route of administration for medication is the one best tolerated by the patient. As long as the patient is able to swallow, pain can be routinely managed with oral medications. Transmucosal, transdermal, rectal, and parenteral routes may be utilized when swallowing is compromised. The important premise that oral medication is the preferred route of administration for a patient able to eat and take fluids orally, leads to the recommendation that practitioners follow the guidelines of the WHO guidelines, as well as the Agency for Health Care Policy and Research (AHCPR), reorganized as the Agency for Healthcare Research and Quality (AHRQ) in 1999, and systematically progress (1) from an oral non-steroidal anti-inflammatory medication or acetaminophen, (2) to a weak, or lower potency, oral opioid analgesic and then, if necessary, (3) to a strong, or higher potency, oral opioid analgesic (WHO, 1986; AHCPR, 1994). These three steps best describe the management of mild, moderate, and severe intensities of pain. At each of these steps, adjunctive, or additional, medications may be added, but similar analgesic products of the same step are unnecessary for the majority of patients. Ultimately, instead of trying to fit patients to the medications, the medications are adjusted to fit the patients. The right dose of any medication becomes the dose that produces comfort and minimal toxicity.

Acetaminophen, often part of combination medications, has no anti-inflammatory effects and thus affords little benefit beyond mild pain relief and a real risk of hepatotoxicity when daily doses exceed 3 to 4 grams. Patients with chronic alcoholism and liver disease, or those who are fasting can develop hepatotoxicity at standard doses (APS, 1999).

Starting with the nonsteroidal anti-inflammatory drugs makes good sense for most pain problems, as these medications work to relieve pain in the periphery, where the nociceptive experience originates (Kanner, 1987). Nonsteroidal anti-inflammatory agents interfere with the manufacture of local pain-sensitizing and inflammation-mediating components (prostaglandins) and thereby limit pain transmission from the periphery to the central nervous system and eventual consciousness (Insel, 1996). While aspirin significantly interferes with platelet aggregation

irreversibly, most of the other nonsteroidal anti-inflammatory medications decrease platelet aggregation only while therapeutic levels are maintained (APS, 1989). Notable exceptions are the COX-2 selective inhibiting agents celecoxib and rofecoxib, nabumetone, and choline magnesium trisalicylate. Choline magnesium trisalicylate is a non-acetylated aspirin derivative that does not appear to have effects on the aggregation of platelets (APS, 1989; Kanner, 1987). Choline magnesium trisalicylate is a generic medication that can be used orally, as tablets or a liquid suspension (helpful for those with swallowing difficulties), with the same general side-effects profile as aspirin and the ability to follow salicylate levels. Celecoxib is available in capsules and rofecoxib is available in tablet and suspension (helpful for those with swallowing difficulties) forms.

The nonsteroidal anti-inflammatory medications in general may produce gastric upset and the potential gastrointestinal bleeding; however, nabumetone, celecoxib, and rofecoxib have lower event rates for these problems (Insel, 1996; Medical Economics Company, 2000) but they do have the potential for renal problems. It is a common occurrence in the hospice setting to encounter patients with pain that is controlled quite poorly despite high-dose opioid analgesics at the time of their admission. These patients benefit significantly from the late addition of nonsteroidal anti-inflammatory agents (if they are not already taking such medications) without further increases in the opioid analgesics when pain is due to bone metastases (Foley, 1985; Walsh, 1985).

Case Example

> Mr. H was a 75-year-old gentleman with advanced prostate cancer with extensive bone metastases. He was initially able to control his pain with 2 mg hydromorphone orally every 4 hours. He later experienced high levels of localized pain in his lower back and pelvis. Rather than increase his opioid analgesic, he was additionally given 750 mg of the nonsteroidal anti-inflammatory agent choline magnesium trisalicylate four times daily, with significant improvement. As his disease progressed, he eventually required more hydromorphone to remain comfortable. His dose was adjusted to 4 mg orally every 4 hours, and he died comfortably.

If the pain is not controlled with nonsteroidal anti-inflammatory medications, the next step is the addition of an opioid analgesic. Routinely, Drug Enforcement Agency (DEA) schedule three (Ciii) combination medications are prescribed after nonsteroidal agents and before pure opioids. This is not a legal requirement, but one of custom. It is important to remember that all of the combination opioid medications, like the pure opioid medications, are effective analgesics if used at equianalgesic dosages (the amount of one medication that produces the same relief as another medication; see Table 42.1). The limiting factor

TABLE 42.1
Equianalgesic Dosages:

Medication	Equianalgesic Dosage (in mg)			Duration of Action (hours)
	i.m.	p.o.	p.r.	
Opioid agonists:				
Codeine	130	200	N/A	3–4
Fentanyl[a]	0.1–0.2	N/A[b]	N/A	1–2
Hydrocodone	N/A	30	N/A	3–4
Hydromorphone	1.5	7.5	3	3–4
Levorphanol[c]	2	4	N/A	4–5
	(single dose)			
	1	1		
	(repeated doses)			
Meperidine[d]	75	300	N/A	3–5
Methadone[e]	10	20	N/A	4–6
	(single dose)			
	2–4	2–4		
	(repeated doses)			
Morphine[f]	10	60	10–20	4–5
		(single dose)		
		30		
		(repeated doses)		
Oxycodone[g]	10–15[h]	15–20	N/A	4–6
Oxymorphone	1–1.5	N/A	10	4–6
Propoxyphene[i]	N/A	300–400	N/A	4–6
Opioid partial agonist:				
Buprenorphine	0.4	N/A	N/A	4–5
Opioid agonist-antagonists:				
Butorphanol[j]	2[k]	N/A	N/A	4–6
Nalbuphine[j]	10	N/A	N/A	4–6
Pentazocine[j]	60	180	N/A	4–6

[a] Transdermal fentanyl dosage is not calculated as equianalgesic to a single morphine dose. In the steady-state condition, a 25-µg/hour patch is approximately equivalent to 10 mg of oral morphine sulfate every 4 hours.

[b] Oral transmucosal fentanyl citrate absorption is variable due to both immediate transmucosal absorption and slower gastrointestinal absorption.

[c] Levorphanol has a long half-life and accumulates over time.

[d] Meperidine is not appropriate for cancer patients due to the half-life of its metabolite, normeperidine, being 8 to 21 hours. Meperidine should never be administered beyond 400 mg/day as the accumulation of normeperidine leads to agitation, myoclonic twitching, and seizures.

[e] Methadone has a long half-life and accumulates over time.

[f] Morphine-6-glucuronide has a longer half-life than morphine and leads to greater morphine effectiveness over time.

[g] Many equianalgesic tables have oxycodone as either equianalgesic to morphine or 1.5 times more potent than morphine. The product insert for OxyContin indicates that oxycodone is two times more potent than morphine.

[h] Oxycodone is only commercially available as an oral preparation in the U.S. It is used parenterally outside the U.S.

[i] Propoxyphene is so weak that it is rarely effective for cancer pain of any significance.

[j] Mixed agonist-antagonist medications must never be given to patients concomitantly receiving pure opioid agonist medications. Butorphanol and pentazocine produce psychotomimetic effects at higher doses.

[k] Nasal butorphanol is equianalgesic to the intravenous form.

for the schedule three agents used in the U.S. is the presence of the co-analgesic (acetaminophen, aspirin, or ibuprofen). Because of the toxicity associated with the co-analgesic agents (gastrointestinal upset and/or bleeding, hepatotoxicity, platelet aggregation interference, and nephrotoxicity), there is a finite limit for the number of schedule three combination products that may be taken daily. This barrier due to the co-analgesic may result in inadequate pain relief for those experiencing more than moderate pain intensity.

Contributing to some of the confusion about effectively prescribing pure opioid analgesics is the continuing observation that most standard textbooks of pharmacology describe opioid analgesic dosages with respect to acute pain, but few references mention the complexities of chronic pain management. Under-dosing the cancer patient is more commonly the rule than the exception (Hill, 1988), and fear about possible respiratory depression due to opioids is best countered by remembering that the most potent antagonist to opioid-analgesic-induced respiratory depression is pain itself (Johanson, 1988). Respiratory depression is not a problem until the pain is well controlled; no one has died from opioid-induced respiratory depression while awake (APS, 1999).

In general, the relative potency of oral to parenteral opioid analgesics is about three to one, due to the first-pass effect of hepatic metabolism. One must take approximately three times more oral medication to obtain the same level of comfort produced by intramuscular or intravenous medication (Pasero, Portenoy, & McCaffery, 1999). Oxycodone is an exception, with 60 to 87% or more of oral doses being bio-available and escaping the first-pass hepatic metabolism (Kaiko, et al., 1996; Leow, Smith, Williams, & Cramond, 1993; Poyhia, Vainio, & Kalso, 1993).

The most frequent error in working with opioid analgesics is to assume that dosages are constant despite the route of administration (not accounting for first-pass liver effects). It is still common to find opioid orders written for 50 to 75 mg meperidine orally or intramuscularly every 4 to 6 hours as needed for pain. This situation shows pharmacological ignorance in two areas: the equianalgesic difference between oral and parenteral routes of administration (300 mg orally is equivalent to 75 mg parenterally) and the 2- to 3-hour duration of analgesic action (Pasero, et al., 1999).

Most important for properly prescribing opioids is their administration on a time-contingent, by-the-clock (or around-the-clock) basis, rather than a pain-contingent, as-needed basis, so that comfort is constantly maintained instead of being continually sought. The development of sophisticated medication release technology has allowed several opioids (fentanyl, morphine, and oxycodone) to provide sustained analgesic action for 8 to 72 hours with stable blood levels increasing overall comfort and lessening potential toxicity.

By maintaining control of the pain around the clock, most patients experience a better quality of life (lower pain intensity, less medication toxicity, improved sleep, and satisfaction) and use less medication (Reuben, Connelly, & Maciolek, 1999). From a learning theory perspective, the use of as-needed medication may cause the patient to use more medication over time because of the linkage made between having pain, taking medication, and experiencing pain relief, resulting in the development of psychological craving. The time-contingent dosing pattern dissociates pill-taking from pain relief (because medication is taken on a fixed time schedule) and thus may prevent the most feared but least likely complication of opioid analgesic use — addiction.

In reality, very little abuse of opioid medication actually occurs among hospice patients or medical patients with legitimate use of these agents. It is inconceivable that cancer patients would ever be removed from their medications as they died, but studies of nonterminal chronic pain patients show little justification for concern when the probability of iatrogenic addiction is 1/800 to less than 1/10,000 (Medina & Diamond, 1977; Perry & Heidrich, 1982; Porter & Jick, 1980). Although 6 to 15% of the U.S. population may have a substance abuse disorder of some type, only 3% of inpatient and outpatient consultations performed by the Psychiatry Service at Memorial Sloan-Kettering Cancer Center were requested for the management of drug-related issues (Passik & Portenoy, 1998).

Physical dependence does occur over time, but the need to increase analgesic medication doses in cancer patients more often relates to the progression of the underlying disease than the rapid development of pharmacological tolerance. Physical dependence is not addiction (a primarily psychological disorder with eventual physiological and sociological manifestations), and patients should not be identified as addicts just because they manifest tolerance of or physical dependence on opioids. Addiction, psychological dependence, signifies that the medication is compulsively sought and utilized for effects other than pain relief (APS, 1999). Physical dependence simply means that a person needs the medication to prevent distressing symptoms secondary to the absence of the agent, the so-called "withdrawal" or "abstinence" reaction (Hill, 1988). The cancer patient has a constant supply of medication that is used time contingently if administered correctly, and little if any drug-seeking behavior is seen (Passik & Portenoy, 1998). In fact, one of the greatest barriers to compliance with the time-contingent administration of these medications when patients are relatively comfortable is the mistaken belief by patients that they will develop an addictive disorder (Breitbart, et al., 1998; Foley & Inturrisi, 1987; Ward, et al., 1993).

The data related to the risk of addiction have been traditionally obtained by surveying known addicts rather than prospectively following patients receiving legitimately prescribed opioid analgesics. In the past 20 years, it has been observed that the true incidence of opioid

TABLE 42.2
Commonly Used Opioid Analgesics in the United States:

Generic name:	Proprietary name:	Dose Forms:	Manufacturers:
Buprenorphine	Buprenex	i.v./i.m.	Reckitt & Colman
		Epidural	
Butorphanol	Stadol	i.v./i.m.	Bristol-Myers Squibb
		Nasal	
Codeine	Tylenol with codeine	p.o.	Ortho-McNeil
Fentanyl	Actiq	Oral	Abbott
	Duragesic	Transdermal	Janssen
	Sublimaze	i.v./i.m.	AstraZeneca
Hydrocodone	Lortab,	p.o.	UCB
	Vocodin		Knoll
Hydromorphone	Dilaudid	i.v./i.m./p.o.	Knoll
Levorphanol	Levo-Dromoran	p.o./s.c.	ICN
Meperidine	Demerol	i.v./i.m./p.o.	Sanofi, Roxane
Methadone	Dolophine	p.o./i.m./s.c.	Roxane
Morphine	MS Contin,	p.o.	Purdue Pharma
	Oramorph		Roxane
	Kadian		Faulding
		i.v./i.m.	Wyeth-Ayerst, AstraZeneca
		Rectal	Upsher-Smith
		Epidural	Baxter, AstraZeneca
Nalbuphine	Nubain	i.v./i.m./s.c.	Endo
Oxycodone	OxyContin, OxyFast,	p.o.	Purdue Pharma
	Percocet, Percodan,		Endo
	Tylox	Ortho-McNeil	
Oxymorphone	Numorphan	Rectal/i.m.	Endo
Pentazocine	Talwin	p.o./i.m./i.v.	Sanofi
Propoxyphene	Darvon, Darvocet	p.o.	Lilly
	Wygesic		Wyeth-Ayerst
Sufentanil	Sufenta	i.v./i.m.	Taylor
Tramadol	Ultram	p.o.	Ortho-McNeil

analgesic abuse is insignificant among patients with medically justified opioid use, only 1 in 800 for headache sufferers to less than 1 in 10,000 burn patients (Medina & Diamond, 1977; Passik & Portenoy, 1998; Perry & Heidrich, 1982; Portenoy, 1990; Porter & Jick, 1980). Even the U.S. Government has declared the risk of addiction in cancer patients to be "an exceedingly rare event" (AHCPR, 1994).

Once the decision to use opioid analgesics is made, the issue becomes which one of them to use (Table 42.2). For mild to moderate pain, it is customary to start with the lower potency opioid analgesics, such as codeine, hydrocodone, or propoxyphene. Using codeine for pain management poses an interesting problem for some patients because codeine is a prodrug that must be converted to an active analgesic, morphine, via the CPY2D6 component of the hepatic P450 microsomal enzyme system and that system is lacking in 7% of Caucasians, 3% of Blacks, and 1% of Asians (Lurcott, 1999), and generally suppressed in all patients receiving the SSRI medications fluoxetine and paroxetine (Stahl, 2000). In the U.S. these medications are commonly given as combination tablets containing aspirin, acetaminophen, or ibuprofen that often is more effective than the amount of the opioid analgesic involved. Codeine and propoxyphene tend to be quite toxic for some patients (the elderly, those with renal insufficiency or opioid allergies), with hydrocodone products tending to be better tolerated and more effective as analgesics.

Some clinicians erroneously view oxycodone as a weak opioid analgesic, much like codeine, hydrocodone, and propoxyphene; but in reality, the co-administration of acetaminophen and aspirin limits the amount of oxycodone patients can take in the form of a fixed combination medication. This leads to the mistaken belief that oxycodone is not strong enough for cancer patients. Pure immediate-release and sustained-release oxycodone preparations are free of acetaminophen or aspirin and permit further titration of the medication to analgesia without the toxicity associated with the co-analgesics. Uniquely, immediate-release and sustained-release oxycodone, used either alone or after converting from a combination oxycodone-containing product, allow for the continued use of the same initial opioid analgesic from mild through moderate to severe pain. In the American Medical Association's *Project to Educate Physicians on End-of-Life Care*, only oxycodone is listed as both a step 2 (moderate pain) and 3 (severe pain) appropriate agent (Emanuel, et al., 1999).

When the pain is consistently more severe, or when the lower-potency opioid analgesics do not produce adequate relief, high-potency opioid analgesics are recommended. The reference gold standard for these opioid medications is traditionally morphine, because it has the distinct advantage of being available in the widest variety of routes of administration (immediate-release and sustained-release tablets, elixirs of varied strengths, concentrate, suppositories, preservative-containing solutions for intramuscular and intravenous use, and preservative-free solutions for epidural and intraspinal techniques) on a worldwide basis.

Morphine is the historic analgesic "gold standard" because it is an effective, relatively inexpensive opioid analgesic with a reasonable 4-hour duration of action (Twycross & Lack, 1984), a short half-life, and is generally available throughout the world. Unlike opioid analgesics with a long half-life (methadone and levorphanol), morphine-caused complications and toxicity are resolved within a matter of hours. The ability to convert from one route of administration to another is quite simple with an equianalgesic table (Table 42.1). Sustained-release morphine allows the patient to have uninterrupted comfort and allows intact sleep for the patient and the caregiver. Sublingual morphine concentrate, although variable in efficacy, allows those patients for whom it is effective to obtain pain relief without the unpleasantness of parenteral or rectal administration. The metabolite of morphine, morphine-6-glucuronide, is an active analgesic with a longer duration of action and half-life than morphine (Osborne, Joel, & Slevin, 1986). The accumulation of morphine-6-glucuronide probably accounts for the observation that repetitively administered oral morphine is one third as effective as intramuscular, while single-dose-administered morphine is only one sixth as effective (Reisine & Pasternak, 1996). Opioid equianalgesic tables in pharmacology textbooks are generally based on acute pain models rather than pain patients receiving chronic opioids and report the oral to parenteral efficacy of morphine as six to one. Hospice patients are not opioid naïve and should be dosed using the three-to-one conversion factor when estimating the oral-to-parenteral conversion of morphine.

All of the other opioid analgesics are equally effective in controlling pain and are typically used as alternatives when patients are allergic to morphine, experience morphine-related toxicity, or express concern about taking morphine (the drug addicts use). The only opioid analgesic that is best avoided in cancer patients is meperidine, due to the accumulation of the metabolite normeperidine, which is associated with the development of irritability, myoclonic jerking, and generalized tonic-clonic seizures (AHCPR, 1994; APS, 1999; Foley & Inturrisi, 1989). Because most cancer patients require relatively high doses of opioid agonist medication, the additional use of a mixed agonist-antagonist (butorphanol, nalbuphine, and pentazocine) is also strongly discouraged, because of the possible precipitation of opioid withdrawal and severe pain for these patients (APS, 1999; Foley & Inturrisi, 1987). Tramadol hydrochloride (a weak opioid-agonist that also inhibits the reuptake of norepinephrine and serotonin) is generally not used for cancer patients and must not be given in doses greater than 400 mg per day for the relatively "healthy" younger patient, 300 mg per day for the greater than 75-year-old patient, 200 mg per day for the patient with creatinine clearance less than 30 ml/min, and only 100 mg per day for patients with cirrhosis (APS, 1999; Medical Economics, 2000).

Opioid-related myoclonus has been reported for heroin, hydromorphone, meperidine, methadone, and morphine (Mercadante, 1998). Metabolites of these opioids may accumulate with renal insufficiency, leading to irritation of the cortex and brain stem reticular formation. High levels of morphine-3-glucuronide, morphine-6-glucuronide, and normorphine accumulate with renal failure and result in generalized myoclonus when patients receive morphine (Reisine & Pasternak, 1996). The neuroexcitatory metabolites of morphine and hydromorphone may be responsible for the hyperalgesic state seen in cancer patients treated with high doses of these medications (Mercadante, 1998).

Whether or not patients experience significant toxicity with morphine therapy, it is often prudent to change to a semisynthetic opioid analgesic. Many of these are currently available (or soon to become available) as controlled-release preparations. Hydromorphone is frequently selected, as the duration of analgesic action and plasma half-life are the same as morphine (Pasero, et al., 1999). Perhaps relatively less nauseating and (central nervous system (CNS) "toxic" than morphine, hydromorphone is available in immediate-release oral tablets (controlled-release tablets are available in Canada and are in clinical trials in the U.S.), suppositories, and injectable solutions (including a 10 mg/ml solution that is quite useful for end-stage cancer pain management, when high-dose parenteral infusions are common).

Case Example

Mr. C, a 70-year-old gentleman, had advanced lung cancer complicated by sacroiliac and fifth lumbar vertebral metastases. He experienced severe pain in his left thigh with muscular wasting. He had previously tried oral morphine with an unclear "reaction." Although he was able to tolerate oral fluids and solids without any overt difficulty, he was quite anxious about taking any oral analgesics and requested that his medication be provided by intravenous route, a dosing format in which he had great confidence. Because he was cared for by his daughter, who was able to learn the needed skills, it was possible to consider the use of parenteral analgesics. He had been started on intravenous hydromorphone in the hospital before coming home to the hospice program. The hospice nursing staff maintained a patent intravenous access with a saline peripheral port, and his daughter gave him doses of 5 or 6 mg hydromorphone every 3 hours, with good relief of his pain for the first week on the program. He was able to sleep well and developed a good appetite. By the second week, his pain was beginning to bother him much more, and a home pain management evaluation was completed. It was decided to add the anti-inflammatory choline magnesium trisalicylate, at 750 mg orally four times daily with food, and to maintain the intravenous hydromorphone at 6 mg every 3 hours. Through the next week, he felt much better, but he developed the need for increasing doses given at decreasing intervals by the fourth week. When his intravenous hydromorphone reached 11 mg every 2.5 hours, he developed considerable nausea and vomiting, associated with anxiety about the ability to ever control his side effects and pain simultaneously. He was given 1 to 2 mg of sublingual haloperidol every 4 hours as needed, relieving his nausea and vomiting. In the final and fifth week on the program, he continued to increase the use of the hydromorphone, eventually reaching 20 mg every 3 hours, yet remained alert, active, and involved with his family and care needs. His family was grateful that they could maintain meaningful dialog with him and complete much of the anticipatory bereavement work. On the day before he died, he met with the funeral director to plan the details of his own funeral and met with a close friend to help prepare the eulogy that would be delivered. Later that day, he went to sleep and died during the night. Although he had miotic pupils, suggesting an opiate effect, throughout his participation in the hospice program, he never developed any respiratory depression except as an agonal event.

Oxycodone and fentanyl are also commonly used medications and allow for very good pain relief with relatively little toxicity. Both of these medications are available in oral formulations in the U.S. Fentanyl transdermal patches (used as the base analgesic and supplemented with oral transmucosal fentanyl citrate for breakthrough pain) can provide analgesia for 2 to 3 days with each patch. In the chronic steady-state condition, a 25 mg/hr transdermal fentanyl patch is approximately equianalgesic to 10 mg oral morphine sulfate every 4 hours or 30 mg every 12 hours when given as sustained-release tablets (Emanuel, et al., 1999). Fentanyl patches may improve medication compliance because patients only have to change them every 3 days; but patients and staff caring for cancer patients often report that patches are difficult to titrate, require the use of a second medication for breakthrough pain, may cause skin irritation, do not stick very well in hot and humid environments, have erratic blood levels due to nonstandard thermal conditions or body weight less than 110 pounds, and have significant cost. During episodes of fever (temperature >104°F), exertion combined with sunny and warm environments, and exposure to high external temperature sources (heating pad, heated water beds, electric blankets, and car seats in the summer), the actual dose of fentanyl delivered may exceed the dose printed on the patch and lead to potential increases in serum fentanyl levels (Newshan, 1998). Dosing tables for fentanyl transdermal patches (suggesting that 45 to 134 mg per day of morphine is equivalent to 25 mg per hour of transdermal fentanyl) have been based on the 6:1 oral to parenteral morphine ratio, resulting in undershooting the dose when going from oral morphine to the fentanyl patch and overshooting when going from the patch to oral morphine and other opioids (Enck, 1995; Johanson, 1993).

Controlled-release oxycodone has been designed to provide sustained delivery of oxycodone over 12 hours, with an oral bioavailability of 60 to 87% (Medical Economics, 2000). With repeated dosing, steady-state levels are achieved in 24 to 36 hours; however, controlled-release oxycodone exhibits a unique biphasic absorption pattern with two apparent absorption half-times of 0.6 and 6.9 hours (describing the initial release of oxycodone from the outer layer of the tablet, followed by prolonged release from the core of the tablet through the use of a patented technology). This unusual release system allows for prompt establishment of stable blood levels of oxycodone with the first dose and little need to overlap parenteral medications with controlled-release oxycodone. Oxycodone is metabolized primarily to noroxycodone (a considerably weaker opioid than oxycodone) and minimally to oxymorphone (a potent analgesic mediated by the CYP2D6 P450 system). Similar to other controlled-release medications, controlled-release oxycodone must be swallowed whole and never broken, chewed, or crushed, which could lead to rapid release and absorption of a potentially toxic dose of medication. With renal or hepatic failure, initial doses are one third to one half of the usual doses; however, oxycodone is not associated with myoclonus or significant CNS toxicity due to its metabolites (Medical Economics, 2000).

The practice of combining opioid analgesics to provide better patient comfort is confusing for patients, their caregivers, and even the prescribing physicians. It is not justified under most circumstances, and there is often misuse of multiple opioid medications because few appreciate that pill size has little to do with relative potency or that sustained-release tablets do not adequately control pain until proper titration has occurred over 2 to 3 days. When two different molecules are given simultaneously, it is usually because the base medication is not available in more than one or two routes of administration, the base medication has not been titrated to full effect, or there is some toxicity being experienced.

It is routinely necessary to provide additional immediate-release opioid medication for breakthrough pain occurring at certain times (incident pain, movement related pain), especially when the base opioid analgesic is a sustained-release preparation. Unanticipated changes in pain can thus be effectively managed on an immediate basis, with day-to-day tailoring of the overall opioid analgesic medication by observing the use of these additional doses. Monitoring the 24-hour total usage of medication, and readjusting the daily dosage, are essential for keeping up with the oral opioid analgesic medication needs of the patient. The approximate dose of additional medication providing good control of breakthrough pain is 5 to 15% of the total daily amount of base medication (Emanuel, et al., 1999). Using 10% is an easier method, allowing the prescriber to simply move the decimal point one digit to the left (avoiding the need for calculators) to determine the breakthrough dosage. This 10% method of calculating the breakthrough dose assumes that the same route of administration is used for the immediate-release medication as for the base controlled-release medication. After receiving three back-to-back doses of breakthrough medication (every 30 to 60 minutes for oral liquid concentrates, or every 1 to 2 hours for solid tablets and capsules), the patient still having considerable pain must be reassessed.

Oral transmucosal fentanyl citrate (often used for breakthrough pain control when using transdermal fentanyl), a solid form of fentanyl incorporated into a sweetened lozenge on a handle, is partially absorbed rapidly through the oral mucosal and subsequently more slowly absorbed in the gastrointestinal tract (APS, 1999). The blood levels achieved will vary, depending on the fraction of the dose that is absorbed through the oral mucosal and the fraction swallowed and absorbed from the gastrointestinal tract (Medical Economics, 2000). Normally, about 25% of the total dose of oral transmucosal fentanyl citrate is rapidly absorbed from the buccal mucosa, and the remaining 75% is swallowed with the saliva and slowly absorbed; the generally observed 50% bioavailability is divided equally between rapid transmucosal and slower gastrointestinal absorption (Medical Economics, 2000). Because only about one third of the swallowed medication escapes first-pass liver metabolism to become systemically available, patients with impaired swallowing (or those incapable of swallowing) receive only half of the potential analgesic efficacy of oral transmucosal fentanyl citrate.

The major complication of all opioid analgesic therapy is constipation, regardless of the route of administration. Constipation must be vigorously managed from the initiation of treatment (prevention). Constipation not relieved adversely impacts the quality of life and must not be ignored. Failure to correct opioid-induced constipation leads to intractable nausea, vomiting, abdominal discomfort, and bowel perforation, as well as emotional distress. Options for treating constipation include: stimulant laxatives, combination stimulant/stool softeners, prokinetic agents, osmotic agents, lubricants, and enemas. Dietary interventions alone or the use of bulk-forming agents are often inadequate and not recommended for those with advanced disease and poor mobility (Emanuel, et al., 1999). Recalling that dirt and water alone produce mud, a viscous material, but the combination of dirt, water, and fiber (straw, grass) produces brick (as in adobe), should make the admonition to avoid bulk-forming agents more clear.

Case Example

> Mr. F was sent home from the hospital with advanced prostate cancer and widely spread bone metastases, with no bowel movement for 1 week prior to entering the hospice program. He was fairly comfortable from a pain perspective, although he experienced increasing abdominal fullness and discomfort thought to be due to opioid-analgesic-induced constipation. Digital examination of the rectum found significant hard, impacted stool that was manually decompressed. Once free of the impaction, he was started on an oral laxative and stool softener combination, and he developed bowel regularity within 2 days. There were no further episodes of impaction, and his bowel integrity was maintained with the same daily laxative/softener combination.

Although nausea and vomiting are initially common with opioids, once acclimated to these medications (in a matter of days for most patients), nausea and vomiting developing later more often result from unrecognized and ineffectively treated constipation. Early in the use of opioids, nausea and vomiting are usually controlled with dopamine-blocking agents (droperidol, haloperidol, metoclopramide, perphenazine, prochlorperazine, promethazine, or trimethobenzamide), antihistamines (diphenhydramine, hydroxyzine, or meclazine), anticholinergics (scopolamine), and serotonin antagonist (dolasetron, granisetron, or ondansetron) agents (Emanuel, et al., 1999). Respiratory depression, significant central nervous system dysfunction, allergic reactions, and the risk of chemical dependency are insignificant in comparison to constipation or nausea and vomiting.

When opioid analgesics fail to provide relief of significant pain despite clear toxicity (respiratory or central nervous system depression), it is necessary to remember that these agents are not always effective for deafferentation (neuropathic) pain due to nerve involvement, viscus or muscle spasm, or extreme psychological distress. It is the use of the adjunctive medications — with or without further opioid analgesics — that is warranted.

Adjunctive medications include antidepressants, antipsychotics, anticonvulsants, anxiolytics, and psychostimulants. These useful materials can be added at any step in the continuum of cancer pain management and often save patients from unnecessary progression to high-potency opioid analgesics or complex analgesic technologies. The adjunctive medications manipulate the neurochemistry of the nervous system and augment the overall effectiveness of both nonsteroidal anti-inflammatory and opioid analgesic combinations.

The antidepressants are remarkable agents, with the ability to block the presynaptic reuptake of norepinephrine and serotonin, resulting in elevated levels of these important neurotransmitters in the brain (Botney & Fields, 1982; Hendler, 1982). The benefit of enhanced serotonin centrally is the consequent periaquaductal release of endogenous opioid peptides with a dampening effect on pain perception (Frier, 1985). These agents correct the depression (which is so common with persistent pain); stabilize sleep; and improve appetite, energy level, concentration, and the ability to experience pleasure. The ability of antidepressants to relieve pain is independent of the antidepressant effect (Feinmann, 1985). Tricyclic antidepressants are recommended as one of the first-choice medications for painful polyneuropathy (Sindrup & Jensen, 2000) and especially for patients experiencing burning and tingling neuropathic pain (Emanuel, et al., 1999). Although the antidepressants most traditionally used for neuropathic pain management are generally the serotonin-enhancing tricyclic agents (amitriptyline and imipramine), the more norepinephrine-enhancing tricyclic agents (desipramine and nortriptyline) are often particularly useful when patients are intolerant to the serotonin-enhancing products or when psychomotor-retarded depression is present. Antidepressants are not habit forming and have little effect on respiration when used in therapeutic doses. Serotonin-enhancing tricyclic antidepressants are associated with a number of annoying anticholinergic side effects that limit their usefulness unless patients can tolerate them. The newer selective serotonin reuptake inhibitors (SSRIs such as citalopram, fluoxetine, fluvoxamine, paroxetine, and sertraline) are generally free of the anticholinergic adverse effects (having unique side effects of their own), but are disappointing as co-analgesics (Emanuel, et al., 1999). Atypical antidepressants (bupropion, mirtazapine, nefazodone, trazadone, and venlafaxine) are being evaluated for their analgesic usefulness and may provide benefit with less potential toxicity (Emanuel, et al., 1999).

Case Example

Mr. D, a 75-year-old gentleman, had severe lability of affect, impaired sleep, and advanced pulmonary cancer, leaving him short of breath and in need of continuous oxygen therapy. He had used diazepam for many years as a bedtime hypnotic, but the hospice staff was concerned about the cumulative respiratory depression of diazepam and sustained-release morphine. Rather than administer diazepam with the sustained-release morphine at 60 mg twice daily, he was started on 10 mg of doxepin hydrochloride at bedtime, which was eventually adjusted upward to 20 mg the next week with improvement in sleep, stabilization of his mood, loss of affective lability, and better management of his chest wall pain.

Antipsychotic medications still commonly referred to as neuroleptics or major tranquilizers, block the postsynaptic dopamine receptors and prevent the transmission of neuronal information. The consequence of these agents is the functional disconnection of the limbic system (the modern-day equivalent of a noninvasive frontal lobotomy), with the patient relatively unconcerned about the pain problem. This effect often permits the rapid tapering of high-dose opioid analgesic medication, especially intravenous, when a patient is trying to leave the hospital to return to the home setting. With antipsychotic medications, it is possible to significantly decrease the opioid dosage and maintain the patient in a relaxed state. Antipsychotic agents are also powerful antiemetics and control nausea and vomiting (Hanks, 1984; Johanson, 1988). The high-potency medications droperidol and haloperidol are particularly noteworthy because they work with minimal effect on the cardiovascular system. Droperidol is only available as a parenteral agent, but haloperidol is available as oral tablets and an oral concentrate (2 mg/ml)that can be used sublingually (Johanson, 1988). The low-potency medications chlorpromazine and thioridazine are relatively toxic for the cardiovascular system and are best avoided in the seriously ill patient. Extrapyramidal reactions do occur with the high-potency medications, but they can be easily managed with the anticholinergic agents benztropine and diphenhydramine.

Case Example

Ms. M was a 45-year-old woman with end-stage human immunodeficiency virus infection. She did not experience significant pain, but she suffered from intractable nausea and vomiting that were not relieved with standard antiemetics used orally or rectally. She was given 1 mg of sublingual haloperidol every 4 hours, with good control of her symptoms.

In general, the anticonvulsants are frequently the only effective oral medications for deafferentation (neuropathic) pain, nerve injuries, and pain characterized by burning, tingling, or paroxysms (Swerdlow, 1986). Anticonvulsants stabilize nerve cell membranes and inhibit spontaneous discharge by blocking sodium channels unspecifically, resulting in the control of seizures centrally or neuropathic pain peripherally (Sindrup & Jensen, 2000; WHO, 1986). The most commonly used agents (carbamazepine, clonazepam, gabapentin, phenytoin, and valproic acid) have been employed in the management of lancinating or stabbing dysesthetic pain (Emanuel, et al., 1999; Lack, 1984; Sindrup & Jensen, 2000). Recently, Bruera, et al. (1999) reported that most patients with neuropathic pain do improve on opioid analgesics. Based on a prospective open label study in which more than two thirds of patients with neuropathic pain achieved good analgesia with opioids alone, coupled to the expected effectiveness of adjuvants rarely exceeding 30%, Bruera, Walker, and Lawlor (1999) recommended opioids as the first-line treatment for these patients. They advised using the adjuvants when patients reached dose-limiting toxicity.

Clonazepam is a potent benzodiazepine with a relatively greater anticonvulsant effect than its congeners (Hanks, 1984). Clonazepam is one of the least difficult anticonvulsants to use in the home hospice setting due to the ability to use it without the need for blood level monitoring. Because it does tend to accumulate and may cause a moderate degree of sedation, clonezapam is often avoided in severely ill patients. However, the long half-life of clonazepam does allow for effective once-daily dosing for many patients.

Gabapentin has become the more typically utilized oral anticonvulsant for neuropathic pain management (Emanuel, et al., 1999). Gabapentin is generally started in low doses (100 mg, one to three times daily) and titrated upward to clinical effect (the reduction of pain) or the manifestation of dose-limiting toxicity (sedation and ataxia). There are no specific blood levels correlating to pain relief, and patients may require 3600 mg per day or more to obtain pain relief. Based on numbers needed to treat (to obtain more than 50% pain relief) studies, gabapentin is considered to be one of the medications of first choice for the treatment of painful polyneuropathy (Sindrup & Jensen, 2000).

Carbamazepine (with the relative risk of bone marrow suppression) and valproic acid (with the relative risk of gastric upset), coupled to the need for blood level monitoring, are generally unattractive as anticonvulsants for the home hospice patient. Carbamazepine is one of the medications of first choice for the treatment of painful polyneuropathy (Sindrup & Jensen, 2000). Carbamazepine is traditionally a preferred medication for trigeminal neuralgia and for other supraclavicular pain problems (phenytoin having the historical reputation for being the anticonvulsant to treat infraclavicular pain), but carbamezapine and valproic acid have the distinct disadvantage of requiring several days of oral titration before therapeutic improvement is noted. Both blood level monitoring and complete blood counts are recommended for the use of carbamazepine.

Anxiety, depression, fear, sleeplessness, and restlessness may all lower a patient's pain tolerance (Emanuel, et al., 1999; Hanks, 1984). Benzodiazepines, although not thought of as analgesics, have a limited role in the management of cancer pain. Most hospice patients sleep fairly well; but as some of them near the end of their lives, they may have disturbing dreams and recurrent nightmares interfering with the restful quality of their sleep for which benzodiazepines may prove helpful. Additionally, when pain interferes with the normal sleep pattern such that little or no stage four delta-wave sleep occurs, the addition of a short-acting sedative hypnotic agent (estazolam, triazolam, or zolpidem) is beneficial. It appears that without the deepest stage of sleep, muscles do not completely relax, and muscular pain may spontaneously develop, causing the patient widespread discomfort. By improving deep stage four sleep, this diffuse muscular ache that many cancer patients experience, which is also a consequence of their debilitation and malnutrition, can be lessened. When patients are morbidly anxious about their condition, the addition of a benzodiazepine medication may significantly improve their anxiety. The long half-life benzodiazepine medications, with maintained blood levels by time-contingent dosing, are preferable to the short half-life medications, which are more likely to produce wide swings in blood levels and consequent rebound anxiety.

Psychostimulants, such as dextroamphetamine and methylphenidate, are useful for the relief of depression, diminishing excessive sedation due to opioids, potentiating the analgesic effect of opioids in patients with postoperative and cancer pain, improving appetite, promoting a sense of well-being, and lessening feelings of weakness and fatigue (Breitbart, Passik, & Payne, 1998). Doses commonly used are 5 to 10 mg once or twice daily (breakfast and lunch), with few patients requiring more than 30 mg per day (Emanuel, et al., 1999). Although pemoline, a unique alternative to the amphetamine-like medications, lacks abuse potential, has mild sympathomimetic effects, has low DEA scheduling permitting telephone orders, and comes in a chewable tablet form that can be absorbed through the buccal mucosal, it is not established that it potentiates opioids although it counters the sedation of opioids and relieves depression (Breitbart, Passik, & Payne, 1998). Pemoline should be used with caution in patients having underlying liver disease.

ANESTHETIC TECHNIQUES

Certain anesthetic techniques are occasionally needed for the hospice patient. Some of the more useful procedures include the celiac plexus block for abdominal pain, the stellate ganglion block for upper quarter pain, the lumbar sympathetic block for lower extremity pain, the intraspinal neurolytic block for bilateral lower body pain, and the epidural use of opioid analgesics (Cousins & Mather, 1984; Foley, 1985).

Case Example

Ms. N was a 50-year-old woman with ovarian and abdominal carcinomatosis, colectomy, and colostomy. She suffered from extreme abdominal, upper and lower back, and pelvic pain. Despite 10 to 20 mg of intravenous morphine per hour, she was never able to achieve effective control of her pain. She was not convinced that further chemotherapy would help her condition and elected hospice care. After consultation with an anesthesiologist, she received an epidural catheter. After it was placed, she had reasonable control of her abdominal and pelvic pain components using 5 to 10 mg hydromorphone every 5 hours. This was supplemented with 10 mg of oral methadone every 5 hours to control the upper back pain, which was not well managed by the epidural catheter. Later, as her disease spread, she experienced more abdominal pain, and a celiac plexus block was done, giving her very good relief. Her methadone was reduced to just 5 mg every 6 hours, with epidural hydromorphone at 10 mg every 6 hours. Although she was finally comfortable with this complex management, her course was punctuated over the last 2 months of her life by good and bad days, impaired appetite, poor sleep, and then pervasive depression. With the addition of 25 mg amitriptyline at bedtime, these symptoms quickly improved. Although she became more emaciated over time, she tolerated both invasive procedures without significant adverse outcome. As she was actively dying, she spent her final hours in the arms of her husband and communicated her wishes for the music to be played at her funeral.

The celiac plexus block provides good abdominal analgesia for several months and is perhaps the ideal management approach for pancreatic (Parris, 1985), hepatic, and intestinal cancer and abdominal carcinomatosis from ovarian malignancy. A significant reduction in pain after this block is reported by 60 to 90% of patients (Foley, 1985; Verrill, 1989). If survival extends beyond several months, the block can be repeated, although frequently with a less successful outcome.

The stellate ganglion block is useful for sympathetically mediated pain involving the scalp, face, neck, arm, and upper chest (Campbell, 1989). This technique is frequently used in the management of upper quarter pain related to brachial plexus involvement by lung cancer or highly invasive breast cancer. Often, a single block is useful; but commonly, a series of these blocks is performed to modify the discomfort. When effective, the results of this block can be quite impressive and startling.

Case Example

Ms. W, a tragic 37-year-old woman, had suffered from widely metastatic breast cancer for 3 years when she was first seen for pain control. Over many months, she had been tried on several different analgesic medications. A series of hypnotic sessions proved to be useful and allowed her to rest for a short time, but only while she was profoundly relaxed during the sessions. When her right arm began to swell quite rapidly, it was decided to try a stellate ganglion block to see if her pain might be sympathetic in origin. The block was performed late in the afternoon, and upon return to her room, she was smiling and reporting very little overall discomfort. She drifted off to sleep, for the first time in days, and died peacefully a few hours later without awakening. The first reaction of the anesthesiologist upon learning of the sudden demise of Ms. W was to assume that there had been an adverse outcome from the technically well-done stellate ganglion block. However, it was clear that she was finally able to experience comfort for the first time in years and was able to let go and die in her sleep.

Intraspinal neurolysis is a highly destructive technique used for intractable pain when lower-body motor function, along with bowel and bladder control, is lost, usually due to a spinal cord tumor or invasion of the spine by metastatic lesions. It involves the deliberate chemical coagulation of the remaining cord structures by placing alcohol or phenol in the subdural space (Ferrer-Brechner, 1989). The end result is absolute anesthesia below the level of the completed cord destruction.

Case Example

Mr. A, a 65-year-old gentleman, had a widely metastatic prostate cancer that had invaded his lumbar spine anteriorly and left him paralyzed below the level of the lesion, without bowel or bladder control, but in constant excruciating pain in his lower body. Despite adequate trials of nonsteroidal anti-inflammatory medication, low- and high-potency opioid analgesics, and transcutaneous electrical nerve stimulation, nothing seemed to relieve his suffering. After consultation with an anesthesiologist, it was decided to complete his cord lesion with intraspinal alcohol. This was done with the patient's informed consent and quickly produced complete resolution of his lower body pain. He still required some anti-inflammatory and opioid analgesic medication for his upper body pain, but was much improved and relatively comfortable after the spinal neurolysis.

Epidural and spinal administration of opioid analgesics is quite effective when the pain is fairly localized, especially if it is entirely below the level of the nipples. Long-term use of intraspinal opioids is recommended for cancer patients with regionalized pain below T1 failing to achieve pain control after adequate trials of several different systemic opioids (APS, 1999). By placing the opioid analgesic into the epidural space or intraspinal, the patient experiences relatively little cognitive impairment, and while the pain is significantly relieved, normal sensation is preserved. Once the catheter is in place, the opioid (usually fentanyl, hydromorphone, or morphine) is administered by continuous infusion or by bolus injections. The availability of small, lightweight, battery-powered portable infusion pumps allows the hospice nursing staff to provide a 24- to 48-hour supply of medication to the patient without the risk of catheter infection due to poor injection technique by the nonprofessional caregiver. Contraindications (absolute and relative) for epidural and spinal opioids with or without anesthetic agents include: bleeding diathesis, septicemia, local cutaneous infection at the site of catheter insertion, known immune suppression, insulin-dependent diabetics, and lack of appropriate support for the ongoing management of the catheter (Swarm & Cousins, 1998).

SPECIAL CONSIDERATIONS FOR PARENTERAL THERAPIES

Parenteral opioid infusions are used much more frequently than anesthetic procedures, but less frequently than oral medications. They can be extremely beneficial for those patients who have patent intravenous access, swallowing difficulties that prevent the use of oral medications, the need for large dosages of medication, and the lack of other routes of administration of opioids. The common technique for the administration of parenteral opioids is via a portable infusion pump delivering high-potency opioid analgesics through a small needle inserted into the subcutaneous tissue.

Case Example

> Ms. T was a 60-year-old woman with advanced hepatic cancer with pelvic metastases. She had delayed chemotherapy to allow for a long-hoped-for trip to Europe. When she first presented to the hospice program, she was experiencing severe bilateral hip pain with radiation into her thighs. Bothersome muscle spasms complicated her pain problem. She was a suspicious, guarded woman who did not have much faith in her physicians. She did not want to take any medication and desperately wanted to avoid being hospitalized. She was initially treated for her pain with intravenous morphine at 12 mg/hr, but was successfully converted to oral morphine in sustained-release form at 400 mg every 12 hours. Once she went home, she began to need more morphine and was quickly using 150 to 180 mg of immediate-release morphine every day in addition to the sustained-release morphine. The hospice staff observed that she used more morphine when her family

members were present. Due to the wide fluctuations in her comfort level, and her increasing belief that the oral medications would never entirely control her discomfort, she was started on a subcutaneous hydromorphone infusion at 2 mg/hr, with satisfactory pain control within 1 day.

For cancer pain that becomes "out of control," Berger, et al. (2000) have described a technique using intravenous ketamine (2 mg/ml), fentanyl (5 μg/ml), and midazolam (0.1 mg/ml) to control pain after traditional analgesics were unsuccessful. They felt that ketamine, an N-methyl-D-aspartate (NMDA) receptor antagonist, and midazolam, a benzodiazepine useful for myoclonus, nausea, and cognitive disturbances associated with opioid therapy, would enhance the overall opioid therapy with fentanyl. As all nine patient studies exhibited some degree of qualitative improvement in cognitive compromise and agitation associated with previous therapy, as well as in overall pain control, Berger, et al. suggested that subcutaneous infusion or dermoclysis of ketamine/fentanyl/midazolam solution be used if intravenous access is lost.

NON-PHARMACOLOGIC APPROACHES

Cancer pain is also managed by a number of nonpharmacologic methods, including cognitive therapy, hypnosis, relaxation and imagery, distraction, reframing, patient education, peer support groups, transcutaneous electrical nerve stimulation (TENS), radiation therapy, and physical and occupational therapy services (AHCPR, 1994; Emanuel, et al., 1999). For prominent muscle spasm, predictably painful procedures, depression, and anxiety, the cognitive techniques are useful (Cleeland, 1987). Hypnosis can augment pain control but rarely relieves the pain completely. Providing orthotics or prosthetics, assistive devices, range-of-motion exercises, and bedside stretching can keep the remaining activities of daily living accessible for the patient. Radiation therapy and TENS are often effective management for bone metastases and pathologic fractures (Bosch, 1984; Howard-Ruben, McGuire, & Groenwald, 1987). TENS requires the participation of the patient. While a meta-analysis of studies of TENS therapy in postoperative patients found that both TENS and sham TENS significantly reduced pain intensity, with no significant differences found between the two for either analgesic use or pain intensity, suggesting that part of the efficacy of TENS could be attributed to placebo effect, patients with mild pain may benefit from a trial of TENS (AHCPR, 1994).

Radiotherapy

Radiation therapy is perhaps the most effective form of treatment for local metastatic bone pain, spinal cord and cauda equina compression, brain metastasis, mediastinal compression and superior vena cava obstruction, lung collapse due to bronchial obstruction, urinary tract obstruction, and limb edema (Hoskin, 1998). The strategy for palliative radiation therapy differs from the techniques used for active cancer treatment. Protracted regimens of more than ten treatments may be more appropriate for patients with life expectancy longer than 6 months to reduce potential late radiation effects or acute effects such as nausea if critical structures such as the stomach have to be included in the radiation field. However, for patients with a more limited life expectancy, radiation can be administered in fewer fractions (Lawton & Maher, 1991; Maher, Coia, Duncan, & Lawton, 1992). In the hospice setting, a single high dose of radiation is generally as effective as multiple smaller doses for the control of pain from bone metastases. Serious late radiation damage (unlikely when life expectancy is short) is related to both high total doses and the delivery of radiation in large fractions over a relatively short period (Hoskin, 1998). Most retrospective and prospective studies report that 75% or more of patients obtain relief from pain and about half of those who achieve relief become pain-free (Nielsen, Munro, & Tannock, 1991).

Radiopharmaceuticals are used therapeutically for the relief of pain in cancer patients (AHCPR, 1994). Iodine-131 results in bone scan evidence of response in 53% of patients with bone metastases from thyroid cancer (Maxon & Smith, 1990). Strontium-89 is the most extensively evaluated as a treatment for bone pain and compares favorably with hemibody irradition in randomized trials, but is only potentially effective in the treatment of pain due to osteoblastic bone lesions or lesions with an osteoblastic component (Hoskin, 1998). Strontium-89 is reported to provide partial pain relief in 65 to 80% of patients and complete pain relief for 10% of patients (AHCPR, 1994; Hoskin, 1998). Rhenium-186 and samarium-153 phosphonate chelates have demonstrated 65 to 80% efficacy in international trials (Maxon, et al., 1990; Turner, Claringbold, Hetherington, Sorby, & Martindale, 1989). These beta-emitting radiopharmaceuticals, requiring only a single intravenous injection, are used to relieve pain from widespread osteoblastic skeletal metastases visualized with bone scintigraphy; 50% of patients will respond to a second administration if pain recurs (AHCPR, 1994).

Bisphosphonates (previously called diphosphonates) inhibit osteoclast activity and reduce bone resorption. Pamidronate and clodronate produce pain relief and reduce other skeletal morbidity (Hoskin, 1998). Placebo-controlled studies with oral clodronate in women with metastatic breast cancer demonstrated lower numbers of hypercalcemic events, vertebral fractures, rates of vertebral deformity, and combined rates of all morbid skeletal events. Because analgesia often begins weeks after treatment is initiated, the late use of bisphosphonates in hospice patients may not produce significant pain improvement if they are only for agonal pain control (Hoskin, 1998).

FINAL COMMENTS ABOUT CANCER PAIN CONTROL

To successfully manage the terminal cancer pain patient, all of the underlying issues must be globally addressed. The etiology of the pain must be accurately defined to direct the appropriate therapy. The analgesics may progress from nonsteroidal anti-inflammatory agents to opioids and adjuvants, but with the clear understanding that the medications are titrated and used for sufficient time to adequately assess their efficacy. Realistic goals about pain and its management must be set and clear communication maintained with all of the parties involved. Education of the patient and the family regarding the use of resources and decision making for choices of therapy are part of the process (Ferrer-Brechner, 1984). Education about the ability to control pain effectively and correction of myths about the use of opioids must be included as part of the treatment plan (AHCPR, 1994; Emanuel, et al., 1999). The emotional and spiritual needs of the patient are as important, and as aggressively managed, as the somatic needs (Emanuel, et al., 1999). Psychosocial interventions should be introduced early in the course of illness so that patients can learn and practice these strategies while they have sufficient strength and energy (AHCPR, 1994).

PROBLEM SYMPTOMS

In addition to pain, hospice patients — especially those with cancer — are bothered by constipation, nausea and vomiting, poor appetite and weight loss, seizures, difficulties with oral care, hydration, skin integrity, and itching. These symptoms are bothersome and steal quality and comfort from the patient and must be as aggressively managed as pain.

CONSTIPATION

As noted earlier, constipation is the expected consequence of opioid analgesic management and must be anticipated and preventively controlled from the moment pain is treated. Most patients can be given a high-fiber diet or a bulk laxative early on in their illness to prevent constipation. If ineffective, or if the patients are taking opioid analgesics, additional laxative strategies are needed (Emanuel, et al., 1999; Portenoy, 1987). Bowel care products are available in a variety of groups, including stool softeners, which prevent excessive drying; stimulants, which increase mucosal secretion and peristalsis, causing movement of fecal material; and combination products. Osmotic wetting agents, lubricants, and prokinetic medications are also available. The goal of therapy for the prevention of constipation is to maintain bowel regularity and keep the stool texture similar to that of toothpaste. In that way, even the weakest patient remains able to expel stool with little straining or effort.

NAUSEA AND VOMITING

Nausea and resulting vomiting may initially be due to the opioid analgesics, but over time may result from metastases, unrelieved constipation, meningeal irritation, metabolic abnormalities, medications, mucosal irritation, infections, or bowel obstruction (Emanuel, et al., 1999). If a correctable process is the culprit, it is best to manage the symptom by focusing on the pathology. When this is not possible, then the routine use of antiemetics is justified. Metoclopramide improves gastric emptying and affects the central nervous system vomiting center at higher doses (Ventafridda & Caraceni, 1994). The high-potency antipsychotic medications droperidol and haloperidol, either oral, sublingual, or parenteral, are effective for nausea and vomiting (Johanson, 1988). The lower-potency antipsychotic medications, such as the typical antiemetics, are generally more sedating than the high-potency agents and are more likely to produce unpleasant side effects such as dry mouth, constipation, urinary hesitancy, and hypotension. Intractable nausea may respond to serotonin antagonists that are able to suppress the serious chemotherapy-induced nausea associated with even Cisplatin (Johanson, 1993). Until vomiting is well controlled, most patients and their family members experience high levels of discomfort.

LOSS OF APPETITE AND CACHEXIA

Appetite loss and declining weight leave most hospice patients weak, listless, and susceptible to skin breakdown. As a result of chemotherapy, radiation therapy, surgery, and the overall debilitation of chronic illness, many patients experience a reduced level of pleasure associated with eating. Some patients may even become anxious about eating due to swallowing difficulties, the risk of choking, or aspiration. The involvement of a dietitian to assist with food preferences or a communication therapist to improve swallowing may be quite useful. Small, frequent portions of favorite foods are better tolerated than large, traditional meals (Lang & Patt, 1994). If chemotherapy has left the patient with little sense of taste, altering the diet to include highly seasoned or spicy foods or serving meals as colorfully as possible may help to stimulate the appetite (Kaye, 1989). Education for caregivers about loss of appetite as part of the dying process is critical because these caregivers may view the patients' loss of interest in food, and resulting cachexia, as therapeutic failure on their part, as food is tied so closely to nurturing in many cultures (Emanuel, et al., 1999). Ultimately, hospice patients should be permitted to eat whatever might give them enjoyment, not what the caregivers think is best for them to eat.

Case Example

Ms. A was a severely emaciated woman with advanced ovarian and abdominal carcinomatosis. She had undergone extensive surgical resection of her tumor, radiation therapy, and several courses of chemotherapy. She had lost most of her appreciation for taste and consequently found all food to have the taste and texture of oatmeal. It was hard for her to maintain her weight without motivation to eat. She began to experiment with different foods and found that spicy Mexican and Chinese meals were satisfying and helped her remain motivated to eat, whereas the more traditional oral nutrition supplements were refused. She enjoyed the cold and creamy quality of vanilla ice cream over any other dessert-type food.

Pharmacologic strategies for stimulating appetite include the use of alcohol, corticosteroids, megestrol, androgens, and the marijuana derivative dronabinol (Emanuel, et al., 1999). Preliminary research suggests that treatment with medications stimulates appetite with relatively low risk of serious side effects (Lang & Patt, 1994).

SEIZURES

Seizures are a significant concern for patients with metastatic brain lesions and cause a great deal of distress for their family members who must witness seemingly unrelenting convulsions. Although fairly easy to control with oral anticonvulsant and steroidal medication, seizures occurring near the end of life are problematic because the patients often are no longer able to swallow effectively. An alternative to the use of crushed tablets or liquid suspensions via a feeding tube is the injectable form of the benzodiazepine lorazepam. Lorazepam provides seizure control for 3 to 4 hours (Leppik, 1983), does not significantly accumulate because it has no active metabolites, and is rapidly absorbed from intramuscular injection sites, unlike the other benzodiazepines. As seizures are often an agonal event, giving a few intramuscular injections is rarely a problem for caregivers once they understand that patients are not going to experience significant pain. Other possible seizure management alternatives include valproate sodium injection (if intravenous access is present), given at less than 20 mg per minute and over 60 minutes per dose; diazepam, 20 mg per rectum once or twice daily; midazolam, 30 to 60 mg per day by continuous infusion; and phenobarbital, 200 to 600 mg per day by continuous infusion (Twycross & Lichter, 1998).

Case Example

Ms. H was a 65-year-old woman with ovarian cancer that had metastasized to her right brain, producing a left hemiplegia and motor seizures. Her pain involved her right hip. She was a remarkably angry woman who, while mildly dysphasic in her speech, was actually electively mute at times. Initially, 300 mg phenytoin at bedtime controlled her seizures, and 250 mg oral naproxen three times daily managed her hip discomfort. Later, 1 mg clonazepam was added at bedtime to control sleep and reported spasm, along with 30 mg sustained-release morphine twice daily. This produced marked daytime agitation, which was felt to be due to the benzodiazepine, and it was replaced by 2 mg oral haloperidol every 2 hours as needed. She lost control of swallowing and stopped taking any oral medications, fluids, or foods in the last week of her life. This resulted in more frequent and severe motor seizures that resulted in secondary generalization. As her daughter was able to administer intramuscular injections, she was managed for the last 2 days of her life with 1 to 2 mg of intramuscular lorazepam every 4 hours, with good control of her seizures. Although she steadily deteriorated, she did not appear to experience significant pain and was able to remain seizure-free with the lorazepam.

SKIN CARE

Skin care is vitally important for hospice patients, especially those who are bed bound. Minor and usually reversible skin disorders may become a major problem in the chronically sick patient, where healing powers are limited (Mortimer, 1993). Changes in body position, with frequent turning, proper padding with heel and ankle protectors, and a thick foam mattress cover should be utilized to prevent decubitus ulceration. There must always be 1 inch of foam between the lowest point of the patient and the surface of the bed (Emanuel, et al., 1999). Once ulcers are established, they are difficult to treat due to the poor wound healing of malnourished and debilitated patients. Bowel and bladder incontinence will produce skin breakdown if the patient is not kept relatively clean and dry. While powders and absorbent surfaces are helpful in keeping the patient dry, the use of urinary catheters and rectal tubes may be of assistance if soiling is constant and/or the patient is highly debilitated. The application of a "barrier" ointment can be quite effective once the skin is irritated.

Case Example

Ms. K, an 80-year-old woman with pancreatic cancer and secondary liver failure, had developed skin breakdown of her buttocks due to frequent diarrhea. Cleansing of her buttocks and perineum was associated with burning pain due to extensive irritation. She became progressively more fearful of any type of bowel activity and would allow herself to remain in a fecal- and urine-soaked bed rather than request appropriate care. To relieve her condition, and her

resulting anxiety about hygiene, she was given a topical material made from equal parts of zinc oxide ointment, vitamin A and D ointment, and 1% dibucaine, to be applied to the involved area every 4 to 6 hours. Within the first few applications, immediate comfort was obtained, and significant healing occurred over the next week.

ITCHING

Itching can be quite serious for patients with extremely dry skin and is often a complication of hepatic failure. Applying topical moisturizers may be helpful for skin dryness, but for protracted distressing itch, use of the antihistamines diphenhydramine and hydroxyzine or low-dose antidepressants may provide relief (Johanson, 1988; Kaye, 1989). One particularly useful agent for itching is the antidepressant doxepin hydrochloride, a potent antihistamine (about 800 times more antihistaminic than diphenhydramine) that produces moderate sedation (Richelson, 1979).

MOUTH CARE

Oral care is routinely performed by healthy individuals and sadly forgotten in some terminal patients. With dehydration due to decreased oral intake, coupled with mouth-breathing as death approaches, it is common for the oral membranes to become dry and caked with debris. Cleansing the mouth with small quantities of water, giving ice chips, wiping the mouth with a lemon-flavored glycerine swab, and applying a lip balm are soothing for the dying patient (Kaye, 1989).

CONCLUSION

Hospice care should be a choice for every person coping with the end of life. It requires a special commitment on the part of the caregiver and the support of a skilled hospice team. Personal illustrations from actual cases effectively managed by the hospice program were presented in this chapter. The stories are human experiences, and they serve as the best teachers. Hospice work with pain and symptom management is enriched by the patients who believe in the hospice philosophy and provide the opportunity to participate in their living and in their deaths. There is no single or best way to control any particular symptom, but the coordinated efforts of the interdisciplinary team bring effective relief for physical, emotional, and spiritual discomfort. Although the team members are important for a successful outcome, the patients remind us that hospice management is not finite. It is evolving, and individualized care must be absolute. Only the patients and their families are able to judge the effectiveness of the hospice team.

REFERENCES

Agency for Health Care Policy and Research. (1994). *Management of cancer pain: Clinical practice guideline.* AHCPR Publication No. 94-0592. Rockville, MD: Agency for Health Care Policy and Research, U.S. Department of Health and Human Services.

American Pain Society. (1989). *Principles of analgesic use in the treatment of acute pain and chronic cancer pain: A concise guide to medical practice* (2nd ed.). Skokie, IL: American Pain Society.

American Pain Society. (1995). Quality improvement guidelines for the treatment of acute pain and cancer pain. *Journal of the American Medical Association, 274,* 1874–1880.

American Pain Society. (1999). *Principles of analgesic use in the treatment of acute pain and chronic cancer pain: A concise guide to medical practice* (4th Ed.). Glenview, IL: American Pain Society.

Appleton, M. (1996). Hospice medicine: A different perspective. *The American Journal of Hospice & Palliative Care, 13,* 7–9.

Beckwith, B.E., Kanaan-Beckwith, S., Gray, T.L., Miscko, M.M., Holm, J.E., Plummer, V.H., & Flaa, S.L. (1990). Identification of spouses at high risk during bereavement: A preliminary assessment of Parkes and Weiss' Risk Index. *The Hospice Journal, 6,* 35–36.

Berger, J.M., Ryan, A., Vadivelu, N., Merriam, P., Rever, L., & Harrison, P. (2000). Ketamine-fentanyl-midazolam infusion for the control of symptoms in terminal life care. *American Journal of Hospice and Palliative Care, 17,* 127–132.

Bonica, J.J. (1985). Treatment of cancer pain: Current status and future needs. In H. L. Fields, et al. (Eds.), *Advances in pain research and therapy* (Vol. 9, pp. 589–616). New York: Raven Press.

Bonica, J.J. (1987). Preface: A short course on the management of cancer pain. *Journal of Pain and Symptom Management, 2,* S3–4.

Bosch, A. (1984). Radiotherapy. *Clinics in Oncology, 3,* 47–53.

Botney, M., & Fields, H.L. (1982). Amitriptyline potentiates morphine analgesia by a direct action on the central nervous system. *Annals of Neurology, 13,* 160–164.

Breitbart, W., Passik, S., McDonald, M.V., Rosenfeld, B., Smith, M., Kaim, M., & Funesti-Esch, J. (1998). Patient-related barriers to pain management in ambulatory AIDS patients. *Pain, 76,* 9–16.

Breitbart, W., Passik, S., & Payne, D. (1998). Psychological and psychiatric interventions in pain control. In D. Doyle, G. W. C. Hanks, & N. MacDonald (Eds.), *Oxford textbook of palliative medicine* (2nd ed., pp.437–454). New York, NY: Oxford University Press.

Brescia, F.J. (1987). An overview of pain and symptom management in advanced cancer. *Journal of Pain and Symptom Management, 2,* S7–11.

Bruera, E., Walker, P., & Lawlor, P. (1999). Opioids in cancer pain. In C. Stein (Ed.), *Opioids in pain control: Basic and clinical aspects* (pp 309–324). Cambridge, UK: Cambridge University Press.

Burnell, G.M., & Burnell, A.L. (1989). *Clinical management of bereavement.* New York: Human Sciences Press.

Campbell, J.N. (1989). Pain from peripheral nerve injury. In K. M. Foley & R. M. Payne (Eds.), *Current therapy of pain* (pp. 158–169). Toronto: B.C. Decker.

Cleeland, C.S. (1987). Nonpharmacological management of cancer pain. *Journal of Pain and Symptom Management, 2,* S23–28.

Cook, A.S., & Dworkin, D.S. (1992). *Helping the bereaved: Therapeutic interventions for children, adolescents, and adults.* New York: Basic Books.

Cosh, R. (1995). Spiritual care of the dying. In I.B. Corless, et al. (Eds.), *A challenge for living* (pp. 131–143). Boston: Jones and Bartlett.

Cousins, M.J., & Mather, L.E. (1984). Intrathecal and epidural administration of opioids. *Anesthesiology, 61,* 276–310.

Emanuel, L.L., von Gunten, C.F., & Ferris, F.D. (1999). *The education for physicians on end-of-life care (EPEC) curriculum.* Chicago, IL: American Medical Association.

Enck, R.E. (1995). Current concepts: Pain management and parenteral opioids: An update. *The American Journal of Hospice & Palliative Care, 12,* 8–15.

Feinmann, C. (1985). Pain relief by antidepressants: Possible modes of action. *Pain, 23,* 1–8.

Ferrer-Brechner, T. (1984). Treating cancer pain as a disease. In C. Benedetti, et al. (Eds.), *Advances in pain research and therapy* (Vol. 7, pp. 575–591). New York: Raven Press.

Ferrer-Brechner, T. (1989). Anesthetic techniques for the management of cancer pain. *Cancer, 63,* 2343–2347.

Foley, K.M. (1985). The treatment of cancer pain. *New England Journal of Medicine, 313,* 84–95.

Foley, K.M. (1988). Pain syndromes and pharmacologic management of pancreatic cancer pain. *Journal of Pain and Symptom Management, 3,* 176–187.

Foley, K.M., & Inturrisi, C.E. (1987). Analgesic drug therapy in cancer pain: Principles and practice. *Medical Clinics of North America, 71,* 207–232.

Foley, K.M., & Inturrisi, C.E. (1989). Pain of malignant origin. In K.M. Foley & R.M. Payne (Eds.), *Current therapy of pain.* Toronto: B.C. Decker.

Frier, J.W. (1985, January/February). Therapeutic implications of modifying endogenous serotonergic analgesic systems. *Anesthesia Progress,* 19–22.

Hanks, G.W. (1984). Psychotropic drugs. *Clinics in Oncology, 3,* 135–151.

Helig, S. (1988). The San Francisco Medical Society euthanasia survey: Results and analysis. *San Francisco Medicine, 61,* 24–34.

Hendler, N. (1982). The anatomy and psychopharmacology of chronic pain. *Journal of Clinical Psychiatry, 43,* 15–21.

Hill, C.S. (1988). Narcotics and cancer pain control. *Ca: A Cancer Journal for Clinicians, 38,* 322–326.

Hill, T.P., & Shirley, D. (1992). *A good death.* Menlo Park, CA: Addison-Wesley.

Hoskin, P.J. (1998). Radiotherapy in symptom management. In D. Doyle, G.W.C. Hanks & N. MacDonald (Eds.), *Oxford textbook of palliative medicine* (2nd ed., pp. 267–282). New York: Oxford University Press.

Howard-Ruben, J., McGuire, L., & Groenwald, S.L. (1987). Pain. In S. L. Groenwald (Ed.), *Cancer nursing principles and practice.* Boston: Jones & Bartlett.

Humphry, D. (1991). *Final exit.* Eugene, OR: Hemlock Society.

Insel, P.A. (1996). Analgesic-antipyretic and anti-inflammatory agents and drugs employed in the treatment of gout. In J.G. Hardman & L.E. Limbird (Eds.), *Goodman & Gilman's the pharmacological basis of therapeutics* (9th ed., pp. 617–657). New York: McGraw-Hill.

Johanson, G.A. (1988). *Physicians handbook of symptom relief in terminal care* (2nd ed.). Sebastopol, CA: Home Hospice of Sonoma County.

Johanson, G.A. (1993). *Physicians handbook of symptom relief in terminal care* (4th ed.). Santa Rosa, CA: Sonoma County Academic Foundation for Excellence in Medicine.

Kaiko, R.F., Benziger, D.P., Fitzmartin, R.D., Burke, B.E., Reder, R.F., & Goldenheim, P.D. (1996). Pharmacokinetic-pharmacodynamic relationships of controlled-release oxycodone. *Clinical Pharmacology and Therapeutics, 59,* 52–61.

Kanner, R.M. (1987). Pharmacological management of pain and symptom control in cancer. *Journal of Pain and Symptom Management, 2,* S19–S21.

Kaye, P. (1989). *Notes on symptom control in hospice and palliative care.* Essex, CT: Hospice Education Institute.

Lack, S. (1984). Total pain. *Clinics in Oncology, 3,* 33–44.

Lang, S.S., & Patt, R.B. (1994). *You don't have to suffer.* New York: Oxford University Press.

Lawton, P.A., & Maher, E.J. (1991). Treatment strategies for advanced and metastatic cancer in Europe. *Radiotherapeutic Oncology, 22,* 1–6.

Leow, K.P., Smith, M.T., Williams, B., & Cramond, T. (1993). Single-dose and steady-state pharmacokinetics and pharmacodynamics of oxycodone in patients with cancer. *Clinical Pharmacology and Therapeutics, 52,* 487–495.

Leppik, I.E. (1983). Double-blind study of lorazepam and diazepam in status epilepticus. *Journal of the American Medical Association, 249,* 1452–1454.

Levin, D.N., Cleeland, C.S., & Dar, R. (1985). Public attitudes toward cancer pain. *Cancer, 56,* 2337–2339.

Lurcott, G. (1999). The effects of the genetic absence and inhibition of CYP2D6 on the metabolism of codeine and its derivatives, hydrocodone and oxycodone. *Anesthesia Progress, 45,* 154–156.

Maher, E.J., Coia, L., Duncan, G., & Lawton, P.A. (1992). Treatment strategies in advanced and metastatic cancer: Differences in attitude between the USA, Canada and Europe. *International Journal of Radiation Oncology and Biological Physics, 23,* 239–244.

Maxon, H.R. III, & Smith, H.S. (1990). Radioiodine-131 in the diagnosis and treatment of metastatic well-differentiated thyroid cancer. *Endocrinologic and Metabolic Clinics of North America, 19,* 685–718.

Maxon, H.R. III, Schroder, L.E., Thomas, S.R., Hertzberg, V. S., Deutsch, E.A., Scher, H.I., Samaratunga, R.C., Libson, K.F., Williams, C.C., Moulton, J.S., & Schneider, H.J. (1990). Re-186 (Sn) HEDP for treatment of osseous metastases: Initial clinical experience in 20 patients with hormone-resistant prostate cancer. *Radiology, 176,* 155–159.

McCaffery, M., & Beebe, A. (1989). *Pain: Clinical manual for nursing practice.* St. Louis: Mosby.

McCaffery, M., & Pasero, C. (1999). Assessment: Underlying complexities, misconceptions, and practical tools. In M. McCaffery & C. Pasero (Eds.), *Pain: Clinical manual* (2nd ed., pp. 35–102). St. Louis, MO: Mosby.

Medical Economics Company (2000). *Physicians' desk reference* (54th ed.). Montvale, NJ: Medical Economics.

Medina, J.L., & Diamond, S. (1977). Drug dependency in patients with chronic headaches. *Headache, 17,* 12–14.

Mercadante, S. (1998). Pathophysiology and treatment of opioid-related myoclonus in cancer patients. *Pain, 74,* 5–9.

Mortimer, P.S. (1993). Skin problems in palliative care: Medical aspects. In D. Doyle, et al. (Eds.), *Oxford textbook of palliative medicine* (pp. 384–395). New York: Oxford University Press.

National Hospice Organization. (1996). *Resource manual for providing hospice care to people living with AIDS.* Arlington, VA: National Hospice Organization.

Newshan, G. (1998). Heat-related toxicity with the fentanyl transdermal patch. *Journal of Pain and Symptom Management, 16*(5), 277–278.

Nielsen, O.S., Munro, A.J., & Tannock, I.F. (1991). Bone metastases: Pathophysiology and management policy. *Journal of Clinical Oncology, 9,* 509–524.

Osborne, R.J., Joel, S.P., & Slevin, M.L. (1986). Morphine intoxication in renal failure: The role of morphine-6-glucuronide. *British Medical Journal, 292,* 1548–1549.

Parris, W.C.V. (1985). Nerve block therapy. *Clinics in Anesthesiology, 3,* 93–109.

Pasero, C., Portenoy, R.K. & McCaffery, M. (1999). Opioid analgesics. In M. McCaffery & C. Pasero (Eds.), *Pain Clinical Manual* (2nd ed., pp. 161–299). St. Louis: Mosby.

Passik, S.D., & Portenoy, R.K. (1998). Substance abuse issues in palliative care. In A. Berger (Ed.), *Principles and practice of supportive care* (pp. 513–529). Philadelphia, PA: Lippincott-Raven Publishers.

Patt, R.B., & Isaacson, S.A. (1996). Cancer pain syndromes. In P.P. Raj (Ed.), *Pain medicine: A comprehensive review* (pp. 502–520). St. Louis: Mosby-Year Book.

Perry, S., & Heidrich, G. (1982). Management of pain during debridement: A survey of U.S. burn units. *Pain, 13,* 267–280.

Portenoy, R.K. (1987). Constipation in the cancer patient. *Medical Clinics of North America, 71,* 303–311.

Portenoy, R.K. (1988). Practical aspects of pain control in the patient with cancer. *Ca: A Cancer Journal for Clinicians, 38,* 327–352.

Portenoy, R.K. (1990). Chronic opioid therapy in nonmalignant pain. *Journal of Pain and Symptom Management, 5,* S46–62.

Porter, J., & Jick, H. (1980). Addiction rare in patients treated with narcotics. *New England Journal of Medicine, 302,* 123.

Poyhia, R., Vainio, A., & Kalso, E. (1993). A review of oxycodone's clinical pharmacokinetics and pharmacodynamics. *Journal of Pain and Symptom Management, 8,* 63–67.

Reisine, T., & Pasternak, G. (1996). Opioid analgesics and antagonists. In J. G. Hardman & L. E. Limbird (Eds.), *Goodman & Gilman's The pharmacological basis of therapeutics* (9th ed., pp. 521–555). New York: McGraw-Hill.

Reuben, S.S., Connelly, N.R., & Maciolek, H. (1999). Postoperative analgesia with controlled-release oxycodone for outpatient anterior cruciate ligament surgery. *Anesthesia & Analgesia, 88,* 1286–1291.

Richelson, E. (1979). Tricyclic antidepressants and histamine H1 receptors. *Mayo Clinic Proceedings, 54,* 669–674.

Rummans, T.A., Bostwick, J.M., & Clark, M.M. (2000). Maintaining quality of life at the end of life. *Mayo Clinic Proceedings, 75,* 1305–1310.

Ryder, B.G. (1993). *The alpha book on cancer and living.* Alameda, CA: The Alpha Institute.

Sindrup, S.H., & Jensen, T.S. (2000). Pharmacologic treatment of pain in polyneuropathy. *Neurology, 55,* 915–920.

Stahl, S.M. (2000). *Essential psychopharmacology: Neuroscientific basis and practical applications* (2nd ed.). New York: Cambridge University Press.

Swarm, R.A., and Cousins, M.J. (1998). Anesthetic techniques for pain control. In D. Doyle, G.W.C. Hanks & N. MacDonald (Eds.), *Oxford textbook of palliative medicine* (2nd ed., pp. 390–414). New York: Oxford University Press.

Swerdlow, M. (1986). Anticonvulsants in the therapy of neuralgic pain. *The Pain Clinic, 1,* 9–19.

Turner, J.H., Claringbold, P.G., Hetherington, E.L., Sorby, P., & Martindale, A.A. (1989). A phase I study of samarium-153 ethylenediaminetetramethylene phosphonate therapy for disseminated skeletal metastases. *Journal of Clinical Oncology, 7,* 1926–1931.

Twycross, R., & Lack, S. (1984). *Oral morphine in advanced cancer.* Beaconsfield, Bucks, England: Beaconsfield Publishers.

Twycross, R., & Lichter, I. (1998). The terminal phase. In D. Doyle, G.W.C. Hanks, & N. MacDonald (Eds.), *Oxford textbook of palliative medicine* (2nd ed., pp. 977–992). New York: Oxford University Press.

Ventafridda V., & Caraceni, A. (1994). Cancer pain. In P.P. Raj (Ed.), *Current review of pain* (pp. 155–178). Philadelphia: Current Medicine.

Verrill, P. (1989). Sympathetic ganglion lesions. In P.D. Walls & R. Melzac (Eds.), *Textbook of pain* (2nd ed., pp. 773–783). Edinburgh: Churchill Livingstone.

Walsh, T.D. (1985). Common misunderstandings about the use of morphine for chronic pain in advanced cancer. *Ca: A Cancer Journal for Clinicians, 35*(3), 164–169.

Ward, S.E., Goldberg, N., Miller-McCauley, C., Mueller, C., Nolan, A., Pawlik-Plank, D., Robbins, A., Stormoen, D., & Weissman, D.E. (1993). Patient-related barriers to management of cancer pain. *Pain, 53,* 319–324.

World Health Organization. (1986). *Cancer pain relief.* Geneva: World Health Organization.

Section VII

Work Disability and Return to Work

43

Postinjury: The Return-to-Work Challenge

Stephen A. Lawson, M.S., C.R.C., C.I.R.S.

CASE STUDY

"I don't give a damn about you people ... and I especially don't give a damn about my insurance company. When they took my arm, they took my ability to work ... they took everything. Everything!"

When I first met Gary, I found a man who had incurred a very serious work injury. Gary had suffered two levels of ruptured discs and damage to the nerves of the dominant hand/arm. In addition, the C-spine laminectomy surgical procedure caused more damage to his dominant side and left Gary with severe pain. Unfortunately, Gary developed degenerative disc disease with scarring and spondylolisthesis at the injury site. In essence, he lost practically all function, his ability to lift, his fine finger dexterity, and his ability to perform anything but extremely limited range of motion with his dominant arm/hand. As a result of the loss of function, Gary also developed a partially frozen shoulder, adding to the pain and frustration with which he was already trying to cope.

Perhaps more disabling, though, was Gary's response, emotionally and psychologically, to his injury. Gary had been a plumber for 15 years and took tremendous pride in his work. He also established his work identity as a plumber, and this was the only thing that he desired to do in life, or, for that matter, saw himself doing throughout the course of his life. Gary once informed me in a counseling session, "I've always shown my family that I love them by working so hard. Before my injury, I worked 12 to 15 hours a day, 6 days a week, and that's how I told my family that I loved them."

Gary is a strapping six-footer whose well-muscled arms come from a lifetime of hard, physical labor. He possesses a high school diploma with no further education.

His work has been strictly in the areas of residential, commercial, and industrial plumbing, and he worked his way up at certain jobs performing supervision and job estimating. Therefore, when his dominant arm became affected because of the cervical injury, Gary was left totally unable to perform his usual and customary work as a plumber. It should also be mentioned that Gary was in constant moderate to severe pain at rest, and he was having an extremely difficult time coping with all the losses he had incurred.

Another complication is that Gary did not look injured whatsoever (unseen disability), yet Gary was very seriously impaired. His friends and acquaintances oftentimes would say, "You look pretty good, Gary," but, in fact, Gary was not well at all. Had he experienced a disability others could see, perhaps a different social phenomenon would have occurred. That is usually the case.

This contributed to Gary's denial and "as-if" behavior. The latter refers to when individuals act "as if" they are able-bodied with no limitations and generally wind up hurting themselves all the more. This is a form of denial and results in working or playing outside their physical limitations. This is generally a fairly common phenomenon in the early stages of disablement and is especially pervasive in men who are gainfully employed and derive much of their masculinity from work.

Upon background examination, I learned that Gary was of Native American descent and had lived in a number of foster homes until he ran away at age 14 to live on his own. His home life had consisted of an alcoholic mother and a father who abandoned him. Gary was the oldest of several children, and from an early age, he took it upon himself to be responsible for the entire family. To him, working was the way he expressed his self-worth and

0-8493-0926-3/02/$0.00+$1.50
© 2002 by CRC Press LLC

validated his existence and manhood. Gary's full range of psychological and emotional expression was dependent upon his ability to perform work and gain the proper recognition from significant others.

Throughout my years of experience as a vocational rehabilitation counselor, Gary stands out as an individual to whom I feel particularly close. By the same token, Gary was certainly one of the most challenging clients I have ever had.

Postinjury, Gary began to isolate himself from his "work friends" and began an emotional landslide that culminated in extreme marital problems and a fragmented relationship with his children. As he says in his soft Georgia drawl, "I felt as bad as a sore-tailed cat in a room full of rocking chairs."

Eventually, Gary's emotional and physical pain led him to the point where he did not care about anyone, including himself, and this led to suicidal and homicidal ideations and actions. In fact, Gary informed me in a counseling session that each day he would put an unloaded rifle barrel in his mouth and pull the trigger to "practice." One day, he actually loaded the rifle and was preparing to kill himself when he had an adverse reaction to the heavy medications he was taking and blacked out. The following day, he woke up in jail, after an apparent scrape with the law. Later, Gary was hospitalized for major depression and substance abuse and was referred to a pain clinic.

These events precipitated the referral to a multidisciplinary program, and Gary was provided with the help that he desperately needed.

OPERATIONAL DIAGNOSIS

Even though Gary's physical condition had stabilized, for the most part, his emotional and psychological life was deteriorating rapidly.

Clinically speaking, Gary became depressed, anxious, suicidal, and even homicidal. Gary basically became a man who lost contact with the world he valued so much and lost touch with himself in the process.

Gary was in constant pain, and this affected his moods, and, as he put it, he found that "sleeping was a luxury." But even more significant was Gary's adverse reaction to his inability to work. As a result, he took his hostility out on everyone, including himself. He literally gave up on life. He was living a nightmare with a life crisis on his hands.

Clinically, I saw Gary as being stuck in the early phases of adjustment to his disability. Yet, there was more going on. Upon closer examination, I began to find a number of complexities in Gary's case that needed sorting out. Fortunately, Gary responded well to the counseling I provided and to the other treatment modalities that made up the multidisciplinary approach.

As an aside, Gary underwent a full course of medical treatment before being referred to a pain management center for approximately 2 years; he was treated at the pain center for another year thereafter. During this time, his vocational rehabilitation case was interrupted on several occasions for prolonged periods. I also testified at a Social Security hearing as an expert witness on his behalf and he was awarded benefits.

Later, he asked to return to me for further vocational rehabilitation evaluation efforts, and because of the very fine efforts provided by the multidisciplinary team, we were able to bring Gary to a physical and mental work-ready status.

Gary's case ultimately became a success; he is now self-employed as a plumber, a rehabilitation plan I recently developed on his behalf. However, in Gary's case, there was no possible way I could have handled all of the complexities involved in his situation, and I desperately needed a multidisciplinary approach. Because of the multidisciplinary approach, his life was saved, and he returned to a productive work effort. (A multidisciplinary team is not needed for every injured person, but can be very beneficial in certain cases.)

There are millions of individuals like Gary who, after the course of injury, have experienced emotional traumatization, accompanied by injury/illness, resulting in low self-esteem, confusion, frustration, depression, loss of meaning and masculinity or femininity, feelings of withdrawal and isolation, and fear. Generally, if an individual is injured to the point that he or she is unable to work because of increased symptomatology, most people will begin an "emotional landslide" unless they are able to find a support group, a professional helper, or they locate someone other than themselves who can assist them in any number of ways to adjust to their disablement and particular life situations.

As practitioners, we should keep in mind that emotional trauma after injury is a very real phenomenon, and if ignored, it can increase pain symptomatology (pain magnification) and also weaken an individual's coping mechanisms. Psychological and physical destruction can occur, such as in Gary's case, but bear in mind that there is hope for salvaging the injured person's remaining assets and maximizing potential through proper case management.

SERVICES RENDERED

- After Gary had completed a full course of medical evaluation and treatment through the normal channels, he was still left with numerous problems and was referred to a pain management center that utilized a multidisciplinary approach. Because all other studies and treatment procedures had failed, a pain center became his last hope. He had new studies performed, such as an

MRI, myelography, and EEG. The studies revealed a second ruptured disc above the prior cervical surgical site, spinal stenosis, cervical spondylolisthesis, and an increase in degenerative disc disease.

- Gary was also referred for psychiatric help. He entered a self-help group with individuals experiencing similar problems with work-related injuries. A Minnesota Multiphasic Inventory revealed major depression and an adjustment disorder. Gary was prescribed tranquilizers and began a program of psychotherapy.
- Gary began a pain management program, which included biofeedback, relaxation, visualization, and transcutaneous electrical nerve stimulation.
- Gary was also referred to an anesthesiologist, and he was evaluated for an implant, although this was not actually performed. He was provided with a program of epidural blocks.
- He began a marriage and family counseling program.
- After completing the pain program, Gary was better able to attempt a return-to-work effort through vocational rehabilitation services. This was ultimately accomplished and he is now a self-employed plumber, is able to control the hours he works and the type of jobs he can physically handle. He farms out work that he cannot perform.

Gary had the courage to press on in a return-to-work effort because of the importance he ascribes to being productive and gainfully employed. What he needed the most was help from people who cared about him, who were proficient in their specialties, and who were truthful with him. After proper treatment and therapy, he took it from there, and now is in control of his life again.

FACTORS OF VOCATIONAL REHABILITATION

Let's examine some factors of vocational rehabilitation that are within the scope and service delivery of the profession. An overview of the profession follows.

HISTORY OF VOCATIONAL REHABILITATION

Vocational rehabilitation had its birth following the Industrial Revolution and World War I (1908 Workman's Comp and 1916 National Defense Act), after society began to realize that injured workers can be productive again when given a chance.

A number of programs on the federal, state, and private levels were developed to assist injured workers in their plight to adjust to their disablements, reach within themselves and identify potential, and then make use of that potential to become productive once again in a work setting.

As such, vocational rehabilitation counselors came on the scene, and vocational rehabilitation became a professional entity within its own specialty.

Over the years, millions of individuals have received help from vocational rehabilitation counselors, and the cost/benefit ratio has certainly proved worthwhile from a monetary view, but more than that, individuals who otherwise probably would have been unable to return to work have experienced and realized their intrinsic right to work with the help of vocational rehabilitation programs.

The basis for vocational rehabilitation programs is twofold:

1. Individuals have an inherent right to work.
2. Individuals have worth, and work opportunities should be extended to them.

Vocational rehabilitation offers professional services to assist injured workers to readapt and restore themselves to a new occupation postinjury that is within their physical and mental limitations. A target goal is to help individuals adjust to their disablement through proper counseling and guidance and to help them adjust to their new self-image and limitations.

Counselors must take on the roles of:

- Counselor
- Teacher
- Medical interpreter
- Legal interpreter
- Friend
- Guide
- Evaluator
- Job specialist
- Negotiator
- Service coordinator
- Case manager

COUNSELING RELATIONSHIP

A trusting relationship between counselor and client generally must occur for maximum benefit to be realized. The counselor will provide insight and help for the injured to struggle, survive, and succeed with the many complexities that stem from disablement. Vocational rehabilitation is a specialty of its own and blends with the medical, psychological, legal, occupational, educational, training, counseling, psychometric, and work-hardening specialties.

The most critical factor in vocational rehabilitation affecting change in the injured worker is the counselor–client rapport. Other strong factors include the skill and expertise of the counselor and the motivation and aptitudes/abilities of the client to work together to develop new opportunities.

EFFECTIVENESS

Vocational rehabilitation has been found to be an extremely valuable benefit for injured individuals. Studies of various vocational rehabilitation programs vary, but all show that the benefit is worthwhile in returning the injured to suitable, gainful employment.

Perhaps not as well publicized or noted is the emotional stabilization provided by the rehabilitation counselor in helping a person to became work ready and self-actualized to maximum potential. This author personally feels that greater appreciation should be focused on this aspect of vocational rehabilitation as a service component. In some cases, rehabilitation success can only be achieved by individuals "working through" their emotional deficits and emotional/psychological adjustment phases before they can reach a work-ready state. One would not expect to construct a building without first laying a foundation, and in many cases, counseling to help the individual adjust to his or her disablement becomes the foundation to the remaining steps of service delivery.

There are cases in which individuals are totally unable to attempt a return-to-work effort because of the severity of their problems. However, these same people may benefit from participating in vocational rehabilitation because of the counseling they receive. Therefore, vocational rehabilitation can still be partially successful without the injured worker returning to work if, in fact, he or she learns to readapt and cope with the imposed limitations of the disablement. Unfortunately, there is a segment of disabled individuals who will never be able to return to either a part-time or full-time occupation because of their limitations, but the same persons may, in fact, benefit from counseling to better cope with their life situation and limitations.

Because of the unpredictable nature of disablement, there are cases in which an individual can adjust to disablement, become work ready via his or her skill level, and yet not enter the work world at that time. However, it is also this author's opinion that in these cases, rehabilitation can still be considered successful as long as the individual is competitive for work even though it comes at a later time.

WORK IS IMPORTANT — THAT'S WHY WE DO IT

WORK MOTIVATIONS

Work can provide healthy therapy in a number of ways. It provides us with a sense of meaning and identity (work identity). When we meet a new person, most often the second question asked after learning the person's name is, "What do you do for a living?" Therefore, we ascribe much of our personal meaning and self-worth to what we do for work.

Societal Expectations

A number of societal expectations and rewards accompany work as well. More often than not, people who do not work or cannot work do not find the same favor as those who do. It also seems that in society as a whole we place a strata of significance and importance on different jobs. For example, an individual who is a professional athlete is generally viewed differently than someone who is a typist. Value has been ascribed by members of society not only to those who do work, but also to those who can work and to the various occupations within the given populace.

Cultural Expectations

Work also has a number of cultural expectations and meanings. Some cultures place tremendous pressure on the individual to perform, either in an educational or work setting or both. Consider the Japanese work ethic. In this culture, failure to achieve could result in ostracization and other levels of rejection.

Conversely, other cultures do not place the same pressure and expectations on the individual to work. Living within this type of culture has a totally different meaning than the former. For example, while on vacation in Mexico, I had to adjust to the slower pace and lesser work demand while there. The point is that our culture can affect how we grow in the work world as we develop over the years.

There are also various types of subcultures that exist within the work world. This means that in order for the individual to be successful and accepted in certain jobs, he or she must conform to the expectations within the subculture pertinent to that occupation.

As an example, the mental picture one draws of an iron worker is certainly different from the mental picture one draws of a florist, and the expectations of each of these individuals to be accepted by their peers within their subcultures of work are different.

Personal Values

As individuals, we place value and meaning on our ability to work and also on the occupation in which we participate.

Work has a way of helping us feel worthwhile, productive, and useful. Work also provides us with the chance to make friends, pass time, face challenges, and assert our opportunity to remain in control. The workplace also provides us with the ability to concentrate on something other than ourselves by way of on-task situations, and gives us a sense of purpose, duty, belonging, and obligation. These factors allow us to benefit from accomplishing job tasks and, hopefully, reap intrinsic and extrinsic reward as a result. Our work personality develops from the above factors.

WORK AS THERAPY

Physical and mental pain can be unusual and confusing phenomena. A fact often overlooked is that physical pain can expose emotional deficits that can overshadow the original physical problem. In essence, a work-related illness/injury known as a disability can evolve into an entire life problem in certain instances.

It has been my experience that doctors typically are not equipped, trained, or otherwise have time to deal with many of the emotional aspects of disablement because their primary focus tends to be on diagnoses, treatment, and seeking a cure within the organic and physical realm. This does not, however, diminish the injured person's need to talk about his or her feelings about the injury, residual limitations, his or her present situation and resulting losses, and hope for the future.

Pain behaviors also can be expressed in a variety of ways, have a number of social and cultural and even moral implications (some see injury as a result of sin) and, at the very least, if severe enough, can wear down even the most stoic person over time.

Pain can magnify as well. It can spread and cause debilitating problems in the most sensitive and precious areas of an individual's life. Over time, mood changes can occur, bitterness and anger can set in, and confusion and frustration with outbursts of anger can become commonplace and wreak havoc on the injured person's family and friends. Injured persons may isolate themselves from relationships, and this will only create more problems.

An individual experiencing unmanaged pain syndromes may find himself or herself feeling as though the pain is "all in their mind." This phenomenon may be perpetuated by treating physicians, family members, friends, and insurance companies to the extent that they feel the problem is in the person's mind. Unfortunately, this may leave the individual feeling as if he or she is "mentally ill," which may not be the case at all. I have seen a number of cases over the years where this phenomenon has occurred and later medical studies revealed a legitimate injury that would validate symptomatology expressed by the person. These individuals may feel ugly, useless, worthless, depressed, unwanted, punished, victimized, withdrawn, angry, fearful, discouraged, unable to sleep restfully, and suicidal or even homicidal. Their behaviors may appear to others as argumentative, unsociable, irresponsible, irrational, hostile, unusually quiet, timid, tired, short-tempered, and with an inability to concentrate.

There is often a significant loss of income, loss of body capabilities to participate in preinjury activities, loss of esteem, loss of personal power, loss of friends, loss of pos-

sessions, loss of resources, and perhaps loss of spouse and family. In essence, these individuals begin to collapse, both in their inside world (psyche) and in their outside world, which may have been supportive of them but no longer is.

It is unfortunate, but oftentimes when individuals drop to the bottom of themselves, they push the outside world away with an ulterior thought that says, "I'm no good. I'm not adequate. You'd be better off without me, and I have no control over myself or over my world any longer."

Indeed, injuries/illnesses can become tragic and devastating, and a disability problem can spread to become a life problem. Therefore, if an injury, mental or physical, occurs, more dynamics within the person's life come into play, and this is where a good rehabilitation counselor can step in and help the person to sort out problems, deal with them emotionally and intellectually, and look for hope to face the challenges. The experienced counselor knows that work can become therapy, as we attach many of our emotions, perceptions of self-worth, and attitudes to how we are at work, and this can help us become better within ourselves.

WORK PERSONALITY

We all know that everyone wears a variety of masks as we have a number of roles we must play, both at home and in the workplace. As such, we develop two different types of personalities. The first type involves our personhood and provides us with our own set of characteristics, traits, identity, and value systems. By the same token, we develop a work personality over our life span with many of the same features, only associated with work.

From a clinical standpoint, whereas the psychiatrist is concerned with rebuilding and restructuring the personality, the vocational rehabilitation counselor is concerned with rebuilding and restructuring the work personality of the client.

Some of the foundational blocks the rehabilitation counselor may wish to explore are worker personality, identity, values, traits, characteristics, and ethics.

In addition, the counselor will consider both the verbal and tested interests of the client to ascertain information of occupational value. Medical information and residual limitations, as well as the individual's work personality type, the labor market, and tested aptitudes and abilities, along with other factors, will be considered in helping the individual and counselor make an intelligent and informed occupational choice.

The vocational exploration phase of developing a plan is critical and instrumental in helping individuals not only to test their own limits, but also to provide them with a vehicle to come to grips with their potential, assuming responsibility, undergoing a new vocational choice, and working their way toward maximizing their potential and earning strength.

A great deal of resource material is available from various publications, computer software, labor market surveys, tests, and the like to help the client and counselor in vocational exploration. Job trials, job analyses, on-site informational interviews, and work tolerance evaluations are also helpful in assessing vocational choices. Many techniques and resources exist to help individuals in their exposure and study of the many jobs in the competitive work world. The counselor will act as a teacher, guide, and advisor to the injured in their job and career planning. Factors considered are the client's limitations, aptitudes and abilities, skill level and general learning ability, the labor market, occupational trends, and the client's interest and work personality type.

Work Adjustment

Work adjustment is a training process designed to help individuals and groups understand the meaning, value, and demands of work and to modify and develop their attitudes, personal characteristics, work behaviors, and functional capacities as required for achieving their optimal level of vocational development. A number of techniques and modalities will work as an adjunct. These consist of job trials or simulated work to help the injured worker make the adjustments necessary to become work ready. Work adjustment takes place not by chance, but rather by careful and professional planning and execution by the counselor and client.

Psychological Adjustment

Considering the many negative effects of disability, it is only natural that the onset of a major disability will often be accompanied by significant emotional reactions (Shontz, 1965). A useful way of describing reactions would be as follows.

Shock

During the first few hours or days after onset of disability, the individual is usually feeling and reacting minimally and may have little awareness of what has happened. This initial phase is called shock and usually involves only muted emotional reactions of the individual.

Realization

Realization is the phase in which some recognition of the reality and seriousness of disability begins to develop. Anxiety, possibly even panic, may be the predominant emotional reaction. This fear is based on anticipation of possible death, critical losses, or unpredictable change. Its extent may or may not be consistent with the seriousness of the disability, but it is important for the counselor to recognize that the client typically feels great fear. Depression and anger also may occasionally appear during this phase.

Defensive Retreat

The anxiety that normally follows onset of disability could easily overwhelm the individual if there were no defense mechanisms available to help him or her cope with the situation. Predominant among these defenses is denial. Such denial may persist or reappear occasionally, long after onset of disability, usually in the form of the individual refusing to make reasonable or realistic allowances for the disability or to accept the limitations imposed.

Acknowledgment

Acknowledgment refers to the phase in which the individual achieves an accurate understanding of the nature of the disability and the imposed limitations. Some persons may demonstrate a very thorough intellectual understanding of the disability prior to the disability, but still not display full appreciation of its implications. Acknowledgment is usually marked by the onset of some degree of depression. The depression that often accompanies recognition of the reality and seriousness of a disability is a very natural grief reaction to the losses that result.

Adaptation

Adaptation is the final phase of adjustment to disability. The term simply means the individual has worked through any major emotional reaction to the disability, is realistic about his or her limitation, and is psychologically ready to make use of his or her potential. This is sometimes referred to as the acceptance phase, but it should be noted that accepting a disability does not imply a willingness to accept a diminished life or to be happy about being disabled. Rather, acceptance or adaptation means learning to live with certain limitations and to make the best use of the remaining assets.

Facilitation of Adjustment to Disability

The emotional reactions and efforts to cope with disability shown by an individual will be determined by a combination of personal characteristics, learning history, and current circumstances. Helping individuals to establish new hope, new goals, and self-actualize to restore their work personality becomes an important factor for readjustment to occur. Helping individuals to resocialize and gain knowledge of how to compete for new employment opportunities, develop new skills, deal with their problems and pain thresholds, and gain insight into their remaining assets allows the injured to develop the confidence and courage they need for restoration to occur.

QUALIFICATIONS OF COUNSELORS

Counseling practitioners within vocational rehabilitation programs generally have a minimum of a bachelor's degree, ranging up to a Ph.D. In most programs, however, this author believes education alone is not enough. A sincere desire to help individuals, the ability to work within a multidisciplinary (or interdisciplinary) approach, to provide guidance and counseling, to politic on behalf of another, to coordinate and synthesize a number of factors, and to develop vocational plans all become pertinent considerations regarding a practitioner's ability and skills.

It is also the author's opinion that counselors should be able to provide counseling to help empower the injured by way of encouragement and hope, to redevelop meaning; recreate simulated work environments and expectations; reactivate such qualities as work ethics, worker values, worker traits, and characteristics; and create a desire to seek out meaningful work effort, as well as to work through crises.

In addition, practitioners should have a strong handle on the medical aspects of disability, a working knowledge of the various stages of adjustment to disability within the injured/ill client, a strong background in and knowledge of psychometric measurement and interest testing, a full range of knowledge about work tolerance evaluation and work-hardening programs, an understanding of the work personality and how to develop and help people make commitments for vocational rehabilitation plans, and a working knowledge of the psychological implications of primary and secondary illness/injury.

Vocational rehabilitation has an interest in many disciplines. It is generally one of the last services offered to an injured person and is best begun after the medical treatment is concluded.

Like other disciplines, vocational rehabilitation is becoming more sophisticated and technological. The human element of interaction and restoration developed between client and counselor is not to be overlooked.

CONCLUSION

In the case study discussed earlier, Gary was successful. He has been able to psychologically and emotionally adjust to his injury and has learned to work within his physical limitations. The price tag for this success was very high and required a number of professional helpers to assist him in the return-to-work process.

Gary still lives with his pain and is fully aware of all of the losses that he has incurred, but as he puts it, "It hurts more when I work, but I feel great."

TABLE 43.1
Steps of Service

Referral	
Initial Evaluation	**Generally Includes**
Benefits review	Vocational counseling
Examination of relevant socioeconomic factors	Vocational exploration
Examination of medical work restrictions	Adjustment to disability
Work history/transferable skills analysis	Counseling recommendations
Testing	**Generally Includes**
Intelligence and aptitude/ability testing	Reading development
Examination of vocational interests	Vocabulary development
Spatial relations assessment	Arithmetic skills inventory
Numerical reasoning assessment	Test review assessment

**Job-Seeking Skills Training/Work Readiness/
Skills Assessment/Job Analysis**

Return to work via

Vocational training	(Same employer)
	Self-employment
Academic training	Modified work
On-the-job training	Alternate work

Postemployment Monitoring (30–60 Days)
Case Closure

It is a very pleasant sight to see Gary when he talks about his work. As he speaks, a slow smile crosses his face: "I have trophies of the work I do everywhere around me. When I drive down a street and see a house or an apartment complex or a laundromat that I worked on — those are my trophies." Gary calls these buildings his trophies because he says that no one can take them away from him. In fact, he signs his plumbing somewhere on every project he finishes.

The change in Gary has been dramatic. This man has gone from an "all or nothing" personality, as his psychiatrist calls it, to a man who is, each day, able to "thank God for the tender mercies," as Gary states softly.

It was a very special moment for me when in one of my last counseling sessions with Gary he reached into his wallet and pulled out a small card with the following scripture, "All as God wills, who wisely heeds to give or to withhold: and knoweth more of all my needs than all my prayers have told."

Gary told me that he had carried this scripture in his wallet for many years, and now he wanted me to have it.

I now carry the scripture in my wallet.

REFERENCE

Shontz, F.C. (1965). Reactions of crisis. *Volta Review, 67,* 364–370.

44

Neuro-Orthopedic Impairment Rating

Gabriel E. Sella, M.D., M.P.H., M.Sc., Ph.D. (Hon. C.), F.A.A.D.E.P.,
S.D.A.B.D.A., F.A.C.F.E., F.A.C.F.M., D.A.A.P.M.

DEFINITIONS: IMPAIRMENT VS. DISABILITY IN THE NEURO-ORTHOPEDIC EVALUATION DOMAIN

The independent medical examiner (IME) deals frequently with injuries or pathologies of the neuro-orthopedic systems. These systems comprise nerves, muscles, tendons, ligaments, fascia, capsules, and bones. These tissues are of primary concern in impairment evaluation. However, the evaluation of these tissues should not exclude the evaluation of other systems within the realm of a comprehensive physical exam and objective investigations.

The *AMA Guides* have established by consensus a number of impairment values that could be granted for permanent injuries under specific sets of conditions. The present chapter is written within the framework of the *AMA Guides* system of granting percentages. In addition to the general description, there is a section on the strengths and limitations of the granting modality according to the author's 10-year experience in the realm of impairment evaluation.

Within the framework of neuro-orthopedic impairment, it should be clear to the reader that this is a medical issue. By definition, impairment is "any loss or abnormality of psychological, or anatomical structure or function." Within the neuro-orthopedic field, this may refer to one or a combination of the following factors described in Table 44.1.

By definition, disability is a legal conclusion related to a permanent impairment. It is a resulting reduction or loss of an ability to perform an activity. Within the

TABLE 44.1
The Neuro-Orthopedic Systems: Structural and Functional Pathology Considered in Impairment Evaluation

Tissue	Structural Dysfunction	Functional Disruption
Nerves: Motor	Hypotonus	Loss of agility, strength, and endurance
Sensory	Loss of sensory fibers (A, δ, C)	Paraesthesia
Muscles	Atrophy	Loss of strength
Tendons	Rupture	Loss of agility
Ligaments	Inflammation	Loss of joint ROM
Fascia	Myofascial scar	Myofascial pain syndrome
Capsules	Capsulitis	Loss of joint ROM
Bursae	Bursitis	Pain, loss of joint ROM
Bones	Fracture	Loss of ROM

neuro-orthopedic framework it refers to a permanent impairment related to one or more tissue components described in Table 44.1. Whereas the IME can grant a given percentage for a permanent loss of a neuro-orthopedic structure/function, the actual final consideration of the relevance of that number in economic, legal, administrative, and other matters is beyond the evaluative aim and lies purely within the realm of the administration and law authorities involved in the case.

0-8493-0926-3/02/$0.00+$1.50
© 2002 by CRC Press LLC

In concrete terms, the loss of the right index finger because of amputation could be granted a permanent percentage value, i.e., 11% WPP (whole person partial impairment). However, the meaning of the loss to a person whose vocation does not rely to a great extent on the right index finger is not the same as that of a surgeon, pianist, or other professional who would have to renounce his or her given profession and no longer be able to practice it. Therefore, whereas the 11% WPP granted by the IME is the same for any person who suffered the amputation of the right index finger, the disability factor granted by the other authorities will depend on a number of factors, not the least of which is the relevance to one's vocation and livelihood.

It is relevant, therefore, for the reader to understand from the beginning the differences between granting an impairment percentage for a permanent injury/body damage and that of disability evaluation and final granting of monies or other social and economic benefits to the sufferer.

BASIC PRINCIPLES OF IMPAIRMENT EVALUATION OF THE NEURO-ORTHOPEDIC SYSTEMS

CAUSATION

The definition of causation within this realm is the factor(s) that are known to have caused the structural or functional impairment. Causation may need to be proven in many cases where there may have been pre-existing or post-existing conditions.

Within this framework, the IME needs to investigate whether the claimant has any history of a pre-existing neuro-orthopedic condition, which should not be confused with that possibly or plausibly created by the accident/injury under claim. The post-existing condition also may be possible/plausible. In other words, the claimant may have had some other injury of a neuro-orthopedic nature after the date of the injury under claim. Therefore, the IME needs to carefully investigate these two possibilities in order to rule out the "purity" of the probable permanent injury as related to the claimed injury factor. At times, the IME has to deal with a multiple causation and is asked to apportion the final impairment(s) to each one of the injury dates.

Therefore, the causation factor is very relevant in the impairment granting process of the neuro-orthopedic systems.

MAXIMUM MEDICAL IMPROVEMENT (MMI)

By definition, this is the factor that allows or rules out the granting of permanent percentage of impairment. There are two types of MMI. The first type refers to an irreversible situation, such as an amputation. The second one refers to a medically or surgically rehabilitative state that was rather constant within the 6 months prior to the evaluation and may be considered rather constant and unchanging within the foreseeable 24 months without major medical/ surgical discoveries. For instance, rehabilitation may improve muscle strength, which can be measured objectively with dynamometry. If it can be demonstrated that the structural damage and the subsequent physical rehabilitation rendered a muscle strength only at 50% of the original or normal for that individual for at least 6 months prior to the evaluation, barring unforeseen medical discoveries, the IME may decide that there is no foreseeable change in the forthcoming 24 months and the loss of muscle strength is permanent at 50% of the original. In this case, the MMI can be granted under those conditions.

PERMANENCY OF INJURY/PATHOLOGY

As described in the paragraph above on MMI, no impairment percentage can be granted if the injury or pathology is not of a permanent nature and has not attained MMI. In other words, an injury, no matter how severe, may not be granted the status of permanency if it is considered to be temporary. For instance, an acute brain concussion, no matter how severe, cannot be granted the status of permanency. The injured party needs to be evaluated in terms of permanency after at least 6 months of treatment. The stability of the post-concussion symptoms, if present, needs to be assessed. Only when those symptoms have been present in a stable form for at least 6 months and foreseeably the forthcoming 24 months could a permanent percentage of impairment be granted.

GRANTING OF PERMANENT PERCENTAGE OF IMPAIRMENT

The granting of the whole person permanent percentage of impairment (%WPP) is a process of clinical evaluation and diagnostic objective investigation that can be done by an experienced IME. The granting takes into consideration the presence of MMI and permanency of impairment.

A number of considerations apply:

In the case of an injury to a limb, if the %WPP is only one, i.e., dependent on only one injury to one tissue or system, the value will have to be transformed from a *partial limb* value to a *whole person* value. In the case of injury to the axial skeleton, the percentage values given in the *AMA Guides* or similar texts are already in the *whole person* format.

When granting a %WPP to a person who already had another permanent injury and percentage of impairment, the new impairment percentage has to be calculated from the vantage point of (100% – previous percentage value). In other words, the primary assumption behind granting percentages of impairment is that the whole person without any permanent injury is considered 100%. Once a permanent percentage of injury is granted, the whole person is no longer 100% but less than that. If the amputation of the right index finger discussed above pre-exists a new amputation, the original value is 11% WPP. The new WPP% has to be calculated from the equation (100 – 11 = 89%). Therefore, should the new amputation have an equal value of 11% from the original 100%, it would only be validated at 10% because it is calculated now as 11/89%. Of course, a new %WPP would have to be calculated from (100 – 11 – 10 = 79%) because the whole-person concept prevails only within 79% that is not permanently damaged in this condition.

The granting of several partial percentages of permanent impairment may be needed in many medical evaluations. If the IME uses the *AMA Guides*, the percentages are to be found in the appropriate sections and the final granting value has to be done in accordance with the mathematical results of the combined values chart.

A further complication occurs in areas that are stipulated as "may be added" or "need to be combined." Herein lies the experience and ongoing education of the IME.

ISSUES OF SYMPTOM MAGNIFICATION AND/OR MALINGERING

Symptom magnification and/ or malingering are prevailing questions in the minds of defense attorneys or defense insurance. They prevail in any system but especially in the neuro-orthopedic systems because of the prevalence of permanent injuries within their realm.

By definition, malingering is a rather unique situation whereby the claimant presents with a number of symptoms stated to be the result of a given injury. When one investigates the causation, one finds there was no such injury event or the claimant was not physically present at the location of an injury. The IME needs to be very careful to rule out somatoform disorders from malingering. In the first case, the claimant may have psychiatric symptoms and, within that realm, truly believes that he/she was injured. An example of this may be a person who watches the news on TV and sees a train accident with several hundred people injured. Believing that he/she was present at the site of the accident and was injured, the person may present to the emergency section of a hospital and give details of symptoms compatible with concussion, etc. The accident may have occurred in Seattle and the somatoform patient may be in New York.

The somatoform condition of actual belief of being injured at the site of the accident may become reality until medical and other investigations determine that there is no causation to the symptoms but they are the offspring of a psychiatric disorder.

True malingering is the situation whereby a person with a clear secondary agenda, most usually monetary or other gain, invents an accident and presents with very well-defined symptoms, asking eventually for a permanent percentage of impairment and disability rights. A good investigation finds out there was no causation. Furthermore, photographic or other documentation prove that the claimant does not have the symptoms/signs of neuro-orthopedic suffering that would allow any believability. For instance, one may see pictures of the sufferer using a walker in the physician's office and playing baseball in a park with friends. In a number of instances, the IME may request a psychiatric evaluation. However, barring the findings of somatoform disorders, the IME may discover true malingering. Within the evaluative process, the IME is alerted to any degree of symptom magnification/malingering/somatoform presentation because the performance of a number of objective tests of neuro-orthopedic evaluation is done in an inconsistent manner. Furthermore, the inconsistency is the trademark of any one or all of these tests.

RATINGS OF PERMANENT PERCENTAGE OF IMPAIRMENT

TEMPORARY VS. PERMANENT IMPAIRMENT/DISABILITY

The definition of temporary vs. permanent neuro-orthopedic impairment has been given above. In terms of the disability concept, it may be relevant to note that the disability grantors need a wider basis of information in their calculation, above and beyond that given by the IME-derived % WPP. That calculation presumes the attainment MMI status of and permanency of structural or functional impairment as defined above. Pain is usually a relevant factor, associated with suffering and described only fractionally in the *AMA Guides*. The disability grantor has to consider pain and suffering, most usually in addition to the % WPP. The monetary award considered by the disability grantors has to take into account not only the parameters described above, but also future costs related to the the neuro-orthopedic impairments. Vocational retraining may be one consideration of disability granting. A retrained individual would by definition be far less dependent on society, family, or employer.

PERMANENCY OF ANATOMIC (NEURO-OSTHEOPATHIC) PATHOLOGY

The permanency of pathology beyond the foreseeable 24 months past the evaluation period is the *sine qua non* of impairment granting. The IME needs to be careful to report that if medical progress is made within 24 months and what appears to be a permanent impairment reduced or annulled related to new medical discoveries/treatments, the percentage granted may not apply under such new circumstances.

PERMANENCY OF FUNCTIONAL NEURO-ORTHOPEDIC PATHOLOGY

The principle of application of new medical treatment with regard to functional neuro-orthopedic pathology applies as above. However, the functional pathology of these two systems is usually of such amplitude that it is relevant to consider increasing the overall percentage value consensually described in the *AMA Guides*. Part of this consideration is related to the subject of chronic pain as discussed in the *Guides*. The main premise is that of dysfunctional, depression-related chronic pain. In reality, the *Guides* need to consider more the corollary relationship between pain of neuro-orthopedic origin and difficulty with accomplishing activities of daily living (ADLs) as well as vocation-related activities.

PERMANENCY OF EFFECTS ON THE ABILITY TO PERFORM ADLs

Impairment of the neuro-orthopedic systems may affect most ADLs as described in any text. This holds true for the neurologic system including CNS activities involved in mentation, sensory and motor function, as well as ANS activities involved in emotion and autonomic functions. The osteopathic system is, of course, involved directly in any motion activity. This includes standing, sitting, walking, squating, reaching, bending, twisting, leaning, and hand functions. The functional pathologies of both systems affect self-care, communication, travel, sexual functions, sleep, and social and recreational activities. Again, chronic pain related to either system pathology may be an underlying reality in the overall ADL accomplishment dysfunction.

NEURO-ORTHOPEDIC-RELATED VOCATIONAL CONSIDERATIONS

1. Ability to perform the main task of a given vocation
2. The concept of reasonable accommodations
3. The concept of undue hardship

The neuro-orthopedic systems contribute to all vocational tasks. The Americans with Disabilities Act stipulates the definitions of "the main task" of a given vocation as compared to secondary tasks. It also defines the concepts of "reasonable accommodations" and "undue hardship."

Within the context of the neuro-orthopedic systems, the individual needs to be rehabilitated in order to perform mentally or physically demanding acts required at a professional level within the work environment. Thus, a person with sequalae of motor dysfunction may be able to return to work to do tasks of a sedentary nature or light duty activities. It also is possible to enact *reasonable accommodations*, such as new equipment that does the actual heavy task while the injured person works on it by controlling buttons, etc. The actual heavy task is still accomplished by the person with permanent neurologic disability; however, it is done so with the help of additional equipment.

Permanent orthopedic impairment may result in the need for prosthetic equipment. Many times, the working environment can be modified to allow for the use of prostheses enabling walking at a slower speed, etc. Thus, the possibility of reasonable accommodations for orthopedic disability may return many people injured in the course of their vocation to work, even if a modified environment is necessary.

Work reality may be such that it is not possible to accommodate for disability. When that is demonstrated by the principle of undue hardship, the ADA parameter of reasonable accommodations may not apply. An example is a work environment where a worker may need to walk up and down one to two flights of stairs several times every hour every day. If the structure of the building and the stairs is such that electric stairways or an elevator cannot be installed or that the cost of such installation could not be a reasonably supported or affordable business expense, it would be considered an undue hardship.

In that case, the neuro-orthopedic pathology would be considered as incompatible with the working environment. New vocational training may be offered to the disabled individual for other types of vocation or opportunity.

THE NEURO-ORTHOPEDIC SYSTEMS AND INSURANCE ISSUES

There are several work-related insurance categories. A partial list includes the social security system, workers compensation systems, federal or state insurances, and finally, private insurance companies with policies related to disability.

Each of the entities mentioned above is regulated by a variety of rules and regulations.

In general, though, they consider remuneration for disability either under an all or none or as a partial system. Furthermore, what may be the rule for one level of insurance, may be the exception or exclusion for another.

In terms of the neuro-orthopedic systems, it is very important for the IME to consider the final impairment conclusions within the legal and regulations framework of the claim.

A careful consideration may help both the needs of the injured claimant and those of the insurance entity, which only considers the claim in light of contractual obligations and the legal requirements.

STEPS OF THE NEURO-ORTHOPEDIC SYSTEMS EVALUATION

MEDICAL HISTORY

1. The medical history needs to be focused on the injury under claim. However, the IME must inquire about and report any other relevant histories. These include prior work-related neuro-orthopedic or other injuries, prior non-work conditions, as well as any other current injuries or diseases.
2. General medical history with special relevance to pre-existing conditions and especially conditions related to the neuro-orthopedic systems must be taken. The general medical history allows the IME to place any neuro-orthopedic system injury/ pathology within the framework of the overall body function. It is very relevant to take an accurate medical history, which can be done effectively and reliably with the use of a comprehensive general health questionnaire. Of special relevance is any prior or concurrent history of pathology affecting the neuro-orthopedic systems. Pre-existing conditions are a relevant factor in terms of the intensity and/or frequency of the symptoms and/or signs presented within the context of the neuro-orthopedic systems pathology under claim.
3. Focus on the causation vs. association with symptoms. The topic of causation has been described above. The IME needs to take a good history of the injury- or disease-causing event in order to rule out any association or lack of association of such event with the neuro-orthopedic presentation under claim. It is more likely than not that a severe fracture of the back, witnessed and well documented, may produce chronic low back pain. It is not likely that the advent of a pneumonia within 2 months of the actual injury would contribute such pain. Just because pathology occurs it does not mean that it is causal or associated with a presentation for permanent impairment evaluation in front of the IME.
4. There should be compatibility and consistency of the medical history with the course

of treatment and current symptomatic presentation. Whereas the causation is the primary event in the course of a neuro-orthopedic pathology, the diagnostic follow-up and rehabilitation treatment are the most relevant subsequent events. One should not wonder why a neuro-orthopedic dysfunction does not heal in time if not treated. This currently is affecting the diagnosing of myofascial pain syndrome months or years after the injurious event. The claimant may suffer from classic trigger-point related pains and dysfunctions and yet the insurance authorities question why the person is not healed. Can one heal necessarily without adequate diagnostic recognition and treatment?

Therefore, the IME needs to follow closely the chronologic course of the diagnostic work-up and treatment. If there was failure in either of them, the claimant may suffer from pathology related to that failure to a relative extent. At times, because of this, the IME may not be able to grant MMI or permanent percentage at the time of the evaluation and may need to suggest appropriate diagnostic and treatment follow-up for a period of 6 to 12 months before a new and final evaluation.

EXAMINEE'S PERCEPTION OF THE NEURO-ORTHOPEDIC CONDITION UNDER CLAIM

It is relevant for the IME to investigate the examinee's perception of the condition and, related to this, the motivation for further improvement. At times, people may be influenced by the medical authorities in an iatrogenic sense and believe that their overall condition is far worse than it actually is. This perception needs to be investigated or ruled out by the IME.

Self-Perceived Functional Limitations

The IME needs to provide a questionnaire including all regular ADLs. Of special relevance are the ADLs related to the neuro-orthopedic systems, such as described above. The ability to fulfill such ADLs on a regular basis is highly relevant in determining the %WPP by the IME and especially the extent of disability by the administrative/legal bodies that grant such disability and monetary and other awards.

Perceived Pain/Discomfort

Pain is possibly the single most relevant factor in determining the ability and will to fulfill ADLs as well as vocational activities. The intensity and frequency of the neuro-orthopedic-related pain must be investigated by the IME. A more complete discussion of this subject is found in Chapter 84 of this text. Suffice it to say that the IME needs to use a "pain grid" which compares and correlates the neuro-orthopedic pain with the ability to function in terms of accomplishment of ADLs.

Perceived Effect on Ability to Achieve/Accomplish the Normal ADLs

The IME may ask about this subject as described above. It may be of relevance to utilize/ask for a functional capacities examination, usually performed by specialized physical therapists. It is not possible most of the time to assess in a consistent manner the perceived and actual abilities of a claimant to perform ADLs in the office. Therefore, the claimant's history, examiner's observations and, when necessary, the functional capacity exam may confirm the extent of the perceived vs. actual ability to perform ADLs.

Self-Perceived Emotional Status and Stress Level

A number of neuro-psychological tests may fit a variety of neuro-orthopedic systems pathologies. The tests may work in terms of ruling out perception of stress and negative emotions (anxiety/depression) vs. actual test scores. More often than not, the IME may need to rely on a neuropsychologist or psychiatrist to assess the emotional component related to post-traumatic conditions of the neuro-orthopedic systems. It is important to note that this may grant further permanent percentage of impairment in cases documented to warrant such additional percentage by psychiatrists or neuropsychologists.

REVIEW OF SYSTEMS

A comprehensive review of systems allows the IME to place the neuro-orthopedic pathology within the overall systematic review. In addition to the general review, one may utilize more specialized questionnaires to rule out the extent of the neuro-orthopedic dysfunction in terms of the claimant's overall pathology.

ASSESSMENT OF CURRENT NEURO-ORTHOPEDIC CLINICAL PATHOLOGY AND STATUS

The IME needs to perform a comprehensive physical examination. If the IME is a specialist who no longer performs such a comprehensive examination, one should state that and refer the claimant to an IME who can do it.

Above and beyond the comprehensive examination, the IME needs to perform a very detailed neurologic and/or orthopedic evaluation such as required by the pathology under claim. In addition to the physical examination, one usually must perform a number of appropriate objective tests.

More often than not, the IME would have available at the time of the examination previous evaluations or investigations done by the treating physicians and/or by prior IMEs. It is very important for the IME to note if there are chronologic symptomatic/signs changes in the claimant's presentation and especially if such changes became stable within the 6-month period prior to the evaluation. This allows for the granting of MMI to all or part of the presentation.

There are times, however, when the IME notices significant discrepancies between the symptomatic presentation, including chronology between one or more previous examinations. The same may apply to the results obtained at different times on objective tests, which creates questions of further pathology unrelated to the event under claim or symptom magnification, malingering, or functional overlay. These issues need to be resolved in terms of clear notification in the examination report.

One of the most relevant factors for the IME to present in the report is consistency of presentation of neuro-orthopedic symptoms/signs within the chronological framework. The question of consistency is the "most consistent question" asked by the opposing counsel or insurance authorities. It is fraudulent for a person to fake symptoms and gain monetarily and otherwise from it. Therefore, the IME needs to rule out this factor not only in the previous exams but also through the objective testing done from the day of injury to the day of the present evaluation.

The neuro-orthopedic physical examination should include the following.

A number of body expressions related to pain or other emotions needed to be observed during the examination. Was any body expression found frequently?

Did the examinee exhibit any behavioral signs of pain or other suffering?

Testing for behavioral consistency vs. symptoms magnification. The Waddell signs were not originally meant to define symptom magnification but can be used within this context when necessary. Did the eight Waddell signs show any overt inconsistency, compatible with the definition of symptom magnification?

Hoover test. Was the normal response of straight leg raising in the supine position observed?

Trochanter pressure test. Was there any low back pain while pressing inward on both greater trochanters?

Were the reflexes normal or abnormal? Name the abnormal reflexes. (See Table 44.2.)

The Babinski reflex is an abnormal reflex. Was the Babinski negative bilaterally?

Posture and gait are assessed with the Romberg and Tandem walk (eyes opened and closed) tests.

Were the Romberg and Tandem walks positive and nondirectional, positive, or negative?

TABLE 44.2
Deep Tendon Reflexes (DTR)

DTR ×3	Brachialis	Radialis	Tricipital	Patellar	Achilles
Right					
Left					

Toe walking, heel walking, everted and inverted foot walking, and squatting represent the testing for L4-L5 roots. Were toe walking, heel walking, everted and inverted foot walking on either foot, squatting, standing from a squatting position, and hopping normal and not antalgic?

Cranial nerves. Nerves I through XII have to be tested bilaterally for the motor and sensory (where applicable) components.

CN I: Olfactory. Does the examinee present with an intact sense of smell for coffee, vinegar, musk, and lemon juice?

CN II: Optic. Does the examinee present with intact vision in both eyes (20/20) without correction? Does the examinee need correction on either eye? What are the Snellen testing results with/without correction? Does the examinee present with intact color vision for green and red, yellow and blue? Does the examinee present with photophobia or blurriness of vision during the examination?

CN III, IV, and VI: Oculomotor (Motor and Parasympathetic), Trochlear, Abducens. Does the examinee present with normal extra-ocular muscle motion with no lateralization, normal ciliary and iris sphincter muscles?

CN V: Trigeminal Motor. Does the examinee present with normal masticatory ability? Sensory. Does the examinee present with normal tactile sensation to the facial skin and trigeminal mucosa of the nose and mouth?

CN VII: Facial, Motor/Parasympathetic. Does the examinee present with normal facial expression, with no asymmetry or lateralization, normal lacrimation and mucous membranes of the mouth and nose, and normal sublingual and submandibular salivation? Sensory. Does the examinee present with normal tactile sensation to the external ear and auditory canal? Does the examinee present with normal taste sensation to the anterior two thirds of the tongue?

CN VIII: Vestibulo-Cochlear, Vestibular N. Does the examinee present with normal equilibrium on Rhomberg and Tandem walks with the eyes opened and closed? Cochlear N. Does the examinee present with normal hearing ability regarding the spoken voice? Does the examinee present with hypoacusia with regard to the spoken voice?

CN IX: Glossopharyngeal Motor. Does the examinee present with normal pharyngeal function, with no asymmetry or lateralization? Parasympathetic. Does the examinee present with normal parotid gland salivation, with no asymmetry or lateralization? Sensory. Does the examinee present with normal tactile and taste sensation to the posterior one third of the tongue?

CN X: Vagus Motor. Does the examinee present with normal pharyngeal and laryngeal function, with no asymmetry or lateralization? Sensory. Does the examinee present with normal tactile sensation to the auditory canal?

CN XI: Accessory. Does the examinee present with normal laryngeal function, with no asymmetry or lateralization? Does the examinee present with normal sternocleidomastoid and trapezius functions, with no asymmetry or lateralization of shoulder shrugging?

CN XII: Hypoglossal. Does the examinee present with normal tongue movements, with no asymmetry or lateralization?

Testing of the brachial plexus and the lumbosacral plexus. The testing needs to be done for each salient nerve which represents more than one particular root while being aware that there is no nerve that comes from only one root.

Was there any brachial plexus root or trunk abnormality?

Was there any brachial plexus nerve motor or sensory abnormality?

Was there any lumbosacral plexus abnormality?

Was there any lumbosacral nerve motor or sensory abnormality?

Cerebellar Function. The finger-to-nose-to-hammer test denotes normal or abnormal cerebellar function. What was the examinee's "finger-to-nose-to-hammer" response? Does the examinee present with normal sensation to light touch, pinwheel, heat, cold, vibration, proprioception, topognosis, and stereognosis as well as pain with no asymmetry or lateralization on head and neck, trunk and limbs? Is there any evidence of focused anesthesia, hypoesthesia, hyperesthesia, or dysesthesia?

Normal range of two-point discrimination on different parts of the body. Does the examinee show any two-point discrimination loss?

Joint position and vibratory loss denote probable compression of peripheral nerves or nerve roots. Was there any joint position or vibratory loss found?

Vibration. Vibratory sense to a tuning fork #256 should be normal bilaterally on the forehead, elbows, wrists, knees, ankles, and first toe. Was the vibratory sense normal?

Positional sense. A normal position sense is tested on the ability to perceive passive extension and flexion on the big toe bilaterally. Did the examinee present with normal, equivocal, or abnormal extension and flexion recognition on the big toe bilaterally?

Speech. Did the examinee present with expressive aphasia or speech impairment? Could the speech be understood and sustained within normal limits? Did the examinee have a good vocabulary and command of language?

Autonomic Nervous System. Vasomotor changes. Did the examinee present with any vasomotor changes such as abnormal skin temperature and edema?

Sweat changes. Did the examinee present with any area of hypohydrosis, anhydrosis, or hyperhydrosis?

Trophic changes. Did the examinee present with abnormality of the skin such as indentations, lack of elasticity, unusual smoothness or shine? Did the finger nails present clubbing, transverse stripes, brittleness, or increased thickness? Did the skin present alopecia or hypertrichosis?

This chapter does not discuss traumatic brain injury affecting any component of the brain.

Mentation. The mental status examination may be simple or complex according to the physical needs and symptomatic presentation of any changes of mentation. A summary of the commonly utilized parameters of the mental status exam is given below.

a. Orientation. Did the examinee present with any orientation problems with regard to time, space, and person?

b. Memory. Did the examinee present with any recent or remote memory loss events?

c. Ability to concentrate. Did the examinee present with any inability to concentrate and maintain attention?

d. Ability to communicate. Did the examinee present with any problems of communication with the examiner and assistant?

e. Appearance. Did the examinee appear anxious or distressed about the evaluation?

f. Restriction of activities of daily living. The examinee needs to be questioned on the subject with relation to the ADLs described below. There may be need to investigate further with regard to other ADLs as necessary.

i. Self-care and personal hygiene. Is there any deficiency in the ability to fulfill the ADLs related to self-care, dressing/undressing, and personal hygiene?

ii. Communication. Is there any deficiency in the ability to fulfill the ADLs related to verbal or written communication? Is there any deficiency in the ability to fulfill the ADLs related to the ability to use a telephone or a computer for communication?

iii. Normal living postures. Is there any deficiency in the ability to fulfill the ADLs related to normal living postures including recumbency, sitting, reclining, standing, bending, twisting, pushing, pulling, lifting, and carrying?

iv. Ambulation. Is there any deficiency in the ability to fulfill the ADLs related to walking including climbing and descending stairs?

v. Travel. Is there any deficiency in the ability to fulfill the ADLs related to travel including driving or getting into and out a public transportation vehicle?

vi. Sexual functions. Is there any deficiency in the ability to fulfill the ADLs related to sexual functions?

vii. Sleep. Is there any deficiency in the ability to fulfill the ADLs related to falling asleep, staying asleep, or waking up? Is there any history of sleep apnea or narcolepsy?

viii. Social and recreational activities. Is there any deficiency in the ability to fulfill the ADLs related to social and recreational activities on an individual or family basis?

Is intellectual functioning at the estimated level compatible with the examinee's education level and age?

TABLE 44.3
Examination of the Skeletal Structures

Bones	Normal	Normal	Hypertrophy	Hypertrophy	Ankylosis	Ankylosis
	Right	Left	Right	Left	Right	Left
Cranium					N/A	N/A
Cervical column						
Thoracic column						
Lumbar column						
Sacrum						
Coccyx						
Thoracic cage						
Ilium						
Ischium						
Pubis						
Scapula						
Clavicle						
Humerus						
Radius						
Ulna						
Metacarpals						
Phalanges						
Femur						
Tibia						
Ankle						
Metatarsals						
Toe phalanges						

Personal financial affairs. Are there grounds to believe that the examinee cannot manage personal financial affairs?

Zung testing for anxiety is a useful test. If done, does it reveal a normal score or one that indicates minimal to moderate anxiety/moderate to high anxiety?

Musculo-skeletal testing (Table 44.3).

    a. Body type. Is the examinee of ectomorphic, mesomorphic, endomorphic, or mixed body type? Is the body well proportioned?

    b. Gait. Does the examinee present with an abnormal gait for body size, age, and sex? Are there any complaints of lower back and limb antalgia?

    c. Two scales, double weighing. Double scale weighing is a methodology for identifying and ruling out unilateral postural defects. It is especially useful in lower limb pain/dysfunction as well as in low back and hip pain/dysfunction. The method can also be used to rule out symptom magnification in presentations of these body sections. The examinee is weighed four times on identical scales in order to determine any significant inequality of weight placement. The results are indicated in Table 44.4. The

TABLE 44.4
Double Weighing Method for Static Gait

Scale (lbs)	Weight Trial I	Weight Trial II	Weight Trial III	Weight Trial IV	Average
Right Foot					
Left Foot					

results indicate that the examinee places % of his weight on the left foot and % of his weight on the right foot. Is there a significant trend in unilateral weight placement, i.e., > 10% placement on one foot vs. the other?

    i. Antalgia. Does the examinee exhibit an antalgic gait characterized by a short stance phase on the painful side? If the gait is not antalgic, does it exhibit a stance phase approx. 60% of the time and a swing phase approx. 40% of the time?

    ii. Lower extremities size. Are the lower limbs equal and proportional to the body size? (See Table 44.5.)

    iii. Short leg gait. Is one lower limb shorter than the other by > 2 cm? Does the gait

TABLE 44.5
Circumferences

Limbs (cm)	Right	Left		Right	Left
Arm			Thigh		
Elbow			Knees		
Forearm			Calves		
Wrists			Ankles		
Hands across			Leg		
MP joints			length		

Joint	Right	Left	Joint	Right	Left
PIP 1			DIP 1		
PIP 2			DIP 2		
PIP 3			DIP 3		
PIP 4			DIP 4		
PIP 5			DIP 5		

TABLE 44.6
Back Length Standing and Flexed

Back (cm)	Level	Normal	Examinee
Straight			
Flexed	C7–S5		
Maximal	C7–T12	2.5	
Flexion	T12–S5	7.5	

Note: Normal extension is approx. 10 cm with spine flexion.

show signs of oblique pelvic and flexion deformity on either knee?

    iv. Coxalgia. Does the examinee complain of, or exhibit, any pain or abnormal stance related to the coccyx?

    v. Coxalgic gait. Does the examinee exhibit an antalgic gait with a lurch toward the painful hip?

    vi. Metatarsalgia. Does the examinee complain of, or exhibit, any pain or abnormal stance related to the forefeet?

    vii. Metatarsalgic gait. Does the examinee attempt to avoid bearing weight on the painful forefoot?

Standing position

    a. Posture. Does postural examination show that the examinee presents with cervical lordosis, scoliosis, dorsal kyphosis, or lumbar lordosis? Are the posterior superior iliac spines proportional? Is the back excursion normal with mild laxity of the sacrum?

    b. Alignment of the lower extremities. Does the examinee present with any alignment deformities of the lower limbs? Which alignment deformities are observed for flexion deformity of knees, genu varum, genu valgum?

    c. Ankles and feet position. Does the examinee present with any alignment deformities of the feet? Does the position of ankles and feet show varus/valgus, heels, flat feet, inversion/eversion of the feet?

    d. Back motion. Does the examinee present with normal back motion for body size, age, and sex? Is there any complaint of pain or ankylosis on the motions of flexion, extension, and lateral rotation? (See Table 44.6.)

    e. Range of motion of back. Does the examinee present with a normal range of motion of the back for body size, age, and sex? The lumbosacral column ROM examination needs to be done with inclinometry, as per protocol.

Seated position

    a. Head and neck motion. Does the examinee present with a normal range of motion of the neck for body size, age, and sex? Are the head and neck motions restricted in flexion, extension, lateral bend to the right, left, rotation to the right or left, or restricted by ankylosis? The cervical column examination done with inclinometry is presented below.

    b. Motion of the thoracolumbar spine. Is the thoraco-lumbar spine motion with the pelvis fixed observed to be within normal limits? Does the motion of the thoraco-lumbar spine in the seated position with the pelvis fixed show rounding, straightening of the back, lateral flexion or rotation abnormalities?

    c. Temporomandibular joints. Does palpation and examination of the lower jaw motion show a normal aperture with the mouth fully open? Is there any crepitus or asymmetry of mouth aperture?

Upper extremities

    a. Shoulders. Does the examinee present with a normal contour and range of motion of the shoulders for the body size, age, and sex?

    b. Contour. Does the examinee present with a normal contour of both shoulders and no asymmetry? Is there any deltoid atrophy on either side? Is there any tissue swelling? (See Table 44.5.)

    c. Range of motion. The shoulder ROM examination needs to be done with inclinometry, as per protocol.

    d. Glenohumeral joint motion. Is there restriction of the glenohumeral joint motion on either shoulder? Is there ankylosis of either glenohumeral joint?

e. Elbows. Does the examinee present with a normal contour and range of motion of the elbows for the body size, age, and sex?

f. Inspection. Do the elbows appear equal and normal on inspection? Does either elbow appear swollen or ankylosed?

g. Palpation. Is there any olecranon bursitis or synovitis noted on palpation of either elbow? Are there any subcutaneous nodules and tophi noted in the olecranon bursa or over the extensor surfaces of the elbows?

h. Range of motion. The elbow ROM examination needs to be done with inclinometry, as per protocol.

Wrists and hands. Does the examinee present with a normal contour and range of motion of the wrists and hands for the body size, age, and sex? (See Table 44.5.)

a. Inspection. Does inspection of the wrists and hands find any deformities or edema? Does inspection and palpation of the wrist find any deformities of the metacarpal phalangeal (MCP), proximal interphalangeal (PIP), and the distal interphalangeal (DIP) joints of the fingers and carpometacarpal (CMC), MCP and interphalangeal (IP) joints of thumbs? Were there any deformities such as boutonniere, swan neck, or radial or ulnar deviation noted on either wrist?

b. Soft tissue swelling. Did the dorsum of either wrist distal to the ulna and over the radiocarpal joint show any soft tissue swelling? Was any soft tissue swelling (volar synovitis) noted on the palmar surface? Was thenar atrophy noted on either palmar area?

c. Finger joints. Did inspection and palpation of the finger joints reveal soft tissue swelling, capsular thickening, or bony enlargement?

d. Fists. By definition a fist is described as 100% when all fingers reach the palm and the thumb reaches and closes over the fingers. Was the examinee able to form both fists at 100%?

e. Range of motion. The range of motion of the wrist, hand and fingers has to be done with goniometry, as per protocol.

f. Grip. Gripometer testing. Is the examinee left/right hand dominant? Was the ability to grasp and manipulate with each hand within normal limits? The strengths of the grip and pinch are assessed in Table 44.7 using the highest of three readings.

g. Pronation and supination. Both are considered as combined functions of the elbow and

TABLE 44.7
Grip and Pinch Strength

Hand Grip (kg)	Right	Left	Finger Pinch (lbs)	Right	Left
1 cm			Key		
3 cm			Thumb and index		
5 cm			Thumb and fifth digit		

TABLE 44.8
Anthropometry

Chest and Abdomen	Measurement (cm)
Across nipples	
Maximum inspiration	
Maximum expiration	
Across umbilicus	

wrists. Did the examinee show normal pronation and supination?

h. Neck and chest inspection. Does the examinee present with a normal contour of the neck and chest for body size, age, and sex? Were the sternoclavicular joints noted to be equal and symmetrical? The measurements of the chest expansion are described in Table 44.8. By definition, normal expansion at the nipple line is above 4 cm in deep inspiration.

Prone and supine positions

a. Knees alignment. Was the alignment compared to that noted on weight bearing different or abnormal?

b. Back. Did inspection and palpation of the back reveal normal paraspinal musculature with the dorsal spines not visible from the cervical to the sacral area? Was kyphosis, scoliosis, or abnormal lumbar lordosis noted? Were there any sudomotor changes in the affected area?

c. Traction maneuvers. Does any straight leg raising maneuver show any symptoms? (See Table 44.9.)

TABLE 44.9
Straight Leg Raising

Straight Leg Raising	Normal°	Right°	Left°
Standing	90		
Sitting	90		
Supine	90		

d. The Gaenslen maneuver. This maneuver detects sacroiliac (SI) joint inflammation. Did the examinee have any pain in the SI joint ipsilateral to the extended hip? Was SI joint inflammation diagnosed with this maneuver?

Hips. Does the examinee present with a normal contour and range of motion of the hips for body size, age, and sex? Does internal and external rotation of the hip joint in extension have a normal range of motion? Do abduction and adduction of the hips in extension have a normal range of motion? Does flexion of the hips have a normal range of motion when the knees are flexed and the hips are carried toward the chest? Is extension of the hips normal (–30°) with the examinee in prone position? The hip ROM examination needs to be done with inclinometry, as per protocol.

Leg lengths measurements. Are the leg lengths as measured from the umbilicus to the medial malleolus found to be equal? Are any joint contractures are present?

Knees. Does the examinee present with a normal contour and range of motion of the knees for body size, age, and sex? Are the patellar position and mobility found to be normal on inspection and palpation bilaterally? Could soft tissue swelling be observed on bimanual evaluation? Was a patellar click sign indicative of intra-articular fluid demonstrated on either knee? Was a bulge sign indicative of a small amount of effusion demonstrated on either knee? Is the popliteal area normal? Is a synovial cyst present on sitting or standing? Is the knee stability demonstrated to be normal bilaterally on stressing the medial and lateral collateral ligament? Is the anteroposterior stability of both knees assessed to be intact by the maneuver of the drawer sign? The knee ROM examination needs to be done with inclinometry, as per protocol.

a. Maneuvers for medial and lateral meniscus testing. Did the testing show negative findings bilaterally of the medial/lateral meniscus tear clinically on either knee?

Ankles and feet. Does the examinee present with a normal contour and range of motion of the ankles and feet for body size, age, and sex? Is there any synovial soft tissue swelling noted on either ankle? Was subtalar motion, which assesses inversion and eversion of the foot, found to be 100% normal? The ankle ROM examination needs to be done with inclinometry, as per protocol.

Toes. Did inspection and palpation of the toes note any deformities of alignment or soft tissue swelling? Were any of the following toe deformities noted: hammer toes, claw toes, hallux valgus?

Joints. Did inspection and palpation of all joints demonstrate any abnormality at rest or in motion? Did inspection and palpation of all joints at rest or in motion show any swelling, tenderness, temperature and color changes over any joint with or without crepitation and deformity? Was any joint tenderness noted? Are warmth and erythema over any joint noted? Is stress pain produced on any joint at any degree of motion from extension? Is crepitation of any joint palpable and audible at rest and in motion? Is any deformity of any joint noted? Is it assessed to be caused by bony enlargement/subluxation/and ankylosis in a normal or abnormal position? Extra-articular, fibromyalgia, and myofascial testing are not discussed in this chapter.

Manual muscle testing. Neck, back, and limbs muscle testing is done actively. It is suggested that passive movements testing should be done only with the expressed permission of the evaluee. The testing is classically scored on a 0-to-5 scale with 5 showing good strength and 0 showing no ability whatsoever to resist any motion.

OBJECTIVE TESTING

Objective testing of the neuro-orthopedic systems may be done with a variety of equipment either during the evaluation and/or referred outside the office. Whatever methodology is utilized, it has to follow statistical protocol rules whereby the test in question is repeated at least five times with resting intervals in order to allow the computation of appropriate averages, standard deviations, and coefficients of variation.

Any methodology needs to be done in a standardized manner so that the IME can compare the results done in previous testing proceed with the same protocol if any testing is done during the evaluation. Many times IMEs are asked to compare apples and oranges. This may be the case especially with range of motion measurements.

In terms of disability evaluations, the usual neurologic system objective tests are the following (but are not exclusive): MRI; CT scan; X-rays; ultrasound; and electrophysiological tests such as nerve conduction, current perception threshold, needle EMG, surface EMG, somato-sensory evoked potentials, EEG, PET scanning, SPECT scanning, vibration testing, and autonomic nervous modalities testing (electrodermal response, CPT, PTM, and TCM).

In terms of disability evaluations, the usual orthopedic system objective tests are MRI, CT scan, X-rays, ultrasound, goniometry (inclinometry), and dynamometry.

CONSIDERATIONS OF TREATMENT FROM THE TIME OF INJURY

The IME needs to study carefully the chronology of investigation and treatment of the injuries of the neuro-orthopedic systems under claim from the time of injury to the time of the evaluation, including giving advice for further appropriateness of treatment.

The IME needs to summarize the positive and negative aspects of the treatment in the terms of chronology appropriateness, fitness to the symptoms, frequency, intensity.

The aim of neuro-orthopedic rehabilitation treatment is to reduce and, if possible, get rid of any symptoms/signs of pathology related to the injury under claim. The evaluee must make a statement regarding the overall reduction of symptoms as perceived by him or herself. The IME needs to take that statement into consideration and compare it with the notes of the various treatments. A conclusion regarding the fit between the clinical file and the evaluee's perception should be part of the report.

Whether the evaluee has achieved the status of MMI and a %WPP is granted, the question of the need for future treatment remains. If there is such a need, the IME is usually asked to provide a plan for short- and long-term neuro-orthopedic rehabilitation.

DIAGNOSIS(SES)

The IME needs to report on the diagnosis(ses) pertinent to the injury/pathology under claim found at the time of the examination. Should the diagnosis not fit the previous one(s), the IME has to give an explanation. The explanation may allow the disability grantors to understand if the original diagnosis may have changed over time because of the treatment or lack of it.

The IME must describe any concurrent pathologies unrelated to the claim there are and explain if any structural or functional associations with the neuro-orthopedic diagnoses under claim.

PROGNOSIS

The IME needs to describe the clinical prognosis pertinent to the injury/pathology under claim for the foreseeable 24

months in terms such as good, conservative, poor, or very poor. This needs to be done in relation to the granting of the MMI and the %WPP.

The IME may need to write a statement if a concurrent unrelated pathology may change or affect the prognosis of the condition under claim.

CONCLUSIONS AND RECOMMENDATIONS

The IME may be asked to provide advice on future treatment or consultation. Unless clearly stated, it should not be assumed that the IME is the treating physician for the condition under claim.

Vocational rehabilitation is the desired goal in most neuro-orthopedic injuries. The IME may suggest a future need for physical or vocational rehabilitation with the goal of returning the injured party back to work with the original vocation or a new one.

GENERAL REFERENCES

AMA (1993). *AMA Guides to Evaluation of Permanent Impairment* (4th ed.). Chicago: American Medical Association.

Gerhardt, J.J. (1992). *Documentation of joint motion* (4th ed.). Portland, OR: Oregon Medical Association Print Shop.

Sella, G.E. (1999). Disability analysis in practice. In K. Anchor & T.C. Felicetti (Eds.) (pp. 279–314). Dubuque, Iowa: Kendall/ Hunt Publishing Co.

Sella, G.E., & Donaldson, C.C.S. (1998). *Soft tissue injury evaluation: Forensic criteria. A practical manual.* Martins Ferry, OH: GENMED Publishing.

Sella, G.E. (1993). A primer for impairment evaluations. American College of Forensic Examiners, Correspondence Course.

Sella, G.E. (1994). *Muscles in motion: Surface EMG analysis of the human body range of motion.* Martins Ferry, OH: GENMED Publishing.

Sella, G.E. (2000). Internal consistency, reproducibility and reliability of S-EMG testing, *Europa Medicophysica, 36*(1), 31–38.

Sella, G.E. (1996). How much do they weigh? Bilateral comparisons of weight placement among symptomatic, asymptomatic individuals and symptom magnifiers. *Disability. The International Journal of the American Academy of Disability Evaluating Physicians, 5*(2), 15–25.

45

Ergonomics for the Pain Practitioner

Hal S. Blatman, M.D.

INTRODUCTION

Ergonomics comes from the Greek *ergos*, meaning work, and *nomos*, meaning laws. It has become a "buzzword" that describes a variety of conditions and objects from specific tasks in the work environment to tool design and seating. The term ergonomics and the term human factors are sometimes used interchangeably. Most people probably recognize use of the term ergonomics in relation to seating and task analysis. The term also is used in relation to lighting and the psychology of shift work. Practically speaking, ergonomics relates to the interface between people and their environment. In the academic setting, the ergonomist may be found in the biomechanics, engineering, medicine, and psychology departments.

The medical professional treating pain patients often hears about physical activities that cause exacerbation of pain symptoms. These activities may be job related, involving materials handling (lifting and placing objects), awkward or sustained postures, repetitive motion, and keyboard data entry. Sometimes, it is the activities at home or away from the workplace that cause significant problems.

When treating pain patients, an awareness of basic ergonomic principles will serve the practitioner well. With an understanding of these principles, the caregiver can be more effective in helping impaired people function in their environment more effectively and with less discomfort.

SUPPLY AND DEMAND

One important concept to understand is nutrient supply and demand with respect to muscle tissue. When a muscle is resting, the cells require less nutritional support than when it is contracting. A resting muscle is softer and blood flow through the muscle is relatively unobstructed. When muscles contract to perform work, the cells of the muscle require nutrients at a level in proportion to the work that is being performed.

A muscle that is contracting requires more nutrients. When a muscle is alternately contracting and relaxing, blood flow through the muscle is enhanced by a pumping action of the muscle. This pumping helps keep the muscle cells supplied with nutrients at the increased level required for the work being performed.

When a muscle is contracting to maintain a posture or position, this sustained contraction requires even more nutrients than does a muscle alternately contracting and relaxing. With this sustained contraction, blood flow is hampered by increased pressure within the contracting muscle tissue. In this case, the nutrient requirements of the muscle are increased and the blood supply is relatively decreased. This leads to a significant imbalance with respect to nutrient supply and demand. It therefore costs the body more to stay in one position (sustained posture) than it costs to move.

This concept can be simply illustrated by trying to hold one arm straight out in front of the body, keeping it perfectly still. Before long, a feeling of fatigue is noticed, and the arm seems to get very heavy. Later, after a few minutes of rest, hold the arm straight out in front of the body again. This time move the hand and arm in small circles. This slight movement of the arm and shoulder results in some degree of alternate relaxing and contracting of the deltoid and trapezius muscles. Even small motions will facilitate blood flow and nutrient supply. Usually with the arm making small motions, the feeling of fatigue is noticed more slowly, and the length of time this posture/motion can be maintained is significantly

0-8493-0926-3/02/$0.00+$1.50
© 2002 by CRC Press LLC

longer. If nutrient supply and metabolic by-product removal are facilitated by muscular contraction and relaxation, the physical activity can be maintained for a longer period of time and with less fatigue.

The concept of muscle tissue nutrient supply and demand has clinical relevance with pain patients. Many pain patients relate that they do better when they are moving, and that they have problems sitting or standing in one position for any length of time. Sometimes maintaining one position causes stiffness, and sometimes it causes an increase in pain. For many people, even 15 minutes of a sustained posture is considered to be a prolonged period of time. It should be realized that even sitting in a relaxed position might require significant static contraction of supportive and balancing musculature. This relaxation may translate to increased stiffness and pain. Instructing patients with low back pain to slightly wiggle or otherwise move their hips every few minutes while sitting can greatly increase the length of time that seated posture can be maintained. This is likely to be important when sitting at the office as well as when riding in a car.

REPETITIVE MOTION INJURY

Repetitive motion injury (RMI) was previously termed both repetitive strain injury (RSI) and cumulative trauma disorder (CTD). Nationally, the Bureau of Labor Statistics calls these conditions illnesses and not injuries. The Occupational Safety and Health Administration (OSHA), the National Institute of Occupational Safety and Health (NIOSH), and the National Academy of Science have replaced these terms with the more neutral Work-Related Musculo-Skeletal Disorders.

Tissue pathology with respect to repetitive motion injuries is generally believed to primarily involve inflammation. Typical diagnoses that fall into this definition include tennis elbow, shoulder bursitis, tendonitis, and carpal tunnel syndrome. Treatment protocols for these conditions may include splinting, physical therapy modalities, anti-inflammatory medication, cortisone injections, and surgery.

For many people, these treatments are not effective. One reason is that pathology of repetitive strain injury (RSI) is not simply inflammation. Indeed, the primary pathology may be trigger points and myofascial pain. Tennis elbow, for example, is always associated with myofascial trigger points in the muscles that dorsiflex and supinate the wrist. Shoulder bursitis is always associated with myofascial trigger points in various shoulder girdle muscles.

Myofascial Trigger Points with Repetitive Strain Injury

It is important to examine pain patients for myofascial trigger points in muscle groups that cause and/or refer pain to the area of complaint. Repetitive motion activities will cause formation of new trigger points, as well as activation of latent trigger points. As myofascial trigger points become more active, they generate more pain.

Sustained posture activities will cause tightening of the active muscles, as well as generalized tightening of the fascia through the muscle tissue. In addition, myofascial trigger points within the muscle will become more active. This increase in trigger point activity will cause an increase in pain, both localized and referred.

Carpal Tunnel Syndrome

Carpal tunnel syndrome (CTS) is usually suspected when there is numbness and/or tingling in the thumb, index, long finger, and the thumb-side half (radial aspect) of the ring finger. People may also be awakened at night by pain in the wrist and forearm. When symptoms progress, people experience forearm and hand weakness, and even light objects such as coffee cups may be dropped.

The condition is often job or activity related, and people who use their hands a lot may be at risk for developing the problem. CTS has been associated with wrist and hand positioning, repetitive wrist use, use of heavy or vibrating tools, trauma, as well as light work such as typing.

In order to better understand what happens in the body in developing symptoms of CTS, it is helpful to understand the anatomy of the wrist. The carpal tunnel is bordered on the top of the wrist by the wrist bones and on the palm side by thick connective tissue. This thick connective tissue is called the transverse carpal ligament. These bone and ligament borders are thought to be relatively fixed and unchanging. Inside the tunnel created by the ligament and bones are the flexor tendons that curl the fingers, and the nerve (median nerve) that enables one to feel the thumb, index finger, long finger, and half of the ring finger.

Carpal tunnel syndrome has traditionally and mistakenly been thought of as a condition resulting from flexor tendon inflammation or swelling that is caused by repetitive motion of the forearm, wrist, and hand. It is thought that when people use their fingers and bend their wrists a lot, the tendons in the tunnel become inflamed, thereby causing them to swell. Because the borders of the tunnel are fixed and there is no extra room in the tunnel for this swelling, the median nerve gets squished, and some of the fingers go numb.

Moreover, the size of the carpal canal is not constant. The canal is largest when the wrist is in neutral (dorsiflexed 15°) position. It gets smaller when the wrist is bent in any direction. When bent positioning compromises canal size, an already marginal situation can be made worse, and this may induce symptoms of numbness and tingling. To evaluate this, a Phalens test can be performed. To perform a Phalens test, compromise the size of the carpal tunnel by palmar flexing the wrist approximately 90°. The test is considered to be positive if the radial fingers start to tingle. Usually the positive result is recorded as well as the time (in seconds) required for the numbness to be appreciated. Some examiners prefer the test to be positive within 10 to 20 seconds, while others wait until 60 seconds before calling the test negative.

In accordance with this inflammation model, the treatment for CTS traditionally involves keeping the wrist in a neutral posture and taking anti-inflammatory medication. Wrist braces are often recommended to ensure that the wrist remains straight, especially during work and sleep. To further aid in reducing the theorized inflammation, cortisone may be injected into the canal. When these treatments do not work well enough, surgeons will cut the transverse carpal ligament so the tunnel can expand to make room for the swollen tendons.

Unfortunately, the results from these treatments may be less than satisfactory. When this is the case, people take their medications and struggle in their braces to continue their jobs. Many experience continued weakness, numbness, and pain. When surgery is helpful, the condition will usually worsen or recur when people go back to their same jobs. Work modification is often an important part of returning these people to gainful employment.

Fortunately, there is a very different way to think about CTS. Recent research has demonstrated that the theorized inflammation of the wrist tendons may not occur. Other research has indicated that there are exercises that can be done to treat and prevent CTS and that this treatment may be more successful than the traditionally prescribed medication and surgery.

New Theory

A more modern idea to explain the pathophysiology of carpal tunnel syndrome is that it actually starts in the biceps muscle of the arm, and not in the wrist. People who use their wrists and fingers a lot, steady and support their forearms and hands with a sustained contraction of the biceps muscle. This continuous contraction of the biceps muscle eventually causes tightening of the connective tissue in the arm, called fascia. The biceps muscle crosses the elbow joint and attaches to the radius bone in the forearm. Because the biceps muscle is a part of the forearm, it also pulls on the fascia of the forearm. With time and continued sustained biceps contractions, the fascia in both the arm and forearm tightens. As this process continues, the transverse carpal ligament (fascia) also tightens. When this ligament tightens, the carpal tunnel gets smaller! In other words, CTS is not caused as much by the tendons of the wrist swelling and becoming larger, but rather by the canal itself getting smaller.

This theory provides a mechanism by which to understand why cortisone injections and anti-inflammatory medicines may not be helpful. It also sheds light on why surgery may initially provide relief and upon resumption of activity the symptoms may return. This theory also provides a mechanism to help understand why various stretching techniques have been effective in the treatment of carpal tunnel syndrome.

TOOLS

Tool design is an important consideration when a job or task needs to be made more "body friendly." There are catalogs of ergonomic tools for many different jobs and functions. In examining the use of tools and considering their modification, basic ergonomic principles provide important guidance.

One very important rule is that, wherever possible, the tool should be bent, and not the wrist. The wrist should be kept in a neutral position as much as possible. As a general rule, the less the wrist deviates from neutral posture, the better. Bent-handled pliers, hammers, and power tools are examples of commercially available alternatives to standard gripped models. These tool modifications allow the worker leverage and mechanical strength while keeping the wrist in a neutral position.

Another consideration in evaluating tools is to investigate the quality of the surface that comes in contact with the body. Bare metal is cold. In tools run by compressed air, the surface gets even cooler with use. In addition, sharp edges can put significant pressure on the skin and body part of contact. An example of poor tool handle design is a pair of metal-handled pliers where the handle has sharp square edges. Design improvements would include rounding the handles and covering them with a thin, tacky, cushioned and insulated material. In checking for factors that contribute to CTS, notice whether the tool handle presses directly upon the carpal canal. A cold hard surface that pounds or vibrates against the wrist can be problematic.

HEADSETS AND PHONE USE

Telephone use can be a significant factor in perpetuation of myofascial pain of the head and neck. There are three major muscular forces that are applied during ordinary phone use. First, the handpiece is held up to the level of the ear and mouth. This requires sustained postural contraction of the upper trapezius muscle. Second, most people push the earpiece into the ear in an effort to hear better and drown out external noise. This activity demands an even more forceful contraction of muscles that raise the arm. Finally, the lateral neck muscles must contract to push back against the force of the earpiece pushing against the ear. In summary, the upper trapezius and lateral neck muscles contract more forcefully and remain contracted in order to keep this posture.

An even worse scenario occurs when a patient attempts to hold the phone receiver by pinching it between the shoulder and ear. This activity requires the upper shoulder and lateral neck muscles to contract and maintain a posture with the muscles shortened. The ingredients of postural contraction and shortened muscles are very strong perpetuators for activation of myofascial trigger points and myofascial pain. Sometimes even 30 seconds of holding the phone in this manner can cause a stiff neck the next day.

A headset can significantly minimize the effect of phone use as a perpetuating factor in cases of myofascial head and neck pain. The set should be comfortable, have variable amplification, and perhaps block out some outside noise. The treating physician should be sensitive to this, and not hesitate to prescribe a headset for job modification when phone use is a suspected cause of a patient's head and neck pain.

POSTURE FOR KEYBOARD WORK

It used to be thought that typists should be seated in an upright position with the typewriter at desk level and the copy flat on the desk. For some people, this posture may require significant energy expenditure, and a partial relaxed slouch may be more comfortable. Efficient posture depends upon the particular typing task being performed. Most computer typists prefer the copy to be propped up on a stand next to the monitor.

Most importantly, the body should be well supported and, for the most part, in a position of rest. When using a computer, the eyes should be able to look slightly downward at the monitor. Tearing is important for nutrition and lubrication of the cornea, and it is increased with downward gaze angle. In addition, the neck should be comfortable, and not in a forward leaning posture.

Other more recent introductions into office furniture concepts place the monitor inside the desk under a glass surface. If desk or counter space constraints are of primary importance, this may be optimal for the particular situation. However, this hardware positioning may be aggravating to the musculoskeletal system of the operator.

Sometimes the most comfortable and best-supported posture will be slouching. This posture may be optimal when typing from copy that is propped up so that the typist can look out with only a slight downward angle. While perhaps more comfortable, this posture may restrict the operator's reach envelope, making it more difficult to answer the phone, refer to other materials, and open a drawer. When typing without copy, it may be most comfortable to lie back, as in a dentist's chair, keyboard in the lap, with the monitor suspended above at a comfortable

distance. This posture may be limited to young hackers who can tolerate decreased tearing.

Upright posture seems to be more appropriate when typing from copy that is flat on the desk. Ergonomic seating should be adjustable so that the body can be well supported in the best position of function for the task.

APPLICATION OF ERGONOMIC PRINCIPLES IN MEDICAL PAIN PRACTICE

During initial interviews and as patients progress in treatment, it will become evident that certain activities seem to be associated with an increase in pain symptoms. The activities may vary from specific job tasks to the use of tools and even posture, such as riding in a car or standing at a counter.

One of the most important considerations for the practitioner is the need to accurately understand the particular task or job environment involved. Obviously, the most direct way is to perform a site visit and see the activity in question on a firsthand basis. This, however, may be logistically difficult.

A much less expensive and often suitably effective method for performing a "site" visit is to ask the patient to bring pictures or a video of his or her work site and activities. Two sets of pictures, each with two or three different perspectives, should be obtained. One set should include the chair and furniture layout without the patient in the pictures. Other sets of pictures should also be obtained, with the patient posed in each of the positions/postures in which he or she spends significant time. It is important to see the patient lift, stoop, answer the phone, type on the keyboard, go into the file, lean on the counter, etc. The patient should be instructed not to pose, just to act naturally. It is important to capture on film bad posture, poor lifting techniques, and true phone habits.

The task of taking pictures involves people in their own medical care and makes them start to think about the possibility of changing their environment. It also demonstrates that the medical practitioner is willing to go the extra mile in an effort to help them.

These pictures are usually reviewed during the context of an office visit. The practitioner can see where basic ergonomic principles can be applied to support the body and minimize sustained posture, repetitive strain, and poor lifting habits.

When giving professional advice regarding changing aspects of the work environment, it is important to make suggestions that are not costly and can easily be tried. These suggestions should be based upon basic ergonomic principles and common sense. Follow-up is also very important, as the success or failure of these suggestions cannot be accurately predicted. Review of corrective actions and results of these efforts provides an environment for continued modification and refinement that is important in any ergonomic safety program. If the situation becomes too complicated and modifications do not work out as hoped, it may be time to consult with a professional ergonomist.

SUGGESTED READING

Chaffin, D.B., & Anderson, G. (1984). *Occupational biomechanics.* New York: John Wiley & Sons.

Dainoff, M.J. (1998). Ergonomics of seating and chairs. In W. Karwowski, & W. Marras (Eds.), *The occupational ergonomics handbook.* Boca Raton: CRC Press.

Eastman Kodak Company (1983). *Ergonomic design for people at work* (Vol. 1, *Workplace, equipment, and environmental design and information transfer*). New York: Van Nostrand Reinhold.

Eastman Kodak Company (1986). *Ergonomic design for people at work* (Vol. 2, *The design of jobs, including work patterns, hours of work, manual materials handling tasks, methods to evaluate job demands, and the physiological basis of work*). New York: Van Nostrand Reinhold.

Grandjean, E. (1986). *Fitting the task to the man. An ergonomic approach.* Philadelphia: Taylor & Francis.

Karwowski, W., & Marras, W. (1999). *The occupational ergonomics handbook.* Boca Raton: CRC Press.

Karwowski, W., & Salvendy, G. (1998). *Ergonomics in manufacturing. Raising productivity through workplace improvement.* Dearborn, MI: Society of Manufacturing Engineers, Engineering & Management Press.

Konz, S., & Johnson, S. (2000). *Work design industrial ergonomics* (5th ed.). Scottsdale: Holcomb Hathaway.

Pelmear, P., Taylor, W., & Wasserman, D. (1992). *Hand-arm vibration. A comprehensive guide for occupational health professionals.* New York: Van Nostrand Reinhold.

Pulat, B., & Alexander, D. (1991). *Industrial ergonomics case studies.* New York: McGraw-Hill, Inc.

Putz-Anderson, V. (1988). *Cumulative trauma disorders. A manual for musculoskeletal diseases of the upper limbs.* New York: Taylor & Francis.

Sanders, M., & McCormick, E. (1987). *Human factors in engineering and design.* New York: McGraw-Hill, Inc.

Section VIII

Physical Therapy, Manual Medicine, Imaging, Electromedicine, and Oriental Medicine

46

Axiologic Disorders — The Missing Outcome Dimension: Innovations in Pain Management

Richard S. Materson, M.D. and C. Stephen Byrum, Ph.D.

> We must look at the value orientation of individuals. Treatment must be of the person, not just the disease.
>
> **C. Stephen Byrum, Ph.D.**

In the new world of interdisciplinary pain management, many advances have been made to assure the correct holistic approach to evaluation and treatment. Medical holism requires attention to the four main pillars of wellness: physical, social, psychological, and spiritual. Other chapters in this book direct the reader to innovations in physical, social, and psychological domains. More controversial and unfortunately quite rare is adequate attention devoted to spiritual domains. Even with the pioneering work of Dossey (1991, 1993) and others who have explored the crossroads of medicine and spirituality, attention to this element of care evokes spirited discussion among care givers. Patients and their families, and an increasing number of healthcare workers, however, have evidenced their interest by attending mind–body medicine courses and spirituality and healing presentations such as those offered under the direction of Harvard's Herbert Benson, M.D. (1975, 1984; Benson & Stark, 1996), and his colleagues. The Center for Complementary and Alternative Medicine at the National Institutes of Health is now supporting investigations into the biologic substrate of the effects of a number of complementary and alternative modalities (CAM). In fact, evidence suggests a strong role for the hypothalamic-pituitary-adrenal axis in this effect likening the process to the relaxation response. The relaxation response is the opposite of the fight–flight response coined earlier at Harvard. The field of psychoneuro-immunology was born of these findings.

AXIOLOGY

The entire discussion of innovations in pain management can be advanced by the introduction of the term *axiology*, a word that undoubtedly is new to most people involved in these discussions. However, the term is extremely old, reaching back into Greek philosophy and Plato's attention to better understanding of the idea of goodness, stretching into the modern age in the thought of the English philosopher G. E. Moore, and finding its epitome in the work of Robert S. Hartman (1967). The term derives from the Greek *axio*, which means "value," so axiology becomes the study of the significance of the valuing process to human existence.

Basically, we human beings are, indeed, rational and emotional, but this often stereotyped dichotomy (right brain/left brain—men from Mars/women from Venus, etc.) may be a less-than-adequate mechanism for understanding human interactions with self, world, and others. A higher-order activity unique to human beings, an activity that stands at the peak of consciousness and beyond and at the same time encompasses the rational and emotional, is the capacity to value, to make value judgments, to evaluate, to weigh, assess, and discern. There is, for example, a distinct difference in the range of consciousness involved when one speaks of wisdom as compared, for example, to speaking of thinking. Wisdom, in this context, is an axiological phenomenon, a value reality.

0-8493-0926-3/02/$0.00+$1.50
© 2002 by CRC Press LLC

Exploring the axiological/value dimension may be the avenue to begin to open the complexities and subtleties of the spiritual arena that is commanding legitimate attention in the healing arts.

Axiological phenomena find many diverse expressions. For example, a pain patient presents to the medical practitioner presumably because of sickness and the *suffering* and pain associated with that sickness. A detailed history and directed physical examination, imaging, and laboratory investigation lead to a diagnostic hypothesis and a treatment regiment is suggested to cure the sickness and its associated pain or at least control it. Pain patients, especially those with chronic pain, along with other chronically ill patients, are rightly described as suffering.

Moving toward an axiological expression, in the ancient world, at least, suffering represented one level of the human response to pain. Beyond this there was—for want of a better word—the acknowledgment of a deeper level of pain that, to use more modern expressions, developed from within the self (the soul, the spirit, the heart, etc) more than from the body. This deeper pain, which could be brought on by bodily suffering, accompany bodily suffering, or cause bodily suffering (sickness, pain, depression, or even death), was acknowledged with such terms as (in our English translation) *ailing*. The ancient Hebrews, for example, frequently used the word *mahleka* to describe this ailing, and felt it could only be responded to—and here the language is dealing with a phenomenon of such depth that the very language itself is defied—by something that would "lift people up," give people a "lift," or even "lift spirits." Therefore, the term ailing points to the spiritual or axiological dimensions of pain, suffering, and sickness; there is great distinctiveness in describing axiological disorders or value disorders.

THE SYMPTOMS OF AXIOLOGIC DISORDERS: AILING

How does one recognize the symptoms of ailing? The overriding issue is that something valued by the person is lost or threatened. This produces the second symptom ailing. The third is a diminished capacity to be touched by the beautiful, to be loved, and to experience goodness. And, the final symptom is a value malaise (general weakness, lack of direction, disorientation, the inability to experience, or the loss of a sense of worth). This loss of a sense of worth can be experienced in numerous dimensions of human loss. As only a limited example, the loss could be *internal*—a loss of the sense of my worth as a individual. There is also *external* loss of worth and value—a loved one who dies, the loss of a job including the losses that occur at normal retirement, the loss of important possessions, or financial reversal. The possibilities are endless, and there are often combinations of axiological/value loss that exponentially compound themselves. Yet, seldom are practitioners attune to developing conversations that will

specifically involve an exploration of valuables lost that have been become causative factors in lack of health and well-being or valuables present that can be capitalized upon to advance the healing processes. We may not have to know about unique, individual value packages possessed by our patients — which *are* our patients on a fundamental level — in order to move in the direction of cures, but the axiological dimension is perhaps a cornerstone to any practice that promotes and sustains healing.

To explore the deeper meaning of loss or the threat of losing something of personal value, one must understand various levels of cognition, i.e., the way we think about things. The reader is invited to follow this exercise.

Consider that most humans are aware about thinking about things in a rational vs. an emotional manner. The rational mind follows the laws of science, physics, mathematics, and logical reasoning. The emotional mind follows a more psychosocial model and feeling tones, moods, and the like. An example might be the birth of a child. Rationally, the birth is the final result of an impregnation, usually a 9-month gestation, and can be described with precise anatomic and physiologic terms. Observed from an emotional perspective, love, pride, elation, beauty, fulfillment, trepidation, and anxiety are potential terms. But there is still a higher level of thinking, the value judgment or spiritual level. This level is often laden with more universal intonations that are frequently "religious like" (Figure 46.1). (To say "spiritual like" would be more consistent with the force of our discussion; religion relates to more institutional and parochial expressions.)

The late Abraham Maslow (1962, 1963) described these phenomena as peak experiences. Maslow would invite a group of learners to "think of the most wonderful experiences of your life; happiest moments, ecstatic moments, moments of rapture, perhaps from being in love, or from listening to music, or suddenly being 'hit' by a book or a painting or from some other great creative moment." He then invited his group to "first list these and then try to tell me how you feel in such acute moments; how you feel differently from the way you feel at other times; how you are at the moment a different person in some ways." The reader is encouraged to create such a memory in your own mind now. What is being recalled are value experiences, experiences that add value to life.

Dr. Maslow discovered an initial resistance among those he challenged, even among those who later admitted to having such experiences. The subjects feared being stigmatized as unsophisticated squares or being exposed as possessing abnormal personalities if, in this climate of scientific rationalism, they shared their true thoughts. Once the resistance was overcome, however, a large number reported what in Maslow's terms were basically religious experiences — for our purposes, axiologic experiences.

Maslow described these peak experiences associated with great moments of love (a mother fondling a newborn infant), moments of asthetic appreciation (observing the spray of the sea on rocks at dawn or dusk), moments of peak creativity (some meaningful and difficult task adequately performed), or great moments of insight and discovery.

Adjectives used to describe the associated feelings were wonder, awe, reverence, humility, surrender, and worship. Subjects recalled feeling that they were recipients of gifts, owe for what they have been given, and are under obligation to repay acts of goodness. The whole universe is perceived as a meaningful and integrated whole. "One feels that he has a place in it, that he belongs in it." Connected is another frequently used term.

Answering the question about how different the world looked at such times, participants replied that love and justice and all the values we commonly call religious or spiritual appear to be part of the very structure of the world. The world is not just there; it is essentially good. Such experiences are "valu-able;" that is, value-enable-ing/axiologically en-able-ing, with able constituting the polar opposite of ailing.

Ordinary cognition, in contrast to peak experiences, is highly volitional, demanding, prearranged, and preconceived. In peak experiences, the will does not interfere, it is held in abeyance. It receives and does not demand. We cannot command the peak experience. It happens to us (that is, unless we are suffering an axiologic disorder). One is reminded of philosopher Martin Buber's (1970) two attitudes by which man can and does relate to the world: "I–It" and I–Thou." "I–Thou" relations are characterized by immediacy, present-ness, subjectivity, spontaneity, unpredictability, and uniqueness. The person confronted by such a relation is not a passive object but an active subject to be confirmed in other-ness. By contrast, "I–It" relations are characterized by detachment, impersonalism, analysis, objectivity, and the search for an ordered, predictable structure of experience.

Leland Kaiser (1999), a well-recognized futurist, advises us, when looking at the unlimited parallel possibilities of future, to engage in precognition. We are advised to give up the bounds of worldly order, such as the rules of physics and mathematics, and to envision the future as it would be at its very best. We temporarily get out of our left-brain mode and into our right-brain function thus expanding our consciousness. Then, he suggests, we can grasp the future as it should be and as we wish it to occur in a perfect world, then come back to cognition in a real world and get about making the future happen by aligning with like-minded thinkers and doers. Kaiser's precognition is probably reflective of a transient shift from "I–It" to "I–Thou" and back again having enjoyed a peak experience.

Armed with an appreciation of "Things We Value," one can observe the great loss if we are deprived by this high order of experiencing reality. In fact, this loss leads to *ailing*, the failure to be able to tune in to this higher level of cognition when we wish to, and later the loss of desire to experience these peak experiences.

There are various degrees of this diminished capacity to be touched by the valuable, the beautiful, love, or goodness: from less frequent and more difficulty attaining this level of cognition to complete absence of the capacity.

Values malaise is the way this is commonly expressed to others. "I don't care any more." " No one cares." There is a loss of focus, a loss of what to care about. "It doesn't matter." "Nothing matters!" "It is not worth it!" There is a surrender to this negative mode of existence, a willingness to give up. Self-value and self-worth are depleted or gone. There seems to be no worth or value in anything. The sufferer is observed to have a loss of motivation. There seems to be little tenacity or stamina. Hope is lost. The mindset is so negative it seems "catchable" Others wish to avoid persons with values malaise, compounding the problem with isolation and loneliness, a self-fulfilling prophecy of the cognitive state. Finally, the sufferer experiences little evidence of joy or fun in life.

Therefore, it is not surprising that a patient whose illness is cured but who remains unrelieved of ailing or suffering associated with being sick has had incomplete treatment outcome (and, therefore, doesn't feel well or able to function efficiently or meaningfully). Adding to proper medical treatments, the relief of axiologic disorders brings a nearly immediate feeling of positive well-being, uplifting, and enormous gratitude; a patient is en-abled.

TREATMENT OF AXIOLOGIC DISORDERS: EXPOSURE TO BEAUTIFUL THINGS

The axiologically disordered patient is deprived of the ability to appreciate the good and beautiful things of this universe, the good and beautiful in others, and the good and beautiful with the aspects of the self. Treatment is by concerted effort of exposure to those realities. Ultimately, the loss of appreciation makes the sufferer detached from others and lonely. As studies of marasmus demonstrated in orphaned infants, love, affection, touching, and being touched are absolutely necessary for normal human growth and development. Just as the affected infants who were malnourished, maladapted, and slightly responsive, the sufferer has to one degree or another the same sparse repertoire of healthy engagement. After cuddling, rocking, touching, and communication response in an atmosphere of loving returns, those infants experience healthy growth and development and response patterns. Similarly, the sufferer ends the isolation and gains happy and productive engagement, thus finding some added base of potential for movement to health and a sense of well-being.

Meaningful Attachment

The first step necessary is that the suffer be cajoled, led, or otherwise influenced to form at least one deep meaningful attachment to another human being. This will require that the sufferer engage in doing kind, loving, and caring things needed by the person to whom he attaches. This can be a giant step for a sufferer whose every impulse is to maintain the isolated world, but it is the key event in returning to a healthy lifestyle and cannot be put off or neglected. There is always someone who can become that object of attachment. Someone on the clinical team must assume responsibility for assisting the identification of the right person and facilitating the introduction or contact. There is a sufficient supply of children, elderly, handicapped, impoverished, or simply unlucky who can be found. Social organizations, family members, and religious service groups have a great abundance of need so the sufferer always will be able to find a rich potential list of beneficiaries.

Acts of Compassion

Conscious acts of compassion is the second sufferer's penicillin. This is different from the attachment discussed above and more than a warm fuzzy feeling. In the recipient, it fulfills the desire not to hurt but to be happy. The natural right to pursue happiness is reinforced for both the giver and the receiver. This forces an affinity with persons who lack the opportunity not to be hurt and not to be happy. This concept goes far beyond feeling sorry for someone, but rather requires the performance of specific actions as a duty and obligation to create an environment for diminished hurt and increased happiness. While some sufferers possess the innate skills to produce conscious acts of compassion toward others, some will require significant coaching of the deeds and the necessary attitudes. Charles Dickens certainly caught the flavor of this in his inspiring story *A Christmas Carol*, when the reformed Ebenezer Scrooge accumulates profound and extraordinary personal benefits exceeding even those given to the Cratchit family and Tiny Tim by his conscious acts of compassion. In order for me to feel good, someone else will have to feel good because of my conscious actions first!

Diminishing the Comparing Mind

Diminishing of the Comparing Mind is the next hurdle on the road to end ailing. The mind in its left-brain cognitive function is exclusive, comparing, and competitive. More right-brained spiritual thinking is inclusive, noncomparing, and noncompetitive. In a connected universe there are ample good things for all of us and each of our portions is equally meaningful. A person is more than his or her job title, rank, salary, or social class. We must not value persons based on their economic achievements but rather value each person for who they are and how they uniquely contribute. This causes us to be more open and accepting of others and to value them. In this fashion we abandon living our life between the "I wish I were" and "I'm glad I'm not" sort of thinking.

Calming the Mind

Conscious Disciplines That Lead to Calming of the Mind is the next therapy required. This concept derives from Thales "Know yourself" and from *Qualb*, Muslim for "mind within the mind." Methods vary, but they require conscious exposure to the beautiful, peaceful, relaxing, rhythmic, and calming. The sufferer must seek out his best space to achieve this renewal. Often nature provides the environment, a walk in the woods, a garden, the beach, a sunset over mountains or waves crashing on rocks, a stream trickling through a mossy ravine. One can go to his/her place through meditation, by blocking out the external, turning consciousness inward. This can be assisted by attention to breathing, contract–relax types of progressive relaxation, listening to music with relaxation-inducing harmonics, or paying attention to a work of art. One need not actually go to the woods or the sea, because having identified a safe place, one can envision it during meditation and transform oneself virtually. Guided imagery assists persons to find a theme or environment most conducive to achieving the desired result.

Bensen and others have identified effective means of evoking the "relaxation response" which not only lead to the calming of the mind but also engage the psycho-neuro-immune system in a positive direction mediated in part by the hypothalamic-pituitary-adrenal axis. These techniques can be successfully achieved by nearly everyone. They require practice and repetition to become automatic and, therefore, easy to engage, much like learning to drive a stick-shift car. In the beginning, the task appears so formidable, and in the end, so ridiculously easy. Persistence pays and is rewarded by recharged batteries and renewed appreciation for those beautiful things of our universe, a profound sense of gratitude for the gifts we have been given. In other words, the renewed ability to enjoy peak experiences.

Conscious Depersonalization

Conscious Depersonalization becomes the next step on the path to healing. Grief and loss are universal conditions. The sufferer feels alone but is not. The suffering is not personal or a punishment for a misdeed or failure.

Bad things happen to good people all of the time; this is the nature of life. We must get over the inclination to believe that we are the ones selected for whatever bad happenstance. All others have experienced grief and loss, and will again. This is part of the life cycle and part of the human condition. However, it is unfortunately easy to slip back into the "it's just me" mindset, and so conscious depersonalization repetition is required.

Rejection of Regret

Conscious Rejection of Regret is the final pill in the bottle of recovery but is as important as each of its predecessors. Regret leads to guilt, which is a major cause of axiologic disorders; guilt and blame becoming automatic powers of devaluation. One needs to put material satisfaction into perspective. Who you are is not what you have! This method of viewing life must be changed consciously to an uplifting approach.. Therefore, one must view a partly completed work as a celebration of the effort to date rather than regret or guilt that it is incomplete. The glass must be viewed as half filled rather than half empty. Obviously, both statements are true, but the former carries with it optimism and hope, and the latter, regret — "What have I achieved so far?" rather than "How far am I behind?" What are the positive qualities we possess rather than enumerating the negatives? Perhaps most importantly, "What significant actions have I taken to help others?" rather than "What have I failed to do?"

WHO DOES WHAT?

Each pain practitioner must decide the mechanism by which the treatment team will assess the axiologic information and assure provision of therapeutic interventions. The reasons for the inquiries and the goals of the interventions must be shared with the patient and his family or support group. Insistence on addressing these issues is probably one of the few forgivable paternalistic actions left in medicine. Obviously, the best methodology requires patient agreement, yet the value of success is so great that the representation of data should be persistent even for the most reluctant. Remember that you are not imposing your own belief system on the patient. No proselytizing for any religion is permitted here. Rather, universal spiritual issues are involved which are backed by bio-psycho-social literature. Each treatment team will of necessity decide who does what. Certainly, if a chaplain well versed in the material is available, that person should be invited to contribute. But the tasks can be accomplished by physician, nurse, social worker, psychologist, and/or some therapists sensitive to and trained in the techniques. One always finds outcome measures helpful when applying a treatment. The Medical Outcome Study short form-36 (MOS-SF-36), the Sickness Impact Profile (SIP), and others may be useful. Less formal measures include clinical observations that document the patient's emergence from his or her isolated shell, their celebrations of doing meaningful things for others, brighter colors and happier subjects in their art work, success in their meditation and visualization, and their developed capacity to describe peak experiences.

The Spiritual Tendencies Inventory© published by Byrum is available in the Appendix at the end of this chapter. This instrument, which is directly related to axiologic assessment, is a very useful self-help device for those persons wishing to better understand themselves on a spiritual matrix. It is designed to be private (not included in a medical record), nor should it be used as a measurement instrument to document a clinical outcome. Rather, it assists the taker inventory his status vs. a control group for feedback which can be used or ignored as desired in the search for added information about the self. In the inventory's ten "domains," there are indications of both spiritual strengths and obstacles which can impact the axiological dimensions of health, well-being, and the associated phenomena of ailing, suffering, and pain. There is no correct score. There is, however, a perceptive mirror which reflects an individual's attitudes and self-judgments and values, with some helpful generalized feedback supplied to advance conversation and consideration. If a patient desires professional advice regarding the data acquired via this route, the treatment team should be prepared to supply it.

In summary, the relief of "ailing," a fundamental component and contributing cause of "suffering," has been one of the most neglected areas in pain medicine, yet one of near universal need. Familiarity with the very simple and pragmatic diagnostic criteria, and implementation of the treatment protocols will provide both the patient and the treatment team with a warm glow of mutually celebratory success.

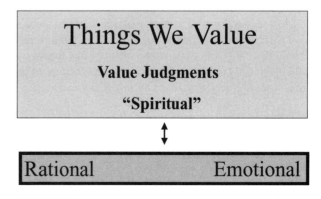

FIGURE 46.1

REFERENCES

Benson, H. (1975). *The relaxation response*. New York: Morrow.

Benson, H. (1984). *Beyond the relaxation response*. New York: Times Books.

Benson, H., & Stark, M. (1996). *Timeless healing*. New York: Scribner.

Buber, M. (1970). *I and Thou*. New York: Charles Scribner's Sons.

Dossey, L. (1991). *Meaning & Medicine. A Doctor's Tales of Breakthrough and Healing*. New York: Bantam.

Dossey, L. (1993). *Healing words. The power of prayer and the practice of medicine*. San Francisco: Harper.

Hartman, R. (1967). *The structure of value: The foundations of scientific axiology*. Carbondale: University of Southern Illinois Press.

Kaiser, L. (1999). The Kaiser Institute. Brighton, CO.

Maslow, A. (1962). Lessons from the peak experiences. *Journal of Humanistic Psychology*, II, 9–18.

Maslow, A. (1963). The scientific study of values, *Proceedings of the 7th Congress of Inter-American Society of Psychology*. Mexico City.

SPIRITUAL TENDENCIES INVENTORY©

The insights gained from this unique instrument can provide important information about the level of *spiritual strength* available to a person, which can be of significant help in situations of illness, stress, trauma, or high-demand challenges of daily life. The instrument will also provide a comprehensive picture of obstacles that inhibit and diminish spiritual strength.*

INTRODUCTION

During the past decade, numerous studies have addressed the relationship of spiritual tendencies to health and well-being. A fairly large body of anecdotal data and several controlled studies have concluded, somewhat persuasively, that such tendencies can make a positive contribution to a person's sense of well-being and impact physical health in a positive manner. Most of the anecdotal data have been compiled in situations in which persons are facing substantial challenges to personal health, and the conclusion has been advanced that spiritual tendencies have helped people cope and sustained them through difficult times. The sole purpose and intent of this Inventory is to gain insight into and establish some conversation about your spiritual tendencies in this regard.

---

* ©C. Stephen Byrum, Ph.D., The Byrum Consulting Group, LLC, 17 Grayswood Hill Road, Signal Mountain, Tennessee 37377. Phone/Fax (423) 886-5587.

DISCLAIMER

The above-noted studies and collections of anecdotal evidence have **not** succeeded in two areas. First, they have not defined in a scientific manner the word *spiritual*. It should be assumed that the word is not a synonym for *religious,* that religious refers to conventional, institutional, traditional expressions that arise in specific cultures, and that being religious does not necessarily mean that a person is spiritual. The term spiritual refers to a deeper core experience that is highly personal, ultimately incapable of being defined, and part of the unique essence of an individual's character and personality.

Second, there is no scientifically validated profiling instrument that relates to spirituality. In the most widely used profiling instruments, the issue of scientific validity is vague and open to debate. Simply realize that the instrument you are using here, which is an evolved form of the best instruments available, is seen as a mechanism for insight, conversation, and contemplation; it does not present itself as a scientific instrument, although its practical usefulness is strongly and confidently asserted.

In conclusion, the following questions are highly personal, are not intended as invasive, will result in absolutely no value judgment about an individual person, and are designed to be of personal benefit. The great benefit will be establishing a conversation from which individuals can gain important insights that will impact their own self-understanding, health, and well-being.

DIRECTIONS

Please contemplate the following questions and give your own personal answers in the spaces provided with each question. Keep in mind that there are no right or wrong answers, no answers that are better than others. To the extent that you are totally honest, the findings will be of more meaning and benefit to you.

PART I INVENTORY OF POTENTIAL STRENGTHS

1. To what extent do you feel that you have a *sense of purpose* in life?

   __Never __Seldom __Randomly __Regularly __Often

2. To what extent is it important to you to have what you would call *meaningful life experiences?*

   __Never __Seldom __Randomly __Regularly __Often

3. To what extent do you feel a *sense of connectedness* to others?

   __Never __Seldom __Randomly __Regularly __Often

4. To what extent do you feel a *sense of connectedness* to nature?

   __Never __Seldom __Randomly __Regularly __Often

5. To what extent do you feel a *sense of connectedness* to your own personal self?

   __Never __Seldom __Randomly __Regularly __Often

6. To what extent do you feel a *sense of connectedness* to that which you personally identify as God/The Divine/The Creator/The Source/or whatever name/idea/concept is meaningful to you personally?

   __Never __Seldom __Randomly __Regularly __Often

7. To what extent is *wholeness* a meaningful concept to you or a word you use in regard to your life or the lives of others?

   __Never __Seldom __Randomly __Regularly __Often

8. To what extent do you use the terms *higher* or *deeper* to describe levels or dimensions of life you believe you can or do experience?

   __Never __Seldom __Randomly __Regularly __Often

9. To what extent do *compassion, empathy, sympathy,* and *caring* describe experiences/feelings that are part of your life and are directed at others?

   __Never __Seldom __Randomly __Regularly __Often

10. To what extent do you feel that something you are doing is what you are supposed to do, something about which you have a *sense of calling?*

    __Never __Seldom __Randomly __Regularly __Often

11. To what extent do you feel attracted to, captivated by, even startled by some reality which is *beautiful* to you?

    __Never __Seldom __Randomly __Regularly __Often

12. To what extent do you feel part of a larger community, if that community is defined by the word *family?*

    __Never __Seldom __Randomly __Regularly __Often

13. To what extent do you feel part of a larger community, if that community is defined by the word *humankind?*

    __Never __Seldom __Randomly __Regularly __Often

14. To what extent do you feel part of a larger community, if that community is defined by the words *cosmic universe?*

    __Never __Seldom __Randomly __Regularly __Often

15. To what extent do you feel that there are "Truths" that can be conveyed by inspiration, revelation, or messengers such as prophets, wise teachers, or holy scriptures?

    __Never __Seldom __Randomly __Regularly __Often

16. To what extent do you experience what you might call a deep sense of *personal satisfaction* in regard to some action, decision, involvement, or activity you have participated in?

    __Never __Seldom __Randomly __Regularly __Often

17. To what extent is the phenomenon of *hope* a personal lens through which you relate to life?

    __Never __Seldom __Randomly __Regularly __Often

18. To what extent is the word *transcendent* a part of your vocabulary?

    __Never __Seldom __Randomly __Regularly __Often

19. To what extent, in spite of the negative realities that are invariably a part of life, are you able to sustain an attitude of *optimism?*

    __Never __Seldom __Randomly __Regularly __Often

20. To what extent are you able to live/act on what you personally would refer to as *faith* when there is no scientific evidence that is available?

    __Never __Seldom __Randomly __Regularly __Often

21. To what extent are you engaged in attendance at religious services conducted in a formal setting (church, synagogue, mosque, etc.)?

    __Never __Seldom __Randomly __Regularly __Often

22. To what extent do you participate in what you would personally define as prayer?

    __Never __Seldom __Randomly __Regularly __Often

23. To what extent do you spend time in what you would personally define as devotional time /meditation/contemplation/reflection?

    __Never __Seldom __Randomly __Regularly __Often

24. To what extent do you spend time reading spiritual/religious writings?

    __Never __Seldom __Randomly __Regularly __Often

25. To what extent to you become engaged in religious activities designed to help others in situations of need?

    __Never __Seldom __Randomly __Regularly __Often

PART II INVENTORY OF POTENTIAL OBSTACLES

1. To what extent do you experience a *sense of anger* as a primary response to people and circumstances that come into your life in a negative way?

   __Never __Seldom __Randomly __Regularly __Often

2. To what extent do you experience a *sense of hate* as a primary response to people and circumstances that come into your life in a negative way?

   __Never __Seldom __Randomly __Regularly __Often

3. To what extent do you have to deal with problems of *financial debt* in your life that make you feel vulnerable or jeopardized in some way?

   __Never __Seldom __Randomly __Regularly __Often

4. To what extent do you have what you would identify as problems with *sleep* or a *lack of adequate rest*?

   __Never __Seldom __Randomly __Regularly __Often

5. To what extent do you experience what you would identify as *impatience* as a primary response to people and circumstances that come into your life in a negative way?

   __Never __Seldom __Randomly __Regularly __Often

6. To what extent do you experience what you would identify as *a desire to win* as a primary motivation in your life?

   __Never __Seldom __Randomly __Regularly __Often

7. To what extent do you find yourself *dwelling on negative events* that have occurred in your past?

   __Never __Seldom __Randomly __Regularly __Often

8. To what extent do you experience a *sense of blame* that you direct toward other people or circumstances in your life?

   __Never __Seldom __Randomly __Regularly __Often

9. To what extent do you feel that you have spent significant parts of your life in circumstances of *criticism and complaint* directed at you personally?

   __Never __Seldom __Randomly __Regularly __Often

10. To what extent do you feel that you have a tendency to *hold grudges* or to think about *retribution or revenge* in regard to what you perceive as negative events that have been directed toward you by others?

    __Never __Seldom __Randomly __Regularly __Often

11. To follow an old saying, to what extent do you feel that you have a tendency to *forgive but not forget*?

    __Never __Seldom __Randomly __Regularly __Often

12. How often do you *lose your temper*?

    __Never __Seldom __Randomly __Regularly __Often

13. To what extent do you experience what you would identify as a *sense of worry (foreboding, impending harm)* about people and circumstances in your life?

    __Never __Seldom __Randomly __Regularly __Often

14. To what extent are meaningful events of *intimacy* and *affection* a part of your life that is absent or insufficient to the needs you feel?

    __Never __Seldom __Randomly __Regularly __Often

15. To what extent do you experience what you would describe as *down, depression, lethargy,* a bad case of the don't cares?

    __Never __Seldom __Randomly __Regularly __Often

16. To what extent do you feel that you are the victim of *bad luck* or the fates being against you?

    __Never __Seldom __Randomly __Regularly __Often

17. To what extent do you feel that you *need to be in control*?

    __Never __Seldom __Randomly __Regularly __Often

18. To what extent are there times in your life that you feel that the use of alcohol or drugs has become excessive?

    __Never __Seldom __Randomly __Regularly __Often

19. To what extent do you feel that you *have to be right*?

    __Never __Seldom __Randomly __Regularly __Often

20. To what extent do you have times in your life during which you feel that you cannot get *caught up,* that you are always behind?

    __Never __Seldom __Randomly __Regularly __Often

21. To what extent do you believe that there is a personal power of evil in the world that desires to do you harm?

    __Never __Seldom __Randomly __Regularly __Often

22. To what extent do you feel that you are unable to successfully meet the expectations of others?

    __Never __Seldom __Randomly __Regularly __Often

23. To what extent do you feel that your life is complicated and diminished by the amount of *clutter* that surrounds you?

    __Never __Seldom __Randomly __Regularly __Often

24. To what extent do you experience what you would define as *fear*?

    __Never __Seldom __Randomly __Regularly __Often

25. To what extent are you dissatisfied and fail to find contentment with the role of the *sexual* experiences in your life?

    __Never __Seldom __Randomly __Regularly __Often

Scoring

While there are no right or wrong answers for this inventory and the scoring is not designed to be any kind of contest with stronger or weaker scores, the following scoring system can establish beneficial implications. Please assign the following points:

Never = 1
Seldom = 2
Randomly = 3
Regularly = 4
Often = 5

Totaling your overall score will create a number between 25 and 125 on Parts I and II.

Your total score on the inventory for Part I is _____ .
Your total score on the inventory for Part II is _____ .

Possible General Implications Part I

1. For a score of 25–59

   The spiritual arena is not of high importance to you in terms of your present tendencies and activities. Why this is the case is unique to your own personal background, but it may be important for you to reflect on the causative influences that have produced this score.

   The arena of the spiritual may be of little benefit as a positive influence on situations of personal health and well-being. The spiritual may not be an active part of your personal coping mechanisms.

   It may be that exploratory inquiries or study in the spiritual area might be of interest and benefit. If such exposures in the past have been blatantly negative to you for whatever reason, exposures of some new variety might be more helpful. Try not to let any negative experiences from the past close doors of possible insight and discovery for you.

2. For a score of 60–94

   The arena of the spiritual is of moderate importance to you in terms of your present tendencies and activities. Why this is the case is unique to your own personal background, but it may be important for you to reflect on the causative influences that have produced these scores.

   The spiritual arena may be of more than passing adequate benefit as a positive influence on situations of personal health and well-being. The spiritual may be of reasonable importance as an active part of your personal coping mechanisms.

   Because you already have some taste for spiritual inquiry, further explorations in this area may deepen the strengths you are finding. Perhaps exposures to new areas of inquiry would enhance the experiences you are already having. Try to hold open a sense of discovery and enlightenment as new dimensions of spirituality are experienced.

3. For a score of 95–125

   The arena of the spiritual is of high importance to you in terms of your present tendencies and activities. Why this is the case is unique to your own personal background, but it may be important for you to reflect on the causative influences that have produced these scores.

   The spiritual arena will be of highly important benefit as a positive influence on situations of personal health and well-being. The spiritual will be an active part of your personal coping mechanisms.

   The present strength of your involvement in spiritual inquiry is likely to be a platform upon which a good deal of your overall-life is built. Continued experiences of growth may be of further benefit. Try not to feel that you have arrived and have no additional dimensions of growth to explore.

Possible General Implications Part II

1. For a score of 25–59

   While you should pay attention to any individual question(s) that you marked often, in general you do not have great obstacles that stand in the way of what can be defined as spiritual.

   Often we are challenged to give attention to correcting negative indicators or solving problems, but we are also challenged by strong, positive indicators. Your challenge may be to understand what you are doing well with regard to these obstacles to the spiritual and keep following and building on those patterns. It also will be important to understand why you have done well in these areas, what personal history has contributed to this, and who may have helped you in making this level of scoring possible.

2. For a score of 60–94

   These scores give evidence of a substantial number of obstacles to the strengths which can be derived from the spiritual. In all likelihood, these obstacles will be having a general impact on quality of life and general happiness. No matter how strong your spiritual strengths might be, they will be compromised to some extent by these obstacles.

   Begin by looking at the areas you have marked "often" and "regularly." Then, give consideration to the various domains, and see if you have a concentration of obstacles in any one or two domains.

   Try to establish personal strategies designed to create conversations; seek input from trusted colleagues and friends, and actions that might reduce the impact of these obstacles.

3. For a score of 95–125

   These scores give evidence of an unusually high number of obstacles to the strengths that can be derived from the spiritual. In all likelihood, the obstacles are having a profound impact on quality of life and general happiness. No matter how strong your spiritual strengths might be, they will be substantially compromised and eroded by these obstacles.

   Calculate your domain scores, and then take note of these scores from the most negative to the most positive. Clearly, the domains with the most negative scores indicate the area where most work is needed. Think about past influences in your personal history, the impact of people who presently populate your life. Can these negative, causative factors find any resolution? Think about the powerful role that your perception of events and people can also play. What is the relationship of your perceptions and responses to reality? These negative obstacles should be approached with great seriousness as they constitute a real threat to personal happiness, success in relationships, general health, and a sense of emotional well-being.

PART I/DOMAIN 1 THE ROLE OF COMPASSION, EMPATHY, AND CARING

YOUR SCORE FOR QUESTIONS 9 AND 25

Scoring Range: 2 --- 10

weaker --------------------------------- stronger

Our ability to get outside of ourselves is enhanced and accelerated by direct actions of compassion and a spirit of empathy and caring that is directed at other people, particularly when other people are in situations of need, pain, or hurt.

Most people report a genuinely positive feeling of meaning and happiness that rises within them when they extend help and care to others. This feeling, while incapable of being logically defined, is a powerful indication of our own humanity at its best, our almost innate connection to others, and a catalyst for positive self-esteem.

Individuals who deal with depression, both as persons afflicted by the malady and professionals involved in treatment, have found that direct involvement with actions of compassion and empathy tend to diminish the intensity of all but the most severe forms of chemical depression. Without question, the positive feelings gained from actions of care can contribute remarkably to human health and well-being. If nothing else, when we are exposed to deep needs of others, we may gain a better perspective on the way that our own lives — in spite of very real challenges — are indeed blessed.

Unfortunately, the positive, spiritual feelings that are the result of actions of compassion and empathy too often occur by accident and coincidence. Is it possible to construct positive strategies of spiritual health and well-being by consciously incorporating into our daily lives actions of care and compassion? Is it possible to create personal spiritual projects designed to help others that may, in the end, have more of a positive impact on us as helpers than on anyone we reach out to help?

PART I/DOMAIN 2 A SENSE OF CONNECTEDNESS

Your Score for Questions 3–5, 12–14

Scoring Range: 6 --30

weaker ----------------------------------stronger

When those first astronauts who walked on the moon sent back those amazing pictures of Earth, most human beings were stilled, if not stunned, by the images. No one who has ever lived on this planet has been afforded exactly that particular perspective. How beautiful our blue and white globe was hanging there almost like a cosmic ornament in outer space. How small we seemed, certainly not the egotistical center of the universe assumed by some past generations. But, more than anything else, how much we who inhabit this planet are interconnected, mutually dependent, in this together. We are not alone!

Loneliness is emotionally and then physically destructive. While we all need moments of personal privacy — "Calgon take me away!" — isolation will destroy us. We need connectivity of any and all varieties; so much so that healthy human beings consciously seek ways to promote and pursue healthy relationships.

Connectivity can be experienced in many dimensions, and the dimensions enhance one another and are mutually reinforcing. The experience of connection in one dimension will exponentially add to the experience in other dimensions; a lack of, antipathy for, or cynicism about connection in any dimension will have a limiting impact on the entire field of potential.

The experience of connectivity can find expression most simply with other people, and then potentially with nature, with what some identify as the Divine/the Holy, perhaps with animals, and even with inanimate objects of personal worth and value.

Although it is not given sufficient attention, the experience of connectivity with self/one's best self/one's ideal self/one's essence is also of deep meaning. The *experience*, not the intellectual concept, of wholeness is the experience of connection with self, and usually is buoyant, with personal meaning and positive consequences for health and well-being.

PART I/DOMAIN 3 THE ROLE OF TRADITIONAL RELIGIOUS ACTIVITIES

Your Score for Questions 6, 15, 20–24

Scoring Range: 7 --35

weaker ----------------------------------stronger

It has been difficult for people to be nonjudgmental about many traditional religious activities. For some, due to the negative excesses in the history of traditional religion and negative personal experiences, there is a deep cynicism about anything that smacks of traditional religion. For others dealing with their own comfort zones and sometimes defensive exclusivism, if some religious practice is not exactly like their religious practice, it is suspect and illegitimate.

If it is possible to get beyond these two invalidating predispositions, there remains a distinct and expansive field of evidence that convincingly suggests that traditional, religious-like activities can be of real positive consequence for health and a sense of well-being.

Whether a person prays or meditates is not the issue; the value of prayer-like or meditation-like states of consciousness for health is almost beyond question. Whether a person recites a Hindu mantra, works rosary beads through his or her fingers, or enjoys joining in the rhythmic singing of congregational hymns is simply a mater of upbringing and personal taste, not an occasion for some competitive debate set on determining who is closer to God or whose practices are right or wrong. The calming rhythms established in activities is the key to health, not the traditions that give rise to the different expressions. It is the quietness and beauty of the holy place that promotes a sense of rest and personal revitalization; that the place is a synagogue, mosque, or church is of very secondary importance.

There is an amazingly diverse world of religious activities in the world today and across centuries of human culture. Within these complex and often curious expressions, legions of human beings have gained deep and lasting meaning for their lives. If we could set aside some of our stereotypes and caricatures and open some of the limiting boxes we live in, there is no telling what we might find that would benefit our lives and contribute in a positive manner to our health and well-being. Who knows, it might be worth a serious look!

PART I/DOMAIN 4 A SENSE OF PURPOSE, CALLING, AND MEANING

Your Scores for Questions 1, 2, 10, 16

Scoring Range: 4 --20

weaker---------------------------------- stronger

The survival instinct has often made the vital difference between life and death. This instinct has guided human lives through a maze of dangers, difficulties, and threats. Now, as times have changed and, following Maslow, basic survival needs have become more easily met, the survival instinct has evolved into a more sophisticated form.

The sense of purpose and calling, the core of our search for meaning, is an advanced, evolved form of the old survival instinct. On levels of basic living, there must be survival; on levels of self-actualization and self-realization, there must be purpose and calling. Purpose and calling promote survival on a more essential, more intrinsic level. Purpose and calling contribute to authentic living today as profoundly as basic survival.

Too often we have added our own dimensions of competition and judgment to purpose and calling. One purpose or calling is seen as being somehow better than another. Suddenly, there are artificial hierarchies that end up prescribing who is of value and what work has worth. People make choices on the basis of culturally defined roles that may not be fulfilling at all without honoring the clues of their own uniqueness.

Purpose and calling need to be defined in concert with cultural precedents and suggestions, but the motivation of experiencing personal happiness must become a high indication of where personal meaning is to be found. Under no circumstances should economics or social status be the only determinative factor in narrowing the range of life choices which may produce purpose and calling.

Finally, be sure to keep in mind that any sense has an intuitive dimension that cannot be reduced to pure logic or rationality. Just as a survival *instinct* must be trusted and acted on to some extent by *faith,* so a sense of purpose and calling must intuitively and instinctively be responded to with a substantial degree of self-trust, trust in others, and perhaps even a trust in a power of beneficence at the core of existence.

PART I/DOMAIN 5 A SENSE OF THAT WHICH IS BEYOND

YOUR SCORE FOR QUESTIONS 7, 8, 11, 17–19

Scoring Range: 6--30

weaker ----------------------------------stronger

The brilliance of Albert Einstein is usually associated with relativity theory and the famous axiom $E = MC^2$. However, for Einstein, before there was math or physics — or any *thinking* pursuit — there was something more fundamental. The great genius put it this way:

> At the core of all of the sciences and humanities there is a common experience—a sense of mystery. That person who is unable to stand in **wonder**, rapt in a sense of **awe**, is as good as dead. His mind and his eyes are blind (Byrum, 1991).

So, the critical component to life in many respect is *wonder.* For Einstein, everyone has the capacity for this experience, but for one reason or another, does not exercise this capacity. They may be too busy to take long walks in a beautiful place. The aesthetic experience of beautiful objects or the appreciation of something of goodness/quality may escape their notice. So, there is little of the wonderful, and what does occur in this domain is more by accident than intentional design.

Without experiences of wonder and awe, life becomes sterile and one-dimensional. When the capacity for wonder is not exercised, we get caught up within ourselves and lose perspective. As children, we have a gift of wonder, and it is exercised constantly; unfortunately, too many of us become all-business, serious adults, put away our childish things, and think that our grown-up status is somehow superior. In fact, we have lost our best selves.

An ancient holy text says, "He who does not believe is condemned already." The text is not claiming some absolute that unaccepted and affirmed brings damnation. Rather, it is saying that without the exercised capacity of an advanced dimension of consciousness, here called believing, an entire level of potential for life is closed off. When this self-limiting occurs, sickness, depression, loss of emotional well-being cannot be far behind. We must watch children caught up in play and filled with an awesome enthusiasm of just living. As adults, we must reclaim this wonder and joyfulness. To do so is to create a context for getting better.

PART II/DOMAIN 1 PERSONAL LIFESTYLE ISSUES

YOUR SCORE FOR QUESTIONS 3, 4, 14, 18, 25

Scoring Range: 5--25

more positive ------------------- more negative

This domain involves a kind of catchall of personal lifestyle issues that may be obvious. However, because so many people have their potentials for good health and balanced well-being lessened because of these issues, perhaps reassertion and reaffirmation are important.

Rest is nature's way of recharging the batteries of our lives. There is no substitute for rest, no potion we can take that does for us what rest does. Health, well-being, clarity of judgment, and facility of performance are all impaired by lack of rest. Part of knowing who we are in our uniqueness is knowing how much rest we require. Intimacy and affection are survival needs, pure and simple.

Intimacy and affection are survival needs, pure and simple. Intimacy needs are a part of the unique core of our humanity. Deprivation or abuse in these areas will eventually become destructive, even to the point of impairing our immune systems and brain chemistry. Healthy sexuality is a divine gift.

Alcohol and drugs can be part of a nexus of unresolved personal and interpersonal problems. While not intrinsically wrong, they often challenge an individual's ability to be in control of his or her own life and destiny. Too harsh a judgmental condemnation of alcohol and drugs may actually encourage abuse. A laid-back, it-doesn't-matter tolerance defies the fact that powerful chemicals will create powerful, often unpredictable interactions with complex body chemistry. A middle ground of absolute control and honest temperance may be the key, all the time knowing that self-honesty in these areas can be very difficult. (Similar assessments of diet and exercise issues can easily be made and have parallel relevance.)

Debt must become part of this set of lifestyle issues. The burden of the debt being assumed by many Americans is a direct, causative factor in health problems. A careful line must be drawn between needs and wants, what we might like, and what we can afford. We must resist allowing *who we are* to be defined in terms of *what we have*.

The person who juggles these issues is like a skilled, highwire artist. Balance and good judgment in these areas give a spiritual gracefulness to life.

PART II/DOMAIN 2 THE POWER OF STRONG, NEGATIVE EMOTIONS

YOUR SCORES FOR QUESTIONS 1, 2, 12, 13, 15, 24

Scoring Range: 6--30

more positive ------------------ more negative

When the ancient religious texts called upon people not to worry, they were not simply trying to give us another rule that we can feel badly about when we fall short. Nor is there an empty-headed, Alfred E. Newman/*Mad Magazine* "What, Me Worry" attitude or a Pollyanna-ish "Don't Worry, Be Happy" platitude being advanced. Real, practical advice is being offered.

The ancient texts advise that the problem with worry about the future (or other realities over which we have little control) is that the realities we will face today will require all of the personal energy we can assemble.

Worry, fear, anger, hate—all of our strong, negative emotions—are powerful realities of personal evaluation that drain us of personal energy at a profound speed. To become obsessively and compulsively consumed with "what ifs," with fits of temper, with fear of worst-case scenarios diminishes our ability to energetically, creatively, and productively deal with what demands our focus today.

If worry and fear or other negative emotions are painful, and if pain is naturally avoided, is it possible that on some level we *choose* to embrace these negative emotions? Do their manifestation give us attention, gain us some kind of emotional leverage with others, or create some kind of self-punishment that we feel we deserve? If any of this is true, we certainly need to work on why we allow the negative emotions to be taken to such dangerous extremes.

On the other hand, involvement with negative emotions may simply be the result of unexamined habits that have come to dominate in our lives. Maybe there are actions of the will that can help us break habits of worry or temper that are just as real, and work with similar tactics, as actions of the will that allow us to break bad habits of eating, drinking, smoking, etc. Habits can take on a life of their own, be in charge of our lives, and destroy us. So, it becomes time for us to take control of ourselves, even in regard to the expression of emotions.

PART II/DOMAIN 3 WHAT HAVE WE DONE WITH TIME?

YOUR SCORE FOR QUESTIONS 5, 9, 20, 22, 23

Scoring Range: 5---25

more positive -------------------more negative

With all of the expectations that assault our lives, we have no option — or so it seems — but to whittle away, a little more and a little more, at the time we have for rest, our free time, or the time we have to really carefully fashion something into a finished, complete project in which we can take real pride. We are continually frustrated by there not being enough time and feeling tired and worn out during much of the time that we do have.

All of our wiggle room is used up. We leave for meetings at the very last moment possible, depending on traffic to cooperate with our need to be somewhere across town by a certain time. We schedule last possible flights or close connections, depending on airlines to run on announced schedules so that we can make the pieces of our lives work. And, when the traffic slows toward gridlock or the planes are late, we find ourselves in fits of emotion that move from nervous anxiety to full-fledged rage. A significant fear that has asserted itself in modern life is the vulnerability we feel in the face of travel rage; road rage has become a penetrating symbol of our modern lives.

What we do to our health and well-being because of the stress of time, expectation, and general accumulating clutter is altogether frightening. Feeling like we will never get caught up can kill us. Thinking that we can perfectly meet the expectations of everyone else and, therefore, becoming "Super-worker" or "Super-parent" can kill us.

The old axiom about the person who cannot manage time well cannot manage anything well, the ultimate test of our ability to cope becoming how we manage time, is exactly right. Managing time begins by making an absolutely *uncompromising* commitment to downtime that is built into every day, every week of our lives. Mark out downtime on schedules in the same way that you would schedule the most important appointment. Build in wiggle room. There are no compromises here. The compromises will be in personal health and relational health.

PART II/DOMAIN 4 HAVING TO BE IN CONTROL

YOUR SCORE FOR QUESTIONS 6, 16, 17, 19, 21

Scoring Range: 5 --- 25

more positive ------------------ more negative

Believing that we have control is like sending a new, teenage driver out the door with the injunction, "Be careful," and thinking that simply because we have said the words the reality will happen. Perhaps the greatest myth of human life is the myth of control. Yet, we crave control, we convince ourselves that we must have it, and even become obsessive and compulsive in our drive to make sure that we possess it. The old phrase from the Beatles, "Let it be, let it be, let it be," is so far from the way we actually approach life that it is amazing; in our push for control, we can't leave anything alone, allowing it to find its own way — we micromanage everything and create situations of amazing stress and self-destruction in the process.

One of the most powerful ways that we try to exert control is in our unending pursuit of winning. We have created a culture in which winning is everything and coming in second conveys a personal weakness or a lack of virtue. Everything becomes a contest, and someone who would attempt to kill a child's parent to distract that child from a cheerleader competition ceases to seem all that strange or outlandish. We become so caught up in being the best we can be that we distort reality and create a world of expectations that no one could accomplish.

Finally, we raise the ante on this whole issue of control by complicating life with over-personalizations that make no sense. We bring into play the phenomenon of bad luck; we feel like the fates are against us, or even that some metaphysical power has it in for us and has picked us out of the masses for some cruel temptation

or test. Do our egos really believe that we are so much the focal point of creation?

The Janice Joplin/Kris Kristofferson song, "Me and Bobby McGee," has the line "Freedom's just another word for nothing left to lose" (Kristofferson, 1971). Maybe that is the key. Maybe it's okay to lose sometimes, to come in second, not to be in control. Maybe there is real freedom in consciously setting aside our need to be in control, to be right, to be No. 1.

PART II/DOMAIN 5 THE POWER OF THE PAST

YOUR SCORE FOR QUESTIONS 7, 8, 10, 11

Scoring Range: 4 --- 20

more positive ------------------ more negative

We have all kinds of clichés: "Nothing is as old as yesterday's newspaper;" "It's over and done;" "What's done is done." Yet, few of these old sayings, as true as they are, really work for us. Instead, what took place yesterday, or years of yesterdays ago, can hold power in the present tense of our lives in astounding ways. Perhaps, it is we human beings and not elephants who are incapable of forgetting. The past can create a reign of terror in our lives.

We hold onto past events with a destructive passion. We clearly remember past mistakes and rehearse over and over again how we might have done something different or better. We place blame, hold grudges, say we can forgive but not forget, and simply add to our already overburdened lives realities that cannot be changed or altered no matter how much emotional energy we give to them.

A major part of authentic human maturity is the ability to write off those negative issues from the past. Sure, we can learn from them, but how often do they have to be in the forefront of our minds for the lesson to really take hold. Everyone has bad things that have happened to them. No one has perfect parents. No one's track record is without blemish. Okay. So, what else is new? Let's move on!

Some psychologists believe that people hold onto the past as a way of exerting additional punishment for some old mistake or lapse in judgment. We have not whipped ourselves enough, so we keeping bringing up the past painfulness. Or, we believe that someone else has not been punished enough, so we keep bringing up negatives from their lives. Do we not have anything better or more constructive to do with our time?

It is the *present* that is the only real possession of life that we have. To the extent that we find ways to focus attention on the past or become obsessed with the future, we diminish and undermine the real time we do actually have. One of the greatest blessings of life is *to forget,* but we have to want to forget, to practice forgetting, and let the past go away.

OTHER CRITICAL REFERENCES ON AXIOLOGY

Byrum, C.S. (1991). *The value structure of theology* (8th ed.) Acton, MA: Tapestry Press.

Dickens, C. (1843). *A Christmas carol.*

Edwards, R.B., & Davis, J.W. (Eds.). (1991). *Forms of value and valuation: Theory and applications.* Lanham, MD: University Press of America.

Hartman, R.S. (1959). The science of value. In A.H. Maslow, (Ed.), *New knowledge of human values.* New York: Harper & Bros.

Hartman, R.S. (1994). *Freedom to live: the Robert Hartman story.* Amsterdam/Atlanta: Editions Rodopi Press. 1972. (Also includes extensive bibliographic references for use in further study.)

Kristofferson, K. (1971). Me and Bobby McGee (Recorded by Janice Joplin). Barre, VT: Kris Kristofferson Guitar Collection. (1999).

47

Surface Electromyography in the Assessment and Treatment of Muscle Impairment Syndromes in Pain Management

Jeffrey R. Cram, Ph.D.

INTRODUCTION

Despite an extensive armamentarium of electrophysiological tools available practitioners in the field of pain management, many limitations exist. Without doubt, it is extremely difficult to evaluate patients suffering from pain using traditional electrophysiological technology. While surface electromyography is not a new technique, recent developments have shown it to be a valuable diagnostic tool and one that allows for the development of precise neuromuscular treatment protocols. The purpose of this chapter is to briefly review the limitations of traditional electrodiagnostic tools in pain management, while providing an overview of the role which surface electromyography (sEMG) can play in the assessment and treatment for muscle impairment syndromes. Specifically, seven muscle impairment syndromes will be reviewed, along with 15 sEMG retraining strategies that attempt to address neuromuscular contributions to chronic pain.

Despite major advances in the field of medicine, knowledge of the causes and mechanisms of pain continues to be limited. Because of the seemingly apparent subjectivity of the clinical evaluation, pain disorders are extremely difficult to document. In order to develop appropriate treatment methods, assessment protocols are necessary which can provide objectivity and reproducibility. Practitioners today are faced with many individuals suffering from a variety of ongoing refractory painful conditions.

Utilizing traditional electrophysiological techniques, it can be impossible to quantify or to substantiate a patient's claim. Throughout this chapter, examples are provided that focus on specific applications of sEMG, thus giving considerable insights into the nature of a chronic pain disorder that entails muscle impairment as a component.

With the recent evolution of the understanding of pain, most clinicians believe that a person can truly suffer from a specific painful disorder without traditional objective correlation. In the past, it was believed that an individual was not truly experiencing pain if certain clinical criteria were not fulfilled. For the most part, this contention may have merit for acute pain syndromes. However, the experienced pain practitioner knows well that often one cannot depend purely on clinical acumen to establish an accurate diagnosis or to document or record the basis for a patient's complaint of chronic pain.

The medical practitioner, psychologist, physical and occupational therapist, or chiropractor who provides ongoing therapy is expected to substantiate the degree of patient improvement. Unfortunately, with many of the present-day technologies available, this can be impossible. The third-party payer or insurance carrier may discontinue or refuse to pay for further treatment based upon lack of substantiation of progress. In accordance with the rising costs of healthcare in the present economic climate, it is essential for third-party payers to limit unnecessary ongoing medical care. Without doubt,

0-8493-0926-3/02/$0.00+$1.50
© 2002 by CRC Press LLC

this is a reasonable approach. Unfortunately, many honest patients continue to suffer from pain throughout their lives, because they had not received proper care for an unsubstantiated disorder that was thought to reflect an expression of malingering.

From a medical perspective, physicians have become dependent on neuroimaging studies, such as MRI scans, CT scans, or bone scans, as well as needle EMG (electromyography) or nerve conduction studies and EPs, evoked potentials. (See Table 47.1.) The clinical practitioner may not be aware of the precise applications and limitations of these studies in the context of attempting to establish the basis for a chronic pain disorder. The correlation between symptoms and neuroimaging findings is limited. It is sometimes believed that a normal needle electromyogram (EMG) may rule out the existence of a pain disorder. Based upon negative findings from these tests, the patient's complaints may be disregarded or assumed to be a product of deception. The pain sufferer, thereafter, is labeled a malingerer and is deprived of appropriate medical care. Of utmost concern is the fact that failure to establish a correct diagnosis at onset may lead not only to ongoing suffering but may also augment the overall cost of medical care. Often, the longer a pain syndrome is left untreated, the more refractory and difficult is the solution.

In the early years of medicine, medical practitioners depended on their primary senses to evaluate an individual and to provide an accurate diagnosis. As technology evolved, instrumentation was developed to enhance those senses. The stethoscope, although still used today as a diagnostic instrument, is known to have certain limitations that have been surpassed in an extraordinary manner by the use of echocardiography. Rather than simply auscultating the chest with a simple diaphragm and bell, computer technology utilizing an advanced electronic interface has provided exceptional insights into cardiac physiology. In a similar manner, physicians in many specialty fields have learned that their abilities to recognize disorders by pure physical examination are most certainly limited.

Surface electromyography can provide the information necessary to evaluate and follow pain sufferers with muscle impairments, as well as to establish selective treatment protocols in a scientific manner. It is well known that muscular tension maintains a substantial role in the development of the pain–spasm circuit, which can be treated using techniques of self-regulation in the form of biofeedback. Traditionally, biofeedback has been associated with relaxation training as a means to lower the emotional arousal component involved in pain. However, based upon limited knowledge of the precise muscles involved in given syndromes, coupled with the lack of generalization of relaxation-oriented protocols, the development of effective biofeedback-assisted relaxation treatment protocols has

TABLE 47.1
Electrophysiological Applications in Pain Management

If the History and Physical Examination Suggest	Select
Local nerve injury Entrapment syndrome Neuropathy	Nerve conduction studies
Radiculopathy Plexopathy Myopathy Neuropathy	Needle electromyography
Central pain	Somatosensory-evoked potentials
Muscle injury Disuse syndrome Muscle spasm Myofascial syndrome Fibromyalgia Postural disorder Psychophysiological state	Surface electromyography

been limited. The development of "static muscle scanning" techniques in the 1980s (Cram & Steger, 1983) allowed the practitioner to precisely map areas of chronic asymmetric muscle tension, better describing one of the characteristic of the pain syndromes. In addition, studies of the recruitment patterns (amplitude and timing) of selected muscles may show asymmetries of muscle function among synergists and antagonists, providing a stronger description of how pain creates and is associated with disordered movement patterns. Both the static and dynamic sEMG findings can serve as landmarks for potential biofeedback-assisted relaxation or muscle retraining sites, thus enhancing the efficacy of these endeavors.

The scientific community has always maintained the responsibility for providing objectivity in its endeavors. The techniques available utilizing surface electrodes can truly improve understanding of the functioning of the muscular system in a precisely documentable and reproducible fashion. The use of objective measures of muscular function can provide insights and direction for the treatment of the many millions of patients with syndromes ranging from headaches and temporomandibular joint dysfunction to diffuse, poorly understood myofascial syndromes.

Clinicians in the pain management arena recognize that more individuals today are suffering from myofascial disorders than in the past. An enhanced understanding of these disorders can greatly reduce the performance of surgical procedures that have always been considered acceptable treatment alternatives despite relatively poor success rates. Without doubt, knowledge of these disorders, derived through surface electromyographic studies, can enhance the quality of medical care and can provide important diagnostic insights for the development of improved treatment protocols. The morbidity associated with invasive treatment approaches can be avoided.

SURFACE ELECTROMYOGRAPHY

Surface electromyography was not developed as an alternative or substitute for needle electromyography studies. It is erroneously believed by some that surface electromyography is a simpler, faster, and more cost-effective alternative to the performance of needle EMG. This, in fact, is not the case. The two technologies differ considerably. Needle electromyography is a procedure characteristically performed by neurologists, physical medicine specialists, and certain physical therapists and chiropractors. The technique involves the placement of needles, either bipolar (with two electrodes) or mono-polar (one electrode) into selected muscle regions for the recording of electrical data in a relatively narrow circumscribed area. These techniques have little applicability for pain management unless one is treating a radiculopathic, neuropathic, or myopathic disorder. The most common application for needle electromyography in pain management today is for the documentation or correlation of a suspected radiculopathy. The typical parameters a needle electromyographer studies are based upon characteristic electrophysiological potentials that are recorded at or about the immediate region of the needle tip.

Needle EMGs study the topology of a single motor unit, while sEMG studies populations of motor units. By studying the muscular energy at this grosser level, the practitioner may begin to see the contributions and perpetrating factors in chronic pain through the quantification of muscle spasm, objective analysis of posture, assessment of emotional contributions, and the identification of faulty motor schemas and imbalances which become involved in the perpetuation of the disorder.

The clinical use of sEMG in the assessment of pain-related disorders was originally introduced by Edmund Jacobson in the 1930 as he began to study the effect of imagination on a variety of muscles. Janet Price in 1948 utilized multisite recording procedures and noted that muscle bracing patterns associated with chronic pain seemed to be asymmetrical, and eventually migrated to areas other than those of the original site of pain. Later, George Whatmore (1974), one of the students of Edmund Jacobson, saw disease as resulting from "dysponesis" or inappropriate muscular efforts. He conceptualized EMG activation patterns from the point of view of excessive bracing, the overrepresentation of emotional events, inefficient movements, or inappropriate attentional efforts. Wolf and Basmajian (1978) were one of the first teams

to document a specific neuromuscular deficit in low back pain patients. Here, they noted the lack of a flexion relaxation response in the erector spinae muscles of back pain patients. More recently, the work of DeLuca and his colleagues (1984) has focused on changes in the energy spectrum of the muscles in back pain patients. Using spectral technique, they have noted that these individuals tend to demonstrate a higher level of muscle fatigue compared to normals.

Surface EMG represents the summation of all of the alpha motor unit activity that reaches the recording electrodes. Typically, the electrodes are placed close together and the recording area is relatively small and specific. Rather than considering these recordings as representing innervations from specific nerve roots, it is more appropriate to think of this activity in terms of motor or muscle function. Such function is organized at multiple levels, including a segmental level.

Also, one should consider the dynamic interplay between the excitation associated with muscle spindle activity vs. the inhibitory influences of the golgi tendon organ. The gamma motor system modulates much of the sensitivity of this interaction and is partially regulated by the cerebellum. It also is excited by nocioception. These afferent fibers give rise to an excitatory push on the gamma motor system, providing the basis for "muscle splinting" around the injured area or joint. This also may modulate posture, potentially leading to learned alpha and gamma motor behavior and antalgic postures. If this postural adjustment is maintained over an extended period of time, trigger points as well as changes in the resting lengths of muscles will ensue. The patient will eventually learn to move differently, usually restricting his or her movement, while substituting inappropriate muscle groups (Lewit, 1985). Last, the pain patient may experience changes in emotional tone associated with pain. Recent evidence (McNutty et al. 1994) has demonstrated that the muscle spindle is activated by ANS activity associated with stress. Fear of pain may increase the resting tone in the muscle due to increased sympathetic tone. In addition, the patient may become anxious about his or her pain, and avoidant behavior patterns may develop. Problems of learned disuse of injured muscles or muscles associated with an injured or fixated joint may need to be addressed. All of the above-described changes in muscle function associated with pain can be documented using surface electromyographic techniques.

While needle EMG studies are very specific, it is now known that the recordings from one motor unit within a muscle are not a valid or general indicator of the status of the muscle itself. Thus, it is very difficult to accurately and reliably assess muscle function using needle EMG recording techniques. On the other hand, surface EMG seems to suffer from a lack of specificity to the precise motor units contributing to the recording.

This volume-conducted sEMG activity from distant muscles is thought to contaminate our confidence in the surface EMG recording.

However, careful placement of closely spaced electrodes, along with close observation of movement patterns associated with the EMG activity, can shed light on the source of the EMG signal. Specific isolated muscle testing may also clarify which muscles are contributing to the surface EMG recording.

An additional problem encountered in surface EMG is that of adipose tissue. The thickness of the adipose tissue may account for alterations of up to 20% of the EMG signal in the resting muscle and 15% in an active muscle. Careful assessment of skinfold thickness at the recording site to help quantify this factor should become part of the standard clinical procedure associated with surface EMG.

One should think of surface EMG as a gross motor rather than a fine motor assessment. Static assessments focus upon patterns of (antalgic) posture, while dynamic, movement-oriented sEMG evaluations explore the general firing patterns at the site(s) of the recording electrodes. Dynamic assessments can be performed to evaluate the neuromuscular system for synergy patterns, co-contractions, asymmetries, irritability, flexion–relaxation, muscle fatigue, faulty motor schemas, and associated emotional responses.

Finally, from an instrumentation point of view, the sEMG signal is processed using a differential amplifier.

Only energy is unique to each recording electrode sites is passed on for amplification, while all common energy (i.e., 60 Hz noise) is rejected. A bandpass filter is utilized to define the energy spectrum of interest. This commonly falls between 15 and 1000 Hz. It is important to note that the major portion of the EMG spectrum is below 80 Hz, and 97% of the signal lies between 5 and 500 Hz. Some commercial EMG biofeedback instruments utilize a very narrow 100- to 200-Hz filter. These filters were designed to facilitate clean, noiseless recordings, avoiding 60-Hz external interference and the biological artifacts of the heart. Bandpass filter considerations are of particular importance in the study of pain-related disorders because chronically fatigued muscles, such as those seen in chronic pain patients, tend to show a preponderance of low frequency signals. The very narrow bandpass 100- to 200-Hz filter would produce an underestimate of the actual level of muscle activity in these patients. In static evaluation procedures (muscle scanning), a narrow filter has been noted to lead to false negative conclusions (Cram, 1990).

SURFACE EMG ASSESSMENTS OF MUSCLE IMPAIRMENT SYNDROMES

The concepts presented below may be studied in greater depth in *Clinical Applications in Surface EMG* by Kasman, Cram, and Wolf (1998). The seven clinical frameworks presented in Figure 47.1 all feed into a self-per-

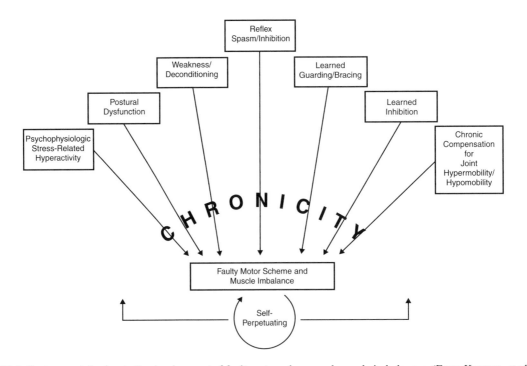

FIGURE 47.1 Factors contributing to the development of fault motor schema and muscle imbalances. (From Kasman, et al., *Clinical Applications in Surface EMG*, Gaithersburg, MD: Aspen Publishers, 1998. With permission.)

petuating faulty motor schema. And, just like elevations in blood pressure do not suggest the origin or etiology of the problem, alterations in sEMG activity need to be understood in a broader context. This chapter explores the possible contribution of each of the seven muscle impairment syndromes.

Elevation in sEMG Due to	Type of Impairment Syndrome
Phobic responses to stairs	Psychophysiological stress
Head forward position	Postural dysfunction
Fear of movement	Learned guarding
Herniated cervical discs	Reflex spasm
Facet blocks	Hypermobility of the cervical joints
Tightness of the upper trapezius relative to lower trapezius	Muscle imbalances

As an example, consider elevations in sEMG levels at rest in the upper trapezius of a patient after a fall down some stairs 6 months prior. These elevations may be due to one or more of the following elements:

Because the clinical syndromes presented here are not mutually exclusive, patients may exhibit qualities of one or more of the syndromes. But, once the etiology is better understood, sEMG retraining procedures (biofeedback) may become one of the treatment elements, one which may help restore the normal motor program that has been altered.

Muscle Impairment Syndrome 1: The Role of Psychophysiological, Stress-Related Hyperactivity

Here, sEMG activity at rest or during movement is elevated either due to general maladaptive coping to stressful situations or a conditioned emotional response to a traumatic event (Post-Traumatic Stress Syndrome).

For example, a patient 4 weeks post motor vehicle accident (MVA) who sustained a flexion extension injury to the neck and shoulder region provides a convenient example. Due to the emotional feature (PTSD) associated with the accident, traditional medical and physical therapies offered to the patient do not produce long-term gains. Clinically, a stress-profiling procedure may be conducted in which the offending muscle is monitored during a baseline recording (Figure 47.2), followed by a period of time in which the patient recalls in detail the events of the MVA. Changes in sEMG recruitment patterns noted during recall of the MVA scene (dysponesis, to use Whatmore's term) provide evidence as to this emotional component.

Once identified, a combination of sEMG "downtraining" and psychological therapy to treat the post-traumatic stress disorder should precede the more physically based

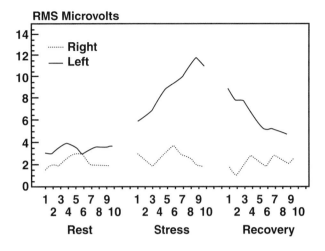

FIGURE 47.2 Stress response pattern in right upper trapezius. Note how the left aspect reacts to the stressor.

therapeutic regimes. Such an approach would enhance the efficient use of clinical time and would greatly facilitate the clinical outcome.

Muscle Impairment Syndrome Type 2: Simple Postural Dysfunction

Here, aberrant motor activity is shown to be a direct function of posture. An example of head posture may be seen in Figure 47.3. The increased paraspinal muscle activity seen in this tracing is reduced as the head is moved from a head forward position to one in which the head is well positioned over its center of gravity. The initial sEMG elevation is associated with a head-forward position and is likely due to the increased load placed on the muscles due to the head being forward of its center of gravity. This increased load would also place untoward loading of the articular structures and chronically place the ligaments on stretch.

According to McKenzie (1981), this chronic physical stress on the soft tissue creates the foundations for pain. In addition, muscle length–tension relationships become inefficient. As the load moments are increased by lengthening the lever arm through which gravity acts, the normal force couples are disrupted and some muscles may recruit at an increased level, while the antagonists takes on a lesser role.

A typical clinical example would be a patient with headache and tension myalgia of the upper quarter and neck associated with work as a keyboard entry person. A postural examination of the patient showed that the patient sits with a head-forward position and with the arms extended slightly while typing. Retraining the patient to type with her head aligned over the spine, and with the elbows closer to her torso resulted in lower sEMG levels and, thus, less tension myalgia.

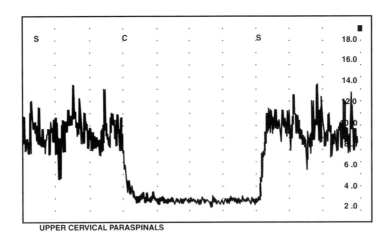

FIGURE 47.3 sEMG activity of the upper cervical paraspinal muscle recorded during a patient's spontaneous forward head posture (S) and corrected postural alignment (C). (From Kasman, et al., *Clinical Applications in Surface EMG*, Gaithersburg, MD: Aspen Publishers, 1998. With permission.)

Muscle Impairment Syndrome Type 3: Weakness and Deconditioning

While muscle weakness may be associated with radiculopathies, plexopathies, neuropathies, or myopathies, the weakness/deconditioning syndrome referred to here involves simple muscle disuse due to immobilization after injury or surgery, or as the cumulative effect of poor motor habits and decreased activity. The condition may include atrophic loss of muscle cross-sectional area, inefficient vascularization, and compromised biochemical and physiological function (Davies & Sargent, 1975). There also may be a change or diminution in neural drive which accompanies changes in muscle tissue. The patterns of dysponetic sEMG activity may include decrements in peak torque, power deficits (i.e., inability to sustain force through ROM arcs), and impaired fatigue resistance.

Consider the case of a patient who has had his knee immobilized and weight-bearing restricted for 6 weeks after sustaining a leg fracture. The quadriceps will undergo disuse atrophy during the period of immobilization. Range of motion, strength, endurance, and functional mobility become impaired during the rehabilitation period. When the knee patient is cleared for active strengthening and is examined, obvious findings of weakness and deconditioning on the involved side are noted during physical examination. With sEMG monitoring, the quadriceps sEMG activity will differ between the involved and uninvolved lower extremities, with maximal effort sEMG activity decreased on the involved side. However, one should be aware that submaximal contractions may show increased activity on the involved side, presumably reflecting decreased neuromuscular efficiency. SEMG biofeedback training could be utilized to enhance the strengthening of the involved side.

Dysfunction Type 4: Acute Reflexive Spasm and Inhibition

Spasm is defined as an involuntary hypertonicity induced by the spinal reflex system (Kraus, 1988). Spasm is commonly triggered by noxious mechanical or chemical stimulation of the pain receptors within the muscle or the associated joint. Inhibition is a neurological suppression of muscle activity induced by pain and/or effusion (deAndrade, et al., 1965). It is driven, in part, by the golgi tendon organ and designed to protect the tendonous attachments and the joint.

Take an example of a low back pain patient with a bulging or herniated disc with pain in the right aspect of the low back, radiating down into the right hip and leg. A back patient with a known bulging or herniated disc has decreased range of motion of the torso and poor sitting tolerance. The patient might present with a flexed and laterally shifted trunk posture, and visibly and palpably elevated lumbar paraspinal tone. Pain is on the same side as the bulging disc. The pain is increased with sitting (supported or not), and the sEMG activation level also increases. Any movements, active or passive, of the lower extremity lead to an activation of the right erector spinae muscles. The pattern of spasm/activation during rest in the seated posture may be easily seen in Table 47.2, reflected in the "muscle scanning" procedure developed by Cram (1990).

An example of acute reflexive inhibition might be seen in a patient with a recent history of trauma and physical examination findings of swelling, tenderness, and inability to tolerate vigorous manual muscle testing of the lower extremity. sEMG monitoring would show a discrete focal drop in sEMG amplitude recorded from the quadriceps during a painful portion of the knee range of motion arc. The focal drop in sEMG activity in this case would be a consequence of neurophysiologic inhibition.

TABLE 47.2
Reflexive Muscle Spasm as Noted in a Muscle Scanning Protocol on a Low Back Pain Patient with Herniated Disk

Muscle Site	Sit		Stand	
	Left	Right	Left	Stand
Cervical	1.2	1.5	1.5	1.7
Trapezius	2.2	3.3	3.2	3.5
T1 Paraspinals	1.2	1.3	1.2	1.2
T6 Paraspinals	3.7	3.8	5.2	5.4
T10 Paraspinals	10.3*	17.1*	4.4	5.9
L3 Paraspinals	10.4*	15.2*	4.2	5.1
Abdominals	1.3	1.5	1.6	1.8

Note: Pain is worse upon sitting.

* Indicates values are outside the normal and expected limits. (From Cram and Engstrom, 1986, *Clinical Biofeedback and Health, 9*(2), 106–116. With permission.)

(From Cram, J.R. (Ed.), 1990, *Clinical EMG for Surface Recording,* Nevada City, CA: Clinical Resources. With permission.)

TABLE 47.3
Protective Guarding Pattern Seen in a Muscle Scanning Finding on a Low Back Pain Patient

Muscle Site	Sit		Stand	
	Left	Right	Left	Stand
Frontal	3.5	3.8	1.2	1.3
Temporal	3.5	3.5	4.6	3.6
Masseter	1.3	1.5	1.5	1.6
Scm	1.2	1.5	0.8	0.9
Cervical	1.6	1.7	1.9	1.9
Trapezius	2.2	2.3	3.0	2.5
T1 Paraspinals	1.5	1.5	1.3	1.1
T6 Paraspinals	3.7	3.5	4.7	4.4
T10 Paraspinals	9.6*	19.2*	44.8*	59.2*
L3 Paraspinals	2.2	11.2*	19.2*	30.4*
Abdominals	1.3	1.5	1.6	1.8

Note: The patient's pain is perceived on the left side of the back and hip.

* Indicates values are outside the normal and expected limits. (From Cram and Engstrom, 1986, *Clinical Biofeedback and Health, 9*(2), 106–116. With permission.)

(From Cram, J.R. (Ed.), 1990, *Clinical EMG for Surface Recording,* Nevada City, CA: Clinical Resources. With permission.)

Muscle Impairment Syndrome Type 5:
Learned Guarding or Bracing

This pattern of neuromuscular activity differs from the reflex spasm model in that the pattern of muscle activity is learned or operantly conditioned rather than being strictly mandated by a reflex. The heightened muscle activity usually occurs upon movement or postural loading and is done in an attempt to avoid pain and the possibility of further injury. The activation pattern is seen on the side opposite the pain (contralateral) as the patient exhibits a learned disuse and inhibition of the painful side and a hyperactivity of the nonpainful side. This is one of the features which differentiates protective guarding from splinting or reflex spasm.

Consider the pattern of muscle activity for a patient with low back pain shown in Table 47.3. These sEMG data were collected done using the muscle scanning procedure mentioned above, in which the right and left aspects of multiple muscle groups were quickly sampled in the seated and standing postures. The patient has left-sided back pain which radiated down into the left hip and leg. Disc herniation is known not to exist. The pattern of activity shows increased sEMG activation on the side opposite of the pain, suggesting a protective guarding pattern. Here, the patient has learned to weight shift away from the pain (antalgic posture).

Muscle Impairment Syndrome Type 6:
Learned Inhibition and Weakness

This syndrome is similar to the protective guarding and bracing model presented above. It differs in that it focuses on the "inhibition" side of the perspective. It is not uncommon, for example, for patients to learn not to move an injured or painful site. The less they move the muscle or joint, the less pain they feel. And through an operant process of negative reinforcement, they learn disuse. It is actually quite common in a unilateral neck/shoulder injury to see the injured side have normal resting tone while the uninvolved side is hyperactive at rest (protective guarding). But when the shoulders are elevated, for example, the injured side shows a hypoactive recruitment pattern, not reaching the same level of activation as the uninvolved side. It is this hypoactivity during strong recruitment that is referred to here as learned inhibition.

Here is another example. An otherwise healthy patient sustains recurrent strains of the hip adductor muscles while playing racquetball. The pain becomes severe and exacerbated whenever the adductor muscles vigorously contract during functional activities. To avoid the contraction-induced pain, the patient learns to reduce firing of the adductors while performing stressful physical activities. Over a period of time the altered patterns become unconsciously incorporated into the patient's selection of motor programs. Interestingly enough, the adductor sEMG amplitude of this patient appears symmetrical on both the involved and uninvolved side during walking and low level activities. In fact, when the patient is subjected to an unanticipated postural perturbation, the adductors are noted to recruit normally. The muscles are normally recruited with postural reactions to help prevent a fall. However, during higher velocity and loading conditions such as sustained unilateral stance, lunging, or formal manual muscle testing, activity on the involved side appears to be markedly decreased and impaired.

Muscle Impairment Syndrome Type 7: Direct Compensation for Joint Hypermobility or Hypomobility

In this syndrome, the neuromuscular system compensates by attempting to stabilize lax joint structures, by affecting movement against joint stiffness, or by subserving linked compensatory movements over kinetic chains (Hertling and Kessler, 1990). Although sEMG activity is aberrant, the primary problem is a biomechanical articular fault. The articular fault is causal to a compensatory motor control pattern, which may spontaneously resolve upon improvement in joint mechanics. Chronic joint dysfunction may lead to motor control problems that, themselves, contribute to deterioration of the kinetic segment and persist even after joint mobility improves. The distinction is made because if aberrant motor activity is felt to be directly compensatory to articular dysfunction, then biofeedback is not a first choice of treatment. The joint dysfunction should be addressed and then sEMG activity re-assessed.

An example of this may be seen in Figure 47.4. Here, a patient with jaw pain is found on physical examination to display hypomobility at the left temporomandibular joint (TMJ). There is a deviation of the midline of the jaw during opening and closing, and a palpable difference between the motions of the left and right mandibular condyles. As opening is initiated (or closing completed), the condyles are felt to spin in place. The condyles are then felt to translate forward as opening continues. This rolling/gliding relationship is necessary for normal jaw range of motion and is expected to be symmetrical at the left and right TMJs. In our case example, sEMG activity shows greater recruitment at the right masseter during jaw opening/closing range of motion. In this case, the right mandibular condyle translates a greater distance along the articular surface of the zygomatic process. The right masseter is activated to a greater degree to subserve the greater range of movement than the right TMJ. The fundamental problem, however, is not one of the right greater than left masseter sEMG activity, but one of the left less than right joint mobility. sEMG spontaneously becomes symmetrical once the left TMJ is mobilized with manual techniques or exercises.

The Final Common Pathway: Chronic Faulty Motor Programs

The final syndrome is an amalgamation and a perpetuation of all of the above syndromes. Here, we assume that the central nervous system learns to cope with pain, muscle

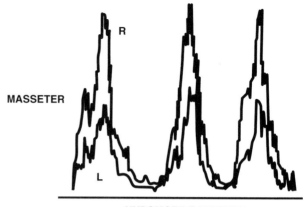

FIGURE 47.4 sEMG activity of the left (L) and right (R) masseter muscles recorded from a patient with left TMJ pain durig three repetitions of jaw opening and closing. Decreased left-side muscle activity was associated with hypomobility of the left joint. (From Kasman, et al., *Clinical Applications in Surface EMG*, Gaithersburg, MD: Aspen Publishers, 1998. With permission.)

weakness, joint instabilities, trigger points, myofascial extensibility issues, etc. As a result of this, there is a learned disruption of the normal agonist–antagonist–synergist relationships. The assessment (and treatment) of this broad syndrome requires sEMG monitoring along with assessment of coincident joint segment dysfunction, soft tissue dysfunction, and behavioral analysis.

Consider Figure 47.5. Here, a patient with chronic cervical paraspinal and suprascapular pain is examined. Motion takes place throughout the shoulder girdle to elevate the arms to the side (abduction). This includes upward rotation of the scapula, achieved by the coordinated actions of the upper trapezius, the lower trapezius, the lower fibers of the serratus anterior, and numerous other muscles with direct and indirect stabilizing roles. A motor program is a planned set of commands from the central nervous system that serves to coordinate the actions of muscles so that a specific goal is achieved, in this case shoulder abduction.

If an inefficient motor program is selected, then one muscle might contract with excessive or reduced tension relative to its synergist, resulting in abnormal loading patterns of both myofascial and articular tissue. With our patient example, it is observed that the sEMG activity of the upper trapezius is considered hyperactive, whereas the activity of the lower trapezius is inhibited. In addition, the patient has a poor ability to recognize these patterns of activation and tension and is unable to voluntarily activate the lower trapezius. Biofeedback may be used to re-educate the patient about his muscle function, and to develop a more appropriate motor program, one which includes the scapular stabilizers (lower trapezius) in arm movement patterns.

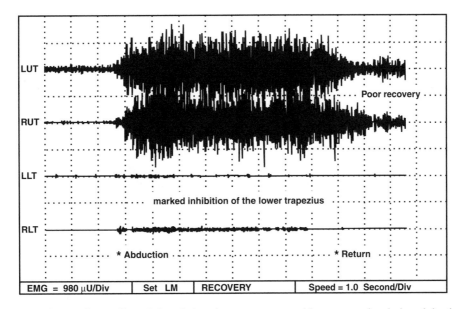

FIGURE 47.5 A grossly abnormal recording of the relations between upper and lower trapezius during abduction to 90°, in which the upper trapezius dominated over lower trapezius. (From Cram, J.R. and Kasman, G.S., *Introduction to Surface EMG*, Gaithersburg, MD: Aspen Publishers, 1990. With permission.)

sEMG RETRAINING AND BIOFEEDBACK TECHNIQUES

Once you understand how potential muscle impairment syndromes may be assessed using sEMG biofeedback techniques, it is useful to consider how the sEMG instrument may be used to treat these disorders. sEMG retraining or biofeedback techniques roughly fall into three clinical entities: downtraining (systemic relaxation), uptraining, and coordination training.

In the broadest sense, downtraining techniques are used to facilitate a reduction in muscles that are overactive. As noted above, they may be overactive for many reasons. If the etiology includes an element of emotions, then the downtraining usually falls under the rubric of systemic relaxation. But please note that some postural training procedures utilize downtraining, as do some ergonomic applications. Ettare and Ettare (1990), for example, have documented the benefits of a dynamic relaxation in which they teach patients to quiet their muscles quickly after every use.

Uptraining is actually easier to teach than downtraining, primarily because the patient is being asked to do something, to learn how to turn on or isolate a particular muscle or muscle group. This type of training is commonly done when working with inhibited muscles, or muscles weakened due to disuse or injury.

Coordination training is considered an advanced level of training and usually follows successful up- or downtraining. It entails trying to teach the patient how to obtain the correct balance of agonists/antagonists. This is more difficult because the cooperation of muscles may involve all three domains of posture, movement, and emotions.

Below, I describe some of the more common sEMG biofeedback procedures. Further examples and explanations of these biofeedback strategies can be found in Kasman, et al. (1998) *Clinical Applications for Surface EMG*, as well as Cram and Kasman (1998) *Introduction to Surface EMG*.

Training Technique 1: Isolation of Target Muscle Activity

Most sEMG biofeedback training strategies begin with assisting the patient to locate, proprioceptively, the dysfunctional muscle. The goal, here, is to learn to isolate it from other muscles. This means learning to contract it alone, and not in concert with surrounding or synergistic muscles. Visual feedback using time series displays of either a raw or processed sEMG signal is usually used to guide the patient's efforts. Figure 47.6 shows an example of training a patient to selectively contract the left lower trapezius (LLT) without creating a co-contraction in the right lower trapezius. As can be seen, the first four contractions are effective, but the fifth one begins to overgeneralize to the contralateral muscle. Through successive training attempts, the patient is taught to produce more and more effort to activate the muscle of interest, while simultaneously inhibiting associated or surrounding muscles. This task may involve open isometric contractions, resisted isometric contractions, open movement, and postural adjustments. After the patient has learned to isolate a particular muscle, then isolation training would proceed to other muscles. In the above example, once the left lower trapezius had been isolated, then the right lower trapezius would be attempted, followed by the left upper trapezius

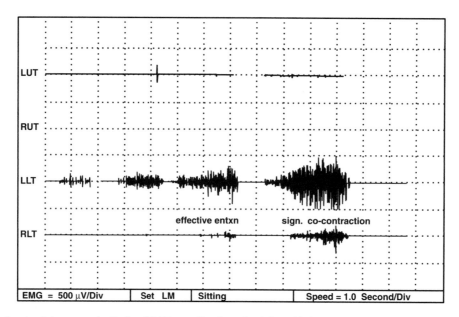

FIGURE 47.6 Isolated training example. Surface EMG recording from the right and left upper and lower trapezius during increasing efforts to recruit and isolate the left lower trapezius. Note that by the fourth attempted recruitment, the patient begins to contract the right lower trapezius along with the left. (From J.R. Cram and G.S. Kasman, *Introduction to Surface EMG*, Gaithersburg, MD: Aspen Publishers, 1990. With permission.)

and finally the right upper trapezius. After isolation is possible, then more advanced coordination training strategies may be employed.

TRAINING TECHNIQUE 2: RELAXATION-BASED DOWNTRAINING

Historically, sEMG biofeedback training was primarily used to assist in the cultivation of low arousal and relaxation (Basmajian, 1989; Gaarder and Montgomery (1977); Schwartz, 1995). Here, sEMG biofeedback is used primarily to treat the emotional layer of neuromuscular dysfunction. In general, the strategy is to use a general or systemic relaxation technique which is assisted by sEMG biofeedback. The feedback, then, is used to guide the success of the relaxation technique. Usually, broad regions or muscles involved in emotional displays (i.e., widely spaced frontal or trapezius placements) are monitored. Such placements take advantage of volume-conducted sEMG activity. However, it is not uncommon also to monitor the injured site and to assess and treat the emotional aspects of trauma. Patients are commonly provided with auditory feedback so that they can close their eyes during the relaxation procedure. Like a beacon, the tone is used to guide them to a more relaxed state on a moment to moment basis. In addition, a time series graph display, usually with a very long sweep time, may be used to see how the relaxation technique has worked over time. The goal is to see a general diminution of resting tone as the patient relaxes.

The selection of the specific relaxation technique depends upon the practitioner's training and the patient's

tendencies. A patient who understands best the physical, concrete world might enjoy the systematic exploration of relaxation using "Progressive Relaxation" introduced by Edmund Jacobson (1976). Here, the patient is taught to tense and release muscles using a systematic step by step, muscle by muscle process. A patient who is more interested in how the mind affects the body might better enjoy an "Autogenics Training" program developed by Luthe (1969). Here, the patient is taught a series of very specific phrases or formulas to repeat. The autogenic phrases have been extensively studied and are known to specifically alter physiological functions. Or, a patient whose strongest attribute is visual representation might best enjoy a guided imagery such as those suggested in the writings of Peper and Holt (1993). Here, patients are asked to close their eyes and the therapist guides them through a relaxing experience, such as laying on the beach on a sunny day soaking in the warmth of the sun and the sand.

Training Technique 3: Threshold-Based Uptraining or Downtraining

Threshold-oriented sEMG biofeedback training utilizes a goal attainment model of training. This technique may be used to teach the patient to either turn on or off a particular muscle or general region. Here, the patient is presented with a highly smoothed and processed sEMG signal along with a visual and/or auditory marker set by the therapist. The marker or threshold is either a colorful line strategically placed within the time series scroll, or an audio event (midi-tone or music), which is turned on or off when the patient meets the specified microvolt level or threshold.

The patient is instructed and shown strategies on how to exceed or fall below this marker. If the patient succeeds in his or her attempts to meet or exceed the threshold, the audio event is played, or the color of the sEMG tracing changes, or the therapist who is attending the training says "good" to reinforce the performance. Once the patient can meet or exceed the criterion set by the therapist 80 to 90% of the time, the therapist raises the threshold in the case of uptraining so that the patient must go to an even higher level of sEMG activity to obtain the threshold-oriented feedback reward. The opposite would be true, of course, for a downtraining protocol. If the patient is having a difficult time meeting the threshold at least 50% of the time, the therapist would change the threshold to afford a higher level of success.

This technique is well steeped in operant or behavioral psychology techniques. The threshold is systematically set and changed to shape and reinforce the patient's sEMG activity to the desired levels. Many computer-based biofeedback systems have been programmed to do this shaping strategy automatically.

Training Technique 4: Threshold-Based Tension Recognition Training

Threshold markers may be used in a variety of ways to shape desired sEMG behaviors. One of these behaviors is the ability to accurately perceive how tense or active the patient's muscle really is. As it turns out, chronic pain patients who have problems with muscle-oriented pain and tension, commonly have lost touch with the proprio-

ceptive nature of what muscle tension feels like. In other words, they commonly don't know what normal feels like, or whether or not a muscle is tense.

The tension recognition technique differs from the uptraining and downtraining approach in that the threshold line now represents the targeted level of sEMG activity the patient is trying to match, rather than the point to exceed or fall below. Here, the patient is systematically trained to go to 5 microvolts, say, over and over and over again. The goal is to train the patient to know proprioceptively where 5 microvolts are from various resting levels and in a variety of postures. Such threshold training is thought to act like an anchor, allowing the patient to more accurately perceive whether his or her muscle activity is elevated above or relaxed below this threshold. Such sensory-based discrimination is very powerful. In one study on headaches (Cram, 1980), such a discrimination training approach was demonstrated to promoted longer-term therapeutic gains than did the downtraining or general relaxation approach described above.

Training Technique 6: Tension Discrimination Training

This procedure is a more advanced form of the threshold-based tension recognition training procedure. It differs only in that the patient is trained to discriminate multiple levels of sEMG activity rather than one. Figure 47.7 demonstrates the use of a visual template in the form of a staircase. Here, the patient is trained using a step template to systematically recognize five equally graded steps of sEMG activity. From a systems model, such

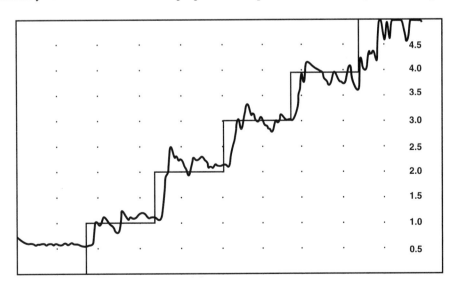

FIGURE 47.7 Tension discrimination training with the use of sEMG feedback from the upper trapezius, with an increase in task complexity from the single threshold model. The "staircase" template shown here is overlaid onto the graphic display. The patient is instructed to match the template as closely as possible. (From Kasman, et al., *Clinical Applications in Surface EMG,* Gaithersburg, MD: Aspen Publishers, 1998. With permission.)

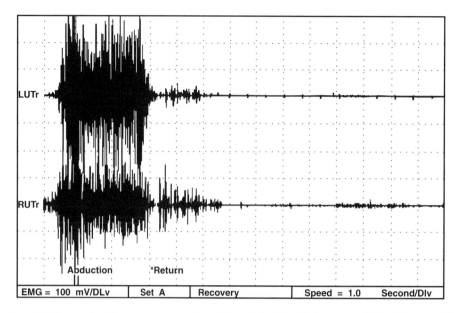

FIGURE 47.8 Surface EMG recording from upper trapezius during abduction of the arm to 90° and return. Note the presence of activity for 2 seconds following the return of the arm to the side. (From Cram and Kasman, *Introduction to Surface EMG*, Gaithersburg, MD: Aspen Publishers, 1990. With permission.)

proprioceptive knowledge of different levels of sEMG activity should allow the muscle to be regulated over a wider range of amplitudes.

Training Technique 7: Deactivation Training

Deactivation training is basic to all sEMG training procedures. In essence, it trains the patient to turn off the sEMG activity following activation. Figure 47.8 show a time series graph in which the patient exhibits spontaneous

sEMG discharge for two seconds following the cessation of a movement. Figure 47.9 shows how the patient was trained using visually guided feedback to turn off the post-movement discharge immediately following the cessation of the movement.

As is well known, many repetitive strain disorders (RSI) are due to overuse. But what probably isn't realized is that overuse is amplified by not letting the muscles rest between repetitions. Teaching a patient to turn off the muscle after each and every use has been found to be an effective method

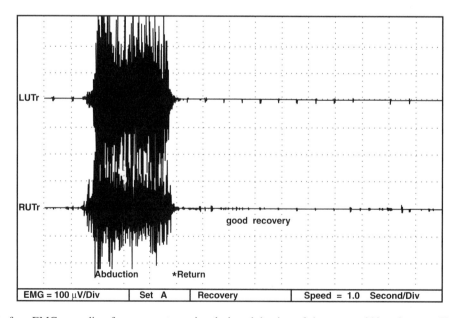

FIGURE 47.9 Surface EMG recording from upper trapezius during abduction of the arm to 90° and return. Here, the patient has been trained to quiet the muscles as quickly as possible following the cessation of movement. (From J.R. Cram and G.S. Kasman, *Introduction to Surface EMG*, Gaithersburg, MD: Aspen Publishers, 1990. With permission.)

for treating RSI. For a broader discussion of this type of procedure in clinical see Ettare and Ettare (1990).

Training Technique 8: Generalization to Progressively Dynamic Movement

Training in muscle control procedures usually begins in a static state. Isometric contractions are easier to produce and replicate than fully dynamic ones. But once they have been mastered, it is important to attempt to generalize them. This generalization typically involves larger and larger contractions, and faster and faster movements.

Training Technique 9: sEMG-Triggered Neuromuscular Electrical Stimulation (NMES)

This is a very sophisticated and powerful procedure which involves not only an sEMG instrument to monitor the electrical activity of the muscle, but also a microcurrent device to activate the muscle indirectly through the stimulation of the peripheral motor nerves (Baker, 1991). The procedure is very similar to the

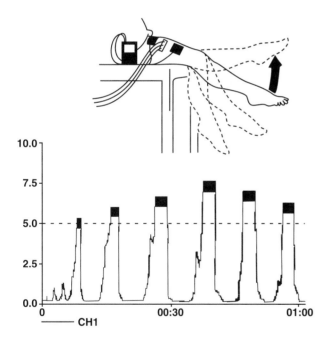

FIGURE 47.10 Standard sEMG-triggered NMES setup. EMG electrodes detect a voltage sum derived from muscle action potentials. The EMG signal is processed in a routine manner, and when the display magnitude exceeds a predetermined value, a relay causes a neuromuscular electrical stimulator to deliver current to the same muscle. The EMG display is nullified during the electrical stimulation because the device would record voltage associated with injection of artificial current, masking the small muscle action potentials. (From Kasman et al., *Clinical Applications in Surface EMG*, Gaithersburg, MD: Aspen Publishers, 1998. With permission.)

threshold-based uptraining one. The only difference is that when the patient reaches a predetermined (threshold) level of activity, the stimulation device is activated and full muscle recruitment is thereby electrically mandated. Usually this technique is used in very weak muscles. The threshold is initially set at a level which the patient can easily reach, but which is nonfunctional. When that threshold is met, a fully functional muscle contraction is created with the microcurrent device. Figure 47.10 shows an example of NMES training of the quadriceps muscle.

Training Technique 10: Left/Right Equilibration Training

Equilibration training is performed when the left and right aspects of homologous muscle pairs are observed to recruit in an asymmetrical fashion during a symmetrical tasks. For example, a symmetrical movement such as forward flexion of the head should bring about a symmetrical recruitment of the sternocliedomastoid muscles. An asymmetry of recruitment might come about due to a hyperextension injury to one side of the neck associated with a motor vehicle accident and the resultant flexion extension injury. The hyperextension injury leads to disruption of muscle spindle activity and long-term inhibited recruitment patterns within the injured muscle.

Equilibration training is designed to restore symmetrical sEMG recruitment patterns. It typically involves simultaneous recording from the right and left aspects of the homologous muscle pair. A processed sEMG signal is displayed on a time series display with the two channels of sEMG aggregated on the same screen using the same sensitivities and sweep times. In this way the symmetry of the activity of the two muscles can be easily seen. A skilled therapist will use a variety of therapeutic skills, such as uptraining the lower, more inhibited side to create greater symmetry of recruitment. The sEMG feedback guides that effort.

Training Technique 11: Motor Copy Training

This is a more advanced coordination training protocol. Here an sEMG recruitment pattern is created during movement. It is stored and later placed on the screen as a background template. The patient is then asked to use his or her own muscle effort during a live sEMG display to copy or follow the template.

Typically these types of procedures are done with patients who have unilateral weaknesses, such as stroke. The uninvolved side is then used during the desired movement to generate the template. The template from the uninvolved side is used teach how to use the involved side in a normalized fashion.

Training Technique 12: Postural Training with sEMG Feedback

This is a fairly straightforward procedure. Typically a time series scroll of the postural muscles of interest is provided. The therapist then assists the patient in obtaining a more natural or correct posture, and the sEMG feedback display demonstrates how the improved posture provides less work and stress on the musculoskeletal activity. In more complicated cases, the therapist might need to uptrain a weakened or unused set of muscles so that they may better play their roles in postural support.

Training Technique 13: Body Mechanics Instruction

This procedure is very similar to the postural training procedure, except this time the patient is doing more vigorous work. It usually involves a time series scroll of a processed signal from muscles that are either prime movers or stabilizers. Commonly, the patient is asked to do a task, such as lifting an object from the ground, and the therapist teaches standard body mechanics and observes how well the muscles recruit during the movement. Corrections and suggestions about the lifting technique might be given, and the lift tried again. The sEMG recording may be used to demonstrate how the new technique for lifting will reduce the probability of injury to the involved muscles.

Training Technique 14: Therapeutic Exercise Validated with sEMG Feedback

In physical medicine, patients are commonly given exercises by the therapist to strengthen a given muscle or muscle grouping. Occasionally, when given a therapeutic exercise, the patient inadvertently uses a muscle substitution pattern to create the desired movement pattern. When sEMG is used, a time series scroll showing the recruitment pattern of the prime movers and stabilizers of the exercise may be used to verify that the exercise is working on the desired muscles. If a muscle substitution pattern is noted, the patient may then be trained using the sEMG feedback to recruit the desired muscles for the given exercise.

Training Technique 15: Functional Activity Performance with sEMG Feedback

All of the prior training techniques lead to this procedure. It is essential to take an isolated training procedure and introduce it into real and varied life activities. Refinements of movement, posture, and emotional tone may be done during this time.

SUMMARY

In summary, we introduced sEMG as a procedure that may provide more beneficial information concerning chronic pain disorders than traditional electrodiagnostic tools. This is particularly true when the pain disorder involves muscles or myofascial pain. Seven muscle impairment syndromes were described, and the role of sEMG in their description and diagnosis was explored. A partial list of disorders with potential neuromuscular or musculoskeletal components includes tension headache, TMJ and myofacial pain disorders, post-traumatic stress disorder, cervical dysfunctions, shoulder girdle and upper extremity dysfunctions, low back dysfunctions, hip dysfunctions, knee dysfunctions, stroke, and urinary incontinence. These disorders are ones in which an sEMG assessment should be considered. In addition, these disorders may also be treatable, in part, using sEMG biofeedback. This chapter provided a description of 15 different sEMG treatment strategies relevant to the chronic pain patient. Formal "Application Guides" that describe clinical protocols for assessment and treatment of many of these disorders are available in Kasman et al. (1998). Please refer to this volume to understand these clinical concepts in further depth.

REFERENCES

Baker, L.L. (1991). Clinical uses of neuromuscular electrical stimulation. In R.P. Nelson and D.P. Currier (Eds.), *Clinical electrotherapy* (2nd ed.) New York: McGraw-Hill.

Basmajian, J.V. (Ed.). (1989). *Biofeedback: Practice and principles for clinicians*. Baltimore: Williams & Wilkins.

Basmajian, J.V., & DeLuca, C. (1985). *Muscles alive*. Baltimore: Williams & Wilkins.

Cram, J.R. (1980). EMG Biofeedback and the treatment of tension headaches: A systematic analysis of treatment components. *Behavior Therapy*, 11, 699–710.

Cram, J.R. (1990). EMG muscle scanning and diagnostic manual for surface recordings. In J.R. Cram (Ed.), *Clinical EMG for surface recordings* (Vol. 2). Nevada City: Clinical Resources,

Cram, J.R., & Engstrom, D. (1986). Patterns of neuromuscular activity in pain and non-pain patients. *Clinical Biofeedback and Health*, 9(2), 106–116.

Cram, J.R., & Kasman, G.S. (1998). *Introduction to surface EMG*, Gaithersburg, MD: Aspen Publishing.

Cram, J.R., and Steger, J.C. (1983). EMG diagnostic scanning for pain related disorder. *Biofeedback and Self-Regulation*, 8(2), 229–241.

Davies, C.T.M., & Sargeant, A.G. (1975). Effects of exercise therapy on total and component tissue leg volumes or patients undergoing rehabilitation from lower limb injury. *Annals of Human Biology*, 2, 327–335.

deAndrade, J.R., Grant, C., & Dixon, A. (1965). Joint distention and reflex muscle inhibition in the knee. *Journal of Bone and Joint Surgery (U.S. Volume)*, 47, 313–322.

DeLuca, C. (1984). Myoelectric manifestations of localized muscular fatigue in humans. *CRC Critical Reviews in Biomedical Engineering, 11*(4), 251.

Donaldson, S. (1991). Multi-channel EMG Assessment and Treatment Techniques. In J.R. Cram (Ed.), *Clinical EMG for surface recordings* (Vol. 2). Nevada City: Clinical Resources.

Donaldson, S., Clasby, B., Skubick, D., & Cram, J.R. (1994). The evaluation of trigger point activity using dynamic sEMG techniques. *American Journal of Pain Management, 4*(3), 118–122.

Ettare, D., & Ettare, R. (1990). Muscle learning therapy: A treatment protocol. In J.R. Cram (Ed.), *Clinical EMG for surface recordings* (Vol. 2). Nevada City: Clinical Resources.

Gaarder, K.R., & Montgomery, P.S. (1977). *Clinical biofeedback: A procedural manual.* Baltimore: Williams & Wilkins.

Hertling, D., & Kessler, R.M. (1990). *Management of common musculoskeletal disorders* (2nd ed.). Philadelphia: J.B. Lippincott Co.

Hubbard, D., & Berkoff, G. (1993). Myofascial trigger points show spontaneous needle EMG activity. *Spine, 18,* 1803–1807.

Jacobson, E. (1976). *You must relax.* New York: McGraw-Hill.

Jacobson, E. (1932). Electrophysiology of mental activities. *American Journal of Psychology, 108,* 573–580.

Kasman, G., Cram, J.R., & Wolf, S. (1998). *Clinical applications in surface EMG.* Gaithersburg, MD: Aspen Publishers.

Kraus, H. (1988). Muscle spasm. In H. Kraus (Ed.), *Diagnosis and treatment of muscle pain.* Chicago: Quintessence Publishing Co.

Lewit, K. (1985). *Manipulative therapy in rehabilitation of locomotor system.* Boston: Butterworth.

Luthe, W. (Ed.). (1969). *Autogenics therapy.* (Vols. 1–4). New York: Grune & Stratton.

McKenzie, R. (1981). *The lumbar spine: mechanical diagnosis and therapy.* Waikanae, New Zealand: Spinal Publications.

McNutty, W., Gervitz, R., Berkoff, G., & Hubbard, D. (1994). Needle EMG evaluation of trigger point responses to psycholophysiological stressors. *Psychophysiology, 31,* 313–316.

Peper, E., & Holt, C. (1993). *Creating wholeness: A self-healing workbook using dynamic relaxation, imagery, and thoughts.* New York: Plenum Press.

Price, J.P., Clare, M.H., & Ewerhardt, R.H. (1948). Studies in low backache with persistent muscle spasm. *Archives of Physical Medicine and Rehabilitation, 29,* 703–709.

Schwartz, M. (Ed.) (1995). *Biofeedback: A practitioner's guide.* New York: Guilford Press.

Sihovenen, T., Partanim, J., Osmo, H., & Soimankalio, A. (1991). Electric behavior of low back muscles during lumbar pelvic rhythm in low back pain patients and healthy controls. *Archives of Physical Medicine and Rehabilitation, 72,* 1080–1087.

Taylor, W. Dynamic EMG biofeedback in assessment and treatment using a neuromuscular re-education model. In J.R. Cram (Ed.). *Clinical EMG for surface recordings* (Vol. 2). Nevada City: Clinical Resources.

Travell, J. (1976). Myofacial trigger points: Clinical review. In J.J. Bonica & D. Albe-Fassard (Eds.). *Advances in pain research,* (Vol. 1). (p. 919). New York: Raven Press.

Veiersted, K.B., Westgaard, R.H., & Andersen, P. (1993). Eletromyographic evaluation of muscular work pattern as a predictor of trapezius myalgia. *Scandanavian Journal of Work Environment and Health, 19,* 284–290.

Whatmore, G., & Kohli, D. (1974). *The physiopathology and treatment of functional disorders.* New York: Grune & Stratton.

Wolf, S., & Basmajian, J. (1978). Assessment of paraspinal electromyographic activity in normal subjects and chronic back pain patients using a muscle biofeedback device. In E. Asmussen & K. Jorgensen (Eds.), *International series on biomechanics* (Vol. 6B). Baltimore: University Park Press.

48

Six Diverse Acupuncture Techniques Useful in Pain Management

William D. Skelton, D.Ac.

INTRODUCTION

Acupuncture is a therapeutic modality that originated in China approximately 3000 years ago. It is the main component of traditional Chinese medicine, and serves as the basis of the physical and rehabilitative side of that system, one that is remarkable not only for acupuncture but in other areas as well. For example, a complete pharmacology was developed in the Sung Dynasty (960–1270 A.D.); a system of preventative medicine, including a nasal-inhaled small-pox immunization, was created in the 17th century; and a sophisticated form of forensic medicine was developed during the Warring States Period (475–221 B.C.).

Over the millennia the understanding and application of acupuncture have changed radically. At various times in China, this therapy has been adapted and modified to fit political structures, populist theories, philosophies, and belief systems. Various cultures have exerted their own influences to modify the practice of acupuncture, which is why there is Japanese acupuncture, French acupuncture, and others. In addition, the ongoing creative and experimental adaptations individuals have contributed to the practice of this therapy furthered the momentum of acupuncture's development. The result is a rich diversity of acupuncture styles and techniques.

The use of acupuncture in the United States has added its own unique mark on the profession and practice of acupuncture. While U.S. acupuncture can be traced back to the early 1800s, it was not until 1972 that the country as a whole became familiar acupuncture and its application. Since that time, acupuncture has steadily become less of an alternative to traditional Western medical treatment and more of a vital component of the U.S. healthcare system, particularly in pain management.

In this chapter I provide a short discussion of the use of acupuncture for the treatment of pain, followed by overviews of six specialized acupuncture techniques that are well suited for use in pain management programs. Although each of these techniques differs from what is typically thought of as a traditional acupuncture treatment, each can fit easily into a pain management program and yield impressive results. None of them rely as heavily on the Chinese biopsychosocial model for diagnosis; they do not try to treat the "whole" person, nor do they require the level of knowledge and skill that is needed to practice acupuncture as an independent approach to healthcare.

Following each overview is an example, or examples, of individual points that might be used in each technique for the treatment of an occipital headache and low back pain. The points listed do not constitute a treatment and are only examples of possible points. The point name or number is followed by a description of the location simply to orient the reader. For the sake of brevity and clarity, I have taken the liberty of selecting common points, giving a general location, and omitting mention of any special needle techniques such as angle, direction, insertion, or method of manipulation that might be indicated, because trained practitioners already have that knowledge.

Each of the acupuncture techniques described in this chapter is simple, effective, safe, and can be incorporated into virtually any program as either a stand-alone modality or as an adjunct to other traditional medical therapies.

0-8493-0926-3/02/$0.00+$1.50
© 2002 by CRC Press LLC

Because of the variety of treatment options possible with these techniques, they easily accommodate the idiosyncrasies of a typical pain management program and those of the patients.

TREATING PAIN WITH ACUPUNCTURE

It is estimated that over 10 million acupuncture treatments are administered in the United States yearly. Acupuncture therapy has moved into the healthcare system on many levels, ranging from integrative health clinics to substance abuse treatment centers. The most common use, however, is in the treatment and management of pain.

Across the country, pain management clinics and pain treatment centers serving a wide variety of specialties, major hospitals, and medical school teaching clinics have added acupuncture therapy to treat pain associated with arthritis, headaches, back and spine problems, and other ailments. Besides being highly effective and clearly popular with patients, there are many advantages to using acupuncture in a pain management program. Two of the most important are that acupuncture is easily adapted to the needs of the program and patient and it is suitable for use in conjunction with the traditional therapies the program offers.

EFFICACY

Studies have demonstrated that acupuncture is effective in treating pain. The 1997 National Institute of Health consensus statement on acupuncture stated that acupuncture may be useful as an adjunct treatment or an acceptable alternative or be included in a comprehensive management program for conditions including myofascial pain, fibromyalgia, osteoarthritis, low back pain, carpal tunnel syndrome, tennis elbow, and others.

ADAPTABILITY

The diversity of acupuncture techniques, such as the ones detailed in this chapter, enable a practitioner to treat a patient regardless of most limitations or restrictions such as implants, braces, wheelchairs, bandages, difficulty sitting or lying down, modesty, or any other barrier that might restrict treatment.

These techniques are easily adapted to the limitations of the pain management program. Often, programs are unable to provide the space or time required for a traditional acupuncture treatment, where a patient might occupy a room for 30 to 60 minutes. These techniques are ideal for group treatment settings, in which the shared results and a group dynamic can enhance the morale and response of the program participants. To reduce scheduling burdens and offer a wider variety of therapies, these techniques can be coupled with other therapies, such as

physical therapy, occupational therapy, and counseling. This multimodality approach can produce impressive results, enabling patients to function at improved levels.

Acupuncture demonstrates additional benefits in pain management programs by treating the acute problems such as muscle aches, headaches, etc. that arise normally or from the rigors of the program. On a more subtle level, acupuncture helps decrease depression, increase a sense of well-being, and improve patients' compliance with the requirements of their treatment programs.

CHOOSING A TECHNIQUE

Effective practitioners of acupuncture in pain management programs demonstrate a repertoire of techniques that range from those of modern acupuncture to those of traditional Chinese acupuncture. The treatment is tailored to the patient, the treatment setting, and the other therapies being administered to the patient. Because of these variables patients presenting with the same condition would typically receive very different treatments, even though the practitioner will probably be biased toward, and more comfortable with, particular treatment techniques.

The practitioner chooses an acupuncture technique or techniques based on the patient's constitution, physical condition, associated symptoms, emotions, and other biopsychosocial factors. Each treatment is also oriented to the disorder, the point in time of treatment, how chronic the condition is, the level or depth of the disorder, and the way the symptoms and signs change. The practitioner takes into consideration the depth, strength, and direction of the treatment techniques to determine which is appropriate.

Each of the techniques described in this chapter works on a different depth and requires a different perspective from the practitioner. In addition, each technique represents the practitioner's orientation to the patient; the choice of technique will also, in part, reflect the level of the practitioner's knowledge and understanding of the attributes that compose acupuncture.

THE SIX TECHNIQUES

AURICULAR ACUPUNCTURE

Auricular acupuncture is a refined and highly effective microsystem based on a somatotopic representation of the ear as an inverted fetus (Figure 48.1). Thus, points on the earlobe correlate to the patient's head, and points on other parts of the ear correlate to the other parts of the patient's body.

Although auricular acupuncture treatment has been a part of traditional acupuncture therapy, it developed as a comprehensive system of diagnosis and treatment in the late 1950s. At that time a French physician, Paul

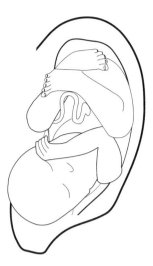

FIGURE 48.1 Somatotopic representation of the ear as an inverted fetus. (Courtesy of Carl L. Milton.)

Nogier, published his findings correlating specific sites on the ear to parts of the body. Now, throughout the world, there are many acupuncturists who only use auricular points for their treatments. The advantages of this system are that acupuncture points for only a small terrain need to be learned, and that the treatment procedure is simple and safe.

Auricular therapy can also be effective without needles, using a technique that involves taping a small surgical steel bead, resembling a BB pellet, onto various auricular points. The patient gently stimulates the bead by pressing on it periodically. Beads can be left in place for days, enhancing and extending the treatment. Self-application of the bead is not practical with auricular points, as it is with some of the techniques that follow, because the precise self-location of auricular points is difficult.

Auricular acupuncture is also amenable to other noninvasive treatment techniques that rely on the electrical stimulation of the points. Electric stimulation devices can assist practitioners in locating and electrically stimulating the auricular points as the therapy. These devices are widely available in the medical marketplace.

As with traditional acupuncture there are different levels of treatment possible with auricular acupuncture, ranging from symptomatic pain management to more complete utilization of the complex theories, techniques, and systems of acupuncture. In pain management, auricular points are very effective, simple to apply, and well tolerated by the patient. Additionally, using a deeper level of understanding of auricular therapy, points can be selected to treat mood, stress, emotions, and functional disorders. Such a wide variety of benefits is of significant value in a pain management program.

There are over 200 auricular acupuncture points that have been identified on each ear (Figure 48.2). They can be located by noting states of tenderness, measuring levels

of electrical resistance, and noting abnormalities in coloration and morphological states.

In a pain management setting it is often most suitable to first select the appropriate points based on the pain being treated. The treatment technique for auricular therapy should produce a sensation of local soreness, warmth, or distention. Periodically, during the treatment, the needles are manually rotated or manipulated to reproduce these sensations. Electrostimulation applied to the inserted needle also can be beneficial for pain management.

Point Examples

- To treat occipital headache
  Point Name: *Occiput* (Figure 48.3)
  Point Location: Posterior and superior to the lateral aspect of the antitragus
  Point Name: *Sympathetic nerve* (Figure 48.3)
  Point Location: At the junction of the medial border of the helix and the infra-antihelix crus
  Point Name: *Subcortex* (Figure 48.3)
  Point Location: Anterior aspect of the inner wall of the antitragus
- To treat low back pain
  Point Name: *Shenmen* (Figure 48.4)
  Point Location: Medial and superior to the lateral angle of the triangular fossa
  Point Name: *Lumbosacral* (Figure 48.4)
  Point Location: On the medial border of the antihelix and level with the lumbar point
  Point Name: *Adrenal* (Figure 48.4)
  Point Location: On the inferior prominence of the tragus

HAND ACUPUNCTURE

There are two distinct systems of hand acupuncture: the Chinese system and the Korean system. They are both microsystems that reflect the anatomy of the patient and have points that influence all parts of the anatomy. Each system is distinguished by the point location, point indications, techniques of needle insertion, and the type of needles used.

The Chinese system of hand acupuncture is the oldest and easiest to use in a pain management program but it has limited application, because there are a limited number of points and areas of the body that it influences. The Korean system has far greater flexibility and scope, requires a deeper understanding of the system, and is more complicated to apply.

Both systems can easily be taught to patients for self-application of an acupressure device that stimulates the appropriate points without penetrating the skin. This approach can give patients a safe way to control their pain to some degree.

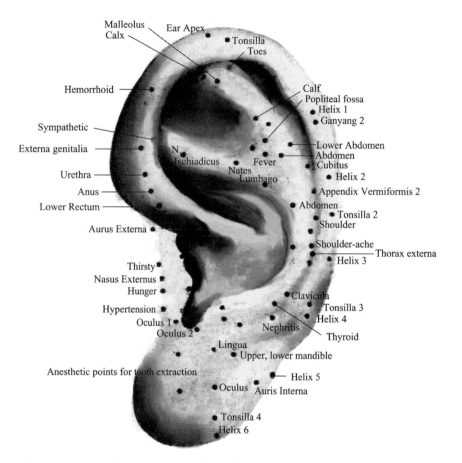

FIGURE 48.2 Auricular acupuncture points. (Courtesy of Carl L. Milton.)

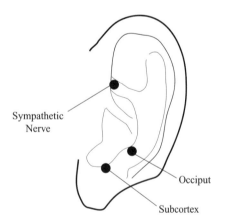

FIGURE 48.3 Auricular points for occipital headache. (Courtesy of Carl L. Milton.)

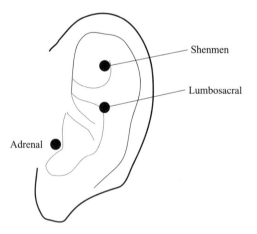

FIGURE 48.4 Auricular points for backache. (Courtesy of Carl L. Milton.)

The Chinese System of Hand Acupuncture

In this system there are specific acupuncture points for the treatment of areas and functions of the body. The locations of points are easily found by using anatomical landmarks on the hand. The points are named according to the part of the body or a specific function or disorder that they affect or control.

In a pain management setting hand acupuncture techniques can be very effective and well tolerated by the patient. In general, point selection is symptomatically based. The treatments are usually contralateral, that is, left-hand points are used for right-sided problems. The needle is manipulated following insertion to generate a moderate to strong sensation. While the needles are *in situ*, the patient is instructed to move and gently flex the area that is in pain or being treated. Electrostimulation of the hand acupuncture points can be appropriate for many cases.

Point Examples

- To treat occipital headache
- Point Name: *Occiput* (Figure 48.5)
  Point Location: On the midpoint of the ulnar side of the fifth finger at the level of the first interphalangeal joint
  Point Name: *Lateral head* (Figure 48.5)
  Point Location: On the midpoint of the ulnar side of the fourth finger at the level of the first interphalangeal joint
- To treat low back pain
  Point Name: *Lumbar and leg #1* (Figure 48.5)
  Point Location: At the radial aspect of the tendon of the second extensor digitorum manus

Point Name: *Lumbar and leg #2* (Figure 48.5)
Point Location: At the ulnar side of the fourth extensor digitorum manus
Point Name: *Vertebrae* (Figure 48.5)
Point Location: On the midpoint of the ulnar side of the fifth finger at the level of the metacarpophalangeal joint

The Korean System of Hand Acupuncture

Korean hand acupuncture was developed in the 1970s. It is a microsystem providing both a somatotopic representation of the human anatomy (Figure 48.6) and a representation of the traditional acupuncture system of points and meridians.

This system consists of a network of 14 micromeridians and 345 micropoints on each hand. The micromeridians and

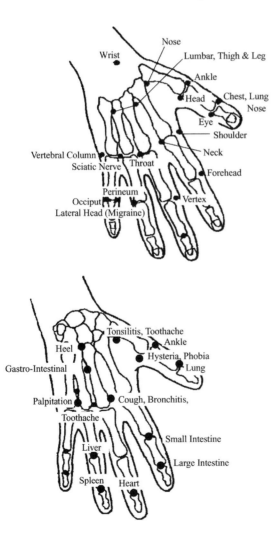

FIGURE 48.5 Chinese hand acupuncture. (Courtesy of Carl L. Milton.)

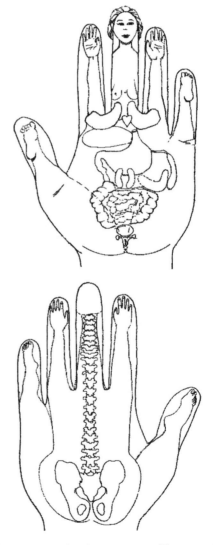

FIGURE 48.6 Korean hand acupuncture. (Courtesy of Carl L. Milton.)

the micropoints are, with some variations, analogous to the traditional acupuncture meridians, or channels.

As with traditional acupuncture there are different levels of treatment possible with Korean hand acupuncture. These range from a purely symptomatic treatment to ones that incorporate all of the complex theories and philosophies and point selections of traditional acupuncture treatment.

The easiest and most suitable level of applying Korean hand acupuncture for use in a pain management program is based on the somatotopic relationship of the hand and the whole body. Points are selected according to the anatomical location of the pain. Tiny needles, made specifically for this system, are inserted into the points and left for the duration of the treatment.

Point Examples

- To treat occipital headache
  Point Name: *#3 Korean I micromeridian* (Figure 48.7)
  Point Location: On the dorsal side of the hand lateral and medial to the midpoint of the crease of the distal interphalangeal joint of the third finger
  Point Name: *#24 Korean B micromeridian* (Figure 48.8)
  Point Location: On the dorsal side of the hand at the midpoint of the crease of the distal interphalangeal joint of the third finger
- To treat low back pain
  Point Name: *#17–20 Korean I micromeridian* (Figure 48.7)
  Point Location: On the dorsal side of the hand on the lateral and medial border of the distal half of the third metacarpal bone
  Point Name: *#7 Korean B micromeridian* (Figure 48.8)
  Point Location: On the dorsal side of the hand, over the third metacarpal bone near the delineation of the distal quarter of its length

HEAD ACUPUNCTURE

Head acupuncture, also known as scalp needling therapy, was developed during the Chinese Cultural Revolution (1966–1976) and incorporates acupuncture techniques popularized during that period of history. The point locations and indications were developed in accord with the representative areas on the cerebral cortex.

In this technique a practitioner first identifies landmark lines along the scalp of the patient. The midline of the head is identified as going from the midpoint between the eyebrows and over the top of the head to the external occipital protuberance. The eyebrow-occipital line is

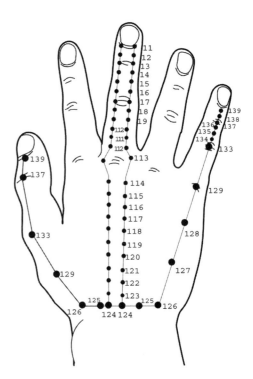

FIGURE 48.7 Points on the Korean I micromeridian. (Courtesy of Carl L. Milton.)

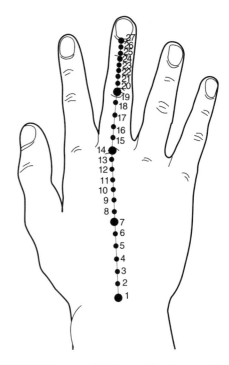

FIGURE 48.8 Points on the Korean B micromeridian. (Courtesy of Carl L. Milton.)

identified as going from the midpoint of the eyebrow and across the temple to the external occipital protuberance (Figure 48.9). The motor area line is identified as going from a point located 0.5 cm posterior to the midpoint of

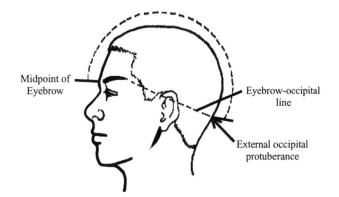

FIGURE 48.9 The eyebrow-occipital line. (Courtesy of Carl L. Milton.)

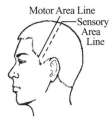

FIGURE 48.10 The motor area and sensory area lines. (Courtesy of Carl L. Milton.)

the midline across to the juncture of the eyebrow-occipital line and the temporal hairline (Figure 48.10). All measurements for other scalp acupuncture lines and point locations are made from these lines.

Typically, a treatment involves selecting the point located over the area of the cerebral cortex that corresponds to the problem. Additional points that have a related effect are often added to the treatment. Contralateral points are used for conditions affecting one side of the patient's body, while bilateral points are used for more general, bilateral, or systemic conditions.

After the appropriate point is located, the scalp over the point is lifted slightly using a pinching method and a needle is inserted under and almost horizontal to the scalp. The needle path follows the lines as measured from the landmarks. Once the needle is inserted to the proper depth, it is rotated 200 to 400 times per minute while maintaining its position at the desired depth. When the needle is applied properly a patient often notices sensations of heat, paresthesia, throbbing, or an involuntary movement in the limb that is being treated. Because there is a possibility that the patient will feel faint or light-headed from this treatment, it is best applied when the patient is in a fully supported position.

Head acupuncture therapy is the most difficult of the techniques discussed here to fit into a pain management program. It is time- and labor-intensive, and it requires precise point location and attention to needle technique. The sensations noted by the patient can be very strong.

Patients tend to be less comfortable with this technique than the others discussed in this chapter, and therefore the technique is best suited for motor and sensory disorders of the limbs. The advantage to head acupuncture, however, is that it can produce results when the other techniques failed.

Point Examples

- To treat occipital headache
  Line Name: *Sensory area line* (Figure 48.10)
  Line Location: 1.5 cm posterior to the motor area line
  Needle Insertion: Upper fifth of the sensory area line
- To treat low back pain
  Line Name: *Sensory area line* (Figure 48.10)
  Line Location: 1.5 cm posterior to the motor area line
  Needle Insertion: Upper two fifths of the sensory area line
  Line Name: *Leg and motor sensory area line* (Figure 48.11)
  Line Location: 1 cm lateral to, and parallel with, the midpoint of the midline
  Approximately 3 cm in length
  Needle Insertion: The entire line

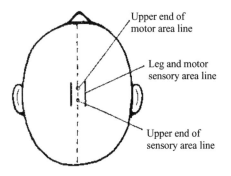

FIGURE 48.11 Leg and motor sensory area line. (Courtesy of Carl L. Milton.)

DISTAL RELEASE ACUPUNCTURE POINTS

Distal release acupuncture points consist of traditional acupuncture points and also of special or extra acupuncture points that have a known effect on a specific area or function of the body. They are part of the aggregate body of knowledge of acupuncture and are used unconventionally, not following the traditional theories and rules of acupuncture. A skilled acupuncturist, over time, develops a repertoire of points that can be used in conjunction with the other levels of therapy.

These points are usually located on the opposite part of the body from the side being treated and are applied symptomatically. They are usually very tender when palpated, which is how most practitioners determine if the point is appropriate. The stimulation of these points is effective in relieving pain, releasing muscle tension, and improving range of motion. Patients are asked to move and stretch the area of pain while the needles are in place. The needles are periodically rotated to evoke a mild distension at the site of insertion.

In a pain management program these points can be utilized to provide fast relief of discomfort and limitations of movement brought on by the activities of the program. They are also useful when a practitioner is unable to treat an area due to the sensitivity of the area. These points can be used to sufficiently relieve discomfort so that a local treatment can be administered. These specialized points are especially useful when the patient is combining acupuncture with another therapy such as physical therapy or occupational therapy.

Point Examples

- To treat occipital headache
   Point Name: *GB 40* (Figure 48.12)
   Point Location: Anterior and inferior to the lateral malleolus, in the depression lateral to the tendon
   Point Name: *BL 60* (Figure 48.12)
   Point Location: At the midpoint of the space between the lateral malleolus and the tendon calcaneus
   Point Name: *S 13* (Figure 48.13)
   Point Location: Proximal to the fifth metacarpal bone, on the medial edge of the palm where a crease forms when the hand is made into a fist
- To treat low back pain
- Point Name: *Yaotongxue* (Figure 48.16)
   Point Location: On the dorsum of the hand between the second and third, and between the fourth and fifth, metacarpal bones, half way between the transverse crease of the wrist and the metacarpophalangeal joint
   Point Name: *SI 6* (Figure 48.14)

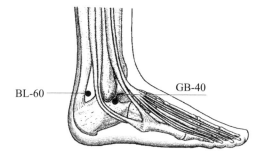

FIGURE 48.12 Acupuncture points GB 40, BL 60. Used to treat occipital headache. (Courtesy of Carl L. Milton.)

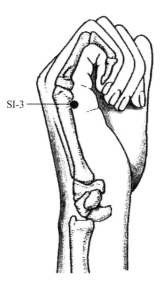

FIGURE 48.13 Acupuncture point S 13. Used to treat occipital headache. (Courtesy of Carl L. Milton.)

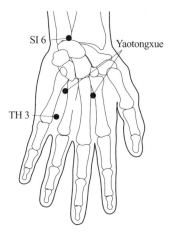

FIGURE 48.14 Acupuncture points Yaotongxue S 6. Used to treat low back pain. (Courtesy of Carl L. Milton.)

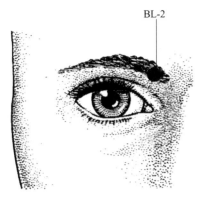

FIGURE 48.15 Acupuncture points B 12. (Courtesy of Carl L. Milton.)

Point Location: Found with the palm facing the chest, just above the styloid process of the ulna, and on its radial side

Point Name: *BL 2* (Figure 48.15)

Point Location: At the medial aspect of the eyebrow, in the supraorbital notch

MYOFASCIAL ACUPUNCTURE

Myofascial acupuncture uses the complex network of acupuncture meridians as the primary basis for treating the body and relies strongly on a physical evaluation of the connective tissue of the body to assess how to go about treating the patient.

The physical evaluation frames the patient's condition in terms of myofascial causal chains that are broader in scope than referred pain patterns. These chains reflect the symptoms and expressions of the connective tissue and give insight to the assorted disorders that have been recorded as meridian symptomology in traditional acupuncture.

A skilled practitioner, using the image of the meridians as an overlay, evaluates a patient, visually noting factors such as gait, posture, and muscle tone. The practitioner manually examines muscle and tissue for indications of tension, painful loci, range of motion limitations, and any other unusual state. By adding the knowledge of the terrain of the meridians, the symptoms and signs from the evaluation are understood in the greater context of a multidimensional model of the body.

This model expands the practitioner's understanding of the interrelationship of the various regions of the body, specifically the upper and lower, front and back, left and right, and internal and external regions, and increases treatment options. More importantly, it provides a framework to understand the expressive paths of the complex emotional, visceral, and somatic interplay. This model has remained a valuable contribution to this style of therapy.

Myofascial acupuncture is exceptionally effective in a pain management program. It is very hands-on and dem-

onstrates to the patient that the practitioner is in touch with the pain syndrome as a whole. During treatment, muscles are isolated and stimulated with needles to produce reactions that either mimic or radiate to the pain. Patients typically find it reassuring to know that their pain can be reached. In addition, the evaluation process takes into account the myriad physical, functional, and emotional symptoms that, while very real to the patient, have often been considered unrelated by other systems of thought. Consequently, this technique works extremely well as a strong adjunct to all other therapies, including counseling and psychotherapy.

In practice, this system bears a similarity to trigger point therapy in the selection of points according to muscle involvement. Many of these points tend to be spatially close to trigger points, and some of the muscle points are stimulated to release tension and pain. However, different from trigger point therapy, other acupuncture points relating to the involved meridians are included in various areas of the body as an integral part of the treatment plan.

Point Examples

- To treat occipital headache
- Point Name: *GB 20* (Figure 48.16)
  Point Location: Between depression below the external occipital protuberance of the occipital bone and the mastoid process, between the trapezius and the sternocleidomastoid muscles, in the splenius capitis and the semispinalis capitis muscles
  Point Name: *GB 21* (Figure 48.16)
  Point Location: In the trapezius muscle at the midpoint between the acromion of the scap-

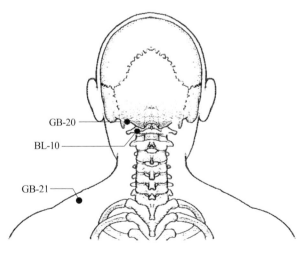

FIGURE 48.16 Acupuncture points GB 20, GB 21, BL 10. Used to treat occipital headache. (Courtesy of Carl L. Milton.)

ula and a point on the midline between the spinous processes of the seventh cervical and first thoracic vertebrae

Point Name: *BL 10* (Figure 48.16)

Point Location: At the margin of the trapezius muscle and over the semispinalis capitis and splenius capitis muscles, aproximately 1.3 in. lateral to a point on the midline between the first and second cervical vertebrae

Point Name: *TH 3* (Figure 48.14)

Point Location: Located on the dorsal side of the hand proximal to the metacarpophalangeal joint between the fourth and fifth metacarpal bones, in the fourth dorsal interosseous muscle

Point Name: *BL 58* (Figure 48.17)

Point Location: In the gastrocnemius and soleus muscles, 1 in. inferior and lateral to the site where the two bellies of the gastrocnemius muscle separate when a patient is fully extending the foot

Additional Points: Various points that influence the posterior cervical muscles, occipitofrontalis muscle, the levator scapulae muscle and the trapezius muscle.

• To treat low back pain

Point Name: *BL 23* (Figure 48.18)

Point Location: In the erector spinae muscles, 1.5 in. lateral to the lower border of the spinous process of the second lumbar vertebra

Point Name: *BL 47* (Figure 48.18)

Point Location: In the latissimus dorsi and iliocostalis muscles, 3 in. lateral to the spinous process of the lower border of the second lumbar vertebra

Point Name: *BL 60* (Figure 48.12)

Point Location: At the midpoint of the space between the lateral malleolus and the tendon calcaneus

Point Name: *S 13* (Figure 48.13)

Point Location: Proximal to the fifth metacarpal bone, on the medial edge of the palm where a crease forms when the hand is made into a fist, in the abductor digiti minimi muscle

Additional points: Various points that influence the superficial and deep paraspinal muscles

CONCLUSION

It is likely that the use of acupuncture in pain management will continue to grow as a result of new research in the

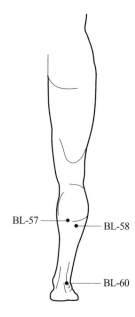

FIGURE 48.17 Acupuncture points BL 57, BL 58, BL 60. (Courtesy of Carl L. Milton.)

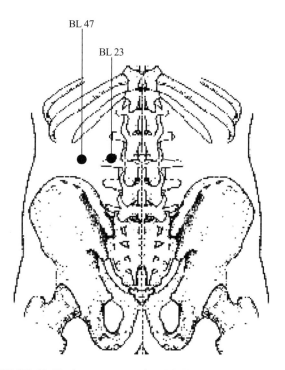

FIGURE 48.18 Acupuncture points BL 23, BL 47. Used to treat low back pain. (Courtesy of Carl L. Milton.)

field, public awareness and acceptance, and its therapeutic flexibility. The techniques discussed in this chapter are a sampling of the ones being used in clinical practice. They serve to exemplify the breadth of the field of acupuncture and to demonstrate, by the nature of the technique, ways the therapy can be added to a pain management program or other treatment programs.

REFERENCES

Chaitow, L. (1977). *The acupuncture treatment of pain.* New York: Arco Publishing Company.

Chen, E. (1995). *Cross-sectional anatomy of acupoints.* Edinburgh: Churchill Livingstone.

Chen, Y. (Ed.). (1989). *Essentials of contemporary Chinese acupuncturists' clinical experience.* Beijing: Foreign Languages Press.

Cheng, Xinnong. (Ed.). (1987). *Chinese acupuncture and moxibustion.* Beijing: Foreign Languages Press.

Dale, R. (1990). The holograms of hand micro-acupuncture: A study in systems of correspondence. *American Journal of Acupuncture, 11*(2), 141–162.

Denmai, S. (Brown, S. (trans.)). (1990). *Introduction to meridian therapy.* Seattle: Eastland Press.

Eckman, P. (1990). An introduction to Koryo Sooji Chim: Korean hand acupuncture. *American Journal of Acupuncture, 18*(2), 135–139.

Ellis, A., & Wiseman, B. K. (1988). *Fundamentals of Chinese acupuncture.* Brookline, MA: Paradigm Publications.

Gunn, C. (1989). *The Gunn approach to the treatment of chronic pain.* Edinburgh: Churchill Livingstone.

Jiao, S. (ca. 1970). *Head acupuncture.* Taiwan: Sanxi Publishing House.

Kailin, D. (1983). On the mastery of acupuncture. *American Journal of Acupuncture, 11*(2), 157–162.

Maciocia, G. (1989). *The foundations of Chinese medicine.* Edinburgh: Churchill Livingstone.

Matsumoto, K., & Birch, S. (1988). *Hara diagnosis: Reflections on the sea.* Brookline, MA: Paradigm Publications.

National Institute of Health. (1997). *NIT consensus statement, 15*(5), 3–5.

Nogier, P. (1983). *From auriculotherapy to auriculomedicine.* Paris: Maisonneuve.

O'Connor, J., & Bensky, D. (Ed.) (1981). *Acupuncture – A comprehensive text.* Chicago: Eastland Press.

Oleson, T., & Kroening, R. (1983). A comparison of Chinese and Nogier auricular points. *American Journal of Acupuncture,* 11(3), 205–223.

Ross, J. (1985). *Zang Fu — The organ systems of traditional Chinese medicine.* Edinburgh: Churchill Livingstone.

Seem, M. (1993). *A new American acupuncture: Acupuncture osteopathy: Myofascial release of the body-mind's holding patterns.* Boulder: Blue Poppy Press.

Seem, M. (2000). *Acupuncture physical medicine.* Boulder: Blue Poppy Press.

Soulié de Morant, French Edition (1972), Maloine, Paris. English Edition (1994), Brookline, MA: Paradigm Publications.

Tan, R. (1994). *Twenty-four more in acupuncture.* San Diego: Richard Tan.

Travell, J. (1983). *Myofascial pain and dysfunction, The trigger point manual.* Baltimore: Williams & Wilkins.

49

Tai Chi Chuan
for Pain Management

Richard A. Peck, L.Ac., M.B.A. and Iva Lim Peck, L.Ac., Dipl.Ac., R.N.

INTRODUCTION

Tai Chi Chuan (a.k.a. T'ai Chi Ch'uan, Taijiquan) is an ancient Chinese martial art/exercise originally developed in the 13th century by Chang San Fang. Because of its underlying concepts of energy and its effect on the body, it has been incorporated into the overall system of Traditional Chinese Medicine (TCM). In the West it is often referred to merely as Tai Chi. This is somewhat erroneous because Tai Chi in Chinese refers to the symbols for Yin and Yang. It is more accurate to refer to it as Tai Chi Chuan, which means Grand Ultimate Boxing or Grand Ultimate Fist.

Originally, Tai Chi Chuan was a closely guarded secret reserved only for those within the Chen family. Since the 1800s it has evolved from the original Chen Style into many different styles (Yang, Wu, Sun, Hao) and is practiced by millions of people all over the world. Tai Chi Chuan is considered by many as one of the best low-impact exercises. Even though it is ancient, it fits well into our modern society. It can be practiced by anyone whether young or old, large or small, male or female. It does not require any special clothing nor does it require any special equipment. It is ideally suited for those with chronic pain.

ORIENTAL MEDICINE: BACKGROUND

To understand the underlying concepts of Tai Chi Chuan, and how this ancient Chinese exercise is useful in pain management, one needs to have some understanding of the concepts of TCM.

Traditional Chinese Medicine is an energetically focused system of healing that dates back over 3000 years. One of the oldest references is the *Huang Ti Nei Ching* (Yellow Emperor's Internal Classic) which is composed of two separate books. The first is the *Su Wen*, which deals with physiology and pathology, and the second is the *Ling Shu*, which deals with the subject of anatomy and acupuncture. The estimated date of the writing is around 1000 B.C.

Most people in the West think of TCM as acupuncture. Acupuncture is only one part of Oriental Medicine. It is really a complex system of healthcare that includes acupuncture, moxibustion, dietary therapy, Chinese herbology, Tui Na (similar to massage), and exercises such as Tai Chi Chuan and Qi Gong (breathing exercises). For a traditionally trained Doctor of Oriental Medicine each of these modalities is as important as the other in the overall health of the patient.

Historically, the development of Oriental Medicine has been an evolutionary process. Ancient texts indicate and suggest that each part of TCM originated in a different part of China. Acupuncture originated in northern China, Chinese herbology began in the southern part, and Tai Chi Chuan originated in the central region.

It is believed that acupuncture was discovered quite by accident. There are numerous legends as to its discovery. The most popular one is an incident of an altercation between two groups of clansmen. One individual was struck in the shoulder by an arrow and his headache went away. The Chinese are great observers of nature. If there is one point that can relieve a physical problem, then there

0-8493-0926-3/02/$0.00+$1.50
© 2002 by CRC Press LLC

must be more. Similar cause-and-effect situations were observed over the years and different pain problems were relieved. Initially, the development of acupuncture was limited to knowledge within a family that was passed down from father to son and generation to generation. Gradually, the knowledge was expanded and there were ancient writers like Chang Chung-Ching, who wrote the *Shang Han Lun* (Essay on Typhoid) (available in English) and Huang Fu-Mi, who wrote the *Chia I Ching*. These and many other well-known physicians and historians throughout the centuries wrote manuscripts on the accumulated knowledge based on the observation and outcome experiences of their time. Many of these texts are still in existence today and have been translated, revised, or modified and are being used as text books in the teaching of Oriental Medicine.

ORIENTAL MEDICINE: CONCEPTS

The Chinese believe that there is an energy or vital life force in our bodies. This life force flows along predetermined pathways, which for our purposes we refer to as meridians. This vital life force is called Qi. It assumes many different forms. It comes to us genetically from our parents in what is referred to as Original Qi. It is in the food we eat and the air we breathe. It can also be enhanced by the exercise we do. For our purposes, we think of this life force collectively as that which gives energy to the various muscles, bones, and organs. The Chinese believe this is the vital energy that keeps us alive.

In a normal healthy person this vital energy flows continuously from one meridian to another and from one part of the body to another. The Chinese also believe that when the energy becomes blocked disease or pain problems occur. Let's think of the energy as a stream of water that runs continuously through the forest. If a tree or log falls over the stream, then the water is blocked and backs up forming a pond or a lake. In the human body, when there is an imbalance of energy flowing along the meridian it can be due to an internal problem or an external injury to a specific area of the body. The energy becomes blocked and backed up, quite often forming a tender point. If the problem is of short duration or is in an acute stage, the energy is probably no more than a small pond with minor consequences to the body. If the log across the stream or the energy is being blocked for an extended period of time, then the problem becomes chronic and we can think of this as a lake. It takes longer for the water to be drained out of a lake than a small pond. The same is said for energy blockage. In general, it may take longer to treat the chronic conditions than the acute conditions. The main objective of the Oriental Medicine practitioner is to identify and relieve the blockage of energy. This can be done by acupuncture, Chinese herbs, Tai Chi Chuan, etc.

ENERGY PATHWAYS

Each of our internal organs is associated with an energy pathway. For example, the heart has a meridian we can call the Primary Heart Meridian. The energy of the Primary Heart Meridian originates in the heart and branches internally in three directions. The first branch travels from the heart internally downward into the abdomen to connect with the small intestine meridian. The second branch travels upward and runs alongside the esophagus to connect with the eye. The third branch leaves the heart, enters the lung, and emerges through its external pathway at a point in the center of the axilla on the medial side of the axillary artery. This is the first acupuncture point of the Primary Heart Meridian system. From there it travels along the posterior and medial aspects of the upper arm down to the cubital fossa. From there it descends along the posterior and medial aspects of the forearm to the pisiform region and enters into the palm, and then goes to the tip of the medial aspect of the little finger, where it ends.

In addition to the Primary Meridian systems, there are two distinct secondary meridian systems. The first is the Connecting Meridian system, which connects one meridian to another, and the second is the Muscle Meridian system, which does not have acupuncture points but connects the energy along the muscular system. It is the Muscle Meridian system that is of primary importance to us. Each Primary Meridian has a Muscle Meridian. Thus, the Primary Heart Meridian has a Heart Muscle Meridian. The Heart Muscle Meridian follows along the same pathway as the Primary Heart Meridian system. It begins from the medial aspect of the small finger inserts at the wrist, then travels upward to the elbow where it again constricts. It flows upward across the chest where it constricts in the center of the chest before it descends into the abdomen. This Muscle Meridian system is the important factor in pain points, muscle pain, and the benefit of practicing Tai Chi Chuan.

TAI CHI CHUAN: DEVELOPMENT

Legend has it that Tai Chi Chuan and Qi Gong originated in the central part of China and more specifically on Wu Tang Mountain. Legends further attribute the creation of Tai Chi Chuan to more than one source. One of the most popular traditions is that in the 13th century a Taoist monk by the name of Chang San Fang watched an altercation between a snake and a crane and created the rudimentary basis of Tai Chi Chuan. Many of the movements of Tai Chi Chuan mimic the movements of animals or forces in nature and thus are named after the animal or natural occurrences. Within the various styles of Tai Chi Chuan there are individual postures in the exercise routine with names such as "Snake Creeps Down," "White Crane

Spreading Its Wings," "Carry Tiger to the Mountain," and "Wave Hands Like Clouds." Each of these movements mimics an animal or force in nature.

In performing the Tai Chi Chuan routine the whole body is slowly and gently stimulated along all the muscle groups, one after the other. The primary method of stimulating these muscle groups is through stretching that alternately contracts and relaxes specific muscles groups and balances the muscular activity throughout the body. The Muscle Meridian system of the body is continually being stretched. Because the Muscle Meridian system follows along the Pathway of the Primary Meridian System any movement will affect the energy flow along the various meridians. The movements of Tai Chi Chuan activate all the Muscle and Primary Meridians. The stimulation of one part of the body has an effect on another part of the body. This follows the concept of Oriental Medicine where an experienced practitioner will balance the energy flow in one part of the body knowing that it has an impact on another part of the body.

To further understand the role that Tai Chi Chuan plays in pain management, it is helpful for one to also understand some of the work done by Dr. Janet Travell and those who followed after her, and their continued work on the development and understanding of trigger points in myofascial release.

Briefly stated, Travell believed and demonstrated that within a muscle or muscle group one or more areas in the muscle group may be tender. The tenderness can be due to different reasons; however, the most common is from an injury to the muscle group. The injury causes the muscle to constrict or shorten causing a tender point. The tightness or spasm on a tender point in the muscle group can affect one or more areas of the body in the form of pain. This pain area usually is in close proximity to the Primary Meridian System and the Muscle Meridian System. If the tenderness can be relieved, it will have a positive and beneficial effect on the constricted muscle and pain pattern problem. The relief of the pain pattern through stimulation of the trigger point can come about through exercises (Tai Chi Chuan), massage, heat therapy, acupuncture, etc.

TAI CHI CHUAN: MOVEMENT AND PAIN RELIEF

In Oriental Medicine spontaneous points that become sore are referred to as Ah Shi Points. The concept of Ah Shi Points was first put forth by Sun Si Mao (561–682) during the Tang dynasty. He believed that when soreness was felt as pressure was applied to a muscle an acupuncture point existed. The Ah Shi Points were used both for diagnostic purposes and for treatment. Many acupuncturists use the concept of Ah Shi Points to treat pain problems that lie along the pathway of the corresponding meridians. The Trigger Points of

Travell in many instances correspond with the Ah Shi Points of Acupuncture.

Tai Chi Chuan is sometimes referred to as "land swimming" because the movements of Tai Chi Chuan resemble very closely the continuous movements of swimming. These continuous movements work differently than physical therapy. In physical therapy there is movement of one or more muscle groups; however, the Muscle Meridian and the Primary Meridian are not always stretched in their entirety. Physical therapy is often for an isolated area where the problem exists. When you look at the stretching movements of Tai Chi Chuan, there is a distinct difference. The movements stretch both the arms and legs along the entire pathway of the Muscle Meridian and Primary Meridian. The constant and smooth flowing movements of Tai Chi Chuan release the tender points identified by Dr. Travell and the Ah Shi Points of Traditional Chinese Medicine. When the tender points can be stretched and relaxed, the pain associated with these tender points will diminish or go away.

Research is now being done here in the United States and overseas to prove the benefits of daily Tai Chi Chuan practice. As one watches the graceful movements of Tai Chi Chuan it appears to be effortless, yet the slow and deliberate exercise has proven to reduce falls in the elderly. Those who practice the art find that their muscles become strong and they acquire substantial flexibility. The mind–body effects of Tai Chi Chuan provide an added boost to both the physical and mental health of an individual.

CONCLUSION

In conclusion, integrating daily Tai Chi Chuan practice into a pain management program will provide the stretching needed to relax the muscles and reduce the pain of many chronic pain patients. Like any form of therapeutic exercise, the only way to achieve optimum outcome is to learn the art from a qualified instructor, and practice it on a daily basis.

REFERENCES

Huang ti nei ching (Yellow emperor's internal classic) (1000 B.C.).

Jou, Tsung Hwa (1981). *The tao of tai-chi chuan.* Warwick, NY: Tai Chi Foundation.

Liang, Shou-Yu, & Wen-Ching, Wu. (1993). *A guide To taijiquan: 24 & 48 postures with applications.* Jamaica Plains. NY: Yangs Martial Arts Association.

Yang, Jwing-Ming. (1987). *Advanced yang style tai chi chuan.* Jamaica Plains, NY: Yang Martial Arts Association.

—50—

Energetic Medicine

Diane H. Polasky, M.A., M.H., D.O.M., Dipl.Ac., D.A.A.P.M.

HISTORICAL OVERVIEW

It is commonly believed that some form of medicine was practiced by all cultures on the planet throughout the course of human history. Initially, however, it was not an isolated methodology. Rather, the promotion of health and the healing and cure of illness and disease were part of a larger system—a working and living portion of a culture's entire cosmological system that interwove spiritual beliefs, an explanation of the universe, the norms and values of the society of which it was a part, and even tasks of daily living.

Cosmological views such as these were often associated with the first form of religion known as *animism* (Harner, 1987). Animism as a religion is based on the belief that all things, living and nonliving, are alive and have a vital essence or a spirit that can be contacted. It is the view that there is more than just the physical self; an individual is part of a giant cosmic web in which all aspects are interconnected and the universe consists of a complex network of forms, energies, and vibrations. This animistic worldview was not contained to any one part of the world, nor to any specific indigenous culture. Each cosmological system acknowledged and called this vital essence, life force, or universal energy by a different name, including *ruach* by the ancient Hebrews, *chi/ki* in the Orient, *mana* in Hawaii, *prana* in India, *huaca* in Peru, and *wakonda* and *manitou* among some of the Native American tribes of North America (White & Krippner, 1997).

By the beginning of written history, several civilizations were practicing a form of energy medicine in which electrical and magnetic forces were employed to influence internal energy systems in the body. These energy systems were extensively documented, especially in India with the study of the chakra system and in China with detailed descriptions of the meridians. The use of energy fields in healing also was described in spiritual texts throughout the world, including the New Testament, where Jesus and others performed healings by a *laying-on-of-hands*.

Classical literature indicates that the use of energy fields continued to be studied and named. In 500 B.C., Pythagoras called it *vital energy* (Brennen, 1993); Hippocrates, in his explorations, pointed out that "nature heals and not the physician," and referenced a vital energy force called the *speira*. Paracelsus took this concept further, applying the principle of the *archeus*, or healing force, in his practice of medicine (Pierrakos, 1975). For the most part, to this point in history, medical paradigms and spiritual beliefs intermingled, and the belief in the existence of this vital energy held potential answers to the mysteries of both body and soul. However, with the advent of the Renaissance, a separation between religion and medicine began to develop, and the concept of animism as a cosmological framework was left to the uncivilized and heathen tribal people.

As the Age of Science and Reason blossomed during the 1600s, a greater understanding evolved in regard to electricity, magnetism, and biological processes. During this time two opposing schools of thought became recognizable. The first, *mechanism*, believed that life obeyed the laws of chemistry and physics and viewed living organisms as complex machines that were completely understandable by means of physical principles. The second school, *vitalism*, believed that life would never be explained by these physical principles alone and that there was a mysterious life force that was separate from the physical but impacted upon it (Becker & Marino, 1982).

0-8493-0926-3/02/$0.00+$1.50
© 2002 by CRC Press LLC

In spite of this controversy, vitalists, including such individuals as Franz Mesmer, Samuel Hahnemann, and Luigi Galvani, continued to issue their findings that indicated the existence of a life force. With the discovery of electricity, some vitalists associated electrical fields with this life force and, between the late 1700s and the early 1900s, a variety of electrical healing devices were developed and widely used to treat a range of ailments (Geddes, 1984). Although broad-reaching claims were made, studies demonstrating their positive effects on health were inconclusive, resulting in condemnation by both the medical and scientific communities. During this same period, as research in biology, chemistry, and physics increased, vitalism as a school of science was dismissed as mere philosophical and esoteric speculation.

Even though vitalism was now on the fringe of the approved scientific paradigm, it never died out completely. Vitalistic-oriented beliefs and practices continued, often based on ancient beliefs, under such names as theosophy, metaphysics, and spiritual healing. Research also proceeded, although for the most part unacknowledged, in such areas as parapsychology and consciousness studies.

VARIANT SCHOOLS OF MEDICAL THOUGHT

Historically, then, it appears that our culture has evolved two seemingly opposing philosophical schools of thought in regard to medicine: Biomedicine and Energetic medicine.

Biomedicine is the formal name given for our current healthcare system in which the primary practitioners earn the degree of Medical Doctor (M.D.) or Doctor of Osteopathy (D.O.). Other names include *western, modern, orthodox, mainstream*, and *conventional*. As a school of thought, Biomedicine emphasizes that knowledge about the world, including nature and human nature, must be pursued by the following criteria:

Objectivism. The observer is separate from the observed;
Reductionism. Complex phenomena are explainable in terms of simpler, component phenomena;
Positivism. All information can be derived from physically measurable data; and
Determinism. Phenomena can be predicted from a knowledge of scientific law and initial conditions (Micozzi, 1996).

Within biomedical philosophy, illness and disease are viewed in the framework of what is known as "The Doctrine of Specific Etiology," or more simply, "The Biomedical Model." This model consists of two major postulates: first, that illness can be categorized into specific diseases characterized by identifiable organic pathology,

and second, that each such disease has a unique primary cause (Werbach, 1986). In this medical paradigm, it is accepted that illness occurs due to organ malfunction, damage, or disturbance in the machinery of the body, and it is the physician's job to repair that machine. It utilizes, and is often also called, *allopathic medicine,* a term coined by Samuel Hahnemann and derived from the Greek *allo,* meaning "other" and *pathos,* meaning "feeling," to denote the standard practice of using medicines either to counteract symptoms or to produce an action unrelated to symptoms (Jacobs & Maskowitz, 1996).

A seeming dialectic to this approach is that of Energetic medicine, also known as Bioenergetic medicine, which has been defined in various ways. One definition states that "Energy medicine refers to therapies that use an energy field—electrical, magnetic, sonic, acoustic, microwave, infrared—to screen for and treat health conditions by detecting imbalances in the body's energy fields … balance can then be restored using holistic therapies, or with treatment devices that rebalance the energy levels of the various fields" (Goldberg, 1993). Another viewpoint explains that "Energetic medicine can be considered to be a general term used to refer to many ancient and some modern medical practices which encompasses many different therapeutic disciplines but which views each as a separate entity with different mechanisms of action" (Becker, 1990).

According to these definitions, Energetic medicine can be considered an umbrella term to cover the wide variety of approaches to healing generally thought by Biomedicine to be vitalistic in theory and which are currently called *alternative, unorthodox, integrative, complementary,* or *holistic*. It also would include other approaches whose methodologies are based on Energetic medicine concepts, including spiritual healing, long-distance healing, laying-on-of-hands, psychic healing, shamanic healing, and specific ethnomedical traditions such as Kahuna, Curanderismo, and Native American healing.

Generally speaking, proponents of Energetic medicine believe that the body is more than a machine and that it is capable of healing itself. They also believe that the body also is capable of performing other actions that lie completely outside the realm of established science (Becker, 1990).

More specifically, utilizing the works of Lewis Mehl (1988) and Marc Micozzi (1996) as a basis, I have formulated what I consider to be essential aspects of an Energetic medical model. It consists of the following postulates:

1. The Body is an Energetic System.
   There exists, within the human body, a coherent and homeodynamic energetic system. Disruptions in the balance and flow of this bioenergy can potentially create an imbalance, and the system's response to energetic

imbalance over time can lead to perceptible disease within the body. Facilitating the body to restore its own energetic balance often can ameliorate symptoms and restore health.

2. Causal Factors of Energetic Imbalance are Multidimensional.

Individuals do not exist in isolation but in relationship with the living universe around them. Understanding that potential causative factors exist that may be outside the realm of normal human perception, and that which is imperceptible to the human senses, are as important in illness and healing as that which can be measured and validated through the senses and current modes of research.

3. The Primary Focus is on the Individual.

There is an emphasis on the whole person as a unique individual with his or her inner resources as well as his or her unique manifestation of imbalances.

4. Self-Healing is the Basis for All Healing.

Treatment modalities utilized simply mobilize the body's inner healing resources. The ability to be well or be sick is largely tied to inner resources, but it is understood that other factors such as time and the external environment can impact on this ability in varying degrees.

5. Emphasis is on Wellness.

Wellness is a focus on engaging the inner resources of each individual as an active and conscious participant in the maintenance of his/her own health. By the same token, the property of being healthy is not conferred upon an individual solely by an outside agency or entity, but results from the balance of internal resources with the external natural and social environment.

6. Health and Healing are Multifaceted.

Awareness that health is more than the absence of disease and the potential for healing exists, and can impact upon, all levels of an individual's existence. Healing does not equal curing and, in this regard, it is possible for an individual to even approach death "healthy."

In general, "Energetic medical therapies focus either on energy fields originating within the body (biofields) or those from other sources (electromagnetic fields), and these therapies are intended to affect the energy fields … that surround and penetrate the human body" (National Center for Complementary & Alternative Medicine Website). Practitioners believe, then, that an appropriate therapy is one that either encourages the body's

own energetic systems or adds external energy to these systems (Becker, 1990).

THE EVOLUTION OF BIOMEDICINE

It is agreed that some of the information derived from the Biomedical model has been both beneficial and effective, providing, for instance, an understanding of the basis of heredity and the ability to see on a cellular level as well as eliminating many major diseases that previously have been lethal. But this mechanistic approach has also fueled a growing tide of dissatisfaction, especially in medicine, where, in spite of all its benefits, its reductionistic approaches have the potential to demean and diminish the complexity of an individual. In this model, by identifying the patient as a diseased body, the whole does not even begin to equal the sum of its parts. Also, as Dr. William Tiller of Stanford University states: "For most of this century, science and medicine have seen health as being dependent upon the balance of body chemistry and the functioning of physical structures. However, attempts to treat illnesses and imbalances chemically often lead to unwanted side effects or the body becoming insensitive to the chemicals" (Goldberg, 1993). In addition, according to the United Nations World Health Organization (WHO), more than 70% of the world's population relies on nonallopathic systems of healing (Krippner, 1999), and Biomedicine is often ill prepared to meet the challenge posed by its encounter with different cultures and their systems of health and healing. These facts, among others, have created a growing interest in nonorthodox medical approaches and have led many health professionals to look beyond conventional drug-based therapies to the field of Energetic medicine.

Initially, medical interest focused on the magnetic fields around the body, but interest in biomagnetism spread widely in the Biomedical research community encouraging exploration of the role of other fields, including electricity, light, heat, gravity, kinetic energy, and sound. This expanding interest has led to the new emerging scientific discipline of *Bioelectromagnetics* or BEM. BEM is defined as "an interdisciplinary science at the interface of physics, biology, and medicine that deals with the effects of low-level electricity, magnetism and electromagnetic fields on life" (Rubik, 2001).

As inquiry led to a greater understanding about how electricity, magnetism, and other energy fields are created and utilized by living organisms, methods have been developed to measure energy fields within and around the human body. Contemporary medicine currently uses a number of electromagnetically sensitive instruments for diagnostic purposes, many of which are commonly known, including electrocardiogram for the heart

(ECG/EKG), electroencephalogram for the brain (EEG), electromylogram for muscles (EMG), electro-retinogram for eye movements, and magnetic resonance imaging for specific body parts (MRI). In addition, the S.Q.U.I.D. (superconducting quantum interference device) magnetometer is now widely used to map the biomagnetic fields produced by various organs and has led to new clinical instruments such as magnetocardiography and magnetoencephalography. Other diagnostic advances include the use of sensitive photometers and thermographic imaging techniques that can map the patterns of light and heat emitted by cells, tissues, organs, and the whole body, and the use of spectroscopy to reveal the energy emissions and absorptions of molecules, thereby revealing the roles of energy fields in molecular processes including hormone–receptor, antibody–antigen and allergic interactions (Oschman, 2000).

BEM FINDINGS AND THEIR POTENTIAL SIGNIFICANCE TO ENERGETIC MEDICINE

More recently, studies in the area of BEM have yielded significant findings potentially relevant to Energetic medicine. Some of the most pertinent are summarized below:

- Electrical currents flowing through tissues produce a magnetic field in the space around it, and changing, pulsing, or moving magnetic fields, in turn, produce an electrical current flow (Becker, 1990).
- Magnetic and electromagnetic fields have energy, carry information, and are the basis of many of the underlying control systems that regulate the complex chemical mechanisms within the body (Becker, 1990).
- Living organisms have biomagnetic fields around them that change from moment to moment in relation to events taking place inside the body (Oschman, 2000).
- Organisms are fundamentally bioelectric and emit low-level fields (Rubik, 2001).
- Organisms are sensitive to extremely low-level fields of electromagnetism (Rubik, 2001).
- The biomagnetic field of an organism extends some distance from the body surface and, therefore, the fields of two adjacent organisms will interact with each other (Chaitow, 1987).
- All electromagnetic fields are force fields that carry energy and are capable of producing an action at a distance (Becker, 1990).
- Living systems respond to external energy fields (Bialek, 1987).

ADDITIONAL VARIABLES RELATED TO ENERGETIC MEDICINE

THE LIVING MATRIX

Studies in both BEM and cellular biology indicate that an overall field also exists within the human body and that internal regulation mechanisms involve more than merely nerve impulses and hormones. Such research indicates that, from the skin to the innermost part of each cell, our entire system is covered with connective tissue internally linking it all together. This field, most commonly known as the *living matrix*, has no central aspect or part that is most basic; rather, it is "a continuous and dynamic supramolecular webwork extending into every nook and cranny of the body: a nuclear matrix within a cellular matrix within a connective tissue matrix. The properties of the whole network depend upon the integrated activities of all of the components, and effects on any one part of the system can, and do, spread to others" (Oschman, 2000).

An understanding of these integrative reactions may shed new light on some of the processes involved with various forms of Energetic medicine. This living matrix has been found to be simultaneously a mechanical, vibrational or oscillatory, energetic, electronic, and informational network (Pienta & Coffey, 1991), it being scientifically understood that vibratory properties include light, electric, magnetic, and electromagnetic energy, heat, gravity, kinetic (motion), chemical, and sound. Given this premise, restrictions in one part have consequences for the entire organism. For example, the structural system cannot be influenced without influencing the energetic/informational system and vice versa. In addition, it is well known that, in the body, each electron, atom, chemical bond, molecule, cell, tissue, and organ has its own vibratory character, with each molecule emitting a specific and precise characteristic energy spectrum creating, in effect, an electromagnetic "signature" or "fingerprint" unique to that molecule (Oschman & Oschman, 1988).

In lieu of these findings, it can be surmised that whenever the body is impacted upon, whether through touch, manipulation of the spine or soft tissue, movement, sound, light, heat, or application of a needle, magnet, laser beam, or electronic/electromagnetic device, this information is absorbed and transmitted through the matrix, creating an effect within the entire system. Also, because every substance contains unique electromagnetic and vibratory qualities, it would follow that the application or ingestion of any herb, essential oil, food, nutritional supplement, homeopathic formula, or even prescription drug would impact the system energetically.

GEOMAGNETIC INTERACTIONS

It has long been accepted by indigenous cultures that an individual exists in relation to the surrounding world. In some instances, such as with Oriental medicine, this concept forms the basis for treatment in which humans are considered as microcosms of the greater macrocosm with energetic interactions between the two influencing homeodynamic functioning.

The influence of external magnetic fields has been, and continues to be, controversial among scientists. However, as BEM findings indicate that organisms are sensitive to low-level electromagnetic fields and that they respond to external energy fields, there is a growing acceptance of the plausibility of these interactions. To date, a variety of physical and behavioral disturbances in the human population have been statistically related to disturbances in the Earth's electromagnetic field or to manmade interferences. Some physical disorders include cardiovascular problems, seizures, headaches, vestibular problems, intraocular pressure, and sleep disorders; behavioral changes have also been noted, including an increase in crime and aggression, anxiety, depression, and loss of attention and memory (Oschman, 2000; Becker, 1990).

THE HEART, EMOTIONS, AND IMMUNE FUNCTION

The heart has been shown to produce the strongest electrical and magnetic activity of any tissue in the body, and the biomagnetic field of the heart can be detected up to 15 ft away from the body (Baule & McFee, 1963). As such, it is the main source of our body's energy. In this regard, perhaps some of the most significant recent discoveries made in BEM research pertain to the relationships that have been found to exist in regard to electrical energy changes of the heart, emotions, and immune function.

It is known that the two branches of the autonomic nervous system, the sympathetic and the parasympathetic, regulate heart rate. Research has shown that mental stress and negative emotions, such as anger, increase the energy in the sympathetic nervous system and positive emotions, such as caring and compassion, increase the energy in the parasympathetic nervous system (Kamada, et al., 1992; Sloan, et al., 1994; Williams, et al., 1982). Along similar lines, particular emotional states have been correlated with measurable changes in the electrical energy spectrum of the heart. For instance, with the feeling of frustration, the heart rate varies somewhat randomly, a condition referred to as "incoherence." Various practices that intentionally focus attention on the area of the heart, while invoking sincere feelings of love and appreciation, lead to a more regular variation in heart rate, a condition referred to as "coherence." This regular variation reflects a balance and coherence between the heart rate and the rhythm of the sympathetic and parasympathetic nervous systems. With appropriate intention and training, a third state can be achieved that is referred to as "internal coherence." Here, the variation in heart rate decreases almost to zero. It is a calm, peaceful, harmonious, and highly intuitive feeling state, in which one becomes aware of one's electrical body and of the minute currents flowing throughout it (McCraty, et al., 1993; Rein & McCraty, 1993).

Additionally, studies in the field of psychoneuroimmunology, which explores the interactions and relationships between emotional states, behavior, neural and endocrine functioning, and immune processes, indicate that immune responses can be influenced by emotions. Research done over the last several decades, including a study published by Solomon and Moos as early as 1964, shows that a correlation exists between immunologic incompetence and specific emotional states such as anxiety and depression (Solomon & Moos, 1964). Based upon this research, it now becomes possible to see how emotional states, the heart, and the immune system are interrelated, and how emotional changes can affect multilevel functioning of not only an individual's internal system, but also his or her bioenergetic output due to the heart's extensive biomagnetic field, thus potentially affecting those around them.

CONSIDERATION OF BEM FINDINGS

If we consider the findings that have just been presented, we can begin to create an image of the human organism that differs from that of the biomedical model. What we have is a living energetic system existing within, and in relationship to, an energetic universe where everything is alive with its own unique vibration, where energy is being emitted and received, and where we are impacting and being impacted upon by all other energy sources in our midst or at an intentioned distance. It is a universe where each individual with whom we come in contact, whether we touch them or not, has an effect on us in a slightly different way, because what they are energetically emitting issues from their subjective emotional states, just as what we are emitting comes from ours—and these energy emissions can be consciously moderated.

If these BEM findings are indeed valid, then it appears that we may very well be circling back and are not truly at theoretical odds with the animistic-based cosmological systems of our ancestors and indigenous cultures the world over. In accordance with this view, we are, indeed, energetic beings living in a world of energy where everything is interconnected and interrelated. Following this, then, in considering the concept of Energetic medicine, we can see that Energetic medicine is not merely the use of electromagnetically sensitive methods and tools; we can see that, in a broad sense, all medicine is Energetic medicine. Whether it be those modalities deemed complementary or alternative or those considered biomedical and conventional, every physical interaction and intervention will have corresponding energetic repercussions.

PAIN AND ENERGETIC MEDICINE

Pain is a high-priority symptom related to many illnesses, disorders, and injuries. In 1995, the U.S. Department of Health and Human Services found that more than 120 million persons were affected by pain with a cost of more than $100 billion in lost productivity and healthcare (Erickson, Wilson, & Shannon, 1995; Turk & Melzack, 1992).

In its definition of pain, the International Association for the Study of Pain includes actual or potential tissue damage as well as the emotional experience of pain. Understanding the multifaceted experience of pain becomes important in treatment. To mitigate their suffering, patients may turn to (other) therapies (incorporated within the realm of Energetic medicine) to reduce feelings of stress, anxiety, nervousness, agitation, despondency, lack of motivation, enjoyment, and lethargy (as well as physical symptoms). In this regard, one recent study indicated that from 30 to 70% of patients use alternative or complementary (energetic) therapies in hope of a cure or palliation of their pain [(Loitman, 2000).

The results of this study would indicate that Energetic medical modalities are being utilized within our population in the search for pain management or relief, and exploration of this field is both warranted and timely.

However, prior to further discussion, the following points must be made:

1. It is important to realize that, within the parameters of the Energetic medical model presented earlier, pain in and of itself is not the primary focus of treatment; rather, it is pain in the context of that specific and unique individual who is presenting.

2. In utilizing the definitions for Energetic medicine listed previously, it is clear to see that a vast array of techniques and modalities exist that potentially can be considered when treating pain. In addition, as a number of these have been utilized for many years, the literature and research findings are voluminous. Due to these facts, it should be noted that the approaches discussed are far from exhaustive and in-depth coverage of each modality/technique is beyond the scope of this chapter. The reader is recommended to explore references at the end of this chapter for further reading in this area.

3. Energetic medicine does not have to be viewed necessarily as an alternative to good conven-

tional care, nor should it be in all cases. However, studies related to each of the techniques shown below indicate that these modalities can enhance positive patient responses, and many of them are often used either alone or in combination with one another as complements to conventional care. As in the utilization of any form of treatment, patients are advised to seek qualified and competent caregivers.

CATEGORIZATION OF ENERGETIC MEDICAL TECHNIQUES

In an attempt to present energetic treatment approaches in a coherent format, Dr. Robert Becker has provided a broad-based classification of techniques that are dependent upon the energy levels used, labeling them *Minimal Energy Techniques, Energy-Reinforcement Techniques, and High-Energy Transfer Techniques* (Becker, 1990). However, given the expansive nature of Energetic medicine, any attempt at categorization can be problematic, as not every technique can be accurately categorized this way and much overlapping can exist.

MINIMAL ENERGY TECHNIQUES

Minimal Energy techniques are defined as "techniques in which no external energy is administered to the body and in which the treatment methods attempt only to activate preexisting energetic control systems" (Becker, 1990).

Generally speaking, the purpose of these techniques is to facilitate the mind's capacity to affect bodily function and symptoms, and the one aspect common to all is that the conscious mind is being influenced in a desired direction, with the body then following (Becker, 1990). During the course of this process, commonly known as *self-regulation,* the conscious mind can control the autonomic nervous system. Self-regulatory techniques are based scientifically on psychophysiology, the study of relations between psychologic manipulations and resulting physiologic responses measured in the body (Sabo & Giorgi, 2000). In many cases, practitioners work with their patients, often explaining to them that they are going to facilitate their own healing by learning methods that will give them control over their own bodies. Strong evidence exists that such strategies can be useful in pain management (Patterson, et al., 1992). A number of these techniques, however, are based on ancient religious and cultural practices, still often used today, in which individuals attain an altered state of consciousness, unlocking healing powers within the mind and body.

Some examples of minimal energy techniques, and their potential benefits in the areas of pain management, are described below.

Relaxation Techniques

A variety of relaxation methods have been developed in the last century, and they typically fall into two categories: *somatic relaxation* refers to a method that emphasizes muscle relaxation through detailed observation and introspection of the body's kinesthetic sensations (i.e., purposeful relaxation of the muscles); *cognitive relaxation* refers to the use of a mental device (e.g., word, thought, sound, breathing) and the practice of a passive or nonjudgmental attitude to induce relaxation in the mind and body (Freeman, 2001). Clinical findings indicate that, as a group, relaxation methods can alter sympathetic activity and are effective in reducing chronic pain in a variety of medical conditions (Freeman, 2001). It is possible, too, that in acute pain situations, highly anxious patients might find some level of reduction not only in their anxiety, but also in response to their pain, although more research in this area is necessary.

Meditation

Meditation is defined as "the intentional self-regulation of attention, and a systematic focus on particular aspects of inner or outer experience" (Astin, Shapiro, & Schwartz, 2000). Many forms of meditation exist, both religion and nonreligion based, and in some cases it can fall under the designation of a cognitive relaxation technique (see above). Research indicates that meditation may be particularly effective in the treatment of chronic pain, and significant reductions have been seen in inhibition of activity due to pain, pain symptoms, psychological symptoms, and pain-related drug use (Kabat-Zinn, Lipworth, & Burney, 1985; 1987). Findings also suggest that meditation is effective in reducing symptoms of anxiety and treating anxiety-related disorders (Eppley, Abrams, & Shear, 1989; Edwards, 1991).

Biofeedback

Biofeedback is an operational term "that refers to a group of experimental procedures in which an external sensor is used to provide the organism with an indication of a state of bodily process, usually in an attempt to affect a change in the measured quantity" (Seifer & Lubar, 1975). The effects of this self-regulation have probably best been demonstrated in studies with yogis from India who were able to slow down respiration, control pain, stop bleeding, raise body temperatures, and speedily heal wounds with their wills alone. Biofeedback research at the Menninger Foundation and elsewhere has shown that some of this same power can be tapped in people with no yogic training (Becker & Selden, 1985).

Biofeedback principles have been used with different instruments to measure changes in muscle contraction, body temperature, skin conductivity, and brain waves. Studies conducted in a variety of settings indicate that biofeedback therapy may be beneficial in the management of chronic and acute pain and stress reduction (Lawlis, 2001a).

Hypnosis/Hypnotherapy

Hypnosis can be defined as "a state of attentive, focused concentration with suspension of some peripheral awareness" (Spiegel & Spiegel, 1978). Hypnotic techniques are said to induce states of selective attentional focusing or diffusion combined with enhanced imagery (NIH Technology Assessment, 1995). The history of the use of hypnosis and trance states is a long one, and there are currently a variety of schools of thought both as to its mechanisms of action and its therapeutic usage.

In general, it has been found that hypnotherapy can be used medically by helping a patient deal with the symptoms of disease, including his/her physiologic or emotional reaction to it, and it can also directly affect the illness and its course through the body. Research demonstrates effectiveness in reducing analgesic dependency, offering an alternative to anesthesia, and treating biologic mechanisms associated with such diseases as hypertension and terminal illness (Saicheck, 2000). Also, based on a review of research in the area of pain management and hypnosis, it can be concluded that hypnosis can be a valuable adjuvant therapy for the treatment of pain due to a variety of causes, including cancer, burns, and surgery (Freeman, 2001b).

Imagery/Guided Imagery/Visualization

Imagery is the thought process that invokes and uses the senses, including vision, sound, smell, and taste, and the senses of movement, position, and touch (Achterberg, 1985). Guided imagery refers to a wide variety of techniques, including simple visualization and direct suggestion using imagery, metaphor and storytelling, fantasy exploration and game playing, dream interpretation, drawing, and active imagination where elements of the unconscious are invited to appear as images that can communicate with the conscious mind (Rossman & Bresler, 2000). Also, in one visualization technique commonly used in healing, a patient is instructed to look inward into his or her body and, in the case of illness, to visualize the disease that is there, then visualize the body's defense system attacking, or affecting changes in, the diseased tissues.

The use of imagery is demonstrated to have definite effects on physiology, biochemistry, immune function, and brain-wave frequencies and, although clinical use of the many imagery techniques available varies, research studies have shown that imagery can impact positively on pain reactions and tolerance in cases of both acute and chronic pain (Freeman, 2001b). Imagery methods have also been shown to facilitate psychophysiological relaxation (Zahourek, 1988) and alleviate anxiety and depression (King, 1988; McDonald & Hilgendorf, 1986; Schaub, B.G. & Schaub, R., 1990). Additionally, a specific imagery technique, known as mental rehearsal, has been utilized to help prepare patients for medical procedures, tolerate them more comfortably, and to relieve pain and secondary side effects, perhaps exacerbated due to heightened emotional states. Published outcomes are almost uniformly positive and include significant reductions in pain and anxiety, length of hospital stays, use of pain medication, and reported side effects (Freeman, 2001b).

Trauma Energetics/Energy Psychology

Energy psychology is based on the concept that while psychological and/or psychosomatic dysfunctions entail chemical, neurological, cognitive, and situational components, most fundamentally they are manifestations of specific biotic energy information or energy configurations that are expressed as diagnosable psychological or physical symptoms. In diagnosis and treatment, the energy psychotherapist relies on isolating where aberrant or destructive energy patterns are encoded within the cellular structures of the body, and then employs procedures to decode those bioenergetic patterns (McClaskey, 1999). Procedurally, a number of techniques are available for the energy psychotherapist to utilize to attain this end; these procedures include, but are not limited to, Eye Movement Desensitization and Reprocessing (EMDR), Traumatic Incident Reduction (TIR), Neuroemotional Technique (NET), Thought Field Therapy (TFT), and Visual/Kinesthetic Dissociation (V/KD).

Research findings in this area are currently insufficient to establish efficacy; however, both clinicians and patients have reported beneficial outcomes not only in the reduction of addictive behavior, anxiety, trauma-related stress, and psychological disorders, but also in the relief of acute and chronic pain. In instances of chronic pain, it has been found that the pain relief frequently improves over time, such that the treatments work faster and the therapeutic effects last longer (Gallo, 1999).

ENERGY-REINFORCEMENT TECHNIQUES

Energy-reinforcement techniques are defined as "techniques in which external energies are administered to the body, but in amounts similar to those that the body itself uses in its energetic control systems; as such, they are seen as reinforcing an inactive or inadequate energetic control system" (Becker, 1990). According to Becker, the body's internal energetic control systems are subtle, and they operate with minute amounts of electromagnetic energy. The techniques in this category appear to work, then, by adding to or reinforcing the existing internal bioenergetic

systems through the application of small amounts of external energy, enhancing the intrinsic energy-controlled systems of the body" (Becker, 1990).

It is within this category that the majority of research in Energetic medicine is found, and many Energetic medical approaches are considered to be energy reinforcing. It should also be noted that many other traditional medical systems have evolved over time, including Native American, Aboriginal, African, Middle Eastern, Tibetan, and Central and South American cultures, all of which have energetically based foundations of belief and healing practices; however, discussion of these systems lies beyond the confines of this chapter.

Below is a partial listing of more commonly utilized energy-reinforcing modalities and pain-related research findings.

Acupuncture/Traditional Oriental Medicine

This ancient system of healing emphasizes the creation, re-creation, and/or homeodynamic maintenance of the vital energy within an individual, known as *chi (qi)* or *ki*. It is based on the concept that imbalances of this energy, due to a variety of causes, can lead to illness and disease; diagnosis involves, among other things, the "reading" of this energy by palpation of radial pulses. Traditional Oriental medicine is an encompassing term that involves the use of methods and techniques including acupuncture, herbal medicine, Oriental massage, and various movement therapies, such as Tai chi and Qi gong. Acupuncture is the best known of these, and treatment consists of the stimulation of specific points in the body on specific pathways, primarily through use of a needle, although practitioners also utilize heat, pressure, friction, suction, or impulses of electromagnetic energy to stimulate the points. (Note: Electroacupuncture involves the use of external applications of electroenergy by means of various devices. It is considered at greater length in the next category.)

Some of the most important findings on the role of energy fields in health and disease have come from acupuncture research. Dr. Robert Becker's work in the area of bioelectromagnetism during the 1980s performed research on acupuncture points and meridians. He found that acupuncture points existed and that they had specific, reproducible, and significant elecrical parameters; he also found that acupuncture meridians had the electrical characteristics of transmission lines, while non-meridian skin did not (Becker, 1990). Further research also showed that acupuncture meridians are low resistance pathways for the flow of electricity (Reichmanis, Marino, & Becker, 1975).

Pain management is considered to be a major area for the application of acupuncture. However, a comprehensive acupuncture bibliography, prepared in response to the 1997 NIH consensus development conference on its use, spanned the literature from 1970 to 1997 and identified 2302 citations in various categories. These categories, which encompassed a wide range of systems and disorders, included general pain, addictions, and psychiatric disorders; cardiovascular system; gastroenterology; genitourinary, pelvic, and reproductive systems; headache; low back, sciatica; lower extremities; neck and shoulders; nervous system; nausea, vomiting, and postoperative problems (Dean, Mullins, & Yuen, 2000). Acupuncture also has been shown to play an extremely important role in the prevention of illness and is utilized to facilitate personal transformational and spiritual growth processes as well.

Ayurveda

Considered India's traditional system of medicine, Ayurveda (meaning "the science or knowledge of life") is a comprehensive system of medicine that places equal emphasis on body, mind, and spirit. It is based on the premise that disease is caused by living out of harmony with our environment and each individual uniquely responds to this disharmony energetically; part of the diagnostic process includes "reading" of this energy in a way similar to Oriental medicine, although what is being read is considerably different. Treatment strives to restore this innate energetic harmony primarily through the use of diet, exercise, meditation, herbs, massage, chromotherapy, and controlled breathing techniques specific to each patient. Although little or no formal research has been conducted, there are many articles and studies in support of its efficacy, especially in cases of chronic conditions (Lad, 1999).

Homeopathy

Homeopathy is a systematic approach to healing formulated by Samuel Hahnemann in the 1790s that uses dilute or energetic forms of medicines to trigger an individual's innate capacity to heal. It works holistically, maintaining that disease is secondary to disharmony within the individual's system and that mental, emotional, and physical symptoms reflect this disharmony. Theoretically, it is based on the "Law of Similars," meaning that the same substance in large doses will produce the symptoms of an illness, but in very minute doses will cure it. In lieu of this, it is understood that the more dilute the remedy, the greater its potency. Homeopaths, therefore, utilize varying potencies of specially prepared plant extracts and minerals to stimulate the body's defense mechanisms and healing processes on whatever level is necessary to treat the specific illness. It is of interest to note that according to the World Health Organization, homeopathy is the second most used healthcare system in the world, primarily utilized in Europe; however, even in the United States, prior to the rise of allopathic medicine as a standard of care around the 1900s, 20 homeopathic medical schools were known to exist, with approximately 8% of all physicians utilizing it in their practices (Chapman, 1999).

Homeopathy is also often considered to be a form of what has been called *Vibrational medicine*, and BEM findings may begin to provide an explanation of its mechanism of action. Diseases and disorders can alter the balance of the electromagnetic properties of molecules, cells, tissues, and organs. When this occurs, use of a specific drug sometimes can restore normal functioning; this is the basis for pharmacology (Oschman, 2000). However, vibrational medicines such as homeopathy demonstrate that similar or even better results can be obtained by providing the specific electromagnetic fingerprint or signature of a natural substance (Smith, 1994). In doing so, they can initiate a response in the defense and repair systems of the body and restore balance to the system without potential pharmaceutical side effects.

A review of clinical trials in homeopathy included 107 controlled trials that were published between 1990 and 1996. Although most trials were of poor quality, there was a positive trend; of the 107 trials, 81 demonstrated improvements in the treatment of headaches, respiratory infections, diseases of the digestive tract, postoperative infections and symptoms, as well as other disorders (Kleijnen, Knipschild, & ter Reit, 1991).

Biologically Based Therapies

This category encompasses a variety of naturally, pharmacologically, and biologically based products, practices, and interventions, many of which overlap with conventional medical usage, but which, by their nature, are appropriately considered as energy reinforcing. Examples of these include, but are not limited to, herbal therapies, orthomolecular and nutritional supplementation, chelation therapy, and special dietary therapies. Despite their diversity in historical usage, mechanisms of action, and clinical approaches, common aims are to control symptoms, promote health, and prevent illness. As therapies in this category have amassed volumes of literature, discussion of detailed findings is not possible, and the reader is invited to explore specifics in texts referenced at the conclusion of this chapter.

Chiropractic and Other Manipulative and Body-Based Therapies

Chiropractic is considered to be one of the major branches of Western medicine. The major difference between chiropractic and other forms of Western medicine is that chiropractic focuses on the spine as integrally involved in maintaining health, providing primacy to the nervous system as the primary coordinator for function, and thus health, in the body. The goal of chiropractic is the maintenance of optimal neurophysiological balance in the body, which is accomplished by correcting structural or biomechanical abnormalities or disrelationships, and the primary method for accomplishing this balance is spinal manipulation, also known as the chiropractic adjustment" (Lawrence, 1999). Although the use of manipulation is primary, chiropractic treatment also can include soft tissue techniques such as massage, and the use of ice, heat, ultrasound, traction, and electrical stimulation. A review of the research literature indicates that chiropractic treatment can be efficacious in treating low back, neck, and headache pain, although it is often utilized, with success, for some nonmusculoskeletal conditions as well (Freeman, 2001a).

Myriad other body-based techniques and methods also exist including, but not limited to, therapeutic massage, Shiatsu, acupressure, myofascial release, Feldenkrais, Alexander method, and Rolfing. Extensive subjective and clinical reports indicate that these and other methods can be beneficial not only for pain and stress reduction, but also to facilitate positive changes in body structure, associated soft tissue, and overall physiological functioning. (Please refer to the specific method in referenced texts for more detailed findings.)

Just as many forms of body-based therapies include the understanding that the whole system is impacted upon during treatment, body-oriented psychotherapies also have been developed that expand on the notion that the body–mind is interconnected and cannot be separated during the course of treatment. Candace Pert further explains this, incorporating bioenergetic aspects, when she states that "most bodyworkers and body psychotherapists take as fact that trauma is absorbed and stored in the body and can be unblocked by some corrective energy flow. Therapeutic massage can be so much more than increasing blood circulation in sore muscles; our concept of the psychosomatic network envisions memories stored in the body (the subconscious mind) in the form of alterations at receptor molecules which transduce chemical changes into ionic fluxes and thus the propagation of electromagnetic waves throughout the network which joins the nervous system, immune cells, gut, glands skin, etc." (Pert, 1999).

Spiritual Healing/Prayer

Spiritual healing is probably the oldest recognized form of energy-based healing and is defined as "the systematic purposeful intervention by one or more persons aiming to help (an)other living being (person, animal, plant, or other living system) or beings by means of focused intention, by touch, or by holding the hands near the other being, without application of physical, chemical, or conventional energetic means of intervention" (Benor, 1999). Prayer may be differentiated from spiritual healing in that, in most cases, it is performed singularly, and might instead be considered as a minimal energy technique. However, in those cases where group prayer is utilized as a healing modality, mechanisms of bioenergetic exchanges may occur.

Although efficacy is unpredictable, healers and those being healed report that pain is the symptom most responsive to spiritual healing, and emotional conditions, such as anxiety and depression, also often respond well (Benor, 1999). A number of studies have examined the effects of religion and prayer on health outcomes and results indicate that these factors were helpful for patients in coping with health problems, illness, and chronic disability that are unresponsive to medical treatment (Koenig, 2000). In addition, Elizabeth Targ and Fred Sicher (1998) published the results of a pilot study showing that advanced AIDS patients who received long-distance intercessory prayer improved their medical outcomes (Springer & Eicher, 1999). Other studies also indicate statistically significant effects of intercessory and remote prayer (Springer & Eicher, 1999).

"Hand-Mediated Energetic Healing Modalities" (HMEHM)

Victoria Slater has coined this phrase to refer to "all healing methods in which a practitioner's hands are the medium of transfer or exchange of something that subjectively feels like energy, although there are some reports of feeling heat" (Slater, 1996). These modalities include new techniques, as well as modern variations of ancient indigenous practices found around the world, such as healing touch, therapeutic touch, polarity, touch for health, Reiki, and external Qi gong. Considered similar to spiritual healing in many aspects, these modalities generally are based on the belief in a universal healing energy flow with the premise being that it is either this healing force moving through the practitioner, or the individual healing force of the practitioner, that affects the patient. Practitioners are able to identify energy imbalances, often by passing their hands over the patient, and healing is promoted when the body's energies become balanced. Another similarity is that these techniques do not require direct physical contact, merely clear, focused intention. They do differ, however, from spiritual healing in that their effectiveness does not require professed faith or belief by either the practitioner or patient, and they are not typically performed within any religious context.

Although research on the objective physiologic causes and effects of these modalities is inconclusive, a review of related literature indicates that these practices can be effective in reducing pain, decreasing stress, depression, and anxiety, positively affecting blood level values, increasing healing rates and immune responses, and promoting relaxation (Slater, 1996). Due to the extensive research in this area, the reader is referred to related chapters in referenced books on complementary/alternative medicine for detailed studies.

Static Magnetic Field Therapy

Research by Robert Becker demonstrated that every nerve fiber in the body is completely encased in perineural cells and that this perineural system is sensitive to magnetic fields. This discovery helped to provide a basis for the use of magnets and biomagnetic fields in healing (Becker, 1990; 1991). In this category, a differentiation is made between the therapeutic use of static or permanent magnetic fields and other forms of electromagnetic therapies. Although theoretically the latter might be placed in this category as their usage is dependent upon devices that issue current, it is more appropriate that they be considered within the next category.

Static magnets have been used in a variety of ways, from placing small magnets over acupuncture points to the use of magnetic insoles, blankets, and beds—all aimed at balancing the body's electromagnetic fields, and thus affecting the functioning of the nervous system, organs, and cells. In regard to pain management, very little research has been documented. In one of the few double-blind studies with static magnetic fields, active and placebo magnets were applied over trigger points on 50 patients with pain; results showed significant reductions in pain (Vallbona, et al., 1997). Another study of fibromyalgia patients using tectonic magnetic mattress pads showed a significant improvement in physical functioning, decreased pain, and improvement in sleep (Colbert, et al., 1998).

Music/Sound Vibrations

In many cultures the use of music and sound has been found to create altered states and to promote healing, and it is now well known that the human body does respond to vibratory stimuli. Research shows that varying frequency, amplitude, and rhythm can elicit physiologic responses, affecting changes in heart rate, blood pressure, brain waves, the nervous system, and in muscles and other body tissues. Recent studies also indicate the efficacy of vibration and vibratory responses within the body to music or other sound waves in relief of both acute and chronic pain (Taylor, 1999).

Light Therapy/Phototherapy/Chronobiology

This energetic modality is defined as "the therapeutic application of electromagnetic energy in the visible spectrum, using ultraviolet, bright white, colored, monochrome, or laser light, to treat a wide range of health disorders" (Wallace, 2000). Based on the concept that varying colors and frequencies can affect the bioenergetic system and thus a number of bodily functions, treatment usually involves using various instrumentation that produces specific frequencies of light energy. It is performed most often by shining light/color on a person's entire body or specific parts; injecting specific irradiated pigments into cells, organs, or tissues that are then, in turn, irradiated with certain frequencies of light (photodynamic therapy); visualization of certain colors either within the body or as part of meditation to apply color to areas of the body; and/or irradiating water with a specific color for drinking (Wallace, 2000).

Research-based findings are currently somewhat limited; however, use of different forms of light therapy has been reported to yield positive results in the treatment of chronic and acute pain and inflammation, headaches, depression, immune and endocrine disorders, as well as in the areas of oncology and dermatology (Goldberg, 1993).

Aromatherapy

Aromatherapy is the therapeutic use of essential oils, absorbed via the skin or olfactory system. Essential oils are defined as steam distillates obtained from aromatic plants, or expressions from the peel of citrus fruits (Evans,1994). Research indicates that aromatic molecules give off signals that travel to the limbic system that, in turn, is directly connected to those parts of the brain that control heart rate, blood pressure, breathing, memory, stress levels, and hormone balance. Findings show that essential oils, when inhaled, affect brain waves. Specific oils have a tranquilizing effect and work by altering the brain waves into a rhythm that produces calmness and a sense of well-being, while others work by producing a heightened energy response (Goldberg, 1993; 1997).

Although the properties of each individual oil appear to be understood, few studies have been done on the analgesic effects of essential oils. However, essential oils are frequently used for the topical treatment of various types of pain, including arthritis, cephalgia, and cancer, and can play a role in altering the perception of chronic pain. In a study, HIV-infected hospitalized children responded well to the chosen blends, helping to decrease the need for analgesic drugs. Some of the children said their pain had been relieved completely; in others, symptoms of chronic chest pain, muscle spasm, and peripheral neuropathy were eased (Buckle, 1999).

RELATED RESEARCH FINDINGS

Although the scientific validity has been, and continues to be, questioned, studies of several of these energy transfer modalities have brought forth interesting results, as shown below:

> Extremely large frequency-pulsing biomagnetic fields were discovered emanating from hands of therapeutic touch practitioners during therapy as determined by SQUID measurements. The signal pulsed at a variable frequency (i.e., sweeping or scanning through a range of frequencies) ranging from 0.3 to 30 Hz, with most of the activity in the range of 7 to 8 Hz. Nonpractitioners were unable to produce the same biomagnetic pulses (Zimmerman, 1990).

> Another study confirmed that an extraordinarily large biomagnetic field emanates from the hands of practitioners of a variety of healing and martial arts techniques, including yoga, meditation, and Qigong. The fields were measured with a simple magnetometer that indicated that these fields were approximately 1000 times stronger than the strongest human biomagnetic fields and the biomagnetic field pulsed with a variable frequency centered around 8 to 10 Hz (Seto, et al., 1992).

> The brain wave activities of various "healers" from around the world were studied and recorded by Robert C. Beck. Utilizing an EEG, he found that all the healers produced similar brain wave patterns when they were in their altered states and performing healings. Regardless of their beliefs and customs, all of these healers produced nearly identical EEG signatures with brain wave activity averaging about 7.8 to 8 Hz (Beck, 1996).

Although these studies did not document any clinical healing effects taking place during this projection of energy, the evidence does show that practitioners, in a variety of settings and using different modalities, emit powerful pulsing biomagnetic fields within a common, specific frequency. This frequency range corresponds to similar frequencies being tested in medical research laboratories for use in facilitating the healing process of certain biological tissues, with initial positive results (Sisken & Walker, 1995).

Additional studies on the effects of Qi gong also yielded notable results:

> A study of *Qigong* masters shows that they can project measurable amounts of heat from their palms, in addition to biomagnetic fields, which increases cell growth, DNA and protein synthesis, and cell respiration. They can also produce inhibiting *qi*, in which infrared energy is absorbed from the environment. This kind of *qi* slows metabolism (Muehsam, et al., 1994).

> Research has been performed employing a Qi gong master emitting external *qi* to a human being or a nonhuman organism while the effects are monitored under controlled scientific conditions. The results of these controlled Chinese trials demonstrated unexpected and unexplainable variations in the basic characteristics of most substances tested, ranging from radioactive materials to simple tap water. In addition, these external *qi* effects were noted at significant distances; for example, more than 10,000 miles between *qi* transmitter and receptor have been recorded, indicating that the matter–energy manipulation phenomenon is not limited to close proximity (Benford, et al., 2000).

> In regard to this latter finding, clinical research and other laboratory and cross-cultural studies also have demonstrated the ability to effect various physiological changes over long distances. Consistent with BEM findings that electromagnetic fields are capable of producing an action at a distance, bioenergetic effects appear to extend beyond hand-mediated practices. Findings such as these would support further clinical exploration of such well-known practices as remote visualization techniques and long-distance prayer.

HIGH-ENERGY TRANSFER TECHNIQUES

High-energy transfer techniques are defined as those "in which electromagnetic energy is introduced or administered to the body in amounts that exceed those that naturally occur, in the sense that the normal system is replaced by this externally derived energy" (Becker, 1990). This category includes the use of a variety of diagnostic and treatment devices. For treatment purposes, the majority of electromagnetic (EM) therapeutic methods used in the United States are nonthermal in nature (causing no significant heating of the tissue) and generally utilize either pulsed electromagnetic fields (PEMFs), pulsed radiofrequency (PRF), or low-frequency sine waves, although others have also been utilized (Taylor, 1999).

Many electrical devices have been demonstrated over time to have beneficial medical applications. For instance, studies during the last several decades show that the use of transcutaneous electrical nerve stimulation (TENS), in which controlled, low-voltage electrical impulses are applied to the nervous system through electrodes, is beneficial for the control of acute and chronic pain. One of the accepted mechanisms of pain relief with the TENS unit is based on research indicating that increased endorphin production is derived from its use (Kahn, 1987).

It is estimated that there are more than 100 types of FDA-approved TENS units currently available, with each device offering some variances of wave forms and frequencies, although all operate on the same basis (Rubik, et al., 1992). Along similar lines, transcranial electrostimulation devices (TCES) and neuromagnetic stimulation techniques are being used to treat symptoms of depression, anxiety, seizures, and insomnia (Rubik, et al., 1992).

While traditional acupuncture is considered an energy-reinforcement technique, electroacupuncture—where either the needles are stimulated with varying frequencies/intensities of electricity or the acupuncture points are stimulated by electrical devices without the use of needles—is considered to be a high-energy transfer technique. Electroacupuncture is frequently used to enhance the analgesic effect in the course of a treatment, but is also utilized to create an anesthetic effect on specific body parts based on where the electrodes are placed. Studies utilizing electroacupuncture have shown it to be beneficial in the treatment of postoperative pain (Christensen & Noreng, 1989), renal colic (Lee, et al., 1992), and in the treatment of chemotherapy-induced sickness in cancer patients (Dundee & Ghaly, 1989).

Recently, medical research has revealed that magnetic fields can convert a stalled healing process into active repair. In regard to nonunion bone fractures, three types of applied electromagnetic fields are now known to promote healing: pulsed EM fields (PEMF) and sinusoidal EM fields (AC fields), DC fields, and combined AC–DC magnetic fields (Rubik, et al., 1992). Efficacy of EM bone repair treatment has been confirmed in double-blind clinical trials (Barker, et al., 1984; Sharrard, 1990), and clinical tests prove that PEMF therapy will jump-start bone repair (Bassett, 1995). In addition, PEMF therapy was found to be effective in reducing pain and improving function in osteoarthritis patients (Track, et al., 1994).

Research employing electric and magnetic fields on soft tissues has been reviewed by Sisken and Walker who observed that PEMF pulses not only accelerated the healing of soft tissue injuries, but also reduced swelling, diminished pain, increased tensile strength of ligaments, and accelerated nerve regeneration and functional recovery, among other findings. They found that to be effective PEMF pulses must be of low energy and extremely low frequency (ELF) (the ELF range is arbitrarily defined as frequencies below 100 hz) (Sisken & Walker, 1995). Short-wave pulsed radiofrequency (PRF) therapeutic applications have also been reported for the reduction of posttraumatic and postoperative pain and edema in soft tissue, wound healing, burn treatment, sprains and strains of the ankle, hand injuries, and nerve regeneration (Markoy & Pilla, 1995).

The use of electromagnetism is being studied for other medical benefits as well, including treatment of autoimmune diseases, immune restoration, additional areas of pain management, and in neurology. However, according to biomedical standards, there is currently no commonly accepted mechanism for electromagnetic field bioeffects, and analgesic action of electromagnetic frequencies is explained through enhanced endorphin production, as well as by anti-inflammatory and anti-edema activity and reduction in spasms (Serabek & Pawluk, 1998).

In addition to those electromagnetic devices currently either approved or pending approval by regulatory agencies, many others also exist that claim to perform a variety of procedures, including the diagnosis of energetic imbalances and the rebalancing of energy fields within the body, as well as facilitating healing in various ways. Despite claims regarding their efficacy, however, definitive documentation is lacking at this time, and clinical studies are continuing.

FUTURE IMPLICATIONS

As research accumulates in the areas of BEM, cellular biology, and quantum physics, new doors of understanding are opening, and work in the areas of energetics and bioenergetics may hold potential answers for continued expansion in the field of medicine. Some future implications of the use of Energetic medicine are considered below.

PREVENTION

In 1996, data showed that disease states can be detected by measuring changes in the electrical conductances of tissues, long before any structural abnormalities have occurred (Brewitt, 1996). In lieu of these data and similar research coming to light, we can begin to see the importance of Energetic medicine in the area of prevention. As Dr. Julian Kenyon states: "If pathological changes can be detected at the energetic stage, then diagnosis can be much earlier and also pathology at this stage is more easily reversible than when a lump has already appeared … " (Kenyon, 1984).

While the current focus is on the healing of injuries and management of pain, it has also been found throughout time that Energetic medical techniques can be of profound significance even if no specific problem is present, and that the free flow of energy through tissues is essential not only for prevention of disease, but also for the promotion of optimal health. An individual who is healthy will not only be happier, but also less likely to have an injury or disease. Energetic medicine has shown that, in many cases, if problems arise, a person will be apt to recover more rapidly. Likewise, athletic, artistic, and intellectual performance can be enhanced when all of the body's communication channels are open and balanced. This point is well understood in many Energetic medicine practices, and people will often come in on a regular basis for what are called *maintenance treatments* or *tune-ups.*

PALLIATIVE CARE

Both patients and physicians have reported dissatisfaction at what currently are often seen as the only answers to the question of how best to provide comfort at the end of life. When a cure is not possible, healing can still take place, and comfort comes in many forms. Energetic medical modalities are becoming viable options not only in pain management for the terminally ill, but also in reducing anxiety, creating a more peaceful outlook, and facilitating empowerment as death approaches.

NEW MEDICAL PARADIGM

Some researchers believe that Energetic medicine may be an important next step in medicine because it takes into account the entire individual. If utilized as a medical model, it would necessitate consideration of all bodily systems, including consciousness, as part of a patient's total experience in both the disease and the healing process (Lawlis, 2001a). In appropriate situations, specific energetic-based modalities also may be desirable over chemically based treatment because they can be generally safer to use, require less time for beneficial action, and dosage adjustment potentially could be determined with less risk of side effects. In addition, as research is beginning to indicate, specific forms of electromagnetic stimulation may be utilized for the regeneration of damaged tissue and bodily structures, for benefit in ameliorating specific symptoms, and for enhancing immunological functioning (Lawlis, 2001b).

CHALLENGES FACING ENERGETIC MEDICINE

Just as it has been established that extremely small amounts of electromagnetism have a variety of positive biological effects, some researchers make the argument that exogenous fields of energy administered to the body may have side effects of an undesirable nature. For example, as mentioned previously, research has shown that electrotherapy can be effective in some cases for chronic pain, to increase endorphin output, and to stimulate the healing of human bone fractures. Experimentation also has shown that exposing cancer cells to specific levels of DC current caused them to grow "at least 300% faster than the controls" (Becker, 1990). Findings such as these indicate the need for further inquiry and, as in the case of any new therapeutic modality, time must be afforded for the slow progression of discovery of benefits, consequences, and parameters. As clinical research of the properties, actions, effects, and interactions of both bioelectromagnetism and electromagnetic therapy continues, it is becoming evident that questions such as these are being addressed.

Even with the advent of extensive research of energy fields and their potential for medical benefits, there continues to be a great deal of criticism. The literature indicates that most criticism is centered around the fact that the human energy field cannot be adequately measured and, in many cases, the mechanisms of action and beneficial effects of energetic modalities have not been sufficiently explained, documented, and validated using current biomedical research standards. Study replication also has been found to be difficult, often yielding inconsistent findings; this may be because individuals are unique, and response to identical stimuli or testing methods may vary among individuals or over time with the same individual.

It is true that challenges exist in attempting to use conventional biomedical research methods to study Energetic medicine. A number of its practitioners and researchers feel that the randomized controlled trial is not always the most appropriate research methodology for energetically based treatments (Gatchel & Maddrey, 1998), many of which are based upon long-standing ethnomedical systems of knowledge. Clearly, it does not fit either the models of etiology and treatment or the current research models found in Western biomedicine. However, rather than dismissing the study of Energetic medicine, as has been suggested by some, consideration of alternative research methodologies is being initiated, including the use of case studies, experiential reports, and observational findings, all of which may provide valuable insights for both practice and research.

The study of biomedicine has been and continues to be an evolutionary process, changing as it embraces each new discovery. In the same regard, many BEM researchers are now beginning to expand what perhaps might be considered a limited and outmoded approach to scientific inquiry by suggesting the incorporation of a systems theory approach to the study of Energetic medicine. They believe that it may offer a plausible and acceptable scientific framework while accommodating the unique aspects inherently found in this form of medicine (Benford, et al., 2000). By definition, "systems at any level, whether physical, biological, social, and/or ecological, are open to information, energy, and matter to varying degrees and, therefore, interact with other systems to varying degrees" (Schwartz & Russek, 1997).

The core of systems theory, then, is dynamic interaction: systems do not simply act on systems; they interact with them in complex ways. As living systems are found to interact with other systems in ways previously uncomprehended, their study requires a focus to incorporate this information. Utilization of the systems approach to the study of Energetic medicine, then, may offer an exciting alternative to the current Biomedical model and an opportunity to begin to understand those aspects of life that exist outside of a reductionistic and mechanistic framework.

REFERENCES

Achterberg, J. (1985). *Imagery in healing: Shamanism and modern medicine.* Boston: Shambala Press.

Astin, J.A., Shapiro, S.L., & Schwartz, G.E.R. (2000). Meditation. In D.W. Novey (Ed.), *Clinician's complete reference to complementary and alternative medicine* (p. 73). St. Louis: Mosby.

Barker, A.T., et al. (1984). Pulsed magnetic field therapy for tibial nonunion: Interim results of a double-blind trial. *Lancet, 1,* (8384), 994–996.

Bassett, C.A.L. (1995). Bioelectromagnetics in the service of medicine. In M. Blank (Ed.), *Electromagnetic fields: Biological interactions and mechanisms,* (261–275). Advances I chemistry series 250, Washington, D.C.: American Chemical Society,

Baule, G.M., & McFee, R. (1963). Detection of the magnetic field of the heart. *American Heart Journal, 66,* 95–96.

Beck, R. (1986). Mood modification with ELF magnetic fields: A preliminary exploration. *Archaeus, 4,* 48.

Becker, R.O. (1991). Evidence for a primitive DC electrical analog system controlling brain function. *Subtle Energies, 2*(1), 71–88.

Becker R.O. (1990). The machine brain and properties of the mind. *Subtle Energies, 113,* 79–97.

Becker, R.O. (1990). *Cross currents.* Los Angeles: Jeremy Tarcher.

Becker, R.O., & Marino A.A. (1982). *Electromagnetism and life.* Albany: State University of New York Press.

Becker, R.O., & Selden, G. (1985). *The body electric* (p. 27). New York: William Morrow and Company.

Benford, M.S., et al. (2000). Exploring the concept of energy in touch-based healing. In D.W. Novey (Ed.), *Clinician's complete reference to complementary and alternative medicine.*

Benor, D., Spiritual healing. In W.B. Jonas and J.S. Levin (Eds.), *Essentials of complementary and alternative medicine,* (pp. 374–375). Baltimore: Lippincott, Williams and Wilkins.

Benor, D.J. (1999). Spiritual healing: does it work? Science says, yes! *Healing research,* 1. Southfield, MI: Vision Publishers.

Bialek, W. (1987). Physical limits to sensation and perception. *Annual Review of Biophysics and Biophysical Chemistry, 16,* 455–478.

Brennen, B. (1993). *Light emerging: The journey of personal healing.* New York: Bantam.

Brewitt, B. (1996). Quantitative analysis of electrical skin conductance in diagnosis: Historical and current views of bioelectric medicine. *Journal of Naturopathic Medicine, 6*(1), 66–75.

Buckle, J. (1999). Use of aromatherapy as a complementary treatment for chronic pain, *Alternative Therapies in Health and Medicine, 5,* 5, 44.

Chaitow, L. (1987). *Soft tissue manipulation.* Wellingborough, U.K.: Thorson.

Chapman, E.H. (1999). Homeopathy. In W.B. Jonas & J.S. Levin, (Eds.), *Essentials of complementary and alternative medicine,* (pp. 472–473). Baltimore: Lippincott, Williams, & Wilkins.

Christensen, P.A., & Noreng, M. (1989). Electroacupuncture and postoperative pain. *British Journal of Anaesthesia, 62,* 258–262.

Colbert, A.P., et al. (1998). Use of tectonic magnetic mattress pad in patient with fibromyalgia. 20th Annual meeting, Bioelectromagnetic Society, St. Petersburg Beach, FL.

Dean, C.F.A., Mullins, M., & Yuen, J. (2000). Acupuncture. In D.W. Novey (Ed.), *Clinician's complete reference to complementary and alternative medicine* (pp. 196–197).

Dundee, J.W., & Ghaly, R.G. (1989). Acupuncture prophylaxis of cancer chemotherapy-induced sickness. *Journal Royal Society of Medicine, 82,* 268–271.

Edwards, D.L (1991). A meta-analysis of the effects of meditation and hypnosis on measures of anxiety. *Dissertation Abstract International, 52,* 2B, 1039.

Eppley, K.R., Abrams, A.I., & Shear, J. (1989). Differential effects of relaxation techniques on trait anxiety: A meta-analysis. *Journal of Clinical Psychology, 45,* 957–974.

Erickson, P., Wilson, R., & Shannon, I. (1995). *Healthy people 2000: Statistical notes: Years of healthy life,* Washington, D.C.: U.S. Dept of Health and Human Services, Report 7, Center for Disease Control and Prevention and National Center for Health Statistics.

Evans, W.C. (1994). *Trease and Evans pharmacognosy.* London: Balliere Tindall,

Freeman, L.W. (2001). Chiropractic. In L.W. Freeman. & G.F. Lawlis, (Eds.), *Complementary and alternative medicine: A research-based approach* (298–303). St. Louis: Mosby,

Freeman, L.W. (2001a) Imagery. In L.W. Freeman & G.F. Lawlis (Eds.), *Complementary and alternative medicine: A research-based approach* (p. 265). St. Louis: Mosby.

Freeman, L.W. (2001b). Relaxation therapy. In L.W. Freeman and G.F. Lawlis (Eds.), *Complementary and alternative medicine: A research-based approach* (p. 140). St. Louis: Mosby.

Gallo, F.P. (1999). *Energy psychology* (pp. 227–228). Boca Raton: CRC Press.

Gatchel, R.J., & Maddrey, A.M. (1998). Clinical outcome research in complementary and alternative medicine: An overview of experimental design and analysis. *Alternative Therapies in Health and Medicine, 4,* 5, 39.

Geddes, L.A. (1984). A short history of the electrical stimulation of excitable tissue including electrotherapeutic applications. *Physiologist 27*(1), S1–S47.

Goldberg, B. (1993). *Alternative medicine: The definitive guide.* Tiburon, CA: Future Medicine Publishing.

Harner, M. (1987). The ancient wisdom in shamanic cultures, interview conducted by Gary Doore. In S. Nicholson, (Ed.), *Shamanism.* Wheaton, IL: The Theosophical Publishing House.

Jacobs, J., & Moskowitz, R. (1996). Homeopathy. In M.S. Micozzi (Ed.), *Fundamentals of complementary and alternative medicine.* New York: Churchill Livingstone.

Jerabek, J., & Pawluk, W. (1998). Magnetic therapy: The eastern European research. Availability: wpawluk@compuserve.com.

Kabat-Zinn, J., Lipworth, L., & Burney, R. (1987). Four-year followup of a meditation-based program for the self-regulation of chronic pain: treatment outcomes and compliance. *Clinical Journal of Pain, 2,* 159–173.

Kabat-Zinn, J., Lipworth, L., & Burney, R. (1985). The clinical use of mindfulness meditation for the self-regulation of chronic pain. *Journal of Behavior and Medicine, 8,* 163–190.

Kahn, J. (1987). *Principles and practices of electrotherapy.* New York: Churchill Livingstone, 127–131.

Kamada, T., et al. (1992). Power spectral analysis of heart rate variability in type As and type Bs during mental workload. *Psychosomatic Medicine, 54,* 462–470.

Kenyon, J. (1984). The segmental electrogram: A non-invasive early diagnostic scanning technique. *British Journal of Holistic Medicine, 1,* 2.

King, J.V. (1988). A holistic technique to lower anxiety: Relaxation with guided imagery. *Journal of Holistic Nursing, 6,* 1, 16–20.

Kleijnen J., Knipschild, P., & ter Reit, G. (1991). Clinical trials of homeopathy. *British Medical Journal, 302,* 6772, 316.

Koenig, H.G. (2000). Spiritual healing and prayer. In D.W. Novey (Ed.). *Clinician's complete reference to complementary and alternative medicine* (p. 136). St. Louis: Mosby.

Krippner, S. (1999). Introduction: Common aspects of traditional healing systems across cultures. In W.B. Jonas and J.S. Levin (Eds.), (pp. 181–182). *Essentials of complementary and alternative medicine.* Baltimore: Lippincott Williams & Wilkins.

Lad, D.V. (1999). Ayurvedic medicine, In W.B. Jonas and J.S. Levin (Eds.). *Essentials of complementary and alternative medicine* (p. 211). Baltimore: Lippincott Williams & Wilkins.

Lawlis, G.F. (2001a). Biofeedback. In L.W. Freeman and G.F. Lawlis (Eds.). *Complementary and alternative medicine: A research-based approach* (chap. 7). St. Louis: Mosby.

Lawlis, G.F. (2001b). Electromagnetic medicine, In L.W. Freeman and G.F. Lawlis (Eds.). *Complementary and alternative medicine: A research-based approach* (p. 470). St. Louis: Mosby.

Lawrence, D.J., Chiropractic Medicine, In W.B. Jonas & J.S. Levin (Eds.), *Essentials of complementary and alternative medicine* (p. 275). Baltimore: J. Lippincott Williams & Wilkins.

Lee, Y.H., et al. (1992). Acupuncture in the treatment of renal colic. *Journal of Urology, 147,* 16–18.

Loitman, J. (2000). Pain management: beyond pharmacology to acupuncture and hypnosis. *Medical Student Journal of the American Medical Association, 283,* 118–119.

Markoy, M.S., & Pilla, A.A. (1995). Electromagnetic field stimulation of soft tissues. *Wounds, 7,* 143.

McClaskey, T. (1999). Trauma intervention and the emerging field of energy psychology. *Trauma Response Pub., 5,* 2, 29, Spring/Summer.

McCraty, R., et al. (1993). New electrophysiological correlates associated with intentional heart focus. *Subtle Energies 4,* 3, 251–268.

McDonald, R.T., & Hilgendorf, W.A. (1986). Death imagery and death anxiety. *Journal of Clinical Psychology, 42,* 1, 87–91.

Mehl, L.E. (1998). Modern shamanism: Integration of biomedicine with traditional world views. In G. Doore (Ed.), *Shaman's path* (p. 129). Boston: Shambhala Publications.

Micozzi, M.S. (1996). Characteristics of complementary and alternative medicine. In M.S. Micozzi (Ed.), *Fundamentals of complementary and alternative medicine* (p. 3). New York: Churchill Livingstone.

Muehsam, D.J., et. al. (1994). Effects of qigong on cell-free myosin phosphorylation: preliminary experiments. *Subtle Energies, 5,* 93–108.

National Center for Complementary & Alternative Medicine website: http://nccam.nih.gov/

NIH Technology Assessment Statement (1995). *Integration of behavioral and relaxation approaches into the treatment of chronic pain and insomnia,* NIH Technology Assessment Statement, Oct 16–18, 1–34.

Oschman, J.L. (2000). *Energy medicine: The scientific basis* (p. 218).

Oschman, J.L., & Oschman N.H. (1994). Book review and commentary [on]: *Biological coherence and response to external stimuli,* Herbert Frohlich, Ed., Springer-Verlag, Berlin, 1988. NORA Press, Dover NH.

Patterson, D.R., et al. (1992). Hypnosis for treatment of burn pain. *Journal of Consulting and Clinical Psychology, 60,* 5, 713.

Pert, C.B. (1999). *Molecules of emotion: The science behind mind-body medicine.* New York: Simon & Schuster.

Pienta, K.J., & Coffey, D.S. (1991). Cellular harmonic information transfer through a tissue tensegrity-matrix system. *Medical Hypotheses, 34,* 88–95.

Pierrakos, J.C. (1975). Psychiatric implications of energy fields in man and nature. In S.R. Dean (Ed.), *Psychiatry and mysticism.* Chicago: Nelson-Hall, 145.

Reichmanis, M., Marino, A., & Becker, R.O. (1975). Electrical correlates of acupuncture points. *Transactions on Biomedical Engineering, 22,* 11, 533–535.

Rein, G., & McCraty, R. (1993). Modulation of DNA by coherent heart frequencies, presented at the 3rd Annual conference of the International Society for the Study of Subtle Energies and Energy Medicine, Monterey, CA, June.

Rossman, M.L. & Bresler, D.E. (2000). Interactive guided imagery, In D.W. Novey (Ed.). *Clinician's complete reference to complementary and alternative medicine* (p. 64). St. Louis: Mosby.

Rubik, B., et al. (1992, September). Bioelectromagnetics applications in medicine. In *Alternative medicine: Expanding medical horizons* (p. 51). A Report to NIH on Alternative Medical Systems and Practices in the U.S., prepared under the auspices of the Workshop on Alternative Medicine, Chantilly, VA.

Rubik, B. (2001). Electromagnetic medicine, interview conducted by G.F. Lawlis. In L.W. Freeman & G.F. Lawlis (Eds.), *Complementary and alternative medicine: A research-based approach* (p. 468). St. Louis: Mosby.

Sabo, M.J., & Giorgi, J. (2000). Biofeedback. In D. W. Novey, (Ed.), *Clinician's complete reference to complementary and alternative medicine* (p. 32). St. Louis: Mosby.

Saichek, K.I. (2000). Hypnotherapy. In D.W. Novey, (Ed.), *Clinician's complete reference to complementary and alternative medicine* (p. 56). St. Louis: Mosby.

Schaub, B.G., & Schaub, R. (1990). The use of mental imagery techniques in psychodynamic psychotherapy. *Journal of Mental Health Counseling, 12,* 4, 405–415.

Schlitz, M., & Lewis, N. (2000, Sept.–Nov.). Frontiers of research: Consciousness, science, and society. *IONS-Noetic Sciences Review,* 33.

Schwartz, G.E., & Russek, L.G. (1997). Dynamical energy systems and modern physics: Fostering the science and spirit of complementary and alternative medicine, *Alternative Therapies in Health and Medicine, 3,* 3, 46–56.

Seifer, A.R., & Lubar, J.F. (1975). Reduction of epileptic seizures through EEG biofeedback training. *Biological Psychology, 3,* 157.

Seto A., et al. (1992). Detection of extraordinary large biomagnetic field strength from human hands. *Acupuncture & Electro-Therapeutics Research International Journal, 17,* 75–94.

Sharrard, W.J.W. (1990). A double-blind trial of pulsed electromagnetic fields for delayed union of tibial fractures. *Journal of Bone and Joint Surgery, 72B,* 347–355.

Sisken, B.F., & Walker, J. (1995). Therapeutic aspects of electromagnetic fields for soft tissue healing. In M. Blank (Ed.), *Electromagnetic fields: Biological interactions and mechanisms* (pp. 277–285). Advances I chemistry series 250, Washington, D.C.: American Chemical Society.

Slater, V.E. (1996). Healing touch. In M.S. Micozzi (Ed.), *Fundamentals of complementary and alternative medicine* (p. 121). New York: Churchill Livingstone.

Sloan, R.P., et al. (1994). Effect of mental stress throughout the day on cardiac autonomic control. *Biological Psychology, 37,* 89–99.

Smith, C.W. (1994). Biological effects of weak electromagnetic fields. In M-W. Ho, F-A. Popp, & U. Warnke (Eds.). *Bioelectrodynamics and biocommunication* (pp. 81–107). Singapore: World Scientific.

Solomon, G.F., & Moos R.H. (1964). Emotions, immunity and disease: a speculative theoretical integration. *Archives of General Psychiatry 11,* 657.

Spiegel, H., & Spiegel, D. (1978). *Trance and treatment: Clinical uses of hypnosis.* New York: Basic Books.

Springer, S., & Eicher, D. (1999). Effects of a prayer circle on a moribund premature infant. *Alternative Therapies in Health and Medicine, 5,* 2, 115–120.

Taylor, A.G. (1999). Complementary/alternative therapies in the treatment of pain. In J. W. Spencer & J. J. Jacobs (Eds.). *Complementary/alternative medicine: An evidence-based approach* (p. 326). St. Louis: Mosby.

Taylor, A.G. (1999). Complementary/alternative therapies in the treatment of pain. In J.W. Spencer & J.J. Jacobs (Eds.), *Complementary/alternative medicine: An evidence-based approach* (p. 328). St. Louis: Mosby.

Trock, D.H., et al. (1994). The effect of pulsed electromagnetic fields in the treatment of osteoarthritis of the knee and cervical spine: Report of randomized, double blind, placebo controlled trials. *Journal of Rheumatology, 21,* 10, 1903.

Turk, D.C., & Melzack, R.D. (1992). The measurement of pain and the assessment of people experiencing pain. In D.C. Turk, & R. Melzack (Eds.). *Handbook of pain assessment.* New York: Guilford Press.

Vallbona, C., et al. (1997). Response of pain to static magnetic fields in postpolio patients: Double-blind pilot study. *Archives of Physical Medicine and Rehabilitation, 87,* 11, 1200.

Wallace, L.B. (2000). Light therapy. In D.W. Novey, (Ed.), *Clinician's complete reference to complementary and alternative medicine* (pp. 154–157). St. Louis: Mosby.

Werbach, M. (1986). *Third line medicine: Modern treatment for persistent symptoms.* Tarzana, CA: Third Line Press.

White, J., & Krippner, S. (Eds.). (1977). *Future science* (pp. 550–551. New York: Anchor Books.

Williams, R., et al. (1982). Type A behaviour and elevated physiological responses to cognitive tasks. *Science, 212,* 483–485.

Zahourek, R.P. (Ed.). *Relaxation and imagery: Tools for therapeutic communication and intervention.* Philadelphia: W.B. Saunders.

Zimmerman, J. (1990). Laying-on-of-hands healing and therapeutic touch: A testable theory. *Bemi Currents, Journal Bio-Electro-Magnetics Institute, 2,* 8, 17.

51

Qigong: A Paradigm Shift Tool for Pain Management

Linda C. Hole, M.D.

Each person carries his own doctor inside him. They come to us not knowing the truth. We are our best when we give the doctor who resides within each patient a chance to go to work.

Albert Schweitzer, M.D.

When you have a disease, do not try to cure it — Find your center, and you will be healed.

Chinese Proverb

INTRODUCTION: WHAT IS QIGONG?

Qigong is a 5000-year-old energy healing practice, an integral part of Chinese medicine, and is practiced by over 80 million people in China. For pain management practitioners in the New Millennium, Qigong is a paradigm shift tool that empowers both the patient and practitioner toward freedom from pain.

Clinical studies document that Qigong is remarkably effective in the treatment of pain, both acute and chronic. In the hands of a skilled practitioner, Qigong often gives dramatic, sometimes near miraculous results in pain relief, especially for those where all else has failed. Qigong not only empowers and frees the patient from pain, it is also simple to learn, practice, and apply, and is available to all.

Qigong is aligned with what Larry Dossey, M.D. heralds as New Era "non-local," "eternal" medicine vs. "internal" medicine (Dossey, 1999). Qigong takes mind–body medicine to the next step. Qi energy medicine is beyond mind, beyond body, beyond space, beyond matter, and transcends time. Qi healing may be long distance, spontaneous, and at times instantaneous.

Qi, pronounced "chee," is your breath, or your universal vital life force energy. Gong, pronounced "gung," is work, or practice.

As one of my Qi masters teaches, Qi is Greek for the letter *chi*, or the cross. Qigong is, thus, also the practice of standing centered between heaven and earth, and at the same time open to the universal "Christ force" healing energy, known in different cultures as *prana*, *shakti*, or *ki*. For some, Qi is simply the breath of God. Christ, of course, is the greatest Qigong master who ever lived.

Nearly every culture has some form of Qi energy healing practice. Modern day practices range from reiki, guided imagery, hypnotherapy, mindfulness stress reduction, reiki, and therapeutic touch, to shamanism and faith healing.

Qigong, however, is not a religion, is nondenominational, requires no particular set of beliefs, and again, is freely available to all. Qigong itself is simply the practice of gentle breathing, movement, stretching, and meditative exercises — exercises that open your body, mind, and spirit to the healing power and life-changing miracles of Qi.

Besides pain relief, Qigong strengthens your immune system, prevents aging and disease, relieves stress, reverses paralysis, increases energy, and promotes peak performance (Chow & McGee, 1994). Qigong practitioners routinely report profound healing and transformation on many levels: in health, relationships, personal and professional growth,

0-8493-0926-3/02/$0.00+$1.50
© 2002 by CRC Press LLC

sense of well-being, plus a life of more love, light, joy, peace, abundance, laughter, freedom, and self-acceptance, qualities that in themselves help relieve pain.

Qigong, furthermore, potentiates the effectiveness of Western medications, alleviates side effects, and allows reductions in dosages (Sancier, 1999).

"Hard" Qigong includes performance miracles such as Qigong masters who light fluorescent bulbs and fires, bend steel, break concrete slabs,and charge batteries with their bare hands. Some also can affect scientific instrument measurements, petri plate growth cultures, and kill laboratory cancer cells across a room (Eisenberg, 1987; Lee, 1999).

"Soft" Qigong superpower phenomena common to masters include medical X-ray vision, uncanny intuition, precognition, fingertip diagnosis, long-distance healing, and the ability to direct or emit Qi, with measurable physical results (Wen, 1998).

Medical Qi miracles include Qi-induced surgical anesthesia, spontaneous cancer remissions, reversal of paralysis, and Qi-induced changes in subjects' blood pressure, EEG, and blood levels of various neurotransmitters and hormones (Chow & McGee, 1994; Lee, 1999).

Wai Qi or "outer Qi," in the context of pain management, is when the practitioner brings about pain relief in the subject by emitting Qi. Qi may be emitted via your hand chakra *Lao Gong* points, fingertips, and via mind over matter intention or *Yi Nian*.

Nei Qi or "inner Qi" is healing by cultivating your own internal Qi via simple breath, movement, and meditation exercises.

The discipline of *Nei Qi* is necessary for the practice of *Wai Qi*.

A Qigong master is someone who has cultivated both *Wai Qi* (outer) and *Nei Qi* (inner), and demonstrated significant Qi healing ability. One of our goals in this chapter is to take the mystique out of Qi healing. The miracles of Qigong are freely available to all. Within each and every one of you is a Qigong master.

THE SCIENCE OF QI

Does Qi really work? Is Qi real? How does Qi work? Cloaked in secrecy for centuries, and outlawed during the Cultural Revolution, Qigong underwent rigorous scientific scrutiny with the post-Cultural Revolution resurgence of traditional Chinese medicine as one possible solution to China's overwhelming health demands. Although the quality of the research is admittedly uneven, the data still clearly document that Qigong is remarkably effective in pain relief, and is real.

DOES QI REALLY WORK?

A survey of clinical studies documents the effectiveness of Qigong, sometimes in combination with Chinese herbal

medicine and/or acupuncture, in both acute and chronic diseases for relieving pain in arthritis (He, 1989), rheumatoid (Chen) and osteoarthritis (Omura et al., 1989); cancer (Chen, G.; Wang, S.; Wang, Ying); chest pain (Kazhuda); diabetic peripheral neuropathy (Feng et al.); disc disease (Lim, 1993; Lin, 1988; Noda, 1993); dysmenorrhea (Huang, Cai, & Zhang, 1996); fibromyalgia (Singh, Berman, Hadhazy, & Creamer, 1998); knee pain (Nakagawa, 1988); low back pain (Lim, 1993); migraines (Pavek, 1988); neck pain (Liu, L., 1998); post-herpetic neuralgia (Omura, Losco, Omura, Takeshige, et al., 1992); trigeminal neuralgia (Tong, 1989); reflex sympathetic dystrophy (Wu, W., Bandilla, Ciccone, Yang, et al., 1999); shoulder pain (Shi, 1998; Wang, F., 1989), including frozen shoulder (Gao, Q., 1996); sciatica (He, 1989), soft tissue injuries such as sprains, strains (Enrico, K. & Enrico, D., 1993; Huang, R., 1989; Huang, X. & Cao, Q., 1993; Huang, Y., 1996); sports injuries (Cui, W., 1998); and pain secondary to surgical and/or traumatic scars (Ma, 1988), and pain secondary to vascular disease (Agish, 1998; Omura, 1990).

Studies also document the efficacy of Qigong in surgical anesthesia (Lin, H., 1988), and in pain relief of organic diseases such as cholelithiasis (Wang, D., et al., 1989) chronic atrophic gastritis (Qigong Science Research Group, 1988); coronary heart disease angina (Sun, Yuan, & Yang, 1988); gastritis (Wang, Y., 1989); irritable bowel (Pavek, 1988); gastric ulcer (Tong, 1989); and prostatitis (Tong, 1989). Omura and Sha report that Qigong is effective also in intractable pain (Omura, et al., 1992), and chronic pain syndromes (Sha, 1998). Quan notes that Qigong, used together with acupuncture, is significantly more effective than acupuncture alone, 94% vs. 55% for acupuncture alone for successful relief of pain (Quan, 1996).

Back and Disc Disease

Noda (1993) reports a 90% success rate in using a body manipulation Qigong approach to treat 2000 patients suffering herniated discs: 70% successful within one to two treatments, 15% with four to five treatments, and 5% requiring more than five treatments. For more than 600 patients suffering back pain, Lim (1993) reports a 98% success rate using Qi music tapes and Qi healing through the mind. Several of the patients avoided surgery. In a series of 292 patients treated with Qigong combined with Chinese and Western medicine, 274 for disc disease and 18 for chronic lumbrosacral pain, Liu (1988) reports a 97.7% success rate for cure and/or significant relief of symptoms.

Fibromyalgia

In 20 fibromyalgia patients who completed an 8-week mind–body protocol including weekly Qigong movement therapy sessions, Singh et al. (1998) report significant pain reduction.

Frozen Shoulder and Tennis Elbow

Gao (1996) reported an overall effective rate using Qigong treatment for relief of symptoms 81.2% in 32 patients suffering a 1-week to 2-year history of frozen shoulder and tennis elbow: 6 patients (18.8%) with the first treatment, 7 patients (21.9%) with 2 to 5 treatments, 13 patients (40.6%) within 6 to 15 treatments.

Migraines

Pavek (1988) reports that in more than 40 patients suffering migraines, successful treatment with the psycho-emotional Qi approach reduced frequency from biweekly to episode intervals of over a year or more.

Coronary Heart Disease Chest Pain

In China, Qigong also is used to treat the pain of organic disease. Sun, Yuan, and Yang (1988) report a 100% success rate in relieving angina pain in 51 patients with diagnosed coronary heart disease, with documented electrocardiogram improvements in 94.12%.

Arteriosclerotic Lower Extremity Pain

Agishi (1996; 1998) in 37 patients with documented arteriosclerotic obstruction of their lower extremities reports that 93.8% experienced improvement in subjective symptoms; 89.6% experienced an "instantaneous" rise in lower extremity temperature following Qi treatments as documented by thermography; 75.6% experienced improvement in pulse amplitude documented by plethysmography; and 88.9% experienced increased dorsalis pedis and tibialis posterior blood flow documented by ultrasound.

Surgical Qi

Inosuke (1993) defines Qigong anesthesia as "the patient loses his consciousness when the Qigong master emits his qi to him." Lin (1988) reports 91.8% success in Qigong surgical anesthesia in 34 cases for thyroid tumor and cyst resections. Johnson (1998) finds that using Qigong pre-, post-, and intra-operatively reduces bleeding, enhances immune function, minimizes infections, accelerates recovery, and reduces pain. Of note, Machi and Chu (1996) report the synchronization between the subject and Qi master in stimulated Qi anesthesia of alpha and beta brain waves, and heart rate.

Is Qi Real?

Subjects may experience Qi as sensations of heat, electric current, pressure, pulsing energy, involuntary movement, perspiration, tingling, relaxation of both body and mind, and pain relief; with simultaneous measurable changes in body temperature, skin temperature, blood pressure, heart rate, body secretions (Enrico, B., & Enrico, D., 1993; Lin, 1988; Nishimoto, 1996; Wu, 1989; Zhao et al., 1996), and over time, healthy weight loss (Wang, Y., 1995). Sancier (1994) reports in a pilot study of electrical conductivity of acupuncture meridians (EAV) that active Qi practice balances acupuncture meridians and internal organs.

Qi masters may experience in addition to the above a measurable increase in temperature of their Lao Gong hand points, an immediate increase in blood levels of ATP with the practice of Qigong exercises, and an immediate decrease in blood levels of ATP upon emitting Qi (Lee, 1999; Lin, H., 1988).

Emitted Qi from a Qigong master's hands has been documented in scientific laboratories to change the color of crystals, light fluorescent bulbs, increase the fluorescence of organisms by 68% (Lin, H., 1999), kill *in vitro* laboratory cancer cells, expose light-sensitive plates, and change magnetic fields (Lee, 1999).

Machi and Chi (1996) measured simultaneous physiologic changes in the subject and a Qi master emitting Qi to the subject. They report changes in electroencephalogram (EEG), electrocardiogram (EKG), galvanic skin resistance (GSR), and skin temperature, In both subject and Qi master, alpha waves increased, and beta decreased. Of note is that the heart rates became synchronized as well.

Non-local Qi, or Qi treatment at a distance, is possible by *Yi Nian* intention, or by inert materials, such as Qi-energized audiotapes, paper, metal, glass, stone, clothes, etc., into which a Qi master has emitted Qi. Omura (1990) reports that placing a (+) Qi stored material on an indicated

TABLE 51.1
Efficacy of Qigong in the Treatment of Pain
Survey World Scientific Literature

	Author	No.	% Reporting Improvement in Symptoms
Back pain	Lim (1993)	600	98
Disc disease	Noda (1993)	2000	90
Disc disease and back pain	Liu (1989)	292	97.7
Fibromyalgia	Singh (1998)	20	Significant
Frozen shoulder and tennis elbow	Gao (1996)	32	81.2
CHD chest pain	Sun (1988)	51	100
ASCVD lower extremity pain	Agishi (1996; 1998)	37	93.8

body area improves circulation, relaxes spastic muscles and vasoconstriction, reduces or eliminates pain, and enhances drug uptake. Lim (1993) and Nishimoto (1996) both use Qi-energized audiotapes in the treatment of pain, with positive results.

Prestigious scientific laboratories in China, such as the National Atomic Energy Lab in Shanghai and the Space Science and National Electro-Acoustics Institute in Beijing, demonstrate that the Qi energy the Qigong masters emit is measurable as infrared, magnetic, static electric, and acoustical energy. Seto (1994) measured the magnetic field between the hands of healers to be in the range of 1 milligaus. Niu, et al. (1988) measured infratonic sound waves emitted by a Qi master in the range of 45 to 76 decibels, or 100 to 1000 times stronger than that emitted by an ordinary person's (45 to 50 decibels). Via Kirilian photography, Lee (1999) exquisitely visually documents the effects of Qi.

The "How" of Qi

Zhang and other scientists document that emitted Qi raises potassium-medicated human skin pain threshold (Lin, 1988; Zhang, 1990). In a double-blind placebo-controlled study of 57 subjects. Lee and Wang (1993) demonstrate that infratonic Qi emitted by a Qigong Machine (QGM) significantly lowers the electrical activity of muscles, as measured by surface electromyelogram. Lin demonstrates increased immune activity with emitted Qi (Lin, H., 1988). Feng (1998) documents Qi-induced decreases in blood sugar levels in diabetics. Higuchi, et al. (1997) found that Qi meditation decreases blood levels of plasma cortisol, adrenalin, and dopamine, and changes levels of endorphins, suggesting that Qi meditation decreases sympathetic nervous system activity.

A number of studies document that Qigong increases blood circulation to the brain, to diseased or stressed tissue (Omura, Losco, et al., 1992), and to the nail folds of Qigong practitioners (Sancier, 1999). Liu reports that in 68 subjects Qigong exercises decrease blood levels of vasoconstrictor 5-hydroxy-tryptamine (5HT), and increases levels of norepinephrine and dopamine, with resulting vasodilation and increased blood flow. Increased blood flow both increases the delivery of oxygen, nutrients, and endorphins and the removal of metabolic waste products for pain relief (Lin, M., 1988).

Animal studies reveal that Qi is independent of placebo effect and provide more clues to the "how" of Qi. In rabbit experiments, emitted Qi induced a change in pulse, an increase in temperature (Lin, H., 1988), increases in osteogenesis osteoblast and osteoclast activity in bone injuries, increases in blood level of antibodies in infection, and changes in electroencephalogram (EEG) (Jia, Jia, & Lu, 1988; Lee, 1999). In guinea pigs, Ryu, et al. (1996) conclude that Qi somehow induces

enhanced release of acetylcholine in the relief of muscle pain, possibly by a somato-autonomic reflex from the anterior hypothalamus. In anesthetized cats, Liu demonstrates that emitted Qi still produces a change in ABER (Lee, 1999). Zhang, Chen, et al. (1990) also find that emitted Qi also depressed the cortical-evoked potential amplitudes elicited by c-fiber inputs as an index of response of the somatosensory cortex to pain in cats. In rats, Yang (1988a, 1988b) demonstrates that the analgesic effect of emitted Qi was inhibited by peri-aqueductal grey lesions (Yang, Xu, 1988; Yang, Guo, 1988). Both Zhang and Yang independently found inhibition of Qi analgesia by nalaxone, suggesting the involvement of endogenous opiates (Yang, Xu, et al., 1988; Yang, Guo, et al., 1988; Zhang, Chen, et al., 1990).

In a series of more than 20 subjects and with Qi masters Kong and Estes, we measured brain wave activity via interactive brain wave analysis (IBVA) induced by emitted Qi, and with Qigong exercises. We found that externally emitted Qi immediately decreases the subject's beta waves (12 to 30 Hz), which are associated with higher cognitive brain activity such as stress and/or concentration, and simultaneously increases alpha (8 to 12 Hz) and theta (4 to 8 Hz) waves. According to Dr. Kong, alpha waves are associated with a Qi healing state of mind, and theta waves indicate enhanced immune activity. An internal Qi state induced by the active practice of Qigong on the part of the subject gives like results (Hole, 1998a).

M. Liu (1988) in both controlled human and animal studies finds that emitted Qi enhances and synchronizes the subject's electroencephalogram (EEG) alpha rhythm. He also notes an increase in the EEG power spectrum with the most pronounced increase in the frontal lobe, inhibition of the cerebral cortex, excitation of the somatosensory cortex, and facilitation of the brainstem medulla and hypothalamus as measured by acoustic brainstem evoked response (ABER). Qi thus induces an alpha-state of deep relaxation, frontal lobe integration of autonomic function, and brainstem regulation of internal organs (Lee, 1999).

These studies clearly demonstrate that Qigong masters, without any voice, touch, or eye contact, can by Qi, induce changes in their subjects' brain wave activity for healing.

How does Qi work? Besides documented endocrine, immune, neurotransmitter, and circulatory changes, and deep relaxation, how does Qi work? The science of energy medicine is rapidly evolving. Gough (1999) suggests that nonlocal inputs, such as a healer's intention, has an impact on the DNA molecules themselves and on intercellular communication. Lee (1999) suggests that the DNA helix itself acts as a superconductor magnetic field detector and amplifier, and that this perhaps is how healers produce bioelectromagnetic energy.

How does Qi bring about healing? How does non-local external medicine work? How does prayer work? As with external medicine and prayer, the biophysics of exactly how Qi works is still somewhat of mystery.

SOME QI CLINICAL EXAMPLES

As with any Qigong practitioner, we see many miracles in our practice, especially with those who have found little or no relief elsewhere. A miracle, however, may be as ordinary as a smile or a teardrop.

Although Qi itself is still somewhat of a mystery, one of the goals of this chapter is to take the mystery out of the *practice* of Qi. Even with little or no previous experience, it is surprisingly possible to use Qigong to successfully relieve pain. While the discipline of daily Qi practice is mandatory for any serious practitioner, there are a number of easy-to-learn and apply Qi tools for pain relief. We present here some case studies and examples from our own experience in hopes of inspiring you to see for yourself that "Qi happens!"

SCANNING AND DIRECTING QI

Chronic back pain in an elderly man. Years ago, I brought my then-12-year-old son to his first introductory 2-hour Qigong workshop. He worked with an elderly gentleman suffering longstanding back pain. When I asked my son how the workshop was for him, to my astonishment he innocently replied, "Oh, you know that old man I worked with? Well, he was hot up top, nothing at the waist, then cold from the waist down … .. So I brushed him off up top, and packed him in at the waist. Then he was warm all over, and his back pain went away."

I have since attended and taught introductory Qigong workshops in which neophytes with no previous Qi training successfully treat those suffering chronic pain. The miracles of Qigong are available to you as well, for the asking.

QI BREATH

Headache in 49-year-old white male VA vet. I remember with fondness my first official Qigong patient. He was a steak-and-potatoes VA vet. He had suffered years of severe intermittent headaches, which had increased in severity and become constant over the last 5 weeks, to the point of waking him from sleep, and they were no longer relieved by narcotic pain medication.

I had just attended my first introductory 1-day Qigong workshop. I considered an MRI to rule out a brain mass, and decided in the meantime to teach him the simple mechanics of Qi breathing. Within minutes, he broke out in a grin, "What'd you do? My headache's gone!" That

was nearly 5 years ago. The headaches he first presented with are still gone.

Migraines in 47-year-old white male blue collar worker. He complained of a lifelong history of constant pressure with episodes of spiking pain, nausea, vomiting, lachcrimation, and aura, growing progressively worse over the past year to the point of being unable to work for the last 1 to 2 months. He had no relief with demerol, stadol, codeine, norgesic forte, morphine, and neurology consult. With Qi breathing, his pain level went from a 10 to a 2 within minutes.

TMJ pain in a 45-year-old white female artist. One of my Qigong exercise class students found relief from her longstanding TMJ, unrelieved by dental consult, in the simple mechanics of Qi breathing. Specifically, she remembered on the in breath to connect her meridians, or energy circuits, by holding her tongue to the roof of her mouth.

QI CENTERING

Cervical strain with radiculopathy in a 47-year-old singer status post-multiple injuries, including a motor vehicle accident (MVA) 3 years ago and a Labor and Industries claim as well. She complained of constant right upper extremity (RUE) pain and paresthesias, with no relief from medications or chiropractic treatment. With proper Qi posture and centering, she had her first night of sleep pain free.

QI EXERCISES AND MEDITATION

Radiculopathy in 49-year-old white female graphic artist with over a 7-year history C5–6 disc disease documented by MRI and neurology consult. She complained of several days of a "pinched nerve in my neck history," decreased mobility of right upper extremity (RUE), with paresthesias and pain radiating to RUE. With in-office Qi exercises and meditation, her mobility was restored and pain relieved within minutes.

Degenerative disc disease in a 30-year-old white female law professional. One of my Qigong students wrote, "For years I suffered constant chronic back pain from degenerative disc disease… With one Qigong class and a 2-minute treatment, I am pain free." That was over a year ago. Where she once was a regular visitor to her chiropractor and the emergency room, she learned to control and relieve her pain with Qigong exercises and breathing.

QI PAIN PICTURES

Arthritic toe pain in a 37-year-old white female ballroom dancer, documented by X-ray, unrelieved for years by NSAIDS and steroid injections. While working with her, images of a "steam roller truck" and a "dragon" came up, which she identified as her mother. By identifying the pain pictures, and moving the pictures of her toe, her pain was immediately relieved, and has not returned for months.

Qi Intention

Shoulder pain in Vietnam veteran with 20 years of no relief. My first experience of healing by intention was in a class with Prof. Tae Woo Yoo, O.M.D. Ph.D., internationally recognized as the founder of the Koryo Hand Therapy (KHT) acupuncture microsystem. Speaking no English, Professor Yoo drew the correct prescription on the chalk board, stroked the meridian *on the chalk board* in the correct direction, and the vet's pain was relieved. Professor Yoo then stroked the meridian on the chalk board in the opposite direction, and the vet's pain immediately returned. With the professor stroked the meridian on the chalk board once again in the correct direction, the veteran's pain was once again relieved.

Back pain in a middle-aged white female health professional. Once, after presenting at a medical headache symposium, a number of people lined up afterward for treatment. Short on time, I instructed a woman in line just to breath, and imagine or intend her pain away. Within minutes she thanked me, her pain gone.

Qi Nonlocal Healing

Frozen shoulder in 45-year-old Oriental female golfer with a 5-month history of progressive pain with little relief from orthopedic consult and physical therapy. Driving home from her appointment, she felt an incredible wave of energy freeing her shoulder from pain, and restoring her range of motion. Within days, she was discharged from orthopedic and physical therapy and went on to play tournament golf.

Qi Acupuncture

Cervical disc disease and Raynaud's syndrome in a disabled white female health professional. I "ran Qi" into her Koryo Hand Therapy correspondence neck area. Within minutes her pain was relieved, and for the first time in years, her hands were warm and pink. Months later, she thanked me because she'd been pain free since that one single treatment.

Sciatic pain for months in a renowned Native American female author. I applied fingertip Qi along her KHT bladder meridian. For the first time in months, she was pain free, and with the addition of a copper ring continued to be pain free for months afterward.

Eye pain in a 50-year-old Greek teacher. She complained of a 3-week history of eye pain with visual disturbance. Applying Qi to her KHT eye point, her pain was gone, and vision clear in minutes.

Qi, Intuition, and the Five Elements

Chest pain and pulmonary interstitial fibrosis with dyspnea in a 67-year-old retired white male. By KHT diagnosis, his element was metal. The element metal has to do with the emotions of grief, loss, regret, and giving too much of yourself away. In helping him intuitively recognize in himself the pain pictures of the element metal, he burst into tears, and both his chest pain and dyspnea were relieved within minutes.

Qi Love, Touch, and Hugs

Polymyalgic rheumatica and osteoarthritis in a 58-year-old white female chronic pain sufferer. With just a waiting room hug, her pain on three occasions was totally relieved.

THE WAY OF QI: SOME PRACTICAL PAIN RELIEF TOOLS FOR YOUR PRACTICE

There are hundreds of different Qigong schools, teachers, masters, and exercises. Following are some basic Qi tools and teachings that you can apply to your life and practice for immediate results.

Activating Your Qi

> Stressed is just desserts spelled backwards.
>
> **Unknown**

At the center of your palm is your hand-healing chakra Lao Gong point, or "old worker." It often appears as a contrasting lighter area at the center of your palm. In some paintings of saints, not only do the saints have halos, they also have golden beams of light, or Qi, coming out of their Lao Gong hand points.

To activate your Qi, rub your palms together back and forth at the Lao Gong points as if you're about to start a fire. What you feel between your hands is Qi. You may feel tingling, warmth, a magnetic force, or a palpable live ball of energy. The more you practice Qigong, the more open and clear you become, the bigger your healing ball of Qi grows, and the greater the miracles of Qi come through you.

Qi Centering: Standing Your Ground between Heaven and Earth

> Be still and know that I am
>
> **Psalms 46:10**

As in the Chinese character for emperor, or master, the Qi posture is standing centered and open, between heaven and earth, open to the heavens above and grounded to the earth below. Many people stand hunched over, carrying heavy burdens with the weight of the world on their shoulders and back. Correct Qi posture is vital for the flow and release of Qi.

For Qi posture, plant your feet on the ground about shoulder width apart; roll your shoulders down and back to both open your heart chakra, and to allow your burdens to roll off your back; stand open and grounded between heaven and earth, then imagine a *silver thread* aligning, supporting, and stretching your spine between heaven and earth. Drop your center of gravity to your *Dan Tian*, the seat of energy 2 in. below your navel.

At your *Hui Yin*, or by the tip of your tail bone, give yourself a *grounding cord* to the center of the earth. "Turn on" your grounding cord, and ask it to draw out, like a magnet, and absorb whatever no longer serves you, whatever is keeping you from being who you truly are, and whatever is stopping you from being free of pain.

Open your *Bai Hui,* or crown, to the heavens above. Imagine a divine waterfall of light, or Qi, washing away and freeing you from whatever no longer serves you, keeping you from being who you are and without pain. Feel the silver thread aligning, supporting, and stretching your spine between heaven and earth, and feel the waterfall of light flowing down your back, to wash away your burdens, your past, and your pain.

Qi Breath: Open Heart of Compassion, Soft Belly of Letting Go

One joy shatters a thousand griefs.

Chinese Proverb

The Qi breath is going back to breathing as a baby breaths—open heart, soft belly via the diaphragm, and relaxing into the breath of God. Note that the words "inspire" and "spirit" both come from the same root *spiritus*. Notice how many people breathe very shallowly. Nonpermission and repressed pain such as anger, grief, and fear are among the causes of shallow breathing. Besides obviously providing the body more oxygen, and greater release of toxins, the deep diaphragm breathing of Qigong also facilitates the release of the emotional and spiritual pain underlying physical pain.

The Qi breath is with the open heart of compassion and soft belly of letting go. First remember to stand centered between heaven and earth in correct Qi posture. On the in breath, allow your soft belly to expand out, so that your diaphragm can *fully* open your lungs for a full deep breath. Draw the breath in through your nostrils down to your *Dan Tian*, again the center of energy 2 in. below your umbilicus. On the in breath, remember to hold your tongue to the roof of your mouth to complete the meridian energy circuits. Chest and shoulders remain still throughout the breath cycle. On the out breath, relax your tongue and belly. With a gentle smile of self-love and self-acceptance, breathe out through your mouth.

Energetically, for beginners, it's simplest to visualize breathing in and out of your heart. On the in breath, breathe in Qi as light and love. On the out breath, breathe out whatever no longer serves you, whatever is keeping you from being who you fully are, whatever is keeping you from being fully alive, and free of pain. As you breathe, imagine the Qi expanding in a golden ball of light to fill your heart, then your body, then your spirit, and continue expanding to protect and surround you throughout the universe.

Qi Exercises: Awaken Your Body, Awaken Your Spirit

A day without dancing is a day lost.

Unknown

Of the hundreds of different Qigong movement and stretching exercises, my favorite is free-form Qi dancing, or moving as the Qi moves you. For medical Qigong, the basic Chow Qigong set, is superb (Chow & McGee, 1994). The purpose of Qi exercises is to awaken your body and spirit; and to clear, open, and bring into harmony your energy channels for greater Qi, greater energy, greater awareness, greater healing, and greater healing ability.

A very effective and simple beginning Qi exercise is "shaking" Qigong, as the Quakers used to do. In Qi posture with the silver thread aligning and stretching your spine heaven to earth, grounding cord rooted to the center of earth, and crown open to the heavens, simply shake your body from head to toe, vertebrate by vertebrate. With a gentle smile of self-love, shake out all your worries, troubles, pain, and tension, … and feel yourself becoming lighter.

Qi Meditation and Awareness

99% is awareness, the rest is gratitude, amusement, and letting go.

Jim Self, Qi Master

Qi meditation centers on the breath; it quiets and stills the mind, body, and spirit; it is key to Qi healing and encompasses many of the same principles taught in Western schools of mindfulness stress reduction, visualization, focusing, hypnosis, transcendental meditation, and centering prayer. As in centering prayer, Qigong calls upon a greater energy, or universal Qi, for healing. The Qi exercises themselves prepare the body for the healing of Qi meditation.

With Qigong practice and meditation comes increased awareness, and the Qi meltdown effect. The walls burying unconscious pain melt, and you eventually become aware of the wound to the psyche beneath the physical pain. With the release of the underlying pain picture, the physical pain is no longer necessary, and may clear as well.

In Qigong, bad, stagnant, or blocked Qi is the root cause of pain and *dis*-ease. One way of dispelling bad Qi is to simply replace it with good Qi. On the in breath, send a golden ball of Qi, of love and light, from your heart to any painful area, and breathe in good Qi. On the out breath, breathe out the bad, stagnant, or blocked Qi, and breathe out the pain. To prevent the bad Qi from reentering, always remember to fill the space where the pain and bad Qi used to be with good Qi.

Self-love, self-acceptance, self-forgiveness, and self-worth are core to Qi meditation and Qi healing. True self-love frees you to release pain, and to love, accept, forgive first yourself and then others. With each breath, give yourself a gentle smile of self-love and self-acceptance.

Other benefits of Qi meditation include learning how to stay centered amidst the chaos and stress of day to day living; the freedom to be who you truly are; inner peace, inner knowing, harmony with oneself and the universe; and the ability to move from your center with clarity and power — all of which help dispel pain.

The MicroCosmic Cycle and the Five Element meditations below are specific and fundamental to Qigong, and are both effective in pain relief.

QI AND THE MICROCOSMIC CYCLE

Pain is removed when the block is eliminated.

Traditional Chinese Medicine Principle

When practicing Qigong, visualize your Qi circulating in a MicroCosmic Cycle. On the in breath, visualize the Qi as light flowing from your *Dan Tian*, the seat of energy 2 in. below your umbilicus, down to your *Hui Yin*, or perineum, then up the Governing vessel energy channel along your spine, through the Three Gates, and up to your crown or *Bai Hui*. On the out breath, visualize the Qi flowing down the front of your body along the Conception vessel back to your *Dan Tian*.

The pelvic Lower Gate relates to fear, survival, sexuality, will power, and pelvic organs. The abdominal Middle Gate relates to power, control, resistance, judgment, empowerment, and abdominal organs. The thoracic Upper Gate relates to heart sadness and joy, speaking your truth, surrender to divine will, and thoracic organs. The *Bai Hui* or crown is your divine knowing and connection to the heavens.

As the Qi flows through the Three Gates, visualize the release of bad, stagnant, and blocked Qi, and see "good" Qi clearing, cleansing, healing, and filling all your energy channels, gates, chakras, and centers with light.

QI AND THE FIVE ELEMENTS: FREE YOUR BODY, FREE YOUR SPIRIT

The root of all disease is spiritual … in the mind and the emotions.

Tae Woo Yoo, O.M.D., Ph.D.

Patients often present with a purely somatic pain complaint, in stubborn denial of any possible underlying wound to the psyche. The physical pain points to a deeper psychospiritual pain, and is a call for help.

The body is about the five senses. The spirit is about the Five Elements: Fire, Earth, Metal, Water, and Wood. Each of the five elements governs a coupled yin–yang organ pair, each with a specific energy channel meridian map on the body. Each of the five elements also is associated with a specific set of emotions, and a whole set of other characteristics specific to the particular element as well—color, taste, season, etc. (see Table 53.1 in Chapter 53). The Five-Element location of the physical pain, the Five-Element color your patient chooses to wear, etc. all give you clues to the wound to the psyche underlying the physical pain.

The Five Element meditation helps release any pain associated with each particular element. Working with the Five Elements helps free the spirit to free the body, and is one of the most powerful, gentle, and effective tools in Qi healing.

QI, EGO, INTUITION, AND PAIN PICTURES: PHYSICIAN HEAL THYSELF

E.G.O. stands for "Easing God Out"

Unknown

The practice of Qigong brings increased awareness and intuition. Qigong masters commonly have "X-ray" medical intuitive vision, and in a moment know far more about the nuances of your life than an ordinary person could possibly know.

To clear the way for Qi, for your own inner knowing, or intuition, Qigong requires that you surrender all ego, both the big ego of arrogance and conceit, and the small ego of fear, unworthiness, and inadequacy. One also must surrender the judgment of ego: all negative thoughts, feelings, limiting beliefs, and pictures. Surrendering ego, judgment, fear, and negativity frees you to be an empty vessel for greater Qi and knowing.

Another way of opening to your intuition is simply asking. For example, ask what the pain means. We commonly say that something or someone is a "headache" or "pain in the neck." Ask who or what is the pain underlying the head ache or neck ache. Ask what the pain in the body represents. For example, back pain may be about getting someone or something "off my back." A pain in the hip may be about fear of stepping forward. Pay attention also to the clues of the Five Elements. The Five Element location of your pain, the Five Element color you choose to wear, all point to the deeper Five Element wound to the psyche beneath the presenting physical pain.

As in guided imagery, we also call upon the inner knowing of the patients. Ask your patients who or what their physical pain is about. They may reveal a sometimes surprising self-realization and/or underlying "pain picture."

As you yourself become more intuitive and start "seeing" pain pictures in others, know that on some level every patient is a mirror for you. For every pain picture you recognize in someone else, you have within you a matching picture for your own pain. This is especially true for those to whom you feel a strong reaction. Know that every patient is a teacher, a mirror, a messenger, and a reminder of your own pain pictures asking for healing.

As Confucius taught, first you take care of yourself, then your neighbor, then your community, then the world. "Physician heal thyself" must come first. The freer and clearer you are of bad, stagnant, blocked Qi, and of your own pain pictures, the freer, clearer, and greater a vessel you become for Qi and healing.

Qi Dx, Rx, and Acupuncture: Scanning and Directing Qi

The Way that can be spoken is not the Way.

Lao Tze

For a more mechanical approach to Qigong relief of pain, "scanning" and "directing" Qi, and Qi acupuncture are easy to learn and apply, effective, and fun.

Scanning Qi. To scan or "diagnose" a patient's Qi, simply run your hands about 6 to 12 in. over the patient's body, and feel their energy field. Areas that seem hot and push your hands out have excess Qi. Areas that seem cold and pull in your hands have deficient Qi. Excess and deficient Qi are signs of pain, illness, or injury. As you scan, allow yourself to intuitively "see" pictures and "feel" emotions that have to do with the patient.

Directing Qi. For treatment, "brush away" the excess Qi, again the areas that feel hot, and/or push your hands out. "Pack in" with good Qi the deficient areas, again those which feel cold, empty, or pull your hands in. Simply brushing away and packing in Qi as indicated often give significant pain relief. The patient also may feel other sensations with the movement of Qi, such as warmth and tingling.

Qi Acupuncture. In our own practice, transmitting Qi via fingertips, or Wai Qi, to indicated acupuncture points and meridians for needleless Qi acupuncture can profoundly enhance treatment.

Qi, Love, Laughter, Hugs, Touch, Gratitude, Reframing, and the Inner Smile

Love is the most important ingredient in healing.

Effie Poy Yew Chow, Ph.D.

Qigong is an attitude. In Qigong, we reframe the challenges of life's day-by-day stresses and crises as opportunities to grow. The Chinese word for crisis translates as either "danger" or as "opportunity." In Qigong, we intentionally choose to reframe the challenges of life in a positive light, look for blessings in disguise, and simply give thanks.

"Negative thoughts can negate all healing" is a corollary Qigong teaching. One key in Qigong healing is moving from the Western left-brain problem-oriented approach of analyzing what's wrong to a more heart-centered approach of remembering, acknowledging, and giving thanks for the good. Rather than dwelling on and thereby reinforcing the negative, Qigong reframes life, and instead focuses attention and gives energy to the positive, thereby making way for healing and blessings to come.

On this level, Qigong is about looking for and affirming the good, giving thanks for the good, and cultivating right thoughts and a positive mental attitude (PMA). Right PMA thoughts do not imply any judgment or condemnation. Right PMA thoughts are those that make your heart sing, give you something to live for, raise your Qi, help move your immune system toward healing, and melt away pain. In Qigong, an attitude of gratitude clears the way for healing and dispelling pain.

For parents, these concepts are obvious. Focusing on a child's negative attention-seeking behavior reinforces the behavior. Giving the child unconditional love, positive attention, and gratitude, within limits of heaven and earth, obviates the child's need for negative attention-seeking behavior, and plants the seed for the positive and good.

Pain is thus your body's negative attention-seeking behavior cry for help. Your symptoms are your friends. Instead of reacting in denial, fear, and/or resistance, what about thanking your body for asking for help, and asking your body what is it telling you? In Qigong, remember to give yourself an inner smile of self-love for you, for your pain, for your body, for your spirit. Unconditional love, and self-love, are vital in Qigong for healing and releasing pain.

Psychoneuroimmunology documents well the mind–body connection, and how your thoughts and emotions affect your immune system. Other important Qigong PMA tools include laughter, hugs, touch, clear intention, letting go, and joy. As taught by Qi Master Effie Chow, Ph.D., we demonstrate via kinesiology and teach our patients the power of these PMA tools for their own self-healing and empowerment.

EMPTY VESSEL, BE STILL, BE PRESENT, AND INTENTION

> Your body is the vessel of your spirit—Honor It

For greater Qi healing, one must become a clear *Empty Vessel* through which greater love, light, Qi, and healing can flow.

One must Be Still, Be Present, and Be in his/her body. Healing does not occur in the past or in the future. Healing usually does not occur out of body. Qi healing occurs in the stillness of the present moment. One must let go of both the past and future, and be truly present in body in the still moment of now. Qi healing also requires that you honor your body with proper nourishment, rest, exercise, etc.

One must hold a *clear intention*, or "Yi Nian," of what he/she would like to create, whether it be wholeness, wellness, happiness, healing… or moving mountains. Hold your intention *lightly* and innocently, without ego or attachments. And lightly, with Qi, expect miracles.

True Qigong masters come from such a grounded empty vessel space of centeredness, clarity, and surrender that the intention of their thoughts shapes reality. They simply command the universe and heal.

LIVING A LIFE FULL OF QI

> Start the day with Love. Fill the day with Love. End the day with Love.
>
> **Sai Baba**

For committed Qigong students, Qigong is far more than simply a set of exercises. Qigong, at its highest, is a Way of Life.

The Way you think, the Way you relate to your loved ones, the Way you relate to your community, the Way you relate to the world, the Way you handle your emotions, the Way you care for your body, the Way you earn a living, the Way you stand in the universe, the Way you commune with nature, the Way you commune with God, the Way you Love — all determine your peace of mind, your state of health, pain, and Qi. The choices you make about the *Way* you live determine *how* you live, *how* you age, *how* you love, and *how* healthy, happy, pain free, and well you are.

In the context of pain management and Qi, pain is a wake-up call to take an inventory of your life. For health,

longevity, well-being, and a life free of pain and full of Qi, one must practice right living: right thoughts, relationships, love, livelihood, nutrition, exercise, practice, service, communion, etc.

The paradox, however, is that right living is about *being* rather than *doing*. The Qi practice of Right Living, or *doing Qi*, comes from the Qi practice of *being in Qi: being* centered, *being* still, *being* present, *being* true to your inner knowing, and *being* true to who you really are. Doing Qi without being in Qi is empty Qi. First be, then do.

INTEGRATING QIGONG INTO WESTERN MEDICINE: LOCAL VS. NONLOCAL MEDICINE

> White man get headache, take aspirin, get stomach ache.
>
> **Unknown Medicine Man**

Qigong is a paradigm shift tool for new era medicine. The traditional Western local medicine model is problem focused, problem solving, deductive, and defined by time and space. The Qigong nonlocal eternal medicine model is focused on remembering the good, giving thanks for the good, raising the Qi, inductive, and beyond time and space. Local medicine is organ centered, with some outside intervention as the cure. Qigong eternal medicine is Qi centered, and about one's relationship with oneself and the Universe.

In the Western local medicine, the power to heal is outside the individual. In the Qigong nonlocal eternal medicine model, we honor the individual's own inner knowing and power to heal. In local medicine, the cup is half empty. In Qigong eternal medicine, the cup is half full. Local medicine gives attention and energy to time and space limited problems. Qigong eternal medicine focuses attention and energy on the beyond time and space positive.

In Qigong, we simply "raise Qi," so that the problems simply melt away, and make room for the miracles to unfold.

There are many ways of integrating Qigong into your life, from the practice of simply remembering the breath to truly living a life full of Qi. The Qigong masters I most admire are full of light, love, joy, and amusement, and at the same time, are extraordinarily powerful healers. Teachers are valuable, and "When the student is ready, the master appears." Ultimately, however, Qigong is about you yourself connecting to your own "Be still and know that I am" healer within and universal Qi.

What more is there to say? Qigong changes lives and has made a tremendous difference in my life and in my practice of medicine. We humbly share these simple yet profound tools with you.

What words are there to express the look on a patient's face when, with a tool as simple as the breath, pain is relieved? What words are there to express how Qigong can transform your life, your practice, and the lives of your patients as well?

We invite you to take a minute to be still, go within, and see for yourself.

ACKNOWLEDGMENTS

Thanks to Effie Chow, Ph.D., Roger Estes; Richard Lee, P.E.; Charles McGee, M.D.; Ken Sancier, Ph.D.; Ron Roth; Jim Self; my children, Ben Fredrick, Tara, and Christopher; parents; family; staff; patients; teachers; and loved ones, Baba, Chuck, Ibriham, and Sidi.

REFERENCE

Agishi, T. (1996). Evaluation of therapeutic external Qigong from a viewpoint of western medicine, *Journal International Society of Information Sciences 14*, (1)102–103.

Agishi, T. (1998). The Modern treatment strategy for arteriosclerotic obstruction. *Artificial Organs 22*, 707–710.

Aoki, T., & Aoki, W. (1997). *Journal International Society of Information Sciences 15*, 235–246.

*Ballentine, R. (1999). *Radical healing*, New York: Harmony Books.

*Beinfield, H., & Korngold, E. (1991). *Between heaven & earth, a guide to Chinese medicine*, New York: Ballantine Books.

Chang, C. (1988). *Study of strength feat concerning human self-curative power*. First World Conference for Academic Exchange of Medical Qigong, 75.

Chen, G. (1988). *The curative effect observed for 24 (cancer) cases under my emitted Qigong treatment*. Second International Conference on Qigong, 141.

Chen, J. (1998a). *Benign tumours treated by Qigong digital pressure*. Fourth World Conference for Academic Exchange of Medical Qigong, *151*, 8–22.

Chen, J. (1998b). *Rheumatoid arthritis treated by emitted qi*. Fourth World Conference for Academic Exchange of Medical Qigong, 124.

Chen, K. (1998). *Cholelithiasis treated by Qigong*. Fourth World Conference for Academic Exchange of Medical Qigong, 158–159.

Chow, E. (1998a). *Chow Qigong: An antidote for modern day stress*. Second World Congress on Qigong, 37.

Chow, E. (1998b). *The miracles of medical Qigong: Directed energy for healing of self and others*. Second World Congress on Qigong, 37.

*Chow, E., & McGee, C. (1994). *Qigong miracle healing from China*, Coeur D'Alene: Medipress.

Chu, W. (1992). *Effect of emitted qi on the electric activities of the parafascicular nucleus pain sensitive neurocyte of big mice*. Fourth International Symposium on Qigong, 35.

*Cohen, K. (1997). *The way of Qigong*, New York: Random House.

Cui, W. (1998). *Reduction of closed fracture with Qigong, integrated Chinese and Western theory*. Fourth World Conference for Academic Exchange of Medical Qigong, 139–140.

Cui, X. (1998). *Qigong's medical effect on the injured athletes during sports games*. Fourth World Conference for Academic Exchange of Medical Qigong, 139–140.

Dockstader, S.B., & Barrett, S.B. (1998). *Stress management through an integrative program of Qigong and psychoneuroimmunology*, Second World Congress on Qigong, 36.

*Dossey, L. (1997). *Reinventing medicine: Beyond mind body to a new era of healing*. New York: Harper Collins.

*Eisenberg, D. (1988). *Encounters with Qi*. New York: W.W. Norton,

Enrico, B.K., & Enrico, D.R. (1993). *Chronic soft tissue injury response to Qigong therapy*. Second World Conference for Academic Exchange of Medical Qigong, 146.

Evans, F.J. (1999). The specific applications of hypnosis in pain management. *Journal International Society of Information Sciences 17*, 273–282.

Feng, L., et al. (1996). *Observations of effect of gallstone elimination by means of qigong therapy*. Third World Conference for Academic Exchange of Medical Qigong, 150.

Feng, L., et al. (1998). *Clinical observation of Qigong on treatment of diabetes mellitus*. Fourth World Conference for Academic Exchange of Medical Qigong, 129–130.

Ferraro, D. (1998). *Medical Qigong teaching experience in Italy and France*. Fourth World Conference for Academic Exchange of Medical Qigong, 209–211.

Fu, Q. (1998). *Digital acupuncture*. Fourth World Conference for Academic Exchange of Medical Qigong, 216–217.

Fukuzaki, K. *Some experiences about Qigong therapy*. Third World Conference for Academic Exchange of Medical Qigong, 165.

Gao, Q. (1996). Qigong's curative effect on frozen shoulder and tennis elbow. Third World Conference for Academic Exchange of Medical Qigong, 144.

Gao, Z., Zhang, S., and Bi, Y. (1990). *Effect of emitted qi acting on zusanli point of rabbits on myoelectric signals of Oddi's sphincter*. Third Nationl Academic Conference on Qigong Science, 52.

Garcia, G. (1998). *The microcosmic orbit or small heavenly cycle in the luohan gong*. Fourth World Conference for Academic Exchange of Medical Qigong, 237–239.

Gauthier-Hernberg, G. (1996). *Doctors must be teachers-not repairmen*. Third World Conference for Academic Exchange of Medical Qigong, 169.

*Gerber, R. (1996). *Vibrational medicine, new choices for healing ourselves*, Santa Fe. NM: Bear & Co.

Gough W.C. (1999). The cellular communication p process and alternative modes of healing, *Subtle Energy Medicine 8*(2), 67–101,

He, J. (1989). *Qigong acupuncture therapy*. Second International Conference on Qigong, 196.

Higuchi, Y., et al. (1997). Endocrine and immune response during guolin new Qigong, *Journal of International Society, Life, and Information Science 15*(1), 138,

Hole, L.C. (1998a). *Chow Qigong, KHT, and God for pain relief.* Second World Congress on Qigong, 41.

Hole, L.C, (1998b). *IBVA a powerful qi assessment tool.* Second World Congress on Qigong, 41.

Huang, C. (1998). *Effective energy accumulation in the human body.* Fourth World Conference for Academic Exchange of Medical Qigong, 191–192.

Huang, H. (1990). *Clinical applications of Chinese Qigong therapy and its mechanism.* First Interntional Congress of Qigong, 100.

Huang, M. (1988). *Effect of the emitted qi combined with self practice of Qigong in treating paralysis.* Beijing, China: First Conference for Academic Exchange of Medical Qigong.

Huang, R. (1989). *Relationship between jinyuan Qigong physiomedicine.* Second International Conference on Qigong, 272.

Huang, X., & Cao, Q. (1993). *Qigong's curative effect on lumbago and joint pain.* Second World Conference for Academic Exchange of Medical Qigong, 137.

Huang, X., Cai, Q., & Zhang, Shiyin. (1996). *Gynepathic diseases treated by Qigong.* Third World Conference for Academic Exchange of Medical Qigong, 153.

Huang, Y. (1996). *Clinical observation of 50 cases of ankle joint sprain treated by Qigong.* Third World Conference for Academic Exchange of Medical Qigong, 151.

Inosuke, Y. (1993). *Fundamentals of Qigong anesthesia and examples.* Second World Conference for Academic Exchange of Medical Qigong, 117.

Inosuke, Y. (1996). *Effectiveness of Qigong therapy.* Third World Conference for Academic Exchange of Medical Qigong, 163.

Jia, L., Jia, J., & Lu, D. (1988). *Effects of emitted qi on ultrastructural changes of the overstrained muscle of rabbits.* First World Conference for Academic Exchange of Medical Qigong, 14.

Johnson, J.A. (1998). *Medical Qigong therapy and surgery.* Fourth World Conference for Academic Exchange of Medical Qigong, 163–164.

*Kabat-Zinn, J. (1994). *Wherever you go, there you are, mindfulness meditation in everyday life.* New York: Hyperion.

*Kaptchuk, T. (1983). *The web that has no weaver,* Chicago: Congen & Weed.

Kazhuda, M. (1988). *An idea of inner diagnostic method.* First World Conference for Academic Exchange of Medical Qigong, 147.

Kono, T., Hoshino, M., & Yamabe, Y. (1988). *Analysis of qi by KinShindan-ho (muscular diagnosing therapy) and manipulative treatment.* First World Conference for Academic Exchange of Medical Qigong, 142.

*Kushi, M. (1980). *How to see your health: Book of oriental diagnosis,* New York: Japan Publications.

Lee, E.F. (1988). *Treatment effect and tentative working theories of autonomous Qigong exercise.* First World Conference for Academic Exchange of Medical Qigong, 74.

*Lee, P.E., & Richard, H. (1997). *Bioelectric vitality: Exploring the science of human energy,* San Clemente, CA: China Healthways Institute, 50-(71).

Lee, P.E., & Richard, H. (1999). *Scientific investigation into Chinese qi-gong.* San Clemente, CA: China Healthways Institute.

Lee, R.H. (1996). *Emitted qi and the freuency of consciousness,* Third World Conference for Academic Exchange of Medical Qigong, 120.

Lee, R.H., & Fu, Y. (1996). *Demonstrating the existence of qi to western doctors.* Third World Conference for Academic Exchange of Medical Qigong, 117.

Lee, R.H., & Wang, X. (1993). *Use of surface electromyogram to examine the effects of the infratonic QGM on electrical activity of muscles, a double blind, placebo-controlled study.* Second World Conference for Academic Exchange of Medical Qigong, 87.

Li, J. (1993). *Bioholographic Qigong digital pressure therapy in the treatment of acute cases.* Second World Conference for Academic Exchange of Medical Qigong, 139.

Lim, J. (1993). *Healing with qi magnetic tape -- a new development in Qigong healing.* Second World Conference for Academic Exchange of Medical Qigong, 143.

Lin, H. (1988). *Clinical and laboratory study of the effect of Qigong anaesthesia on thyroidectomy.* First World Conference for Academic Exchange of Medical Qigong, 84.

Lin, M. (1988). *Observation on skin thermography during Qigong needling.* First World Conference for Academic Exchange of Medical Qigong, 147.

Liu, B., Jiao, K., Chen, Q., Li, Y., & Shang, L. (1988). *Effect of Qigong exercise on the content of monoamine neur0-transmitters in blood.* First World Conference for Academic Exchange of Medical Qigong, 67.

*Liu, H. (1997). *Mastering miracles: The healing art of Qigong,* New York: Warner Press.

Liu, L. (1998). *Clinical research in treating spine-related diseases with Qigong combined with Chinese and Western medicine.* Fourth World Conference for Academic Exchange of Medical Qigong, 131–133.

Liu, S. (1998). *Treatment and clinical research of hypertension.* Fourth World Conference for Academic Exchange of Medical Qigong, 161–162.

Liu, X. (1989). *Treatment of 19 cases of cerebral thrombosis by Qigong therapy of insertion points and whole leading.* Second International Conference on Qigong, 179.

Liu, Y., He, S., & Xie, S. (1993). *Clinical observation of the treatment of 158 cased of cerebral arteriosclerosis by Qigong.* Beijing, China: Second Conference for Academic Exchange of Medical Qigong,

Lu, L., Liu, Y., & Zhuang, Y. (1996). *The clinical study of coronary heart disease treated by Qigong with music.* Third World Conference for Academic Exchange of Medical Qigong, 135.

Ma, D. (1988). *Oral facial scar softened by Qigong therapy.* First World Conference for Academic Exchange of Medical Qigong, 108.

Machi, Y., & Chu, W.Z. (1996). Physiological measurement for Qigong anesthesia, *J Int Soc Life Inf Sci 14*(2):129–145.

Machi, Y., & Yamamoto, M. (1996). *A physiological measuring method of exercise effect for Qigong.* Third World Conference for Academic Exchange of Medical Qigong, 117.

Machi, Y., & Yamamoto, M. (1996). *Students of Qigong want to know.* Sixth International Symposium on Qigong, 89–95.

Mayer, M. (1996–1997). *Journal of Traditional Eastern Health & Fitness 6,* 20–31.

Moon, B.L. (1998). *Chow Qigong & physiotherapy at an american hospital.* Second World Congress on Qigong, 45.

Mori, K., Chai, J.Y., & Endo, T. (1998). *Interdisciplinary approach to Qigong scientific study on principle of healing by Qigong.* Second World Congress on Qigong, 46.

Mori, K., Ikemi, Y., & Chai, J. (1993). *A scientific study of the principle of healing by Qigong.* Second World Conference for Academic Exchange of Medical Qigong, 71.

*Moyers, B. (1993). *Healing & the mind.* New York: Doubleday.

Nagura, O., & Sakai, K. (1996). *A study on the scientification of Qigong for the purpose of establishing a preventive medical science.* Third World Conference for Academic Exchange of Medical Qigong, 161.

Nakagawa, S. (1988). *Treatment method towards functional disease of the knee joint.* First World Conference for Academic Exchange of Medical Qigong. 146.

Nishimoto, S. (1996). *Report on the changing of the autonomic nervous system reducing pain of patients treated by external qi with alpha wave 1/F music.* Third World Conference for Academic Exchange of Medical Qigong, 147.

Niu, X., et al. (1988). *Measurement and analysis of infrasonic waves from emitted Qi.* First World Conference for Academic Exchange of Medical Qigong, Beijing.

Noda, K. (1993). *Study of the treatment of slipped disk.* Second World Conference for Academic Exchange of Medical Qigong, 145.

Omura, Y. (1990). Effects of external Qigong on inanimate substances, *Acupuncture and Electrotherapeutics Research, International Journal 15,* 137–157.

Omura, Y., Lin, T.L., Debreceni, L., Losco, B.M., Freed, S., Muteki, T., & Lin, C.H. (1989). Changes taking place in both Qigong masters and their patients during Qigong treatment. *Acupuncture and Electrotherapeutics Research, International Journal 14,* 61–89.

Omura, Y., Losco, B.M., Omura, A.K., Takeshige, C., et al. (1992). Common factors contributing t intractable pain and medical problems ... (+) Qigong energy stored material, *Acupuncture and Electrotherapeutics Research, International Journal 17,* 107–48.

Pavek, R.R. (1988). *Effects of Qigong on psychosomatic and other emotionally rooted disorders.* First World Conference for Academic Exchange of Medical Qigong, 150.

Qigong Science Research Group. (1988). *Observations of the curative effect in cases of chronic atrophic gastritis treated with daoying (inducing) or tuina (releasing) therapy.* First World Conference for Academic Exchange of Medical Qigong, 103.

Quan, F. (1996). *Observations of effect of Qigong and acupuncture in treatment of lumbar sprain.* Third World Conference for Academic Exchange of Medical Qigong, 152.

Ryu, H., Lee, H., Shin, Y., Chung, S., Lee, M., Kim, H., & Chung, H. (1996). Pain relief, application of a static magnetic field or external qigong. *Acupuncture and Electrotherapeutics Research, International Journal 24,* 119.

Sancier, K.M. (1999). Therapeutic benefits of Qigong exercises in combination with drugs, *International Society for Lifevand Information Science 5*(4), 383–389.

Sancier, K.M. (1994). The effect of Qigong on therapeutic balancing measured by Electroacupuncture According to Voll (EAV): A preliminary study. *Acupuncture and Electrotherapeutics Research, International Journal, 9* (2/3):119–127.

Seto, A., et al. (1992). Detection of extraordinarily large biomagnetic field strength from the human hand. *Acupuncture & Electrotherapeutics Research Journal 17,* 75–94.

*Sha, Z.G. (1997). *Zhi neng medicine.* Vancouver, BC: Zhi Neng Press.

Sha, Z.G. (1998). *Chronic pain solutions at the physical, emotional, mental and spiritual levels.* Second World Congress on Qigong, 48.

Shi, Y. (1998). Research on scapulohumeral periarthritis treated by Qigong. Fourth World Conference for Academic Exchange of Medical Qigong, 136–137.

Singh, B., Berman, B., Hadhazy, V., & Creamer, P. (1998). A pilot study of cognitive behavioral therapy in fibromyalgia, *Alternative Therapies and Health Medicine 24*(2) 67–70.

Sulikowski, R. *Qigong increases productivity.* Third World Conference for Academic Exchange of Medical Qigong, 168.

Sun, J., Yuan, R., & Yang, C. (1988). *Analysis of 51 cases with coronary heart disease treated by Qigong.* First World Conference for Academic Exchange of Medical Qigong, 135.

Suzuki, M., Kamiya, N., Kojima, K., & Kojima, K. (1997). The effectiveness of treatment of the painful shoulder, *Japanese Mind-Body Science 6,* 67

Takeshige, C., & Sato, M. (1996). Pain relief mechanisms. *Acupuncture and Electrotherapeutics Research Journal 24,* 119–131.

Tian, Y. (1998). *Prevention and cure diseases of the cardiovascular and cerebrovascular system.* Fourth World Conference for Academic Exchange of Medical Qigong, 159–161.

Tong, P. (1989). *Acupuncture of mixture unity of energy stream.* Second International Conference on Qigong, 138.

Wang, D., Zhao, J., Chen, K., Ma, K., Zhou, G., Lu, J., Mao, Z., & Shong, J. (1989). *The analysis of treatment of gallstone by emitted qi.* Second International Conference on Qigong, 121.

Wang, F. (1989). *Reports of treatments of shoulder inflammation by Qigong tapping of insertion points and artificial bleeding methods.* Second International Conference on Qigong, 153.

Wang, J., Li, D., & Zhao, J. (1989). *Experimental research on compound analgesia by Qigong information treating instrument and acupuncture.* Second International Conference on Qigong, 135.

Wang, S., Wang, B., Shao, M., & Li, Z. (1993). *Clinical study of the routine treatment of cancer coordinated by Qigong.* Second World Conference for Academic Exchange of Medical Qigong, 129.

Wang, Y. (1989). *Treatment of gastritis with Qigong and xinxi water. Analysis of 33 cases.* Second International Conference on Qigong, 145.

Wang, Y. (1993). *Clinical observation on 30 cases of cancer treated by Qigong therapy.* Second World Conference for Academic Exchange of Medical Qigong, 131. 93.

Wang, Y. (1995). *Miraculous Qigong for slimming down.* Fourth International Conference on Qigong, 30–31.

Wen, R. (1998). *Lumbar problems treated by Qigong.* Fourth World Conference for Academic Exchange of Medical Qigong, 16.

Wu, H. (1989). *Chinese super power meditation — The experiment, healing effort, and theory of a new technique for training "qi-energy."* Second International Conference on Qigong, 267.

Wu, T., & Wu, J. (1998a). *Increase the immune system naturally.* Second World Congress on Qigong, 51.

Wu, T., & Wu, J. (1998b). *Qigong - Oriental medicine without medication.* Second World Congress on Qigong, 52.

Wu, W., Bandilla, E., Ciccone, D., Wu, Y., & Shen, R. (1998). *Qigong and late-stage teflex sympathetic dystrophy (RSD).* Second World Congress on Qigong, 52.

Wu, W., Bandilla, E., Ciccone, D., Yang, J., et al. (1999). The effects of Qigong treatment on patients with treatment resistant RSD. *Alternative Therapies and Health in Medicine 5*, 45–54.

Yan, B. (1989). *Functions of Qigong (breathing exercise) in clinical practice.* Second International Conference on Qigong, 209.

Yang, K., Xu, H., Guo, Z., Zhao, B., & Li, Z. (1988a). *Analgesic effect of emitted qi on white rats.* First World Conference for Academic Exchange of Medical Qigong, 45.

Yang, K., Guo, Z., Xu, H., Lin, H., et al. (1988b). *Influence of electrical lesion of the periaqueductal gray (PAG) on the analgesic effect of emitted qi in rats.* First World Conference for Academic Exchange of Medical Qigong, 43.

Yao, S. (1989). *The application of the air needle and the eight methods of Linggui to the Qigong theory.* Second International Conference on Qigong, 242.

Yennie, R. (1998). *From ancient to modern man, secrets of the body electric.* Fourth World Conference for Academic Exchange of Medical Qigong, 223–224.

Yuan, Z. (1993). *Survey of 100 doctors using simulated Qigong in the USA.* Second World Conference for Academic Exchange of Medical Qigong, 144.

Yuen, K. (1996). *Qigong for the rehabilitation of acute and chronic pain.* Third World Conference for Academic Exchange of Medical Qigong, 145.

Yumiko, K. (1998). *Aesthetic Qigong.* Fourth World Conference for Academic Exchange of Medical Qigong, 175–176.

Zhang, J., Chen, Y., He, J., Xian, T., & Yi, Y. (1990). *Analgesic effect of emitted qi and the preliminary study of its mechanism.* Third National Academic Conference on Qigong Science, 37.

Zhang, J., Hu, D., & Ye, Z. (1990). *Effect of waiqi (emitted qi) on experimental bone fracture in mice.* Third Nationl Academic Conference on Qigong Science, 57.

Zhang, Y. (1998). *Huolong zhengjing-gong (fire-dragon Qigong).* Fourth World Conference for Academic Exchange of Medical Qigong, 241–242.

Zhao, M., He, M., & Li, S. (1996). *Studies of dynamic meridian transmission of qi circulation therapy and its clinical effect.* Third World Conference for Academic Exchange of Medical Qigong, 124.

Zhou, D., Li, Z., & Zhang, J. (1989). *An experimental observation on the effect of Qigong on improvement of body flexibility.* Second International Conference on Qigong, 111.

52

Koryo Hand Therapy: Modern Pain Management

Daniel C. Lobash, Ph.D., L.Ac.

Koryo Hand Therapy (KHT) is a natural, fast, effective, and safe energetic medicine system for reducing and eliminating pain. KHT is one of many increasingly popular microsystems for resolving pain and other functional problems. The microsystems commonly applied for the resolution of pain include the hand, ear, foot, scalp, iris, nose, and along the second metacarpal bone, among others.

Korean traditional medicine doctor, Tae Woo Yoo, O.M.D., Ph.D. developed the KHT system between 1971 and 1975. It is practiced throughout South Korea and the major text has been translated into six languages. It is a complete energetic medicine system based on the theory, principles, and methods of traditional body acupuncture. Each hand contains the information for the whole organism; that is, all of the structures of the body are represented on each hand. For example, the little finger on the right hand is related to the right leg.

In addition to body representation, all of the acupuncture meridians of the whole body are represented in a miniature but analogous form on each hand. Due to the relationship of the hand and the body, the hand can be used to access information about the condition of the systems of the body as well as provide a means to transmit information to the brain that will result in immediate or near immediate pain reduction.

SCOPE OF APPLICATION

KHT can be applied to any problem traditionally treated with body acupuncture. For purposes of this chapter, the materials presented are confined to pain reduction applications. Any pain, whether severe or low level, chronic or acute, can be successfully treated with KHT Correspondence Therapy. In fact, correspondence therapy is especially effective in creating near instantaneous pain relief. Examples of treatable conditions include neck pain ranging from that caused by accidents to sleeping in a draft; gallbladder-induced pain; pain due to stomach ulcers, gastritis, gas; back, shoulder, wrist, any joint pain, and in fact any pain anywhere in the body due to any cause.

SAMPLE CLINICAL CASES DEMONSTRATING THE EFFECTIVENESS OF CORRESPONDENCE THERAPY

Case 1. A 30-year-old patient had severe pain in the jaw, as shown in Figure 52.1, from dental work the previous day. Searching with a small probe located an exquisitely sensitive point on the jaw's corresponding area. Massage stimulation with the probe tip and a small metal pellet fixed to the skin with adhesive tape immediately reduced the pain 70% and the swelling by 50% within 10 minutes.

Case 2. An 80-year-old patient had suffered for 3 months with lower back pain resulting from twisting as she reached toward a top shelf. She had tried physical therapy and chiropractic, but had only temporary relief. One treatment relieved the pain immediately and it did not return. Shown in Figure 52.2 is the corresponding search area for the lower back.

Case 3. Migraine headache pain of a young woman was reduced by 50% through a simple instruction of where to press and self-massage on the corresponding area of the middle finger, as shown in Figure 52.3.

0-8493-0926-3/02/$0.00+$1.50
© 2002 by CRC Press LLC

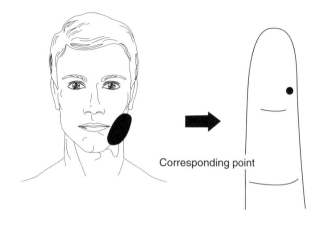

Pain in the Jaw   Middle finger

FIGURE 52.1 Patient with severe pain in the jaw and where to press on the corresponding point of the middle finger.

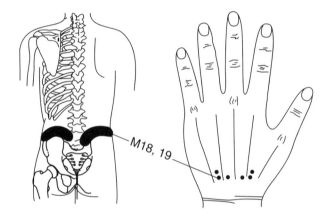

FIGURE 52.2 Patient with low back pain and where to press on the corresponding points of the hand.

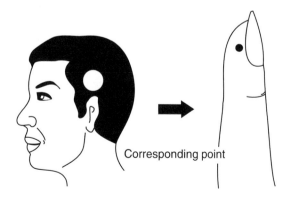

Pain on the side of the head   Middle finger

FIGURE 52.3 Patient with pain on the side of the head and where to press on the corresponding point of the middle finger.

UNIQUE CHARACTERISTICS OF THE HAND MICROSYSTEM

There are several characteristics of the hands that are useful to know and understand as diagnostic and treatment access points. Some of these characteristics also apply to other microsystems of the body.

1. Every pain or discomfort in the body is registered in the related microsystem of the hand.
2. Two common forms of registration that can be detected are reduced pain threshold to mechanical palpation and increased electrical conductance at the corresponding point.
3. Stimulation of the corresponding point has a unique capacity to signal the brain that, in turn, initiates a biochemical chain of events resulting in reduction of pain and inflammation at the corresponding point/area of the body. The action in most cases occurs instantaneously or within minutes. Shown in Figure 52.4 are several instruments used in corresponding point location and treatment.
4. A precise proportional relationship exists between the body structure and the image of the body as it is projected on the hand. Identification of the exact location on the body of pain enables finding the precise corresponding point on the hand.
5. Stimulation of corresponding points can be by means of mechanical pressure, electricity, and specially designed hand acupuncture needles; heat from burning moxa, tiny aluminum disks fixed over the corresponding points with adhesive tape; and several other appliances specially designed to stimulate hand points.
6. Mild stimulation of corresponding hand points results in effective body response. The degree of stimulation of corresponding hand points is minimal compared to that required for similar effects through body stimulation.
7. Areas of the body that are difficult or forbidden to treat in traditional body acupuncture can easily be treated on the hands. For example, it is possible to stimulate corresponding eye points on the hands but not on the body.

RELATIONSHIP OF THE HAND AND THE BODY

In Koryo Hand Therapy the hand is related to the body in a very precise pattern as shown in Figures 52.5 to 52.9 and as described below.

Each hand contains the information and structure for the whole body. This means that diagnosis and treatment

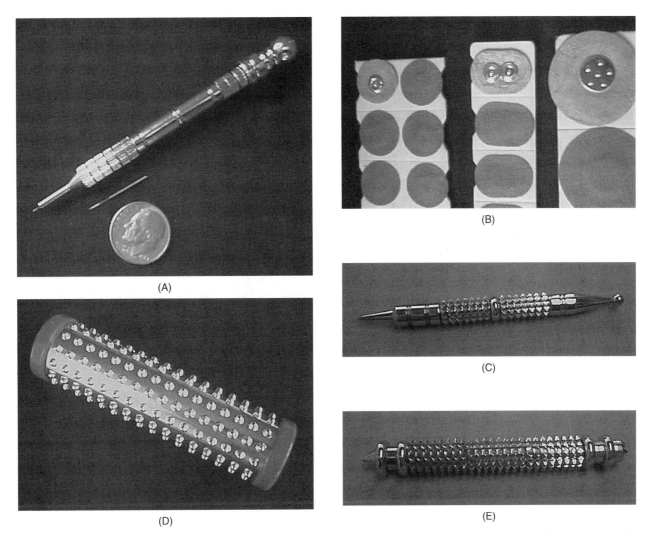

FIGURE 52.4 Instruments used in corresponding point location and treatment. (A) Needle inserter; (B) pellets; (C) point finder; (D) hand roller; (E) heavy duty hand massager.

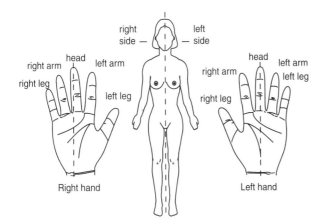

FIGURE 52.5 Frontal relationships. In the frontal view, the midline of the body is represented as the midline of the hands.

FIGURE 52.6 Pains on the anterior surface of the body are treated on the palm side of the hands. The arms correspond to the ring and index fingers.

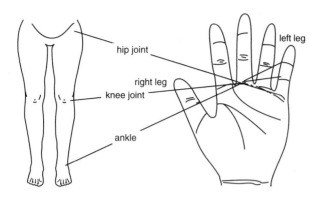

FIGURE 52.7 Pains on the anterior surface of the body are treated on the palm side of the hands. The legs correspond to the ring and little finger.

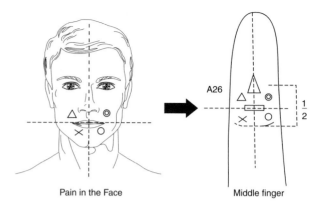

FIGURE 52.8 Pain in the face corresponds to the most distal phalange of the middle finger.

affecting the body could be done on either hand. The preferred treatment pattern, however, is to diagnose and apply stimulation to the hand on the problem side of the body. In the frontal view, the midline of the body is represented as the midline of the hands. The frontal relationships are shown in Figure 52.5.

Pains on the right side of the midline of the body are diagnosed and treated on the right side of the midline of the right hand and vice versa. The midline of the hand bisects the middle finger from the top to the base of the palm just above the wrist.

Pains on the anterior of the body are diagnosed and treated on the palm side of the hands. Pains on dorsal side of the body are diagnosed and treated on the dorsal surface of the hand. Pains on the sides of the body have correspondences on the sides of the hands and fingers.

The arms and legs correspond to the ring and little fingers, respectively, as shown in Figures 52.6 and 52.7. With reference to Figures 52.6 and 52.7, pains on the opposite surface of the body from that shown in the illustrations are found on the opposite surface of the hand. Pain in the face corresponds to the most distal phalange of the middle finger, as shown in Figure 52.8. Pain along the spine corresponds to the dorsal surface of the hand, as shown in the illustration of Figure 52.9.

These illustrations provide guidelines for locating the approximate area on the hands corresponding to pains in the body. The next section describes the process of locating corresponding points with precision.

LOCATING PRECISE CORRESPONDING POINTS

In order to achieve the maximum possible pain reduction, corresponding points must be located with great precision. This means that the maps of the body as shown above merely serve as guides to locating the approximately correct area. Then the precise points must be found exactly with a pressure probe and/or electrical point finder. Apply

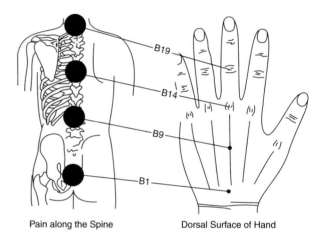

FIGURE 52.9 Pain along the spine corresponds to the dorsal surface of the hands.

the following steps to locate the correct corresponding points:

1. Determine the exact locations of pain in the body. Ask the patient to be very precise in locating and pointing to the painful area. Then ask the patient to rate the discomfort level on a 10-point scale, where 0 is no pain and 10 is excruciating pain. If appropriate, establish range-of-motion limitations and ask the patient to notice the limitation, as well as noting it yourself.
2. Locate the approximate corresponding area on the hand where greater sensitivity is expected. Squeezing the client's hand at the expected corresponding area between your thumb and forefinger can do this. When the correct corresponding area is found, the client will tell you. Note that this is still only the approximate area. Now the search must be refined to locate the exact corresponding point.

3. To locate the exact corresponding point, a metal probe with rounded tips is desirable (Figure 52.4C). The reason for this is that the correct corresponding point can be located even a thousandth of an inch adjacent to the point currently being palpated. You must search in a very fine grid pattern until the exact point is located. When the correct point is stimulated, the client will definitely experience a sharp pain that is quite different from other points being probed.

4. As previously mentioned, the client will reflexively jerk a hand, lift a leg, grimace, squint, say "ahhh, ahhh, ahhh," etc.

5. There may be more than one corresponding point. All that are related to the current painful syndrome should be located and treated.

6. If the point cannot be located, then consider probing with more pressure. Consider that if there is a pain in the body, then there will necessarily be a corresponding point of greater sensitivity on the hand. Another strategy to locate difficult-to-find points is first to stress the painful body part by pressing, or having the client stress, the corresponding body part. This is generally only required in cases of low level, chronic pain.

STIMULATING CORRESPONDING POINTS

The choice and application of the best treatment method are the next steps. The major consideration is to stimulate the corresponding point. There are many strategies available.

1. Mechanical stimulation with a round-tipped, but pointed, probe is simple but does not have as long lasting an effect as other methods. However, the process of searching for and finding the corresponding point also stimulates the point. After this procedure, metal pellets, needles, electricity, and moxa can be added to enhance the effect.

2. Micro hand needles have been created that are thinner and shorter than typical 1/2-inch ear needles. The small size makes insertion nearly painless. The needles are typically inserted with a specially designed mechanical inserter that further reduces discomfort (Figure 52.4A). Needles are typically used for high-level, acute pain. The rule of thumb is that the more intense and acute the pain, the stronger the stimulation desired for greatest effect.

3. Metal pellets can be applied for most conditions. The general rule is to use pellets for chronic conditions, when a milder stimulation is desired, or if the client rejects the needle option, and with children. The pellet is actually shaped more like a small (1/8-inch diameter, approximately) flat disk made of aluminum with an antioxidizing coating. When it is affixed with tape over a corresponding point, it has a similar effect to a needle. The application is painless and the effect excellent. In KHT there are three sizes to accommodate larger corresponding areas, such as for lower back or stomach pain (Figure 52.4B).

4. Moxabustion is a traditional method of applying heat to acupuncture points as the method of stimulation. A small tube of either loose herbs prepared to a consistency similar to a cigarette or a special smokeless cylinder with the consistency of chalk is lit and burned. A cardboard insulator through which the heat penetrates through a small hole in the base limits direct contact with skin. Moxa on the corresponding points has the effect of increasing and evenly distributing blood circulation in the corresponding areas of the body. Moxa treatment is particularly indicated for "cold" diseases commonly found in gynecological conditions and where fatigue is a major factor, such as chronic fatigue and related immune-deficiency syndromes.

5. Microcurrent stimulation through an electronic point locator/stimulator designed for hand therapy is an excellent and fast method of treatment. One pole of the device, commonly the negative one, is held against the corresponding point and the positive pole is held opposite it on the hand. This treatment is commonly combined with pellet and or moxa treatment. First the microcurrent is applied and then the moxa and /or pellets are added.

DURATION OF EFFECTS AND FREQUENCY OF TREATMENT REQUIRED

Exact parameters here are difficult to establish, as each case is unique. However, this much can be said. With correspondence therapy, there is an immediate reduction of pain ranging from 40 to 100%. In acute pain conditions, such as a strained ankle, the effect is dramatic and one treatment may suffice. However, the effect, similar to body acupuncture, may begin to deteriorate in 12 to 48 hours. However, the pain level does not typically return to even close to its original level. In chronic conditions, the pain reduction may be only 20 to 40% and may require extended treatments. If sufficient structural change is the precipitating cause, such as stenosis, treatments may be only palliative and repeated treatments will be required. It is impossible to state any reliable predictive conclusions. As a general rule, beginning treatments should occur two to three times per week for the first week, then two times per week and then once per week until the problem is fully resolved. The prognosis is more predictable after one treatment. The second and additional treatments yield less dramatic drops in pain level because the problem begins an immediate resolution with the first treatment. A course of treatment may be from one to ten treatments.

SELF-CARE

A benefit to the practitioner and the client is that many treatment strategies can be self-applied. Individuals can easily be taught to apply moxabustion in the form practiced in KHT. This is perhaps the number one effective home treatment. Moxa can be self-applied once or even twice per day and the additional benefit to the healing process is dramatic. This is especially helpful if the clients cannot see the practitioner more than once per week. Moxabustion in the original form, which evolved over time with body acupuncture, consists of loose, finely shredded herbs rolled into a ball and placed on the top of a needle. The herb is lit and burns with an even and consistent heat that is transferred to the patient via the needle shaft. That same concept has been adapted to hand therapy, but in a smokeless, modern form.

Also, clients can be instructed about where to place pellets and where to apply mechanical stimulation and even simple massage. All of these forms of self-treatment supplement the work of the practitioner.

GOING BEYOND CORRESPONDENCE THERAPY

Correspondence Therapy is very effective but it does have limitations and in some cases stronger treatments are required. As was mentioned earlier in this chapter, in addition to the hand representing the entire body, each hand contains a set of micromeridians that is parallel, but not identical to, the body meridians in name and function. Often a pain in the body will reflect an energetic imbalance in the flow of energy through the organ–meridian complex. In order to affect the root cause of the pain, the energetic balance in the meridian flow must be reestablished. To accomplish this, the meridians must be stimulated in a specific way, as well as stimulation of the corresponding organ. In this case, most of the principles of meridian treatment common to whole body acupuncture can be applied to the hand micromeridians. By virtue of the existence of micromeridians, many treatment strategies can be applied that include

1. Simple meridian stimulation
2. Tonification and sedation of the energetics of specific meridians
3. Application of the principles of the eight extra meridians
4. Treatment plans based on the inborn constitutional patterns and other strategies unique to KHT.

All of the available options are not covered in this chapter due to space limitations.

RESEARCH STUDIES ON KHT

Many case studies and anecdotal studies have been conducted in Korea but none of them is available in English. In Japan, research was published by Professor Imura of the Department of Health that reported on the use of KHT for injuries. The results showed that there was a 19.5% placebo response to the stimulation of randomly selected points on the hand vs. a 69.5% positive response to the stimulation of the KHT corresponding points on the hands.

Dr. Roberto Jodorkovsky, M.D. recently conducted a pilot study. It showed a 96% positive response in a pediatric population. He diagnosed, treated, and followed a group of 106 of his pediatric patients over a 6-month period. The results of his study were reported in the *Medical Acupuncture Journal 11(1)*, Spring/Summer 1999. The question he sought to answer was if Koryo Hand Therapy could be an effective therapeutic treatment approach in a suburban pediatric practice where standard Western medicine was combined with Koryo Hand Therapy.

The study group consisted of 106 pediatric patients who were a regular part of his practice and who ranged from 3 to 20 years of age. The kinds of conditions presenting included pain in the neck, shoulder, knee, hip, wrist–hand, back, ankle–foot, viral sore throat, head, nose, chest, ear, as well as sinusitis, allergic rhinitis, recurrent abdominal pain, and asthma. Symptoms ranged from less than 1 day to greater than 6 months. The criteria for the success of a treatment for pain syndromes were that the condition resolved completely or was judged at least 50% better. The criteria for success of chronic nonpain syndromes were that specific medication usage was voluntarily reduced 50% and duration and frequency of relapses decreased.

The total number of treatments needed to meet these criteria was 132 for all 106 patients. The recovery rate was notable: 70% saw the improvement within 3 days and 52% saw improvement within 24 hours. For many, relief was virtually immediate.

Dr. Jodorkovsky reported that despite the limitations of an uncontrolled study of this nature, the results were so overwhelmingly positive that they more than made up for methodological and design deficiencies. At the present time he is analyzing data from a more narrowly focused, blinded study of enuresis.

MAJOR BENEFITS OF KHT IN A PAIN MANAGEMENT PRACTICE

There are many obvious benefits to applying KHT in a pain management practice, including

1. Correspondence Therapy is very easy to learn; even children have been taught the fundamentals.
2. It is efficient, as diagnosis and treatment can take as little as 5 minutes.
3. Treatment can be completely painless, and in the case of the microthin needles inserted only 1 mm, nearly painless.
4. It is safe as needles in the hand cannot penetrate vital organs.
5. It is convenient to patients and practitioners, as clothing is not removed.
6. Pain reduction is immediate and is virtually guaranteed for a positive response.
7. It is acceptable to children, the needle phobic, and literally all ages.
8. KHT is an ideal adjunct to any other healing modality or it can stand alone as a complete energetic medicine practice.

HOW TO LEARN KHT

The Correspondence Therapy level or application can be learned in a variety of formats. In a 1-day seminar, with distance learning including a videotaped seminar, and eventually via the Internet. After 1 day of practice and learning the basics, practitioners are ready to treat patients.

Learning the entire scope of KHT requires attendance at a series of seminars on theory and practice. Learning the theory and concepts of KHT beyond Correspondence Therapy is made easier with a basic knowledge of Traditional Chinese Medicine theory. The entire scope of KHT includes

1. Micromeridian therapy
2. Eight Extraordinary meridian therapy
3. Five Element therapy
4. Hot/Cold therapy
5. Ring therapy
6. Designer Food therapy
7. Moxabustion therapy
8. Birth Constitution therapy

Included in the aforementioned are many different treatment and combination treatment strategies.

WHO PRACTICES KHT

At the present time in the United States, practitioners include physicians in many specialties, nurse practitioners, nurses, acupuncturists, chiropractors, physical therapists, massage therapists, holistic health practitioners, and at the basic level even interested lay people. KHT has been taught throughout the world and the basic text has been translated into six languages including English, German, Russian, Japanese, French, and Spanish.

In summary, the key words that exemplify Korean Hand Therapy are effective, efficient, safe, acceptable, and economical.

53

Koryo Hand Therapy for Pain Relief

Linda C. Hole, M.D.

A wise man should consider that health is the greatest of human blessings, and learn how by his own thoughts to derive benefit from his illness.

Hippocrates

INTRODUCTION

Koryo Hand Therapy (KHT), a hand acupuncture microsystem developed by Dr. Tae Woo Yoo, O.M.D., Ph.D. of Korea, is a remarkably effective and powerful tool for pain management that is based on a simple systematic relationship between your body's acupuncture meridians and corresponding hand "map."

KHT is noninvasive, *painless and effective without needles*, has no significant side effects, often gives immediate and dramatic results within minutes, and is easy to both learn and apply. KHT is recognized worldwide for its elegant methodical simplicity, immediate onset of action, and often instantaneous, near-miraculous results. KHT is especially a godsend for those who have found little or no relief elsewhere.

Qi is your breath, your universal vital life force, or the healing energy transmitted via Qigong, a 5000-year-old energy medicine healing system from China. Qi enhances your KHT treatment, and gives even more remarkable results in pain relief.

Dr. Yoo, the internationally renowned acupuncturist who discovered KHT, considers KHT a gift of God. In his own words, he describes the birth of KHT:

> One autumn night in 1971 I was awakened from sleep by a severe pain in the back of my head … For some reason, I found myself staring at the back of my middle finger, and it occurred to me that there might be a point there to treat the pain. I proceeded to stick my finger with the tip of a ballpoint pen, and indeed found a particularly painful area. I then proceeded to insert a needle in this sensitive spot, and my God the headache was gone. The speed and degree of pain relief was overwhelming. I mentally visualized the tip of my finger as possibly representing the head of the human body, and wondered whether there was a relationship of the rest of the hand with the whole of the human body.

In this chapter, we focus on KHT, and build on Chapter 52, the introductory chapter on Koryo Hand Therapy by Dan Lobash Ph.D., L.Ac. and on Chapter 51 on Qigong by this author.

Although KHT is based on the same principles as Traditional Chinese Medicine (TCM) acupuncture, KHT requires no TCM, acupuncture, or Qigong training to learn or apply. For those with TCM experience, practitioners find KHT superior for:

- Greater efficacy, depth, and breath, with results even when all else has failed
- Immediate onset of action, with results usually within minutes
- Far more efficient in the amount of time required for treatment
- Far simpler to learn and apply
- Essentially no side effects
- Noninvasive and painless; no needles are required
- Empowers patients in self-care, and to become free of dependence on habit-forming medications

0-8493-0926-3/02/$0.00+$1.50
© 2002 by CRC Press LLC

One great advantage of KHT is its simplicity. We routinely teach KHT to our patients for self-care. We've even taught children how to effectively use KHT to successfully treat family and friends. In this chapter, we hope you will be inspired to see for yourself what KHT can do to ameliorate pain.

CLINICAL SCOPE AND STUDIES

In our medical practice, we have found KHT effective in the treatment of a wide range of pain disorders including acute injuries, arthritis, bone pain, cancer, carpal tunnel syndrome, chest pain, disc disease, dysmennorhea, fibromyalgia, fractures, hypothalamic syndrome, headaches, migraines, myopathies, neuralgias, pelvic pain, peripheral neuropathies, radiculopathies, RSD reflex sympathetic dystrophy, RSI repetitive stress injury, sciatica, shingles, shoulder pain, frozen shoulder, soft tissue and sports injuries, surgical postoperative pain, chronic pain, and intractable pain.

Roberto Jordokovsky, M.D., a pediatrician, reports in a 1999 pilot study for the AAMA and the *Journal of Physical Medicine* on 106 children and adolescents treated with KHT. For the 65% with painful acute conditions, e.g., sprains, back pain, headache, etc., he observed a nearly 100% positive response within one treatment session, and no side effects. For the 35% with chronic conditions, he noted significant improvement over time with repeated follow-up treatments.

Patrick Mok, M.D., anesthesiologist and pain management specialist, reports his findings on the treatment of neuralgia and myopathy. "Practically all patients will have positive results with KHT to different degrees, usually within 3–4 treatments … (with) significant pain alleviation of varying degrees and duration, abolishment of acute exacerbations, and enhanced medication effect, with decreased doses of medication required … and a documented case of return to normal levels of CPK."

With controlled studies in English in progress, KHT medical doctors and practitioners across the country report similar results.

THE SCIENCE OF KHT

A punch biopsy of any part of your body gives a hologram of your body. Cells, by their embryological cellular "memory," remember their origins and how they relate to the whole. Other well-documented acupuncture microsystems include the scalp, eyes, ears, tongue, face, and foot. For every body pain, there is a sensitive correspondence KHT point on the hand. The KHT hand microsystem is one of the most powerful for pain relief.

Studies by Dr. M.H. Cho and Dr. Y. Mitsuo demonstrate that stimulation of KHT hand points induces an increase in temperature of predicted KHT corresponding body parts. Professor Yoo (1976, 1977) further reports that stimulation of KHT hand points increases electroencephalogram alpha waves.

In acupuncture, Dr. Bruce Pomeranz, professor of physiology at the University of Toronto, did the classic studies demonstrating that acupuncture stimulates the release of endorphins, dinorphins, serotonin, and norepinephrine. Acupuncture research also documents vasodilatation, and increased blood levels of enkephalins, mRNA, prostaglandins, and other anti-inflammatory agents.

KHT TO GO: SOME CASE EXAMPLES

KHT is so simple and fun to apply, with such immediate results, that we routinely give impromptu "curbside" treatments almost everywhere we go. With KHT, it is not uncommon for patients to require only a single treatment for long-standing relief. In hopes of inspiring you to explore KHT for yourself, we share here some case examples, with more clinical examples and treatment details to follow in the "How" section of this chapter (see also, Qigong Chapter 51, Qi Acupuncture section).

HEADACHE

A middle-aged blue-collar worker complained of severe headaches. As I applied needles to his sensitive KHT correspondence hand points, he burst out with a series of very loud vocal four-letter expletives, for the whole office and waiting room to hear. Then with a sigh of relief, "Whew! That sucker did it! — My headache's gone."

SURGICAL PAIN

At the registration tables of a medical meeting, a fellow attendee complained of acute incisional postoperative pain. When we found the corresponding hand KHT painful point, he literally dropped to his knees in surprise. We applied simple fingertip Qi and pressure to the KHT correspondence hand point, and his incisional pain was relieved.

DISC DISEASE

We visited a family friend the night before his scheduled surgery for his herniated disc. We found him at home lying on the floor, with porta-potty at side, having signed himself out of the hospital against medical advice. With a single several minute treatment, he returned to work within 2 weeks.

KHT LEVELS OF TREATMENT

KHT levels of treatment range from simple to elegant. The most straightforward for beginners are the Correspondence, Basic, and Meridian levels of treatment. The Mo and Yu points, and Dr. Yoo's Formulary are also helpful. For more complex and chronic pain disorders, deeper treatment is necessary, such as the Three Constitutions, Five Elements, or Birth Constitution Biorhythmic approach. Combining different levels of treatment gives even more effective results.

- **Correspondence**. This is the simplest level of treatment to learn, usually gives immediate and effective results, and when augmented with Qi, at times even long-lasting results. Simply find the corresponding or sensitive points on the hand to ease the body pain.
- **Basic**. This basic set of points energizes the three vital "heaters" or "burners," upper, middle, and lower, and may be used as a foundation for any KHT treatment.
- **Meridian**. Use an acupuncture atlas to find the acupuncture meridian location of the pain. Balancing the meridians balances the internal organs, and thereby helps dispel the pain.
- **Three Constitutions**. There are three fundamental "Constitutions" in KHT theory: Yang, Yin, and Kidney. The "Extraordinary" points free constitution-level blockages, and thus also pain. Use in combination with Correspondence, Meridian, and Five Elements treatments.
- **Five Elements**. Each yin–yang organ pair has an Element. Balancing the Five Elements gives a deeper level of treatment for pain relief.
- **Mo and Yu Points**. Each organ has a control gathering front Yin "Mo" and back Yang "Yu" point. These points in combination with other levels of treatment potentiate pain relief.
- **Biorhythmic and Birth Constitution**. Each person's date and time of birth determine his or her Five Element "core" Three Constitutions diagnosis.
- **Formulary**. A cookbook approach, which includes specific prescriptions based on Dr. Yoo's years of experience, is especially useful for those new to KHT.
- **More KHT Tools**. Connecting Meridians, Four Gates, Hot vs. Cold, Long vs. Short Lever, Long Distance, Pendulum, Upside Down points, the Four Lifesaving points, Three Emergency Points, Four Gate points, Four Spiritual Points, Eight Extraordinary points, Twelve Source points, Five Su points, and Special Points for Nervous Disease are more KHT tools available—all superbly effective for pain relief, and simple to learn.

KHT METHODS OF TREATMENT

Ways of stimulating KHT hand points include

- *Mechanical pressure*, e.g., with a ball point pen, or special KHT probe
- *Pressure pellets*, with negative silver- and positive gold-colored pellets
- *Magnets*, with negative north poles, and positive south poles
- *E-Beam microcurrent* electrical stimulation, with negative and positive leads
- *Needles*, with polarity by color, and/or slant of needle
- *Moxa*, or heat stimulation—a must for those with deep or chronic illness
- Qi-KHT fingertip pressure with Qi
- *Five Element ring therapy*, silver and gold colored
- *Five Element food therapy* formulas for each element
- *Yi Nian*, or "Clear Intention," or simply visualizing the correct treatment.

Negative, or silver-colored, pellets, magnets, needles, and rings sedate and calm. Positive, or gold-colored, materials tonify and strengthen.

Five Element ring therapy, and Five Element food therapy are deeper methods of balancing the internal organs of the Five Elements. Just holding the correct specially formulated Five Element food packet, or wearing the Five Element ring on the correct finger may relieve the pain.

Simultaneous Qi emission with any method potentiates the treatment results.

Some Precautions

Bad effects may occur if one overtreats, especially with magnets. Pressure points left too long, and or applied with overzealous pressure may damage the skin. Misdiagnosing and applying the entirely wrong prescription, especially when using the Three Constitutions Extraordinary Points, may rarely cause dizziness, nausea, and even fainting, for which the antidote is to immediately remove the points. There are also the obvious precautions with pregnancy, and possible burns with moxa. KHT, however, is by and large very forgiving, and when practiced correctly, has essentially no side effects.

How Do I Learn and Apply KHT?

The best way to learn KHT is to simply start experimenting with the hand points. Sometimes when we teach an introductory workshop, we invite an audience participant to find the KHT pain relief points on a volunteer. The incredulous looks on their faces when the pain disappears are priceless.

THE HOW OF KHT: SOME KHT PAIN RELIEF TOOLS

The practice of KHT is simple. KHT hand points become sensitive in correlation to the pain in the body and internal organ imbalance. Simply stimulating the indicated Correspondence, Basic, Meridian, Three Constitutions, Five Element, and/or Mo and Yu points gives pain relief.

Incorporating Qi into the treatment augments the pain relief, regardless of the specific method of stimulating the indicated hand points. When you apply Qi to indicated KHT hand points, your patient may experience an electric tingling or warm sensation in the corresponding body part, and sometimes even break out laughing.

We usually use the ipsilateral hand to treat pain. Treat the right hand for a right-sided pain, the left hand for a left-sided pain. For severe conditions, we sometimes use the contralateral hand, or "long lever." The contralateral long lever applies more healing force than the ipsilateral short lever.

The more sensitive distal points on the fingers are used for the acute conditions. The more proximal points on the fingers are used for chronic conditions.

CORRESPONDENCE THERAPY

The Correspondence Level of treatment is the most direct first-step KHT approach to pain. For a step-by-step guide to the Correspondence Therapy, see Dr. Lobash's introductory Chapter 52.

In general, the palmar surface of your hand corresponds to the anterior or "Yin" surface of your body: face, chest, abdomen, knees, etc. The dorsal surface of your hand corresponds to the posterior or "Yang" surface of your body: occiput, spine, buttocks, achilles tendon, etc. Each finger corresponds to a limb, with the middle finger representing the spine and head. Each finger joint corresponds to a body joint.

The sensitivity of the correspondence point is in direct relation to the severity pain of the affected body area. Stimulating the correspondence point alleviates the presenting pain. The correspondence point itself will become less sensitive as the body pain is dispelled.

Correspondence Therapy Clinical Example

Chronic Pain in a 42-year-old C6–7 quadriplegic, who complained of long-standing neck, shoulder, and lower extremities unrelieved by opiates. Simple fingertip Qi

applied to his KHT correspondence point for his trapezius muscles gave immediate relief of his shoulder pain.

YI NIAN CLEAR INTENTION

Yi Nian clear intention is visualizing the specific KHT prescription itself, and the pain-free result you'd like to achieve. The mere clear intention of seeing your patient free from pain may give remarkable results. This level of treatment is an example of what Larry Dossey, M.D. heralds as New Era "nonlocal" medicine.

Yi Nian Clear Intention Clinical Example

For a veteran who complained of over 20 years of intractable shoulder pain, Professor Yoo drew the correct KHT prescription on the blackboard, a simple arrow, then stroked the arrow *on the blackboard* in the correct direction of the meridian flow necessary to relieve the pain—and the patient's pain was immediately relieved. To prove the phenomenon, Professor Yoo then erased the blackboard, drew the prescription again, stroked the arrow on the blackboard in the opposite direction, and the his pain returned. Professor Yoo then erased the blackboard one last time, drew the correct prescription once again, stroked the arrow on blackboard in the correct direction, and the veteran's pain was gone.

BASIC THERAPY

The Basic points may serve as a foundation for any KHT pain relief treatment, in that they energize and balance the three "heaters" and the internal organs. The Lower Heater controls pelvic excretion and reproduction. The Middle Heater controls abdominal organs and digestion. The Upper Heater controls the heart and lungs, circulation, and respiration. Regular use of the Basic Treatment points for health maintenance results in more restful sleep, increased energy, vitality, alertness, sexual energy, and overall sense of well-being.

THREE CONSTITUTIONS THERAPY

There are three basic "constitution" "excess syndromes" in KHT theory: Yang Excess, Yin Excess, and Kidney Excess. Constitution Level treatment is appropriate for both acute and chronic pain, and is usually necessary for organic and chronic pain. An imbalance or blockage at a Constitution Level may contribute to pain. Freeing the imbalance and blockage frees the pain.

Within each constitution, there are two types: Yang and Yin. In Yang types, the excess organ is a hollow Yang organ, and the carotid pulse is greater than the radial. In Yin types, the excess organ is a solid Yin organ, and the radial pulse is greater than the carotid.

One way of diagnosing the constitution is by palpating the abdomen. For each syndrome, there is a specific tender abdominal TCM point: Stomach 25 for Yang Excess Syndrome, Spleen 15 for Yin Excess Syndrome, and Conception Vessel 4 for Kidney Excess Syndrome. Kidney Excess Syndromes also may be tender at Stomach 25 and Spleen 15 as well. For each of the three syndromes, there are specific sets of Extraordinary points for treatment: one set for Yang types, and another for Yin types.

Yang Excess Syndrome

Patients are characteristically thin, conciliatory, kind, and are the most responsive to treatment. The major excess organs are the large intestine, liver, and heart. They are prone to dizziness, headaches, nervousness, fatigue, low back pain, sciatica, hemiplegia, and impotence. Their conditions are aggravated by excessive drinking, sexual indulgence, emotional stress, imbalanced diet, and overeating.

Yin Excess Syndrome

Patients are usually overweight, often "greedy," tend to be big eaters and sleepers, and are slower to respond to treatment. The primary excess organ is the spleen. They are especially prone to neuralgias: trigeminal neuralgia, intercostal neuralgia, and lower extremity neuralgias, progressing to loss of sensation. They are also prone to headaches, especially migraines, seizures, paralysis, and stroke.

Kidney Excess Syndrome

These patients by nature like to save and spare, are preoccupied with their own troubles, tend to right-sided disorders, and are prone to disc disease and paralysis, plus allergic, rheumatic, and autoimmune disorders. The excess organ is the kidney, and they are the most difficult to treat.

Three Constitutions Clinical Example

Once when I was presenting at a medical symposium, a young woman with a 6-month history of a constant headache volunteered herself before the full audience for pain relief. I applied only the four indicated Three Constitutions Extraordinary points, and her headache was gone.

MERIDIAN THERAPY

Meridian therapy is a safe and gentle method of controlling the six solid Yin, and six hollow Yang organs of TCM. Each meridian governs one organ of a pair of coupled solid Yin and hollow Yang organs, each with its own specific body surface dermatome-like area.

With hands raised up to the heavens and the palm Yin surface facing forward, the Yang meridians run on the lateral and posterior Yang back surface of the body, and flow from heaven to earth. The Yin meridians run on the medial and anterior Yin surface of the body, and flow from earth to heaven.

Upper extremity pain may result from imbalances in the coupled Yin–Yang organs: lung–large intestine, heart–small intestine, pericardium–triple heater. Lower extremity pains results from imbalances in the coupled Yin–Yang organs: liver–gall bladder, spleen–stomach, and kidney–bladder.

The imbalances are excess or deficient organs. In the coupled pairs of organs, excess in the yang organ means deficiency in the coupled yin organ. Pain is usually secondary to the excess organ.

For meridian level treatment of pain, first determine the location of the pain on the body, then which meridian controls the specific body area, and the meridian's organ. Next, sedate the excess organ via its meridian, or tonify the coupled deficient organ. Sedate by running microcurrent or Qi against the flow of the meridian. You may use Qi to sedate by simply stroking your fingertip against the direction of the meridian flow. Tonify by running microcurrent or Qi in the same direction as the flow of the meridian. Tonify via fingertip Qi by stroking the KHT micromeridian in the same direction as meridian flow.

Current runs negative to positive with pellets, and north to south with magnets. Thus, one may also use pellets and magnets to tonify and sedate. Gold- or silver-colored rings on the correct fingers continue the tonification or sedation.

For pain, simple sedation of the indicated meridian usually gives some immediate relief. For a depleted patient with a low energy level, for example, someone suffering cancer pain, tonifying the coupled deficient organ is a better choice.

As a practitioner, you can almost simply show your patient an acupuncture atlas, ask the patient to point to the affected body area, then treat the indicated meridian according to the diagram.

Meridian Therapy Clinical Examples

Sciatica for months in a renowned author. I applied fingertip Qi to sedate her bladder meridian. I stroked her 5th finger dorsal midline along her KHT bladder micromeridian, from distal tip to proximal metacarpal joint, then gave her a pinky copper ring to continue bladder sedation tonification at home. For the first time in months, she was pain free, and continued to be pain free for months afterward.

Carpal tunnel in a young woman with adult-onset diabetes. Carpal tunnel in KHT is often a pericardium meridian imbalance. With a single KHT treatment, her

TABLE 53.1
The Five Elements

Element	Wood	Fire	Earth	Metal	Water
Color	Green	Red	Yellow	White	Black
Emotion	Anger	Joy	Thinking	Grief	Fear
Direction	East	South	Center	West	North
Climate	Wind	Hot	Damp	Dry	Cold
Taste	Sour	Bitter	Sweet	Pungent	Salt
Orifice	Eyes	Tongue	Mouth	Nose	Ear
Tissue	Tendon Vessels	Blood	Muscle	Skin	Bone
Yin/Yang	Liver	Heart	Spleen	Lung	Kidney
Organ	Gall Bladder	Small Intestine	Stomach	Large Intestine	Bladder

physical therapist noted an increase in both muscle strength and mass.

Headache in a 23-year-old computer wizard camp director, who complained of long-standing frontal headache radiating to vertex. Dx: Gall bladder deficiency. Rx: Sedate liver. Result: Headache relieved.

FIVE ELEMENT THERAPY (SEE TABLE 53.1)

We introduced the Five Elements in Chapter 51 on Qigong. When other levels of KHT treatment are insufficient to fully alleviate the pain, go to the Five Elements, a deeper more profound level of treatment.

There are Five Elements: Fire, Earth, Metal, Water, and Wood, each of which governs a pair of coupled Yin and Yang organs. Each element has a whole set of element-specific characteristics: color, emotions, sound, taste, direction, etc.

The Five Elements themselves are governed by a "Mother Son" Nourishing Cycle, and by a Control Cycle. For each meridian there are specific Five Element points. In Five Element therapy, we pick tonifying and sedating points according to the principles of the Mother–Son Nourishing and Control cycles. Five Element therapy may bring to light the deeper psychospiritual pain picture underlying the surface physical pain.

When patients present with a physical pain, they often deny any related deeper pain. Five Element therapy dispels the physical pain in part by addressing the underlying psychospiritual pain as well. Giving patients feedback on their Five Element diagnosis helps them become aware of the deeper wound underlying their physical pain. With this awareness, there are often tears of release, signifying a more profound, and sometimes life-changing, healing.

Five Element Clinical Examples

Intercostal neuralgia in a 46-year-old female professional artist. Heart sedation relieved her pain. The Fire, or

Heart, emotion is sadness. Her underlying pain was deeply suppressed *Heart* Sadness over the death of her father.

Left sciatica in a 30-year-old health professional. Left bladder sedation relieved her pain. On the right, she had large intestine excess. Water, with the emotion fear, is the bladder element. Metal, with the emotion grief, is the large intestine element. Her underlying issues were grief over her father's illness, and fear that he may die.

COMBINED LEVELS OF TREATMENT

Although simple Correspondence Therapy may give immediate and dramatic results, and is adequate for simple and/or acute pain, other levels of treatment are necessary for deeper pain. For organic and/or chronic pain, our approach is to first diagnose and balance the Three Constitutions, then address the Five Element organ imbalance underlying the presenting pain.

Chronic and Organic Pain Clinical Examples

Diabetic Peripheral Neuropathy in a 53-year-old white CEO with constant pain and numbness, especially of left upper extremity, sleepless even with medication. Dx: Left and right Yang syndrome, with large intestine and bladder excess. Rx: Sedate large intestine and bladder excesses. Result: pain relieved, and sensation returned.

Herpetic Neuralgia in a 29-year-old health professional with acute herpetic trigeminal neuralgia, onset after death of a loved one, in tears with pain, unable to open mouth, chew, or smile. Dx: Left Yin syndrome with spleen and lung excess, right Yin syndrome with gall bladder and bladder excess. Rx: Sedate excess organs. Result: Left office with full range of motion of mouth, and happy smile as well.

CONCLUSION

KHT is a truly effective, easy-to-learn, rewarding, and paradigm shift tool for empowering New Era medicine pain management. The look on a patient's face, with the realization that the presenting symptom is suddenly gone, is again priceless—sometimes amazement, sometimes disbelief, sometimes pure relief, sometimes laughter, sometimes tears of release and gratitude.

My hope in sharing these tools with you is to give you a taste of what's possible, and encourage you to explore KHT for yourself, and see what a tremendous difference KHT can make in your own life, in your practice, and in the lives of your patients.

ACKNOWLEDGMENTS

Thanks to Peter Eckman, M.D., Gene Liu, Greg, Dan Lobash, L.Ac., and Prof. You, Ph.D., O.M.D.

REFERENCES

KHT literature available in English is scarce. Texts and articles available include

Eckman, P. (1995). Ayruveda and Korean hand acupuncture: A brief introduction to some similarities between constitutional typologies. *American Journal of Acupuncture, 23*(2).

Eckman, P. (1990a). The Daoist concept of alarm points. *The AAMA Review 3*(1), 13–17.

Eckman, P. (1990b). An introduction to Koryo Sooji Chi: Korean hand acupuncture. *American Journal of Acupuncture 18*(2).

Eckman, P. (1993). The physiologic basis of acupuncture micro-systems. *The AAMA Review 1*(2), 7–11.

Helms, J. (1995). *Medical acupuncture for physicians.* Berkeley, CA: Medical Acupuncture Publishers.

Jordokovsky, R. (1999). Hand acupuncture experience in pediatric patients. *AAMA Medical Journal of Acupuncture 11*(1), 25-28.

Yoo, T. (1976). *Lectures on Koryo hand therapy.* Seoul Korea: Eum Yang Maek Jin Publishing Co., translated into English 1993.

Yoo, T. (1977). In P. Eckman (Ed.), *Lectures on Koryo hand acupuncture: Vol. I.* Seoul Korea: Eum Yang Maek Jin Publishing Co.

54

ETPS Neuropathic Acupuncture

Bruce Hocking, D.Ac.

FOREWORD

The social and human costs of chronic pain are staggering. During the 20th century, chronic pain has disabled millions of people, costing hundreds of billions of dollars in rehabilitation and lost productivity in addition to untold human suffering (Statistics Canada, 1992). According to some statistics, 80% of these payments have been made for patients with neuromyofascial pain. For the future, there is little evidence to suggest that the rate of growth of chronic soft tissue pain conditions will decrease or even plateau.

Today, doctors and patients can choose from a variety of treatments, though surgery and prescription drugs are the most popular avenues in the United States. The major disadvantage associated with drugs or surgery is that they do not always solve the root problems; rather, they mask pain or surgically remove local pathology. Pharmaceuticals occasionally are effective, but can result in unpleasant interactions and side effects to a degree that reduces the quality of life for those who ingest them on a long-term basis. Moreover, the risks associated with drugs and surgery are not always outweighed by the benefits, as many patients actually feel worse.

A number of complementary and alternative modalities (CAMs) have been promoted as solutions to fill the void left by allopathic medicine. However, their relative efficaciousness may be regarded as sporadic. Progress in identifying a broader range of therapeutic benefits of CAMs has been hindered by considerable infighting among different disciplines, to a degree reminiscent of a quest to be the first to race up the hill, plant a flag, and claim victory in a winner-takes-all contest. While natural solutions do offer some relief in the battle

against chronic pain, long-term victory appears elusive when approaching a patient with a single modality or treatment philosophy.

The development of Electro-Therapeutic Point Stimulation (ETPS) therapy represents a turning point in the fight against chronic pain. Where surgery and prescription drugs fall short, ETPS provides nonsurgical, noninvasive treatment of chronic neuromyofascial pain. ETPS does not replace, nor does it dispute the validity of conventional medicinal approaches. Rather, ETPS recognizes that all therapeutic approaches must be examined to determine the most efficacious treatment for the patient. ETPS also recognizes that different therapies produce different responses and that the key to understanding the source of a patient's chronic pain is to perform an overall mechanical and neuropathic analysis of the body. This analysis helps to identify problematic areas that contort the body, resulting in asymmetrical posture and motion, physical conditions that ETPS therapy believes can lead to degenerative changes and chronic pain throughout the body.

INTRODUCTION

ETPS neuropathic therapy is a hybrid modality used in the treatment of neuromyofascial pain. In its most basic form, ETPS therapy applies brief, staged, concentrated stimulation to points relating to different therapeutic systems. Patient assessments are performed at the end of each stage to determine therapeutic effectiveness. Through a series of systematic and reproducible protocols, the diagnosis and treatment of root causes of soft tissue pain can be completed with a high degree of accuracy.

0-8493-0926-3/02/$0.00+$1.50
© 2002 by CRC Press LLC

The theoretical underpinnings of ETPS therapy are based on sound medicine, firmly grounded on the principles of acupuncture, osteopathic trigger points, neuromuscular and neural therapies. As such, the constituent elements of ETPS therapy are not new. Its unique contribution to pain relief, however, comes from the synthesis of different approaches, combining the therapeutic "pearls" of trigger, motor, and acupuncture points with a mechanical analysis of the body. The result is a simple, easy-to-use series of protocols.

By following the recommended protocols, physicians are able to identify which stage(s) is/are most responsible for contributing to a patient's pain condition. Stages deemed ineffective in producing positive therapeutic responses are eliminated from future treatments. Those stages producing positive responses are examined diagnostically to determine interrelationship(s) with the patient's condition and are integrated into future protocols.

ETPS therapy does not isolate or treat a pain condition; rather, it is used to determine how the patient's overall body mechanics and neuropathic/radiculopathic manifestations can be combined with acupuncture and trigger points to produce unique protocols. These protocols bridge many different treatment philosophies to provide therapeutic responses where other modalities fail to achieve successful results. Because it is effective in the diagnosis of root causes of pain, ETPS therapy can serve as an invaluable tool for all types of physicians in their efforts to substantiate current treatment and as an integrative tool for current protocols.

The therapeutic benefits of ETPS are based on four different physiological principles.

1. Circulation response. Increasing or decreasing circulation (called "chi" in Eastern therapies) can benefit the patient in a manner similar to the application of heat (vaso dilation) and ice (vasoconstriction) in Western medicine.
2. Autonomic/parasympathetic response. A medium for chronic pain, the Autonomic Nervous System (ANS) covers over 90% of the body and consists of the sympathetic and parasympathetic nervous systems. ETPS stimulation of parasympathetic "gates" can have a calming effect on the body, providing the patient with immediate and long-lasting relief from pain, anxiety, and insomnia.
3. Endorphin response. Endorphins are similar to morphine in their ability to reduce pain, but are thousands of times stronger and do not produce harmful side effects. Endorphins may be released through concentrated low-frequency ETPS stimulation of neural points causing the pituitary to secrete endorphins, thereby releasing adrenal cortico-atrophic

hormone (ACTH) and hydrocortisols for acceleration of soft tissue repair.
4. Myofascial release. Chronic pain is known to originate in neuropathy, or functional alterations of the peripheral nervous system (PNS). Neuropathy is always caused by muscle contraction, while radiculopathy is neuropathy at the spinal root. Relaxing contracted muscles relieves impingement of the nerves, reduces heightened sensitivity of pathways, and improves the patient's ROM.

The balance of this chapter, divided into two main sections, provides an overview of ETPS therapy. Part A describes the six pillars of ETPS therapy, the core foundation of knowledge upon which the synthesis of different modalities is built. They are (1) acupuncture; (2) the relationship between radiculopathy and neuropathy and chronic pain; (3) the relationship between dermatomes and chronic pain; (4) the relationship between gait and chronic pain; (5) the relationship between scar therapy (neural) and chronic pain; and (6) ETPS stimulation. Based on this body of knowledge, Part B describes five ETPS protocols, all of which use an approach to treatment that allows therapists to diagnostically isolate and treat chronic pain concurrently.

ETPS therapy has proven successful in the treatment of various indications. These include back and neck pain, whiplash, TMJ, fibromyalgia, neuropathies, migraines, headaches, sport injuries, carpal tunnel, failed backs, postoperative radiculopathy, plantar fasciitis, frozen shoulder and shoulder pain, tennis elbow, and most other neuromyofascial pain syndromes. Due to the limitations of this forum, the description of ETPS therapy and related treatments will focus on back and neck pain, fibromyalgia, and plantar fasciitis protocols.

PART A: THE SIX PILLARS OF ETPS THERAPY

ACUPUNCTURE

In order to utilize ETPS protocols effectively, therapists must have a basic, practical understanding of acupuncture. Long regarded as an effective modality for the treatment of pain, acupuncture contributes four key dimensions to the development of ETPS protocols: the release of endorphins, key acupuncture points, a numbering system for point location, and the movement of circulation and energy. Each dimension is discussed below.

The Release of Endorphins

Acupuncture has been scientifically proven to release endogenous morphines from the anterior pituitary (Andersson,

1999; Augustinsson, et al., 1977; Cheng, McKibbon, Roy, & Pomeranz, 1980; Fisher, 1992; Martelete & Fiori, 1985; Pomeranz, 1981). Once released, internal morphines stimulate the release of ACTH and glucocorticoids, natural hormones that accelerate soft tissue healing. These powerful nonaddictive opiates are circulated throughout the body to relieve pain and remain elevated for a period of 12 to 72 hours. All acupuncture points can release endorphins as long as a proper therapeutic response is achieved with needles or low frequency stimulation. ETPS therapy activates endorphin response for overall pain relief through the application of low-frequency endorphin-releasing parameters to ETPS protocols (Christopher, Lorenzo, Zirbs, Chantraine, & Visher, 1992; Lehmann, Russell, Spratt, Liu, Fairchild, & Christensen, 1986; Pomeranz & Niziak, 1987).

Key Acupuncture Points

Key acupuncture points are utilized for their beneficial therapeutic effects on the body. Distal points located on the extremities are stimulated to produce proximal pain relief and have been integrated into ETPS protocols to enhance pain relieving benefits. Four examples of distal points related to the treatment of back pain are described below.

- B 40 (Figure 54.1). An effective low back pain point integrated into circuits with ETPS back pain protocols to produce a highly effective therapeutic stage. Located on the midline of the transverse knee crease.
- K 3 (Figure 54.2). Is circulated with L4-L5 segmental levels for back pain that is worse in the morning. Located halfway between the apex of the medial malleolus and the Achilles tendon.
- B 60 (Figure 54.3). A powerful sciatic point circuited with L4-L5 segmental levels for afternoon back pain. Located halfway between the apex of the lateral malleolus and the Achilles tendon.
- Gb 34 (Figure 54.4). An influential point for muscles, tendons, and tissues that should always be incorporated into the first stage of a standard protocol because of its ability to reduce muscular hypertonicity and spasticity throughout the entire body. Applying ETPS therapy to this acupuncture point is an absolute must for therapists who perform manual or soft tissue therapy on patients. Located inferior and posterior to the head of the fibula.

Meridian Numbering System for Point Location

Soft tissue research suggests that there is a strong therapeutic connection between trigger, motor, and acupuncture points and a low level of skin resistance (Gunn & Mil-

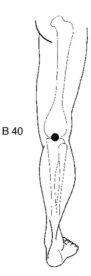

FIGURE 54.1 B 40 is a distal acupuncture point that influences proximal low back pain.

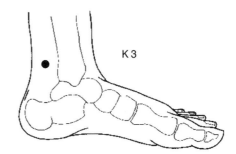

FIGURE 54.2 K 3 is a distal acupuncture point for low back pain. Very effective for sciatica patients with pain aggravated in the morning.

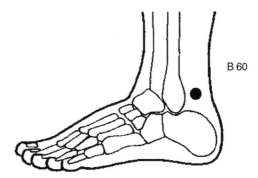

FIGURE 54.3 B 60 is a distal acupuncture point for low back pain. Effective for sciatica patients reporting aggravation in the evening.

brandt, 1976; Hartley, 1989; Low & Reed, 1994; Robinson, MacKler, & Snyder, 1995; Travell & Simons, 1992). For this reason, ETPS therapy uses the acupuncture meridian numbering system to assist in point location. In addition, the meridian system facilitates greater anatomic specificity when locating trigger points compared to palpation.

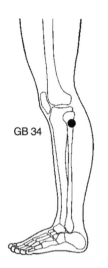

FIGURE 54.4 GB 34 is the myofascial release point, also known as the physical therapy point in acupuncture. Applied in circuits for myofascial release of receptor muscles.

To demonstrate the advantages of the meridian numbering system, consider acupuncture point Gb 21 and the upper trapezius trigger point. Although physically the same point, locating Gb 21 through the acupuncture meridian system is generally easier and will result in a more exact positioning compared to efforts to identify the upper trapezius trigger point through palpation alone.

Circulation and Energy

Blood and circulation in ETPS therapy are assumed to be in line with the concept of *chi* in acupuncture. Chi is a difficult concept to translate into English, but can be described as flowing energy, vitality, or life force. In the Oriental concept of medicine and the human body, the maintenance of health is achieved by releasing blocks, often caused by muscular tension, that restrict the flow of positive (yang) and negative (yin) energy. Many ailments, including neuromyofascial pain, are thought to be symptomatic of restricted or unbalanced chi.

Much of the skepticism with chi in Western culture largely centers on the inability of modern science to quantify this energy force. Rather than casting doubt on the existence of chi, the lack of recognition reflects the inflexibility and underlying hubris of modern Western paradigms. Acceptance of chi is not a prerequisite for practicing ETPS therapy; however, an open mind to its potential healing power is necessary.

ETPS adopts a simplified approach to chi. Positive or negative polarity (vasodilative or vasoconstrictive therapy) may be applied to trigger or acupuncture points depending on the historical response of the condition to heat and ice. Excessive or hyperfunctioning conditions usually respond better to vasoconstrictive therapy, while deficient or hypofunctioning conditions respond better to vasodilative therapy.

The circulatory setting is especially important with some chronic pain categories, such as fibromyalgia and reflex sympathetic dystrophy, where the traditional vasoconstrictive approach to pain therapy is poorly tolerated by patients. The therapeutic versatility necessary to treat positive and negative polarity is accomplished with ETPS' neuropoint stimulator, which has a current reversal function.

The importance of polarity in the treatment of pain should not be discounted. Based on our clinical experience, there appears to be a 70:30 split in the chronic pain population; approximately 70% of patients respond better to vasoconstrictive therapy (sedation), while 30% respond better to vasodilative therapy (tonification). With ETPS stimulation, therapists have the option of easily incorporating these ancient, but powerful healing philosophies into treatment protocols increasing flexibility and individualizing the therapy to better suit patient needs.

THE RELATIONSHIP BETWEEN RADICULOPATHY, AND NEUROPATHY AND CHRONIC PAIN

Neuropathic Therapy

ETPS therapy has achieved significant success in relieving pain by integrating acupuncture philosophies into pain protocols. However, a singular reliance on acupuncture for treatment was found to be insufficient in addressing a number of neuropathic and mechanical issues. For instance, acupuncture offers no clear direction for the treatment of impinged nerves, nor does it integrate dermatomes and neuropathic pain patterns into protocols. Through years of experience, ETPS therapy has found that neuropathy plays a role in chronic pain and that its treatment through ETPS therapy can, in some cases, reduce or eliminate the need for drugs and surgery.

The introduction of neuropathic pain therapies into ETPS protocols greatly enhanced the understanding and therapeutic outcomes of chronic pain syndromes. The theories of radiculopathy and neuropathy suggest that nociception and inflammation are not the catalysts for chronic pain syndromes. Instead, the root of many chronic pain syndromes appears to be neuropathy and the muscular contractions causing neuropathy.

The cause of neuropathy is thought to be severe muscular contraction, that is, muscles that have contracted and remain contracted in the absence of action potential. Radiculopathy, defined as neuropathy at the nerve root, seems to have the strongest influence on chronic pain syndromes. Radiculopathy impinges nerves at the root and causing abnormal functioning of the pathways as well as the muscle tissue they innervate. In this way, radiculopathy creates an increased susceptibility to injuries along the dermatomes to the nerve endings.

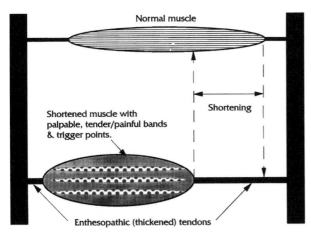

FIGURE 54.5 Top muscle illustrates muscular homeostasis. Lower muscle indicates muscle shortening, stretching of the tendons, and straining of the joints.

ETPS electrical stimulation produces a myofascial release of contracted muscles. When muscles contract and remain contracted, there is an electrical depolarization within the muscle (Fambrough, Hartzell, Powell, Rash, & Joseph, 1974; Becker & Selden, 1987). ETPS direct current stimulus creates an electrical loop within the muscles, enabling electrical repolarization and thus relaxation of the muscles (Figure 54.5).

Radiculopathy and Chronic Pain

Poor postural lifestyle and repetitive strain motions, usually occurring while playing sports or in the workplace, contribute to a pooling of "micro" injuries in the paraspinal muscles. If a sufficient number of micro injuries build up over time, a relatively minor movement by the patient can initiate paraspinal muscular contraction severe enough to produce radiculopathy and chronic pain (Bradley, 1974; Gunn, 1980; Gunn, et al., 1976; Gunn, et al., 1978; Gunn & Milbrandt, 1976; Loh & Nathan, 1978; Sola, 1981; 1984; Thomas and Ochoa, 1993).

Radiculopathy caused by paraspinal muscular contraction is believed to affect the ANS by impinging nerves at the nerve root, usually proximal to the dorsal/ventral rami juncture. Nerve impingement reduces the flow of motor impulses throughout the nerve pathway. According to Cannon's Law of Denervation (Cannon & Rosenbluth, 1949), a reduction of motor impulses through a nerve pathway produces disuse sensitivity and abnormal behavior within the receptor organ or tissue.

Radiculopathy influences tissue throughout the entire dermatome by reducing the flow of motor impulses at the nerve root. Nerve impingement and radiculopathy also influence distal pain by elevating acetycholine (ACH) and adrenaline levels throughout the pathways (Cannon & Rosenbluth, 1949), thereby increasing susceptibility to extremity muscular contraction (i.e., neuropathy). The environment created by increasing susceptibility to extremity neuropathy also increases susceptibility to distal injuries. Based on this series of relationships, it should be apparent that the treatment of most distal injuries must include an examination of the spine. In other words, if the spine significantly contributes to distal injuries, it should be a focus in pain therapy.

If paraspinal muscular contractions (radiculopathy) contribute significantly to distal pain and/or disease, then the release of paraspinal muscles through ETPS therapy should provide relief to distal pain disorders. Therefore, stimulating the paraspinal "Back Shu" points, which directly influence radiculopathic segments, can relax contracted muscles to a degree sufficient to reduce nerve impingement and allow the increase of motor impulses throughout the nerve pathways.

Manifestations of Radiculopathy and Neuropathy

Back Shu points are located paraspinally at the level of the spinous process interspace. Segmental levels with radiculopathy should be selected according to the following manifestations:

  Bilateral signs of trophedema are usually located at segmental levels L1–S3. Trophedema is a collagenic change in the skin that occurs when impinged nerves reduce the flow of motor impulses through pathways. Trophedema may be located with the "skin rolling" test, which will clearly identify the location in relation to nontrophic skin (Figure 54.6). Another manifestation, sudomotor, can be identified visually because it produces general warmth and sweating in the vicinity of radiculopathy. Trophedema and sudomotor manifestations are commonly located in the lumbar sacral segmental levels of L1–S3. Once the radiculopathic segments have been identified, they are correlated via dermatomes to distal injuries/pain conditions to determine root involvement in chronic pain conditions.

  Motor bands may be palpated paraspinally throughout contracted muscles, usually T2–T12. Cross-fiber palpation will easily identify thick, ropy bands within paraspinal muscle bellies that often run the entire length of the muscle.

  Posterior and lateral neck creasing at segmental levels, usually C2–T1 (Figure 54.7). Skin creasing suggests that some degenerative changes have occurred in the neck at the related segmental level. Occasionally, major creases will occur at every correlating segmental level on the neck.

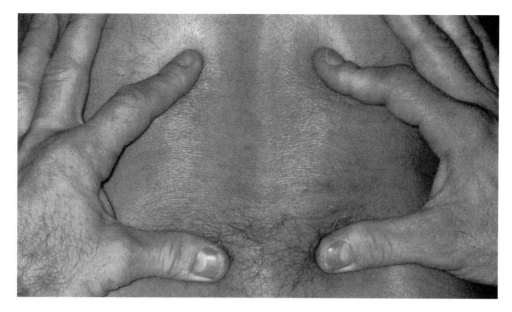

FIGURE 54.6 Illustration of trophedma (physical manifestation of nerve impingement, called radiculopathy) as demonstrated using the "skin rolling" test.

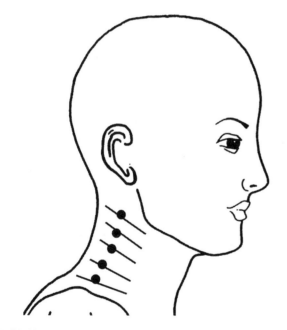

FIGURE 54.7 Illustrates lateral creasing in the neck and the suggested location of myofascial release points throughout tight motor bands. DO NOT apply microcurrent stimulation anterior to the corner of the jaw (over the carotid sinus).

Sympathetic Deregulation with Parasympathetic Points

The ANS comprises the sympathetic and parasympathetic nervous systems. Both neuropathy and radiculopathy stress the ANS by producing nerve impingement. Nerve impingement blocks the flow of motor impulses and deprives an organ or tissue of excitatory input (e.g., neural impulses) for a period of time causing disuse supersen-

sitivity. Supersensitive nerve pathways and innervated structures react abnormally to stimuli, causing patients to perceive more pain than is actually being created (Bradley, 1974; Gunn, 1980; Gunn, et al., 1976; Gunn, et al., 1978; Gunn & Milbrandt, 1976; Loh & Nathan, 1978; Sola, 1981; 1984; Thomas and Ochoa, 1993).

Neuropathy, and radiculopathy in particular, increases the upregulation of the sympathetic nervous system by reducing the flow of motor impulses, making treatment difficult due to the patient's high sensitivity levels. Parasympathetic points treated with vasoconstrictive therapy deregulate the sympathetic nervous system, thereby permitting a more aggressive and proactive approach to patient treatment. Key parasympathetic points are as follows:

- Lu 9 (Figure 54.8). A powerful vascular/parasympathetic point. Located on the transverse wrist crease, in the hollow on the ulnar side of the radius bone.
- P 6. A good nausea and parasympathetic point. Located three fingers proximal from the most distal wrist crease, deep between the palmaris longus and flexor carpi tendons.
- H 7. A good mind-calming and parasympathetic point. Located on the transverse wrist crease, in a hollow on the radial side of the thick, flexor carpi ulnaris tendon.
- Sp 6 (Figure 54.9). An immune, parasympathetic, and distal pain point for perineum. Located four fingers superior to the medial malleolus and posterior to the tibia bone. Press against the posterior edge of the tibia bone to find this tender point properly.

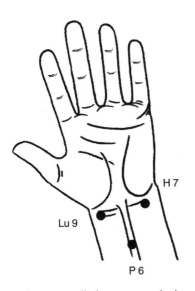

FIGURE 54.8 Three upper limb parasympathetic points Lu 9, P 6, and H 7, used to deregulate the autonomic nervous system (ANS), permitting continued therapy on supersensitive patients.

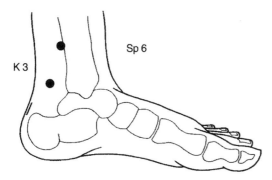

FIGURE 54.9 Sp 6 and K 3 are lower limb parasympathetic points for deregulation of lower viscera, again, permitting continued therapy on sensitive patients.

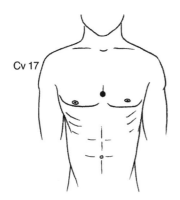

FIGURE 54.10 Acupuncture point for body calming. Also called "sea of tranquility." CV 17 should ONLY be treated on severe pain patients, and only AFTER all the above points have been treated.

- K 3. A low back pain, congenital energy, and parasympathetic point. Located in the hollow midway between the medial malleolus and the Achilles tendon. Used for morning back pain, circuited with B 25 (L 4–L 5 interspace).
- Cv 17 (Figure 54.10). A respiratory and parasympathetic point. Located on the midline of the sternum, horizontal with the fourth intercostal space.

THE RELATIONSHIP BETWEEN DERMATOMES AND CHRONIC PAIN

The application of ETPS therapy requires an inspection of dermatomes for their interrelationship with segmental levels. This important inspection will provide evidence in determining if radiculopathy is contributing to a pain condition. Distal injuries are correlated first with their dermatomes and second proximally to the segmental levels that innervate the dermatomes. ETPS stimulation to paraspinal points that influence the dermatomes and nerve pathways will relax contracted muscles, allowing for increased motor impulses throughout pathways, improved nerve regeneration, and reduced pain levels (Figure 54.11).

There are three ways to integrate the nerve root with pathways and dermatomes: segmental nerve root and paraspinal stimulation, nerve pathway treatment, and integrative circuits and nerve ending treatment using distal dermatome and acupuncture points.

Paraspinal Point Location

Radiculopathy and nerve impingements often occur paraspinally at the segmental nerve root and innervate the injury or pain area. Locating and treating paraspinal points corresponding to radiculopathic segmental levels is an important step in the application of ETPS protocols.

These paraspinal points are located approximately 1 in. bilateral to the midline on the medial border of the erector spinal muscles ridge. When stimulated, they provide a relaxing effect on the deep paraspinal muscles of semispinalis, longissimus, and iliocostalis, all of which influence the entire spinal column and the extremities through the dermatomes. One of the most successful applications of this ETPS paraspinal therapy is at the L 4–S 2 segmental levels, which innervate the lower limbs and feet. Paraspinal stimulation of L 4–S 2 segmental levels can provide significant pain relief to the vast majority of patients suffering from lower extremity pain such as plantar fasciitis, peripheral neuropathy, metatarsalgia, and heel spurs.

The integration of paraspinal segmental points into the clinical pain setting is an effective therapy. Pain must travel through the pathways and all pathways are connected to the spinal cord. Spinal Back Shu points are selected according to neuropathic manifestations

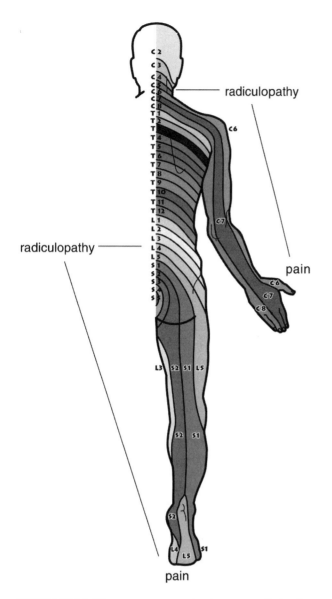

FIGURE 54.11 Illustrates nerve root impingement called radiculopathy, influences distal pain throughout the extremities.

observed at the segmental levels that innervate the injury or pain syndrome. Different manifestations will affect different segmental levels. Brief stimulation of these spinal points with ETPS therapy provides an easily integrated, diagnostic, and effective approach to chronic pain management.

Integrative Neural Circuits

Circuits have been used in acupuncture therapy for centuries. A circuit consists of a series of stimulated points integrated into a single treatment to produce enhanced therapeutic benefits. In ETPS therapy, selected acupuncture, trigger, and motor points are circuited for their ability to isolate nerve pathways and relax specific muscles and groups of muscles. Segmental level L 2–L 3 has, for

instance, a strong analgesic relationship with the lumbar region. In traditional acupuncture, this segmental level relates to the kidneys, widely regarded as powerful organs in pain therapy, which indirectly influence the spinal column. Paraspinal points at segmental level L 2–L 3 (B 23 in acupuncture) are circuited with B 40 (a distal acupuncture point for the lower back) to produce a powerful analgesic response for lower back pain.

Another circuit combines segmental levels L 4–L 5 (B 25 in acupuncture) with the important low back pain point B 60 (lateral malleolus). B 60 strongly influences the L 5 dermatome, and produces a strong analgesic response in sciatic patients when circuited with the L 4–L 5 nerve roots. This circuit is ideal for patients whose pain gets progressively worse throughout the day.

The circuit L 4–L 5 (B 25) and K 3 (medial malleolus, opposite B 60) provides another opportunity to individualize pain treatment to meet patients' needs. This circuit is ideal when sciatic/low back patients display morning pain and stiffness that may or may not improve throughout the day. Recognizing that patients with morning back pain and stiffness often display weak kidneys, circuiting B 25 and K 3 treats the kidneys by helping to relieve stiffness and stimulate nerve roots, thereby addressing radiculopathic and energetic contributions to injury. (See Figure 54.12.)

In ETPS therapy, there are numerous circuits that produce outstanding responses. A therapist who possesses a working knowledge of dermatomal patterns and extremity acupuncture points may use this understanding to create integrative circuits. Circuits are created between the dermatomal nerve root (spinal points) and any major trigger/acupuncture points located distal to the injury. These circuits permit therapists to release individual or groups of muscles in one application, ultimately saving manual therapists time and effort.

Integrating Dermatome Points

The final approach to integrating segmental/dermal therapy is the treatment of dermatome points located on the lateral and medial side of the nail base at the tips of the fingers and toes. All dermatomes and meridians connect the extremities with the midline. Therefore, if stimulation is applied at the nerve root to alleviate distal pain, stimulation may also be applied to the extremities to alleviate proximal pain. Stimulation is applied to dermal points on the fingers and toes relating to pain along dermatomes and meridians. In our experience dermatome point stimulation has been found to be a successful treatment for a significant percentage of patients who are unresponsive to nerve root and pathway treatments and an integrative adjunct to improve outcomes. (See Figure 54.13.)

Successful applications of this circuit are often applied on the feet. Segmental levels L 4–S 2 innervate the feet

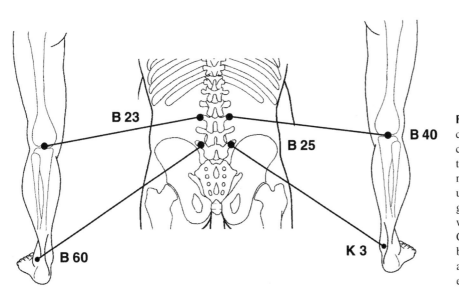

FIGURE 54.12 Illustrates neural circuits performed in ETPS therapy. Circuits B 23–B 40 are treated bilaterally to reduce upper leg pain and calm nerve pathways resulting from radiculopathy. Circuits B 25–K 3 are integrated bilaterally for back patients with pain aggravation in the morning. Circuits B 25–B 60 are integrated bilaterally for back patients with pain aggravation in the afternoon or evening.

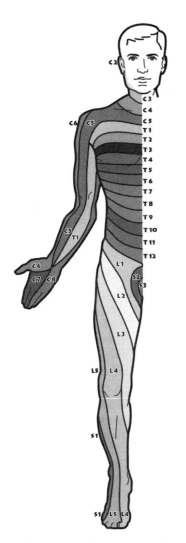

FIGURE 54.13 Illustration of the segmental dermatomes.

ETPS individually to produce an effective analgesic response in the lower back. More importantly, these dermal points also represent the end of the two acupuncture meridians, the gallbladder and the bladder, both of which have a strong influence over hip and back pain. Gb 44 is located on the fourth toe and B 67 is located on the fifth "baby" toe. Proximally following the meridians, the gallbladder meridian influences the lateral leg and hip region, while the bladder meridian influences the spine. Therefore, these two points may be used to diagnostically determine root causes of low back or hip pain. If Gb 44 is more sensitive than B 67, the piriformis–iliotibial fascial muscles (and, therefore, the gait) are more likely to be responsible for a patient's back pain. If B 67 is more sensitive, local spinal pathology, such as a bulging disc, is most likely responsible. Through years of ETPS experience, the sensitivity of these two points has proven to be an accurate diagnostic indicator of pain, mechanical imbalances, or neuropathy along the meridian or the muscles that intersect the meridian. (See Figure 54.14.)

Myofascial Release with Dermatome Therapy Points

The cross integration of dermatomal points with acupuncture meridians displays the flexibility of ETPS therapy. Dermatome points correspond strongly with jing well points, acupuncture points used to treat acute diseases in related organs. Dermatome point stimulation also is an effective treatment for myofascial release of muscles relating to, or intersecting with, correlating meridians. The integration of dermatomal and jing well points has proven successful in the treatment of hard to reach muscles, such as the psoas, and difficult injuries, such as adductor groin. Far from experimental, this technique has been applied for decades in many therapies, including Electro Acupuncture According to Voll (EAV) therapy, with much reported

with the fourth and fifth toes representing the L 5 and S 1 dermatomes. These two points may be stimulated with

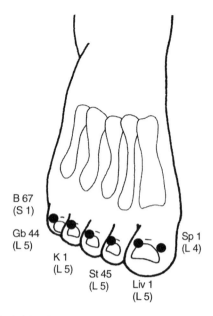

FIGURE 54.14 Distal acupuncture points that correspond to the segmental dermatomes. Located at the base of the nail, on the illustrated side.

success. The example described below, focusing on the stomach meridian and the psoas muscle, demonstrates an effective application of this approach.

There is a strong myofascial/therapeutic relationship between the psoas muscle, the stomach meridian and the corresponding jing well point. If the stomach meridian is followed proximally from the distal end at St 45 (located on the lateral base of the second toenail), the meridian travels through the quadriceps and intersects the psoas muscle (Figures 54.15 and 54.16). Stimulation of St 45 provides effective myofascial release of the corresponding ipsilateral psoas muscle. Widespread success of this technique has been witnessed at ETPS workshops and reported through clinical feedback, with approximately 80% myofascial release occurring within minutes of treatment. This unique ETPS response can save manual therapists a significant number of hours of therapeutic work in addition to rescuing patients from the agony of deep manual therapy.

Another therapeutic pearl is the stimulation of Sp1 (L 4 dermatome point located at the medial nail base of the first toe) for groin pain. Traditionally used for acute menstrual cramping, this technique has proven successful in relieving pain associated with difficult to treat adductor groin injuries in ETPS therapy. In many cases, successful results have been achieved within minutes of treatment.

The integration of dermatome points provides one of the simplest approaches to the treatment of pain. With a working knowledge of dermatomal patterns and acupuncture meridians, a therapist can quickly treat any proximal segment or muscle with the related dermal points.

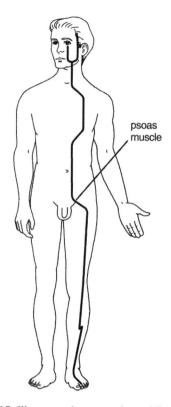

FIGURE 54.15 Illustrates the stomach meridian and the anatomical location of the psoas muscle.

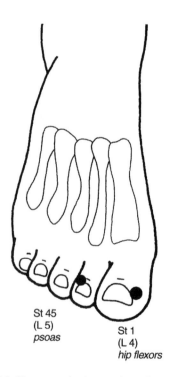

FIGURE 54.16 Illustrates the integration of acupuncture "jing well" points with meridians for myofascial release of psoas and hip flexor muscles.

The Relationship between the Gait and Chronic Pain

For many years, different fields of science and meridian research have studied the mechanics of the human body in order to identify potential relationships with chronic pain. Based on our experience with ETPS therapy, there appears to be a causal relationship between the gait and several chronic pain syndromes. In more precise terms, body asymmetry produces an irregular gait that stresses the ANS, which in turn causes pain (Figure 54.17).

"Gait" refers to the postural positioning of the iliac crest and its subsequent relationship to the spine and lower limbs. A positive right gait will, for instance, produce a shortened right leg and a length discrepancy between the two legs. Leg length discrepancy (LLD) leads to asymmetrical movement with a disproportional amount of body weight shifted to the longer and often weaker leg (Figures 54.18 and 54.19).

Positive gait irregularities also stress the spine to produce misalignment of the segments, asymmetrical movement, and paraspinal degenerative changes. These mechanical imbalances precipitate muscular contractions and radiculopathy (Friberg, 1983; Yochum & Barry, 1994). Radiculopathy leads to denervation supersensitivity of the nerves and an upregulation of the sympathetic nervous system. Thus, radiculopathy not only contributes to and perpetuates chronic pain, but also can serve as the major precipitator of chronic pain syndromes in many cases.

After studying hip positioning and mechanical relationships to the gait, there appears to be a neuropathic and, therefore, myofascial component to asymmetrical positioning. If contracted, the piriformis muscle, and its specific attachments, may be responsible for gait misalignments. Viewed through the ETPS framework of analysis, the trochanter will be pulled upward (superiorly) in the acetabulum if the piriformis contracts, thereby producing a positive, or higher, hip on one side. This imbalance in turn pulls up the femur to create a LLD. Therefore, the first step in treating gait imbalances should be a manual correction of the gait and LLD after a visual inspection has been completed.

Current therapeutic solutions to LLD include lifts and orthotics. The problem with these solutions is that they do not specifically address the root causes of LLD. The dominant one-sided nature of the human body, combined with the prevalence of repetitive-action lifestyles, places stress on the piriformis muscle resulting in contraction. If true, leg length corrections that do not address the gait may actually contribute to poor body mechanics and a continued stressing of the ANS.

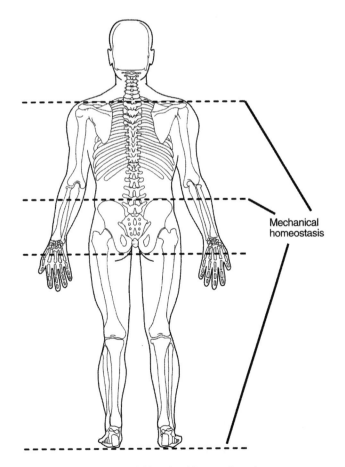

FIGURE 54.17 Mechanical homeostasis, as seen by level hip, shoulders, and trochanters.

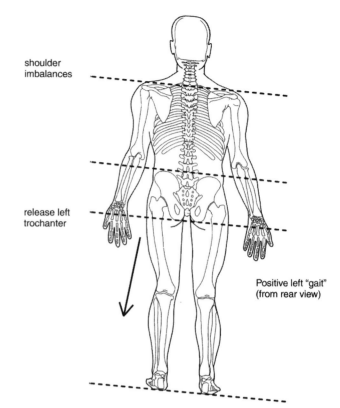

FIGURE 54.18 Illustrates superior movement of left trochanter in the actetablum. This is often due to contraction of the piriformis muscle, which precipitates mechanical imbalances of the shoulders and hips, and leg length discrepancy of the left leg. Called a positive "left" gait.

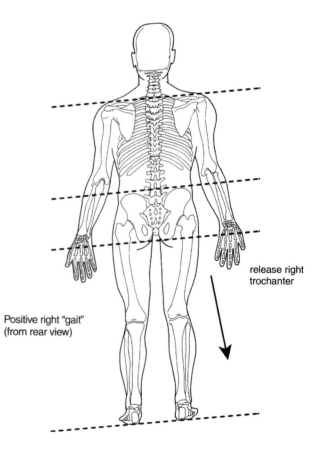

FIGURE 54.19 Illustrates superior movement of right trochanter in the acetablum. This is often due to contraction of the piriformis muscle, which precipitates mechanical imbalances of the shoulders and hips, and leg length discrepancy of the right leg. Called a positive "right" gait.

Manual Piriformis Stretch

In ETPS therapy, a specific manual therapy called a piriformis stretch is performed in order to properly reposition the trochanter in the acetabulum; in other words, realign the hip and pelvis. Stretching the piriformis until the trochanter and acetabulum restore proper gait balance will produce symmetrical leg lengths and mechanical homeostasis throughout the body. With the patient in the prone position, approach from the right (R) side, place your R hand on the superior angle of the trochanter at a 45% angle. Lift the leg 6 in. above the knee with the left (L) hand and abduct the leg to a 30% angle or until trochanter becomes prominent on the R hand.

In one motion, rotate your R hand medially and use the L hand to gently lift the R leg on midline (beside the L leg). If properly executed, this piriformis stretch places the trochanter in the proper anatomical location creating hip, spine, and mechanical symmetry throughout the body. In some cases, the shortened leg is so badly displaced in the trochanter that this realignment technique will make the shorter leg longer than the other one. For this reason, the piriformis stretch should always be performed bilaterally to ensure symmetry of the hip and pelvis. The importance of symmetry throughout the hip and pelvis region in general, and the piriformis stretch in particular, cannot be understated in the fight against chronic pain.

Myofascial Release of Piriformis Using Circuits

After achieving mechanical repositioning, a myofascial release on the piriformis must be completed to prevent the leg from recontracting and producing the same positive gait and LLD. Without this release, a repetitive lifestyle would constantly pressure the piriformis to recontract, thereby misaligning the gait and creating the conditions for the cycle to reappear.

Two circuits will release the piriformis, hip, and lateral thigh muscles (Figure 54.20). The first is the piriformis–IT circuit. To start, palpate cross-fiber at the superior angle of the piriformis muscle. Thick motor bands are often easily palpated where piriformis glute min/medius meet. Apply one circuit to the most tender trigger point found within the motor bands; the other circuit should be applied to the trigger point of the iliotibial band (found at the end of main rae with hands at the side (Gb 31 in acupuncture). Simultaneous stimulation of these two points often provides a strong myofascial response between the hip and lateral thigh muscles, creating immediate pain relief. It also allows the piriformis muscle to relax and facilitates proper positioning of the trochanter in the acetabulum.

Piriformis–Gb 34 is the second circuit. For this treatment, keep one modality on the same tender piriformis trigger point as above. The other modality is placed on Gb 34, the acupuncture point responsible for relaxing muscle tissue (inferior and posterior to the head of the fibula). This circuit performs an overall myofascial release and often relaxes muscular tissue not released in the first circuit.

To perform a myofascial release, two circuits must be created. The first is a circuit between the superior angle of the piriformis trigger point and the middle of the IT band (acupuncture point Gb 31). The second circuit is performed between the superior angle of the piriformis trigger point and the myofascial acupuncture point Gb 34 (inferior/posterior to head of fibula). These two circuits, performed bilaterally, are effective in maintaining a myofascial release of the piriformis and related gluteal and hip muscles responsible for gait misalignment.

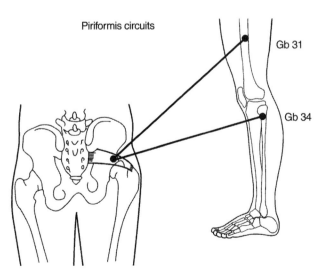

FIGURE 54.20 Piriformis circuits are performed to produce myofascial release of hip and leg muscles responsible for gait imbalances. They are applied bilaterally after mechanical realignment for optimal, lasting results.

The integration of a piriformis stretch/release is an important part of ETPS protocols. Its introduction can significantly improve soft tissue and mechanically based therapeutic outcomes of any pain program. Once learned, the stretch can be applied in seconds and should be integrated into any pain management protocol.

THE RELATIONSHIP BETWEEN SCAR THERAPY AND CHRONIC PAIN

Occasionally, patients may continue to suffer from pain after receiving treatment based on the above-mentioned therapeutic steps addressing the mechanical and myofascial components of chronic pain. Therefore, other sources of pain, such as neural therapy, have been included in ETPS protocols to treat scars throughout the dermatomes and meridians.

Neural therapy, the stimulation of scars for pain reduction and homeostasis, has been an accepted and proven form of neuromyofascial pain therapy for years. Neural therapy theory suggests that scarring restricts the flow of energy, disrupts the lymphatic and circulatory systems, and interferes with muscle energy and mechanical stability of the body. All of these systems are affected adversely when a scar influences the dermatome or meridian to which it is connected.

For unresponsive pain conditions, inspection for distal scarring along the dermatomes or distal/proximal scarring along the meridian can be helpful in determining where to treat the pain condition next. If a scar is located in the corresponding dermatome or meridian, ETPS stimulation along the scar perimeter can provide immense relief to suffering patients. This approach is especially effective if there is extremity joint scarring, especially around the ankle and knees.

Based on current medical knowledge, it is not clear why scar stimulation is an effective form of treatment for some patients. One leading theory suggests that neural therapy "breaks up" the collagenic tissue surrounding the scar. Intermittent stimulation of the scar perimeter, sometimes called "surrounding the dragon," is thought to break up scars, thereby permitting an increase in the functioning and homeostasis of the lymphatic, energetic, neural, and circulatory systems. Irrespective of the pathology, scar treatment has been found to reduce local pain. The stimulation of scars relative to the injury via dermatomes and meridians has produced impressive therapeutic responses with some hard-to-treat chronic local pain as well as discomfort along the dermatome and meridians

APPLICATION OF ETPS STIMULATION

Traditional stimulation of trigger motor and acupuncture points includes invasive techniques such as acupuncture and hypodermic needles and noninvasive modalities such as TENS and microcurrent stimulation. Both TENS and microcurrent stimulation may be applied with traditional pads or via point stimulation. Truly integrative therapies, such as ETPS, employ potent, versatile, and patient-friendly stimulation. Based on these criteria, an initial treatment utilizing invasive needles is relatively less productive because it damages tissue and requires a recovery and/or an incubation period of 20 to 30 minutes to determine therapeutic efficacy. In contrast, ETPS therapy often can generate positive results in a matter of minutes.

ETPS therapy is best applied with noninvasive direct current (DC) stimulation. Alternating current (AC) is ineffective because it does not produce the square wave necessary for the stimulation of an endorphin response (Christopher, et al., 1992; Lehman, et al., 1986; Pomeranz et al., 1988; Pomeranz & Niziak, 1987). Furthermore, AC cannot by definition produce a monophasic pulse, a form of stimulation that can be reversed in order to produce the highly sought after vasodilative and vasoconstrictive responses (Bronzino, 1998). DC also is favored for its ability to repolarize contracted muscle tissue, a necessary physiological response for the release of myofascial tension. Finally, DC stimulation is preferred because it produces few, if any, adverse side effects. With no significant iatrogenic responses, noninvasive and concentrated DC stimulation can be used to treat multiple systems at one sitting, thereby creating an opportunity to outperform traditional needle therapies that concentrate on one system in each treatment. The result is greater therapeutic versatility and productivity.

ETPS applies DC microstimulation in stages to determine the root cause of chronic pain syndromes. Concentrated DC microstimulation, applied by a point stimulator, is the only modality that can produce therapeutic responses quickly enough to eliminate or include therapeutic systems in future treatment protocols. Traditional TENS, applied by pads, is far too inefficient a stimulation to produce beneficial therapeutic response in a short period of time (Cheng & Pomeranz, 1986; Gadsby & Flowerdew, 2000). Therefore, pad stimulation is not the desirable modality for ETPS therapy.

PART B: ETPS INTEGRATIVE PROTOCOLS

ETPS integrative protocols combine the therapeutic efficacy of acupuncture, intramuscular therapy, and neural therapies. As a rule, a mechanical neuropathic assessment is performed and stimulation is applied in stages in order to isolate fascial, neural, or meridian systems and to determine and treat the root cause(s) of neuromyofascial pain. The application of these different integrative therapies, methodically and in stages, to isolate different therapeutic systems provides a window of opportunity for healthcare practitioners (HCP) to diagnose soft tissue pain.

The first step in the treatment of any chronic pain condition is to assess and apply the ETPS Standard Protocol. The ETPS Standard Protocol is designed to address body mechanics, radiculopathy, and spine therapy as well as fascial contractions responsible for positive gait and body misalignment. ETPS therapy initially assumes that chronic pain syndromes have a precipitory influence from the hip misalignment and lower back radiculopathy. Therefore, the Standard Protocol will identify or eliminate the nerve root, gait, and body mechanics as major contributors to the chronic pain condition.

Depending on the results of the initial assessment, one or more specific sets of protocols may be performed. The Standard Protocol is described below as well as protocols for back pain, neck pain, fibromyalgia, and plantar fasciitis.

STANDARD PROTOCOL

1. Assess patient for gait and radiculopathic irregularities.

   The first step in standard protocol is to assess the patient in order to determine the degree of discomfort, range of motion or injury, degree of disability, and level of pain. Identify gait imbalances through iliac crest levels and leg length discrepancies. Select vertebral segments that display radiculopathic manifestations of trophedema and sudomotor responses.

2. Manually release gait and stretch piriformis.

   Manually release the gait using the piriformis stretch (as described in Part A). Start with the side with the positive (or higher) gait and the shorter leg. Perform stretch bilaterally.

3. Treat radiculopathy at levels identified in Step 1 with a paraspinal release using Back Shu points.

   These points are located at each segmental level at the spinous process interspace (SPI), approximately 1 in. bilateral at the medial border of the erector spinal muscle ridge (two fingers bilateral from midline).

   The simultaneous application of two ETPS modalities to these bilateral spinal points provides an exceptional myofascial release of the paraspinal muscles that precipitate radiculopathy and nerve impingement. If ETPS therapy is applied to a series of spinal points correlating to an area of radiculopathy that innervates distal pain or injuries, the entire pain condition may be treated (Figure 54.21).

4. Release piriformis with fascial circuit Piriformis–IT band, Piriformis–Gb 34.

   Release fascia responsible for gait misalignment by performing a fascial circuit between any tender motor bands palpated throughout the piriformis muscle, the IT band point (Gb 31), and the myofascial point Gb 34 (Figure 54.22). Ask the patient to sit up slowly and then slide off the table, placing both feet on the ground at the same time (to prolong treatment outcome).

   The Standard Protocol effectively treats lower back radiculopathy and fascial components of gait and overall mechanical imbalances. Many pain conditions throughout the body may be effectively treated with the Standard Protocol, suggesting that radiculopathy and gait imbalances are major contributors to the chronic pain cycle.

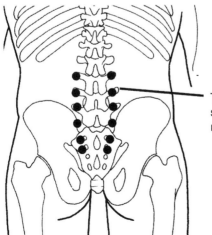

Treat spinal points at segmental levels where radiculopathy is found

FIGURE 54.21 Illustrates paraspinal points treated in areas of trophedema (nerve root impingement), identified during skin rolling test (see Figure 54.6).

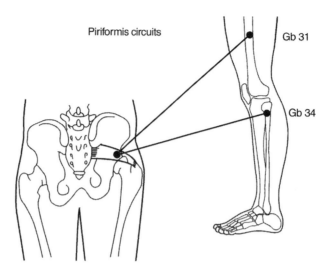

FIGURE 54.22 Piriformis circuits are performed to produce myofascial release of hip and leg muscles responsible for gait imbalances. Applied bilaterally after mechanical realignment for optimal, lasting results.

Other Integrative Protocols

ETPS integrative protocols go beyond standard procedures with the inclusion of segmental levels, fascial planes, and acupuncture-trigger points that work well for individual pain conditions. Additional circuits, fascial groups, and modalities are included on a step-by-step basis with an assessment performed at the end of each step or stage.

ETPS protocols are designed to integrate different philosophies and apply treatments in stages to determine the root cause of pain. Once the root causes have been determined, continued treatment may be applied to areas known to produce therapeutic responses. If applied properly, ETPS therapy can diagnose the root cause of pain with a significant degree of accuracy, thus assisting all HCP in the treatment of chronic soft tissue pain.

In ETPS therapy, the patient is assessed before and after each therapeutic stage to determine the degree of success. With several therapeutic stages in back pain, it is possible to determine which segmental levels, muscle dermatomes, and meridians are responsible for the patient's pain in approximately 10 to 15 minutes. Generally, one or more stages will produce pain relief for the majority of patients, thus indicating which dermatomes, segments, muscles, and meridians should be investigated further as the source of chronic pain. Stages that produce minimal or negative responses (i.e., the patient and pain are noticeably worse after treatment) should be eliminated in future treatment episodes. Using this therapeutic process of elimination, therapists can investigate and treat patients at the same time, ultimately producing faster and more effective outcomes. After assessing the exact points and therapeutic systems using the ETPS elimination process, concentrate only on those stages that produce positive therapeutic benefits.

Presented below are four additional protocols for the diagnosis and treatment of back pain, neck pain, fibromyalgia and plantar fasciitis.

Back Pain Protocol

Step 1 Apply Standard Protocol.
Assess patient after each of the following stages.
- Check gait–piriformis.
- Inspect for signs of neuropathy and radiculopathy, especially between L 2–S 2.
- Manually release gait.
- Perform paraspinal release at segments with trophedema (–ve).
- Circuit piriformis–IT Band (–ve) and piriformis–Gb 34.

Step 2 Stimulate circuits designed to treat the nerve pathway or meridian involved with injury.
Perform these circuits bilaterally with patient lying in the prone position. Ask patient to sit up and dismount with both feet landing on the floor at the same time. (See Figure 54.23.)
- Circuit L 2–L 3. Interspace with B 40 (low back pain distal point) and treat with negative (vasoconstrictive) polarity.
- Circuit L 4–L 5. Interspace with B 60 (anatomic and acupuncture trigger point) for patients whose pain becomes more severe throughout the day.
- Circuit L 4–L 5 with K 3 (kidney source point) for patients with back pain and stiffness that is most severe in the morning.

Step 3 Stimulate sacral triangle and dermatomal points for lateral hip release and spinal pain.

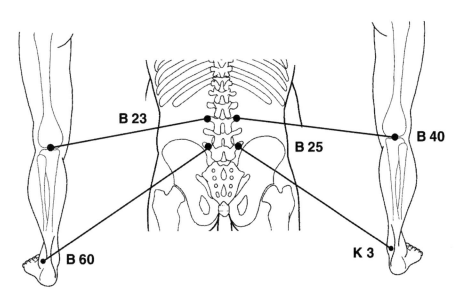

FIGURE 54.23 Neural circuits performed between paraspinal nerve root points and key distal acupuncture points to reduce upper leg pain and calm nerve pathways resulting from radiculopathy. Circuits B 23–B 40 are treated bilaterally. Circuits B 25–K 3 are integrated bilaterally for back patients with pain aggravation in the morning. Circuits B 25–B 60 are integrated bilaterally for back patients with pain aggravation in the afternoon and evening. Apply vasoconstrictive ETPS therapy.

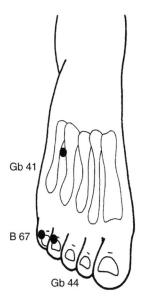

FIGURE 54.24 Distal acupuncture points B 67 and Gb 44 are combined with GB 41 to produce "sacral triangle." These points are treated to reduce proximal nerve root pain and for myofascial release of hips in stage three (3) of back pain protocol. Apply vasoconstrictive ETPS Therapy.

If success is limited in the first two steps, Step 3 can often provide immense relief to patients. Stimulation need only be applied for 20 to 30 seconds on the proper dermatome point in order to provide relief. Based on our experience using ETPS therapy, a significant number of patients with back pain will respond only to Step 3. Treat the distal dermatome points involved with painful or

radiculopathic vertebral segments, and the posterior/lateral muscles believed to be involved with mechanical gait imbalances.

- Sacral triangle includes B 67, Gb 44, and Gb 41. B 67 (located at the base of fifth toenail on the lateral side) and Gb 44 (located at the base of the fourth toenail lateral side) correlate to S 1 and L 5 dermatomes and nerve roots. Gb 41 is located at proximal end of the fourth and fifth tendons (Figure 54.24).

The application of ETPS dermatome points can produce useful information.

i. Are stimulated nerve endings most efficacious in the treatment of proximal pain?

ii. Are the hip and gluteal muscles responsible for back pain? If true, Gb 41 and Gb 44 will be sensitive.

iii. Is spinal injury or disc bulge responsible for back pain B 67? If true, the spine will be tender.

Step 4   Dermatomal points for anterior hip flexors.

Located at the lateral side of the base of the second toenail, St 45 isolates the treatment release of the psoas and hip flexor muscles (Figure 54.25). With some pain patients, the psoas muscle may be contracted alone or with the piriformis muscle. If pain continues to persist after Steps 1 to 3, a quick stimulation of St45 (second toe base nail lateral side) will reveal if the psoas muscle is contributing to the pain condition. Patients

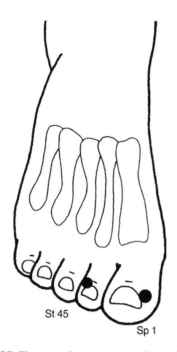

FIGURE 54.25 Illustrates the acupuncture jing well points Sp 1 and St 45 used ipsilaterally for the myofascial release of the psoas and hip flexor muscles. Apply vasoconstrictive ETPS therapy.

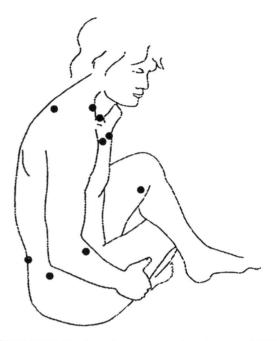

FIGURE 54.26 Tender points are treated at the end of ETPS protocols for additional pain relief. They are identified by the patient and treated in short intense bursts with ETPS stimulation. Apply vasoconstrictive ETPS therapy.

should be assessed between treatments of both the R and L points to determine which psoas muscle is most involved in the injury. This step is integrated to include both posterior and anterior hip stabilizing muscles in order to determine if they individually or collectively contribute to the patient's chronic pain state.

Step 5 Neural therapy.

Application of ETPS stimulation to scars that intersect with, or are located in, the dermatomes or on meridians that relate to pain is an effective approach to more complex pain conditions. Inspect for scarring, either surgical or injury related, distal in the dermatomes to the injury and distal proximal to the injury/pain along the meridian. For back pain, inspect for scars along the lateral anterior knees and paraspinal back. If scars exist, stimulate briefly (10 to 15 seconds) at 1/8-inch intervals surrounding the scar. This process has produced effective responses with many patients.

Step 6 Tender points.

Tender trigger points are treated as a last step in the therapy because ETPS assumes that all pain is referred from another anatomical area of the body. Therefore, the treatment of local pathology is secondary to root sources of pain (i.e., body mechanics and radiculopa-

thy). However, local pathology can exist and the tender trigger point(s) may be identified by the patient and treated by the therapist after Steps 1 through 5. After identification, apply brief ETPS stimulation of 15 to 20 seconds per point. This technique has proven successful in alleviating the majority of any pain that remains. (See Figure 54.26.)

NECK PAIN PROTOCOL

Step 1 Apply Standard Protocol.

Pay special attention to radiculopathy at the L 2–L 3 interspace levels, as they have a strong influence on neck pain.

Assess patient after each of the following stages.

- Check gait–piriformis.
- Look for signs of neuropathy and radiculopathy, especially at the L 2–L 3 level.
- Manually release gait.
- Perform paraspinal release at segments with trophedema (-ve)
- Circuit pirformis–IT Band (–ve) and piriformis–Gb 34.

Step 2 Posterior neck and trapezius release.

- Paraspinally release cervical neck at level of crease identified in Step 1. This step is designed to diagnose and treat the posterior muscles of the neck involved with injury.

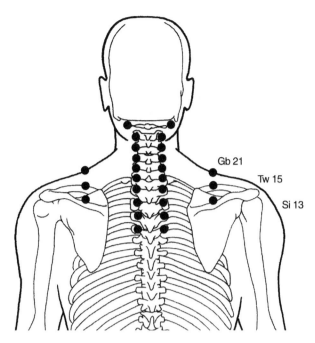

FIGURE 54.27 Illustrates the posterior paraspinal neck points and the trapezius myofascial release points. A positive therapeutic response indicates involvement of these segments and muscles with the injury. Apply vasoconstrictive ETPS therapy.

- Stimulate Gb 21, Tw 15, and Si 13, designed to release the trapezius, rhomboid, and supraspinatis muscles (Figure 54.27).

Step 3 Lateral neck release.
- Laterally release neck, palpating for motor bands. Stimulate the motor bands at the level of the horizontal neck creases. All contributors to neck and limb disorders, stimulation of these areas is designed to release the scalenes, levator scapula, and splenius capitus muscles (Figure 54.28).

Step 4 Distal point for the neck.
- Si 3: Posterior muscles of the neck. Located at the medial end of the distal transverse palm crease. Note: locate and treat this point with the fist clenched (Figure 54.29). This is the first point to treat when there is a wry neck or torticollis. Treat bilaterally.

Step 5 Dermal points for the neck.
Treat these points first if patient's neck is hypersensitive (i.e., postaccident/whiplash or postoperative). If not hypersensitive, follow protocol order.
- Li 1: Designed to release SCM ipsilaterally. Located at the radial side of the base of the index fingernail (Figure 54.30).
- Si 1: Designed to release ipsilateral scalenes. Located at the lateral side of the base of the little fingernail (fifth metacarpal).

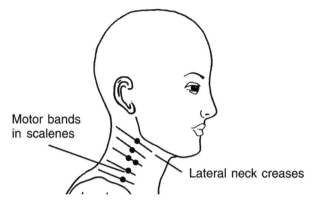

FIGURE 54.28 Illustrates lateral neck muscles and suggested location of myofascial release points throughout tight motor bands points. Release these with ETPS stimulation for highly effective relief of upper extremity pain. DO NOT apply microcurrent stimulation anterior to the corner of the jaw (over the carotid sinus). Apply vasoconstrictive ETPS therapy.

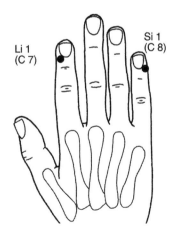

FIGURE 54.29 Confluent acupuncture point Si3 displays influence over the posterior neck and spine. Often highly sensitive on patients with posterior disc problems. Treat bilaterally, apply vasoconstrictive ETPS therapy.

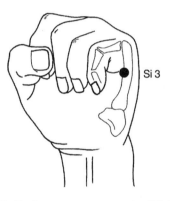

FIGURE 54.30 The hand illustrates the integration of acupuncture jing well points for myofascial release of Sterno Cliedo Mastoid (SCM) using Li 1 and the scalene muscles using Si 1. Treat bilaterally, applying vasoconstrictive ETPS therapy.

Step 6 Neural therapy.

Inspect for scarring, either surgical or injury, distal in the dermatomes from C 5–T 1 or along any upper limb meridians. For neck pain, inspect for scars around the elbow and wrist.

Step 7 Tender trigger points.

Ask the patient to identify any local tender points remaining in the cervical region. Apply ETPS therapy to these points, usually trigger points (TPs) or acupuncture points (APs) throughout injured tissue. Brief stimulation of 15 to 20 seconds per point has been successful in alleviating the majority of any pain that remains.

FIBROMYALGIA PROTOCOL

Step 1 Treat the parasympathetic points (-ve).

Treat the following parasympathetic points. Assess the patient after each stage.

- Lu 9 (Figure 54.31): A powerful vascular and parasympathetic point. Located on the transverse wrist crease, in a hollow on the ulnar side of the radial bone.
- P 6: A good nausea and parasympathetic point. Located three fingers proximal from the most distal wrist crease, deep between the palmaris and flexor carpi tendons.
- H 7: An excellent mind-calming and parasympathetic point. Located on the transverse wrist crease, in a hollow on the radial side of the thick flexor carpi ulnaris tendon.
- Sp 6 (Figure 54.32): An immune, parasympathetic, and distal pain point for perineum. Located four fingers superior to the medial malleolus and posterior to the tibia bone. Note: Press directly against the bone to find this point.
- K 3: A low back pain, congenital energy, and parasympathetic point. Located in the hollow midway between the medial malleolus and Achilles tendon. Also used for morning back pain and circuited with B 25 (L 4–L 5 interspace).
- Cv 17 (Figure 54.33): A respiratory and parasympathetic point. Located on the midline of the sternum, horizontal with the fourth intercostal space.

Step 2 Apply Standard Protocol.

Assess patient after each stage.

- Check gait–piriformis.
- Look for signs of radiculopathy (motor bands), especially at T 9–10 levels.
- Manually release gait.

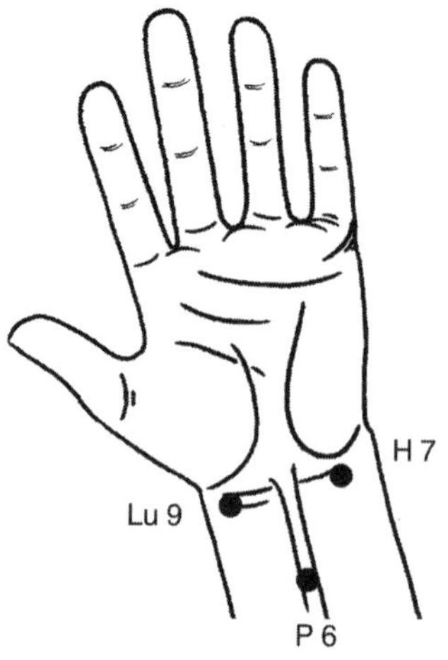

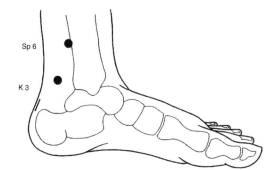

FIGURE 54.31 Three upper limb parasympathetic points Lu 9, P 6, and H 7, used to deregulate the Autonomic Nervous System (ANS), permitting continued therapy on supersensitive patients. Treat bilaterally, applying vasoconstrictive ETPS therapy.

FIGURE 54.32 Sp 6 and K 3 are lower limb parasympathetic points, used for deregulation of lower viscera, permitting continued therapy on sensitive patients. Treat bilaterally, applying vasoconstrictive ETPS therapy.

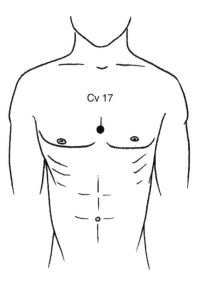

FIGURE 54.33 Acupuncture point for body calming. Also known as "sea of tranquility," Cv 17 should ONLY be treated on severe patients, and only AFTER all the above points have been treated.

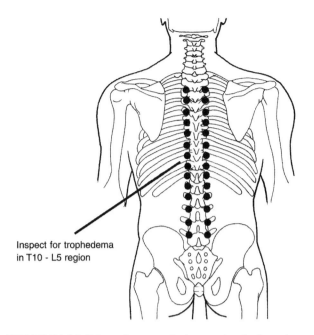

FIGURE 54.34 Palpate for paraspinal motor bands throughout the thoracic region. Release identified motor bands with paraspinal points. Apply vasodilative ETPS therapy.

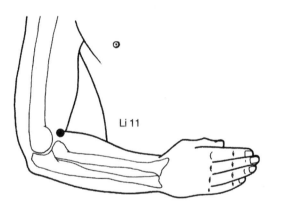

FIGURE 54.35 Homeostatic acupuncture point Li 11. Apply vasoconstrictive therapy to right arm and vasodilative therapy to left arm.

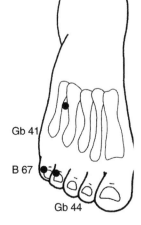

FIGURE 54.36 Sacral triangle may be treated with vasoconstrictive ETPS stimulation for additional relief beyond steps 1 to 3. Note the audible differences between B 67 and GB 44. A high pitch with GB 44 denotes hip and fascial pain root, and a high pitch with B 67 denotes spinal radiculopathic involvement in pain cycle.

- Perform paraspinal release from T 10–S 2 (+ ve) encompassing segments with trophedema (Figure 54.34). Note: Use positive polarity for paraspinal stimulation.
- Circuit pirformis–IT Band (–ve) and piriformis–Gb 34.

Step 3 Homeostatic point Li 11 (–ve).

If success is limited in the first two steps, Step 3 can often provide relief to the patient. Stimulation needs to be applied only for 20 to 30 seconds on the proper dermatome point in order to provide relief. It is located at the lateral end of the transverse elbow crease, with the elbow semiflexed (Figure 54.35).

Step 4 Sacral triangle B 67, Gb 44, Gb 41 (–ve) (Figure 54.36).

Isolate the treatment release of the psoas muscles. With some patients, the psoas muscle may be contracted alone or with the piriformis muscle. If pain still exists after Steps 1 through 3, a quick stimulation of St 45 (second toe base nail lateral side) will reveal if the psoas muscle is contributing to the pain condition.

Patients should be assessed between treatments of both the R and L points to determine which psoas muscle is most involved in the injury. This step is integrated into this protocol to include both posterior and anterior hip stabilizing muscles to determine if they individually or collectively contribute to the patient's chronic pain state.

Step 5 Release tender trigger points.

As noted earlier, tender trigger areas are treated as a last step in ETPS therapy because it is assumed that all pain is referred from another anatomical area of the body (Figure 54.37).

Ask the patient to identify tender points and apply ETPS therapy to these points (usually TPs or APs throughout injured tissue). Brief stimulation of 15 to 20 seconds per point has proven successful in alleviating the majority of any pain that remains. After each stage, stop and assess patient. Treat all points bilaterally.

PLANTAR FASCIITIS PROTOCOL

Step 1 Apply Standard Protocol.
Assess patient after each stage.
- Check gai–piriformis.
- Look for signs of neuropathy and radiculopathy.
- Manually release gait.

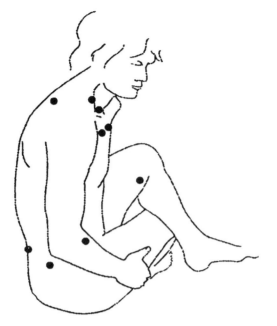

FIGURE 54.37 Two to three tender points may be identified by patient and treated AFTER the previous steps are completed. *Note:* Do not apply stimulation to more than three tender points, as aggravation of symptoms is common with excessive stimulation.

- Perform paraspinal release from L4–S2 (encompassing segments with trophedema) (Figure 54.38).
- Circuit pirformis–IT Band and piriformis–Gb34

Step 2 Myofascial release of fascial overlay throughout calf muscles.

B57 (Figure 54.39): Located at the muscular junction of the Achilles tendon, this is an excellent point for releasing the entire calf area.

Step 3 Treat local points for pain relief.

- K 3 (Figure 54.40): The best point to treat for patients who display a stiff back in the morning. Located in the hollow between the medial malleolus and the Achilles tendon.
- K 5: Located one thumb's width below K 3.
- K 6: Located in the hollow just below the medial malleolus.
- B 60 (Figure 54.41): Located in the hollow between the lateral malleolus and the Achilles tendon. Very tender on sciatica patients.
- B 62: Located in the hollow just below the lateral malleolus.

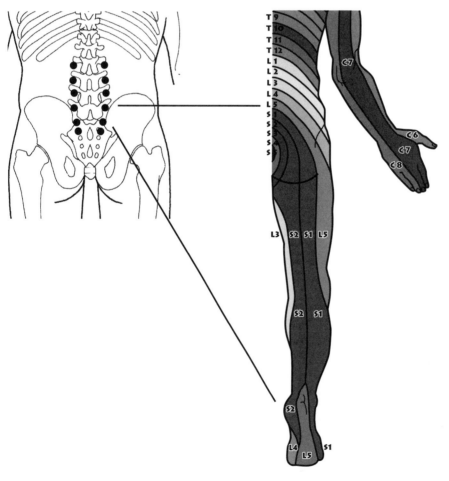

FIGURE 54.38 Inspect for trophedema at segmental levels L 4–S 2, as identified with skin rolling test (see Figure 54.6). Paraspinal release with vasoconstrictive ETPS therapy.

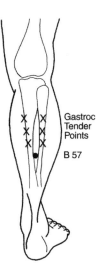

FIGURE 54.39 Release acupuncture point B 57 and tender points located throughout motor bands (identified through palpation) using vasoconstrictive ETPS therapy.

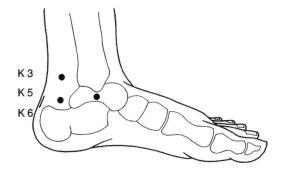

FIGURE 54.40 Local medial acupuncture points K 3, K 5, and K 6, which are treated for additional relief from plantar fasciitis pain. Treat with vasoconstrictive ETPS therapy.

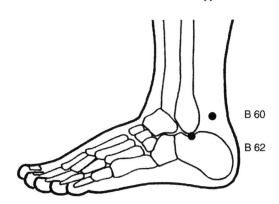

FIGURE 54.41 Local lateral acupuncture points B60 and B62, which are treated for additional relief from plantar fasciitis pain. Treat with vasoconstrictive ETPS therapy.

Step 4 Treat dermatome points.
- B 67 (Figure 54.42): At the base of the baby toenail, on the lateral side. Innervation, S 1
- Gb 44: At the base of the fourth toenail, on the lateral side. Innervation, L 5.

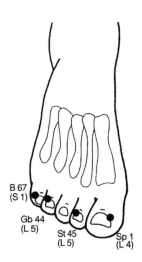

FIGURE 54.42 Distal jing well acupuncture points Sp 1, St 45, Gb 44, and B 67. Treat for additional relief of plantar fasciitis pain using vasoconstrictive ETPS therapy. *Note:* Audible differences between points and correlate to dermatomes for clues to root causes of pain.

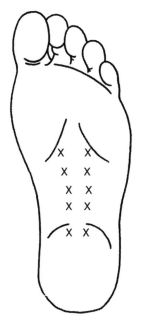

FIGURE 54.43 Apply vasoconstrictive ETPS therapy to tender points identified by patient on plantar region of foot.

- St 45: At the base of the second toenail, on the lateral side. Innervation, L5.
- Sp 1: At the base of the big toenail, on the medial side. Innervation, L 4.

Step 5 Tender trigger points.

Ask the patient to identify tender points and apply ETPS therapy to these points, (usually TPs or APs throughout injured tissue). Apply brief stimulation of 15 to 20 seconds per point (Figure 54.43).

CLINICAL RESEARCH STUDY

In a pilot study on carpal tunnel syndrome recently completed at the Canadian Centre for Integrative Medicine, Markham, Ontario, Dr. Gordon Ko (physiatrist, American Association of Electrodiagnostic Medicine) recorded improvements in five consecutive patients who completed ETPS (one time per week for 4 to 6 weeks). Using the Neuromax 1004 (including skin temperature measurements), the pre- and post-treatment median nerve latencies and amplitudes improved (9 hands). The mean scores are listed below with range in brackets.

Mean Values	Pre-Treatment	Post-Treatment
Distal motor latency	4.61 msec	4.22 msec
	(3.8 to 6.0)	(3.7 to 5.9)
Sensory onset latency		
Palmar	1.98 msec	1.81 msec
	(1.5 to 3.0)	(1.5 to 2.9)
2nd and 3rd digits	3.13 msec	2.93 msec
	(2.5 to 4.2)	(2.5 to 3.6)
Sensory amplitudes		
Palmar	37.0 uV	44.5 uV
	(19.3 to 99.0)	(29.3 to 120.3)
2nd and 3rd digits	13.6 uV	16.7 uV
	(5.0 to 22.7)	(5.3 to 26.0)

Clinical improvement was reported in all patients without any significant adverse effects. One patient with severe CTS who completed the "Dash" (Disabilities of the arm, shoulder, hand) survey demonstrated marked improvement with a pre-score of 20/100 and a post-score of 1.7/100 (a higher score indicates increased functional limitations). Prior to treatment, the patient's right-hand sensory responses were absent. After treatment, palmar and third digit responses were measurable.

Further research is required to verify the efficacy of treatment and supporting data. A call for patients is now under way to proceed with a larger controlled study with Dr. Gordon Ko at the University of Toronto.

ETPS NEUROPATHIC THERAPY CASE STUDY

A case study of the benefits of ETPS neuropathic therapy on 345 chronic pain patients was performed. Patients were all over the age of 65, and divided into two groups: one group treated daily for 3 weeks; one group treated themselves weekly for 3 months. Assessments were performed at the beginning and end of each time frame.

Mean scores improved in both groups without any adverse side effects. A significant improvement was reported in the mean score with patients listed below:

Mean Values	Pre-Treatment	Post-Treatment
Average pain score: Daily n = 293	7.48/10 (9.9 to 5.8)	2.99/10 (6.3 to 1.5)
Average pain score: Weekly n = 52	6.13/10 (8.5 to 4.2)	2.35/10 (6.8 to 0.5)

Clinical improvement was reported in all patients without any adverse side effects. Further research is required to verify the efficacy of treatment and the accuracy of the supporting data.

CONCLUSION

ETPS therapy incorporates acupuncture, osteopathic, trigger point, neuromuscular, and neural therapies into simple, easy-to-use protocols. With this approach, it is possible to integrate different philosophies and access a wide variety of soft tissue pains using one modality. With back pain, an exceptionally common condition, each stage in an ETPS protocol treats a specific pathway, group of muscles, segmental levels, acupuncture meridian, or scar. Through this step-by-step elimination process, it is possible to identify and treat those levels, muscles, or meridians at the root of a patient's pain.

Although ETPS therapy has been able to make modest breakthroughs in the diagnosis and treatment of chronic pain through its synthesis of different modalities, additional research is required to advance the body of knowledge. Perhaps an even greater challenge than pure research is the need for competing disciplines to work cooperatively by reducing the barriers that compartmentalize medicine. Drawing from the Oriental paradigm, the advancement of knowledge and the pursuit of truth begin with questions, rather than proclamations of answers. This paradigm is the foundation of ETPS therapy, "How can the constituent elements of medicine be combined to advance the treatment of chronic pain?"

ACKNOWLEDGMENT

The author wishes to thank Chris Stillinger for the artwork in this chapter.

REFERENCES

Andersson, S.A. (1979). Pain control by sensory stimulation. In J.J. Bonica (Ed.), *Advances in pain research and therapy* (Vol. 3) (pp. 561–585). New York: Raven Press.

Augustinsson, L.E., et al. (1977). Pain relief during delivery by transcutaneous electrical nerve stimulation. *Pain, 4,* 59–65.

Becker, R.O., & Selden, G. (1987). *The body electric, electromagnetism and the foundation of life.* New York: Quill Press.

Bradley, W.G. (1974). *Disorders of peripheral nerves.* Oxford: Blackwell Scientific Publications.

Bronzino, J.D. (1998). *The biomedical engineering handbook.* Boca Raton: CRC Press.

Cannon, W.B., & Rosenbluth, A. (1949). *The supersensitivity of denervated structures.* New York: Macmillan.

Cheng, R., & Pomeranz, B. (1986). Electrotherapy of chronic musculoskeletal pain: comparison of electroacupuncture acupuncture-like TENS. *Clinical Journal of Pain, 2,* 142.

Cheng, R., McKibbon, L., Roy, B., & Pomeranz, B. (1980). Electroacupuncture elevates blood cortisol levels in naive horses; sham treatment has no effect. *International Journal of Neuroscience, 10*(2–3), 95–97.

Christopher, D., Lorenzo, B., Zirbs, A., Chantraine, A., & Visher, T.L. (1992). Electroacupuncture in fibromyalgia: Results of a controlled trial. *British Medical Journal, 305,* 1249–1252.

Fambrough, D.M., Hartzell, H.C., Powell, J.A., Rash, J.E., & Joseph, N. (1974). *Differentiation and organization of a post-synaptic cell — the skeletal muscle fiber, synaptic transmission and neuronal interaction.* New York: Raven Press.

Fisher, H.W. (1992). Acute low back pain treated by spinal manipulation and electronic acupuncture. *Journal of Manipulative and Physiological Therapeutics 15*(3), 199–202.

Friberg, O. (1983). Clinical symptoms and biomechanics of lumbar spine and hip joint in leg length inequality. *Spine 8*(6), 643–651.

Gadsby, J.G., & Flowerdew, M.W. (2000) The effectiveness of transcutaneous electrical nerve stimulation (TENS) and acupuncture-like transcutaneous electrical nerve stimulation (ALTENS) in the treatment of patients with chronic low back pain. *Cochrane Database System Review, 2,* CD2000210.

Gunn, C.C. (1980). "Prespondylosis" and some pain syndromes following denervation. *Supersensitivity 5*(2), 185–192.

Gunn, C.C., et al. (1976). Tenderness at motor points: A diagnostic and prognostic aid for low-back injury. *Journal of Bone and Joint Surgery, 58A*(6), 815–825.

Gunn, C.C., et al. (1978). Early and subtle signs in low-back sprain. *Spine 3*(3), 267–281.

Gunn, C.C., & Milbrandt, W.E. (1976). Acupuncture loci: A proposal for their classification according to their relationship to known neural structures. *American Journal of Chinese Medicine, 4*(2), 183–195.

Gunn, C.C., & Milbrandt, W.W. (1997). Utilizing trigger points. *Osteopathic Physiology, 44*(3), 29–52.

Hartley, A. (1989). *A pain control manual: Point locations for musculoskeletal injuries and transelectrical nerve stimulation techniques.* Toronto: Anne Hartley.

Lehmann, T.R., Russell, D.W., Spratt, K.F., Liu, Y.K., Fairchild, M.L., & Christensen, S. (1986). Efficacy of electroacupuncture and TENS in the rehabilitation of chronic low back pain patients. *Pain, 26*(3), 277–290.

Loh, L., & Nathan, P.W. (1978). Painful peripheral states and sympathetic blocks. *Journal of Neurology, Neurosurgery, and Psychiatry, 41,* 664–671.

Low, J., & Reed, A. (1994). *Electrotherapy explained: Principles and practice* (2nd ed.). Woburn, MA: Butterworth Heinemann.

Martelete, M., & Fiori, A.M. (1985). Comparative study of the analgesic effect of transcutaneous nerve stimulation (TNS), electroacupuncture (EA), and meperdine in the treatment of post operative pain. *Acupuncture Electrotherapeutics Research, 10,* 183–193.

Pomeranz, B. (1981). Neural mechanisms of acupuncture analgesia. In Lipton, S. (Ed.), *Persistent pain (*Vol. 3, pp. 241–257). New York: Academic Press.

Pomeranz, B., & Niziak, G. (1987). Codetron, a new electrotherapy device overcomes the habituation problems of conventional TENS devices. *American Journal of Electromedicine,* first quarter, 22–26.

Pomeranz, B., et al. (1988). Electroacupuncture suppression of a nociceptive reflex is potentiated by two repeated electroacupuncture treatments: The first opioid effect postulates a second nonopioid effect. *Brain Research, 452*(1–2), 232–236.

Robinson, A.J., & Mackler, L.S. (1995). *Clinical electrophysiology: Electrotherapy and electrophysiologic testing.* Baltimore: Lippincott, Williams & Wilkins.

Shriber, W.J. (1981). *A Manual of Electrotherapy* (4th ed.).

Sola, A.E. (1981). Myofascial trigger point therapy. *Resident and Staff Physician, 27*(8), 38–46.

Sola, A.E. (1984). Treatment of myofascial pain syndromes. In C. Benedetti, C.R. Chapman, & G. Morrica (Eds.), *Advances in pain research and therapy,* Vol. 7. New York: Raven Press.

Statistics Canada, Canadian social trends, absenteeism at work. *Perspectives,* Spring 1992.

Thomas, P.K., & Ochoa, J. (1993). Symptomatology and differential diagnosis of peripheral neuropathy: clinical features and differential diagnosis. In P.J. Dyck & P.K. Thomas (Eds.), Peripheral neuropathy (pp. 749–774). Philadelphia: Saunders.

Travell, J.G., & Simons, D.G. (1998). Myofascial pain and dysfunction: The trigger point manual (Vol. 1 & 2). Baltimore: Lippincott, Williams & Wilkins.

Yochum T., & Barry, M. (1994). Examination and treatment of the short leg. *Year-end Clinical Compendium. American Chiropractic Association Journal of Chiropractic.*

55

Magnetic Biostimulation in Peripheral Neuropathy

Michael I. Weintraub, M.D., F.A.C.P., F.A.A.N.

INTRODUCTION

For more than 2000 years, interest in the health effects of magnets on biological processes has been explored and debated in the scientific community. The public has perceived that magnets are an important source of natural energy and good health and has created a worldwide demand, spending more than $500 million in the United States and Canada and $5 billion worldwide in sales last year. Anecdotal endorsements by more than 70 sports figures in golf, baseball, tennis, football, etc. have also enhanced utilization. As we enter the new millennium, there has been a shift in focus. Rather than ignoring it, the public's and medical community's interest and curiosity about the subject of alternative medicine has heightened. What are the facts and what is fantasy? This chapter explores the topic of magnetic therapy in terms of static magnets, mechanisms of biological effects, and current investigations. While time-varying magnetic field (electromagnetic) devices are mentioned, a comprehensive discussion is beyond the scope of this chapter.

HISTORICAL PERSPECTIVE:

Man's fascination with magnetism is a historical blend of science, sensationalism, quackery, fashion, and controversy. However, it is a story worth telling because it provides insights into how contemporary American society deals with the current surge of interest in alternative medical therapies.

For an excellent review of the background history, the article by Mourino is exceptionally informative (Mourino, 1990). Claims of magnetic healing have been traced for more than 2000 years. The term "magnet" was probably derived from Magnes, a shepherd, who legend states was walking on Mount Ida and was suddenly drawn to the Earth by the metallic tacks in his sandals. He dug to ascertain a cause, and in the process, discovered magnetite, the mineral lodestone containing a magnetic oxide of iron (Fe_3O_4). The ancients also called these Herculean stones, lodestones, or live stones as they were meant to "lead the way." The observations that lodestones could attract iron filings and that amber rods rubbed with fur could attract paper and other objects were considered manifestations of the same phenomena. Thus, magnetism and electrostatic attraction were considered similar mechanisms and this closeness is reproduced throughout subsequent history of the subjects (Mourino, 1991; Geddes, 1991; MacKlis, 1993; Armstrong & Armstrong, 1991). Because history has a way of repeating itself, distinct footprints can be easily traced.

Briefly, the ideas expressed by the ancient Greek and Roman civilizations represent the historical origins of "invisible movement of matter." Plato, Euripides, and other individuals attributed various powers to magnets and sensed that the lodestones could be put to practical use, e.g., building boats with iron nails and also destroying them by closely putting them against the magnetic mountains of rocks, etc. Healing properties of lodestones and amber were attributed to a "soul" and by 200 A.D., Greek physicians were prescribing amber pills to stop

0-8493-0926-3/02/$0.00+$1.50
© 2002 by CRC Press LLC

hemorrhage and magnetic rings were sold in the markets of Samothrace in an attempt to cure arthritis. In 1289, Peter Peregrinus is credited with writing the first major treatise on magnetism. Lodestones were thought to have strong aphrodisiac powers, curative powers for gout, baldness, arthritis, and even the power to draw poison from wounds. His work also contains the first drawing and description of the compass in the Western world.

The Middle Ages was a dark period for science and an astounding number of beliefs and myths were attributed to magnets. For example, it was stated that magnets could draw gold from wells and that an antidote for magnets was garlic. In the 16th century, Paracelsus investigated the medical properties of lodestones in the treatment of diseases such as epilepsy, hemorrhage, and diarrhea. Paracelsus was a physician and alchemist who denounced Galenic medicine and made public displays of burning books, etc. He combined mysticism with practical issues and became very controversial. One of his major points was "that every person is a magnet" that can attract good and evil and is an important "elixir of life." By the middle of the 16th century, attempts were made to separate the magnetic phenomena from the "amber effect." William Gilbert, physician to Queen Elizabeth I of England (1533–1603), wrote his classic text "deMagnete" in 1600, describing hundreds of detailed experiments on electricity by using amber and electrons. He also described terrestrial magnetism by using the compass and the Earth as a magnet. He debunked many quack medical uses of magnets and was responsible for laying the groundwork for future research and study.

Thomas Brown continued this attack on popular magnetic salves and remedies and suggested that their putative healing power was due only to the incorporated herbal and mineral compounds. He performed experiments demonstrating that lodestones retained their magnetism and that garlic could not destroy them and that diamonds did not impede them. It should be noted that in the nearly 100 years after the publication of Gilbert's book, no major advancements were made in the study of magnetism. In the early 18th century, significant interest in electricity and magnetism arose. An electrostatic engine was invented in 1705 by Francis Hauksbee. He mounted a glass globe on a spindle and rotated it with great speed while a woolen cloth was pressed against it by a strong, brass spring. Hauksbee discovered that this apparatus could produce a strong, electric charge that could be transferred to other objects by means of a metal chain (wire) connected to fine metal points suspended just above the surface of the glass globe. This produced electrical shocks, and by 1743 showmen were traveling throughout Europe with their electrical machines and even went to the English New World (American colonies), giving people shocks for a small fee. Fortuitously, in that year in Boston, Benjamin Franklin observed an

electrified boy exhibition by an itinerant electrician that roused Franklin's interest in electrical and magnetic phenomena. In fact, much of the current nomenclature of electrical terminology, such as charge, discharge, condenser, electrical shock, electrician, positive, negative, plus, and minus, originated with Franklin. Magnetism was not Franklin's major research area; and he distinguished himself in his studies of electrical fluid and charges. According to him, all matter contains a magnetic field that is uniformly distributed throughout it. When an object is magnetized, the fluid condenses in one of its extremities. That extremity becomes positively magnetized while the donor region of the objects becomes negatively magnetized. The degree to which an object can be magnetized depends on the force necessary to start the fluid moving within it.

Across the continent in Europe, Father Maximilian Hell was effecting medical cures with artificial lodestones, i.e., pieces of iron that had been strongly magnetized through a process developed during the period 1743–1751. His student, Anton Mesmer, obtained a supply of these magnets and began to apply them to his patients. Many patients were experiencing hysterical or psychosomatic symptomatology and, consequently, Mesmer's cures were "astounding" and spectacular. His results were principally due to the power of suggestion, and he began to experiment with other objects such as nonmagnetic materials, e.g., paper, wool, silk, and stone. Mesmer reasoned that he was not dealing with ordinary mineral magnetism but with a special kind that he named "animal magnetism." He theorized that ill people could overcome a disease by "mesmerizing" their body's magnetic poles to induce a crisis, often in the form of convulsions "so as to restore their health and harmony." In a single, short year, mesmerism and mesmeric cures became the rage of Vienna. In 1775, Mesmer published his first medical treatise on the medicinal uses of the magnet. Mesmer's exaggerated claims of success bordered on the theatrical and forced the Royal French Academy of Science to convene a special study in 1784. This panel included Anton Lavoisier, J.R. Guillotin, and Benjamin Franklin. In a controlled set of blind experiments in which patients were exposed alternatively to a series of magnetic or sham-magnetic objects and were asked to describe their sensations, the Committee decided that the efficacy of the magnetic healings seemed to reside entirely within the mind of the patient, i.e., power of suggestion in susceptible or naive individuals. Based on these findings in France, mesmerism soon came to symbolize medical quackery and was scorned. Mesmer's theories were declared fraudulent. The French Revolution subsequently occurred in 1789 and Mesmer left France in disgrace.

Credit for discovering the true nature of electromagnetism goes to Hans Christian Oersted (1777–1851). He noted that a compass needle was deflected when a current flowed through a nearby wire. He carried out some experiments and found to his astonishment that not only did a current-carrying wire exert a force on a magnet, but a magnet also exerted a force on a coil of wire carrying electric current. The coil acted like a magnet, behaving as if it possessed magnetic north and south poles. Magnetism and electricity were somehow connected. It was Oersted who was instrumental in creating the proper scientific environment that led to further progress. Subsequently, the pace of scientific research on magnetism skyrocketed. Society embraced the application in the treatment of illness which led to commercial enterprises. The alleged benefits of magnetotherapy were summarized in a mail-order pamphlet printed in 1886 and distributed by Dr. C. J. Thatcher. He explained how magnetic healing provided a "plain road to health without the use of medicine and dependent upon the magnetic energy of the Sun." He believed that the iron content of the blood made it the primary magnetic conductor of the body. The most efficient way to recharged the blood's magnetic field was through the use of magnetic garments, and Thatcher's Chicago Magnetic Company produced over 700 individual magnetic devices and garments. The complete set was said to "furnish full and complete protection of all the vital organs of the body."

He was dubbed by *Collier's Magazine* "The King of Magnetic Quacks." By the late 19th Century and early 20th Century, the medical establishment was beginning to accept the role of electromagnetic approaches to the treatment of some diseases. In fact, one of the standard medical textbooks from the period devotes an entire chapter to the use of galvanism and electromagnetic fields in the treatment of neurologic disease. However, there were numerous skeptics who provided contradictory data making it difficult for the medical establishment to either restrict or condone the practice of magnetic healing. Thus, magnetic devices were sold without regulation. In 1896, D'Arsonval placed his head inside a magnetic coil which caused phosphenes (stimulation of the retina). However, many people date the era of modern magnetic stimulation from the clinical reports of Bickford and Fremming (1965) who were able to twitch skeletal muscles by magnetic stimulation of peripheral nerves. Subsequently, Barker (1975) and McLean, Holcomb, Wamil, et al. (1995) at the University of Sheffield (1986) developed the first commercial magnetic stimulator. As might be expected, stimulation using magnetic coils for the central and peripheral nervous systems, has been worldwide for more than a decade and has created a new discipline both for diagnosis and therapy. Similarly, the development of Nuclear Magnetic Resonance (MRI) led to imaging research applied to biological systems. Hydrogen, sodium, and phosphorous were studied. Tissues have a specific "signature" and these techniques

have been further refined and are used by the neurological community on a daily basis.

The use of pulsed electromagnetic fields (PEMF) is another form of electromagnetic energy that influences biological changes. This has been investigated specifically at the cellular membrane level with ionic flux as well as stimulating osteoblasts in nonunion fractures. It also has been approved by the FDA for incontinence and healing of nonunion fractures. Exposure to various EMF, i.e., high-voltage power lines, microwaves, has generated fears of lymphoblastic leukemia and other malignancies. This issue was discussed in the *Archives of Physical Medicine and Rehabilitation* by Vallbona, Hazelwood, and Jurida (1997).

DEFINITIONS

TYPES OF MAGNETIC FIELDS

There are two broad groups of magnetic fields: static and time-varying. In time-varying suprathreshold magnets high-current electrical pulses pass through a coil of wires inducing a magnetic flux which does not attenuate as it passes through tissues. The magnetic pulse then induces a proportional electrical field in an opposite direction to the current in the coil. Repetitive electrical stimulation of the cerebral cortex has long been known to interfere with cerebral processing and is the basis for electroshock therapy. Similarly, single-pulse transmagnetic stimulation (TMS) of the motor cortex can disrupt neural function. Thus, noninvasive stimulation of the human cortex and peripheral nervous system can be safely utilized to measure function and may have a profound impact therapeutically. Depending upon the pulse frequency (1 to 5 Hz), the excited axons may have excitatory or inhibitory effects which may be distant or local. While it is beyond the scope of this chapter, suffice it to say that TMS is a young science that is being explored in movement disorders, psychiatric disease, epilepsy, speech disorders, behavior and spinal cord dysfunction, etc. (Pascual-Leone, Valls-Sole, & Brasil-Neto, et al., 1994; George, Lisanby, & Sackheim, 1999). This is a painless and reliable approach that does not require direct skin contact and produces the same results as standard electrical stimulation. Because of the strengths of these suprathreshold magnetic fields, numerous biological reactions can occur and are described later.

Static or permanent magnets for the management of pain are commercially available in various magnetic configurations, sizes, and compositions. Manufacturers have created devices from neodymium, ceramic, iron, plastiform, barium ferrite, etc. These are weak devices usually measured in gauss or Tesla. There are two specific types of magnets described as unipolar (north or south) or bipolar. The term "bipolar" refers to magnets that at the surface have alternating north and south poles in a concentric pattern or grid. Other patterns developed are called multipolar with triangular arrangements of alternating north and south poles. Each proponent of their configuration has made claims as to "best and most efficacious design," but no large-scale clinical studies exist comparing one design to another. However, laboratory analysis explored and tested this issue in a 1995 study at Vanderbilt University. McClean and co-workers (1995) demonstrated an enhanced effect of multipolar magnets on sensory afferent firing (pain axons) compared to unipolar or bipolar designs. Beneficial effects from permanent magnets have been attributed to penetration of the field which is proportional to the strength of the magnetic field at the surface. It is also a function of the size of the magnet. It is well-known that magnetic fields lose their intensity as they penetrate body tissue. Thus, it is important to keep these devices firmly affixed to the skin surface for maximal penetration. Gaussmeter recordings taken at increasing distances from a magnetic surface demonstrate a rapid decrease in gauss strength and penetration with distance. Thus, the flux density at the target area is probably more clinically relevant than the magnetic reading at the surface of the skin. The strength and force of any magnet are designated as its gauss rating. This represents the energy field at the topmost center of the magnet, the energy field declines with distance. Most commercial magnets have 300 to 600 gauss strength but not all brand of magnets are equivalent in depth penetration and each manufacturer makes its own claim. Specifically, in the utilization of bipolar magnets, it has been suggested that there is spatial cancellation from the adjacent opposite poles producing no active magnetic field penetration to the target region.

DURATION OF CONTACT

This has not been scientifically confirmed. Valbonna, et al., (1997) utilized bipolar magnets for 45 minutes in post-polio syndrome whereas Collacott, Zimmerman, White, and Rindone (2000) used bipolar magnets for 18 hours per week. Weintraub (1998; 1999), utilized multipolar magnetic devices (475 gauss) constantly 24 hours per day. One manufacturer, Magnetherapy, Inc., recommends using a unipolar magnet for a minimum of 8 hours per day with continuous application until pain has been relieved.

PRECAUTIONS

Static magnets are thought to be safe and are not regulated by the FDA. However, all manufacturers have cautioned about their use during pregnancy because there is no available information regarding the role of magnetic fields in pregnancy and/or on the fetus. Individuals who wear a pacemaker or electronic implants also should not use these devices. Patients with open and fresh wounds also are cautioned against wearing these devices.

MECHANISMS OF THE BIOLOGICAL EFFECTS OF MAGNETIC FIELDS:

The exact mechanisms of the interaction of magnetic fields with biological tissues resulting in functional changes are presently unknown. Electromagnetic fields (EMF) are known to alter biomolecular DNA synthesis, cell proliferation, membrane calcium fluxes, and cell surface properties *in vitro* (Cleary, 1995). The principle site of biophysical interaction leading to cell functional alterations is most likely the lipid membrane surface where EMF may affect the ability of ion pump enzymes to move calcium, sodium, and potassium ions across the cell membrane (Blank & Soo, 1993). Magnetic fields also may alter the equilibrium between cell death and proliferation via modulation of calcium influx (Fanelli, Coppola, Barone, et al., 1999). An excellent overview of the biological effects of electromagnetic fields is found in a two-volume publication edited by Carpenter and Ayrapetyan (1994). Adey (1981) demonstrated that at the cell surface, ionic phenomena arise producing transmembrane signaling. Thus, at the atomic level, there are disordered free radicals which reflect the level of involvement with generation of electromagnetic signals (Adey & Chopart, 1987). Adey also has identified glycoprotein strands protruding through cell membranes, which he feels act as antennae or tissue components of electromagnetic fields traveling along cell surfaces. This produces transduction with an intracellular cascade of metabolic, messenger, and cell-growth regulating enzymes. This is an athermal interaction at the atomic level. He has noted that disordered, free radicals are associated with oxidative stress, diseases including Parkinson's, Alzheimer's, and coronary artery disease, aging, cancer, and diabetes mellitus. Observed bioeffects of imposed fields point to a needed mechanistic basis, beyond the fabric of biomolecules in physical processes at the atomic level. It is well-known that free radicals are usually unstable and highly reactive and are capable of abstracting electrons from surrounding lipids, proteins, or DNA molecules, thus inducing cellular changes and damage. Adey further suggests that nitrous oxide is the specific agent involved and further theorizes that magnetic benefit occurs at the level of free radicals with the splitting of nitrous–oxygen bond (NO). Thus, ion parametric resonance theory has been attributed to biological effect.

Cope (1973) also indicates that at the atomic and subatomic levels there have been changes in biological systems. It is his premise that microregions exist within cells and molecules and are sensitive to external magnetic fields (both low and high). Such interactions can lead to changes in enzymatic reactions, cellular potentials, conduction velocity, etc. Nordenstrom (1983) proposed that the endothelial lining of the cardiovascular system serves as a conduit for the transmission of electrical energy throughout large regions of the body. Thus, it is not inconceivable that a magnetic field from either a permanent magnet or electromagnetic device can induce electric current in vascular elements in one region of the body, etc., which in turn could be transferred to other regions.

The biologic phenomenon that is responsible for altering rates of wound healing with pulsed electromagnetic fields (PEMF) exposure as well as improvement in stress incontinence is not well understood. However, the FDA has approved its utilization. Both human and animal studies indicate increased peripheral blood flow resulting from such an exposure. Specifically, changes occur in fibroblast concentration, fibrin fibers, and collagen at wound sites, again attributed to increased blood flow (Bassett, Mitchell, Norton, et al., 1979; Pujol, Pascual, Bolz, et al., 1998). Some authors feel that water plays a major role in explaining the therapeutic effects of magnetic fields. While this mechanism is clearly applicable in MRI, it also needs further assessment in the laboratory. Beall, Hazlewood, and Rao (1976) demonstrated cyclical changes in the physical state of water, with water being most organized in an S-phase due to exposure to magnetic fields.

Jacobson and Yamanashi (1995) explored biophysical interactions that might explain electromagnetic inducement of oncogenes. The final product of the study was the production of a testable theoretical model with a magnetotherapy mechanism wherein physiologic magnetic fields may be directed from an exogenous source through the patient, producing changes in the lattice structure of normal genes. This research suggests effects of magnetic therapy that go well beyond changes in blood flow.

A blockade of action potentials of cultured sensorineurons by small static magnetic fields has been previously reported by McLean, et al. (1995). The exact mechanism of the interaction of magnetic fields with biological tissues resulting in functional changes is unknown. Previously, Weintraub (1998; 1999) hypothesized that C-fibers are influenced by constant contact with static magnets leading to a reduction of burning and painful symptoms in the feet. This probably involves the potassium (K +) internal rectifying channel (Horn, Quasthoff, & Grafe, et al., 1996). Thus, there is a repolarization or a hyperpolarization that develops due to constant exposure.

Currently, blood flow studies in response to static magnetic fields (unipolar, bipolar, and multipolar) utilizing laser-Doppler perfusion measurements are currently in progress. Thus, from a clinical perspective, objective data may be obtained that can be extrapolated to look at specific dosing of magnetic fields, frequency and duration of utilization, as well as a spatial coverage.

Despite laboratory attempts to identify a mode of action, a large clinical study of cohorts with detection of biological markers ultimately will determine if there is a legitimate role of magnetic therapy in pain medicine.

The safe application of electromagnetic fields has been attested by the World Health Organization (WHO) (1987) which reported that all the available evidence indicated the absence of any adverse effects on human health due to exposure to static magnetic fields up to 2 Tesla.

As we enter the 21st Century, we see that history has indeed repeated itself, but with more progress. Previous applications of permanent magnets have been utilized by Weintraub (1998; 1999) as well as Vallbona, et al. (1997) and Collacott, et al. (2000) with varying results. To any serious student of medicine and neurology, skepticism should be maintained in view of the absence of large longitudinal, randomized, placebo-controlled trials. An open mind is necessary. Science still does not have all the answers!

MAGNETIC STIMULATION IN DIABETIC PERIPHERAL NEUROPATHY: A NOVEL APPROACH

It has been estimated that 16 million Americans suffer from diabetes mellitus. Most represent adult-onset Type II noninsulin-dependent (90%) and 10% have Type I insulin-dependent diabetes mellitus. The Diabetes Control and Complications Trial (1988) identified risk factors associated with the development of diabetic neuropathy that include degree of hyperglycemia, duration of diabetes, age, male sex, and height. Other complications of retinopathy and nephropathy also are associated with these same risk factors and may coexist with neuropathy. Thus, over 60% of individuals with diabetes mellitus suffer some form of neuropathy (peripheral and/or autonomic or combination) and in most, the ensuing symptoms are serious enough to interfere with daily activities. Diabetic peripheral neuropathy represents a spectrum from clinically silent to a progressive axonopathy of the dying-back type characterized by myelinated fiber loss and reduced fiber regeneration with sprouting. Usually, the neurological examination reveals blunted sensation to pin prick, vibration, position, and temperature, and usually blunting and/or absence of deep tendon reflex response. Motor weakness may also be present. Neurological complications occur equally in Type I and Type II diabetes mellitus. Quantification of the above process by nerve conduction velocity and quantified sensory testing (QST) (Dyck, O'Brien, Kosambre, et al., 1993) identifies if the symptomatology is primarily secondary to small unmyelinated C-fibers (dysesthetic pain, warm thermal perception, autonomic function) or large-fiber damage (deep-seeded gnawing pain, altered position, and vibration). Also, loss of sympathetic regulation of sweat glands and local blood flow leads to skin dryness, cracking, and ultimately secondary local infections leading to amputation (Low, Caskey, Tuck, et al., 1983).

Dysesthetic symptoms remain a refractory problem and are notoriously difficult to treat with conventional pharmacologic agents and the patient often becomes disabled. Disappearance of pain occurs and is misinterpreted by patients as improvement, whereas it signifies that the neuropathy is progressing. This should serve as a warning sign for more frequent foot care because this scenario often leads to amputation.

Numerous pathogenic mechanisms have been offered including metabolic, vascular, autoimmune, sorbitol toxicity, etc. Despite hundreds of millions of dollars of research, there is no specific etiology accepted. Presently, it is considered a heterogenous disease with various aspects of pathology and pathogenic mechanisms.

A number of treatments have been used in an attempt to reverse and halt diabetic peripheral neuropathy, but only strict glycemic control has been found effective (Low & Dotson, 1999). Similarly, despite hundreds of millions of research dollars, associated peripheral vascular disease and impaired wound-healing results in more than 200,000 cases of foot ulcers and about 100,000 amputations per year. Despite over $1 billion in research, effective therapy for the prevention and treatment of diabetic peripheral neuropathy is not currently available.

Most research has focused on pharmacologic approaches for pain relief by blocking central or peripheral transmission pathways. But, the optimal drug has yet to be developed. Troublesome side effects also are a significant problem. Therapeutic options with conventional pharmacologic agents are, therefore, limited. Thus, alternative therapies directed at slowing or halting the process become attractive. Anecdotal reports over the past 2000 years have suggested that the application of static magnets in painful areas of the body can reduce discomfort; however, these claims have not been scientifically validated. As we enter this new millennium, a great opportunity exists to critically evaluate new and novel therapeutic approaches.

Prior pilot studies using commercially available multipolar magnets (475 gauss) resulted in unexpected pain relief in individuals with diabetic peripheral neuropathy and peripheral neuropathy from other etiologies. A follow-up pilot study looked at the potential role of placebo response and the results indicated that the pain relief benefit was not placebo. The fact that nerve conduction studies and SSEP, which measured large A-fiber conduction serially over 4 months, did not demonstrate any significant change, suggested that the pain modifying benefit was secondary to C-polymodal receptor afferent modulation. In view of the fact that burning was extremely sensitive to magnetic application, it only reinforced this as a theory. Consequently, a larger longitudinal study was required in an attempt to statistically determine if magnetic stimulation is a legitimate therapy.

NATIONWIDE RANDOMIZED PLACEBO-CONTROLLED STUDY

In July 1999, a multicenter, randomized, double-blind placebo-controlled study was started in the United States. A cohort of 300 cases with Stage II/III DPN (Dyck, Kratz, Karnes, et al., 1993) was enrolled and observed for a 4-month period. Both examiners and patients were blinded. One group wore magnetic foot devices (475 gauss) constantly over a 24-hour period whereas a control group wore a similar appearing sham device. Baseline parameters of numbness, tingling, and pain were measured three times per day on a VAS scale of 0 to 10 as well as nocturnal interruption secondary to foot pain and foot discomfort after a standardized 10-minute exercise. Baseline nerve conduction velocity and/or Quantified Sensory Testing (QST) of C- and A-fibers or sympathetic skin response (SSR) are to be taken.

Several sites with special interest in autonomic functions, blood flow, intraepidermal nerve fiber assessment, microneurography, and threshold electrotonus are also being performed serially. Currently, there are 115 sites in all 50 states including Washington, D.C. and Puerto Rico. All seven Podiatric Medical Centers in the United States are participating as well as the five largest foot and ankle centers. Of the neurological university centers, over 60% of the examiners are Chairpersons, Professors, or Chiefs of Neuromuscular Division. In an attempt to complete the study by March 2001, additional community investigative sites of practicing Board Certified Neurologists with expertise in electrodiagnostic studies were added. There also is close community collaboration with endocrinologists and physical medicine and rehabilitation specialists. This diabetic cohort of 300 patients represents the mosaic of the United States population as regards racial representation with Native Americans, Asiatics, Hispanics, African-Americans, and Caucasians. It also will demonstrate how university and community investigators from several disciplines can work together and produce a quality study. Biological markers are actively being sought in an attempt to identify the proposed mechanism of effectiveness. It is hoped that this study will validate the two prior pilot studies. But, irrespective of the results (positive or negative), it needs to be published. The public spent $500 million in the United States and Canada in 1999 and over \$5 billion worldwide for magnetic devices. Thus, the legitimacy of their use needs to be determined from a scientific standpoint. This study also will determine the role of placebo as well as the role of A- and C-fibers in response to constant magnetic field stimulation. The results may also suggest, too, that further clinical improvement can arise with increased Gaussian strength or improved steep field penetration or combination therapy with drugs.

If indeed this study is positive, it suggests the need to prophylactically wear these devices when diagnosed with diabetes mellitus prior to the emergence of clinical symptoms. It also would suggest a positive effect on wound healing.

Magnetic therapy is currently riding the crest of the tidal wave of public enthusiasm for alternative medicine. This current scientific endeavor will definitively determine if there is a legitimacy to static magnetic fields in diabetic peripheral neuropathy (DPN).

In conclusion, at this time, the best defense against DPN is maintaining optimal glucose control. This slows the onset and progression not only of neuropathy but other complications. Despite the functional benefits and dramatic pain relief reported with the two prior studies (75 to 90%), it is important to underscore that while these results are provocative, they must be considered anecdotal due to small sample size. The current nationwide initiative and its results will be eagerly anticipated because this will be a definitive study. Also important is that this study considers C- and A-fiber function over a 4-month period. Several blinded cases have demonstrated significant electrophysiological changes correlating with improved clinical status. These results must be duplicated. Healthy skepticism by the medical community still needs to prevail until the results of this definitive, randomized placebo-controlled study is completed.

REFERENCES

Adey, W.R. (1981). Tissue interactions with non-ionizing electromagnetic fields. *Physiological Review, 61*, 435–514.

Adey, W.R. (1996–1999). Cell and molecular biology associated with radiation fields of mobile telephone. In R. Stone (Ed.), *Review of radio science*. Oxford: Oxford University.

Adey, W.R., & Chopart, A. (1987). Cell surface ionic phenomena in transmembrane signaling to intracellular enzyme systems. In N. Blank & E. Findl (Eds.), *Mechanistic approaches to interactions of electromagnetic fields with living systems* (pp. 365–387). New York: Plenum Press.

Armstrong, D., & Armstrong, E.M. (1991). *The great American medicine show* (185–194). New York: Prentice Hall.

Barker, A.T., Freeston, I.L., et al. (1987). Magnetic stimulation of the human brain and peripheral nervous system: An introduction and the results of an initial clinical evaluation. *Neurosurgery, 20*, 100–109.

Bassett, C.A., Mitchell, S.N., Norton, L., et al. (1979). Electromagnetic repairs of non-unions. In C.I. Brighton, J. Black, & S.R. Pollack (Eds.), *Electrical properties of bone and cartilage* (pp. 605–630). New York: Gruen & Stratton.

Beall, P.T., Hazelwood, C.F., & Rao, P.N. (1976). Nuclear magnetic resonance of intracellular water as a function of HeLa cell cycle. *Science, 192*, 904–907.

Bickford, R.G., & Fremming, B.D. (1965). Neuronal stimulation by pulsed magnetic fields in animals and man. In *Digest of the Sixth International Conference on Medical Electronics and Biological Engineering* (p. 112).

Blank, M., & Soo, L. (1993). The NA, K-ATPase as a model for electromagnetic field effects on cells. *Bioelectrochemistry and Bioenergetics, 30*, 85–92.

Carpenter, D.O., & Ayrapetyan, S. (1994). *Biological effects of electric and magnetic fields: Sources and mechanisms.* San Diego: Academic Press.

Cleary, S.F. (1995). Biophysical aspects of electromagnetic field effects on mammalian cells. In A.H. Frey (Ed.). *On the nature of electromagnetic field interactions with biological systems* (pp. 29–42). Austin, TX: RG Landes Co.

Collacott, E.A., Zimmerman, J.T., White, D.W., & Rindone, J.P. (2000). Bipolar permanent magnets for the treatment of chronic low back pain: A pilot study. *Journal American Medical Association, 283*, 1322–1325.

Consensus Statement of the American Diabetes Association and The American Academy of Neurology. (1988). Report and recommendations of the San Antonio Conference on Diabetic Neuropathy. *Diabetes, 3*, 1000–1004.

Cope, F.W. (1973). Biological sensitivity to weak magnetic fields due to biological superconductive Josephson junctions. *Physiological Chemistry and Physics, 5*, 173–176.

Dyck, P.J., O'Brien, P.C., Kosambre, J.L., et al. (1993). A 4, 2 + 1 stepping algorithm for quick and accurate estimation of cutaneous sensation threshold. *Neurology, 43*, 1508–1512.

Dyck, P.T., Kratz, K.M., Karnes, J.L., et al. (1993). The prevalence by staged severity of various types of diabetic neuropathy, retinopathy and nephropathy, in a population-based cohort: The Rochester diabetic neuropathy study. *Neurology, 43*, 817–824.

Fanelli, C., Coppola, S., Barone, R., et al. (1999). Magnetic fields increase cell survival by inhibiting apoptosis via modulation of Ca 2 + Influx. *FASEB Journal, 13*, 95–102.

Geddes, L. (1991). History of magnetic stimulation of the nervous system. *Journal of Clinical Neurophysiology, 8*, 3–9.

George, M.S., Lisanby, S.H., & Sackheim, H.A. (1999). Transcranial magnetic stimulation: application in neuropsychiatry. *Archives of General Psychiatry, 56*, 315–320.

Horn, S., Quasthoff, S., Grafe, P., et al. (1996). Abnormal axonal inward rectification in diabetic neuropathy. *Muscle Nerve, 19*, 1268–1275.

Jacobson, J.I., & Yamanashi, W.S. (1995). An initial physical mechanism in the treatment of neurologic disorders with externally applied pico Tesla magnetic fields. *Neurological Research, 17,* 144–148.

Low, P.A., & Dotson, R.N. (1999). Symptomatic treatment of painful neuropathy (Editorial). *Journal American Medical Association, 280,* 1863–1864.

Low, P.A., Caskey, P.E., Tuck, R.R., et al. (1983). Quantitative sudomotor axon reflex test in normal and neuropathic subjects. *Annals of Neurology, 58,* 573–580.

Macklis, R.M. (1993). Magnetic healing, quackery and the debate about the health effects of electromagnetic fields. *Annals of Internal Medicine, 118,* 376–383.

McLean, M.J., Holcomb, R.R., Wamil, A.W., et al. (1995). Blockade of sensory neuron action potentials by a static magnetic field in the 10 mT range. *Bioelectromagnetics, 18,* 20–32.

Mourino, M.R. (1991). From Thales to Lauterbur, or from the lodestone to MR imaging: Magnetism and medicine. *Radiology, 180,* 593–612.

Nordenstrom, B.E.W. (1983). *Biologically closed electric circuits. Clinical, experimental, and theoretical evidence for an additional circulatory system.* Stockholm, Sweden: Nordic Medical Publications.

Pascual-Leone, L.A., Valls-Sole, J., Brasil-Neto, J.P., et al. (1994). Akinesia in Parkinson's Disease: II. Effects of subthreshold repetitive transcranial motor cortex stimulation. *Neurology, 44,* 892–898.

Pujol, J., Pascual-Leone, A., Bolz, C., et al. (1998). The effect of repetitive magnetic stimulation on localized musculoskeletal pain. *NeuroReport, 9*:1745–1748.

United Nations Environment Programme MF. (1987). The International Labour Organization. World Health Organization.

Vallbona, C., Hazelwood, C.F., & Jurida, G. (1997). Response of pain to static magnetic fields in post-polio patients: A double-blind pilot study. *Archives of Physical Medicine and Rehabilitation, 78,* 1200–1203.

Weintraub, M.I. (1998). Chronic submaximal magnetic stimulation in peripheral neuropathy. Is there a beneficial therapeutic relationship? Pilot study. *American Journal of Pain Management, 8,* 9–13.

Weintraub, M.I. (1999). Magnetic bio-stimulation in painful diabetic peripheral neuropathy: A novel intervention. A randomized double-placebo crossover study. *American Journal of Pain Management, 9,* 8–17.

56

Manipulation under Anesthesia: An Anthology of Past, Present, and Future Use

Robert C. Gordon, B.S. (Ed.), B.S. (Bio.), D.C., D.A.A.P.M., Anthony Rogers, M.D., Daniel T. West, D.C., Robert S. Matthews, M.D., and Mathew R. Miller, P.Ac.

The purpose of this chapter is to enlighten the reader about the treatment of manipulation under anesthesia (MUA). The chapter covers the anthology of MUA from the historical past to its present day usage. We present a basis for using the MUA procedure when manipulative therapy is the therapy of choice, but when conservative office manipulative therapy has had only minimal effect. The focus is on adaptation of this modality into pain management practice when neuromusculoskeletal conditions are being treated. We do not hold MUA out as an all-inclusive treatment modality that is going to replace all forms of treatment for neuromusculoskeletal conditions. We also make no implied reference to any guarantees that if you use MUA you will obtain the same results as have been historically achieved by other MUA practitioners. We do, however, suggest that this modality has been successful with certain types of conditions, later referenced, when other modalities have not. Because this modality has had some success during the years it has been used, this form of therapy needs to be considered as part of the pain management algorithms being considered for neuromusculoskeletal conditions when manual therapy is the therapy of choice.

HISTORICAL PERSPECTIVE

MUA has been used with great success by osteopathic, chiropractic, and orthopedic professionals since the late 1930s. Siehl and Bradford (1952) speak of Persol's International Clinic, which reported 200 cases treated with this modality in 1938. Results indicated that there was a 94 to 97% recovery rate for the conditions treated with the MUA technique. But we can really go back to some of the earliest times when we consider both manipulation and anesthesia. Early Egyptian scrolls and drawings depicted manipulation being used along with herbs to relax the body. Even the earliest of cave drawings showed forms of manipulation being used to "cast out evil spirits." The point is that the use of manipulation and anesthesia predate many of the medical models referenced for the time when manipulation and medicine were first reported. In this section we present a historical anthology of the MUA procedure to lend support to the concept that this procedure has been used for many years. It is not meant to document every article written about this procedure, but instead to give a validated perspective from many sources concerning the multidisciplinary approach of this procedure.

Over the past 60 years, the MUA procedure has come under scrutiny from both the scientific community and insurance carriers. The words "safe" and "effective" have been thrown about with little regard to their full meanings in interpreting the procedure they are discussing. A new procedure that has very little history of use certainly would be classified as having questionable clinical validity. In the medical field, any potential procedure must undergo months of testing with controlled studies to validate its clinical therapeutic value. This is especially true when new procedures that may mean life or death for patients are found to be clinically significant. It is important to investigate these new procedures so that the patients we treat may benefit from everything available

0-8493-0926-3/02/$0.00+$1.50
© 2002 by CRC Press LLC

to them, especially if the new procedures may save their lives. An investigational trial of all procedures must take place to determine if a procedure has clinical significance and whether it is safe for use and effective in procuring results. To become safe and effective, the new procedure must show a record of success, must be able to be duplicated by other practitioners, and must obtain clinically satisfactory results from patients undergoing the procedure. It must have been used by practitioners throughout the country for conditions shown to respond similarly to the procedure, and it must have been used with enough success to warrant its use as an alternative to other procedures if it is used as an intervention rather than other forms of therapy. This sounds much like the same requirements for inclusion in the AMA CPT codes of reimbursable procedures ("Introduction and Instruction for Use," 2000).

Because manipulation under anesthesia has been used as an alternative to prolonged conservative manual therapy and surgical intervention since the late 1930s, and because MUA has been completed on well over 20,000 patients since that same time (number of procedures is based on literature review and clinician interview throughout the United States and United Kingdom), and because the procedure has been used with regularity on the same types of conditions with similar results over that same time period, it falls within the parameters for being both a safe and an effective procedure (Hunter, 1974).

Literature reviews, which have been completed on numerous occasions by many authors, indicate that a considerable body of material has been written on the subject of manipulation under anesthesia, including references in manual therapy texts. I quote from some of these original articles. Clybourne (1948) states:

> I have had the opportunity to use manipulation under anesthesia on a sufficiently large number of cases to realize its scope and limitations. The type of case most amenable to treatment by manipulation is that in which the main pathological cause is the interference with joint motion by the presence of adhesions.

According to Siehl and Bradford (1952), a review of 100 MUA procedures on 87 cases indicated "the method was first used on those cases which were not responding or were responding very slowly to usual manipulative management."

Siehl (1963) states

> A conservative regime which includes manipulative treatment of the lower lumbar intervertebral disc syndrome under anesthesia eventuates in a significantly high percentage of satisfactory results to warrant its use as an essential part of conservative therapy.

Siehl presented an 11-year study of 723 cases treated with MUA at the annual meeting of the American Osteopathic Academy of Orthopedics, Bal Harbour, Florida, October 31, 1962.

Lindemann and Rossak (1959) concluded in the same paper presented by Siehl (1962):

> In our opinion, it is not permissible to regard the reposition under anesthesia without further ado as technical blunders. ... It deserves its place in the scale of the orthopedic therapeutic measures for the treatment of the protrusion and the dorso-lateral prolapse in the lumbar region. For the forms of the sciatic syndrome which are evoked through the dorso-lateral compression working on the nerve roots, the reposition under anesthesia is harmless and presents absolutely an acknowledged and trustworthy procedure in treatment.

In an early presentation at the 39th Annual Session of The American Congress of Physical Medicine and Rehabilitation (1962) Ronald Barbor, M.D. of London, England expressed the essence of the controversy surrounding the use of the MUA procedures we use today when he wrote:

> Manipulation is a word used to mean passive movement, forced movement, mobilization, or stretching. Manipulation carried out while the patient is anesthetized, as done by orthopedic surgeons is reputable, but manipulation done on a conscious patient is disreputable in the eyes of the medical profession, because this is the method used by osteopaths and chiropractors.

Because this concept of the right professional providing the right procedure is still employed today by most insurance companies, the MUA procedure has not been given the proper opportunity to prove its efficacy with the frequency that it should, based on the data from the clinical outcomes seen throughout the country (West, Mathews, Miller, & Kent, 1999). Documentation of the safe and effective use of MUA was evident early when Soden (1949), described the reason for the use of anesthesia during manipulative therapy by writing:

> The answer to the question of "why anesthesia" lies not only in the successful clinical results, but also in the physiology of anesthesia. According to Dr. William Baldwin (Professor of Physiology at the Philadelphia College of Osteopathy), general anesthesia carried well into the surgical stage causes the abolition of reflex response due to a slowing of the reflex arc, and an accompanying change in the graded synaptic resistance at the segmental level. Therefore, due to these factors, postural tonus of the muscles is abolished. With the removal of this postural tonus, there is lost the muscle function of joint stabilization

and the splinting action of the muscles of the joint structures. The loss of these factors of muscular function is desirable in producing joint motion by manipulative procedures, especially when there has been present, previously, a reflexly maintained increase in the postural tonus.

This theory has been the foundation of the MUA technique for many years, but, of course, now with the advancement and use of new medicines, anesthesiologists are able to place patients in conscious sedation, which, when performed properly, can allow the joint to be mobilized without putting the patient under general anesthesia, which also allows for end range appreciation in joints, joint capsules, and appeneuroses (Ettema & Huijing, 1990). In fact, there are really no facilities that I know of in the country that are still inducing general anesthesia for this procedure. That change alone makes for a safer physiological environment for the procedure to be completed.

Krumhansl and Nowacek in Grieve (1986) make the following comment:

> The importance of fascial lengthening, tendon stretching and ligamentous mobilization are as important as the realignment of joints. Patients with long-standing, intense pain resulting from motor vehicle accidents, industrial accidents and severe falls gradually compensate. Eventually even the 'normal' joints of the spine and proximal extremities become involved. Most frequently there develops a zig-zag pattern of muscle tightness and locked facets, either in individual segments or in groups. Manipulation under anesthesia is a final step in a long sequence of medical and physical treatments for patients who have endured prolonged and intractable pain and who have not responded to the more conventional methods of treatment. It is neither new nor revolutionary. Orthopaedic surgeons in the United Kingdom have practiced it for many years. Osteopaths in the United States have relied on its efficacy. A few American orthopaedists have incorporated this approach into their treatment regimes (Stoddard, 1969; Fisher, 1948; Mennell, 1960).

Rumney (1968) states

> Manipulative therapy to the musculoskeletal system under anesthesia has a definite place as an elective modality. Manipulation of the joints of the spine and the appendages under anesthesia has been carried out by orthopedic surgeons for many years, in both the osteopathic and allopathic professions.

Beckett and Francis (1994) reported on a controlled study of MUA completed by Chrisman, Mittnacht, and Snook (1964) that included 39 patients who all had low back pain, sciatica, and positive findings on at least one sciatic nerve stretch with at least one reflex, motor, or

sensory deficit finding. Using guidelines from an earlier study by Mensor (1955), 27 of the 39 patients had positive myelograms for disc herniation. The average duration of the symptoms was 6 years, with a range of 10 days to 25 years. For their last attacks of back pain, these patients had received conservative management including heat, analgesics, muscle relaxants, bracing, flexion exercises, and rest. These patients then received MUA. A similar group of 22 patients received the same conservative care but no MUA. Chrisman, et al. (1964) reported that "the effects of the MUA were frequently dramatic and more than one half of the patients reported their sciatic symptoms lessened within 24 hours." Using Mensor's criteria (1955), Chrisman, et al. (1964) reported that 21 of the MUA patients had excellent or good outcomes at 5 to 10 months follow up, 4 patients had fair outcomes, and 14 patients had unsatisfactory results. Overall, they reported that 51% of the patients with an unequivocal picture of ruptured intervertebral disc unrelieved by conservative care had good or excellent results after MUA (Beckett & Francis, 1994). The 22 non-MUA patients did poorly (no mention of specific results or testing methods) and 16 eventually required surgery (Chrisman, et al., 1964). The findings of Chrisman, et al. (1964) were consistent with the findings of Mensor (1955) in the earlier study.

H.A. Williams (1998), past president, Council on Chiropractic Orthopedics, ACA, states the following in a three-part article in the *ACA Journal of Chiropractic*:

> Manipulation under anesthesia as a procedure appears to be well within the province of chiropractic. Traditionally, chiropractics' goal has been to restore and maintain the welfare of the human body. In my opinion, MUA fits within that goal since the responsible chiropractor is concerned with appropriateness, necessity, utility, identifiable goals and objectives, utilization standards, protocols, indications, contraindications, patient needs, patient selection, patient safety, defensive practices, collaboration and a (currently limited) scientific basis (Bilkey, 1993)

P.E. Greenman (1992) observes that

> manipulation while the patient is under anesthesia is an old widely recognized procedure in musculoskeletal medicine. It is used for treating acute and chronic musculoskeletal conditions with significant biomechanical dysfunction unresponsive to conservative therapy.

C.G. Davis (1996) states:

> Manipulation under anesthesia (MUA) has been used successfully for many years in treating acute and chronic musculoskeletal conditions that have been unresponsive to other types of care. The purpose of anesthesia is to obliterate the responses to pain and the

muscle spasm that may limit other forms of conservative care from being successful.

In the same article as above, Davis quotes Morey (1975): "manipulation with the patient under anesthesia should be performed by graduate manual medicine practitioners who have a high level of skill and have been trained in structural diagnosis and manipulative treatment." Davis goes on to expand upon the concept of being trained in manipulative therapy by specifically relating to his state of California and its interpretations of those practitioners who are educated to perform manipulations of any kind:

The capacity to perform manipulative therapy is defined by statute and in California, manipulative therapy can be performed by a physician, including a medical doctor, an osteopath, or a chiropractor. Additionally in the state of California the Attorney General has stated that the adjustment in manipulation of hard tissue, that is bones and bony structure, is particularly a chiropractic technique. Shekelle, Adams, Chassin, Hurwitz, and Brook (1992) report from a RAND study found that 94% of the manipulative therapy performed in the United States is by chiropractors. As part of the chiropractic education there are over 600 hours of basic instruction for manipulative therapy with an additional 8 months of internship (LACC Class Catalog, 1982) with additional training in proctoring requirements to perform manipulation under anesthesia (Davis, 1996).

This statement is true relative to all chiropractic colleges and most states with regard to application by professionals who perform manipulative therapy.

Gordon (1995) wrote:

Standard Chiropractic services include procedures which specifically move articulations to promote the healing process, increase flexibility, correct a subluxation complex and provide holistic concepts in healthcare. Chiropractic care has been healing the world for the past 100 years and has literally cured the world of many of its ills. With the introduction of MUA, we have another avenue to try if the patient falls into MUA categories before referral is necessary. The basic concept behind mobilization, manipulation, and adjusting procedures while the patient is under a sedative/hypnotic is to increase articular, ligamentus, tendenous and muscular flexibility that has not been achieved in the office routine. Standard chiropractic techniques are used but the physiological state of the patient is changed, and the procedure is done in a different environment. Even with the enhancement of physiotherapy, many cases don't respond in the office, and it's only with the physiological change that the body can respond and the fixation be altered so the patient receives relief. Many chronic cases are candidates for the MUA procedures and they tend to respond extremely well.

Gordon, Hickman, & Gray (1999) state:

MUA has been recorded to have been successful as far back as the late 30's by the osteopathic profession. The anesthetics used were not as sophisticated, and the techniques were not what has been considered by manipulative therapy literature as site specific (Kleyhans, Terrett, Glasglow, Twomey, & Schull, 1985). The purpose of using MUA is to provide mobilization, manipulation and adjustments of the spinal motion units and the surrounding soft tissue in an atmosphere where there is a decrease in muscle splinting and contracture and where the patient's apprehension about the maneuver lessens. It is also used because the patient is more responsive to manipulative procedures than in an office setting. When used on properly selected patients it is more cost effective and more productive to the patient's return to normal lifestyle than prolonged conservative care or possible surgical intervention (Gordon, 1993).

West, et al. (1999) wrote:

Manipulation under anesthesia (MUA) is the use of manual manipulation of the spine combined with the use of general anesthetic. The addition of anesthetic allows for the benefits of manipulation to be shared with those patients who cannot tolerate manual techniques because of pain response, spasm, muscle contractures, and guarding. MUA uses a combination of specific short lever arm manipulations, passive stretches, and specific articular and postural kinesthetic integrations to obtain a desired outcome (Gordon, 1993; Wiesel, Boden, & Feffer, 1994; Wyke, 1972).

West, et al. continue the discussion on manipulation under anesthesia by describing the anesthesiology part of MUA.

There has been much discussion regarding the use of general anesthetic in the performance of MUA. Issues discussed include the depth of consciousness associated with general anesthesia, the inability of the patient to give pain feedback or resist over zealous manipulation, and the intrinsic guarding mechanism of voluntary/involuntary muscle fibers, which protect the elastic barrier in the conscious patient.

To address these concerns West, et al. make the following points:

First, only highly skilled graduate practitioners who have trained in structural diagnosis and manipulative treatments should perform these procedures. And secondly, the advent of newer, short-acting, highly titratable, and completely reversible intravenous anesthetics allow for controlled anesthesia depths, preservation of patient pain response, as well as significantly reduce morbidity and mortality rates.

Several references in the above literature have related to the use of general anesthetics with the MUA procedure. As this procedure has evolved into what is practiced today, we have found that the same or better response to MUA could be achieved using conscious sedation. Most of the procedures currently done in the United States use conscious sedation. (See the "Conscious Sedation" section of this chapter.) The anesthetics utilized are short acting and can be titered to allow for patient response, yet allow for a protective level that permits the doctor to complete the manipulative technique without putting the patient at a point where tissue damage will occur. All of the articles that have been reviewed point to the fact that manipulation under anesthesia has been not only used for a number of years, but also has been investigated both clinically and scientifically. Today, with the advent of newer medications employed with anesthesia and the formation of a national association, the National Academy of MUA Physicians (1995), in October of 1995, the procedure of manipulation under anesthesia is being recognized as a real alternative to prolonged conservative care and possible surgical intervention (Gordon, et al., 1999). The National Academy of MUA Physicians has established standards and protocols for the primary practitioner doing the manipulation under anesthesia (who, in most instances, is a chiropractic physician), has established standards for anesthesia, for nursing, and for the facilities where MUA is performed. These standards and protocols have started to be endorsed throughout the United States primarily by state boards. Most of the state boards of chiropractic have adhered to the provisions in their state laws, which state that procedures taught by CCE-accredited chiropractic colleges fall within the scope of practice of a chiropractic physician. A couple of the states have adopted a policy relative to manipulation under anesthesia, directing specific language to their scope of the practice. The North Carolina Board of Chiropractic Examiners released a position statement in August 1994 that stated:

> Manipulation of a patient under anesthesia by an MUA trained chiropractor is within the scope of chiropractic in North Carolina. MUA is an exceptional combination of effective pain management procedures that has expanded the options to help relieve persistent pain. MUA is not an experimental procedure. It is well established within the chiropractic and medical communities and the utilization of MUA has been enhanced by the professional cooperation of these two procedures (Williams, 1998).

SCIENTIFIC SUPPORT

The MUA procedure is used to alter adhesions and correct joint dysfunction caused by chronic connective tissue scarring and/or joint fixation from disuse following injury or repetitive trauma causing pain. The procedure also is being employed in acute care with medical intervention to decrease the time it takes to overcome certain neuromusculoskeletal conditions. The procedure is directed at altering adhesions by stretching tissues while the patient is under conscious sedation or in concert with joint injection. The most widely accepted theory for the results obtained by using this technique is that as the practitioner uses the MUA techniques, the forces and concurrent responses to those forces cause desired changes in mechanoreceptors and, thus, neurological changes through the joints and joint capsules. By stretching the muscle fibers surrounding the joints, adhesions that are built up in the muscle fibers from disuse in the injured area are altered to give the connective tissues and joints more mobility and, secondarily, increase flexibility. References indicate that if continuous linear force is used to prolong a period of sustained stretch, the stretch reflex in the muscle spindle, the Golgi tendon response, is reversed so that instead of an immediate counter-reaction contraction called a bolistic response stretch, the muscle can be stretched into an altered disuse plastic deformans state (Alter, 1988). If the disuse or altered plastic deformans state is attained in the disuse range of the injured elastic range of the muscle(s) being stretched, there is a good chance that permanent change will occur. If this same range was achieved in the normal muscle and joint end range, plastic deformans would result in strain and potential fiber tearing of the muscle. But, if we consider that most muscle fibers are in a shortened state from disuse after an injury, and that the cross-bridging normally responsible for creating muscle contraction is in a state of contracture, the ability to stretch the muscle beyond this state is a considerably significant part of the MUA technique. We feel this is occurring because the patient who undergoes the MUA procedure has a definite increase in range of motion with very little, if any, microtrauma. And if proper follow-up post-MUA therapy is performed (Gordon, 1993), the increase in range of motion is permanent in 85 to 95% of the cases (Gordon, 1993; Lindemann & Rossak, 1959; West, et al., 1999). If completed properly with the properly selected patients, MUA is one of the more gentle forms of manipulative techniques.

Reference has always been made to properly selected patients and those same references have also stressed the importance of properly trained practitioners.

> No amount of experience in the office setting will qualify a physician for manipulation of the patient under anesthesia. No hospital should permit the physician to perform such manipulation until he has been observed and has received supervision and the approval of an experienced operator who himself has been previously approved by certification and hospital proficiency standards (Siehl-Bradford, 1952).

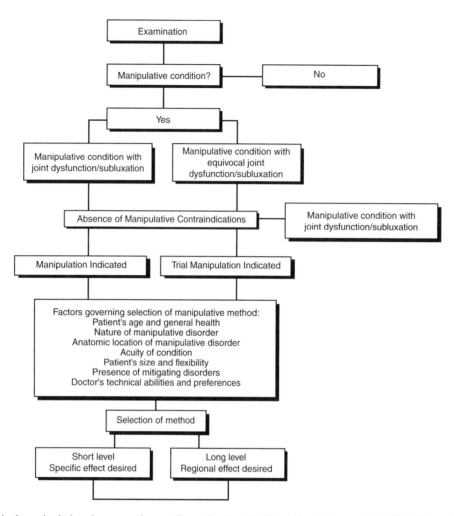

FIGURE 56.1 Spinal manipulation therapy pathway. (From Gordon, R., West, D., Mathews, R., Miller, M., and Kent, G. (1995). *Standards and Protocols*. Manchester, MO: The National Academy of MUA Physicians. With permission.)

The basis of change achieved when using the MUA technique makes it mandatory that the practitioner be properly trained to perform this technique. It is not a technique that just anyone can perform with success and the more training the practitioner has in the art of manipulation, the better prepared he or she is to successfully complete this procedure. In the past 40 years or so, chiropractors have had more education in manipulation than other professionals and, therefore, have also been the practitioners of choice for those considering MUA.

MUA has been used historically for both acute and chronic conditions. The concept of acute care, however, takes on a different meaning when we speak of MUA. Acute refers to severity, not time, as it pertains to MUA. By this we mean that many conditions have recurrent acute exacerbations over the course of the treatment period. This is determined by the patient's perception of pain, and is measured subjectively by the doctor using a visual analogue scale and patient questionnaire instruments. Measurement in improvement in many

facilities is objectively obtained by using MRI, EMG, Functional Capacity testing, and video fluoroscopy.

The use of MUA is in itself traumatic on a microtrauma scale, and increasing the inflammation by stretching and articular manipulations during the MUA procedure would tend to increase this inflammatory response, so we don't normally use MUA on acute traumatic cases. There are instances, however, when the patient has unrelenting pain that is interfering with activities of daily living (ADLs). In these instances, the team that would provide the MUA procedure might evaluate whether the patient could be brought into the MUA program using MUJA (manipulation under joint anesthesia) to gently stretch out the areas to try and give the patient some relief through the benefit of increased circulation from passive stretching, injectable medications, and decreased inflammatory response.

The National Academy of MUA Physicians (1995) has established parameters for acute care MUA that state that MUA/MUJA is a proper progressive alternative if forms of manipulative treatment and medical

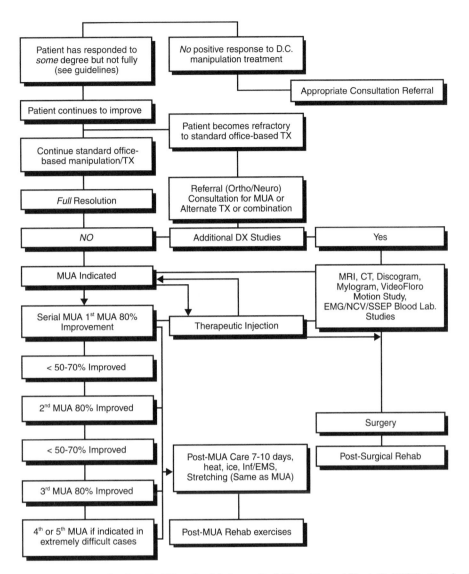

FIGURE 56.2 MUA pathway. (From Gordon, R., West, D., Mathews, R., Miller, M., and Kent, G. (1995). *Standards and Protocols.* Manchester, MO: The National Academy of MUA Physicians. With permission.)

pharmocologic intervention for a period of 2 weeks have been tried and had little effect with minimal change and progressive deterioration. This treatment would vary from the normal MUA and involve coordination with the medical team member and involve pain management combined with manipulative therapeutics. It has been established that when this acute traumatic care stage has been reached, it usually takes only one MUJA to bring the patient back to the conservative office program (Gordon, 1993).

MUA vs. MUJA

The use of these techniques has advanced the broader-based MUA technique even more in the last 4 to 5 years. MUA is a common technique for alteration of joints, joint capsules, and muscle tissue using stretching and articular manipulation under conscious sedation.

MUJA, or manipulation under joint anesthesia/analgesia, has advanced into the field in the past 4 or 5 years as an alternative to conscious sedation by using joint injection to decrease the inflammation in the joint, anesthetize the joint, and manipulate the joint to provide mobilization and flexibility while decreasing joint irritation.

ACUTE CARE MUA

MUJA is used for acute care MUA and is being put forward by the concept that relief from intractable pain (pain, neuromusculoskeletal in origin, with no relief) could be provided by injection into the affected joint, with mobilization and manipulation used secondarily to diffuse the injected medicine and help eliminate the inflammatory reaction in the affected joints (Dreyfuss, Michaelsen, & Horne, 1995).

REASONS FOR MUJA

Early mobilization of the involved joints, despite otherwise intractable pain and/or muscle spasm, reduces compressive forces on the discs, facet capsules, and nerve roots (which would cause additional scar tissue if left untreated), thereby allowing nutrients and fluids into the area of the lesion and helping the body heal itself more naturally and rapidly.

MUJA RESULTS

In Acute Care MUA, MUJA reduces:

- Excessive scar tissue build-up
- The chance for muscle contracture
- Duration and frequency of regular outpatient spinal manipulative therapy
- The percentage of resultant permanent impairment

MUJA IN CHRONIC CARE

MUJA has been used to affect joint involvement in chronic neuromusculoskeletal conditions. Injection into the involved joint to determine the pain location has been utilized for many years as both an objective diagnostic tool and a therapeutic tool. It is employed in conjunction with the injection to improve joint mobility. The same standards of care and protocols are followed when patients are chosen for the MUJA procedure as for the MUA procedure. The conditions treated with MUJA are somewhat the same as MUA, with the exception being more joint involvement as compared to myofascial and/or muscular involvement.

The majority of MUA candidates historically have been those patients who suffer from chronic joint restriction due to fixation from disuse following trauma. This syndrome sets up a vicious cycle that Michael Alter (1988) calls the "self-perpetuating cycle of muscle spasm." In this cycle, the patient undergoes a form of trauma, which can be caused by direct contact or through repetitive incremental injuries. These injuries then set up pain stimuli, inflammation, emotional tension, sometimes infection, temperature variations, and eventual immobilization from disuse. As the cycle proceeds, it sets up reflex muscle contraction which, if gone untreated, progresses to muscle contracture. This, in turn, progresses to restricted movement and fixation in the joints, which has a direct effect on what Wyke (1972) calls "dysfunctional postural kinesthetics." Wyke refers to a disturbance in postural kinesthetics resulting in altered mechanoreceptor response.

Typically, Types I, II, and IV mechanoreceptors are concurrently involved, setting up a cycle of trauma-induced altered posture affecting movement, which then stimulates nociceptive response.

Using the MUA technique, we complete stretching maneuvers and mobilization techniques coupled with specific adjustive techniques to help alter adhesion accumulation that has been laid down by the body as connective tissue protective mechanisms to prevent further damage to the areas involved. Because new medications allow us to perform this technique while the patient is in conscious sedation, we can provide progressive linear forces to these areas and alter these adhesions without tearing tissue in the process. Because these medications allow the patient to relax and not respond with immediate muscle contraction when pain is perceived, we are able to perform these maneuvers so that end range is not lost. The natural protective mechanisms are present but are slowed down temporarily, and pain is perceived, but not remembered (Gordon, 1993). By completing the MUA procedure as a team, with the anesthesiologist as a very valuable member who provides just the right medications to allow this physiological change from the normal office manipulative therapy program, the certified MUA doctor is able to accomplish considerably more with MUA than if the same patient were to undergo these procedures in the office setting without the conscious sedation. The most important concept here is that if the patient were able to recover in the office setting without the use of conscious sedation, the patient would not have been a candidate for the MUA procedure in the first place.

SERIAL MUA

MUA as performed today is completed in a 2- to 4-day continuous program. The procedure is repeated every day with same-day follow-up care given in the facility or the doctor's office 1 to 2 hours after the actual procedure. The reason for doing the procedure in a serial fashion is to alter the adhesion formation present during the remodeling phase of the inflammatory cycle into a phase where permanent change is made. The procedure is done in small increments each day to effect change rather than in 1 day and possibly causing inflammatory exacerbation. Kotlke (1971) indicates that if altered, an adhesion will begin to re-form in 24 to 48 hours. Serial MUA and post-MUA therapy are performed every day to prevent re-formation of connective tissue adhesions after alteration.

THE MUA PROCEDURE (GORDON, 1993)

The patient is draped in the appropriate gowning and is taken by gurney or led walking to the operative area and asked to lie supine on the operating table. The patient is then placed on the appropriate monitors for conscious sedation as established by ASA standards. When the patient and doctor are ready, the anesthesiologist will administer the appropriate medications to assist the patient into conscious sedation using medications that allow the stretching, mobilization, and adjustments necessary for the completion of the outcome the doctor desires.

The Cervical Spine

The patient's arms are crossed and he or she is approached from the cephalad end of the table. Long-axis axial traction is applied to the patient's cervical spine and musculature while counter-traction is applied by the first assistant, who then is positioned to stabilize the patient's shoulders in order to use the counter-traction maneuver. Traction in the same manner is then applied in a controlled lateral coronal plane bilaterally, and then in an oblique manner by rotating the patient's head to 45° and elevating the head toward the patient's chest. This is also accomplished bilaterally. The patient's head is then brought into a neutral posture and cervical flexion is achieved to traction the cervical paravertebral muscles. The cervical spine is then taken into a rotatory/lateral (bone setting) traction maneuver to achieve specific closed reduction manipulation of the vertebral elements at the level of articular abnormality on one side and again using the same technique on the opposite side, if indicated, at the level of articular abnormality. During this maneuver, a low velocity thrust is achieved after taking the vertebrae slightly past the elastic barrier of resistance, and into the paraphysiologic space. (Cavitation may or may not be achieved.)

The Thoracic Spine

With the patient in the supine position on the operating table, the upper extremities are flexed at the elbow and crossed over the patient's chest to achieve maximum traction of the patient's thoracic spine. The first assistant holds the patient's arms in the proper position and assists in rolling the patient for the adjustive procedure. With the help of the first assistant, the patient is rolled to his/her left/right side, selection is made for the contact point, and the patient is rolled back over the doctor's hand. The elastic barrier of resistance is found and a low velocity thrust is achieved using a specific closed reduction anterior to posterior/superior manipulative procedure. This maneuver is referred to as an anteriority adjustment.

The Lumbar Spine

With the patient supine on the procedure table the primary physician addresses the patient's lower extremities, which are elevated alternatively in a straight leg-raising manner to approximately 90° from the horizontal. Linear force is used to gradually increase the hip flexion during this maneuver. Simultaneously, the first assistant applies a myofascial release technique to the calf and posterior thigh musculature. Each lower extremity is independently bent at the knee and tractioned cephalad in a neutral saggital plane, lateral oblique cephalad traction, and medial oblique cephalad traction maneuver. The primary physician then approximates the opposite single knee from his/her position from neutral to medial slightly beyond the elastic barrier of resistance. (A piriformis myofascial release may be accomplished at this time.) This is repeated with the opposite lower extremity. Following this, a Patrick-Fabere maneuver is performed up to and slightly beyond the elastic barrier of resistance.

With the assisting physician stabilizing the pelvis and femoral head (as necessary), the primary physician extends the right lower extremity in the saggital plane, and while applying controlled traction gradually stretches the para-articular holding elements of the right hip by means of gradually describing an approximately 30 to 35° horizontal arc. The lower extremity is then tractioned straight caudad and internal rotation is accomplished. Using traction, the lower extremity is gradually stretched into a horizontal arch to approximately 30°. This procedure is then repeated using external rotation to stretch the para-articular holding elements of the hips bilaterally. These procedures are then repeated on the opposite lower extremity.

By approximating the patient's knees to the abdomen in a knee–chest fashion with the knees separated to avoid abdominal pressure, the lumbo-pelvic musculature is stretched in the saggital plane, by both the primary and first assistant, contacting the base of the sacrum and raising the lower torso cephalad, resulting in passive flexion of the entire lumbar spine and its holding elements beyond the elastic barrier of resistance. With the patient's lower extremities kept in hip/knee flexion, the patient's torso is secured by the first assistant and the lumbar fasciae/musculature elongated obliquely to the right of midline, in a controlled manner up to and beyond the elastic barrier of resistance. (Cavitation may be noted.) This is repeated on the opposite side.

With the use of the undersheets, the patient is carefully placed in the left/right decubitus position and positioned so that the lumbar spine overlays the kidney plate to the point where the lumbar spine attains the horizontal, and is de-rotated to avoid facet imbrication. The patient's body is stabilized by the first assistant. The knee and hip of the upper leg are flexed and the lower leg stabilized in the extended position by the first assistant. Segmental localization of the appropriate lumbar motion units is made by the primary physician and the elastic barrier of resistance found. A low-velocity impulse thrust is applied to achieve cavitation. (If desired, the PSIS is then adjusted on the opposite side with the patient in the same position as above.)

The patient is then repositioned supine by means of the undersheets. With appropriate assistance, the patient is transferred from the procedure table to the gurney and is returned to the recovery room, where appropriate equipment is utilized to monitor vital signs. The IV is maintained up to the point where the patient is fully alert and stable, and the patient is then transferred to a sitting recovery position and given fluids and a light snack. Following this, the patient is discharged with appropriate home instructions (Gordon, et al., 1999; Gordon, 1993). (Note: It must be emphasized that all pathology has been ruled out, and proper patient selection has taken place.)

CONSCIOUS SEDATION*

This is a brief overview of conscious sedation, which is used in the MUA and MUJA procedures. It is not intended as an anesthesia "how to" course but instead provides an understanding of the term "conscious sedation" and the usual medications used in delivering this type of anesthesia.

PRE-OPERATIVE CONSIDERATIONS

Anesthesia can be divided into 3 classifications: general anesthesia, MAC (monitored anesthesia care), and local. General anesthesia is placing the patient into an altered level of consciousness so that his/her vital reflexes are severely depressed or absent. The patient is usually unconscious, cannot cooperate, and is prone to airway obstruction. Local anesthesia consists of injecting local anesthetic agents into the area to be operated on. MAC can be both conscious or unconscious sedation and can be a continuum between the two; however, the goal for MU(J)A is conscious sedation.

Conscious sedation is produced by the administration of pharmacologic agents. A patient undergoing conscious sedation has a depressed level of consciousness but retains the ability to independently and continuously maintain a patent airway and respond appropriately to physical stimulation and/or verbal commands. The medications and dosages utilized for conscious sedation are not intended to produce deep sedation or loss of consciousness. Practitioners of conscious sedation should be ACLS trained and comfortable with airway management and resuscitation.

The objectives of conscious sedation are altering of the level of consciousness and mood, maintaining consciousness and cooperation, providing relaxation and amnesia, and elevating the pain threshold, with minimal variation of the patient's vital signs. The patient should be easily aroused from sleep, have purposeful responses to verbal communication and tactile stimulation, and should be able to return to ambulation in a short period

of time, with the duration of amnesia also falling within the duration of the procedure.

The undesirable effects that one is trying to avoid are a deep unarousable sleep, respiratory depression, airway obstruction, apnea, decrease in vital signs (bradycardia, hypotension, etc.), agitation and combativeness, and loss of pain reflexes.

Pre-procedural evaluation of each patient is mandatory and can be done by the patient's primary care physician and/or anesthesiologist. Acute, unforeseen medical problems can arise previous to the procedure or even the day of the procedure and may necessitate postponement. However, standard pre-operative practices should be in place that allow for the identification of chronic conditions or significant items in the patient's medical history, which can then be addressed prior to the day of the procedure. The patient should have a complete medical history and physical including drug allergies, previous experience with sedation and/or anesthesia, pertinent laboratory and X-ray results, and medications the patient is taking. The patient will then be given an ASA (American Society of Anesthesia) classification, which ranges from Class 1 to Class 6. Most patients will fall between Classes 1 to 3 (1 = normal health, 2 = mild systemic disease, and 3 = severe systemic disease).

The day of the procedure, the patient will be seen by the anesthesiologist and all data will be reviewed including the patient's NPO status. If everything is in order, the patient will be taken to the operating or procedure room and placed on the procedure table. Monitors including blood pressure, EKG, and pulse oximetry will be placed. IV access will be established so that the sedating agents can be given. After baseline vital signs have been established, the patient will begin to be sedated and the procedure can then begin. The sedation is usually accomplished by a combination of benzodiazepines, narcotics, and ultrashort-acting hypnotic agents. Variability in pain tolerance and medication requirements is great, and the range of responses to the various medications can be dramatic; therefore, titration of the various agents is the key to optimum sedation.

PHARMACOLOGY OF MEDICATIONS (COMMONLY USED SEDATING AGENTS)

Benzodiazepines provide sedation and amnesia but are not analgesic or anti-emetic. The common medications in this class in order of duration are midazolam (Versed), diazepam (Valium) and lorazepam (Ativan). The adverse effects are respiratory depression, hypotension, bradycardia, and hypoventilation and are potentiated by narcotics.

Narcotics provide analgesia and this is more pronounced if given before a painful stimulus. The common medications in this class in order of duration are Alfentanil, fentanyl (sublimaze), meperidine (Dem-

---

* Contributed by Anthony Rogers, M.D.

erol), and morphine. The adverse effects are respiratory depression, apnea (potentiated by benzodiazepines), bradycardia, hypotension, pruritis, nausea/vomiting, and urinary retention.

Barbiturates provide sedation and hypnosis. The common medications in this class are propofol (diprivan), methohexital (brevital), and ketamine (dissociative agent). The adverse affects are respiratory depression, apnea, tachy/bradycardia, hypotension, and pain on injection.

There are two reversal agents in use, one for the narcotics and one for the benzodiazepines. The duration of action is usually shorter than those being reversed, so caution should be given to resedation and the patient should be closely monitored. The agents are naloxone (narcan), which is used in the reversal of narcotics and flumazenil (romazicon), which is used in the reversal of benzodiazepines. There is no reversal agent for the barbiturates.

The post-operative course should be short if the sedation was titrated and the shorter-acting agents were used. With a combination of versed and propofol most patients are awake and alert within 5 minutes after the procedure and are able to be discharged within the shortest period of time, usually a half hour, but this may vary from center to center.

ANESTHESIA RECORD[*]

A standard example of a medication dose record might be

Sex: Male	Chief Complaint: Cervicogenic Headaches
Age: 44	Paracervical myospasm
Wt.: 187 lbs.	Paralumbar myospasm
	Lumbar disc dysfunction
Nonsmoker	Nature of Condition: Chronic
N K A Treatment Modalities:	SMPT; PT; Pharmacological intervention; 3 Epidurals
No Prescription or OTC Meds	
ASA Class 1	
No Relative Med. Hist.	
Onset: MVA– 4/20/96	
Anesthesia Record:	40 mg propofol
	50 mcg fentanyl
	2 mg versed

Patient was supplemented with 20 mg propofol one time during the 15-minute procedure.

The usual initial dosage range for MUA at this facility has been

25–50 mg propofol
50–100 mcg fentanyl
0–2 mg versed

Supplemental doses of propofol vary depending on patient's weight and response and are titered accordingly.

INDICATIONS AND CONTRAINDICATIONS

The indications and contraindications for MUA are based on conditions that would ordinarily be indicated for manipulation or contraindicated for manipulation. The addition of contraindications for anesthesia becomes part of the equation because of the use of manipulation with conscious sedation. The following list is composed of conditions that have been recorded historically as successfully treated with MUA, or have been contraindicated for the use of MUA. The list is evolutionary; as more becomes known about this procedure, both parts of the list will grow in length.

Indications	Contraindications
1. Bulging protruded, prolapsed, or herniated discs without free fragment and not surgical candidates	1. Any form of malignancy
	2. Metastatic bone disease
	3. TB of the bone
2. Frozen or fixated articulations	4. Acute bone fractures
3. Failed low back surgery	5. Direct manipulation of old compression fractures
4. Compression syndromes with or without radiculopathies caused from adhesion formation, but not associated with osteophytic entrapment	6. Acute inflammatory arthritis
	7. Acute inflammatory gout.
	8. Uncontrolled diabetic neuropathy
5. Restricted motion, which causes the patient pain and apprehension, but manipulation is the therapy of choice	9. Syphilitic articular or periarticular lesions
	10. Gonorrheal spinal arthritis
	11. Advanced osteoporosis (as indicated diagnostically)
6. Unresponsive to manipulation and adjustment when they are the treatment of choice	12. Evidence of cord or caudal compression by tumor or disc herniation (Note: Use a 5–8 mm in L/S bulge or 3–5 mm in C/S as a guide for further investigation prior to recommending MUA in these areas.)
7. Unresponsive pain, which interferes with the function of daily life and sleep patterns but falls within the parameters for manipulative treatment	
8. Unresponsive muscle contracture that is preventing normal daily activities and function	13. Osteomyelitis
	14. Widespread staph/strep infection

[*] Case presented courtesy of The Center for Special Surgery at Hawthorne, John Tauber, Administrator; Dave Hershan, M.D., Anesthesiologist.

9. Post-traumatic syndrome injuries from acceleration/deceleration or acceleration/deceleration types of injuries which result in painful exacerbation of chronic fixations

10. Chronic recurrent neuromusculoskeletal dysfunction syndromes, which result in a regular periodic treatment series and are always exacerbation of the same condition

11. Neuromusculoskeletal conditions that are not surgical candidates but have reached maximum medical improvement (MMI), especially with occupational injuries

15. Sign/symptom of aneurysm

16. Unstable spondylolysis

COMPLICATIONS

As with any procedure, when addressing the safe and effective nature of the procedure, it is also necessary to discuss complications from that procedure as well as concern regarding those complications. Phil Greenman (1992) states that

> temporary flare-ups of symptoms after the procedure have been reported by several patients. This flare-up is attributed to stretching of the adhesion and mobilization of inflamed soft tissue joints. It is easily controlled with appropriate post-operative care. Serious complications have been rare.

He quotes Poppen (1945) who reported in 1945

> two cases of paralysis after manipulation by competent orthopedic surgeons with the patient under anesthesia. This complication occurred in a population of 400 cases of intervertebral disc disease. It appears that serious complications can be avoided by appropriate patient selection, suitable operative technique by a competent practitioner, and consideration for the contraindications and potential complications.

Davis (1996) notes:

> because of the range of possible adverse reactions, cases must be carefully selected. (Referring to cervical MUA) Success is directly related to the skill of the anesthesiologist in providing the appropriate sedation and the operator's manipulative skills. Data on complications from cervical MUA are not available. However, the relevant values for severe complications for all cervical

manipulations have been estimated at between 1 in 380,000 to over 1 in one million (Eder & Tilscher, 1990; Terrett & Kleynhans, 1992). Deaths from chiropractic cervical manipulations are rare (Terrett, 1988). General anesthesia has a higher risk of about 1 death per 200,000 for ambulatory surgery (Liu, 1992). Though it is possible that the vertebral artery can be compressed or damaged with manipulation throughout the cervical spine this has generally been reported in the first three segments. Between the C1-C2 transverse process the vertebral arteries are relatively fixed at the C1-C2 transverse foramen, therefore rotation will produce stretching of the vertebral artery. At C2-C3 level, compression may be due to superior articular facet of C3 on the ipsilateral side of head rotation, and the C1 transverse process can compress the internal carotid artery. An important point to make here is that lateral flexion on the neck apparently has little effect on vertebral artery blood flow in most cases suggesting little stress on the artery.

The procedure of manipulation under anesthesia of the cervical spine is completed with low-velocity, high-amplitude thrusting procedures that put very little torsion into the cervical spine. The primary focus of MUA in the cervical spine is axial and lateral tractioning and oblique tractioning with articular cavitation occurring generally during the stretching maneuvers (Gordon, et al., 1999; Gordon, 1993). Also, currently, with the use of conscious sedation rather than general anesthesia the patient is able to discern pain, although neuro-perception is slowed down, and retain end range of muscles and joints during the MUA procedure. This allows for full stretching maneuvers and articular cavitation without the inherent risk of vertebrovascular accident, tissue rupture, or joint dislocation. Patients also have undergone prerequisite conservative care for at least 4 to 6 weeks and usually several months prior to having an MUA. Because the office form of manipulation is high velocity, low amplitude, if damage to the spinal segments, vertebral arteries, or tissue were going to occur, it certainly would have happened during the office manipulative therapy program. Again, this is why a regime of conservative manipulative therapy before considering the MUA procedure is recommended and also why there are very few recorded instances of tissue damage, injury, or CVAs from MUA. As with any technique using forms of anesthesia, there are inherent risks that are part of this procedure. But historically there have been very few reports of damage from the MUA procedure and most of those were either from medication reaction or because the procedure was performed by uncertified, unskilled practitioners.

The safety and the effectiveness of manipulation under anesthesia have been widely proven by clinical documentation. The above-referenced articles and information all relate to the educational standards necessary to perform this procedure, proper patient selection for the procedure, and then proper follow-up care once the procedure has been completed. The standards also apply to physician training to provide proper diagnostic and examination procedures prior to having the patient undergo manipulation under anesthesia. If all of these areas are followed properly, the MUA procedure is safe to perform. It has been completed on several thousand patients and the effectiveness has greatly outweighed any minimal risks from the types of anesthesia used. All of the malpractice insurance carriers for the chiropractic profession, the osteopathic profession, and the medical profession cover these types of physicians for MUA. If there were any question regarding the safety and effectiveness of this procedure, insurance carriers would not cover physicians under malpractice parameters.

REFERENCES

Alter, M. (1988). *The science of stretching* (2nd ed., pp. 13). Champaign, IL: Human Kinetics Pub., Inc.

Anderson, Jr., E.R. (2000). Introduction and instruction for use. In *AMA current procedural terminology*, (CPT), (4th ed.) Ix.

Barbor, R. (1962). Rationale of manipulation of joints. Paper read at the 39th annual session of The American Congress of Physical Medicine and Rehabilitation, Cleveland, OH.

Beckett, R.H., & Francis, R. (1994). *Spinal manipulation under anesthesia. Advances in chiropractic* (p. 325). Arlington, VA: ACA.

Chrisman, O.D., Mittnacht, A., & Snook, G.A. (1964). A study of the results following rotatory manipulation in the lumbar intervertebral disc syndrome. *Journal of Bone and Joint Surgery, 46*, 517.

Clybourne, H.E. (1948). Manipulation of low back region under anesthesia. *Journal of American Osteopathic Association*, Sept., 10.

Davis, C.G. (1996). Chronic cervical spine pain treated with manipulation under anesthesia. *Journal of Neuromuscloskeletal Systems, 4*, 102.

Dreyfuss, P., Michaelsen, M., & Horne, M. (1995). Manipulation under joint anesthesia/analgesia: a treatment approach for recalcitrant low back pain of synovial joint origin. *Journal of Manipulative and Physiological Therapeutics*, April, 17.

Eder, M., & Tilscher, H. (1990). *Chiropractic therapy: Diagnosis and treatment* (p. 60). In M.S. Gengenbach (Ed.). Gaithersburg: Aspen.

Ettema, G., & Huijing, P.A. (1990). Architecture and elastic properties of the series elastic element of muscle-tendon complex. In J. Winters (Ed.), *Multiple muscle systems, biomechanics and movement organization*. New York: Springer-Verlag.

Fisher, A.G.T. (1948). *Manipulative treatment, general principles treatment by manipulation* (5th ed., p. 66). New York: Hoeber.

Fung, Y.C.B. (1967). Elasticity of soft tissues in simple elongation. *American Journal of Physiology, 213*, 1532.

Gilkey, D.P. (1993). Issues concerning chiropractic standards of practice. In J. Sweere (Ed.), *Chiropractic practice: A clinical manual* (p. 41). Gaithersburg: Aspen.

Gordon, R. (1993). *Syllabus on MUA for the course sponsored by The National College of Chiropractic* (4th ed., p. 25). Salisbury, NC: Cornerstone Professional Education.

Gordon, R. (1995). Justifying MUA within the standard chiropractic scope of practice. *Florida Chiropracters Association Journal*, Nov.–Dec., 16.

Gordon, R., Hickman, G., & Gray, J. (1999). Proprioception as a prerequisite to SG cell response in inhibiting musculoskeletal pain using manipulation under anesthesia. *Dynamic Chiropractic*, May, 8.

Gordon, R., West, D., Mathews, R., Miller, M., & Kent, G. (1995). *Standards and protocols*, Manchester, MO: The National Academy of MUA Physicians

Greenman, P.E. (1992). Manipulation with the patient under anesthesia. *Journal of the American Osteopathic Association, 92*, 1159.

Hunter, P. (1994). District Judge, The State of Wyoming. 5th Judicial District. Consolidated Park Co. Civil Case. Workers Compensation Case Appeal. Attorneys Bancroft, T.C., Kahl, D.L. For the plaintiffs: Stickney, C.L., Dunn, E.L., Helmey, J.E., Ivie, J., Messick, W.L., et al. Aug. 3.

Kleyhans, A.M., Terrett, A.G.J., Glasglow, E.F., Twomey, L.T., & Schull, E.R. (Eds.). (1985). The preventing of complications from spinal manipulative therapy. In *Aspects of manipulative therapy* (p. 116). New York: Churchill Livingstone.

Kotlke, F.J. (1971). Therapeutic exercise to maintain mobility. In F.J. Kotlke & P.M. Elwood (Eds.), *Handbook of physical medicine and rehabilitation* (p. 389). Philadelphia: W.B. Saunders.

Krumhansl, B., & Nowacek, C. (1986). Manipulation under anesthesia. In G.P. Grieve (Ed.), *Modern manual therapy of the vertebral column*, Edinburgh: Churchill Livingstone.

Los Angeles Chiropractic College Class Catalog, 1982.

Lindemann, V.K., & Rossak, K. (1959). Indications, contraindications and complications of reposition in lumbago and sciatic syndrome. (Trans. by L. Siehl and D. Siehl.) *Zeitschrift für* (Orthop.) *91*, 335.

Liu, P. (1992). *Principles and procedures in anesthesiology* (p. 7). Philadelphia: J.B. Lippincott.

Mennell, J. (1960) *Therapeutic manipulation: Back pain* (p. 114). Boston: Little Brown Co.

Mensor, M.C. (1955). Nonoperative treatment, including manipulation for lumbar intervertebral disc syndrome. *American Journal of Bone and Joint Surgery, 5*, 925.

Morey, L.W., Jr. (1975). Manipulation under general anesthesia. *Osteopathic Annals*, March, 127.

North Carolina Board of Chiropractic Examiners position statement. (1997, December). From H. Williams. Manipulation under Anesthesia: Part I. Review of the literature and discussion of the state of the art. *American Chiropractic Association Journal of Chiropractic*.

Poppen, J.L. (1945). The herniated intervertebral disk-an analysis of 400 verified cases. *New England Journal of Medicine, 232*, 211.

Rumney, I.C. (1968). Manipulation of the spine and appendages under anesthesia: An evaluation. *Journal of the American Osteopathic Association, 63,* 235.

Shekelle, P.G., Adams, A.H., Chassin, M.R., Hurwitz, E.L., & Brook, R.H. (1992). Spinal manipulation for low back pain. *Annals of Internal Medicine 117,* 590.

Siehl, D. (1963). Manipulation of the spine under general anesthesia. *Journal of American Osteopathic Association, 62,* 881.

Siehl, D., & Bradford, W. (1952). Manipulation of the low back under general anesthesia (Persol's International Med. Clinic Case Study 1938). *Journal of American Osteopathic Association,* Dec., 239.

Soden, C.H. (1949). Osteopathic manipulative therapy under general anesthesia. In *Academy of Applied Osteopathics 1949 Yearbook* (p. 188). Carmel, CA: Academy of Applied Osteopathics.

Stoddard, A. (1969). Clinical spinal syndromes and their management. *Manual of Osteopathic Practice, 3,* 174.

Terrett, A.G.J. (1988). Vascular accidents from cervical spine manipulation: the mechanisms. *American Chiropractic Association Journal of Chiropractic 22,* 59.

Terrett, A.G.J., & Kleynhans, A.M. (1992). Cerebrovascular complications of manipulation. In S. Haldeman (Ed.). *Modern development in the principles and practice of chiropractic* (2nd ed., p. 579). New York: Appleton-Century-Crofts.

West, D., Mathews, R., Miller, M.R., & Kent, G.M. (1999). Effective management of spinal pain in one hundred seventy-seven patients evaluated for manipulation under anesthesia. *Journal of Manipulative and Physiological Therapeutics 22,* 299.

Wiesel, S.W., Boden, S.C., & Feffer, H.L. (1994). A quality-based protocol for management of musculoskeletal injuries: A ten-year prospective outcome study. *Clinical Orthopaedics, 301,* 164.

Williams, H.A. (1998). Manipulation under anesthesia, Part III, Discussion/critique. *American Chiropractic Association Journal of Chiropractic,* Feb.

Wyke, B. (1972). Articular neurology, a review. *Physiotherapy Journal of the Chartered Society of Physiotherapy, 58,* 94.

57

Pulsed Signal Therapy: A Practical Guide for Clinicians*

Richard Markoll, M.D., Ph.D.

Before the next century is out of its infancy, physics will be as important in the treatment of disease as pharmacology and biotechnology are today. ... The future holds exciting and rewarding prospects for those ... who use their diverse knowledge and skills as teams to forge the principles for a new era of medical therapeutics. Without interdisciplinary effort, however, success will be elusive. ... Herein lies our challenge.

C. Andrew L. Bassett

A DESCRIPTION OF THE SERVICE

The development of Pulsed Signal Therapy (PST™) was initiated 3 decades ago following proof that pulsed electromagnetic fields (PEMF) could promote the healing of bone fractures and reports that they could also relieve pain due to osteoarthritis and traumatic joint damage. Because most of these latter claims were based on anecdotal observations and different PEMF devices had varied characteristics, an effort was made to determine whether a pulsed electromagnetic field with specific parameters might provide superior and more consistent results. The normal stimulus for cartilage production and bone formation results from piezoelectric signals that generate a "streaming potential" in the extracellular matrix when skeletal structures are subjected to physical pressure. Bones that are immobilized in a cast for long periods of time become

demineralized, and conversely, it has been shown that regular exercise helps build stronger bones. Because this restorative electrical signal is impaired in osteoarthritic joints, it seemed logical to attempt to define and accurately reproduce this natural physiologic stimulus so that similar benefits could be achieved in affected tissues not subjected to any load. Basic science research that focused on physical chemistry as well as clinical trials conducted between 1973 and 1988 confirmed the validity of this approach. Since then, the ability of PST to relieve osteoarthritic pain and improve mobility has been unequivocally verified in double-blind and open label clinical trials of over 100,000 patients with osteoarthritis of the knee and other joints. This noninvasive treatment is not associated with any pain or discomfort and long-term follow-up confirms sustained efficacy as well as an absence of any adverse side effects.

More recently, PST has been found to be effective in temporomandibular joint syndrome (TMJ), tinnitus, which is difficult to cure, and periodontal disease, an established risk factor for heart attack and stroke. PST is currently administered at over 500 sites in 16 countries, where it is reimbursed by fiscal intermediaries and governmental agencies because of its proven cost effectiveness and safety record. Many facilities are located in clinics associated with academic medical institutions or respected hospitals, such as The American Hospital in Paris. PST presently is approved only for veterinary use in the United States.

---

*The Publisher and American Academy of Pain Management cannot assume responsibility for the validity of all materials contained in this chapter or for the consequences of their use. Pulsed Signal Therapy is presently approved only for veterinary use in the United States.

0-8493-0926-3/02/$0.00+$1.50
© 2002 by CRC Press LLC

The PST device consists of a control box connected to a ring-shaped coil that emits a proprietary pulsed electromagnetic field. Different coil sizes have been developed to treat peripheral joints (knees, shoulders, and wrists), the spine (cervical, thoracic, and lumbar vertebral bodies), tinnitus and dental disorders, and for veterinary applications as illustrated in Figures 57.1 through 57.4.

The joint to be treated is placed inside the coil and exposed to PST, usually for 1 hour on 9 consecutive days, interrupted only by a weekend. It is important to emphasize that PST is a patented procedure that should not be confused with PEMF devices that make similar claims but have scant supportive scientific clinical or basic research data.

THE HISTORY OF THE SCIENCE

The Yellow Emperor's Canon of Internal Medicine, which dates back 4000 years, describes how lodestones applied to acupuncture points could be used to relieve pain. Cleopatra allegedly wore one on her forehead while sleeping to prevent aging. In the Middle Ages, lodestones were also ground up to make powders to be applied as a magnetic salve to promote wound healing. Paracelsus believed they could be ingested to treat everything from diarrhea and epilepsy to various types of hemorrhage. By the middle of the 18th century, more powerful carbon-steel magnets that could be made in different shapes corresponding to any organ or structure in the body that required treatment became available. Magnet mania swept through Europe and France due to Mesmer, who used various magnetic paraphernalia in his salon to increase the flow of "animal magnetism," which could cure anything. Although Mesmer was discredited, the popularity of magnets steadily increased in the United States. By the beginning of the 20th century, magnetic insoles, rings, belts, girdles, caps, and other apparel were sold to cure everything from athletes' feet and baldness to menstrual cramps and impotency. The use of magnets to relieve pain declined with the advent of drugs and surgical procedures that could provide proven benefits. Over the past decade, they have become popular again because of stronger and smaller neodymium products that are easier to apply, and aggressive marketing by manufacturers eager to capture part of the estimated billion dollar worldwide market. While some studies do suggest that permanent magnets may relieve the pain of diabetic neuropathy, post-polio syndrome, and carpal tunnel syndrome, the action mechanism is obscure and there is little evidence of sustained benefits.

It is not clear when electricity was initially used to treat illness, but the electric catfish, which is indigenous to the Nile, is portrayed in Egyptian mural paintings that date back to 4000 B.C. The first recorded medical application was in 46 A.D. by Scribonius Largus, a Roman physician who used

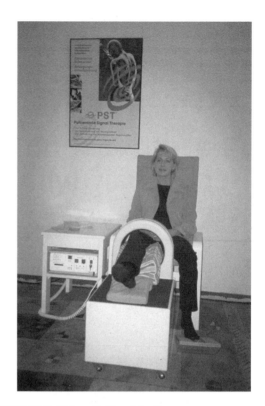

FIGURE 57.1 Osteoarthritis of the knee.

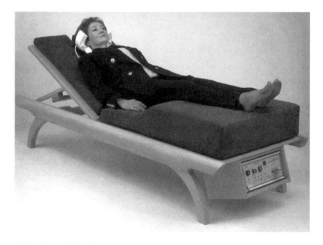

FIGURE 57.2 Tinnitis.

a live torpedo fish to treat a patient with gout, and who also wrote that headaches and other pains could be cured by standing in shallow water near these electric fish. The powerful South American electric eel was introduced in Europe in 1750 and people flocked to be treated with its "natural" electricity. The invention of the Leyden jar around the same time dramatically demonstrated the ability of stored electricity to produce muscle contractions, and as batteries were progressively improved during the 19th and early 20th centuries, numerous types of "medical coils" increasingly appeared. Electromagnetic therapy was viewed as a legitimate subspecialty, much like the rapidly growing fields of

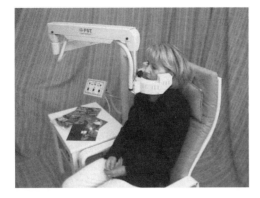

FIGURE 57.3 TMJ and periodontal disease.

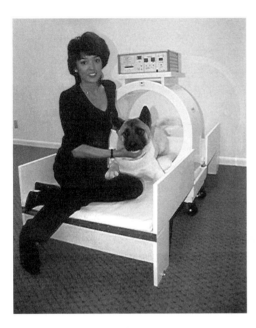

FIGURE 57.4 Veterinary applications.

radiology and radium therapy and was used by over 10,000 physicians and countless others to treat almost every type of pain or functional complaint. There were numerous instruments with names like "The Dynamiser" and "Oscilloclast," based on theories that each organ and person were "tuned" to a specific wavelength that could rejuvenate them. Claims were frequently made by charlatans to promote the sale of worthless devices. The 1910 Flexner report, which stated that there was no scientific basis for any of these outlandish and fraudulent claims, and the introduction of X-ray and electrocautery instrumentation that provided proven benefits, led to their gradual demise. However, as with permanent magnets, there also has been a recent resurgence of various types of "electromedical" devices that continue to make unsupported claims.

Pulsed electromagnetic fields have been used to treat nonunion bone fractures for several decades, with a relatively consistent success rate of 70 to 80% in several

countries. (Bassett, Pilla, & Pawluk, 1977; Brighton & Pollack, 1985). In 1979, the FDA approved certain PEMF devices for the treatment of fractures that failed to unite satisfactorily within 9 months. This approach has benefited hundreds of thousands of patients including some where nonunion had persisted for 15 or more years despite surgical and other interventions. In 1990, approval was granted for failed spinal fusions of any age.

PST is based on the application of a very specific type of pulsed electromagnetic field to bone and adjacent tissues. The PST device generates a pure magnetic field output signal that employs direct current with unidirectional biological frequencies below 30 Hz. The "waveform" is quasi-rectangular with measured field strengths generally below 2 mT or 20 Gauss. The system is controlled through a pulsed unidirectional magnetic DC field with multiple output frequencies implemented via a free-wheeling diode to optimize the inductance characteristics. Various frequency/amplitude combinations are switched over automatically and transmitted under continuous control during the treatment period. Induction of treatment takes place during the first 10 minutes, followed by a combination of pulsed signals that delivers the therapy over the remaining 50 minutes. PST differs from conventional alternating-current magnetic field therapies such as the Krause-Lechner type system as illustrated in Figure 57.5.

This system coil delivers an alternating-current magnetic field that generates a sinusoidal waveform. This signal does not conform with what normally takes place in the body, because electrical activities in all living organisms follow only direct-current-oriented processes. PST also differs from other pulsed electromagnetic field (PEMF) approaches that utilize a direct-current-oriented signal transmitted at a specific intensity and a particular frequency that remains constant during treatment, as illustrated in Figure 57.6.

Intensity

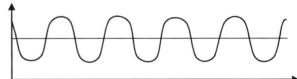

Kraus-Lechner Type System with Alternating-Current Oriented Magnetic Field

FIGURE 57.5 Krause-Lechner type system.

Intensity

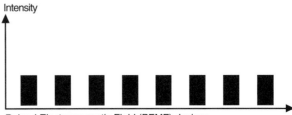

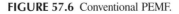

Pulsed Electromagnetic Field (PEMF) devices

FIGURE 57.6 Conventional PEMF.

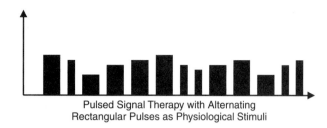

FIGURE 57.7 Pulsed signal therapy (PST).

While standard pulsed electromagnetic field devices do deliver a direct current signal, it never varies in either amplitude or frequency, which is also inconsistent with electrical signaling in living organisms. In contrast, pulsed signal therapy delivers changing pulsed electromagnetic signals in an alternating fashion that mimics signals generated in the body that are known to stimulate chondrocyte activity. The intensity of these rectangular pulses lies predominantly in the range of 0.5 to 1.5 milliTesla with relatively low frequencies that range from 10 to 20 Hz, as shown in Figure 57.7. The low biological frequencies and energy field strength at which PST operates is in a physiologic range, which helps explain why treatment is both effective and safe.

The most important distinction between patented PST and other electromagnetic therapies that are often in the public domain lies in proprietary specific amplitude, frequency, and repetition parameters. These have been designed to simulate physiological electrical signals in order to reproduce their biological benefits. PST's patented signal (pulsed DC magnetic field: 0.28 W., max. 20 gauss; 5–24 Hz; quasi-rectangular waveform) is the only electromagnetic stimulus with proof of efficacy in rigorously controlled clinical trials, as well as safety based on long-term follow-up. In sharp contrast to other devices making similar claims, the proposed mechanisms of action also are supported by extensive *in vitro* and other basic science research studies. The studies of Gierse, Breul, Faensen, and Markoll (in prep.). demonstrated that human chondrocyte cell cultures exposed to the specific electromagnetic fields generated by PST attained statistically significant higher mitosis rates than chondrocytes in untreated cultures (nearly twice that of the control group). Nerucci, Marcolongo, and Markoll (2000) demonstrated that PST enhances proteoglycan concentration in human chondrocyte cultures. These *in vitro* findings support one of the proposed action mechanisms believed to be responsible for the benefits of PST as illustrated in Figure 57.8.

NEED FOR THE THERAPY

Osteoarthritis currently affects 20.7 million Americans and its prevalence is expected to increase to 40 million within the next 20 years. It is responsible for 7 million physician visits and 3 million hospitalizations per year,

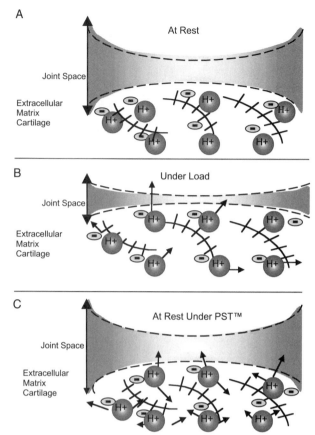

FIGURE 57.8 Action mechanism of PST. (A) Extracellular matrix at rest. An equilibrium exists between hydrogen and negative charges in the extracellular matrix, and there is no streaming potential of ionic flux as in (B) and (C). (B) Extracellular matrix under pressure. When the joint space is compressed as a result of physical pressure, a streaming potential is created as fixed negative charges in fluid are forced out of hydrogen protons to move into the joint space. (C) Extracellular matrix, as in (A), with PST. A similar streaming potential can be generated in the resting state by PST. This is from the forced movement of hydrogen protons, which results in alternating energies stimulating chondrocytes in matrix connective tissue. PST stimulates physiological streaming potentials as in (B).

with annual medical costs averaging $2655.00 (Gabriel, Crowson, Campion, & O'Fallon, 1997). Sales of products to treat osteoarthritis in the world's seven major pharmaceutical markets (United States, France, Germany, Italy, Spain, United Kingdom, and Japan) totaled approximately $1.6 billion in 1998, and according to one recent report, are forecast to leap to more than $4 billion in 2008 (The Marketletter, 1999). Nonsteroidal anti-inflammatory drugs (NSAIDs) are among the most commonly prescribed medications in the United States, accounting for more than 70 million prescriptions per year. Approximately 14 to 20 million patients take an NSAID on a daily basis (Statistical Bulletin, 1992). This figure is not inclusive of over-the-counter use of nonsteroidal anti-inflammatory drugs, estimated to be greater than 26 billion tablets per year. This number has grown steadily since NSAIDs first became available without a prescription in 1983, and as the use of aspirin as a cardioprotective agent has increased.

According to the Food and Drug Administration, NSAIDs cause more adverse drug reactions than any other class of drugs. Harmful kidney, central nervous system, and hematologic effects can occur, but gastrointestinal (GI) complications are far and away the most common and serious. The prevalence of endoscopic evidence of gastric ulceration is estimated at 10 to 20% and most of these patients have no prodromal symptoms or warnings that there is any problem (Hochberg, et al., 1995; Henrietta, 1999). There are approximately 200,000 hospitalizations a year due to NSAID-related GI bleeding and ulcer complaints. Up to one in ten patients taking NSAIDs will suffer some serious gastrointestinal complication causing 70,000 hospitalizations and 10,000 to 20,000 deaths each year (Fries, 1991). The economic impact of these complications has been estimated at approximately $1.5 to 4 billion annually (Smalley & Griffin, 1996; Smalley, et al., 1996). The significance of this is underscored by the advent of COX-2 inhibitor NSAIDs, which have fewer GI complications but are not significantly more effective in relieving pain and are much more expensive. Both Celebrex® and Vioxx®, the only two currently approved in the United States, easily surpassed Viagra® as the best-selling medication within the first 12 months of their introduction.

Numerous nonprescription drugs and nutritional supplements for the treatment of osteoarthritis are popular and a variety of medical and surgical approaches are also available. Some of these are summarized and compared to PST in Table 57.1.

This is not intended to be a comprehensive list of therapies for osteoarthritis but rather an indication of the diverse treatments available. For example, as this chapter was being completed, there was a report that Cat's Claw, a popular herbal treatment, had been shown to be equally or more effective than a prescription NSAID for osteoarthritis in a European double-blind study. However, the drug is not available in the United States and there are other questions about the validity of the study. Similarly, permanent magnets are widely used to treat pain but I am not aware of any studies showing them to be effective in osteoarthritis. It is important to emphasize that unlike PST, most of these and other popular remedies provide inconsistent benefits and must be used on an ongoing basis.

Joint and adjacent soft tissue damage due to trauma is also a huge and growing problem that responds to PST. According to the Institute for Preventive Medicine in Ann Arbor, Michigan, "Sports injury is the most under-recognized major public health problem facing the world community. In addition to being an enormous public health issue, injuries continue to usurp our limited healthcare financial resources" (Nicholl, Coleman, & Williams, 1995). Numerous reports confirm that joint pain resulting from some sport injury affects millions of people of all ages all over the world. In England and Wales alone, there are 29 million sports incidents per year that require new or ongoing treatment (Bijur, 1995). An Albert Einstein College of Medicine study estimates that every year there are close to 4.5 million sports and recreation injuries to American children and adolescents alone (Madhok, 1993).

INDICATIONS AND CONTRAINDICATIONS

While the vast majority of clinical trials have been devoted to osteoarthritis, PST also has been found to be effective in relieving pain and disability due to trauma, temporomandibular joint disease, tinnitus, periodontal disease, carpal tunnel syndrome, osteoporosis, tendonitis and convalescence following surgical repair of ligaments, fresh bone fractures, aseptic necrosis, fibromyalgia, sciatica, post-polio syndrome, migraine, metatarsalgia, acute burns, immune deficiency disorders, drug resistant epilepsy, diabetic neuropathy, herniated disc and Dupuytren's Contracture, as are discussed in the following section. There are no known contraindications to pulsed signal therapy, and it has been used successfully in hemophiliacs with joint problems. Although there are no reported adverse effects in patients who are pregnant or have implanted pacemakers, treatment is avoided because of potential medical-legal problems.

RESULTS TO DATE

Double-blind clinical trials and other open label randomized studies conducted in the United States, Canada, France, Italy, and Germany over the past decade are summarized in Table 57.2. The protocol initially used 30-minute treatment periods for 18 days, but it was subsequently found that a 1-hour treatment for 9 days was more effective. Administering therapy for 1-hour twice a day for 5 successive days because of time constraints also has had good results, but there are insufficient data to determine whether this might be a satisfactory option.

The initial double-blind studies in the United States were conducted in three treatment centers and reported in the *Journal of Rheumatology* (Trock, et al., 1993; Trock, Bollet, & Markoll, 1994). Pain was evaluated using WOMAC and later OMERACT III validated instruments of outcome measures. Functionality was measured using WOMAC and modified Ritchie scales, as well as global evaluations of improvement by the patient and examining

TABLE 57.1
Osteoarthritis Treatment Modalities Compared with PST

Treatment Common Home Remedies	Duration of Relief	Adverse Side Effects
External Application		
Heat	Several hours	None
Heat and cold	Several hours	None
Paraffin baths	Several hours	None
Rest and exercise	Several hours	None
Capsaicin (hot pepper)	Variable duration when effective	Burning sensation at site of application
Dimethyl sulfoxide (DMSO)	A few hours	Garlic odor to breath
Oral Administration		
Glucosamine; chondroitin sulfate preparations	Effective for several hours in some double-blind studies but not others; must be taken continuously	Concerns about possible development of insulin resistance and/or diabetes
Methyl sulfonyl methane (MSM) and various herbal products	Variable and no good double-blind studies; must be taken continuously	None
Homeopathic preparations	Unknown; no good double-blind studies	None
Nonprescription NSAIDs and analgesics	2–8 hours; requires chronic administration	Gastrointestinal ulcerations, bleeding, kidney, and liver complications
Prescription Medications		
NSAIDs	3–12 hours; requires chronic administration	Gatrointestinal ulceration, bleeding not uncommon (see text); may also affect the rate at which damaged cartilage regenerates
Glucocorticoid steroids	4–8 hours depending on dose; requires chronic administration	Fluid retention, gastric ulceration, diabetes
Codeine and its congeners	4–6 hours; requires chronic administration	Dependency and addiction
Viscosupplementation-hyaluronic acid (HA) injection	Up to 6 months	Long-term effects not known and benefits are controversial
Chondrocyte culture implantation	Variable and still experimental	Very expensive and long-term benefits or complications not known
Surgical Procedures		
Arthroscopy	Variable depending on condition	Soft tissue, bone, and articular complications, as well as unexplained pain occur; in one study of 71 patients, there were 82 complications in 50 wrists
Osteotomy	Variable depending on condition	Negative side effects often outweigh benefits Decrease in muscle mass
Resection	Variable depending on condition	Negative side effects often outweigh benefits; rehabilitation required
Arthrodesis	Variable depending on condition	Negative side effects often outweigh benefits; loss of flexibility
Total joint replacement (Arthroplasty)	Approximately 10 years, but may be risky if done more than once	Long rehabilitation, not long lasting enough for younger people
Electrical Stimulation		
Transcutaneous electric nerve stimulation (TENS) and cranioelectricalstimulation (CES)	Variable and requires multiple treatments if effective	None; does not affect cartilage loss which will cause pain to recur
High voltage pulsed galvanic stimulation (HVPGS), interferential electrical stimulation, MENS (minimal electrical noninvasive stimulation)	Variable but not long lasting and requires repeated treatment	None; does not affect cartilage loss which will cause pain to recur
Pulsed signal therapy	Sustained pain relief and cartilage growth continues after treatment	None

TABLE 57.2
Documented PST Clinical Studies

Study Design	Facility	Study Director(s)	Publication	Results/Notes
A double-blind trial of the clinical effects of pulsed electromagnetic fields in osteoarthritis	Yale University School of Medicine Teaching Hospital, Waterbury, CT	Thomas P. Greco Richard Markoll	*Journal of Rheumatology,* 20 (3), 1993	Pilot study
A double-blind trial of the clinical effects of pulsed electro-magnetic fields in osteoarthritis	Yale University School of Medicine Teaching Hospital, Waterbury, CT	David H. Trock Alfred Jay Bollet Richard H. Dyer L. Peter Fielding W. Kenneth Miner Richard Markoll	*Journal of Rheumatology,* 20 (3), 1993	Good to very good results, with high statistical significance
The effect of pulsed electromagnetic fields in the treatment of osteoarthritis of knee and cervical spine	Yale University School of Medicine Teaching Hospital, Melville, NY	David H. Trock Alfred Jay Bollet Richard Markoll	*Journal of Rheumatology,* 21 (3), 1994	Good to very good results, with high statistical significance
Treatment of painful osteoarthritis with pulsed electro-magnetic fields	Yale University School of Medicine Teaching Hospital, Danbury, CT	David H. Trock Alfred Jay Bollet Susan H. DeWitt Richard Roseff Michel Spiegel Richard Markoll	*Yale Danbury Clinical Journal*	Good to very good results, with high statistical significance
Comprehensive report of all patients treated with magnetic therapy	Yale University School of Medicine Teaching Hospital, Waterbury, CT	Alfred Jay Bollet David H. Trock	*Yale Clinical Presentations*	Good to very good results, with high statistical significance
Diagnostic profile of pulsed signal therapy patient population treatment of degenerative joint disease, muscle/ligament/tendon injuries, disc degeneration-herniation	McGill University, Vancouver, Canada	Cecil Hershler	*Canadian Presentation,* Vancouver, Montreal	High statistical significance

Completed Clinical Studies/Europe

Study Design	Facility	Study Director(s)	Publication	Results/Notes
Ètude de vérification de l'efficacité anatalgique des champs électromagnétiques pulsés (PST) dans la gonarthrose	Cochin Hospital, Paris, France	C.-J. Menkés Serge Perrot	American College of Rheumatology (Presentation) Nov. 1998. Submitted to *Journal of Rheumatology*	Good to very good results, with high statistical significance
Prospective clinical study of osteoarthritis of the knee	Niguarda Hospital, Milano, Italy	M. Cossu N. Portale	*La Riabilitazione – Rivista di Medicina Fisca e Riabilitazione* April–June 31, 1998.	High statistical significance
Prospective, clinical verification study of PST in osteoarthritis of the knee and hip and degenerative LWS changes	PST Treatment Center, Munich, Germany Technische Universität, Munich, Germany	Stephan Frhr. Von Gumppenberg Knut Pfeiffer Harald Martin	The British Institute of Musculoskeletal Medicine (in press)	High statistical significance
Multicenter study of the clinical effect of PST in osteoarthrosis of the knee (Grade II and III, Kellgren)	Ludwig-Maximilian University, Munich, Germany	Rainer Breul Stephan Frhr. Von Gumppenberg Michael Faensen Horst Cotta	*Journal of Orthopaedic Medicine* (in press)	Further documentation and analysis of patient data

(continued)

TABLE 57.2 (CONTINUED)
Documented PST Clinical Studies

Study Design	Facility	Study Director(s)	Publication	Results/Notes
Perpetual prospective study (VITAL: Visual Therapy Log, see below)	Ludwig-Maximilian University, Munich, Germany	Rainer Breul Friedrich Hahn Dieter Rost	The Scoeity of Orthopaedic Medicine (in press)	High statistical significance. Further documentation and analysis of patient data
Procedural proposal for patients suffering with osteoarthritis of the knee by means of PST vs. placebo	University of Siena, Siena, Italy	Roberto Marcolongo	*Journal of Rheumatology* (in press)	High statistical significance

physician. It should be emphasized that only qualified physicians and health professionals are licensed to administer PST and only after they have satisfactorily completed training in our treatment protocol with each specific device. This includes detailed instructions on how to conduct a double-blind trial, as well as obtain an accurate history, and perform a thorough physical examination before and after treatment. For the past decade, all therapists also have been required to use our specially developed computer software program called "VITAL" (Visual Therapy Log) which captures all relevant follow-up details using a form of WOMAC evaluation criteria. A recent analysis of data obtained from monitoring 70,000 patients through our VITAL program confirms sustained benefits and no evidence of long-term adverse effects. Ongoing clinical studies are outlined in Table 57.3.

It should be noted that Tables 57.2 and 57.3 refer only to clinical trials dealing with osteoarthritis. Numerous studies have been performed or are in progress for a variety of the disorders.

Because PST was designed to repair and restore any type of connective tissue damage, we have explored its use in a variety of disorders including.

TRAUMA

In May 1990, we initiated a 4-year study of 1000 patients under the auspices of a Yale University teaching hospital in Connecticut. Several hundred patients with various sport injuries resulting from swimming, bowling, bicycling, jogging, tennis, basketball, baseball, golf, skiing, ice skating, boxing, gymnastics, handball, hockey, karate, mountain climbing, soccer, track and field, wrestling, as well as others sustained by fire and police personnel were included. Because most of the patients were relatively young and healthy, they responded very rapidly to PST compared to our experience with elderly patients with chronic diseases. Since 1996, we have developed a large number of sports-type injury clinics in Europe and Asia. Currently, PST is available to most European soccer players within their clubs' medical facilities. Following a request, PST also was made available for German Field and Track athletes at the Sydney 2000 Olympic Games.

TINNITUS

Tinnitus is a common disorder characterized by a ringing, buzzing, or other persistent sound described as everything from a teakettle's whistle to the test tone for the Emergency Broadcast System. It can have many causes, is sometimes associated with dizziness or other neurological complaints, and it is estimated that more than 50 million Americans are affected. While there is no cure, one authority believes that tinnitus patients should be treated as if they had chronic pain. In a study of 160 adults with severe tinnitus reported at a recent meeting of the American Academy of Otolaryngology, it was emphasized that subjects additionally complained of stress, anxiety, fatigue, and depression, symptoms also common in patients suffering from chronic pain, and our experience has been similar. We conducted three prospective clinical trials in Berlin, Nuremberg, and Munich, Germany using untreated patients (population at large) as a control. A total of 199 patients were treated, 128 females and 71 males ranging in age from 17 to 78 years (mean age 57 years). Patients suffering from long-standing chronic tinnitus (Grades, II, III, or IV) who had failed to respond to various types of therapies were randomly selected. Treatment consisted of 12 1-hour PST sessions conducted over a 2-week period. Using validated measurement instruments based on the accepted Goebel-Hiller Protocol developed at the University of Tüebingen, all patients were evaluated before and at the end of treatment, and 6 and 12 weeks after the treatment. Data on hearing loss and other relevant parameters were also obtained. A gratifying and progressive trend of improvement was reported at the end of treatment and 6 weeks later. Final evaluation 12 weeks following treatment revealed that 26% were unchanged, 52% were very significantly improved, and 22% were now completely symptom free. No adverse side effects were reported or noted. Almost three out of

TABLE 57.3
Clinical Studies Currently in Progress

Study Design	Facility	Study Director(s)	Size	Publication	Results/Notes
Study of the clinical effect of PST in trials of the synovial liquid in osteoarthritis of the knee	Auguste-Victoria-Hospital Berlin, University of Erlangen	Detlef Schuppan Michael Faensen Richard Markoll	40	Study in progress, to be submitted for publication	Study began: December 1998 End date: December 2001
Trial of the medium-term effect of PST therapy vs. placebo in osteoarthritis of the knee	Prof. Kahan, Hospital Rangueil, Toulouse E. Vignon, Hospital E. Herriot Lyon	André Kahan	230	Study in progress, to be submitted for publication	Study began: September 2001 End date: Spring 2002

four stated that they were very satisfied and would definitely recommend PST, including some in the group who reported no change. Many in the significantly improved cohort reported a loss or diminution of high-frequency pitch ringing or replacement by a low-frequency hum that was much less disturbing.

Much larger European studies are in progress and a pilot study of 100 patients has been agreed upon in the United States. Presently, an extended multiphase clinical study, under the auspices of the Medical Director of the German Tinnitus League, is in progress. The first phase of the study was completed and evaluated at the end of 2000 and demonstrated significant results in the same etiology domain as previously observed.

TEMPOROMANDIBULAR JOINT DISORDER (TMJ)

During follow-up evaluation of patients who were treated for osteoarthritis of the cervical spine, it was noted that a significant number of patients indicated that their temporomandibular joint disorder (TMJ) complaint also improved. Based on these observations, we completed a pilot study of 30 patients who reported an 80% improvement in their TMJ symptoms. Based on these encouraging results, a randomized prospective, double-blind study of 120 patients was undertaken in patients with varied TMJ complaints at five European centers. Statistically significant improvement in pain and mandibular mobility was confirmed. Another double-blind study of 102 patients at the University Dental Clinic in Greifswald, Germany, and a third study at the Freie Universität in Berlin reported similar improvement. As a result of the above studies, PST was recently approved for the treatment of tinnitus and TMJ disorders by appropriate European regulatory bodies in accordance with the International Medical Device Directive and the International Organization for Standardization (ISO) 9000. I should add that following a detailed audit of our Munich facility, PST received ISO 9001 and EN 46002 certifications for standards for quality. The company also received the CE mark in 1998 after demonstrating compliance with the

Medical Device Directive. The ISO 9000 is a required certification for medical devices that corresponds to FDA approval in the United States.

PERIODONTAL DISEASE

An open label clinical study was undertaken in 1999 at the Rothlauf Dental Clinic in Munich, Germany. Sixty patients with chronic periodontal gum disease were enrolled. Significant improvement was documented clinically and objectively with X-ray studies in all patients. Gingival pockets were not as deep and periodontal tissue became thicker. A subgroup of patients who had a routine scraping and cleaning procedure within 2 years of receiving PST showed the greatest improvement. The objective video and/or X-ray has been described as "remarkable." A clinical study of human patients at the University of Milan is now in progress and will be completed toward the end of 2001. Ongoing studies at the University of Modena have confirmed efficacy in an animal model of periodontal disease.

CARPAL TUNNEL SYNDROME

A pilot study involving 45 patients with intractable symptoms demonstrated relief of pain and a full return to all normal activities within 3 weeks of completing a series of treatments, thus avoiding surgery. A clinical study in the United States of patients with intractable pain is currently underway to document improvement and explore possible mechanisms of action.

TENDINITIS AND LIGAMENTOUS DAMAGE

Our experience has consistently been that tendinitis due to rotator cuff injury or golfer's elbow responds dramatically within 3 weeks. A surgical procedure is the treatment of choice for repairing a torn anterior cruciate ligament in the knee, and full recovery generally requires 6 to 8 months of rehabilitation. In more than two dozen patients who received PST immediately after such surgery, full recovery was obtained within 3 months. Meniscal tears also respond well.

Osteoporosis

In one controlled study of 100 women aged 55 to 75 with X-ray evidence of moderate to advanced osteoporosis, the mean increase in bone density was greater than 25% following PST treatment.

Fresh Bone Fractures

While most bone fractures heal within a few weeks, spiral and various compound fractures may require casting and extensive rehabilitation for more than 3 months. We have treated a wide variety of fresh fractures, and our experience has been that the time required for casting is reduced by more than half.

Aseptic Necrosis

Aseptic necrosis of bone is a painful problem that does not respond to medication. Surgery is costly, usually only partially effective, and entails a long period of convalescence. We have treated aseptic necrosis since 1990, and in one study of 17 patients, 15 showed marked improvement, particularly with respect to relief of pain.

Fibromyalgia

Fibromyalgia is characterized by the constant presence of widespread pain so severe that it often is incapacitating. Signs and symptoms include muscle pain, aches, stiffness, disturbed sleep, depression, and fatigue. In the United States, 5 million people may be afflicted with its symptoms. It has been estimated that 15 to 20% of patients seen by U.S. rheumatologists may have fibromyalgia. The disorder shares many of the symptoms of myofascial and chronic fatigue syndrome and primarily affects women aged 25 to 50 years. Our experience has been that PST treatment relieves the signs and symptoms of fibromyalgia in over 80% of severe cases.

Post-Poliomyelitis Syndrome

Post-poliomyelitis syndrome is manifested by complaints of joint pain and difficulty walking that may surface decades after an attack of poliomyelitis. In a study of five such patients who received a course of 18 PST treatments, all had relief of pain and ambulation was significantly improved. In one patient who had not been able to bend her ankle or walk without a marked limp for 62 years, range-of-ankle-motion returned to 60% of normal, her limp disappeared, and she was able to discard her cane and return to an active social life, including dancing.

Sciatica

Sciatica is a term used to describe severe referred pain in the leg and often due to pressure on the sciatic nerve from pathology in the lumbar region. Our experience has been that PST treatment can provide significant improvement within 2 or 3 weeks.

Metatarsalalgia

Metatarsalalgia is a general term used to describe pain in the ball of the foot due to a variety of disorders such as Morton's neuroma, or atrophy of the plantar fat pad. In more than 50 patients with metatarsalgia who had received 15 to 18 PST treatments, over 80% were pain free or only "had a slight twinge once in a while."

Plantar Fasciitis

This problem is due to soft tissue inflammation in the foot which also causes severe pain when attempting to walk. Our experience in over 40 patients with nonspecific fascitiis shows dramatic improvement with complete recovery and an absence of pain following a standard course of PST treatment.

Acute Burns

A European study of 23 acute burn patients demonstrated that reepithelialization occurred in less than 50% of the anticipated time following a course of PST treatment.

Immune Deficiency Disorders

An open-label European study of 25 patients with neutropenia or pancytopenia due to immune system dysfunction showed significant improvement that persisted for up to 1 year in some instances. While anecdotal, treating hematologists were impressed with these results.

Drug-Resistant Epilepsy

Three patients with drug-resistant epilepsy were treated in an uncontrolled study. Complete neurological evaluation was obtained prior to and 1 and 3 months following PST treatment. All the neurologists concluded that their patients had experienced such significant improvement that a large pilot study is planned with a more specific protocol and parameters.

Diabetic Neuropathy

Diabetic Neuropathy is a serious complication of diabetes mellitus manifested by pain and tingling and a loss of sensation. There is no treatment for this disorder, which often leads to severe foot infections and amputation of various portions of the lower extremities. In one study of 17 patients with well-documented diabetic neuropathy, 16 reported marked improvement and an increase in quality of life following PST treatment because they had regained the ability to engage in many daily activities that were previously difficult or impossible.

MIGRAINE

In a pilot study of seven patients with a long history of migraine headaches, 15 PST treatments were administered over a 3-week period. A 9-month follow-up of five patients revealed a mean average of less than one attack per month per patient over this time period. These results were so impressive that a larger double-blind study is planned.

AVASCULAR NECROSIS AND ANKYLOSING SPONDYLITIS

This disorder also respond well to PST. We have treated 100 patients with bilateral avascular necrosis of the neck of the femur in the past 2 years, with remarkable relief of symptoms as well as objective evidence of radiological improvement. Ankylosing spondylitis is another indication for PST and treatment is targeted to the source of the referred pain rather than its location.

BACK AND NECK PAIN

Due to herniated disk, spondylolisthesis, and other lumbosacral problems can improve significantly following PST treatment. A double-blind study of 176 patients, 81 with cervical spine and 86 with knee complaints reported in the *Journal of Rheumatology* (Trock, Bollet, & Markoll, 1994) reported marked improvement following nine PST sessions with an absence of pain and a return to normal activities 4 to 6 weeks following treatment.

DUPUYTREN'S CONTRACTURE

In its early stages Dupuytren's Contracture responds to PST and can significantly shorten the recovery period following surgical procedures.

In addition to the above, a variety of other disorders have responded to PST. In 1996, we treated a 15-year-old girl with a tentative diagnosis of osteochondritis dissecans who was unable to walk without assistance or crutches. She received the standard program of nine consecutive sessions over a 10-day period. On the 14th day, she was able to walk for short periods without crutches and progressively improved so that 3 weeks later, she was able to join a walking tour in Greece. Although advised not to participate in any strenuous hiking activities, she was able to keep up with the group

climbing hills and tough terrain with no difficulty. She has not received any additional treatment, and she was able to enter a course in karate training later in 1996, and subsequently achieved Black Belt status. At present, she continues to pursue an unusually active life with no orthopedic complaints.

PREDICTIONS

This chapter began with C. Andrew L. Bassett's emphasis on the "vast interdisciplinary gap between biophysics and medicine" and the need for physicians to have more basic science education. The importance of this component has now been recognized, as relevant courses in physics are increasingly being integrated and introduced into the medical curriculum. This is vividly illustrated by the clinical benefits of PST, which is based entirely on solid physical chemistry research.

In a 1993 article, Bassett also made the following prediction:

> Against this background, it is clear that the physical control of certain pathologic states with selected time-varying magnetic fields can be highly effective, safe and economic in comparison to present treatment methods. As *in vitro* (tissue culture) and *in vivo* (animal) studies progress, substantial biomechanistic data support a rational expansion for clinical investigation to include PEMF use for speedng nerve repair for benefiting cardiac ischaemia (i.e. heart attacks), and for controlling loss of function following a cerebral vascular accident (stroke). Experimental results, also, suggest that conditions as diverse as adult onset diabetes and cancer deserve the concerted research attention of the bioelectromagnetics community.

C. Andrew L. Bassett, 1993

Andy Bassett, a good friend who was very supportive of our research, unfortunately did not live long enough to see his prophecy fulfilled well ahead of schedule. Along with Bob Becker and others, he pioneered the use of electromagnetic fields for the treatment of fractures that failed to unite, and stimulated many others to explore the use of electromagnetic fields for diverse clinical disorders. Pasche (1999) has proven the efficacy and safety of low energy emission fields (LEET) for the treatment of insomnia and anxiety disorders in rigidly controlled double-blind polysomnography studies at major sleep centers. Other forms of cranioelectrical stimulation can markedly improve depression and repetitive transcranial magnetic stimulation (rTMS) has been particularly effective in patients resistant to medication. Sodi Pallares (2000) has demonstrated remarkable reversal of metastatic malignancies and terminal cardiomyopathy with a combined magnetotherapy–metabolic regimen.

These and other observations, such as Liboff's (1985) ion cyclotron resonance studies, are difficult to explain in terms of Newtonian physics. They appear to defy the laws of thermodynamics because these feeble forces produce nonthermal effects that do not appear to involve caloric exchange. However, as Rosch and Adey (1999) have proposed, they do become comprehensible from a quantum physics perspective, and are consistent with an emerging paradigm of energy medicine that views communication in the body at a physical/atomic level rather than the current chemical/molecular model.

Life on earth evolved under constant geomagnetic influences, so it should not be surprising that all living cells, tissues, and organs are sensitive "electromagnetic systems" with specific electrical or magnetic resonance characteristics. Becker (1990) has shown that our bodies exhibit a positive polarity along the central axis, and a negative polarity in peripheral structures. He also has demonstrated that this polarity is reversed in hypnosis and anesthesia, as well as following an injury that creates a positive potential at the trauma site. He believes that this reversal of polarity generates a microcurrent of injury that is conducted through Schwann and glial cell sheaths surrounding neurons, which act to initiate repair and regenerative processes. Nordenström (2000) has proposed that there is a local build-up of positively charged ions following injury that creates an electrical voltage potential between opposite ions that are separated. Much as occurs in a battery, this energy can be tapped once the circuit is closed to permit the flow of electricity between these charged areas. The speed, versatility, and integration of these activities suggest the existence of the biologic equivalent of electrical systems composed of electrodes, switches, amplifiers, resistors, and capacitors that can store and regulate energy flow, which he refers to as "Biologically Closed Electrical Circuits" (BCEC). Based on this, he has developed a very effective treatment program for metastatic lung tumors that has now been replicated by others in tens of thousands of patients all over the world.

As enthusiasm for "electroceuticals" grows, there will undoubtedly be claims of other therapeutic triumphs. There are already reports of benefits for patients with everything from Alzheimer's and Parkinson's disease to multiple sclerosis, migraine, and epilepsy. Unfortunately, it may be difficult to distinguish between approaches that are authentic and promising and are supported by a scientific rationale, and others based on anecdotal reports and speculation by well-meaning but misinformed zealots. In addition, entrepreneurs and charlatans eager to cash in on the growing popularity of bioelectromagnetic medicine who may take advantage of desperate patients for whom conventional medicine has little to offer. As their efforts

---

TABLE 57.4
Questions to Ask When Evaluating Electromagnetic Devices Claiming to Relieve Pain or Provide Other Benefits

1. Have rigidly supervised double-blind studies been conducted in a clearly defined and properly selected patient cohort under the auspices of a university medical center or affiliated teaching facility?
YES___
2. Are the individuals conducting the study and the supervising Scientific Director of the organization offering the therapy qualified scientists with appropriate academic or other medical credentials, as opposed to salespeople or engineers?
YES___
3. Have follow-up studies been performed that demonstrate long-term sustained benefits, safety, and absence of adverse side effects?
YES___
4. Have any supportive basic science studies been performed at university-affiliated or recognized research centers by appropriately qualified scientists?
YES___
5. Have the results of clinical trials and supportive basic science studies been published in established peer reviewed medical and scientific journals as opposed to popular lay publications, other media presentations, or self-serving press releases?
YES___
6. In addition to Institutional Review Board approval, has an academic or other appropriate teaching facility reviewed and signed off on the study protocol and the results that were obtained?
YES___
7. Has the device or procedure been patented, and if so, are these merely simple design patents as opposed to process patents that cover the technology?
YES___
8. Is there a definitive database that can be made available to provide background information that explains the biological effects of the therapy being offered?
YES___

---

are shown to be worthless, there is apt to be a rising tide of resentment from the public as well as the scientific community, with the danger that the baby will be thrown out with the bathwater.

One way to prevent this when evaluating various claims is to ask the questions in Table 57.4 and compare the responses with PST.

PST can answer a resounding YES to all of these. Our experience has been that others can respond satisfactorily to only one or two, and in some cases none. There is little doubt in my mind that bioelectromagnetic therapies will be increasingly incorporated into mainstream medicine in the millennium, *if we can separate the wheat from the chaff.* As Andy Bassett predicted, this has already started to occur and some current standard treatments are likely to be supplanted.

This "energy medicine" paradigm also may provide important insights into how acupuncture, homeopathy, the laying on of hands, faith healing, placebos, as well as prayer can relieve pain and provide other rewards. Pfeiffer (2000) has already demonstrated with Kirlian photography that there are marked differences in energy levels before and after treatment with PST. Similar approaches may lead to a greater understanding of how we can communicate with other living systems to improve health and harmony in nature. As Jules Henri Poincaré noted this should be the goal of the true scientist:

> The scientist does not study nature because it is useful; he studies it because he delights in it, and he delights in it because it is beautiful. If it were not beautiful, it would not be worth knowing, and if nature were not worth knowing, life would not be worth living.

ACKNOWLEDGMENT

The author wishes to acknowledge with gratitude the cooperation and participation of Professor Paul J. Rosch, M.D., President, The American Institute of Stress; Theresa K. Toohil, Ph.D., Information Management Consultant, and Stacy L. Candia, Administrative Associate.

REFERENCES

Adey, W.R. (1999). Whispering among cells. The American Institute of Stress. Proceedings Tenth International Montreux Congress on Stress, Switzerland.

Antiarthritis medication usage, United States, 1991, *Statistical Bulletin, Metropolitan Insurance Companies 73*, 25, 1992.

Bassett, C.A.L. (1993). Applications of electromagnetic fields in medicine. *Bioelectromagnetic Society Newsletter, 110*, 1,4.

Bassett, C.A.L., Pilla, A.A., & Pawluk, R.J. (1997). A non-operative salvage of surgically resistant pseudoarthrosis and non-unions by pulsing electromagnetic fields. A preliminary report. *Clinical Orthopaedics, 124*, 128.

Becker, R.O. (1990). *Cross currents. The perils of electropollution. The promise of electromedicine*. Los Angeles: Jeremy Tarcher.

Bijur, P.E., et al. (1995). Sports and recreation injuries in U.S. children and adolescents. *Archives of Pediatric and Adolescent Medicine, 149*, 1009.

Brighton C.T., & Pollack, S.R. (1985). Treatment of recalcitrant non-union with a capacitively coupled electrical field. A preliminary report. *Journal of Bone and Joint Surgery, 67A*, 577.

Carbone, C. (1999). Treatments "set to surpass $4 billion in 2008." TPRNewswire/ via NewsEdge Corporation, Decision Resources, Inc., October 14, 1999. Online data.

Fries, J.F. (1991). NSAID gastropathy: the second most deadly rheumatic disease? Epidemiology and risk appraisal. *Journal of Rheumatology, 18*(suppl. 28), 6.

Gabriel, S.E., Crowson, C.S., Campion, M.E., & O'Fallon, W.M. (1997). Direct medical costs unique to people with arthritis. *Journal of Rheumatology, 24*, 719.

Gierse, H., Breul, R., Faensen, M., & Markoll, R. (in preparation, 2000). Pulsed signal therapy (PST) stimulates mitosis of human chondrocytes in culture. Proceedings Tenth International Conference on Biomedical Engineering, Singapore 2000, 473–474.

Henrietta, G. (1999). Advances in the treatment of the elderly arthritic patient. American Society of Consultant Pharmacists Annual Meeting. *Medscape*. Online data.

Hochberg, M.C., et al. (1995). Guidelines for the medical management of osteoarthritis. Part I. Osteoarthritis of the hip. *Arthritis and Rheumatism, 38*, 1535.

Liboff, A. R. (1985). Cyclotron resonance in membrane transport. In A. Chiabrera, C. Nicolini, C., & H.P. Schwan (Eds.), Interactions between electromagnetic fields and cells. New York: Plenum Press.

Madhok, R., et al. (1993). Trends in the utilization of primary total hip arthroplasty 1969 through 1990: A population-based study in Olmsted County, Minnesota. *Mayo Clinic Proceedings, 68*, 11.

Nerucci, A., Marcolongo, R., & Markoll, R. (2000). Pulsed signal therapy (PST) enhances the proteoglycans concentration in human chondrocyte cultures. In *Biomedical and Environmental Mass Spectrometry Twenty-Second Annual Meeting Abstract Book (*p. 48). Frederic, MD: The Bioelectromagnetics Society.

Nicholl, J.P., Coleman, P., & Williams, B.T. (1995). The epidemiology of sports and exercise related injury in the United Kingdom, *British Journal of Sports Medicine, 29*, 232.

Nordenström, B. (2000). Do biologically closed electricl circuits conduct Q1? The American Institute of Stress. Proceedings Eleventh International Congress on Stress, Hawaii.

Pallares, D.S. (2000). Magnetotherapy - metabolic - thermodynamic reversal of advanced malignancy and cariomyopathy. The American Institute of Stress. Proceeding Eleventh International Congress on Stress, Hawaii, 2000.

Pasche, B. (2000). Low energy emission therapy (LEET) for the treatment of insomnia and anxiety. The American Institute of Stress. Proceedings Tenth International Montreux Congress on Stress, Switzerland, 1999.

Pfeiffer, K. (2000). Changes in Kirlian photography energy fields following puled signal therapy. The American Institute of Stress. Proceedings Eleventh Internation al Congress on Stress, Hawaii.

Rosch, P.J., & Adey, W.R. (1999). The American Institute of Stress. Proceedings Tenth Internaitonal Montreaux Congress on Stress, Switzerland.

Smalley, W.E., & Griffin, M.R. (1996). The risks and costs of upper gastrointestinal disease attributable to NSAIDs, *Gastroenterology Clinics of North America, 25*, 373.

Smalley, W.E., et al. (1996). Excess costs from gastrointestinal disease associated with nonsteroidal anti-inflammatory drugs, *Journal of General Internal Medicine, 11*, 461.

Trock, D.H., Bollet, A.J., & Markoll, R. (1994). The effects of pulsed electromagnetic fields in the treatment of OA of the knee and cervical spine. Report of randomized, double blind, placebo controlled trials, *Journal of Rheumatology, 21,* 1903.

Trock, D.H., et al. (1993). A double-blind trial of the clinical effects of pulsed electromagnetic fields in OA. *Journal of Rheumatology, 20,* 456.

58

Infrared Photon Stimulation: A New Form of Chronic Pain Therapy

Jacob Green, M.D., Ph.D., Deborah Fralicker, R.N., D.C., William Clewell, Ph.D., Earl Horowitz, D.P.M., Timothy Lucey, B.S., Victor John Yannacone, Jr., J.D., and Constance Haber, D.C.

INTRODUCTION

In this chapter we report our experiences with the subjective amelioration of diverse painful conditions by means of infrared photon stimulation. The use of infrared photon stimulation devices at classical acupuncture treatment points and directly over the painful areas was successful in several diverse groups of patients suffering chronic pain. No deleterious effects were detected in more than 500 infrared exposures among any of the normal control subjects and diverse patient groups.

BACKGROUND

In one study of 25 patients complaining of painful feet, 21 with chronic painful diabetic neuropathy, and 4 with painful nondiabetic neuropathy (Green, Horwitz, Fralicker, Ossi, Briley, & Lucey, 1999), infrared photon stimulation resulted in significant amelioration of pain according to a patient visual analog scale. Warming of previously cold painful feet as a result of infrared photon therapy was identified in a large percentage of cases with neuropathy. Participating patients also assessed infrared photon stimulation treatment to be significantly beneficial on a Likert (Leikert) Scale evaluation.

Infrared photon stimulation was first applied to asymptomatic volunteer subjects in single sessions repeated over a period of 3 to 6 weeks at a dedicated multidisciplinary neurologic/pain rehabilitation center.

Recordings of any neurovascular change of each sham or infrared energy application session in the control subject group were made by high-resolution dynamic digital infrared imaging (Green, 1989; Green, 1993; Green, Leon-Barth, Kohli, & Green, 1989).

Seven normal control subjects did not have any immediate or delayed deleterious effects attributable to the infrared photon therapy.

Those patients with positive assessment of the infrared photon therapy by patient visual analog pain scale correlated most closely with those who had the most profound physiological changes demonstrated on high-resolution, dynamic digital infrared imaging (Figures 58.1a,b).

In a second study (Fralicker, Green, Clewell, Ossi, & Briley, unpublished), 74 chronic myofascial pain patients who on high-resolution, dynamic digital infrared imaging initially exhibited a significant increase in infrared radiation from a focal area of the skin were observed to have less infrared radiation from the skin at those sites, and a more harmonious and congruous pattern of infrared radiation on side-to-side comparison following infrared photon therapy. The change in infrared radiation pattern was an objective measure of positive effect attributable to the infrared photon stimulation treatment (Figure 58.2)

Similarly, almost all patients reported a significant decrease in pain on their visual analog pain scales and also a positive assessment of the procedure by Likert (Leikert) scale assessment. Independent chart review

0-8493-0926-3/02/$0.00+$1.50
© 2002 by CRC Press LLC

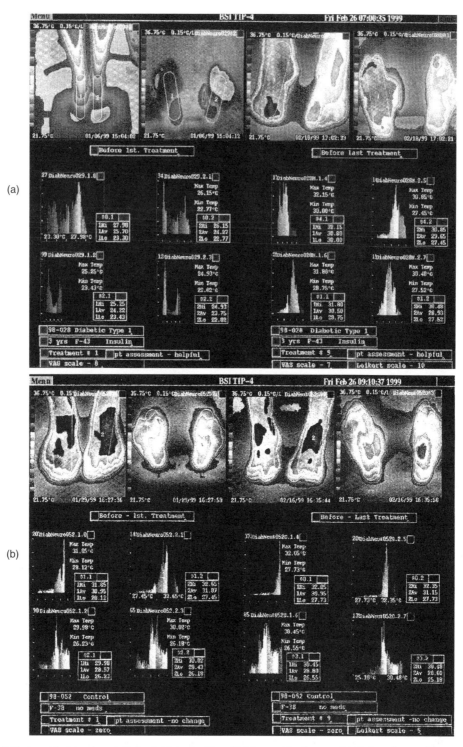

FIGURE 58.1 (a) First and last treatment: Patient. Note significant histographic change. (b) Before first and last treatment: Control. Note no change in histographic pictures.

showed no increase in pain medicine use occurred in this patient study group.

Patients afflicted with complex regional pain syndrome, type I (previously known as reflex sympathetic dystrophy) (Rowbotham, 1998) have been notoriously difficult to treat. Current theory hypothesizes that the common pathophysiologic process is reduction of the regional vascular supply with resultant tissue ischemia, which, in turn, leads to continued nociception.

One recent consideration for the change in nomenclature from RSD to CRPS (complex regional pain syndrome) was microangiopathy. M. Stanton-Hicks, Janig,

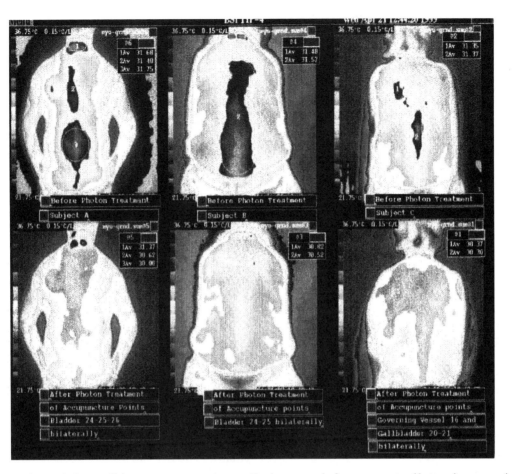

FIGURE 58.2 Before and after needleless acupuncture treatment. Top images are before treatment and bottom images are immediately after treatment.

Hassenbusch, Haddox, Boas, and Wilson (1995) reported that microangiopathy of the affected limbs (van der Laan, ter Laak, Gabreels-Feston, Gabreels, & Goris, 1998) was pathologically verified in amputations done on a number of RSD patients.

A significant clinical review of 824 patients was done by Hooshmand and Hashmi (1999) who found that the complex regional pain syndrome is characterized by hyperpathic allodynic pain, vasomotor dysfunction, flexor spasms, inflammation, and limbic system dysfunction. They concluded that casting, amputation, and elective surgery are high on the list of aggravating factors.

We report here the use of infrared photon stimulation in chronic regional pain syndrome (Green, Fralicker, Clewell, Horowitz, & Lucey, 1999). In a single patient with reflex sympathetic dystrophy (complex regional pain syndrome) (Green, 1993), we observed progress toward more normal symmetry in the infrared energy radiation signature. Although a single patient's report, it appears to be significant in that we have again corrected the autonomic-sympathetic dysfunction characterized by a well-defined asymmetrical infrared energy radiation pattern with documented change toward a more normal infrared radiation signature following infrared photon therapy.

MODE OF ACTION

Our observations suggest that the bioelectrochemical physiological reactions proceeding continuously in living creatures at all levels from their electron transfer during oxidative phosphorylation in intracellular organelles to the conduction of signals along axons and the transfer of physiologically active materials throughout the entire body by means of the vascular and lymphatic systems acquire information from and transfer information to the autonomic-sympathetic nervous system (Yannacone, personal commun.). That information can be monitored in real time as it modulates the radiation of infrared energy from the skin to the environment (Christoph, Strasser, Eiswirth, & Ertl, 1999).

Our experience with the use of infrared photon stimulation in treating chronic pain has created a bridge between the qualitative and almost mystical character of Eastern medical practices such as acupuncture, acupressure, and *Nei Qong*, and the more quantitative technologically driven traditions of Western medicine.

It appears that application of infrared energy at classical acupuncture points can, under appropriate conditions, have significant impact on autonomic-sympathetic activity and that application of infrared energy to the surface of the skin may influence bioelectrochemical physiological processes far removed from the site of application.

Our observations indicate that the meridians or great channels for rapid transfer of energy within the human body that are at the heart of Chinese medical theory, seem to actually exist and, at least in the functional sense, may behave as a kind of biological "superconducting pathway" or physiological "wormhole" linking organs and organelles to expedite physiological processes (Yannacone, personal commun.).

Our observations also suggest that infrared energy radiated from the skin is subject to modulation by physiological processes far removed from the site of the radiation and that the skin behaves as a kind of antenna transferring information from organs and organelles deep within the body during the process of radiating infrared energy (Yannacone, personal commun.). Observing such infrared radiation can provide a means of monitoring physiological function in real time (Yannacone, personal commun.).

It appears that portions of the infrared energy absorbed by or transmitted through tissue can affect bioelectrochemical physiological processes locally, regionally, and at a distance, resulting in clinical improvement (Karu, 1987). Infrared photon stimulation appears to be of significant value in the treatment of chronic pain of a neuropathic and neuromuscular character and represents an alternative to opioid analgesics (Figures 58.3 and 58.4).

It has been suggested that neuromodulation or neuroaugmentation may well be more effective in pain relief than direct electrical stimulation by means of implanted or external electrical stimulators (Melzack & Wall, 1965; Melzack, Stillwell, & Fox, 1977). Consideration of acupuncture as a neuromodulation technique for pain control was described in 1992 by Ng, Katims, and Lee, and by Helms in 1998.

Our observations have begun to establish a theoretical foundation for consideration of effects attributable to acupuncture and acupressure (Yannacone, Green, & Hobbins, private commun.).

DATA PRESENTATION AND REVIEW

Better overall Likert (Leikert) scale assessment of treatment effectiveness was noted in those patients whose infrared energy radiation signatures became more coherent. Note, however, high-resolution, dynamic digital infrared imaging revealed that not all treated patients demonstrated "normal" infrared energy radiation signatures, indicating that underlying pathophysiological processes may still be continuing.

Clinical outcomes of infrared photon therapy in patients with neuropathy involving the lower extremities are summarized according to patient judgment in Table 58.1 (21 patients with diabetic neuropathy, 4 with nondiabetic neuropathy, and 7 control subjects without neuropathic features or pathognomonic infrared energy radiation signatures). Statistically significant decreases in the patients' reported levels of pain were achieved, along with patient assessment that the treatment was effective. Infrared energy radiation signatures became more coherent and moved dramatically toward the normal controls.

Seventy-four patients with myofascial pain treated with infrared photon stimulation, first at established acupuncture treatment sites and then over the painful region identified by the patients, experienced significant changes in the asymmetry of their infrared energy radiation signatures (Green, 1993). Statistically significant changes were attributed to infrared photon stimulation therapy.

While suggesting that infrared photon stimulation at classical acupuncture points is effective in myofascial pain therapy, we have taken the liberty of identifying those classical acupuncture points in a manner we believe to be more consistent with the conventional anatomical nomenclature of Western medicine (see Figure 58.5).

DISCUSSION

Many patients complaining of chronic pain (lasting longer than 6 months) are seen by physicians each day. Despite myriad scientific advances and new invasive procedures, minimal improvement has been noted in many of those suffering chronic painful conditions. These patients often turn to alternative medicine and seek unconventional treatment.

Our prior unsuccessful attempts to treat chronic painful conditions by means of early commercial photon stimulators were described previously (Green, 1998). In this chapter, we summarize our success with infrared photon stimulation in conjunction with high-resolution, dynamic digital infrared imaging. We consider this technology along with real-time monitoring suitable for effective outpatient treatment of chronic pain. We are satisfied that by careful and thoughtful application of infrared photon stimulation we can significantly influence the autonomic-sympathetic nervous system and visualize and document these changes using high-resolution dynamic digital infrared imaging.

Successful therapy for chronic pain is economically important. In 1994 Liberty Mutual received 119,000 claims for back pain alone (Webster & Snook, 1994). Multidisciplinary pain clinics are expensive with an estimated outpatient therapy cost in 1995 of $4746 per patient. Outpatient treatment appears to be less expensive, however (Kee, Middaugh, Pawlick, & Nicholson, 1997). Medical costs directly and indirectly attributable

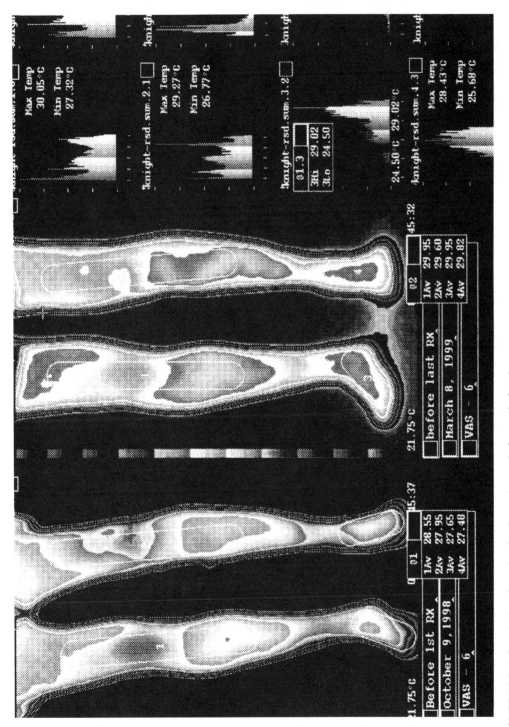

FIGURE 58.3 Infrared, chronic regional pain syndrome, before and after therapy.

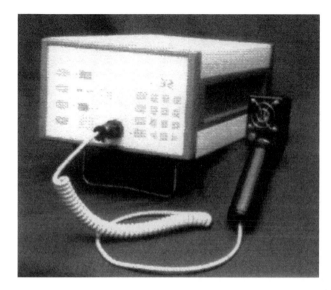

FIGURE 58.4 Typical photon stimulator.

to chronic, episodic, and recurrent back pain treatment are estimated to be $50 billion a year (Frymoyer, Katz, and Bahril, 1991).

The effectiveness of longer-term treatments, including supervised education in a back school, objectively led to significantly fewer re-injuries (Brown, Sirles, & Hilyer, 1992). Alternative adjunctive treatments including back belts to reduce injuries have also been (minimally) effective (Mitchell, Lawler, Bowden, Mote, Asundi, & Purswell, 1994). Various and sundry treatment programs for chronic back pain including exercise (Feine, Widmer, & Lund, 1997), and splinting (McMillas & Blasberg, 1994; Wright & Schiffmn, 1995) have been evaluated. Continued excitability of peripheral tissue and central neural excitability together may contribute to the persistence of soft tissue pain (treatment failures) in post-trigger point injection cases. Electrical stimulation of myofascial trigger points has also been used successfully as still another treatment for chronic recurrent back pain (Airaksinen & Pontinen, 1992). Any improvement in chronic recurrent back-pain treatment will be of great economic significance.

LASER THERAPY

It is important to recognize that the infrared photon therapy discussed in this chapter is not laser therapy. It is not the low-level laser therapy (LLLT) reported in the literature (Gam, Thorsen, & Lonnberg, 1993). The mode of action of infrared photon therapy seems to be significantly different and the results have been considerably more promising.

An assessment of laser therapy for musculoskeletal disorders was carried out in a meta analysis of randomized clinical trials and reported by Beckerman, de Bie, Bouter, De Cuyper, and Oostendorp (1992) who found no clear relationship between laser energy dosage and outcome in the 36 reviewed and published clinical trials involving a large number of patients. On average, however, laser treatment was more effective than just placebo. The conclusion was that laser seemed to have a substantial therapeutic impact on rheumatoid arthritis, post-traumatic joint disorder, and myofascial pain.

TMJ and degenerative joint disease therapy with laser have been studied and laser therapy was found to be effective in the management of the pain associated with rheumatoid arthritis and degenerative TMJ disease (Bertolucci & Grey, 1995). Mulcahy and others, however, believe that no therapeutic effect of laser treatment exist and that the positive outcomes reported were merely placebo (Mulcahy, McCormack, McElwain, Wagstaff, & Conroy, 1995).

Alternative therapies including Qi Gong energy and electrical fields were reported by Omura and Beckman (1995); however, improved circulation and enhanced drug uptake were thought responsible for the positive outcomes.

Yang, Guyuang, and Chang (1995) successfully utilized an assessment of brain magnetic field changes evoked by acupuncture treatments using a SQUID (superconducting quantum interference device) biomagnetometer to assess 12 subjects. Posterior neck treatments using 100-W LLLT in another study (Wong, Lee, Zucherman, & Mason, 1995) reported rapid alleviation of pain and tingling in the arms.

A subjective positive result, i.e., decreased symptomatology, was reported following acupuncture therapy in

TABLE 58.1
Clinical Outcomes via Patient Judgment

Number of Patients	Type of Group	Appointment VAS (pain)	Leikert Scale (overall opinion)	
			First	Last
23	Diabetic neuropathy (all types)	5.6	4	8.1
4	Nondiabetic neuropathy	5.1	2.5	7
7	Control Group	1.7	0.7	5

Scale: 5 = Neutral

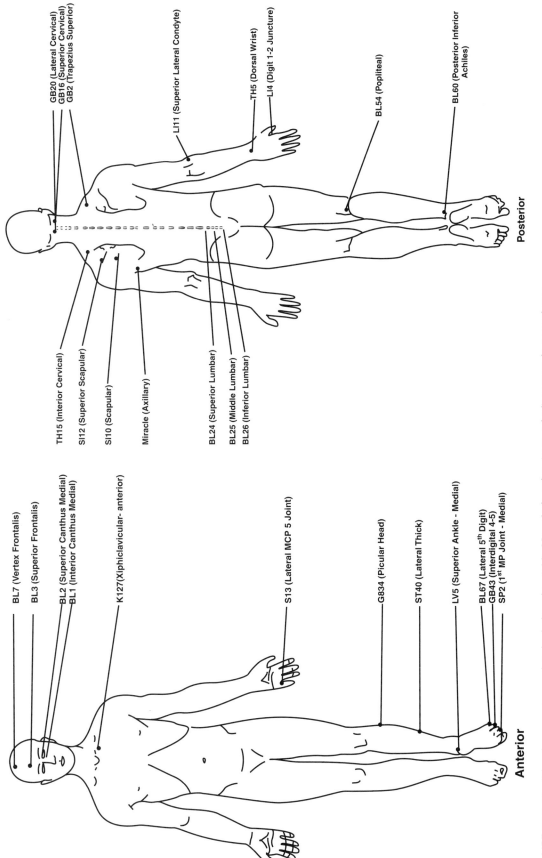

FIGURE 58.5 Traditional acupuncture points in designation (old). New designation (anatomical) appears in parentheses.

temperomandibular joint (TMJ) pain, myofascial pain, and occlusal splint (Johansson, Wenneberg, Wagersten, & Haraldson, 1991). Occlusal lifting (a TMJ treatment) did alleviate muscle tension in a study of silver spike joint electrotherapy and other modalities (Sugimoto, Konda, & Shimahara, 1995).

A number of studies involving lasers as surgical instruments for removal of tattoos have been published (Alfelberg, Bailin, & Rosenberg, 1986; Fitzpatrick & Goldman, 1994; Reid, Miller, Murphy, Paul, & Evens, 1990; Taylor, et al., 1990). Others have treated and reported on the treatment of Nevus of Ota with therapeutic lasers (Geronemus, 1992; Watanabe, et al., 1994). Cutaneous pigmented human lesions have been successfully destroyed by lasers (Anderson & Parrish, 1983; Kilmer, Goldberg, & Anderson, 1994; Tan, Morelli, & Kurban, 1992). Port-wine nevi have been treated by various laser techniques (Garden, Polla, & Tan, 1988; Tan, et al., 1989).

Other articles describe the application of physical modeling for optimal treatment protocol development and the application of various wavelengths for more specific laser treatment (Van Gemert, 1991): Q-switched ruby laser and Q-switched YAG laser (Alster, 1995; Gonzalez, Gange, & Momtaz, 1992), cool lasers and flash pump-pulsed dye laser in the treatment of various skin lesions (Chess & Chess, 1993; Fitzpatrick, Lowe, Goldman, Borden, Behr, & Ruiz-Esparza, 1994), and various precise laser treatments using specific identified tissue parameters (Svaasand, Norvang, Fiskerstrand, Stopps, Berns, & Nelson, 1995).

The diffusion of light in turbid material and reflections has been considered in other laser treatment protocols (Ishimaru, 1990). Major international symposia have been held on the diagnostic and therapeutic uses of lasers (Steiner, 1989).

Treatment by means of lasers of different wavelengths and variable energy output characteristics have been considered in several literature reviews (Fitzpatrick, Goldman, & Ruiz-Esparza, 1993; Polla, Tan, Garden, & Parrish, 1987). Similar diverse technical considerations of light distribution in the skin were made for therapeutic sources of infrared light emission therapy (Miller & Veitch, 1993).

In the search for other modalities in the treatment of chronic pain, Waylonis, Wilke, O'Toole, Waylonis, and Waylonis (1988) reported on the clinical responses to various therapy modes (utilizing a McGill Pain Questionnaire), but no particular advantage of neon laser therapy was reported in this single study.

Innovative considerations for photon therapy included skin-contact monochromatic infrared irradiation therapy (Thomasson, 1996) and photothermal sclerosis of leg vein problems (Goldman & Eckhouse, 1996).

Various proton and photon energy beams have been used along with a so-called Monte Carlo model for photon irradiation for cancer patients (Hug, Fitzek, Liebsch, & Munzerider, 1995; Lovelock, Chui, & Monahan, 1995).

REVIEW SUMMARY AND CONCLUSIONS:

It appears that infrared photon stimulation carries with it a significant potential for amelioration of the chronic pain characterized by autonomic and neurovascular abnormalities demonstrable by means of high-resolution dynamic digital infrared imaging. Further research and continued treatment of patients with infrared photon stimulation are clearly indicated and warranted. We are now exploring applications of infrared photon stimulation for treatment of chronic myofascial back pain conditions.

REFERENCES

Airaksinen, O., & Pontinen, P.J., (1992). Effects of the electrical stimulation of myofascial trigger points with tension headaches. *Acupuncture Electro-Therapeutics Research, 17*(4), 285–290.

Alster, T., (1995). Q-switched alexandrite laser treatment (755 nm) of professional and amateur tattoos. *Journal of the American Academy of Dermatology, 33*, 69–73.

Apfelberg, D.B., Bailin, P., & Rosenberg, H., (1986). Preliminary investigation of KTP/532 laser light in the treatment of hemangiomas and tattoos. *Lasers in Surgery and Medicine, 6*(1)38–42, 56–77.

Baldwin, F.D., (1996). Unconventional therapy in Pennsylvania practices. *Pennsylvania Medicine, 99*(1), 9–11.

Beckerman, H., de Bie, R.A., Bouter, L.M., De Cuyper, H.J., & Oostendorp, R.A. (1992). The efficacy of laser therapy for musculoskeletal and skin disorders; a criteria-based meta-analysis of randomized clinical trials. *Physical Therapy, 72*(7), 483–491.

Bertolucci, L.E,, & Grey, T., (1995). Clinical analysis of mid laser vs. placebo treatment of arthralgic TMJ degenerative joints. *Cranio, 13*(1), 26–29.

Brown, K.C., Sirles, A.T., & Hilyer, T.M.J. (1992). Cost-effectiveness of a back school intervention for municipal employees. *Spine, 17*(10), 1224–1228.

Cary, T.S., Garrett, J., Jackman, A., McLaughlin, C., Fryer, J., & Smucker, D.R. (1995). The outcomes and costs of care for acute low back pain among patients seen by primary care practitioners, chiropractors, and orthopedic surgeons. The North Carolina back pain project. *New England Journal of Medicine, 333*(14), 913–917.

Chess, C., & Chess, Q. (1993). Cool laser optics treatment of large telangiactasia of the lower extremities. *Journal of Dermatologic Oncology, 19*, 74–80.

Cristoph, J., Strasser, P., Eiswirth, M., & Ertl, G. (1999). Remote triggering of waves in an electrochemical system. *Science, 284*(5412), 291–293.

Davis, A.E. (1996). Primary care management of chronic musculoskeletal pain. *Nurse Practitioner, 21*(8), 72, 75, 79–82.

Feine, J.S., Widmer, C.J., & Lund, J.P. (1997). Physical therapy: A critique. *Oral Surgery, Oral Medicine, Oral Pathology, Oral Radiology and Endodontics 83*(1), 123–127.

Fitzpatrick, R.E. & Goldman, M.P. (1994). Tattoo removal using the alexandrite laser. *Archives of Dermatology, 130*(12)1508–1514.

Fitzpatrick, R.E., Goldman, M.P., & Ruiz-Esparza, J. (1993). Laser treatment of benign pigmented epidermal lesions using a 300 nsecond pulse and 510 nm wavelength. *Journal of Dermatologic Surgery and Oncology, 19*(4), 341–347.

Fitzpatrick, R.E., Lowe, N.J., Goldman, M.P., Borden, H., Behr, K.L., & Ruiz-Esparza, J. (1994). Flashlamp-pumped pulsed dye laser treatment of port-wine stains. *Journal of Dermatologic Surgery and Oncology, 20*(1), 743–748.

Fralicker, D., Green, J., Clewell, W., Ossi, G., & Briley, M. (Unpublished observation). Chronic myofascial pain treated with a new device: The photon stimulator — Physiological and clinical assessment.

Frymoyer, J.W., Katz, and Bahril W. (1991). An overview of the incidences and costs of low back pain. *Orthopedic Clinics of North America, 22*(2), 263–271.

Gam, A.N., Thorsen, H., & Lonnberg, F. (1993). The effect of low-level laser therapy on musculoskeletal pain: A meta-analysis. *Pain, 52*(1), 63–66.

Geronemus, R. G. (1992). Q-switched ruby laser therapy of Nevus of Ota. *Archives of Dermatology, 128*(12), 1618–1622.

Goldman, M.P. & Eckhouse, S. (1993). Photothermal sclerosis of leg veins. *Journal for Dermatologic Surgery, 22*(4), 323–330.

Gonzalez, E., Gange, R.W., & Momtaz, K.T. (1992). Treatment of telangiactases and other benign vascular lesions with the 577 nm pulsed dye laser. *Journal of the American Academy of Dermatology, 27*(2 Pt. 1), 220–226.

Gray, R.J.M., Quails, A.A., Hall, C.A., & Schofield, M.A. (1995). Temporomandibular pain dysfuction: Can electrotherapy help? *Physiotherapy, 81*(1), 47–51.

Green, J. (1998). Poster Presentation: Use of over-the-counter infrared emitter for the treatment of myofascial pain syndrome. American Academy of Pain Management, Atlanta, Georgia, September 10.

Green, J. (1993). Tutorial 12. Thermography — Medical infrared imaging. *Pain Digest, 3*, 268–272.

Green, J. (1989, August). A preliminary note: Dynamic thermography may offer a key to the early recognition of reflex sympathetic dystrophy. Clinical Thermography. *Journal of the Academy of Neuromuscular Thermography*, 104–105.

Green, J., Fralicker, D., Clewell, W., Horowitz, E., & Lucey, T., (1999). Photon stimulation therapy for chronic regional pain syndrome: a new technique. *Disability, 8*(3), 47–51.

Green, J., Horowitz, E., Fralicker, D., Ossi, G., Briley, M., & Lucey, T. (1999). A photon stimulation: A new form of therapy for chronic diabetic painful neuropathy of the feet. *Pain Digest, 9*, 286–291.

Green, J., Leon-Barth, C., Kohli, H., & Green, S. (1989, August). The pathophysiology of reflex sympathetic dystrophy as demonstrated by dynamic thermography. Clinical Thermography. *Journal of the Academy of Neuromuscular Thermography*, 121–125.

Haber, C., & Bales, M. (1998, November). Bales photonic stimulator, Bales Scientific, Inc. 1620 Tice Valley Blvd., Walnut Creek, CA 94595.

Hay, L.R., &, Helewa, A. (1994). Myofascial pain syndrome: A critical review of literature. *Physiotherapy Canada, 46*(1), 28–36.

Helms, J.M. (1998). An overview of medical acupuncture alternative therapies. In *Essentials of Complementary and Alternative Medicine*. Baltimore: Williams and Wilkins.

Hooshmand, H., & Hashmi, M. (1999). Complex regional pain syndrome (reflex sympathetic dystrophy syndrome): Diagnosis and therapy — A review of 824 patients. *Pain Digest, 9*, 1–24.

Hug, E.G., Fitzek, M.M., Liebsch, N.J., & Munzenrider, J.E. (1995). Locally challenging osteo- and chondrogenic tumors of the axial skeleton, results of combined proton and photon radiation therapy using three-dimensional treatment planning. *International Journal of Radiation: Oncology–Biology–Physics, 32*(3), 467–476.

Ishimaru, A. (1989). Diffusion of light in turbid material. *Applied Optics, 29*, 2210–2215.

Johansson, A., Wenneberg, B., Wagersten, C., & Haraldson, T. (1991). Acupuncture in treatment of facial muscular pain. *Acta Odontologica Scandinavia, 49*(3), 153–158.

Karu, T. (1987). Photobiological fundamentals of low power laser therapy. *Journal of Quantum Electronics, 23*, 1707–1713.

Kee, W.G., Middaugh, S., Pawlick, K., & Nicholson, J. (1997). Cost benefit analysis of a multidisciplinary chronic pain program. *American Journal of Pain Medicine, 7*(2), 59–62.

Kilmer, S.K., Wheeland, R.G., Goldberg, D.J., & Anderson, R.R. (1994). Treatment of epidermal pigmented lesions with teh frequency-doubled q-switched ND: YAG laser. *Archives of Dermatology, 130*(12), 1515–1519.

Lovelock, D.M., Chui, C.S., & Mohan, R. (1995). Monte Carlo model of photon beams used in radiation therapy. *Medical Physics, 22*(9), 1387–1394.

McMillas, A.N., & Blasberg, B. (1994). Pain-pressure threshold in painful jaw muscles following trigger point injection. *Orofacial Pain, 8*(4), 384–390.

Melzack, R., & Wall, P.D. (1965). Pain mechanisms, a new theory. *Science, 150*, 971–979.

Melzack, R., Stillwell, D.M., & Fox, E.J. (1997). Trigger points and acupuncture points for pain: Correlations and implicaitons. *Pain, 3*, 3–23.

Miller, I.D., & Veitch, A.R. (1993). Optical modeling of light distributions in skin tissue following laser irradiation. *Lasers in Surgery and Medicine, 3*(5), 565–571.

Miner, M.A., & Sanford, M.K. (1993). Physical interventions in the management of pain in arthritis: An overview for research and practice. *Arthritis Care and Research, 6*(4), 197-206.

Mitchell, L.V., Lawler, F.H., Bowden, D., Mote, W., Asundi, P., & Purswell, J. (1994). Effectiveness and cost-effectiveness of employer-issued back belts in areas of high risk for back injury. *Journal of Occupational Medicine, 36*(1), 90–94.

Mulcahy, D., McCormack, D., McElwain, J., Wagstaff, S., & Conroy, C. (1995). Low level laser therapy: A prospective double blind trial of its use in an orthopaedic population. *Injury, 26*(5), 315–317.

Nelson, J.S. (1991). Selective photothermolysis and removal of cutaneous vasculopathies and tattoos by pulsed laser. *Plastic and Reconstructive Surgery, 99*(4), 723–731.

Ng, L.K.Y., Katims, J.J., & Lee, M.H.M. (1992). Acupuncture: A neuromodulation technique for pain control. In G.M. Arnoff (Ed.), *Evaluation and treatment of chronic pain,* (2nd ed.). Baltimore: Williams and Wilkins.

Omura, Y. & Bechman, S.L. (1995). Application of intensified Qui Gong energy, electrical field, magnetic field, elecrical pulses, strong Shiatsu massage or acupuncture on the accurate organ representation areas of the hands to improve circulation, special emphasis on enhanced chlamydia, uric acid syndrome. *Acupuncture and Electro-Therapeutics Research, 20*(1), 21–72.

Polla, L.L., Tan, O.T., Garden, J.M., & Parrish, J.A. (1987). Turnable pulsed dye laser for the treatment of benign cutaneous vascular extasia. *Dermatologica, 174*(1), 11–17.

Reid, W.H., Miller, I.D., Murphy, M.J., Paul, J.P., & Evans J.H. (1990). Q-switched ruby laser treatment of tatoos: 9-year experience. *British Journal of Plastic Surgery, 43*(6), 663–669.

Rowbotham, M.C. (1998). Complex regional pain syndrome type I (reflex sympathetic dystrophy) more than a myth. *Neurology, 51,* 4–5.

Shekelle, P.G., Markovich, M., & Louis, R. (1995). Comparing the costs between provider types of episodes of back pain care. *Spine, 20*(2), 221–226.

Stanton-Hicks, M., Janig, W., Hassenbusch, S., Haddox, J.D., Boas, R., & Wilson, P. (1995). Reflex sympathetic dystrophy, changing concepts and taxonomy. Review. *Pain, 63,* 127–133.

Steiner, R. (1989, September). Lasers in dermatology. Proceedings of the International Symposium, Ulm, 26 September 1989: The role of skin optics in diagnostic and therapeutic use of lasers. Laser Biology Research Laboratory, University of Texas, D.M. Anderson Cancer Center, 1365–1374.

Sugimoto, K., Konda, T., Shimahara, M., Hyodo, M., & Kitade, T. (1995). A clinical study on SSP (silver spike point) electrotherapy combined with splint therapy for temporomandibular joint dysfunction. *Acupuncture and Electro-Therapeutics Research, 20*(1), 7–13.

Svaasand, L.O., Norvang, L.T., Fiskerstrand, E.J., Stopps, E.K.S., Berns, M.W., & Nelson, J.S. (1995). Tissue parameters determining the visual appearance of normal skin and port-wine stains. *Lasers in Medical Science, 10*(1), 55–65.

Tan, O.T., Morelli, J.G., & Kurban, A.K. (1992). Pulsed dye laser treatment of benign cutaneous pigmented lesions. *Lasers in Surgery and Medicine, 12,* 538–542.

Taylor, C.R., Gange, R.W., Dover, J.S., Flotte, T.J., Gonzalez, E., Michaud, N., & Anderson, R.R. (1990). Treatment of tattoos by Q-switched ruby laser. *Archives of Dermatology, 126*(7), 893–899.

Thomasson, T.L. (1996). Effects of skin-contact monochromatic infrared irradiation on tendonitis, capsulitis, and myofascial pain. *Journal of Neurology, Orthopedics, and Medicine & Surgery, 16,* 242–245.

van der Laan, L., ter Laak, H.J., Gabreels-Festen, A., Gabreels, F., & Goris, R.J. (1998). Complex regional pain syndrome type I (RSD): Pathology of skeletal muscle and peripheral nerve. *Neurology, 51*(1), 20–25.

Van Gemert, M. (1991). Can physical modeling lead to an optimal laser treatment strategy for port-wine stains? *Laser Applications in Medicine and Biology, 5,* 221–256.

Yang, Z.L., Guyuang, Z., & Chang, Y.G. (1995). A neuromagnetic study of acupuncturing L1-4 (Hegu). *Acupuncture and Electro-Therapeutics Research, 20*(1), 15–20.

Watanabe, T.H. (1994). Treatment of Nevus of Ota with the Q-switched ruby laser. *New England Journal of Medicine, 331*(26), 1745–1750.

Waylonis, G.W., Wilke, S., O'Toole, D., Waylonis, D.A., & Waylonis, D.B. (1998). Chronic myofascial pain: Management by low-output helium-neon laser therapy. *Archives of Physiology, Medicine and Rehabilitation, 69*(12), 1017–1020.

Webster, B.S., & Snook, S.H. (1994). The cost of 1989 workers' compensation low back pain claims. *Spine, 19*(10), 1115.

Wilson, B.C., & Jacques, S.L. (1990). Optical reflectance and transmittance of tissues: Principles and applications. *IEEE Journal of Quantum Electronics, 26*(12), 2186–2199.

Wong, E., Lee, G., Zucherman, J., & Mason, D.T. (1995). Successful management of female office workers with a repetitive stress injury or a carpal tunnel syndrome by a new treatment modality — Application of low level laser. *International Journal of Clininical Pharmacology Therapeutics, 33*(4), 208–211.

Wright, F.F., & Schiffman, E.L. (1995). Treatment alternatives for patients with masticatory myofascial pain. *Journal of American Dental Association, 126*(7), 1030–1039.

59

Physical Therapy and Pain Management

C. Kumarlal Fernando, M.A., L.P.T.

Physical agents such as sunlight, water, mud baths, and mineral baths have been used as therapeutic agents for the management of pain since ancient times. Today, in the modern world, physical therapists trained in the use of physical agents such as electricity, sound, magnetism, water, and exercises use sophisticated equipment for pain management and the treatment of musculoskeletal and neurological problems. However, the physical agents and modalities themselves are not the complete answer to the problem. Physical exercises, combined with other modalities, help the whole patient and return the patient to normal activities of daily living.

Pain is as old as life itself. It is subjective and defies description. The concept of pain includes, first of all, a sensation evoked by harmful or potentially harmful stimuli, and second, a reaction to this primary sensation. These reactions are threefold: physical, rational, and emotional.

Individual biorhythms, changing continuously during the day, the month, and the year, have an effect on the experience of pain. Women tolerate potentially painful stimuli when ovulating or when they are premenstrual. Most pain is worse in the evenings, perhaps partly due to absence of the distractions of the day, but also due to increased activity of the sympathetic nervous system, which is highest in the evening when body temperature is highest. In controlled experiments, where the stimuli are kept constant, the experience and presence of pain vary from person to person. According to Mersky (1979), "Pain is an unpleasant sensory and emotional experience associated with actual or potential tissue damage, or described in terms of such damage." According to this definition, pain has psychological as well as physiological aspects and, therefore, the whole person, rather than a body part, must be treated. Otherwise, only a part of the pain will be eased.

Physical therapy treatment for pain is designed to combat the physiological aspects of pain such as tissue damage, inflammation, ischemia, edema, defects of reduced physical and metabolic activity, and trauma.

But if strategies in the management of pain are to be truly effective, it is important for physical therapists to understand that both physical and psychological components are needed. Melzack (1973) states, "The puzzle of pain, as we have seen, is far from solved and there are few problems more worthy of human endeavor than the relief of pain and suffering."

However, in treating the acute stages of pain, techniques aimed at the physiological aspects are very effective. It is important to realize that the optimal management is entirely different for acute and for chronic pain. Acute pain is the kind of severe pain that, for classification purposes, lasts less than 7 days. Subacute pain lasts from 1 week to 3 months; chronic pain, longer than 3 months (Mooney, Modic, & Brown, et al., 1988).

Prior to the treatment process, and before the application of any physical agent, a thorough evaluation of the patient must be performed. This chapter describes the various modalities that I employ and how I combine them in the management of pain. The physical agents involved are interference current (medium frequency), transcutaneous electrical stimulation, iontophoresis, superficial heat and cold, ultrasound, phonophoresis, shortwave therapy, therapeutic exercises, deep friction, and traction techniques. Each of these modalities is described in the section on Treatments.

0-8493-0926-3/02/$0.00+$1.50
© 2002 by CRC Press LLC

EVALUATION OF THE PATIENT

Prior to treatment of any patient, the physical therapist must evaluate that patient with regard to the pain problem. As a part of the general examination, a thorough history is taken with attention directed to the particular part of the body involved. A majority of the patients will have had their problems diagnosed by their referring physician. But if the diagnosis has not yet been made, a physical evaluation and general history are recorded. The first step is to map out the painful area as accurately as possible. For this, the patient is given a diagram of the body and asked to mark the places where pain is present. Then further examination focuses on skin changes, muscle changes (such as guarding, spasms, and tenderness), joint changes, temperature changes, soft tissue swelling, crepitus, range of motion measurements, limitation of activities, and weakened muscles. Maneuvers that cause pain, pressure on trigger points, neck movements, and maneuvers that relieve pain are considered. Such clinical measurements as straight leg raise, range of motion, and joint and muscle strength are obtained. From these studies a decision is made regarding the goals of treatment and appropriate techniques to meet those goals.

The evaluation of a patient is carried out according to the following protocol: patient history, observation, examination, special tests of reflexes, joint movements, and muscle strength. The patient history must include a complete medical history. The emphasis in the case must be placed on that portion of the assessment having the greatest clinical relevance. Important data in the history are the age and occupation of the patient; whether the problem began gradually or suddenly; whether the patient experienced this condition previously; whether the patient experienced any trauma; the intensity, duration, and frequency of pain; whether the pain is constant, periodic, or occasional; whether it has moved or spread; whether it is associated with rest, certain postures, certain functions, or time of day. Is the pain nerve pain, which tends to be sharp, bright, and burning in quality and usually runs along the nerve? Is it bone pain, which tends to be deep, boring, and very localized? Or is it muscular pain, which tends to be diffused, aching, poorly localized, and may refer to other areas of the body. Muscle pain is usually dull and hard to localize, and is often aggravated by injury.

Some of the questions asked during the patient's history taking are: What type of sensation does the patient feel? Are there pins and needles, abnormal sensations, or tingling? Do the joints lock or are they unlocking? Are there changes in the color of the limb, ischemic changes, loss of hair, or abnormal nails of the hand or foot? In observing the patient, the physical therapist must look for any fractures, scoliosis, kyphosis, muscle wasting, size of the limbs, shape, color, temperature, any scars, texture of the skin, any crepitus on movement, any swelling, any heat or redness, the patient's facial expression, lack of sleep, and whether the patient moves around or walks abnormally.

EXAMINATION

First, the patient's active movements, then passive movements, and last, resistive movements are each tested several times to see whether the symptoms increase or decrease and whether there is weakness. Muscles are tested manually and range of motion noted. The patient's active movements help in diagnosing any problems with the contractile substance, and passive movements helping diagnose problems with the ligaments and the inert substances. Finally, special tests are done to check on the particular system that is at fault. For instance, straight leg raise is performed for back problems and draw testing is performed for knee problems.

After the examination is evaluated, goals of treatment and a treatment plan are established and the patient is treated accordingly. I wish to stress that a single treatment modality is very rarely the answer in the management of pain. The treatment procedure entails modalities, exercises, and home programs, combined to help the patient get better. It is important to know that a single modality, even if it gets rid of the pain, is not a treatment by itself if the patient is not able to return to normal activities of daily living. For instance, a patient with tennis elbow may be treated with ultrasound or phonophoresis and the pain relieved. But when the patient returns to playing tennis, this again causes microtrauma in the common extensor tendon and the condition recurs. Therefore, the treatment must first eliminate the pain by using ultrasound or phonophoresis and cold packs, and then exercises must be started in order for the patient to strengthen the muscles to ensure that they are not torn again. The various modalities are explained in the following section.

TREATMENTS

Hippocrates cautioned his students and colleagues to observe carefully, proceed slowly, and exercise restraint in treatment, a philosophy expounded in the injunction: "First, do no harm" (Gordon, 1949). With this in mind, physical therapists treat patients conservatively and cautiously with much restraint. Most patients treated for pain by physical therapy are patients with low back pain. It is particularly important in view of the multiplicity of possible causes of backache that an exact diagnosis be established prior to treatment, if possible. Today, with MRI, CAT scan, and myelography, disc disease can be diagnosed very easily. Most back pain is due to disc lesions, which, properly treated with physical therapy, can be helped. Indications for the use of physical modalities are symptomatic pain relief, relief of muscle spasm, strengthening and endurance training, increase of spinal mobility or joint mobility, and postural re-education.

REST

The first modality of treatment is rest. For sufferers of acute pain, bed rest is the most frequently prescribed treatment. It must specifically entail rest for the affected body part. Relief is obtained by unloading the spinal segment or the joint involved. If it is the spine, the intradiscal pressure is decreased. In the case of compression of a spinal nerve, edema of the perineural sheath is thought to be the reason for the pain (Bell, et al., 1984), and bed rest allows the edema to subside, thus contributing to the relief of pain. The required length of bed rest is disputed for patients with acute backache. Many practitioners believe a minimum of 2 weeks is needed, but some maintain that 2 days may be sufficient in some cases. Deyo and Rosenthal (1986), for example, have shown that 2 days of bed rest can be just as effective as 7 days. But to push a patient who is in severe pain with only 2 days of bed rest could, in fact, cause harm. Most authorities still advocate 2 weeks of bed rest initially, followed by gradual movements and strengthening. The length of bed rest prescribed — from 2 to 14 days — depends mostly upon the patient, the symptoms, and the severity of the pain. In chronic pain, however, bed rest is not the solution because it may result in muscle atrophy and generalized deconditioning.

HEAT THERAPY

Heat therapy is used as an adjunct to other types of treatment. Superficial moist heat is relaxing, soothing, and pleasant. Moist heat produces vasodilatation that allows rapid removal of cell metabolites from the tonically contracted muscles, thereby achieving therapeutic effects (DeLateur, 1982). A nonspecific counter-irritant, moist heat also contributes to analgesia, which, according to Lehman, et al. (1958), is produced by an increase in the pain threshold.

The rationale for using moist heat is mainly to relax superficial muscles and also to prepare the skin for subsequent physical agents. In addition to hot packs, moist warm towels, water bottles, infrared lamps, and paraffin wax baths are used for acute and chronic pain conditions.

In chronic pain conditions, hydrotherapy can be effective because of the buoyancy of the water and the counter-irritant phenomenon. The buoyancy of the water counteracts the effects of gravity which diminish the weight-bearing stress on the lumbar spine, thereby reducing pain. The temperature of the water also relaxes and sedates muscles and joints so that the patient can much more easily perform the exercises in the water.

CRYOTHERAPY

Ice cools the superficial layer of the muscle, which decreases muscle spasms and elevates the pain threshold. Because of this, the analgesia and muscle relaxation will last longer. Also, the counter-irritant effect of ice further contributes to the analgesia (Lipold, et al., 1960).

DEEP HEAT

Shortwave diathermy and ultrasound are two methods of applying effective deep heat therapy in the treatment of pain conditions.

ULTRASOUND

The ultrasound generated in the United States produces sound waves at the frequency of one megacycle per second. For clinical application, a transmission medium is always required. Generally, the ultrasound waves are transmitted via water, oil, or transmission gel. It has been suggested that about 50% of the ultrasound is transmitted to a depth of 5 cm (Goldman & Heuter, 1956).

Deep tissues, such as joint capsules and deep muscles, can be treated with ultrasound. Homogeneous substances, like subcutaneous fat and metal implants, absorb less energy than muscle, so ultrasound produces very little increase in the temperature of these materials. Therefore, patients with implants can be treated with ultrasound in the kinds of treatment situations where one must be very careful. A physiological effect of ultrasound is to decrease the level of cortisol. Painful nerves and nerve plexors have been found to increase the level of cortisol, and because ultrasound is a strong anti-inflammatory substance, its use decreases inflammation due to trauma. Ultrasound, therefore, can be used in the treatment of lumbosacral nerve root irritation, nerve root impingement, and various types of neuritis (Touchstone, et al., 1963). Ultrasound also affects joint capsules and ligaments, increasing their range of motion. Muscle spasms of a localized nature can be effectively treated with ultrasound, which increases temperature in the muscles, by about 1 to 2°C. Ultrasound is contraindicated in pregnancy, in malignancies, in bone overgrowth, and in patients who cannot perceive pain and heat.

SHORTWAVE DIATHERMY

Large body parts such as the back and thigh, and deep areas such as the hip, can be treated with shortwave diathermy. Shortwave equipment produces high-frequency electromagnetic waves, having a length of 11 m and a frequency of 27 megacycles. Shortwave diathermy with condenser electrodes uses the electrical components of the electromagnetic waves, and shortwave diathermy with induction electrodes uses the magnetic components of the electromagnetic waves. The effect is deep tissue penetration and heating. Greater heating of fat or muscle is achieved with condenser electrodes. When heat is needed in deep joints such as the hip, condenser shortwave therapy is more effective. Induction electrodes are used for superficial heating and muscle tends to become warmer than fatty tissue. Therefore, induction coils are used for the treatment of superficial muscles and joints. The thermal physiological effects of shortwave diathermy are elevation of muscle temperature to 42°C after a 20-min application, and increased blood flow into the heated muscle. A concurrent increase in metabolism and relaxation of contracted fiber is experienced. In Reynaud's disease and other vascular conditions of the extremities, an increase of blood flow can be brought about by heating the abdominal area. Shortwave diathermy is used mainly for reduction of effusion in arthroscopic surgical knees and for osteoarthritis of the knee, where it is very effective. It is contraindicated if the patient is pregnant or has a pacemaker or a metal implant.

IONTOPHORESIS AND PHONOPHORESIS

The introduction of various ions into the tissues beneath the skin via electricity is called iontophoresis. Phonophoresis is the driving of ions into the tissues via ultrasound. Using a sound applicator, various medications can be driven into the tissues to a depth of about 5 cm (Griffin & Karselis, 1997).

Hydrocortisone and Lidocaine

Hydrocortisone and lidocaine are two medications used in phonophoresis to treat the pain of musculoskeletal conditions. Hydrocortisone in a 1 or 10% concentration is used in both acute and chronic pain conditions such as bursitis, tendonitis, and neuritis. Before phonophoresis or iontophoresis is applied, the patient's complete history must be reviewed to avoid choosing any medication to which the patient is allergic. Iontophoresis is used in cases of neck and back pain, arthritic conditions, bursitis, rotator cuff, and tendonitis. Physiological effects of the direct current alone are known and are utilized in the technique of iontophoresis. The positive pole alone produces an acid reaction and tends to decrease nerve irritability. The negative pole cathode is alkaline and tends to increase nerve irritability.

INTERFERENCE CURRENT THERAPY (ICT)

Medium Frequency Electrical Therapy

Interference current therapy was developed by the Austrian physicist, Nemec. Two electrical currents, each with a different frequency, 4000 and 4100 Hz, are applied to the skin through surface electrodes and an interference

pattern is established at the intersection of the two currents, The result of this interference pattern is that the targeted tissue receives a net frequency of 100 Hz of low frequency current. The main advantage of this type of current is that is penetrates the skin with very little resistance and, hence, less intensity output is required. Also, this low frequency current produces superficial muscle contractions and tends to depolarize the muscle membrane to a great extent. Moreover, motor nerves and sensory nerves are more readily depolarized at lower frequencies. Therefore, deep stimulation of muscle and nerve is possible by the selective application of ICT using from 1 to 100 Hz. At frequencies of 0 to 10 Hz, motor nerves are readily depolarized and muscle contractions initiated. This frequency can be used muscle contraction, for muscle relaxation, muscle strengthening, and muscle reeducation. Also, smooth muscles surrounding blood vessels reportedly respond well to stimulation at these lower levels, which can be used in such situations as sympathetic reflex dystrophy. ICT also allows the therapist to effectively reduce and treat edema in acute conditions, and pain relief is possible from frequencies of 1 to 100 Hz. The specific features of interference current are no polar effects, as pure sinusoidal current is used; stimulation of cell division; increased adenosine released through depolarization of the cell membrane leading to adenosine triphosphate; improved microcirculation due to increased adenosine release; and ATP splitting, which results in an increase of free phosphate ions beneficial for mineralization (Hausner, 1982).

TRANSCUTANEOUS ELECTRICAL NERVE STIMULATION (TENS)

In 46 A.D., Scribonius Largus described the use of the torpedo fish, an electric eel, to control pain. This was the beginning of the technique of electrical stimulation for the relief of pain. TENS uses electrodes to stimulate the skin in the treatment of acute and chronic pain conditions. In 1967, Drs. Shealy and Mortimer (1970) developed a dorsal column stimulator for surgical implantation in patients with chronic intractable pain. At the time, they used TENS as a screening device for their patients. Eventually, they eliminated the surgery because they found that the screening process alone brought relief. At that point, TENS, as an alternative method of pain management, became a reality. In addition, Drs. Melzack and Wall's Control Therapy of Pain Perception convinced the medical community of the benefits of electrical neuromodulation of pain. The physiological basis for the treatment is the stimulation of large myelinated afferent fibers, which at the level of the spinal cord tend to block the passage of painful impulses carried by smaller unmyelenated afferent fibers. TENS can be used with a pulsed alternative current wave of 0.1-ms duration, frequency of approximately 100 Hz, and variable voltage to the point of tingling or parasthesia, but not pain. In my practice, 75% of patients require a high width with a low rate for about 2 to 6 pulses per second, and the other 25% require a high width with a high rate, with an amplitude such that they can feel the tingling on the muscle contraction. Obviously, TENS is not used alone. TENS is used with other modalities described later in this chapter. A great many studies are known to have proven the effectiveness of TENS in acute and chronic conditions.

ULTRASOUND IN CONJUNCTION WITH MUSCLE STIMULATION

Ultrasound is used in conjunction with muscle stimulation to treat muscle spasms, softened scar tissues, and microscopic fibrous tissue adhesions. Electrical stimulation by mechanically pumping the muscle being treated promotes the removal of the products of that muscle's increased metabolism. Ultrasound with muscle stimulation is mainly used in muscle splinting, guarding, or muscle spasms to help restore the muscle to its normal function, thereby breaking the cycle of muscle spasm and pain.

AUDIOVISUAL NEUROMUSCULAR RE-EDUCATION AND ELECTROMYOGRAPHIC BIOFEEDBACK

Audiovisual neuromuscular re-education and electromyographic biofeedback are techniques used for the evaluation and treatment of patients as well as for muscle re-education. These techniques are adjuncts to therapies commonly used in rehabilitation medicine. For two of the problems treated, the three main techniques are inhibition of spasticity, recruitment of motor units, and muscle relaxation. These three techniques are used in combination or alone, depending on the problem. EMG feedback is used for patients with muscle spasms of unknown etiology causing pain. In physical therapy, these are usually chronic back pain problems. The management of chronic pain with EMG feedback can be effective for those patients who are in severe pain due to muscle spasms. These spasms aggravate pain and set up a vicious cycle of muscle spasm, pain, and movement (Fernando & Basmajian, 1978).

LUMBAR TRACTION

This system involves positioning the patient with knees and hips bent at 90° and pelvis tilted to decrease lumbar lordosis. A rope attached to a belt around the patient's pelvis is draped over the top of a triangular frame. The patient pulls on the rope to lift the pelvis off the floor. This system can be used in the hospital as well as in outpatient programs. According to Cottrell (1981), relief is experienced in 97% of acute and 94% of chronic low back pain.

Twomey applied 9 kg of traction to L1, S2 cadavers spines and measured an average overall increase in spine length of 8.7 mm (Cottrell, 1985; Twomey, 1985). In addition to the relief of back pain due to bulging disks or protrusion of the nucleus pulposus, there are other benefits. For instance, when the facet joint has become restricted in motion by impingement of the meniscus, capsulitis, or free bodies, traction can release the impinged facet joint and help relieve the muscle spasm. Also, as rapid stretching of skeletal muscles causes reflex excitation, the more prolonged stretching produced by traction is relaxing. This is one of the reasons for using traction. It has been said that stretching by traction stretches the mechanical receptors of the disc, which exerts a beneficial effect on some patients (Cyriax).

Studies by Ramos and Martin (1994) of the Department of Neurosurgery of McAllen Texas, studied intradiscal physical pressure during vertebrae decompression. Transducers were placed in the L4, L5 disc under A-P and lateral fluoroscopy. With the catheter in place, the patient was placed prone on a VAX-D table. Various decompression tensions from 50 to 100 lb were applied. The distraction tensions and intradiscal pressure changes were noted.

Intradiscal pressure was significantly reduced to minus 150 to 160 mm of Hg.

In numerous studies, this was not shown in conventional tractions studies; on the contrary, many traction devices actually increase intradiscal pressure.

The capillary pressure in the vertebral body is greater than the intradiscal pressure; it negates oxygen diffusion to the disc, which, in turn, impedes healing.

Contraindications for Traction

Contraindications for traction include spine infections, spine malignancies, cord completion from central disc herniation, vascular disease, acute inflammatory arthritis, pregnancy, uncontrolled hypertension, and claustrophobia. It also is contraindicated in patients with ligament disruption or dislocation fractures.

DEEP FRICTION

A penetrating massage technique is required to treat deep seating lesions. Given properly, deep friction has a fourfold effect. It induces (1) traumatic hyperemia, (2) movement, (3) increased tissue perfusion, and (4) mechanoreceptor stimulation. For deep friction to be effective the right spot must be found, and the friction must be given across the fibers composing the affected structure. The friction must be given with sufficient sweep and must reach deeply enough. In the case of tendons around a sheath, the tendons must be kept taut. The ideal treatment lasts from about 2 to 20 min daily and from 2 to 7 days depending on the condition. The ordinary conditions treated by deep friction are muscular lesions, tenderness sheaths, long-standing scars, muscular tendinous junction lesions, tendons without a sheath (as in tendonitis or tennis elbow where the short tendon or the supraspinatus tendon is strained), recent strains, and chronic sprains. Contraindications include inflammation due to bacteria, traumatic arthritis of the elbow joint, ossification or calcification (in soft structures), bursitis, rheumatoid types of arthritis, and pressure on nerves. According to Dr. Cyriax (1975), deep friction is very effective and when properly used with other techniques, the results are excellent. I have used deep friction with success in tennis elbow, muscular tendinous lesion, rotator cuff lesions, and other muscle conditions.

EXERCISE THERAPY

The many types of exercise therapy are divided into active and passive. The active are divided into assisted, resistive, and free. It is very important that exercise therapy be prescribed properly and administered by those who know the treatment protocols and programs. It is useless to give a patient a list of exercises to be done at home, or to tell the patient to walk or swim, with no direction or teaching by a physical therapist. In the overall management of pain, exercise therapy is the most important part of the treatment program. The modalities only lower the pain threshold or minimize the pain, but it is up to the physical therapist to strengthen muscles, increase joint range, and by the use of prescribed exercises and therapeutic programs, to get the patient back to normal activities of daily living and to a normal holistic state as soon as possible. Therefore, the management of pain is really exercise therapy in combination with modalities, not modalities alone. There are many different kinds of exercises including isometric, isotonic, isokinetic, etc. Sophisticated equipment may be used. As mentioned, low back pain is the condition seen by physical therapists in at least 70% of the cases of pain management. Exercise therapy to minimize back pain aims to improve flexible strength and endurance, and to return the patient to activities of daily living and normal functions. Exercises can reduce pain by stretching muscles in spasm and also can minimize the possibility of recurrence of low back problems. Various exercise programs can help the back by helping its nutrition, which will modulate pain and improve spinal biomechanics. The three most commonly used types of exercises are hyperextension, extension, and flexion.

PRINCIPLES OF MUSCLE REHABILITATION

The three major principles of muscle rehabilitation are (1) specificity, (2) overload, and (3) provision of optimal condition for performance (Malone, 1988).

Specificity

If a muscle is trained for strength, then improvement is only in strength and not in other parameters. If the training is limited to a specific range, then the strength gains are significant only in that range. If the strength gains are obtained by isometric exercise, then the strength during dynamic exercise is minimal. And, if the strength gains are obtained by dynamic exercise that is concentric and eccentric, then the isometric improvements are minimal (Lindh, 1979).

Slow speed exercises do not stimulate muscles to the extent that fast speed exercises do. During fast contractions, firing rates of motor units are greater than in slow contractions (Sale, 1987).

Overload

Muscle strength improvement is directly proportional to the overload applied to the muscle. Maximum loading increases maximal activation of prime movers and, hence, produces muscle hypertrophy. A muscle can be overloaded in two ways: (1) by increasing resistance, and (2) by performing submaximum contractions to the point of fatigue.

EXTENSION AND FLEXION EXERCISES IN THE MANAGEMENT OF LOW BACK PAIN DUE TO INTERVERTEBRAL DISC LESIONS

Clinicians have held widely diverse views on which therapeutic exercises should be prescribed to patients with low back pain. Authorities such as Williams (1965), Cailliet (1966), and Rowe (1960) emphasized exercises that strengthen the flexors of the spine, while others, such as Mock and Armstrong, advocated exercising the flexors as well as the extensors of the lumbar spine.

Although advocates of the different procedures claimed success with their particular techniques, no studies were published to verify their claims. Then Sarno and I studied various techniques, and based on our studies, recommended that for people with this problem, all muscle groups, including the iliopsoas, should be strengthened. I developed exercises and techniques based on my studies and those of numerous investigators all over the world. I have been giving these exercises—extension as well as flexion—to back patients since 1968 (Fernando and Sarno, 1970).

Rationale for Exercise Treatment for Low Back Pain

Where backache is due to intervertebral disc lesions, as soon as the acute episode subsides, exercise therapy should be commenced. The aim of treatment is to minimize intradiscal pressures by using nonweight-bearing positions within the patient's pain-free range of movement. This is important, as a rise in intradiscal pressure in patients with a herniation could lead to protrusion of the nucleus pulposus, which could then impinge on the sinuvertebral nerve or its branches that innervate the posterior longitudinal ligament, the outer layer of the annulus, and the synovial joints, thereby giving rise to pain and its resulting clinical syndrome. Nearly 50% of all intervertebral disc lesions are posterior. Only about 10 to 12% of such lesions are posterolateral, which type can give rise to a radiating pain in the lower extremities. The aim of treatment is to stabilize the lumbar spine so as to avoid recurrence of herniation, irritation, pain, and muscle spasm. This rationale was originally expounded by Morris and Bressler (1961), and then by Armstrong (1964), and later by Lucas (1973). I expanded their ideas based on my studies and the reports of other investigators all over the world (Fernando & Sarno, 1970; Fernando, 1974).

By itself, an isolated ligamentous spine fixed at its base will collapse under a force as small as 4.5 lb. The stability of the lumbar spine is dependent upon two muscle systems: the extrinsic stabilizers and the intrinsic stabilizers.

The extrinsic stabilizers of the lumbar spine are comprised of all the muscles surrounding it. Its intrinsic stabilizers are the ligaments and intraabdominal pressures. To improve these systems and thus stabilize the lumbar spine, several important physical therapeutic measures can be undertaken:

- Strengthen the abdominal muscles
- Strengthen the back extensor muscles
- Strengthen the iliopsoas group

By strengthening the abdominal and back extensor muscles we not only strengthen the extrinsic stabilizers, but also increase the integrity of the intrinsic stabilizers, namely, intraabdominal pressure, which opposes the forces on the lumbar spine and, thus, minimizes them.

By strengthening the iliopsoas group, the extrinsic stabilizers are strengthened. The fact that this group of muscles weakens in patients with low back pain indicates that this procedure is necessary.

The majority of patients treated by physical therapists have low back pain, and at least 90% of back problems referred to physical therapy are due to intervertebral disc lesions. These patients can be divided into three categories: (1) back pain alone, (2) back pain with referred pain into the buttock and thigh, and (3) pain below the knee with or without back pain or neurological signs. In addition to the disc, other structures produce back and leg pain, such as tendons, ligaments, fascia, and facet joints. However, on the basis of current information, the disc remains the primary structure thought to be responsible for low back pain, particularly when sciatica is present (Mooney, Modick, & Brown, 1988).

In addition to these three categories, patients can also be divided according to the duration of the pain:

(1) acute pain of 7 days or less, (2) subacute pain of 1 week to 3 months, and (3) chronic pain of longer than 3 months (Mooney, et al.). I believe that the majority of patients referred to physical therapy who linger longer than 3 months have pain due to disc lesions and not chronic pain due to unknown or idiopathic conditions. New studies clearly show that chronic pain is due mainly to disc problems that have gone undetected (Grubb, et al., 1987). For many years, practitioners have manipulated and immobilized backs for the facet joint. But again, studies show that manipulating the facet joint does not open up the facet nor relieve the pain. The facet phenomenon (McFadden & Taylor, 1986) is secondary to the disc; therefore, it is dangerous to manipulate or mobilize the patient (Butler, et al., 1990). Furthermore, no studies indicate that manipulation is effective in disc disease (Doran & Newell, 1975; Glover, Morris, & Kholsa, 1974; Godfrey, Morgan, & Schatzker, 1984; Hoehler, Tobeis, & Buerger, 1981; Paris, 1983; Sims-Williams & Young, 1978).

All exercises are performed in nonweight-bearing positions, and within the patient's pain-free range of movement. This is important, as in nonweight-bearing positions, intradiscal pressures are kept low, and thus the chances of the nucleus pulposus protruding and irritating sensitive structures are minimized. In the beginning, all exercises are performed isometrically, and then later, progress is made to isotonic movements still within the patient's pain-free range of movement. If complete rehabilitation is the goal, the patient eventually should be able to perform through the entire normal range of motion (Fernando, 1974).

The treatment plan for category 1A is bed rest for 2 to 7 days or more, depending on the severity of the pain, followed by hot packs, neurostimulation if there is muscle spasm or listing, back exercises, and a TENS electrical stimulator. At the end of 7 days, when the pain subsides,

---

TABLE 59.1

Classification of Clinical Categories of Lumbar Disc Disease

1A) Acute low back pain
2A) Acute low back pain with thigh pain referred
3A) Acute low back pain with lower leg pain nerve root irritation
1B) Subacute low back pain
2B) Subacute low back pain and thigh pain referred
3B) Subacute low back pain and leg pain nerve root irritation
1C) Chronic low back pain
2C) Chronic low back pain and thigh pain referred
3C) Chronic low back and lower leg pain nerve root irritation

From Mooney, et al. (1988). In Frymoyer, J. & Gord, F.L. (Eds.). *New perspectives on low back pain*. (With permission.)

strengthening exercises can begin for abdominals, back extensors, leg musculature, etc. For category 1B, after 7 days the treatment is the same as for 1A, with increasing activity on bicycle and treadmill. All the exercises should be done in the patient's pain-free range. In category 1C, patients have pain of 3 months duration, and strengthening exercises, endurance exercises, and range-of-motion exercises continue. However, patients properly treated in the A and B stages should not reach stage C or the 3-month period. Hence, the chronic low back pain due to a disc lesion can be cut short if the patient is treated adequately in stages 1A and 1B. I have seen many patients in the 1C stage who were not treated properly in 1A and 1B. At this point, modalities can be used to break the vicious cycle of spasm and pain and then the strengthening exercises can be continued. In addition to the treatment programs, the patient must be taught correct techniques for lifting and performing other activities of daily living to avoid back problems. Instruction in the proper use of tables, chairs, and beds should be included.

1A) Acute Low Back Pain

The patient rests from 2 to 7 days, or longer, depending on the pain. While the patient rests, hot packs, ultrasound, or neurostimulation, depending on muscle spasm and list, can be used. A TENS unit for 6 to 8 hours per day also can be used. When the pain subsides, which may be on the 3rd, 4th, or 5th day, pelvis tilt and back extension exercises can be started, depending on the evaluation. If flexion exercises are painful, they must not be done. If extension exercises are painful, they must not be done. Whatever is NOT painful is done. It is also important to begin with isometric rather than isotonic exercises in the early stages, then gradually to build up to isotonic and isokinetic, again depending on the pain. All exercises are performed within the pain-free range and in reclining positions to minimize intradiscal pressures. As the patient progresses, exercises can be done sitting or standing. As part of the program, patients should be taught back-protective techniques, back school techniques, walking, and swimming.

2A) Acute Low Back and Thigh Pain Referred

The program is much the same as in 1A, but back traction is also used. In the Cottrell System, a very simple positional device is used for 30 minutes twice a day in the early stages. As time goes on, when the pain down the thigh subsides, its use is decreased to once a day. Exercises are then performed and modalities applied, depending on pain and spasm. If no spasm is present, ultrasound can be used. If spasm is present, neurostimulation or interferential therapy can be used. Both are effective in reducing spasm. TENS also is used 6 to 8 hours daily and the patient is cautioned not to use the unit while driving, lifting heavy objects, or performing other activities of daily living.

3A) Acute Low Back Pain, Lower Leg Pain, Nerve Root Irritation

Again, bed rest, back traction, (90/90 Cottrell System), TENS, cold packs, interferential therapy, or neurostimulation are used, then exercises are begun depending on whether pain is present. The object is to minimize positions that increase intradiscal pressures and cause protrusions of the nucleus pulposus that impinge on nerve or pain sensory structures.

In my experience over the last 32 years, I have used this technique to treat thousands of patients with excellent results. Rarely was there a need for surgical intervention. In the subacute and acute stages, the treatments are much the same. As I mentioned, no patient should ever become chronic if treated in the manner described. The patients who come for treatment after 6 months of pain are patients with disc lesions that have not been diagnosed properly, and have not been treated properly (Grubb, et al., 1983). As with a subacute patient, we progress toward strengthening, back-protection techniques, back school, and the modalities mentioned, with emphasis on walking and relaxation exercises.

Treating disc lesions is simple and effective and I have found no need for esoteric treatment techniques such as mobilization or manipulation. These can be dangerous and have no place in the treatment of disc lesions. If something goes wrong, paraplegia, further disc lesions, or exacerbation of present problems could ensue.

Surgery is a last resort for a disc lesion. Studies by Weber (1983) show that 10 years after treatment, whether the treatment is conservative or surgical, the results are the same. Now, one may well question: Why have surgery with its attendant risks if, at the end of 10 years, the results are the same whether surgically treated or conservatively treated with physical therapy?

The latest data as presented by Taylor, Deyo, Cherkin, et al. (1994) revealed that in 1990, the rate for surgery in the United States was 131 per 100,000 patients. Another study comparing the rates of back surgery in 13 countries reveals that the U.S. rate is at least 40% higher than any other country, and more than 5 times that of Scotland and England. The reason for this was explained as cultural differences and practice patterns.

REFERENCES

Andersson, G.B., Schults, A.S., & Nachemson, A.L. (1983). Intervertebral disc pressures during traction. *Scandinavian Journal of Rehabilitation, 9,* 88–91.

Armstrong, J.R. (1964, September). Lumbar disk lesions.

Bell, G.R., et al. (1984). The conservative treatment of sciatica. *Spine, 9,* 54–56.

Butler, D., et al. (1990). Discs degenerate before facets. *Spine, 15*(2), 111.

Cailliet, R. (1966). *Low back pain syndrome*. Philadelphia: Davis.

Cherkin, D.C., Deyo, R.A, Loeser, J.D., et al. (1994). An international comparison of back surgery rates. *Spine, 19*, 1201–1206.

Cottrell, G.W. (1981). The treatment of low back pain. *Orthopedic Transactions, 1*, 80.

Cyriax, J. *Textbook of orthopedic medicine (*Vol. 2, 10th ed.). London: Bailliére Tindall.

DeLateur, B.J. (1982). *Therapeutic heat.* In J. F. Lehman (Ed.), *Therapeutic heat & cold* (3rd ed.) (pp. 404–562). Baltimore: Williams & Wilkins.

Deyo, D., & Rosenthal, K. (1986). How many days of bed rest for acute low back pain. *New England Medical Journal, 316*, 1064.

Doran, D.M.L., & Newell, D.J. (1975). Manipulation in the treatment of low back pain: A multicentre study. *British Medical Journal, 2*, 161–164.

Fernando, C.K. (1968). Thesis: *Conservative management of low back pain in the chronic stage.* New York University, New York.

Fernando, C.K. (1974). *Treatment of low back pain* (pp. 304–314). World Conference of Physical Therapy. Montreal.

Fernando, C.K. (1978). EMG biofeedback in physical therapy. In E. Peper, F. Ancoli, & M. Quinn (Eds.), *Mind/body integration* (p. 453). San Francisco: Plenum Press.

Fernando, C.K. (1989). Some supplementary equipment needs in the rehabilitation setting. In J.V. Basmajian (Ed.), *Biofeedback: Principles and practices for clinicians.* Baltimore: Williams & Wilkins.

Fernando, C.K., & Basmajian, J.V. (1978). Task force study section report. The use of biofeedback in physical medicine and rehabilitation. Prepared for the Biofeedback Society of America.

Fernando, C.K., & Sarno, J. (1970). *Low back pain: a new rationale and technique of treatment by therapeutic exercises.* Proceedings of the First National Assembly, Asian Pacific League of Physical Medicine and Rehabilitation.

Frymoyer, J.W. (1991). *The adult spine. Principles and practice.* New York: Raven Press.

Glover, J.R., Morris, J.G., & Kholsa, T. (1974). Back pain: A randomized clinical trial of rotational manipulation of the trunk. *British Journal of Industrial Medicine, 31*, 39–64.

Godfrey, C.M., Morgan, P. P., & Schatzker, J. (1984). A randomized trial of manipulation for low back pain in a medical setting. *Spine, 9*, 301–304.

Goldman, D.E., & Heuter, T.F. (1956). Tabulated data on velocity and absorption of high frequency sound in tissues. *American Acoustics Society, 28*, 35.

Gordon, F.L. (1949). *Medicine throughout antiquity*. Philadelphia: F.A. Davis.

Griffin, J., & Karselis, T. (1997). *Physical agents for physical therapy* (Vol. 97). Springfield, IL: Charles C Thomas Publishers.

Grubb, S.A., et al. (1983). The relative value of lumbar roentgenograms, metrizamide myelography, and discography in the assessment of patients with chronic low back syndrome. *Spine, 12*(3), 282–283.

Hausner, K. (1982). Interferential electrotherapy enhances wound and fracture healing. *American Journal of Electromedicine, 2*(1).

Hoehler, F.K., Tobeis, J.S., & Buerger, A.A. (1981). Spinal manipulation for low back pain. *Journal of the American Medical Association, 245*, 1835–1838.

Lehman, J.F., et al. (1958). Pain threshold measurements after therapeutic application of ultrasound, microwaves and infrared. *Archives of Physical Medicine Rehabilitation, 39*, 560–565.

Lindh, L.M. (1979). Increase of muscle strength from isometric quadriceps exercises at different knee angles. *Scandinavian Journal of Rehabilitation Medicine, 11*(33) , 33–36.

Lipold, O.C.J., et al. (1960). A study of the aphrodesia produced by cooling muscles. *Journal of Physiology, 153*, 218–231.

Luca, G.L. (1973). Comparative analysis of lumbar disc disease. *Clinical Orthopedics.*

Malone, T.M. (1978, September). Rehabilitation of sports injuries. *Muscle Injury & Rehabilitation, 1*(3), 54.

McFadden, K.D., & Taylor, J.R. Axial rotation in the lumbar spine and gaping of the zygapophyseal joints. *Spine, 15*(4).

Melzack, R. (1973). *The puzzle of pain.* (p. 232). New York: Williams and Wilkins.

Mooney, V., Modic, M., & Brown, M. (1988). *New perspectives on low back pain.* (p. 134). J.W. Frymoyer & S.L. Gordon (Eds.). American Academy of Orthopedic Surgeons Symposium.

Morris, J.M., & Bressler, K. (1961). Role of the trunk in stability of the spine. *Journal of Bone and Joint Surgery.*

Paris, S.V. (1983). Spinal manipulative therapy. *Clinical Orthopedics and Related Research, 179*, 55–61.

Ramos, G., & Martin, W. (1994). Effects of vertebral axial decompression on intradiscal pressure, *Journal of Neurosurgery, 81*, 350–353.

Rowe, M.L. (1960). *Newer concepts of low back pain.*

Sale, D.G. (1987). Influence of exercises and training in motor activation. *Exercise Sports Scientific, 15*, 95–151.

Shealy, C.N., & Mortimer, J.T. (1970). Dorsal column electrical analgesia. *General Neurosurgy, 32*, 560.

Sims-Williams, R.W., & Young, G.L. (1978). Controlled trial of mobilization and manipulation for patients with low back pain in general practice. *British Medical Journal,* 1338–1340.

Tasuma, T., et al. (1986). Historological development of intervertebral disc herniation. *Journal of Bone and Joint Surgery, 68*, 1066–1072.

Taylor, V.M., Deyo, R.A., Cherkin, D.C., et al. (1994). Low back pain hospitalization: Recent United States trends and regional variations. *Spine, 19*, 1207–1213.

Touchstone, J.C., et al. (1963). Cortisol in peripheral nerves. *Science, 142*, 1275.

Twomey, L.T. (1985). Sustained lumbar traction. An experimental study of long spine segments. *Spine, 10*(2), 146–149.

Weber, H. (1983). Lumbar disc herniation: A controlled perspective study with ten years of observation. *Spine, 8*, 131–140.

Williams, P.C. (1965). *The lumbosacral spine.* New York: McGraw-Hill.

60

Electromedicine: The Other Side of Physiology

Daniel L. Kirsch, Ph.D., D.A.A.P.M.

A fresh look at physiology is needed to better understand the primary medical complaint of pain. Universities are still teaching their students that life is based on a chemical model. Rather than view life processes on a chemical basis alone, it is more realistic to view them on an *electrochemical* basis. All atoms are bonded electrically. This is a basic foundation necessary to understand electromedicine that is taught during the most elementary training in the basic sciences. Further in our rudimentary training we learned that there are voltage potentials across the membrane of all cells. All standard physiology textbooks define the Nernst and Goldman Equations to determine membrane and action potentials. They do not, however, speculate on the staggering significance of these facts.

If batteries are placed in series, their voltage potentials are combined. A simple remote-control device may use three 1.5-V batteries to produce the 4.5 V needed to operate a television. The human body has trillions of cells, each having a 10- to 200-mV potential across their membranes. The overall electrical potential in humans is 2×10^4 V/mm (Kitchen & Bazin, 1996). All good scientists should ask themselves why we find electricity so prevalent in biological systems.

It is already established that bioelectricity plays a major role in physiology. Robert O. Becker, M.D. has spent more than 30 years attempting to determine how trillions of cells with hundreds of subtypes can function harmoniously in the form we call human. The result of that inquiry is a complete revolution in our previous concepts of biology (Becker, 1983).

Becker (1982) found that electromagnetic fields control all living processes. The earliest concept of such field effects can be traced back to ancient China. Traditional Oriental medicine is based on the controlling power of *ch'i* (Qi) or *ki* energy; a concept that predates electricity but appears to be analogous (Kirsch, 1978). Chiropractic also developed based on a similar observation termed *innate intelligence* by Daniel David Palmer in 1895 (Palmer, 1910). Indians use the term *prana* to represent the same concept. Allopathic practitioners are limited to the vague notion of *homeostasis*.

In Western civilization, the first documented use of electricity to manage pain was by the physician Scribonius Largus in 46 A.D. (Tapio and Hymes, 1987). He claimed that just about everything from headaches to gout could be controlled by standing on a wet beach near an electric eel. Not surprisingly, attempts at producing pharmaceutical preparations from dead eels proved ineffective. In 1791, Luigi Galvani discovered that electrical impulses could cause muscle contraction (Smith, 1981). By 1800, Carlo Matteucci showed that injured tissue generates an electric current (Becker and Marino, 1982). The discovery of alternating current by Michael Faraday in 1830 opened the door to the development of manmade devices as sources of electricity. Over 10,000 medical practitioners in the United States alone made use of electrotherapeutic modalities until publication of the 1910 Flexner report, which stated that there was no scientific basis for electromedicine at that time. Flexner's report was originally prepared by the American Medical Association and sponsored by the Carnegie Endowment for the Advancement of Teaching (Walker, 1993). Since the Carnegie family was heavily invested in the young pharmaceutical industry, it is no wonder their report declared allopathic medicine superior.

Since then, arguably the greatest development in the field of electromedicine was when Becker (1981) *electrically induced limb regeneration* in frogs and rats as a model

0-8493-0926-3/02/$0.00+$1.50
© 2002 by CRC Press LLC

to study bioelectrical forces as a controlling morphogenetic field. Regeneration represents a return to embryonic control systems and cellular activities within a localized area. It can, therefore, be considered a more accessible and more observable form of morphogenesis. The complexity of instructions required to designate all of the details to recreate a finished extremity is impossible to transmit by previously understood biochemical processes alone.

Becker (1983) proposed that a primitive direct current data transmission and control system exists in biological systems for the regulation of growth and healing. His studies of extraneuronal analog electrical morphogenetic fields have eliminated any rational arguments against the importance of bioelectricity for *all* life processes. Becker has laid the groundwork for the medical professions to start to evolve toward a more reasonable integrated view of biology incorporating our understanding of both biochemistry and biophysics.

Björn Nordenström, M.D. (1983, 1998), former Chairman of the Nobel Assembly, also has proposed a model of bioelectrical control systems he calls *biologically closed electric circuits* (BCEC). The principle is analogous to closed circuits in electronic technology. Nordenström's theory is that the mechanical blood circulation system is closely integrated anatomically and physiologically with a bioelectrical system.

Nordenström hypothesizes that ionic and nonionic compounds interact in a way that makes selective distribution and modulation of electrical and other forms of energy possible throughout the body, even over long distances. The biological circuits are switched on by both normal electrical activities of the organs and pathological changes, such as tumor, injury, or infection. Like Becker, Nordenström views bioelectricity as the primary catalyst of the healing process.

Using the vascular interstitial system as an example, Nordenström postulates two branches of this system. The first branch, the intravascular system, proposes that walls of blood vessels act as insulators, much like cables in a battery system. The electrical resistance of the walls of the arteries and veins is 200 to 300 times greater than the blood within.

Delayed available energy, or potential energy, is carried by blood cells that bind oxygen, as well as other chemicals such as glucose, neutral fat, nonpolar amino acids, etc. These are all noncharged packages of energy that arrive at specific sites and are released primarily by reduction/oxidation. Nordenström terms these *ergonars*. The intravascular plasma acts as the conductor, where ions such as sodium, calcium, and chloride supply immediately available energy to the system, primarily by electrophoresis. Nordenström calls these *ionars*.

The second branch addresses the interstitial system. The tissue matrix acts as an insulator while the interstitial fluid acts as a conductor.

Capillary membranes are the main components that close the system. These membranes act as junctions between the interstitial and vascular fluids allowing exchange of ionars and ergonars along gradients of electrical potential.

This theory represents a comprehensive attempt to describe functions of anatomical components in terms of electromagnetic forces, rather than limiting them to chemical interactions. Nordenström further theorizes that similar closed circuit systems exist in the urinary and gastrointestinal systems. Using electrical intervention, Nordenström (1984, 1989) reversed terminal cancer in most of his patients as clinical proof of his theories. Several other researchers are confirming the value of electromedicine for the treatment of cancer (Pallares, 1998; Lyte, et al., 1991; Morris, et al., 1992; Sersa, et al., 1992; and Belehradek, et al., 1981).

The medical community has barely taken notice of these remarkable theories. Few practitioners are even aware of the works of Becker or Nordenström. Nordenström is familiar with this type of ignorance. In the 1950s he pioneered a series of remarkable innovations in clinical radiology (including percutaneous needle biopsy) that were considered radical at the time, but are routinely employed by every major hospital in the world today.

Lack of updated education of healthcare professionals is the main stumbling block to acceptance of the modern theories and practice of electromedicine. The other problem is the wide variety of technologies available. At present, there are well over 100 different models of transcutaneous electrical nerve stimulation (TENS) devices in the marketplace and an increasing number of other electrical devices. Most healthcare practitioners who want to utilize such technology have received little or no training in electrobiology or electrical technology. Hence, when it comes to making an educated decision on what type of instrument to choose for a practice or a particular patient, practitioners are often overwhelmed when meeting with an electromedical sales representative. Purchase decisions are frequently made based on lack of knowledge, misinformation, unsubstantiated claims such as testimonials not backed by solid research, or price. If a device is effective in only 2% of the population, treatment of 1000 patients can result in 20 testimonials. The plural of anecdote is not data. Accordingly, healthcare professionals should rely only on evidence-based technologies supported by double-blind research.

BASIC PRINCIPLES

The basic unit of energy is the electron. In 1600, William Gilbert coined the word *electricity* (Bauer, 1983). Using sulfur and friction to generate electricity, Guericke found that it had several properties in common with magnetic forces, such as repulsion/attraction, transference of properties, and opposite poles. Faraday termed the positive pole the *anode*, meaning "upper route" and the negative pole *cathode*, or "lower route." Electrons flow from negative to positive, or cathode to anode.

Fluid-based biological systems are conductive media. Blood, water, and lymph all conduct electricity. Various molecular ions, such as calcium, sodium, and chlorides, carry current. When current is carried by ions, electrolysis occurs. In this process, electricity breaks the conducting fluid down into its components. In the case of water, electricity reduces the H_2O molecule into its components of two atoms of hydrogen and one of oxygen. The half-reaction for the formation of water is $1/2 O_2 + 2H^+ + 2e^- \rightarrow H_2O$. The resultant voltage released at a pH of 7.0 is 0.816 V (Segel, 1975). This process occurs within all types of tissue (e.g., nerves, muscle, bone, etc.) throughout the body.

Many interactions of this nature are highly complex and not yet thoroughly understood. Certain types of electrical stimulation have caused neurotransmitters to be manufactured and released. Some of these treatments are even considered to be frequency specific, but there is still a lot to learn before we can specify the biochemical effects of frequencies, or any other individual aspect of a waveform.

WAVES AND PULSES

In fluids, such as water, the sinusoidal wave is the only basic waveform. However, with electrical technology, different shaped waveforms can be built. These are often referred to as *square, rectangular, triangular, sawtooth,* etc. In actuality, they are composed of thousands of waves known as harmonics. A collection of harmonics within a single electrical activity is called a *pulse*.

Frequencies (Hz) and Pulse Repetition Rates (PRR)

Pulses are measured in cycles moving through a medium in 1 second. One cycle per second is also called a *Hertz* (Hz). In electrical devices, pulses have frequencies. Just as the collection of harmonics is called a pulse, total frequencies (built by the resonance of harmonics) is referred to as the *pulse repetition rate* (PRR). It is the speed at which the pulse moves. For example, a 1 Hz pulse will have harmonic frequencies that build the pulse, ranging from 1 Hz to hundreds of thousands of Hz and beyond, theoretically to infinity. This is often a source of confusion, not only among practitioners, but also among manufacturers of devices as well. In engineering terms, the term *frequency* should only be used with a pure sinewave. Only in this one case, frequency is the same as the pulse repetition rate. With any other

waveform (e.g., square, rectangular, triangular, etc.) there is an infinite number of harmonic frequencies generated within each pulse.

The interplay of harmonics identifies a given musical instrument as a particular aural experience. Some people prefer the sound of a specific note on a piano, while others would rather hear the same note played on a violin. Although the note is the same in each case, the harmonics vary. The interplay of harmonics in electromedicine is essential in affecting the results of a given treatment. With this in mind, we can begin to understand why one electromedical device may work for one patient, yet provide poor results for another. If we could predict what harmonics each tissue needed at a given time, we could design devices that would provide more consistent results in pain management, healing, altering consciousness, and regulating biological processes in general.

The body accepts frequencies and pulse repetition rates in a nonlinear, differential manner. For example, low frequencies penetrate greater depths of tissue than high frequencies. Higher frequencies are auto-shielding; that is, they are limited in penetration because the resistance of tissue acts like a faraday cage, forming eddy–repulsion. This eddy current produces a back electromotive force and blocks the penetration. The reflection of input signals in any conductor (in this case the body) is a mirror image of the opposite phase. The higher the frequency, the greater the rejection and the shallower the penetration. Complex frequencies interact in the body causing a diffuse spread of current.

A nonlinear electrical device is called a *diode*. A diode conducts current of one polarity far greater than the opposite polarity. Most living tissue exhibits nonlinear characteristics, functioning somewhat like diodes.

With square and rectangular waves, a shotgun-like distribution of thousands of frequencies occurs simultaneously within each pulse, like buckshot scattering over a wide area. A sinewave, on the other hand, is more like a bullet from a rifle, which must strike a target accurately to be of use. Our present knowledge of electrophysiology is not sufficient to determine the optimum frequencies for specific tissue responses; therefore, the use of sinewaves is not recommended.

Pulse Width

The length of time a pulse lasts is called the *width*. This is usually measured in microseconds. Pulse width really refers to the time the wave is active. This is important with respect to how a given tissue may be affected, and is part of a hypothetical window of optimal electric stimulation.

The body responds to the peak of electrical signals and to the number of electrons in that signal. The maximum charge per pulse is measured in microcoulombs, which is the total energy of each pulse. The definition of a coulomb is the quantity of electric charge carried by 6.25×10^{18} electrons. Returning to our bullet analogy, we can see that a .22 bullet has less energy than a .45 bullet because it is lighter. While the .22 might go faster, the .45 can knock down a bigger target with its increased energy. Consider each spike a bullet and the pulse width the energy carried by that bullet. Taking our analogy a step further, the velocity of the bullet is the voltage, while the mass of the bullet is the energy, measured in microcoulombs.

Biphasic Signals

Because ions dissociate by electrolysis in the presence of electrical current, living tissue can become polarized in a direct current field. This can cause conflict in neural tissues. Therefore, modern stimulators usually provide alternating or biphasic (also known as bipolar) current. That is, current that reverses polarity each half cycle. This is called a zero net current. If the current continued to flow in the same direction, polarity stress could result in irreversible tissue damage.

As an analogy, picture a group of soldiers marching across a bridge. Before they get to one side, an about-face order is given and they return. Before they reach the opposite side, another about-face order is given, and so on, so that they never actually reach a side. By going back and forth, biphasically, there is no net electron flow across the bridge and no soldiers are added or subtracted. They never get across the bridge to cause an irreversible balance in the status quo. Accordingly, a biphasic current does not add electrons to the body; it simply moves them back and forth.

Amperage, Voltage, and Resistance

Electricity travels in a *circuit*. The number of electrons moving per unit of time is called *amperage*. Amperage is a measure of the amount of *current*. *Voltage* is a measure of the pressure in the circuit. *Resistance* to the electron flow in the circuit is measured in *ohms*. A classic analogy of this is water flowing through a garden hose. The amount of water in the hose corresponds to the amperage. The water pressure corresponds to the voltage. The hose can take only so much water pressure at a given time. Any more pressure or water will be met by more resistance from the hose. This concept is mathematically stated by Ohm's law of $E = IR$, where E (electromotive force) is the voltage, I is the current, and R is the resistance. One can increase the current and decrease the voltage by decreasing resistance, just as more water can pass with a lower pressure through a fire hose than through a garden hose. Similarly, more current can pass through a larger diameter wire or through a highly conductive metal such as copper. In both cases, the thicker wire and more conductive metal have lower resistance.

In the case of a human body, resistance is determined by factors such as fluid content, general health, skin thickness, amount of oil on the skin, temperature and humidity in the air, etc. If a person has a higher resistance, less current will flow through. However, voltage can be increased to maintain the desired level of current. The better electromedical devices deliver a constant current by self-adjusting voltage as skin resistance changes.

Conductivity

Skin resistance is several thousand ohms (as high as $100,000 \ \Omega$ when dry). Wet skin can be as low as $1000 \ \Omega$. Resistance between the hand and foot excluding skin resistance is as low as $500 \ \Omega$. Overall, tissue conductivity is proportional to its water content as can be seen in Table 60.1.

TABLE 60.1
Water Content of Various Tissues

Tissue	Water Content
Skin	5–16%
Bone	5–16%
Fat	14–15%
Brain	~68%
Muscle	72–75%

CLINICAL ASPECTS OF ELECTROMEDICINE

The correct form of electromedical intervention will often have a profound and usually immediate effect on pain. Although caution is advised during pregnancy for liability purposes and the possibility of inducing a miscarriage, and electrical stimulation should not be used on patients with demand-type cardiac pacemakers manufactured prior to the electromagnetic compatibility standards that went into effect in 1998, there are no known significant lasting adverse side effects to therapeutic electromedical technology. There are, however, a number of contraindications as listed below.

GENERAL OVERVIEW OF BENEFITS

1. Low incidence of adverse effects.
2. Relatively easy to learn.
3. Can be administered by paramedical personnel.
4. Expands the practitioner's clinical capability.
5. Enhances the total efficacy of clinical efforts.
6. An alternative therapy in cases refractive to conventional methods.
7. Eliminates or reduces the need for addictive medications in chronic pain syndromes.

8. May be applied on a scheduled basis or PRN.

9. Some modalities produce cumulative effects.

10. May be self-administered by patients for palliative care.

11. Noninvasive therapies are less liable to result in malpractice claims than many conventional procedures.

12. Highly cost effective.

GENERAL OVERVIEW OF CONTRAINDICATIONS, PRECAUTIONS, AND ADVERSE EFFECTS

1. Possible interference with pre-1998 demand-type pacemakers. Also, other implanted devices such as defibrillators, morphine pumps, artificial joints, joint screws, etc.

2. Strong stimulation or pressure from probes placed directly on the carotid sinus could result in vaso–vagal syncopé.

3. Some modalities may cause skin reactions (redness through actual burns) due to excessive stimulation, prolonged use of direct current (or polarity imbalance), or simply sensitive skin.

4. Direct currents can cause electrochemical damage (i.e., chemical burns).

5. Contact dermatitis or disease transmission due to unclean electrodes.

6. Electric shock hazard due to device malfunction or improper use.

7. Many modalities contraindicated for use around heart.

8. Most modalities contraindicated for use on head.

9. Excessive stimulation may produce muscular soreness or spasm, or exceptionally vigorous muscle stimulation can cause muscle or joint damage.

10. Some modalities can cause cardiac fibrillation.

11. Shock hazard from sudden interruption of current in some modalities.

12. The use of most modalities has not been researched in pregnancy (possible physiological implications, such as miscarriage; and unsubstantiated legal arguments in case of developmental defects).

13. Masking of pain that may serve as a protective mechanism.

14. Masking of pain that may hinder or delay diagnosis.

15. Some devices can raise or lower blood pressure.

16. Patients may not be able to drive or operate heavy machinery during or after use.

17. Some devices may cause headaches, vertigo, or nausea.

18. Sensations experienced by the patient can cause anxiety, or panic attacks due to fear of electricity.

19. Some devices may cause vasodilation which would be contraindicated in some people due to hemophilia or thrombosis (may detach thrombus).

20. Spreading of acute inflammation due to muscle pumping action.

21. Some devices may increase injury if used for recent traumatic injuries.

22. Some modalities must not be used over the spine.

23. Some devices may be contraindicated in malignancy (while others are designed to treat cancer).

24. As in drugs, tolerance is the biggest problem of most modalities, such as TENS.

25. Metal electrodes may be toxic. Electrode materials may be driven through the skin through iontophoresis.

26. Electricity passing through any substance produces heat. For human skin 1 mA/cm^2 is just below the level at which cell damage due to heat is produced. Higher currents may damage cells (Becker, 1990).

INDICATIONS AND CONTRAINDICATIONS FOR SPECIFIC ELECTROTHERAPY MODALITIES

The following tables may be used as general guides to determine which modality might be prescribed for a given diagnosis. However, this information is far from complete, and certainly will not, in itself, suffice as a complete course in electromedicine. The reader should keep in mind the above list of general contraindications, precautions, and adverse effects, and that quality, consistency of the outputs, and other factors vary widely among products. This information is culled from the author's 3 decades of training and experience in electromedicine as well as that of several other leading authorities (Becker, 1990; Benton, Baker, Bowman, & Waters, 1981; Jaskoviak & Schafer, 1993; Kirsch, 1999; Kitchen & Bazin, 1996; Low & Reed, 1994; Nelson & Currier, 1991; Thuile & Kirsch, 2000).

Auriculotherapy

Treatment of ear acupuncture points for pain management and systemic disorders (all acupuncture applications).

Uses low frequency 0.5–320 Hz, < 2 S, < 500 mA.

Cranial Electrotherapy Stimulation (CES)

Treatment of the brain for pain, stress, anxiety, depression, insomnia, and addictions when treated at lower or mid-brain levels (ear lobes). Also may be useful to treat organic brain disorders (e.g., stroke, Parkinson's disease, multiple sclerosis, etc.) when treated on top or above ears. Remove earrings and hearing aids.

Uses low-frequency biphasic currents of 0.5–100 Hz, < 2 S, < 1.0 mA.

Indications		Contraindications
Addictions (alcoholism, cigarette withdrawal, cocaine, heroin, marijuana, methadone, opiates, polysubstance abuse, withdrawal)	Learning disorders Multiple sclerosis Muscle tone/movement/tremor Obsessive-compulsive disorders Pain (systemic, idiopathic, delusionary or hallucinatory)	Patients prone to vertigo Pregnancy
Anxiety	Phobia	
Attention deficit disorder	Parkinson's disease Phantom limb syndrome	
Bronchial asthma		
Cerebral palsy		
Chronic fatigue syndrome	Raynaud's disease Reaction time, vigilance	
Closed head injuries		
Cognitive dysfunction	Reflex sympathetic dystrophy	
Dental analgesia	Rehabilitation (systemic disorders)	
Depression		
Eating disorders		
Fibromyalgia syndrome	Stress Stroke	
Headaches	Temporomandibular joint disorder	
Insomnia		

Cryotherapy

Ice, cold packs, vapocoolant sprays, cold therapy, cold immersions, and cryokinetics. This is included here in opposition to hyperthermia treatment that is a given therapeutic factor of some electromedical modalities.

It takes about 15 minutes for ice to reduce skin temperature from 84 to 43°F, 60 minutes to decrease subcutaneous tissue from 94 to 70°F, and about 2 hours to decrease intramuscular temperature from 98 to 79°F. Use of cold for more than 30 minutes may cause temporary nerve palsy.

Indications		Contraindications
Inhibits bleeding after acute trauma	Angiomas Boils and carbuncles	Raynaud's disease Coma
Reduces pain and reduces the accompanying reflex muscle spasm in acute musculoskeletal injuries	Febrile states Herpes blisters Sprains and strains Tumors Varicose ulcers Warts	Rheumatoid arthritis and gout Cryesthesia (e.g., tooth decay) Paroxysmal cold hemoglobinuria

Decreases blood flow to areas of acute inflammation
Spasticity
Burns
Closed pressure sores
Reduces adverse tissue changes and relieves pain in the first-aid treatment of insect and snake bites

Electroacupuncture

Pain management, vasodilation, nausea, healing (all acupuncture applications).

Uses low frequency 0.5–100 Hz, 0.2 mS, at microcurrent to TENS-like amplitudes.

Faradic

Functional electrical stimulation (FES) provides tetanic contractions of denervated muscles. Used for impaired movement, muscle strengthening.

Uses low frequency 30–100 Hz, 0.1–1 mS, biphasic currents applied to motor points.

Indications	Contraindications
Brachial plexus injury	Areas of diminished sensation
Difficulty in voluntary movement (post-stroke or head trauma)	Beyond the flexibility of implanted prosthesis
Facilitation of voluntary motor function	Metastatic carcinoma Over metallic implants
Guillian-Barré syndrome	Over open wounds
Maintaining or increasing range of motion	Over or through heart Pacemakers
Muscle spasticity	Pregnancy
Muscle strengthening	Transcranially
Orthotic training	
Rehabilitation of muscles (post-orthopedic surgery, spinal injuries)	

Galvanic

Neuralgia, circulation disorders, myalgia (denervated muscle), alleviates pain, promotes healing. Used for forcing chemicals through the skin via iontophoresis.

Negative electrode (cathode) is generally thought to promote healing; however, recent evidence indicates that the driving electric force of the degrading, energy-liberating, catabolic process of injury fluctuates from anodic into cathodic phases, attenuating toward a state of equilibrium ("healing") as is the case with all spontaneous reactions (Nordenström, 1983). Biphasic devices are safer and may actually be better for promoting healing.

Galvanic currents are continuous direct currents of < 0.33 mA/cm^2.

Primary Effects of Direct Currents

Type of Effect	Anode (+)	Cathode (–)
Physiochemical	Attracts acids	Attracts alkaloids
	Repels alkaloids	Repels acids
	Attracts oxygen	Attracts hydrogen
	Corrodes metals by oxidation	Does not corrode metals
Physiological	Hardens scar tissue	Softens tissues
	Decreases nerve irritability	Increases nerve irritability
	Dehydrates tissue	Congests tissues
	Produces vasoconstriction	Produces vasodilation
	Retards bleeding	Enhances bleeding
	Produces ischemia	Produces hyperemia
	Tends to be analgesic	Tends to increase pain at low intensities
		Germicidal effects

Indications	Contraindications
Acute trauma	Carotid sinus area
Adhesions	Impaired cutaneous sensation
Arthritis	Near the heart
Intervetebral disc syndromes	Over any metallic implant (e.g., joints, pins, or IUD)
Joint pain	Over scars and adhesions
Neuritis	Pacemakers
Myalgia	Pregnancy
Sciatica	Transcranially
Sprains and strains	Treatment on a metallic table

High Voltage Pulsed Galvanic

Vasodilation, healing of superficial wounds, reduction of edema, pain management, muscle stimulation.

Uses low frequency 2–200 Hz typical (< 1 kHz), < 500 V, 1.2–1.5 mA, 1–600 mS.

Indications	Contraindications
Adhesions	Areas of diminished sensation
Circulatory stasis	Metallic implants
Edema	Metastatic carcinoma
Muscle spasm	Over or through heart
Muscular atrophy	Over open wounds
Pain	Pacemakers
Passive exercise	Pregnancy
Restricted joint movement	Transcranially
Trigger points	

Interferential

Pain due to traumatic injuries, post-operative pain, joint conditions, myalgia and tendinitis, bursitis, edema, hematoma. Nerve blocks via Wedensky Inhibition occur when the frequency of the stimulation is faster than the frequency of the action potential (due to its shorter wavelength), because the nerve cannot recover. With continued stimulation, the nerve becomes partially insensitive. The maximum frequency of an action potential lasting 10 mS is 100 Hz.

Generally uses medium frequency combination of 4000 and 4100 Hz = 100 Hz, at 4–15 mA.

Indications		Contraindications
Anterior tibial syndrome	Myositis	Abscess
Bursitis	Neuralgia	Anxiety
Bronchial asthma	Neuroma	Carotid sinus area
Capsulitis	Osteoarthritis	Circulation block
Causalgia	Pain	Heart area
Cholecyctitis (chronic)	Periarthritis	Hyperpyrexia
Effusions	Phantom limb pain	Menstruation
Epicondylitis	Post-traumatic edema	Metastatic carcinoma
Facial palsy	Prostatitis	Pacemakers
Fibrositis	Psoas syndrome	Pregnancy
Frozen shoulder	Rheumatic disorders	Thrombophlebitis
Hematoma calcification	Sciatica	Transcranially
Hemiplegia	Shoulder–arm syndrome	Tuberculosis
Herpes zoster	Spasm	Varicosities
Incontinence	Spondylitis	
Intermittent claudication	Sprains and strains	
Intervertebral disc syndrome	Spurs	
	Stiffness	
Ischialgia	Sudeck's atrophy	
Joint deformity	Synovitis	
Low back pain	Thoracodynia	
Lymphedema	Trigger points	
Myalgia	Vasospasm	

Laser ("Cold Laser")

Nanosecond pulse widths, usually 500–5000 Hz, 15–25 W (< 25 mW actual). *Avoid eyes.*

Indications	Contraindications
Bursitis	Near eyes
Degenerative joints	Over thyroid gland
Diseases of the oral cavity (stomatitis, post-extraction problems, ulcers, herpes labialis)	Over pacemakers
	Pregnancy
	Tumors
Post-operative or -traumatic musculoskeletal complaints	
Scars	
Ulcers (decubitus and herpetic)	

Microcurrent Electrical Therapy (MET)

Acute, chronic, and post-operative pain, initiating and accelerating healing.

Often references Arndt's Law: Weak stimuli excite physiological activity, moderate stimuli favor it, strong stimuli retard it, and very strong stimuli arrest physiological activity. At 500 µA adenosine triphosphate (ATP) increases by 500%, but drops below baseline above 5 mA (Chang, Van Hoff, Bockx, et al., 1982). At 100–500 mA, amino acid transport rises 30 to 40% above controls.

Uses low-frequency biphasic currents of < 2 S, 0.3–100 Hz, < 1 mA.

Indications

Systemic Pain	Head and Neck Pain	Abdominal Pain
Arthritis	Cervicogenic	Bladder pain
Bursitis	headache	Bowel stasis
Cancer	Cluster headache	Diverticulosis
Causalgia	Dental disorders	Dysmenorrhea
Cholecyctitis	(periodontal and	Labor
(chronic)	orthodontic pain)	Post-operative pain
Decubital ulcers	Facial palsy	Prostatitis
Effusions	Migraine	
Fibrositis	Sinusitis	
Hematoma	Sprains and strains	
calcification	Subocciptal	
Hemiplegia	headaches	
Herpes zoster	Tinnitus	
Ischialgia	Temporomandibular	
Lymphedema	joint disorder	
Multiple sclerosis	Tension headache	
Myalgia	Torticollis	
Myositis	Trigeminal	
Neuralgia	neuralgia	
Neuroma	Whiplash	
Osteoarthritis		
Pain (systemic and		
idiopathic)		
Phantom limb		
syndrome		
Post-traumatic		
edema		
Raynaud's disease		
Rheumatoid		
arthritis		
Scars		
Synovitis		
Trigger points		

Back Pain	Lower Extremity Pain	Upper Extremity Pain
Coccydynia	Ankle pain	Carpal tunnel
Failed back surgery	Anterior tibial	syndrome
Intercostal neuralgia	syndrome	Epicondylitis
Intervetebral disc	Foot pain	Frozen shoulder
syndrome	Fractures	Hand pain
Low back pain	Joint mobilization	Peripheral nerve
Lumbrosacral pain	Knee pain	injury
Radiculitis	Passive stretch pain	Shoulder–arm
Spasm	Sciatica	syndrome
Sprains and strains	Sprains and strains	Sprains and strains
Thoracodynia	Spurs	Subdeltoid bursitis
Whole back pain	Tendonitis	Wrist pain
	Thrombophlebitis	

Contraindications

Carotid sinus area	Demand type	Pregnancy
	pacemakers	

Russian Stimulation

Muscle stimulation primarily for post-operative rehabilitation.

Uses medium frequency 2500–4000 Hz, 50 Hz, 0.2–0.4 mS

Shortwave Therapy (Diathermy)

Increases elasticity in connective tissue (particularly skin), muscles, ligaments, and joint capsules. Generally used for vasodilation, wound healing (use only after 2 to 4 days), arthritis, bursitis, sinusitis, tendonitis, contusion, rupture, fracture, hematoma, herpes zoster, neuropathy, deep muscle pain and spasm.

Diathermy creates heat but does not depolarize nerves. *Remove all metals to a distance of at least 1 m. Contraindicated if there is any implanted metal. Patients should be dressed in a gown with a towel under the electrodes.*

Uses high-frequency >300 kHz, short wavelengths 3–30 m. Typically, 27.12 MHz, 65–400 mS, 32 W average (< 200 W).

Indications	Absolute Contraindications	Relative Contraindications
Amenorrhea	Fractures (recent)	Areas of decreased
Brachial plexus	Hearing aids	vascularity
neuritis	Hemoptysis,	Arteriosclerosis
Bronchiectasis	epitaxis, melena,	(advanced)
Bronchitis	and other	Hypothermesthesia
Bursitis (subacute	hemorrhagic	Infants and
and chronic)	tendencies	debilitated elderly
Colic	Malignancy	Intrauterine device
Contusions	Menstruation	(metallic)
Dislocations	Metallic dental	Metallic buttons,
Diverticulitis	appliances and	zippers, hairpins,
Dysmenorrhea	fillings	buckles, clasps,
Epicondylitis	Metallic implants	keys, knives, etc.
Fibrositis	On a metal table	Nondraining
Fibrous	Over adhesive	cellulitis
fixation/ankylosis	strapping	Osteomyelitis

Furuncle/carbuncle
Hypertonia
Intercostal neuralgia
Ischialgia (chronic)
Intervetebral disc
  syndrome
Low back pain
Mastitis
Myalgia
Myositis
Neuritis
Osteoarthritis
Pelvic inflammatory
  disease (subacute,
  chronic)
Pleurisy
Prostatitis
Pyelitis (subacute,
  chronic)
Rheumatoid
  arthritis (subacute,
  chronic)
Sprains and strains
Tenosynovitis

Over casts
Over moist
  dressings
Pacemakers
Peptic ulcers
Pregnancy
Pyretic states
Rheumatoid
  arthritis (acute)
Septic arthritis
  (acute)
Tuberculosis
  (pulmonary or
  joint)

Osteoporosis
  (advanced)
Over growing
  epiphyseal plate
Patients on
  anticoagulants,
  cortisone, gold
  therapy
Peripheral vascular
  disease (occlusive)
Poliomyelitis (acute
  stage)
Polyneuritis with
  impaired
  circulation
Suppurating
  inflammatory
  process
Thrombosis
Transcranially
Varicose veins

Transcutaneous Electrical Nerve Stimulation (TENS)

Acute, chronic, and post-operative pain.

Uses low-frequency biphasic currents of 75–400 mS, 50–150 Hz, < 100 mA.

Indications

Systemic Pain	Abdominal Pain	Back Pain
Bursitis	Bladder pain	Coccydynia
Cancer	Bowel stasis	Intercostal neuralgia
Causalgia	Diverticulosis	Intervertebral disc
Ischialgia	Dysmenorrhea	syndrome
Neuralgia	Labor	Low back pain
Osteoarthritis	Post-operative pain	Lumbrosacral pain
Passive stretch pain		Radiculitis
Rheumatoid arthritis		Sprains and strains
Synovitis		Thoracodynia
		Whole back pain

Lower Extremity Pain	Upper Extremity Pain	Contraindications
Ankle pain	Carpal tunnel	Metallic implants
Foot pain	syndrome	Metastatic
Fractures	Epicondylitis	carcinoma
Joint mobilization	Frozen shoulder	Near carotid sinus
Knee pain	Hand pain	area
Sciatica	Peripheral nerve	Over or through
Sprains and strains	injury	heart
Tendonitis	Sprains and strains	Pacemakers
Thrombophlebitis	Subdeltoid bursitis	Pregnancy
	Wrist pain	Transcranially

Ultrasound

Promotes blood circulation; improves metabolism, muscle relaxation, pain control; increases elasticity of connective tissues. Used to treat tendon adhesions and scars, post-traumatic injuries, binding tissue contractions (scars), Dupuytren's Contracture, bursitis, capsulitis, tendonitis, and chronic open wounds. Micromassage, microdestruction, and heat generation.

May cause mechanical or thermal tissue damage. Overdose may decrease blood sugar levels, cause fatigue, nervousness, irritability, constipation, and a tendency to catch cold. Do not use over pregnant uterus, heart, testicles, spine, areas of thrombophlebitis, infections.

High frequency mechanical vibrations using piezo-electricity > 20 kHz (typically between 0.8 and 3 Mhz) and 0.1–3 W/cm^2.

Indications		Contraindications
Bursitis (subacute, chronic)	Sprains and strains (subacute, chronic)	Acute infection
Calcific bursitis	Sudeck's atrophy	Areas of thermohypersthesia
Causalgia	Tendonitis	Near hearing aid
Decubital ulcers	(subacute, chronic)	Near malignant
Fibrositis (subacute, chronic)	Trigger points	lesions
Fibrotic	Varicose ulcers (chronic)	Near metallic
polymylosis		implants
Herpes zoster		Near pacemakers
Joint contractures		Occlusive vascular
Myalgia		disease
Neuralgia		Over bony
Osteoarthritis		prominences
Painful neuroma		Over epiphyseal
Periarthritis (nonseptic)		plates of growing children
Radiculitis (subacute, chronic)		Over nerve plexuses
Raynaud's disease		Over suspected embolus
Rheumatoid arthritis (subacute, chronic)		Over the eye
		Over the heart
Scars		Over a pregnant uterus
Shoulder–hand syndrome		Over the reproductive organs
Spondylitis		Over spinal cord after laminectomy
		Radiculitis (acute)
		Tendency to hemorrhage
		Transcranially

SUMMARY

One must stray from the routine procedures of today in order to create the advances of tomorrow. There is still a lot to learn about bioelectricity and electromedicine. In order to do so, we must first acknowledge that there is another side of physiology. Everyone concerned about health should demand widespread access to conservative, safe, alternative care. To lessen human suffering is a notable goal. That we have not been able to achieve enough of this to date without causing undo harm is a good indication that the answers must lie elsewhere. Biophysics must be better understood to realize the actual basis for the control of the regulatory processes of life.

Even at its present state of evolution, electromedicine offers an unprecedented conservative, cost-effective, fast, safe, and powerful tool in the management of the pain patient. As such, it should be the first priority on the list of treatment options.

REFERENCES

Bauer, W. (1983). Neuroelectric medicine. *Journal of Bioelectricity, 2,* 2–3. 159.

Becker, R.O. (1981). *Mechanisms of growth control.* Springfield, IL: Charles C Thomas Co.

Becker, R.O. (1982). Electrical control systems and regenerative growth. *Journal of Bioelectricity, 1*(2), 239–264.

Becker, R.O. (1983). The role of the orthopaedic surgeon in the development of bioconductivity. *Journal of Bioelectricity, 2*(1), 77–81.

Becker, R.O. (1990). *Cross Currents: The perils of electropollution, the promise of electromedicine.* Los Angeles, CA: Jeremy P. Tarcher, Inc.

Becker, R.O., & Marino, A.A. (1982). Electromagnetism and life. Albany: State University of New York Press.

Belehradek, J., Orlowski, S., Poddevin, B., et al. (1981). Electrotherapy of spontaneous mammary tumors in mice. *European Journal of Cancer, 27,* 73–76.

Benton, L.A., Baker, L.L., Bowman, B.R., & Waters, R.L. (1981). *Functional Electrical Stimulation: A Practical Clinical Guide* (2nd ed.). Downey, CA: Rancho Los Amigos Hospital.

Chang, N., Van Hoff, H., & Bockx, E., et al. (1982). The effect of electric currents on ATP generation, protein synthesis, and membrane transport in rat skin. *Clinical Orthopedics, 171,* 264–272.

Jaskoviak, P.A., & Schafer, R.C. (1993). *Applied physiotherapy* (2nd ed.). Arlington, VA: The American Chiropractic Association.

Kirsch, D.L. (1978). *The complete clinical guide to electroacutherapy* (2nd ed.). Glendale, CA: National Electro-Acutherapy Foundation.

Kirsch, D.L. (1999). *The science behind cranial electrotherapy stimulation.* Edmonton, Alberta, Canada: Medical Scope Publishing.

Kitchen, S., & Bazin, S. (1996). *Clayton's electrotherapy* (10th ed.). London: W.B. Saunders Company, Ltd.

Low, J., & Reed, A. (1994). *Electrotherapy explained: principles and practice* (2nd ed.). Oxford: Butterworth Heinemann.

Lyte, M., et al. (1991). Effects of *in vitro* electrical stimulation on enhancement and suppression of malignant lymphoma proliferation. *Journal National Cancer Institute, 83,* 116–119.

Morris, D.M., et al. (1992). Electrochemical modification of tumor growth in mice. *Journal of Surgical Research 53,* 306–309.

Nelson, R.M., & Currier, D.P. (1991). *Clinical electrotherapy* (2nd ed.). Norwalk, CT: Appleton & Lange.

Nordenström, B.E.W. (1983). *Biologically closed electric circuits: Clinical, experimental and theoretical evidence for an additional circulatory system.* Stockholm: Nordic Medical Publications.

Nordenström, B.E.W. (1984). Biologically closed electrical circuits: Activation of vascular interstitial closed electric circuits for treatment of inoperable cancers. *Journal of Bioelectricity, 3,* 137–153.

Nordenström, B.E.W. (1989). Electrochemical treatment of cancer. Variable response to anodic and cathodic fields. *American Journal of Clinical Oncology* (CCT), *12,* 530–36.

Nordenström, B.E.W. (1998). *Exploring biologically closed electric circuits.* Stockholm, Sweden: Nordic Medical Publications.

Pallares, D.S. (1998). *Lo que he descubierto en el tejido canceroso.* Col. Pedregal de San Nicolás, Tlalpan, Mexico (in Spanish), 1–275.

Palmer, D.D. (1910). *The science, art and philosophy of chiropractic: The chiropractor's adjuster.* Portland, OR: Portland Printing House.

Segel, I.H. (1975) *Biochemical calculations,* (2nd ed.). New York: Wiley, 414–415.

Sersa, G., et al. (1992). Anti-tumor effect of electrotherapy alone or in combination with interleukin-2 in mice with sarcoma and melanoma tumors. *Anti-Cancer Drugs, 3,* 253–260.

Smith, S.D. (1981). Biological control of growth – A retrospective look. In Becker, R.O. (Ed.), *Mechanisms of growth control.* Springfield, IL: Charles C Thomas.

Tapio, D. & Hymes, A.C. (1987). *New frontiers in transcutaneous electrical nerve stimulation.* Minnetonka, MN: LecTec Corp.

Thuile, C., & Kirsch, D.L. (2000). *Schmerzen Linden ohne Chemie: CES, die Revolution in der Schmerztherapie.* IGEM, Austria (in German).

Walker, M.J. (1993). *Dirty medicine: Science, big business, and the assault on natural health care.* London: Slingshot Publications.

61

A Practical Protocol for Electromedical Treatment of Pain

Daniel L. Kirsch, Ph.D., D.A.A.P.M.

If there were pharmaceutical products that could control people's physical pains more than 90% of the time and were safe enough to use as often as necessary without causing any significant side effects, physicians would prescribe them often. If those drugs could also calm people who were seriously clinically anxious or depressed, while being safe enough for people who are only a bit stressed, they would be the most widely prescribed drugs on Earth. If those same drugs could also heal broken bones and close wounds, the pharmacies could not possibly stock enough of them.

What if there is something that could do all these things and so much more, but is not a drug? What if there is a treatment that is so safe it could be used daily to control pain and stress-related diseases. What if it is also so inexpensive that once purchased for a fraction of the cost of conventional care, it will cost almost nothing to use? There is. New forms of electromedicine offer all this and more.

Change has always fought its way into the healthcare system slowly. A mere 100 years ago it would have been considered quackery to propose that invisible little germs could cause disease. Even after the discovery of bacteria, for 35 more years most doctors refused to believe that washing their hands before surgery would make much of a difference. Yet progress in medicine occurred as we developed tools to look deeper into the body, and to see smaller particles. We even speak of subatomic particles, such as electrons, which could both cause disease in the form of free radicals and cure known diseases as well as functional disturbances of the body and mind. We have

learned to appreciate the power of physics in our lives with convenient technologies such as microwave ovens and cellular telephones. Today, our daily lives are increasingly more influenced by electronics than chemistry.

As we begin this new millennium, we rely on various forms of technology to diagnose our patients, both locally through an ever-increasing armamentarium of devices, and even over long distance with telemedicine. But we also can treat our patients with new technologies for a variety of disorders with remarkable and unprecedented safety and efficacy.

Most systems of healthcare have historically been based on biophysics. Acupuncture is an obvious example. Chinese call the electrical properties of life *Chi* energy, Japanese call it *Ki*, Indians call it *Prana*, and chiropractors call it "innate intelligence." Even homeopathy is based on the energetic residual of the chemical after it has been so diluted that chemists question its continued existence. Western allopathic medicine stands alone in reliance on synthetic chemical treatments and invasive procedures, many of which impose a risk worse than the disease for which it is offered. In fact, conventional medical care is the third leading cause of death in the United States with at least 225,000 people dying annually from iatrogenic conditions (Starfield, 2000).

Change takes time in medicine as in any established system. There are strong controlling economic influences and long-standing institutions that will always argue for the status quo. Yet people are more educated and informed about healthcare than ever before. With that comes concern over side effects of dangerous treatments. Why do

0-8493-0926-3/02/$0.00+$1.50
© 2002 by CRC Press LLC

we not try the most inexpensive and conservative treatments first, instead of last? When that treatment is based on sound electromagnetic principles, most physicians are surprised to discover that, while not a drug, the results are often more immediate and spectacular than one can imagine. Also, unlike drugs, the results are usually long lasting and cumulative.

While electromedicine has been practiced in some form for thousands of years, research and clinical usage in electromedicine are expanding as never before in history. Perhaps even more than any other therapeutic option, electromedicine is now used routinely by a growing number of practitioners from all of the healthcare professions, as well as by patients themselves at home. Only the United States Food and Drug Administration (FDA) restricts the sale of electromedical devices for use by or on the order of licensed healthcare practitioners. All other countries allow people to purchase therapeutic electromedical devices over the counter for their own personal use. Electromedical modalities are easy to use, relatively safe, and the newer technologies, such as microcurrent electrical therapy and cranial electrotherapy stimulation, have proven efficacy unprecedented by any prior form of medical intervention.

One word of caution, though: Medicine is still a science. Modern electromagnetic therapies have attracted many charlatans. Simply said, not everything is equally safe and effective. Rely only on evidence-based technologies.

MICROCURRENT ELECTRICAL THERAPY

Joseph M. Mercola and Daniel L. Kirsch (1995) coined the term "microcurrent electrical therapy" (MET) to define a new form of electromedical intervention using biocompatible waveforms.

Patrick DeBock (2000), a physiotherapist at the University of Antwerp in Belgium, recently compared MET with TENS based on the Eight Parameter Law which covers every possible influence in electrotherapy. In his conclusion, DeBock states, "MET has a completely different mechanism, which at this time is not fully understood, but works on a cellular level ... It looks as if TENS is going to lose this competition ... MET will, in most cases, be much more satisfying than TENS because of the longer lasting and more intense effects."

A growing body of research shows the effectiveness of MET to do more than control pain. It can actually accelerate and even induce healing. When a wound is dry, its bioelectric current flow is shut off. Eaglstein and Mertz (1978) have shown moist wounds to resurface up to 40% faster than air-exposed wounds. Falanga (1988) found that certain types of occlusive dressings, like Duoderm, accelerate the healing of wounds. It is probable that these dressings achieve their effects by promoting a

moist environment (Kulig, Jarski, Drewek, et al., 1991). The moisture may allow endogenously produced current to flow more readily through the injury, and thus promote wound healing. Electrical stimulation of the wound has a similar effect, and also tends to increase the amount of growth factor receptors, which increases the amount of collagen formation (Falanga, et al., 1987).

Electricity was first used to treat surface wounds over 300 years ago when charged gold leaf was found to prevent smallpox scars (Robinson, 1925). There are several recent studies supporting the beneficial effects of treating wounds with an artificial current (Goldin, et al., 1981; Ieran, et al., 1990; Jeran, et al., 1987; Mulder, 1991). Experimental animal wound models in the 1960s demonstrated that electrical intervention results in accelerated healing with skin wounds resurfacing faster, and with stronger scar tissue formation (Assimacopoulos, 1968; Carey & Lepley, 1962).

Assimacopoulos (1968a) published the first human study using direct current for wound healing. He documented complete healing in three patients with chronic leg ulcers due to venous stasis after six weeks of electrical therapy. One year later Wolcott, Wheeler, and Hardwicke (1969) published the most frequently cited work in the history of electrical wound healing. They used direct currents of 200 to 1000 μA on 67 patients. Gault and Gatesn (1976) repeated the Wolcott and Wheeler protocol on 76 additional patients with 106 ischemic skin ulcers. Rowley, McKenna, Chase, and Wolcott (1974) studied a group of patients having 250 ischemic ulcers of various types. These included 14 symmetrical control ulcers. The electrically stimulated ulcers had a fourfold acceleration in healing response compared to the controls. Carley and Wainapel (1985) performed one of the only studies on this subject with equal and randomized active and control groups. All of these studies documented significant accelerated healing from electrical stimulation.

One additional consistent observation in these studies was a reversal of contamination in the wounds. Wounds that were initially contaminated with *Pseudomonas* and/or *Proteus* were usually sterile after several days of MET. Other investigators also have noticed similar improvements and encourage the use of this therapy as the preferred treatment for indolent ulcers (Alvarez et al., 1983; Barron & Jacobson, 1985; Kaada, Flatheim, & Woie, 1991; Lundeberg, Eriksson, & Malm, 1992). Additionally, no significant adverse effects resulting from electrotherapy on wounds have been documented (Weiss, et al., 1990). A review of the literature by Dayton and Palladino (1989) shows that MET is clearly an effective and safe supplement to the nonsurgical management of recalcitrant leg ulcers.

Some of these studies used unipolar currents that were alternated between negative and positive based on various criteria. Some researchers initially used negative current to inhibit bacterial growth and then switched to positive current to promote healing. To date no study has compared this variable of MET. However, there is some compelling basic science research, and one animal study, suggesting that a biphasic waveform, which provides both negative and positive current, may be better in that it both sterilizes the wound and promotes wound healing (Stromberg, 1988; Windsor, Lester, & Herring, 1993).

In the 1960s Robert O. Becker (1985) demonstrated that electrical current is the trigger that stimulates healing, growth, and regeneration in all living organisms. He found that repair of injury occurs in response to signals that come from an electrical control system, and suggested that this system became less efficient as we age.

Becker developed his theory of biological control systems based on concepts derived from physics, electronics, and biology. He postulated that the first living organisms must have been capable of self-repair, otherwise they never would have survived. The repair process requires a closed-loop system. A specific signal is generated, called the current of injury, which causes another signal to start repair. The injury signal gradually decreases over time with the repair process, until it finally stops when the repair is complete. Such a primitive system does not require demonstrable consciousness or intelligence. In fact, many animals actually have a greater capacity for healing than humans.

Science has amassed a vast amount of information on how the brain and nervous system work. Most of this research involves the action potential as the sole mechanism of the nerve impulse. This is a very sophisticated and complex system for the transfer of information. It is helpful to compare this conceptualized concept of the nervous system to a computer.

The fundamental signal in both the computer and the nervous system is a digital one. Both systems transfer information represented by the number of pulses per unit of time. Information also is coded according to where the pulses originate, where they go, and whether or not there is more than one channel of pulses feeding into an area. All our senses (e.g., smell, taste, hearing, sight, and touch) are based on this type of pulse system. Like a computer, the nervous system operates remarkably fast and can transfer large amounts of information as digital on-and-off data.

It is unlikely that the first living organisms had such a sophisticated system. Becker believes they must have had a much simpler mechanism for communicating information because they did not need to transmit large amounts of sophisticated data. Accordingly, they probably used an *analog* system. An analog system works by means of simple DC currents. Information in an analog system is represented by the strength of the current, its direction of flow, and slow wavelength variations in its strength. This is a much slower system than the digital model. However, the analog system is extremely precise and works well for its intended purpose.

Becker theorizes that primitive organisms used this analog type of data transmission and control system for repair. He postulates that we still have this primitive nervous system in the perineural cells of the central nervous system. These cells comprise 90% of the nervous system. The perineural cells have semiconductor properties that allow them to produce and transmit nonpropagating DC signals. This system functions so vastly differently from the "all or none" law of propagation of the nerve action potentials that Becker called this the fourth nervous system.

This analog system senses injury and controls repair. It controls the activity of cells by producing specific DC electrical environments in their vicinity. It also appears to be the primary primitive system in the brain, controlling the actions of the neurons in their generation and receipt of nerve impulses. Accordingly, as knowledge of this aspect of our nervous system is uncovered, another mystery of brain physiology may be explained, including the regulation of our consciousness and decision-making processes. Given this understanding, the application of the correct form of electrical intervention is a powerful tool for treating pain, initiating the endogenous mechanisms for healing, and altering states of consciousness.

Chang, Van Hoff, Bockx, et al. (1982) proposed another mechanism for MET. Their research showed that microcurrent stimulation increased adenosine triphosphate (ATP) generation by almost 500%. Increasing the level of current to milliampere levels actually decreased the results. Microcurrent also was shown to enhance amino acid transport and protein synthesis in the treated area 30 to 40% above controls.

It would be helpful to review the cellular nature of an injury to fully appreciate the importance of Chang's research. Becker (1985) has shown that trauma will affect the electrical potential of cells in damaged tissues. Initially the injured site has a much higher resistance than that of the surrounding tissue. Basic physics dictates that electricity tends to flow toward the path of least resistance. Therefore, endogenous bioelectricity avoids areas of high resistance and takes the easiest path, generally around the injury. The decreased electrical flow through the injured area decreases the cellular capacitance (Windsor, et al., 1993). As a result, healing is actually impaired. This may be one of the reasons for inflammatory reactions. Pain, heat, swelling, and redness are the characteristics of inflamed tissues. Electricity flows more readily through these hot inflammatory fluids.

The correct microcurrent application to an injured site augments the endogenous current flow. This allows the traumatized area to regain its capacitance. The resistance of the injured tissue is then reduced, allowing bioelectricity to enter the area to reestablish homeostasis. Therefore, microcurrent electrical therapy can be viewed as a catalyst helpful in initiating and sustaining the numerous chemical and electrical reactions that occur in the healing process.

When a muscle experiences trauma it goes into spasm to protect itself. This decreases its blood supply, reducing the amount of oxygen and nutrients that reach it. The decreased circulation causes an accumulation of metabolic waste products. This acts as noxious input resulting in pain.

Adenosine triphosphate is an essential factor in the healing process. Large amounts of ATP, the cell's main energy source, are required to control primary functions such as the movement of vital minerals, like sodium, potassium, magnesium, and calcium, into and out of the cell. It also sustains the movement of waste products out of the cell. Injured tissues are deficient in ATP.

As MET restores circulation and replenishes ATP, nutrients can again flow into injured cells and waste products can flow out. This is necessary for the development of healthy tissues. As ATP provides the energy tissues require for building new proteins, it also increases protein synthesis and membrane transport of ions.

SURVEY RESULTS

Two surveys were recently conducted on a total of 3000 people using Alpha-Stim™ technology employing the combined treatment protocols of MET and CES as presented here.

Healthcare practitioners completed a post-marketing survey of 500 patients in 1998 (Kirsch, 1999). There were 174 males, and 326 females, ranging from 5 to 92 years old. Outpatients accounted for 479 of the forms, while 21 were hospitalized at the time of treatment. Treatment was satisfactorily completed by 197 (41%) of the patients with 207 (43%) still receiving treatment at the time of the survey.

Ten patients discontinued treatment because they thought it was not helping them, and three more discontinued due to undesirable side effects. An additional 13 terminated treatment when their insurance ran out and they could no longer pay for treatment; 20 patients moved out of the area while treatment was in progress or discontinued treatment for other, unstated reasons.

Negative adverse effects were all rare, mild, and self-limiting, with 472 (94.4%) reporting none. Six (1.2%) reported vertigo as a side effect and 2 (0.4%) reported nausea, either of which normally occurs when the current is set too high or in patients with a history of vertigo. Only 3 (0.6%) reported skin irritation, and 1 (0.2%) each reported anger, a metallic taste, a heavy feeling, or intensified tinnitus. These generally receded or disappeared as soon as the current was reduced.

The most important aspect of this survey was the results reported as a degree of improvement in the seven symptoms present in most patients for which MET and/or CES is prescribed; i.e., pain, anxiety, depression, stress, insomnia, headache, and muscle tension. The treatment outcome was broken down into response categories beginning with [it made the condition] "Worse," and progressing up to "Complete" improvement or cure. As in pharmaceutical studies, a degree of improvement of 25% or more was considered to be clinically significant. The data for all 500 patients reporting on multiple symptoms are summarized in Table 61.1.

In addition, 2500 patients were surveyed through a form attached to warranty cards (Smith, 2001); 1411 (72.40%) of the patients were female; ages ranged from 15 to 92 years old with a mean of 50.07 years. The length of use ranged from the minimum of 3 weeks which was

TABLE 61.1
Results of Using Alpha-Stim™ Technology for MET and CES as Reported by Healthcare Practitioners

Condition	N	Worse	No Change	Slight < 24%	Fair 25–49%	Moderate 50–74%	Marked 75–99%	Complete 100%	Significant > 25%
Pain	286	1 0.35%	5 1.75%	20 6.99%	48 16.78%	77 26.92%	108 37.76%	27 9.44%	260 90.91%
Anxiety	349	0 0.00%	8 2.29%	14 4.01%	39 11.17%	89 25.50%	181 51.86%	18 5.16%	327 93.70%
Depression	184	0 0.00%	8 4.35%	11 5.98%	31 16.85%	38 20.65%	82 44.57%	14 7.61%	165 89.67%
Stress	259	0 0.00%	6 2.32%	12 4.63%	37 14.29%	70 27.03%	124 47.88%	10 3.86%	241 93.05%
Insomnia	135	0 0.00%	16 11.85%	12 8.89%	17 12.59%	34 25.19%	45 33.33%	11 8.15%	107 79.26%
Headache	151	1 0.66%	8 5.30%	6 3.97%	25 16.56%	32 21.19%	63 41.72%	16 10.60%	136 90.07%
Muscle tension	259	2 0.77%	6 2.32%	6 2.32%	42 16.22%	76 29.34%	111 42.86%	16 6.18%	245 94.59%

Note: Total N = 500 patients with multiple symptoms.

the only inclusion criterion, to a maximum of 5 years in two cases. The average period of use reported was 14.68 weeks or approximately 3.5 months. Of 1949 primary pain patients, 1813, or 93.02% rated their improvement as significant, and these findings correlate well with the physicians' survey of 500 patients where 90.91% of 286 pain patients were observed to have significant improvement. The data for all 2500 patients reporting on multiple symptoms are summarized in Table 61.2.

BASIC TREATMENT PROTOCOL FOR MICROCURRENT ELECTRICAL THERAPY (MET)

The following section is intended as a practical guide for clinicians to utilize the principles discussed in this chapter. The methods of treatment provided herein have been developed by the author based on 3 decades of experience in electromedicine. The reader is cautioned to remember that not all brands of microcurrent devices are equally efficacious. Always check the manufacturer's specific instructions before using a medical device. As medicine is not an exact science, the author cannot assume responsibility for the clinical efficacy of, or liability for, the methods and treatments found in this text.

STEP ONE: HISTORY AND BRIEF EXAM

It is important to take a comprehensive history and do a brief analysis of the patient's current condition before beginning each session of MET treatment. A diagnosis is not enough. One should determine when the pain first presented, its frequency, duration, intensity, limitations-of-motion, positions which exacerbate the pain, and any precipitating factors. Ask about the specifics of previous treatments and details of *all* surgical scars and traumatic injuries. Microcurrent electrical therapy is a very holistic procedure. It may be necessary to clear the body of any and all electrical "blocks" in order to achieve the best results. Even brief 10- to 20-second treatments of other problems and/or old injuries may reverse a refractory case.

Immediately before each treatment determine the patient's *present* pain level, and positions that exacerbate the pain. Ask the patient to rate his or her present pain on a scale of 0 (no pain) to 10, with 10 being excruciating, debilitating pain. Tell the patient to consider 10 as "the worst *this condition* has been." Also note any immediate limitations-of-motion, positive orthopedic and neurologic test findings, and objective signs of psychological distress. Because the results of MET can be seen after only a minute or so of treatment in most people, these indicators are necessary reference parameters to determine effectiveness throughout a single treatment session.

ADJUST THE SETTINGS

Use 0.5 Hz frequency most of the time. It is unusual ever to need other frequency settings. However, if 0.5 Hz does not work, and a number of electrode placements sites have been attempted, try 1.5 Hz; 100 Hz sometimes produces faster results when treating inflammatory articular problems (e.g., arthritis, bursitis, tendonitis, etc.). However, 100 Hz does not contribute much to long-term results so treatment should always be completed using a low frequency. Set the current intensity level at the highest comfortable position, which is usually 500 to 600 µA for probes, although sometimes less for the silver electrodes used with MET. Do not use standard TENS electrodes except in the initial treatment of hypersensitive patients. Carbon TENS electrodes have a resistance of about 200 ohms, while silver electrodes have a resistance of about 20 ohms. Only silver electrodes will work effectively with MET devices.

When using probes, first affix new felt electrodes and saturate them with an appropriate electromedical conducting solution. Then apply firm pressure, but less than what would cause more pain. Tap water does not work well in some places anymore because of recent advances in desalination during water processing. Saline solution may be used if a conducting solution is not available.

For extremely hypersensitive people, such as fibromyalgia patients, it is better to start with a minimal amount of current. Even low-level MET currents may be uncomfortable in some patients. For these patients it may be necessary to initially reduce the conductivity by using more resistive electrodes. Over the course of a few weeks, the therapeutic dosage of electricity can gradually be increased. Start with standard carbon electrodes, followed by silver electrodes, then probes with tap water, until the area is desensitized enough to use probes with conducting solution. Fortunately, this is rarely necessary. Most people will not even feel MET stimulation at a current of 600 µA.

BASIC TREATMENT STRATEGY

There are only a few principles one must remember when treating patients with MET. The patient should be in a relaxed position to receive maximum beneficial effects. For example, do not let patients help with the treatment of their hands by holding up their arms, which would cause the arm muscles to tense. In this case, it is better to place both hands on a table.

The most important variable is the position of the probes, or silver electrode pads. Place the probes, or pads, in such a way that if a line were drawn between them, the line would travel through the problem area. Keep in mind that the body is three-dimensional. Therefore, many possible lines can be drawn through the problem area. Some lines will work much better than others. *The correct electrode location is the one that works!* However, the one

TABLE 61.2
Results of Using Alpha-Stim™ Technology for MET and CES for at Least 3 Weeks as Reported by Patients

Condition	N	Slight < 24%	Fair 25–49%	Moderate 50–74%	Marked 75–100%	Significant > 25%
Pain (all cases)	1949	136 6.98%	623 31.97%	741 38.02%	449 23.04%	1813 93.02%
Back pain	403	20 4.96%	109 27.05%	157 38.96%	117 29.03%	383 95.04%
Cervical pain	265	18 6.79%	69 26.04%	125 47.17%	53 20.00%	247 93.21%
Hip/leg/foot pain	160	6 3.75%	43 26.88%	53 33.13%	58 36.25%	154 96.25%
Shoulder/arm/hand pain	150	13 8.67%	41 27.33%	63 42.00%	33 22.00%	137 91.33%
Carpal tunnel syndrome	25	0 0.00%	5 20.00%	17 68.00%	3 12.00%	25 100.00%
Arthritis pain	188	11 5.85%	51 27.13%	88 46.81%	38 20.21%	177 94.15%
TMJ pain	158	17 10.76%	60 37.97%	60 37.97%	21 13.29%	141 89.24%
Myofascial pain	62	6 9.68%	18 29.03%	18 29.03%	20 32.26%	56 90.32%
RSD	55	10 18.18%	16 29.09%	19 34.55%	10 18.18%	45 81.82%
Fibromyalgia (alone)	142	13 9.15%	53 37.32%	52 36.62%	24 16.90%	129 90.85%
Fibromyalgia (with other)	363	33 9.09%	131 36.09%	152 41.87%	47 12.95%	330 90.91%
Migraine	118	2 1.69%	49 41.53%	30 25.42%	37 31.36%	116 98.31%
Headaches (all other)	112	20 17.86%	30 26.79%	24 21.43%	38 33.93%	92 82.14%
Psychological (all cases)	723	61 8.44%	175 24.20%	237 32.78%	250 34.58%	662 91.56%
Anxiety (alone)	128	13 10.16%	29 22.66%	42 32.81%	44 34.38%	115 89.84%
Anxiety (with other)	370	33 8.92%	85 22.97%	122 32.97%	130 35.14%	337 91.08%
Anxiety/depression	58	3 5.17%	19 32.76%	19 32.76%	17 29.31%	55 94.83%
Depression (alone)	53	7 13.21%	11 20.75%	23 43.40%	12 22.64%	46 86.79%
Depression (with other)	265	29 10.94%	61 23.02%	93 35.09%	82 30.94%	236 89.06%
Stress	123	6 4.88%	30 24.39%	39 31.71%	48 39.02%	117 95.12%
Chronic fatigue	50	3 6.00%	30 60.00%	10 20.00%	7 14.00%	47 94.00%
Insomnia	163	10 6.13%	47 28.83%	47 28.83%	59 36.20%	153 93.87%

Note: Total N = 2500 patients with multiple symptoms. From consecutive warranty cards analyzed as of July 2000.

that works may be transient, working well one day, but ineffective another day. As the problem begins to resolve, the electrode locations may require frequent adjustments.

A common mistake made by clinicians familiar with traditional TENS is placing the electrodes on each side of the spine for back pain. This is a two-dimensional approach. With such a placement, microcurrent will travel just under the skin between the electrodes and never reach the spine. Nor can the electrodes be effectively placed "between the pain and the brain." These are common placements for TENS electrodes, but MET is not TENS. A better way is to place one electrode next to the spine at the level where the problem is, and the other on the contralateral side, anteriolaterally (front and opposite side). A line drawn between those will go right through the spinal nerves. Next, reverse the sides. Then follow up by doing another set of contralateral placements one spinal level above, and one below the problem to accommodate overlap in the dorsolateral fasciculus.

Always treat bilaterally. Bilateral treatment includes the spinal cord, thereby involving dermatomes, myotomes, and sclerotomes. Also, if the problem is within the axial skeleton and the contralateral side is ignored, there is a good chance that the primary location of a pain problem will be missed. Pain often presents itself on the tense side, which may be compensating for muscular weakness on the other side.

QUICK PROBE TREATMENTS

When using probes, set the timer on a probe setting, or if one is not available, treat about 10 seconds per site. In other words, move the probes to the next location every 10 seconds. Consider one treatment "set" to be 12 to 20 of these 10-second stimulations, each at a different angle of approach. The first set should take about 2 minutes, but then additional treatment may be done at 1-minute intervals. The patient should be reevaluated between each set.

The protocol involves four steps:

1. First treat in a large "X" manner over a wide area holding the probes so that the current is directed through the problem area. An example of this strategy for knee pain would be to first make the large X by treating from the medial, superior thigh to the lateral foot, then lateral at the hip to the medial foot.
2. Treat with smaller Xs, or a "star" (*) closer and directly around the involved knee (e.g., two obliques, one or two medial–lateral, one or two anterior–posterior, etc.).
3. Treat the opposite knee for at least 20 seconds (one X), even if it is asymptomatic.
4. Connect the two knees by placing a probe on each knee at least four times.

The above example takes 2 minutes. A big X beyond the area (20 seconds), a star through the chief complaint (40 seconds), treat the opposite side with one small X (20 seconds), and connect the two sides (40 seconds). Then reevaluate the pain based on the original criteria.

If the pain is gone, stop for the day. If it is reduced, ask the patient to point to where it hurts with one finger and treat for another minute or so directly through the area of pain, which may have moved after the original 2-minute treatment.

Think in terms of symmetry. Look, palpate, and otherwise examine areas above, below, and to the left and right of the primary area undergoing treatment. Always treat the opposite side and connect both sides.

SILVER SELF-ADHESIVE ELECTRODES

These are used following the same strategy as the probes, except for a longer period of time. The probes and brief electrode treatments assume MET is working as a catalyst for the patient's own bioelectrical system, whereas keeping electrodes in place can be viewed as using MET to augment endogenous bioelectricity. For optimum results, silver electrodes also may be moved around the problem area. Whereas the probes are used for 10 seconds a site, silver electrodes should be left at each location for *at least* 5 to 10 minutes. Some cases will require an hour or even several hours of stimulation daily. Accordingly, silver electrodes are best used for home care. However, if brief stimulation works, do not continue treatment at that session. More is not better when using MET technology to manage pain!

WHEN TO STOP

Reevaluate the patient after the 2-minute protocol using the original criteria. It is not enough to ask if the patient feels better, ask for a specific percentage of how much better. If the patient has difficulty with a 0-to-10 scale, to facilitate communication, ask, "If you had a dollar's worth of pain when we began, how many cents do you have left?" Also, reexamine for improvement in objective signs, such as range-of-motion increases, etc. Stop when the pain is completely gone, or when the improvement has reached a plateau after several treatment sets. Continuing to treat the area at this time may cause the pain to return! If the pain is gone, it is far better to stop treatment for that day even if the patient only had 1 or 2 minutes of treatment.

If the patient can no longer identify any pain, but complains of stiffness, this indicates that it is time to stop treatment for the day. Microcurrent may not reduce residual stiffness. Post-pain stiffness usually wears off by itself. Yoga, Tai Chi, or simple stretching exercises are good means of controlling chronic stiffness.

Although most patients will have an immediate response to treatment, in some the effects will be delayed, continuing to improve over a day or two after the treatment. In these patients relief will generally occur 1 to 3 hours post-treatment or even as late as the next morning. Some patients will experience a cumulative effect, continuing to improve over time. Patients who experience a delayed effect are more difficult to treat due to lack of immediate feedback. Usually, patients who experience a delayed effect from microcurrent treatment also have a delayed effect with anesthetics. Ask the nonresponsive patient if his or her dentist had to wait more than 10 minutes after injecting anesthetic prior to doing dental procedures. Because treating patients who exhibit delayed responses can be viewed as a type of "blind" treatment, one must rely on experience with other patients who exhibited an immediate response in order to develop the skills to treat those few who have a delayed response. A post-treatment diary is also helpful in analyzing the response of these patients.

FOLLOW-UP

Most patients should be given at least three to seven treatments before evaluating their responses to microcurrent electrical therapy. It helps to explain to the patient that the effects of MET treatment are cumulative. Like antibiotics, one must take several doses over a period of time to get results. Although results will usually be seen during or subsequent to the first treatment, the longevity of the results can only be evaluated after a series of treatments. Fortunately, most patients will experience long-lasting results. However, in some cases the results will plateau to a similar time period regardless of treatment. For example, a patient may only get 1 or 2 days of relief no matter what combination of treatment strategies is employed. For these, and cases of severe pathology, the effectiveness may be only short-lived, so a MET device should be prescribed for home care. After an initial series of up to ten clinical treatments, a good rule of thumb is to prescribe a unit for anyone with a chronic condition who requires more than one or two palliative treatments per month, and for patients who have progressive pathologies. When used at home, after an initial series of 1 or 2 weeks of daily treatments, treatment every other day usually provides better results than daily treatment.

TIPS FOR LIMITED OR POOR RESULTS

While a good MET device will be at least somewhat efficacious on more than 90% of the population when used correctly, MET will not work for everyone. In cases where there are no results at all, a few things should be considered. Dehydrated patients may not respond well. Patients should be advised to drink at least eight to ten glasses of water daily. Nutrition is certainly a factor. A poor diet does not provide the necessary building blocks to reinstate homeostasis.

Also, preliminary observations suggest that people who have had a significant exposure to strong electrical current may be poor candidates for MET. This means that they either have been held by electrical current at some time in their life, or have been treated with mA TENS or similar modalities for a prolonged period of time, usually years. There have even been a few reports of failures in patients who were struck by lightning. Brief exposure to very high levels of electricity is not as bad as longer exposure to any level of electricity. Such patients need to be treated for a longer period of time.

Aside from hydration and nutrition and electrical shock, the primary reversible reason patients fail to respond to treatment is that they have some sort of a blockage somewhere on or in their body that is resisting endogenous electrical flow. This is usually something superficial, like a scar or old injury. It need not be anywhere near the patient's primary problem. Identify *all* scars by taking a very thorough, persistent history, and examining the patient completely. All scars are important no matter how old or how far they are from the chief complaint. Scar tissue impedes the systemic flow of endogenous bioelectricity because it is a poor conductor of electricity. Accordingly, scar tissue may interfere with the patient's entire bioelectrical system. If scars are present they should be treated with silver electrodes for 10 minutes per scar, at least four times. Simply cover the scars with the electrodes, or for large scars, place the electrodes on the ends of the scars. This may be done 4 days in a row or there can be a short interval of up to a few days between the treatments. Some people report that it helps to repeat this procedure after a month or so.

During treatment for scars the person may experience a significant surge of energy. This can be viewed as if an electrical "bioresistor" has broken down, reestablishing the normal flow of bioelectricity. After scar therapy, patients will often report feeling half their age. Because people have nothing with which to compare their life experiences, they usually attribute the subtle effects of scars on their electrical system as normal aging. Be aware that this treatment will often also increase pain, because the whole body and mind "wake up," including the painful part. However, in nearly all cases, when this happens the painful area can then be successfully treated. Always schedule enough time to treat the pain after a scar treatment, so the patient will not need to endure even a temporary increase in pain.

If all the scars are treated and there are still no results, or if there are poor results, a few other options still exit. Question the patient about old injuries that may not have healed properly. These also could be electrical blocks and should be approached in the same way as scars. Consider treating the primary complaint at a lower current setting of 100 μA with silver electrodes for 60 minutes or more. Slightly higher pulse repetition rates (e.g., 1.5 Hz) may produce results in some people when the 0.5 Hz fails, but this is rare. For more information about treating scars, or how to determine which scars to treat, physicians and dentists may contact the American Academy of Neural Therapy through their Web site at www.neuraltherapy.com.

SAMPLE PROTOCOLS

The following illustrated sample protocols may be used as a guide for treatment using MET.

HEAD PAIN PROTOCOL

SAMPLE 1 (See Figure 61.1): Head Pain

Include the temporomandibular joint (TMJ), neck, and shoulders.

1. Above the ear to the tip of the contralateral shoulder. Reverse sides.
2. Across the shoulders by treating bilaterally across the distal tips of the acromions.
3. A few "X" patterns across back of neck.
4. From one TMJ to the other.
5. Temple to ipsilateral masseter muscle. Reverse sides.
6. About 1 minute through the primary area of involvement.

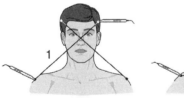
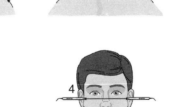
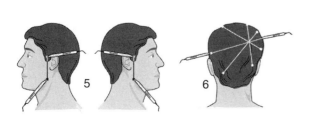

FIGURE 61.1 Head pain protocol.

Balance out contralateral side by treating any mirror areas not already covered.

Note: Reduce the current as necessary to avoid vertigo. Treating near the eyes may cause the patient to see flashing lights due to stimulation of optic nerve. Patient may also taste metal fillings when treating across oral cavity. None of these conditions is harmful.

SINUS AND OCULAR PAIN

SAMPLE 2 (See Figure 61.2): Sinus and Ocular Pain

Begin sinus and ocular pain treatment using the above protocol for head pain.

7. Treat sinuses when indicated, above and below eyes, or from side to side (see notes in head pain section). The patient should be able to breathe more clearly immediately after treatment.
8. For ocular headaches, treat behind eyes by placing probes on each temple, lateral to the lateral canthus of the eyes, and across each eye (one at a time) at the bridge of the nose to the lateral canthus.

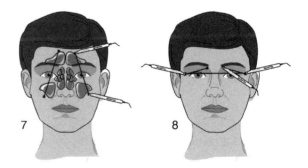

FIGURE 61.2 Sinus and ocular pain protocol.

TEMPOROMANDIBULAR DISORDER

SAMPLE 3 (See Figure 61.3): Temporomandibular Disorder (TMD)

Begin temporomandibular disorder treatment using the above protocol for head pain.

7. A star pattern across TMJ. Reverse sides.
8. Connect the TMJ with the sternocleidomastoideus (SCM) muscles, below the mastoid, and along the clavicular and sternal branches. Reverse sides.

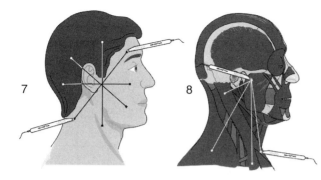

FIGURE 61.3 Temporomandibular disorder (TMD) pain protocol.

UPPER EXTREMITY PAIN PROTOCOL

SAMPLE 4 (See Figure 61.4): Upper Extremity

1. First make the large "X" by treating from the anterior shoulder to the posterior hand, and the posterior shoulder to the anterior hand.
2. Complete 40 seconds to 1 minute of smaller Xs closer to and directly around the shoulder, elbow, wrist, hand, or other area of pain. For carpal tunnel syndrome (CTS) or repetitive strain injury (RSI), treat superior to the elbow

to the webs between the fingers in addition to local treatment at the wrist.
3. Treat the area corresponding to the area of pain on the other upper extremity for 20 to 40 seconds.
4. Connect the two upper extremities by placing one probe on each in several symmetrical places encompassing the pain area for 40 seconds to 1 minute.

LOWER EXTREMITY PAIN PROTOCOL

SAMPLE 5 (See Figure 61.5): Lower Extremity

1. First make the large "X" by treating from the medial, superior thigh to the lateral foot, then the lateral hip to the medial foot.
2. Complete 40 seconds to 1 minute of smaller Xs closer to and directly around the hip, knee, ankle, foot, or other area of pain.
3. Treat the area corresponding to the area of pain on the other lower extremity for 20 to 40 seconds.
4. Connect the two lower extremities by placing one probe on each in several symmetrical places encompassing the pain area for 40 seconds to 1 minute.

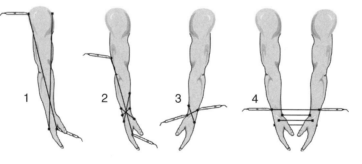

FIGURE 61.4 Upper extremity pain protocol.

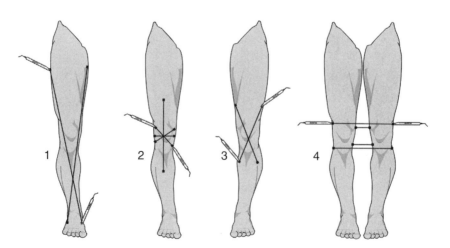

FIGURE 61.5 Lower extremity pain protocol.

BACK PAIN PROTOCOL

SAMPLE 6 (See Figure 61.6): Back Pain

1. Anterior between the trapezius muscle and the clavicle connected to the contralateral posterior hip. Reverse sides.
2. Then place one probe next to the spine at the level where the problem is, and the other on the contralateral side, anteriolaterally (front and opposite side). A line drawn between those will go right through the spinal nerves. Reverse the sides. Repeat contralateral placements one spinal level above, and one below the problem.
3. Also treat across the vertebrae, from each side of the body through the problem area, above, and below.
4. For low back pain with sciatic radiculitis, connect various levels from L3 to L5 about 1 inch lateral to the spine with the ipsilateral, posterior

leg at 4- to 6-inch intervals with the last, most inferior placement at the lateral foot (or just past where the pain radiates).

CRANIAL ELECTROTHERAPY STIMULATION

Cranial electrotherapy stimulation (CES) is the application of low-level, pulsed electrical currents (usually not exceeding 1 mA), applied to the head for medical and/or psychological purposes. It is used primarily to treat both state (situational) and trait (chronic) anxiety, depression, insomnia, stress-related and drug addiction disorders, but it is also proving indispensable for treating pain patients (Kirsch & Smith, 2000; Lichtbroun, Raicer, & Smith, 2001; Thuile & Kirsch, 2000).

Drs. Leduc and Rouxeau of France were the first to experiment with low-intensity electrical stimulation of the brain in 1902. Initially, this method was called electrosleep

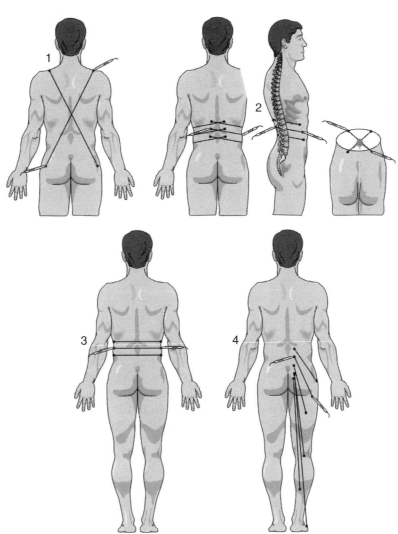

FIGURE 61.6 Back pain protocol.

as it was thought to be able to induce sleep. Since then, it has been referred to by many other names, the most popular being transcranial electrotherapy (TCET) and neuroelectric therapy (NET). Research on using what is now referred to as cranial electrotherapy stimulation (CES) began in the Soviet Union during the 1950s.

Cranial electrotherapy stimulation is a simple treatment that can easily be administered at any time. The current is applied by easy-to-use clip electrodes that attach on the ear lobes, or by stethoscope-type electrodes placed behind the ears. In the 1960s and early 1970s, electrodes were placed directly on the eyes because it was thought that the low level of current used in CES could not otherwise penetrate the cranium. This electrode placement was abandoned more than 20 years ago. Recent research has shown that from 1 mA of current, about 5 μA/cm^2 of CES reach the thalamic area at a radius of 13.30 mm which is sufficient to affect the manufacture and release of neurotransmitters (Ferdjallah, Bostick, Jr., Francis, Jr., & Barr, 1996).

Anxiety reduction is usually experienced during a treatment, but may be seen hours later, or as late as 1 day after treatment. Although in some people it may require a series of 5 to 10 daily treatments to be effective. Severe depression often takes up to 3 weeks to establish a therapeutic effect.

Cranial electrotherapy stimulation leaves the user alert while inducing a relaxed state. Psychologists call this an *alpha state*. The effect differs from pharmaceutical treatment in that people usually report feeling that their bodies are more relaxed, while their minds are more alert. Most people experience a feeling that their bodies are lighter, while thinking is clearer and more creative. A mild tingling sensation at the electrode sites also may be experienced during treatment. The current should never be raised to a level that is uncomfortable. One 20-minute session is often all that is needed to effectively control anxiety for at least a day, and the effects are usually cumulative. If the patient can only tolerate a small amount of current (< 200 μA) due to vertigo or nausea, more time is required. Cranial electrotherapy stimulation also may be used as an adjunct to anxiolytic or antidepressive medication, but the dosage of medication should then be reduced by approximately one third. It is also proven to be an effective complimentary treatment along with psychotherapy, biofeedback training, and surgical anesthesia (Kirsch, 1999). For people who have difficulty falling asleep, CES should be used in the morning to avoid the possibility of increased alertness that may interfere with sleep.

Most people can resume normal activities immediately after treatment. Some people may experience a euphoric feeling, or a state of deep relaxation that may temporarily impair their mental and/or physical abilities for the performance of potentially hazardous tasks, such as operating a motor vehicle or heavy machinery, for up to several hours after treatment.

At present, there are over 100 research studies on CES in humans and 20 experimental animal studies (Kirsch, 1999). No significant lasting side effects have ever been reported. Occasional self-limiting headache (1 out of 450), discomfort or skin irritation under the electrodes (1 out of 811), or lightheadedness may occur. A rare patient with a history of vertigo may experience dizziness for hours or days after treatment.

Most cranial electrotherapy stimulators are limited to 600 μA. To put this into perspective, it takes one half of an ampere to light an ordinary 60-watt light bulb. To truly compare the work done per second by these two different currents, we must multiply the currents by the respective voltages that drive them. The product of current × voltage is a measure of the rate of generation of energy, and is referred to as the power output. By definition, when a device outputs 1 ampere of current with a 1-volt driving force, the power output of the device is 1 watt. Therefore, a device producing a maximum output of 600 μA is limited to about 11,000 times less power than the light bulb: (600/1,000,000) amperes × 9 volts = 0.0054 watts. Some people do not even feel this amount of current.

As in many areas of biology and therapy, the evidence of CES effectiveness is empirical. It is generally believed that the effects are primarily mediated through a direct action on the brain at the limbic system, the hypothalamus and/or reticular activating system (Brotman, 1989; Gibson & O'Hair, 1987; Madden & Kirsch, 1987). The primary role of the reticular activating system is the regulation of electrocortical activity. These are primitive brainstem structures. The functions of these areas and their influence on our emotional states were mapped using electrical stimulation. Electrical stimulation of the periaqueductal gray matter has been shown to activate descending inhibitory pathways from the medial brainstem to the dorsal horn of the spinal cord, in a manner similar to β-endorphins (Ng, Douthitt, et al., 1975; Pert, Dionne, Ng, et al., 1981; Salar, Sob, et al., 1981). Cortical inhibition is a factor in the Melzack-Wall Gate Control theory (Melzack, 1975). Toriyama (1975) suggested it is possible that CES may produce its effects through parasympathetic autonomic nervous system dominance via stimulation of the vagus nerve (CN X). Taylor (1991) added other cranial nerves such as the trigeminal (CN V), facial (CN VII), and glossopharyngeal (CN IX). Fields, Tacke, and Savana (1975) showed that electrocortical activity produced by stimulation of the trigeminal nerve is implicated in the function of the limbic region of the midbrain affecting emotions. Substance P and enkephalin have been found in the trigeminal nucleus, and are postulated to be involved in limbic emotional brain structures (Hokfelt, Ljungdahl, et al., 1977). The auditory-vertigo nerve (CN VIII) must also be affected by CES, accounting for the dizziness one experiences when the current is too high. Ideally, CES electrodes are placed on the ear lobes because that is a convenient way to direct current through the midbrain and brain stem structures.

From studies of CES in monkeys, Jarzembski, Sanford, and Sances, Jr. (1970) measured 42 to 46% of the current entering the brain, with the highest concentration in the limbic region. Rat studies by Krupisky (1991) showed as much as a threefold increase in β-endorphin concentration after just one CES treatment. Pozos, Richardson, and Kaplan (1971) conducted mongrel dog research that suggests CES releases dopamine in the basal ganglia, and that the overall physiological effects appear to be anticholinergic and catecholamine-like in action. Richter, Zouhar, Tatsuno, et al. (1972) found the size, location, and distribution of synaptic vesicles were all within normal limits after a series of ten, 1-hour treatments in Rhesus monkeys. Several studies in stump-tailed macaques and humans revealed a temporary reduction in gastric hypersecretion (Kotter, Henschel, Hogan, et al., 1975; Reigel, Dallmann, Christman, et al., 1970; Reigel, Larson, Sances, Jr., et al., 1971; Wilson, Reigel, Unger, et al., 1970).

A recent review by Kirsch (1999) of 106 human studies involving 5439 subjects (4058 receiving cranial electrotherapy stimulation, while the remainder served as sham-treated or placebo controls) revealed significant changes associated with anxiolytic relaxation responses, such as lowered reading on electromyograms (Forster, Post, & Benton, 1963; Gibson, & O'Hair, 1987; Heffernan, 1995; Overcash, & Siebenthall, 1989; Voris, 1995), slowing on electroencephalograms (Braverman, Smith, Smayda, & Blum, 1990; Cox, & Heath, 1975; Heffernan, 1996; Heffernan, 1997; Krupitsky, 1991; McKenzie, Rosenthal, & Driessner, 1971; Singh, Chhina, Anand, et al., 1971), increased peripheral temperature, an indicator of vasodilatation (Brotman, 1989; Heffernan, 1995), reductions in gastric acid output (Kotter, Henschel, Hogan, et al., 1975), and in blood pressure, pulse, respiration, and heart rate (Heffernan, 1995; Taylor, 1991).

The efficacy of CES has also been clinically confirmed through the use of 27 different psychometric tests. The significance of CES research for treating anxiety has been reconfirmed through meta-analyses conducted at the University of Tulsa by O'Connor, Bianco, and Nicholson (1991), and by Klawansky, Yeung, Berkey, Shah, et al. (1995) at the Department of Health Policy and Management, Harvard School of Public Health.

Seventeen studies conducted follow-up investigations from 1 week to 2 years after treatment (Brotman, 1989; Brovar, 1984; Cartwright, & Weiss, 1975; Flemenbaum, 1974; Forster, et al., 1963; Hearst, Cloninger, Crews, & Cadoret, 1974; Heffernan, 1995; Hochman, 1988; Koegler, Hicks, & Barger, 1971; Magora, Beller, Assael, & Kenazi, 1967; Matteson, & Ivancevich, 1986;

Moore, Mellor, Standage, & Strong, 1975; Overcash, 1999; Patterson, 1988; Smith, 1999; Turaeva, 1967; Weiss, 1973). Sixteen of 16 (100%) reported that at least some of the subjects had continued improvement after a single CES treatment, or a series of CES treatments. The other follow-up report only commented on safety (Forster, et al., 1963). None of the 17 studies revealed any long-term harmful effects.

When restricted to anxiety populations or studies that measured for physiological and/or psychological changes in anxiety, there are 40 scientific studies of CES involving 1835 patients. Thirty-four of the 40 (85%) studies reported efficacious results in the treatment of anxiety. Five of the studies on CES (all using the Alpha-Stim) support the effectiveness for managing anxiety during or after a single treatment (Gibson, & O'Hair, 1987; Heffernan, 1995; Smith, 1999; Voris, 1995; Winick, 1999).

None of the 6 of 40 (15%) anxiety studies categorized by the authors as having negative or indeterminate results were recent; 5 were done in the 1970s, and one in 1980. Three showed both actual treatment and sham groups to improve significantly, most likely because both groups were also taking medications (Levitt, James, & Flavell, 1975; Passini, Watson, & Herder, 1976; Von Richtofen, & Mellor, 1980). One was a depression study in which the author noted that acute anxiety was not relieved and again, the study did not control for medications (Hearst, et al., 1974). One reported no significant change on anxiety or depression scales, but subjective insomnia improved (P < .05) during active treatment (Moore, et al., 1975). Only one study conducted on a population of insomniacs, with an average duration of symptoms for almost 20 years, did not show any significant change at all in any parameters (Frankel, Buchbinder, & Snyder, 1973). [Perhaps the device used in Frankel's study was defective.]

Cranial electrotherapy stimulation has been well researched and clearly proven to be the most effective, and safest method of treatment for anxiety, and anxiety-related disorders. It is also highly effective for depression and insomnia, muscle tension, fibromyalgia, and headaches. As an increasing number of patients seek alternatives to the side sfects and potential addiction to mood-altering pharmaceuticals and controlled substances, CES offers a viable solution. It is easy enough to offer CES in a psychologist's, dentist's or physician's office, clinic, or hospital, and chronically stressed patients will find it cost-effective over time to own their own CES device.

INDICATIONS

In addition to the primary claims for anxiety, depression insomnia, and pain, CES has been researched with significant results for many other conditions. Smith and Shiromoto (1992) showed it to be highly effective in blocking fear perception in phobic patients. Favorable results also have been reported for labor, epilepsy, hypertension, surgery, spinal cord injuries, chronic pain, arthritis, cerebral atherosclerosis, eczema, dental pain, asthma, ischemic heart disease, stroke, motion sickness, digestive disorders as well as various addictive disorders including cocaine, marijuana, heroin and alcohol abuse (Brovar, 1984; Daulouede, 1980; Feighner, Brown, & Olivier, 1973; Gomez & Mikhail, 1978; Overcash & Siebenthall, 1989; Patterson, 1983; Schmitt, Capo, Frazier, & Boren, 1984; Smith, 1975; Smith, 1982; Wharton, McCoy, & Cofer, 1982).

Reflex sympathetic dystrophy (RSD) and fibromyalgia syndrome (FS) are two significant pain diagnoses from primary central and autonomic nervous system etiologies that respond best to CES (Alpher & Kirsch, 1998; Lichtbroun, Racier, & Smith, 1999). Adding somatic treatment with MET to these two conditions does not seem to improve the outcomes.

Besides specific pathological disorders, there are a growing number of studies being conducted that show increases in cognitive functions. Michael Hutchison (1986) discussed several mind-enhancement techniques in his book *Megabrain,* devoting Chapter 9 to CES as a tool for attaining higher levels of consciousness. Sparked by Hutchison, Madden and Kirsch (1987) completed a study that demonstrated CES is a useful tool for improving psychomotor abilities. Smith (1999) demonstrated that CES significantly improved stress-related cognitive dysfunction, such as attention deficit disorder (ADD), after only 3 weeks of treatment, and maintained the effect through an 18-month follow-up assessment.

METHODOLOGY

Cranial electrotherapy stimulation devices are generally similar in size and appearance to TENS units, but produce very different waveforms. *Standard mA-current TENS devices must never be applied transcranially.* CES electrodes can be placed bitemporally, forehead to posterior neck, bilaterally in the hollow just anterior to the mastoid processes, or through electrodes clipped to the earlobes. The ear clip method, developed by the author, is the easiest and possibly most effective electrode placement.

The electrodes must first be wet with an appropriate conducting solution. When using ear clip electrodes, apply them to the superior aspect of the ear lobes, as close to the jaw as possible. Start with a low current and gradually increase it. If the current is too high the patient may experience a painful stinging sensation at the electrodes, dizziness, or nausea. If any of these three symptoms arise, *immediately* reduce the current and the symptoms will subside in a few moments. After a minute or two, try increasing the current again, but keep it at a comfortable level. It is okay for the patient to feel the current as long as it is not uncomfortable.

The ideal treatment time is 20 to 60 minutes, but some patients may achieve the full benefits of a CES treatment within 10 minutes. Many dentists use it instead of nitrous oxide gas to help relax patients during dental procedures (Winick, 1999). Sometimes these dental procedures last for hours with the patient undergoing CES treatment the entire time.

Although CES treatment is indicated for insomnia, because of the increased alertness some patients find it difficult to fall asleep immediately after a treatment. Accordingly, it is recommended that CES be used at least 3 hours before going to bed. Also, in most cases after daily treatments for the first week or two, treating every other day is usually more effective than daily treatment.

THE CES EXPERIENCE

During the treatment, most patients will experience a subjective change in body weight. They may feel heavier at first and then lighter, or they may feel lighter initially. The patient may feel worse during the heavy cycle and this feeling can last for hours or even days in rare cases unless extra treatment time is given. Therefore, it is important to continue the treatment if the patient feels heavier at the end of the allotted time, even if it has already been 20 minutes or more. Continue for at least 2 to 5 minutes after the patient feels lighter. Not all patients will be aware of these weight-perception changes.

Following CES, most people feel better, less distressed, and more focused on mental tasks. They generally sleep better and report improved concentration, increased learning abilities, enhanced recall, and a heightened state of well-being.

Psychologists first described these general feelings during the 1970s as an *alpha state* of consciousness. Meditation, biofeedback training, relaxation instructions, chanting, hypnotherapy, and certain religious rituals also produce such states. This is not the same as the alpha brain wave frequency of 8 to 13 Hz. Often, practitioners are confused by device representatives who claim that their particular devices will output and entrain a brain to the alpha *frequency.* There is no evidence to support that CES devices work on an entrainment principle.

CONTRAINDICATIONS

There have not been any significant lasting harmful side effects reported in any of the research literature from either MET or CES. As with all electrical devices, caution is advised during pregnancy, and with patients using an older model (pre-1998) demand-type pacemaker. In addition, it is recommended that patients do not operate complex machinery or drive automobiles during and shortly after a CES treatment.

SUMMARY

Microcurrent electrical therapy and cranial electrotherapy stimulation are electromedical modalities that use low level currents that usually do not exceed 1 mA. Beneficial effects have been reported for a wide variety of pain, psychological distress, and addiction-related disorders.

Pain is a complex process encompassing the entire nervous system. To achieve optimal results through electromedical intervention, the peripheral and central nervous systems should both be treated. Cranial electrotherapy stimulation induces a relaxed, alert state. It is a primary modality effective for controlling anxiety, depression, insomnia, and generalized stress ubiquitous in pain patients. In addition, there is mounting evidence that CES can enhance cognitive functions. Because of its safety and effectiveness, the combination of MET and CES used with the protocols described here is highly recommended for a broad range of pain and stress-related disorders.

REFERENCES

Alpher, E.J., & Kirsch, D.L. (1998). Traumatic brain injury and full body reflex sympathetic dystrophy patient treated with cranial electrotherapy stimulation. *American Journal of Pain Management, 8*(4), 124–128.

Alvarez, O.M., et al. (1983). The healing of superficial skin wounds is stimulated by external electrical current. *Journal of Investigative Dermatology, 81*, 144–148.

Andersson, et al. (1976). Effects of conditioning electrical stimulation in the perception of pain. *ACTA Orthopaedica Scandinavica, 47*, 149–162.

Assimacopoulos, D. (1968). Low intensity negative electric current in treatment of ulcers of leg due to chronic venous insufficiency: Preliminary report of three cases. *American Journal of Surgery, 115*, 683–687.

Assimacopoulos, D. (1968a). Wound healing promotion by the use of negative electric current. *Annals of Surgery, 34*, 423–431.

Barron, J.J., & Jacobson, W.E. (1985). Treatment of decubitus ulcers: A new approach. *Minnesota Medicine, 68*, 103–105.

Becker, R.O. (1985). *The body electric.* New York: William Morrow and Co.

Braverman, E., Smith, R., Smayda, R., & Blum, K. (1990). Modification of P300 amplitude and other electrophysiological parameters of drug abuse by cranial electrical stimulation. *Current Therapeutic Research, 48*(4), 586–596.

Brotman, P. (1989). Low-intensity transcranial electrostimulation improves the efficacy of thermal biofeedback and quieting reflex training in the treatment of classical migraine headache. *American Journal of Electromedicine, 6*(5), 120–123.

Brovar, A. (1984). Cocaine detoxification with cranial electrotherapy stimulation (CES): A preliminary appraisal. *International Electromedicine Institute Newsletter, 1*(4).

Carey, L.C., & Lepley, D. (1962). Effect of continuous direct electric current on healing wounds. *Surgical Forum, 13*, 33–35.

Carley, P.J., & Wainapel, S.F. (1985). Electrotherapy for acceleration of wound healing: Low intensity direct current. *Archives of Physical Medicine and Rehabilitation, 66*, 443–446.

Cartwright, R.D., & Weiss, M.F. (1975). The effects of electrosleep on insomnia revisited. *Journal of Nervous and Mental Disease, 164*(2), 134.

Chang, N., Van Hoff, H., Bockx, E., et al. (1982). The effect of electric currents on ATP generation, protein synthesis, and membrane transport in rat skin. *Clinical Orthopedics, 171*, 264–272.

Cox, A., & Heath, R.G. (1975). Neurotone therapy: A preliminary report of its effect on electrical activity of forebrain structures. *Diseases of the Nervous System, 36*, 245–247.

Daulouede, J. (1980). Une nouvelle methode de sevrage des toxicomanes par utilisation du courant de Limoge (A new method of eliminating drug addiction using Limoge's current). *Annales Medic-Psychologiques, 138*(3), 359–370.

Dayton, P.D., & Palladino, S.J. (1989). Electrical stimulation of cutaneous ulcerations: A literature review. *Journal of the American Podiatric Medical Association, 79*, 318–321.

DeBock, P. (2000). A comparison between TENS and MET. *Physical Therapy Products*, September, 28–33.

Eaglstein, W.H., & Mertz, P.M. (1978). New method for assessing epidermal wound healing: The effects of triamcinolone acetonide and polyethylene film occlusion. *Journal of Investigative Dermatology, 71*, 382–384.

Falanga, V., et al. (1987). Electrical stimulation increases the expression of fibroblast receptors for transforming growth factor-beta (abstracted). *Journal of Investigative Dermatology, 88*, 488.

Falanga, V. (1988). Occlusive wound dressings. *Archives of Dermatology, 124*, 872–877.

Feighner, J.P., Brown, S.L., & Olivier, J.E. (1973). Electrosleep therapy: A controlled double-blind study. *Journal of Nervous and Mental Disorders, 157*, 121.

Ferdjallah, M., Bostick, F.X., Jr., & Barr, R.E. (1996). Potential and current density distributions of cranial electrotherapy stimulation (CES) in a four-concentric-spheres model. *IEEE Transactions on Biomedical Engineering, 43*(9), 939–943.

Fields, W.R., Tacke, R.B., & Savana, B.S. (1975). Pulpal anodal blockade of trigeminal field potentials elicited by tooth stimulation in the cat. *Experimental Neurology, 47*, 229–239.

Flemenbaum, A. (1974). Cerebral Electrotherapy (Electrosleep): An open clinical study with a six month follow-up, *Psychosomatics, 15*, 20–24.

Forster, S., Post, B.S., & Benton, J.G. (1963). Preliminary observations on electrosleep. *Archives of Physical and Medical Rehabilitation, 44*, 81–89.

Frankel, B.L., Buchbinder, R., & Snyder, F. (1973). Ineffectiveness of electrosleep in chronic primary insomnia. *Archives of General Psychiatry, 29,* 563–568.

Gault, W.R., & Gatesn, P.F. (1976). Use of low intensity direct current in management of ischemic skin ulcers. *Physical Therapy, 56,* 265–269.

Gibson, T.H., & O'Hair, D.E. (1987). Cranial application of low level transcranial electrotherapy vs. relaxation instruction in anxious patients. *American Journal of Electromedicine, 4*(1), 18–21.

Goldin, H., et al. (1981). The effects of Diapulse on the healing of wounds: A double-blind randomized controlled trial in man. *British Journal of Plastic Surgery, 34,* 267–270.

Gomez, E., & Mikhail, A.R. (1978). Treatment of methadone withdrawal with cerebral electrotherapy (electrosleep). *British Journal of Psychiatry, 134,* 111–113.

Hearst, E.D., Cloninger, R., Crews, E.L., & Cadoret, R.J. (1974). Electrosleep therapy: A double-blind trial. *Archives of General Psychiatry, 30,* 463–466.

Heffernan, M. (1995). The effect of a single cranial electrotherapy stimulation on multiple stress measures. *The Townsend Letter for Doctors and Patients, 147,* 60–64.

Heffernan, M. (1996). Comparative effects of microcurrent stimulation on EEG spectrum and correlation dimension. *Integrative Physiological and Behavioral Science, 31*(3), 202–209.

Heffernan, M. (1997). The effect of variable microcurrents on EEG spectrum and pain control. *Canadian Journal of Clinical Medicine. 4*(10), 4–11.

Hochman, R. (1988). Neurotransmitter modulation (TENS) for control of dental operative pain. *Journal of the American Dental Association, 116,* 208–212.

Hokfelt, T., et al. (1977). Immunohistological analysis of peptide pathways possibly related to pain and analgesia: Enkephalin and substance P. *Proceedings of the National Academy of Science, 74,* 3081–3085.

Hutchison, M. (1986). *Megabrain.* New York: Beech Tree Books, William Morrow.

Ieran, M., et al. (1990). Effect of low frequency pulsing electromagnetic fields on skin ulcers of venous origin in humans: A double blind study. *Journal of Orthopedic Research, 8,* 276–282.

Jarzembski, W.B., Sanford, J.L., & Sances, A., Jr. (1970). Evaluation of specific cerebral impedance and cerebral current density. *Annals of the New York Academy of Sciences, 170,* 476–490.

Jeran, M., et al. (1987). PEMF stimulation of skin ulcers of venous origin in humans: Preliminary report of a double blind study. *Journal of Bioelectricity, 6,* 181–188.

Kaada, B., Flatheim, E., & Woie, L. (1991). Low-frequency transcutaneous nerve stimulation in mild/moderate hypertension. *Clinical Physiology, 11,* 161–168.

Kirsch, D.L. (1999). *The science behind cranial electrotherapy stimulation.* Edmonton, Alberta, Canada: Medical Scope Publishing.

Kirsch, D.L., & Smith, R.B. (2000). The use of cranial electrotherapy stimulation in the management of chronic pain: A review. *NeuroRehabilitation, 14,* 85–94.

Klawansky, S., Yeung, A., Berkey, C., & Shah, N., et al. (1995). Meta-analysis of randomized controlled trials of cranial electrotherapy stimulation: Efficacy in treating selected psychological and physiological conditions. *Journal of Nervous and Mental Diseases, 183*(7), 478–485.

Koegler, R.R., Hick, S.M., & Barger, J. (1971). Medical and psychiatric use of electrosleep (transcerebral electrotherapy). *Diseases of the Nervous System, 32*(2), 100–104.

Kotter, G.S., Henschel, E.O., Hogan, Walter J., et al. (1975). Inhibition of gastric acid secretion in man by the transcranial application of low intensity pulsed current. *Gastroenterology, 69,* 359–363.

Krupitsky, E.M., Burakov, G.B., Karandashova, JaS., et al. (1991). The administration of transcranial electric treatment for affective disturbances therapy in alcoholic patients. *Drug and Alcohol Dependence, 27,* 1–6.

Krupisky, E.M., Katznelson, Ya.S., Lebedev, V.P., et al. (1991). Transcranial electrostimulation (TES) of brain opioid structures (BOS): Experimental treatment of alcohol withdrawal syndrome (AWS) and clinical application. Presented at the Society for Neuroscience Annual Meeting, New Orleans, November 10–15.

Kulig, K., Jarski, R., Drewek, E., et al. (1991). The effect of microcurrent stimulation on CPK and delayed onset muscle soreness. *Physical Therapy, 71,* 6(suppl.).

Levitt, E.A., James, N., & Flavell, P. (1975). A clinical trial of electrosleep therapy with a psychiatric inpatient sample. *Australia and New Zealand Journal of Psychiatry, 9,* 287–290.

Lichtbroun, A.S., Raicer, M.S., & Smith, R.B. (1999). The use of Alpha-Stim cranial electrotherapy stimulation in the treatment of fibromyalgia. Presented at the 15th annual International Symposium on Acupuncture and Electro-Therapeutics, Columbia University, New York City, October 21–24.

Lichtbroun, A.S., Raicer, M.S., & Smith, R.B. (2001). The treatment of fibromyalgia with cranial electrotherapy stimulation. *Journal of Clinical Rheumatology, 7*(2), 72–78.

Lundeberg, T.C., Eriksson, S.V., & Malm, M. (1992). Electrical nerve stimulation improves healing of diabetic ulcers. *Annals of Plastic Surgery, 29*(4), 328–331.

Madden, R.E., & Kirsch, D.L. (1987). Low intensity transcranial electrostimulation improves human learning of a psychomotor task. *American Journal of Electromedicine, 2*(2/3), 41–45.

Magora, F., Beller, A., Assael, M.I., & Askenazi, A. (1967). Some aspects of electrical sleep and its therapeutic value. In F.M. Wageneder, & St. Schuy (Eds.) (pp. 129–135). *Electrotherapeutic sleep and electroanaesthesia.* Amsterdam: Excerpta Medica Foundation, International Congress Series No. 136.

Matteson, M.T., & Ivancevich, J.M. (1986). An exploratory investigation of CES as an employee stress management technique. *Journal of Health and Human Resource Administration, 9,* 93–109.

McKenzie, R.E., Rosenthal, S.H., & Driessner, J.S. (1971). Some psychophysiologic effects of electrical transcranial stimulation (electrosleep). American Psychiatric Association, *Scientific Proceedings Summary*. Also in *The nervous system and electric currents* (1976). N.L. Wulfsohn, and A. Sances, (Eds.). New York: Plenum. 163–167.

Melzack, R. (1975). Prolonged pain relief by brief, intense transcutaneous somatic stimulation. *Pain, 1*, 373–375.

Mercola, J.M., & Kirsch, D.L. (1995). The basis for microcurrent electrical therapy (MET) in conventional medical practice. *Journal of Advancement in Medicine, 8*(2), 107–120.

Moore, J.A., Mellor, C.S., Standage, K.F., & Strong, H. (1975). A double-blind study of electrosleep for anxiety and insomnia. *Biological Psychiatry, 10*(1), 59–63.

Mulder, G.D. (1991). Treatment of open-skin wounds with electric stimulation. *Archives of Physical Medicine and Rehabilitation, 72*, 375–377.

Ng, L.K.Y., Douthitt, T., et al. (1975). Modification of morphine-withdrawal syndrome in rats following transauricular electrostimulation: An experimental paradigm for auricular electroacupuncture. *Biological Psychiatry, 10*, 575–580.

O'Connor, M.E., Bianco, F., & Nicholson, R. (1991). Meta-analysis of cranial electrostimulation in relation to the primary and secondary symptoms of substance withdrawal. Presented at the 12th Annual Meeting of the Bioelectromagnetics Society, June 14.

Overcash, S.J. (1999). A retrospective study to determine the effect of cranial electrotherapy stimulation (CES) on patients suffering from anxiety disorders. *American Journal of Electromedicine, 16*(1), 49–51.

Overcash, S.J., & Siebenthall, A. (1989). The effects of cranial electrotherapy stimulation and multisensory cognitive therapy on the personality and anxiety levels of substance abuse patients. *American Journal of Electromedicine, 6*(2), 105–111.

Passini, F.G., Watson, C.G., & Herder, J. (1976). The effects of cerebral electric therapy (electrosleep) on anxiety, depression, and hostility in psychiatric patients. *Journal of Nervous and Mental Disease, 163*(4), 263–266.

Patterson, M. (1983). *Getting off the hook*. Wheaton, IL: Harold Shaw Publishers.

Patterson, M., Firth, J., & Gardiner, R. (1984). Treatment of drug, alcohol and nicotine addiction by neuroelectric therapy: Analysis of results over 7 years. *Journal of Bioelectricity, 3*(1/2), 193–221.

Pert, A., Dionne, R., & Ng, L.K.Y., et al. (1981). Alterations in rat central nervous system endorphins following transauricular electroacupuncture. *Brain Research, 224*, 83–94.

Pozos, R.S., Richardson, A.W., & Kaplan, H.M. (1971). Electroanesthesia: A proposed physiologic mechanism. In D.V. Reynolds & A. Sjoberg (Eds.), *Neuroelectric research* (pp. 110–113). Springfield, IL: Charles C Thomas.

Reigel, D.H., Dallmann, D.E., Christman, N.T., et al. (1970). Physiological effects of electrotherapeutic currents in the primate and man. In F.M. Wageneder & St. Schuy (Eds.). *Electrotherapeutic sleep and electroanesthesia*. (Vol. II) pp. 158–165). Amsterdam: Excerpta Medica.

Reigel, D.H., Larson, S.J., Sances, A., Jr., et al. (1971). Effects of electrosleep currents on gastric physiology. In D.V. Reynolds & A. Sjoberg (Eds.). *Neuroelectric research*. Springfield, IL: Charles C Thomas.

Richter, W.R., Zouhar, R.L., Tatsuno, J., et al. (1972). Electron microscopy of the macaca mulatta brain after repeated applications of electric current. *Anesthesiology, 36*(4), 374–377.

Robinson, K.R. (1925). Digby's receipts. *Annals of Medical History, 7*, 216–219.

Rowley, B.A., McKenna, J.M., Chase, G.R., & Wolcott, L.E. (1974). The influence of electrical current on an infecting microorganism in wounds. *Annals of the New York Academy of Science, 238*, 543–551.

Salar, G., et al. (1981). Effect of transcutaneous electrotherapy on CSF β-endorphin content in patients without pain problems. *Pain, 10*, 169–172.

Schmitt, R., Capo, T., Frazier, H., & Boren, D. (1984). Cranial electrotherapy stimulation treatment of cognitive brain dysfunction in chemical dependence. *Journal of Clinical Psychiatry, 45*, 60.

Singh, B., China, G.S., Anand, B.K., et al. (1971). Sleep and consciousness mechanism with special reference to electrosleep. *Armed Forces Medical Journal* (New Delhi), *27*(3), 292–297.

Smith, R.B. (1975). Electrosleep in the management of alcoholism. *Biological Psychiatry, 10*, 675.

Smith, R.B. (1982). Confirming evidence of an effective treatment for brain dysfunction in alcoholic patients. *Journal of Nervous and Mental Disorders, 170*(5), 275–278.

Smith, R.B. (1999). Cranial electrotherapy stimulation in the treatment of stress related cognitive dysfunction with an eighteen month follow-up. *Journal of Cognitive Rehabilitation, 17*(6), 14–18.

Smith, R.B. (2001). Is microcurrent stimulation effective in pain management? An additional perspective. *American Journal of Pain Management, 11*(2), 62–66.

Smith, R.B., & Shiromoto, F.N. (1992). The use of cranial electrotherapy stimulation to block fear perception in phobic patients. *Current Therapeutic Research, 51*(2), 249–253.

Starfield, B. (2000). Is U.S. health really the best in the world? *Journal of the American Medical Association, 284*(4), 483–485.

Stromberg, B.V. (1988). Effects of electrical currents on wound contraction. *Annals of Plastic Surgery, 21*, 121–23.

Taylor, D.N. (1991). Effects of cranial transcutaneous electrical nerve stimulation in normal subjects at rest and during stress. Doctoral dissertation, Brooklyn College of the City University of New York.

Thuile, C., & Kirsch, D.L. (2000). *Schmerzen Linden ohne Chemie: CES, die Revolution in der Schmerztherapie* (in German). IGEM, Austria.

Toriyama, M. (1975). Ear acupuncture anesthesia. *Ear Throat, 47*, 497–501.

Turaeva, V.A. (1967). Treatment of eczema and neurodermatitis by electrosleep. In F.M. Wageneder, & St. Schuy (Eds.). *Electrotherapeutic sleep and electroanaesthesia.* (pp. 203–204). Amsterdam: Excerpta Medica Foundation.

Von Richthofen, C.L., & Mellor, C.S. (1980). Electrosleep therapy: A controlled study of its effects in anxiety neurosis. *Canadian Journal of Psychiatry, 25*(3), 213–229.

Voris, M.D. (1995). *An investigation of the effectiveness of cranial electrotherapy stimulation in the treatment of anxiety disorders among outpatient psychiatric patients, impulse control parolees and pedophiles* (pp. 1–19). Dallas: Delos Mind/Body Institute.

Weiss, D.S., et al. (1990). Electrical stimulation and wound healing. *Archives of Dermatology, 126,* 222–225.

Weiss, M.F. (1973). The treatment of insomnia through use of electrosleep: An EEG study. *Journal of Nervous and Mental Disease, 157*(2), 108–120.

Wharton, G.W., et al. (1982; 1983). The use of cranial electrotherapy stimulation in spinal cord injury patients. A poster study presented at the American Spinal Injury Association Meeting, New York, and at the Texas ASIA meeting in Houston.

Wilson, A.S., Reigel, D., Unger, G.F., et al. (1970). Gastric secretion before and after electrotherapeutic sleep in executive monkeys. In F.M. Wageneder & St. Schuy (Eds.). *Electrotherapeutic sleep and electroanesthesia.* (Vol. II, pp. 198–206). Amsterdam: Excerpta Medica.

Windsor, R.E., Lester, J.P., & Herring, S.A. (1993). Electrical stimulation in clinical practice. *Physician and Sports Medicine, 21,* 85–93.

Winick, R.L. (1999). Cranial electrotherapy stimulation (CES): A safe and effective low cost means of anxiety control in dental practice. *General Dentistry, 47*(1), 50–55.

Wolcott, L.E., Wheeler, P.C., & Hardwicke, H.M. (1969). Accelerated healing of skin ulcers by electrotherapy. *Southern Medical Journal, 62,* 795–801.

Section IX

Behavioral, Social, and Spiritual Concerns and Aspects of Pain Management

62

Pain, Disease, and Suicide

Blake H. Tearnan, Ph.D.

NATURE OF THE PROBLEM

INCIDENCE

There are over 30,000 completed suicides in the United States each year. Most successful suicides are carried out by men, but women attempt suicide more often (National Center for Injury Prevention and Control, 1999). Suicide is currently the third leading cause of death among young adults ages 15 to 34, and in the United Kingdom, suicide is the second most common cause of death in this age group after motor vehicle accidents (Williams, 1997). Recently, the Surgeon General identified suicide as one of the top public health concerns in the United States (Parker, 1998). Overall, suicide accounts for nearly 9% of males and 4% of females in loss of years of life before the age of 65. This figure is similar for most Western countries (Williams, 1997). Clearly, suicide represents a major health concern.

RISK FACTORS

Extensive research has been done to identify risk factors associated with suicide in the general population. Some of the more consistent findings include increased rates for men by a factor of nearly 2 to 1 in most countries and 5 to 1 in Finland (Sainsbury, Jenkins, & Baert, 1981). Whites in the United States are also approximately twice as likely to commit suicide as blacks or other nonwhite groups, and this difference is particularly associated with the older age group. The exception to this finding is that suicide is particularly high in young Native Americans (Williams, 1997).

Most studies have found the presence of psychiatric disturbance and/or substance abuse increases the risk of suicide in all populations (Williams, 1997). For example, it is a well-established fact that suicidal behavior is particularly associated with major depression. Other findings have shown suicidal risk is greater in Protestants than other religious affiliations including Catholics and Jews. However, in general, churchgoing is associated with decreased risk of suicide, possibly related to increased social supports (Williams, 1997).

The incidence of suicide in various social classes also has been studied. One investigation of social classes in England and Wales found the risk of suicide was greater in the professional and unskilled classes (Charlton, Kelly, Dunnell, Evans, Jenkins, & Wallis, 1992). Comparatively fewer suicides were found in lower-level professional and executive, skilled and partially skilled classes. However, the highest risk was found among individuals who had no occupation at all. Studies conducted in the United States have shown that people in the lower classes living in substandard housing have proportionately higher rates of suicide (Charlton, et al., 1992). The exception is African-Americans living in poor communities. Williams (1997) concluded that this result was possibly related to the strong social ties within the African-American community.

It is clear economic conditions, particularly unemployment, increase the risk of suicide. Generally, men who are unemployed and seeking employment are at two to three times greater risk. Boor (1980) found that among suicide victims, the rate of unemployment was 50% across several studies.

There have been numerous studies on suicide related to lifespan issues. In most all Western countries, suicide is extremely uncommon in young children but rises steadily after puberty with the risk increasing with age (Buda & Tsuang, 1990). Recent studies have confirmed

0-8493-0926-3/02/$0.00+$1.50
© 2002 by CRC Press LLC

earlier investigations, but in men rather than women, where the rates actually have decreased in recent years (Kaplan & Sadock, 1996). The rates of suicide in younger men appear to be rising, and recent studies have shown a slight decline in the suicide rate among older people. Williams (1997) explains the rise in suicide in young males as caused by the increase of working class men who are unemployed and may be experiencing significant economic hardship. This group is also most likely to abuse alcohol and other drugs.

MEDICAL ILLNESS AS A RISK FACTOR

Perhaps more than any other factor, medical illness is associated with an increased risk of suicide (Druss & Pincus, 2000). Psychological autopsies performed on completed suicides have found general medical disorders substantially raise the risk for completed suicide. Several other studies have shown certain medical illnesses are associated with unusually high rates of suicide. For example, the risk of suicide among epileptic patients is 4 times greater than the general population and 25 times greater for temporal lobe epileptics (e.g., Rosenfeld, Breitbart, Stein, et al., 1999; Chochinov, Wilson, Enns, & Lander, 1998). Also, people suffering from peptic ulcer, Huntington's chorea, spinal cord injuries, AIDS, and those undergoing renal dialysis experience higher rates of suicide compared to the general medical population.

Cancer is particularly associated with an increase in suicide. Although the overall incidence is low, patients with cancer are at two times increased risk for committing suicide when compared to the population at large (Fox, Stanek, Boyd, et al., 1982). One study examining male cancer patients (Marshall, Burnett, & Brasure, 1983) showed there was a 50 to 100% greater likelihood of suicide among male cancer patients when compared to the general population. For women, the risk was increased by 30 to 50%. Suicidal behavior is particularly prevalent immediately following the diagnosis of cancer and in the beginning of treatment for men (Fox, Burnett, & Brasure, 1983). Apparently this difference in sexes disappears roughly 2 years after the diagnosis.

Investigations have identified several factors that are likely to increase the risk of suicide in cancer patients. These include significant disability, delirium, prognosis, disfigurement, feelings of hopelessness, and pain (e.g., Allebeck & Bolund, 1991; Hietanen & Lonnqvist, 1991; Chochinov, et al., 1998). History of psychiatric disturbance, poor family support, psychological disorder, especially depression, substance abuse, pain, and family history of suicide all may be additional risk factors for cancer patients but are not specific to cancer.

In a recent study, Henderson and Ord (1997) studied 241 patients who were diagnosed with head and neck cancer. They studied these patients over a 5-year period between 1991 and 1996. The patients' medical charts were examined to identify patients who had committed suicide, had expressed suicidal intent, or refused therapy preferring to die. The results showed 1.2% of their sample committed suicide. Two patients admitted to suicidal intent and an additional four patients refused treatment. They concluded that head and neck cancer patients have some of the same risk factors as other cancer patients but appear particularly prone to suicide because there is often significant disfigurement after treatment, and many of these patients use alcohol, have poor social support and may become socially isolated because their speech apparatus interferes with speaking. In addition, these patients also report other changes in quality of life including decreased smell, interference in taste for foods, and inability to chew foods and swallow.

It is interesting to speculate that some somatic diseases, like cancer, may pose a greater risk of suicide because of the alteration of certain neurochemical processes such as the availability of serotonin or by some other mechanism (Stenager, Stenager, & Jensen, 1994). The problem is compounded by the use of various medications that can precipitate mood disturbance and cognitive impairment and by various medical illnesses that can cause an organic mood disturbance, not necessarily by altering brain chemicals but by some other pathway.

Studies have shown the risk of suicide rises in patients with a general medical illness, even when co-morbid factors, such as depression or pain, are controlled for. In one study, Druss and Pincus (2000) showed a significant association between various medical conditions and suicidality that persisted after adjusting for depressive illness and alcohol use. In this investigation, the authors examined the presence of a medical illness in more than 7500 individuals, ages 17 to 39 years of age. They administered the Diagnostic Interview Schedule as part of a national survey. The information collected from this survey included any incidence of lifetime suicidal ideation and suicide attempts. Also assessed were common medical illnesses, presence of major depression and alcohol usage. One purpose of the study was to determine if there was a relationship between medical illness and suicidality after controlling for psychiatric morbidity. The results show 16% of the respondents without medical illness described suicidal ideation at some point in their lives; whereas, individuals with a general medical condition reported a 25% lifetime incidence of suicidal ideation. The figure was as high as 35% in those individuals who reported two or more medical illnesses. The sample on the whole reported a 5.5% incidence of attempted suicide whereas 9% of the respondents with a medical illness made a suicide attempt and 16% of those with two or more medical conditions had attempted suicide. After controlling for major depression and alcohol use as well as certain demographic characteristics, the results showed that the presence of a medical condition predicted a 1.3 times increase in the likelihood of suicidal ideation. Certain medical illnesses showed a much higher increase in the incidence of suicidal ideation. For example, cancer and asthma were each associated with more than a fourfold increase in the likelihood of a suicide attempt.

Although medical illness by itself is associated with an increased risk of suicidality, clearly when co-morbid psychiatric conditions, such as depression and substance abuse are present, along with a number of demographic and lifespan issues, the risk increases dramatically (Williams, 1997). Persistent pain is another factor in the medically ill patient that can raise suicidal risk. This was demonstrated clearly by Stenager et al. (1994) who examined a sample of suicide attempters admitted to a department of psychiatry. Each patient underwent a structured interview examining a multitude of factors that may have led up to the suicide attempt. The results show 52% of the patients were shown to have a somatic disease, and 21% were taking analgesics daily for pain. The patients experiencing a physical illness differed from other suicide attempters on a variety of measures including depression scores, age, pain, and the presence of psychoses. The authors noted fewer of the physically ill subjects reported significant psychopathology, and those with significant pain were more often depressed and abused medications. They concluded the risk of parasuicide for subjects with a physical illness, but without depression, was significantly less. In a smaller sample of successful suicides, they noted the subjects were older and there was also a tendency toward painful somatic diseases and depression, increasing the risk for suicidality.

Venkoba (1990) reviewed the literature on the relationship between somatic disease and suicide. The investigation included examining the association between pain from physical illnesses, like duodenal ulcer, and suicide. Some of the conclusions reached indicated patients suffering from physical illnesses associated with pain, especially when scores on depression and hopelessness were high, were associated with significantly increased suicidal behavior.

In a 5-year follow-up study, Nielsen, Wang, and Bille-Brahe (1990) also concluded that depression and physical illness represented the greatest risk for suicide. In addition, they showed that subjects reporting no depression and pain contacted their primary care providers more often before attempting suicide. Obviously, patients with a somatic illness and depression are especially susceptible to suicidal behavior. This is particularly true for older patients with painful somatic diseases and depression.

The relationship between somatic disease and suicidality is clear. Patients with a variety of illnesses are at increased risk, and the problem is compounded by a number of factors including depression, pain, and lifespan. These findings also extend to chronic, nonmalignant pain

patients. Studies have shown that these patients are at greater risk for depression and suicide than the general population. Fishbain, Cutler, Rosomoff, and Rosomoff (1997) examined 18 studies that looked at the association of chronic pain and suicide. He concluded that suicidal ideation, suicidal attempts, and suicide completions are commonly found in chronic pain populations. He also noted that chronic pain patients usually show other suicidal risk factors, especially depression. He concluded that chronic pain is a significant suicide risk factor. He cautioned that a careful search for co-morbid risk factors needs to be accomplished when evaluating the chronic pain patient.

In summary, it is well-established that one of the most significant risk factors for suicide is somatic illness. Medical illness is associated with 30 to 50% of attempted and successful suicides. Certain medical conditions such as cancer epilepsy, AIDS, spinal cord injuries, and chronic pain pose increased risk. In most cases, the co-occurrence of depression, especially associated with feelings of hopelessness, increases the risk of suicide. Evidence from various studies indicates that although medical illness poses a significant risk factor for suicide, rarely does the patient attempt or commit suicide in the absence of a psychiatric disorder.

UNDERSTANDING PAIN, SUFFERING, AND SUICIDE

Medical illness increases the risk for suicide. There are a number of factors that appear to compound the problem including pain, especially chronic pain, and depression associated with feelings of hopelessness. Efforts to understand the relationships among pain, depression, and suicide have traditionally relied upon the biomedical model. This disease model of pain has been useful for promoting the development of various analgesic medications and neuroablative techniques that have shown some success in pain management.

BIOMEDICAL MODEL

In the strictest sense, the biomedical model posits that pain results from a disturbance in nerve pathways, and pain intensity is presumed to be a function of the degree of physical damage. Pain is conceived as a closed, unmodulated, unidirectional system. The affective quality of pain is thought to be incidental to the underlying disease and strongly correlated to the signal intensity of pain. The degree of disability associated with pain is considered directly proportional to the underlying impairment, and changes in disability, depression, and suffering occur by reducing the signal intensity of pain. Dramatic displays of pain behavior associated with few physical findings are often attributable to psychological overlay, and pain is viewed as symptomatic and never a problem in and of itself.

Limitations of the biomedical approach are numerous, especially when applied to the understanding of persistent pain of a nonmalignant nature. Studies conducted as far as back as the 1950s show pain and the disability and suffering associated with it, are often poorly correlated to biological disturbance (Melzack & Wall, 1983). How patients interpret and apply meaning to their pain, and the social and environmental factors with which they come in contact also have been shown to affect pain and the suffering associated with it (Melzack & Wall, 1983).

BIOPSYCHOSOCIAL MODEL

The biopsychosocial model (Turk & Waddell, 1992) maintains that pain usually is initiated by nociception with accompanying sensory perception, but pain is also influenced by emotional, social, and environmental factors. In this conceptualization, each factor interacts in complex ways to affect pain. It carries with it the overriding assumption that changing the pain experience requires attention to multiple influences.

The biopsychosocial model also assumes that the affective quality of pain is not simply an incidental response to pain, but is related to multiple factors such as how the pain is interpreted, the social consequences of the pain, pre-morbid psychological vulnerabilities, perceived loss of self, and so forth.

DISABILITY AND SUFFERING DEFINED

Disability and suffering are often poorly related to underlying physical impairment, especially in chronic pain (Turk & Waddell, 1992). According to the biopsychosocial model, this finding can be easily assimilated because non-physiologic influences are recognized to affect disability and suffering, such as fear of pain or type of job. Clearly, reducing pain does not always decrease disability and suffering. Because physical disturbance, disability, and suffering are often poorly related due to multiple physical, environmental, and social factors, it is erroneous to attribute the lack of any clear relationship to so-called psychological overlay.

Suffering and the disability associated with pain from the perspective of the biopsychosocial model exert independent influences on pain and, as emphasized above, are not incidental to physical impairment. This has important implications for the understanding of pain and in the treatment of depression and prediction of suicidal risk associated with pain. If suffering and disability are simply consequences of underlying organic pathology and related proportionally to the degree of physical disturbance, then treatment efforts directed at symptomatic relief of pain to affect a change in suffering and disability would be effective. However, clearly this has been shown not to be the case (Turk & Waddell, 1992).

Suffering is defined as "a state of severe distress associated with events that threaten the intactness of the person. It occurs when an impending destruction of the person is perceived; suffering continues until the threat has passed" (Cassell, 1982). According to Fordyce (1988), this definition emphasizes the anticipatory nature of suffering and events that are likely to precipitate threats to the self or the intactness of the person. In other words, suffering is an emotional experience triggered in anticipation of events the person perceives as potentially threatening. Although related to the signal intensity of pain, suffering is independent. For example, a patient with chronic pain may experience persistent pain related to a number of underlying pain mechanisms, including disc disruption. The suffering expressed by the patient is related to the sensory experience of pain triggered by the disc pathology, but is also affected by the understanding the patient has about the pain, fear of pain and re-injury, possibly the type of job to which the patient is expected to return, and what the patient thinks may happen in the future as long as the pain persists. Suffering is diminished not simply by affecting a change in pain intensity, which is often not possible, but by reducing the perceived threat associated with pain the patient is experiencing. This could be as direct as educating the patient more effectively about the underlying nature of the pain problem and offering reassurances that being bound to a wheelchair is not likely to happen if a modicum of activities are initiated.

Fordyce (1988) observed that clinicians often confound pain and suffering. This carries with it important implications because it places paramount importance on correcting the physical disturbance before the relief of pain, as well as suffering, can occur. As Fordyce wrote, "Suffering behaviors may occur for many reasons and may have little or no relationship to nociception."

Like suffering, disability, or the patient's diminished capacity, is frequently unrelated to nociception, especially in chronic pain (Turk & Waddell, 1992). Patients are disabled for a variety of reasons including physical impairment. But, patients are also disabled because of fear, uncertainty associated with pain, and co-morbid factors such as depression. Turk and Waddell (1992) in a series of studies showed that the correlation coefficients were minimal to modest at best among various medical conditions and expressed disability. In lower back pain, they found a 0.5 correlation and in arthritic conditions only a 0.3 correlation between underlying damage and disability.

THE ROLE OF COGNITIONS AND EMOTIONS

It should be clear by now that cognitive factors play an important role mediating in pain perception and the expression of suffering and disability. One of the first studies demonstrating the influence of beliefs, including attributions in pain, was conducted by Henry Beecher

(1959). He showed wounded soldiers requested far fewer narcotics and reported less intense pain experiences when compared to civilian post-surgery patients. Beecher concluded after interviews with the soldiers that the meaning of pain was entirely different for them. If they survived the battle, it meant a ticket home and out of the range of danger. In other words, they attached a different meaning to the pain experience than civilians who may have interpreted the pain as a nuisance and a disruption of daily activities (Fordyce, 1988).

There are countless other studies showing how patients interpret their pain experiences and that the meaning they give to their pain affects not only pain perception, but also disability and suffering levels (c.f., Wall, 2000). In particular, patients who perceive greater levels of threat, more ambiguity, and feel more vulnerable, possibly related to a loss of self-control and the inability to cope, express more distress. This can translate into heightened levels of pain-related suffering and disability (Chapman & Gavrin, 1999).

Underlying the experience of pain and influencing in part all the different facets of the pain experience, especially levels of suffering, is the emotional tone of the patient. Patients who are more anxious and depressed cope more poorly with pain and with the problems a medical illness presents. Depression is a common consequence of persistent pain (Fishbain, 1999). It compounds the problem of pain by heightening a sense of threat leading to increased levels of suffering (Tearnan & Lewandowski, 1992). Depression also increases fatigue and contributes to lowered self-confidence for managing day-to-day problems.

CONCEPTUAL FRAMEWORK

Medical illness raises the risk for suicide because somatic disease, especially associated with persistent pain, strains coping abilities. This increases the likelihood that the patient will attribute failures to cope to personal inadequacies, and uncertainty about the future and worries about the medical condition will cause further loss and deterioration of the self. This often leads to feelings of depression, especially in individuals sensitive to loss of control (Duggleby, 2000). Depression heightens the sense of vulnerability because a failure to cope is thought to be more probable. Threat is judged more significantly when a sense of vulnerability increases, leading to increased suffering. Feelings of hopelessness result from the belief that suffering will never stop and, as a result, nothing positive will ever come of the future. Suicide is in response to a belief of hopelessness (Chochinov, et al., 1998). Death is seen as an option to end the suffering and prevent a future without hope.

Evidence for this conceptual understanding of how suicide may result from a medical illness is based on a number of studies including investigations showing a strong link between pain and the later development of depression (Fishbain, et al., 1997). Suffering as it relates to the expectation of threat was first talked about in the pain literature by Fordyce (1988), but was borrowed originally from social psychology (Higgins, Bond, Klein, & Strauman, 1986) and work by Cassell (1982) suggesting psychological distress and emotional upheaval occur when events threaten the intactness of the person.

The relationship between psychological distress and suffering also was demonstrated by Tearnan and Lewandowski (1992). They showed that chronic pain patients consistently identified certain factors when asked to report what they were most concerned about when their pain increases. These included the expectation that the pain will negatively impact others, contribute to a loss of productivity, cause physical harm, lead to psychological problems, and cause more pain. These five groupings were supported in factor analytic studies sampling over 600 pain patients. The patients scoring high on all concerns, conceptualized collectively as pain suffering, expressed more depression and distress in general. They also reported more problems associated with overall pain and disability, especially activity interference.

According to Chapman and Gavrin (1999), suffering represents "a disparity between what one expects of oneself and what one does or is. A serious disruption in the psychosocial trajectory of human life, such as the onset of uncontrolled pain, can cause such a disparity and thereby compel changes in a sense of self." For example, the development of a painful shoulder would probably have little impact on a man working in a sedentary capacity but could be devastating to a professional football player "because it affects what he or she is and can hope to be in the future" (Chapman and Gavrin, 1999).

Patients with persistent pain, largely as a result of trying to cope with the various stressors a somatic illness can cause, can become consumed by negative events they anticipate will occur in the future (Fordyce, 1988). This is fueled by the often ambiguous nature of physical illness and the inability of the medical system to assist patients in coping more effectively with a pain problem that is unlikely to dissipate completely.

The suffering that results from medical illnesses with persistent pain occurs as a consequence of self-blame for failure to adequately cope and for trying to fight against the onslaught of numerous stressors patients frequently feel ill equipped to manage (Chapman & Gavrin, 1999), particularly those patients prone to feel out of control.

It should be mentioned that even though depression resembles suffering because both are associated with negative thoughts, feelings of exhaustion, and general psychological impairment, suffering is not a pathologic state (Chapman & Garvin, 1999). Depression, unlike suffering, is associated with self-blame and self-depreciation.

A considerable body of research has shown that hope-lessness is correlated highly with suicidal ideation in general medical patients and is a significant predictor of eventual completed suicide (Chochinov, et al., 1998). Physical disease by itself is seldom decisive for the suicidal act (Williams, 1997). Also, depression has been defined differently by various investigators but is generally associated with measures of discouragement and pessimism and is not based fully on medical prognosis. Chochinov et al. (1998) defined hopelessness as encompassing the capacity to find purpose in living. Patients experiencing medical illnesses who have lost the capacity to believe the future will change will generally express hopelessness and are at increased risk for suicide.

In an important review by Hall, Platt, and Hall (1999), 100 patients who made severe suicide attempts were studied. They were interviewed by the authors, and their charts carefully reviewed. All patients required treatment in the emergency room or were admitted to intensive care or a surgical unit of a large urban hospital. Results from the study suggested that the symptoms most predictive of severe suicide attempts were beliefs of hopelessness and insomnia; severe, relentless anxiety, often with intermittent panic attacks, depressed mood, recent conflict or loss, and alcohol abuse. The majority of the patients developed symptoms within 3 months before the suicide attempt, and most had experienced a significant loss. The majority of the patients attempted suicide impulsively. Interestingly, the majority of the patients described fleeting, intermittent, transient but not disturbing thoughts of suicide and no persistent thoughts of a plan. Particularly relevant to this discussion was that 41% of patients had some type of chronic medical illness. Most of the patients had never attempted suicide before and 88% had sought counseling from a healthcare provider in the month prior to the attempt.

PHYSICIAN-ASSISTED SUICIDE

End-of-life issues have become increasingly important as attention shifts from curative to palliative care for patients nearing the end of life. Issues of withdrawing or withholding life support treatment and the legalization of physician-assisted suicide in Oregon have stimulated discussions among many health professionals and represent a significant challenge to groups traditionally concerned with preserving rather than facilitating death. The ethical and moral dilemmas faced by healthcare professionals are outside the scope of this discussion. Instead, a brief review of issues important to pain, depression, and hopelessness are presented as explanations for why patients request assistance from the physician to end their lives prematurely.

Physician-assisted suicide remains a controversial issue, but one that has been discussed more openly in the

past decade (Cohen, Steinberg, Hails, Dobscha, & Fischel, 2000). Disagreements largely revolve around whether patients who request end-of-life measures have reached this decision through rational thought processes or are their requests triggered by pathological depression (Cohen, et al., 2000). The available data are not conclusive enough to settle the issues physicians must confront in deciding whether or not to actively end a patient's life or discontinue treatment. However, several well-controlled studies have recently shown that patients who request physician-assisted suicide score high on formal measures of depression and hopelessness (Shuster, Breitbart, & Chochinov, 1999). Unfortunately, physicians often place very little emphasis on ruling out depressive illness, considering depression a natural consequence to terminal illness (Haghbin, Streltzer, & Danko, 1998). This is particularly disconcerting because a substantial minority of physicians report a lack of confidence in diagnosing depression, and many admit to discomfort making a psychological referral (Haghbin, et al., 1998).

There are many healthcare professionals who believe the rational decision to end life occurs in only a minority of patients and palliative care efforts need to be made before any decision to hasten death is reached. This includes assessment of depression and hopelessness. Studies in Oregon show that patients who died through physician-assisted suicide were 7.3 times more likely than controlled patients to be concerned about loss of independence and 9 times more concerned about loss of bodily function, suggesting anxiety and possibly depression in the generation of decisions to end life (Cohen, et al., 2000).

In the area of pain control, studies have shown patients who request physician-assisted suicide do so because of depression and helplessness rather than from physical pain (e.g., Emanuel, Fairclough, & Emanuel, 2000; Emanuel, 1997). Depression can be caused in part by poor pain control but is often related to a multitude of other factors supporting discussions made earlier on pain, suffering, and disability. In one large study van der Maas, van Delden, and Pijnenborg (1992) showed only 5% of the euthanasia cases were motivated solely by pain. Another study by Emanuel and Emanuel (1998) found patients experiencing pain were no more likely to request euthanasia than those without pain.

DISCUSSION AND TREATMENT IMPLICATIONS

Medical illness is a significant risk factor for suicide, particularly in patients who are depressed and expressing beliefs of hopelessness. The presence of pain compounds the problem and may increase the likelihood of suicide.

It is important healthcare providers learn to formally assess and screen for depression and beliefs of hopelessness in general medical populations, particularly in patients with medical conditions where persistent pain is present. Studies have shown that when less formal screening is provided, even professionally trained mental health professionals often have difficulty recognizing the presence of depressive symptoms and hopelessness (Haghbin, 1998).

It is important to also recognize in the assessment process that a general medical illness increases the likelihood of suicide but having more than one physical illness raises the risk of suicide substantially (Druss & Pincus, 2000). Even when depression and alcohol use are adjusted, the relationship between medical illness and suicidality persists. As Druss and Pincus suggest, perhaps depression and alcohol use do not necessarily mediate the relationship between suicide and medical illness. Possibly other intermediate factors, such as disability, disruption of social supports, and chronic pain, may make an individual regard his life as no longer worth living.

It is worth emphasizing that while studies have shown that depression and suicide are related, most patients admitting to suicidal behavior do not meet criteria for major depression. This strongly suggests assessing for suicidal ideation and intent, aside from examining for signs of depression (Druss & Pincus, 2000).

It is imperative that healthcare professionals, not just mental health professionals, talk openly about depression, death, and suicide with their patients. There is no evidence these discussions will trigger suicidal behavior (Henderson & Ord, 1997). In fact, more evidence exists that these discussions help correct misconceptions, establish a strong rapport between the clinician and patient, and improve a patient's sense of personal control (Henderson & Ord, 1997).

In cases where a patient admits to thoughts of suicide, either through formal screening or in discussions with the patient, referral to a psychologist, psychiatrist, or other appropriate mental health professional should be made. The discomfort many health professionals feel about initiating this type of referral needs to be addressed, mostly by the professional, because, as the author generally has found, if talked about in an open and honest manner, patients are not offended or upset but generally see the importance of addressing psychosocial issues.

Thoughts of suicide and the risk of suicide should be assumed by the clinician when working with the medical patient experiencing persistent pain. Addressing the problem directly, assessing for it aggressively in an open and honest manner, and applying solid pain management techniques in an interdisciplinary setting, including attention to behavioral medicine issues, are appropriate measures for dealing with the potential problem of suicide. This requires attention to effective pain management practices including educating the patient about better ways to manage and cope with pain, reducing the ambiguity and uncertainty about the future and the medical illness associated with the pain, eliminating medications likely to precipitate depression and confusion, and encouraging the patient to increase levels of activity using the skills of pacing.

It is important that under certain circumstances extraordinary measures be taken to prevent the possibility of suicide, particularly when patients express depression, beliefs of hopelessness, excessive alcohol use, and are reporting severe levels of anxiety and/or panic attacks. Recent losses of close personal relationships, global insomnia, and a sense that the medical condition is deteriorating are signs of which the clinician needs to be particularly aware. In addition, patients out of work and unable to find jobs, patients who are unskilled and feel disenfranchised, and mothers with few social supports are particularly prone to attempt suicide (Williams, 1997).

An examination of the many risk factors for suicide reveals the prevalence of these signs within the pain population. Although single-modality, unidimensional treatment approaches might be appropriate for short-term transient pain, they are inappropriate for persistent pain, especially because pain is rarely a symptom that exists in isolation. For the nonmalignant chronic pain patient, education, attention to emotional factors, focus on function rather than cure, and attention to other problems such as sleep disturbance, are important in managing pain and should reduce the risk of suicide. These same general treatment recommendations are suitable for the cancer patient, except the physician should make every effort to prevent the pain and to relieve it promptly. Also, fears about cancer need to be addressed and, like the nonmalignant pain patient, what patients think about is important, especially in efforts to alleviate their fears and correct misconceptions.

It is helpful to conceptualize pain as a stressor that can promote a destructive stress response, leading to a variety of physiologic, cognitive, and behavioral consequences such as fatigue, myalgia, and impaired cognitive functioning (Chapman & Gavrin, 1999). Addressing the pain problem by reducing the stress of pain and its consequences can involve reducing the unpleasant sensation of pain, altering the perception of unpleasantness or the consequences of loss that are associated with pain, and modifying the body's response to the stress through medications or relaxation. Developing skills to manage the stressors more effectively, including pacing of activities, interacting more effectively with physicians to participate in care, and understanding the mechanism of pain also may be important.

The essential focus of treatment, however, starts with the recognition that the problems medical patients in pain present with are not alleviated by attention just to the sensation of pain. They are best dealt with when attention is directed to a multitude of other factors. It is up to the clinician to formulate what problems are best managed to affect a change in patients. For example, in certain patients, treating the depression and beliefs of hopelessness with cognitive restructuring techniques might be the most effective approach, whereas other patients might benefit more from reducing their fears through simple physical therapy activities. Still, in other patients, attention to social factors and isolation might be the best approach to affect change in mood, pain, sleep, and hopefully suicidal risk.

Whatever specific treatment measures are applied to affect change, it is important that they sustain hope, reduce uncertainty, contribute to pain acceptance and, in some cases, encourage patients to turn their attention to spiritual needs (Duggleby, 2000).

REFERENCES

Allebeck, P., & Bolund, C. (1991). Suicides and suicide attempts in cancer patients. *Psychological Medicine, 21,* 979–984.

Beecher, H.K. (1959). *Measurement of subjective responses.* New York: Oxford University Press.

Boor, M. (1980). Relationship between employment rates and suicide rates in eight countries: 1962–1967. *Psychological Reports, 47,* 1095–1101.

Buda, M., & Tsuang, M.T. (1990). The epidemiology of suicide: Implications for clinical practice. In S. Blumenthal & D. Kupfer (Eds.), *Suicide over the life cycle: Risk factors, assessment and treatment of suicidal patients.* Washington, D.C.: American Psychiatric Press.

Cassell, E.J. (1982). The nature of suffering and the goals of medicine. *New England Journal of Medicine, 306,* 639–645.

Chapman, C.R., & Gavrin, J. (1999). Suffering: The contributions of persistent pain. *Lancet, 353,* 2233–2237.

Charlton, J., Kelly, J.S., Dunnell, R., Evans, B., Jenkins, R., & Wallis, R. (1992). Trends in (factors associated with) suicide deaths in England and Wales. *Population Trends (London),* 10–16 and 34–42.

Chochinov, H.M., Wilson, K.G., Enns, M., & Lander S. (1998). Depression, hopelessness, and suicidal ideation in the terminally ill. *Psychosomatics, 39,* 366–370.

Cohen, L., Steinberg, M., Hails, K., Dobscha, S., & Fischel, S. (2000). Psychiatric evaluation of death-hastening requests: Lessons from dialysis discontinuation. *Psychosomatics, 41,* 3, 195.

Druss, B., & Pincus, H. (2000). Suicidal ideation and suicide attempts in general medical illnesses. *Archives of Internal Medicine, 160,* 1522.

Duggleby, W. (2000). Enduring suffering: A grounded theory analysis of the pain experience of elderly hospice patients with cancer. *Oncology Nursing Forum, 27* (5), 825.

Emanuel, E. (1997). The painful truth about euthanasia. *Wall Street Journal, 23,* 1, 123.

Emanuel, E.J., Fairclough, D.L., & Emanuel, L.L. (2000). Attitudes and desires related to euthanasia and physician-assisted suicide among terminally ill patients and their caregivers. *Journal American Medical Association, 284* (19), 2460–2468.

Emanuel, E.J., & Emanuel, L.L. (1998). The promise of a good death. *Lancet, Suppl. 2,* SII21–9.

Fishbain, D.A. (1999). The association of chronic pain and suicide. *Seminars in Clinical Neuropsychiatry, 4* (3), 221–227.

Fishbain, D.A., Cutler, R., Rosomoff, H.L., & Rosomoff, R.S. (1997). Chronic pain-associated depression: Antecedent or consequence of chronic pain? A review. *Clinical Journal of Pain, 13* (2), 116–137.

Fordyce, W. (1988). Pain and suffering: A reappraisal. *American Psychologist, 43* (4), 276–283.

Fox, B.H., Stanek, E.J., Boyd, S.C., et al. (1982). Suicide rates among cancer patients in Connecticut. *Journal of Chronic Disease, 35,* 89.

Haghbin, Z., Streltzer, J., & Danko, G. (1998). Assisted suicide and AIDS patients: A survey of physicians' attitudes. *Psychosomatics, 39,* 1, 18.

Hall, R., Platt, D., & Hall, R. (1999). Suicide risk assessment: A review of risk factors for suicide in 100 patients who made severe suicide attempts. *Psychosomatics, 40:*1, 18.

Henderson, J., & Ord, R. (1997). Suicide in head and neck cancer. *Journal of Oral and Maxillofacial Surgery, 55,* 1217–1221.

Hietanen, P., & Lonnqvist, J. (1991). Cancer and suicide. *Annals of Oncology, 2,* 19–23.

Higgins, E.T., Bond, R.N., Klein, R., & Strauman, T. (1986). Self-discrepancies and emotional vulnerability: How magnitude, accessibility, and type of discrepancy influence affect. *Journal of Personality and Social Psychology, 51,* 5–15.

Kaplan, H.I., & Sadock, B.J. (1996). *Pocket handbook of clinical psychiatry* (2nd ed.). Baltimore, MD: Williams & Wilkins.

Marshall, J.R., Burnett, W., & Brasure, J. (1983). On precipitating factors: Cancer as a cause of suicide. *Suicide and Life-Threatening Behavior, 13,* 15.

Melzac, R., & Wall, P.D. (1983). *The challenge of pain.* New York: Basic Books.

National Center for Injury Prevention and Control. (1999). Ten leading causes of death by age group. Atlanta: Centers for Disease Control and Prevention.

Nielsen, B., Wang, G.A., & Bille-Brahe, U. (1990). Attempted suicide in Denmark: Five years follow-up. *Acta Psychiatrica Scandinavica, 81,* 250–254.

Parker, S. (1998, October). Seeing suicide as preventable: A national strategy emerges. *Christian Science Monitor, 3.*

Rosenfeld, B., Breitbart W., Stein K., et al. (1999). Measuring desire for death among patients with HIV/AIDS: The schedule of attitudes toward hastened death. *American Journal of Psychiatry, 156,* 94–100.

Sainsbury, J., Jenkins, J., & Baert, A.E. (1981). *Suicide trends in Europe.* Copenhagen: World Health Organization,

Shuster, J., Breitbart, W., & Chochinov, H. (1999). Psychiatric aspects of excellent end-of-life care. *Psychosomatics, 40:*1, 1.

Stenager, E.N., Stenager, E., & Jensen, K. (1994). Attempted suicide, depression and physical diseases: A 1-year follow-up study. *Psychotherapy and Psychosomatics, 61,* 65–73.

Tearnan, B.H., & Lewandowski, M.J. (1992). The Behavioral Assessment of Pain Questionnaire. *Journal of the American Academy of Pain Management, 2*(4), 181–191.

Turk, D.C., & Waddell, G. (1992). Clinical assessment of low back pain. In D.C. Turk & R. Melzack (Eds.), *Handbook of pain assessment* (pp. 15–36). New York: Guilford.

van der Maas, P., van Delden, J., & Pijnenborg, L. (1992). Euthanasia and other medical decisions concerning the end of life. Amsterdam: Elsevier.

Venkoba, R. (1990). Physical illness, pain, and suicidal behavior. *Crisis, 11*(2), 48–56.

Wall, P. (2000). *Pain: The science of suffering.* New York: Columbia University Press.

Williams, M. (1997). *Cry of pain: Understanding suicide and self-harm.* London: Penguin Books.

63

Assessing the Veracity of Pain Complaints and Associated Disability

Michael F. Martelli, Ph.D., Nathan D. Zasler, M.D., F.A.A.P.M.&R., F.A.A.D.E.P., C.I.M.E., D.A.A.P.M., Keith Nicholson, Ph.D., Treven C. Pickett, A.B.D., Psy.D., and V. Robert May, Rh.D.

INTRODUCTION

Evaluation of pain complaints and pain-related disabilities presents a significant diagnostic challenge. In cases of clear, severe, and/or functionally disabling physical pathology and pain, the evaluations and opinions of most healthcare practitioners are fairly consistent. In most cases, however, where physical findings are less clear, practitioners who specialize in pain and disability assessments may express widely varying opinions. Medical evidence is often problematic or disputable and the relationship between physical findings and subjective report is frequently weak. Pain, ultimately, is a subjective complaint that is difficult to verify or refute (Hall & Pritchard, 1996; Merskey, 1986). Finally, despite recent biopsychosocial and psychophysiologic advances in terms of understanding, simplistic and dichotomous conceptualizations remain overly represented (Martelli, 2000).

Traditionally, pain and pain-related disability evaluations have been conducted by such specialists as physiatrists, orthopedists, neurologists, neurosurgeons, psychiatrists, psychologists, and neuropsychologists. Further, diagnosis and treatment are the presumed reasons for assessment, and the estimation of frank malingering, as well as significant exaggeration of symptoms, is generally estimated to be less than 20% (Martelli, Zasler, Mancini, & MacMillan, 1999). A recent review by Fishbain, Cutler, Rosomoff, and Rosomoff (1999) indicates that malingering might be present in between 1 and 10% of chronic

pain patients, but there are significant problems with the reliability of any such estimates and an absence of reliable methodologies for detecting malingering in chronic pain patients. However, it should be noted that pain evaluation referrals also frequently involve such contexts as healthcare insurance policy coverage, disability insurance policy application, social security disability application, personal injury litigation, worker's compensation claims, functional capacity evaluations, and determination of capacity for work. In these medicolegal situations, the incidence of symptom exaggeration and malingering may be significantly higher (Rohling & Binder, 1995; Binder & Rohling, 1996).

Importantly, the evaluation of pain complaint and pain-associated functional impairment and disability may be one of the more confounded and misunderstood areas of healthcare-related work. The task of making determinations regarding pain severity, impact, and related functional impairment and disability is fraught with potential obstacles and pitfalls. This is, of course, due to the poorly understood and complex nature of the deficits involved, as well as the lack of formal, scientifically validated conceptual models and "rating systems." Disentangling the multiple contributors to subjective pain experience and associated functional disability requires careful scrutiny.

Chronic pain patients may present with some response bias to report pain or related disability. In the present chapter, response bias is defined as a class of behaviors that reflects less than fully truthful, accurate, or valid symptom report and presentation. Importantly, response bias is a ubiquitous phenomenon affecting almost any domain of human self-report. However, in the context of medicolegal or insurance presentations, with which this chapter is primarily concerned, the prevalence or importance of such bias becomes more acute (Rohling & Binder, 1995; Binder & Rohling, 1996; Youngjohn, Burrows, & Erdal, 1995). Given frequent financial and other incentives to distort symptoms and performance during examinations conducted in medicolegal or insurance contexts (i.e., healthcare policy coverage, disability insurance, social security disability, personal injury litigation, worker's compensation claims, functional capacity, and work evaluations), assessment of examinee veracity and motivation to provide accurate and full effort during assessment becomes critical. The importance of detecting response biases or invalid symptoms is crucial with regard to increasing the likelihood of diagnostic accuracy. Accurate diagnosis is prerequisite to provision of appropriate and timely treatment and prevention of iatrogenic impairment and disability reinforcement; it is also critical to appropriate legal compensation decisions.

Medicolegal and insurance assessments, with their significant consequences of determination decisions regarding impairment and disability, require the following in order to ensure validity: (a) an accurate assessment of possible response bias to report pain or related disability; (b) an accurate assessment of attribution, i.e., whether pain and related problems are correctly being attributed to the compensable cause; and (c) sensitivity, specificity, utility, and ecological validity of assessment measures.

Blau (1984; 1992) has expounded on the importance of determining response biases and measuring true levels of impairment in medicolegal situations. Essentially, in this arena, an alleged victim of a wrongful act or omission attempts to establish (a) causality in order to demonstrate entitlement to compensation for damages, which is awarded based on (b) level of damages suffered. In cases of less obvious, clear-cut, and significant trauma with psychologic, neurologic, or soft tissue damage, causality and level of current and future damages are more difficult to prove and expert evaluation and opinion are heavily relied upon for making legal determinations. In the parallel insurance situation, the insured attempts to access entitlements to healthcare treatment and disability benefits, and expert evaluation and opinion are relied upon for making policy determinations. In both cases, financial and other incentives clearly represent motivational factors that increase the likelihood of response bias in the form of exaggerated or feigned symptoms.

EXAMINING PATIENT RESPONSE BIASES

Examinee response bias, or predilections toward less than fully valid, accurate, and effortful behavioral responses, can take several forms. Bias ranges from interpretations of symptoms that may be minimized to exaggerated or feigned, and that may be accurately or inaccurately attributed to different events. For instance, pre-existing symptoms may suddenly be attributed to an accident, symptoms previously not noticed suddenly may be given such vigilant attention that attention and anxiety alone produce significant increases, or an accident may cause an aging person to do a self-inventory of health that reveals symptoms due to aging that were present but previously minimized. Further, a heightened awareness or vigilance effect can lead to focusing and sensitization to problems which would otherwise be innocuous. In addition, environmental realities also exert influence over response to injury and symptoms. For example, the vastly different consequences for diagnoses of cancer vs. mild traumatic brain injury or back injury produce differential reinforcement; the former is clearly undesirable and negative, while the latter can result in highly desirable monetary compensation.

Martelli et al. (1999) reviewed the literature and found that the following injury context variables were associated with poorer post-injury adaptation and recovery, and increased likelihood of response bias.

1. Anger or resentment or perceived mistreatment
2. Fear of failure or rejection (e.g., damaged goods; fear of being fired after injury)
3. Loss of self-confidence and self-efficacy associated with residual impairments
4. External (health, pain) locus of control
5. Irrational fear of injury extension, reinjury, or pain
6. Discrepancies between personality/coping style and injury consequences (e.g., very physically active person with few intellectual resources who has a back injury)
7. Insufficient residual coping resources and skills
8. Prolonged inactivity resulting in disuse atrophy
9. Fear of losing disability status, benefits, and safety net
10. Perceptions of high compensability for injury
11. Preinjury job (task, work environment) dissatisfaction
12. Collateral (especially if "silent")
13. Inadequate and/or inaccurate medical information
14. Misdiagnosis, late diagnosis, or delays in instituting treatment
15. Insurance resistance to authorizing treatment or delays in paying bills
16. Retention of an attorney
17. Greater reinforcement for "illness" vs. "wellness" behavior
18. Dichotomous (organic vs. psychologic) conceptualizations of injury and symptoms

These variables represent vulnerability factors that can reduce effective coping with post-injury impairments and increase the likelihood of maladaptive coping and response bias.

Importantly, these variables are not mutually exclusive, and, as with the variables presented below, more than one can contribute to symptom report and presentation

Additional review of the literature, balanced with clinical experience, identifies the following significant sources of response bias that can be seen during examinations (Martelli, 2000).

1. Cultural Differences. For example, many non-Western cultures mix emotional and physical pain and symptoms at a conceptual and phenomenological level. Also, some cultures see failure to impose severe penalty/extract significant compensation for harm as a sign of weakness and disgrace in God's eyes.

2. Reactive Adversarial Malingering (RAM) based on fear, mistrust of the opposing side's honesty, or mistreatment (e.g., from assumed "facts" in many work settings and cultures, including plaintiff attorney groups) resulting in a deliberate pendulum-like overplaying of symptoms. This may be especially characteristic in persons/groups with tendencies toward suspiciousness, including immigrants, outsiders, or those who feel chronically underprivileged.

3. Conditioned Avoidance Pain-Related Disability (CAPRD), or, roughly, phobic or extreme anxiety reactions wherein activity (mental or physical) is associated with anticipation of an exacerbation of pain, with such stress possibly resulting in an actual exacerbation. Kinesiophobia and cogniphobia are two types.

4. Desperation Induced Malingering (DIM) or Desperation Induced Symptom Exaggeration (DISE), e.g., insecure immigrant workers, aging workers, tired workers, workers insecure about work changes, immigrants who tried introjection and feel resentful that they were not rewarded, persons who recently climbed back on the horse only to get knocked off again without belief they can climb back in the saddle one more time, workers fearing their own limited or declining abilities, real or imagined abuse from employers, family, etc., immigrants who feel rejected by the culture and feel entitled, immigrants who feel disillusioned because the new land was not everything they had hoped — i.e., those who believe this to be a viable solution to a desperate situation. Probably also included are those making desperate pleas for help and who, upon confronting tests that seem different and maybe easier than the real-life situations where they have problems, reduce effort to highlight their problems.

5. Sociopathic, Manipulative, and Opportunistic (SMO) types. These rather self-explanatory styles can be found in all groups.

6. Passive Aggressive or Impatient or Rebellious types, representative of those who resent others not listening to them and believing them at face value, and resent imposed evaluations or doctor's visits, especially ones that examine psychological function or motivation. They may play games with doctors by withholding or undermining procedures or treatments, and may especially alter performance or play games on tests that seem nonchallenging or unrelated to real life situations.

7. Psychologically Decompensated types, i.e., the extremely dysfunctional patient who is usually easily recognizable.

8. Those who don't take our examinations or tests as seriously as we do. The authors have some very limited but relevant survey data suggesting that plaintiffs may take our examinations a little more seriously than defendants. In contrast, weathermen seem to be taken more seriously than independent examiners by persons who have not graduated high school, while independent examiners seem to fare better with those who have been to college.

Importantly, a too often overlooked form of bias is one that is iatrogenic to the nature of the insurance and adversarial legal system. In an effort to elucidate expectancy influences and bias for persons sustaining injuries, Martelli, Zasler, and Grayson (2000) collected survey attitudinal data from professionals who work with injured Worker's Compensation (WC) patients. A summary of the preliminary data is offered in Table 63.1, broken down by the three sample groups: (1) disability evaluators, comprised of physicians, chiropractors, physical therapists, and vocational evaluators; (2) staff from a rehabilitation neuropsychology service; (3) attendees at a case management conference, including over 50% WC case managers. These data are quite compelling. Overall, approximately 25% of WC patients are believed to be exaggerating or malingering, with higher rates evidenced by WC case managers. This suggests a general skepticism and distrust faced by injured persons during evaluations. In contrast, the majority of professionals filling out the survey believed they would be treated unfairly by the WC system if they were injured, suggesting a general skepticism and distrust of the extant systems that fund evaluation and treatment of injury and disability.

TABLE 63.1
Survey of Attitudes Regarding Worker's Compensation (WC)

Question	Respondent Sample (%)		
	Disability Evaluating Professionals (N = 17)	Medical Psychology Service Staff (N = 7)	Case Managers (N = 16) (including 7 WC employees)
% Injured workers who fake/exaggerate/malinger	19.2	24.7	28.5
% Injured workers that WC insurance treats < fairly	49.2	62.5	23.2
% Employers who treat injured workers < fairly	53.5	41.2	32.7
Likelihood your employer would treat you < fairly	43.75	54.2	46.4
Likelihood WC would treat you if injured < fairly	60.0	65.9	48.9

Despite the preliminary nature of these data derived from small samples and the fact that generalizability across situations cannot be assumed, they nonetheless seem compatible with the levels of diffuse distrust observed by the authors in medicolegal situations. These data highlight the importance of considering the much different set of motivational factors that operate on examinees that present to independent evaluation. In addition, they strongly argue for deliberate and thorough preparation of examinees prior to the examination.

In an interesting theory about a major type of response bias in chronically disabled workers, Matheson (1988; 1990; 1991a; 1991b) conceptualized a "symptom magnification syndrome" based on a careful analysis of injured industrial workers. He defined this syndrome as a conscious or unconscious self-destructive (e.g., blocks return to productive activity) and socially reinforced pattern of symptoms, which are intended to control life circumstances of the sufferer, but which impede healthcare efforts. He further defines three major subtypes, and provides classification guidelines for evaluation via observation during performance of simulated work tasks completed within functional capacity evaluations. The Type I "refugee" is defined as displaying illness behavior that provides escape or avoidance of life situations perceived as unsolvable. Somatization, conversion, psychogenic pain, and hypochondriacal disorders are conceptualized as extreme subcategories for this type. The Type II "game player" employs symptoms for positive gain. Although this type seems associated with the psychiatric diagnosis of malingering, Matheson argues that true malingering is a medicolegal concept, while Type II symptom magnifying is a treatable self-destructive syndrome. The Type III "identified patient" is motivated by maintenance of the patient role as a means of life survival. Associated psychiatric diagnoses include factitious disorder (May, 1999).

Main and Spanswick (1995) also examined simulated or exaggerated incapacity in persons claiming physical disability. They identified a list of features associated with simulated or exaggerated incapacity. Features identified as primarily suggestive of simulated or exaggerated incapacity included

1. Failure to comply with reasonable treatment
2. Report of severe pain with no associated psychological effects
3. Marked inconsistencies in effects of pain on general activities
4. Poor work record; history of persistent appeals against awards
5. Previous litigation

Features identified as not primarily suggestive included

1. Mismatch between physical findings and reported symptoms
2. Report of severe or continuous pain
3. Anger
4. Poor response to treatment
5. Behavioral signs/symptoms

A brief review of important sources of bias, or threats to objectivity, which require assessment during evaluation of physical, sensory, and neurocognitive impairments follows.

ATTRIBUTION AND BIAS

Examinee attribution bias can confound accurate diagnosis. Examples include mistaking clinical entities like depression or sleep disturbance and concomitant physical, memory, or motivational problems for physical injury and pain-related sequelae. This can occur due to misattribution or over-attribution or retrospective attribution, or illusory correlation, or heightened awareness due to vigilance biases. Importantly, conditions like depression and sleep disturbance are reversible and may have even been present pre-injury without producing significant limitations. Furthermore, these factors may be interacting with true physical injury symptoms to increase distress, prolong impairment, and interfere with recovery. Finally, such factors as presence of vigilance to symptoms can increase physiologic arousal and lead to increased symptomatology and perceptions of impairment, in a vicious cycle.

Examiner misattribution can similarly occur. Only methodical medical and psychological assessment can differentiate sequelae secondary to, for example, brain injury from chronic pain. Tendencies toward over-diagnosis of brain injury-related disorders by brain injury specialists given abnormal neurocognitive findings and/or nonspecific somatic complaints not exclusively pathognomonic of brain injury can be avoided only through careful differential diagnosis. Brain injury specialists sensitized to neurologic symptoms have been observed by the authors to misdiagnose chronic pain sequelae as post-concussive symptoms, which may result in iatrogenic impairment associated with an escalation of medical costs, prolongation of inappropriate treatment, and eventual failure that produces helplessness and chronic disability (e.g., nonresolving post-concussive disorders) and misperceptions in the injured person. Conversely, similar observations have been made for psychiatrists and psychologists prone to infer psychiatric etiologies for all pathology, including pain and physical injury sequelae (Main & Spanswick, 1995; Martelli, Zasler, & Grayson, 1999a).

THE RESPONSE BIAS CONTINUUM

As indicated above, for the purposes of this chapter, response bias is defined as any behavioral predisposition involving less than fully truthful, accurate, and valid symptom report and presentation. This includes less than fully effortful behavioral responses displayed on formal and informal interview and examination procedures. Formal assessment of response bias, which is frequently lacking or only haphazardly attended to in most clinical examinations, represents the only assurance that clinical exam findings are accurate and valid reflections of pain severity, frequency, and functional impairment levels. Response bias appears best conceptualized on a continuum that extends from

1. Denial and unawareness of impairments,
2. Symptom minimization,
3. Symptom magnification/exaggeration to
4. Frank malingering.

Denial and unawareness refer to either psychologic or organic phenomenon wherein impairments are underappreciated due to dysfunction of brain operations subserving awareness or psychological repression to guard against distressful realizations. Symptom minimization is a related, but more consciously motivated desire, and usually involves an attempt to minimize the impact of undesirable functional restrictions or distress (Martelli, et al., 1999a).

Symptom magnification, in contrast, refers to exaggeration of impairment and can occur in relation to multiple factors and serves a wide range of psychological needs (e.g., efforts to legitimize latent dependency needs, resolve pre-existing life conflicts, retaliate against employer or spouse or other, reduce anxiety, exert a "plea for help," or solicit acknowledgment of perceived difficulties). Symptom exaggeration always promotes passivity and helplessness and an external locus of control and is a significant impediment to rehabilitation (Martelli, Zasler, & Grayson, 1999b).

Symptom exaggeration also can occur in patients with premorbid histories of psychologic problems who "latch on" to a specific diagnosis that not only becomes responsible for all life problems, but also promotes passivity and helplessness and an external locus of control. When patients are assessed for claims of major disability following uncomplicated mild whiplash or soft tissue injuries, nonorganic contributors should be closely scrutinized. Depression, post-traumatic stress disorders, anxiety conditions, and other psychiatric syndromes generally have a favorable psychological and functional prognosis given timely and appropriate assessment and treatment. Misdiagnosis of these conditions serves to promulgate misperceptions and amplify functional disability and healthcare costs.

Malingering, as defined in the DSM-IV (p. 683) (American Psychiatric Association, 1994) is "...the intentional production of false or grossly exaggerated physical or psychological symptoms, motivated by external incentives such as avoiding military duty, avoiding work, obtaining financial compensation, evading criminal prosecution, or obtaining drugs." Malingering should be suspected if any combination of the following is noted:

1. Medicolegal context of presentation
2. Marked discrepancies between claimed stress or disability and objective findings
3. The presence of Antisocial Personality Disorder

Therefore, measures of malingering, or deliberate symptom production for purposes of secondary gain, should always be administered in cases of medicolegal presentation, suspicion of any disincentive to exhibit full effort, or suspicion of sociopathic personality disorders.

According to Lipman's typology (1962), malingering can be categorized into four categories: (1) fabrication of nonexistent symptoms; (2) exaggeration of symptoms that are presented as worse than in actuality; (3) extension of symptoms that have actually improved or resolved; and (4) misattribution or fraudulent attribution of symptoms to an injury when they actually preceded, postdated, or are otherwise unrelated. Notably, exaggeration is considered much more frequent than fabrication, while more than one category can occur in a single person. Finally, as Miller (2001) notes, different combinations of types can occur in persons with more than one problem (e.g., chronic pain, PTSD, post-concussion syndrome), which can further co-occur with other psychological syndromes (e.g., somatoform and personality disorders).

IDENTIFYING RESPONSE BIAS

The difficulty with defining pain, actual accentuation of the pain response (e.g., hyperpathia) seen in some chronic pain problems, response bias to reported pain, and its possible deception, makes the assessment of pain-related complaints extremely challenging. Pain, defined as an unpleasant sensory and emotional experience associated with actual or potential tissue damage (Merskey, 1986), is a complex multidimensional subjective experience mediated by emotion, attitude, and perception. Unlike other modalities, it is not possible to devise simple signal detection paradigms for the evaluation of response bias given that this is a subjective experience with no clear objective referents, especially in the case of chronic pain associated with actual injury and nociception or abnormal function of the nervous system. Clearly, multiple variables may impact on pain reporting and behavior. For example, arousal, stress, tension, and anger all may exacerbate subjective reporting of pain and pain behavior, as may depression, through effect on physiologic function. Psychoemotional and psychosocial concomitants of chronic pain must also be appreciated, including loss of self-esteem, lowered frustration tolerance, depression, sexual dysfunction and decreased libido, and anger and guilt. Further, situational factors make additional contributions to pain-related complaints. The context of an exam, however, typically requires that psychological and physical pain factors be addressed individually, despite the fact that these components are typically inextricably intertwined with one another, as well as such affective conditions as depression and anxiety.

Physicians should be familiar with exam strategies designed to evaluate disorders with (a) probable "functional" components, or symptoms that seem more strongly associated with psychosocial vs. structural factors, as well as (b) feigned symptoms, including bedside exam techniques for physical and cognitive "malingering." Examples include such strategies as Hoover's test for evaluation of malingered lower extremity weakness, sideways/backward walking for assessment of feigned gait disturbance, and a positive Stenger's test on audiologic assessment for nonorganic hearing loss. Other tests that might be of value in the context of response bias detection on the physical examination include Mankopf's maneuver, strength reflex test, arm and/or wrist drop test, hip adductor test, axial loading test, Gordon-Welberry toe test, Bowlus and Currier test, Burns bench test, Magnuson's test, among others [(Babitsky, Brigham, & Mangraviti, 2000); see also Table 63.3 for a relatively comprehensive listing].

Some major exam findings that are inconsistent with structural lesions include patchy sensory loss, pain in a nondermatomal distribution, nonpronator drift, and/or astasia-abasia. Motor and other impairment inconsistencies that fluctuate or disappear under hypnosis, drug-assisted interviews or "presumed" nonobservation may certainly increase the index of suspicion regarding nonorganicity, although exceptions to this rule do exist. Faked hemiparesis is typically more common on the left side, perhaps due to the fact that most persons are right-hand dominant. Consistency regarding laterality of symptoms, particularly with referred pain and/or neurologic impairment, should be evaluated.

Clinicians evaluating chronic pain must be familiar with psychosocial syndromes that may present as pain, including

1. *Factitious disorder*, or the intentional production or feigning of physical symptoms, or exaggerated expression of physical conditions in order to adopt a sick role
2. *Somatoform disorders*, characterized by preoccupation with physical symptoms and pain that exceeds possible organic pathology
3. *Hypochondriasis*, or preoccupation with pain as part of a conviction that it is a part of a pernicious disease process
4. *Conversion disorder*, or the expression of frank psychiatric disorder via some symbolic transformation

Clinicians should also be familiar with symptoms related to pain imperception. Pain complaints should be assessed, in part, when of CNS origin as opposed to psychogenic, by concurrently assessing temperature perception, given that the same neural pathways mediate these sensations. When temperature sensation is preserved in the presence of a loss of pain sensation, after either brain or spinal cord injury, the deficit is not likely to be organic (the loss should occur contralateral to and below the level of the lesion). This point also belabors the fact of understanding the neuropathology/pathology of the lesion based on imaging studies and the implications that these findings have for anticipated clinical exam findings. Alleged pain imperception can be evaluated, as can any impairment for that matter, with appropriately designed forced choice testing. Additionally, examiners should realize that alleged pain imperception or loss of sensation is difficult to fake upon repeated bilateral stimulation. This is due to the fact that examinees who exaggerate rely on subjective strategies rather than truly responding to the strength of the stimuli. Therefore, assessments such as Von Frey hairs could be utilized in the aforementioned scenario to provide further objective evidence of feigned sensory deficits.

It is worth emphasizing that the presence of structural inconsistencies, a nonorganic syndrome and/or response bias does not necessarily exclude the diagnosis of another organic syndrome. This certainly complicates the process of disentangling multiple clinical entities that sometimes coexist. Unfortunately, the science and art of methodic differential diagnosis are too often underappreciated in the evaluation process (Martelli, et al., 2000).

A relevant screening procedure frequently used by physical therapists, doctors, and chiropractors for estimating when psychological factors are significantly influencing pain-related responses is the assessment for Waddell's Nonorganic signs (Waddell & Main, 1984; Waddell, Main, Morris, Paoloa, & Gray, 1984; Waddell, 1999). These are listed below:

Screening for Nonorganic Response Bias: Waddell Signs

1. Overreaction
   Guarding/limping, bracing, rubbing affected area, grimacing, sighing.
2. Tenderness
   Widespread sensitivity to light touch of superficial tissue.
3. Axial loading
   Light pressure to skull of standing patient should not significantly increase low back symptoms.
4. Rotation
   Back pain is reported when shoulders and pelvis are passively rotated in the same plane.
5. Straight leg raising
   Marked difference between leg raising in the supine and seated position.
6. Motor and sensory
   Giving way or cog wheeling to motor testing or regional sensory loss in a stocking or nondermatomal distribution (rule out peripheral nerve dysfunction).

Additional nonorganic signs include lower extremity giving way, no pain-free spells in the past year, intolerance of treatments; and emergency admissions to hospital with back trouble.

Importantly, the presence of Waddell's or other nonorganic signs does not exclude physical components as the cause of low back pain. Rather, they suggest only that psychological factors appear to be influencing the patient's responses and behavior. Notably, physical and psychological findings are not mutually exclusive, and psychological factors may more often be a result of low back pain than a cause (Simmonds, Kumar, & Lechelt, 1998). Further, recent reports strongly demonstrate the relationship between high levels of anxiety and nonorganic responses during physical exams in chronic low back pain (Hadjistauropoulos & LaChapelle, 2000). As such, the importance of minimizing anxiety-related response bias during exams should, therefore, be emphasized with regard to optimizing accurate performance and assessment. Clinicians should familiarize themselves with the wide variety of simple yet effective anxiety management interventions.

With regard to assessment of psychological/psychiatric, somatic, and neuropsychological impairments, including chronic pain, response bias represents an especially important threat to validity. Because these assessments usually begin with an interview about self-reported symptoms and subsequently rely heavily on standardized measures of performance on tests which are variably normed, their validity requires the veracity, cooperation, and motivation of the patient for obtaining valid performance measures. Recent evidence, however, strongly suggests that patients seen for presumptive injury-related impairments over-report preinjury functional status (Lees-Haley, Wil-liams, Zasler, Margulies, English, & Steven, 1997). This is especially true with post-concussive and pain related deficits because these symptoms often appear with similar frequency in the general population (Lees-Haley & Brown, 1993). In addition, the demonstrated ability of physicians and psychologists to accurately detect malingering in examinations and test protocols has been less than impressive (Hall & Pritchard, 1996; Loring, 1995). Nonetheless, various instruments, techniques, and strategies are available that have demonstrated at least some utility in detecting response bias, especially malingering, as a means of increasing confidence in appropriate motivation during examination, and hence the validity of assessment findings.

In Table 63.2, a general summary of hallmark and selected signs of response bias are presented. The signs are predicated on examination of inconsistencies and can certainly be applied to most aspects of comprehensive medical and psychological evaluations for chronic pain.

In Table 63.3, a summary of some very specific response bias detection measures and strategies, along with guidelines, is presented in an integrated format. Importantly, these strategies are presented as illustrations of indicators of important information for interpreting examination findings and test data within a larger context of multidisciplinary evaluation for chronic pain. This approach integrates contextual information, history, behavioral observation, interview data, collaborative data, and personality data with measures of effort or performance (or symptom exaggeration or malingering) and physical examination, medical and neuropsychological examination performance data. This approach potentially offers increased reliability with regard to estimating the degree to which an examinee is responding truthfully and exerting full effort or withholding or distorting effort or performance, and the degree to which specific and general test results from multiple assessment areas are reliable and valid and reflect true abilities.

TABLE 63.2
Response Bias: Hallmark Signs

1. Inconsistencies within and between the following (given absence of significant psychiatric, attentional, comprehension, or other disorders where inconsistencies are not uncommon):
   a. Reported symptoms
   b. Examination/test performance
   c. Clinical presentation
   d. Known diagnostic patterns
   e. Observed behavior (in another setting)
   f. Reported symptoms and exam/test performance
   g. Measures of similar abilities
   h. Similar tasks or tasks within the same exam or test (especially when difficult tasks are performed more easily than easy ones)
   i. Different examination sessions
2. Grossly impaired performance and extreme complaints
   a. Poorer performance and more extreme complaints vs. established expectancies or normative data for similar injury/illness
   b. Very poor performance on easy tasks (especially when presented as difficult)
   c. Failing tasks that all but severely impaired perform easily
3. Lack of specific diagnostic signs of impairment
4. Specific signs of exaggeration/dissimulation/malingering on psychological testing
   a. Minnesota Multiphasic Personality Inventory (MMPI/MMPI-2) Original and additional validity scales: L, F, Fb, Fp, Ds, K, VRIN, TRIN, F-K, Fake Bad, etc.
   b. Personality Assessment Inventory (PAI) Validity scales (inconsistency, infrequency, positive and negative impression management) and 8 malingering and 6 suspected malingering patterns
   c. Pain Assessment Battery (PAB): Symptom magnification, extreme beliefs frequency and other "validity" indicators
   d. Millon Behavioral Health Inventory (MBHI) validity scales (3)
   e. Hendler (i.e., Mensana Clinic) Back Pain Test: scores of 21–31 (exaggerating)
   f. Cognitive malingering detection tests (e.g., memorization of 15 items test, Digit Recognition Tests, Computerized Assessment of Response Bias, Word Memory Tests, Word Memory Test, Word Completion Memory Test, etc.).
5. Interview evidence
   a. Nonorganic temporal relationship of symptoms to injury
   b. Nonorganic symptoms, or symptoms that are improbable, absurd, overly specific or of unusual frequency or severity (e.g., triple vision)
   c. Disparate examinee history/complaints across interview or examiners
   d. Disparate corroboratory interview data vs. examinee report
6. Physical exam findings
   a. Nonorganic sensory findings
   b. Nonorganic motor findings
   c. Pseudoneurologic findings in the absence of anticipated associated pathologic findings
   d. Inconsistent exam findings
   e. Failure on physical exam procedures designed to specifically assess malingering

Empirical support exists indicating that each of these indicators has some utility in detecting dissimulation or suboptimal effort.* Examining the pitfalls and limitations of each of these procedures, both conceptual and methodological, is well beyond the scope of this chapter. However, increasing evidence exists for improved discrimination and increased reliability when multiple measures are employed. The conceptual approach offered by the proposed Motivation Assessment Profiling (MAP) is one where behavioral observation, interview, collaborative, historical, personality, and contextual data with neuropsychological and medical performance data and measures of effort or performance (or response bias) are integrated

as an optimal method for estimating the degree of effort or performance and the degree to which test results are reliable and valid and reflect actual abilities. Notably, in evaluation of response bias and malingering, as in evaluation of pre- and post-injury status, the following investigative tools may be used in conjunction with interviews and examination and testing: (1) school records; (2) medical records; (3) driver records; (4) service and criminal records; (5) employment records; (6) psychological/psychiatric records and reports; (7) interviews with family members, friends, teachers, and employers, etc.; (8) any other available materials (e.g., from attorneys through formal discovery).

Importantly, the strategies and guidelines offered in Table 63.3 are presented as important indicators for

* See starred references.

TABLE 63.3
Response Bias Detection Measures and Strategies

Pain Assessment Measures with Built-In Response Bias Indicators

Pain Assessment Battery (PAB), Research Edition	Symptom Magnification Frequency (SMF) > 40%
Proposed clinical hypothesis procedure evaluating	Extreme Beliefs Frequency (EBF) > 35%
	Four other "validity" indicators (i.e., alienation, rating percent of max, % extreme ratings (2 scales))
Millon Behavioral Health Inventory (MBHI)	Elevations on 3-item validity scale
Hendler (i.e., Mensana Clinic) Back Pain Test	Scores of 21–31 (Exaggerating)
	Scores > 31 (Primary psychological influence)

Medical Indicators

Hoover's test	Test for malingered lower extremity weakness associated with normal crossed extensor response
Astasia-abasia	"Drunken type" gait with near-falls but no actual falls to ground
Nonorganic sensory loss	Patchy sensory loss, midline sensory loss, large scotoma in visual field, tunnel vision
Nonorganic upper extremity drift	Long tract involvement results in pronator type drift; proximal shoulder girdle weakness and malingering typically present with downward drift while in supination
Stenger's Test	Test for malingered hearing loss during audiologic evaluation
Gait discrepancies when observed vs. not observed	If organic, should be consistent regardless of whether observed or not
Gait discrepancies relative to direction of requested ambulation	Gait for a patient with hemiparesis should present similarly in all directions; malingerers do not as a rule practice a feigned gait in all directions
Forearm pronation, hand clasping, and forearm supination test for digit/finger sensory loss	Malingered finger sensory loss is difficult to maintain in this perceptually confusing, intertwined hand/finger position
Pain vs. temperature discrepancies	Because both sensory modalities run in the spinothalamic tract, they should be found to be commensurately impaired contralateral to the side of the CNS lesion
Lack of atrophy in a chronically paretic/paralytic limb	Lack of atrophy in a paralyzed/paretic limb suggests the limb is being used or is getting regular electrical stimulation to maintain mass
Impairment diminishes under influence of sodium amytal, hypnosis or lack of observation	All these observations are most consistent with nonorganic presentations including consideration of malingering or conversion disorder
Incongruence between neuroanatomical imaging and neurologic examination	Lack of any static imaging findings on brain CT or MRI in the presence of a dense motor or sensory deficit suggests nonorganicity
Arm drop test	An aware patient malingering profound alteration in consciousness or significant arm paresis will not let his own hand, when held over his head, drop onto his face
Presence of ipsilateral findings when implied neuroanatomy would dictate contralateral findings	An examinee claiming severe right-brain damage who claims right-eye blindness and right-sided weakness and sensory loss
Tell me "when I'm not touching" responses	An examinee with claimed sensory loss who endorses that he does not feel you touch him when you ask him to tell you "if you do not feel this."
Lack of shoe wear in presence of gait disturbance	An examinee with claimed longer term gait deviation due to orthopedic or neurologic causes should demonstrate commensurate wear on shoes (if worn with any frequency)
Calluses on hands in "totally disabled" examinee	An examinee who is unable to work should not present with signs of ongoing evidence of physical labor
Assistive device "wear-and-tear" signs	In any examinee using assistive devices for any period of time, e.g., cane, crutches, there should be commensurate wear on the device consistent with the claimed impairment and disability
Mankopf's maneuver	Increase in heart rate commensurate with nociceptive stimulation during exam (some controversy exists on whether this always occurs)
Lack of atrophy in a limb that is claimed to be significantly impaired	If side-to-side measurements and/or inspection do not bear out atrophy consider other causes aside from one being claimed

---

continued

TABLE 63.3 (CONTINUED)
Response Bias Detection Measures and Strategies

Sudden motor give-away or ratchitiness on manual strength testing	Considered to normally be a sign of incomplete effort or symptom exaggeration
Weakness on manual muscle testing without commensurate asymmetry of DTRs or muscle bulk	Suggests simulated muscle weakness if longstanding
Toe test for simulated low back pain	Flexion of hip and knee with movement only of toes should not produce an increase in low back pain
Magnuson's test	Have examinee point to area several times over period of examination; inconsistencies suggest increased potential for nonorganicity
Delayed response sign	Pain reaction temporally delayed relative to application of perceived nociceptive stimulus
Wrist drop test	In an examinee with claimed wrist extensor loss, have him pronate forearm, extend elbow, and flex shoulder … if upon making a fist in this position he also extends wrist, then nonorganicity should be suspected
Object drop test	Examinee claims inability to bend down yet does so to pick up a light object "inadvertently" dropped by examiner
Hip adductor test	Test for claimed paralysis of lower extremity, similar to Hoover's test yet looks for crossed adductor response
Disparity between tested range of motion (ROM) and observed range of motion of any joint	When ROM under testing is significantly disparate (e.g., less) from observed, spontaneous ROM, suspect functional contributors
Straight leg raise (SLR) disparities dependent on examinee positioning	Differences in SLR between sitting, standing, and/or bending may suggest a functional overlay to low back complaints
Grip strength testing via dynamometer	Three repetitions at any given setting should not vary more than 20% and/or bell-shaped curve should be generated if all 5 positions are tested
Sensory "flip" test	Sensory findings should be the same if testing upper extremity in supination or pronation or lower extremity in internal vs. external rotation, differences may suggest a functional overlay
Pinch test for low back pain	Pinching the lumbar fat pad should not reproduce pain due to axial structure involvement; if test is positive, suspect a functional overlay

Personality Instruments with Built-In Response Bias Designs

Personality Assessment Inventory (PAI)	Inconsistency (INC), Infrequency (INF), Positive Impression Management (PIM), and Negative Impression Management (NIM) scales.
	8 score patterns thought to comprise a Malingering Index (Morey, 1996).
	> 2 patterns malingering suspected
	> 4 patterns likely malingering
Minnesota Multiphasic Personality Inventory (MMPI-2)	Validity indices (L, F, Fb, Fp, Ds, K, VRIN, TRIN), F-K (Gough, 1954)
	The Fake Bad Scale (Lees-Haley, 1991)
	Compare subtle to obvious items
	Rogers et al. (1994) – cutoff scores:
	Liberal:
	1. F-scale raw score > 23
	2. F-scale T-score > 81
	3. F-K index > 10
	4. Obvious – subtle score > 83
	Conservative:
	1. F-scale raw > 30
	2. F-K index > 25
	3. Obvious – subtle score > 190

Qualitative Variables in Assessing Response Bias

Time/response latency comparisons across similar tasks	Inconsistencies across tasks
Performance on easy tasks presented as hard	Low scores or unusual errors
Remote memory report	Difficulties, especially if less than recent memory, or severely impaired in absence of gross amnesia

TABLE 63.3 (CONTINUED)
Response Bias Detection Measures and Strategies

Personal information	Very poor personal information in absence of gross amnesia
Comparison between test performance and behavioral observations	Discrepancies
Inconsistencies in history and/or complaints, performance	Inconsistencies across time, setting, interviewer, etc.
Comparisons for inconsistencies within testing session (quantitative and qualitative)	A. Within tasks (e.g., easy vs. hard items)
	B. Between tasks (e.g., easy vs. hard)
	C. Across repetitions of same/parallel tasks (rule out fatigue)
	D. Across similar tasks under different motivational sets
Comparisons across testing sessions (qualitative, quantitative)	Poorer/inconsistent performance on re-testing
Symptom self-report: complaints	High frequency, severity of complaints and higher frequency, severity vs. significant other report or other collaborative report
Main & Spanswick, 1995	Failure to comply with reasonable treatment
	Report of severe pain with no associated psychological effects
	Marked inconsistencies in effects of pain on general activities
	Poor work record and history of persistent appeals against awards
	Previous litigation
Symptom self-report: early/acute vs. late/chronic symptom complaint	Early symptoms reported late or acute symptoms reported as chronic
Response to typically helpful pain interventions	Failure to show any pain relief to at least one of the following: biofeedback, hypnosis, mild analgesics, psychotherapy, relaxation exercises, heat and ice, mild exercise
	Failure to show any pain relief in response to TENS

Assessment of Cognitive Effort:
Performance Patterns on Existing Psychological/Neuropsychological Tests

Full scale IQ	Low (vs. expected, estimated, etc.)
Arithmetic and orientation scale performance	"Near-miss" (Ganser errors)
WMS-R Malingering Index: Attention/Concentration Index vs. Memory Index	Attention–concentration index score < general memory index (AC-GMI)
Grip strength	Unusually low w/o gross motor deficit
Recognition memory (California Verbal Learning Test (CVLT))	< 13
Rey Complex Figure and Recognition Trial	Atypical recognition errors (> = 2); recognition failure errors
Word Stem Priming Task Performance	Poor or unusual performance
Specific Cognitive Effort/Response Bias Measures	
Word Memory Test (WMT)	< 50% chance responding
Test of Memory Malingering (TOMM)	< 50% chance level responding
Dot Counting Test (DCT)	Correct/incorrect responses
Computer Assessment of Response Bias (CARB)	< 89% raises suspicion
Rey Memory for 15 Items Test (MFIT)	Lezak (1983), < 3 complete sets, < 9 items
Symptom validity testing (SVT)	< 50% chance level responding

interpreting examinee data. Integration of contextual information, history, behavioral observation, interview data, collaborative data, personality data, with measures of effort or performance (or symptom exaggeration or malingering) and examination and test performance data provides the best information for estimating, for instance, the degree to which a person was responding truthfully and exerting full effort, and the degree to which test results are reliable and valid and reflect actual abilities and current status.

It also should be noted that the necessary recent increase in attention to response bias assessment has been accompanied by frequently haphazard and overzealous application of poorly validated detection models and single

assessment procedures regarding malingering. Further, some alarming trends have appeared that do not objectively or critically evaluate the weaknesses, as well as strengths, of these procedures. Based on a critical evaluation of the current state of the art, it appears that many common assumptions about response bias detection and malingering measures should be considered myths (Martelli, Zasler, Mancini, et al., 1999). Importantly, malingering (1) should not be considered dichotomous, or EITHER/OR (i.e., present/not; malingering/not); (2) should not be considered something that clinicians can reliably or validly assess with any high degree of certainty, even when serious efforts are made; and (3) should not be considered a discrete entity that symptom validity tests (SVT) measure.

TABLE 63.4
General Weaknesses of Response Bias Assessment Measures

1. Psychometric research inadequacies (e.g., basic test construction issues such as reliability, validity, as well as convergent and divergent validity studies are poorly addressed).
2. Limited generalizability of analogue research (i.e., simulated malingerers vs. externally or criterion-validated malingerers, unknown differences between simulated and real malingerers; cf. studying serial killers this way), as well as tendencies for measures with good discrimination to show less effectiveness in cross-validation and follow-up studies.
3. Variable group membership (i.e., wide variability in samples for both simulators and symptom/disorder groups).
4. Differential vulnerability to response bias (i.e., some tests are more obvious while others are more subtle).
5. Questionable generalizability of findings (i.e., from one measure to any other (response bias or real) test, or to actual symptoms, or across time; conversely, good effort on a response bias measure does not necessarily predict response on any other measure).
6. Absence of mutual exclusivity (i.e., poor effort can occur in presence of real disorder, symptoms).
7. "Law of the instrument" operational definitions wherein malingering becomes what malingering tests measure. Specifically, the definitions of "effort," and validation studies to examine the construct are missing. Further effort cannot be assumed uniform for mild traumatic brain injury (TBI), chronic pain, and depression diagnoses, for nonlitigating and litigating, etc.
8. Effects of fatigue, pain, disinterest, non-attended (computer) administration, mixing real tests and SVTs in a battery with unknown face validity, and other factors, on response bias tests, are not understood and have not been addressed.
9. Exclusive or even primary reliance on any current SVT/Index or combination potentially violates APA ethics and *APA Standards for Educational and Psychological Tests* with regard to making a diagnosis of malingered pain or n making decisions about recommending treatment termination, due to limited reliability and validity data.
10. Frequently high misclassification rates (i.e., false positive) when these are assessed through record review and detailed analysis.
11. Problems associated with inaccurate assumptions of nonorganic conditions based on inconsistencies or absence of peripheral findings. Notably, recent advances in our relatively poor understanding of pain and its mechanisms and associated sequelae have implicated central nervous system effects in many such cases. A growing body of evidence strongly associates central nervous system effects, especially central sensitization phenomenon, in cases where peripheral findings are inconsistent, weak, or even apparently nonexistent (Jay, Krusz, Longmire, & McLain, 2000; Miller, 2000; Nicholson, 2000; Nicholson, in review; Mailis, Papagapiou, Umana, Cohodarevic, Nowak, & Nicholson, in press).

A specific method of response bias assessment that is worth mentioning is SVT, which typically refers to a forced-choice technique originally designed for assessing effort or symptom validity with respect to nonorganic blindness (Pankratz, 1988). This technique has been extended to assess effort in purported sensory loss and, more recently, memory complaints (Colby, 2000). The typical SVT paradigm involves presentation of a stimulus, followed by a distraction, and then presentation of the original stimulus with a novel stimulus with instruction to identify the original stimulus. With regard to memory assessment, a series of words is presented for recall and, following a delay, each word is presented with a sham, with the subject instructed to select the previously presented word. In the case of visual or sensory assessment, the simplest procedure entails exposing the subject to a series of visual or sensory stimuli (e.g., pinpricks while blindfolded, asking whether or not he or she perceived each. Performance is then compared with chance, which is the worst possible expected performance if sensory function or ability is completely absent. Below chance (i.e., below 50%) performance across a sample of numerous trials indicates negative bias and indicates that the symptom is feigned. Such performance provides strong and unambiguous evidence of conscious dissimulation or symptom malingering, because worse- than-chance performance requires recognition and suppression of true responses.

A summary of some of the major problems with extant response bias procedures is offered in Table 63.4 to (1) emphasize the necessary caution with regard to overinterpretation of response bias procedures; (2) emphasize the importance of employing multiple data sources and making thoughtful inferences only after integration of thorough historical information, interview, assessment, behavioral observations, collaborative interview, and data sources, and so on (Martelli, 2000).

Table 63.5 is presented to further caution against simplistic and dichotomous conceptualizations with regard to diagnosis, Table 63.5 is presented. Notably, this table represents just 64 of the possibilities with regard to injury-related presentations. The range of possibilities represented span from (a) persons with real, uncomplicated disorders with impairments on exam and in functional status, without exaggeration on either (but possibly minimization or denial) to (b) persons with no real physical pathology or impairments, but who exaggerate or feign impairments on exam and functional status.

Necessarily, a cautious approach is indicated with regard to estimating the probabilities regarding presence or absence of physical impairment and response bias. However, in many cases, it is not sufficient to integrate data from multiple sources and make inferences about which of the 64 possible combinations is most likely. Descriptive characterization is often relevant. For

TABLE 63.5
Diagnostic Realities in Assessment of Chronic Pain

Real Physical Pathology	Residual Functional Impairments	Residual Impairments On Exam, Testing	
1. Yes	1. Yes, and exaggerated	1. Yes, and not exaggerated	
2. Mixed	2. Yes, and not exaggerated	2. Yes, and exaggerated	
3. Indeterminate	3. No, and exaggerated	3. No, and exaggerated	
4. No	4. No, and not exaggerated	4. No, and not exaggerated	=
4	× 4	× 4	64

instance, if a person has both physical pathology and exaggeration, inferences must be generated about not only the degree of physical impairment, but also the degree of awareness of exaggeration on the part of the subject. Has the person adopted a sick role, and talked themselves into believing they cannot perform certain tasks or lack certain abilities (e.g., somatoform disorder), with conscious withholding of effort due to intending to demonstrating what they believe to be true disabilities? Or, are they less conscious and aware, as in a conversion disorder? Or are they completely aware, but coping in a way that may be adaptive as in the case of an aging worker with a chronic history of back failures who may be shy, have low self-esteem and self-confidence; be disconnected from or less than well liked by his/her employer, against the backdrop of believing that another back injury is inevitable and cumulatively painful and disabling, that uncomfortable interactions with others may be required, that the company sometimes fires previously injured workers, that the company did not make obvious safety precautions to prevent the individual's injury; and that no other job options are realistic?

CONCLUSIONS

To summarize, the major response bias detection strategies presented in Table 63.3 provide an illustrative summary of a constellation or profiling approach to response bias detection strategy use that relies on assessing relevant information for interpreting examination data. This conceptual model is also a methodological approach for constructing a profile of motivation and response bias, which (a) incorporates a wide array of findings from common instruments and procedures during evaluation; (b) summarizes empirically supported indicators with at least some purported utility in detecting suboptimal effort; (c) despite numerous pitfalls and limitations of each of these procedures, both conceptual and methodological, offers improved discrimination and increased reliability given multiple measures; (d) integrates behavioral observation, interview, and collaborative, historical, personality, and contextual data with medical examination and psychological performance data and measures of response bias, as

an optimal method for estimating the degree of effort or performance and the degree to which examination findings are reliable and valid and reflect actual abilities; and (e) allows estimation of motivation by incorporating currently available instruments and methods and the available published research for direct and indirect measurement of motivation and response bias.

Notably, these strategies are not offered individually and, again, are not intended to support a simple dualistic model that assumes examinees either try hard or malinger, or that evidence of less-than-full effort on any one test necessarily implies absence of impairment in other areas of examination or in real world abilities. Although they also are not offered with specific guidelines (e.g., failure on any one, or any two, or any three, etc. represents inadequate performance, or symptom exaggeration or malingering), they are offered with the suggestion that (a) examination performance can be influenced by multiple factors including a desire to be completely truthful and perform with full effort; (b) the degree of truthfulness and effort exerted on examinations exists on a continuum (vs. a dichotomy) and can be estimated by the extent to which indicators of unreliable report and poor/inconsistent effort are present; (c) reliability and validity of examination findings are dependent on relative assurances of full effort; and (d) interpretation and diagnostic impressions are dependent upon reliable and valid examination results.

It should be emphasized that "failure" on one measure of response bias or malingering does not mean that the entire set of complaints is biased or malingered. Ethical guidelines universally caution against overzealous interpretation of limited test data. In fact, the only reasonable evidence of certain or definite malingering is confession or admission. A secondary form of evidence, although somewhat less than perfectly reliable, is when the person or examinee is detected, via surveillance, performing an act he or she reported was absolutely impossible to perform under any circumstance.

It should be noted further that a great disparity exists between the adversarial legal process and the responsibility of attorneys to be client advocates vs. the dispassionate, objective scientific ethics expected and required of psychologists and physicians. The danger of attorney "coaching" based on utilization of this material cannot be underestimated. This, of course, would then represent a form of "stealth" threat to the validity of examination data. This threat, or expected consequence of collision between disparate legal and scientific ethics, has recently been documented in a national publication noting a case of attorney–client coaching (Youngjohn, 1995). However, compared to simpler models where only a couple of isolated response bias measures are used, it seems extremely unlikely that the multiple measures, such as those outlined in the MAP approach, could be understood and manipulated.

Finally, enhancing response bias detection as a means of optimizing interpretability of examination results, critical as it is, should not be considered the final step. Decreasing response bias must certainly be considered a more efficacious and economic approach to enhancing utility of medical and psychological assessments.

The following explicit and comprehensive recommendations for enhancing motivation, assessing response bias, and increasing efficiency, utility, and ecological validity of examination procedures are offered (Martelli, et al., 1999b).

RECOMMENDATIONS FOR ENHANCING VALIDITY IN CHRONIC PAIN ASSESSMENTS

1. Establish rapport and attempt to establish a working relationship with patients. Even in cases of independent examinations where the referral source and expectation are extremely adversarial, valid data collection requires a collaborative effort. Be on guard by addressing potential sources of bias directly, and providing feedback, education, and clarification.

2. Prepare patients and examinees before beginning examination and testing. Employ understanding, as well as education, in order for examinees to be prepared to respond truthfully and to the best of their abilities. Emphasize that the procedures and tests don't always measure everything, but that they do assess poor motivation or effort. Emphasize that interview data, corroborative data, and functional abilities are just as important as examination data.

3. Spend time with patients/examinees and try to get to know them from a motivational, emotional status, personality, and coping style perspective. If motivation seems poor, confront and attempt to elicit more valid responses vs. ignore and/or proceed with collecting invalid data and/or attempting to interpret data of questionable validity. Such questioning of motivation/effort should not involve a "gotcha"

attitude. We can't assume that everyone takes our tests seriously, will be as forthcoming, honest, or effortful as we would like, will not doubt our procedures or try to emphasize their problems, or that we won't have to work at getting them optimally motivated.

4. Ensure that important general situational and psychosocial variables affecting motivation are adequately assessed during an interview that is concluded prior to examination procedures. Specifically, assess the impact of anger or blame and feelings of resentment or victimization (Rutherford, 1989), as well as the other variables shown in the literature to be associated with poor recovery and adaptation to impairments (Martelli, Zasler, & Grayson, 2000).

5. In addition to emotional and motivational issues, always assess interest/disinterest in the examination and testing procedures process, and any obstacles or impediments to optimal effort and performance. Always assess anxiety level and ensure that measures are taken to minimize its effect and potential interference with valid assessment.

6. Rely primarily on M.D.s and Ph.D.s for all aspects of examination, including interviewing and testing, with limited use and reliance on technicians. Experienced M.D.s and Ph.D.s who conduct interviews, examinations, and test administration are infinitely more capable of

   a. Integrating history, interview, personality, and emotional assessment data and inferences, with more sophisticated clinical observations during examination;

   b. Adapting more creative modifications of testing procedures given suspicion of low motivation, as well as modifications to the testing process (e.g., provision of corrective feedback, instruction, anxiety reduction interventions) to increase motivation and optimize effort;

   c. Benefiting from the probability that examinees will be less likely to believe they can "fake out the doctor";

   d. Avoiding the possibility of symptom exaggeration owing to fear that a technician or inexperienced clinician will miss legitimate problems.

7. Differentially utilize instruments with built-in response bias or symptom validity measures. Most major objective personality measures, some of the newer domain-specific pain assessment measures, and some neuropsychological measures (e.g., Memory Assessment Scales (Williams, 1992), and the Rey Complex Figure Test and

Recognition Trial (Meyers & Meyers, 1995)) provide simulator performance data.

8. Apply multiple strategies for assessing motivation, especially when cutoff score approaches are employed, and include qualitative and qualitative measures. Integration of contextual information, history, behavioral observations, interview and collaborative data, and personality and coping data with measures of effort or performance and current test data, provides the best information for estimating the degree of effort exerted, and the degree to which test results are reliable and valid.

9. Vary the response bias measures and procedures that are employed in order to prevent dilution of utility. Notably, publicizing of these tests has led to increased recognition by potential defendant attorneys, litigants, support groups, Internet groups, etc.

10. Promote development of assessment procedures with built-in response bias or symptom validity measures and develop built-in measures for existing assessment procedures.

11. Employ more sophisticated and less dichotomous continuous conceptualizations of motivation and response bias using multiple independent measures and estimated effort. Employ a reasonably sophisticated model that conceptualizes motivation and effort as continuous variables that can vary across tests, settings, and occasions. Utilize and devise models that measure degree of apparent motivation and effort, using multiple data sources, and estimate confidence levels in inferences given consideration of the multiple factors that contribute to test results. Employ similarly sophisticated models for assessing persistent impairments, adaptation to impairments, disability, and so on. Probability statements based on multiple meas-ures are probably best.

12. Do not freely share relevant trade secrets (e.g., information about response bias tests, or known patterns of performance on procedures and instruments) with referral sources, attorneys, and nonphysicians and nonpsychologists. They often adhere to a completely different set of professional ethics.

13. Remain aware that in science and medicine things are rarely either–or, clear cut, or unidimensional. Avoid simplistic conceptual models that are compatible with dichotomous approaches to assessing motivation/effort and malingering. Such approaches usually rely on cutting scores for one or two measures. Note that cutting scores by their nature (Dwyer, 1996) always entail judgment, inherently result in misclassification, impose an artificial dichotomy on essentially continuous variables, and "true" cut scores do not exist.

14. Promote utilization of independent examinations by clinicians who actually spend a significant portion of their time treating the type of patient being assessed. This helps assure more adequate clinical skills for accurate diagnosis and understanding, including detection and appreciation of suboptimal performance, as well as collection of internalized tracking data to validate previous inferences across time, and continuous self-correction and increased collection of internalized norms regarding ecological and predictive validity of available assessment measures.

REFERENCES

* Allen, C.C., & Ruff, R.M. (1990). Self-rating versus neuropsychological performance of moderate versus severe head-injured patients. *Brain Injury, 4*(1), 7.

* Allen, L.M., & Cox, D.R. (1995). *Computerized assessment of response bias* (revised ed.). Durham, NC: CogniSyst, Inc.

* Allen, M. (1985). Review of Millon Behavioral Health Inventory. In J.V. Mitchell (Ed.), *The ninth mental measurements handbook* (p. 1521). Lincoln, NE: University of Nebraska Press.

American Psychiatric Association (1994). Committee on Nomenclature and Statistics. *Diagnostic and statistical manual of mental disorders* (4th ed.). Washington, D.C.: American Psychiatric Association.

* American Psychiatric Association (1994). *Diagnostic and statistical manual of mental disorders,* (4th ed. revised). Washington, D.C.: American Psychiatric Press.

* Arnett, P.A., Hammeke, T.A., & Schwartz, L. (1995). Quantitative and qualitative performance on Rey's 15-Item Test in neurological patients and dissimulators. *Clinical Neuropsychologist, 9*(1), 17.

Babitsky, S., Brigham C.R., & Mangraviti, J.J. (2000). Symptom magnification, deception and malingering: Identification through distraction and other tests and techniques (VHS video). Falmouth, MA: SEAK, Inc.

* Beetar, J.T., & Williams, J.M. (1995). Malingering response styles on the memory assessment scales and symptom validity tests. *Archives of Clinical Neuropsychology, 10*(1), 57.

* Bernard, L.C., Houston, W., & Natoli, L. (1993a). Malingering on neuropsychological memory tests: Potential objective indicators. *Journal of Clinical Psychology, 49*(1), 45.

* Bernard, L.C., McGrath, M.J., & Houston, W. (1993b). Discriminating between simulated malingering and closed head injury on the Wechsler memory scale–revised. *Archives of Clinical Neuropsychology, 8*(6), 539.

* Berry, D.T., Baer, R.A., & Harris, M.J. (1991). Detection of malingering on the MMPI: A meta-analysis. *Clinical Psychology Review,* 11, 585.

Binder, L.M., & Rohling M.L. (1996). Money matters: A meta-analytic review of the effects of financial incentives on recovery after closed-head injury. *American Journal of Psychiatry, 153*(1), 7.

* Binder, L.M., & Pankratz, L. (1987). Neuropsychological evidence of a factitious memory complaint. *Journal of Clinical & Experimental Neuropsychology, 9*(2), 167.

Blau, T. (1984). *The psychologist as expert witness.* New York: John Wiley & Sons.

Blau, T. (1992). The psychologist as expert witness. Presented at the National Academy of Neuropsychology annual meeting, Reno, Nevada.

* Brandt, J. (1988). Malingered amnesia. In R. Rogers (Ed.), *Clinical assessment of malingering and deception* (pp. 65–83). New York: Guilford Press.

Colby, F. (2000). Does the binomial distribution stand falsely accused? *Brain Injury Source, 4*(4), 18–21.

* Cullum, C., Heaton, R., & Grant, I. (1991). Psychogenic factors influencing neuropsychological performance: Somatoform disorders, factitious disorders and malingering. In H.O. Doerr, & A.S. Carlin (Eds.), *Forensic neuropsychology.* New York: Guilford Press.

Dwyer, C.A. (1996). Cut scores & testing: statistics, judgment, truth, and error. *Psychological Assessment, 8*(4), 360.

* Elmer, B.N., & Allen, L.M. (1995). *User's guide to the pain assessment battery* (Research ed.). Durham, NC: CogniSyst, Inc.

* Faust, D. (1995a). The detection of deception. Special issue: Malingering and conversion reactions. *Neurologic Clinics, 13*(2), 255.

Fishbain, D.A., Cutler, R.B., Rosomoff, H.L., & Rosomoff, R.S. (1999). Chronic pain and disability exaggeration/malingering research and the application of submaximal effort research to this area: A review. Poster presented at International Association of Pain 9th World Congress, Vienna, Austria.

* Franzen, M.D., & Iverson, G.L. (1998). Detecting negative response bias and diagnosing malingering: The dissimulation exam. In P.J. Snyder & P.D. Nussbaum (Eds.), *Clinical neuropsychology – A pocket handbook for assessment* (pp. 88–101). Washington, D.C.: American Psychological Association.

* Green, P., Iverson, G., & Allen, L. (1999). Detecting malingering in head injury litigation with the Word Memory Test. *Brain Injury, 13*(10), 813.

Hadjistavropoulos, H.D., & LaChapelle, D.L. (2000). Extent and nature of anxiety experience during physical examination of chronic low back pain. *Behavior Research and Therapy, 38*(1), 13.

Hall, H.V., & Pritchard, D.A. (1996). *Detecting malingering and deception: Forensic distortion analysis.* Delray Beach, FL: St. Lucie Press.

* Hayes, J.S., Hilsabeck, R.C., & Gouvier, W.D. (1999). Malingering traumatic brain injury: current issues and caveats in assessment and classification. In N.R. Varney, and R.J. Roberts (Eds.), *The evaluation and treatment of mild traumatic brain injury.* Mahwah, NJ: Lawrence Erlbaum Associates.

* Hendler, H.H., & Eimer, B.N. (in press). Psychological tests for assessing chronic pain and disability.

* Hendler, N.H., Viernstein, M., Gucer, P., & Long, D. (1979). A preoperative screening test for chronic back pain patients. *Psychosomatics, 20*(12), 301.

* Iverson, G.L. Qualitative aspects of malingered memory deficits. *Brain Injury, 9*(1), 35, 1995.

Jay, G.W., Krusz, J.C., Longmire, D.R., & McLain, D.A. (2000). *Current trends in the diagnosis and treatment of chronic neuromuscular pain syndromes.* Las Vegas: American Academy of Pain Management and Elan Pharmaceuticals.

Lees-Haley, P., & Brown, R.S. (1993). Neuropsychological complaint base rates of 170 personal injury claimants. *Archives of Clinical Neuropsychology, 8,* 203.

Lees-Haley, P.R, Williams, C.W., Zasler, N.D., Margulies, S., English, L.T., & Steven, K.B. (1997). Response bias in plaintiff's histories. *Brain Injury, 11*(11), 79–99.

Lezak, M. (1965). *Neuropsychological assessment,* (3rd ed.). New York: Oxford University Press.

Lipman, F.D. (1962). Malingering in personal injury cases. *Temple Law Quarterly, 35,* 141.

Loring, D.W. (1995). Psychometric detection of malingering. Presented at the annual meeting of the American Academy of Neurology, Seattle.

Mailis, A., Papagapiou, M., Umana, M., Cohodarevic, T., Nowak, J., & Nicholson, K. (in press). Unexplainable widespread somatosensory deficits in patients with chronic nonmalignant pain in the context of litigation/compensation: A role for involvement of central factors. *Journal of Rheumatology.*

Main, C.J., & Spanswick, C.C. (1995). Functional overlay, and illness behaviour in chronic pain: distress or malingering? Conceptual difficulties in medico-legal assessment of personal injury claims. *Journal of Psychosomatic Research, 39*(6), 737.

Martelli, M.F. (2000). Psychological Assessment of Response Bias in Impairment and Disability Ratings. Presentation as part of Symposium #2031 (The Psychologist's Role in the Social Security Disability Process) at the American Psychological Association 2000 Convention, Washington, D.C.

Martelli, M.F., Zasler, N.D., & Grayson, R. (1999a). Ethical considerations in medicolegal evaluation of neurologic injury and impairment. *NeuroRehabilitation: An Interdisciplinary Journal, 13,* 1, 45.

Martelli, M.F., Zasler, N.D. & Grayson, R. (1999b). Ethical considerations in impairment and disability evaluations following injury. In R.V. May & M.F. Martelli (Eds.), *Guide to functional capacity evaluation with impairment rating applications.* Richmond: NADEP Publications.

Martelli, M.F., Zasler, N.D., & Grayson, R. (2000). Ethics and medicolegal evaluation of impairment after brain injury. In M. Schiffman (Ed.), *Attorney's guide to ethics in forensic science and medicine*. Springfield, IL: Charles C Thomas.

Martelli, M.F., Zasler, N.D., Mancini, A.M., & MacMillan, P. (1999). Psychological assessment and applications in impairment and disability evaluations. In R.V. May & M.F. Martelli (Eds.), *Guide to functional capacity evaluation with impairment rating applications*. Richmond: NADEP Publications.

Matheson, L. (1988). Symptom magnification syndrome. In S. Isernhagen (Ed.), *Work injury*, Rockville, MD: Aspen Publishers.

Matheson, L. (1990). Symptom magnification syndrome: A modern tragedy and its treatment. Part one: Description and definition. *Industrial Rehabilitation Quarterly, 3*(3), 1, 5, 8–9, 12, 23.

Matheson, L. (1991a). Symptom magnification syndrome: A modern tragedy and its treatment. Part two: Techniques of identification. *Industrial Rehabilitation Quarterly, 4*(1), 1–17.

Matheson, L. (1991b). Symptom magnification syndrome: A modern tragedy and its treatment. Part three: Techniques of treatment. *Industrial Rehabilitation Quarterly, 4*(2), 5–6, 22–24.

May, R.V. (1999). Symptom magnification syndrome. In R.V. May & M.F. Martelli (Eds.), *Guide to functional capacity evaluation with impairment rating applications*. Richmond: NADEP Publications.

Merskey, H. (1986). Classification of chronic pain, descriptions of chronic pain syndromes and definitions of pain terms. *Pain, 3*, S10–S11, S13–S24.

* Meyers, J., & Volbrecht, M. (1999). Detection of malingerers using the Rey complex figure and recognition trial. *Applied Neuropsychology, 6*, 4, 201.

* Meyers, J.E., & Meyers, K.R. (1995). *Rey complex figure and recognition trial*. Odessa, FL: Psychological Assessment Resources.

Miller, L. (2000) Neurosensitization: A model for persistent disability in chronic pain, depression, and posttraumatic stress disorder following injury. *NeuroRehabilitation, 14*(1), 25–32.

Miller, L. (2001). Not just malingering: Syndrome diagnosis in traumatic brain injury litigation. *NeuroRehabilitation, 16*, 1–14.

* Millis, S. R. (1994). Assessment of motivation and memory with the recognition memory test after financially compensable mild head injury. *Journal of Clinical Psychology, 50*(4), 601.

* Mittenberg, W., Arzin, R., Millsaps, C., & Heilbronner, R. (1993). Identification of malingered head injury on the Wechsler Memory Scale. *Psychological Assessment, 5*, 34.

* Morey, L.C. (1996). *An interpretive guide to the personality assessment inventory (PAI)*. Odessa, FL: Psychological Assessment Resources.

Nicholson, K. (2000). At the crossroads: Pain in the 21st century. *NeuroRehabilitation, 14*, 57.

Nicholson, K., Psychogenic pain: Review of the construct, a novel taxonomy and neuropsychobiological model (in review).

* Nies, K.J., & Sweets, J.J. (1994). Neuropsychological assessment and malingering: A critical review of past and present strategies. *Archives of Clinical Neuropsychology, 9*(6), 501.

Pankratz, L. (1988). Malingering on intellectual and neuropsychological measures. In R. Rogers (Ed.), *Clinical assessment of malingering and deception*. New York: Guilford Press.

* Rogers, R. (Ed.). (1988). *Clinical assessment of malingering and deception*. New York: Guilford Press.

Rohling, M.L., & Binder, L.M. (1995). Money matters: A meta-analytic review of the association between financial compensation and the experience and treatment of chronic pain. *Health Psychology, 14*(6), 537.

Rutherford, W. (1989). Postconcussion symptoms: Relationship to acute neurological indices, individual differences, and circumstances of injury. In H.S. Levin, H.M. Eisenberg, and A.L. Benson (Eds.). *Mild head injury* (p. 229). New York: Oxford University Press.

Simmonds, M.J., Kumar, S., & Lechelt, E. (1998). Psychosocial factors in disabling low back pain: Causes or consequences? *Disability and Rehabilitation, 18*, 161.

Waddell, G. (1999). Nonorganic signs or behavioral responses to examination in low back pain. *Hippocrates' Lantern, 6*(3), 1.

Waddell, G., & Main, C.J. (1984). Assessment of severity in low back disorders. *Spine, 9*, 204–208.

Waddell, G., Main, C.J., Morris, E.W., Paoloa, M.D., & Gray, I.C. (1984). Chronic low back pain, psychologic distress, and illness behavior. *Spine, 9*, 209.

* Williams, J.M. (1992). *The memory assessment scales*. Odessa, FL: Psychological Assessment Resources.

* Youngjohn, J.R. (1995). Confirmed attorney coaching prior to neuropsychological evaluation. *Assessment, 2*(3) 279.

Youngjohn, J.R., Burrows, L., & Erdal, K. (1995). Brain damage or compensation neurosis? The controversial post-concussion syndrome. *Clinical Neuropsychologist, 9*(2), 112.

64

Psychoneuroimmunology

Jan M. Burte, Ph.D., D.A.A.P.M.

Historically, the study of mind/body interaction can be traced to early Greek physicians. Indeed, when one begins a search of its earliest origins, one inevitably is led to Hippocrates and Galen of ancient Greece. To the ancient Greeks, emotions were seen to play a significant role in the progress and maintenance of diseases. What today is known as tuberculosis was described symptomologically by Hippocrates and prescribed to have its etiology in stress. However, the importance of the role of the mind in maintaining health has passed through many significant perceptions since that time. Until recently, post-Descartian thinking resulted in the mind's role in immune functioning being allocated to the periphery of medicine.

Masek, Petrovicky, Sevcik, Zidek, and Frankova (2000) pointed out that psychoneuroimmunology (PNI) was comprehensively described only as recently as 20 years ago. They go on to define PNI as the bidirectional communication between the central nervous system (CNS), neuro-endocrine system, and immune system. With a return to examination of the interactive role of the central nervous system, the endocrine and immune systems came a new field currently labeled PNI. Many definitions of PNI are available, depending on the emphasis or direction of the pathways particular fields of researchers choose to emphasize.

One definition offered by Paul Martin (1998) is "the field of scientific research that is concerned with the complex interrelationship between the psychological and emotional factors, the brain, hormones and immunity and disease."

The purpose of the chapter is to offer the following: First, a basic understanding of precisely which pathways are considered in PNI. For example, what are the biological immune responses (cortisol levels, cytokines levels,

natural killer-cell levels, etc.) that are affected by environmental and internally mediated stress? Second, to restate the question often raised by clinicians, "Does statistical significance (i.e., changes in hormone levels) assume clinical relevance (i.e., a clinical change in the immune system's protective potential)?" Third, if we accept that stressors experienced through conscious awareness and judgment impact the immune system, what can be done to reduce those stressors?

A discussion of treatment modalities is offered, and finally, hope for a united direction for future research unifying the basic sciences (statistical analyses) and the applied sciences (clinical relevance). What then do we know about the integrative reaction of the CNS and the immune response?

Stress, via bidirectional interactions between the central nervous system, endocrine system, and immune system, impacts the hypothalamic, pituitary, adrenal (HPA), and the sympathetic adrenal medullary (SAM) axes, can induce modulation of the immune system and, thereby, defense against infectious agents and health (Yang & Glaser, 2000).

In a review of research articles, Sali (1997) notes that stress increases the risk of viral infection. Stress and depression can depress immunity, whereas stress reduction enhances immunity. Sali points to outcome data on improved cancer prognosis by enhanced immunity resulting from stress reduction. Spiegel (1999) found increased survival rates in breast cancer patients who attended stress reduction groups or programs. Further, Van der Pompe, Anoni, Visser, and Garsseri (1986) suggested the importance of psychotherapy and psychological resiliency in breast cancer survival. Utilizing a twin study model (124 normal adult twin pairs; Hickie, Bennet, Lloyd, Heath,

0-8493-0926-3/02/$0.00+$1.50
© 2002 by CRC Press LLC

and Martin 1999) found a positive genetic relationship between psychological distress and immunity. They concluded that genotype may play a significant role in the reactivity of the immune system to stress. Garssen and Goodkin (1999) suggest that some evidence has been found that a low level of social support and a tendency toward helplessness and repression of negative emotions are factors that promote cancer progression but not cancer initiation. These same factors are also symptoms commonly associated with depression. Further, Christiansen, Edwards, Wiebe, Bonotsch, McKelvey, Andrews, and Lubaroff (1996) found that immunosuppression (NKC activity) could be positively impacted by self-disclosure of traumatic or stressful experiences.

A question is then raised: "Does a correlation exist between depression, suppressed immunological functioning, and the elevation of underlying disease processes to a level above threshold (i.e., the symptomatic expression of herpes or the increase in joint counts in rheumatoid arthritic patient)?" Research continues to support the concept that stress plays a significant role in exacerbating pathophysiology. Berin and Perdue (1997) note that reported stress often precedes relapses in patients with inflammatory bowel disease or irritable bowel syndrome and that CNS and immune-mediated pathophysiology as expressed by changes in the epithelium may exist.

Stress and pain also have been demonstrated to adversely affect endocrine and immune function in regard to postsurgical wound healing, with greater fear or distress prior to surgery being associated with slower and more complicated postoperative recovery (Kiecolt, Glaser, Page, Marucha, MacCallum, & Glaser, 1998) and to small punch biopsy wound healing in caregivers as demonstrated by increased healing time and lower cytokines (IL–1) levels (Glaser, 1996). In regard to posttraumatic patients, Klapheke (2000) suggested that their depression should be seen as a contributory factor to the net state of immunosuppression in transplant patients

PSYCHONEUROIMMUNOLOGY AND PAIN

The impact of pain on immune functioning has been studied extensively in animals, but more recently the role of various types of pain on immune function has been examined. Kremer (1999) notes that surgery negatively affects immune function, and that pain has a deleterious effect on immune function. Via neuroendocrine pathways, depression, stress, and pain can be viewed as psychoneurological phenomena. He suggests that treatment of postoperative pain must be included in the recovery process because of its psychoneural immunological impact on the patient.

In a study to assess acute pain impact on immune levels in 10 HIV+ and 10 HIV- patients, Eller (1998) found no significant difference between groups. However, significant

changes in state anxiety, systolic blood pressure, diastolic blood pressure, and CD4+ lymphocyte numbers were associated with levels of perceived pain intensity to a cold pressor test.

In extreme situations where physical trauma and pain are severe, the body releases endogenous opioids which reduce the perception of pain and have pain-relieving actions. However, as a result, the immune activity of natural killer cells and lymphocytes is reduced.

This raises the issues of placebos and other treatments that work by altering the individual's perception of pain without actually providing an external source of analgesia. If, in fact, they operate as some believe by triggering pain-relieving opioids, do they then represent a two-edge sword which offers pain relief, thus, diminishing the immuno-suppressant levels of IL-6 and cortisol while possibly decreasing tumor suppression by lowering NKC and certain lymphocyte activities?

Another issue about pain is its controllability. Laudenslager (1983) found that lack of control vs. control over pain induced by electric shock determined lymphocyte responsiveness of rats. This may also explain the more recent findings of researchers that depression (learned helplessness) with regard to pain may be significantly related to dysfunctional reciprocal relations between neuroendocrine and immune function (Geiss, Varodi, Steinback, Bauer, & Anton, 1997).

The patient's perception of the controllability of pain and level of optimism may also play a significant role in the impact that pain has on immune functioning. In an examination of pain patients suffering with temporomandibular pain and dysfunction syndrome, immune functioning was not impacted compared to controls. However, patients who scored high on measures of "demoralization" (low self-esteem and perceptions of helplessness and hopelessness) demonstrated significant decreases on measures (Marbach, Schleifer, & Keller, 1990).

In a review article, Page and Ben-Eliyahu (1997) note that the immune system plays a role in controlling the spread of cancer and that perio-operative pain relief improves immune status and health outcomes. They suggest that sufficient evidence exists to view pain as a pathogen in and of itself that is capable of facilitating the progression of metastatic disease via immunosuppression.

Along similar lines, a study by Parker, Smarr, Anglone, Mothersead, Lee, Walker, Bridgers, and Caldwell (1992) utilizing the Beck Depression Inventory, the Arthritis Helplessness Index, and the Arthritis Impact Measurement Scales (AIMS) pain score in conjunction with immunophenotypic analyses of peripheral blood lymphocytes found that the percentage of HLA-DR + cells in the peripheral blood and helplessness related to joint count in rheumatoid arthritis (RA) patients. Further, joint count had an effect upon depression and depression affected the perception of pain, demonstrating the interrelationship among psychological factors, immunologic activation, and disease activity in RA. Zautra, Hoffman, Potter, Matt, Yocum, and Castro (1997) also found that interpersonal stressors were associated with increased disease activity in a study of 41 rheumatoid arthritic women.

Affleck, Urrows, Tennen, Higgins, Pav, and Aloisi (1997) examined sedimentation rates, an indication of systemic inflammation and soluble interleukin-II receptors (a marker of immune system activation known to correlate with the RA disease activity). For RA patients, they found that daily event stressors were associated with increased joint pain (regardless of mood) and decreased joint inflammation (reduced levels of soluble interleukin-II receptors).

Another issue that often is raised is the impact of acute stressors on individuals who are experiencing chronic life stressors. It would seem that individuals who are experiencing chronic life stress might be more vulnerable to the impact of acute stressors. The importance of this is apparent when we look at disease onset rates in more vulnerable populations, such as the infirmed, ill, or impoverished, who may be experiencing higher levels of chronic life stress. Indeed, Pike, Smith, Hauger, Nicassio, Patterson, McClintick, Costlow, and Irwin (1997) found that individuals experiencing chronic life stress demonstrated greater subjective stress, higher peak levels of epinephrine, lower peak levels of beta endorphin and of NK cell lysis and NK cell distribution to a mild acute stressor than did controls. These changes persisted beyond termination of the stressor and sympathomedullary recovery. It reinforces the concept that those already suffering, often the case in chronic illness or injury patients, are most vulnerable to further immunosuppression from acute stressors. In the case of traumatic injury, Schrader (1996) suggests that the individual's psychologic and physiologic states may alter the immune system and decrease immunity as measured by serum cortisol levels, and further, that the perception of diminished control and subjective stress may contribute to immune changes when combined with the immunosuppressive effects noted with regard to pain, suggesting that the state of significantly decreased immunity needs to be addressed from a psychological, controlled coping skill, and pain management approach.

Interestingly, research suggests when the stress is consistent with the stressor (perhaps demonstrating better coping skills by the individual), immunological changes are less severe than when the stress experienced is greater than expected from the trauma. Solomon, Segerstrom, Grohr, Kemeny, and Fahey (1997) found that earthquake survivors who manifested acute psychological reactions to a realistic degree given the life stress experienced less disruption of an aspect of immunity (lymphocyte subsets – total T[CD3+] helper T[CD4+] cytotoxic T[CD3+ and CD8+] 19+) and natural killer cell (NK; CD3–, CD16+ sign CD56+) as well as lymphoid cell mitogenesis (PHA and DWM) and NK cell cytotoxicity than those who had more severe reactions or who repressed their stress reactions.

Adaption to stress and its impact on the immune system may be somewhat more complicated. Kelly, Hertzman, and Daniels (1997) have suggested that PNI measures may act as markers to adaption to socioeconomic and psychosocial stressors.

There appears to be significant evidence that psychological stress contributes to immunological suppression (Biondi & Annino, 1997). However, there is less compelling evidence suggesting that immunosuppression may result in mental disease. However, recent research identifies the hypersecretion of IL-2 in schizophrenia and IL-6 in depression. Muller (1997) suggests that cytokine changes resulting from stress impacting the immune system may play a role in psychiatric disorders. Further, Dabkowska and Rybakowski (1994) suggest that the immune system may play a role in increasing vulnerability to psychiatric disorders.

Given the interactive nature of PNI, it is evident that a relationship exists between emotional disorders such as depression and alterations in the response of the immune system. However, as Kaye, Morton, Bowcutt, and Maupin (2000) point out, the associations and relevance of these alterations with regard to health and illness are not yet fully determined.

Anyone who has spent a night in pain or stressed knows the impact that either can have on sleep. Hall, Baum, Buysse, Prigerson, Kupfer, and Reynolds III (1998) report that sleep has been demonstrated to be a significant factor in the stress/immune relationship of NKC number and functions.

Severity of pain was also a factor. This suggests that clinicians must be aware of the patient's mental state and take into account immunological susceptibilities in those patients who present with significant levels of emotional demoralization (chronic pain syndrome) when invasive potentially immunosuppressant interventions are considered.

In fact, an optimistic outlook may protect the immune system from the negative impact of stress. First-year law students evaluated at the onset of the semester who were found to manifest a more optimistic attitude had more helper T-cells (T-cell increased 13%) and higher natural-killer cell cytotoxicity mid-semester than their pessimistic peers (T-cell dropped 3%). This led to the suggestion that the optimist's attitude protected their immune functioning (Segerstrom, 1998).

Another important question often asked is, "Does stress impact sufficiently enough on the immune system to create a health risk?" Glaser (1996) found studying antibody responses to flu-vaccinated Alzheimer's disease patients' caregivers and to Hepatitis B-vaccinated medical students that the findings indicated psychological stress may be able to alter a person's response to a vaccine and, therefore by implication, his or her risk to infection by a live virus. Koenker (2000) states that psychological stress sufficiently impacts the immune system to raise catecholamine and CD9 levels and increases the risk of viral infection-released histamines which trigger severe bronchoconstriction in asthmatics. It also alters insulin needs, increasing the risk for diabetes mellitus; alters acid concentrations in the stomach contributing to peptic and stress-ulcers and ulcerative colitis; and increases plaque buildup in arteries thus adding to the risk of angina and heart attack. (Elliott & Eisdorfer, 1982; Lieberman, 1974).

As we continue to learn about complex PNI interactions our views of the forms of intervention and pharmocotherapies may significantly change. Masekt, Petrovicky, Sevcik, and Zidek (2000) point out that the data strongly suggest that in the very near future we will not only better understand the very complex communication between mind and body, but also have completely new types of compounds become available.

Vedhara, Fox, and Wang (1999) raised the question as to whether *in vitro* statistically significant results can be equated to *in vivo* immune outcomes. Although not yet completely answered, significant *in vivo* research is present, as evidenced by the plethora of treatment outcome studies represented in the literature. These studies suggest the presence of a PNI effect.

TREATMENT

Having reviewed the mechanisms and correlations between the psyche (mind), and neuro (brain/endocrine) and immune system, and seeing that a bidirectional relationship exists, we next should review what forms of intervention have been applied in treating various conditions. One might feel initially tempted simply to try to correlate treatments with conditions/diseases, but this would undermine the very essence of the psychoneuroimmunological model which seeks to approach immunosuppression from a more holistic framework. Perhaps the best title for all interventions which utilize this model is the one proposed by Biondi and Zannino (1997) who refer to such interventions as psychoimmunotherapy, namely, the application of conjoint psychological intervention in pathologies such as tuberculosis, herpes simplex virus, and HIV. Coyle (1996) offers a similar concept of psychoneuroimmunology in the treatment of multiple sclerosis.

An important issue rises, however, but the point of intervention. Hiramoto, Solvason, Hsueh, Rogers, Demissie, Hiramoto, Gauthier, Lorden, and Ghanta (1999) state

Psychoimmunology has been credited with using the mind as a way to alter immunity. The problem with this concept is that many of the current psychoimmu-

nology techniques in use are aimed at alleviating stress effects on the immune system rather than at direct augmentation of immunity by the brain. They raise the question as to whether the mind can, via conditioning, be trained to remember an output pathway to raise immunity.

If so, then it lends increased credibility to the mind-control components promoted in Eastern philosophies and healing arts.

Further, as we break down the concept of training pathways, one is presented again with questioning to what extent conditioning is behaviorally mediated via the build-up of neural pathways or unconsciously mediated via imagery-based internal experiences.

Let us first examine the different modalities utilized and presented in the literature concerning stress reduction as a means of enhancing immune function. Stress management represents a broadly defined treatment orientation encompassing a huge variety of treatments. The singular underlying common goal is to bring about either objectively or subjectively reported changes in the patient's experience of stress. However, as has been frequently noted in the literature from Selye (1956; 1976) to the present, not all stress is negative, and although general stress values have been numerically quantified (Holmes and Rahe 1967), not all events maintain equal stress values for all individuals. In addition, factors such as the ability to control the stressors (Schrader, 1996; Kiecolt, et al., 1998; Kaye, et al., 2000; Laudenslager, 1983), support systems (Spiegel, 1999), chronicity of the stressor (Pike, et al., 1997), and adaptation to the stressors (Kelly, et al., 1997) may play a significant role in the impact of stress on immunological functioning and responsiveness to treatment.

Some of the treatments that have sought to address the effects of stress include biofeedback, hypnosis, cognitive behavioral, behavioral approaches, exercise, nutrition, physical manipulation, yoga, and a host of other techniques including laughter therapy, dance, and the arts. What almost all of these approaches have in common is that they seek to change the patient's (assuming he or she is ill at this point) appraisal of the stressors that preceded the influence of immunodepression, the stressors associated with his/her appraisal of the illness and treatment. This typically includes the patient's ability to control pain and the degree to which he or she is limited or disabled by the illness or pain, as well as the stressors associated with the patient's appraisal of future functioning and/or mortality.

In essence, stress combined with a stress-prone personality leads to physiological and hormonal consequences which deplete the immune system. This opens the door for possibly increased susceptibility to or maintenance of illness. Ultimately, the presence and impact of that consequent illness, especially if pain is concomitant, can easily become a stressor unto itself and further mitigate stress-induced immunosuppression. In this model then, a downward spiral of health requiring significant multimodal intervention is required if we are to reverse its direction.

BASIC STRATEGIES OF CHANGE

BIOFEEDBACK

Biofeedback as a form of intervention provides the patient with an increased sense of control over physiological responsivity to stressors. Through monitoring their EMG, EEG, and/or thermal responsiveness to covert and/or overt stimuli, patients can learn to significantly reduce physiological reactivity. Biofeedback can be especially useful in reducing arousal responses to conditioned stressors such as finger sticks, nausea associated with chemotherapy, and stress-induced cervical headaches associated with environmental queues (i.e., entering a hospital).

In addition, by experiencing feedback on their physiological functioning, patients who have been educated about the concept of PNI can gain an increased sense of control (previously noted as extremely important) over their physiological responsiveness and, thereby, over their environmental stressors. It provides for the generally positively perceived concept of "learning and master" to be placed back into the patient's hands. For example, even patients who feel little control over their illness and/or pain can gain some emotional and/or pain relief by focusing on minor successes in controlling physiological changes during biofeedback. Immediate biological biofeedback may be especially helpful with patients who evidence low to moderate levels of hypnotizability, whereas highly hypnotizable patients appear to benefit more from delayed biological feedback. In delayed biofeedback, information is provided after several minutes of self-hypnosis training in order to shape and confirm the efficacy of the self-hypnosis training (Wickramasekera, 1999).

Within the thermal biofeedback approach, one goal is to teach the patient to lower sympathetic nervous system activity level through autogenic hand warming. Additionally, a quieting of the muscular armoring through EMG biofeedback can benefit patients by reducing stress-induced pain as well as pain-induced stress. The relaxing of the physiology and musculature is then enhanced with EEG biofeedback where patients can induce increased alpha and beta wave activity, thereby seeking to incur a quieter mental and emotional state. Alterations of cognitions, beliefs, and perceptions can be achieved via the association of altered physiological states with new concepts and coping thoughts. Bibliotherapy in conjunction with the biofeedback, which includes educating the patient about the benefits controlling stress responses has upon their limbic system (increasing

NKC activity and possibly reducing mutagenic effects), helps the patient tangibly connect with intervening in his or her own treatment (Davis, 1986).

CRANIAL ELECTROTHERAPY STIMULATION (CES)

With patients having difficulty achieving therapeutic levels of alpha states, even with biofeedback, cranial electrotherapy can assist by passing microcurrents through the cranial area via electrodes attached to the earlobes. CES stimulation has been shown to be helpful when utilized for emotional distress such as depression and anxiety by teaching the patient how to achieve a relaxed, quieted but alert state. While CES has not been found traditionally to be useful in treating stress-related disorders, recent studies have begun to demonstrate its effectiveness. Research has also demonstrated utility in pain management. By passing microcurrents through affected pain regions, patients report significant reductions at the sites of their pain. By combining CES with microcurrent stimulation at pain sites patients can reduce emotional distress and physical discomfort (Kirsch, 1999), thereby positively impacting upon the pain and emotional components of the PNI triad. The pain relief associated with microcurrent stimulation may provide the patient with an increased sense of control over pain and a smoothing of EEG peaks (associated with pain) when emotional and physical complaints are conjointly present (Hefferman, 1997). Because this treatment can often be self administered by the patient, it further enhances their sense of self-efficacy. It has little or no documented negative interactions with other forms of treatment.

VISUALIZATION/IMAGERY

Visualization has been conceived as the active process by which we "voluntarily and intentionally instruct the body." Whereas imagery is the spontaneously occurring "appearing in unconsciousness" modifier, qualifier, or belief emerging from the unconscious (Norris, 2000). Visualization represents how we ingest the world around us and what we then transfer to our unconscious or cognitive processing mind. Imagery represents how we interpret that information from the perspective of our internal beliefs and knowledge base. It represents, "What does that visualization mean to me?" Perhaps more succinctly stated, as clinicians, we can guide patients into varying visualizations but the imagery is the process within them, their "experience" of the visualization. Through the use of imagery, patients can learn to change their outlooks for the future, and for the illness process. This has been shown to be tremendously helpful in improving clinical outcomes.

Pioneering in the use of imagery in fighting cancer in works such as *Love, Medicine, and Miracles* (Siegel, 1986) helps patients develop a sense of personal efficacy in dealing with their illnesses, and enhancing the PNI triad. Visualization can help patients focus on the events they are experiencing in the process of working through their illnesses.

An excellent example of the use of imagery applied to the treatment of severe and chronic illness, especially cancer, is the program developed by Mitchell Gaynor, M.D. In his book, *Healing E.S.S.E.N.C.E.*, he details the use of imagery throughout seven steps toward healing: experiences, see, surrender, empower, nurture, create, embody (Gaynor, 1995). Even patients with no prior experience with imagery can develop a practical and useful means of controlling illness and enhance the healing process.

Whatever the name, mental imagery (Moye, Richardson, Post-White, & Justice, 1995), guided imagery (Giedt, 1997), relaxation imagery (Andrews and Hall, 1990), and autogenic training (Benor, 1996) have been shown to be immuno-enhancing. In a somewhat more extreme example of drug-induced imagery states, Roberts (1999) found that entheogen-induced mystical and peak experiences may boost the immune system.

HYPNOSIS

Hypnosis is arguably the most effective approach in unifying the different aspects of the PNI triad. In ways, hypnosis may encompass many of the other approaches previously mentioned. Hypnosis can have a positive effect on illness by intervening at several levels including symptom alleviation, emotional stabilization, stress reduction, self-image enhancing, and self-efficacy empowering. It also can be employed in directly attempting to enhance endocrine responsiveness and CNS reactivity as well as pain control. Kalt (2000) states that "techniques which attempt to influence the mind fall into the theoretical categories of passive, active, or targeted approaches, each of which may carry varying degrees of importance in immuno-enhancement."

Hypnosis has often been segregated into three general orientations. These include direct, indirect, and nondirective approaches. The following is a brief discription of each approach and its utility in PNI intervention.

Traditional Approaches of Direct Suggestion with Formal Induction

In these approaches, general trance depth is considered to be important in symptomological change, or behavioral changes are given as a directive from the therapist. Although imagery may be employed, it is often the hypnotherapist's conceptualizations that direct the patient's internal experience. Direct hypnotic approaches have been effectively used, especially in situations where the patient either is strongly invested

in turning over control to the therapist (i.e., pain management) or where the patient enters the therapeutic setting with significantly impaired feelings of self-empowerment or self-efficacy.

The need to feel that "the therapist is hypnotizing them" provides an initial sense of being taken care of, which may be critical to some patients, especially those deeply ingrained in the medical model. Issues of suggestibility and susceptibility are often raised when arguing the effectiveness of traditional hypnotherapeutic interventions.

With regard to pain management, significant support exists for the importance of the hypnotic suggestibility of patients. Highly suggestible patients demonstrate significantly greater pain tolerance (DePascalis, Magurano, & Bellusci, 1999; Farthing, Venturino, Brown, & Lazer, 1997; Rainville, Carrier, Hofbauer, Bushnell, & Duncan, 1999; Sandrini et al., 2000; Zachariae, Anderson, Bjerring, Jorgensen, & Arendt-Nielsen, 1998) and postoperative recovery than less suggestible patients (Defechereuz, Meurisse, Hamior, Gollogly, Jorus, & Faymonville, 1999; Mauer, Burnett, Oullette, Ironson, & Dandes, 1999). Other studies have demonstrated that the ability to be hypnotized may be less of a factor especially in emergency room settings where an increase in hypnotic susceptibility may be induced by the trauma (Pebbles-Kleiger, 2000).

Indirect Approaches

Currently, one of the most commonly utilized indirect hypnotic approaches is Ericksonian hypnosis. Ericksonian hypnosis promotes the idea of trusting in the patient's unconscious to deal with issues that arise. By its very nature, Ericksonian hypnosis employs a psychoimmunotherapeutic bent. Through the use of metaphor, storytelling techniques, and indirect suggestion, the patient is asked to seek what internal images or associations arise while in a hypnotic state in order to bring about emotional and psychotherapeutic change (Erickson, 1980). Distraction and dissociative suggestions have been utilized with pain patients within the Ericksonian model (Burte, Burte, & Aroaz, 1994). The therapist often acts in a reflective manner, guiding the patient into a deepening understanding of the spontaneously generated images by applying metaphors or stories to relay the hypnotic suggestion while allowing the patient to integrate the message into his or her own schema. The therapist helps the patient to understand the nature and origin of his or her symptoms, whether emotional, physical, or physiological. Ericksonian approaches have been extensively employed in the treatment of medical illness both symptomologically and etiologically (Erickson, 1986).

Simonton and Henson (1992) utilize hypnotic approaches in helping patients learn how to increase their ability to heal (enhance their PNI triad). Visualizing their bodies fighting illness by generating increased T-cells (i.e., little white Pac men eating the cancer) or visualizing bronchial dilation or shunting off blood flow to a tumor are examples of but a few of the plethora of indirect hypnotic applications patients can utilize.

Nondirective Approaches

The new hypnosis initially developed by Araoz (1985) presents a somewhat different model than either the traditional (direct suggestion) or Eriksonian models (indirect suggestion). The new hypnosis utilizes the symptoms brought to the session by the patient as the means of entering the patient's "inner state." A process of observing the patient's somatopsychic behaviors (i.e., hair twirling, fist clenching), and psychosemantic expressions (i.e., "he turns my stomach") within the framework of how these actions are manifested through the visual, auditory, olfactory/taste, proprioceptive, and kinesthetic senses is initiated. Patients are then led into their own inner awarenesses. They are encouraged not to judge or critique what arises. Often the patients gain new insights into the process, which affects their interpretations or reactions to stressors.

At this point, patients are given the opportunity to "visualize and introduce changes that promote greater well being." Perhaps most critical in the PNI framework is the concept of negative self-hypnosis (NSH). Patients often find that they maintain negative self-hypnotic statements such as broad concepts of "I can never overcome this illness, it is going to kill me" to more minute specific beliefs about their illnesses or stressors.

The goal in applying the new hypnosis or any hypnotic intervention is to be able to intervene and exchange those negative self-hypnotic beliefs for positive self-hypnotic beliefs (PSH). This is best accomplished when, through the hypnotic experience, the patient feels a change that comes from changes in his or her inner awareness and belief system. For example, a patient who was experiencing chest pain of a nonorganically based nature, reported that in trance, due to unresolved issues with his father he became aware of the pain as an image of his father's fist squeezing his heart. Upon imaging a conversation where he resolved these issues and could see his father's hand stroking his heart, the pain abated (Burte, 1989).

In situations where pain or stress has a clear etiological basis, the new hypnosis has been employed in developing coping skills, visualizing analgesia, or promoting positive internal representation for changes in biophysiology (Burte et al., 1994).

Eye Movement Desensitization and Reprocessing (EMDR)

An interesting new approach, known as EMDR, has been employed with trauma patients. It demonstrates some promising results. Perhaps of most significance in PNI is the concept of repressed trauma as a possible precursor to immunosuppression.

Group Therapy

Extensive work has been conducted on the impact of group therapy and stress management on immunosuppression. David Speigel's (1999) work with breast cancer patients demonstrates the efficacy of group support as does the work of other researchers who have found subsequently that group therapy can enhance life expectancy and functioning of patients with HIV and other immunosuppressant disorders. It appears that group therapy offers patients a sense of cohesiveness and an opportunity to express their negative emotions and beliefs while simultaneously helping them develop a better mental attitude and coping skills which, in turn, appears to enhance immune system functions.

Societal isolation and self-imposed feelings of family isolation (even at times when under the best of supportive conditions) negatively impact the PNI triad in the chronic pain and chronically ill patient (Hitchcock, 1998). Lack of family coherence, at times present with severely ill patients, emphasizes the importance of group therapy as an outlet for these patients. It provided a sense of coherence and support that they cannot obtain from their families or personal support networks. A review of the literature appears to suggest that a diverse range of therapeutic/support groups may be effective, and, in fact, it may be merely the intangible element of not facing adversity alone that enhances immune functioning. Stress management, pain management, coping skills development, dance, acting "as if," group laughter, supportive nondirective groups, all appear to contribute positively to patient well-being and demonstrate PNI enhancement.

Meditation

Role Play and Dance

Another technique found to impact the immune system includes meditation, which via the pineal gland influences melatonin levels, which, in turn, have been shown to modulate the progression of breast and prostate tumors (Coker, 1999). In addition to covert techniques such as meditation, the mere outward expression or "acting/modeling of happy behaviors have been found to stimulate endorphins and enhance immune system function" (Anderson, 1997). This may be especially helpful when it is difficult to convince patients of the impact of their negativistic thinking. At such times, perhaps we can encourage them to "act as if" they were happy in order to bring about immunological changes. Still other researchers have found that dance therapy (Hanna, 1995) may improve patient immune functioning possibly by providing proprioceptive feedback and feelings of self-efficacy and physical self-control during those times.

A variety of other modalities too far reaching to encompass in this brief chapter also deserve mentioning as they are represented in the PNI literature. Behavioral approaches (Caudell, 1996; Cottraux, 1993;), diet and psychological health (Miller, 1996; Norris, 2000), healing energy (Wright & Sayre-Adams, 1999), laughter and music (Bittman, 2000; Strickland, 1993), and exercise (LaPierriere, Ironson, Antoni, Schneiderman, Klimas, & Fletcher, 1994) have been demonstrated to provide positive changes, although further investigation of their mechanisms is necessary.

Physical manipulative techniques that directly affect the physiology and nerve transmission, such as chiropractic massage therapy (Homewood, 1981; Rich, 1999) may bring physical and restorative relief and provide pain control (with or without opioids). These are but a few approaches that may promote healing via reducing stress, reducing pain, or enhancing patient efficacy.

A word of caution is raised by Greer (1991), who notes that within the PNI model of intervention, one must be on guard that a "blaming the victim" mentality is not promulgated inadvertently. Emphasis should be on positive change, not responsibility for creating one's own impaired status. Any intervention that increases the individual's sense of control of his or her environment or pain level reduces stress, enhances optimism and self-efficacy, impacts the PNI triad proactively, and may promote increased health by reducing immunosuppression (Burte, 2000).

"Goodbye" said the fox. "And now here is my secret, a very simple secret. It is only with the heart that one can see rightly. What is essential is invisible to the eye." "What is essential is invisible to the eye" the little prince repeated so that he would be sure to remember (Antoine de Saint-Exupéry, 1943).

ACKNOWLEDGMENTS

I would like to acknowledge Michele Underwood, Steve Bonomo, and Theresa Barle for their assistance.

REFERENCES

Affleck, G., Urrows, S., Tennen, H., Higgins, P., Pav, D., & Aloisi, R. (1997). The dual pathway model of daily stressor effects on rheumatoid arthritis. *Annals of Behavioral Medicine, 19*(2), 161–170.

Altman, F. (1997). Where is the "neuro" in psychoneuroimmunology? A commentary on increasing research on the "neuro" component of psychoneuroimmunology. *Brain, Behavior, and Immunity, 11*(1), 1–8.

Andersen, D.L. (1997). Nurses: act now! *Journal of Practical Nursing, 47*(1), 16–18.

Andrews, V.H., & Hall, H.R. (1990). The effects or relaxation/imagery training on recurrent aphthous stomatitis: a preliminary study. *Psychosomatic Medicine, 52*(5), 526–535.

Araoz, D.L. (1985). *The new hypnosis.* New York: Brunner/Mazel Inc.

Benor, R. (1996). Autogenic training. *Complementary Therapy in Nursing and Midwifery, 2*(5), 134–138.

Berin, M.C., & Perdue, M.H. (1997). Effect of psychoneural factors on intestinal epithelial function. *Canadian Journal of Gastroenterology, 11*(4), 353–357.

Biondi, M., & Zannino, L.G. (1997). Psychological stress, neuro-immune-modulation and susceptibility to infectious diseases in animal and man: A review. *Psychotherapy and Psychosomatics, 66*(1), 3–26.

Bittman, B. (2000, September) Psychoneuroimmunology of laughter and music. Paper presented at the 11th annual clinical meeting of the American Academy of Pain Management.

Burte, J.M. (1989, October). *Internally directed hypnosis.* S. Rosenberg (Ed.), New York Society of Clinical Hypnosis course workbook.

Burte, J.M., Burte, W., & Aroaz, D.L. (1994). Hypnosis in the treatment of back pain. *Australian Journal of Clinical Hypnotherapy and Hypnosis, 15*(2), 93–115.

Burte, J.M., & Aroaz, D.L. (1994). Cognitive hypnotherapy with sexual disorders. *Journal of Cognitive Psychotherapy Winter, 8,* 299–311.

Burte, J.M. (2000). Psychoneuroimmunology. Paper presented at the 11th annual meeting of the American Academy of Pain Management, Sept. 21, 2000.

Caudell, K.A. (1996). Psychoneuroimmunology and innovative behavioral interventions with leukemia. *Oncology Nursing Forum, 23*(3), 493–502.

Christensen, A.J., Edwards, D.L., Wiebe, J.S., Benotsch, E.G., McKelvey, L., Andrews, M., & Lubaroff, D.M. (1996). Effect of verbal self-disclosure on natural killer cell activity: Moderating influence of cynical hostility. *Psychosomatic Medicine, 58*(2), 150–155.

Coker, K.H. (1999). Meditation and Prostate Cancer: integrating a mind/body intervention with traditional therapies. *Seminars in Urologic Oncology, 17*(2), 111–118.

Cottraux, J. (1993). Behavioral psychotherapy applications in medically ill. *Psychotherapy and Psychosomatics, 60*(3–4), 116–128.

Coyle, P.K. (1996). The neuroimmunology of multiple sclerosis. *Advances in Neuroimmunology, 6*(2), 143–154.

Dabkowska, M., & Rybakowski, J. (1994). Stress, depression and schizophrenia in view of psycho-immunology. *Psychiatria Polska, 28*(3 Suppl.), 23–32.

Davis, H. (1986). Effects of biofeedback and cognitive therapy on stress in patients with breast cancer. *Psychological Reports, 59*(2), 967–974.

Defechereux, T., Meurisse, M., Hamoir, E., Gollogly, L., Joris, J., & Faymonville, M.E. (1999). Hypnoanesthesia for endocrine cervical surgery: A statement of practice. *Journal of Alternative Complementary Medicine, 5*(6), 509–520.

DePascalis, V., Magurano, M.R., & Bellusci, A. (1999). Pain perception, somato-sensory event related potentials and skin conductance responses to painful stimuli in high, mid, and low hypnotizable strategies. *Pain, 82*(2), 159–171.

de Saint-Exupéry, A. (1943). *The Little Prince.* New York: Harcourt Brace (reprinted 1982).

Eller, L.S. (1998). Testing a model: Effects of pain on immunity in HIV+ and HIV− participants. *Scholarly Inquiry for Nursing Practice, 12*(3), 191–124.

Erickson, M.H. (1980). Hypnotic alteration of sensory perceptual and psychological process. In E. Rossi (Ed.), *The collected papers of Milton H. Erickson on hypnosis* (Vol. II). New York: Irvington Press.

Erickson, M.H. (1986). Mind-body communication in hypnosis. In E. Rossi & M. Ryan (Eds.), *The seminar, workshops and lectures of Milton H. Erickson* (Vol. 1). New York: Irvington Press.

Farthing, G.W., Venturino, M., Brown, S.W., & Lazar, J.D. (1997). Internal and external distraction in the control of cold pressor pain as a function of hypnotizability. *International Journal of Clinical Experimental Hypnosis, 45*(4), 433–446.

Garssen, B., & Goodkin, K. (1999). On the role of immunological factors as mediators between psychosocial factors and cancer progression. *Psychiatry Research, 85*(1), 51–61.

Gaynor, M. (1994). *Healing E.S.S.E.N.C.E. A cancer doctor's practical program for hope and recovery.* New York: Kodansha International.

Geiss, A., Varodi, E., Steinbach, K., Bauer, H.W., & Anton, F. (1997). Psychoneuroimmunological correlates of persisting sciatic pain in patients who underwent discectomy. *Neuroscience Letters, 237*(2–3), 65–68.

Giedt, J.F. (1997). Guided imagery. A psychoneuroimmunological intervention in holistic nursing practice. *Journal of Holistic Nursing, 15*(2), 112–127.

Glaser, R. (1996). The effects of stress on the immune system: Implications for health. Summary of presentation on Dec. 17, Science Writers Briefings, OBSSR and APA. http://www/.od.nih.gov/obssr/stresimn.htm

Greer, S. (1991). Psychological response to cancer survival. *Psychological Medicine, 21*(1), 43–49.

Hall, M., Baum, A., Buysse, D.J., Prigerson, H.G., Kupfer, D.J., & Reynolds, C.F. III. (1998). Sleep as a mediator of the stress-immune relationship. *Psychosomatic Medicine, 60*(1), 48–51.

Hanna, J.L. (1995). The power of dance: health and healing. *Journal of Alternative and Complementary Medicine, 1*(4), 323–331.

Hefferman, M. (1997). The effect of microcurrent of EEG spectrum and pain control. *Canadian Journal of Clinical Medicine, 4*(10), 4–11.

Hickie, I., Bennet, B., Lloyd, A., Heath, A., & Martin, N. (1999). Complex genetic and environmental relationships between psychological distress, fatigue and immune functioning: A twin study. *Psychological Medicine, 29*(2), 269–277.

Hiramoto, R.N., Solvason, H.B., Hsueh, C.M., Rogers, C.F., Demissie, S., Hiramoto, N.S., Gauthier, D.K., Lorden, J.F., & Ghanta, V.K. (1999). Psychoneuro-endocrine immunology: perception of stress can alter body temperature and natural killer cell activity. *International Journal of Neuroscience, 98*(1–2), 95–129.

Hitchcock, L.S. (1998). The role of self-help groups in easing chronic pain. In R. Weiner (Ed.). *Pain management: A practical guide.* Boca Raton: CRC Press.

Holmes, T.H., & Rahe, R.H. (1967). The social readjustment rating scale. *Journal of Psychosomatic Research, 11*(2), 213–218.

Homewood, A.E. (1981). *The neurodynamics of vertebral sublaxation.* St. Petersburg, FL: Valkyrie Press.

Kalt, H.W. (2000). Psychoneuroimmunology: An interpretation of experimental and case study evidence towards a paradigm of predictable results. *American Journal of Hypnosis, 43*(1), 41–52.

Kaye, J., Morton, J., Bowcutt, M., & Maupin, D. (2000). Stress, depression and psychoneuroimmunology. *Journal of Neuroscience Nursing, 32*(2), 93–100.

Kelly, S., Hertzman, C., & Daniels, M. (1997). Searching for the biological nature of pain. *Seminars in Oncology Nursing, 13*(1), 10–15.

Kiecolt-Glaser, J.K., Page, G.G., Marucha, P.T., MacCallum, R.C., & Glaser, R. (1998). Psychological influences on surgical recovery. Perspectives from psychoneuroimmunology. *American Psychologist, 53*(11), 11209–11218.

Kirsch, D. (1999). *The science behind cranial electrotherapy stimulation: An annotated bibliography.* Edmonton, Canada: Medical Scope Publishing Company.

Klapheke, M.M. (2000). Transplantation psychoneuroimmunology: Building hypotheses. *Medical Hypotheses, 54*(6), 969–978.

Koenker, H. Stress and the Immune System. http://www.econ.uiuc.edu/~hanko/bio/stress.html.

Kremer, M.J. (1999). Surgery, pain and immune function. *The Clinical Forum for Nurse Anesthetists, 10*(3), 94–100.

LaPerriere, A., Ironson, G., Antoni, M.H., Schneiderman, N., Klimas, N., & Fletcher, M.A. (1994). Exercise and psychoneuroimmunology. *Medicine and Science in Sports and Exercise, 26*(2), 182–190.

Laudenslager, M.L. (1983). Coping and Immunosuppression. *Science, 221*, 568.

Marbach, J.J., Schleifer, S.J., & Keller, S.E. (1990). Facial pain, distress, and immune function. *Brain, Behavior, and Immunity, 4*(3), 243–254.

Martin, P. (1998). *The healing mind: The vital links between brain and behavior, immunity and disease.* New York: St. Martin's Press.

Masek, K., Petrovicky, P., Seucik, J., Zidek, Z., & Frankova, D. (2000). Past, present and future of psychoneuroimmunology. *Toxicology, 142*(3), 179–188.

Mauer, M.H., Burnett, K.F., Oullette, E.A., Ironson, G.H., & Dandes, H.M. (1999). Medical hypnosis and orthopedic hand surgery: Pain perception, postoperative recovery and therapeutic comfort. *International Journal of Clinical and Experimental Hypnosis, 47*(2), 144–161.

Miller, M. (1996). Diet and psychological health. *Alternative Therapies in Health and Medicine, 2*(5), 40–48.

Moye, L.A., Richardson, M.A., & Post-White, J.B. (1995). Research methodology in psychoneuroimmunology: rationale and design of the IMAGES-P clinical trial. *Alternative Therapies in Health and Medicine, 1*(2), 34–39.

Muller, N. (1997). Role of the cytokine network in the CNS and psychiatric disorders. *Nervenarzt, 68*(1), 11–20.

Norris, P. (2000). Self-regulation for immune system disorders. http://www.cjnetworks.com/~lifesci/immu.htm

Overcash, S.J. (1999). A retrospective study to determine efficacy of cranial electrotherapy stimulation (CES) on patients suffering from anxiety disorders. *American Journal of Electromedicine, 16*(1), 49–51.

Page, G.G., & Ben-Eliyahu, S. (1997). The immune-suppressive nature of pain. *Seminars in Oncology Nursing, 13*(1), 10–15.

Parker, J.C., Smarr, K.L., Angelone, E.O., Mothersead, P.K., Lee, B.S., Walker, S.E., Bridges, A.J., Caldwell, C.W. (1992). Psychological factors, immunologic activation and disease activity in rheumatoid arthritis. *Arthritis Care Research, 5*(4), 196–201.

Peebles-Kleiger, M.J. (2000). The use of hypnosis in emergency medicine. *Emergency Medicine Clinics of North America, 18*(2), 327–338.

Pike, J.L., Smith, T.L., Hauger, R.L., Nicassio, P.M., Patterson, T.L., McClintick, J., Costlow, C., & Irwin, M.R. (1997). Chronic life stress alters sympathetic, neuroendocrine and immune responsibility to an acute psychological stressor in humans. *Psychosomatic Medicine, 59*(4), 447–457.

Rainville, P., Carrier, B., Hofbauer, R.K., Bushnell, M.C., & Duncan, G.H. (1999). Dissociation of sensory and affective dimensions of pain using hypnotic modulation. *Pain, 8*(2), 159–171.

Rich, G.J. (1999). Healing hands. *Psychology Today, 32*(2), 23.

Roberts, T.B. (1999). Do entheogen-induced mystical experiences boost the immune system? Psychedelics, peak experiences and wellness. *Advanced Mind and Body Medicine, 5*(2), 139–147.

Sali, A. (1997). Psychoneuroimmunology: Fact or fiction. *Journal of the Family Physician, 26*(11), 1291–1294, 1296–1299.

Sandrini, G., Mianov, I., Malaguti, S., Nigvelli, M.P., Moglia, A., & Napp, G. (2000). Effects of hypnosis on diffuse noxious inhibitory controls. *Physiological Behavior, 69*(3), 295–300.

Schrader, K.A. (1996). Stress and immunity after traumatic injury: The mind-body link. *American Association of Clinical Nursing Clinical Issues, 7*(3), 351–358.

Segerstrom, S. (1998). Optimism is associated with mood, coping and change in response to stress. *Journal of Personality and Social Psychology, 74*(6), 1646–1655.

Selye, H. (1956). *The stress of life.* New York: McGraw Hill.

Selye, H. (1976). *Stress in health and disease.* Woburn, MA: Butterworth.

Siegel, B. (1998). *Love, medicine and miracles.* New York: Harper and Row.

Simonton, O.C., & Henson, R. (1992). *The healing journey.* New York: Bantam.

Solomon, G.F., Segerstrom, S.C., Grohr, P., Kemeny, M., & Fahey, J. (1997). Shaking up immunity: psychological and immunologic changes after a natural disaster. *Psychosomatic Medicine, 59*(2), 114–127.

Spiegel, D. (1999). Embodying the mind in psycho-oncology research. *Advances in Mind and Body Medicine, 15*(4), 267–273.

Strickland, D. (1993). Seriously, laughter matters. *Today's OR Nurse, 15*(6), 19–24.

Turk, D., Merchenbaum, D., & Genest, M. (1983). *Pain and behavioral medicine: A cognitive-behavioral perspective.* New York: Guilford Press.

Van der Pompe, G., Antoni, M., Visser, A., & Garssen, B. (1996). Adjustment to breast cancer: The psychobiological effects of psychosocial interventions. *Patient Education and Counseling, 28*(2), 209–219.

Vedhara, K., Fox, J.D., & Wang, E.C. (1999). The measurement of stress-related immune dysfunction in psychoneuroimmunology. *Neuroscience and Biobehavior Reviews, 23*(5), 699–715.

Watt, D., Verma, S., & Flynn, L. (1998). Wellness programs: A review of the evidence. *Canadian Medical Association Journal, 158*(2), 224–230.

Wickramasekera, I. (1999). How does biofeedback reduce clinical symptoms and do memories and beliefs have biological consequences? Toward a model of mind–body healing. *Applied Psychophysiology and Biofeedback, 24*(2), 91–105.

Wright, S.G., & Sayer-Adams, J. (1999). Healing energy and the complementary therapies. *Complementary Therapy in Nursing and Midwifery, 5*(4), 95–97.

Yang, E.V., & Glaser, R. (2000). Stress induced immunomodulation: Impact on immune defenses against infectious disease. *Biomedicine and Pharmacotherapy, 54*(5), 245–250.

Zachariae, R., Andersen, O.K., Bjerring, P., Jorgensen, M.M., & Arendt-Nielsen, L. (1998). Effects of opioid antagonist on pain intensity and withdrawal reflexes during induction of hypnotic analgesia in high and low hypnotizable volunteers. *European Journal of Pain, 2*(1), 25–34.

Zautra, A.J., Hoffman, J., Potter, P., Matt, K.S., Yocum, D., & Castro, L. (1997). Examination of changes in interpersonal stress as a factor in disease exacerbation among women with rheumatoid arthritis. *Annals of Behavior Medicine, 19*(3), 279–286.

65

Variables in the Sensation and Perception of Pain

Richard H. Cox, M.D., Ph.D., D.Min. and John Essman, M.A., R.E.E.G./E.P.T., R.P.S.G.T.

Whosoever is spared personal pain must feel himself called to help in diminishing the pain of others.

Albert Schweitzer

INTRODUCTION

Pain is doubtless one of the most illusive and complicated aspects of life, particularly for the practicing health professional. From the inception of recorded human history everyone from the afflicted to sages, philosophers, theologians, and magicians have attempted to enlighten us regarding this condition. We are now wise enough to know that what we are currently recording will no doubt also be shown to be just as naive in years to come. Yet, despite this, we must try to consolidate what we know in an attempt to help those living in this era of history. We now know enough to see pain as more than a result and more than a syndrome. It is doubtless an illness all its own. Portenoy (1996) conceptualized longstanding pain associated with tissue damage as far more disabling than the injury itself.

Whereas "pain" has traditionally been thought of as a result of distress, usually with physical etiology, we now recognize many kinds of pain arising from multiple, singular, and combined sources. Whereas physical pain continues to be our greatest challenge in the medical world, other disciplines have joined to remind us of emotional pain and spiritual pain. We have come to recognize the interconnection of these kinds of pain and the reciprocal nature of the origins and amplifiers of pain. We have come to see that physical pain can be reduced or increased by emotional and spiritual pain and vice versa. The latest version (1995) of *Roget's Thesaurus* classifies pain as a physical experience, as does the Sixth Edition (2000) of *The Columbia Encyclopedia.* Our definitional literature has not caught up with the experiential world.

Practitioners are now challenged to preserve *good* pain while attempting to eliminate *bad* pain. Someone has said that without pain we could die without knowing that we were sick. Therefore, there is good pain, i.e., that pain which triggers action to protect the body and mind. However, there is also bad pain that produces more pain and suffering. Sometimes the signals of these two kinds of pain become confused and produce even greater suffering and actually escalate simple neuropathic pain into allodynia, the normally nonpainful stimulus that is perceived as painful, and is probably psychologically mediated. The possibility that such pain is psychologically mediated does not, however, mean that the pain is psychosomatic (psychologically induced) or only imagined. The etiology of pain and the mediation of pain are not the same. The origin of a neurological message and the transmission of that message are not the same thing. Pain may be *caused* by psychological stimuli or the stimulus may be transmitted neurologically, or in variations and combinations. Allodynia may truly be somatopsychic and real regardless of the mechanism that produced the final perceived sensation (Iadarola & Caudle, 1997).

Because pain is highly individualized and individually reported, it is possible that a practitioner could unwittingly create a state for future serious injury

0-8493-0926-3/02/$0.00+$1.50
© 2002 by CRC Press LLC

because of neuropathic reporting and the subsequent alleviation of good pain. Illustrative of this are the persons who have been delivered from headache only to die from undiagnosed brain tumors. When healers are instructed by the Oath of Hippocrates to "do no harm," they must first recognize that the remediation of pain, in and of itself, although seemingly a noble gesture, may in truth not always be the most beneficial goal of treatment. Every quadriplegic knows that the absence of pain is a serious detriment to one's health.

Pain is a multichannel warning system within the human body. It is transmitted via many different pathways and culminates in the body's awareness that something is wrong. However, pain is more than a warning system. It is frequently an entity in itself that precludes normal thought and physiological functions. Illustrative of this are conditions such as post-herpetic neuralgia, a condition in which the nervous system continues to emit painful messages long after the actual viral infection has been arrested. When this is the case, the pain becomes both the etiology and the result of a condition that is definable as a separate and distinct illness.

THE CHALLENGE OF PAIN MEASUREMENT AND ASSESSMENT

One of our greatest unsolved problems in dealing with pain is our inability to see or measure it. We are getting closer to understanding substance P and its binding receptor NK-1. The release of neuroactive substances such as glutamate, calcitonin, along with substance P and substance K combines with biochemical mediation of nociceptive neurons, producing a perceived and probable actual change in the neurogenic recognition and transmission of the stimulus, which is ultimately experienced as pain. Good pain and bad pain are by all probability "attenuated by different toxin-ligand molecules" (Iadarola & Caudle, 1997).

There have been several attempts to measure pain; however, none has proven valid. The Gaston-Johansson Pain-O-Meter and the Gaston-Johansson Pain-O-Meter Visual Analogue Scale are attempts to quantify and identify levels of pain (Sittner, Hudson, Grossman, & Gaston-Johansson, 1998). In the final analysis, the only reliable measurer of pain is the person experiencing it. Pain is most accurately measured by descriptors such as "burning," "lancinating," "stabbing," "aching," "throbbing," etc. The perception of pain measurement on a scale of one to ten is probably as beneficial to most practitioners as anything. The patient can then indicate if the remediation is providing a lesser or greater scale score. Perception, in truth, is everything when it comes to the phenomenon of pain.

Doubtless one's level of consciousness is related to one's perception of pain. Qualia are the philosophically designated intrinsic properties of conscious experience. However, any health service provider who has worked with unconscious patients knows that even in the state of deep coma patients respond to deep pain, proving that consciousness is not a necessary requirement for pain perception. The qualia become beneficial in diagnosis and treatment of illness because they provide us with the descriptors, and the descriptors have common and frequent relationships to certain physiological conditions. Certainly the more accurately a patient can describe the pain, the more likely the physician will be able to provide the correct remedy.

Descarte believed that pain was a simple mechanism of action–reaction. As simplistic as this description is, the vast majority of persons who adhere to Western medical thought maintain a view that is not very different. The rapidly growing body of literature regarding pain is proving that pain is not simply an action–reaction phenomenon but a complex neural, chemical, anatomical, emotional, and cultural mixture. Most health service providers, even in the Western world, have given up the Cartesian mind/body separation, but we as yet have insufficient practitioner understood knowledge of the complex mechanisms we know are present but as yet unexplained.

Pain and *suffering* are not synonymous although often companions. Culturally mediated experiences of the same kind of stimuli produce different levels of perceived suffering. Athletes, martyrs, and mentally ill and hypervigilant persons have been reported to experience severe traumatic stimuli that under other conditions and in other cultures are reported as very different levels of suffering. There is no absolute correlation between the actual stimulus of pain and the reported level of suffering. Persons experiencing coma, yoga, hypnosis, and other states of altered consciousness have shown the presence of pain stimulus without the recognition of such by the person experiencing it. The attempt to measure pain by its consequent manifestations of suffering are, therefore, without scientific or experiential bases (McQuillen, 1991).

The aspect of suffering has been coupled with the degree to which the etiology of the pain is perceived to be a threat to the patient as a person. This has also been called one's "Total pain" (Cassel, 1982). It stands to reason that a threat of change or loss of life can markedly impact the meaning and, therefore, the attention paid to said stimulus, with the ultimate stakes of an impaired quality of life, which could result in social isolation, occupational difficulties, and financial hardship to name but a few. This can stand as a true test of a person's character, possibly adding kindling to underlying dysfunctional character traits, which could lead to a multitude of poor choices.

INDIVIDUAL DIFFERENCES IN PERCEPTION

There are only minor and poorly substantiated differences in each gender's perception of pain. These vague and nonscientifically based reports tend to indicate that much additional study is needed before one can conjecture regarding gender-related pain (Marble, 1999). Kelly (1999) asserts that because women probably experience pain more frequently than most men, they feel pain more keenly, yet women have a lower threshold for pain than men. The research is scant and far from scientifically based on this subject.

Children are most interesting in their reactions to pain. They tend to relate pain to various actions done to them, and they tend to see all pain as bad. As children mature, differentiate pain and its severity into various categories. Young children see pain as having an "owie," or being "stuck or poked," or simply that it "stings" or "burns." We, of course, know that young children do not relate causality to consequence in the same fashion as do older children or adults. It only goes to reason that they would perceive pain as whatever is present in the end state. Much the same as the child who spills the milk says, "the milk spilled," the child in pain says simply that "it hurts" (Woodgate & Kristjianson, 1996).

The same ambiguity is present in attempting to differentiate the experience of pain by ethnicity. A recent study reported that white persons reported "less severe disabling pain and withstood more pain for longer intervals than blacks" (Pirisi, 2000). Numerous studies have demonstrated that responses and expressions differ greatly from one ethnicity to another; however, studies do not exist that clearly demonstrate that the variations of response are due solely or primarily to ethnicity (Chapman, Toru, Martin, Tanaka, Okazaki, Colpitts, Mayero, & Gaghardi, 1982; Clark & Clark,1980; Morse & Morse, 1988; Woodrow, Friedman, Seigelaub, & Collen, 1972). Generalizations abound regarding certain ethnic responses to pain, however, solid research is lacking to establish any such claims.

There is an emerging literature regarding the responses of older people to pain. Ruzicka (1998) reports that the beliefs of elders modify the experience of pain considerably. She found that "Pain is common and older people are expected to put up with it," and "Searching for the meaning in the pain experience is important, and often a review of past personal experience is the method used to attach meaning to the experience," and that elders are reluctant to express pain. There is doubtless a critical element present regarding the experience of pain and the willingness to complain about it. This is most probably a result of culture rather than age.

CHANGING PERCEPTIONS

Pain is more strongly linked with emotion than any other area of perception (Matlin, 1988). A visual perception, such as a beautiful sunset, exists out there in the environment and, therefore, can be a common or shared experience with another individual. In contrast, a perception of pain, such as a toothache, is a much more in here experience, within the confines of our bodies; therefore, such an experience is difficult to convey to others (Verillo, 1975).

Pain is a subjective experience depending on the nature of the perception of the individual; therefore, the experience of and response to a given painful stimuli can change as the perception changes. Cornock (1996) pointed out a few of the many factors that may affect a person's perception of any given painful stimulation. He included cultural factors, the context in which the pain occurs, expectations, emotions, motivations, personality, past experiences, and preparations. To understand these as some of the contributing influences of the net experience a person has provides the clinician with key elements for addressing a person's past experiences to help change the present perception of a painful process.

Interestingly, pain research has investigated essentially every aspect covered in a basic college psychology course, including learning and motivation, psychophysics and perception, brain and behavior, memory and cognition, individual differences, development, personality, psychological disorders, and social behavior (Craig & Rollman, 1999). To truly understand a pain process holistically, one must understand physiology, psychology, sociology, and spirituality. Since Melzack and Wall (1965) published their Gate Control theory, a watershed of different types of nontraditional treatment methods has been forthcoming because of the suggestion of efficacious modulation of pain in concert with traditional allopathic medicine. For the first time, it became apparent that the sufferer had some degree of control over the pain processes associated with his/her given affliction, with proper education and work.

A greater sense of personal control over one's body can have great influence on the impact of his/her perception. Much like the elephant who has learned he can't break free from his shackles, even though the claims are oftentimes much smaller chains than what were originally used, the individual with an external locus of control, dependent on others to take care of his/her ills, often will lack the confidence to break free from the confines of the condition. This often will lead to a less proactive and sedentary, unhealthy lifestyle, which does not promote healing.

Likewise, a sense of self-efficacy is closely related to an internal sense of control. Self-efficacy originated with Albert Bandura and is defined as "an individual's sense of their abilities, of their capacity to deal with the particular sets of conditions that life puts before them" (Reber, 1995). Obviously, learned helplessness can be the net result of a poor sense of self-efficacy. Knowing this may be a normal reaction of individuals suffering from painful conditions, work geared toward self-confidence, personal controllability, and an internal locus of control may prove fruitful for many patients. It is important to remember, however, that some individuals *need* their pain. It gives them focus, attention, and reinforcement that may be beyond the scope of the clinician to understand.

Cornock (1996) outlined four major nonpharmaceutical approaches that can be used to help alter the pain patient's perception of pain. Please refer to the psychological technique chapter of this text for a more comprehensive understanding of these concepts. These include

1. Information control. Through open communication of pain and its underlying conditions, some of the mystery is eliminated, thus alleviating the fear of the unknown.
2. Behavior methods. Through operant models of conditioning, desirable behavior is reinforced and positive change is rewarded. Relaxation and biofeedback also may be used to reduce tension and stress that may contribute to pain.
3. Cognitive approaches. These work to replace maladaptive thoughts, provide nonpain imagery, and refocus attention.
4. Hypnosis. A modality used for many different problems through relaxation, the placebo effect, and possibly the effect of the clinician on the patient.

With the successful use of one or several of these techniques, pain can be managed effectively by changing the perception of the ongoing physiological pain.

TWO MAJOR TYPES OF PAIN

Nociceptive pain was defined by Pasero, Paice, and McCaffery (1999) as "pain resulting from the ongoing activation of primary afferent neurons by noxious stimuli. The nervous system is intact." Furthermore, Portenoy (1996) added, it tends to be "commensurate with the degree of ongoing tissue damage from an identifiable peripheral lesion that involves either somatic or visceral structures." Somatic pain is generated from muscle, skin, joint, connective tissue or bone, oftentimes has an achy or throbbing quality and is often easily localized. Visceral pain arises from visceral organs such as the pancreas and the GI tract.

Nociceptive pain (visceral or somatic in nature) has four basic processes. *Transduction* is the conversion from one energy to another. This is a peripheral process that begins with a mechanical, thermal, or chemical stimulus,

and causes some degree of tissue damage. This injury to tissues produces the release of algogenic (pain-causing) substances that promote immune functioning and inflammation responses, and activate pain receptors. The algogenic substances include serotonin, bradykinin, and histamine, but this process also involves the production of other substances such as substance P and prostaglandin.

This nociceptive pain process triggers an action potential, sending messages toward the central nervous system. *Transmission* is the movement of pain impulses from the site of transduction to the brain. This phase begins in the dorsal horn of the spinal cord, triggers the release of substance P among other chemicals, sending this impulse to the brain. *Perception* is the process of recognizing, defining, and responding to pain, our conscious experience of the pain. Last, *modulation* is the activation of descending pathways that exert inhibitory effects on the cells responsible for pain transmission. This occurs, in part, with the release of endogenous opioids, serotonin, and norepinephrine (Pasero, et al., 1999).

The second major type of pain is neuropathic pain, defined as pain initiated or caused by a primary lesion or dysfunction in the nervous system. Within neuropathic pain, there are two distinctive types: centrally generated pain, initiated or caused by a primary lesion or dysfunction in the central nervous system, and peripherally generated pain, caused by primary lesion or dysfunction in the peripheral nervous system (Pasero, et al., 1999). Science has explained fairly effectively the physiology of pain processes, although work is certainly not complete in this area. Modern theories such as Melzack's Neuromatrix theory may be more thoroughly understood through a working knowledge of preceding basic theories.

THEORIES OF PAIN

SPECIFICITY THEORY

The specificity theory was greatly influenced by the writings of René Descartes. Pain and touch sensors on the skin are wired to a pain center in the brain through specific receptors and pathways, similar to the visual system (Matlin, 1988). The painful stimulus was theorized to travel directly to the brain, and any emotions displayed as part of the experience were in response to the original stimulus. The theory assumes the intensity of the pain is directly proportional to the amount of damage and because pain is neural, it results in triggering irritation of specific neural pathways.

There is a fundamental fault with this theory regarding the denial of the emotional aspect of the pain experience, and considers only biological factors. Chemical blocking and surgical severing of nerve tracts oftentimes fail to eliminate pain. Additionally, the existence of pain in conditions with no apparent physiological bases cannot be explained. For example, there is no way to account for the soldier who feels no pain from injuries until after an intense battle. There is an organic basis for pain; there is just no conscious awareness until the person has time to focus on it.

PATTERN THEORY

This theory suggests that the pattern of nerve endings determines sensation due to pain spots in the tissue which, through summation, produce nerve activation. The intensity and frequency of a stimulus (known as pattern of the stimulation) determine to what extent (if at all) it will consciously be perceived as painful. Each receptor does respond to many different types of stimulation, but that response is greater to some stimuli than others. Therefore, a receptor, which responds vigorously to touch, may still respond to a hot stimulus, but less vigorously, even less so to painful stimuli and very little to cold stimuli. Ultimately, the brain was thought able to interpret a code in terms of the relative strengths of the receptors' responses (Matlin, 1988). The weakness of this theory has to do with the fact the focus was on sensation, while ignoring the variables of the perception of pain.

OPERANT BEHAVIOR MODEL

Fordyce (1976) introduced this new mindset by describing the operant factors that occur in chronic pain. Central to this theory are behavioral manifestations rather than the sensation of pain. It suggests pain behavior, such as excessive rest, overuse of pain medications, verbal complaints, protective behaviors, limping and bracing, although initially useful in combating pain, may be positively reinforced by spouses and healthcare providers. The behavior may be maintained further by the avoidance of activity which may test the waters too much, putting the individual at risk of having the noxious stimulation return.

Well behaviors, such as exercise and work, may not be sufficiently reinforcing and the pain behaviors may, therefore, be maintained. "The operant conditioning model focuses on overt manifestation of pain and suffering expressed as pain behaviors such as limping, moaning and avoiding activity. Emphasis is placed on the communicative function of these behaviors" (Turk & Gatchel, 1999). The psychological factors involved in the chronic pain patient are considered only reactions to painful stimuli, rather than affecting the perception directly.

COGNITIVE BEHAVIOR-TRANSACTIONAL MODEL/STRESS–DIATHESIS MODEL

This more recent theory is heavily influenced by social learning and cognitive theories and the great importance the family or support system plays in the manifestation of a chronic pain condition. The major emphasis concerns the social context in general and the family context in particular. Just as in the Stress–Diathesis model, a framework exists in every individual, including the biological (CNS neurobiological), behavioral, cognitive, and affective domains, that results in coping techniques by the individual that may be positively or negatively reinforced by the family or support system. This is similar to the operant conditioning model regarding the importance of significant others, but the family is viewed as a more active participant in the evaluative response to the adequacy of coping strategies and the individual's ability to effectively meet the challenges of his or her given condition.

Schemas, described as relatively fixed beliefs about the world, develop in family systems. These have a significant effect in specific appraisals regarding the pain patient's condition, and may affect the individual's ability to deal effectively with the condition and help determine the level of adaptation. Past failure to deal effectively with one's condition can enhance the perceived threat of the condition, which could lead to intensified focus on the symptoms, heightening the level of perceived pain, and increasing disability and affective distress (Turk & Gatchel, 1996).

The cornerstone of the Stress–Diathesis model, as previously mentioned, includes biological, psychological, and social factors. Simply put, preexisting personality features place the individual at risk of maladaptive response to a painful condition. This places stress on the person, thus influencing the interrelationship between the neurobiological and psychological variables, which can lead to vulnerability. This vulnerability can result from the crossover of several domains, including cognitive perceptions of control/efficacy, affective depression which leads to anxiety and fear, behavioral declines in functional activity and, finally, family and social interactions that may significantly influence pain expression.

STIMULATION-PRODUCED ANALGESIA (SPA)

This is a pain modulation theory largely based on stimulation-produced analgesia through the production and utilization of endogenous opiates, such as endorphins and enkephalins, for the modulation of pain. The opioid peptides largely associated with pain are enkephalins, beta-endorphins, and dynorphins. It is thought SPA as well as opiate analgesia operate in part through descending control of spinal and trigeminal nociceptors (Basbaum, 1983). With discovery of these endogenous opiate-like substances, the scientifically based suggestion could be made that the brain itself can produce substances that can act to modulate the perception of pain.

Gate Control Theory and Three Dimensions of Pain

A multitude of different theories about pain and its processes has existed since antiquity. It was not until Melzack and Wall published their Gate Control Theory in 1965 that science could understand the pain process from the perspective of descending nerve pathways originating from higher regions and acting via the midbrain and medulla, affecting the perception of pain by inhibiting the transmission of signals through the substantia gelatinosa of the dorsal horn in the spinal cord.

They considered pain to have three dimensions: sensory-discriminative (thought to provide information regarding the nature of the noxious stimulus), motivational-affective (the reactive component of the process, with importance in both acute and chronic pain and medicated by polysynaptic afferent pathways thought to be interconnected between the brain stem's reticular activating system and the limbic system), and cognitive-evaluative (the meaning of a given pain can profoundly alter its sensory experience) (Portenoy, 1996). It is these three areas that are the bases of the widely used McGill Pain questionnaire.

Physiologically, three variables control the gate. A-δ fibers (sharp pain), are small fibers and travel at a slower conduction velocity than those of the A-β fibers. C fibers (dull pain) are unmyelinated afferent neurons, with slow conduction velocity. Both the C and A-δ fibers tend to open the gate by obstructing or inhibiting the special gate neurons of the substantia gelatinosa. Finally, A-β fibers (messages of light touch) are large fibers with much faster conduction velocities than the previous two.

It is theorized that besides the modulation of the pain signal by the stimulated A-β nerve fibers our conscious experience of pain intensity is affected not only by the magnitude of the pain stimulus but also by concentrations of chemical regulators, namely, the endogenous opiates in two major classes: enkephalins and endorphins (Coren, Ward, & Enns, 1999). Willer, Dehen, and Cambier (1981) found the effects of psychological stress when subjects anticipating painful shocks triggered the endogenous opiate system to protect the individual from the forthcoming pain. Similarly, it has been that found women have an increased pain tolerance in the last 2 weeks of pregnancy, presumably to ready them for the upcoming painful events (Cogan & Spinnato, 1986).

Neuromatrix

Neuromatrix as proposed by Ronald Melzack in the 1990s expounded upon the influential gate control theory. It considers pain a multidimensional experience characterized by the "body–self neuromatrix" in the brain, which are considered genetically (but modified by sensory experience) determined neurosignature patterns of nerve impulses. These patterns may be triggered with or without actual sensory inputs; therefore, providing an explanation for the mystery of the perception of pain sometimes present in individuals devoid of pathology or injury.

It proposes that "the output patterns of the neuromatrix activate perceptual, homeostatic, and behavioral programs after injury or pathology or as a result of multiple other inputs that act on the neuromatrix" (Melzack, 1999b). Pain then can be viewed as an output of an extensive neural network in the brain instead of as a much more complicated process than simple injury, inflammation, or other pathology. Stress is a major triggering factor in this theory, due to the complex processes required for the body to restore homeostasis. Chrousos (1992) defined stress as a state of threatened homeostasis, that is, a disruption by stressors of physiological processes such as blood sugar level and body temperature that are normally maintained at a fixed, delicately balanced set point. Therefore, a disruption of homeostasis due to a stressor (physical or psychological) activates programs of neural, hormonal, and behavioral activity.

Indeed, the neuromatrix theory considers five basic types of inputs that produce the unique neurosignature outputs. These include "(1) sensory inputs (cutaneous, visceral and other somatic receptors); (2) visual and other sensory inputs that influence the cognitive interpretation of the situation; (3) phasic and tonic cognitive and emotional inputs from others areas of the brain; (4) intrinsic neural inhibitory modulation inherent in all brain function; (5) the activity of the body's stress-regulation systems, including cytokines as well as the endocrine, autonomic, immune and opioid systems" (Melzack, 1999a).

PAIN THRESHOLD VS. PAIN TOLERANCE

There is no denying the subjectivity of pain. The response a given individual has is an intensely personal experience, and therefore, cannot be predicted with certainty. There are times when seemingly innocuous stimuli are perceived as excruciating, whereas quite severe injuries can produce almost no perceived sensation to the individual.

Obviously, this poses a great challenge to the healthcare professional during the assessment. It is important to be mindful of the inherent difference of pain *threshold* vs. pain *tolerance*. When considering pain and sensation as a process, there are many aspects, which are fairly consistent and reproducible from person to person, and from the same person over time. Pain threshold is scientifically based, quantifiable and reliable. It has been defined as the intensity of a stimulation at which a subject says, "It's painful" half the time and "It's not painful" half the time (Matlin, 1988). Threshold is variable across the body as evidenced by neurologists' two point discrimination test. More pain receptors means greater discrimination of the presented stimulus, and a lower pain threshold.

The great challenge is that pain tolerance has so many variables and elements. Not only does it vary between individuals, but within the same individual at different times. What possible factors can account for the high variability in the tolerance of pain over time? Turk and Flor (1999) point out that an injury to the nociceptive transmission system or to the activity of the modulatory system can lower pain intensity. There may also be abnormal neural activity, which may produce hypersensitivity creating a self-sustaining process started by the original injury. Examples of such processes may be seen in phantom limb pain, neuropathic pain, or complex regional pain.

Finally, psychological factors may affect normal responses to pain, and yield quite variable and unpredictable responses. One of the most important factors when considering the tolerance and general perception of pain is the *meaning* of the pain to the sufferer. Needless to say, a painful condition associated with a minor injury or temporary illness will likely be a much different experience than similar pain levels associated with more severe life-altering conditions.

CONCLUSION

There is considerable evidence that the expression of pain follows social modeling, cultural expectations, and religious beliefs. Stoicism, hysteria, athletic endurance, and numerous other designations of discomfort accompany lifestyles and life expectations. It has been observed that wealthy persons expect to be able to "buy relief" from pain, and that athletes view pain as the only way to gain. Winners in athletic endeavors often express the pain of overexertion or injury differently if they win or lose the contest. The pain from muscular irritation and other physical states resulting from "practice" becomes dissociated a part of their experience. Religious persons have been known to welcome pain as a believed prelude to rewards in the after life. Pain is not universally perceived the same, expressed the same, nor is it treated the same. For these and myriad other reasons, pain continues to be our most illusive encounter with human existence.

REFERENCES

American Heritage Publishing Staff. (1995). *Roget II: The new thesaurus*. Boston, MA: Houghton Mifflin.

Basbaum, A.I. (1983). The generation and control of pain. In R.N. Rosenberg & W.D. Willis (Eds.), *The clinical neurosciences: Neurobiology* (Vol. V, p. 313). New York: Churchill Livingstone.

Cassel, E.J. (1982). The nature of suffering and the goals of medicine. *New England Journal of Medicine, 306*, 639–645.

Chrousos, G.P. (1992). Regulation and dysregulation of hypothalmic-pituitary-adrenal axis. *Endocrinology and Metabolism Clinics of North America, 21*, 833–858.

Clark, W.C., & Clark, S. (1980). Pain responses in Nepalese porters, *Science, 209*, 410–412.

Cogan, R., & Spinnato, J.A. (1986). Pain and discomfort thresholds in late pregnancy. *Pain, 27*, 63–68.

Coren, S., Ward, L.M., & Enns, J.T. (1999). *Sensation and perception* (5th ed., p. 248). New York: Harcourt Brace.

Chapman, C., Toru, S., Martin, R., Tanaka, A., Okazaki, N., Colpitts, Y., Mayero, J., & Gaghardi, G. (1982). Comparative effects of acupuncture in Japan and the United States on dental pain perception. *Pain, 12*, 319–328.

Cornock, M.A. (1996). Psychological approaches to cardiac pain. *Nursing Standard, 11*, 34–38.

Craig, J.C., & Rollman, G.B. (1999). Somesthesis. *Annual Review of Psychology, 50*, 305–331.

Fordyce, W.E. (1976). *Behavioral methods for chronic pain and illness*. St. Louis: Mosby.

Gale Group Staff (Eds.). (2000) *The Columbia encyclopedia* (6th ed.). Mt Kisco, NY: Visible Ink Press.

Iadarola, M.J., & Caudle, R.M. (1997). Good pain, bad pain. *Science, 278*, 5336, 239.

Kelly, A.L. (1999). The painful truth. *Walking Magazine, 14*, 2, 30.

Kerns, R.D., & Payne, A. (1996). Treating families of chronic pain patients. In R.J. Gatchel & D.C. Turk (Eds.), *Psychological approaches to pain management, a practitioner's handbook*. New York: Guilford.

Marble, M. (1999). Gender differences (pain response). *Women's Health Weekly*, October, 19.

Matlin, M.W. (1988). *Sensation and perception* (2nd ed.). Boston: Allyn & Bacon.

McQuillen, M.P. (1991). Can people who are unconscious or in the 'vegetative state' perceive pain. *Law and Medicine, 6*, 4, 373.

Melzack, R. (1999a). Pain and stress: A new perspective. In R.J. Gatchel & D.C. Turk (Eds.), *Psychosocial factors in pain: Critical perspectives*. New York: Guilford.

Melzack, R., (1999b). Abstract. From the gate to the neuromatrix. *Pain* (Suppl. 6), S121–126.

Melzack, R., & Wall, P.D. (1965). Pain mechanisms: A new theory. *Science, 150*, 971–979.

Morse, J.M., & Morse, R.M. (1998). Cultural variation in the inference of pain. *Journal of Cross-Cultural Psychology, 19*(2), 232–242.

Pasero, C., Paice, J.A., & McCaffery, M. Basic mechanisms underlying the causes and effects of pain. *Pain, clinical manual* (2nd ed.). St. Louis: Mosby.

Pirisi, A. (2000). The color of pain. *Psychology Today, 32*, 4, 22.

Portenoy, R.K. (1996). Control of pathological pain. In L. Kruger (Ed.), *Pain and touch* (pp. 343–386). San Diego, CA: Academic Press.

Reber, A.S. (1995). *Penguin dictionary of psychology* (2nd ed.). New York: Penguin Books.

Ruzicka, S.A. (1998). Pain beliefs. *Journal of Holistic Nursing, 16*, 3, 369.

Sittner, B., Hudson, D., Grossman, C., & Gaston-Johansson, F. (1998). Adolescents perceptions of pain during labor. *Clinical Nursing Research, 7*(1), 82.

Turk, D.C., & Flor, H. (1999). Chronic pain: A biobehavioral Perspective. In R.J. Gatchel & D.C. Turk (Eds.), *Psychosocial factors in pain critical perspectives* (p. 28). New York: Guilford.

Turk, D.C., & Gatchel, R.J. (1996). *Psychological approaches to pain management: A practitioner's handbook.* New York: Guilford.

Turk, D.C., & Gatchel, R.J. (1999). *Psychosocial factors in pain: Critical perspectives.* New York: Guilford.

Verillo, R.T. (1975). Cutaneous sensations. In B. Scharf (Ed.), *Experimental sensory psychology.* Glenview, IL: Scott, Foresman.

Willer, J.C., Dehen, H., & Cambier, J. (1981). Stress-induced analgesia in humans: Endogenous opioids and naloxone-reversible depression of pain reflexes. *Science, 212,* 689–690.

Woodgate, R. & Kristjianson, L.J. (1996). My hurts: Hospitalized young children's perceptions of acute pain. *Qualitative Health Research, 6,* 2, 184.

Woodrow, K., Friedman, G., Seigelaub, M., & Collen, M. (1972). Pain tolerance: Differences according to age, sex, and race. *Psychosomatic Medicine, 34,* 548–556.

66

Screening for Alcohol and Other Substance Use Disorders*

Nick J. Piazza, Ph.D.

Alcohol and other drug use are primarily or secondarily implicated in a large number of medical problems, including pain (Kitchens, 1994). Undetected and untreated alcohol or other substance use disorders can have a significant effect on a patient's response to treatment as well as treatment compliance. Adger and Werner (1994) stated that healthcare professionals "should screen all patients for [substance] use and determine the need for further assessment and intervention." Failure to at least screen for a substance use problem could lead to misdiagnosis, and failure to provide the patient with the most appropriate care.

Adger and Werner state that the goal of screening is to determine the likelihood that a problem exists and whether further assessment is needed. They believe that all patients should undergo screening for alcohol or other drug problems. If a screen is positive, then the Health Care Provider (HCP) should refer the patient for a detailed substance use assessment, and initiate prevention or treatment measures where appropriate.

Assessment is a lengthier, more involved process usually conducted by personnel specifically trained in substance use disorders. The purpose of assessment is to "determine the extent of the problem, explore coexisting medical and psychiatric conditions, and assist in treatment planning" (Adger & Werner, 1994). Most HCPs feel competent to screen for a substance use disorder; however, they may prefer to refer the patient to a specialist for assessment.

CHARACTERISTICS OF A GOOD SCREEN

There are a number of characteristics that help determine whether a screening procedure is of value. The most important characteristics are sensitivity, specificity, validity, reliability, and cost-efficiency.

SENSITIVITY AND SPECIFICITY

Sensitivity refers to the proportion of individuals correctly identified as positive for a particular condition or disorder. In this case, sensitivity would refer to the percent of individuals correctly identified by a particular screen as having a substance use disorder. A screen with good sensitivity is important because it can tell us who needs to be referred for a more complete evaluation, who may not respond to medications or therapies as expected, or who may be malingering or drug-seeking.

Specificity refers to the proportion of individuals correctly identified as negative or as not having a substance use disorder. The value of a highly specific screen is that it can tell us who is least likely to have a substance use disorder. A screen with good specificity can tell us when it is unnecessary to expend valuable time or resources evaluating patients for a condition they most likely do not have.

Salaspuro (1994) noted that a good screen should not overidentify individuals as having a problem (i.e., false positives) nor should it overidentify individuals as being problem-free (i.e., false negatives). A high false-positive

---

* Portions of this chapter were excerpted from Piazza, N.J., Martin, N., & Dildine, R. (2000). Screening instruments for alcohol and other drug problems. *Journal of Mental Health Counseling, 22,* 218–227. With permission.

0-8493-0926-3/02/$0.00+$1.50
© 2002 by CRC Press LLC

rate would mean that valuable time and resources were expended on individuals who, in fact, did not have a substance use disorder, while a high false negative rate means that individuals went untreated because they were not detected by screening.

VALIDITY AND RELIABILITY

Validity refers to a screening instrument's ability to measure what it purports to measure. Valid screening procedures for substance use disorders should accurately discriminate true positives and true negatives from false positives and false negatives. A number of threats to validity exist including standardization on a too small sample, using a screen on individuals who were not part of the standardization group, using a screen for purposes other than those for which it was developed. A perfectly valid instrument would achieve a value of 1.0. Screening instruments for substance use disorders can range from lows of about 0.4 to highs of 0.9 or better.

Reliability refers to the consistency with which an instrument measures the variable or condition of interest. A reliable screen will yield consistent results across individuals and, more importantly, across time. Conversely, an unreliable instrument yields different results each time it is administered. Technically, it is not possible to have an unreliable screening procedure that is valid. Validity is dependent on the stability of the results obtained.

As with validity, reliable screens should approach a value of 1.0. Most screening instruments report test–retest reliability because this measures the stability of results over repeated administrations of the procedure. Questionnaire-based screens often will report internal consistency or alpha reliability. High internal consistency or alpha values mean that the items on the questionnaire are highly intercorrelated and most likely measure the same variable or condition.

COST-EFFICIENCY

Cost-efficiency implies that the benefits of using the screening procedure are greater than the costs. Using an inexpensive but poorly constructed screen with low sensitivity and specificity may prove to be more costly over time because resources are wasted on false positives and false-negative patients go undetected and untreated. In addition, screening all persons in a population for a low prevalence disorder may add considerable cost to treatment while benefiting only a few individuals.

LABORATORY OR BIOLOGICAL SCREENING PROCEDURES

LABORATORY TESTS

Laboratory tests, especially liver enzyme tests, have long been used as a means to screen for potential alcohol abuse.

Fleming (1993) identified four useful laboratory measures. These include measuring levels of gamma-glutamyl transferase (GGT), mean corpuscular volume (MCV), alanine aminotransferase (ALT), and aspartate aminotransferase (AST). Fleming (1993, p. 231) selected these tests because they "measured direct hepatic and hematopoietic cellular alcohol toxicity." Fleming notes that the sensitivity of these screens ranges from 20 to 90%, with GGT levels the most sensitive of the four measures.

O'Connor and Schottenfeld (1998) recommend testing for carbohydrate-deficient transferrin in addition to the measures listed above. They report that carbohydrate-deficient transferrin levels have a "sensitivity of 58 percent to 70 percent and a specificity of 82 percent to 98 percent for the detection of heavy drinking or alcohol abuse" (O'Connor & Schottenfeld, 1998).

BLOOD-ALCOHOL CONCENTRATION (BAC)

BAC is a measure of the percent of alcohol concentrated in a volume of blood. The BAC is sometimes alternatively referred to as the blood-alcohol level or BAL. The procedure involves drawing a sample of blood and analyzing the sample to determine how much alcohol is present. Persons with a BAC of 0.1% or higher are considered too intoxicated to drive in 34 states, the District of Columbia, and Puerto Rico; 16 states and all the provinces in Canada have set their legal intoxication limit at 0.8% (Harley Owners Group, 2000). The validity and reliability for this test are sufficiently high that BAC is accepted as evidentiary of intoxication in a court of law. It has been the author's experience that any BAC over 0.15% in an adult is suggestive of alcohol abuse or dependence, while a BAC of 0.2% is almost always associated with alcohol dependence.

URINALYSIS

Many drugs are broken down or metabolized in the liver. The by-products of liver metabolism are called metabolites. The kidneys filter these metabolites from the blood supply, and then dump them in the urine where they are expelled during urination. It is possible to determine whether a patient has recently ingested a drug by examining the urine for the presence of these metabolites. This procedure is commonly known as urinalysis.

Urinalysis actually consists of two tests. The first test is known as the enzyme multiplied immunoassay technique or EMIT. The strength of an EMIT is its specificity. A negative EMIT fairly conclusively indicates that the patient's urine is relatively free of drug metabolites. An EMIT's sensitivity, however, is sufficiently poor that a significant proportion of individuals will be false positives. Consequently, it is necessary to run a second measure—a gas chromatography/mass spectrometry (GC/MS)—to confirm the results of the EMIT. GC/MS accuracy approaches 100% and is considered evidentiary in courts of law. It is possible that a patient may test positive on urinalysis because he or she is taking a legitimately prescribed medication (e.g., meperidine [Demerol®]). These individuals should be considered false positives, and many urinalysis laboratories employ Medical Review Officers (MROs) to eliminate these cases.

OTHER BIOLOGICAL SCREENS

Procedures have been developed to test a patient's hair, breath, sweat, and saliva for the presence of alcohol, drugs, or their metabolites. The best known is probably the Breath-a-lyzer® test, which provides a highly accurate estimate of BAC. Instruments that look like a child's sucker change color when exposed to saliva containing traces of drugs. Finally, hair analysis can determine if an individual has used drugs any time in the weeks or months prior to testing. Obviously, the longer the individual's hair, the farther back in time detection will be possible.

ADVANTAGES AND DISADVANTAGES OF LABORATORY OR BIOLOGICAL SCREENS

ADVANTAGES

Biological and laboratory screens are most useful and most valid for those situations where evidence of substance use or impairment is required. Urinalysis, especially when combined with a GC/MS and an MRO, has an especially high sensitivity rate with almost no false positives. Because of the high sensitivity combined with a low false-positive rate, urinalysis is most often employed in situations where it is important to determine if an individual is drug-free. Examples of such situations include following an accident or injury in the workplace; compliance with drug-free workplace policies; fitness for work determinations; and compliance with the terms of abstinence-based treatment programs, probation, or parole.

DISADVANTAGES

A number of limitations exist to using biological screens to determine who may or may not have a substance use disorder. The principle disadvantage is that individuals need only abstain for a few days to test negative on urinalysis. Conversely, some procedures such as hair analysis will yield positive results weeks or even months after use has stopped. Liver enzyme tests often have high false-negative rates for young, healthy, or early stage users who do not have a many-year history of heavy or abusive drinking. Laboratory procedures also can be expensive and time consuming. Finally, laboratory and biological screens cannot differentiate legitimate users from recreational or problem users. All a biological

screen can tell the HCP is that the individual has recently used; biological screens cannot determine why the drug is present or the nature of the use. This led Fleming (1993) to recommend that laboratory testing be limited to assessing toxicity, while questionnaires and patient reports were more valid for differentiating problem from nonproblem users.

PSYCHOSOCIAL SCREENING INSTRUMENTS

Piazza, Martin, and Dildine (2000) noted that psychosocial screening instruments for detecting substance use disorders fall into one of two categories. The first category consists of so-called *logically derived* instruments. Logically derived screens typically have good *content* or *face validity* in that the items obviously measure substance use-related behaviors and problems. The greatest asset of logically derived screens is that a positive result is a strong indication that a problem is present. The greatest liability for logically derived screens is that the items are so obvious that anyone motivated to deny or conceal a problem can easily "fake good." In fact, it can be said that logically derived screens are best at detecting those individuals who wish to be identified. Despite this inherent weakness, however, O'Connor and Schottenfeld (1998) noted that self-reported information regarding substance use is "reliable and reproducible."

A second category described by Piazza et al. (2000) is comprised of what are known as empirically derived instruments. Empirically derived instruments use research and statistical analysis to identify items that can discriminate individuals with substance use disorders from individuals who are problem-free. Generally, the content of the item is unimportant. What is important is that the item correctly identifies who is a member of the criterion group (i.e., that group of individuals with a substance use disorder). Items on empirically derived screens often have poor content or face validity; however, they should have good to excellent *predictive* or *criterion validity*. Empirically derived screens appear to be best at identifying individuals who are motivated to deny or minimize a substance use disorder because item content appears unrelated to substance use. Unfortunately, because most empirically derived screens do not ask questions related to substance use, they frequently do not give any indication of the severity or extent of a drinking or other drug problem.

MICHIGAN ALCOHOLISM SCREENING TEST (MAST)

The MAST was originally developed by Selzer (1971) and consists of 24 face valid items. Pokorny, Miller, and Kaplan (1972) and Selzer, Vinokur, and van Rooijen (1975) later developed abbreviated versions of the questionnaire with 13 items each. The most discriminating items are

1. Have you ever attended a meeting of AA?
2. Have you ever sought help about your drinking?
3. Have you ever been in a hospital because of your drinking?

Items are scored 1, 2, or 5 points according to their diagnostic utility. The MAST is designed to assign respondents into one of three categories: no drinking problem (score of 0 to 3), possible problem (score of 4 to 6), and alcohol dependent (score of 7 or higher).

The MAST is one of the best known and most widely used logically derived screens. Its wide acceptance and use, however, are inconsistent with the problems associated with the instrument. Selzer (1971) acknowledged that because the items are so obvious, alcoholics wishing to avoid detection could easily do so. To correct for this, Selzer set the cutoff scores lower to improve sensitivity. This resulted in a false-positive rate of about 33% and lowered the overall accuracy rate to about 75% (Jacobson, 1983; Creager, 1989). Correlations between MAST results and counselor diagnoses reveal a concurrent validity of r = .65 (Mischke and Venneri, 1987). Finally, the MAST only assesses for alcoholism and cannot discriminate between alcohol abuse and problems with other drugs.

The MAST's applicability to women and minorities is also questionable. Jacobson (1983) reports that there is little information on female norms, and nothing in the literature addressing minority norms.

The high false-positive rate and low overall accuracy led Popkin, Kannenberg, Lacey, and Waller (1988) to conclude that the MAST "may be useful in detecting persons who acknowledge having an alcohol problem." Russell (1994, p. 58) described the MAST as lengthy, difficult to score, and "impractical for clinical use."

SELF-ADMINISTERED MICHIGAN ALCOHOLISM SCREENING TEST (SAAST)

This is a modified version of the MAST that has been developed for self-administration. The SAAST is a 35-item questionnaire that correlates highly (r = .83) with the MAST. Davis, Hurt, Morse, and O'Brien (1987) reported that the SAAST correctly identified 92.1% of 520 alcoholic participants and only incorrectly classified 1.3% of 636 controls. It was not clear in the Davis, et al. study, however, whether the alcoholic group contained individuals who were attempting to deny a problem on the instrument. A 92.1% accuracy rate should not be surprising in a group of alcoholics who are being open and honest about their drinking experiences. A

final concern is that like the MAST questions on the SAAST are specific to alcohol and do not address problems with other drugs.

CAGE, T-ACE, AND TWEAK

These three logically derived instruments were developed as brief screens that could be administered orally during a clinical interview. All three are very similar and share many of the same strengths and weaknesses. The CAGE was specifically developed for use by primary care physicians. Kitchens (1994) noted, however, that the CAGE had not been standardized for use with pregnant women. The T-ACE and the TWEAK are variations of the CAGE that were specifically developed to "ascertain drinking in pregnant women" (Nilssen & Cone, 1994).

THE CAGE

Nilssen and Cone (1994) report that the CAGE is probably the "most widely used test in clinical practice." It consists of four items, answered with either yes or no:

1. Have you ever felt you should *C*ut down on your drinking?
2. Have people *A*nnoyed you by criticizing your drinking?
3. Have you ever felt bad or *G*uilty about your drinking?
4. Have you ever had a drink first thing in the morning to steady your nerves or get rid of a hangover (*E*ye opener)?

Two or more yes answers are interpreted as a positive screen, suggesting the need for further assessment. The principle advantages of the CAGE are that it is easy to remember, easy to administer during a clinical interview, and takes only about a minute to complete. The reported accuracy rates of the CAGE are quite variable, ranging anywhere from 40 to 95% (Sokol, Martier, & Ager, 1989). O'Connor and Schottenfeld (1998) reported that lifetime sensitivity for patients with an alcohol problem ranges from 60 to 95%.

Despite its advantages, a number of problems have been associated with using the CAGE. Nilssen and Cone (1994) noted that the CAGE is specific to alcoholism and does not assess for problems with drug use. They also note that the CAGE assesses lifetime use instead of focusing on current drinking history. Fleming (1993) reports that the CAGE's lifetime approach results in a false-positive rate of over 50%. Kitchens (1994) pointed out that while the CAGE is "reasonably accurate at identifying those individuals who are alcohol dependent or heavy drinkers," the CAGE is "not at all sensitive to detecting the lower levels of consumption that may be dangerous." In addition, the items on the CAGE are very obvious and can be easily denied by someone motivated to do so.

THE T-ACE

The T-ACE is similar to the CAGE, except that it drops the CAGE question on guilt and replaces it with a question on alcohol tolerance (Sokol, et al., 1989). Russell (1994) reported finding sensitivity and specificity rates for the T-ACE of about 79%. Russell stated that the T-ACE performed about the same as the MAST and slightly better than the CAGE with a sample of pregnant women. Despite the improvement in performance, the T-ACE still suffers from the same limitations as the CAGE, i.e., specificity to alcohol, lifetime focus, inability to detect early stage problems, and easy deniability. Another problem is that it has only been standardized on pregnant women and not on the general population.

THE TWEAK

The TWEAK "combines questions from the MAST, CAGE, and T-ACE tests that have been found most effective" (see Table 66.1) (Russell, 1994). Russell reports that the TWEAK is superior to the CAGE or the MAST and equivalent to the T-ACE when used with pregnant women. Because the TWEAK is a derivative of the MAST, CAGE, and T-ACE, it shares the same liabilities as these instruments. In addition, the TWEAK is more complicated to score.

THE ALCOHOL USE DISORDERS IDENTIFICATION TEST (AUDIT)

The AUDIT was developed under the auspices of the World Health Organization (WHO) to serve as a multicultural screening instrument (Babor & Grant, 1989). The AUDIT "was specifically designed to be used in primary care settings to screen for alcohol problems at earlier stages" (Nilssen & Cone, 1994). The developers intended for the AUDIT to be used to identify harmful drinking rather than alcohol use disorders. However, Russell (1994) believes that the AUDIT "also can detect alcohol disorders with a high degree of accuracy."

The AUDIT is a logically derived, paper-and-pencil screen consisting of ten items. The items relate to three areas of harmful drinking: (a) amount and frequency of alcohol consumption, (b) dependency symptoms, and (c) harmful effects. Items are scored on a scale from 0 to 4, with a maximum possible score of 40. A score of 8 or higher is positive for harmful drinking. Russell (1994) claims the AUDIT has a sensitivity rate of 92% and a specificity rate of 93% for identifying harmful drinking. Isaacson, Butler, Zacharek, and Tzelepis (1994) reported sensitivity and specificity rates of 96% for patients in a general medical clinic. The AUDIT would appear to be a very strong instrument for identifying harmful or at-risk drinkers within a multicultural population.

SUBSTANCE ABUSE LIFE CIRCUMSTANCES EVALUATION (SALCE)

The SALCE was developed to use with people arrested for driving under the influence (DUI). The intended use for the SALCE is to differentiate those individuals needing to alter their use of alcohol or other drugs from individuals who may have a more serious substance use disorder. Popkin, et al. (1988) report that the SALCE "was not designed to differentiate alcoholics from nonalcoholics." The SALCE is a logically derived screen consisting of an 85-item questionnaire that is to be used in conjunction with a 20-minute interview. Total screening time is estimated to be approximately 40 minutes.

Applicability of the SALCE is probably limited to use with DUI offenders as it has never been standardized on other populations. Internal consistency reliability for the SALCE is reported to be r = .93; no test–retest reliability

---

TABLE 66.1
Tweak

T	*T*olerance: How many drinks can you hold?
W	Have close friends or relatives *W*orried or complained about your drinking in the past year?
E	*E*ye-opener: Do you sometimes take a drink in the morning when you first get up?
A	*A*mnesia: Has a friend or family member ever told you about things you said or did while you were drinking that you could not remember?
K(C)	Do you sometimes feel the need to *C*ut down on your drinking?

The TWEAK uses a 7-point scale. The Tolerance item scores 2 points if the respondent reports she can consume five or more drinks without falling asleep or becoming unconscious. A positive response to the Worry item scores 2 points. Positive responses to the remaining items are scored 1 point each. A total of 2 or more points indicates a positive screen. (Adapted by permission from Russell, M. (1994). *Alcohol Health and Research World, 18,* 55–61.)

was reported (Popkin, et al., 1988). Popkin, et al. (1988) report a 61% agreement rate between the SALCE and assessment based on professional interviews.

Popkin, et al. (1988) noted that the SALCE "appears to be reasonably well constructed, includes a measure of response bias (truthfulness), and has the automated capability for updating norms specific to DUI offenders." Popkin, et al. (1988) felt the SALCE had considerable potential for use in DUI programs. They did note, however, that no independently published evaluations of the SALCE exist and that the publishers consider their data to be proprietary and not available for independent evaluation.

THE MACANDREW SCALE

The MacAndrew Scale (MAC) and the MacAndrew Scale-Revised (MAC-R) consist of 49 true/false items embedded in the Minnesota Multiphasic Personality Inventory (MMPI) and the Minnesota Multiphasic Personality Inventory-2 (MMPI-2), respectively. Greene (1991) wrote that the MAC scale was originally developed to differentiate alcoholic outpatients from nonalcoholic psychiatric outpatients. The MAC and MAC-R are empirically derived scales designed to be indirect measures of alcoholism, because neither version of the scales contains any questions obviously related to actual alcohol consumption or alcohol-related problems.

Butcher, Dahlstrom, Graham, Tellegen, and Kaemmer (1989) stated that "raw scores of 28 or above strongly suggest substance abuse. Scores between 24 and 27 are somewhat suggestive of substance abuse, … [and] scores below 24 contraindicate a substance-abuse problem." Graham (1990) also noted that drug addicts and alcoholics obtained similar scores on the MAC.

Reliability and validity are problems for both the MAC and the MAC-R. Graham (1990) observed that "No internal consistency data were reported for the original MAC scale, but the MAC-R scale does not seem to have particularly good internal consistency." Butcher, et al. (1989) reported coefficient alphas of .56 for males and .45 for females. One week test–retest reliability coefficients for the MAC-R were .62 for males and .78 for females (Graham, 1990). Sensitivity rates for white males ranged around 80%, with false positive rates approximating 20% (Greene, 1991). Accuracy rates for the MAC and the MAC-R scales for adolescents, women, and minorities can be much poorer. Greene (1991) reported that true positive and false positive rates for African-American males were both nearly 60%, while true positive rates for white adolescents and women "ranged around 75%, with approximately 35% false positives."

Another validity problem common to both the MAC and the MAC-R is that the scales are not independent of other personality characteristics or psychopathology. Butcher, et al. (1989) noted that high scores on these scales

"are suggestive of persons who are socially extroverted [sic], exhibitionistic, and willing to take risks." There is no mechanism for determining if a high score has been produced by a respondent's substance use or these confounding personality and behavioral variables.

Greene (1991), Butcher et al. (1989), and Graham (1990) all state that validity, reliability, and accuracy problems preclude using the MAC and the MAC-R to diagnose substance-related disorders. Graham (1990) stated that an elevated MAC-R score is only indicative of the "possibility of substance abuse," while Butcher, et al. (1989) believed that high scores are "associated with addiction-proneness rather than with alcoholic tendencies alone." Greene (1991) went so far as to suggest that professionals might want to "avoid using the MAC scale to predict whether a client will abuse substances, which has been the standard use of the MAC scale since it was first developed."

SUBSTANCE ABUSE SUBTLE SCREENING INVENTORY (SASSI)

The SASSI has gone through two revisions since its release in 1985 (Miller, 1985). The current version is referred to as the SASSI-3 (Miller, Roberts, Brooks, & Lazowski, 1997). The SASSI-3 actually consists of two separate screens: one logically derived, the other empirically derived. The logically derived portion is comprised of 26 face valid items formerly known as the Risk Prediction Scales (RPS). Items on the RPS are scored on a scale from 0 to 3. The second portion is made up of 67 true/false empirically derived items. The 93 items of the SASSI-3 are divided into five clinical subscales, two defensiveness subscales, one validity scale, and two supplementary scales. The SASSI-3 is written on a sixth-grade reading level and takes 15 to 20 minutes to complete. Hand scoring takes an additional 5 to 10 minutes.

The SASSI-3 is interpreted using decision rules for a configural analysis of the scores on the different subscales. The publisher claims a 93.8% correspondence rate between the SASSI-3 and a professional diagnosis, with a sensitivity rate of 94.1% and a specificity rate of 92.7% (F. Miller, personal communication, May, 1997). A separate study (Piazza, 1996) found that the adolescent version of the SASSI had similar accuracy rates. A plus for the SASSI-3 is that accuracy rates are about the same whether respondents are being honest about their substance use or are attempting to deny or conceal a problem. Additionally, the norm sample of 2800 individuals was comprised of about 30% African- and Native-Americans. This means that the SASSI-3 should be valid for these groups.

Reliability coefficients are equally impressive. Test–retest reliability coefficients for the clinical and defensiveness scales ranged from .92 to 1.00, while the

Cronbach alpha coefficient for the overall SASSI-3 was 0.94 (F. Miller, personal communication, May, 1997).

The SASSI-3 appears to be a compact and efficient marriage of the advantages to the two types of screens. Persons who are motivated to provide an honest report of their alcohol and drug use can reveal this on the Risk Prediction Scales. These data can be very useful in assessing the severity of a substance use disorder and for treatment planning. Persons who are in denial or who are deliberately being deceptive are typically identified through a configural analysis of the clinical and defensiveness scales. While information on the severity of the problem is lost, the SASSI can provide information on the degree of denial or defensiveness exhibited by the examinee.

DISCUSSION

Logically and empirically derived screens each have their own strengths and limitations. Choosing a screen involves trading off between ease of administration and accuracy. Selecting a screen should be based on the provider's needs, patient factors, and the circumstances under which the screen is to be used.

Logically derived screens seem to be best employed in situations where the motivation to provide an honest self-report is high. Typically, this means a situation where the patient is well known to the provider and a good working relationship exists. A positive relationship can lower defensiveness and denial, which should lead to a more honest self-appraisal. When these conditions are met, using an instrument like the CAGE, T-ACE, TWEAK, or AUDIT can be productive. All four of these screens are brief and easily administered, scored, and interpreted. It should be noted, however, that denial is a defining characteristic of alcohol and other drug use disorders. The motivation to deny or minimize a substance-related disorder may be strong even in the presence of a positive relationship.

Empirically derived screens should probably be employed in situations where the client is unknown to the provider, where there is a diverse client population, or where clients are likely to be motivated to conceal their problems. Generally, this would include situations such as intake, diagnostic, or evaluative interviews where clients may be motivated to present themselves in the most favorable light. It is probably best to use the SASSI 3, or a comparable instrument, in these circumstances. Using the SASSI-3 should yield valid and reliable results even if the examinee is trying to defeat the screen. The disadvantage to using any of the empirically derived screens, however, is they are more complicated to administer, score, and interpret. In fact, we would recommend completing the 3- to 4-hour training program before attempting to use the SASSI-3. The advantage of improved accuracy, however, would appear to make the cost of additional training well worth it.

REFERENCES

Adger, H., & Werner, M.J. (1994). The pediatrician. *Alcohol Health and Research World, 18,* 121–126.

Babor, T.F., & Grant, M. (1989). From clinical research to secondary prevention: International collaboration in the development of the Alcohol Use Disorders Identification Test (AUDIT). *Alcohol Health and Research World, 13,* 371–374.

Butcher, J.N., Dahlstrom, W.G., Graham, J.R., Tellegen, A., & Kaemmer, B. (1989). *Minnesota Multiphasic Personality Inventory-2: Manual for administration and scoring.* Minneapolis: University of Minnesota Press.

Creager, C. (1989). SASSI test breaks through denial. *Professional Counselor,* 65.

Davis, L.J., Hurt, R.D., Morse, R.M., & O'Brien, P.C. (1987). Discriminant analysis of the self-administered alcoholism screening test. *Alcoholism: Clinical & Experimental Research, 11,* 269–273.

Fleming, M.F. (1993). Screening and brief intervention for alcohol disorders. *The Journal of Family Practice, 37,* 231–234.

Graham, J.R. (1990). *MMPI-2: Assessing personality and psychopathology.* New York: Oxford University Press.

Greene, R.L. (1991). *The MMPI/MMPI-2: An interpretive manual.* Boston: Allyn & Bacon.

Harley Owners Group. (2000). *America's touring handbook.* Milwaukee, WI: Harley Owners Group.

Isaacson, J.H., Butler, R., Zacharek, M., & Tzelepis, A. (1994). Screening with the Alcohol Use Disorders Identification Test (AUDIT) in an inner-city population. *Journal of General Internal Medicine, 9,* 550–553.

Jacobson, G.R. (1983). Detection, assessment, and diagnosis of alcoholism: Current techniques. In M. Galanter (Ed.), *Recent developments in alcoholism:* (Vol. 1, pp. 377–413). New York: Plenum Press.

Kitchens, J.M. (1994). Does this patient have an alcohol problem? *Journal of the American Medical Association, 272,* 1782–1787.

Miller, G.A. (1985). *The substance abuse subtle screening inventory manual.* Bloomington, IN: The SASSI Institute.

Miller, G.A., Roberts, J., Brooks, M.K., & Lazowski, L.E. (1997). SASSI-3: A quick reference for administration and scoring. Bloomington, IN: Baugh Enterprises, Inc.

Mischke, H.D., & Venneri, R.L. (1987). Reliability and validity of the MAST, Mortimer-Filkins questionnaire, and CAGE in DWI assessment. *Journal of Studies on Alcohol, 48,* 492–501.

Nilssen, O., & Cone, H. (1994). Screening patients for alcohol problems in primary health care settings. *Alcohol Health and Research World, 18,* 136–139.

O'Connor, P.G., & Schottenfeld, R.S. (1998). Patients with alcohol problems. *The New England Journal of Medicine,* 592–602.

Piazza, N.J. (1996). Dual diagnosis and adolescent psychiatric inpatients. *International Journal of the Addictions, 31,* 215–223

Piazza, N.J., Martin, N., & Dildine, R.J. (2000). Screening instruments for alcohol and other drug problems. *Journal of Mental Health Counseling, 22,* 218–227.

Pokorny, A.D., Miller, B.A., & Kaplan, H.B. (1972). The brief MAST: A shortened version of the Michigan Alcoholism Screening Test. *American Journal of Psychiatry, 129,* 342–345.

Popkin, C.L., Kannenberg, C.H., Lacey, J.H., and Waller, P.F. (1988). Assessment of classification instruments designed to detect alcohol abuse (DOT Publication No. HS 807 475). Springfield, VA: National Technical Information Service.

Russell, M. (1994). New assessment tools for risk drinking during pregnancy. *Alcohol Health and Research World, 18,* 55–61.

Russell, M. (1994). New assessment tools for risk drinking during pregnancy. *Alcohol Health and Research World, 18,* 55–61.

Salaspuro, M. (1994). Biological state markers of alcohol abuse. *Alcohol Health and Research World, 18,* 131–135.

Selzer, M.L. (1971). The Michigan Alcoholism Screening Test: The quest for a new diagnostic instrument. *American Journal of Psychiatry, 127,* 1653–1658.

Selzer, M.L., Vinokur, A., & van Rooijen, M.A. (1975). A self-administered Short Michigan Alcoholism Screening Test (SMAST). *Journal of Studies on Alcoholism, 36,* 117–126.

Sokol, R.J., Martier, S.S., & Ager, J.W. (1989). The T-ACE questions: Practical prenatal detection of risk-drinking. *American Journal of Obstetrics and Gynecology, 160,* 863–870.

67

Interactive Guided Imagery in Treating Chronic Pain

David E. Bresler, Ph.D., L.Ac. and Martin L. Rossman, M.D.

Chronic pain has become the Western world's most expensive, disabling, and common disorder. It is estimated that 8 to 10% of the population of most Western countries suffer from chronic headaches. Arthritis afflicts over 50 million Americans, of whom 20 million require medical care. Low back pain generates nearly 20 million doctor visits per year and has disabled 7 million Americans (National Center for Health Statistics). Add facial and dental pain, neuralgia, cancer pain, chronic neck and shoulder pain, fibromyalgia, and other common pain syndromes, and it's easy to understand why chronic pain is estimated to cost the nation's economy $60 billion dollars per year. The cost in human suffering is incalculable.

Our focus in this chapter is on the uses of a particular form of mental imagery, called Interactive Guided Imagery, to relieve chronic pain, increase pain tolerance, reduce the emotional toll and amplification of pain, and relieve suffering. In the past 30 years of treating patients with chronic pain and other chronic illnesses, we have found Interactive Guided Imagery to be unusually effective in relieving symptoms, enhancing tolerance, relieving feelings of hopelessness and helplessness, promoting healing, and increasing functional abilities in our patients.

WHAT IS INTERACTIVE GUIDED IMAGERY?

Mental images, formed long before we learn to understand and use words, lie at the core of who we think we are, what we believe the world is like, what we feel we deserve, and how motivated we are to take care of ourselves. They strongly influence our beliefs and attitudes about how we fall ill, what will help us get better, and whether or not any medical and/or psychological interventions will be effective.

Imagery has powerful physiological consequences that are directly related to the healing systems of the body. Research on the omnipresent placebo effect, the standard to which we compare all other modalities (and find relatively few more powerful), has provided some of the strongest evidence for the power of the imagination and positive expectant faith in healing. It is well documented that 30 to 55% of all patients given inactive placebos respond as well or better than those given active treatments or agents (Frank, 1974).

If people can derive not only symptomatic relief, but actual physiologic healing in response to treatments that primarily work through beliefs and attitudes about an imagined reality, then learning how to better mobilize and amplify this phenomenon in a purposeful, conscious way becomes an important, if not critical, area of investigation for modern medicine.

In addition to its potential for stimulating physical healing, imagery provides a powerful window of insight into unconscious processes, rapidly and graphically revealing underlying psychological dynamics that may support either health or illness. To the clinician, this "window" is invaluable for quickly identifying opportunities for positive change, manifestations of resistance to change, and ways to work effectively with both.

Guided imagery is a term variously used to describe a range of techniques from simple visualization and direct

0-8493-0926-3/02/$0.00+$1.50
© 2002 by CRC Press LLC

imagery-based suggestion, through metaphor and story-telling. Guided imagery is used to help teach psychophysiologic relaxation, to relieve symptoms, to stimulate healing responses in the body, and to enhance tolerance to procedures and treatments.

Interactive Guided Imagery (IGI) is a service-marked term coined by the Academy for Guided Imagery to represent its highly interactive, nonjudgmental, content-free style of using guided imagery to evoke patient autonomy. This approach allows patients to draw upon their own inner resources to support healing, to choose the most appropriate adaptations to changes in health, and to find creative solutions to challenges that they previously thought were insoluble. IGI is particularly useful in our current healthcare climate, where cost-effective mind/body medicine, improved medical self-care, and briefer yet more empowering approaches to healthcare are becoming more highly valued by patients, providers, and insurers alike.

Before explaining the principles and practices of IGI, let's briefly examine some of the unique aspects of chronic pain that demonstrate why a sophisticated mind/body approach that utilizes techniques such as IGI is critical to long-term success.

CHRONIC PAIN DEMANDS DIFFERENT TREATMENT THAN ACUTE PAIN

Modern technology has created a huge variety of pharmaceutical products for pain relief, many of which are available over the counter. For acute or self-limiting pain, these agents are usually highly effective, for they provide temporary relief while the body heals itself. With the development of neural blockade and other modern anesthetic techniques, patients who undergo operative or other invasive procedures are generally spared all but the slightest degree of pre- or post-surgical discomfort.

Yet, the pharmacological approaches that have proven so successful in the management of acute pain are often ineffective or even counter-intentional for controlling chronic or long-term pain. Although acute pain usually gets better by itself as the body heals, chronic pain typically becomes worse with time. As a rough rule of thumb, chronic pain refers to any pain problem that lasts longer than 6 months. Victims are referred endlessly from doctor to doctor, for even if temporary relief can be obtained, the pain inevitably returns.

For example, when analgesic medications are used over a prolonged period of time, pharmacologic tolerance begins to develop and effectiveness is progressively reduced. As tolerance develops, patients typically increase their dosages with the idea that "if a little is good, a lot will be even better." Unfortunately, higher dosages only produce greater amounts of side effects, for tolerance continues to develop. In addition, most of the more effective analgesic agents also carry a high risk of dependency.

As a result, it is common to find patients with chronic pain taking large amounts of ineffective medications that produce significant side effects, many of which even contribute to the pain experience. When patients or their doctors attempt to reduce these medications, withdrawal symptoms make pain even less tolerable, and they return in desperation to their former regimes.

When medications fail, patients are often told, "Nothing more can be done. You'll have to learn to live with it." But in our opinion, there is *always* hope for someone in pain. Until *every* therapeutic approach has been attempted, no one should ever be told, "Nothing more can be done."

This statement has two iatrogenic implications: First, it destroys the most significant healing asset that victims of chronic pain (or other chronic illnesses) possess, namely, hope or positive expectant faith. Second, it conveys the subtle message that if you "have to learn to live with it," the only time you won't have it is when you are no longer alive. This may add to the significant suicidal ideation already experienced by many people in chronic pain.

The way we communicate with patients in pain has important effects and implications. As we discuss below, such negative communications may actually retard the body's intrinsic healing abilities, while more positive, imagery-based suggestions may enable patients to unlock the door to the most potent and varied pharmacy yet discovered — the one in our own brain.

THE IMPORTANCE OF THE PAIN EXPERIENCE

One of the greatest challenges in researching and treating chronic pain is to resolve ambiguity in the terms and concepts we use to describe it. For example, it is helpful to distinguish between a painful *sensation* (mental awareness of an unpleasant stimulus) and the pain *experience* (the total subjective experience of pain). Furthermore, it is important to recognize that there is not necessarily any direct relationship between the sensation and experience of pain.

This is seen in a study reported by Beecher, who found that soldiers seriously wounded in battle reported only mild discomfort compared to civilians with similar injuries because they were elated to learn that the war was over for them and they were to be sent home. In contrast, patients with phantom limb pain often report agonizing discomfort even though the entire stump has been anesthetized.

Many individuals think of pain primarily as a tangible thing, much like a splinter is a thing, that is, an object or substance from outside that infiltrates the body. Thus, if you accidentally strike your thumb with a hammer, you might say that you "feel pain in your thumb that is radiating to your hand."

Such a notion is totally inaccurate, for there is no pain "in" your thumb, any more than there is pleasure "in" your mouth when you eat something that tastes good. You probably wouldn't say, "Umm. My mouth is full of pleasure that is radiating to my stomach."

When you injure your thumb, you stimulate neural receptors that send a barrage of electrical and chemical messages up through the nerves in your hand and arm to your spinal cord and brain. Whether or not a given sensation becomes "painful" depends upon the way it is interpreted by the nervous system. If you've ever scratched an itch really hard, you know that sometimes it's hard to tell if something hurts or feels good. If, for all sorts of reasons, the nervous system decides that the messages from the thumb are urgent and require immediate action, it creates an experience of pain that is identified with the thumb so that you'll give it proper attention. However, it is important to note that the main pain receptor is between the ears, and that's where pain resides.

Like many perceptions, pain is well known to be influenced by learning and early developmental predispositions. For example, animals raised in a pain-free environment show insensitivity to noxious stimuli in later life. Social, cultural, and ethnic differences in the experience of pain also are well documented. A vivid example is the elective initiation rituals of many primitive tribes, which would be considered nothing short of torture if practiced by members of Western cultures.

Aristotle was the first to suggest that "pain is an emotion," as pervasive as anger, terror, or joy. The emotional component of pain is inexorably bound to other aspects of the pain experience, for anxiety and agitation are the natural consequences of a painful sensation that tells higher cognitive centers that something is wrong. If the "something" can be clearly identified and appropriate corrective action can be taken, the (acute) pain experience is terminated.

However, for most patients with chronic pain, the "something" is vague, and fear of continued pain in an unknown future produces even greater anxiety. On a physiologic level, sympathetic hyperactivity develops, as manifested by increased heart rate, blood pressure, respiration, palmar sweating, and muscle tension. In patients with musculoskeletal pain, this increased muscle tension often augments the sensation of pain, which further increases anxiety, which, in turn, produces even greater muscular tension and more pain. The amplifying relationship between pain and anxiety is well known to clinicians, for treatment of one frequently provides relief of the other as well.

Over time, exhaustion of sympathetic hyperactivity is inevitable, and more vegetative signs and symptoms soon emerge, such as feelings of helplessness, hopelessness, and despair, sleep and appetite disturbances, irritability, decreased interests and libido, erosion of personal relationships with family and friends, as well as increased somatization of complaints. Thus, acute pain and anxiety become chronic pain and depression.

It is well known that the most notable emotional change in patients with chronic pain is the development of depression. This may be overt or masked to both patient and health practitioner. In a sense, depression can be considered a type of emotional pain, and when it is effectively treated, the chronic pain experience is also often relieved.

It is important to emphasize the psychophysiological basis of chronic pain, for it is a complex subjective experience that involves physical, perceptual, cognitive, emotional, and spiritual factors. When a patient with low back pain complains that "my back hurts," his/her pain experience also may involve anxiety or depression (producing insomnia, loss of appetite, and decreased sexual desire), drug dependence or addiction, separation from work, family, and friends, loss of avocational interests and hobbies, numerous secondary gains, and a host of other problems. These may remain indelibly associated with the experience of back pain, even after the entire spine has been chemically anesthetized.

Thus, it is easy to see why no simple pill or shot can cure chronic pain. The most common error made by clinicians is to evaluate and treat only the physical aspect of the problem, for they assume that the objective of therapy is to treat pain in people. To us, however, the objective of therapy is to treat people in pain, which takes a much broader perspective. From this point of view, it is nonsensical to wonder if a patient has real vs. unreal pain, organic vs. psychologic pain, or legitimate vs. hysterical pain. Pain is an intensely subjective and personal experience, and even if no physical explanation for it can be found, *all pain is real*.

PAIN VS. SUFFERING

In our culture, pain is usually considered an enemy to be fought and overcome, and our first approach is to search for a pain killer. This approach overlooks and ignores the survival value of pain, which can be a warning signal, a protector, a potential teacher, guide, motivator, or even an incentive for change. While some believe that chronic pain is a symptom that has lost its meaning, this is the result of our healthcare system's tendency to medicalize and externalize symptoms rather than to examine their meaning in a holistic context.

Whatever the cause, when one cannot tolerate or cope effectively with pain, he or she suffers, which is manifested as an inability to sleep, eat, work, or fully enjoy one's life. Life, in the most personal, meaningful sense, stops. As we discuss below, suffering is primarily an epiphenomenon of one's attitude and beliefs, and we are convinced that it is possible to have pain, and yet not suffer, depending upon how we relate to the pain we experience.

In the more traditional psychological literature, a distinction is often made between pain sensitivity and pain tolerance. To illustrate the clinical importance of pain tolerance when teaching fellows and residents at UCLA, one of us (DB) found it helpful to compare X-ray films of two patients with knee pain.

The first patient was a professional football player who had undergone six prior knee surgeries. While reviewing his films, we wondered how this individual could walk, much less continue to play football. However, he reported little pain or discomfort, took no pain medications (they made him "feel less ferocious"), and only desired treatment that would increase stability and range of motion in his knees.

The second patient was injured on the job and had filed extensive worker's compensation litigation. Although his knee X-rays were completely normal, he suffered greatly and was unable to climb stairs, drive a car, or sleep for more than 2 to 3 hours at a time. He was totally disabled, despondent and depressed, and dependent on his family, four medical doctors, and seven different pain medications.

The first patient had significant pathology but high tolerance and barely complained of pain. The second had minimal if any pathology, but little tolerance to the pain he experienced.

In the clinical situation, we often confront limitations in our ability to reverse severe physical pathology (e.g., degeneration of cartilage in a joint). However, our ability to help patients enhance their tolerance of pain seems to have no upper limit. Thus, practitioners who help patients embrace a more positive belief or attitude about pain can be successful in helping to reduce suffering and enhance tolerance, even when nothing more (medically) can be done.

Increasing pain tolerance is, after all, the basis of effectiveness of our most potent pain medications. When a patient is given an injection of morphine (which mimics the effects of endorphins), he or she will often state. "It still hurts, but it doesn't bother me." This represents enhanced central tolerance, not reduced sensation, yet it enables the patient to become more highly functional.

The extent to which a patient's suffering can be reduced through psychophysiological approaches such as IGI depends upon many complex variables including the patient's belief systems and attitudes, early life experiences, the degree of physical pathology, and perhaps most importantly, the meaning of pain in the context of the patient's life.

THE MEANING OF PAIN

Since the dawn of creation, pain has provided critically important information concerning our relationship to our inner and outer environments. Pain strongly conveys the message that something is wrong, and it encourages the body to take action to prevent further injury. From an evolutionary point of view, it is one of the most powerful ways to insure the survival of an organism in a dangerous world.

While most authorities acknowledge the positive aspects of acute pain, many believe that chronic pain is a biological mistake or obsolete symptom that serves no useful purpose. In order to correct this mistake, they recommend strong drugs or surgical procedures to obliterate the sensation of pain. It is interesting to note that the exact technique utilized will depend more upon the type of specialist consulted than upon the patient's unique needs.

For example, an internist may prescribe medication; a psychologist, psychotherapy; an acupuncturist, needles; a chiropractor, manipulation; and so forth. Abraham Maslow used to say, "When all you have is a hammer, you tend to look for nails."

In our opinion, the best long-term interests of the patient often are not served when the major goal of therapy is to artificially mask or suppress pain without attempting to understand its ultimate message. To do so is like responding to a ringing fire alarm by cutting its wires to stop the annoying clamor, rather than by leaving the burning building.

We invite patients to consider the notion that like the oil light in a car, their nervous systems are generating the experience of pain for a reason. We invite them to explore the possibility that chronic pain is usually not a disease or mistake but a symptom generated through the wisdom of the body.

We then teach them about the extraordinary self-balancing, regeneration, and repair systems of the body and remind them that symptoms are the way that the body tries to heal itself or prevent further injury. Like the oil light and the fire alarm, once their message is heard and appropriate action is taken, symptoms usually will disappear, for they are no longer needed.

Much of contemporary medicine is based on an symptomatic adjustment model of therapy designed to reduce or suppress symptoms. If a patient has high blood pressure, antihypertensives are prescribed to reduce it. If a patient is unable to sleep, medications are given for sedation at night. If a patient has excessive anxiety, tranquilizers are often utilized. But *why* does a given patient have hypertension, sleep disorders, or anxiety neurosis? What is the message that the symptoms are trying to convey? Exploring this question in a nonjudgmental way can be the key to relieving or modulating many symptoms, including chronic pain.

Pain is a message that alerts us to danger. Through the primitive, survival-oriented wisdom of the nervous system, it motivates us to correct the situation by changing and adapting to the shifting demands of the world in which we live. Through pain, we are warned about all of the dangers we face, and if we continue to ignore them, the intensity of pain will increase in an attempt to get our attention and/or elicit some change.

Perhaps this is why many chronic pain patients receive only temporary relief after symptomatic treatment. Although the nervous system can be fooled for a short time by drugs or surgical treatment, if it believes that some subtle danger still remains, pain will attempt to break through and, over time, continue to return until the message is heard and properly responded to.

PRINCIPLES OF INTERACTIVE GUIDED IMAGERY (IGI)

HEALING BENEFITS FROM RESPECTFUL ATTENTION

Although no one really knows what *consciousness* is, we believe that it is critically related to the process of attention, for we only experience what we attend to. There is an old saying that "whatever you give your attention to grows," whether it be your garden, your children, your worries and fears, or your pain.

Over the years, most of us learn to give our attention to the conscious, verbal part of our mind that narrates a linear logical, rational, analytic monologue describing its perspective of the world and how we think about it. It's the little voice inside your head that talks all the time, the person most of us think we are.

However, who we really are is much more than just what we think. We are also the richness of our intuitions, emotions, feelings, memories, drives, fantasies, goals, appetites, aspirations, expectations, ambitions, values, passions, beliefs, perceptions, and sensations. Any or all of these aspects of self may require and even demand attention, finding ways to compete by intruding on everyday consciousness through physical, cognitive, emotional, or even behavioral symptoms, if need be.

Rather than suffer the results of neglecting these parts of ourselves, we can focus attention on them in a relaxed state of mind and invite images that represent them to come to mind. By properly dialoguing interactively with these images, we can reconnect with important and powerful inner resources that are deeply dedicated to protecting us and improving the quality of our lives.

IMAGERY IS THE PRIMARY ENCODING LANGUAGE OF THE BODY'S HEALING SYSTEMS

Imagery can be thought of as one of the brain's two higher-order information processing and encoding systems. The system we are most familiar with is that which uses *sequential information processing*, and it underlies linear, analytic, and conscious verbal thinking. Most health professionals are highly educated and highly rewarded for their abilities in using this mode of information processing.

Imagery serves a *simultaneous information processing* system, which underlies the holistic, synthetic, pattern thinking of the unconscious mind, and can reveal to us how seemingly disparate areas of our lives are intimately related.

A brief clinical example from Dr. Bresler's practice serves to focus on the importance of this relational quality to life.

A 52-year-old cardiologist named John was suffering from excruciating low back pain following treatment for rectal cancer. Although surgery and radiation therapy apparently had eradicated the cancer, he described the pain that remained as unbearable. Because the area had been so heavily irradiated, neither repeated nerve blocks nor further surgery could be used to help relieve his terrible discomfort, and he had long ago developed tolerance to his pain medications.

When John first came in, he already had narrowed down his personal alternatives to three: (1) successful treatment, (2) voluntary commitment to a mental institution, or (3) suicide. John was convinced that under no circumstances could he continue to live with pain and, at the same time, maintain his sanity.

In reviewing his medical records, I noticed that during a psychiatric workup, John had described his pain as "a dog chewing on my spine." This image was so vivid that I suggested we make contact with the dog, using guided imagery. With his training in traditional medicine, he thought the idea was silly, but he was willing to give it a try.

In John's case, our initial goal was to have the dog stop chewing on his spine. Over the next few sessions, the dog began to reveal critically important information. According to the dog (named Skippy), John never had wanted to be a physician, his own career choice was architecture, but he had been pressured into medical school by his mother. Consequently, he felt resentment not only toward his mother, but also toward his patients and colleagues. Skippy suggested that this hostility had, in turn, contributed to the development of his cancer and to the subsequent pain problem as well.

During one session, Skippy told John, "You're a damn good doctor. It may not be the career you wanted, but it's time you recognized how good you are at what you do. When you stop being so resentful and start accepting yourself, I'll stop chewing on your spine." These insights were accompanied by an immediate alleviation of the pain, and in only a few weeks' time, John became a new person, and his pain progressively subsided.

This type of experience demonstrates how powerfully the imagery process can reveal meaning in a supposedly meaningless symptom, and show the way to healing. While imagery does not always lead so dramatically to relief, and disease remission from such dialogues does not always occur, they almost always lead to better self-understanding and enhanced coping skills for dealing with a chronic illness or condition.

IMAGERY HAS PHYSIOLOGICAL CONSEQUENCES

Numerous research studies have shown that imagery is able to affect almost all major physiologic control systems of the body, including respiration, heart rate, blood pressure, metabolic rates in cells, gastrointestinal mobility and secretion, sexual function, and even immune responsiveness (Sheikh & Kunzendorf, 1984).

Imagery is essentially a way of thinking that uses sensory attributes, and in the absence of competing sensory cues, the body tends to respond to imagery as it would to a genuine external experience. For example, imagine that you have a big, fresh, yellow, juicy lemon in your hand. Experience it in your mind's eye until you sense its heaviness and fresh tartness. Now, imagine taking a knife and slicing into the lemon. Carefully cut out a thick, juicy section. Now take a deep bite of the lemon slice and imagine tasting the sour lemon juice, saturating every taste bud of your tongue so fully that your lips pucker and your tongue begins to curl.

If you were able to imagine this vividly in your mind's eye, the image probably produced substantial salivation, for the autonomic nervous system easily understands and responds automatically to the language of imagery.

Here is the crux of the matter: If imagining a lemon makes you salivate, what happens when you imagine you're a hopeless, helpless victim of chronic pain? Doesn't it tell your nervous system to give up? Isn't it likely to create neural and biochemical signals that go along with being defeated rather than actively healing? And, in the other direction, might not resolving serious life problems, improving communications and relationships, and learning to modulate pain create a healthier and more functional physiology in the body?

IMAGERY IS THE LANGUAGE OF THE EMOTIONS

Imagery also is a powerful tool in the healing arts because of its close relationship to the emotions. Imagery is the expressive language of the arts — poetry, drama, painting, sculpture, music, and dance, and thus of the emotional self. Emotions show us what's personally important to us and they can be either potent motivators or barriers to changing lifestyle habits. As clinicians, we have concluded that, by and large, if an issue doesn't affect you emotionally, it probably won't make you sick nor is it likely to help you get well.

Emotions motivate us to action and they also produce characteristic physiologic changes in the body, including varying patterns of muscle tension, blood flow, respiration, metabolism, and neurologically and immunologically reactive peptide secretions. Modern research in psychoneuroimmunology points to the emotions as key modulators of neuroactive peptides secreted by the brain, gut, and immune systems (Pert & Chopra, 1997).

PATIENT AUTONOMY IS MOST SUPPORTED BY USING A TWO-WAY INTERACTIVE GUIDING STYLE

One key to the extraordinary clinical effectiveness of Interactive Guided Imagery is the unique interactive communications component that it incorporates. By working interactively instead of simply reading an imagery script, the Interactive Imagery Guide ensures that the experience has personal meaning for the client, and that it proceeds at a pace determined by the client's actual needs and abilities rather than the guide's best guess estimate.

For example, an Interactive Imagery Guide might ask, "Of all the different problems, symptoms, and challenges now going on in your life, allow an image to form that represents the single most important and critical issue for us to work on now, and then describe it to me." The guide can then facilitate a dialogue between the client and the image to find out what the image wants, needs, and has to offer.

Because the content, direction, and pace are set by the client, not the guide, it is the client who actually (unconsciously) guides the process to the resources most needed to support healing, change, and positive therapeutic results.

PATIENT AUTONOMY IS MOST ENCOURAGED BY USING CONTENT-FREE LANGUAGE AND NONJUDGMENTAL GUIDING

We often like to say that "the guide provides the setting, while the client provides the jewel." Whenever possible, the Interactive Imagery Guide uses nonjudgmental, content-free language, because it encourages clients to tap their own inner resources to find solutions for solving their own problems.

At a time when there is so much concern about false memory syndrome (Pope, 1996), this type of content-free guiding also insures that the client's experience is not unduly contaminated or influenced by the suggestions of the guide.

PATIENT AUTONOMY IS ENCOURAGED BY SPECIFIC QUALITIES AND SKILLS UTILIZED BY THE GUIDE

There are important personal qualities that the Interactive Imagery Guide brings to the therapeutic experience, including a nonjudgmental attitude, patience, and trust in the client's own abilities. The consistent emphasis on resources and solutions, the repetitive inner focus as a source for solutions and strengths, and the modeling provided by the guide's belief that the clients have within them more resources than they had imagined, leads to minimal transference, greater opportunities for effective client self-care, an enhanced sense of self-efficacy, and the rapid development of patient autonomy.

PROVIDER–PATIENT/CLIENT INTERACTIONS

PATIENT ASSESSMENT PROCEDURES

The Interactive Imagery Guide must first decide whether there are any contraindications to introducing imagery to the patient, such as a medical or surgical condition requiring emergency treatment, or mental illness precluding its use. Having decided that imagery may offer benefit, a history is taken regarding the client's prior experience with imagery, hypnosis, relaxation, meditation, or related approaches. This allows the guide to utilize prior positive experiences or to address relevant issues in the case of negative experiences.

If the client has no prior experience with relaxation or imagery, the guide usually invites the client to relax while being guided through a brief relaxation technique. The client is then invited to imagine him or herself in a beautiful, safe, and peaceful place and then to describe what he or she sees, heasr, smells, and feels there. The guide may suggest that this special place has other qualities that also might be uniquely helpful to the client. For example, a fearful client might be encouraged to imagine hi or herself in a powerful place, a sanctuary, or a place where you are completely safe and beyond harm. A client who feels he or she is too exhausted to deal with a situation might be encouraged to imagine a place of great energy and vitality, or a place of rest, renewal, and refreshment.

Imagining a quiet, safe place is one of the quickest ways to teach most people to relax and it powerfully illustrates the profound effects a simple imagery experience can have.

Occasionally, a client cannot imagine such a place, or gets more anxious as the eyes close and he or she begins to relax. If this anxiety doesn't respond to reassurance that the person is in control, and gentle encouragement to see what comes next, it may be a signal that the person has not experienced such a place or that relaxing may be psychologically dangerous to them. Relaxation-induced anxiety may also be a marker for early trauma, as is the experience of having an imaginary safe place suddenly turn dangerous or foreboding.

Alternatively, clients may be invited to turn their attention to specific symptoms, to allow images to form for them, and to invite healing imagery to come to mind. They may be invited to have an imaginary dialogue with an image of a symptom, or with a kind, wise "Inner Advisor" who can provide previously inaccessible information about their issues or illness.

In this relaxed state, we can invite images to form for almost anything we want to know more about, and systematically explore the images to expand awareness and identify new options that promote healing.

Typically, patients are initially seen one to three times to explore the potential benefits of working with IGI. After three sessions, clients may have solved the problem, may have found a successful way to work it out by themselves, may have identified an issue that will require additional work, or may have found that the method or practitioner is not suitable for them.

While imagery may bring psychological material to light that was not previously perceived to be part of the medical equation, it also can provide ways to work with this material that do not create unnecessary dependence on a therapist. Many medical or nursing professionals will work with patients if the situation appears it will yield to a brief course of teaching and counseling, while referring those with more complex issues to therapists who are more highly trained in the method.

TREATMENT OPTIONS

Because imagery is a natural way we think, and can almost always be helpful, there are virtually an unlimited number of situations where it can be used in healthcare settings. For simplicity, it may be helpful to consider three major categories of use:

1. Relaxation and stress reduction, which are easy to teach, easy to learn, and almost universally helpful.
2. Visualization, or directed imagery, where the client/patient is encouraged to imagine desired outcomes in a relaxed state of mind. This affords the patient a sense of participation and control in his or her own healing, which itself is of significant value. In addition, it also may relieve or reduce symptoms, stimulate healing responses in the body, and/or provide effective motivation for making positive lifestyle changes.
3. Receptive or insight-oriented imagery, where images are invited into awareness and explored to gather more information about a symptom, illness, mood, situation, or solution.

Another set of options to consider is whether the client will be able to use imagery most effectively as a self-care technique, in a group or class, or as part of an individual counseling or therapy relationship. Self-help books and tapes are another inexpensive option for many clients who are capable of utilizing these techniques on their own.

In practice, most patients and practitioners will explore all of the above options and utilize the ones that suit a given client the best, given the unique nature of the issue, patient coping responses and approach to life, and the amount of time, energy, and funds the patient is willing or able to invest in the process.

DESCRIPTION OF COMMONLY USED TREATMENT TECHNIQUES

The list of techniques utilized in IGI is quite extensive, and this approach has been applied to problems ranging from severe depression and chronic pain, to post-traumatic stress, to relationship conflicts, to enhance creativity, to the search for life purpose. However, some of the more basic techniques include the following.

Conditioned Relaxation

This powerful, relaxation technique is based on Pavlovian classical conditioning techniques and utilizes imagery-linked breathing and body awareness techniques to train the patient to relax automatically by taking a special "signal breath." Instead of tensing when pain starts to flare, patients become conditioned to relax and gently move the painful symptoms out of their bodies.

Symptom Suppression Techniques

Symptomatic imagery techniques reduce the physical symptoms of pain without concern for their causes. They are a useful alternative to analgesic medications, and are particularly helpful when discomfort is so intense that the patient cannot concentrate enough to use other guided-imagery approaches. They include a wide variety of scenarios and techniques, such as "glove anesthesia," a two-step imagery exercise in which patients first are taught to image developing feelings of numbness in the hand, as if it were being placed into an imaginary anesthetic glove. Next, they learn to transfer these feelings of numbness to any part of the body that hurts, simply by placing the "anesthetized" hand on it. Glove anesthesia often helps to take the edge off the pain sensation, thus permitting patients to explore other aspects of the pain experience more fully. In addition, glove anesthesia provides a dramatic illustration of the power of self-control. When patients realize that they can produce feelings of numbness in their hands at will, they recognize that they may be able to control their discomfort, too. This is profoundly therapeutic for pain sufferers who feel totally helpless and unable to affect their discomfort.

Symptom Substitution Techniques

Symptom substitution is another symptomatic technique that permits the nervous system to move the discomfort to a new area of the body where it will be less disruptive. For example, patients can learn to experience their headaches in, say, their little finger instead of their head. This technique does not ask the nervous system to stop the experience of pain (or to cover up the message it is trying to communicate). Rather, it moves the symptom to a less traumatized area so that patients can work more effectively to identify what is wrong.

Interactive Imagery Dialogue

This interactive technique can be used with an image that represents anything the client or therapist wants to know more about, and in many ways, it is the quintessential insight technique. We use it to explore an image of a symptom (whether physical, emotional, or behavioral), an image representing resistance that arises anywhere in the process, an image for an inner resource that can help the client deal with the current problem, or an image of the solution.

When using Interactive Imagery, the point is not to analyze the images, but to communicate with them as if they are alive (which of course, they are). This is not to say they have an existence apart from the client, but rather that the images represent complexes of thoughts, beliefs, attitudes, feelings, body sensations, expectations, and values that at times can function as relatively autonomous aspects of the personality. These constellations have been referred to as subpersonalities by Assagioli, or ego states by Watkins and Watkins.

The Inner Advisor

After relaxing in his or her own safe place, a client is invited to dialogue with an imaginary figure who is designed to be both wise and loving, or as characterized in analytic terms, an "Ego Ideal." We call this figure the "Inner Advisor," and it is often referred to as the "Inner Guide," "Inner Healer," "Inner Wisdom," "Inner Helper," "Inner Physician," "Higher Self," or any other term that is meaningful and comfortable for the client. As the client is invited to imagine a figure with these qualities, a dialogue with whatever figure arises is usually meaningful and helpful.

Evocative Imagery

This state-dependent technique helps clients shift moods and affective states at will, thus making new behaviors and insights more accessible to consciousness. Through the structured use of memory, fantasy, and sensory recruitment, the client is encouraged to identify a personal quality or qualities that would serve him or her especially well in the current situation. For instance, a client may need more calmness or peace of mind in order to deal more effectively with pain.

The guide then invites clients to relax and recall a time when peace of mind was actually experienced. Through the use of sensory recruitment and present tense recall, the clients are encouraged to imagine they are there again now, feeling that peace of mind. Once this peaceful feeling state has been well established and amplified, the patients are invited to let the past images go, but to come back to the present, bringing the feelings of peace of mind. As they now become aware of their pain problems while strongly in touch with this feeling, they are usually able to tolerate it far more effectively.

Evocative imagery was researched by Dr. Sheldon Cohen at Carnegie-Mellon University (personal communication) and found to be highly effective in shifting affective states. Research aimed at assessing the effects of those altered affective states on subsequent behavior, problem-solving, and self-efficacy remain to be done and offers a fertile field for future psychological and behavioral research.

Grounding: Moving from Insight to Action

This is the process by which the insights evoked by imagery are turned into actions, and increased awareness and motivation are focused into a specific plan for attitudinal, emotional, and/or behavioral change. This process of adding the will to the imagination involves clarification of insights, brainstorming, choosing the best option, affirmations, action planning, imagery rehearsal, and constant reformulation of the plan until it actually succeeds. It is often the missing link in insight-oriented therapies, for it connects the new awareness to a specific action plan. It's where the "rubber meets the road," and imagery can be used to enhance this process by providing creative options for action and by utilizing imagery rehearsal to troubleshoot and anticipate obstacles to success.

TREATMENT EVALUATION

We refer to the time spent before entering into a formal guided imagery exploration as the "foresight" part of the process. Along with evaluating the appropriateness of using imagery with the client or patient, the guide works with the client to establish the desired goals and objectives for their work together.

As with any medical or psychological situation, goals can be defined in physical, emotional, or behavioral terms, and a reasonable trial period of exploration is agreed upon. We often ask patients to do three exploratory sessions and then decide whether this approach seems useful to them, whether they can best use it as self-care in a brief, time-limited period of work (10 to 15 sessions), or whether it looks like a longer-term piece of work will be needed.

Many physicians and nurses work for a defined period of time with patients in a psycho-educational or counseling model, with well-defined symptomatic or behavioral goals, and refer patients to mental health practitioners if their work becomes psychologically complex. At the same time, we urge that mental health practitioners take precautions to ascertain the medical status of any patient to make certain they are also aware of the medical options.

At the end of each session, and at the end the agreed-upon time period, the goals of the work are reviewed and progress assessed (we call this phase "hindsight").

After this evaluation, an agreement is made to terminate treatment, to continue for another period of time, to refer to another practitioner, or to define a period of time in which the client will do "ownwork" and then return to report progress.

TREATMENT APPLICATIONS IN ADDITION TO PAIN

Since imagery is a natural language of the unconscious and the human nervous system, its potential uses in the healing professions are protean. We think that imagery is essentially a way of working with the patient, rather than a way of treating particular disease entities. Thus, it is almost always useful as an adjunctive therapy, while it is rarely, if ever, utilized as a sole therapy.

Table 67.1 lists some of the major applications of imagery in the healing professions.

TABLE 67.1
Applications of Interactive Guided Imagery in the Health Professions

In Medicine
- Relaxation and stress reduction
- Pain reduction and symptom relief
- Increasing compliance with treatment regimens
- Tolerating difficult procedures
- Preparing patients for surgery
- Stimulating healing responses (immunity, blood flow)
- Insight and affect recognition
- Engaging patients in their own self-care
- Finding meaning in illness

In Psychotherapy
- Relaxation and stress reduction
- Systematic hyposensitization for phobias
- Conflict clarification and resolution
- Shift of locus and control and relief of powerlessness
- Positive suggestion, affirmation, and enhanced self-esteem
- Finding vision and meaning
- Action planning
- Values clarification
- Increased creativity and enhance problem-solving
- Modulation of mood and affect
- Insight and awareness development
- Grieving

In Nursing
- Relaxation and stress reduction
- Deepening rapport
- Enhancing compliance
- Tolerating procedures
- Pain and symptom relief
- Engaging patients in self-care
- Addressing emotional needs of patients

CONTRAINDICATIONS AND PRECAUTIONS

1. Do not substitute imagery for necessary medical or surgical interventions.

   The primary danger in using imagery to augment healing in medical situations is when it is used in lieu of appropriate medical diagnosis and/or treatment. We emphasize the necessity of an accurate diagnosis prior to using any psychophysiologic approach so that the patient also is aware of the medical options for treatment. At times, patients may decide that they do not have acceptable medical options available and will then choose to use imagery and mind/body/spirit approaches as their first-line treatment. Although there are some situations in which this makes perfect sense, each situation must be evaluated individually to ascertain the patient's ability to judge for him or herself and to make such choices.

2. Do not use imagery inappropriately with patients with unstable or unmanaged psychopathology.

   There are several diagnostic categories of mental illness where the practitioner must use extreme care when utilizing exploratory receptive imagery techniques. In particular, patients who are psychotic or who are on the verge of psychotic breaks, patients with dissociative identity disorders, and patients with borderline personality disorders must be handled with care, and only by well-trained and experienced practitioners.

   While these diagnoses do not represent absolute contraindications for imagery work, they absolutely require treating health professionals to have appropriate training and expertise in these areas. While many clients with these diagnoses may benefit from certain uses of imagery (usually directed imagery scripts focusing on centering, calmness, self-control, safety, etc.), great caution should be taken when using potentially disorganizing receptive imagery techniques.

   In proper therapeutic hands, imagery techniques can be one of the most effective ways to work with clients who are survivors of traumatic abuse and who tend to pathologically dissociate. However, such treating practitioners must be well trained and experienced in working with both survivors of abuse and with exploratory IGI approaches.

3. Do not confuse responsibility with blame.

   The fact that an illness can be helped through mental processes does not necessarily suggest that it was caused by mental means. When using exploratory techniques such as imagery dialogue with symptoms, or working with an inner advisor, there is a tendency to confuse the ability to learn from illness with blame for causing the illness.

   This issue needs to be handled with skill and sensitivity, and while the practitioner may not be able to prevent certain clients from self-blaming (this may be an important issue to address with them), they can help most people realize that using positive images to stimulate healing does not necessarily mean that their negative images caused their illness.

4. Do not underestimate the holotropic principle and the innate resources of the patient.

   Imagery is a potent form of communication and suggestion. Whenever possible, we advocate using the patient's own imagery and an interactive guiding style because we are convinced that the client has within him- or herself a great deal of information, experience, knowledge and problem-solving resources that have not yet been used most effectively.

   While there are certainly places and situations where a guide needs to supply suggestions and images, these are relatively rare when utilizing IGI, and may even rob clients of the opportunity to learn an important way to help themselves. This creates or sustains a sense of dependency on the expertise of the guide, rather than attention to the inner abilities that have always been available to help them to help themselves.

SCOPE OF PRACTICE FOR INTERACTIVE GUIDED IMAGERY

This has been an important and problematic area for the Academy for Guided Imagery. As we considered the criteria for formal certification in IGI, we decided to exercise caution and restrict certification eligibility to professionals licensed to provide counseling services in their states of residence.

We soon found out that many states have no such licensing for therapists, and people of various levels of quality were providing counseling, psychotherapy, hypnosis, and guided imagery. As a result, we evaluate each candidate on an individual basis, assessing him or her for both competence and ethical standards as we observe them in clinical supervision as part of the Academy's training.

Health professionals must practice within the scope of their licensure, education, experience, and competence. Within these guidelines, certification in IGI can significantly help make professionals more effective at what they already do. Using guided imagery or IGI does not turn a physician into a psychotherapist, or a psychotherapist into a physician.

Instead, it gives each a greater range of skillfulness in working with issues that involve both mind and body, and with issues involving emotions and behavioral change.

Certified IGI practitioners must discriminate between psychotherapy and psychoeducation, and between enhancing healing responses and the practice of medicine. They must ethically practice each within their scope of licensure, training, experience, and competence.

Because our approach is holistic, there is more cross-over in these areas than is immediately apparent. If we can effectively activate healing responses through essentially psychological means, how does this affect the scope of practice of mental health practitioners who are well-versed in IGI? Shouldn't they be critical members of every primary healthcare team? We believe so.

TRAINING, CERTIFICATION, AND ISSUES OF COMPETENCE

Many health professionals utilize guided imagery in their work, although they may have only learned to lead someone by reciting a noninteractive script. The quality of their training and competence with this approach is highly variable. Because the potential for doing harm always exists when these techniques are used inappropriately or without adequate skills, standards of practice and quality control are an issue of critical importance.

The Academy for Guided Imagery has established specific standards of competence and ethical behavior that must be met before Certification in Interactive Guided Imagery is awarded. Quality assurance is based largely upon direct observation of clinical work in small group and individual supervision sessions during the training program. Over 52 hours of supervision, four to six different faculty members carefully observe each candidate, and provide specific feedback to enhance his or her skills. We know of no other such standards of quality assurance established for imagery practitioners.

REIMBURSEMENT STATUS

Imagery practitioners usually bill and are reimbursed for their work in the same way as for other professional services they render. Sessions are usually billed as psychotherapy, counseling, stress reduction training, or medical hypnosis. When applied for medical purposes, medical practitioners may ethically bill for medical services, although insurance companies may challenge this if services are lengthy and repetitive. There are currently no separate billing codes for guided imagery or IGI.

PROSPECTS FOR THE FUTURE

When you look closely at almost every form of human therapeutic interaction and communication, imagery is usually centrally involved, primarily because it is a fundamental language of the body's healing systems. As this is better recognized, we are hopeful that health professionals will learn more about the best ways to utilize this potent form of thinking to support optimal health and healing.

Feedback from the thousands of health professionals who have taken IGI training confirms that it is a rapid route to insight, growth, and change. One constant piece of feedback we get is that learning to use imagery interactively has improved the listening, communicating, and therapeutic skills of our graduates, whether they are mental health professionals, physicians, or nurses.

We feel that competence in effectively yet respectfully guiding the imagery process should be a fundamental part of every health professional's education and training, and the Academy for Guided Imagery is working toward that goal by co-sponsoring many of its professional training programs with well-established schools of medicine, nursing, and psychology.

In addition to professional training and Certification in Interactive Guided Imagery, the Academy for Guided Imagery is a resource for self-help books and tapes and reliable information on imagery. The Academy also is participating in research studies exploring the uses of imagery in pain control, surgical preparation and recovery, and cancer chemotherapy, and it recently established the nonprofit Imagination Foundation to support further research in these and other areas. The Imagination Foundation is currently soliciting both funds and research proposals investigating imagery in healing.

Humans have always used their imaginations to solve problems that threatened their survival. Our times demand that we now learn to use this powerful information-processing and problem-solving mechanism even more effectively to help heal ourselves, our families, our communities, and our planet. A sustainable future depends in part on our ability to imagine it in both personal and global terms, and we are committed to supporting the healing potential of this much under-utilized resource — the human imagination.

RESOURCES

PROFESSIONAL TRAINING

The Academy for Guided Imagery
Martin Rossman, M.D. and David Bresler, Ph.D.
Professional Certification Training in Interactive Guided Imagery™, Public Education, Healthcare Consulting, Speakers, Books, and Tapes
P.O. Box 2070
Mill Valley, CA 94942
1-800-726-2070; FAX 415-389-9342
http://www.interactiveimagery.com

Imagery for Health and Healing
Jeanne Achterberg, Ph.D.
369 Montezuma, Ste. 342
Santa Fe, NM 87501-2626
505-986-826

PROFESSIONAL ASSOCIATIONS

International Association for Interactive Imagery™
P.O. Box 124
Villa Grande, CA 95486

Imagination Foundation
P.O. Box 2070
Mill Valley, CA, 94942
1-800-726-2070; FAX 415-389-9342

TAPES, VIDEOS, BOOKS, AND RELATED MATERIALS

The Imagery Store (Academy for Guided Imagery)
P.O. Box 2070
Mill Valley, CA 94942
1-800-726-2070

Health Journeys (BelleRuth Naparstek, Ph.D.)
891 Moe Drive, Suite C
Akron, OH 44310
1-800-800-8661

Source Cassettes (Emmett Miller, M.D.)
P.O. Box W
Stanford, CA 94309
1-800-528-2737

REFERENCES

Academy for Guided Imagery, 1-800-726-2070. www.interactiveimagery.com

Cohen, S. Personal communication.

Frank, J. (1974). *Persuasion and healing*. New York: Schocken Books.

Imagination Foundation, POB 2070, Mill Valley, CA 94942. www.imaginationfoundation.org

Inventory of Pain Data from the National Center for Health Statistics. Washington, D.C.: U.S. Government Printing Office.

Pert, C.B., & Chopra, D. (1997). *Molecules of emotion: Why you feel the way you feel*. New York: Scribner.

Pope, K.S. (1996). Memory, abuse, and science. *American Psychologist*, 957–974.

Sheikh, A., & Kunzendorf, R.G. (1984). Imagery, physiology and psychosomatic illness. In A. Sheikh (Ed.), *International review of mental imagery*. (Vol. 1, pp. 95–138). New York: Human Services Press.

Vargiu, J. (1974). *Subpersonalities, synthesis 1* (pp. 57–90). Redwood City, CA: Synthesis Press.

Watkins, J.G., & Watkins, H.H. (1979). The theory and practice of ego-state therapy. In H. Grayson (Ed.). *Short-term approaches to psychotherapy*. New York: Human Sciences Press

68

Behavioral Protocols for Burning and Cramping Phantom Limb Pain*

Richard A. Sherman, Ph.D.

CONCEPTUAL INTRODUCTION

Behaviorally oriented treatments for phantom limb pain have been in use at least since the late 1970s (e.g., Sherman, 1976). Use of behavioral interventions is predicated on the supposition that amputees can learn to recognize and then control incorrect levels of physiological functions related to their phantom pain.

This idea requires that (1) there are specific physiological parameters which are directly related to specific descriptors of phantom pain and (2) people can, indeed, learn to control them. Over the past several decades, data have accrued that strongly infer that the extent of near-surface blood flow in the residual limb is inversely correlated with intensity of burning/tingling descriptions of phantom limb pain and that many amputees can learn to control blood flow in the residual limb sufficiently to reduce or eliminate these sensations. Data also show that cramping/twisting descriptions of phantom limb pain are related to increased muscle tension and spikes/spasms of the major muscles in the residual limb and that amputees learning to eliminate these abnormalities also eliminate their cramping phantom pain. There are no known physiological correlates of shocking shooting phantom pain and none of the behavioral interventions appears to be effective for this description of phantom pain.

RELATIONSHIPS BETWEEN PHANTOM LIMB PAIN AND MUSCLE TENSION

Chronholm (1951) quotes Amyot, Livingston, and others as having noted increased muscle tension and spasms in the stumps of amputees. He found that 51 of 99 amputees questioned about stump muscular activity reported spontaneous hyperactivity.

Onset and intensity of cramping and squeezing descriptions of phantom pain are related to muscle tension in the residual limb. A variety of studies have demonstrated that intensity of cramping phantom pain and amount of muscle tension in the residual limb change together from day to day (Sherman & Arena, 1992) and from moment to moment (Sherman, Griffin, Evans, & Arena, 1992).

Changes in surface electromyographic (sEMG) representations of muscle tension in the residual limb precede changes in cramping and squeezing phantom pain by up to several seconds. This relationship does not hold for any other descriptions of phantom pain. The critical point is that the amputee only shows changes in muscle tension in the painful residual limb. Surface EMG in the pain-free residual limb does not change significantly. If the change in EMG was simply a reaction to the change in pain, the change in EMG would have followed, rather than preceded, the change in pain and at least some change in

---

* Adapted from *Phantom Pain*, Sherman, Devor, Jones, Katz, and Marbach (1997).

0-8493-0926-3/02/$0.00+$1.50
© 2002 by CRC Press LLC

muscle tension in the pain-free limb should have been observed as would be expected from a generalized withdrawal reflex from pain.

Relationships between overall muscle tension in the residual limb and cramping phantom pain have also been shown to hold throughout the day in subjects' normal environments (Sherman, Evans, & Arena, 1993). The device used to establish the relationship was capable of recording surface EMG from the residual limb and button press representations of pain intensity (Sherman, Arena, Searle, & Ginther, 1991). The relationship between cramping phantom pain and muscle tension in the residual limb is supported by the consistent success of treatments resulting in reduction of residual limb muscle tension for cramping phantom pain but not for other descriptions (Sherman 1976; Sherman et al., 1991; Sherman et al., 1992).

Numerous amputees report that cramping phantom pain decreases with any activity that tends to decrease muscle contraction levels in the residual limb and increases with activities increasing overall levels of contraction. Thus, such activities as phantom exercises, which result in changes in muscle tension in the residual limb, can result in temporary changes in intensity of phantom pain. Gessler (1984) reported that when the muscles of the residual limb of 10 amputees with chronic cramping phantom pain were relaxed, the phantoms felt as though they were opening.

BURNING-TINGLING-THROBBING PHANTOM LIMB PAIN

Reduced near-surface blood flow to a limb has been implicated as a predictive physiological correlate (first cousin to a cause) in many pain conditions including causalgia and reflex sympathetic dystrophy (Karstetter & Sherman, 1991). Return of blood flow to normal patterns through any intervention, including time alone, usually results in either the complete cessation or significant decrease of the pain (Sherman et al., 1991). If phantom limb pain is a referred pain syndrome, anything affecting the nerve endings in the residual limb is likely to affect phantom pain as well. A number of excellent studies have demonstrated that (a) the ends of the nerves that used to serve the amputated limb are still sensitive to stimuli; (b) cooling the nerve ends causes increased firing rates; and (c) reducing blood flow to the extremity results in cooling it (Campbell, 1987; Harber, 1955; Janig, 1987; Koschorke, Meyer, & Campbell, 1987; Matzner & Devor, 1987; Sherman & Arena, 1992).

Chronholm (1951) quotes Pitres (1897) as having stated that the perceived temperature of the phantom is related to the temperature of the stump. Measurements of skin temperature in amputees have been made since at least 1952 (Berkeley Medical School, 1952). The study found that amputees' residual limbs were cooler at the distal end than paired points on the opposite extremity and that the cooler areas did not warm up when attempts were made in increase cutaneous blood flow through such mechanisms as giving the subjects whiskey to drink. Wahren (1990) reviewed the propensity of finger amputees to be very sensitive to the cold and for their pain to be aggravated by cold environments. They found that the residual areas of the fingers were cooler than corresponding areas on the intact hand and were more sensitive to pain in response to cooling. Kristen, et al. (1984) reported using videothermographic recordings of temperatures in the residual limbs of 50 amputees to detect phantom pain. They found that most amputees having phantom pain showed different patterns of temperature than those who had none.

Consistent, inverse relationships between intensity of phantom limb pain and temperature in the residual limb relative to that of the intact limb have been demonstrated for burning, throbbing, and tingling descriptions of phantom pain but not for any other descriptions (Sherman & Bruno, 1987).

It has also been established that (a) for these descriptors of phantom pain there is a day to day relationship between the relative amount of blood flow in the stump and pain intensity and that (b) there is an immediate change in pain when blood flow changes. However, this does not mean that the changes in blood flow cause the change in pain. It is possible that a change in pain intensity causes a physiological chain reaction which eventually causes a decrease in blood flow to the stump. This is improbable for several reasons. Although videothermographs normally record only near-surface blood flow patterns, hands are thin enough so that thermographs can record blood flow patterns throughout the hand. In four cases of burning or tingling phantom pain following a finger amputation, blood flow changed only in the area just proximal to the amputation site. The rest of the hand was essentially unchanged and there were no changes in the paired area of the intact hand. If blood flow was changing as a result of a reflex, we would have expected a bilateral change or, if unilateral, a change related to dermatomal distribution patterns in which an entire dermatome would have cooled off. This was not the case so we conclude that a reflex reaction is not likely. The subjects were taught to increase blood flow in the stump by using temperature feedback to relax, and thus dilate, the peripheral blood vessels. Increasing peripheral blood flow to the cool area of the stump resulted in a decrease in the pain intensity. If the decrease in blood flow was due to an increase in pain, blood flow would decrease for all descriptors of phantom pain, not just a consistent few (Sherman & Arena, 1992).

Numerous thermograms form the key evidence that the decreased blood flow associated with burning phantom pain is not the subsequent result of a general sympathetic reaction because only the painful residual limb shows decreased blood flow—the other residual limb maintains its temperature. This tight, progressive relationship has been replicated numerous times (e.g., Sherman & Bruno, 1987) and indicates that there is more than a casual relationship between the two.

"The existence of a vascular related mechanism for burning phantom pain is also supported by the short term effectiveness of those invasive procedures, such as sympathetic blocks and sympathectomies, which increase blood flow to the limb and reduce the intensity of burning phantom and stump pain but not other descriptors (Sherman 1980; Wall, 1981). It is indirectly supported by the virtual ineffectiveness of every surgical procedure involving severing nerves either in the spinal cord or running between the amputation site and the spinal cord (Sherman & Sherman, 1985; Wall 1981). Beta blockers such as propranolol cause dilation of peripheral blood vessels and have been reported to be successful in ameliorating phantom pain at least in the short term (Marsland, Weekes, Atkinson, & Leong, 1982)" (Sherman & Arena, 1992). Relationships between muscle tension and burning phantom limb pain (Sherman & Bruno, 1987) have been shown to be due largely to the change in near-surface blood flow that accompanies increased muscle tension (Laughlin & Armstrong 1985; Richardson, Schmitz, & Borchers, 1986).

RECOMMENDED PROCEDURE FOR BEHAVIORAL INTERVENTIONS TO PATIENTS WITH CHRONIC PHANTOM LIMB PAIN*

As early as 1979 it became apparent that different descriptions of phantom pain responded to different treatments (Sherman, Gall, & Gormly, 1979). Initial attempts to treat phantom limb pain with a combination of biofeedback and relaxation techniques showed excellent success up to 6-month to 3-year follow-ups with 14 of 16 successive phantom pain patients. The major difference between those patients who succeeded in learning to control their pain and those who did not was the ability to control their physiology in any measurable way. The two failures never (a) demonstrated the ability to relax or (b) reported subjective feelings which would be associated with learning to relax or to control their muscle tensions.

In an attempt to align behavioral and medical treatments of phantom pain with underlying physiological correlates, amputees who showed increased burning phantom limb pain in response to decreased blood flow in the residual limb were treated with peripheral vasodilators and temperature biofeedback. When increased muscle tension

---

* Modified from Sherman & Arena, 1992 and Sherman, et al., 1997.

and spasms in the stump were related to episodes of cramping phantom pain, muscle relaxants and muscle tension biofeedback were used to control the pain (Sherman et al., 1997).

In the most recent cases, EMG biofeedback was effective for 13 of 14 trials for cramping phantom pain. EMG biofeedback had minimal success with 2 and no success with 10 of 12 trials for burning phantom pain. It had no success with 8 trials of shocking phantom pain. Temperature biofeedback was ineffective for 4 trials of cramping phantom pain, was effective for 6 of 7 trials with burning phantom pain, and had no success with 3 trials for shocking phantom pain. Nitroglycerine ointment (a topical vasodilator) was ineffective for 1 trial of cramping phantom pain and 1 trial of shocking phantom pain but successful for 2 trials of burning phantom pain. Trental (a blood viscosity enhancer) was ineffective for 2 trials of cramping phantom pain and 1 trial of shocking phantom pain. Nifedipine (a systemic vasodilator) was effective for 3 trials of burning phantom pain but ineffective for 1 trial of cramping and 2 trials of shocking phantom pain. Flexeril (a muscle relaxant) was effective for 2 trials of cramping phantom pain but ineffective for 1 trial of shocking phantom pain. Indocin (an anti-inflammatory agent) was ineffective for 2 trials of cramping phantom pain. These medications have potential side effects and cannot be used by patients with a variety of medical problems. Thus, the use of "self-control"-oriented strategies is encouraged to avoid these limitations.

It is clear that burning phantom pain responds to interventions that increase blood flow to the residual limb while cramping phantom pain responds to interventions that decrease tension and spasms in major muscles of the residual limb. Shocking–shooting phantom pain does not respond well or consistently to either type of intervention.

It is strongly recommended that biofeedback of appropriate parameters be used in conjunction with other self-control training strategies to treat cramping/squeezing and burning/tingling phantom limb pain. It is important for clinicians to recognize that biofeedback as utilized for control of phantom limb pain is not some kind of black box psycho-magic. Rather, it is simply the process of recording the physiological parameters (such as muscle tension in the residual limb) that precede changes in phantom pain, and showing the signals to patients. The patient uses the information to change the signal. The patient also learns to associate sensations related to onset of phantom pain with tension in the muscle, decreased blood flow, etc. and to use the learned ability to control the parameter to prevent the onset of or to stop it if it has already begun.

Unfortunately, the large, controlled studies with long-term follow-ups needed to clearly show that burning and cramping phantom pain are amenable to behavioral interventions have not been conducted.

SUMMARY

CRAMPING PHANTOM PAIN

The existent data (e.g., Sherman, 1994) support the contention that nearly all amputees with cramping phantom limb pain, who can learn to recognize the relationship between their pain and spikes in the surface EMG of the residual limb and can learn to prevent the spikes from occurring, can prevent their phantom pain to the extent they can prevent the spikes. If the spikes continue, so will the cramping phantom pain. If the spikes can be voluntarily stopped once an episode of phantom pain begins, the episode can nearly always be almost entirely aborted. The small studies showed that the vast majority of people can learn to control nearly all of their cramping phantom pain. Again, no learning, no control. Follow-ups of 1 to several years showed that the results are sustained.

BURNING PHANTOM PAIN

The same premise holds true for burning as for cramping phantom pain. If patients can learn to increase blood flow to the residual limb, burning phantom pain will decrease to the extent that blood flow is normalized. The burning will remain away as long as blood flow remains normal. Unfortunately, about half of the patients have not been able to learn to raise the blood flow in their residual limbs to a significant extent.

REFERENCES

Campbell, J. (1987). Painful sequelae of nerve injury. *Pain, 34*, 334.

Cronholm, B. (1951). Phantom limbs in amputees. *Acta Psychiatrica et Neurologica Scandinavica, 72*(Suppl), 1–310.

Gessler, M. (1984). Relief of phantom pain by stimulation of the nerve supplying the corresponding extensor-muscles. Proceedings of the International Society for the Study of Pain, meeting held in Hamburg, Germany.

Haber, W.B. (1955). Effects of loss of limb on sensory function. *Journal of Psychology, 40*, 115–123.

Janig, W. (1987). Pathophysiology of nerve following mechanical and ischemic injury. *Pain, S4*, 335.

Karstetter, K., & Sherman, R. (1991). Use of thermography for initial detection of early Reflex Sympathetic Dystrophy. *Journal of the American Podiatric Medical Association, 81*, 198.

Kristen, H., Lukeschitsch, G., Plattner, F., Sigmund, R., & Resch, P. (1984). Thermography as a means for quanititative assessment of stump and phantom pains. *Prosthetics and Orthotics International, 8*, 76–81.

Koschorke, G., Meyer, R., & Campbell, J. (1987). Myelinated afferents that innervate neuromas display marked sensitivity to stimuli. *Pain, S4*, 281.

Laughlin, M.H., & Armstrong, R.B. (1985) Muscle blood flow during locomotory exercise. *Exercise and Sport Sciences Reviews, 13*, 95–136.

Marsland, A.R., Weekes, J.W.N., Atkinson, R., & Leong, M.G. (1982). Phantom limb pain: a case for beta blockers? *Pain, 12*, 295–297.

Matzner, O., & Devor, M. (1987). Contrasting thermal sensitivity of spontaneously active A- and C-fibers in experimental nerve-end neuromas. *Pain, 30*, 373–384.

McKechnie, R. (1975). Relief from phantom limb pain by relaxation exercises. *Journal of Behavior Therapy and Experimental Psychiatry 6*, 262–263.

Richardson, D., Schmitz, M., & Borchers, N. (1986). Relative effects of static muscle contraction on digital artery capillary blood flow velocities. *Microvascular Research, 31*, 157–169.

Sherman, R.A. (1976). Case reports of treatment of phantom limb pain with a combination of electromyographic biofeedback and verbal relaxation techniques. *Biofeedback and Self Regulation, 1*, 353.

Sherman, R.A. (1980). Special review: Published treatments of phantom limb pain. *American Journal of Physical Medicine, 59*, 232–244.

Sherman, R.A. (1994). What do we really know about phantom limb pain? *Pain Reviews, 1*(3), 261–274.

Sherman, R.A., & Arena, J.G. (1992). Phantom limb pain: Mechanisms, incidence, and treatment. *Critical Reviews in Physical and Rehabilitation Medicine, 4*, 1–26.

Sherman, R., Arena, J., Searle, J., & Ginther, J. (1991). Development of an ambulatory recorder for evaluation of muscle tension and movement in soldiers' normal environments. *Military Medicine, 156*, 245–248.

Sherman, R.A., & Bruno, G.M. (1987). Concurrent variation of burning phantom limb and stump pain with near surface blood flow in the stump. *Orthopedics, 10*, 1395–1402.

Sherman, R., Devor, M., Jones, C., Katz, J., & Marbach, J. (1997) *Phantom pain*, New York, Plenum Press.

Sherman, R., Evans, C., & Arena, J. (1993). Environmental-temporal relationships between pain and muscle tension: Ramifications for the future of biofeedback treatment. In M. Shtark & T. Sokhadze (Eds.), *Biofeedback: Theory and practice*. Novosibirsk: Nauka Publishers.

Sherman, R., Gall, N., & Gormly, J. (1979). Treatment of phantom limb pain with muscular relaxation training to disrupt the pain-anxiety-tension cycle. *Pain, 6*, 47–55.

Sherman, R., Griffin, R., Evans, C., & Grana, A. (1992). Temporal relationships between changes in phantom limb pain intensity and changes in surface electromyogram of the residual limb. *International Journal of Psychophysiology, 13*, 71–77.

Sherman, R., & Sherman, C. (1985). A comparison of phantom sensations among amputees whose amputations were of civilian and military origins. *Pain, 21*, 91–97.

Studies relating to pain in the amputee. (1952). A progress report from the prosthetic devices research project at the Institute of Engineering Research, Department of Engineering, U of C Berkeley Medical School, Series II, Issue 23.

Tsushima, W. (1982). Treatment of phantom limb pain with EMG and temperature biofeedback: A case study. *American Journal of Clinical Biofeedback, 5*, 150 - 153.

Wahren, L. (1990). Changes in thermal and mechanical pain thresholds in hand amputees. A clinical and physiological long-term follow-up. *Pain, 42,* 269–277.

Wall, P.D. (1981). On the origin of pain associated with amputation. In J. Siegfried & M. Zimmermann (Eds.). *Phantom and stump pain,* (pp. 2–14). New York: Springer-Verlag.

69

Hypnotherapeutic Advances in Pain Management

Jan M. Burte, Ph.D., D.A.A.P.M.

There is little doubt that the induction of hypnoidal states utilizing chanting and breathing exercises dates back to earliest history. The earliest clinical records of hypnosis are attributed to John Elliotson (1792 to 1869), an English surgeon, who used hypnosis for pain management in his practice. James A. Esdaile (1808 to 1859) performed more than 300 operations using hypnosis as analgesia while practicing in India (Bassman & Wester, 1992). One such operation reportedly entailed the removal of a 103-pound tumor (Jackson, 1999). Hypnosis and trance represent an age-old treatment for a variety of conditions including pain; hypnosis has been embraced as a legitimate therapy consequent to continuing research only over the past 50 years (Hrezo, 1998).

Hypnosis as a form of pain management fell in and out of favor from the early 1940s until the 1960s when Milton H. Erickson demonstrated its utility with acute and chronic pain control (Erickson, 1986). The application of hypnosis within the medical and pain setting has continued to develop from the work of Hilgard and Hilgard (1975), Hilgard and LeBarron (1982), Barber and Adrian (1982), and Melzack and Wall (1965; 1983).

Zohaurek (1985) points out two historical misconceptions of pain that have affected the role of hypnosis in treating pain.

1. Pain was considered only to be a symptom of an underlying disease or trauma. Therefore, research and treatment focused on the etiological cause and ignored the pain, assuming it would disappear when the cause was addressed.

Historically, pain reporting was by necessity heavily relied upon as part of the initial diagnostic procedure, where severity, location, and nature of the pain often assisted in proper diagnosis. Although pain reporting maintains a significant role in diagnosis, the advent of additional diagnostic procedures (i.e., CAT, MRI scans) goes beyond pain reports and reduces their unique significance. The reliance on pain reports was especially true in certain acute pain situations although not as much in chronic pain situations where a diagnosis had been reached (Bonica, 1990). It was postulated that hypnosis could mask the symptoms of pain and might interfere with obtaining a proper diagnosis and treatment (i.e., hypnosis utilized to mask pain associated with appendicitis could result in delaying care until the appendix had ruptured).

2. Pain was seen as evolving from either a physical or a psychological origin rather than from both. Pain was perceived to have either a "real/organic" basis or a "functional/imaginary" basis (Fordyce, 1976, Sternbach, 1978). Current thinking might view the impact of pain as an etiological factor that by its bidirectional psychoneuroimmunological role (on the psychological, endocrinological, and immunological systems) may contribute to the maintenance of illness (Burte, 2000) or enhance the progression or metastasis of certain illnesses (Paige and Ben-Eliyahu, 1997).

0-8493-0926-3/02/$0.00+$1.50
© 2002 by CRC Press LLC

Since 1958, hypnosis has been recognized by the American Medical Association as a legitimate form of medical treatment when administered by an appropriately trained practitioner (Simon & James, 1999). Fortunately, with the resurgence of integrative, mind/body, psychoneuroimmunological approaches, current thought and research have begun to view hypnosis as a potentially significant modality in the treatment of pain and illness.

In this section, I focus on the hypnotherapeutic advances in pain management. In the next section, I discuss the applicability of hypnosis in the treatment of specific illnesses. Due in part to its historical misportrayal in the popular media, patients referred for hypnosis often ask, "But does it really work?" Contemporary popular media portray hypnosis as an effective means of pain control (Foderaro, 1996). Currently, sufficient experimental and clinical research exists to allow clinicians to respond affirmatively to the question. However, certain caveats, discussed later, still exist.

What then is medical or clinical hypnosis and what are the contemporary views of both practitioners and the public, especially within the realm of pain management? One recent survey indicates, "that most people have a positive view of the therapeutic benefits with a vast majority of respondents believing that it reduces the time that is usually required to uncover causes of a person's problems, and that hypnotized persons can undergo dental and medical procedures without pain" (Johnson and Hauck, 1999).

Retrospectively, it is important to recognize that "pain," until the 20th century, was considered an untreatable consequence of illness or injury. Indeed, Chaves and Dworkin (1997) astutely point out that hypnoanalgesia did not fully emerge until the 19th century, due largely in part to the societal belief that, at that time, did not define pain relief and reduced suffering as the primary goal in treatment. Prior to effective clinical techniques for pain management, pain was an accepted aspect of life. One might wonder whether the introduction of pharmacological forms of pain relief such as analgesia and anesthesia altered patients' perceptions and ultimately their thresholds for pain.

If pain can act as a mediator in trance production with pain patients, then did our progenitors and do perhaps third world cultures who had/have limited access to various forms of pain relief intuitively rely on hypnosis and self-hypnosis to alter their pain thresholds? For these individuals, pain, whether from childbirth, dental procedures, illness, or injury, was anticipated.

Today, the application of hypnotic analgesia in acute and chronic pain treatment has grown substantially. Both patients and clinicians are demonstrating increased knowledge and experience with hypnosis. In many cases, patients bring clinical experiences with hypnosis for related or unrelated issues to the treating physician (Lynch, 1999), thereby opening a door to increased complementary approaches to standard interventions.

Where this may be significantly prevalent is in the nonpharmacological strategies employed in managing cancer pain. As Zaza, Sellick, Willan, Reyno, and Browman (1999) point out, while pharmacological treatments are appropriately the central component of cancer pain management, the under-utilization of effective nonpharmacological strategies may contribute to the problem of pain and suffering among cancer patients. In a study of 214 health professionals, Zaza, et al. (1999) found that the healthcare professionals recommended "imagery" exercises 54% of the time and meditation 43% of the time. They expressed interest in learning more about hypnosis and other nonpharmacological strategies suggesting its under-utilization as a complementary or adjunctive treatment to standard care. In a critical review of the literature, Sellick and Zaza (1998) found that in randomized controlled studies of hypnosis in managing cancer pain, substantial evidence exists for its effectiveness when nonpharmacological pain management approaches are being sought.

This concept, then, of unifying both the confidence of the practitioner and the trust and belief of the patient, may represent the components necessary to obtain efficacious pain relief. Barber (1998) aptly delineates a two-component model as to why hypnosis may work for pain management. He suggests that in the first component the "clinician communicates specific ideas that strengthen the patient's ability to derive therapeutic support and to develop a sense of openness to the unexplored possibilities of pain relief within the security of a nurturing therapeutic relationship." In so doing, the patient is led to relax in the clinician's confidence in hypnosis. In the second component, "the clinician employs posthypnotic suggestions that capitalize on the patient's particular pain experiences which simultaneously ameliorate the pain experience and which, in small repetitive increments, tend to maintain persistent pain relief over increasing periods of time." This second component offers the patient a sense of voluntary learned control over his or her pain, thereby reducing anxiety and learned helplessness.

A somewhat more constructionistic view is offered by Chapman and Nakamura (1998) who suggest that hypnosis alters the learned pain experience (pain schemata) by interacting with feedback processes that prime the associations and memories tied to the pain, thereby shaping the formation of pain expectations and processes and ultimately reducing the experience of pain.

As mentioned previously, hypnosis has fallen in and out of favor over the years due in part to arguments concerning the lack of hard scientific data to support its efficacy or pathophysiology. With increasing frequency studies are demonstrating the impact of hypnosis on pain from the perspective of changes occurring in the brain itself. Rainville, et al. (1997) demonstrated that positron emission tomography revealed significant changes in pain-evoked activity within the anterior cingulate cortex consistent with the encoding of perceived unpleasantness, thereby linking frontal lobe limbic activity with pain susceptible to hypnotic suggestion.

In an examination of exposure to noxious stimuli presented to subjects, Faymonville, Laureys, Degueldre, DelFiore, Luxen, Franck, Lamy, and Maguet (2000) found that hypnosis could reduce the intensity and unpleasantness of the exposure. By examining cerebral blood flow of subjects both with and without hypnotic intervention, they concluded that hypnotic modulation of pain appears to be mediated by the anterior cingulate cortex.

Rainville (1999a) in their examination of cerebral blood flow utilizing PET scans found that the hypnotic experience may result in increased occipital regional cerebral blood flow (RCBF) and delta activity (EEG) by altering the consciousness associated with decreased arousal via facilitation of visual imagery. Frontal increases in RCBF may be associated with verbal mediation of suggestions, working memory, and top–down processes involved in re-interpreting the perceptual experience of the noxious stimuli. They concluded that specific patterns of cerebral activation appear to be associated with the hypnotic state.

Other researchers have demonstrated the effectiveness of hypnotic analgesia on raising pain thresholds by examining the nociceptive flexion (RIII) reflex and EEG patterns (Danziger, et al., 1998).

However, the real question for clinicians is, "Can learning to develop hypnoanalgesia to noxious stimuli in a laboratory (an acute short-term artificial environment) be generalized to a patient's ability to control real nociceptive acute or chronic pain. Crawford (1998) found that chronic back pain patients could be trained to utilize hypnotic analgesia on a noxious stimulus and then generalize the hypnotic analgesia to their back pain. They concluded that "hypnotic analgesia is an active process that requires an inhibitory effort dissociated from conscious awareness where the anterior frontal cortex participates in a topographically specific inhibitory feedback circuit that cooperates in the allocation of the thalamocortical activities." They further point out that the subjects could successfully transfer the experimental pain reduction to reduction of their own chronic pain and, in so doing, also experience increased well-being and increased sleep quality.

Utilizing a modulated form of pain, patients can learn the hypnotic skill of pain control or the raising of their pain thresholds. They can then be taught to generalize this skill to pain situations that are more a function of their illness or injuries.

Hypnotic analgesia has also been shown to reduce subjective pain perceptions and the nociceptive flexion reflex in high-hypnotizable subjects (Sandrini, Mianov, Malaguti, Nigrelli, Moglia, & Nappi, 2000). This raises yet another question. If pain can be unlearned via hypnoanalgesia, does it imply that at least to some degree it

is a psychoneurologically learned behavior? The concept of the existence of a "neural signature of pain" that acts as a progenitor of subsequent pain experiences is offered by Melzack (1983). If this is so, we should teach patients how to communicate more positively when in acute pain stages before they develop chronic pain. Meta-analyses of 18 studies revealed a moderate-to-large hypnoanalgesia effect supporting the efficacy of hypnotic technique for pain management in both clinical and experimental pain settings (Montgomery, Dultamel, & Redd, 2000).

When we speak of pain patients and hypnosis, another important question is raised. Does hypnosis work equally well for all patients? The literature seems to suggest that numerous variables must be considered in drawing any conclusions. Issues of patients' hypnotic susceptibility, chronic vs. acute pain, and the origin and etiology of the pain are relevant factors.

In the realm of hypnosis, the question of the importance of hypnotic susceptibility and trance depth has long been debated (Frankel, Apfel, Kelly, et al., 1979; Hilgard & Hilgard 1979; Perry, Gelfand, & Marcovitch, 1979) especially with regard to pain (Hilgard and LeBaron 1982). Recent studies that have examined the importance of hypnotic susceptibility of pain patients (as opposed to non-pain patients) appear to indicate that when dealing with acute pain issues, hypnotic susceptibility is very important. Sandrini, et al. (2000) examined subjects rated as either high or low susceptibles on the Harvard Group Scale of Hypnotic Susceptibility (Shor & Orne, 1963) and the Stanford Hypnotic Susceptibility Scale (Weitzenhoffer & Hilgard, 1959). Utilizing a noxious stimulus, they concluded that, "the susceptibility of the subject is critical in hypnotically induced analgesia. Similarly, high hypnotic but not low hypnotic subjects demonstrated significant reductions in pain intensity and reduced nociceptive receptive reflexes during hypnotic analgesia (Zachariae, et al., 1998).

Increased hypnotizability was also found to positively affect sensory and pain thresholds during dissociated imagery and focused analgesia as measured by skin conductance responses, somatosensory event-related potentials, and pain perceptions (De Pascalis, Maguarano, & Belluschi, 1999). The ability to modulate pain was greater when subjects demonstrated higher hypnotic suggestibility (Rainville, 1999b). Controlled associative ability (Agargun, Tegeoglu, Kara, Adak, & Ercan, 1998) and the ability to utilize internal (guided imagery), and external distractors (word memory and pursuit of motor tasks) were also found to be effective only in high susceptibility subjects fulfilling analgesic suggestions (Farthing, Vonturino, Brown, & Lazar, 1997).

Is then the low suggestibility patient subjugated to not being able to utilize hypnosis or is suggestibility trainable? In a brief training experience Milling, Kirsh, and Burgess (1999), utilizing the Carlton Skill Training Program, found that training failed to increase overall suggestibility scores or to enhance the effects of a suggestion for pain reduction. However, pain reduction was more highly correlated with post-traumatic levels of suggestibility than to pre-treatment suggestibility.

Many authors have thought that hypnotizability is a skill that is enhanced with practice but occurring at a rate set by the patient. It has been further suggested that "hypnosis may be best conceived as a set of skills to be deployed by the individual rather than as a state" (Alden and Heep, 1998). Others have suggested that hypnotic susceptibility may not be a factor in treatment. In a study of hypnotic susceptibility and the treatment of irritable bowel syndrome, hypnotic susceptibility to suggestion was not a factor in the positive effect found for hypnosis (Galovski and Blanchard, 1998). Utilizing the Hypnotic Induction Profile as part of the hypnotic experience, clinicians can within 5 to 10 minutes assess a patient's hypnotic response capabilities and provide the patient with an initial first-hand experience (skill acquisition trial) of what hypnosis is like (Spiegel and Spiegel, 1978/87). Any patient, but especially pain patients, may spontaneously shift to an altered state of awareness increasing their suggestibility merely as a function of their motivation to develop rapid rapport and trust in the clinician in an effort to escape the pain (Araoz, 1985).

A simple but effective means of incorporating the patient's willingness to accept suggestion is presented by Eimer (2000) who, at the end of an induction concludes, "As you go deeper and deeper into relaxation and hypnosis, the door way to your unconscious opens and, with your permission, I have the opportunity to talk directly to your unconscious and give it the information it needs to help you make the changes you want to make"(p. 20).

A review of the literature points to an increasingly broadening range of applications of hypnosis in treating medical conditions with associated pain. One area where hypnosis has been utilized for both acute pain and healing is with burn victims. Hypnosis has been shown to reduce pain even in situations where opioids fail to bring relief (Ohrbach, Patterson, Carroughen, & Gilbram, 1998). Treatment and dressing changes can be an extremely painful part of burn care. Wright and Drummond (2000) found that rapid induction analgesia (RIA) was effective in reducing pain and anxiety associated with dressing changes, and Ewin (1986) found that hypnosis positively reduced pain in adults during debridement. Similar findings were also found with pediatric patients (Foertsch, O'Hara, Stoddard, & Kealey, 1998). Indeed, burn victims may demonstrate enhanced receptivity to hypnotic suggestion secondary to issues of motivation, dissociation, and regression (Patterson, Adcock, & Bobardier, 1997), especially within the subset of burn patients who report high levels of baseline pain (Patterson and Ptacek, 1997).

Another area where hypnosis has been extensively utilized is in the arena of surgical intervention. Hypno-anesthesia, the use of hypnotic suggestion rather than general anesthesia to mediate pain during surgical intervention, has been successfully employed for endocrine cervical surgery (Defechereux, Meurisse, Hamoir, Gollogly, Joris, & Faymonville, 1999; Meurisse, Hamoir, Defechereaux, Gollogly, Derry, Postal, Joris, & Faymonville, 1999). Hypnosedation (hypnosis in combination with conscious IV sedation and local anesthesia) has been employed as an alternative to traditional anesthetic techniques (Faymonville, Meurisse, & Fissette, 1999; Meurisse, et al., 1999).

Hypnosis has also been shown to provide proprioceptive pain and anxiety relief, reduced Alfenta and Midazolam requirements and increased patient satisfaction and surgical conditions when compared to other surgical stress strategies in patient receiving conscious sedation (Faymonville, Mambourg, Joris, Vrijens, Fissette, Albert, & Lamy, 1997). Audiotaped hypnotic instructions produced reduced anxiety (Ghoneim, Block, Sarasin, Davis, & Marchman, 2000) while pre-operative hypnosis resulted in a reduction of consumption of analgesics (Engvist and Fischer, 1997) in third molar surgeries.

Self-hypnosis has been employed as an anesthesia for liposuction surgery (Botta, 1999) and for postoperative levels of pain control and relaxation in coronary artery bypass surgery (Ashton, Whitworth, Seldonridge, Shapiro, Weinberg, Michler, Smith, Rose, Fisher, & Oz, 1997) and arteriotomies (Austan, Polise, & Schultz, 1997). It is attributed to reduced reported pain and anxiety and improved hemodynamic stability during invasive medical interventions such as percutaneous vascular and renal procedures (Lang, Benotsch, Fick, Lutgendorf, Berbaum, Berbaum, Logan, & Spiegel, 2000). In particular, hand surgery that requires painful rapid remobilization of the hand is especially benefited by hypnosis. Hypnosis reduces perceived pain intensity allowing patients to be more compliant and able to withstand physical rehabilitative interventions (Mauer, Burnett, Ouelette, Ironson, & Dandes, 1999), as well as increased rates of anatomical and functional healing (Ginandes & Rosenthal, 1999).

Hypnosis also has demonstrated its efficacy with children dealing with the pain and anxiety associated with invasive medical procedures (Hilgard & LeBaron, 1984), including bone marrow aspiration (Liossi & Hatira, 1999), resulting in lower levels of reported pain, reduced anxiety, and shorter hospital stays (Lambert, 1996; Smith & Barabasz, 1996). Distraction and imagery techniques have been shown to be highly effective in reducing pain in painful procedures (Broome, Lillis, McGahee, & Bates, 1992). Scripts and metaphors for children with painful conditions are readily available to the pediatric pain practitioner (Wester & O'Grady, 1991; Mills & Crowley, 1986).

Another significant area where hypnosis has continued to demonstrate its utility is cancer intervention. Numerous books and articles on the use of imagery and healing (Gaynor, 1994; Siegel, 1998) have discussed the psycho-neuroimmunological benefits of hypnosis (see Chapter 64 on psychoneuroimmunology in this volume). For many years hypnosis has also been shown to provide specific pain relief and reduced suffering for cancer patients (Sacerdote, 1966; Hilgrad & Hilgard, 1975; Hilgard and Le Barron 1984) and more recently, by employing physical relaxation coupled with imagery that provides a substitute focus of attention for painful situations (Spiegel and Moore, 1997). Patients demonstrate an increased awareness of the willingness to employ hypnosis adjunctively to their standard medical care resulting in new programs that incorporate hypnosis into their treatment protocols (Lynch, 1999). As recently as 1996, the NIH Technology Assessment Panel presented its conclusion in *JAMA* that strong evidence exists for the use of hypnosis in alleviating pain associated with cancer.

Vidakovic-Vukic (1999) notes that irritable bowel syndrome (IBS) is a frequently observed painful disorder, but its etiology and pathogenesis are still unknown. However, it is clear that individual perceptions may play an important role in its pathogenesis. Vidakovic-Vukic points out that in recent years hypnotherapy has been shown to be successful in the treatment of IBS, resulting in either reduced or complete disappearance of pain and flatulence and a normalization of bowel habits. Similar results with a hypnotic treatment where the focus of intervention was "gut directed" and "symptom driven" found that abdominal pain, constipation, and flatulence improved, while anxiety scores decreased (Galovski & Blanchard, 1998).

McGrath (1999), based on the studies of P.J. Whorwell and those of O.S. Palsson, presents hypnosis as a significant component in the treatment of IBS with success rates approaching 80% reported in the literature. The focus of hypnosis for IBS should be on the gut-directed and associated symptomology. In a review article, Camilleri (1999) points out that in addition to various medicinal interventions and fiber intake, hypnosis may play an important role in relief of pain in IBS patients.

Hypnosis also has been shown to be effective in acute pain care settings such as emergency room settings with burn pain, pediatric procedures, psychiatric presentations, and obstetric situations (Peebles-Klieger, 2000; Zahourek, 1985). Iserson (1999) describes a simple method of hypnosis utilized in pediatric fracture reduction on four cases of angulated forearm fractures using distraction techniques when no other form of analgesia was available. Interestingly, fracture healing also may be enhanced utilizing hypnosis. Faster edge healing, improved ankle mobility, greater function mobility to descend stairs, lower use of analgesic, and trends toward lower self-reported pain were found in patients who received hypnotic intervention in addition to standard orthopedic emergency room care (Ginandes & Rosenthal, 1999).

Hypnotically induced glove anesthesia with transference to the pain site for acute pain relief is a commonly utilized technique. This is accomplished by using suggestions of creating a numbing sensation in the hand. Patients may be asked to imagine their hands in a bucket of anesthetic gel or a glove or other such images. This numbing or pleasant sensation is then transferred to the pain site with a pleasant increase in numbness. An excellent example of this technique is offered by Basserman and Wester (1984). Other techniques include distraction techniques and dissociative techniques (Burte, 1999; Eastwood, Gaskowski, & Bowers, 1998). In all cases, a trusting rapport with the clinician appears to be a critical factor in achieving the desired goals. In addition, as has been noted earlier, pain may act as a mediator toward an altered state of increased suggestibility to pain alleviation. Acute pain patients may willingly and rapidly transfer their pain to the hypnotherapist or anyone willing to accept the pain. Patients should be reassured that proper medical care is forthcoming and they can let go of their pain. As Schafer (1996) points out, perhaps as many as half the patients in an emergency room may be in spontaneous trance. An alternative approach is to focus on the imagery the patient spontaneously reports associated with the pain. Psycho-semantics and somatopsychic queues are observed when utilizing the patient's perceptions, internal representations, and understandings of the pain to alter the cognitive, emotional, and sensory experience (Burte and Araoz, 1994).

Utilizing the New Hypnosis Model developed by Daniel Araoz (1985), patients are helped to achieve an altered state of internally directed experiencing of their symptomology. By focusing on the way they interpret and communicate their pain through any or all of their five senses, patients are led to a reinterpretation and understanding of their ability to modulate their pain. How patients integrate pain sensations will impact their pain thresholds. Positive suggestions to pain altered the amount of time that patients could keep their hands immersed in ice water (Staats, Hekmat, & Staats, 1998). For example, in the case of an individual with recently cracked ribs, he may be asked to experience or visualize the ribs as they appear to him. He is then asked to visualize ways to soothe, protect, or heal the ribs (i.e., an anesthetic band wrapped around the chest, relaxing, protecting, and healing the area of injury), while communicating calming, relaxing, and possibly "in control of the situation" thoughts. At times, visualizing being in a safe or pleasant situation helps induce a hypnoidal form of relaxation or mild dissociation. Though creating relaxation has often been seen as an important element-inducing trance for the pain patient, it may be a secondary goal with the imaging or individualized experience of the pain as the primary pathway to the hypnotic state.

Acute pediatric pain represents a somewhat different issue in that children often lack clinical insight regarding their condition, an understanding of the etiology, potential longevity, or plausible interventions available for ameliorating their pain, concepts that help adults cope with acute pain more effectively. Patients provided appropriate preoperative information demonstrate less acute pain (Stevensen, 1995). Hypnosis may represent a complementary treatment in conjunction with other forms of intervention such as pharmacological pain management (Rusy & Weisman, 2000). By providing cognitive and behavioral schemata via modalities easily accessed by children (i.e., imagery, fantasy), the acute pediatric pain patient can be empowered similarly to the way adults utilize reason to empower coping ability with pain.

Hypnosis may be a means of reducing both pain and pain-related distress (Chen, Joseph, & Zeltzer, 2000). For example, Adam, a young cancer patient was treated utilizing hypnosis for pain. First he was taught glove anesthesia which he applied to areas where he was to have finger sticks, Broviac changes, and later bone marrow aspirations. He was taught to visualize himself as a cartoon super hero named He-Man. By lifting his crutch and later his finger into the air and reciting the words, "By the power of Grey Skull I am He-Man," Adam was magically (hypnotically) transformed into He-Man, the strongest man in the universe. At such times, he could withstand increased levels of pain and invasive procedures.

Recurrent pediatric headaches appear to show a positive response to hypnotic intervention when relaxation and/or thermal feedback techniques are employed (Holden, Deichman, & Levy, 1999). The use of autogenic training (hand warming) with imagery has also been useful in reducing or eliminating pediatric migraines when done early into the migraine episode at the first signs of visual aura or muscular discomfort.

Crawford, Knebel, Kaplan, Vendermia, Xie, Jamison, and Primbam (1998), in drawing attention to the transition of the acute pain to the chronic pain patient, note that by utilizing hypnosis, patients could alter acute pain experiences. They further suggest that learned hypnotic analgesia resulted in reported chronic pain reductions, increased psychological well-being, and increased sleep quality. The "neurosignature of pain" can influence subsequent pain experiences (Melzack, 1983). Specific pain reduction hypnotic skills may indeed be essential in developing lasting pain relief, especially in situations where chronic pain based on medical conditions (i.e., cancer tumors, herniated discs) is anticipated. In this context, hypnotic pain control may be conceived as a set of skills rather than a state (Alden & Heap, 1998).

Chronic pain patients clearly represent a different population than acute pain patients. The most common form of chronic pain, other than from illness, is chronic low back pain, accounting for $50 to $100 billion dollars a year in lost wages and medical care (Burte, Burte, & Araoz, 1994; Miller & Krauss, 1990). Unlike acute pain, chronic pain may result in significant changes in individuals, personalities, and clinical presentations as evidenced by performance on MMPI profiles (Strassberg, Tilley, Bristone, & Oei, 1992).

Chronic pain patients clinically demonstrate elevated levels of feelings of hopelessness, helplessness, and despair. They often report ongoing struggles with depression, somatic preoccupations, and obsessive concerns with fatal illness (Miller & Krauss, 1990). When chronic pain becomes a central issue in the individual's life, it may function as a coping mechanism altering the patient's capacities, both psychopathophysiologically and etiologically (Kuhn, 1984). In addition to its direct impact on pain alleviation, it is with the depression and hopelessness the chronic pain patient experiences that hypnosis can play a key role. Metaphors and hypnotic scripts can address both the pain and psychological distress (Havens & Walters, 1989). Individuals who are diagnosed with what would today be referred to as chronic pain syndrome (CPS) often are overwhelmed by the impact of their pain. For CPS patients the pain often takes on an all-encompassing life of its own, dictating the patient's quality of life both psychologically and physically. The CPS patient's pain alleviation is often complicated by issues of learned behaviors, conditioned avoidances, and conscious and unconscious secondary gains. Hypnotherapy represents a complementary component in a multidisciplinary approach that should first acknowledge that the CPS patient is not primarily a psychiatric patient but rather a composite of both psychological and physical distress. Melzack (1990) points out the advantages of a multidisciplinary approach inclusive of narcotics, for the purpose of rescuing people in chronic pain. As Hitchcock (1998) points out, there are significant myths and misconceptions about the chronic pain patient that the pain practitioner must address in formulating a treatment plan. She further points out that in many ways the patient is a valuable contributor to the understanding of his or her own condition. As such, hypnosis may assist patients in that understanding via uncovering techniques and experiential insights into various aspects of their pain.

In addition to low back pain, many other conditions can result in CPS. Patients experiencing temporomandibular disorders who underwent hypnotic intervention demonstrated significant decreases in pain severity and frequency which were maintained for at least 6 months after treatment (Simon and Lewis, 2000).

Self-hypnosis has been used adjunctively in dealing with pain associated with sickle-cell anemia (Dinges, Whitehouse, Onre, Bloom, Carlin, Bauer, Gillen, Shapiro, Ohene-Frempong, Dampier, & Orne, 1997). Hypnosis has helped adolescent teens and adults with cystic fibrosis (CF) develop improved attitudes about health and a sense of independence and decreased anxiety (Belsky & Kahanna,

1994; Olness & Kohen, 1996). Utilizing a technique introduced by Bressler (1990), Anbar (2000) taught CF patients to seek an inner advisor while in self-hypnosis to uncover information pertaining to their physical or psychological symptoms. In so doing, they achieved greater levels of physical comfort and reduced anxiety levels.

Hypnotic intervention resulted in improvement in symptoms resulting from multiple sclerosis (Sutcher, 1997); fibromyalgia syndrome, especially when utilized as part of a multidisciplinary treatment (Berman & Swyers, 1999); and phantom limb-pain (Sthalekar, 1993; Muraoka, Komjama, Hosoi, Mine, & Kubo, 1996). The list of illnesses, disease conditions, and injury-induced pain conditions for which hypnosis has historically been utilized and for which its application may apply is beyond the scope of one chapter. A review of the literature suggests that its clinical application is continually expanding.

Another arena where hypnosis may play a significant role in pain management and suffering is with patients experiencing psychogenic and psychosomatic pain. Through the use of the affect bridge (Watkins, 1971) and listening to the patient's somatopsychic language (Burte, Burtre, & Araoz, 1994) patients can gain insight into the range and variety of symptoms they are experiencing. The psychosemantics the patient utilizes in describing his or her life situations or pain offers insight into the nonorganic etiology of the conditions. Queues associated with past trauma may maintain the patient's symptoms, whereas re-associating those symptoms to positive images may result in symptom reduction or alleviation (Burte, 1993). With the psychosomatic patient with no known organic etiological basis for the pain the exploration of the negative self-hypnotic (NSH) statements associated with the condition will lend insight into the symptom output. This is especially relevant with patients experiencing sexual dysfunction associated with pain (Araoz, 1998; Burte & Araoz, 1994).

Techniques and case histories are presented in the above noted works, but the essence of the hypnotherapy is to have the patient, by experiencing these NSH statements in trance, identify the bridges between his or her psychic conflicts (semantic input) and the pain or dysfunctional symptoms (somatic output).

ACKNOWLEDGMENT

I thank Lea Racioppi for her assistance.

REFERENCES

Alden, P., & Heap, M. (1998). Hypnotic pain control: Some theoretical and practical issues. *International Journal of Clinical and Experimental Hypnosis, 46*(1), 62–67.

Anbar, R.D. (2000). Hypnosis, Theodore Roosevelt and the patient with cystic fibrosis. *Pediatrics, 106*(2), 339–346.

Araoz, D.L. (1998). *The new hypnosis in sex therapy.* Northvale, NJ: Jason Aronson Inc.

Araoz, D.L. (1985). *The new hypnosis.* New York: Brunner/Mazel.

Arargun, M.Y., Tegeoglu, I., Kara, H., Adak, B., & Ercan, M. (1998). Hypnotizability, pain threshold and dissociative experiences. *Biological Psychiatry, 44*(1), 69–71.

Ashton, Jr., C., Whitworth, G.C., Seldonridge, J.A., Shapiro, P.A., Weinberg, A.D., Michler, R.E., Smith, C.R., Rose, E.A., Fisher, S., & Oz, M.C. (1997). Self-hypnosis reduces anxiety following coronary artery bypass surgery. A prospective randomized trial. *Journal of Cardiovascular Surgery (Torino), 38*(1), 69–75.

Austan, F., Polise, M., & Schultz, T.R. (1997). The use of verbal expectancy in reducing pain associated with arteriotomies. *American Journal of Clinical Hypnosis, 39*(3), 182–186.

Barber, J. (1998). The mysterious persistence of hypnotic analgesia. *International Journal of Clinical and Experimental Hypnosis, 46*(1), 28–43.

Barber, J. & Adrian, C. (1982). *Psychological approaches to the management of pain.* New York: Brunner/Mazel, Inc.

Basserman, S.W., & Wester, W.C. (1984). In W.C. Wester & A.H. Smith, Jr. (Eds.), *Hypnosis and pain control in clinical hypnosis: A multidisciplinary approach.* Philadelphia: Lippincott.

Bassman, S.W., & Wester, II, W.C. (1992). *Hypnosis, headache and pain control, an integrated approach.* Columbus, OH: Psychology Publications Inc.

Belsky, J., & Kahanna, P. (1994). The effects of self-hypnosis for children with cystic fibrosis: A pilot study. *American Journal of Clinical Hypnosis, 36*, 282–292.

Berman, B.M., & Swyers, J.P. (1999). Complementary medicine treatments for fibromyalgia syndrome. *Baillieres Best Practical Research in Clinical Rheumatology, 13*(93), 487–492.

Bonica, J.J. (1990). *The management of pain* (Vol. 1, 2nd ed.). Philadelphia: Lea & Febiger.

Botta, S.A. (1999). Self-hypnosis as anesthesia for liposuction surgery. *American Journal of Clinical Hypnosis, 41*(4), 299–331.

Bressler, D.E. (1990). Meeting an inner advisor. In D.C. Hammond (Ed.), *Handbook of hypnotic suggestion and metaphors.* New York: W.W. Norton.

Broome, M.E., Lillis, P.P., McGahee, T.W., & Bates, T. (1992). The use of distraction and imagery with children during painful procedures. *Oncology Nursing Forum, 19*, 499–502.

Burte, J.M. (1993). The role of hypnosis in the treatment of tinnitus. *Australian Journal of Clinical Hypnotherapy and Hypnosis, 14*(2), 41–52.

Burte, J.M. (1999). Introduction for creating a dissociative state. In S. Rosenberg, (Ed.), *Course workbook.* New York: New York Society of Clinical Hypnosis.

Burte, J.M. (2002). Psychoneuroimmunology. In R. Weiner (Ed.), *Pain management: A practical guide for clinicians* (6th ed.). Boca Raton, FL: CRC Press.

Burte, J.M. & Araoz, D.L. (1994). Cognitive hypnotherapy with sexual disorders. *Journal of Cognitive Psychotherapy, 8*(4), 299–312.

Burte, J.M., Burte, W., & Araoz, D.L. (1994). Hypnosis in the treatment of back pain. *Australian Journal of Clinical Hypnotherapy and Hypnosis, 15*(2), 93–115.

Camilleri, M. (1999). Review article: Clinical evidence to support current therapies of irritable bowel syndrome. *Alimentary Pharmacology and Therapeutics, 13,* Suppl. (2), 48–53.

Chapman, C.R., & Nakamura, Y. (1998). Hypnotic analgesia: A constructivist framework. *International Journal of Clinical and Experimental Hypnosis, 6*(1), 6–27.

Chaves, J.F., & Dworkin, S.F. (1997). Hypnotic control of pain: historical perspectives and future prospects. *International Journal of Clinical and Experimental Hypnosis, 45*(4), 356–376.

Chen, E., Joseph, M.H., & Zeltzer, L.K. (2000). Behavioral and cognitive interventions in the treatment of pain in children. *Pediatric Clinics of North America, 47*(3), 513–525.

Crawford, M.J., Knebel, T., Kaplan, L., Vendemia, J.M., Xie, M., Jamison, S., & Pribram, K.H. (1998). Hypnotic analgesia: 1. Somatosensory event related potential changes to noxious stimuli and 2. Transfer learning to reduce chronic low back pain. *International Journal of Clinical and Experimental Hypnosis, 46*(1), 92–132.

Danziger, N., Fournier, E., Bouhassira, D., Michaud, D., DeBroucher, T., Santarcangelo, E., Carli, G., Chertock, L., & Willer, J.C. (1998). Different strategies of modulation can be operative during hypnotic analgesia, a neuro-physiological study. *Pain Management, 75*(1), 85–92.

Defochereux, T., Meurisse, M., Hamoir, E., Gollogly, L., Joris, J., & Faymonville, M.E. (1999). Hypnoanesthesia for endocrine cervical surgery: a statement of practice. *Journal of American Complementary Medicine, 5*(6), 509–520.

DePascalis, V., Maguarano, M.R., & Bellusci, A. (1999). Pain perception, somatosensory event related potentials and skin conductance responses to painful stimuli in high, mid, and low hypnotizable subjects: Effects of differential pain reduction strategies. *Pain, 83*(3), 499–508.

Dinges, D.F., Whitehouse, W.G., Onre, E.C., Bloom, P.B., Carlin, M.M., Bauer, N.K., Gillen, K.A., Shapiro, B.S., Ohene-Frempong, K., Dampier, C., & Orne, M.T. (1997). Self-hypnosis training as an adjunct treatment in the management of pain associated with sickle cell disease. *International Journal of Clinical and Experimental Hypnosis, 45*(4), 417–432.

Eastwood, J.D., Gaskowski, P., & Bowers, K.S. (1998). The folly of effort: Ironic effects in the mental control of pain. *International Journal of Clinical and Experimental Hypnosis, 46*(1), 77–91.

Eimer, B.N. (2000). Clinical applications of hypnosis for brief and efficient pain management psychotherapy, *American Journal of Hypnosis, 43*(1), 17–40.

Engvist, B., & Fischer, K. (1997). Preoperative hypnotic techniques reduce consumption of analgesics after surgical removal of third mandibular molars: A brief communication. *International Journal of Clinical and Experimental Hypnosis, 45*(2), 102–108.

Erickson, M.H. (1966). The interspersal hypnotic technique for symptoms correction and pain control. *American Journal of Clinical Hypnosis, 8,* 198–209.

Erickson, M.H. (1986). Mind-body communication in hypnosis. In E. Rossi & M. Ryan (Eds.), *The seminars, workshops and lectures of Milton H. Erickson* (Vol. III). New York: Irvington Publishers Inc.

Ewin, D.M. (1986). The effect of hypnosis and mental sets on major surgery and burns. *Psychiatric Annals, 16*(2) 115–118.

Farthing, G.W., Vonturino, M., Brown, S.W., & Lazar, J.D. (1997). Internal and external distraction in the control of cold pressor pain as a function of hypnotizability. *International Journal of Clinical and Experimental Hypnosis, 45*(4), 433–446.

Faymonville, M.E., Mambourg, P.H., Joris, J., Vrijens, B., Fissette, J., Albert, A., & Lamy, M. (1997). Psychological approaches during conscious sedation. Hypnosis versus stress reducing strategies: A prospective randomized study. *Pain, 73*(3), 361–367.

Faymonville, M.E., Meurisse, M., & Fissette, J. (1999). Hypnosedation: A valuable alternative to traditional anaesthetic techniques. *Acta Chirurgica Belgica, 99*(4), 141–146.

Faymonville, M.E., Laureys, S., Degueldre, C., DelFiore, G., Luxen, A., Franck, G., Lamy, M., & Maguet, P. (2000). Neural mechanisms of antinociceptive effects of hypnosis. *Anesthesiology, 92*(5), 1257–1267.

Foderaro, L.W. (1996). Hypnosis gains credence as influence on the body. *New York Times.* February 24, p. 23.

Foertsch, C.E., O'Hara, M.W., Stoddard, F.J., & Kealey, G.P. (1998). Treatment resistant pain and distress during pediatric burn dressing changes. *Journal of Burn Care and Rehabilitation, 19*(3), 219–224.

Fordyce, W.E. (1976). *Behavioral methods from chronic pain and illness.* St. Louis: C.V. Mosby.

Frankel, F.H., Apfel, R.J., Kelly, S.F., et al. (1979). The use of hypnotizability scales in the clinic: A review after six years. *International Journal of Clinical and Experimental Hypnosis, 27,* 63–67.

Galovski, T.E., & Blanchard, E.B. (1998) The treatment of irritable bowel syndrome with hypnotherapy. *Applied Psychophysiological Biofeedback, 23*(4), 219–32.

Gaynor, M. (1994). *Healing E.S.S.E.N.C.E.: A cancer doctor's practical program for hope and recovery.* New York: Kodansha International.

Ghoneim, M.M., Block, R.I., Sarasin, D.S., Davis, C.S., & Marchman, J.N. (2000). Tape recorded hypnosis instructions as adjuvant in the care of patients scheduled for third molar surgery. *Anesthesia and Analgesia, 90*(1), 64–68.

Ginandes, C.S., & Rosenthal, D.I. (1999). Using hypnosis to accelerate the healing of bone fractures: A randomized controlled pilot study. *Alternative Therapies Health and Medicine, 5*(2), 67–75.

Havens, R.A., & Walters, C. (1989). *Hypnotherapy scripts: A neo-Ericksonian approach to persuasive healing.* New York: Brunner/Mazel.

Hilgard, E.R., & Hilgard, J.R. (1975). *Hypnosis in the relief of pain.* Los Altos, CA: William Kaufman.

Hilgard, J.R., & Hilgard, E.R. (1979). Assessing hypnotic responsiveness in a clinical setting: A multi-item clinical scale and the advantages over single item scales. *International Journal of Clinical and Experimental Hypnosis, 27,* 134–150.

Hilgard, J.R., & LeBaron, S. (1984). *Hypnotherapy of pain in children with cancer*. Los Altos, CA. William Kaufman.

Hilgard, J.R., & LeBaron, S. (1982). Relief of anxiety and pain in children and adolescents with cancer: Quantitative measures and clinical observations. *International Journal of Clinical and Experimental Hypnosis, 30*, 417–442.

Hitchcock, L. (1998). Myths and misconceptions about chronic pain. In R. Weiner (Ed.), *Pain management: A practical guide* (5th ed.). Boca Raton, FL: CRC Press.

Holden, E.W., Deichman, M.M., & Levy, J.D. (1999). Empirically supported treatments in pediatric psychology: Recurrent pediatric headache. *Journal of Pediatric Psychology, 24*(2), 91–109.

Hrezo, R.J. (1998). Hypnosis, an alternative in pain management for nurse practitioners. *Nurse Practical Forum, 9(4)*, 217–226.

Iserson, K.V. (1999). Hypnosis for pediatric fracture reduction. *Journal of Emergency Medicine, 17*(1), 53–56.

Jackson, D.D. (1999). You will feel no pain. *Smithsonian, 29*(12), 126–137.

Johnson, M.E., & Hauck, C. (1999). Beliefs and opinions about hypnosis held by the general public: A systematic evaluation. *American Journal of Clinical Hypnosis, 42*(1), 10–20.

Kuhn, W. (1984). Chronic pain. *Southern Medical Journal, 77*, 1103–1106.

Lambert, S.A. (1996). The effects of hypnosis/guided imagery on the postoperative course of children. *Journal of Developmental and Behavioral Pediatrics, 17*(5), 307–310.

Lang, E.V., Benotsch, E.G., Fick, L.J., Lutgendorf, S., Berbaum, M.L., Berbaum, K.S., Logan, H., & Spiegel, D. (2000). Adjunctive non-pharmacological analgesia for invasive medical procedures: A randomized trial. *Lancet, 29*, 355 (9214), 1486–1490.

Liossi, C., & Hatira, P. (1999). Clinical hypnosis versus cognitive behavioral training for pain management with pediatric cancer patients undergoing bone marrow aspirations. *International Journal of Clinical and Experimental Hypnosis, 47*(2), 104–116.

Lynch, Jr. D.F. (1999). Empowering the Patient: Hypnosis in the Management of Cancer, Surgical Disease and Chronic Pain. *American Journal of Clinical Hypnosis, 42*(2), 122–130.

Mauer, M.H., Burnett, K.F., Ouelette, E.A., Ironson, G.H., & Dandes, H.M. (1999). Medical hypnosis and orthopaedic hand surgery: Pain perception, post-operative recovery and therapeutic comfort. *International Journal of Clinical and Experimental Hypnosis, 47*(2), 144–161.

McGrath, M. (1998). Gimme a break! *Prevention, 50*(6), 98–103.

Melzack, R. (1990). The tragedy of needless pain. *Scientific American, 262*(2), 27–33.

Melzack, R., & Wall, P.D. (1965). Pain mechanisms: A new theory. *Science, 150*, 971–979.

Melzack, R., & Wall, P.D. (1983). *The challenge of pain*. New York: Basic Books.

Meurisse, M., Defechereux, T., Homoir, E., Maweja, S., Marchettini, P., Gollogly, L., Degaugue, C., Joris, J., & Faymonville, M.E. (1999), Hypnosis with conscious sedation instead of general anesthesia? Applications in cervical endocrine surgery. *Acta Chirurgica Belgica, 99*(4), 151–158 .

Meurisse, M., Hamoir, E., Defechereux, T., Gollogly, L., Derry, O., Postal, O., Joris, J., & Faymonville, M.E. (1999). Bilateral neck exploration under hypnosedation: A new standard of care in primary hyperparathyroidism. *Annals of Surgery, 229*(3), 401–408.

Milling, L.S., Kirsch, I., & Burgess, C.A. (1999). Brief modification of suggestibility and hypnotic analgesia: Too good to be true? *International Journal of Clinical and Experimental Hypnosis, 46*(1), 62–67.

Mills, J.C., & Crowley, R.J. (1986). *Therapeutic metaphors for children and the child within*. New York: Bruner/Mazel.

Montgomery, G.H., DuHamel, K.N., & Redd, W.H. (2000). A meta-analysis of hypnotically induced analgesia: How effective is hypnosis? *International Journal of Clinical and Experimental Hypnosis, 48*(2), 138–153.

Muraoka, M., Komiyama, H., Hosoi, M., Mine, K., & Kubo, C. (1996). Psychosomatic treatment of phantom limb pain with post traumatic stress disorder: A case report. *Pain 66*(2–3), 385–388.

NIT Technology Assessment Panel on Integration of Behavioral and Relaxation Approaches into the Treatment of Chronic Pain and Insomnia (1996). Integration of behavioral and relaxation approaches into the treatment of chronic pain and insomnia. *Journal American Medical Association, 276*(4), 313–318.

Ohrback, R., Patterson, D.R., Carroughen, G., & Gibram, N. (1998). Hypnosis after an adverse response to opioids in an ICU burn patient. *Clinical Journal of Pain, 14*(2), 167–175.

Olness, K., & Kohen, D. P. (1996). *Hypnosis and hypnotherapy with children*. (3rd ed.). New York: Guilford Press.

Paige, G.G., & Ben-Eliyahu, S. (1997). The immune-suppressive nature of pain. *Seminars in Oncology Nursing, 13*(1), 10–15.

Palsson, O. (1997). Hypnosis and IBS. Paper presented at the American Gastroenterological Association.

Patterson, D.R., & Ptacek, J.T. (1997). Baseline pain as a moderator of headache hypnotic analgesia for burn injury treatment. *Journal of Consulting and Clinical Psychology, 65*(1), 60–67.

Patterson, D.R., Adcock, R.J., & Bobardier, C.H. (1997). Factors predicting hypnotic analgesia in clinical burn pain. *International Journal of Clinical and Experimental Hypnosis, 45*(4), 377–395.

Peebles-Klieger, M.J. (2000). The use of hypnosis in emergency medicine. *Emergency Medicine Clinics of North America, 18*(2), 327–338.

Perry, C., Gelfand, R., & Marcovitch, P. (1979). The relevance of hypnotic susceptibility in the clinical context. *Journal of Abnormal Psychology, 88*, 592–603.

Rainville, P., Duncan, G.H., Price, D.D., Carrier, B., & Bushnell, M.C. (1997). Pain affect encoded in human anterior cingulate but not somatosensory cortex. *Science, 277*(5328), 968–971.

Rainville, P., Hofbauer, R.K., Paus, T., Duncan, G.H., Bushnell, M.C., & Price, D.D. (1999a). Cerebral mechanisms of hypnotic inductions and suggestions. *Journal of Cognitive Neuroscience, 11*(1), 110–125.

Rainville, P., Carrier, B., Hobauer, R.K., Bushnell, M.C., & Duncan, G.H. (1999b). Dissociation of sensory and affective dimensions of pain using hypnotic modulation. *Pain, 82*(2), 159–171.

Rusy, L.M. & Weisman, S.J. (2000). Complementary therapies for acute pediatric pain management. *Pediatric Clinics of North America, 47*(3), 589–599.

Sacerdote, P. (1966). The uses of hypnosis in cancer patients. *Annals of the New York Academy of Science, 125,* 1011–1019.

Sandrini, G., Mianov, I., Malaguti, S., Nigrelli, M.P., Moglia, A., & Nappi, G. (2000). Effects of hypnosis on diffuse noxious inhibitory controls. *Physiological Behavior, 69*(3), 295–300.

Schafer, D.W. (1996). *Relieving pain: A basic hypnotherapeutic approach.* Northvale, NJ: Jason Aronson Inc..

Sellick, S.M., & Zaza, C. (1998). Critical review of five non-pharmacologic strategies for managing cancer pain. *Cancer Prevention and Control, 2*(1), 7–14.

Shor, R.E., & Orne, E.C. (1963). Norms on the Harvard group scale of hypnotic susceptibility, Form A. *International Journal of Clinical Hypnosis, 11,* 47–49.

Siegel, B. (1998). *Love medicine and miracles.* New York: Harper & Row.

Simon, E.P., & James, L.C. (1999). Clinical applications of hypnotherapy in a medical setting. *Hawaii Medical Journal, 58*(12), 344–347.

Simon, E.P., & Lewis, D.M. (2000). Medical hypnosis for temporomandibular disorders: Treatment efficacy and medical utilization outcome. *Oral Surgery, Oral Medicine, Oral Pathology, Oral Radiology, and Endodontics, 90*(1), 54–63.

Smith, J., & Barabasz, A. (1996). Comparison of hypnosis and distraction in severely ill children. *Journal of Counseling Psychology, 43*(2), 187–193.

Spiegel, D., & Moore, R. (1997). Imagery and hypnosis in the treatment of cancer patients. *Oncology (Huntington), 11*(8), 1179–1189 and 1189–1195.

Spiegel, H., & Spiegel, D. (1978/1987). *Trance and treatment: Clinical uses of hypnosis.* Washington, D.C.: American Psychiatric Press, Inc.

Staats, P., Hekmat, H., & Stats, A. (1998). Suggestion/placebo effects on pain: Negative as well as positive. *Journal of Pain and Symptom Management, 15*(4), 235–243.

Sternbach, R.A. (1978). Clinical aspects of pain. In R.A. Steinbach (Ed.), *The psychology of pain.* New York: Raven Press.

Stevensen, C. (1995). Non-pharmacological aspects of acute pain management. *Complementary Therapy in Nursing and Midwifery, 1*(3), 77–84.

Sthalekar, H. (1993). Hypnosis for relief of chronic phantom pain in a paralyzed limb. *The Australian Journal of Clinical Hypnotherapy and Hypnosis, 14*(2), 75–80.

Strassberg, D.S., Tilley, D., Bristone, S., & Oei, T.P.S. (1992). The MMPI and chronic pain: A cross-cultural view. *Psychiatric Assessment, 4*(4), 493–497.

Sutcher, H. (1997). Hypnosis as adjunctive therapy for multiple sclerosis: A progress report. *American Journal of Clinical Hypnosis, 39*(4), 283–290.

Vidavic-Vukic, M. (1999). Hypnotherapy in the treatment of irritable bowel syndrome: methods and results in Amsterdam. *Scandinavian Journal of Gastroenterology Supplement, 203,* 49–51.

Watkins, J.G. (1971). The affect bridge: A hypnoanalytic technique. *International Journal of Clinical and Experimental Hypnosis, 19,* 21–27.

Weitzenhoffer, M.M., & Hilgard, E.R. (1959). *Stanford hypnotic susceptibility scale: Forms A and B.* Palo Alto, CA: Consulting Psychologist Press.

Wester, W.C., & O'Grady, D.J. (1991). *Clinical hypnosis with children.* New York: Brunner/Mazel.

Whorwell, P.J., Houghton, L.A., Taylor, E.E., & Maxton, D.G. (1992). Physiological effects of emotion assessment via hypnosis. *Lancet, 340*(8811), 69–72.

Wright, B.R., & Drummond, P.D. (2000). Rapid induction analgesia for the alleviation of procedural pain during burn care. *Burns, 26*(3), 275–282.

Zachariae, R., Andersen, O.K., Bjerring, P., Jorgensen, M.M., & Arendt-Nielsen, L. (1998). Effects of opioid antagonist on pain intensity and withdrawal reflexes during induction of hypnotic analgesia in high and low hypnotizable volunteers. *European Journal of Pain, 2*(1), 25–34.

Zaza, C., Sellick, S.M., Willan, A., Reyno, L., & Browman, G.P. (1999). Health care professionals' familiarity with non-pharmacological strategies for managing cancer pain. *Psychooncology, 8*(2), 99–111.

Zohaurek, R. (1985). *Clinical hypnosis and therapeutic suggestion in nursing* New York: Grune & Stratten.

70

Drug Misuse and Detoxification

John Claude Krusz, M.D., Ph.D.

... The use of drugs to alter consciousness is nothing new. It has been a feature of human life in all places on the earth and in all ages of history ... the ubiquity of drug use is so striking that it must represent a basic human appetite...

A. Weil (1972)

INTRODUCTION

The use of drugs that produce powerful effects on mood, affect, and thinking and alter levels and states of consciousness has been a part of our civilization since recorded history. This refers to both illicit substances (e.g., opium, cocaine, cannabis, synthetic psychoactive substances) as well as to licit and commonly available drugs (e.g., alcohol, tobacco, caffeine-containing beverages). Although the latter group of substances raises fewer emotionally heated societal concerns than the former, use and misuse of these substances are also discussed in this chapter.

CONFUSING TERMINOLOGIES

The term "drug abuse" has been used indiscriminately and is confusing and inaccurate. It commonly refers to repetitive usage of drugs that are productive of tolerance and physical dependence in a nonmedical or nontherapeutic context. The author prefers the term "drug misuse" rather than drug abuse for the following reason: On a pharmacologic level, one is not abusing the action of the drug itself. It is merely a molecule with a set of pharmacologic and biochemical activities relating to dosage and concentration, as well as route of administration, but as such no

inherent ability exists to abuse what the drug does pharmacologically. The body that the drug is put into, however, is what is being abused, and in that sense, this author believes that the term drug abuse refers more to the abuse of the person, and when speaking about the drug itself, it is a case of misusing the drug. The other major point about drug misuse is that it tends to portray the idea that the drug involved is one that generally is a nonprescription medication or one upon which social sanctions have been placed. Therefore, the terms drug abuse or drug misuse are confusing and derived mostly from social definitions, as relating to people's behavior with pharmacologic substances. Different cultures consider various substances to be included in what is deemed drug misuse patterns at different times. For instance, although no one would question the drug misuse concept of a person's use of 2 liters of blended spirits per day and the consumption of 80 cigarettes in the same time on a chronic basis, one would hardly call the imbibing or consuming of the same substances for a shorter time drug misuse (e.g., New Year's Eve party, a Mardi Gras celebration). Jaffe (1990) uses the terminology "nonmedical drug use" as a substitute for the older and more confusing term drug abuse, and the author thoroughly agrees that changing the phraseology would be helpful. Terms like drug abuse tend to connote the usage of societally disapproved substances, whereas drug misuse or nonmedical drug use includes a whole spectrum of involvement and usage. This can include very casual or experimental use on a few occasions of even commonly available substances (e.g., nicotine, alcohol) to the use of certain substances for specific kinds of effects (e.g., consumption of large quantities of caffeine by students for the purposes of studying, the use of amphet-

0-8493-0926-3/02/$0.00+$1.50
© 2002 by CRC Press LLC

amines and other central nervous system stimulants by truck drivers to circumvent occupational fatigue). The most extreme example of drug misuse, of course, would include chronic daily usage of large amounts of substances, licit or illicit, as originally conveyed in the more nonspecific term drug abuse.

DRUG ADDICTION

"Addiction" is another very confusing and, unfortunately, often misused term. Many substances are considered to be addicting, and the usual connotation of an addict is a person who is hopelessly and irreconcilably rooted in daily repetitive behaviors that are focused on obtaining and using large amounts of the same drug. In reality, the notion of addiction more properly should connote an extreme degree of drug dependence (see below). The degrees of drug dependence themselves form a large spectrum of usage from very casual to extremely habitual or addictive behaviors and are discussed in a succeeding section in this chapter. Once again, the term addiction has become distorted, and the social definition or notion of an addicted individual conveys a very severely impaired lifestyle with a daily search for, and use of, the substance to which the individual is addicted. The other confusing element for the term addiction relates to the mistaken notion that addiction is synonymous with physical dependence (see below). Physical dependence, as is discussed later, refers more to the occurrence of withdrawal symptoms upon sudden cessation of drug use, whereas addiction does not have the same inference, although, once again, in the minds of many people, the terms are often used interchangeably, and in that sense, imprecisely. It is particularly encouraging that major compendia on psychopharmacologic mechanisms of drugs do not even mention the word addiction once in their very extensive reviews of numerous categories of psychoactive substances (e.g., *Psychopharmacology: Third Generation of Progress*, (Meltzer, 1987)).

DRUG DEPENDENCE

The term "drug dependence" is another confusing term with many different connotations. Unfortunately, it is also confused with physical dependence on drugs, and at the outset, drug dependence fits many of the characteristics of a behavioral syndrome. This implies that an individual who is using a particular psychoactive substance will devote a higher degree of effort to obtaining the substance and will presumably use the drug despite negative social and medical sanctions. The term drug dependence once again refers to a spectrum of usages, although generally it is taken to mean something more than strictly casual or intermittent use of a drug. The individual's behavioral

syndrome suggests that the drug is needed for social or personal well-being and that not using the drug has a greater cost to the individual's well-being and offers a poorer quality of life. Drug dependence typically includes activities designed to procure the drug upon which the patient is dependent, and the seeking and obtaining of the drug will be given a higher priority in the individual's life than other ongoing behaviors or activities. Once again, the continuum of drug dependence is very difficult to sharply demarcate from recurrent drug use on an intermittent basis, which does not have the characteristics of dependence or the behavioral syndrome of preoccupation with attainment, securing of a supply, and repeated, often daily use of the substance. In that sense, drug dependence has the connotations of compulsivity and is behaviorally similar to disorders that are chronic and relapsing in nature (Edwards, Arif, & Hodgson, 1981).

The range of drug-dependent behavior is as extreme as the concept of drug addiction (see above). On one end of the spectrum, it is as nontroubling in most people's minds as daily use of caffeine or tobacco, which certainly meet the criteria for a drug-dependent behavioral syndrome and yet do not have the social connotation of frank drug addiction. The other concept that creates a lot of confusion is the idea that the drug-dependent behavior in some way is disruptive, not only to the life of the person who engages in the drug-acquiring and drug-using behavior, but also that a societal cost exists as a result of that person's repeated search and usage of psychoactive substances.

TOLERANCE

The concept of tolerance to a drug's effect is strictly a pharmacologic issue and yet often also gets intermingled or exchanged with not only physical dependence, but also with drug dependence, as discussed above. Tolerance, in its broadest pharmacologic sense, refers to a smaller effect for any given dose of a medication or drug when given on a repeated basis. Therefore, in order to obtain the same pharmacologic effect, larger and larger doses of the medication or drug have to be administered. The classic example of tolerance to a psychoactive substance is the opiates. In this instance, tolerance includes shortened duration of effect, a decreased intensity of effect (particularly for analgesic, euphoriant, and sedating activities of the drug), as well as an increase in the dose which would be considered lethal.

Two types of acquired pharmacologic tolerance are generally discussed. One is dispositional tolerance, which has to do with increasing the rate of metabolism of the drug over time so that the same dose is more rapidly metabolized and, therefore, the effective concentration on receptors or end organs is reduced, resulting in a smaller effect. Many examples can be cited. Among the more common are the liver enzyme-inducing properties of alcohol, anticonvulsants (e.g., carbamazepine acid, valproic acid), and barbiturates.

Pharmacodynamic tolerance refers to adaptive responses within biologic systems that are affected by the drug itself and result in a reduced response over time to the same dose of a drug. Because many of the effects are biobehavioral in nature, tolerance of the pharmacodynamic type is often noted to develop rapidly. The classic example is tolerance to the effects of opiates, particularly with regard to the euphoriant and sedating properties of the drug. Whereas tolerance to the respiratory depressant or miotic effects of opiates does not follow a similar pattern, a marked pharmacodynamic tolerance exists when the drug is given repeatedly, and this is most obvious with effects such as euphoria. Unfortunately, the escalation of a dose in a tolerant individual in order to produce a desired degree of euphoria or sedation often carries the risk of allowing toxic effects of the drug to occur (e.g., fatal respiratory depression), because tolerance to this effect of opiates does not increase nearly as much as the more behavioral effects of the drug. The underpinning of pharmacodynamic tolerance is always on the basis that the neuronal populations the drug affects become altered in their activity in the presence of continued administration of the drug.

Tolerance to a multitude of substances can occur in perhaps less dramatic ways, although the example of the barbiturates and other sedative drugs also involves pharmacodynamic tolerance. Additionally, dispositional tolerance plays a larger role in permitting the use of escalating doses of these drugs to obtain a desired degree of sedation or "high." Another factor in dispositional tolerance may lead to a decreased dosing interval based on the more rapid metabolism of the drug and excretion from the body. It certainly is conceivable that when a drug is metabolized more rapidly, a tendency to administer the drug more often exists, and in that sense the notion of the reinforcing ability of a drug comes into play. Drugs are notorious reinforcers, particularly if their effects are very profound and relatively short-lived or if their metabolism is increased at a fairly appreciable rate with continued use. The classic example of a powerfully reinforcing drug is cocaine and, to a lesser extent, amphetamines. The former substance has a marked ability to act as a reinforcer, particularly in maintaining drug misuse behaviors, simply because the half-life of cocaine is exquisitely short. Therefore, the behaviorally reinforcing repeated administration of the substance tends to promote a pattern of use which results in a rapid establishment of drug-dependent behavior. This is in the absence of any formal physical dependence on the substance, as might be encountered in the case of opiates, barbiturates, nicotine, or caffeine. This also introduces the topic of drugs as reinforcers of behavior, a powerful basic mechanism implicated in the generation of

drug dependence as a behavioral syndrome (see the following section).

The phenomenon of tolerance also can transcend multiple categories of drugs. This is known as cross tolerance, and chronic exposure to one drug can frequently produce a tolerant state to other categories of drugs. Examples include cross tolerance of barbiturates to other sedative hypnotic compounds. In some cases, cross tolerance to amphetamines and cocaine and other stimulants is fairly easy to demonstrate, and perhaps more rapid enzymatic metabolism of the drugs in common may be a fundamental feature of the phenomenon of cross tolerance (Barrett, 1987).

DRUGS AS BEHAVIORAL REINFORCERS

This section attempts to outline the underpinnings of broader concepts already discussed, such as drug dependence, and some of the conditioning factors which may promote continued drug-seeking behavior. The reinforcing properties of drugs are well known, both in laboratory animals as well as in humans. Indeed, laboratory experiments have been designed to allow animals to perform repetitive tasks, such as lever- or bar-pressing, the running of mazes, and other behavioral tasks. These learned behaviors are reinforced by the reward, a dose of a drug that presumably produces a pleasurable effect and, therefore, promotes continued reinforcement and furthers behavior designed for obtaining more of the same drug. This is true for opioids, barbiturates, ethanol, and central nervous stimulants (e.g., cocaine, amphetamines, nicotine, caffeine). Many factors intervene in the effectiveness of a drug in promoting reinforced behavior, and most important are the properties of the drugs themselves, particularly if their actions are short and their euphoriant or stimulant properties are powerful in the central nervous system (CNS). The most dramatic example of reinforcement is with cocaine and amphetamines. Laboratory animals will continually bar-press, sometimes for thousands of repetitions, to obtain a single dose of the drug, even in the presence of toxic effects from the drug. Animals will literally die in their attempts to obtain more of the presumably pleasurable effects of cocaine. If placebo or saline is substituted for the drug, the furious activities will cease after a time; however, they will return with an even more rapid re-onset of behaviors if a single priming dose is given. A quite similar though less dramatic pattern is noted with morphine and other opioids. The timing and intensity of behaviors needed to raise the dose occurs at a slower rate than it does in the case of cocaine or amphetamines. A lessened pattern of reinforcement is noted in the case of barbiturates and other sedatives, and still less is seen with other drugs (e.g., nicotine), where the behavioral reinforcement is seen under a more restricted set of experimental conditions. Likewise, caffeine, despite being a relatively powerful CNS stimulant in large doses, is a relatively weak reinforcer. A common substance like ethanol is one of the least reinforcing drugs in laboratory experimental situations. In the laboratory setting, many factors determine whether or not an animal will self-administer the drug (e.g., the CNS effects of the drug, the amount of work required to obtain a dose, the time allowed between the actual reinforcing behavior and the actual drug administration). It should be noted that these behaviors are strikingly not in the presence of any physical dependence on the part of the animals (Johanson & Schuster, 1991; Young & Herling, 1986).

The reinforcing properties may occur on both positive and negative bases. The former would be an example of behaviors that are reinforced because the drug induces pleasurable effects. The latter (negative reinforcement) would occur because the drug would terminate unpleasant or anxiety-provoking states, such as pain. Examples of negative reinforcement in a clinical setting occur with dependence on benzodiazepines and sedative hypnotics, as well as opiates, and many people continue to take the former two classes of drugs, not for their positive reinforcing effects, but rather to circumvent the onset of anxiety, panic, or other withdrawal symptoms (Busto, Sellers, Naranjo, Cappell, Sanchez-Craig, & Sykora, 1986; Wickler, 1980; Woods, Katz, & Winger, 1987).

The positive reinforcing effects of centrally acting drugs occur in spite of initially unpleasurable effects associated with initial usage of certain drugs. This is most clearly illustrated by morphine and other narcotic opiates. The initial effects associated with the use of these drugs can often produce severe nausea, vomiting, and other side effects that would appear to be not positively reinforcing. In light of this, the euphoriant and other properties of the drug are sufficiently strong, and as tolerance for the unpleasurable effects develops, the predominant reinforcer remains the euphoriant effect of the drug that promotes continued and escalating usage. Secondary reinforcers are often social factors, such as one's peer group or the perception that usage of the drug permits membership in an elite club or circle of friends. Indeed, peer approval is often a very strong secondary reinforcer, and this social reinforcement often will promote continued usage of a drug even though it initially causes unpleasurable effects. This is often seen in nicotine, marijuana, or alcohol usage, at least in the initial stages. One also has to consider that as physical dependence develops (see below), the onset of any unpleasurable effects associated with discontinuation of regular drug use will automatically promote or reinforce continued administration of the drug. This would then act more as a negative reinforcer, as outlined above in the case of benzodiazepines, although it is most dramatically encountered in the usage of morphine and other narcotics. Often, the cessation of repetitive usage of a drug will induce an anxiety-provoking aversive

state, and this often is in the absence of any effects on the physical well-being of the individual. The perception of dysphoria and the threat of being left in a behaviorally anxious state often are powerful negative reinforcers for continued use of a drug. Even a drug such as nicotine, which does not produce a strong state of physical dependence, often will be extremely difficult to stop using because of very subtle perceived threats to one's well-being in the absence of the drug. This, therefore, promotes continued usage of the substance, presumably because there is an effect on psychological well-being with the nicotine present and a perception that all is not well if one does not continually administer the nicotine in the form of cigarettes or tobacco. Modern approaches to withdrawal from nicotine include use of chewing gum or patches of nicotine in a graded dosage to slowly taper away from the usual blood levels of nicotine, which are self-administered during the day when one smokes (see section on nicotine). These principles of positive and negative reinforcement are based on learning theory, and the issue of continued drug usage can be viewed as behavior which is maintained by the consequences of the drug action on the individual (Jaffe, 1989, 1990; Kaplan & Saddock, 1988).

PHYSICAL DEPENDENCE

The concept of physical dependence, mentioned previously, principally relates to repetitive use of a substance that establishes biochemical and pharmacodynamic tolerance factors in biologic systems (neuroadaptation), such that when drug use is stopped, a state of withdrawal occurs. This withdrawal state is the hallmark of physical dependence and is based strictly on alterations in the neuroadapted state of the organism consequent to repeated drug administration, usually of a drug that demonstrates principally pharmacodynamic tolerance but also may exhibit dispositional and other tolerances. By definition, a strongly positive reinforcement has already occurred, and the existence of a severe degree of drug dependence, together with behaviors that in the past may have been termed addiction, is accompanied by a severely modified neuroadaptive state secondary to the drug use. This neuro-adaptive state is a physiologically, biochemically, and pharmacodynamically changed system, which has been acted upon by the medication used, and these systems have been modified initially by the drug producing the physical dependence. The sine qua non of physical dependence is the expression of a state of withdrawal when the drug is abruptly terminated. It is implicit in the model of withdrawal that CNS functioning has been altered by continued administration of a drug. How rapidly the CNS returns to its baseline state after discontinuance of the drug is different for various medications or drugs, and withdrawal symptoms can be quite severe. Based on long-term usage of drugs like morphine or opium, withdrawal symptoms can be even more profound and onset faster with pharmacologic antagonist medications (e.g., naloxone), and one can demonstrate withdrawal symptoms after a single dose of morphine by administering naloxone or nalorphine (Bickel, Stitzer, Bigelow, Liebson, Jasinski, & Johnson, 1988; Heishman, Stitzer, Bigelow, & Liebson, 1989).

Diagnostic criteria for opioid withdrawal have been developed and published in the DSM-III-R Diagnostic and Statistical Manual of Mental Disorders (American Psychiatric Association, 1987). Some of these criteria involve cessation of prolonged moderate or heavy use of an opioid (this is defined as several weeks or more) or, alternatively, reduction in the amount of opioid used, succeeded by at least three of the following: (1) craving for an opioid, (2) nausea and vomiting, (3) muscle aches, (4) lacrimation or rhinorrhea, (5) pupillary dilation, (6) piloerection or sweating, (7) diarrhea, (8) yawning, (9) fever, and (10) insomnia. These diagnostic criteria, although by no means complete, at least give a list of withdrawal effects that can be seen in the acute phase after discontinuance of chronic or even acute opiate use.

Abstinence syndromes create a spectrum of effects. The immediate syndrome of abstinence is as exemplified in the case above. Less dramatically, withdrawal from alcohol, cocaine, nicotine, or sedative/hypnotics, though productive of many symptoms, is a fairly benign event. The most life-threatening symptom for medical management is the occurrence of seizures. These are usually single in occurrence and rarely require medication. Similarly, even withdrawal from morphine rarely produces any life-threatening sequelae, although the person undergoing withdrawal may be extremely uncomfortable until the neuroadapted state returns to its biologic baseline.

DRUG MISUSE AS PRIMARY PSYCHIATRIC DISEASE

The misuse of psychoactive drugs raises some fundamental questions about whether or not such use can be considered principally a behavioral disorder or principally a psychiatric disorder. The author favors the former, and although a large body of data has been developed to categorize dependence and substance "abuse" (American Psychiatric Association, 1987), the author is by no means certain that the vast majority of tolerant and dependent states consequent to repeated drug use are indeed based on fundamentally psychiatric diseases.

While it is true that patterns of drug misuse can be quite profound and can coexist with well-recognized psychiatric entities like bipolar and manic depressive illness, schizophrenia, schizotypal, and the whole range of affective disorders, the author has noticed a strong pattern of drug misuse by patients who otherwise manifest evidence

of organic brain dysfunction. For example, the author has observed that patients with neurobehavioral seizures (e.g., intermittent explosive disorder, temporal lobe syndromes, other behaviorally aberrant states) often give a history of self-administering psychoactive substances for the purpose of reducing internal anxiety and to produce a sense of calm and relative order insofar as their behavior and thought processes are concerned (unpublished observations). Furthermore, certain individuals will have documentable abnormalities on the electroencephalogram (EEG) and quantitative EEG (brain mapping). Some of these individuals, while they may require traditional psychiatric diagnoses as they are treated in the medical system, actually may have more of a fundamental organic derangement of their thought processes, emotions, and affect, as is often the case in temporal lobe disorders. Some of these patients exhibit features behaviorally compatible with an organic brain disorder, such as a partial complex seizure. This may manifest itself in purely behavioral terms and may be relieved or ameliorated by (self-medicated) psychoactive drug use. Often, patients will give a history of feeling calmer, thinking more clearly, and other positive aspects related to ongoing and repetitive use of amphetamines, cocaine, marijuana, or sedative hypnotics. From a neurologic and neurobehavioral standpoint, this type of history is not, in the author's opinion, fundamentally a psychiatric problem, but rather an organic state relievable by pharmacologic administration of psychoactive substances. This often predisposes an individual to many maladaptive patterns of behavior, and the issues of tolerance, physical dependence, and alteration of lifestyle based on sustained drug-seeking and drug-using behavior often become the primary focus of medical attention, whereas in reality one could postulate that these are secondary spin-offs of an organically aberrant neurologic state. Nevertheless, various psychiatric criteria have been developed for different kinds of drug misuse, and the history and evolution of psychiatric thinking in this area are well summarized by Jaffe (1989). A very nicely summarized and coherently presented chapter on these phenomena is to be found in Dr. Steve Stahl's book *Essential Psychopharmacology*.

The evolution and refinement of biologic and psychiatric criteria regarding psychoactive drug use are very much active processes and continue to progress. Indeed, it will be interesting to see what new revisions are proposed in upcoming DSM versions. One can certainly make a good case for the coexistence of primary psychiatric disorders and concurrent maladaptive drug use patterns as perhaps secondary biologic factors. Concurrent psychiatric treatment of both elements often comes under the rubric of dual diagnoses, wherein a primary psychiatric diagnosis is treated at the same time that one attempts to detoxify or eliminate psychoactive substance misuse patterns.

This portion of the chapter outlines major issues relating to usage of specific categories of psychoactive substances and includes a short synopsis of the scope of the problem. This was very well summarized by Mello and Griffiths (1987). The initial focus is on drugs with the largest societal impact (i.e., alcohol and tobacco), rather than focusing on the more traditional "hard core" items, such as narcotics and stimulants. From a psychiatric viewpoint, the overuse of alcohol and alcohol dependence ranks quite high in relationship to other psychiatric disorders. They outdistance other major psychiatric diseases, such as depressive disorders, phobias, schizophrenias, and phobic disorders, at least in terms of their lifetime prevalence rates. This translates into an enormous impact on public health issues, societal productivity, and the like. It has been estimated that in excess of $100 billion per year is lost in terms of productivity, actual and projected medical costs, and the effects of crime related to the pursuit of psychoactive drugs. This is probably a very conservative estimate, and the author suspects that the above figure, taken from a 1984 estimate, is probably a fifth of the actual cost to society. This is particularly true if one considers including overusage of legal intoxicants, such as alcohol and nicotine.

Major forces and trends have developed in the medical world, and a much greater societal awareness of the impact of repeated use of alcohol and nicotine currently exists. The overall usage of hard liquor has decreased somewhat, although this may be offset by continued and escalating nationwide usage of "softer" forms of alcohol, such as wine and beer. Generally, patterns of nicotine use have diminished somewhat, although this is still a very large problem in the adolescent or teenage population and continues to be a major problem in terms of lung cancer rates, particularly in women. A WHO report cites that 25 to 45% of women are smoking in wealthy nations worldwide. This is the first international study of women and tobacco use, and data suggest that female smokers will outnumber male smokers in the near future (*American Medical News*, 1982).

The 1980s saw an explosion in cocaine usage, both in its usual hydrochloride form as well as in free-base or crack cocaine form. The overall usage of cocaine seems to have decreased somewhat, with an increasing trend seen in the usage rate of addicting opiates, such as morphine and heroin. Indeed, designer-type drug use has been prominent as clandestine chemists seek to modify or improve existing opiate molecules. One unfortunate spin-off of such experimentation resulted in the appearance of a syndrome virtually indistinguishable from idiopathic Parkinson's disease based on the toxic effects of an impurity in the synthesis of illicit meperidine (Langston, Ballard, Tetrud, & Irwin, 1983). The neurotoxin identified destroyed the very same subnucleus in the substantia nigra which is etiologically and pathophysiologically involved in idiopathic Parkinson's disease. A small epidemic of young, opiate-misusing individuals surfaced in a fairly short time in California in the early 1980s. Obviously, this side effect was an unintended one, but is pharmacologically treatable with dopaminergic agents normally used to treat idiopathic Parkinson's disease.

Other "designer" opiates, such as alpha-methylfentanyl, also surface from time to time and speak to the creativity of individuals attempting to use opiate derivatives on a chronic basis. These designer drugs are usually structurally similar to the more regulated pharmaceuticals and represent an attempt to evade regulatory control and legal ramifications. Another so-called designer drug is MDMA ("Ecstasy," "hug drug") (Peroutka, 1987). This is only one representative of a whole family of phenyliso-propylamines, which share CNS stimulant and hallucinogenic properties. Recreational drug use of derivatized substances continued to be very prevalent in the 1990s. A number of items have been enjoyed, including gamma-hydroxybutyrate (GHB), flunitrazepam, and a host of amphetamine analogs, such as MDMA, MDEA, paramethylthioamphetamine, DOET, DMA, TMA, and some of their derivatives, and represent some 50 compounds with potential for widespread illicit use. As noted above, they also bridge pharmacologically distinct categories of psychoactive substances (Glennon, 1987). These designer substances are covered here in more detail.

MDMA (3,4-methylenedioxymethamphetamine) "Ecstasy," XTC, "Adam," "E"

This substance has probably enjoyed more use or, more properly, has been more widely enjoyed in the last decade than virtually all other designer drugs. MDMA was shown to consistently produce, in humans, increases in systolic and diastolic blood pressures, pupillary diameter, heart rate, and rises in plasma cortisol and prolactin (de la Torre et al., 2000). In rats, acute doses produced a hyperthermic response. One week after acute dosing, about 50% of 5HT and 5HIAA were lost in cortex and hippocampus, as were binding sites to SSRI drugs, thus indicating degeneration of 5HT neurons in the brain due to MDMA (Colado, Granados, O'Shea, Esteban, & Green, 1999). This remarkable toxicity to the serotonergic system has been consistently observed and is a peculiar feature of MDMA and related compounds like MDEA ("eve"). One hypothesis relates depletion of intraneuronal 5HT to activation of post-synaptic 5HT2a/c receptors located on GABA interneurons. This then leads to decreased GABA transmission and consequent increased dopamine synthesis and release that then is taken up by the formerly depleted 5HT containing neurons. The excessive dopamine in the 5HT nerve terminal is then deaminated by MAO-B, causing degeneration of 5HT nerve terminals (Sprague, Everman, & Nichols, 1998). Chronic users of MDMA showed depressed serotonergic functions, including reduced pro-lactin and cortisol responses compared to controls, weeks after stopping the use of MDMA (Gerra, Zaimovic, Giu-castro, Maestri, Monica, Sartori, Caccavari, and Delsig-nore, 1998). Cognitive problems have been documented in MDMA users. They had difficulties with sustained attention tasks and verbal and visual memory. Poorer memory performance was associated with lower CSF 5HIAA levels (Bolla, McCann, & Ricaurte, 1998). Parrott and Lasky (1998) described the effects of MDMA ("Ecstasy") on mood and cognition before, during, and after a Saturday night dance. Several days after ingestion of MDMA, users felt more depressed, abnormal, unsocia-ble, and less well tempered than nonusers. They also per-formed more poorly on memory tasks. Criteria for depen-dence were met in several cases of chronic and heavy MDMA users (Jansen, 1999). Attempts have been made by PET scanning techniques to correlate the effects of MDMA on brain 5HT synthesis. In the dog, 5 hours after MDMA infusion, 5HT synthesis was about half of that at baseline and about one thirteenth of the synthesis seen 1 hour after infusion of MDMA, when a large increase was noted. A decrease in 5HT transporter binding was also seen in PET studies (Nishisawa, Mzengeza, & Diksic, 1999). Recently, MR spectroscopy studies (Chang, Ernst, Grob, & Poland, 1999) have shown that the brains of MDMA users have larger myoinositol fractions in parietal white matter, suggesting increased glial content and pos-sibly inferring neuronal damage in these areas. Amphet-amine analogs can cause seizures as one consequence of overuse. The characteristics of stimulant-induced seizures were studied by Hanson, Jensen, Johnson, & White (1990). Methamphetamine-related seizures were influ-enced only by diazepam and valproate whereas other anti-convulsants were ineffective.

MDEA (3,4-methylenedioxyethamphetamine) "Eve"

This is another of the many substituted amphetamine ana-logs; it is not as popular or available as MDMA. However, it, too, has been shown to produce serotonergic deficits and impair memory in rats (Barrionuevo, Aguirre, Del Rio, & Lasheras, 2000). MDEA also produces dose-related hyperthermia, and also affected 5HT transporter density in the frontal cortex and in the hippocampus. The pathol-ogy of fatal toxicity due to MDEA ingestion has been studied in seven males aged 20 to 25 (Milroy, Clark, & Forrest, 1996). Marked changes were identified in the liver with cell necrosis. Changes consistent with catechola-mine-induced myocardial damage were seen in most of the cases. In the brain, perivascular hemorrhagic changes were noted in four cases. The changes were similar to those seen in heat stroke, although only two cases had documented hyperthermia. An additional report (Arimany,

Medallo, Pujol, Vingut, Borondo, & Valverve, 1998) reported intentional overdose and death with MDEA.

2-CB (4-bromo-2,5-dimethoxyphenethylamine) also known as Synergy, Herox, Nexus, Venus

This psychoactive substance is a hallucinogen enjoyed as a designer drug. It is one of a number of psychedelic substances initially created by the libertarian pharmacol-ogist, Dr. Alexander Shulgin. It has been described as an example of an empathogenic agent, as have MDMA, GHB, and other related substances (Velea, Hautefeuille, Vazeille, & Lantran-Davoux, 1999). These agents are overused at all-night parties called "raves," where oblig-atory prolonged social contact is part of the environment. 2-CB itself produces mild confusion, stupor, and a child-like interest in visual phenomena; a typical dose is 20 to 40 mg; the effects last up to 6 hours.

GHB (gamma-hydroxybutyrate) also known as "G"

This fatty acid derivative is structurally similar to GABA and has pharmacologic properties as an inhibitory chem-ical transmitter in the central nervous system. It has pow-erful CNS depressant effects and its actions may be medi-ated through specific receptors for this agent, or via activity on GABA-B receptors. Some of its actions also may involve alterations in dopaminergic transmission in the basal ganglia. It has been used clinically as a general anesthetic and to treat sleep disorders. It induces a state of euphoria, and has been enjoyed recreationally during the last few years (Tunnicliff, 1997). Although initially thought to be safe, recent reports (Reuters Health, 10-27-2000) confirmed 71 cases of death due to ingestion of GHB or its precursor, 1,4–butanediol (also called BD or "pro–G."). BD can be obtained on the Internet and is rapidly metabolized to GHB in the body. BD has been sold as a dietary and body-building supplement and as a sleep aid. It is also an industrial solvent. Fifteen of the deaths had no other intoxicants involved. Another case report (Harrington, Woodward, Hooton, & Horn, 1999) documented near-fatal or prolonged reactions to very small doses of MDMA or GHB in a patient who is HIV-positive and being treated with protease inhibitors. These drugs inhibit the cytochrome P-450 system in the liver and intestines and inhibit the metabolism of GHB and MDMA. GHB is also commonly used at all-night dance parties.

Of particular concern in the last decade is the escalat-ing phenomenon of polydrug misuse. It is well known that alcoholics often abuse tobacco, tranquilizers, antidepres-sants, and caffeine. Similarly, physically dependent nar-cotic users often misuse other categories of drugs in an attempt to stave off withdrawal symptoms (see above). A common substance like marijuana is often used with alco-hol and tobacco. Some of the history of legally prescribed co-intoxicants dates back to the era of laudanum, which was a mixture of wine and opium. The emergence of polydrug use heightens the challenges for medical and other practitioners in terms of successfully reducing or eliminating simultaneous use of psychoactive substances. Also, the risk for medical complications consequent to multiple drug use escalates in parallel with the number of substances used. This poses many new kinds of problems, particularly where intravenous drug use is common. The widespread epidemic of AIDS, syphilis, bacterial endocarditis, and renal, hepatic, cardiac, and pulmonary complications of recurrent drug use add to the total cost to society (Jaffe, 1989, 1990; Mello & Griffiths, 1987).

ALCOHOL

The usage of ethanol is a worldwide phenomenon, somewhat more prevalent in so-called technologically advanced societies, such as North America and Europe. Alcohol is undoubtedly the single most widely used substance on the earth. It has been estimated that the total cost to society for alcohol-related medical issues accounts for 10 to 13% of the nation's total health expenditures. In 1975, the total cost in terms of accidents, crime, health-related problems, and productivity exceeded $45 billion. Obviously, accurate incidence and prevalence measures are extremely difficult to obtain, although population-based statistics show that males age 18 to 64 have the highest lifetime prevalence rate. In women, age 18 to 24, alcohol-related problems rank fourth in terms of prevalence among other psychiatric diseases (Myers, Weissman, Tischler, Holzer, & Leaf, et al., 1984; Robins, Helzer, Weissman, Orvaschel, & Gruenberg, et al., 1984).

Alcohol misuse has been separated in diagnostic criteria (American Psychiatric Association, 1987) from the older term "alcoholism." The latter term has been replaced by alcohol dependence, which implies prolonged excessive use of alcohol such that sudden cessation results in a withdrawal syndrome. The enigma of how alcohol produces its acute CNS depressant effects as well as the larger question of a specific locus of pharmacologic effect for the substance has been studied since the turn of the century. Meyer (1901) first proposed a membrane hypothesis for alcohol's intoxicating and sedating effects. He suggested that alcohol affected neuronal membrane lipids, and over the years many scientists have sought to confirm and extend his theory. Indeed, alcohol has been shown by several lines of experimental evidence to increase the fluidity of lipids in neuronal membranes. These experiments have been performed *in vitro* in membranes obtained from genetically sensitive mice that were predisposed to alcohol sensitivity or insensitivity. Gangliosides were found to be important in allowing alcohol's effects on membrane fluidity. Membrane-bound proteins are affected by their surrounding lipids when alcohol is present. Numerous receptor

protein complexes have been shown to be affected by ethanol, including the GABA-benzodiazepine-barbiturate-chloride ion receptor, the adenylate cyclase system, including the guanine-nucleotide-dependent coupling protein (G protein), sigma opiate receptor, Na+K+-ATPase, as well as monoamine oxidase (Chen & Goldstein, 1976; Liljequist, Culp, & Tabakoff, 1986; Luthin & Tabakoff, 1984; Marks, Smolen, & Collins, 1984; Perlman & Goldstein, 1984; Tabakoff & Hoffman, 1983, 1987). Therefore, although no specific receptor has been found for alcohol, the interactions of the substance with multiple neuromodulating and neurotransmitter systems give additional depth, as well as confusion, to understanding of the basic pharmacology of alcohol.

Equally puzzling is the mechanism(s) that underlies the biochemical pharmacology of tolerance and physical dependence to alcohol. Once again, numerous lines of evidence point to serotoninergic and peptidergic mechanisms in the development of ethanol tolerance. For instance, genetically distinct rodents that self-administer alcohol have been shown to have reduced serotonin (5-HT) concentrations in the brain. Drugs that inhibit 5-HT reuptake into axonal terminals have been shown to decrease self-administration of alcohol by animal as well as human subjects. Turnover of norepinephrine in the CNS also is altered consistently during chronic alcohol ingestion by animals and humans. An association of arginine vasopressin (antidiuretic hormone) with maintenance of the tolerant state to alcohol also has been shown in numerous experiments. This naturally occurring brain peptide has multiple physiologic functions and is somehow involved in learning and memory. The reverse is also true in that antagonists to vasopressin can accentuate the loss of tolerance to alcohol. Genetically distinct rodents that lack this peptide were reported not to develop alcohol tolerance to prolonged administration of the substance (Bloom, 1989; Jaffe, 1990; Tabakoff & Hoffman, 1987).

The pharmacology of tolerance to alcohol includes pharmacodynamic tolerance, together with eventual development of a state of physical dependence when alcohol is maintained in the bloodstream at high concentrations for long periods of time. Withdrawal phenomena begin to occur within 10 to 96 hours after cessation of drinking, and so-called uncomplicated alcohol withdrawal may consist of mild tremors, anxiety, nausea, cramps, elevated blood pressure, hyperreflexia, disturbed sleep, and rebound of REM sleep, as well as hallucinations. Alcohol-offset seizures are also a relatively frequent complication of the withdrawal state and can occur even with alcohol present in the bloodstream. A reduction in blood level is a sufficient trigger to onset of tonic-clonic seizures, which usually occur once or at most in brief flurries ("rum fits"). A cross tolerance demonstrated between ethanol and other sedative hypnotic drugs, including benzodiazepines, barbiturates, and chloral hydrate, although none exist between ethanol and opiate narcotics (Jaffe, 1990).

A more severe abstinence syndrome has been termed alcohol hallucinosis, with continued hallucinations, confusion, disorientation, weakness, and agitation. Hallucinations are often persecutory and have extremely vivid characteristics. This state may last for 3 to 4 days and has been termed delirium tremens or alcohol withdrawal delirium (Jaffe, 1990). Although most alcohol abstinence syndromes are self-limiting, delirium tremens is a medical emergency because of the instability of the cardiovascular system and also the potential for seizures. The larger long-term issue is that of a prolonged abstinent state, which can take many months or even years before normal biochemical equilibrium is established.

Biological risk for alcoholism has been shown to have genetic underpinnings, and multiple factors have been elucidated, including genetically determined differences and isoenzyme patterns for alcohol dehydrogenase, genetically distinct brain proteins, differences in brainwave EEG patterns, and in long-latency cognitive evoked potentials (P300). Two relatively distinct groups of alcoholics have been characterized, namely, type I alcoholics, who exhibit low novelty-seeking and high harm-avoidance behavior, and who drink to alleviate anxiety, and type II alcoholics, who show high novelty-seeking and low harm-avoidance behavior and who mainly drink to experience alcohol's euphoric properties (Cloninger, Dinwiddie, & Reich, 1989; Schuckit, 1987).

Although detoxification from alcohol is a complicated matter, it can be accomplished rapidly with pharmacologic and medical measures instituted to prevent seizures and acute cardiovascular collapse. Detoxification can be accomplished using lorazepam or, more traditionally, the older benzodiazepines (e.g., chlordiazepoxide) administered daily. These compounds reduce the anxiety, tremulousness, and noradrenergic overactivity associated with the acute withdrawal state. Curiously enough, conventional anticonvulsants, such as phenytoin, are ineffective in preventing alcohol-offset tonic-clonic seizures. Benzodiazepines and perhaps sodium valproate and carbamazepine may have a preferential ability to prevent alcohol withdrawal seizures. As noted above, even after the acute withdrawal state to alcohol is finished, extended abstinence features (the so-called prolonged alcohol abstinence syndrome) can occur for years, and persisting neuropsychological and electroencephalographic changes can be seen (Grant, 1987; Mendelson & Mello, 1979). Permanent impairments in brain function also are known to exist, particularly in Wernicke's disease and Korsakoff's psychosis, characterized by structural changes in mammillothalamic tracts with profound disruption of memory, deranged thinking processes, and confusion, often on a permanent basis. Other long-term effects of alcohol have been seen in reproductive function, both in males and

females, and human fetal alcohol syndrome has been well described in alcohol-exposed fetuses (Mello, 1987).

The treatment of alcoholism, both at the time of acute withdrawal as well as on a long-term basis, has taken many different approaches. Acute prevention of withdrawal symptoms can be accomplished readily via use of benzodiazepines, as mentioned above. On a long-term basis, if chronic anxiety is a predisposing factor to continued use of alcoholism, then it makes sense that long-term administration of benzodiazepines and other anxiety-reducing agents may prove useful. Newer agents, such as buspirone (BuSpar), which are serotonin agonists, also may play a role in the long-term treatment of alcohol-prone patients. Serotonin reuptake inhibitors, such as zemelidine and fluoxetine, have been shown to reduce alcohol consumption in alcohol-prone individuals (Jaffe, 1989; 1990).

More traditional pharmacologic approaches that have been used in the past to curb or eliminate alcohol consumption include medications like disulfiram and, to a lesser extent, carbamide. Both of these drugs inhibit the alcohol-metabolizing enzyme, aldehyde oxidoreductase (aldehyde dehydrogenase). This enzyme metabolizes a breakdown product of ethanol, namely, acetaldehyde, which is normally converted to acetic acid. Therefore, by inhibiting acetaldehyde's metabolism, levels of this intermediate build up and are associated with unpleasant side effects, such as tachycardia, flushing, vomiting, pounding in the chest, hypotension, sweating, and dizziness. These side effects are believed to act as deterrents and create a conditioned aversion to the usage of alcohol. Disulfiram was used for a long time, but its use currently has diminished because of lack of efficacy and because of ethical questions regarding its repeated administration. Other less widely used approaches from the past included the use of emetine and lithium, which produce protracted vomiting. It was felt that these agents could help induce conditioned aversion to alcohol. None of these techniques has been found to be useful routinely (Jaffe, 1989). Likewise, apomorphine, a dopaminergic agonist, also has been used as an aversive conditioning agent and is a treatment for the recurrent craving and anxiety surrounding the cessation of drinking. Clonidine has been used to reduce some of the increased central sympathetic tone in numerous drug cessation regimens, including alcohol, opiates, and CNS stimulants.

In large measure, the mainstay of rehabilitation efforts following the acute withdrawal of alcohol has centered on behavioral and cognitive therapies. The Alcoholics Anonymous 12-Step Program remains a useful tool, although the efficacy rate for successful rehabilitation from chronic alcohol use is quite low. Group and individual psychotherapeutic efforts are important concomitants in an overall approach to the rehabilitation from alcohol usage. In the last decade, it has been increasingly recognized that alcohol use is a problem not only from the standpoint of the effects of that molecule on the central and peripheral nervous systems, but also as a worldwide problem with respect to polydrug use of multiple CNS-active agents simultaneously. Indeed, alcohol, nicotine, and marijuana are the top three drugs used in a nonmedical setting according to National Institute on Drug Abuse statistics (National Institute on Drug Abuse, 1983). Since alcohol is readily available, it is often used as a counter-drug to "smooth out" anxiety and dysphoria when other preferred centrally active agents are not immediately available. Heroin addicts in methadone programs and patients in other drug detoxification systems for cocaine and amphetamine abuse often use alcohol as a baseline tranquilizing agent. This underscores the need to search for better pharmacologic methods to treat underlying behavioral anxiety states. Perhaps newer central serotoninergic agents (e.g., selective reuptake blockers) and the buspirone category of medications may prove useful in the future. The author has observed that patients with an organically based predisposition to behavioral instability and consequent dependence on multiple centrally active agents often respond to anticonvulsant therapy in ameliorating or abating drug use (unpublished observations). More research is needed to define the rate and prevalence of CNS instabilities and usage of medications that stabilize organic brain dysfunction and their application in prevention of recurrent alcohol and other drug use (Kreek, 1987).

NICOTINE AND TOBACCO

The practice of consuming nicotine in various forms is an example of a complex social behavior with multifactorial inputs. The initiation and maintenance of this behavior have their roots in social and cultural bases. The entire practice becomes a repeatedly reinforced, overlearned, and, in many cases, reflex or automatic behavior, re-inforced by repeated conditioning. Nicotine in tobacco is a potent psychochemical, with central and peripheral nervous system effects as well as those on cardiovascular, gastrointestinal, skeletal, motor, and endocrine systems (Jaffe, 1990). Nicotine has been demonstrated to produce tolerance as well as physical dependence. Positive effects of nicotine have been demonstrated on various behavioral measures, such as facilitation of memory or attention, decrease in irritability, appetite suppression, and euphoria when administered intravenously. Animals can be taught to self-administer nicotine, although the reinforcing effects are less profound than cocaine or amphetamines. Nevertheless, the pharmacology of nicotine, together with the mode of administration wherein each puff of a cigarette can be considered a single dose of drug, make nicotine an almost ideal reinforcing agent, particularly with respect to its positive or pleasurable effects (as noted above), including behavioral alerting.

The pharmacologic mechanisms of nicotine affect the cholinergic systems of the central and peripheral nervous system with stimulation of nicotinic as well as muscarinic receptors. In addition, a large body of evidence imputes release of serotonin, dopamine, histamine, endorphins, and other neurotransmitters and neuromodulators as additional central effects of nicotine (Jones, 1987). A much more diversified pharmacology of some 4000 compounds has been identified in tobacco (when burned) and tremendously complicates the understanding of not only nicotine effects, but also effects of other potent substances contained in tobacco. Metallic ions, radioactive compounds, alkaloids, tars, cyclic aromatic hydrocarbons, and other substances have been recovered from tobacco that is burned. This makes tobacco the most complex of all misused substances and engenders great concern in terms of the epidemiology of cancers and other serious health complications, including cardiovascular diseases and peripheral vascular disease. Chronic obstructive lung disease, effects on myocardial ischemia, and acceleration of atherogenesis have also been demonstrated (Barry, Mead, Nabel, Rocco, Campbell, Fenton, Mudge, & Selwyn, 1989).

Despite the heightened national societal awareness of the ill effects of chronic tobacco use, increased usage has been reported in the female population in the last 2 decades. National rates of the incidence of lung cancer in women are approaching that in men and may well surpass it in the near future. In general, the nicotine content of individual cigarettes has been reduced, and the average amount of nicotine per cigarette has decreased from 2.3 to 1.2 mg, and the average yield of tars has similarly been reduced from 38 mg to around 10 mg per cigarette. Although the tars are much more associated with serious and even fatal medical complications, it is important to remember that so-called low-yield tar cigarettes do not contain less nicotine than the traditional high-tar preparations (Benowitz, Hall, Herning, Jacob, & Jones, et al., 1983; Jones, 1987). In addition, marked increases in national consumption of other tobacco preparations, such as snuff and chew, contribute to the problems on a national level.

Data accumulated from the literature show that the vast majority of people who have ceased using tobacco do so on their own without any formal help. Therefore, most of the persons studied in the setting of tobacco cessation really represent a minority of tobacco users. Comparatively, only a very small percentage of chronic smokers actually cease using tobacco each year, generally less than 5% (Fielding, 1985; Orleans, 1985). The abrupt cessation of nicotine use will reliably produce a withdrawal syndrome that varies in intensity from person to person. Continued craving is a chronic problem akin to the prolonged abstinence syndrome noted for alcohol and other centrally active drugs of misuse. Irritability, restlessness, difficulty in concentration, headache, and increased appetite, together with insomnia, are frequent features of the nicotine withdrawal syndrome. Indeed, EEG changes have been documented for long periods of time after cessation of nicotine use, as are changes in physiologic parameters and performance on neuropsychological tests (Jaffe, 1990).

A host of treatment approaches have been tried, including behavioral counseling techniques and, more recently, the use of nicotine given in gradually reduced dosages, either as a gum (nicotine polacrilex and Nicorette) and most recently as a patch. Nicotine substitutes, such as lobeline, have been tried in the past, but are not very useful due to the much weaker CNS effect of this compound. Also, nicotine's inherent pharmacodynamic properties, together with the minute-by-minute regulation of dosage obtained via the practice of smoking, make oral forms of nicotine, such as gum, a poor substitute. The behavioral reinforcing effects of the act of smoking, with all of its psychosocial implications, are powerful conditioning stimuli which perpetuate the habit in the first place.

Patch forms of nicotine administration (e.g., Nicoderm™, Habitrol™) offer a continual release of nicotine into the system, such that dosage can be gradually reduced over a matter of 6 to 10 weeks and hopefully withdrawal from nicotine accomplished in a gradual manner so as not to induce negative behavioral phenomena associated with the nicotine withdrawal syndrome. Nicoderm and Habitrol patches offer only one approach to accomplish cessation of nicotine use. Many other behavioral approaches, including hypnosis and acupuncture, aversive conditioning, and other methods have met with partial success. Of prime importance is the degree of motivation on the part of the smoker to end continued usage of tobacco and nicotine. Generally, higher rates of cessation are noted in the setting of serious diseases. Physician advice often will go unheeded unless a concomitant motivator exists for stopping the use of tobacco. Clonidine also has been used in one study and was shown to be promising as an adjunct in reducing use of tobacco and other centrally acting substances.

Aversive conditioning techniques have also been tried, and one of the most effective methods is a so-called rapid smoking technique, wherein a skilled therapist works with the patient one on one. The patient inhales smoke from his or her own cigarette every 5 to 6 seconds, and this continues until the patient asks to stop administration of the nicotine. Presumably, the blood levels of nicotine create negative pharmacologic effects, such as nausea, and the author feels that this may be, in very skilled hands, an appropriate method to create an aversive environment surrounding the use of tobacco. Commercially available programs, which include many behavioral and aversive techniques, together with motivational techniques, have been available and in some ways are more effective, at least in the short term, to produce a higher cessation rate of tobacco use. Behavioral modification techniques can easily be incorporated, as can biofeedback and stress management techniques, to teach patients to substitute other behaviors for repeated use of tobacco and nicotine (Jaffe, 1989).

CAFFEINE

Although far less productive of dependence than many of the other substances discussed in this chapter, caffeine remains one of the most widely used substances in the world. It is a CNS stimulant and a modulator of smooth muscle contraction with pleasurable effects, both physically and psychologically. Caffeine has mood-elevating and antifatiguing properties. An average cup of coffee contains about 100 mg of caffeine, and cola-based soft drinks contain about half that amount. Tea, chocolate, and certain other plants consumed by human beings contain caffeine and other xanthine derivatives (e.g., theophylline, theobromine), which also produce CNS excitation at appropriate doses. It is not unusual to ingest 500 to 700 mg of caffeine per day, and it has been estimated that 25% of the American population does so (Jaffe, 1989).

The establishment of dependence on caffeine is an overlearned social phenomenon and is inextricably woven into many cultural practices (e.g., afternoon tea, morning coffee). From the standpoint of demonstrating withdrawal effects upon cessation of caffeine intake, one of the most prevalent neurologic symptoms is that of headache, together with increased fatigue. Headache, including vascular migraine syndromes, can be precipitated or exacerbated by removing caffeine from the diet. Rarely, headaches will increase and persist for weeks after curtailment of caffeine intake. Complaints of fatigability and decreased alertness also are common after stopping caffeine use. From a pharmacologic viewpoint, caffeine is a much weaker reinforcer of animal behavior in the laboratory than other CNS stimulants, such as cocaine and amphetamines. Chronic users of caffeine rarely report any euphoriant effects. After abstaining from the use of caffeine, reintroduction of the substance will institute pleasurable effects in former chronic caffeine users. Thus, a low level of neuroadaptation occurs with chronic caffeine use. Once again, its short half-life lends itself to repeated administration and thus chronic repetitive dosing, which tends to escalate the daily dose of caffeine. In most cases, caffeine can be withdrawn reasonably slowly without any adverse physiologic effects other than transient fatigue, irritability, and possibly headache. In fact, caffeine is found in many ergotamine preparations and has been used as an adjunctive medication for the treatment of migraine. Many patients with chronic headaches can keep the headache pattern at bay with caffeine dosed repeatedly throughout the day.

Extremely high doses of caffeine can theoretically produce sufficient excitation to allow seizures to occur, particularly in patients with lowered seizure thresholds.

Societally, caffeine overusage tends to be part of programmed behaviors, including concomitant use of nicotine. The DSM-III-R (American Psychiatric Association, 1987) diagnostic criteria for psychiatric disorders include that of caffeine intoxication, usually ingestion of more than 250 mg of caffeine. In special situations, it may contribute to behavioral instability and thus may warrant medical intervention to reduce unwanted side effects often seen with intake of large doses of caffeine.

CANNABIS (MARIJUANA)

This CNS intoxicant has, from a world viewpoint, the highest rates of usage, and it has multiple pharmacologic properties, including euphoriant, mood-stimulating, behavioral, and potent cardiovascular effects. References to usage in Indian and Middle Eastern literature of the forms that are available reveal that cannabis and cannabis products go by many names, from the euphemistic "grass, weed, reefer, and pot" to ganja, bhang, dagga, hashish, and sinsemilla. All cannabis is derived from the flowering tops of hemp plants, and the plant is indigenous to many parts of the world. The plant contains over 400 chemicals, and about 50 of these are cannabinoids. The most abundant psychoactive cannabinoids include cannabinol, cannabidiol, and isomers of tetrahydrocannabinol (THC). The isomer responsible for most of the characteristic effects of ingested or smoked marijuana is D9-THC and it is responsible for many of the psychostimulant, euphoric and, in higher dosages, hallucinogenic properties of the parent plant. Different cultures have extracted the active ingredients in various ways. In most cases, plants are harvested and dried, and dried leaves and flowering tops are usually smoked, ensuring a rapid onset of effect. Extraction of the cannabinoids into solvents also can produce potent pharmacologic effects. The THC content of cultivated marijuana has steadily increased. In the 1960s, average THC content was 1 to 2% in domestically grown marijuana, whereas today it is not uncommon for harvested material to contain 7 to 8% THC. Traditionally, more potent preparations, using only the flowering tops of the plant, often contain in excess of 10 to 15% of THC and are known as hashish or hashish oil.

The pharmacological effects of THC include sedation, decrease of aggressiveness, loss of ability to perform complex motor and psychologic tasks, perceptual and sensory distortions or enhancements and, in larger doses, ataxia, incoordination, stupor, as well as hallucinations. A great deal of energy has been extended in searching for marijuana receptors, and it is highly unlikely that the myriad effects of this substance will be explained by actions in a single particular kind of receptor in the CNS. Effects of chronic marijuana usage include diminished gonadotropin-releasing hormone, luteinizing hormone, and follicle-stimulating hormone levels in both sexes. In women, diminished prolactin levels are seen after smoking marijuana. Numerous lines of evidence point to some interaction of cannabinoids with humeral and cell-mediated immune system components. Of great concern is the obligatory contamination of cannabis products with pesticides, herbicides, and organic and inorganic metals, which may add to the overall CNS toxicity (Jaffe, 1989, 1990; Mendelson, 1987). Persistent levels of cannabinoids and other extremely lipid-soluble substances have been demonstrated in tissues for months after cessation of marijuana use, which raises concerns of long-lasting effects of chronic marijuana use on behavior, cognition, and intellectual functioning.

Statistical surveys of the incidence of marijuana usage show that a declining fraction of adolescents and young adults regularly use the substance, although it remains one of the most commonly used psychoactive substances, and fully 50% of Americans have tried or used marijuana in their lives. Like all behaviorally reinforcing drugs, a small segment of users will have unpleasant behavioral and cardiovascular effects or exacerbation or production of psychiatric abnormalities and on this basis will probably not use the substance repetitively. Anxiety, panic reactions, and paranoid symptoms may be produced or aggravated in susceptible individuals, and many users do not rate these as pleasant effects. In comparison, the anti-anxiety and mild euphoriant properties of marijuana lend themselves to repeated usage as mild intoxicants and relaxants. There is seemingly no tolerance for the pleasurable effects of cannabis and, therefore, continued behavioral reinforcement would be expected to promote repetitive use of marijuana. However, there is tolerance to some of its effects on mood, and it is likely that this is responsible for the escalation of dosage needed to produce the same degree of "high" with repetitive use. Paradoxically, a "reverse tolerance" to the effects of cannabis has been described, in that smaller and smaller doses are needed over time to achieve certain desirable euphoriant effects. A well-described amotivational syndrome exists in cultures where daily usage of marijuana and hashish occurs. This has been described in the Caribbean (Jamaican) peoples, and there has been much debate as to whether or not marijuana directly affects motivation or whether these are indirect effects of the drug (Cohen, 1982). Social usage of marijuana is often impossible to study in its own right because of concomitant usage of tobacco, alcohol, and other commonly used substances, often ingested in close proximity to marijuana itself. This complicates research protocols and epidemiologic studies of marijuana use.

Attempts have been made to look for bona fide pharmacologic uses for marijuana. Trials of oral THC have been used successfully to reduce glaucoma in otherwise refractory patients (Jaffe, 1990). Similarly, a synthetic cannabinoid derivative, nabilone, has been used as an antiemetic. This substance also produces many of the psychoactive effects of natural D9-THC (Jaffe, 1990; Mendelson, 1987).

Because of the production or exacerbation of psychiatric symptoms and behavioral aberrations associated with marijuana use, the DSM-III-R (American Psychiatric Association, 1987) has developed diagnostic criteria for a cannabis delusional order, as well as cannabis intoxication. These are generally utilized in conjunction with approaches to other chemical dependencies, and it is rare that prolonged psychotic or schizophreniform states will result from acute misusage of marijuana or its derivatives. The cannabis withdrawal syndrome has been described with impaired motor performance on discontinuation, associated with insomnia, anxiety, and other symptoms reminiscent of withdrawal from sedative hypnotics. Whether this represents a mere return to the patient's baseline state of behavior is uncertain but remains a possibility. Once again, utilizing the principle that the anxiolytic and psychostimulant properties of marijuana may help correct a baseline state of agitation or internal dysphoria, one might, therefore, search for more appropriate pharmacologic management of individuals who repeatedly use marijuana and its derivatives, thereby circumventing the potential for engagement in illegal and societally disapproved drug-seeking behaviors. Behavioral, affective, and cognitive therapies certainly play a strong role in the overall rehabilitation and management of individuals who have strong histories of chronic marijuana use.

CENTRAL NERVOUS SYSTEM STIMULANTS (COCAINE AND AMPHETAMINES)

The most powerful reinforcers in licit or illicit usage are the CNS stimulants, particularly cocaine. Reference has been made (see above) to its powerful effects on reinforcement of self-stimulating behavior in animals and as clinically observed by usage in people. In the last 10 years, cocaine has emerged as the statistical drug of choice for recreational repeated self-administration. Although traditionally snorted or used intravenously as a soluble hydrochloride salt, free-base or crack cocaine has enjoyed widespread misuse throughout many cultures in the Western Hemisphere in the last decade. A similar phenomenon has been described for misuse of amphetamines, which historically dates back to World War II and to an epidemic of widespread amphetamine usage in post-war Japan in the 1950s. In the next 2 decades, amphetamine compounds were readily available pharmaceutically, and many adolescents and young adults used amphetamines, more so for their stimulant properties and less apparently so for purely recreational purposes (Abelson & Fishburne, 1976). In 1970, the Harrison Act was amended, and amphetamines were placed in Schedule II, with tight controls on distribution and dispensing of the substances. Large quantities of manufactured amphet-

amines were, nonetheless, illicitly diverted. By 1980, usage of amphetamines had declined rather dramatically, in contradistinction to the escalating use of cocaine in our population. Clearly, the inverse relationships are linked, at least in the author's mind, based on the relative availability of cocaine and relative nonavailability of amphetamines. In the 1980s, reports of clandestine manufacturing operations for amphetamines and methamphetamines surfaced, and intranasal and intravenous use of "crank" continues alongside that of cocaine. The population at highest risk for use and abuse of these substances is the 18- to 25-year-old group. Cocaine is the only drug for which increasing risk of usage develops above this age group, although escalating usage of alcohol remains another major problem (Fischman, 1987; O'Malley, Johnston, & Bachman, 1985).

Pharmacological mechanisms subserving repeated self-administration of amphetamines and cocaine relate directly to the effect of these drugs on the dopamine system. In particular, their ability to block reuptake of dopamine and also to act as dopamine agonists produces CNS excitation, and this is coupled with repeated dosing, which becomes a powerful behavioral reinforcer. On a practical level, the effects of amphetamines are indistinguishable from the effects of cocaine, even to seasoned users, with the only major difference being the duration of the drug effect. The patterns of misuse for both substances tend to be similar, with a flurry of administration occurring in "runs" or binges, and that for cocaine generally lasting less than 1 or 2 days, whereas in the case of amphetamine usage, a typical binge may last for several days. Generally, the intense repeated usage of these substances ends when the availability of the drug is curtailed or when the user is exhausted, confused, or disorganized. Users will often inject larger and larger amounts of a drug to obtain the same degree of rush or flash, and the free-base form of cocaine is said to be more profound in this respect. The rush is often described in orgasmic connotations and becomes the principal focus for repeated use during the binge. Following such a binge, the user will often crash, with profound lethargy and often will sleep for up to 24 hours or longer to mitigate the severe CNS exhaustion attendant to prolonged stimulant use. The temporal pattern of binges consists of intense usage punctuated by short periods of abstinence. A phenomenon called sensitization (Fischman, 1987) exists which occurs with repeated psychostimulant usage. This has been demonstrated in both humans and animals and consists of an increased effect of a specific dose of a stimulant with repeated administration. Thus, the repetitive patterns are akin to the stereotypic behaviors elicited in animals with chronic administration of cocaine or amphetamines. Sensitization has been described for numerous variables, namely, local motor activity, stereotypic behaviors, increased seizures and startle responses, and other aspects of CNS stimulation. Post

(1977) compared the effects of repeated usage of psycho-stimulant drugs to animal models of "kindling" wherein repeated low-level stimulation of hippocampal and amygdala preparations resulted in prolonged after-discharges and seizure-like activity in brain preparations.

At the same time that the process of sensitization is occurring, the process of tolerance also occurs with regard to the rush or flash obtained with a single dose of cocaine. Cross tolerance and cross sensitization occur among CNS stimulants, and yet no tolerance occurs to the positive reinforcing effect of this group of substances on behavior. Thus, the ability of cocaine or amphetamines to act as reinforcers occurs consistently whether one has a short history of repeated cocaine use or an intermittent history spanning many years. The effect of sensitization seems to be consistently present, even with long periods of discontinuance of drug use (Post, 1977).

Treatment of dependence on cocaine and amphetamines is extremely difficult, as one can imagine, because of the extremely powerful behavioral and reinforcing effects of these drugs. Nevertheless, the list of severe and potentially fatal medical problems associated with unrestrained use of cocaine mandates very vigorous efforts in detoxification and rehabilitation of individuals who are severely dependent on these substances. In addition, a mixture of cocaine with heroin (so-called "speedballing") adds additional measures of medical risk, and certainly cocaine users are very well known to misuse multiple other substances, such as alcohol, sedative hypnotics, marijuana, and opiates. Long-term serious psychiatric complications of cocaine and amphetamine use include paranoid states and a syndrome virtually indistinguishable from paranoid schizophrenia with extreme hypervigilance. Persistent toxic psychoses, together with hallucinations, have been well described following prolonged amphetamine or cocaine use. More commonly, a briefer state of drug-induced delirium with suspiciousness, paranoia, and visual and tactile hallucinations (formication) occurs following binges or runs of stimulant use. Of great concern are more fatal medical complications (e.g., accelerated hypertension, cerebrovascular infarction, intracerebral hemorrhages, myocardial infarctions, coronary artery spasms, fatal cardiac arrhythmias, seizures, respiratory depression, gastrointestinal and peripheral vascular necrosis) from the prolonged vasoconstrictor effects of CNS stimulants.

Withdrawal from cocaine reliably produces a syndrome that is longer lasting and more pervasive than the typical crash following acute discontinuance of stimulant use. The entire abstinence syndrome occurs over a long period of time in stages. The first stage is rather brief, lasting 3 to 5 days, with anorexia and agitation being replaced by profound exhaustion, depression, hypersomnia, and hyperphagia. A second phase develops over the ensuing 6 to 12 weeks, with improved mood and a better normalization of sleep; however, cocaine craving returns,

and the greatest likelihood of relapsing to former cocaine use occurs during this phase. Whether or not this stage mimics the natural cycle of binge use for amphetamines and cocaine is a point that has been debated (Jaffe, 1989). The third and most prolonged phase of cocaine withdrawal may take up to a year and resembles the prolonged alcohol abstinence syndrome, with establishment of successful conditioned avoidance responses and behaviors based on a combination of behavioral retraining and possibly medication.

Various medications have been utilized to curb cocaine craving, including clonidine and desipramine. Very fragmentary data with Tegretol (unpublished results) also indicate that this agent may be effective in curbing the intense craving for cocaine and amphetamines. In the acute phases of withdrawal, haloperidol or other dopamine blockers may very well be useful. In some cocaine users, particularly with underlying cyclothymic disorders, lithium has been reported to be helpful in reducing relapse to continued use of cocaine. It has been suggested that chronic blockade of dopamine receptors may alter craving for psychostimulants. However, the opposite effect has also been demonstrated, wherein neuroleptics given to recent cocaine users resulted in increased craving for the drug. Studies are in progress to determine which category of medicines may have long-term utility in curbing the nationwide epidemic of cocaine use. Similar treatments for amphetamine dependence have been developed, and tricyclic antidepressants are currently being used, along with dopaminergic blockers to block craving and some of the euphoriant actions of amphetamine. Alpha-methyl-paratyrosine (AMPT) was tried in older studies but is not clinically available. AMPT blocks the formation of dopamine and ultimately norepinephrine and had been found to block amphetamine-induced euphoria. However, it does not have any ability to block the effects of cocaine or methyl-phenidate (Ellinwood, 1979).

Rehabilitative treatment for chronic users of stimulants is rudimentary at this point. Numerous psychological approaches have been attempted, including behavioral, psychodynamic, and supportive psychotherapeutic techniques. In some cases, a contractual agreement by the person in treatment has been beneficial. In this type of arrangement, the person undergoing treatment agrees that the treating professional may inform his or her employer or professional societies if relapse into use of cocaine or amphetamine occurs within a certain time period. Within the boundaries of such an agreement, it has been shown that a significant portion of patients treated do abstain from a relapse into stimulant use. However, much higher relapse rates were noted after expiration of the contractual time period. Combining psychopharmacologic approaches with behavioral and psychotherapeutic techniques gives the best results, because chronic stimulant use is felt to create a relative state of dopamine deficiency by downregulating post-synaptic receptors. This is by no means the only neurotransmitter system involved. Effects on the serotoninergic system also have been described, and at this time tricyclic antidepressants still remain useful in helping to attenuate relapse rates. By blocking the uptake of dopamine, serotonin, and norepinephrine, it is felt that the antidepressant effects would help ameliorate the post-crash fatigue and lassitude that are parts of the second stage of cocaine withdrawal syndrome. At best, success rates are currently limited, and better psychopharmacologic agents have to be developed, although desipramine is now favored among the tricyclic anti-depressants.

Opioids

The history of opiate use dates back to the 1st century A.D. and most likely even earlier. The prototypical opiate, morphine, is found in the opium plant. The advent of pipe smoking ushered in the practice of ingestion by smoking, particularly in the Far East. Morphine and its synthetic derivative, heroin, remain very popular drugs of misuse and are among the most severe tolerance- and physical-dependence-producing substances known in modern pharmacology. There seems to have been a return to more heroin misuse nationally in the last 5 years, and this, in part, reflects availability of natural materials and prevailing market and social forces that wax and wane regarding different drugs of misuse. During the height of the 1980s cocaine era, misuse of opiates had waned somewhat. However, there seems to be a return to the levels of usage seen in the 1970s.

The pharmacology of morphine and other opioids has been progressing steadily since the identification of multiple kinds of opiate receptors in the CNS. These developments in turn sprang forward from the identification of naturally occurring endorphins and enkephalins in the central and peripheral nervous system. The μ receptor subtype is the site of action of the classic opiates, namely, morphine, heroin, and codeine. These drugs are preferentially agonists at this receptor subtype. A second κ receptor is the site of action of numerous other clinically useful drugs, namely, butorphanol and nalbuphine. A Δ receptor has been identified and seems to be the binding site for endogenous met-enkephalin. A σ receptor also has been described, and stimulation of this receptor has hallucinogenic and excitatory effects with very little analgesia. Most of the analgesic effects of opiates are mediated through the μ receptor. The pharmacology of the tolerance and physical dependence to various effects of opiates is quite complicated, and some of the newer agents (e.g., pentazocine, cyclazocine) have agonist effects at one receptor subtype and antagonistic effects at other receptor subtypes. The pharmacology of these receptor subtypes is very well described (Jaffe, 1989; Woods & Winger, 1987).

The pharmacologic actions of opioids that have predominant effects at μ or κ receptors are subclassified into direct effects, dependence-producing effects, discriminative effects, and reinforcing effects. Many of these studies have been done *in vitro* and in animals and have less relevance to the pharmacology of these substances in humans. Much of the pharmacologic subcategorization has been done with agents that are antagonists to various kinds of receptors, such as nalorphine. This was the first substance noted to reverse the effects of morphine acutely, particularly analgesic and euphoriant effects. Although nalorphine antagonized morphine-induced euphoria and precipitated withdrawal symptoms, it, too, could produce analgesia in humans. Unlike the euphoriant-producing morphine, nalorphine generally produces dysphoria in humans. An even more selective opioid antagonist, naloxone, is currently in clinical use to acutely reverse some of the lethal effects of morphine or heroin, namely, those of respiratory depression and some of the effects on the cholinergic system peripherally. Naloxone (Narcan) can rapidly reverse agonist actions of morphine and heroin and can be dramatic in reversing acute life-threatening effects of overdoses in emergency room settings. A concerted effort has been made pharmacologically to elucidate and preserve analgesic properties of opioids with a minimum of euphoriant and physical dependence-producing properties. No ideal molecule exists, although some success with a combination of analgesic effects (by virtue of κ-receptor stimulation) with a minimum of physical dependence-producing properties has been achieved with mixed agonist-antagonist molecules (e.g., nalbuphine, butorphanol, pentazocine) (Woods & Winger, 1987).

With respect to the withdrawal syndrome from opioids and the practical management of detoxification from this category of medication, volumes of literature have been written on opioid maintenance using methadone, and this drug enjoys a prime position in one of the major approaches to treatment of heroin and morphine use in the United States and other countries. The use of methadone was pioneered by Dole and Nyswander in the mid-1960s. Methadone is an opioid with relatively pure μ-receptor agonist properties and has a longer half-life than heroin or morphine. It has proved to be relatively safe in terms daily use and to block the euphoriant effects of subsequent doses of heroin. Other opioid maintenance drugs have been investigated, although none is clinically available. One such medication, l-a-acetylmethadole (L-AAM), is under investigational use. It is similar to methadone in its action but has long-lived metabolites and can be given every other day. In any case, it is now more than 15 years since L-AAM was introduced, and it still remains a controversial and investigational drug. Another investigational drug, buprenorphine, blocks the subjective effects of parenterally administered morphine or heroin (Mello & Mendelson, 1980). Apparently, when given to patients who are self-administering low doses of heroin, buprenorphine suppresses some of the withdrawal symptoms, whereas when given to patients using high doses of opiates, it seems to precipitate abstinence, more like traditional opioid antagonists.

The controversy surrounding use of methadone as a replacement for heroin or morphine has been debated for nearly 30 years. Proponents of methadone maintenance feel that a slowly tapered oral dosing of methadone can successfully achieve detoxification from heroin use. In addition, the methadone can block some of the euphoriant "rush" effects of injected heroin or morphine. Furthermore, one of the objectives of treatment is to prevent severe withdrawal which is associated with far higher relapse rates in return to use of injected opioids. Patients are often initially stabilized on 80 to 100 mg of oral methadone, and a tapering regimen which reduces the methadone dosage by 10% per week has often been employed. A more gradual taper (3% per week) is utilized when the methadone dose falls below 20 mg/day. Opponents of the methadone system cite widespread diversion of methadone itself and the sale of the substance by heroin addicts who are enrolled in oral methadone programs. Attempts have been made to institute oral naltrexone (Trexan) therapy when the methadone taper is nearly finished in order to have an oral opioid antagonist present in the former user's system on a daily basis. The aim of this therapy is hopefully to block euphoriant effects of any subsequently injected opiate should the person return to former usage patterns.

Because the acute opioid withdrawal syndrome is believed to be a state wherein the adrenergic nervous system is hyperactive, centrally acting $\alpha2$ agonists (e.g., clonidine) have been utilized to suppress some of the acute withdrawal reactions. Lacrimation, rhinorrhea, jitteriness, and sweating can be attenuated by the oral administration of clonidine. Clonidine is far less effective against other withdrawal phenomena, such as insomnia, craving, lethargy, and muscle aches, but has been utilized successfully in tapering off oral methadone dosage and institution of oral naltrexone, as discussed above. Blood pressure has to be monitored with clonidine, as it is a centrally acting antihypertensive agent. Sedation also can be a problem, although with regard to the restlessness involved in opioid withdrawal, this side effect may indeed be quite useful.

Other techniques utilized for accomplishing opioid withdrawal seem "hard-nosed" but take advantage of the unpleasant nature of withdrawal as an aversive conditioning technique. Abrupt withdrawal without any pharmacologic supports has been advocated by some as a reasonable way of accomplishing rapid detoxification from opioid dependence. Since clinical withdrawal is rarely life-threatening, it at least has the advantage of accomplishing what can be a lengthy detoxification program in a matter of days. Most oral methadone programs can continue for 3

to 6 months, and the cost of such programs is quite high. There is no evidence to suggest that rapid detoxification has any greater relapse rate than more traditional techniques (Jaffe, 1989). Furthermore, approximately 85% of heroin addicts meet criteria for at least one psychiatric diagnosis, and it is often the more psychiatrically impaired patients who have the lowest rates of success in formal detoxification programs.

Sedative-Hypnotics and Benzodiazepines

Among the most available substances in our society are benzodiazepine anxiolytics and sedatives, and use and misuse of this category of drugs have taken on dramatic proportions in the last 10 to 15 years. In past years, the same kind of problem occurred with use of older hypnotic/sedatives, such as barbiturates, which are much more tightly regulated since implementation of the Controlled Substances Act of 1970. Other nonbarbiturate sedatives, including glutethimide, methyprylon, chloral hydrate, and meprobamate, enjoyed widespread misuse in small segments of the population. An excellent overview of the scope of benzodiazepine usage in the United States is presented in a Task Force Report of the American Psychiatric Association (1990) on benzodiazepine dependence, toxicity, and abuse.

There has been an increasing awareness over the last decade that short half-life benzodiazepines can be problematic, in terms of potential for both dependence and misuse. Withdrawal from benzodiazepines is commonly believed to represent a return of the original anxiety symptoms for which the medication was prescribed (Griffiths & Sannerud, 1987). Benzodiazepines and other sedative hypnotics are known to be fairly strong reinforcers, and much experimental data in humans have provided abundant evidence that a true physical dependence, as well as tolerance, can occur with virtually every benzodiazepine. Those benzodiazepines that are more lipid-soluble tend to be more problematic. Older benzodiazepines, such as diazepam (Valium), together with newer lipid-soluble short half-life preparations, such as alprazolam (Xanax) and triazolam (Halcion), are much more problematic in terms of tolerance- and dependence-producing properties with chronic usage. Withdrawal phenomena, including seizures, have been reported in patients who have misused high doses of benzodiazepines, barbiturates, and other nonbarbiturate sedative-hypnotics. Agitation and restlessness generally occur in a predictable fashion, and the length of time of the withdrawal process can range between several days to several weeks.

The magnitude of the problem of benzodiazepine misuse certainly far exceeds numerically that seen for opiates. It is estimated that 11 to 12% of the population has used benzodiazepines at least intermittently, whereas about 3 or 4% of the population uses benzodiazepines on a chronic basis. Upward of a 100 million prescriptions per year have been written for these substances, and iatrogenic dependence is a very real issue on a national level.

Treatment modalities for benzodiazepine withdrawal have been devised using slow tapers and changes to long-acting, low-potency compounds. In general, avoidance of long half-life compounds for use as nighttime hypnotics, together with avoidance of ultrashort-acting compounds for the same purpose, would be a wise choice in preventing iatrogenic tolerance and dependence on benzodiazepines. Use of drug holidays is another technique that might favor a more rational use of this class of compounds.

Beta blockers (propanolol), clonidine, carbamazepine, and buspirone have been used in the treatment of withdrawal symptoms from benzodiazepines. Because withdrawal effects are related to the uncovering of inhibitory GABA receptor sites in the CNS, drugs such as carbamazepine may prove useful, not only to control benzodiazepine withdrawal seizures, but also to quiet the arousal state often seen in withdrawal (Klein, Uhde, & Post, 1986; Ries, Roy-Burne, & Ward, et al., 1989). Buspirone has been utilized in treating benzodiazepine withdrawal symptoms, and unfortunately does not prevent emergence of such symptoms although clinically it may be useful on its own merit to treat underlying anxiety while benzodiazepine dosage is tapered. Use of short-term phenobarbital also has been advocated in the treatment of benzodiazepine withdrawal symptoms. It is preferred to pentobarbital, which has its own spectrum of dependence-producing effects (Martin, Kapur, Whiteside, & Sellers, 1979).

Of equal concern in selected populations of drug-using individuals is the combined usage of benzodiazepines with alcohol or opiates. In both cases, additive and synergistic respiratory depression is a constant threat, and tolerance to respiratory depression does not develop for any of these substances (Jaffe, 1990). Recommendations from the American Psychiatric Association's Task Force Report (1990) on benzodiazepine prescribing include avoidance of short half-life preparations; discontinuance symptoms can appear even at ordinary therapeutic doses; the immediate discontinuance symptoms are felt to be a rebound presentation of the original anxiety symptoms with more severe withdrawal symptoms, including seizures, being manifestations of bona fide physical dependence; the onset of withdrawal symptoms occurs sooner and is more pronounced with short half-life preparations; tapering for high-potency short half-life preparations should be performed very gradually with additional use of other supportive medication as mentioned above. The task force guidelines also noted interaction of benzodiazepines with alcohol, particularly in terms of daily tasks, such as driving and effects on memory consolidation, and it was believed that benzodiazepines most strongly reinforced their use in patients who have a predisposition to misusing other categories of drugs such as alcohol, other sedative-hypnotics, and opiates. Thus, benzodiazepine misuse continues to be a national phenomenon, and iatrogenic factors clearly contribute to the problem.

A much more recent problem in the United States and in the world in the last few years is the use of flunitrazepam, commonly marketed as Rohypnol. Street names for this drug abound: Rophies, Ropies, Roofies, Ropes, Roches, Rochas, Rochas Dos, Rophs, Ropers, Ribs, R-25s, Roach-2s, Trip and Fall, Remember All, Mind Erasers, Forget Pills, and Date Rape Drug. This benzodiazepine has been implicated in sexual assault (date rape) cases especially when mixed with alcohol and is a cheap form of intoxicant (Saum and Inciardi, 1997). An estimated one in four women will be raped in their lifetimes and approximately 75% of these incidents will be acquaintance rapes. Flunitrazepam is odorless, colorless, and tasteless and produces drowsiness, impaired motor skills, and profound anterograde amnesia. Ultrasensitive techniques are available to detect this drug in urine and blood samples in suspected rape victims (Anglin, Spears, & Hutson, 1997). Flunitrazepam and GHB have become the drugs of choice for date rape situations, as they cause disinhibition and relaxation of voluntary muscles and cause lasting anterograde amnesia for events that occur under the influence of the drug. Alcohol potentiates these effects (Schwartz, Milteer, & LeBeau, 2000). One study in Sweden looked at male juvenile offenders who had used Rohypnol frequently and described its effects in producing feelings of increased power and self-esteem, in reducing fear and and insecurity, and in providing a sense that all was possible. It was also associated with loss of episodic memory and with impulsive violence, especially when used with alcohol (Daderman and Lidberg,1999a). The authors felt that the drug should be classified as a Schedule 1 drug in Sweden and they also pointed out in a second paper (Daderman and Lidberg,1999b) that flunitrazepam abusers became cold-blooded, ruthless, and violent and did not remember their violent actions. They discussed how flunitrazepam could exert profound effects on GABA-ergic systems and thus lower serotonin levels, a state where impulsive execution of violent crimes, including suicides have been well associated. A retrospective study in Prague of intoxicated poisonings over 4 years revealed that Rohypnol was the second most common intoxicant utilized, after alcohol (Rath and Vever, 1998). A survey (between 1995 and 1997) in Dade County, Florida, of benzodiazepines detected in biological samples from drivers arrested while driving under the influence (DUI) showed that 10% of the samples were flunitrazepam, but that these numbers fell dramatically after it became a Schedule 1 drug in 1997 (Raymon, Steele, & Walls, 1999).

HALLUCINOGENS:
LSD, MESCALINE, PSILOCYBIN, AND PHENCYCLIDINE

Perhaps no other psychotropic substance has generated more research and theoretical interest into the mechanisms of mental dysfunction than lysergic acid diethylamide (LSD). This and other substances produce psychedelic effects with perceptual and sensory distortions as well as hallucinations. The discovery in 1943 of LSD's psychedelic effects by Hoffman stimulated a wave of excitement regarding potential use of LSD as a model for schizophrenia and other mental disorders. In the 1960s and early 1970s, the use of LSD-like substances, including psilocybin (extracted from mushrooms) and mescaline (found in the peyote cactus), escalated tremendously in U.S. society. The experimental use of these substances to heighten self-introspection and self-fulfillment created a strong scientific interest scientifically in unlocking the mechanisms for the effects of these drugs on CNS functioning. Resurgence of the pharmacologic mechanisms of these substances yielded abundant evidence that LSD and other psychedelic substances interact with serotonin (5-HT) receptors as well as other neurotransmitter systems in the brain. Actions of psychedelic substances were demonstrated in many brain areas, but in particular, the 5-HT2 receptor was felt to be a fundamental site of action of LSD. Other hallucinogens (e.g., mescaline) were found to have more profound effects on the locus ceruleus in the brainstem, and substances that block norepinephrine and serotonin receptors were found to be useful in preventing the psychedelic effects of hallucinogens (Jaffe, 1990).

Use of phencyclidine (PCP) and other similar substances has supplanted older hallucinogens. It and some of the newer designer drugs, such as MDMA, DOET, and the like (see above), have a plethora of pharmacologic actions in the CNS. Phencyclidine was first developed in the 1950s as an anesthetic for animals, and related substances, such as ketamine (Ketalar), are still used occasionally as anesthetics.

Originally, about 10% of patients anesthetized with phencyclidine would exhibit a state of delirium and aggressive behavior on emergence from the medication. Phencyclidine and some of its related substances have hallucinogenic, analgesic, CNS stimulant, and depressant actions simultaneously. They are bona fide intoxicants, producing slurred speech, nystagmus, and gait ataxia, together with numbness of extremities. Sweating, catatonic postures, rigidity, and a blank stare are often responses to larger doses of the drug. Bizarre behavior, aggressive outbursts, and amnesia can occur. Distortion of sensory input to the CNS occurs, and evidence of CNS stimulation with sweating, fever, salivation, and muscle rigidity are seen. On the street, most of what is passed off as LSD is actually phencyclidine or similar derivatives, because these are easier to manufacture illicitly than LSD itself. PCP goes by a wide range of street names, including "angel dust," "crystal," or "hog." Pharmacologically, PCP affects multiple transmitter systems, but in particular, research has shown that it may antagonize CNS actions of N-methyl-d-aspartate (NMDA), and the receptor for PCP may actually be a part of an NMDA receptor complex controlling calcium and other ionic channels as well as sodium and potassium voltage-regulated channels. This is akin to the GABA-benzodiazepine-chloride ion channel receptor on which benzodiazepines and other drugs are thought to exert their effects (Jaffe, 1989).

One particularly relevant pharmacologic effect of phencyclidine is its agonist effect at the σ opiate receptor site. Why the actions of PCP at the σ receptor site overlap with its effects on NMDA receptors is uncertain. Multiple lines of data suggest the possibility that activation of the σ receptor and NMDA receptor has differential effects on sodium or potassium conductance, which may explain some of the excitatory effects of NMDA itself (Jaffe, 1989).

LSD and PCP are generally used in short runs or binges, with profound exhaustion and lethargy following multiple doses of these drugs. In the case of PCP, it is often smoked with marijuana or misused along with alcohol and other drugs. Toxic psychoses and flashbacks can occur with all hallucinogens, and "bad trips" have been seen in a small percentage of hallucinogen users. These can include states of paranoid ideation and can occur randomly despite repeated "good trips" in past usage of the drug. PCP, in particular, has been likened to a mild psychosis resembling schizophrenia, and although globally chronic misuse of hallucinogens and PCP was less prevalent in our society in the 1990s than it was in the 1960s and 1970s, there does remain a small percentage of people who prefer to misuse these substances on a repeated basis.

Acute treatment of hallucinogen and PCP toxic effects includes use of phenothiazines and dopamine- and norepinephrine-blocking drugs. Treatment with a dopamine blocker may be necessary for a week or longer, as protracted disorientation and toxic psychosis can occur, in particular, after phencyclidine. One unusual property of phencyclidine is its enterohepatic recycling, which can delay excretion of the compound. Urinary acidifiers have been used in the past to hasten renal excretion of the substance.

MDMA (ecstasy) has been mentioned already (see above) and remains a current hallucinogen used by a small fraction of mostly adolescent and college-age individuals. It has mixed pharmacologic actions with CNS stimulant and psychedelic and hallucinogenic properties. The continued wave of popularity of so-called designer hallucinogens continues unabated and will likely remain a problem in a small segment of the drug-misusing population.

Inhalants and Solvents

Drugs of misuse in this category involve a bewildering array of anesthetic gases and organic solvents, including xylene, toluene, benzene, kerosene, and gasoline, together with pressurized propellants like freon and other fluorocarbons. Hexane and some its derivatives are known to produce peripheral neuropathies as well as an agitated, disordered, encephalopathic state. Profound visual hallucinations, feelings of derealization, "spaciness," and distortions in the sense of time all occur. Chronic glue sniffing, in particular, is fraught with long-term effects, including an encephalopathy secondary to widespread brain damage from chronic administration of the volatile substance. Often, inhalant users are extremely young in age, generally come from low income populations, and do not have easy an access to other CNS-active agents. Sniffing of glue or a solvent from a closed container, such as a paper bag, or "huffing" of inhalants is performed generally as a group activity, and often other substances, such as alcohol, marijuana, and nicotine, are used concurrently. There is no specific treatment for acute CNS effects of these substances other than removal of the offending solvent. Typically, chronic users of inhalants tend to be dull in their affect, exhibiting some of the long-term sequelae of subtle, but widespread, encephalopathic process. Neuropsychological testing often confirms problems with memory and problems with motor speed performance on subcategories of neuropsychological testing.

A recent study (Young, Longstaffe, & Tenenbein, 1999) looked at the relationship of inhalant misuse to the use of other substances. This was a survey done in the setting of a juvenile detention facility with 209 children incarcerated over a 3-month period. The study obtained epidemiologic data about mean ages of substance misuse of a number of drugs, including inhalants. Mean age of initial experimentation for inhalants was 9.7 years, as compared to 11.9 years for marijuana, 12.0 years for alcohol inebriation, 11.2 years for cigarette use, and 13.2 to 14.7 years for the remaining substances (opiates, CNS stimulants, and psychedelics). Thus, the implication is made that inhalant misuse in early life may be associated with misuse of other substances.

Iatrogenic Dependence

One of the many tasks of physicians who routinely treat chronic pain patients is the detoxification and redirection of medication usage patterns for chronic pain or headache patients who have been allowed free access to opiate-containing preparations for relief of their symptoms. It is truly regrettable that more emphasis on proper pain management techniques is not offered during the routine medical school or house officer training phases of practitioners. In the author's opinion, too little emphasis is placed on proper pain control management techniques, and unfortunately, most pain is approached as if it were acute pain. Thus, practitioners prescribe opiates and other dependence-producing medications for conditions that are in themselves chronic and not likely to benefit from repeated administration of drugs. This problem is seen by every chronic pain practitioner, regardless of the population of patients he or she treats, and a great deal of effort, redirection, and patient retraining is mandatory in getting most chronic patients to undo the effects of iatrogenic dependence on opiates for chronic pain or headache problems. It is equally curious to the author that terminally ill patients who deserve pharmacologic support in relief of their pain often are, paradoxically, undertreated with pain-relieving medications, with the vain hope of sparing the terminally ill cancer-ridden patient the additional burden of addiction to an opiate. This seems trivial at best and further underscores the general lack of familiarity with proper use of highly addictive substances in the setting of pain control, particularly in terminal diseases.

Treatment approaches to detoxification of codeine, meperidine, and oxycodone preparations are generally accomplished fairly rapidly, and rarely is severe opioid withdrawal a protracted problem. Most detoxification measures utilize progressively smaller dosages of either the same or less addicting opiates, and therapy is often supplemented with anti-inflammatories, antianxiety agents, clonidine, and adequate attention to establishment of a structured sleeping regimen. Substitution of agents like carbamazepine for chronically painful syndromes that involve sharp and burning pain (e.g., reflex sympathetic dystrophy, sympathetically mediated pain syndromes, causalgias, and sharp components of peripheral and other neuropathies) often allows adequate pain management without resorting to dependence-producing medications. The greatest challenge for the pain practitioner is in reeducating the patient not to reach for the next dose of analgesic, and this particularly rings true in the treatment of chronic headache sufferers. Behavioral reorientation, training in biofeedbacking and stress management, and nonpharmacologic approaches to pain (e.g., cranial electrotherapy stimulation and transcutaneous electrical nerve stimulation therapy) offer the potential for adequate pain treatment for chronic conditions.

Ergotamine Dependence

One relatively rare, but nonetheless important, source of iatrogenic dependence occurs in the use of ergotamine to control recurrent headaches. Daily use of ergotamine in as low a dosage as 2 mg can lead to a cycle of dependence on the medication, and often escalating doses are needed to achieve the same headache-free state. In fact, Saper and Jones (1986) found that ergotamine used more than three times per week may also predispose patients to the phenomenon of ergotamine dependency. The use of daily ergotamine can create a situation whereby headaches rebound if ergotamine is not continually administered. Over time, dosage of ergotamine increases, and any attempts to lower the daily dosage result in prompt exacerbation of the headache. After a time, only minimal or transient improvement in the headache pattern is noted, despite escalation of ergotamine dosage. In addition, treatment of the headache using other medication approaches often fails in the setting of ergotamine dependency. Fortunately, detoxification from ergotamine can be accomplished with the use of repetitive intravenous dihydroergotamine (DHE-45), together with intravenous opiates and sedative anxiolytics (e.g., lorazepam), and detoxification management of the ergotamine withdrawal headache will usually occur in 4 to 7 days (Raskin, 1988). After a successful withdrawal from ergotamine, headaches cease to be a problem for some time, but the patient is at risk for return of headaches and, therefore, effective pharmacologic measures must be instituted to prevent relapse into another cycle of ergotamine dependence.

CONCLUSION

This chapter has discussed basic pharmacologic principles, such as tolerance and physical dependence, provided an overview of the many different categories of misused drugs and their patterns of misusage, and outlined elements of detoxification of patients from these drugs. More likely than not, there always will exist personalities who will seek to misuse mind-altering substances, whether for purely recreational purposes or to attain internal states of peace or euphoria, or to counter, likewise, inner states of disquietude, anxiety, restlessness, and ennui. Whatever the specific reason for misusing a psychochemical, hopefully either substitution of licit medication or replacement of drug use by other self-activating behaviors would, in large measure, result in diminished misuse. A better understanding of basic pharmacologic mechanisms also would result hopefully in availability of medications with a minimal potential for production of tolerance and physical dependence. Exciting new prospects in the neurobiology and neuropharmacology of peptides in the CNS are emerging rapidly. Undoubtedly, mind-altering properties of neuropeptides, too, will come to light and be exploited by drug-using experimentalists, as has occurred with drugs discussed in this chapter. It may very well be part of human nature to want to change or alter one's sensorium, hopefully to a place that is more peaceful and less troubled, and thereby achieve a state of relative inner peace. That so many diverse chemicals producing so many different kinds of effects are all capable of achieving what is perceived as inner harmony speaks for the myriad underlying emotional needs of humankind.

In closing, the author would like to quote a passage from Aldous Huxley (1970):

…That humanity at large will ever be able to dispense with Artificial Paradises seems very unlikely. Most men and women lead lives at the worst so painful, at the best so monotonous, poor, and limited that the urge to escape, the longing to transcend themselves if only for a few moments, is and has always been one of the principal appetites of the soul. And for private, for everyday use there have always been chemical intoxicants. All the vegetable sedatives and narcotics, all the euphorics that grow on trees, the hallucinogens that ripen in berries or can be squeezed from roots — all, without exception, have been known and systematically used by human beings from time immemorial. And to these natural modifiers of consciousness, modern science has added its quota of synthetics (p. 62).

REFERENCES

Abelson, H., & Fishburne, P. (1976). National survey — main findings: Nonmedical use of psychoactive substances. Springfield, VA: National Technical Information Service.

Anglin, D., Spears, K.L., & Hutson, H.R. (1997). Flunitrazepam and its involvement in date or acquaintance rape. *Academy Emergency Medicine, 4*, 323–326.

Arimany, J., Medallo, J., Pujol., A., Vingut, A., Borondo, J.C., & Valverve, J.L. (1998) Intentional overdose and death with 3,4-methylenedioxyethamphetamine (MDEA; "Eve"): Case report. *American Journal of Forensic Medicine and Pathology, 19*, 148–151.

Barrett, J.E. (1987). Nonpharmacologic factors determining the behavioral effects of drugs. In H.Y. Meltzer (Ed.), *Psychopharmacology: The third generation of progress* (pp. 1493–1510). New York: Raven Press.

Barrionuevos, M., Aguirre, S., Del Rio, J., & Lasheras, B. (2000). Serotonergic deficits and impaired passive-avoidance learning in rats by MDEA: A comparison with MDMA. *Pharmacology, Biochemistry, and Behavior, 65*, 233–240.

Barry, J., Mead, K., Nabel, E.G., Rocco, M.B., Campbell, S., Fenton, T., Mudge, Jr., G.H., & Selwyn, A. (1989). Effect of smoking on the activity of ischemic heart disease. *Journal of the American Medical Association, 3*, 398–401.

Benowitz, N.L., Hall, S.M., Herning, R.I., Jacob, III, P., Jones, R.T., et al. (1983). *New England Journal of Medicine, 309*, 139–142.

Bickel, W.K., Stitzer, M.L., Bigelow, G.E., Liebson, I.A., Jasinski, D.R., & Johnson, R.E. (1988). Buprenorphine: Dose-related blockade of opioid challenge effects in opioid-dependent subjects. *Journal of Pharmacology and Experimental Therapeutics, 247*, 47–53.

Bolla, K.I., McCann, U.D., & Ricaurte, G.A. (1998). Memory impairment in abstinent MDMA ("Ecstasy") users. *Neurology, 51*, 1532–1537.

Busto, U., Sellers, E.M., Naranjo, C.A., Cappell, H., Sanchez-Craig, M., & Sykora, K. (1986). Withdrawal reaction after long-term therapeutic use of benzodiazepines. *New England Journal of Medicine, 313*, 854–859.

Chang, L., Ernst, T., Grob, C.S., & Poland, R.E. (1999). Cerebral (1)H MRS alterations in recreational 3,4-methylene-dioxymethamphetamine (MDMA, "ecstasy") users. *Journal of Magnetic Resonance, 10*, 521–526.

Chen, J.H., & Goldstein, D.B. (1976). *Science, 196*, 684–685.

Cloninger, C.R., Dinwiddie, S.H., & Reich, T. (1989). Epidemiology and genetics of alcoholism. *Annual Review of Psychiatry, 8*, 331–346.

Cohen, S. (1982). Marijuana and youth: Clinical observations on motivation and learning, ages 2–11. Washington, D.C.: U.S. Government Printing Office.

Colado, M.I., Granados, R., O'Shea, C., Esteban, B., & Green, A.R. (1999). The acute effect in rats of 3,4-methylene-dioxyethamphetamine (MDEA, "Eve") on body temperature and long-term degeneration of 5HT neurones in brain: A comparison with MDMA ("Ecstasy"). *Pharmacology and Toxicology, 84*, 261–266.

Daderman, A.M., & Lidberg, L. (1999a). Flunitrazepam (Rohypnol) abuse in combination with alcohol causes premeditated grievous violence in male juvenile offenders. *J. Am. Acad. Psychiatry Law, 27*, 83–99.

Daderman, A., & Lidberg, L. (1999b) Rohypnol should be classified as a narcotic. *Lakartidningen, 96*, 1005–1007.

de la Torre, R., Farre, M., Roset, P.N., Hernandez Lopez, C., Mas, M., Ortuno, J., Menoyo, E., Pizarro, N., Segura, J., & Cami, J. (2000). Pharmacology of MDMA in humans. *Annals New York Academy of Sciences, 914*, 225–237.

Edwards, G., Arif, A., & Hodgson, R. (1981). Nomenclature and classification of drug and alcohol-related problems: A WHO memorandum. *Bulletin WHO, 59*, 225–242.

Ellinwood, E.H. (1979). In R.I. Dupont, A. Goldstein, & J. O'Donnell (Eds.), *Handbook on drug abuse* (pp. 221–231). Washington, D.C.: U.S. Government Printing Office.

Fielding, J.E. (1985). *New England Journal of Medicine, 313*, 555–561.

Fischman, M.W. (1987). Cocaine and the amphetamines. In H.Y. Meltzer (Ed.), *Psychopharmacology: The third generation of progress*. New York: Raven Press.

Gerra, G., Zaimovic, A., Giucastro, G., Maestri, D., Monica, C., Sartori, R., Caccavari, R., & Delsignore, R. (1998). Serotonergic function after (+/-) 3,4-methylene-dioxymethamphetamine ("Ecstasy") in humans. *International Clinical Psychopharmacology, 13*, 1–9.

Glennon, R.A. (1987). Psychoactive phenylisopropylamines. In H.Y. Meltzer (Ed.), *Psychopharmacology: The third generation of progress* (pp. 1627–1634). New York: Raven Press.

Grant, I. (1987). Alcohol in the brain: Neuropsychological correlates. *Journal of Consulting and Clinical Psychology, 55*, 310–324.

Griffiths, R.R., & Sannerud, C.A. (1987). Abuse of and dependence on benzodiazepines and other anxiolytic-sedative drugs. In H.Y. Meltzer (Ed.). *Psychopharmacology: The third generation of progress* (pp. 1535–1541). New York: Raven Press.

Hanson, G.R., Jensen, M., Johnson, M., & White, H.S., Distinct features of seizures induced by cocaine and amphetamine analogs. *European Journal of Pharmacology, 377*, 167–173.

Harrington, R.D., Woodward, J.A., Hooton, T.M., & Horn, J.R. (1999). Life-threatening interactions between HIV-1 protease inhibitors and the illicit drugs MDMA and gamma-hydroxybutyrate. *Archives of Internal Medicine, 159*, 2221–2224.

Heishman, S.J., Stitzer, M.L., Bigelow, G.E., & Liebson, I.A. (1989). Acute opioid physical dependence in post-addict humans: Naloxone dose effects after brief morphine exposure. *Journal of Pharmacology and Experimental Therapeutics, 248*, 127–134.

Huxley, A. (1970). *The doors of perception*. New York: Perennial Library.

Jaffe, J.H. (1989). Psychoactive substance use disorders. In H.D. Kaplan & B.J. Saddock (Eds.). *The comprehensive textbook of psychiatry*, 5th ed. (pp. 642–686). New York: McMillan.

Jaffe, J.H. (1990). Drug addiction and drug abuse. In A.G. Gilman, E. Goodman, T.W. Rall, & F. Murad (Eds.), *The pharmacological basis of therapeutics*, 8th ed. (pp. 522–573). New York: MacMillan.

Jansen, K.L.R. (1999). Ecstasy (MDMA) dependence, *Drug and Alcohol Dependency, 53*, 121–124.

Johanson, C.E., & Schuster, C.R. (1991). Animal models of drug self-administration. In N.K. Mello (Ed.), *Advances in substance abuse: Behavioral and biological research* (pp. 219–297). Greenwich, CT: JAI Press.

Jones, R.T. (1987). Tobacco dependence. In H.Y. Meltzer (Ed.), *Psychopharmacology: The third generation of progress* (pp. 1589–1595). New York: Raven Press.

Klein, E., Uhde, T.W., & Post, R.M. (1986). Preliminary evidence for the utility of carbamazepine in alprazolam withdrawal. *American Journal of Psychiatry, 143*, 235–236.

Kreek, M.J. (1987). Multiple drug abuse patterns and medical consequences. In H.Y. Meltzer (Ed.), *Psychopharmacology: The third generation of progress* (pp. 1597–1604). New York: Raven Press.

Langston, J.W., Ballard, P., Tetrud, J.W., & Irwin, I. (1983). Chronic Parkinsonism in humans due to a product of meperidine-analog synthesis. *Science, 219*(4587), 979–980.

Liljequist, S., Culp, S., & Tabakoff, B. (1986). *Life Sciences, 38*, 1931–1939.

Luthin, G.R., & Tabakoff, B. (1984). *Journal of Pharmacology and Experimental Therapeutics, 228*, 579–587.

Marks, M.J., Smolen, A., & Collins, A.C. (1984). *Alcoholism Clinical and Experimental Research, 8*, 390–396.

Martin, P.R., Kapur, B.M., Whiteside, E.A., & Sellers, E.M. (1979). *Clinical Pharmacology and Therapeutics, 26*, 256–264.

Mello, N.K. (1987). Alcohol abuse and alcoholism: 1978–1987. In H.Y. Meltzer (Ed.), *Psychopharmacology: The third generation of progress* (pp. 1515–1520). New York: Raven Press.

Mello, N.K., & Griffiths, R.R. (1987). Alcoholism and drug abuse: An overview. In H.Y. Meltzer (Ed.), *Psychopharmacology: The third generation of progress* (pp. 1511–1514). New York: Raven Press.

Mello, N.K., & Mendelson, J.H. (1980). *Science, 207,* 657–659.

Meltzer, H.Y. (Ed.) (1987). *Psychopharmacology: The third generation of progress.* New York: Raven Press.

Mendelson, J.H. (1987). Marijuana. In H.Y. Meltzer (Ed.), *Psychopharmacology: The third generation of progress* (pp. 1565–1571). New York: Raven Press.

Mendelson, J.H., & Mello, N.K. (1979). Biologic concomitants of alcoholism. *New England Journal of Medicine, 301,* 912–921.

Meyer, H.H. (1901). *Archives of Experimental Pathology and Pharmacology, 46,* 338–346.

Milroy, C.M., Clark, J.C., & Forrest, A.R.W. (1996). Pathology of deaths associated with "ecstasy" and "eve" misuse. *Journal of Clinical Pathology, 49,* 149–153.

Myers, J.K., Weissman, M.M., Tischler, G.L., Holzer, C.E., Leaf, P.J., et al. (1984). *Archives of General Psychiatry,* pp. 959–967.

Nishisawa, S., Mzengeza, S., & Diksic, M. (1999). Acute effects of 3,4-methylenedioxymethamphetamine on brain serotonin synthesis in the dog studies by positron emission tomography. *Neurochemistry International, 34,* 33–40.

O'Malley, P.N., Johnston, L.D., & Bachman, J.G. (1985). In N.J. Kozel & E.H. Adams (Eds.). *Cocaine use in America: Epidemiologic and clinical perspectives* (NIDA Research Monograph, 1961). Washington, D.C.: U.S. Government Printing Office.

Orleans, C.T. (1985). Annual reviews. In W.P. Creger (Ed.), *Annual Review of Medicine* (pp. 51–61). Palo Alto, CA:

Parrott, A.C. & Lasky, J. (1998). Ecstasy (MDMA) effects upon mood and cognition: Before, during and after a Saturday night dance. *Psychopharmacology* (Berlin), *139,* 261–268.

Perlman, B.J., & Goldstein, D.B. (1984). *Molecular Pharmacology, 26,* 547–552.

Peroutka, S.J. (1987). Incidence of recreational use of 3,4-methylenedimethoxymethamphetamine (MDMA, "Ecstasy") on an undergraduate campus (Letter). *New England Journal of Medicine, 317*(24), 1542–1543.

Post, R.M. (1977). In E.H. Elloinwood & M.N. Kilbey (Eds.), *Cocaine and other stimulants* (pp. 353–372). New York: Plenum Press.

Rath, D., & Vever, J. (1998). Poisoning in patients treated during 4 years at the Metabolic Unit of the Second Internal Medicine Clinic of the Charles University Medical School in Prague, *Vnitr Lek, 44,* 654–657.

Raymon, L.P., Steele, B.W., & Walls, H.C. (1999). Benzodiazepines in Miami-Dade County, Florida driving under the influence (DUI) cases (1995–8) with emphasis on Rohypnol: GC-MS confirmation, patterns of use, psychomotor impairment, and results of Florida legislation. *Journal of Analytical Toxicology, 23,* 490–499.

Ries, R.K., Roy-Burne, P.P., Ward, N.G., et al. (1989). Carbamazepine treatment for benzodiazepine withdrawal. *American Journal of Psychiatry, 146,* 536–537.

Robins, L.N., Helzer, J.E., Weissman, M.M., Orvaschel, H., Gruenberg, E., et al. (1984). *Archives of General Psychiatry, 41,* 949–958.

Reuters Health Information Services, 10-27-2000, Deaths linked to 1,4-butanediol, a precursor to rave party drug GHB

Saper, J.R., & Jones, J.M. (1986). Ergotamine tartrate dependency: Features and possible mechanisms. *Clinical Pharmacology, 9,* 244–256.

Saum, C.A., & Inciardi, J.A. (1997). Rohypnol misuse in the United States. *Substance Use and Misuse, 32,* 723–731.

Schuckit, M.A. (1987). Biology of risk for alcoholism. In H.Y. Meltzer (Ed.), *Psychopharmacology: The third generation of progress* (pp. 1527–1533). New York: Raven Press.

Sprague, J.E., Everman, S.L., & Nichols, D.E. (1998). An integrated hypothesis for the serotonergic axonal loss induced by 3,4-methylenedioxymethamphetamine. *Neurotoxicology, 19,* 427–442.

Schwartz, R.H., Milteer, R., & LeBeau, M.A. (2000). Drug-facilitated sexual assault ("date rape"). *Southern Medical Journal, 93,* 558–561.

Tabakoff, B., & Hoffman, P.L. (1983). *Life Sciences, 32,* 192–204.

Tabakoff, B., & Hoffman, P.L. (1987). Biochemical pharmacology of alcohol. In H.Y. Meltzer (Ed.), *Psychopharmacology: The third generation of progress* (pp. 1521–1526). New York: Raven Press.

Tunnicliff, G. (1997). Sites of action of gamma-hydroxybutyrate (GHB) — A neuroactive drug with abuse potential. *Clinical Toxicology, 35,* 581–590.

Velea, D., Hautefeuille, M., & Vazeille, G. (1999). Lantran-Davoux, C., New synthesis empathogenic agents. *Encephale, 25,* 508–514.

Weil, A. (1972). *The natural mind: A new way of looking at drugs and the higher consciousness.* Boston: Houghton Mifflin.

Wickler, A. (1980). *Opioid dependence: Mechanisms and treatment.* New York: Plenum Press.

Woods, J.H., & Winger, G. (1987). Opioids, receptors, and abuse liability. In H.Y. Meltzer (Ed.), *Psychopharmacology: The third generation of progress* (pp. 1555–1564). New York: Raven Press.

Woods, J.H., Katz, J.L., & Winger, G. (1987). Abuse liability of benzodiazepines. *Pharmacological Reviews, 39,* 251–419.

Young, A., & Herling, S. (1986). Drugs as reinforcers: Studies in laboratory animals. In S.R. Goldberg & I.P. Stolerman (Eds.), *Behavioral analysis of drug dependence* (pp. 9–67). New York: Academic Press.

Young, G.S.J., Longstaffe, S., & Tenenbein, M. (1999). Inhalant abuse and the abuse of other drugs, *American Journal of Drug and Alcohol Abuse, 25,* 371–375.

MONOGRAPHS AND GENERAL REFERENCES

American Medical News, April 1982, p. 22.

American Psychiatric Association. (1987). Diagnostic and statistical manual of mental disorders (3rd ed.). Washington, D.C.: American Psychiatric Association.

American Psychiatric Association Publications (1990). Benzodiazepine dependence, toxicity, and abuse: A task force report of the American Psychiatric Association. Washington, D.C.: American Psychiatric Association.

Bloom, F.E. (1989). Neurobiology of alcohol action in alcoholism. *Annual Review of Psychiatry, 8,* 347–360.

Gilman, A.G., Goodman, E., Rall, T.W., & Murad, F. (Eds.). (1990). *Pharmacological basis of therapeutics* (8th ed.). New York: MacMillan.

Kaplan, H.D., & Saddock, B.J. (Eds.). (1988). *Synopsis of psychiatry, behavioral sciences, and clinical psychiatry: Psychoactive substance disorders* (5th ed.). Baltimore: Williams & Wilkins.

Kaplan, H.D., & Saddock, B.J. (Eds.) (1989). *Comprehensive textbook of psychiatry* (5th ed.). Baltimore: Williams & Wilkins.

National Institute on Drug Abuse (1983). Highlights from the national survey on drug abuse: 1982. U.S. Department of HHS-DHS-ADAMHA (DHHS Publ. [ADM] 83-1277). Washington, D.C.: U.S. Government Printing Office.

Raskin, N.H. (1988). *Headache* (2nd ed.). Edinburgh: Churchill Livingstone.

Stahl, S.M. (2000). *Essential psychopharmacology — Neuroscientific basis and practical applications* (2nd ed.). Cambridge: Cambridge University Press.

—71—

A Multi-Systems Approach to Behavioral Health and Pain Management

Richard H. Cox, M.D., Ph.D., D.Min.

This chapter approaches behavioral health from a systems point of view rather than the more traditional behavioral medical designation, because it is important to identify with a larger body of information and practice than simply that of medicine. Further, the usual connotation of "multi-disciplinary" is not used because that labeling implies the utilization of skills of more than one professional discipline. Each discipline is more than a body of knowledge and an accumulation of skills. We live in a world of systems. Sociologists recognize at least six such systems: the social system, the political system, the economic system, the educational system, the religious system, and the domestic system. In addition and in permutations, other systems obviously exist as well.

A multi-systems approach to behavioral health allows the essence of many systems to impact the immediate situation. In this discussion we are concerned with the problem of pain management. Any one system offers partial answers; however, in many, perhaps most instances, even several systems offer less than complete answers. It is only in the understanding of multiple systems that we can even begin to understand the complex and vexing problems of pain. However, only the multi-system approach offers the patient and the practitioner a method for dealing with what will frequently be less than what either had hoped would eventuate. It is not only the involvement of several different disciplines working together on a healing team; it is the inherent philosophy, attitude, expectations, modeling, spiritual depth, and many more contributions of each participant. It is the value of

whole systems within a holistic context that allows the team to transcend the skills of the individual's discipline and reach into the depths of who each is as a healing person and who the patient is who wishes to be healed.

The purpose of this chapter is not to be definitive in any area, but rather to further the holistic gestalt of the healing enterprise. Healing is both an art and a science, with no one discipline capable of claiming ownership to any larger part than any other discipline. In the most precise definition of healing, all disciplines and techniques are only adjunctive to the person who has the pain. Healing comes from within the organism, not from the technique or system providing the knowledge. All modalities, disciplines, and specialties assist in the process. More often than not, therapies speed the healing process, help the body's systems to sort out their own mechanisms for repair, and stop any further progress of inflammation, infection, and degeneration. Rarely, if ever, is it possible to designate the specific therapy that single-handedly produced the results.

When the outcome of a diagnosis and treatment is positive, all disciplines stand in line to accept the credit; when the outcome is less than desirable, it is difficult to find a discipline that will accept responsibility. The concept of "turf ownership" by professional disciplines has been a serious detriment to finding methods for the management of pain. Turf ownership has meant economic and power brokerage; hence, the needs of human suffering have been sacrificed because of the unwillingness of the healing disciplines to share their knowledge, admit that

0-8493-0926-3/02/$0.00+$1.50
© 2002 by CRC Press LLC

they have a limited area of knowledge, and work with other professionals in a collegial fashion.

The concept of "systems" is crucial in that every healing philosophy builds upon a system that supports both the ideation and the practice of that particular approach. For instance, Western medicine works within a system that has become highly technical, political, and costly. As in all such healing-art systems, it is not possible to change only one part without disrupting the entire system. Sometimes it is easier and more effective to introduce a third player to integrate, sort out, and use parts of multiple systems as needed to arrive at a desired end. Alternative approaches to healthcare are the third party in human suffering at this time. The combination of many systems formerly not admitted into the healing-art circle have forced Western medicine to examine its system. Further, and probably more importantly, medical practice in the United States has been forced to listen to patients who are no longer willing to trust and pay for the one-system approach.

Eastern as well as Western, and all other healing systems, are steeped in cultural determinants that are not easily changed. Folk medicine systems are bound in a history all their own. The behavioral health system approach allows for picking and choosing from many systems rather than ascribing to any one system in its entirety. However, in order for this to happen, the team leader and all participants must allow themselves a professional degree of freedom and have a healthy enough personal ego to withstand the criticism that can be expected from their more system-bound colleagues.

There is no intent in this writing to deny or diminish the valuable contributions of all disciplines to the process of attaining and maintaining health. However, all health, both the attaining and retaining of such, is in the final analysis "behavioral." The patient who will not think positively, eat responsibly, exercise adequately, comply with health provider prescriptions, and at least to a minimal extent take charge of his/her own life, cannot hope to attain health. By the same token, disciplines that by overt or covert action limit patients to one practice of healing may be potentially harmful. Disciplines that do not recognize the behavioral aspects of health and healing sacrifice their patients' health to the ego of their profession. The simple fact that all disciplines rely upon their patients to be compliant demonstrates the foundation and essential nature of behavior as the primary basis for healing.

Western healing arts have been very slow to recognize the behavioral aspects of health and healing. Eastern systems recognized them and built behavioral components into their healing systems thousands of years ago. The difference lies within the focus of the art. Western healing has focused upon the techniques and abilities of the healer. The patient has been an object that was given pills, operated on, treated, etc. Eastern healing has always been a philosophy first and techniques second. Western healing has emphasized techniques to the near dismissal of philosophy. Only several thousands of years later and in the light of increased technology and failed healing have Western healers (particularly allopathic physicians) been willing to incorporate the behavioral aspects of healing into their practices.

In truth, the majority of medical practitioners still do not incorporate the psychological, environmental, sociological, spiritual, and behavioral components of life into their practices. The name of the game in current Western medicine is "referral," thus further segmenting the body and the mind from the spirit. The patient is left to integrate what differing specialists have prescribed, but ostensibly none of them practices. It is not uncommon for a patient to be tangled in a web of many specialists and suffering from polypharmacy and tremendous confusion, as well as his or her basic illness. Although each specialist is highly trained, each operates within the same system; thus, the patient does not escape the single-system approach even when seeking a second opinion or changing physicians.

Many methods and disciplines that deal with pain exist but are not always administered within the medical system and do not necessarily follow the medical model. Behavioral medicine was originated by L. Birk in 1973 in relation to biofeedback. In 1977 the term was further canonized at the Yale Conference on Behavioral Medicine. The seminal work of Wilbert Fordyce (cf. Fordyce, 1976), utilizing operant conditioning and building on the historical work of Pavlov and Skinner, led the way for understanding the psychological underpinnings and emotional interactions of pain. Behavioral health is used in this discussion to emphasize an even larger concept, namely, that behavior is the key to any and all pain management programs. Understanding the interdisciplinary approach to pain means integrating all management around the firm acceptance that behavior is the major principle regardless of the technique or theoretical approach. Three major innovations sparked the beginning of modern pain theory: behavior modification, neuromodulation, and psycho-neuroimmunology.

The Western world is now ready and requesting another innovation. Healing as practiced in this generation has proven that even with the remarkable advancements of medical technology and scientific interventions, the majority of the population cannot avail themselves of these benefits. Cost factors, bureaucracy, mismanaged care, and inattention to the inner person have made modern healing a vocational trade rather than a professional practice. Increasingly we have machines, laboratories, and technicians to do what professional practitioners formerly did. No one can say that medical science has not advanced. One can, and must say, that medical practice has become less face-to-face patient oriented. Thus, the behavioral component of practice has suffered tremendously. Patients no longer benefit from the wisdom of an experienced practitioner, but are subjected to the statistical, actuarial, third-party pay organizations, whose basic interest is not in health but in profit.

The behavioral component of healing builds upon the concept that healing is much more extensive and deeper than solving the immediate problem of pain or dysfunction. Most ailments and complaints are not the health/illness issue itself but rather the results of that issue. Therefore, relieving symptoms doubtless decreases suffering but may not in truth bring about actual healing. In a multi-systems approach symptoms are seen as the results of dysfunction, not the dysfunction. Therefore, healing is much more than the alleviation of symptoms.

To unite the behavioral elements of healing would require a transformation of the Western mind, and a willingness to subrogate financial gain to the betterment of the individual. Social systems, philosophical ideation, teaching methods, curriculum renovations, administrative approaches, and far more than can be discussed in this short chapter will be needed to allow behavioral systems to bring together what they could and should do. The art and science of medicine in Western thought do not allow for the broadest holistic approach to healing. Larry Dossey, M.D. has helped us to see that healing at its deepest level is primarily behavioral and secondarily technique based (see Dossey, 1993).

We now await a marriage of the marvelous technology of healing to our knowledge of human persons as spiritual beings. Such a union could indeed bring the science and art of healing together. Actually, some small signs of this happening exist in isolated instances. In some places teams of healers are working together within a much more egalitarian system rather than in a pyramidal system with a physician at the top giving orders to the subordinates on the staff. Where systems exist with one profession "on the top," the obvious and practiced approach is that one part of the human is more important than others. It is true that in an emergency situation the hemorrhage must be stopped to save the patient's life; however, if the patient has no will to live, it may all be to no avail.

Relieving pain and building, maintaining, and restoring health belong to many different disciplines. Likewise, dealing with the pain that accompanies human existence is the bailiwick of many professions. Human pain can be classified as physical, emotional/behavioral, and spiritual/existential. This chapter primarily addresses only the emotional/behavioral and the spiritual/existential.

Some of the major professions that most directly assume care for these areas are

- Psychologists
- Psychiatrists
- Social workers
- Counselors
- Marriage/family therapists
- Clergy

Although there are many practitioners of varied sorts within these groups, and some that do not easily fit into any group, for the most part, the mainline professions dealing with human pain of a nonphysical sort are those listed.

Likewise, there are more kinds of intervention than could be listed in a reasonable chapter; however, most treatment modalities dealing with nonphysical pain (and often physical pain) are

- Pharmacology
- Psychotherapy/counseling
- Biofeedback
- Hypnosis/relaxation/guided imagery
- Desensitization
- Group process
- Psychodrama
- Psychoeducation
- Bibliotherapy
- Marriage/family therapy
- Pastoral care
- Social work interventions
- Alternative approaches (see the *Encyclopedia of Alternative Medicine*)

By far the most prevalent current method for controlling human behavior and any resultant pain (both physical and emotional) is medication. Although the profession best trained to manage psychopharmacology is psychiatry, the overwhelming preponderance of psychotropic medications are prescribed by nonpsychiatrist physicians. Clinical psychologists (trained in recent years) are very well equipped to manage psychotropic medication. However, even though the literature is replete regarding the superior efficacy of combined psychotherapy with psychopharmacology, few psychiatrists continue to practice psychotherapy today. In the not-too-distant past psychiatrists practiced both prescriptive medicine and psychotherapy. Psychologists, who are doubtless the broadest-trained professionals in the area of human emotions, and who do continue to practice psychotherapy, are as yet unable to prescribe. Doubtless this fact will change as public knowledge and demand reveal the benefits of the psychologist as a single behavioral practitioner, who can provide both psychotherapy and medication as well as have the skills to work within many healing systems. Now that psychiatry has moved into other areas, largely medicating the severely mentally ill, the masses of persons needing assistance with the emotional problems of normal living are left without a single service source.

This leaves the management of human emotional pain split among numerous professionals to deal with a single emotional problem. Depression, probably the most prevalent of all mental illnesses, is illustrative of this point. The psychiatrist prescribes an antidepressant medication and may or may not refer for psychotherapy, and the psychologist provides psychotherapy and may or may not refer for medication.

Psychiatry is best described divided into three areas. Behavioral psychiatry attempts to deal with emotional pain by combining psychotherapy with medication, with the emphasis on psychotherapy and medication as an adjunctive support. Organic psychiatry manages primarily with psychotropic medications, usually without psychotherapy, while placing the emphasis upon neurochemistry. A third area of modern psychiatry, cosmetic psychiatry, actively attempts to modify the personality and the behaviors resultant therefrom entirely by psychoactive agents (see Hedaya, 1996).

A well-rounded, holistic, human-attentive discipline does not exist. The well-trained clinical psychologist is doubtless the closest to such a model. The clinical psychologist who has been trained in a practitioner-oriented model program is knowledgeable of social systems, learning systems, family systems, biological/physiological systems, psychopharmacological systems, a wide variety of diagnostic systems, and a broad spectrum of treatment systems. Such a well-trained professional still needs to be incorporated within the team rather than attempting to be "all things to all people."

We need to clarify the difference between health and healing. Behavioral approaches have value in attaining and maintaining health. They also have a valuable place in the role of healing. Most health professionals are, in truth, mostly practicing symptom relief, i.e., a part of the healing process. Behavioral practitioners, of course, at times also practice only small parts of the process. However, the literature shows that they are much more prone to refer their patients for the benefits of other disciplines than vice versa.

Although patients dealing with physical pain frequently expect to need the services of more than one health service provider, in the realm of emotional pain, relatively few patients expect that they will need the services of more than one provider. Further, relatively few patients receive the services they need in the treatment of mental illness. Physicians under-utilize psychologists for psychotherapy and psychologists under-utilize physicians for medical management. Recent changes in insurance-based medical practice have prohibited many of the referral benefits previously practiced and which practitioners of all kinds would like to continue to afford their patients.

The changing field of training and practice, combined with the evolving landscape of healthcare, is producing dramatic and traumatic changes. As has been noted, psychiatry has virtually abandoned psychotherapy. Psychologists are now trained in psychopharmacology and may soon have prescription privileges. The American Psychological Association at the 1996 Convention in Toronto, Canada endorsed moving toward prescription privileges for psychologists, and five states are currently entertaining potential legislation.

All healing professions are evolving and only the future will tell us which professions will practice certain specific methods. Most of the helping professions are branching out into areas previously practiced by other disciplines, and more and more there is doubt about the essential training needed for the practice of specific modalities. It seems that turf-building and turf-maintenance have been more important than the actual professional expertise required for the application of a specific modality.

For instance, social workers and counselors are including methods of treatment, such as hypnosis, and the use of psychological tests into their practices that were once believed to be the domain of psychology and psychiatry. Optometrists now prescribe medications, opticians are vying for the right to do refractions and, in some instances, are performing opthalmological functions not previously allowed. Nurses routinely prescribe pharmacologic agents with physician supervision that is sometimes very minimal. Pharmacists are moving toward prescription authority, opticians are gearing up for doing vision examinations, psychologists are now training for psychotropic prescriptive practice, and use of nurse midwives is no longer debated in many communities. In many settings, registered nurse practitioners are for all practical purposes today's family doctors. Physical therapists do spinal adjustments and joint manipulation, once the turf of the chiropractor. Most of these, and many more changes did not take place because of training, but rather grew out of need, economics, and political desires. In some instances, mainline medical practitioners were unwilling to provide services to underprivileged and rural populations.

In most instances, the practice began before the formalized education and training. Educational programs and certification followed the establishment of the practice. Such was the history of midwives. In a similar instance, patients were shown to benefit from manipulation; however, chiropractors were not allowed on hospital staffs. Physical therapists were already on the staff and respected practitioners in their field. Manipulation was a "natural" and with training (sometimes quite minimal) manipulative/adjustment techniques were introduced. Many more illustrations of how patient need has permitted and even mandated changes in the health service system exist. The purpose of noting these changes, and the many not mentioned, is that the pain management not only does not belong to one profession, but also nearly every profession is currently undergoing a tremendous metamorphosis in order to encompass more and more of the problem of human pain.

We must recognize that in the final analysis, it is behavior that counts in society. Humans have illnesses all of the time, but society is usually concerned only when behavior is impacted by pain and/or suffering. Different ages held forth different expectations for what was considered normal health. Furthermore, cultures, ethnicities, and even gender demand and allow differences in what is considered normal. Behavior is the key. It is the key to what is considered acceptable and when the patient changes geographic location, religious beliefs, or even jobs, what is acceptable may change. Although we as individuals may care how others feel, in truth, we as society really only care about how people act, and more specifically, how that action affects us as individuals.

In the final analysis, behavioral health is exactly that: behavioral health. Changing behavior can be done in a variety of ways. Sometimes behavioral changes come about due to internal thought process reorganizations. Other times the changes are due only to social demand and we behave in a given way to avoid the unpleasantness of society's reaction to us. At other times, changes in behavior come about due to physical and/or mental changes of a structural nature, e.g., the loss of a limb or the result of brain (or other) surgery. The most effective behavioral change occurs when the individual has reasoned through his/her actions and by cognitive choice has determined to act differently regardless of how he or she might feel or think.

Personality type and parameters of known past behavior are important indices to the adaptation, use/misuse, and eventual outcome of illness. Although the astute interviewing clinician may have excellent clues and insight into these factors, even with short- or long-term observation, psychological assessment utilizing validated psychological tests is the best single method to obtain documentation for diagnosis and intervention in the behavioral aspects of pain management. It was Hippocrates himself who said, "It is more important to know what sort of person has a disease than to know what sort of disease a person has" (quoted from *Alternative Medicine*, 1995).

Human behavior, including the management of pain, is best influenced by cognitive choices. The compliant, cooperative, consciously participating patient is certainly the best patient for helping find solutions. All professions have recognized the value of cognitive intervention in behavior.

Thus, one common thread prevails throughout almost all the professions, and that is counseling of some sort. The difference is whether the counseling is incidental (as in the case of most medical management) or primary (as in the case of psychotherapy).

In most instances, pain cannot be effectively managed apart from patient cooperation. As we do not have accurate methods to measure pain objectively, it is possible for the physical cause of the pain to be removed and for the patient to continue to report its presence. At differing times in our history, we have identified psychosomatic, somatopsychic, allodynic, histrionic, and other forms of pain that medical science could not diagnose by laboratory or physical examination. Finally, most practitioners now recognize that the single most valuable measurement of pain is that reported by the patient, regardless of what the tests may show. Thus, the labels ascribed to various pain experiences are not important. Behavior intervention is, because it starts with the patient's experience and ends with the patient's experience.

Behavioral health systems offer the most effective methods for "entering the patient's experience" and helping the patient to move out of it. Further, it is rarely possible to determine what aspect of treatment actually produced the result. Many practitioners have found that the techniques psychotherapists believe were helpful and what patients report were actually helpful are often very different. Although this type of dilemma makes statistically controlled research difficult, patient benefits are without doubt.

Behavioral health systems work best within a team setting. The reason they are spoken of as "systems" is that each professional entity recognizes that the combination of several disciplines is greater than the sum of the parts. Pain management when left to disciplines that practice in isolation leaves the patient as the coach of the team and often as the untrained captain of his or her pain. The patient is certainly primary and must be central to the planning and implementation of any pain management program; however, pain management given to a team practice combines the best of several disciplines, includes the patient, and equally important, provides a constant quality control check on the total treatment.

Whether the treatment method is problem-solving counseling, insight-producing psychotherapy, or psychoneuroimmunology, the behaviorally oriented practitioner will insist upon:

1. A thorough and complete history of the patient, including, but not limited to, the pain syndrome. This encompasses religious and spiritual aspects, developmental landmarks and difficulties, emotional problems, family concerns, social history, medical history, occupational history, family systems, and at times a genogram, as well as numerous other informational items that arise in the course of taking a complete history. (Few practitioners obtain a careful, complete history, particularly in the patient's own words rather only than from a preprinted form.)

2. The patient's pre-morbid and morbid personality. Frequently, psychological testing combined with the social history and a careful initial interview

provide these data. Psychological testing is the most cost-effective method for obtaining information of this nature. The Beck Depression Scale, The Hardiness Scale, the 16PF, The Minnesota Multiphasic Personality Inventory, The California Personality Inventory, the Edwards Personal Preference Schedule, and many more tests can be utilized to assess the personality. Those mentioned are considered "pencil and paper" type. Other specific tests are known as "projective techniques," such as the Rorschach Psychodiagnostic Test, the Thematic Apperception Test, Kinetic Drawing tests, and others. Tests in trained hands show how personality factors may be of value in understanding the etiology, process, and treatment of pain. Psychologists are helpful in understanding the meaning of pain, the secondary gains of pain, and the perceived purpose of the pain in a patient. The patient's perception is imperative. Pain, after all, is measured by the patient's perception. Without understanding how the patient perceives his or her world, the treatment of pain may only be a laboratory experiment. The reader is encouraged to review the discussion by Materson in this book.

3. The medical/physical/laboratory examination and diagnosis. Care needs to be given to other than routine blood, urine, and fecal tests. Routine tests frequently provide routine results. Physicians tend to be skeptical of some of the newer alternative-type diagnostic procedures. Further, an old axiom in medicine is still true: "We will not find it, if we don't remember to look for it." Persons with chronic pain usually have been through every routine test known and every common disease entity has been explored. The alternative practitioner often is successful when the traditional one is not because other avenues are being explored and tests considered by the general medical community as out-in-left-field are being pursued. A patient was recently referred to one practitioner who was two years post-CVA with residual hemiparesis and significant depression. Prozac and other SSRI mediations were part of her polypharmacological management by a variety of physicians of different specialties, but her condition was worsening. The use of her right arm and leg was only slightly better after two years of physical therapy, and her depression was severe and sometimes suicidal. Psychotherapy combined with auricular acupuncture produced dramatic results very quickly as two

practitioners worked together. Medications were brought into reasonable control, and her mood was stabilized, with only minor episodic depressions. She is now opening doors with her previously paralyzed hand, utilizing prehensile grasp, and remarkably improved in overall social functioning. She, as well as her primary care physicians, were afraid of trying alternative approaches. Dr. Norman Shealy's book, *Miracles Do Happen* (1995), testifies to the effectiveness of alternative approaches to pain management.

4. Collaborative interviews and networking for diagnostic and treatment information and patient support. No individual practitioner can offer sufficient help in the limited time available. The family (and at times other networking persons) needs to be seen as a primary resource for support. This means family education, inclusion in the treatment plans, in the actual in-home treatment, and follow-up. Pawlicki discusses the role of the family elsewhere is this book. In primitive societies, the patient's family actually assisted the nursing, dietary, and housekeeping staff in hospitals. The emotional, hence healing, support given to the patient is clearly beneficial, to say nothing of the cost factor.

5. The willingness to experiment with different approaches. No one method of treatment suffices for all patients. Practitioners who are unwilling to entertain new ideas and new methods become disappointed in results. Patients who are unfortunately stuck with such practitioners suffer from stagnation and closed-minded thinking.

6. The emotional/existential aspects of human pain frequently require a deeply spiritual intervention. Although it does not require a clergyperson, frequently a clergyperson trusted by the patient can make early interventions very effectively. Rituals, symbols, and highly personal spiritual actions often produce healing. Further, every person has his or her own interpretation of the meaning of pain and why it is being endured. When a patient believes that pain is inflicted by God and must be endured for heavenly reward, it is very difficult to allow anyone to take away the pain and hence take away the reward for faithful endurance!

7. Last, but far from least, listen to the patient. Early labeling does not help. Considering a patient psychosomatic is of no value. Early correct diagnosis is obviously of major importance;

however, we must not lose sight of the many times that the early diagnosis is wrong, but a plan of treatment is in place and not easily interrupted to look for another diagnosis. Because pain is perceived, and perception is reality to the patient, only the patient can tell the practitioner what hurts, what is wrong, and frequently what needs to be done to correct it.

This is particularly true in regard to emotional pain. The concept of behavioral health systems includes the concept of the person as part of a system which includes the family, neighborhood, school, church, club, community organizations, and all other aspects of occupation, society, and the world with which they are closely linked. One cannot overemphasize that to treat the person is to treat the system. To attempt to treat the patient without reference to the system is to assume an overly powerful role and to think that the influence of a few minutes in the practitioner's office can overcome the influence of the many hours during the week with family, friends, and the community.

Sometimes patients must be allowed to live with their pain until they are ready to give it up. The practitioner should not feel discouraged or that he or she has failed when patients do not overcome pain. The reward is real for both the patient and practitioner when pain is relieved; however, if the practitioner is successful in truly entering the patient's world, and if the patient establishes a healthy relationship with the practitioner, healing has begun.

The meaning of the relationship must be underscored. Patients learn to trust when there is genuine caring. Patients know if they are being treated as a person. Transference and counter-transference cannot be avoided; they can only be controlled and utilized productively. Positive transference is to be encouraged. The misuse of the transference phenomenon, which produces a transgression of boundaries, has unfortunately led to "throwing out the baby with the bath." The behavioral health system includes the practitioner as an integral part of the system. The practitioner who wishes to be a technician cannot extend his or her own healing qualities. The patient will respond to a relationship with trust and will respond to a technician as to any machine.

Some therapists take pride in avoiding relationships. To think that one does so is only a figment of the imagination. Whenever two persons meet, let alone work together on pain, an automatic, unavoidable relationship is established. The question does not have to do with whether there will be a relationship; the question only has to do with whether it will be a positive, healing one or a negative, damaging one. Many practitioners employ the healing tools of their trade only to cancel out those benefits with their poor interpersonal relationship ability.

The more one studies psychoneuroimmunology, the more one is forced to recognize the spiritual aspects of healing, including the value and art of touch, attitude, transfer of energy, prayer, meditation, and truly wishing another well. Such aspects of healing are not possible within negative relationships. Researchers who have studied healing in other cultures have documented both the positive and negative effects of psychoneuroimmology as well as the effects of cultural expectation. Voodoo, shamanism, and other psychic manifestations of culture, religion, and ethnicity are not unreal because they are psychic. They are all the more real because they emphasize the underlying behavioral systems that produce and alleviate human suffering.

When behavioral health systems are encouraged to work in harmony, the outcome is always greater. To argue whether the physical pain produces the emotional or vice versa, as is sometimes discussed, is immaterial. It is only when the practitioners of all parts of the human dilemma join the same team that answers to the problem of human pain are found. Behavioral health systems are crucial in understanding, not necessarily explaining, the causes of pain. As part of these systems, the behavioral health scientist utilizes a vast array of techniques and is often the best-equipped professional to be the team leader.

Suffering and pain are not synonymous. We may be better able to assist with suffering than with pain. Persons at peace with themselves and those around them clearly suffer less when in pain than those who are not. Pain is reduced or increased by one's perception of suffering. The narcotics used for pain control are linked to physiology. Pain and suffering may or may not be linked at the same time and/or in the same way to physiology. Suffering may not be reduced simply by the alleviation of pain. Why humans suffer is an age-old question epitomized in the biblical book of Job and doubtless discussed long before that time. We do not hope for understanding of the philosophical, theological, existential, and other esoteric aspects of pain. We do, however, believe that although we may not know why we suffer, we can learn to suffer less and assist others in relieving at least some of their suffering. Suffering, as distinguished from pain, is a learned response, as is the lack of suffering. Suffering occurs both in the presence and the absence of pain. Behavioral responses are not always explainable; however, they may be understandable. We do need to remember that pain is many times a friend, in that without pain we could die without knowing we were even ill. Suffering has its values. The lack of suffering for some, and in some cultures, is in and of itself painful. To relieve one of suffering does not guarantee the relief of pain, nor does the relief of pain guarantee the relief of suffering.

Pain must also be seen as a disease entity in and of itself not simply the result of injury or illness. It is possible that at times pain is the illness. Pain disrupts, brings about dysfunction, produces further illness, and is far more than a combination of symptoms that could be classified as a syndrome. Pain, when diagnosed as a distinct illness, requires a full and complete behavioral and medical team to intervene. Frequently, until pain is seen as the illness rather than the results of an illness, permanent relief is not possible. When pain is recognized as the illness, behavioral approaches are mandatory in unraveling the mystery of pain and suffering.

REFERENCES

Anderson, U. (2000). *Immunology of the soul.* Winter Park, FL: Synchronicity Press.

Birk, L. (1973). *Biofeedback: Behavioral medicine* (p. 362). New York: Grune & Stratton.

Burton, Goldberg Group. (Compiled by). (1995). *Alternative medicine.* Fife, WA: Future Medicine Publishing.

Dossey, L. (1993). *Healing words.* New York: Harper.

Fordyce, W.E. (1976). *Behavioral methods for chronic pain and illness.* St. Louis: Mosby.

Hedaya, R. (1996). *Understanding biological psychiatry.* New York: Norton.

Shealy, C.N. (1995). *Miracles do happen.* Australia: Element Books.

Section X

Legal Considerations

Promoting Ethics and Objectivity in the Medicolegal Arena: Recommendations for Experts

Michael F. Martelli, Ph.D. and Nathan D. Zasler, M.D., F.A.A.P.M.&R., F.A.A.D.E.P., C.I.M.E., D.A.A.P.M.

INTRODUCTION

The skills required for conducting medicolegal evaluations too often exceed the expertise of the professional performing them. This certainly appears true in the personal injury arena, where promises of large financial settlements and higher forensic reimbursement rates have resulted in a proliferation of practitioners choosing this specialization. Too often, this occurs without having procured sufficient specific training in medicolegal evaluations and/or having demonstrated expertise in a clinical specialty independent of forensic practice. It is perhaps more so the case for chronic pain treatment providers who are frequently called into medicolegal proceedings as an incidental and sometimes undesirable consequence of routine clinical treatment.

Importantly, identifying and mitigating ethical conflicts that arise within the medicolegal arena present a formidable challenge for even the most skilled of forensic experts. Clinical training in medical and graduate schools has a customary and usually exclusive focus on training related to advocating for the patient's well-being. In independent examinations (IE) conducted within medicolegal contexts, the distinguishing feature is a requirement for objectivity that requires dissolution of the patient–doctor relationship in favor of a dispassionate examinee–examiner relationship. Collaborative rapport and expectancies of trust and assistance are eschewed. The resulting disparity produces many inherent ethical con-

flicts. Some are easily avoidable and tend to be associated with the unscrupulous practices of a few. Many others, however, relate directly to the medicolegal context itself, where the adversarial nature of the legal process conflicts with the scientific and therapeutic ethics of clinical treatment.

This chapter explicates the professional standards and ethical responsibilities of forensic experts who conduct medicolegal evaluations, with an emphasis on the role of the expert in facilitiating objective evaluations that assist the court in its decision-making process.

PROMOTING OBJECTIVITY AND GUARDING AGAINST BIAS

Without exception, the guiding principle in forensic ethics is the expectancy that the scope and content of an IE, subsequent reports, and testimony offered in depositions and court proceedings would be the same regardless of who retained the professional in question (American Academy of Physical Medicine and Rehabilitation, 1992; American Medical Association, 1997; Committee on Ethical Guidelines for Forensic Psychologists, 1991). However, frequent observations of significant disagreement among professionals, supported by preliminary survey data collected by the authors, indicate that lack of objectivity, or bias, is an all-too-frequent occurrence.

0-8493-0926-3/02/$0.00+$1.50
© 2002 by CRC Press LLC

There are several common sources of bias, most of which can be addressed in terms of general professional ethics.

COMMUNICATIONS IN THE FORENSIC EVALUATION

Clear communications of ethical standards (e.g., informed consent) with both the attorney and examinee prior to commencement of the evaluation are prerequisites for establishing ethical interactions that facilitate objectivity. Examinations from treating clinician vs. the unique intent of the independent examiner, which produce wide discrepancies in terms of the type, scope, and time requirements of the evaluation, should be clarified with the examinee. Explaining that opinions regarding diagnoses, prognoses, and/or recommendations will not be shared directly should be included. The policy of asking the examinee to sign an informed consent form, with a witness present, is an increasingly adopted policy to be considered. Full apprisal of the retaining attorney should also define the scope and extent of the services rendered. These issues will be discussed in greater detail below.

THE "PROFESSIONAL" EXPERT WITNESS

Experts who derive a large part of their income (i.e., 50%) from medicolegal evaluations may be at special risk for compromised objectivity. Medicolegal work incurs fees that are substantially higher than regular clinical fees, with generally much greater reimbursement. Significant pressures to maintain continued highly lucrative medicolegal referrals exert pressure to offer opinions consistent with the views of retaining attorneys, whose primary motivation is client advocacy.

Importantly, courts and attorneys usually prefer black/white opinions and eschew practitioners with less simplistic diagnostic and conceptual viewpoints. Practitioners can be subtly reinforced while garnering much higher reimbursements (vs. standard clinical fees) by employing a more dichotomous and simplistic (and easier) adversarial ethic vs. a scientific (more laborious) ethic in their opinions that are solicited (and paid for) by attorneys.

As is often the case, experts who are strongly invested in medicolegal practice will have an unequal weighting of referrals from defense or plaintiff attorneys, and in extreme cases experts may completely exclude one of these two groups. Further, professionals, like others, only have not biases, but also personal styles better suited for some settings than others.

Based on results of previous ethics surveys (Pope & Vetter, 1992; discussed below), observations of local practitioners, informal surveys and subsequent formal surveys conducted as part of an ethics review project, some preliminary inferences were offered by the first two authors (Martelli, Zasler, & LeFever, 2000a). Based on results of an anonymous survey of brain injury service providers from two southeastern cities, degrees of medicolegal involvement and degree and type of nonobjectivity among fellow professionals were estimated, along with requests for personality descriptors. Bias ratings showed strong positive association with the estimated degree of medicolegal involvement. Further, bias was fairly evenly distributed and discretely categorized into the three bias category options included on the survey: (a) plaintiff slant; (b) defense slant; and (c) retaining attorney slant. Further, there was some association between skeptical or suspicious behavioral traits and compulsive tendencies with practitioners perceived to have diagnostic biases more compatible with defense attorney interests/medicolegal involvements (i.e., defense expert). Histrionic or hypochondriacal and sympathetic personality traits were more associated with practitioners perceived to have diagnostic biases more favorable to plaintiffs (i.e., plaintiff's expert). Descriptions relating social finesse and flexible morals, in contrast, were associated with practitioners perceived by reputation as attorney's experts (i.e., agree with the retaining side, whether defense or plaintiff).

Importantly, a particular medicolegal specialization can be presumed to result in continued reinforcement of the same traits that served as a predisposition to the specializations, further reinforcing bias. Notably, the only protection against bias concerning pressures relating to high reimbursement rates and personal biases is the insistence on striving toward a local reputation for being fair and objective (i.e., a "straight shooter").

Bias also can be associated with exclusive attorney referral patterns. Many attorneys will avoid situations where there is consistent use of the same experts because of the appearance of bias. Nonetheless, the medicolegal community is not without examples of professionals who have been the sole forensic experts for the entire caseload of an attorney over the course of several years. Probitive questions during voir dire (i.e., questioning of an expert to establish the scope and depth of his or her expertise prior to being accepted as an expert) frequently address such questions, along with financial arrangements associated with forensic practice, etc.

ETHICS IN CONDUCTING MEDICOLEGAL EVALUATIONS

As a group, physicians pledge to uphold the Hippocratic oath, which directs that first and foremost, they do no harm. Licensed psychologists, although they take no oath, by virtue of privilege of license, adhere to professional ethics mandating that they promote the welfare of their patients, according to formal, professional, ethical guidelines published by the American Psychological Association (APA) and any regulatory state statutes (American

Psychological Association, 1995). The common thread implicit in all professional interactions is doing no harm to patients and others to whom the expert has responsibility. This ideal extends to professional work in the medicolegal community.

In a membership survey of the American Psychological Association (APA), randomly sampled psychologists were queried regarding ethical concerns in clinical psychological practice (Pope & Vetter, 1992). Forensic psychology ranked as fifth among the 23 categories of reported incidents of ethical dilemmas behind confidentiality, dual relationships, payment concerns, and teaching/training concerns. Major concerns included presentation of false testimony, the attorney's role in procuring desirable (potentially false) testimony, rendering of conclusions not grounded in objective data or scientific principles, and harm from reporting inaccurate data in forensic cases. Truly bitter language (e.g., "whore"), however, was reserved for descriptions of psychologists perceived as willing to present false testimony in court and/or who succumb to alleged attorney pressures or inducements for this kind of testimony.

A more recent membership of the National Academy of Neuropsychology (Brittain, Francis, McSweeney, Fisher, and Barth, 1997) revealed concerns from the majority of 456 respondents regarding examiner competence (64%), inappropriate use of tests (61%), and conflict between the law and ethics (55%). Further, 50% opined that the APA ethics code was insufficient to address ethical problems in neuropsychology, while 57% expressed dissatisfaction with the ability of ethics boards to enforce guidelines.

Clearly, such issues concern professionals practicing in the forensic and medicolegal arenas, the legal system, and those entities that make policy concerning training and certification for professional competency. Unfortunately, most physicians and psychologists acknowledge that they receive insufficient formal training or education with regard to ethics in medicolegal/forensic situations and that guidelines for ethical medicolegal practice have been lacking (Martelli, Zasler, & Grayson, 2000).

Problematic situations are inevitable when medical and psychological ethics are brought into the courtroom, where adversarial client advocacy is the rule. Appreciation and sensitivity to the potential disparities between conflicting interests and ethics seem the most logical approach to protecting the ethics and objectivity of medical and psychological examiners while affording the courts and its representatives benefit of their expertise. In the current chapter, relevant ethical issues are reviewed in order to illustrate ethical behaviors as they relate to many common aspects of medicolegal situations. Although some of the current dilemmas described are unique to the interaction of the American legal and healthcare systems, most have international relevance.

EXPERTISE AND QUALIFICATIONS IN MEDICINE AND PSYCHOLOGY

It has been previously noted that formal guidelines describing the qualifications to serve as an expert witness are only recently being developed. General Principle A of the American Psychological Association's Ethical Code for Psychologists (1995) implicitly addresses this issue:

> Psychologists strive to maintain high standards of competence in their work. They recognize the boundaries of their particular competencies and the limitations of their expertise. They provide only those services and use only those techniques for which they are qualified by education, training, or experience.

This principle is especially relevant to guidelines developed by Binder and Thompson (1995), which cover issues related to maintaining awareness of the relevant neuropsychological literature, seeking rigorous peer review to ensure competence, limiting practice to boundaries of competence, and seeking consultation as appropriate. Parallels certainly can be applied to physicians involved in the same process.

In 1996, the American Medical Association published its Code of Medical Ethics through its Council on Ethical and Judicial Affairs (AMA, 1997). Although this document is relatively general, it does stipulate that "medical experts should have recent and substantive experience in the area in which they testify and should limit testimony to their sphere of medical expertise." The code also notes that the "medical witness must not become an advocate or a partisan in the legal proceeding." Additionally, it encourages witnesses to inform attorneys of "...all favorable and unfavorable information developed by the physician's evaluation of the case."

There have been numerous other specialty organization publications dealing with recommendations for expert witness testimony. The American Academy of Physical Medicine and Rehabilitation's Board of Governors approved a "white paper" on expert witness testimony in April 1992. Central to these guidelines is the concept that the expert witness functions to educate the court as a whole, as opposed to "representing either of the parties involved, even though the expert witness may have been contacted primarily by one party." The guidelines note that the ultimate test for accuracy and impartiality is a willingness to prepare testimony that could be presented unchanged for use by either the plaintiff or defendant. Further review of this document reveals several recommendations which warrant attention: (1) the physician should identify opinions which are personal and not necessarily held by other physicians; (2) a distinction should be made between medical malpractice and medical maloccurrence when analyzing any case; and (3) there should be a willingness to submit transcripts of depositions and/or courtroom testimony for peer review.

Especially relevant are guidelines that have been adopted by the American Academy of Neurology and developed by the American Board of Medical Specialties for the physician expert witness, which include the following two standards:

1. The physician expert witness should be fully trained in a specialty or a diplomate of a specialty board recognized by the American Board of Medical Specialties, and qualified by experience or demonstrated competence in the subject of the case. The specialty of that physician should be appropriate to the subject matter in the case.

2. The physician expert witness should be familiar with the clinical practice of the specialty or the subject matter of the case at the time of the occurrence, and should be actively involved in the clinical practice of the specialty or the subject matter of the case for three of the previous five years at the time of the testimony.

The preceding guidelines are frequently cited as a useful model for guiding expert witness qualification in clinical neuropsychology (Lees-Haley & Cohen, 1999). With regard to the first standard, however, it should be noted that standards of training in neurology are considerably easier to demonstrate than in neuropsychology. Standardized medical school curricula, standardized residencies approved by the American Board of Medical Specialties to insure common standard compliance, written examinations of basic medical information for individuals with degrees from foreign medical schools, and eligibility to sit for board specialty certification examinations all exist as clearly demonstrable criteria.

Clinical neuropsychology, as a profession, has been making greater efforts toward standardization of training, but given greater variability, has tended to rely even more strongly on board eligibility as an independent criterion with which to evaluate education, training, and experience. The APA Division 40 definition of a clinical neuropsychologist describes prerequisite training while suggesting that the attainment of the American Board of Professional Psychology (ABPP)/American Board of Clinical Neuropsychology (ABCN) diploma is the clearest evidence of competence as a Clinical Neuropsychologist (Division 40 Executive Committee (1989). More recently, training guidelines have been defined and accepted by professional organizations in neuropsychology (Hannay, Bieliauskas, Crosson, Hammeke, Hamsher, & Koffler, 1998).

Based on these training guidelines and definitions, Loring (1995) proposed board eligibility as the training standard for expert witness consultations. This requirement would seem to promote standardized practice of neuropsychology while also providing a measure of quality control for those who conduct neuropsychological assessments for forensic cases.

The second standard regarding subject matter competency proscribes the offering of opinions outside areas of a professional's competence. In addition, it requires continuing active clinical practice in the area relevant to expert testimony, for 3 of the previous 5 years from the date of testimony. The failure to define level of "active clinical practice" might seem somewhat problematic, although by implication, greater vs. lesser levels of active practice would be more consistent with this principle. Consistent with APA Standard 1.05, which states that "psychologists … maintain a reasonable level of awareness of current scientific and professional information," Binder and Thompson (1995) offer that psychologists should remain aware of general trends in the relevant neuropsychological literature, use up-to-date neuropsychological tests and norms, rely on current knowledge, consider important demographic characteristics of individuals in making interpretations, and acknowledge limitations in current knowledge. An ability to discuss relevant research literature, accurately, and without notes, would be an obvious measure of this ability.

An additional issue with regard to identification of good expert witnesses in the area of evaluating persons with neurologic disability relates to credibility. Aside from the issues discussed above, it should be noted that many practitioners flaunt multiple certificates hanging on their walls. However, for many organizations, these certificates represent little more that "vanity" boards, where eligibility requirements are hardly stringent. The integrity of the individual should, in part, of course, be measured by the quality of the organizations they belong to, and the thoroughness of the inclusionary process for each organization. Relevant questions include whether the certifying organizations required the individual to take some type of oral and/or written test, what other inclusionary criteria were employed, whether attendance is required at a certain number of approved courses per year, whether the organization is the primary certifying organization, and so on. Inquiries about manner of receipt of board certifications and diplomates are important, given that certifying organizations and clinical specialty boards may have, in their earlier years, allowed "grandfathering" in of persons who were not required to meet current inclusion requirements.

Examination of the individual's publication record, as well as the types of publications should be assessed. Relevant questions would include whether the articles were published in peer-reviewed publications, and their recognized quality. In addition, lectures in one's claimed area of expertise should be reviewed, as should the organizations for whom they have lectured, with an emphasis on looking for those that are nationally or internationally recognized. It is also important to critically examine an expert's qualifications based in part on clinical, scientific, academic, and administrative positions held, and the manner in which they gained appointment (e.g., the individual's historic performance, a voting process, or some less selective process).

Martelli, Zasler, and Grayson (1999) have attempted to summarize the relevant criteria by which professional expert competence can be evaluated. These have been adapted for psychologist and physician specialists in chronic pain assessment and treatment are included in Table 72.1. As can be seen, they are heavily borrowed from ethics in psychology. A qualifications checklist is included for the general knowledge/competency (again, borrowed primarily from psychology). In addition, a selected qualifications checklist is included for Chronic Pain Specialists. Finally, an Expert Opinion Competency/Credibility Weighting summary list is offered, which represents a preliminary framework for evaluating relative credibility of expert witnesses.

DUAL/MULTIPLE RELATIONSHIP CONSIDERATIONS

Multiple relationships potentially constitute an ethical dilemma in the medicolegal context. For example, as indicated in APA Ethics Code, Section 1.17 (1995):

> Psychologists must always be sensitive to the potential harmful effects of other contacts on their work and on those persons with whom they deal. A psychologist refrains from entering into or promising another personal, scientific, professional, financial, or other relationship with such persons if it appears likely that such a relationship reasonably might impair the psychologist's objectivity or otherwise interfere with the psychologist effectively performing his or her functions as a psychologist, or might harm or exploit the other party.

There is a strong tradition in clinical psychological practice relating to proscription of both developing personal relationships with persons who are current or former clients, or providing psychotherapeutic services to persons with whom a prior personal relationship exists. Clearly, this prohibition is intended, in the former situation, to protect a patient from potential exploitation in a relationship predicated on equal status by someone who maintains, or previously maintained, a relationship based on higher power or skills and dependency. In the latter case, the purpose is guarding against problems stemming from the preexisting relationship obligations and biases conflicting with the prerequisite objectivity required by a psychologist for effective diagnosis and treatment.

The latter protection is most relevant in medicolegal work. Consistent deliberate opinion exists that a preexisting professional relationship would represent a potential conflict of interest that interferes with the objectivity required by an expert witnesses. As such, the presence of a preexisting relationship should usually eliminate consideration of serving as an expert witness in the case where any other expert is available. It should be noted that this mandate is often at odds with the conceptualization of experts in the legal community, where "treating clinicians" are often considered to be more credible experts from the standpoint that they have more familiarity with the patient.

Perhaps the only exception might occur when no other expert is or can be made available, or where declining to serve as an expert witness might produce resultant harm to the patient from deprivation of needed service that outweighs threats to objectivity. In such cases, prudence would mandate documentation in the report of both the preexisting relationship and procedures and safeguards employed in order to facilitate the highest possible levels of objectivity. This should, of course, be balanced against potential compromise of the therapeutic relationship if the patient did not receive the desired expert testimony and/or opinions supportive of the patient's legal claim.

In an effort to elucidate ethical conflicts due to potential multiple relationships of medical professionals engaged in standard medicolegal practice, Blau (1984; 1992) differentiated the following professional roles: (1) "Treating Doctor," who has a special (usually empathic) bond with his/her patient, and whose role is to describe the everyday treatment procedures that were employed, and not offer opinions beyond those contained in their reports, or perform evaluations on the basis of anything other than medical necessity; (2) "Expert Witness," who without prior knowledge of the examinee obtains special and extraordinarily complete information and for whom, in order to promote objectivity, no bond with the examinee is permitted; (3) "Trial Consultant," whose function, consistent with the adversarial process, is to assist with critical scrutiny and impeachment of experts and opinions from the opposing side. As Blau notes, these roles represent different interests and obligations. Failure to set limits and avoid mixing of the conflicting interests inherent in these contrasting roles would undoubtedly reduce objectivity and compromise the opposing welfares of the different parties to whom obligations are maintained.

Unfortunately, in a frequently observed occurrence by the authors, treating clinicians accept invitations to serve as "expert" witnesses when other professionals are available. Although understandable, this practice is nonetheless problematic. This practice is appealing to attorneys for several reasons, including ease, as the professional is already involved; inherent time and/or cost savings to the patient and his or her legal representative; and the advantage of natural advocacy inherent in clinician–patient relationships. The problems include mixing of usually incompatible roles. The fact that this frequently occurs may be explained by

TABLE 72.1

Summary Guidelines for Evaluating Professional Expert Qualifications

Professional Expert Qualifications Checklist: General
- **Knowledge Competence Base (derived from APA Ethics and P.M. &R. White Paper):**
  - ❏ Remains aware of general trends in the relevant neuropsychological literature and incorporates current knowledge into regular practice.
  - ❏ Uses up-to-date neuropsychological tests and norms and considers important demographic characteristics of individuals in making interpretations.
  - ❏ Appropriately acknowledges limitations in current knowledge.
  - ❏ Seeks rigorous peer review to ensure competence.
  - ❏ Can discuss relevant research literature accurately, without notes.
  - ❏ Limits practice to boundaries of competence, seeking consultation as appropriate.
  - ❏ Is fully trained in a specialty or has earned a diplomate of a specialty board in spacialty area (i.e., Pain Management), and is qualified by experience or demonstrated competence in the subject of the case.
  - ❏ Is familiar with the clinical practice of the specialty or the subject matter of the case at the time of the occurrence, and has been actively involved in the clinical practice of the specialty or the subject matter of the case for three of the previous five years at the time of testimony.

Professional Expert Qualifications Checklist: Chronic Pain
- **Professional Organizations:**
- (A) Current Memberships
- (B) Current Committee Memberships
  - ❏ American Academy of Pain Management
  - ❏ American Pain Society
  - ❏ American Academy of Pain Medicine
  - ❏ International Association for the Study of Pain
  - ❏ Canadian Pain Society
  - ❏ World Institute of Pain
  - ❏ State or regional chronic pain associations
  - ❏ Special national associations with significant pain management components (e.g., American Chiropractic Association, Assoc. for Applied Psychophysiology and Biofeedback)
  - ❏ Am. Psychological Assoc: Division 22 (1/2 point)
  - ❏ American Academy of Physical Medicine and Rehabilitiation (1/2 point)
- **Specialty Conference Attendances:**
- (A) # Attendances at Last Three Meetings of...?
- (B) # Presentations at Last Three Meetings of...?
  - ❏ American Academy of Pain Management
  - ❏ American Pain Society
  - ❏ American Academy of Pain Medicine
  - ❏ International Association for the Study of Pain
  - ❏ Canadian Pain Society
  - ❏ World Institute of Pain
  - ❏ State or regional dedicated Chronic Pain Conferences
  - ❏ Conferences of specialty national associations with significant pain management components (e.g., American Chiropractic Association, Assoc. for Applied Psychophysiology and Biofeedback)
  - ❏ Am. Psychogolical Assoc.: Division 22 — Rehab. Psychology (1/2 point)
  - ❏ American Academy of Physical Medicine and Rehabilitation (1/2 point)
- **Professional Journal Familiarity:**
- (A) Do You Currently Subscribe to...?
- (B) Have You Read "." (Latest Issue Article in)...?
  - ❏ American Journal ofPain Management
  - ❏ Clinical Journal of Pain
  - ❏ American Journal of Pain
  - ❏ Pain
  - ❏ Cephalgia and/or Headache
  - ❏ Current Review of Pain
  - ❏ Cranio: The Journal of Craniomandibular Practice
  - ❏ Archives of Physical Medicine and Rehabilitation (1/2 point)
  - ❏ The Pain Clinic (1/2 point)
  - ❏ The Pain Practitioner (1/2 point)
  - ❏ Any Specific Pain related newsletter (1/2 credit per)
  - ❏ What specialty dedicated chronic pain assessment and treatment books do you own? (author, pub. date)
- **Specialty Area Clinical Treatment Experience (last 2 years/lifetime):**
  - ❏# Clinical Patients Personally Treated (excluding assessment; ≥ 5 h total time)
  - ❏# Clinical Patients Personally Assessed (not technician; ≥ 4 h total time)

TABLE 72.1 (CONTINUED)
Summary Guidelines for Evaluating Professional Expert Qualifications

- **Publication Record (last 3 years/lifetime):**
  - ❏# Publications in Recognized Specialty Journals
  - ❏# Publications in Books in Specialty Area
  - ❏# of Editorial Positions with Specialty Journals or Organizations
  - ❏Recognized quality of the work
- **Presentations and Talks in Area of Expertise (last 3 years/lifetime):**
  - ❏# Lectures in Specialty Area
  - ❏# Lectures at Relevant National or International Specialty Organization Meetings
  - ❏# of Clinical, Scientific, Academic, and Administrative positions held
  - ❏Manner of gaining appointments in positions held

Additional Disability Evaluator Qualifications Checklist may be Relevant

EXPERT OPINION: COMPETENCY/CREDIBILITY WEIGHTING
(Last 3 Years Total Score and/or Last Year Total Score)
_____ Professional Organization Memberships
_____ Professional Meeting Attendances
_____ Professional Meeting Presentations (Total #)
_____ Professional Journal Subscriptions, Reading (Total #)
_____ Specialty Direct Clinical Treatment Experience
_____ Publication Record
_____ Talks and Presentations in Relevant Area of Expertise
_____ Relative Competence/Credibility Score

the typically greater emphasis in professional ethical codes to proscription of conflicts between professional and non-professional roles and activities than between differing professional roles. Strasburger, Gutheil, and Brodsky (1997) argue that these conflicting professional roles should be avoided by offering the patient's treatment record in lieu of testimony. That is, they recommend that treating doctors maintain strict role boundaries as fact witnesses and decline to perform the functions of an expert witness. In other words, treating clinicians ideally should provide testimony only as fact witnesses, and decline expert witness actvities such as reviewing the reports or depositions of other witnesses. In situations where testifying as an expert witness cannot be avoided, they should acknowledge the inherent conflicts in both testimony and reports.

With regard to the relationships between attorneys and health practitioners, contrasting professional motivations and standards produce frequently conflicting interests. Financial incentives, which are well-recognized threats to objective patient reports, deserve equal consideration as a threat to to medical practitioners. Given the discrepancy between the adversarial client advocacy of attorneys, and the dispassionate, objective scientific ethics required of physicians and psychologists, concern must necessarily be raised when one considers that attorneys are the usual referral source, payers, and consumers of examination findings and reports from experts.

Moreover, medicolegal evaluations tend to be conducted by a limited number of professionals in the community, which fosters the development of social relationships between referring attorneys and medicolegal examiners. At a time when insurance reimbursement severely restricts payments, it would seem naive to think that attorney satisfaction with examiner findings is an irrelevant factor in the development of referral decisions, formal referral relationships, and/or social relationships. Subtle test-interpretation influences and adoption of adversarial and dualistic tendencies (e.g., either–or, black–white) in interpretation of findings may be operative both above and below the level of expert examiner or witness awareness. Such subtle threats to objectivity would seem especially likely in cases of greater ambiguity in either test results, behavioral observations, and/or responses on measures of motivation and response bias.

Importantly, the process of a consulting call to the examiner from the referring plaintiff or defense attorney to discuss initial findings and favorability to the case often represents an invitation to join the client–attorney team. Depending on favorability of findings, additional paid consultations may be scheduled with the expert regarding methods of presenting findings and invariably, juxtaposing the findings against opposing counsel arguments. This practice represents a subtle but incremental team invitation. This veiled invitation to join the client–attorney team seems much less subtle when the issues of validity of findings become equated with winning in court by a favorable jury or judge ruling.

Another important influence of an adversarial legal process is the reinforcement of dichotomous opinions. Uncertainties, shades of gray, and reservations are usually not conducive to an adversarial process and are often eschewed in the legal process. Our experience confirms the expectancy that the initial selection of an expert is influenced by reputation and history with regard to the expert's tendencies to think in "black and white" vs. "shades of gray" and/or to find single causes vs. multiple determinants of behavior. Much less obvious are the tendencies for social reinforcement and subtle increases and decreases of interest or ego approval to potentially influence opinions in borderline situations.

For example, in the case of ambiguous clinical findings where an opinion of either malingered or valid test results is rendered in an attorney consultation, an initially tenuous endorsement could inappreciably become strengthened by confirmatory bias. That is, the tendency to selectively considered evidence in accordance with existing bias could be fueled by the clinician's underlying discomfort with expressing opinions that appear uncertain or displeasing to the retaining attorney.

With regard to the current healthcare environment, Martelli, Zasler, and Grayson (1999) noted that current managed healthcare organizations and practices leave many physicians, psychologists, and other healthcare professionals feeling diminished. Their expertise, opinions, and recommendations are questioned, while their services are constrained. Medical necessity has been redefined by bottom-line business accounting that pays greater attention to cost-effectiveness demands, increased accountability, and a low-leniency, cost-cutting atmosphere. At the same time, reduced insurance coverage and reimbursement create pressures to maintain accustomed standards of living by identifying new income sources for healthcare providers. Clearly, medicolegal work represents one of the last unregulated frontiers. The lucrative attorney referral-driven medicolegal arena clearly poses a real economic opportunity that not only offers financial incentives, but also ego expertise enhancements, which signify pressures for bias that ranges from subtle reinforcement of adversarial- and dualistic-oriented opinions to shaping of perspective. As such, the typical healthcare professional should assume that the maintenance of scientific objectivity will necessarily be difficult.

In a proposed remedy, Brodsky (1991) offers an interesting recommendation for protecting medical professionals from mixing the disparate responsibilities of science and adversarialism. Brodsky offers an *objectivity quotient* that equals the number of cases in which there is agreement with the referring attorney, divided by the total number of cases. He suggests that base rate and referral difference be acknowledged and offers a preliminary cut-off point of 0.8 or greater for suggesting preexisting bias. The present authors consider this a somewhat liberal cut off, and suggest a maximum of 0.75.

ETHICAL ISSUES IN CONDUCTING AND INDEPENDENT EXAMINATION

Informed Consent

Within the context of the actual examination, full disclosure regarding the purpose of examination, as well as the tests and procedures being utilized, is required to optimize examinee compliance. Examiners must be careful about such disclosure in order to promote a balance between accurately representing the purpose of the testing to the examinee, without increasing distrust in a process that is, by its legal nature, adversarial.

As previously noted, many evaluations conducted from more traditional clinical referral sources and not originally performed as medicolegal evaluations become part of subsequent litigation proceedings. This is especially true in cases of injury and impairment. The medicolegal context clearly imposes special obligations and responsibilities for the medical professional. With regard to psychologists, relevant professional ethical principles have been elaborated.

Section 1.21 of the APA Principles (1995) states:

> When a psychologist agrees to provide services to a person or entity at the request of a third party, the psychologist clarifies to the extent feasible, at the outset of the service, the nature of the relationship with each party. This clarification includes the role of the psychologist (such as therapist, organizational consultant, diagnostician, or expert witness), the probable uses of the service provided or the information obtained, and the fact that there may be limits to confidentiality.

Informed consent guidelines have been provided by Johnson-Greene, Hardy-Morais, Adams, Hardy, and Bergloff (1997) for neuropsychological evaluations. They recommend that neuropsychologists explain fully to all patients in language that can be easily understood the purpose of the examination, the reason for referral, and any limitations of confidentiality. In medicolegal evaluations it is also important to indicate who will provide feedback about results, or explain that the circumstances of the independent evaluation dicate that no feedback is provided.

These ethical principles and related guidelines are probably more easily observed for evaluations conducted at the request of the plaintiff's attorney, who functions as patient advocate and usually has communicated the purpose and potential benefit of the evaluation. In addition, the manner in which feedback will be provided is explained. Requests for independent evaluations from defense counsel, however, may be more challenging, given that the referral from the opposing attorney promotes greater distrust, especially when the examinee is informed regarding the nature of the assessment, the examiner's relationship to the opposing attorney or insurance company, and information that feedback will not be provided directly to the examinee.

Third-Party Observers

It has been observed previously that court orders sometimes have permitted attorneys and/or legal representatives to sit in on independent evaluations. In such cases, the independent evaluation process is potentially corrupted as an additional and uncontrolled factor is added that may influence examinee behavior and performance. Less invasive, but possibly still disruptive, is videotaping of the independent examination. Probably least disruptive, although still possibly a threat to the integrity of the process, is the practice of audio taping of independent evaluations.

An additional ethical threat is posed when test material and examination procedures are revealed. Unprotected disclosure of assessment instruments and examination procedures potentially reduces the validity of such procedures in future assessment situations with other persons and, hence, potentially compromises the greater welfare of the public at large.

With regard to psychological and neuropsychological tests instruments and procedures, task force committees of the APA have issued reports with specific guidelines intended to limit the disclosure of tests, in order to protect the integrity and security of test materials, and to avoid misuse of assessment techniques and data (American Psychological Association, 1996). Notably, one of the tenets of the independent examination is that the examiner conveys only information that was garnered within the context of the exam, does not alter exam findings in any way, and does not document things that did not occur. At a less tangible level, the independent examiner's role is to make objective clinical interpretations and inferences based on dispassionate logic that is devoid of personal interest or interests of others. In contrast to the attorney, who explicitly advocates as an adversary for his or her client, the examiner should function only as an advocate for the truth. Too often, however, the adversarial nature of courts, legal proceedings, and attorneys "creeps" into the scientific arena and introduces a significant and powerful threat to objectivity that can produce bias in persons purportedly functioning as scientists. When creeping adversarialism (Martelli, Zasler, & Grayson, 2000b) infiltrates the examinations and opinions of scientists, distrust generated by systems adhering to adversarial principles only increases. Of course, the nature of these systems dictates that they must attempt to discredit even the most objective scientific procedures and findings. Demands to be present and observe independent examinations may be either reactive to fear of adversarial or biased procedures from the examiner, with or without reason, or attempts to collect as much information as possible to build stronger adversarial arguments to impeach opposite opinions.

Available Guidelines and Assessment Procedures

In the medicolegal examination, documentation regarding the evaluation and all procedures administered is usually closely scrutinized by opposing counsel and his/her team of experts. Consequently, tests and assessment procedures selected for medicolegal circumstances usually represent measures with a stronger research database, greater acceptance within the profession, and more established history of use in the courts. With regard to psychology, selection of such tests reflects, in part, anticipation of attacks on the scientific validity of psychological instruments. Section 2.07 of the APA Ethics Code (1995) states:

(a) Psychologists do not base their assessment or intervention decisions or recommendations on data or test results that are dated for the current purpose, and
(b) Similarly, psychologists do not base such decisions or recommendations on tests and measures that are obsolete and not useful for the current purpose.

Examiners are expected to use up-to-date tests and norms, rely on current knowledge, consider important demographic characteristics of individuals in making interpretations, and acknowledge limitations in current knowledge. Examiners are cautioned to interpret test results carefully if experimental procedures are utilized or tests are used with individuals for whom normative data are not available.

Report Content and Related Issues

Necessary and usual parts of a comprehensive assessment physician examiners should use for any examinee include the following: examinee demographic details; referral source and party responsible for payment; basis of report; documents requested and reviewed, including those not received; history of present illness; past medical history; family medical history; psychosocial history; educational history; vocational history; military history, if applicable; legal history, if applicable; review of systems; comprehensive exam findings, including pertinent negative findings; diagnostic impressions; opinions regarding maximal medical improvement (MMI); causality and apportionment opinions; recommendations and relevant appendices.

Specific information relevant to opinions should ideally be delineated when reviewing documents that served as the basis of the report. This provides documentation that not only were the records reviewed, but also demonstrates a more deliberate analysis of the information, temporal relationship of complaints to any injury in question, analysis of symptom profile in correlation with the type of injury or impairment being claimed, consistency of reporting over time, findings suggestive of neurologic recovery pattern over time (or lack thereof), and clear delineation of inferential reasoning, among other purposes.

It should also be considered important to acknowledge potentially relevant information that was unavailable or not provided. For example, as is more often the case for defense-related evaluations, examiners may not be given an opportunity (or make an effort) to interview corroboratory witnesses; this can be frustrating to legitimate examiners trying to do a thorough and objective evaluation.

As part of the analysis of information and examination findings, an examiner's report should ideally include (a) an evaluation of the appropriateness of the diagnostic testing procedures and process; (b) an estimate of the reliability and validity of the findings that served as a basis for impairment claims; (c) an estimation of degree to which the measures used were specific and sensitive to the condition being examined; as well as (d) the degree of confidence in interpretations and opinions offered. Inherent in such testing should be evaluations, both from a physical, as well as mental standpoint, of response bias.

Notably, many examiners feel uncomfortable commenting on the testing procedures and/or conclusions of other clinicians. Objective assessment requires global analysis of opinions. This type of commentary is inherent in performing an adequate and comprehensive evaluation of any case. Meticulous evaluation of pre-injury problems, including prior treatment, medical, psychiatric, and otherwise, developmental difficulties (e.g., attention deficit disorder, or hyperactivity in school), psychoemotional problems during childhood, and learning disabilities, among other variables, must all be evaluated within the context of the clinical presentation. Prior injuries, surgeries, and past use of medication should be assessed, as should the frequency and severity, as well as functional significance, of any complaint that is being claimed post-injury that also was present pre-injury.

The individual's legal history, including police records, should be requested and reviewed, as this may have an impact on understanding current behavior. A history of certain types of legal problems may make an examiner more suspicious of some reported symptoms; nonetheless, ethical imperatives require that the examiner remain unbiased, complete an objective assessment, and not assume that individuals with certain types of background do not incur legitimate injuries.

Ethical Considerations when Submitting Reports

Ethical considerations clearly proscribe altering exam findings, or documenting things that did not occur. They also proscribe leaving out, or altering, potentially salient information from forensic or other reports. Further, the failure to address, and logically explain, inconsistent information or findings, reduces credibility and invites suspicion of bias.

The matter of issuing draft reports prior to the final reports poses an interesting dilemma that represents a potentially great danger to objectivity and ethical conduct. By introducing an opportunity for review and comment, attorneys or other interested parties may issue requests for changes. Requests issued from attorneys or referring parties for changes to reports, often for "legal purposes" (e.g., to clarify technical points for the court) or to clarify grammar, may represent a slippery slope that leads to nonobjective input and possible influence regarding other aspects of the examination findings and report. Recommendations that seem prudent include avoiding draft reports under all circumstances, and in order to avoid temptation or suspicion of impropriety, adopting a policy of refusal of any requested report changes, except for correction of notable grammar or information errors. In the case of true and significant errors occurring in the context of the report, or where important clarification of information is clearly relevant, three options can be advised: (1) attach an amended page to the report; (2) simply mark through (with a line) the incorrect portion of the report, without deleting or whiting out, and insert the correct information; (3) produce a corrected version and document that it is an updated version and the rationale for its production, while maintaining the original version with all other examinee records to produce upon request.

As previously noted, sharing examination results with the examinee are clearly proscribed by existing ethical guidelines and recommendations, as well as legal statues in most states. Signing of an informed consent, noting the potential dangers associated with sharing the information and/or report directly with the examinee, is increasingly recommended as standard procedure. It is also recommended that examiners have a disclaimer at the end of a report which generally reiterates the basis of the report and the opinions as germane to the expert's qualifications and training, and the fact that all opinions are given with "medical probability," unless otherwise stipulated. Finally, it is also advised that examiners include a statement that their conclusions are based, in part, on the assumption that the materials provided for review are true, correct, and complete, and that if more information becomes available at a later date, opinions may be subject to change.

CONCLUSION

RECOMMENDATIONS FOR EXPERTS

Providers of medical information and testimony have ultimate responsibility for ethical conduct as it relates to this information. The authors offer the following recommendations for purposes of enhancing ethical relationships between expert clinicians and the courts.

Avoid or resist attorney efforts at enticement to join the attorney–client team. Such compromises of scientific boundaries and ethical principles exist on a continuum ranging from standard attorney–client advocacy at the beginning of the expert consultation phase (e.g., promotional information when first retaining an expert, with either provision of selective or incomplete records or less than enthusiastic efforts to produce all records) and extending to completion of the evaluation, when requests for changes in reports and/or documentation might be made.

Respect role boundaries and do not mix conflicting roles. Remember that the treating doctor possesses a bond with the patient, but does not as a rule obtain complete pre- and post-injury information in the context of assessing causality and apportionment. In contrast, the expert witness must conduct a thorough and multifaceted case analysis sans the physician–patient relationship in order to facilitate objectivity and allow optimum diagnostic formulations. Finally, the trial consultant's function in this adversarial process is to assist with critically scrutinizing and attacking positions of experts for the opposing side. These roles all represent inherently different interests, and mixing them can only reduce objectivity.

Insist on adequate time for thorough record review, evaluation and report generation, and preparation for deposition and court appearances.

Work at building a reputation for general objectivity and fairness, as well as reliance on multiple data sources, reaching opinions only after reviewing complete information from both sides and completing an unbiased evaluation.

Spend a good part of your time actually treating the patient population being examined or about whom you are offering testimony. This treatment should be current, and with a comparable frequency to that of treating practitioner specialists. Maintain the ability to discuss relevant research and scientific methodology issues competently and without notes.

Arrive at opinions only after reviewing all of the evidence from both sides of the adversarial fence, employing multiple data sources, completing an unbiased evaluation, and interpreting data within the full context of comprehensive historical, behavioral observation, and contextual information. Being otherwise favorable to the retaining attorney's interests suggests endorsement of "opinion prostitute," "scientific perjurer," or "hired gun" status (Martelli, Zasler, & Grayson, 2000b). The only way a practitioner can reduce the likelihood of facing an "opinion prostitute" on the opposing side in future cases is to insist on establishing and maintaining a reputation for scientific objectivity.

Balance cases from plaintiff and defense attorneys. Predilection for one side or the other suggests bias and sets up predisposition to nonobjectivity. For example, a preponderance of plaintiff work suggests a bias toward overdiagnosis and/or uncritical sympathy, while a ratio that favors hiring by the defense suggests an underdiagnosis or skepticism bias. Perhaps Brodsky's (1991) suggested cutoff ratio of 0.80 for favorability findings (or our recommended ratio of 0.75) would represent an initial cutoff for defense vs. plaintiff ratio. That is, experts should do at least 25% of their work for the opposite side of the current case being represented. Further, it might be a reasonable expectation that data on these ratios be collected as an important method for considering the objectivity of opinions.

Ensure against excessive favorability to the side of the retaining attorney or firm. Objectivity demands that scientific opinions not be influenced by the position of the legal advocate. Importantly, Brodsky (1991) recommends using a ratio of 0.8 as a cutoff for detecting excessive bias. That is, practitioners should possess prerequisite objectivity to disagree with the referring attorney at least 20% of the time. We suggest that a more useful cutoff would be 0.75, where experts are expected to generate findings that do not support the referring attorney's position at least 25% of the time (Martelli, et al., 2000b).

Never arrive at opinions that are inconsistent with plaintiff records, exam data, test data, behavioral presentation, etc., especially when such opinions are favorable to the side of the retaining attorney firm. Instead, always:

Consider or mention, in reports and discussion, information not supportive of expressed opinions, including historical or behavioral observation information; exam and test findings; discrepancies between plaintiff's complaints and observed behavior and/or history; discrepancies between the severity of the injury and the severity of the reported symptoms; discrepancies between opinions and known occurrence rates (or base rates) in the general population; opinions and logical arguments of experts from the other side of the case, presented fully and in an objective manner.

Strive to demonstrate objectivity by disputing the opinion of other experts only through a complete and deliberate logical dispute of a full and complete representation of the other expert's findings, inferential reasoning, and conclusions.

Always assess response bias and make efforts to guard against motivational threats to valid assessment.

Avoid cutting corners, be thorough, and rely on standardized, validated, normed, and well-accepted procedures and tests.

Limit use of technicians and non-M.D.s or non-Ph.D.s for evaluation and testing.

Intensively assess the client being evaluated, use only appropriate normative data for comparisons (e.g., persons of similar education or age; comparisons to medical patients vs. psychiatric patients), take into account the symptoms' base rates (i.e., how frequently the symptoms occur in the general population and in the absence of the injury being evaluated), consider the many other explanatory factors for symptoms (e.g., medications, sleep disturbance, depression, etc.), and adjust the interpretations according to medical conditions (e.g., inherent somatic complaints of progressive disorders like M.S. and Parkinson's and chronic pain), relevant situational variables (e.g., attention and other deficits correlated with chronic pain conditions, fatigue, insomnia/sleep deprivation), cultural factors (e.g., rural impoverished backgrounds) etc.

Attempt to devise and employ a formalized quality assurance system that allows for monitoring and assessing (and improving) the validity and reliability of diagnostic and prognostic statements against real world findings. A formalized peer review system or similar mechanism that routinely allows for feedback from peers should be pursued.

Always prepare examinees by emphasizing the importance of accurate/honest performance with full effort on all interview questions, exam-

ination procedures, and tests (e.g., to produce valid and reliable profiles that permit comparison with known symptom patterns). Further emphasize the liabilities associated with exaggerating impairments (e.g., producing invalid profiles, lower the credibility, suspicion of malingering of all symptoms).

Recognize the limitations of medical and psychological data and opinions, and how, in science and medicine, few findings and symptoms are black and white, clean, or attributable to a single event (e.g., Occam's Razor).

Increase attention to issues relating to scientific methodology, objectivity, maintenance of scientific rigor.

Consider promoting increased awareness within the forensic professions of relevant issues relating to ethics and scientific objectivity. Promote utilization of objective data, such as Brodsky's (1991) ratio, in regular clinical practice, and recommend adoption of similar standards by local, state, and national professional organizations. Reinforce those who collate such data. Provide relevant information, including opinions and observations from known experts, as well as copies of relevant information such as this chapter, to colleagues. Promote issues relevant to legal use of medical and scientific evidence and testimony by encouraging courses in law school and programs offered by state bar associations and at annual trial lawyer and other association meetings.

REFERENCES

American Academy of Physical Medicine and Rehabilitation (1992). Expert witness testimony. White Paper.

American Medical Association, Council on Ethical and Judicial Affairs (1996–1997 edition). *Code of medical ethics: Current opinions with annotations.* Washington, D.C.: American Medical Association.

American Psychological Association (1995). *Ethical principles of psychologists and code of conduct.* Washington, D.C.: American Psychological Association.

American Psychological Association, Committee on Legal Issues (1996). Strategies for private practitioners coping with subpoenas or compelled testimony for client records or test data. *Professional Psychology, 27,* 245–251.

Binder, L.M., & Thompson, L.L. (1995). The ethics code and neuropsychological assessment practices. *Archives of Clinical Neuropsychology, 10*(1) 27–46.

Blau, T. (1984). *The psychologist as expert witness.* New York: John Wiley & Sons.

Blau, T. (1992). The psychologist as expert witness. Presented at the National Academy of Neuropsychology annual meeting, Reno, NV.

Brittain, J.L., Francis, J.P., McSweeney, A.J., Fisher, J.M., & Barth, J.T. (1997). Ethics in neuropsychology: Where are we now? Workshop presented at the annual meeting of the National Academy of Neuropsychology, Las Vegas, NV.

Brodsky, S.L. (1991). Testifying in court: Guidelines and maxims for the expert witness. Washington, D.C.: American Psychological Association.

Committee on Ethical Guidelines for Forensic Psychologists (1991). Specialty guidelines for forensic psychologists. *Law and Human Behavior, 15*(6), 655–665.

Division 40 Executive Committee (1989). Definition of a clinical neuropsychologist. *The Clinical Neuropsychologist, 3,* 22.

Hannay, H.J., Bieliauskas, L.A., Crosson, B.A., Hammeke, T.A., Hamsher, K. DeS., & Koffler, S.P. (1998). Proceedings of the Houston Conference on Specialty Education and Training in Clinical Neuropsychology. *Archives of Clinical Neuropsychology, 13.*

Johnson-Greene, D., Hardy-Morais, C., Adams, K.M., Hardy, C., & Bergloff, P. (1997). Informed consent and neuropsychological assessment: Ethical considerations and proposed guidelines. *The Ethical Neuropsychologist, 11*(4), 454–460.

Lees-Haley, P.R., & Cohen, L.J. (1999). The neuropsychologist as expert witness: Toward credible science in the courtroom. In J.J. Sweet (Ed.), *Forensic Neuropsychology.* Lisse: Swets & Zeitlinger.

Loring, D.W. (1995). Psychometric detection of malingering. Paper presented at the annual meeting of the American Academy of Neurology, Seattle, WA.

Martelli, M.F., Zasler, N.D., & Grayson, R. (1999). Ethical considerations in medicolegal evaluation of neurologic injury and impairment. *NeuroRehabilitation: An Interdisciplinary Journal, 13*(1), 45–66.

Martelli, M.F., Zasler, N.D. & Grayson, R. (2000a). Ethics and medicolegal evaluation of impairment after brain injury. In M. Schiffman (Ed.), *Attorney's guide to ethics in forensic science and medicine.* Springfield, IL: Charles C Thomas.

Martelli, M.F., Zasler, N.D., & Grayson, R. (2000b). Ethics and medicolegal evaluation of impairment after brain injury. In M. Schiffman (Ed.), *Attorney's guide to ethics in forensic science and medicine,* Springfield, IL: Charles C Thomas.

Martelli, M.F., Zasler, N.D., & LeFever, F.F. (2000). Preliminary consumer guidelines for choosing a well-suited neuropsychologist for evaluation and treatment of acquired brain injury (ABI). *Brain Injury Source, 4*(4), 36–39.

Pope, K.S., & Vetter, V.A. (1992). Ethical dilemmas encountered by members of the American Psychological Association: A national survey. *American Psychologist, 47*(3), 397–411.

Strasburger, H., Gutheil, T.G., and Brodsky, B.A. (1997). On wearing two hats: Role conflict in serving as both psychotherapist and expert witness. *American Journal of Psychiatry, 154*(4), 448–456.

73

Business Side of Pain Management

Devona Slater, C.M.C.P.

The clinical side of pain management is only half the battle. In today's environment being paid for the professional services you perform can be as complicated as treating your most complex pain patient. There is a wealth of information you must know that really should be classified as nonclinical but is just as important as the clinical information. Business expertise related to pain management is a necessity for every practice. You must recognize that if you do not run the business, the business will run you. This chapter is a place to start building your basic business skills.

PERSONNEL, STAFFING, AND MANAGEMENT STYLES

The first step in determining your staffing is to look realistically at the needs for your practice. A general rule of thumb for pain practitioners would be three or four staff per physician, depending on your mode of practice. The first two individuals would cover administrative duties including, but not limited to, scheduling, answering phones, booking appointments, medical records, billing, insurance collections, credentialing, personnel administration, and accounting functions. If billing, accounting, or payroll is outsourced, personnel will be reduced. You may need one clinical individual to start with, expanding to two or three as your practice grows. Clinical personnel should be an extension of you and used to handle back office duties such as patient phone calls, prescription refills, lab reports, and initial charting for patient visits. A good pain nurse is worth his or her weight in gold, and will truly make or break the profitability of the clinic.

When trying to fill a position in the clinic it is best to define the position and set a salary scale before considering any one person for a position. Many practices make the mistake of knowing "Sally" is the perfect employee because she is a friend or used to work for a competitor. No one sits down and objectively looks at whether "Sally's" skills match what is needed to accomplish the job in the clinic. Choose staff wisely and avoid filling a position with "just a warm body." Finding the correct personnel will make your job easier down the line and patience is important in making the selection.

After finding that perfect employee it always amazes me how little training physicians give to staff on how they want the practice to run. Employees will generally live up to expectations set for them, but rarely succeed when no expectations are communicated. Orientation and training for each employee are very important steps to make the clinic operate smoothly. Personnel files are an essential element of any business and should be treated as confidential information. Documentation in employee files is as important as documentation in a patient's medical chart. The file should contain a current résumé, an emergency contact, specific tax forms (i.e., W-4 & I-9 and state employment), signature sheet from compliance and policy manuals, a current job description that lists expectations, performance evaluations, salary history, incident reports, and any other personal information gathered regarding the employee. Please be aware that incident reports and performance evaluations should be detailed and contain both positive and negative notes. Accurate documentation may be your only defense if you have to defend unemployment claims or wrongful termination suits.

0-8493-0926-3/02/$0.00+$1.50
© 2002 by CRC Press LLC

TABLE 73.1
Sample Table of Contents

Administrative Manual	Clinical Manual
Office hours and schedule	Patient work-ups
Telephone management	Triage
Appointment scheduling	Charting
Medical records management	Patient education
Emergency procedures	Standing orders
Front desk check-out	Procedure set-ups
Patient billing and collections	Narcotics policy
Refund processing	Sterilization guidelines
Accounting and bookkeeping	Inventory control

OPERATIONS MANAGEMENT

Every practice needs a bible of how and why the clinic runs the way it does. In the office setting you will need several. First, you will want an employee manual, which will communicate what you expect from employees, outline benefits, and give some basic but essential information about your office. Some practices may choose to incorporate compliance information in this manual or segregate it into a separate manual. The goal of the manual is to set lines of authority, communicate basic business practices, and define the benefit structure offered. It is necessary that a written acknowledgment be retained in the personnel file of each employee stating that the manual was received, read, and understood by the employee.

The second sets of manuals you will want to complete are policy and procedure manuals. To accommodate personnel and for ease of understanding, I recommend breaking the policy and procedure manual into two separate manuals, one for administrative staff and one for clinical staff. It is even helpful to break them into sections that mirror the tasks assigned to employees. Remember, these manuals are to be very detailed concerning how you want tasks to be accomplished. Table 73.1 is a sample table of contents for each manual. Stop and jot down a brief note if you have strong feelings about how you want areas handled in your practice.

Many practices do not create a set of manuals until something goes wrong. This is a huge mistake. Communication and documentation in the medical office are as important as keeping medical records on patients. Writing things down with specific instructions is a good way for you to establish expectations and goals for your practice. Do not skip this step of creating a road map for the direction of your practice.

FINANCIAL MANAGEMENT

Many physicians make the mistake of believing that financial management is solely the process of recording how you spend the money brought in. In reality, financial management starts with when the patient is scheduled for the appointment. It is important for all of the staff to realize that this is the first step to a successful practice. Explaining financial policies on the phone when the appointment is made sets the tone of the entire process for the patient. The expectation is that the patient understands his or her responsibility for payment, what the office will and will not do regarding insurance, and this allows the patient to be prepared for that first visit. This is not something that should be viewed as greed but instead as a service to inform. The approach is to capitalize on every patient contact to communicate expectations. You inform them to bring in any prescriptions they are taking; why not remind them that you need a copy of the insurance card, precertification, or checkbook for the co-pay.

Registration or the "check-in" process is something that is neglected in many practices and has a huge impact on financial management. I cannot stress enough how important complete and accurate information is from this very point forward. If the registration process breaks down, the entire financial process is in jeopardy. With all the forms and tools in today's society, you would think this step would be easy, but it is the one that needs the most attention in physician offices. Remember how important selecting the right person is for the job. Invariably, I will go into a physician's office and find the least intelligent and lowest paid person in the front desk position. Not to belittle the point, but you get what you pay for and running the front desk is a critical process in the financial health of your practice.

It is recommended that you develop a form that captures not only the patient's information but also information of a close relative or friend. This might be the only way to locate a collection problem, so keep in mind what information is necessary in the process of skip tracing a patient. The registration form should include an assignment of benefits form as well as a financial policy statement. Do not accept registration forms that are not filled out completely. The patient is telling you something by not completing the information, i.e., "I don't care whether you get paid or not." Stop right there and do not allow that patient into your practice. There are no shortages of pain patients; you might as well only see the ones who are interested in paying for your services.

The financial policy for your practice should specifically instruct patients on what administrative procedures will be followed to help them obtain benefits for their healthcare. It should state clearly that patients are expected to pay for medical services regardless of insurance coverage. Payment arrangements or payment options such as credit cards or bank loans may be outlined in the policy. It also should inform the guarantor as to when an account will be referred to a professional collection agency. It is recommended that this be a two-part carbon form signed by the patient. One copy is given to the patient and the other is retained in the chart or billing file for future reference.

Many practices also need to include an ABN, Advanced Beneficiary Notice. This is a form required by Medicare, which tells the patient that Medicare may not pay for the treatment they are requesting. In pain practices this is common, and communicating this message right at the beginning to the patient will help him or her understand what the financial responsibility might be when incurring this treatment option.

This process of registration, precertification, and benefit structure has become so complicated that many practices have hired what I would term as financial counselors. If your practice chooses to hire such a specialist, you must plan for this in your office layout. This individual will need a private place to speak with patients about confidential matters. Again, personnel selection is extremely important.

THE MEDICAL RECORD

The chart has become so important that a chapter should be devoted solely to its contents and organizational structure. I will summarize what should be a review for physicians regarding documentation. You must realize that documentation is not only a communication tool for your own office but also will help you in medical-legal issues as well as provide for a defense in billing. Each visit, yes, every encounter with the patient no matter how brief, should follow the charting guidelines in Table 73.2.

A well-organized chart is like gold, precious, and to be guarded. Do not underestimate the importance of organization. Simple tools will help keep everyone current on the status of the patient if the rules are followed. Pain charts should begin with the left side reflecting a medication and patient visit summary. Separate sections for visits/procedures, radiology findings, and previous medical records are suggested. The chart needs to work for you and be organized so that all clinical staff can quickly identify risk areas for the patient.

CPT/ICD-9 Coding

The Center for Medicare and Medicaid Services (CMS) has adopted a single diagnostic coding system, the International Classification of Diseases, Ninth Revision, Clinical Modification (ICD-9-CM). This coding system is used regardless of the setting in which the services are rendered in accordance with the coding guidelines and reporting requirements. Procedures/services are coded using the Health Care Financing Administration's Common Procedure Coding System (HCPCS), of which the American Medical Association's Physicians' *Current Procedural Terminology*, Fourth Edition (CPT-4) system is a part.

TABLE 73.2
Charting Guides

1. The medical record must be legible and complete.
2. Each visit should include the following:
   a. Date
   b. Reason for the visit
   c. Appropriate history and physical exam
   d. Review of ancillary data, lab or X-ray, as indicated
   e. Physician assessment
   f. Plan of care
3. Past and present diagnosis should be accessible to the treating and/or consulting physician.
4. Rationale for ordering and the results of diagnostic tests, X-ray or lab, should be documented in the medical record.
5. Patient health risk factors noted.
6. Patient's progress, including the response to treatment, change in treatment plan, revision of diagnosis, and patient noncompliance to the plan should be documented.
7. The plan of care should outline specific treatments and medications, specifying frequency and dosage, any referrals or consultations to outside specialists, education given to patient or family, and specific instructions for follow-up with physician.
8. Written support of the complexity of the visit and the physician's medical decision-making process to create the plan for treatment.
9. Medical documentation should not be limited to physician documentation; nursing and other non-physician staff should be dated and signed by the person making the chart entry.
10. CPT/ICD-9 codes reported on the HCFA 1500 form must be reflected in the documentation of the medical record.

The majority of third-party payors also subscribe to this methodology, making coding the industry billing standard. CPT-4 codes tell the payor *what* services were provided and billed, and ICD-9 CM codes provide the *reason* medical services were rendered. Documentation in the patient's medical record to substantiate codes listed on the HCFA-1500 insurance claim form may be reviewed by a payor, pre- or post-payment of benefits. Payors may deny payment or request a refund if documentation does not provide enough information to demonstrate that billed services were performed or that services were medically necessary.

A complete revision of current diagnosis coding systems is underway with a target implementation date of October 2001 in the United States. ICD-10-CM represents the most significant revision of ICD (International Classification of Disease) since its inception. There are thousands more diagnosis codes (more than 50%), with more characters; codes are alphanumeric and the organization has changed. The goal is granularity, i.e., to provide greater detail that will be useful in healthcare policy and outcomes research.

To code accurately, it is necessary to have a working knowledge of medical terminology and to understand the characteristics, terminology, and conventions of the ICD-9-CM. Transforming verbal descriptions of diseases, injuries, conditions, and procedures into numerical designations (coding) is a complex activity and should not be undertaken without proper training.

Originally, coding was accomplished to provide access to medical records by diagnosis and operations through retrieval for medical research, education, and administration. Medical codes today are utilized to facilitate payment of health services, to evaluate utilization patterns, and to study the appropriateness of healthcare costs. Coding provides the basis for studies and research into the quality of healthcare.

Coding must be performed correctly and consistently to produce meaningful statistics to aid in the planning for the health needs of the nation. At the physician/patient encounter, the physician ascertains what is wrong with the patient through evaluation, diagnostic tests, and various forms of treatment. This information is then translated into the language of codes to send to the insurance carrier requesting reimbursement for services and procedures performed based on medical necessity and diagnosis involved.

The government's definition of medical necessity is "a service that is reasonable and necessary for the diagnosis or treatment of illness or injury, or to improve the functioning of a malformed body member" (Medicare Carrier's Manual). In other words:

- Services must be consistent with the symptoms or diagnoses of the illness or injury under treatment;
- Necessary and consistent with generally accepted professional medical standards, i.e., not experimental or investigational;
- Not furnished primarily for the convenience of the patient, the attending physician, or another physician or supplier; and
- The service must be furnished at the most appropriate level, which can be provided safely and effectively to the patient.

Establishing medical necessity is the first step in third-party reimbursement. Justify the care provided by presenting the appropriate facts. These facts must be substantiated by the patient's medical record, which may be requested by the insurance carrier for pre- or post-payment review at any time.

The first diagnostic code referenced on the HCFA-1500 claim form describes the most important reason for the care provided. Often a single ICD-9-CM code adequately identifies the need for care. If additional facts are required to substantiate the care provided that day, list the ICD-9-CM codes in the order of their importance. Be careful to link your diagnosis codes to the proper CPT-4 code, especially when more than one procedure is pro-

vided during a single encounter or on a single date of service.

Physicians and coders often have a dilemma when attempting to code "pain" to the highest degree of specificity. Standard coding requirements are to code to the highest degree of specificity and code the "disease," not the symptom. In a pain management practice, it is often necessary to code the "pain symptom" until the physician is able to make a more specific diagnosis; this may take several visits and diagnostic tests.

Documentation should be reviewed and the patient's current pain diagnosis coded for each visit, independent of prior visits and treatment. Diagnoses change based on treatment outcomes and diagnostic tests; the physician should provide a diagnosis for every encounter and/or procedure performed.

Most Medicare carriers have implemented local medical review policies that list specific medical necessity coverage guidelines determined by the diagnosis code assigned. Policies vary from state to state so it is necessary for each practice to review its own carrier's local medical review policies. This can be done via the Internet. The Web site is www.lmrp.net.

If a remittance advice lists "not medically necessary" as a reason for nonpayment, the patient's medical record and the carrier policy should be carefully reviewed to determine if a different diagnosis would have been more appropriate. Billing personnel may need asistance from physicians to select a more appropriate code. A diagnosis should not be altered unless documentation in the patient's medical record substantiates the change.

Third-party payors differ on coverage and benefits as well as reporting requirements. For example, carriers exist that do not accept CPT-4 codes designated as "unlisted procedure," which makes it very difficult to bill a procedure that does not have a designated CPT-4 code. Carrier representatives should be queried for billing instructions in such instances.

Another approach for carriers that do not accept unlisted codes is to carefully choose a CPT-4 code that is very similar in description and objective and with a relative value unit (RVU) (from the Medicare schedule) that is also similar. Write to your major payors. Your letter should contain information about the procedure (attach a procedure report), what procedure code is thought to be appropriate, and additional explanation of the procedure. Explain that there is no CPT-4 code and that you will submit your changes under xxxxx procedure, and ask them to please notify your office if this is not acceptable or if the company would prefer that you use a different CPT-4 code or its own specifically assigned HCPCS code.

Included with procedure descriptions are common diagnosis codes. This listing of diagnoses is not intended to be exclusive of the indications for a specific procedure or treatment. Diagnoses are a composite of some of the

Medicare carrier policy statements and are intended as guidelines only.

CORRECT CODING INITIATIVE

On December 19, 1989, the Omnibus Budget Reconciliation Act of 1989 (P.L. 101-239) was enacted. Section 6102 of P.L. 101-239 amended Title XVIII of the Social Security Act by adding a new Section 1848, Payment for Physicians' Services. This section of the Act provided for replacing the previous reasonable charge mechanism of actual, customary, and prevailing charges with a resource-based relative value scale (RBRVS) fee schedule, which began in 1992.

Accurate coding and reporting of services by physicians are major concerns of HCFA. Medicare carriers have included in their claims processing system various computerized edits to detect improper coding of procedures. Many of these edits are designed to detect fragmentation, or separate coding of the component parts of a procedure, instead of reporting a single code which includes the entire procedure.

The purpose of the National Correct Coding Council's (AdminiStar Federal) contract was to develop Correct Coding Methodologies for HCFA's Bureau of Program Operations. This manual, termed the Correct Coding Initiative (CCI), is used by all Medicare carrier intermediaries and some commercial payors as well. Commercial payors may have their own version of "CCI," sometimes referred to as "black box edits," that are not published.

Each CCI chapter consists of the Manual divided into two sections:

1. Mutually exclusive procedures are those which cannot be performed during the same operative or patient session;
2. Comprehensive and Compound procedure code combinations, which are divided into Column 1 and Column 2 procedures. The Component procedure (column 2) will not be reimbursed when the same provider renders the procedure on the same date; this is referred to as "unbundling."

Unbundling is essentially the billing of multiple procedure codes for a group of procedures that are covered by a single comprehensive code. Attempting to bill separately for these already bundled charges will constitute a claim for unbundled codes.

There are two types of unbundling: the first is unintentional and results from a misunderstanding of coding, and the second is intentional, when the technique is used by providers to manipulate coding in order to maximize payment. It is important to refer to a current copy of the CCI to avoid billing unbundled codes. This practice of billing unbundled codes is fraud and will be prosecuted as such by the U.S. Attorney General.

A copy of this quarterly publication can be obtained from: HCFA Correct Coding Initiative, AdminiStar Federal, P.O. Box 50469, Indianapolis, IN, 46250-0469.

CHARGE TICKETS

Charge tickets should be designed as a communication tool for your billing staff. It should cover 90 to 95% of the services you perform. Each year the charge ticket should be updated for changes in CPT-4, procedure coding or ICD-9, diagnosis coding. It should always include all levels of evaluation and management services with some type of guideline to remind physicians of the appropriate medical situations that constitute each level.

Most physicians do not have a system for establishing prices for the services they perform. While it is true that many managed care fees are set, you must know your costs and individual statistics in order to evaluate whether you are being paid fairly for your services. It is good to start with some outside resources. Gather the Medicare RBRVS fee schedule, the ASA Relative Value Guide, and any other professional society recommendations regarding fees and put them into a worksheet that identifies the different schedules by CPT code. This will give you a side-by-side comparison so that you can begin to analyze and draft your own fee schedule.

The next critical step is to analyze your individual practice data. Evaluate the demand for pain services in your area and assess your competition. Gather some outside resources from your region's business journal or the Chamber of Commerce regarding the payors in your area and the number of lives that each represents. Finally, look at your utilization of the procedures you perform.

There are publications available for national averages per year on physician charges. The important thing to realize is that the information is on charges submitted, not on payments made. The information is available by region or by specific zip code. Normally, the information shows the average allowable reimbursement paid by commercial payors and 50 to 75% and 95% of what most physicians charge.

The most important element in setting fees is to identify how much it actually costs you to perform a procedure. This can be done in several ways. Activity-based costing looks at the cost of each activity needed while performing a procedure. Because most physician groups do not have accounting expertise to efficiently do this, I recommend estimating the direct costs by procedure, allocating a charge per procedure for overhead, and then adding an acceptable mark-up for profit.

Now go back to your spreadsheet and add the column of cost. You have all the information you need to decide how to set your fees. Profit cannot be realized if costs exceed income. Performing more services does not guarantee profit. You must constantly monitor your payors with regard to the fee schedule that they pay.

- Checks and balances must exist in your system to assure that you capture all charges into the billing system, that the insurance claims are generated, and that the money will come back to the practice within a reasonable time period. The first check and balance should be the schedule to the charge tickets. This should be done every day with no exceptions. Balancing controls by either dollar amount or hash totals of CPTs should be implemented to verify the charge tickets to the computer system. When insurance claims are generated, some verification system as well periodic monitoring of the accuracy of the claims should be done. Payment could come as soon as 14 days if filing electronically or take up to 45 days. If no payment is received by the 45th day, immediate collection follow-up should be started.
- Negotiate contracts that allow at least 90-day timely filing deadlines.
- File electronically.
- Keep track of internal turnaround time.
- Keep track of claims turnaround time.
- Work the mail to discover your problems.

The most important fact you must face is that you are not a bank. Accounts receivables on the books is not cash in the bank. Establishing and adhering to a financial policy will benefit everyone in your practice. You must establish a system to collect co-pays and small balances at the time services are rendered. Your best possible time for collection is when you see the patient for follow-up visits. Remind patients of their balances and that you will help them collect benefits that they have paid for from their insurance carrier. You are entitled to be paid for the services you have performed. Today is a plastic society; accept MasterCard and Visa in your practice.

Probably the best action for your practice is to make it everyone's responsibility to collect money. Knowing how to figure a bill, understanding co-pays and deductibles, and filing secondary insurance immediately all help reduce the practice's accounts receivable. When it comes to patient statements, put a due date on the statement. All individuals pay bills by the day they are due. Physicians make the mistake of not having due dates on statements, which sends the message that it is OK for the patient to pay whenever they can.

Many times office staff avoid collection calls. Collection calls are necessary to keep accounts receivable under control. Many times using a matter-of-fact attitude helps with making staff more comfortable in the process of collection calling. It is important to take the following approach:

- Call the person by proper name.
- Have your facts ready.
- Be pleasant but matter of fact.
- Most importantly, Follow-up... Follow-up...Follow-up.

Many times collections is nothing more than teaching patients about responsibility for their portion of the bill. Continually reminding patients of their payment promises and staying in contact with accounts that have slow payment are necessary for your financial health. Make sure your statements are easy to read and clearly tell the patient what you want them to do. Many times patients believe statements are only informational and have no call to action.

Being in private practice means accepting that a few patients never intend to pay. Identification and early placement of those accounts with a professional collection agency are in the best financial interest of your practice. Staff need to concentrate on those accounts under 90 days in order to have effective collections.

Finally, just a word to the wise: It is important for physicians to recognize and admit when they need help with business issues. Physicians are busy individuals and trusting by nature. They must develop business skills in order to survive. It is never wrong to ask for help or admit that something is not quite right, just do not wait too long before inquiring. Seek advice from well-qualified professionals who have the reputation of being brutally honest.

REFERENCES

American Medical Association. (2000). *Current Procedural Terminology*, Chicago: AMA Press.

Medicode. (2000). *International Classification of Diseases, Ninth Revision, Clinical Modification* (6th ed.). Salt Lake City: Medicode.

74

Pain Management: Medical and Legal Issues of Undertreatment

James S. Lapcevic, D.O., Ph.D., J.D., F.C.L.M.

The American physician is currently faced with a practice paradox (Parran, 1997), demanding a new balance in the prescribing of controlled medications for the treatment of pain. This newly developed clinical dilemma comprises underprescribing narcotic analgesics to a majority of pain patients, while, on the other hand, overprescribing to a minority of patients. To stay the course of quality clinical practice requires physicians to understand both the medical and legal strategies undergirding the forces forging a new paradigm of medical care. Several thematic key issues are considered in this structure.

Pain, an important and serious symptom, is one of the most common reasons for seeking medical care (Weiner, 1993). Nine of ten Americans age 18 years or older report suffering pain at least once a month, and 42% of adults report experiencing pain every day (Gallup, Inc., 1999). Chronic pain is experienced daily by an estimated 75 million people in the United States (Bostrom, Ramberg, Davis, & Fridlund (1997). In the last decade interest in pain management (Rorarius & Baer, 1994; Tittle & McMillan, 1994) has risen largely due to surveys revealing that inadequate pain control is a norm under traditional clinical management, with as many as 75% of postoperative patients unnecessarily suffering unrelieved pain (Shapiro, 1996). In recent years, we have gained a new awareness of pain, its effects on quality of life, and the evaluation and issues involved in its treatment. The increasing number of those experiencing pain and other chronic medical conditions urges physicians to stay abreast of the most current and effective options for pain assessment, evaluation, and management. Yet much pain remains underreported as well as undertreated (Anon., 1998; Dahlman, Dykes, & Elander, 1999). Varying patient populations have been found to receive less than quality treatment of their pain if indeed any treatment at all (Bernabei, Gambassi, Lapane, et al., 1998; Cleeland, Gonin, Baez, Loehrer, & Pandya, 1997; Foley, 1997).

In a survey of physicians, 82% responded that they had not been adequately educated in pain management (Lavies, Hart, Rounsefell, & Runciman, 1992); patient surveys found more than half wanted decision capacity on when more analgesia should be given them.

EDUCATIONAL INTERVENTIONS TARGET EFFECTIVE MANAGEMENT PAIN

Pain is defined as an unpleasant sensory or emotional experience associated with actual or potential tissue damage and described in terms of such damage (Merskey, 1986). Classification of pain is either acute or chronic (see Table 74.1), although acute pain can evolve into chronic pain if not treated fully, promptly, and adequately (Marcus, 2000) to avoid such conversion (Katz, 1996). Effective management requires multifactorial assessment of components that differ only in magnitude from one affected person to the next (Goldstein, 1999). Pain is a dynamic process with a clinical significance (Carr, Jacox, Chapman, et al., 1992) affecting sympathetic nervous system activity, neuroendocrine activity (Kehlet, 1989; Lutz & Lamer, 1990), and it has adverse effects on the immune

0-8493-0926-3/02/$0.00+$1.50
© 2002 by CRC Press LLC

TABLE 74.1
Classification of Pain

	Acute Pain	Chronic Pain	
		Nonmalignant	**Malignant**
Duration	Hours to week	Months; years	Unpredictable
Pathophysiology	Identifiable	Not always identifiable	Identifiable
Prognosis	Predictable	Unpredictable	Multidisciplinary
Treatment	Analgesics	Multidisciplinary	

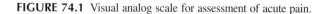

0   1   2   3   4   5   6   7   8   9   10
No pain   Worst pain

FIGURE 74.1 Visual analog scale for assessment of acute pain.

system (Terman & Liebeskind, 1991). The control of pain can influence clinical outcome (Whipple, Lewis, Quebbman, et al., 1995) while unrelieved pain can impair recovery (Brown & Carpenter, 1990; Carr, Jacox, Chapman, et al., 1992) as well as result in anxiety, depression, sleep deprivation, or any combination of these. Pain itself can be clinically assessed by subjective direct and indirect methods utilizing pain scales to chart the pain intensity. Common measures of pain intensity are

1. Categorical scale of pain intensity. A simple descriptive scale representing the oldest approach to pain assessment. Most often, this scale consists of four categories: 0 = no pain, 1 = slight or mild pain, 2 = moderate pain, and 3 = severe pain.

2. Visual analog scale (VAS) (Figure 74.1). The patient is asked to draw a mark somewhere along the line between no pain = 1 and worst pain = 10. Good agreement between descriptive and visual analog ratings has been found (Litman, Walker, & Schneier, 1985). To ensure proper management of pain, healthcare professionals should chart pain as formalized in a report prepared by the American Pain Society (APS) Quality Care Committee (American Pain Society, 1995) (see Table 74.2). Pain assessment should be charted as the "fifth" vital sign (Oncology Nursing Society, 1998) in patient evaluation. The Veterans Administration has made a decision to implement in all its facilities the process of charting pain as a fifth vital sign. Continued assessment of pain should involve evaluating and charting at several critical times in the pain management process (see Table 74.3) (Jacox, Carr, Payne, Berde, Biebart,

TABLE 74.2
Major Recommendations to Include in a Program Designed to Enhance Relief of Pain

- Make sure that a report of unrelieved pain will raise a red flag sufficient to attract the attention of clinicians.
- Make information about analgesics readily available, especially in the area where orders are written.
- Promise patients that they will recieve responsive analgesic care, and urge them to facilitate this process by communicating their pain.
- Define and implement policies (and safeguards) for use of advanced techniques for pain control (such as intraspinal patient-controlled opioid infusion).
- Assess on a continual basis both the process of pain control and procedures used to achieve this clinical outcome.

TABLE 74.3
Instances When Pain Should Be Evaluated and Charted

- Whenever there is a new report of pain
- At regular intervals after initiation of therapy
- At an interval commensurate with the therapy (such as 15 to 30 minutes after administration of parenteral drug therapy; 60 minutes after oral therapy)

Cain, et al., 1994). Distinguishing characteristics of acute and chronic pain (see Table 74.4) are summarized.

Basic tenets (McCarberg, 2000) of pain management are

1. Do not assume a patient's pain is being adequately treated because the patient does not complain.

2. "Pain" should always be considered the fifth vital sign. Ask the patient about pain, prescribe what is needed to relieve that pain (including opioids, if necessary), and follow up with frequent evaluations of the efficacy of the treatment regimen.

TABLE 74.4
Distinguishing Characteristics of Acute and Chronic Pain

Acute Pain	Chronic Pain
A symptom of disease	Is itself the disease
Self-limiting	Persists beyond the usual course of acute disease
Provoked by	Provoked by
• Noxious stimulation	• Chronic pathologic process
• Tissue injury	• Dysfunction of PNS or CNS
• Abnormal function of somatice or visceral structures	• Psychological and learned (environmental) factors
Followed by emotional, psychological, and autonomic responses	May not be followed by autonomic and neuroendocrine responses; vegetative state may emerge
Has a biological function (alerting, warning, resting, healing)	Never has a biological function

3. Modify treatment according to patient response.
4. Make use of both pharmacologic and nonpharmacologic methods for pain relief.
5. Involve the patient as much as possible in pain control strategies, explain options available, and foster a positive attitude in the patient toward dealing with pain.
6. Ensure continuity of pain management once the patient leaves the hospital; pain can and should be controlled in the outpatient setting to the same extent as when the patient is hospitalized.

Over the past decade concerted efforts have been made to educate healthcare providers regarding the need to aggressively treat pain. Reliance on the primary care physician, who is quite capable of treating routine chronic pain conditions, continues due to the relatively small numbers of pain specialists. The American Academy of Pain Management, the American Academy of Pain Medicine, and the American Pain Society, professional organizations for the study of the scientific and clinical aspects of pain, have available membership directories that can help the primary care physician find help through a specialist in his or her area.

Pain is classified as acute or chronic. Acute pain is sometimes defined as pain that persists for less than 3 months and can be understood when associated with an acute injury as cause and effect. Chronic pain, on the other hand, is pain that persists for more than 3 months beyond the normal time of healing (e.g., pain related to chronic back problems or sickle-cell disease). Diseases such as AIDS can cause chronic noncancer pain and demand the same attention to pain relief as given to terminal cancer patients. Cancer pain is either resolved after the cancer is resolved or may continue indefinitely as a complication of otherwise curative therapy.

Pain may also be classified as neuropathic, or nociceptive and visceral. Nociceptive and visceral pain originates in muscle, bone, or visceral structures, whereas neuropathic pain originates in the nerves. Neuropathic pain can be defined as pain resulting from noninflammatory dysfunction of the peripheral or central nervous system without trauma or peripheral nociceptor stimulation, usually described by pain patients as "burning," "shooting," or "lancinating."

To make good pain management decisions, physiology, anatomy, and referred-pain pathways must be considered. There is no substitute for touching the patient. It has been said that the best cheap test for evaluating physiologic change and understanding the origin of a patient's pain is a good neurological physical examination (Saberski, 2000). The weak point in patient evaluation is the patient's complaint; the strong must be the physician's knowledge that pain is complex, and may not be what is expressed (Saberski, 2000).

While it is important to stay abreast of new technologies despite dramatic technological breakthroughs, there can be no replacement for a thorough and complete history and physical examination. Physicians may need assistance in identifying chronic pain patients who are not adequately coping with the experience of pain while making their quality of life independent of the perception of pain. By asking three questions, clinicians can identify patients who are in all probability not coping well and might benefit from psychological intervention that addresses self-efficacy.

The self-efficacy screen (Kores, Murphy, Rosenthal, Elias, & North, 1990) comprises three questions (see Table 74.5) with graded response. While this verbal screen is not sufficiently sensitive to identify all pain patients in need of psychological intervention, it will identify a subset for whom treatment can be expanded to address their psychological and physiological pain management needs. Patients with pain may have an exaggerated response if an underlying depression is also present. In patients using long-term opioids for treatment of chronic pain, some useful questions may be used to screen for signs of addiction (Ewing, 1984) (see Table 74.6). Portenoy (1996a) has classified aberrant drug-related behaviors into those probably more or probably less predictive of addiction (see Table 74.7).

TABLE 74.5
Self-Efficacy Screen

1. Do you feel that by taking care of yourself you can limit your pain?	Yes	No
2. Do you feel that doctors/therapists will control your pain?	Yes	No
3. Despite your best efforts, does your pain prevent you from getting a good night's sleep?	Yes	No

Note: A negative response to questions 1 and 2 and a positive response to question 3 indicate poor coping and need for psychological intervention. Note that question 2 is keyed paradoxically. While one might expect the pathologic answer to question 2 to be a positive response, it is a negative response that is actually interpreted as significant.

TABLE 74.6
CAGE Test

C	Have you ever felt you should *cut* down on your substance use?	Yes	No
A	Have people *annoyed* you by criticizing or complaining about your substance use?	Yes	No
G	Have you ever felt bad or *guilty* about your substance use?	Yes	No
E	Have you ever needed an *eye opener* in the morning to steady your nerves or get rid of a hangover?	Yes	No

Note: Any patient responding yes to two or more of the questions in this simple screening test should be subject to more intense scrutiny for the signs of addiction (Kores, Murphy, Rosenthal, Elias, & North, 1990).

TABLE 74.7
Representative Aberrant Drug-Related Behaviors*

Probably More Predictive
- Selling prescription drugs
- Forging prescription
- Stealing or "borrowing"
- Frequent prescription "loss"
- Injection oral/topical formulations
- Obtaining prescription drugs form nonmedical sources
- Concurrent abuse of related illicit drugs

Probably Less Predictive
- Aggressive demand for more drug
- Drug hoarding
- Unsanctioned dose escalation
- Unapproved use of the drug
- Unkempt appearance

* Empirically divided into those that are assumed to be relatively more predictive and those that are assumed to be relatively less predictive of addiction. (Adapted from Portenoy, R. K. *Journal of Pain and Symptom Management, 11,* 203–217, 1996.)

For pain of terminal disease, pain relief should be provided because easing pain and improving functions are the goals when treating acute and chronic pain patients whether or not there exists a history of addiction. By using questions geared to level of function and behavior, healthcare providers can adequately assess probability of drug abuse or addiction. Fear of addiction in the terminally ill patient is exaggerated as is the likelihood of inducing respiratory depression.

Pain at the end of life can be adequately managed with clearly defined management strategies. The World Health Organization has proposed a three-step analgesic ladder approach to pain management in which nonopioid, opioid, and adjuvant analgesics are used based on the type and intensity of pain (see Table 74.8). The steps are coupled to the Visual Analog Pain Scale assessment (see Figure 74.1). The categories of analgesics and dosages are succinctly noted (see Table 74.9), while comparison of opioids in oral and parenteral dosage conversion (see Table 74.10) shows clearly that dosage adjustments (Education for Physicians, 1999) are necessary when routes of administration or conversion from one opioid to another are considered. Opioids are the mainstays and clearly the agents of choice for treatment of moderate to severe pain. Through appropriate knowledge of opioid dosing intervals and titration of dose, severe pain even at end of life can be managed. Healthcare providers must remain diligent in management of end-of-life pain because unrelieved pain for the terminally ill patient is an ethical issue (Ferrel & Rhiner, 1994) as much as it is dehumanizing. The ethical principle of "double effect" allows for the administration of opioids to control pain even though the dying process may be hastened (Cavanaugh, 1996). Physicians can and should enhance the dying patient's quality of life by enabling the patient to avoid pain (Cavalieri, 1999).

TABLE 74.8
World Health Organization's Three-Step Ladder of Analgesics

Step 3: Severe pain
(7 through 10 on pain scale)
- Morphine
- Hydromorphone
- Methadone
- Oxycodone
- Transdermal fentanyl
- With or without nonopioid analgesics
- With or without adjuvant analgesics

Step 2: Moderate pain
(5 through 6 on pain scale)
- Codeine
- Hydrocodone
- Dihydrocodeine
- Oxycodone
- Tramadol
- With or without nonopioid analgesics
- With or without adjuvant analgesics

Step 1: Mild pain
(1 through 4 on pain scale)
- Aspirin
- Other nonsteroidal anti-inflammatory drugs
- Acetaminophen
- With or without adjuvant analgesics

TABLE 74.9
Categories of Analgesic Dosages Analgesics

Nonopioids

Nonsteroidal Anti-Inflammatory
- Aspirin (650 mg every 4 hours)
- Ibuprofen (400 to 600 mg every 6 hours)
- Diflunisal (500 mg every 12 hours)
- Sulindac (150 to 200 mg every 12 hours)
- Naproxen (250 to 500 mg every 12 hours)
- Diclofenac (50 to 75 mg every 12 hours)
- Salsalate (750 to 1500 mg every 12 hours)

Acetaminophen (60 mg every 4 hours)

Tramadol (50 to 75 mg every 8 hours)

Opioids

Step 2 Opioids
- Codeine (100 mg every 4 hours)
- Dihydrocodeine (50 to 75 mg every 4 hours)
- Hydrocodone (15 mg every 4 hours)
- Oxycodone (7.5 to 10 mg every 4 hours)
- Propoxyphene (180 mg every every 4 hours)

Step 3 Opioids
- Morphine (15 mg every 4 hours)
- Oxycodone (7.5 to 10 mg every 4 hours)
- Hydromorphone (50–150 mg every 4 hours)
- Transdermal fentanyl (50 mg/hour)

Adjuvant Analgesics

Antidepressants
- Amitriptyline (25 to 150 mg at bedtime)
- Notriptyline (25 to 150 mg at bedtime)

Anticonvulsants
- Carbamazepine (100 mg to 200 mg twice or four times daily)
- Valproic acid (200 to 400 mg twice or four times daily)
- Gabapentin (300 to 1800 mg three times daily)

Local Anesthetics
- Lidocaine (1.5 mg/kg IV)
- Mexiletine hydrochloride (400 to 600 mg/d)

Capsaicin (topically three times daily)

Steriods
- Prednisone (20 mg/d to 80 mg/d)
- Dexamethasone (4 mg/d to 16 mg/d)

[a] All dosages are oral unless specified otherwise.
From *Education for Physicians on End-of-Life Care*. Participants handbook, American Medical Association, Chicago, IL, 1999. With permission.

TABLE 74.10
Comparison of Opioids in Oral and Parenteral Dosage Conversions

Oral Dosage	Opiod	Parenteral Dosage
15 mg	Morphine	5 mg
10 mg	Oxycodone	—
4 mg	Hydromorphone	1.5 mg
15 mg	Hydrocodone	—
100 mg	Codeine	60 mg
150 mg	Meperidine hydrochloride	50 mg

Adapted from *Education for Physicians on End-of-Life Care*. Participants handbook. American Medical Association, Chicago, IL, 1999. With permission.

GUIDELINE DEVELOPMENT

Many Americans are now over the age of 60. That segment of the population of the United States over 65 will double in the next 33 years, with the oldest of the old, those over age 85, the fastest growing segment of the entire population. The elderly represent 12.7% of the population or one in every eight Americans (James, 2000). By the year 2030, 20% of our population will be over 65. As the population ages, more conditions causing pain, from arthritis to malignancy, will emerge. A significant proportion of all pharmaceuticals will be analgesic agents (Hill, 1996).

In the past decade, societal and government needs have molded medical practice into a less variable and more standardized activity (Hill, 1996a). Guidelines for pain management have been issued by such diverse groups as the World Health Organization, the American Pain Society, the American Society of Anesthesiologists, the American Academy of Pediatrics, the International Association for the Study of Pain, and the United States Agency for Health Care Policy and Research (AHCPR) (Hill, 1995).

Federal oversight of controlled substances extends into community standards of care. According to the AHCPR guidelines (1992), opioids may be prescribed to treat acute and chronic pain, but the prescribing physician assumes the burden of proving that the prescription falls within normal clinical procedures for pain management. A physician prescriber of a controlled substance is obligated to demonstrate both the medical necessity and adherence to law of such a choice. Many healthcare practice acts do not provide for the interpretation of phrases such as "practicing medicine in a manner inconsistent with public health and welfare" (Hill, 1996b). It is often the legal process that later defines these concepts of "reasonably necessary" and "good faith" that are critical to the justification, and even legal defense, of controlled substance prescribing in an individual case.

Allegations of prescribing too much, too little, or not prescribing a controlled substance that was needed according to the definition outlined in federal or state guidelines may be open to court interpretation through expert witnesses brought in by medical boards, plaintiffs, or the Drug Enforcement Agency (DEA). Claims that prescribing behavior was not in good faith or not reasonably necessary, requirements designed to establish medical necessity which may be redefined ad hoc, can make it difficult for physicians to justify their treatment decisions. To avoid unwittingly running a collision course with these complex issues, better training in proper pain management procedures is necessary for physicians (Carr, 1998). Generally, physicians who prescribe scheduled or nonscheduled analgesic medications believe their patients need them. Physicians must be aware of the immediate medicolegal ramification, including the burden of proof, that must be considered when analgesic medications are prescribed (Clark, 1998).

Ideally, treatment guidelines should be based on data from the medical literature, case law, and clinical experience, although the boards that administer and interpret healthcare practice acts are comprised of state government officials' appointees whose members' biases may be reflected in the guidelines (Hill, 1996b). While not all state medical boards hit the mark, many experts favor state medical policy, issuing from the medical boards rather than from elected officials, directly addressing physicians concerns through medical guidelines. In 1999, The Ohio State Medical Association, in cooperation with the state legislature, distributed a new clinical handbook titled *Pain: The Fifth Vital Sign*. Distributed to all physicians, but directed at primary care physicians, the booklet encouraged better pain management including a step-by-step guide to documentation requirement compliance.

In 40 states, a variety of efforts have been undertaken to improve pain management: lawmakers through specific legislation, regulators through new regulations, and state medical boards through revised or newly adopted guidelines and policy statements on pain treatment as state governments and medical boards focus on pain (see Table 74.11). Good documentation (the virtual flack jacket), despite its hassles, is one way to reduce the likelihood of a routine inquiry mushrooming into a full-blown investigation, although nothing — not the best documentation, the best guidelines, or the most enlightened regulatory attitudes — will reduce physician risk to zero, but that seems the inherent nature of the occupation. The kind of medical documentation adequate for most medical problems is often seen as inadequate in the treatment of pain (Hoover, 1996). The American Medical Association (AMA) and the American Hospital Association (AHA) have formulated criteria, in the development of an increasing number of

TABLE 74.11

State Governments and Medical Boards Focus on Pain

State	Pain Laws	Pain Regulations	Medical Board Guidelines and Policy Statements
Alabama		X	
Alaska			X
Arizona			X
Arkansas		X	
California	X		X
Colorado	X		X
Florida	X		X
Georgia			X
Idaho			X
Iowa		X	
Kansas			X
Louisiana		X	
Maine		X	
Maryland			X
Massachusetts			X
Michigan	X		X
Minnesota	X		X
Mississippi		X	X
Missouri	X		
Montana			X
Nebraska	X		X
Nevada	X	X	
New Jersey		X	
New Mexico	X		X
North Carolina			X
North Dakota	X		
Ohio	X	X	X
Oklahoma	X	X	X
Oregon	X	X	X
Pennsylvania		X	X
Rhode Island	X		X
Tennessee		X	X
Texas	X	X	X
Utah			X
Vermont			X
Virginia	X		X
Washington	X	X	X
West Virginia	X		X
Wisconsin	X		
Wyoming			X

Note: These laws and regulations give physicians immunity when prescribing opioids for intractable pain.

Sources: Health Policy Tracking Service of the National Conferences of State Legislatures, September 1999; and the Pain and Policy Studies Group, University of Wisconsin-Madison, January 2000.

treatment guidelines, to guide policy makers in this area. Primary criteria include the potential to improve individual patient outcome, affect a large patient population, reduce cost either for the individual or in the aggregate, and reduce unexplained variations in medical practice (Carr, Jacox, Chapman, et al., 1995).

AHCPR guidelines for effective pain relief promise patients attentive and effective analgesic care as well as quantification in the medical chart of pain assessment and pain relief. AHCPR has issued recommendations regarding use of medications for management of pain in adults after extensive literature review and evaluation of data. The AHCPR guidelines establish basic principles with which analgesic drug treatment should comply (see Table 74.12) and integrate specialized technology and nonpharamacologic approaches. A systematic review of the literature is used to compile evidence for each mode of pain relief. Type I evidence comes from large trials; Type Ia evidence is derived from multiple, randomized, controlled trials that may be consolidated as meta-analysis. Type Ib data originate from at least one large, randomized, controlled study with statistically significant results. Type II studies involve well-designed but nonrandomized comparisons. Type III evidence is from descriptive studies. Type IV evidence is expert consensus, based on the opinions of prominent practitioners (Carr, Jacox, Chapman, et al., 1992). Balanced Analgesia combines an opioid and a nonopioid to reduce the opioid requirement and has now become standard practice (Joshi, 1994). Certain opioids should be avoided when possible. Meperidine hydrochloride is not recommended for long-term use because of the potential for accumulation of normeperidine, a toxic metabolite, that can cause confusion or seizures. Propoxyphene, for example, is an opiate with a 13-hour half-life. It is metabolized by a mechanism of n-demethylation through a saturable mechanism, forming the metabolite norpropoxyphene. In the elderly, susceptibility to the accumulation of this potential toxic metabolite exists. Additionally, partial and mixed opioid agonists such as buprenophine hydrochloride, pentazocine hydrochloride, butorphanol tartrate, and nalbuphine hydrochloride, because of their limited efficacy and possible toxicity, should be avoided (Cherny & Portenoy, 1994).

The newly found appreciation calling for aggressive action against acute pain resulted in the Federation of State Medical Boards of the United States, Inc. promulgating model guidelines in 1998 for pain management strategies and objectives (Model Guidelines, 1998). Clinicians will be held to those guidelines, and the quality of medical practice will be judged in part by the ability to meet those criteria. Some states have adopted even more stringent guidelines for pain treatment: at present, certain barriers to delivery of adequate analgesia and pain management exist. Members of the healthcare team, patients, and the healthcare system continue impeding the delivery of proper analgesia (see Table 74.13) (Jacox, Carr, Payne, et al., 1994).

TABLE 74.12
Pain Management Guidelines

Medications for Management of Pain in Adults

Medication	Evidence*	Comments	Precautions
Oral NSAIDs	lb, IV	Effective for mild-to-moderate pain. Begin pre-operatively.	Relatively contraindicated in patients with renal disease and risk of or actual coagulopathy. May mask fever.
Oral NSAIDs in conjunction with opioids	la, IV	Potentiating effect resulting in opioid sparing. Begin pre-operatively.	As above.
Parenteral NSAIDs	lb, IV	Effective for moderate-to severe pain. Expensive. Useful if opioids contraindicated, especially to avoid respiratory depression and sedation.	As above.
Oral opioids	IV	Route of choice. As effective as parenteral in appropriate doses. Use as oral medication tolerated.	
Intramuscular	lb, IV	The standard parenteral route, but injections painful and absorption unreliable. Hence, avoid this route when possible.	
Subcutaneous	lb, IV	Preferable to intramuscular route when low-volume continuous infusion is needed and intravenous access if difficult to maintain. Injections painful and absorption unreliable.	Avoid this route for long-term repetitive treatment.
Intravenous	lb, IV	Parenteral route of choice after major surgery. Suitable for titrated bolus or continuous administration but requires special monitoring.	Significant risk of respiratory depression with inappropriate dosing.
PCA (systemic)	la, IV	Intravenous or subcutaneous routes recommended. Good steady level of analgesia. Popular with patients but requires special infusion pumps and staff education.	Significant risk of respiratory depression with inappropriate dosing.
Epidural and intrathecal opioids	la, IV	When suitable, provides good analgesia. Use of infusion pumps requires additional equipment and staff education. Expensive if infusion pumps are used.	Significant risk of respiratory depression sometimes delayed in onset. Requires careful monitoring.

* la = evidence obtained from meta-analysis of randomized controlled trials.

  lb = evidence obtained from at least one randomized controlled trial.

  IV = expert consensus based on the opinions and/or clinical experiences of respected authorities.

  NSAID = nonsteroidal anti-inflammatory drug.

  PCA = patient-controlled analgesia.

TABLE 74.13
Barriers to Delivery of Adequate Analgesia

Healthcare Professionals	Reasons for Patient Reluctance to Report Pain	Healthcare System

• Inadequate knowledge of pain management (especially clinical pharmacology)
• Poor assessment of pain
• Concern about:
  • Regulation of controlled substances
  • Side effects of pain medication
  • Development of tolerance
  • Fear of patient addiction
	• Fear that pain means progression of disease
	• Want to be a "good" patient
	• Do not want to distract physicians from treating underlying disease
	• Reluctant to take pain medication
	• Fear of addiction or of being classified as an addict
	• Concerned about adverse reactions and development of tolerance
		• Low priority given to pain management
		• Inadequate reimbursement
		• Limits availability of treatment
		• Limits access to treatment
		• Restrictive regulation of controlled substances

Modified from Jacox, A., et al. (March 1994). Management of Cancer Pain. Clinical Guideline. Rockville, MD: U.S. Department of Health and Human Services.

FOCUS ON PAIN

In 40 states (see Table 74.11), a variety of efforts have been made to improve pain management. Some of these have been undertaken by lawmakers through specific legislation, or by regulators through new regulations. Others are results of revised or newly adopted guidelines and policy statements on pain treatment from state medical boards. Aimed at making standards uniform across the nation and encouraging better pain management, physicians who prescribe a controlled substance "for a legitimate medical purpose" are reassured not to worry about board action or that of a state regulatory or enforcement agency. The Federation initiative was endorsed by the Drug Enforcement Administration and by advocates for better pain management. The medical use of controlled substances has gained a new legitimacy, but physician fears of regulatory scrutiny linger.

Historically, from the advent of the Victorian era until after World War I, doctors were held largely responsible for the heroin, morphine, opiate, and cocaine problem that swept the United States. The Harrison Narcotic Act of 1914 began the heavy-handed crackdown on narcotics that narrowed the scope of medical practice and interfered with their legitimate medical use, especially in pain management (Guglielmo, 2000). A short decade ago, conventional wisdom in the medical establishment was that physicians treating chronic pain with opioids were at substantial risk of being sanctioned by state medical regulatory boards for overprescribing (Hill, 1993; Joranson, 1992; Portenoy, 1996b). A review of state medical board actions from 1990 to 1996 reveals that the perception of regulatory risk far exceeds the reality (Martino, 1998). A California study (Morrison & Wickersham, 1998) concluded that most offenses of disciplined physicians involved some aspect of patient care (e.g., inappropriate prescribing) and in the face of increasing consumer complaints, medical regulatory boards may have increased dealings with physicians who commit disciplinary offenses. Regulatory risks associated with overprescribing are still perceived as real and far greater (Glanelli, 1999) than those associated with underprescribing despite regulatory relief efforts. The premise of the regulatory relief efforts was that the undertreatment of pain is a public health problem. Ann M. Martino, Ph.D., executive director of Iowa's Board of Medical Examiners, recommends new laws be written to discipline physicians who prescribe too little pain medication. Ironically, she writes, the most immediate means [of achieving good pain management] may not be regulatory relief but more regulation (Martino, 1998).

It has been recommended that physician education is key to better pain management. Knowledge of the best drug and nondrug methods for controlling pain and of the federal and state laws that apply to medical practice is recommended at "should know" levels. State medical boards or medical societies are good resources. Caveat: A potent reminder finds that knowledge alone is insufficient to promote behavioral change (King, Bungard, McAlister, et al., 2000); in the absence of other actions such steps as disseminating a medical guideline or providing continuing medical education are unlikely to significantly, or even measurably, improve the effectiveness of an intervention (Goff, Canely, & Gu, 2000).

For decades, improving the quality of healthcare delivery relied on changing physician behavior. Experience has shown that quality improvement is better achieved through system solutions that support clinicians in providing quality care (Calonge, 2000). The imperative to measure, promote, and improve the quality of medical care continues to be an essential, if not daunting, endeavor. The quality of healthcare is, in the opinion of many, a serious problem (Chassin, & Galvin, 1998). Research demonstrates that physicians overuse healthcare services by ordering unnecessary interventions (Leape, 1992; Nyquist, Gonzales, Steiner, & Sande, 1998), underuse services by failing to provide a standard of care that would produce favorable outcomes (Chasin, 1997), and devise the wrong treatment plan or improperly execute the correct plan (Leape, 1994). Quality assurance in the healthcare system is an important public health objective (Lohr, 1990). The lessons of history confirm that the medical factors that have prompted medical malpractice litigation still continue but are in the public interest: scientific innovation, uniform standards, and liability insurance (Gostin, 2000). From a legal perspective, government directly and indirectly (the tort system) regulates the healthcare system.

Medical malpractice litigation ostensibly seeks higher quality care. Tort law, on the other hand, functions to deter substandard medical conduct, to avoid unnecessary injury, and as a fair method of compensation. Several reform methods are currently under public debate, the most prominent among these proposals being capitation on damages, which has been enacted in some states. Although this approach does not eliminate liability, it is proposed that such action would decrease fear of inordinate damage awards.

EMERGING STANDARD OF CARE IN PAIN MANAGEMENT AND LEGAL IMPLICATIONS

The rapidity of change in the clinical practice of medicine has brought frustration because of decreased autonomy, increased oversight, pressures on reimbursement, and allegations of fraud and abuse. Malpractice and legal complications of care have increased.

Despite the widespread promulgation of the benefits of opioid analgesics in all types of pain states — acute, chronic, and cancer — fear and trepidation remain on

TABLE 74.14
Key Points Included in the Controlled Substances Act

- Opioids are necessary to public health.
- A mechanism is devised for external medical input.
- Drug availability is guaranteed.
- The federal definition of an addict does not include the chronic pain patient.
- Regulations specifically recognize the treatment of intractable pain with opioids
- Prescription size is not restricted.
- Without a special license granted by the DEA, physicians may not provide methadone maintenance for patients with known addiction to controlled substances.

TABLE 74.15
Liability Issues in Pain Management

Liability to Patients

For cost-containment practices that affect pain management (Townsend, 1983)

For inappropriate pain management

Liability to Third Parties

For injury caused by patients treated for pain (Heller, 1992; Vainio, 1995; Wilchinsky, 1989)

Liability to Patients, Healthcare Providers, and Third Parties

For risks and side effects of drugs and pain management devices

the part of physicians prescribing opioids. The Uniform Controlled Substance Act of 1970 provides for the registration of those handling controlled substances, as well as for the labeling, order forms, record keeping, and reporting of substances or their use. Key points included in the Controlled Substances Act are listed in Table 74.14.

The issues of safety, efficacy, and compliance associated with the use of controlled substances invite problems of liability (see Table 74.15). States exercise parallel prohibition on the nonmedical use of controlled substances with most statutes based on the 1970 Model Uniform Controlled Substances Act. It is the intricacies and interrelationships between federal and state laws regulating the prescribing of opioid analgesics that have been repeatedly identified as one of the more significant barriers to the provision of effective pain management and palliative care (Rich, 2000). The barriers to pain management provide plausible reasons for so many patients to experience undertreated pain. Collectively, these barriers have either contributed to or caused an enduring epidemic of pain and suffering trailing in the wake of untreated pain (Rich, 2000). Patient-related barriers to good pain management also exist. The general public is ignorant and fearful of

opioid analgesics, and reluctant to be viewed as too demanding of more in the way of care than has been proffered. Laypersons can hardly be more sophisticated and knowledgeable about an emerging aspect of clinical medical practice than healthcare professionals (Cleeland, 1992). In 1996, an international panel of distinguished healthcare professionals assembled by the Hastings Center (International Project, 1996) identified the goals of medicine as

> The prevention of disease and injury and promotion and maintenance of health;
> The relief of pain and suffering caused by maladies;
> The care and cure of those with a malady, and the care of those who cannot be cured; and
> The avoidance of premature death and the pursuit of a peaceful death.

The stated goals strike a remarkable balance between the curative and the palliative approaches to patient care, strongly suggesting that the hegemony of the curative model that is the hallmark of modern medical education and practice reflects a medical ethos inconsistent with the core values of medicine (Rich, 2000).

EMERGING LIABILITY ISSUES IN THE MANAGEMENT OF PAIN

It is argued that there are three essential duties of a healthcare professional (Edwards, 1984) regarding pain management:

1. The first duty is to minimize iatrogenic (physician-induced) pain; no further pain and suffering are to be inflicted upon a patient beyond the unavoidable consequence of a reasonable effort to effect a cure.
2. The second duty is to be a competent practitioner in pain management. Effective application of state-of-the-art pain relief techniques is required to relieve as much pain as possible without imposition of patient burden that exceeds benefits. This is a duty that can reasonably be placed on all physicians who care for pain patients and not one reserved for pain or palliative care specialists only. It is time for those physicians who are most likely to see chronically ill patients in the first line of duty (general practitioners, oncologists) to make pain control and palliative care a part of routine clinical practice (Stjernsward, et al., 1996).
3. The third duty is to adequately inform the patient of the risks and benefits of alternative pain management strategies, including that of

not pursuing pain relief (Emanuel, 1996). Physicians have a duty to continue their education throughout their professional lives to maintain their practices consistent with advances in science and technology.

The issue of whether physicians should be insulated from ethical or legal responsibility for undertreating pain due to deficiency in this area of medical education (American Medical Association, 1996) was in seemingly direct contradiction with the AMA's Principles of Medical Ethics and the current opinion of the AMA on Professional Rights and Responsibilities (1996).

There is a developing healthcare professional consensus that failure either to effectively manage pain that can be managed or to refer the patient to a professional who can bring state-of-the-art techniques to bear on the problem, constitutes a breach of professional ethics and a departure from an emerging standard of care (Oherney & Catane, 1995). The concept of the patient's legal right to effective pain management and the correlative duty on the part of physicians because of their virtual monopoly on the authority to prescribe narcotics to provide effective pain management to patients has begun to emerge in the last decade. One of the first serious discussions on poor pain management as an example of medical malpractice was conducted by Margaret Sommerville, a Canadian legal scholar and bioethicist (1986). With the prevailing standard of care, it is argued that because it is abundantly clear that physicians traditionally fail to alleviate pain, a patient would find it difficult to establish undertreatment of pain as a departure from the applicable standard of care. The failure of the medical profession to adopt and consistently apply readily available therapeutic modalities that would improve patient care presents precisely a situational scenario ripe for judicial standard setting. With deficiencies in prevailing custom and practice so clearly inconsistent with the traditionally attributable goal of the medical profession, courts appear likely to revert to a past irresistible impulse to find the entire profession negligent (Hooper, 1932).

A primary impetus for the promulgation of clinical practice guidelines for pain assessment and management has been the demonstration, through recent studies, that many healthcare professionals lack, or fail to apply, basic knowledge and skills in this area. A declaration that "not relieving pain brushes dangerously close to the act of willfully inflicting it" has become one of the strongest statements recorded from an objective, nonclinician perspective (Morris, 1991). The willful infliction of pain is torture, which is foreclosed to the government by the Eighth Amendment to the U.S. Constitution, as "cruel and unusual" even in punishment of convicted criminals.

TOWARD A NEWER MEDICAL MODEL

Inadequate pain control appears to be the spur for increased interest in physician-assisted suicide, but one reason for inadequate pain management is an unfounded concern of both patients and healthcare providers that pain control is a form of euthanasia. Euthanasia refers to the intentional act of painlessly putting to death persons with incurable and distressing disease as an act of mercy (*Black's Law Dictionary*, 1979). Appropriate pain management aims to reduce suffering, not cause death.

In January 1998, Kirk Robinson, president, and Kathryn Tucker, director of legal affairs, for the Oregon-based organization Compassion in Dying Federation (CIDF), sent a memorandum to every medical board in the United States arguing that dying patients have a right to adequate pain medications. Although the focus of the memorandum was end-of-life care, it outlined a series of steps for each state board to follow in addressing the perceived risks for overprescribing controlled substances and the absence of any risk real or imagined for underprescribing medications to any patient experiencing pain. The idea that state medical boards should take on the responsibility of scrutinizing licensees for inadequate pain care was urged, as well as the adoption of underprescribing as a ground for discipline. Additionally, the Compassion in Dying Federation (CIDF) put all boards on public notice that it was willing to assist chronic pain patients and their families in making complaints and/or in filing suits against practitioners who fail to provide adequate pain relief through underprescribing.

In July of 1994, the California Medical Board issued a formal statement on "Prescribing Controlled Substances for Pain Management." The Board stated that "principles of quality medical practice dictate that citizens of California who suffer from pain should be able to obtain the relief that is currently available" and that "pain management should be a high priority in California." Concomitantly, the Board issued "Guidelines for Prescribing Controlled Substances for Intractable Pain" (*Webster's Third New International Dictionary*, 1993) which included the following admonition:

> The Board strongly urges physicians to view pain management as a priority in all patients.... Pain should be assessed and treated promptly, effectively and for as long as the pain persists. The medical management of pain should be based on up-to-date knowledge about pain, pain assessment and pain treatment (Medical Board of California, 1994).

The legal theory of negligence in medication error lawsuits can be applied to cases claiming inappropriate management of pain (Frank-Stromborg & Christiansen, 2000). In any allegation of inappropriate pain management, the patient (plaintiff) must prove:

1. that a duty of care was owed to the patient by the defendant (healthcare professional);
2. the duty owed was breached with conduct that violated a standard of care recognized in the profession;
3. that breach of the duty owed was the cause of injury or the suffering; and
4. the patient (plaintiff) suffered damages as a result (Keeton, Dobbs, Keeton, & Owen, 1984).

In cases involving pain control, the professional will be judged according to the expectation of what a reasonable practitioner would have done in similar circumstances (Willis, 1998). In general, the standard of medical care a physician may with reason and fairness be expected to possess is that commonly possessed or reasonably available to minimally competent physicians in the same speciality or general field of practice throughout the United States. A physician should have a realistic understanding of the limitations of his or her knowledge or competence and, in general, exercise minimally adequate medical judgment (*Hall v. Hilbun*, 1985). In litigation, the appropriate specialty is located to provide information through testimony about the standard of care and any deviation from such standard. In most cases involving questionable pain treatment, the standard of care usually is defined and represented by the AHCPR guidelines. A minority of jurisdictions take the position that adherence to customary practice should not insulate a physician from malpractice liability if the patient (plaintiff) can provide persuasive evidence that the physician failed or refused to apply readily available measures that would have prevented harm to the patient. The Wisconsin Supreme Court (*Nowatske v. Osterlok*, 1996) stated that should customary medical practice fail to keep pace with developments and advances in medical science, adherence to custom might constitute a failure to exercise reasonable care. Evidence that a defendant followed customary practice is not the sole test of professional malpractice (*Toth v. Community Hospital*, 1968). The notion that an entire medical specialty (*Helling v. Carey*, 1974), or at least all the members of a particular locale, would never be guilty of negligence by adhering to a substandard standard of care fell to a Louisiana appellate court statement:

> We are firm in the opinion that it is patently absurd, unreasonable, and arbitrary to hold that immunity from tort liability may be predicated upon a degree of care or procedure amounting to negligence not withstanding such procedure is generally followed by other members of the profession in good standing in the same community (*Favalora v. Aetna*, 1962).

Most lawsuits brought by patients against healthcare providers are for medical malpractice, which is defined as a breach of accepted medical practice resulting in injury and legally recognized damage to the patient. Courts are now willing to hold physicians liable for allowing a patient to suffer because of a failure to provide appropriate pain relief under the recognition of improper pain management as a breach of good and acceptable practice. A medical malpractice judgment exceeding $1 million against the Veterans Administration included an award of $125,000 for pain and suffering predicated largely upon the defendants' failure to provide sufficient pain medication in the final days of the patient's life (*Gaddis v. United States*, 1997). The primary claim and bulk of the total award for damages in a South Carolina case was based on a failure to timely and properly diagnose and treat the patient's throat cancer.

In California, William Bergman, a man in his early 80s, wrenched his back pulling a battery out of a car. Over the next few days he developed more and more back pain, which was originally thought to be a strain–sprain until the patient became immobilized due to the pain (Tucker, 2000). He was taken to the emergency room of a northern California hospital whereupon he was hospitalized for severe pain in his back with a diagnostic finding of metastatic lung cancer. The patient indicated he wished no treatment for his cancer but wished only to receive pain medication that would allow him to return to his home and functionality for what time he had left. Dr. Wing Chin became Mr. Bergman's assigned physician for his hospitalization. The patient was reported by nursing to have increasing Visual Analog Pain Scale (VAS) ratings despite receiving Demerol on a prn order for pain relief based on patient request. Bergman was subsequently discharged to his home with the oral pain medication Vicodin. Demerol is inadequate for cancer pain relief and is inappropriate for use in the aged due to nervous system toxicity that may develop as a side effect of metabolite formation. Morphine agents are appropriate for cancer pain relief. Oral Vicodin is indicated for moderate to moderately severe pain. Pain medications for cancer pain relief should be given at specific times, not on a prn basis. Dr. Chin was called regarding Mr. Bergman's pain and when asked about morphine agents for pain relief, the family was told that he (Dr. Chin) did not possess the required multiple prescription form pad to order these pharmaceuticals for patient use. After 2 days at home in what was described as "agonizing pain," a hospice nurse succeeded in contacting William Berman's regular physician, who immediately administered Roxanol achieving pain relief. Mr. Bergman died the next day.

Mr. Bergman's daughter (Beverly Bergman) was so disturbed by her father's suffering that she made formal complaint, supported by independent expert opinion, to the Medical Board of California (MBC), that the pain care provided to an elderly, terminally ill cancer patient was inadequate.

California is among the most progressive states in attempting to improve pain care. In 1994, the MBC adopted an official guideline on pain management, which specifically identifies failure to adequately manage pain as "inappropriate prescribing." The MBC expressly recognized that this is a form of professional misconduct, subject to the full range of sanctions.

The MBC agreed with Beverly Bergman that the physician had failed to provide adequate pain care but declined to take any action against the physician (Letter from MBC, 1998). It was not until after the MBC concluded that inadequate pain relief had been provided but declined to take any disciplinary action that a formal complaint was filed.

In February 1999 what appears to be the first malpractice suit against a physician (*Bergman v. Chin*, 1999) grounded primarily on failure to properly manage a patient's pain, was filed in Superior Court of California (*Gaddis v. United States*, 1997; *Bergman v. Eden Medical Center*, 1999). Cases of inadequate pain treatment may result in civil liability in tort cases with significant financial implications. The unusual aspect of the Bergman case is that a cause of action under the California Elder Abuse Statute is included, which provides heightened remedies to what would be available under a medical malpractice claim, including punitive damages, no cap on damages, and attorney's fees. The defendant physician and hospital agreed that the family was only entitled to the limited remedies available in a malpractice claim, repeatedly disputed the elder abuse claim, and petitioned for it to be dismissed. In January 2000 the court ruled against dismissal of the elder abuse claims, recognizing that inadequate pain care can constitute elder abuse. Kathryn Tucker, Esq., director of legal affairs for the Compassion in Dying Federation, explained that a successful trial means the Bergman family will be able to recover significant damages and as exposure for inadequate pain care becomes more significant, providers will be more motivated to attend and treat pain properly under exposure to significantly greater financial risk (Partners Against Pain, 2000). Dying patients clearly have the right to adequate pain medication; this was recently recognized by the Supreme Court (*Vacco v. Quill*, 1997; *Washington v. Glucksberg*, 1997; Burt, 1997).

Illustrative of the law's recognition that assurance of comfort and appropriate pain control are integral components of appropriate medical care (*State v. McAfee*, 1989) is, in this instance, a quadriplegic who was incapable of spontaneous respiration and sought court approval for discontinuation of his respirator. The Georgia Supreme Court affirmed the patient's right to refuse medical treatment and held that he was also entitled to have a sedative administered at the time:

> Mr. McAfee's right to be free from pain at the time the ventilator is disconnected is inseparable from his right to refuse medical treatment. The record shows that Mr. McAfee has attempted, in the past, to disconnect his ventilator, but has been unable to do so due to the severe pain he suffers when deprived of oxygen. His right to have a sedative (a medication that in no way causes or accelerates death) administered before the ventilator is disconnected is a part of his right to control his medical treatment.

The implication of this ruling is that providers may be held accountable for not providing such measures (Shapiro, 1996).

In a North Carolina negligence law suit, a healthcare provider was held liable for the first time for failure to treat serious pain appropriately (*Estate of Henry James v. Hillhaven Corp.*, 1990).

Henry James, 74 years of age, a retired house painter, was diagnosed with cancer of the prostate for which he was subjected to removal of his testicles. The cancer, however, was metastatic in nature, having spread to his leg and spine. His pain was severe and excruciating. He was placed in a nursing home in February 1987. Almost at once, nursing began cutting his prescription pain medications by giving him on some days mild headache medicines, placebo substituted for morphine, or nothing at all. The nursing supervisor explained to the family he was in danger of becoming a drug addict and because James and his family were Medicare and Medicaid recipients she did not like her tax dollars supporting his drug habit. Eventually, Mr. James became irritable, withdrawn, and bedfast, where he lay sweating and moaning in pain dying 4 months later. His family eventually filed a complaint with a state regulatory agency and went to court. On November 20, 1990, trial began in North Carolina. After 3½ days of testimony, the jury took less than 1 hour to render the verdict that the nursing home had been negligent in failing to provide Mr. James adequate pain relief. At the trial, Catherine Faison, James' great niece, explained that as far as the nursing home was concerned, when he died, it was a closed issue; it was over. "It's not over for me," Faison told the jury. " I can't sleep at night when I think about the fact that he had to lay over there and suffer… I think about him laying there hurting, saying I want my medication, and not being able to get it. I don't want to suffer like that… I don't think anybody would. Somebody needs to say you can't do it."

Safe harbor provisions in intractable pain legislation enacted in many states grant immunity from discipline to physicians who treat intractable pain. These enactments clarify the position that physicians shall not be disciplined for treating intractable pain with large doses of medication, even if such prescriptions hasten the moment of the patient's death, as long as the intent is simply to alleviate pain. Such provisions are designed to clear the confusion that may occur because of the similarity with prescribing medications to end a patient's life.

In 1999, the Oregon Board of Medical Examiners disciplined a physician for the undertreatment of a patient's intractable pain. Dr. Paul Bilder, an Oregon pulmonary specialist, was disciplined for a pattern of failing to treat pain adequately (Goodman, 1999). The physician was reported to have undertreated patients as follows (Mascheri, 1999).

1. Tylenol (Loeb, 1996) was used for an elderly male cancer patient's musculoskeletal pain, denying requests for stronger medications when pain increased. He also denied a nurse's request for catheterization, citing a risk of infection. The patient died the next day.

2. He removed a catheter from an 84-year-old man against the patient's and family's request, directing that he instead use diapers. He further reduced a hospice nurse's requested dose of 5 to 20 mg of Roxanol every 4 hours to 0.25 cc and gave Tylenol (Loeb, 1996) to treat the patient's 102° temperature. The patient died that evening.

3. He refused a request for sedatives and pain control for a 35-year-old intubated, mechanically ventilated woman who became increasingly restless, had increased wheezing, and was fighting the ventilator. After the patient extubated herself, the doctor ordered a paralytic agent but no sedative following reintubation.

4. He used physical restraint to intubate a 33-year-old man without using anxiolytics or narcotics. The patient had been admitted with severe pneumonia associated with hypoxemia. The physician, it is claimed by the board, engaged in "unprofessional or dishonorable conduct" and "gross negligence or repeated negligence," according to a stipulated order released by the board. While the physician will not lose his license, this is the first time a state board has taken this type of actions.

Thus, in addition to potential liability to patients for inappropriate pain management, professional discipline of healthcare professionals also may ensue. As a result of development and growing acceptance of pain management guidelines, medical boards may be more inclined in the future to undertake disciplinary action for inadequate pain management.

Increased use of advanced directives resulting from passage of the federal Patient Self-Determination Act (effective December 1, 1991) also may increase physicians' exposure to professional discipline for inappropriate pain management. In the interests of sustaining protection, physicians are advised to honor appropriate pain management instructions set forth in patients' advanced directives. Where questions or concerns arise about complying with such pain management instruction, ethics committees should be consulted (Shapiro, 1994).

Appropriate pain management aims to reduce suffering, not cause death. When physicians deliberately administer lethal doses of medications — even for reasons of compassion — they risk prosecution for homicide, and when lethal doses of medications are prescribed, they risk prosecution for assisting suicide.

To avoid exposure to criminal prosecution, physicians should (a) prescribe medications in doses in accordance with what is necessary to manage pain with good medical judgment; (b) clearly communicate their rationale for pain medication prescriptions with patients, their families, and other caregivers; and (c) clearly document the intent behind and need for the medication prescribed.

Investigations of physicians for perceived excessive prescribing of pain medication reduces physician willingness to treat pain with strong pain medications. This is one factor contributing to the problem of undertreatment of pain. During the past few years, aggressive educational efforts have begun to correct the undertreatment of pain and other physical suffering in dying patients — a major failing in medical care (Noble, 1999).

A pending federal bill would have significant adverse impact on progress in this area. The Pain Relief Promotion Act of 1999 (PRPA, 2000), should Congress decide to enact it, would increase physician exposure to investigations for prescribing aggressive pain treatment at the end of life. It is the public fear of intolerable suffering that is a major reason for public support of assisted suicide (Blendon, Szalay, & Knox, 1992). In 1994, Oregon became the first state in the nation to pass a law permitting physician-assisted suicide. By November, 1997, all barriers (e.g., legal challenges and ballot measures to rescind the law leading to delays in implementation) were put aside and Oregon's Death with Dignity Act became fully operative.

The legal effect of PRPA is at odds with its appealing title because the act, introduced by Rep. Henry Hyde (R, IL) and Sen. Don Nickles (R, OK), is designed to override Oregon's physician-assisted suicide law (BNA Health Law Reporter, 1999). The primary goal of PRPA is to prevent physicians in Oregon from continuing to implement the Death with Dignity Act (Orentlicher & Caplan, 2000). Title I of the PRPA amends the Controlled Substances Act to nullify Oregon's physician-assisted suicide law. Section 101 of PRPA states opiates, drugs, and other controlled substances may not be intentionally used "for the purpose of causing death or assisting another person in causing death." While rejecting assisted suicide, Title I of PRPA makes a strong statement favoring palliative care as a part of a legitimate medical practice to use a controlled substance with the intent to alleviate patients' pain — "even if the use of such a substance may increase the risk of death" (PRPA, 1999 S102). Educational and training programs for local, state, and federal law enforcement personnel on the legitimate use of controlled substances in pain management and palliative care (PRPA, 1999). In deciding what uses of controlled substances are consistent with the public interest, the U.S. Attorney General "shall give no force and effect to state law authorizing or permitting assisted suicide or euthanasia" (PRPA, 1999).

Title II of PRPA provides for "programs to provide education and training to healthcare professionals in palliative care." The PRPA would potentially expose to criminal prosecution physicians in every state who provide pain management drugs that they knew would or could increase the likelihood of a patient's death. Under Section 101 of PRPA, the line between acceptable palliative care and unacceptable assisted suicide is defined solely by the physician's intents.

Section 401 of the Controlled Substances Act (CSA) contains a broad prohibition on the distribution and dispensing of federally controlled substances, and violation of Section 401 carries criminal penalties. Section 303, however, provides a so-called safe harbor from the broad prohibition (of Section 401) for the medical profession, allowing physicians to use such federally controlled substances, including the drugs necessary to ease the pain of patients, in the course of their practices. When Congress passed the Controlled Substances Act to address trafficking in illicit drugs, it employed language that incidentally covers physicians who use controlled substances to assist a patient in suicide or perform euthanasia. As currently drafted, PRPA adds to the end of that safe-harbor section (Section 803) two new elements of law that when read in the context of the CSA, radically affect the ability of physicians to practice medicine. The amendment first includes a deceptively physician friendly support for aggressive pain management that "may increase the risk of death" and next adds a provision removing from Section 823 the use of such federally controlled substances to intentionally cause or assist in the causing of a patient's death. Without this safe-harbor provision, physicians in Oregon who comply with their patients' wishes pursuant to that state's Death with Dignity Law will be subject to the CSA criminal sanctions. The notion of intent and the unclear manner in which it is used in S.1272 creates trouble for physicians in all states whether or not they plan to engage in physician-assisted suicide. Legally, intent is considered to be established where there is knowledge that the death is substantially certain to occur as a result of the conduct; however, intent also can be found where death should have been reasonably expected to occur as a result of the conduct. When intent is the critical issue, physicians must be concerned that law enforcement officers will see a criminal intent where none existed. The risk of prosecution is exacerbated by the fact that when high doses of medication are utilized in a terminally ill

patient who dies of natural causes, the death may be mistakenly ascribed to the medication. The PRPA would mandate that those difficult, and subjective, questions be resolved by the criminal process, after the fact. Physicians are left exposed to the general criminal penalties associated with Section 841(a) if they potentially should have known that the dosage they prescribed would result in death, even if their subjective intent in fact was to provide palliative care. If the physician uses aggressive doses of opiate drugs to provide palliative care and is charged under the PRPA, a conviction would result in draconian consequences. The intent to cause death can be inferred from the drug or dose ordered, the potential therefore exists for physician incarceration if the local authorities view, in retrospect, the dosage received by the patient as excessive. A physician convicted under PRPA for using a Schedule II drug and causing a patient's death faces a minimum sentence of 20 years in prison and a maximum sentence of life in prison.

The Controlled Substances Act is an anti-drug abuse law enforcement statute administered by the Attorney General (Testimony before Senate, 1998). The Department of Justice was given the authority to prevent and prosecute illicit drug use, a power that has been exercised in large part by the DEA. Under the Pain Relief Promotion Act (PRPA) instead of looking to medical experts and the FDA for guidance on the appropriate use of opioids, barbiturates, and other palliative drugs in end-of-life care, physicians also would have to consider the views of DEA's agents (Testimony before House, 1999).

By using a federal statue to override an Oregon healthcare law, PRPA contravenes the principle of federalism, a fundamental tenet of American law. The regulation of medical practice traditionally has been the province of states and their medical boards, not that of the federal government and its law enforcement agencies. The preamble to the Medicare law expressly prohibits any federal "supervision or control over the practice of medicine or the manner in which medical services are provided" (Iglehart, 1992).

In the past decade, physicians have become more likely to face civil lawsuits as well as criminal prosecutions when charged with substandard medical care. It is likely that the PRPA would induce physicians to avoid the threat of legal liability and again exacerbate the undertreatment of pain causing increased suffering in the patients with pain. Pressure on physicians to undertreat pain will increase under PRPA, yet the risk for so doing is an increasingly punitive reality — truly placing physicians between the rock and the hard place.

CONCLUSION

Pain is one of the most common reasons for seeking medical care, yet it is often inadequately treated. Untreated, the pain accompanying illnesses slows recovery, severely impairs an individual's quality of life, and adds significantly to the healthcare system's financial burden. The Joint Commission on Accreditation of Healthcare Organizations (JCAHO) standards (the new evidence-based pain management standards introduced by JCAHO) (Phillips, 2000) asserts that individuals seeking care at accredited hospitals, behavioral health facilities, and healthcare networks, have the right to appropriate assessment and management of pain. All patients are to be screened for the presence of pain. For those reporting pain, a complete assessment must be conducted to characterize a patient's pain by location, intensity, and cause, including a detailed history, physical examination, psychosocial assessment, and diagnostic evaluation.

The most reliable indicator of pain existence and intensity is the patient's self-report because it is more accurate than others' observations. These standards do not dictate specific pain management procedures nor advocate in any way the use of certain drugs (e.g., opioids).

A discussion of the emerging standards and guidelines (Jacox, Carr, & Payne, 1994) coupled with developing disciplinary and legal consequences to remold physician action and delivery of medical care utilizing the fulcrum of inadequate pain management as inappropriate medical care appears designed to move physicians into fungible units in need of surveillance to assure compliance with all controlling legal authority. The House version of the Pain Relief Promotions Act was passed in October of 1999, although a filibuster is expected when the bill is introduced in the Senate.

REFERENCES

21 USCA § 841(b)(1)(c) (1999).

Agency for Health Care Policy and Research. (1992). Acute Pain Management Guideline Panel. Acute Pain Management: Operative or Medical Procedures and Trauma. Pub. No. 92-0032. Washington, D.C.: U.S. Department of Health & Human Services.

American Academy of Pain Management, 13947 Mono Way #A, Sonora, California 95370; (209) 533-9744, Fax (209) 533-9750.

American Academy of Pain Medicine, 4700 W. Lake Avenue, Glenview, Illinois 60025-1485; (847) 375-4731, Fax (847) 375-4777. The AMA-recognized speciality society of physicians who practice pain medicine.

American Medical Association. (1996). Code of Medical Ethics.

American Medical Association. (1999). Education for Physicians on End-of-Life Care. Participants handbook. Chicago, IL: American Medical Association.

American Pain Society Quality of Care Committee. (1995). Quality improvement guidelines for the treatment of acute pain and cancer pain. Journal of the American Medical Association, 274, 1874–1880.

American Pain Society, 4700 W. Lake Avenue, Glen View, Illinois 60025-1485; (847)375-4715, Fax (847) 375-4777.

Bergman v. Chin, No. H205732-1 (Cal. App. Dep't. Super. Ct. Feb. 16, 1999).

Bergman v. Eden Med. Ctr., No. H205732-1 Cal. Sup. Ct., Alameda Cty. (Medical negligence and elder abuse for failure to adequately treat ain in elderly patient dying of lung cancer) (pending).

Bernabei, R., Gambassi, G., Lapane, K., et al. (1998). Management of pain in elderly patients with cancer. SAGE Study Group. systematic assessment of geriatric drug use via epidemiology. Journal of the American Medical Association, 279, 1877–1882.

Black's Law Dictionary. (1979). (5th ed., p. 497). St. Paul, MN: West Publishing.

Blendon, R.J., Szalay, U.S., & Knox, R.S. (1992). Should physicians aid their patients in dying? The public perspective. Journal of the American Medical Association, 267, 2658–2662.

Bostrom, B.M., Ramberg, T., Davis, B.D., & Fridlund, B. (1997). Survey of post-operative patients' pain management. Journal of Nursing Management, 5, 341–349.

Brown, D.L., & Carpenter, R.L. (1990). Perioperative analgesia: A review of risks and benefits. Journal of Cardiothoracic Anesthesia, 4, 368–383.

Burt, R.A. (1997). The Supreme Court speaks: Not assisted suicide but a constitutional right to palliative care. New England Journal of Medicine, 337, 1234–1236.

Calonge, N. (2000). Processes and targets for improving the quality of healthcare. Preventive Medicine and Managed Care, 1(3), 149–152.

Carr, D.B. (1998). Clinical pain management guidelines. Emergency Medicine, 30(45), S2–S6.

Carr, D.B., Jacox, A.K., Chapman, C.R., et al. (1992). Acute pain management: Operative or medical procedures and trauma. Clinical Practice Guideline. AHCPR Pub. No. 92-0032. Rockville, MD: Agency for Health Care Policy and Research, Public Health Service, U.S. Department of Health & Human Services.

Carr, D.B., Jacox, A.K., Chapman, C.R., et al. (1995). Acute Pain Management. Guideline Technical Report, No. 1. AHCPR Pub. No. 95-0034. Rockville, MD: Agency for Health Care Policy and Research Public Health Care Policy and Research, Public Health Service, U.S. Department of Health and Human Services.

Cavalieri, T.A. (1999). Pain management at the end of life. Journal American Osteopathic Association, 99(6), S16–S21.

Cavanaugh, T.A. (1996). The ethics of death — Hastening or death-causing palliative analgesic administration to the terminally ill. Journal of Pain and Symptom Management, 12, 248–254.

Chasin, M.R. (1997). Assessing strategies for quality improvement. Health Affairs (Millwood, VA). 16, 151–161.

Chassin, M.F., & Galvin, R.W. (1998). The National Roundtable on Health Care Quality: The urgent need to improve healthcare quality. Journal of the American Medical Association, 280, 1000–1005.

Cherny, N.J., & Portenoy, R.K. (1994). The management of cancer pain. CA. *A Cancer Journal for Clinicians, 44,* 263–303.

Clark, H.W. (1998). Legal implications of prescribing opioid controlled substances. *Emergency Medicine, 30*(45), S29–S33.

Cleeland, C.S. (1992). Documenting barriers to cancer pain management. *Current and Emerging Issues in Cancer Pain: Research and Practice, 321,* 325–327.

Cleeland, C.S., Gonin, R., Baez, L., Loehrer, P., & Pandya, K.J. (1997). Pain and treatment of pain in minority patients with cancer. The Eastern Cooperative Oncology Group Minority Outpatient Study. *Annals of Internal Medicine, 127,* 813–816.

Dahlman, G.-B., Dykes, A.-K., & Elander, G. (1999). Patients' evaluation of pain and nurses' management of analgesics after surgery. The effect of a study day on the subject of pain for nurses working at the thorax surgery department. *Journal of Advanced Nursing, 30,* 866–874.

Edwards, R.B. (1984). Pain and the ethics of pain management. *Society of Science and Medicine, 18,* 515–517.

Emanuel, E.J. (1996). Pain and symptom control: patient rights and physician responsibilities. *Hematology and Oncology Clinics of North America, 10,* 41–47.

Estate of Henry James v. Hillhaven Corp. (N.C. Super. Ct., Hertford Cty. 1990). *Faison v. The Hillhaven Corp.,* No. 89 CVS 65 (Hertford Cty. Super. Ct. N.C. Dec. 1990) ($15 million jury award, half of which was punitive, against nursing home nurse's conduct in failing to provide prescribed pain medications to terminally ill patient, settled on appeal for undisclosed amount).

Ewing, J.A. (1984). Detecting alcoholism: The CAGE questionnaire: A critical review. *Journal of the American Medical Association, 252,* 1905–1907.

Favalora v. Aetna Cs. & Sur. Co., 144 So.2d 544, 551 (La. Ct. App. 1962).

Ferrel, B.R., & Rhiner, M. (1994). High-tech comfort: Ethical issues in cancer pain management for the 1990s. *Journal of Clinical Ethics, 2,* 108–112.

Foley, K.M. (1997). Management of cancer pain. In V.T. De Vita, S. Hellman, & S. Rosenberg (Eds.), *Cancer: Principles and practice of oncology* (5th ed., pp. 2807–2841). Philadelphia: Lippincott-Raven Press.

Frank-Stromborg, M., & Christiansen, A. (2000). The untreatment of pain: A liability risk for nurses. *Clinical Journal of Oncology Nursing, 4*(1), 41–44.

Gaddis v. United States, 7 F. Supp. 2d (D.S.C. 1997).

Gallup, Inc. (June 9, 1999). *Pain in America: Highlights from a Gallup survey.*

Glanelli, D.M. (1999). Opioid prescriptions rarely lead to rebuke, study finds. *AMA News (Professional Issues)* February 8.

Goff, D.C., Canely, L.K., & Gu, L. (2000). Increasing the appropriate use of reductase inhibitors among patients with coronary heart disease enrolled in a network — model managed care organization. *Preventive Medicine and Managed Care, 1,* 141–148.

Goldstein, F.J. (1999). Management of acute pain. *Journal American Osteopathic Association, 99*(6), S1–S5.

Goodman, E. (1999). *Charlotte Observer.* September 11.

Gostin, L. (2000). A public approach to reducing error, medical malpractice as a barrier. *Journal of the American Medical Association, 283,* 1742–1743.

Guglielmo, W.J. (2000). Can doctors put their fears to rest? *Medical Economics,* (February 21), 47–59 from David E. Joranson, director of the Pain and Policy Studies Group at the University of Wisconsin — Madison.

Hall v. Hilbun, 466 So.2d 856,871 (Miss. 1985).

Heller, M.B. (1992). Emergency management of acute pain: New options and strategies. *Postgraduate Medicine,* 39–47.

Helling v. Carey, 519 P.2d 981 (Washington, 1974). The most often-cited case in which a court essentially condemned an entire medical speciality.

Hill, C.S. (1993). The Negative Influence of Licensing and Disciplinary Boards and Drug Enforcement Agencies in Pain with Opioid Analgesics. *Journal of Pharmacology Care and Pain Symptom Control, 1,* 43–62.

Hill, Jr., C.S. (1995). When will adequate pain treatment be the norm? *Journal of the American Medical Association, 274,* 1881–1882.

Hill, Jr., C.S. (1996a). Adequate pain treatment: a challenge for medical regulatory boards. *Journal of the Florida Medical Association, 83,* 677–678. Editorial.

Hill, Jr., C.S. (1996b). Government regulatory influences on opioid prescribing and their impact on the treatment of pain of nonmalignant origin. *Journal of Pain and Symptom Management, 11,* 287–298.

Hoover, v. Agency for Health Care Administration, 676 So.2d 1380 (Fla. Dist. Ct. App. 1996) (Florida medical disciplinary board penalized and restricted physician for perceived excessive prescribing of pain medication; action of board reversed by court); Hollabaugh v. Arkansas State Med. Bd., 861 S.W.2d 317 (Ark. Ct. App. 1993)(similar case in Arkansas).

Iglehart, J.K. (1992). The American healthcare system: Introduction. *New England Journal of Medicine, 326,* 962–967 (citing 42 USC § 1395).

International Project of Hastings Center. (1996). The Goals of Medicine: Setting New Priorities. *Hastings Center Report* (Nov.-Dec.), S1.

Jacox, A., Carr, D.B., & Payne, R. (1994). New clinical practice guidelines for the management of pain in patients with cancer. *New England Journal of Medicine, 330,* 651–655.

Jacox, A., Carr, D.B., Payne, R., Berde, C.B., Biebart, W., Cain, J.M., et al. (1994). Guideline Panel. Management of Cancer Pain. Clinical Practice Guideline Number 9. Rockville, MD: Agency for Health Care Policy and Research, U.S. Department of Health and Human Services, Public Health Service; AHCPR Publication No. 94-0592.

James, G. (2000). Addressing barriers to healthcare for our elderly. *Family Physician Journal of American College of Osteopathic Family Practice, 4*(9), 9–13.

Joranson, D.E. (1992). Opioids for chronic cancer and noncancer pain: A survey of state medical board members. federation bulletin. *Journal of Medical Licensure and Discipline, 9,* 15.

Joshi, G.P. (1994). Postoperative pain management. *International Anesthesiology Clinics,* 113–126.

Katz, W.A. (1996). Approach to management of non-malignant pain. *American Journal of Medicine, 101,* 54S–63S.

Keeton, W., Dobbs, D.B., Keeton, R.E., & Owen, D.G. (1984). *Prosser and Keeton on the law of torts.* St. Paul, MN: West Publishing.

Kehlet, H. (1989). Surgical stress: The role of pain and analgesia. *British Journal of Anaesthesia, 63,* 189–195.

King, K.M., Bungard, T.J., McAlister, F.A., et al. (2000). for the CQIN Investigators. Quality Improvement for CQI. *Preventive Medicine and Managed Care, 1,* 129–137.

Kores, R., Murphy, W.D., Rosenthal, T.L., Elias, D., & North, W.C. (1990). Predicting outcome of chronic pain treatment via a modified self-efficacy scale. *Behavior Research and Therapy, 24.*

Lavies, N., Hart, L., Rounsefell, B., & Runciman, W. (1992). Identification of patient, medical and nursing staff attitudes to postoperative opioid analgesia: Stage I of a longitudinal study of postoperative analgesia. *Pain, 48,* 313–319.

Leape, L.L. (1992). Unnecessary surgery. *Annual Review of Public Health, 13,* 363–383.

Leape, L.L. Error in Medicine. (1994). *Journal of the American Medical Association, 272,* 1851–1857.

Letter from Medical Board of California to Beverly Bergman dated August 19, 1998 states in pertinent part: "Our medical consultant did agree with you that pain management for your father was indeed inadequate."

Litman, G.S., Walker, B.R., & Schneier, B.E. (1985). Reassessment of verbal and visual analog ratings in analgesic studies. *Clinical Pharmacology and Therapeutics, 38,* 16–23.

Loeb, J.L. (1996). Pain management in long-term care. *American Journal of Nursing, 99*(2), 48–52. (Recent studies have found that acetamenophen is the most commonly prescribed and appropriate pain relief medication for mild to moderate pain.)

Lohr, K.N. (Ed.) (1990). Medicare: A strategy of quality assurance. Washington, D.C.: National Academy Press.

Lutz, L.J., & Lamer, T.J. (1990). Management of postoperative pain: Review of current techniques and methods. *Mayo Clinic Proceedings, 65,* 584–596.

Marcus, D.A. (2000). Treatment of non-malignant chronic pain. *American Family Physician, 61,* 1331–1338.

Martelli, M.F., Zasler, N.D., & Grayson, R. (1999). Ethical considerations in medicolegal evaluation of neurologic injury and impairment. *NeuroRehabilitation: An Interdisciplinary Journal, 13*(1), 45–66.

Martino, A.M. (1998). In search of a new ethic for treating patients with chronic pain: What can medical boards do? *Journal of Law and Medical Ethics, 26,* 332–349.

Mascheri, L.L. Associate Director, State Government Affairs. Intractable Pain Legislation. AOA Division of State Government Affairs: September, 1999.

McCarberg, B. (2000). Managing the acute pain patient: Alleviating the pain. *Family Practice Research Journal, 22*(9), S4–S7.

Medical Board of California (July 29, 1994). Guideline for prescribing controlled substances for intractable pain.

Medical Board of California Action Report 4 (Oct. 1994).

Merskey, H. (1986). Classification of chronic pain, descriptions of chronic pain syndromes and definitions of pain terms. *Pain, Suppl. 3,* S1–S226.

Model Guidelines for the Use of Controlled Substances for the Treatment of Pain. (1998). Euless, TX: Federation of State Medical Boards of the United States, Inc.

Morris, D.B. (1991). *The culture of pain,* 134.

Morrison, J.M, & Wickersham, M.S. (1998). Physicians disciplined by a state medical board. *Journal of the American Medical Association, 279*(23), 1889–1893.

Nickles proposal opposes legalized assisted suicide. BNA Health Law Reporter June 24, 1999; 8, 1027

Noble, H.B. A shift in the treatment of chronic pain. *New York Times,* August 9, 1999, A13.

Nowatske v. Osterlok, 543 N.W.2d 265,2710272 (Wis. 1996).

Nyquist, A.-C., Gonzales, R., Steiner, J.R., & Sande, M.E. (1998). Antibiotic prescribing for children with colds, upper respiratory tract infections, and bronchitis. *Journal of the American Medical Association, 279,* 875–877.

Oherney, N.I., & Catane, R. (1995). Professional negligence in the management of cancer pain. *Cancer, 76,* 2181.

Oncology Nursing Society. (1998). Oncology Nursing Society position: Cancer pain management. *Oncology Nursing Forum, 25,* 817–818.

Orentlicher, D., & Caplan, A. (2000). The Pain Relief Promotion Act of 1999, A serious threat to palliative care. *Journal of the American Medical Association, 283*(2), 255–258.

Pain Relief Promotion Act of 1999, HR2260, § 101.

Parran, T. (1997). Prescription drug abuse — A question of balance. *Medical Clinics of North America, 81,* 967–978.

Patient Self-Determination Act, 42 U.S.C. sect. 395 *et seq.* (1991).

Phillips, D. (2000). JCAHO pain management standards are unveiled. *Journal of the American Medical Association, 284,* 428–429.

Policy and Practice. (2000, November 1). Pain act provides no relief. *Family Practice News.*

Portenoy, R.K. (1996a). Opioid therapy for chronic nonmalignant pain: Clinicians' perspective. *Journal of Law and Medical Ethics, 24,* 296–309.

Portenoy, R.K. (1996b). Opioid therapy for chronic nonmalignant pain: Medication history review of the critical issues. *Journal of Pain Symptom Management, 11,* 203–217.

Purdue Pharma Limited Partnership. (2000). Undertreatment of pain goes to court as elder abuse. *Partners against Pain, 3*(1), 4.

Rich, B.A. (2000). A prescription for the pain: The emerging standard of care for pain management. *Wm. Mitchell Law Review, 1.*

Rorarius, M.G.F., & Baer, G.A. (1994). Non-steroidal anti-inflammatory drugs for postoperative pain relief. *Current Opinion in Anesthesiology, 7,* 358–362.

Saberski, L.R. (2000, August). Frailty: My name is physician. The weak, the strong link, and the pain evaluation: Not all pain is the same. *The Pain Clinic,* 7–8.

Shapiro, R.S. (1994). Legal bases for the control of analgesic drugs. *Journal of Pain and Symptom Management, 9,* 153–159.

Shapiro, R.S. (1996). Healthcare providers' liability exposure for inappropriate pain management. *Journal of Law and Medical Ethics, 24,* 360–364.

Sommerville, M.A. (1986). Pain and suffering at the interfaces of medicine and law. *University of Toronto Law Journal, 36,* 286.

State v. McAfee, 259 Ga. 579, 385 S.E. 2d 651 (Ga. 1989).

Stjernsward, J., et al. (1996). The World Health Organization cancer pain and palliative care program: Past, present, and future. *Journal of Pain and Symptom Management, 12,* 65–68.

T.J. Hooper, 60 F.2d 737,740(2d Cir. 1932). Judge Learned Hand's words: … a whole calling may have lagged in the adoption of new and available devices. Courts must in the end say what is required; there are precautions so imperative that even their universal disregard will not excuse their omission.

Terman, G., & Liebeskind, J. (1991). Pain can kill. *Pain, 44,* 3–4. Editorial.

Testimony before the House Subcommittee on the Constitution of the Committee on the Judiciary, Hearings on HR220 on the Pain Relief Promotion Act of 1999, 106th Cong. 1st Sess (June 24, 1999) (testimony of David E. Joranson).

Testimony before the Senate Committee on the Judiciary, The Lethal Drug Abuse Prevention Act of 1998," 105th Cong. 2nd Sess. (July 31, 1998) (testimony of Principal Deputy Associate Attorney General Joseph N. Onek). The board's letter stated: "There is insufficient evidence at this time to warrant pursuing further action in this case. Your file shall be maintained with the Medical Board for future reference in the event we receive additional complaints in the future which, along with your complaint, could constitute sufficient evidence for disciplinary action."

The Oregon Death with Dignity Act, Oregon Rev. Stat. § 127.800 (1996).

Tittle, M., & McMillan, S.C. (1994). Pain and pain-related side effects in an ICU and on a surgical unit: Nurses' management. *American Journal of Critical, 3,* 25–30.

Toth v. Community Hosp. at Glen Cove, 239 N. E. 2d 368, 373 (N.Y. 1968).

Townsend, R.J., Spartz, M.E., Fahrenbruch, R.W., et al. (1983). Hospital labor cost savings in dispensing analgesics: Controlled vs. non-controlled. *Hospital Formulary, 18,* 716–720.

Tucker, K.L. (2000). Lecture notes. On Inadequate Treatment of Pain: Accountability, American Academy of Pain Management 11th Annual Clinical Meeting.

Vacco v. Quill, 117 S. Ct. 2293 (1997).

Vainio, A., Ollila, J., Matikainen, E., et al. (1995). Driving ability in cancer patients receiving long-term morphine analgesia. *Lancet, 346,* 667–670.

View cancer pain as a "pathogenic agent" to treated, expert says. (1998). *Oncology News International, 7*(10), 36, 43.

Washington v. Glucksberg, 117 S. Ct. 2258 (1997).

Webster's Third New International Dictionary. (1993). "Intractable" is a term used to describe any situation or condition that is unmanageable or untreatable.

Weiner, S.L. (1993). *Differential diagnosis of acute pain by body region* (pp. 1–2). New York: McGraw-Hill.

Whipple, J.K., Lewis, K.S., Quebbman, E.J., et al. (1995). Analysis of pain management in critically ill patients. *Pharmacotherapy, 15,* 592–599.

Willis, J. (1998). Should nurses start running from patients' complaints? *Nursing Times, 94*(15), 7–12.

Wilschinsky v. Medina, 775 P.2d 713 (NM 1989). The New Mexico Supreme Court ruled that a physician could be held liable to a man who was injured by an automobile driven by his patient to whom he had administered drugs that caused drowsiness. It further held that a physician does have a legal duty to use reasonable care in treating patients, and that this duty extends to the driving public when the physician administers drugs known to cause drowsiness and impairment of judgment.

75

Provider Accountability for Inadequate Pain Management

Kathryn L. Tucker, J.D.

Patients in the United States are routinely undertreated for pain. This problem has been widely recognized and documented in the medical literature. In a seminal medical study of end-of-life care, researchers found that 50% of all patients who died during hospitalization "experienced moderate or severe pain at least half of the time during their last 3 days of life" (SUPPORT, 1995).

Elderly patients are particularly vulnerable to insufficient pain treatment. A recent study in the *Journal of the American Medical Association* found that up to 40% of cancer patients in nursing homes are not appropriately treated for pain. In addition, 26% of those experiencing pain did not receive any pain medication, and 16% were given over-the-counter pain relievers like aspirin or acetaminophen for their pain (Bernabei, et al., 1998). At the same time, it is well established that only perhaps 10% of dying patients have conditions in which alleviation of pain is truly difficult or impossible (Jacox, et al., 2000).

One repeatedly identified cause of this problem is physician concern that prescribing controlled substances will invite regulatory agency oversight (Breaking Down the Barriers, 1998). Other factors inhibiting adequate pain treatment described in the medical literature include the fear that strong pain treatment will hasten death (Schneiderman, 1997), and the concern that the patient will become addicted to the pain medication (Stavish, 1997).

Oversight is triggered in some states by laws that require duplicate or triplicate prescription forms, with copies going to reviewing authorities. These laws were intended to deter illegitimate drug use. Unfortunately, they have had an enormous impact on legitimate use, as well.

It is not uncommon for physicians to be investigated for prescribing controlled substances in amounts that regulators perceive as excessive. Even if the physician's conduct meets relevant guidelines for pain management, such investigations may result in physician discipline, including suspension or revocation of prescribing authority, other limitations on medical practice, and other penalties (Hoover v. Agency for Health Care Administration, 1996). It has become widely recognized that the multiple copy prescription laws deter physicians from writing prescriptions for controlled substances, and thus, create barriers to access to adequate pain medication. In response, some states have, in recent years, eliminated traditional multiple copy laws (N.Y. Public Health Law, 2000). This is a step in the right direction; yet, it is unlikely to correct the serious problem of inadequate treatment of pain on its own.

The American Society of Law, Medicine, and Ethics (ASLME) recently undertook a reform effort, the Project on Legal Constraints on Access to Effective Pain Management. The Project developed a model Pain Relief Act that creates a "safe harbor" for physicians who prescribe pain medication as long as the physician substantially complied with accepted practice and care guidelines for pain management (The Pain Relief Act, 1996). This safe harbor shelters physicians from both disciplinary and criminal action if the physician can "demonstrate by reference to an accepted guideline that his or her practice substantially complied with that guideline." The physician also must have kept appropriate records, written no false prescriptions, obeyed the CSA, and not diverted medications to personal use (The Pain Relief Act, 1996).

0-8493-0926-3/02/$0.00+$1.50
© 2002 by CRC Press LLC

The safe-harbor concept is also encompassed in state laws known as Intractable Pain Treatment Acts (IPTA). The existing state statutes generally provide shelter from disciplinary action, but make no mention of criminal exposure. The California IPTA, for example, provides that "no physician or surgeon shall be subject to disciplinary action by the board for prescribing or administering controlled substances in the course of treatment of a person for intractable pain" (California Business and Professional Code, § 2241.5(c)). To be immune from board discipline this IPTA requires that the patient not be known to have chemical dependency or to be using drugs for nontherapeutic purposes. The physician must prescribe medications for therapeutic purposes, keep appropriate records, not write false prescriptions, and prescribe in a manner consistent with the state and federal CSA (California Business and Professional Code, § 2241.5(c)).

Unfortunately, IPTAs have proven to be largely ineffectual (Rich, 2000). Reports continue to document that undertreatment of pain is pervasive (Rich, 2000). The situation in California exemplifies this failure.

California is among the most progressive states in attempting to improve pain care. The state legislature passed its IPTA in 1990 (Rich, 2000). In 1994 the Medical Board of California (MBC) provided all California physicians with a copy of the clinical guidelines for pain management issued by the U.S. Agency for Health Care Policy and Research (AHCPR), and adopted a policy statement in May 1994 encouraging aggressive pain care. Subsequently, the MBC (1994) adopted an official guideline regarding pain management, which specifically identifies failure to adequately manage pain as "inappropriate prescribing." In explicitly making undertreatment of pain a type of inappropriate prescribing, the MBC has expressly recognized that this is a form of professional misconduct and, thus, subject to the full range of sanctions.

In 1997, the California legislature passed the Pain Patient's Bill of Rights (California Health and Safety Code § 124960). This law provides, in pertinent part, that "a patient suffering from severe chronic intractable pain has the option to request or reject the use of any or all modalities to relieve his or her severe chronic intractable pain." (California Health and Safety Code § 12496(h).

This law explicitly confers a specific right on California citizens to request any and all modalities to relieve pain. Yet, notwithstanding California's official posture of a commitment to ensuring that patients receive adequate pain care, including specifically adequate access to opioid analgesics, we cannot assume that physicians are providing adequate pain care or being held accountable when they do not. A recent specific case demonstrates this.

In 1998, the MBC was presented with a formal complaint, supported by an independent expert opinion, that the pain care provided to an elderly, terminally ill cancer patient was inadequate. The MBC itself *agreed* that the physician had failed to provide adequate pain care (MBC Letter, 1998). Yet the MBC *declined* to take any action against the physician (MBC Letter, 1998). At least one other case of inadequate pain care presented to the MBC, also supported by an expert opinion that the pain care was inadequate, was also closed without any corrective action.

SIGNS OF CHANGE: ACCOUNTABILITY IN THE MEDICAL DISCIPLINARY AND TORT CONTEXTS EMERGE

There are signs, however, that the laissez-faire attitude regarding inadequate treatment of pain is beginning to change. In 1999, a state medical disciplinary board took corrective action against an Oregon physician who failed to treat his patients adequately for pain (Goodman, 1999).

Cases of inadequate pain treatment are beginning to result in civil liability in tort cases, with significant financial implications (*Estate of Henry James v. Hillhaven Corp.*, 1990; *Gaddis v. United States*, 1997; *Bergman v. Eden Med. Ctr.*, 2001). The recent emergence of guidelines and standards governing appropriate pain care permits establishing that, in a specific case, the pain care provided was inadequate and should result in professional discipline. Medical organizations establishing standards or guidelines for pain treatment include the World Health Organization (1986), the American Pain Society (1995), the American Medical Association (McGivney, et al., 1984), AHCPR (1992), the Federation of State Medical Boards (1998), and the Joint Commission on Accreditation of Healthcare Organizations (JCAHO) (2000). These guidelines all indicate the importance of pain management as an essential element of medical treatment.

There are new requirements for mandatory assessment and routine charting of pain, imposed by the VA system, state law, and JCAHO accreditation provisions (California Health and Safety Code § 1254.7). These provisions will increase patient awareness of their right to good pain care, increasing the likelihood that patients will seek accountability for inadequate pain care, and will enable patients and their advocates to establish with a clear documentary record that the pain care provided in a particular case was inadequate and should result in professional discipline. The record developed by the new assessment and charting rules will for the same reasons also make civil liability on various theories, including professional negligence and elder abuse, easier to establish.

This is entirely appropriate and necessary because knowledge of how to treat pain is available. The problem is that without outside motivation, physicians fail to acquire and apply available knowledge. Physicians must be motivated to acquire and apply this available knowledge (Rich, 2000).

As these types of cases become more common, risk managers can be expected to undertake efforts to minimize risk, leading to more attentive and aggressive provision of pain care.

CHANGES IN LAW ON THE HORIZON

Laws such as Intractable Pain Treatment Acts and Pain Relief Acts, which currently provide a safe harbor for physicians who follow guidelines in prescribing medications to relieve pain, may be revised to explicitly create rough waters for physicians who fail to do so. Such revisions would *require* disciplinary action, or provide an explicit tort cause of action, when there is failure to adequately prescribe, order, administer, or dispense pain management therapies, including controlled substances such as opioid analgesics, for pain relief or modulation in accordance with prevailing clinical practice guidelines.

In the wake of the cases involving inadequate pain care presented to the Medical Board of California, discussed above, which resulted in no action by the Board, such legislation has been introduced in the California State Legislature. In its original form, the proposed California legislation would mandate the MBC to, at a minimum, compel physicians shown to have failed to treat pain adequately to receive continuing education in pain management (Assembly Bill 487, 2001). AB487 has been amended and is expected to pass in a form that requires all California physicians to obtain continued education in pain management.

By amending state law relating to pain in this way, essential steps in encouraging and motivating physicians to treat pain appropriately will be accomplished. Such amendments would create rough waters for physicians who fail to treat pain adequately. This is essential because a safe harbor is not enough; the seas outside must be rough. Physicians who presently fail to adequately treat pain are *already* in a safe harbor, in the sense that there is rarely professional accountability for such conduct. There must be a reason to seek the safe harbor. Until physicians are aware that professional consequences and accountability attach if they fail to treat pain adequately, necessary improvement in the provision of pain care will not occur.

REFERENCES AND ANNOTATED BIBLIOGRAPHY

Acute pain management: operative or medical procedures and trauma clinical practice guideline (Clinical Practice Guideline No. 1, Publ. No. 92-0032 (Feb. 1992) (visited 5/31/00) <http://www.ahcpr.gov/clinic/medtep.acute.htm>; AHCPR, Clinical guideline no. 9: Management of cancer pain, Pub. No. 94-0592 (Mar. 1994).

American Pain Society. Quality improvement guidelines for the treatment of acute pain and cancer pain, 274 *Journal of American Medical Association,* 1874 (1995).

Assembly Bill 487 California State Legislature, 2001 Session.

Bergman v. Eden Med. Ctr., No. H205732-1 Cal. Sup. Ct., Alameda Cty. (physician's failure to adequately treat pain in elderly patient dying of lung cancer) found to be reckless conduct violating elder abuse statute. Jury awarded $1.5M to survivors.

Bernabei, R., et al. (1998) *Management of pain in elderly patients with cancer, Journal of American Medical Association, 279,* 1877, 1879.

Breaking down the barriers to effective pain management, Recommendations to improve the assessment and treatment of pain in New York State, Report to the Commissioner of Health, (Jan. 1998) hereinafter "NY Report"; Institute of Medicine, (1997); see also, *Approaching Death, Improving Care at the End of Life,* at 191, 197 (National Academy Press) (1997) (laws designed to prevent diversion of drugs such as triplicate prescriptions and limits on the number of medication dosages prescribed are burdensome and deter legitimate prescribing of opioids to patients at the end of life); David Joranson, State Medical Board Guidelines for Treatment of Intractable Pain, 5, *American Pain Society Bulletin,* 2 (May/June 1995) (citing California study reflecting that physicians avoid prescribing controlled substances including "triplicate" drugs for patients with intractable pain for fear of discipline by the medical board); Robyn S. Shapiro, Health Care Providers' Liability Exposure for Inappropriate Pain Management, 24; *Journal of Law, Medicine, and Ethics,* 360, 363 (Winter 1996) (identifying fear of legal penalties, especially disciplinary action, as one of the most important reasons health professionals undertreat pain. Citing California survey revealing that 69% of physicians stated that the potential for disciplinary action made them more conservative in their use of opioids in pain management).

California Business & Professional Code § 2241.5(c).

California Health & Safety Code § 124960.

California Health & Safety Code § 1254.7; See CAMH Standard RI.1.2.8; CAMLTC Standard RI.2.6; CAMAC Standard RI.1.2.7; CAMHC Standard RI.1.1.8; CAMBHC Standard RI.1.2.7. http://www.jcaho.org/standard/pm_hap.html.

CIDF Letter. (1998). The idea that state medical boards should take on the responsibility of scrutinizing licensees for inadequate pain care was presented to all 50 state medical boards by Compassion in Dying Federation (CIDF) in a letter sent in January 1998. Letter on file at CIDF offices.

Estate of Henry James v. Hillhaven Corp. (N.C. Super. Ct., Hertford Cty. 1990) ($15 million jury award, half of which was punitive, against nursing home for nurse's conduct in failing to provide prescribed pain medications to terminally ill patient, settled on appeal for undisclosed amount).

Gaddis v. United States, 7 F. Supp. 2d 709 (D.S.C. 1997) (damages awarded to deceased patient's estate and to family for failure to treat pain of terminally ill cancer patient adequately). *Guideline for Prescribing Controlled Sub-*

stances for Intractable Pain, Guideline adopted by the MBC July 29, 1994.

Goodman, E. (1999). Reporting that Dr. Paul Bilder, an Oregon pulmonary specialist, was disciplined by the Oregon Medical Board for a pattern of failing to treat pain adequately. *Charlotte Observer.* Sept. 11.

Hoover v. Agency for Health Care Admin., 676 So. 2d 1380 (Fla. Dist. Ct. App. 1996) (Florida medical disciplinary board penalized and restricted physician for perceived excessive prescribing of pain medication; action of board reversed by court); see also, *Hollabaugh v. Arkansas State Med. Bd.*, 861 S.W.2d 317 (Ark. Ct. App. 1993) (similar case in Arkansas). See generally, J. Sullum, *No Relief in Sight*, 28 Reason 22 (Jan. 1997).

Jacox, A., et al. (1994). (Cancer pain can be relieved for up to 90% of patients); American Pain Society, *Treatment of pain at the end of life: A position statement from the American Pain Society* (visited May 30, 2000) <http://www.ampainsoc.org/advocacy/treatment/htm> ("Well-trained clinicians can provide adequate pain relief for more than 90% of dying cancer patients.")

JCAHO, Comprehensive accreditation manual for hospitals: The official handbook (CAMH) (visited 5/31/00) <http://www.jcaho.org/standard/pm_,hap.html>.

MBC Letter to Beverly Bergman dated August 19, 1998. This letter states in pertinent part: "Our medical consultant did agree with you that pain management for your father was indeed inadequate." The board's letter stated: "There is insufficient evidence at this time to warrant pursuing further action in this case. Your file shall be maintained with the Medical Board for future reference in the event we receive additional complaints in the future which, along with your complaint, could constitute sufficient evidence for disciplinary action."

McGivney, W.T., et al., The care of patients with severe chronic pain in terminal illness, 251 *Journal of American Medical Association,* 1182 (1984).

Model guidelines for the use of controlled substances for the treatment of pain, 85 Fed. Bull: *Journal of Medical Licensure & Discipline* 84 (1998) ("[P]rinciples of quality medical practice dictate that … people …have access to appropriate and effective pain relief… The Board encourages physicians to view effective pain management as a part of quality medical practice for all patients with pain, acute or chronic, and it is especially important for patients who experience pain as a result of terminal illness.")

New York Public Law. (2000). Some states have phased out multiple copy prescription programs, substituting electronic data programs, e.g., N.Y. Pub. Health Law §§ 3332-3333 (Consol. 2000); 710 Ill. Comp. Stat. 570 (West 2000) (amended in 1999). It remains to be seen if this substitution will mitigate the problems caused by the multiple copy programs. Proponents assert that elim-

ination of the need for a duplicate or triplicate pad will facilitate prescribing. Others are skeptical, asserting the concern that scrutiny would be applied to prescribing controlled substances is in no way mitigated by a program that enables electronic data sorting and review.

Prescribing Controlled Substances for Intractable Pain, policy statement of the MBC adopted May 6, 1994.

Rich, B. (2000). *A prescription for the pain: The emerging standard of care for pain management*, Wm. Mitchell L. Rev. 1.

Scheiderman, L.J. (1997). *The Family Physician and End-of-Life Care, Journal of Family Practice, 45,* 259 (*citing* Sidney H. Wanzer et al. (1989). *The physician's responsibility toward hopelessly ill patients: A second look, New England Journal of Medicine, 320,* 844–849).

Stavish, S. (1997). HCFA's palliative care study: Is payment incentive enough? *Ann. In. M., 126,* I-55, I-56.

SUPPORT (Study to Understand Prognoses and Preferences for Outcomes and Risks of Treatments) Principal Investigators (1995). A Controlled Trial to Improve Care for Seriously Ill Hospitalized Patients, *Journal of American Medical Association, 274,* 1591, 1594. *See also* Jacox, A., et al. (1994). New clinical-practice guidelines for the management of pain in patients with cancer, *New England Journal of Medicine, 330,* 651 (pain associated with cancer is frequently undertreated); Joranson, D., et al. *Opioids for chronic cancer and non-cancer pain: A survey of state medical board members,* 79 Fed. Bull.: *Journal of Medical Licensure & Discipline,* (4), 15–49 (1992) (reporting on studies that reflect "that adequate pain control is not being achieved in a significant portion of patients, and that patients often do not receive analgesics to match the severity of their pain," notwithstanding that pain can be well controlled for more than 85% of all cancer patients). The systematic undertreatment of pain has been officially recognized by the Agency for Health Care Policy and Research (AHCPR), AHCPR, *Acute pain management: Operative or medical procedures and trauma, clinical practice guideline* ("Half of all patients given conventional therapy for their pain — most of the 23 million surgical cases each year — do not get adequate relief." <http://www.ahcpr.gov/clinic/medtep.acute.htm> *See also* Von Roenn, J.H., Physician attitudes and practice in cancer pain management, 119 *Annals of Internal Medicine,* 121, (1993) (A survey of doctors treating patients with cancer found that 86% of the respondents "felt that the majority of patients with pain were undermedicated.")

The Pain Relief Act. (1996). *Journal of Law, Medicine, & Ethics, 24,* 317 (1996).

World Health Organization, *Cancer pain relief* (1986).

76

Law Enforcement and Regulatory View about Prescribing Controlled Substances for Pain

Dale A. Ferranto, M.S.

A BRIEF HISTORY OF DRUG ABUSE, ENFORCEMENT, AND REGULATION

In order to fully appreciate the law enforcement and regulatory view about prescribing controlled substances for pain, it is valuable to study the history of drug abuse and the resultant parallel development of governmental policy and control. This history is, in fact, the story of pharmaceuticals. Aldous Huxley, the famous British author, succinctly noted that "pharmacology antedated agriculture" (O'Brien & Cohen, 1984, p. IX). Drugs have been used and abused for centuries in medicinal, religious, and recreational settings. One of the earliest mentions of herbal medicines occurs in the Old Testament book The Song of Solomon. In Chapter 4, verses 13 and 14, Solomon sings of "spikenard" and "aloes". The early Chippewa Native Americans used spikenard as a cough medicine, and aloe is still used today as a disinfectant and burn remedy.

Various world events and scientific advances contributed to America's attitude toward drugs and the abuse of drugs through the centuries. The isolation of morphine from opium in 1804, coupled with opium's commercial value demonstrated by two intense Opium Wars between England and China, and the subsequent development of the hypodermic syringe in 1853 were medical breakthroughs of a double-edged nature. Most physicians believed that relieving pain with needle-administered morphine was harmless because the injected drug bypassed the digestive tract. The immediate post-Civil War era would thus find America with 400,000 morphine addicts (O'Brien & Cohen, 1984, p. XV).

Ignorance among medical professionals combined with popularization of hypodermic therapy (Weston, 1952) gave birth to an American drug dependence that has yet to be cured. At the time, opium was perceived as a vice but not a menace, so governmental regulation merely took the form of taxation.

Amidst the dark cloud of drug abuse naïvete that soon engulfed America, two healing arts organizations were founded. The American Medical Association (A.M.A.) began in 1847, and the American Pharmaceutical Association (A.P.A.) was founded in 1852. Though weak and unsupported until 1900, each association would play vital roles in awakening the United States government and the people to the evils of drug abuse. Through legislative influence and sponsorship of model prescribing and pharmacy laws, the medical professionals assumed a major portion of the responsibility to detoxify the nation.

As the twentieth century began, attention toward another drug, alcohol, so consumed the early era prohibitionists that in 1881, to some people, opiate abuse was the favored alternative. The *Catholic World Magazine* of that year reported, "The gentleman who would not be seen in a barroom…procures his supply of morphia and has it in his pocket ready for instantaneous use. It is odorless and occupies but little space" (O'Brien & Cohen, 1984, p. XV). Also, patent medications containing opiates and cocaine deluged America as cure-alls for "misery, general aches, pains, headaches, and that tired feeling" (Weston, 1952, p. 16).

0-8493-0926-3/02/$0.00+$1.50
© 2002 by CRC Press LLC

Physicians, though now organized in a medical association, continued on courses of misguided treatments. Opiate abusers were medicated to keep them comfortable, not clean. Narcotic- and cocaine-based elixirs and cocktails enjoyed thriving "medicinal" markets. Drug abuse had a firm, yet unrecognized, foothold on America. But from all embryonic indicators of this terrible disease, government failed to react and develop policy to confront the problem early, particularly when the commercial production of heroin as diacetylmorphine (1898) emerged on the market.

The evolution of regulatory and enforcement activities started with mere taxation (1864) and research (1886) when Congress announced an act to "Provide for the study of the nature of alcoholic drinks and narcotics, and their effects upon the human system" (Weston, 1952, p. 17). Exercising national intervention in matters previously reserved for the individual states, the Federal Government embarked on a course of codification of narcotic laws (Johnson, 1988). And, while not entirely taboo, "recreational" drug use was coming under greater suspicion, and unless one obtained drugs by prescription, a great deal of negative stereotyping of addicts was attached to opiate consumption.

Americans, though, continued to cherish and readily seek physician prescribed drugs. This patent medicine craze of high opiate content medications and the delayed realization that "dangerously addicting substances were distributed with little worry for their effect" (Musto, 1973, p. 7) caused two major events. The first was a revival of an old form of professional criminality, drug diversion, and the second was a reaction by state and federal agencies to control the first.

The criminal physician and pharmacist seized the opportunity to cash in on the highly lucrative pharmaceutical drug business. Their enterprise, though, was nothing really new. In 1604, Miguel de Cervantes in *Man of Glass* offered his view of the unscrupulous doctor, writing, "Physicians may and do kill without fear or running away and without unsheathing any other sword than that of a prescription" (Cervantes, p. 78). Additionally, Sir Arthur Conan Doyle, himself a physician, allowed Sherlock Holmes to conclude, "When a doctor goes wrong he is the first of criminals. He has nerve and he has knowledge" (Doyle, 1977). So doctors thus inclined and known as "croakers" or gentlemen of high rank who like their base and comfort without earning it (Keegan, 1987, p. 129) emerged as drug diverters and suppliers for drug abusers.

The government's reaction and policy response to the rising epidemic of pharmaceutical drug abuse quickened in the early 1900s. Prescription requirements increased for opiate substances, and curing addiction became a true legal and medical challenge. Federal laws, originally argued as unconstitutional, were then enacted, and they included the Pure Food and Drug Act (1906), The Harrison

Narcotic Law (1914), the Drug Abuse Act (1970), and the Anti-Drug Abuse Act of 1988.

The nexus between drug abuse and prescriptions also led James H. Beal, an outspoken pharmacist/lawyer of the A.P.A., to propose a model state pharmacy law for habit-forming drugs. Though not enthusiastically embraced by his medical and pharmacist colleagues, Beal's model became a turning point in endorsing further narcotic-related healing arts legislation.

The diverse and heterogeneous growth of America during the new twentieth century fragmented our society resulting in more formal sanctions and controls by government on pharmaceutical substances of abuse (Richardson, 1974, p. 86). While the subject of drug abuse temporarily disappeared from government scrutiny during the World Wars, Great Depression, and Korean War, it reemerged with vengeance after the Vietnam conflict. America's appetite for drugs exploded and, simultaneously, drugs were being developed at a tremendous rate: approximately 75% of today's pharmaceuticals were formulated within the last 40 years. The supply–demand equation of this phenomenon has remained so unbalanced that full, complete, and effective enforcement of drug policies could now only be achieved in a police state.

The diversion of pharmaceutical controlled substances presented a unique regulatory and enforcement problem to authorities trying to prevent drug abuse. The Drug Abuse Warning Network (D.A.W.N.) reports that highlight hospital overdose admissions and coroner death reports in over 800 hospitals nationwide consistently indicated that pharmaceutical drugs were involved in approximately 50% of the deaths and, of the top 20 drugs of abuse, 15 were pharmaceuticals. Three sources of these drugs primarily appeared in criminal casework. The first was identified as "doctor shoppers" or patients who successfully scammed prescribers for medications. The second was prescribers themselves who had lost the ability or desire to practice medicine, and consequently decided to merely make a living by writing "script." The third source was prescription forgers

Intermingled among the enforcement and regulatory thrusts to halt drug diversion by unscrupulous patients and prescribers was the increasing concern about pharmaceuticals and pain management. Because many of the drugs of choice being diverted and scammed were opioids, synthetics, and other acute and chronic pain medications, the legitimate medical practice prescribing of these drugs came under the same umbrella of enforcement and regulatory suspicion. Many states enacted multiple copy prescription programs hoping to monitor and control pharmaceutical drug diversion and abuse. In many cases, however, prescribers felt impeded in otherwise legitimate prescribing practices by the increased government oversight. The result was that many patients who truly needed the opiate-strength medications did not receive them. More professionally palatable and patient-friendly prescription drug law and regulation options, particularly in the emerging medical discipline of pain management, would therefore be required as America entered the next millennium.

THE MISSION OF ENFORCEMENT AND REGULATION

There is a great deal of misinformation and misconception about the intended role of law enforcement and regulation in the prescribing, administering, and dispensing of pharmaceutical drugs. Some of the misunderstanding stems from weak investigative casework that resulted in poor administrative decisions and prosecutions. Horror stories are passed from prescriber to prescriber, and the facts are many times distorted. As a result, newly licensed and authorized prescribers begin their careers suspicious and somewhat paranoid about the role of government in the business of medicine.

The enforcement and regulatory mission is not intended to meddle in the practice of medicine. Overzealous and inexperienced investigators occasionally display an interfering, authoritative attitude that regrettably supports allegations of meddling but they are not encouraged by their employers to do so.

Similarly, enforcement and regulatory authorities have no desire to deny patient care and pain relief. However, initial complaints and information received by the investigators, medical consultants, and prosecutors often raise questions as to the type, quality, and quantity of medication treatment the patient is alleged to be receiving or being denied by the prescriber. This concern of authorities may erroneously translate into interfering with specific drug needs of the patient and prescribing actions of the prescriber.

The interest and obligation of enforcement and regulatory authorities, though, are to prevent the diversion of pharmaceutical drugs from legitimate medical practice to illegal uses. Pharmaceutical controlled substances, particularly pain medications, command a very high value on the "street." While the vast majority of prescribers never intentionally divert drugs to illegitimate use, hosts of interested "patients" and other nonlicentiates actively mingle and network in the pharmaceutical drug environment with the sole goal of separating the drugs from the prescriber and pharmacist.

It is also in the public and consumer safety interests for enforcement and regulatory personnel to ensure the highest medical standards of prescribing. Many states have specific guidelines issued by their licensing boards and bureaus to prescribers detailing the criteria used to evaluate prescribing practices. These standards are used as measures to comply with the state and federal prescribing laws, and they are the same foundation from which administrative disciplinary actions, criminal prosecutions, and civil litigations are launched.

Enforcement and regulatory agencies generally establish priorities for investigative case management. Attention toward prescribers has traditionally focused on the "Four Ds": dishonest, duped, dated, and disabled. Nonlicensed individuals (particularly medical clinic owners/operators) involved in pharmaceutical drug diversion and abuse usually manipulate prescribers to achieve illegal, profit-driven goals, and they may also be involved in prescription forgery, pharmaceutical drug smuggling, and billing fraud.

High on the food chain of enforcement and regulatory personnel is the "dishonest" prescriber. This licentiate may have lost the ability or desire to practice within accepted legitimate medical needs. Commonly driven by a get rich-quick greed, the dishonest prescriber makes a good living merely by "writing script" and sale of their signature. Both the public safety and the integrity of the medical profession demand immediate and intense efforts to stop the activities of the dishonest prescriber.

The "duped" prescriber is really a victim of a drug-seeking patient. In most states, a patient who "scams" a prescriber for a controlled substance has committed a crime. Specifically, the patient withholds material facts from the prescriber, i.e., the patient is receiving controlled substances from other prescribers. This obtaining by fraud and deceit is most pronounced by clever patients who are terrific actors, knowledgeable about prescribing practices and the *Physician's Desk Reference,* and present physical ailments that are difficult to confirm, and strike at the most opportune times and vulnerable targets such as weekend emergency departments (Burke, 2000), clinic lunch hours, and on-call medical group partners.

The third of the "Four Ds" is the dated prescriber. This prescriber has simply not kept abreast of current medical prescribing practices and, consequently, either prescribes incorrectly or refuses to prescribe as necessary or becomes an easy drug source to be duped. Continuing medical education is the key to salvaging this prescriber and maintaining contemporary standards of legitimate medical care.

The "disabled" prescriber is a person who has personal dependency problems that interfere with the professional practice of good healthcare for his or her patients. Drug abuse is one of the most common disabling causes for prescribers. Many regulatory boards and bureaus provide rehabilitation to disabled prescribers through impaired practice programs that limit the prescriber's authority while being paired with another prescriber who has legal oversight and reporting responsibility. Successful completion of the impaired practice program can lead to full restoration of prescribing privileges.

Enforcement and regulatory attention toward pain management prescribers could likely be generated by conduct of any one of the "Four Ds." It should be clear, though, that the dishonest prescriber, particularly in the specialty of pain management, would be a very high casework priority. At the same time, educating the police and the prescriber about legitimate and acceptable standards of prescribing for pain would help to better focus limited healthcare, enforcement, and regulatory resources where they will do the most good for the patient.

OPIA PHOBIA AND MULTIPLE COPY PRESCRIPTION PROGRAMS

While the mission of enforcement and regulatory authorities as previously described seems clear and well intentioned, prescribing paranoia, whether real or perceived, has emerged particularly among pain management prescribers. Described as a "chilling effect" or "opia phobia," a serious, sometimes overly cautious reluctance to treat pain patients with appropriately prescribed controlled substances exists throughout this community of prescribers. Affected prescribers maintain that excess governmental oversight and regulation coupled with multiple copy and electronic prescription systems for pharmaceutical drugs drives their inaction. Dr. Russel Portenoy may have described it best, "Laws and regulations intended to curtail illicit opioid use may be an unintended impediment to legitimate prescribing."

No empirical studies have demonstrated this theory of prescribing paranoia but it clearly ranks as an important element in the discussion of pain management. Possibly the closest measure of this chilling effect was observed when the state of New York placed benzodiazepines into its prescription monitoring system. The prescribing of benzodiazepines dramatically decreased. The disturbing effect of this response was quite possibly the undertreatment of conditions requiring sedative, tranquilizing, and hypnotic medications.

In the specialty of pain management, the relational cause and effect of opia phobia may manifest itself more dramatically and tragically. Dr. Brad Stuart, speaking from a hospice perspective, illustrates one such outcome stating, "Even though we know how to treat pain effectively, many physicians consistently undertreat it for a variety of reasons. No wonder sick people are looking for a way out" (Stuart, 1999). Managing legitimate pain by prescribing controlled substances in legitimate medical practice should be immune to any perception of enforcement and regulatory barriers.

Once again, understanding the problem and educating to the communities of regulators as well as the regulated about the solution are key steps in warming the chilling effect and overcoming an opia phobia. Both communities must communicate internally as well as together to discover the middle ground that will allow each to accomplish the prescriber, the police, and, most importantly, the patient's best interests. Dr. Daniel A. Dotson sums up this needed approach writing, "Exacerbating the fundamental misinformation and peer pressure (about prescribing for pain) is the effect of the regulation by various state and federal agencies which have been — historically and, in some cases, still are — unable to distinguish between the self-destructive drug-seeking lifestyle of the addict and the productive and responsible life of the legitimate pain patient consuming the same or greater doses of narcotics" (Dotosn, 2000).

Many states are now in the process of modifying or eliminating the real or perceived barriers to legitimate controlled substance prescribing for pain. In California, model legislation exists regarding the treatment of intractable pain, prescribing for the terminally ill, and a bill of rights for pain patients. Nationally, electronic and paperform multiple copy prescription systems are being reviewed, revised, and in some cases, abandoned. Progress is slowly being made on the monitoring and medical fronts to affect better pain patient care.

LEGITIMATE PRESCRIBING IN GOOD MEDICAL PRACTICE

Through their enforcement and regulatory agencies and in concert with federal prescribing codes a variety of states have published guidelines for prescribers who treat patients for intractable pain. The Medical Board of California guidelines which follow are one example, and they are predicated upon the "position that the public is best served by a healthcare environment where physicians are free to exert their own best medical judgment consistent with accepted community standards of care" (Medical Board of California, 1996):

HISTORY/PHYSICAL EXAMINATION

A thorough medical history and physical examination must be accomplished. Prescribing controlled substances for intractable pain in California also requires evaluation by one or more specialists.

TREATMENT PLAN/OBJECTIVES

The treatment plan should state objectives by which treatment success can be evaluated, such as pain relief and/or improved physical and psychosocial function, and indicate if any further diagnostic evaluations or other treatments are planned. Several treatment modalities or a rehabilitation program may be necessary.

INFORMED CONSENT

The physician should discuss the risks and benefits of the use of controlled substances with the patient or guardian.

PERIODIC REVIEW

The physician should periodically review the course of opioid treatment of the patient and any new information about the etiology of the pain. Continuation or modification of opioid therapy depends on the physician's evaluation of progress toward treatment objectives.

CONSULTATION

The physician should be willing to refer the patient as necessary for additional evaluation and treatment to achieve treatment objectives. Physicians should give special attention to those pain patients who are at risk for misusing their medications. The management of pain in patients with a history of substance abuse requires extra care, monitoring, documentation, and consultation with addiction specialists, and may entail the use of agreements between the provider and the patient to specify rules for medication use.

RECORDS

The physician should keep accurate and complete records, including the medical history and physical examination, other evaluations and consultations, treatment plan objectives, informed consent, treatments, medications, agreements with the patient, and periodic reviews.

COMPLIANCE WITH CONTROLLED SUBSTANCES LAWS AND REGULATIONS

To prescribe substances, the physician must be appropriately licensed in California and comply with federal and state regulations for issuing controlled substances prescriptions. Documented adherence to these guidelines will substantially establish the physician's responsible treatment of patients with intractable pain and will serve to defend that treatment practice in the face of complaints which may be brought.

The identification and acknowledgment of pain-prescribing issues by enforcement and regulatory agencies have been huge steps forward in improving patient care. Legislation and published prescribing guidelines for prescribing controlled substances to pain patients also have contributed to better understanding the responsibilities and limitations of the prescriber, the patient, and the police. Circling this structure of pain management healthcare and regulation, however, is an evolving body of criminal and civil litigation.

Historically, the concern of most enforcement agencies, regulatory boards, and prescribers has been overprescribing of pain medications to patients. The fear was based upon the addiction of patients and subsequent treatment of addicts that resulted in criminal prosecutions, administrative discipline, and lawsuits. Now the courts and administrative law judges are entertaining actions regarding the undertreatment of pain. In at least one such case, the alleged failure to treat pain has been charged as elder abuse (Lazarus & Stanton, 2000). The outcome of such cases may chart new approaches to pain management prescribing and should, therefore, be closely monitored by pain treatment specialists.

THE FIFTH VITAL SIGN: PRESCRIBING FOR PAIN

The medical discipline of pain management has been maturing for decades. Effective procedures and therapies to treat pain are growing in number every year. Pain is now considered a critical vital sign in the medical workup.

Yet, discussion and dilemma about the correct balance between treatment and regulation exist. Perhaps this needed balance can be achieved in an integrated approach by the prescribers, the police, and the public through education, expertise, and teamwork.

It is imperative that the medical community, the enforcement and regulatory authorities, and the patients have open dialog about their missions, responsibilities, and needs. The myths about prescribing practices held by the police and the myths about enforcement practices held by the prescribers need to be eliminated in order that patients can better understand and reap the benefits of their true treatment options and limitations. At the same time, all parties to the pain treatment issues need to stay informed and educated with contemporary knowledge about available care within regulatory boundaries and community standards. And, when such care and/or conditions become obsolete, the same interested parties should collectively see that they are legally discontinued or changed.

Prescribers as well as government regulators also should be experts in their respective fields. Pain management prescribers should be well versed in available treatments, controlled substances, alternative healing (Shannon, 2000) including nutrition (Fox, 2000), and multidisciplinary approaches to integrated therapies. Enforcement and regulatory personnel should understand the limits of legal and administrative standards, acknowledge and appreciate the complexities of pain management, and exercise their authority in fairness and under the spirit of the law to seek justice.

The shared education and expertise of each interest group (prescribers, police, and public) in a teamwork approach will enhance the likelihood of better communication and cooperation in solving pain management issues. Achieving necessary compromises in draft legislation and proposed treatment regimens can speed up bureaucratic processes and advance patient care without undue delay. This common interest approach for improved treatment of the patient will also help to discourage the damaging us vs. them philosophy between prescriber and regulator.

As we begin the new millennium, healthcare providers are on the leading edge of patient driven treatment of pain. The patient's voice supported by new legislation is now an integral component of the decision-making treatment process. While the options available are multidisciplinary ranging from traditional medicine to transdermal magnets, one of the most basic courses of care, prescribing strong controlled substances, remains an action fraught with paranoia of government regulatory oversight and penalty coupled with a perceived addiction consequence for the patient. As a result, the patient suffers needlessly; and, studies have shown that pain can kill (Liebeskind, 1991).

Good prescribing is based upon the practice of good medicine. The prescriber who embraces established treatment guidelines during the initial and all subsequent adjustments to prescribing, dispensing, and administering controlled substances to pain patients will unlikely have any problems with enforcement and regulatory authorities. Legitimate medical indication is the guiding principle for the prescriber.

The laws and regulations that exist to curtail dishonest and dangerous prescribing practices of unscrupulous prescribers are not intended to deny the treatment of legitimate pain. They should not impede legitimate prescribing or allow government authorities to meddle in the practice of medicine. The enforcement and regulatory authorities, with support from the medical community, should be used to their full extent to protect the patient and the public healthcare trust.

REFERENCES

Burke, J. (2000). Emergency room shoppers. In *Partners against pain: E.D. physician, beware the opioid shopper* (5th ed., p. 4). H. Lazarus & M. Stanton (Eds.). Stanford, CT: Purdue Pharma Limited Partnership.

Cervantes, M.D. (1604/1983). *Man of glass.* Franklin Center: The Franklin Library,

Dotson, D.A. (2000). Why not relief?, *Pain Physician, 3,* 65.

Doyle, A.C. (1977). *The adventure of the speckled band.* Franklin Center: The Franklin Library,

Fox, M.C. (2000, Sept./Oct.). Eat this, ache less, *Fitness Swimmer,* 20.

Johnson, H.A. (1988). *History of criminal justice.* Anderson Publishing Company, Cincinnati, 209.

Keegan, J. (1987). *The mask of command.* Viking Penguin, Inc., New York.

Lazarus, H. and Stanton, M., Eds. (2000). Undertreatment of pain goes to court as elder abuse. In *Partners against Pain* (5th ed., p. 1). Stanford, CT: Purdue Pharma Limited Partnership.

Liebeskind, J.C. (1991). Pain can kill, *Pain, 44,* 3.

Medical Board of California. (1996). Treatment of intractable pain: A guideline, Action Report, Sacramento, 57, 1.

Musto, D.F. (1973). *The American disease: Origins of narcotic control.* New Haven, CT: Yale University Press.

O'Brien, R. & Cohen, S. (1984). *The encyclopedia of drug abuse,* New York: Facts on File, Inc.

Richardson, J.F. (1974). *Urban police in the United States.* Port Washington: Kenikat Press.

Shannon, S. (2000, July). Alternative healing: What really works? *Readers Digest,* 45.

Stuart, B. (1999, May). Assisted suicide: The illusion of free choice, *San Jose Mercury News,* San Jose.

Weston, P.B. (Ed.). (1952). *Narcotics U.S.A.,* New York: Greenburg.

77

Ethics of Care:
Pain Management and Spirituality

Myrna C. Tashner, Ed.D.

For an effective discussion of the *ethics of care and pain management and spirituality,* we must reexamine how we view ourselves: body, mind, and spirit.

Since the time of René Descartes, humankind has gradually learned to focus on itself as body (matter) and mind (brain). In general, this is due to a "deal" worked out between Descartes and the Pope. In order to get permission to study the body, Descartes appealed to the Pope for permission to dissect a human corpse. In their agreement, Descartes agreed that he would have nothing to do with the spirit/soul, the mind, or the emotions if he should find them in the body. The soul, mind, and emotions were the exclusive jurisdiction of the church at that time. Descartes claimed the physical body as his realm of study, thus separating the body from the mind. This bargain set the tone and direction of science for the next 200 years. It divided the human into two distinct and separate spheres that could not overlap.

This agreement gave us the Cartesian era with its reductionist methodology, which attempts to understand life by examining the tiniest pieces of it and then extrapolates from those pieces to generalities about the whole.

Human development has been studied formally since the time of St. Augustine, but its beginnings date to the days of Jesus, and even back to the ancients. However, it has only been in the last 100 years or so that psychologists applied scientific methods to the examination of human development. Sigmund Freud was the first. He is credited with the beginning of psychoanalytic theory, a significant study of human development. Later, Jean Piaget contrib-

uted theories of cognitive and social development, including environment and relationships studies. But in the last 25 years, according to the American Psychological Association, society's concerns about adolescence, aging, and life span have become the focus of psychology. At the end of the 19th century, psychology was concerned with the study of mind and consciousness through introspection, thus describing experience. Now at the end of the 20th and beginning of the 21st, the focus of psychology has broadened to a science and practice concerned with human behavior, as well as the mental process that underlies experiences and behavior.

Maybe it is time to put us back together; after all, we are body, mind, and spirit/soul, a whole being. This chapter shows that when we manage our pain, and/or heal, we seem to do it as a whole being using our minds, emotions, and spirits within the body physical.

The establishment of the study of ethics may be considered the result of humankind's movement away from and/or forgetting of the natural laws, or the Laws of the Universe with the primary law: We are all one. Ethics is designed to protect and ensure that we do not harm those who choose to place themselves in our care. We must remember to do no harm to ourselves as well. In primitive cultures, moral principles of conduct and proper actions were part of the expected behavior of a member of the tribe. Only in particular situations, when the member chose to invalidate someone else's personal space, or neglected to respect the rights of his or her fellow tribe members, did the chief or medicine person get involved

0-8493-0926-3/02/$0.00+$1.50
© 2002 by CRC Press LLC

to resolve the matter. For example, in the Mayan culture a tribesman would be expelled from the tribe and sent to live alone in the jungle for lying.

In our complex society, made up of members of many different cultures and backgrounds, we have evolved a specific professional discipline called ethics, or laws of professional conduct for our professional disciplines, such as medicine, psychology, ministry, and law. These are standards of expected behaviors to be considered a member of that group, or professional tribe.

The Dalai Lama, (1999) a respected religious leader, has written a book on the subject of ethics for our new millennium in which he describes ethics as a "universal responsibility" the individual needs to be a responsible person. Responsibility is a word derived from "respond-ere," the Latin word for the ability to answer. It is the ability to answer the urgings of our intuition and our heart, as well as respond with intelligence in the discipline we have chosen to practice. For example, we need to follow our awareness of what is needed to function as a healthy whole person, as well as how to maintain our body–mind–spirit's wellness.

Respect is also paramount. It is so important to respect what our bodies tell us, we need to look again at what our patients/clients are really telling us are their problems, and respect what they say. Although managed care does not like to reimburse for it, nor consider listening a part of care, or consider it appropriate to pay for it, the art of listening and questioning is important before diagnosing and prescribing treatment and medications.

To be a good listener, we need to begin by practicing on ourselves. How often do we listen to ourselves, seriously listen, and then respect what our intuition tells us about our body, mind, and spirit? This is an area of fertile ground for self-study, growth, and development, and possibly for forgiveness of self and/or others. Paying attention and appreciating what we learn about ourselves can only deepen our appreciation for and commitment to ourselves. Experience is a very good teacher.

Compassion is the word used to describe the feeling of empathy (including love, affection, kindness, gentleness, generosity of spirit, and warm-heartedness) toward others, while honoring our limitations to remove their problems or pain from them. Before we can have true compassion for others, we need to be compassionate toward ourselves. To have compassion means to undergo or suffer with a patient or loved one the painful experience in his or her life. Again this study begins with self, being with and going within ourselves, and then learning to live well and in harmony with self. It starts with responsibility for our needs and well-being through respecting what we learn about the self, and living in compassion and harmony with self.

We are involved in and dedicated to the science of medicine and pain management. Currently, it seeks to heal the body without necessarily recognizing the energy of the soul/spirit that lies behind illness and, therefore, cannot heal the body or the soul/spirit. To put it simply, how often do we not pay attention to our inner knowing and excuse it by saying something like, "Oh, well, I just missed it." Then we relieve our guilt and responsibility by telling ourselves that everything will work out okay. And that is true, everything will work out, with or without your cooperation. However, it can be more fun and fulfilling to learn about the beauty of breathing from meditation rather than from emphysema. Medicines aim to relieve the symptoms, but they may or may not heal the body, and medicine probably will not heal the pain of the soul/spirit. I have given up counting the number of patients who have told me, "If only I had stopped smoking or stopped being sexually promiscuous, this would not have happened." The fact is, if we are not responsible, respectful, and compassionate, and if we do not listen to our intuition, eventually we have a good chance of contributing to a body illness.

The science of psychology is in a situation similar to that of the science of medicine. Over time and under the influence of Cartesian philosophy of thought, psychology has come to mean the science of the study of the personality, emotions, and cognitions without recognizing the force and energy of the soul that lie behind the configurations and experiences of the personality. Therefore, psychology cannot heal the soul/spirit either, because the current science is focused on that which is visible to others.

FROM TREATING SYMPTOMS TO TREATING THE WHOLE PERSON FOR WELLNESS

Now we are experiencing a shift in attitude toward the treatment of illness from the Descartes reductionism to holism, considering the body, but also the mind, emotions, soul/spirit. In some medical practices (e.g., Dossey, Chopra, Sheely) healthcare professionals are working with the patient's body and spirit. Dossey's *Reinventing Medicine* (1999) describes the coming era of medicine as including a focus on and use of spiritual energy for healing intervention in hospitals.

There is scientific evidence to support the importance of emotions in pain management and healing. Research by Candice Pert (1997) on the molecular energy of emotions and how these emotions connect and influence the body is described in *Molecules of Emotions*. As a graduate student, Pert laid the foundations for the discovery of endorphins, the body's pain suppressors and ecstasy inducers. Her later discovery of the opiate receptors extended to every field of medicine and contributed to the synthesis of behavior, psychology, and biology. She went on to show that neurotransmitters secreted by the brain change physical activity, including behavior, mood, and emotion. She described stress as information overload, a condition in which the body system is taxed with emotional unprocessed information to the degree that the body shuts down with what we call disease. Stress prevents the molecules of emotion from flowing freely. She discovered for herself the value of meditation practice and the power of visualization.

The scientist and philosopher, Gary Zukav, addressed the issues of the spirit and soul in his book *Seat of the Soul* (1989). He defined the soul as an energy system and described humans as multisensory beings, as opposed to five-sensory beings, capable of perceiving and appreciating beyond the human five-sensory personality. He stated that compassion, clarity, and boundless love are natural to the soul, and life is the opportunity of the soul to learn lessons about the laws of physics and the Universe. Life's experiences are for the purpose of soul growth, power, and energy. The soul has a reverence for all of life. To be reverent is to be spiritual. Reverence creates compassion, kindness, and patience.

In a sense we have come full circle, from the Pope and the Catholic Church maintaining their priority over the whole human, to medicine and science, which were able to study the body, to physicians like Freud and Jung who focus on the "untouchable" psyche or soul, to psychologists taking the soul and studying behavior and personality, to medicine now realizing it needs to consider the person as a whole vs. pieces or parts — body, mind and spirit — in holistic medicine.

RELIGION VS. SPIRITUALITY

For some time religions have focused on the practice of belief and ritual for the purpose of honoring the divine, or God, or Yahweh, or Allah. It can lead to and/or be a spiritual experience, but not necessarily. Religion is a set of doctrines, dogmas, beliefs held by a group of believers who may form a church. That brings to mind the image of people gathering in a building.

Spirituality is not religion. It conjures up a sense of the sacred and the soul. Our patients evolve into exploring what spirituality means for them. Deepak Chopra, M.D., in *How to Know God* (2000) describes spirituality as learning to cooperate with God, learning that there is one reality, the spiritual, that nothing lies outside the mind of God or awareness.

C. Myss, in *Why People Don't Heal and How They Can* (1997), describes spirituality as accepting divine direction, which is an ongoing process of self-discovery. It starts with a quiet, growing dissatisfaction with institutional religion, and an inner sense that there must be more to spirituality, the need to seek it out using meditation and a new path to inner power. It is a journey in self-discovery and an approach to God from a point of view that is not tied to a specific religion, but is more general. Myss sug-

gests that illness possibly may be the means through which God leads us to discover more about ourselves. This could be true of the challenge of disease, or aging. In *Seat of the Soul* (1989), Zukav describes spirituality as the immortal process itself, that pertains to that which is immortal within you, the individual.

I like to think that spirituality gives power back to you as a person and makes you responsible for your life force. Spirituality empowers you as a person. Spirituality places the power where it belongs, in and with you. You are responsible as a person, but by listening to your "inner voice," you can learn much about yourself, your attitudes, and behaviors including your pain. This knowledge can lead to pain management and healing.

This self-awareness reframes you in the world. In the Cartesian concept of you as body, which has many systems that function for living, pain and illness are signs of malfunction in a system of the physical body. But if you consider yourself a spiritual being and the center of the dynamic of living, not your body, then your world looks like this: You are a spiritual being, living in a spiritual world, governed by spiritual laws, having a human experience. The effects and consequences of this change in the order of things are awesome, for each effect follows the Laws of the Universe, which are really simple. For example, as you intend, so it shall be. Or, as you think, so you are.

NATURE OF SPIRITUALITY

Spirituality can be a deep search for the meaning of life. Much of our knowledge of spirituality has come from Eastern traditions (Hindu, Buddhist, etc.), Jesus and Paul, Native Americans, mystics including Ralph Waldo Emerson and Henry David Thoreau, and contemporary ones, such as C. Myss, D. Chopra, N. Walsch, and the Dalai Lama.

Spirituality has an unseen dimension, beyond the five-sense component of energy. Healing of illness and pain has a historical involvement with spirituality. Some suggest that this is what the master teacher Jesus Christ was attuned with his many miracles. Humankind's fascination with this energy was evident in 18th-century Europe in medical societies that were challenged by some of their members to explain the healing process. In 1900 in Vienna the physician Franz Mesmer formulated a theory of healing using the energy of magnets and gravity. His ideas took hold in the United States, and influenced, among others, a New England watchmaker P.P. Quimby. Through his study of mesmerism Quimby produced changes in the mind by use of the mind. Quimby renamed the work "hypnosis," but later came to believe that a Higher Intelligence can work through us to correct thought errors that cooperated to create illness. Belief patterns of patients had to change. Quimby said he thought that was how Jesus

Christ healed and he proceeded to heal using this principle. Quimby attracted students and followers, including Mary Baker Eddy, who experienced her healing through his work, and who later founded Christian Science. She believed that prayer and the power of the mind could bring about healing. It is interesting to note that some insurance companies pay for the services of Christian Science practitioners.

Eddy's student and fellow mystic, Emma Curtis Hopkins, founded the Metaphysical School in Chicago. A New York physician, Dr. H. Emily Cady, and Charles and Myrtle Fillmore, co-founders of Unity School of Christianity, studied in Hopkins' school. Dr. Cady wrote a classic work for Unity School on the power of the mind entitled *Lessons in Truth* (1892), in which she detailed her understanding of the teachings of the master Jesus as practical and applicable for healing, as well as pain management. She explained a relationship with the Almighty One that was personal, practical, and the essential responsibility of the individual. She emphasized discipline of the mind and responsible management of thought. Remembered from these 19th-century metaphysicians are sayings based on the Law of Mind Action theme, i.e., change your thinking and change your life; or, thoughts held in mind produce after their kind.

SPIRITUALITY AND PAIN MANAGEMENT

When we talk about spirituality, pain management, and the power of the mind to heal, we are talking about concepts that have a historic base in our culture. Keep in mind that when we talk about spirituality and pain management, we are not necessarily talking about healing of the physical body, although that is what people in pain want.

Pain is a word that describes the experience of physical pain caused by cancer, surgery, burn; emotional/mental pain that can be situational or chronic; or spiritual pain as in a dark night of the soul or loss of the sense of self. We learn and grow, because pain can be a teacher. It can set up an addiction, not only to medications but also to the experience of pain for the benefits it can give us.

In the following true illustrations, we discuss four pain-filled experiences and the use of the mind and the inner spiritual power to manage the physical pain.

The author's experience with this concept was as a graduate student. I was working three part-time jobs to meet expenses. I also was studying for my licensing boards and doing my dissertation research. I also was very conscious of what I ate as I was just beginning my study of yoga, and learning to breathe correctly and to relax my body. One day I noticed small blisters on my right forearm, but I thought nothing of them

and continued my schedule. I don't remember exactly how long it took, but within a few days, I was aware of a lot of pain in that arm which now had many more blisters. To make a long story short, I went to my physician who diagnosed shingles and prescribed medication for pain.

Of course, the prescribed medication was strong, and I experienced side effects. The pain didn't go away, but got worse. I had a choice: go into the hospital for a morphine drip, or just live with the side effects of the prescription drugs.

Instead, I chose to take aspirin and practice the relaxation technique I had learned in yoga. And I had the bright idea to add the image of white light flowing into my body going to the site of each hurting nerve ending and surrounding it, relieving it of the inflammation. I asked that it relieve me of the pain.

I knew about breathing and relaxation from yoga. My doctor had told me aspirin was the strongest non-prescription painkiller. But the image was something that came from within me. I quickly became aware that when I was in the relaxed state with that image, I was pain free. It was natural to be grateful and I giggled with delight.

The following story was told to the author by a Native American friend.

In the late 1960s, I developed severe pain in my left hand. The fingers were swollen with red speckles. I thought I had been bitten by something. Within days the pain and swelling had gone to my left knee, and my ankle and foot were painful and swollen. After 2 weeks of aspirin and Tylenol, ice and heat, I saw my family doctor. He examined me and ordered blood tests. Several days later I received his diagnosis: rheumatoid arthritis. He told me to expect continued pain and deterioration to the level of being wheelchair bound. I was devastated. I had three small children, a husband, a life. I couldn't be a cripple.

I called my mother in tears. She listened and told me she would study and pray about it. My mother was Native American, of the Choctaw nation. She was raised with both white and Native traditions. My grandfather was English. My sisters and I were raised with a mixture of both cultures. I refer to my mother as Native American, but never referred to myself as such. My father was very white Irish.

The pain continued. I called my mother again. She said she was praying. Nothing happened.

Several days later I went to my mother's house. My dad was out back in his garden. Mother met me at the door. She said she was expecting me. I limped inside. She placed a kitchen chair in the middle of the room, pointed and said, "Sit." I sat.

Mother began by placing her hands on my shoulders, then my head. She began speaking with gut spouch. After a few minutes she began doing a slow native two-step dance around my chair. I had seen the dance many times in my lifetime and I accepted it as "right." I began to relax. My mother's tempo increased. Then she began speaking in another language. Her voice rose and fell. Her feet beat a tempo, and I felt my whole being slip into her chant; although I didn't understand the words, the tempo of her feet beat a chant into my heart. Time passed, maybe hours, I don't know. She finished by placing her hands to my head and shoulders and ordering the spirit of illness to leave my body, never to return. Was the pain gone at that time? No. But the next morning I awoke to less discomfort. By noon I could open and close my left hand. Within 3 days I was working — pain free. The medical community may say I went into spontaneous remission. I say I was healed.

Some 30 years later, I fell up the stairs at work. (Most people fall downstairs; I took a different route.) I hit my right knee on the stair's edge. That evening, it was very sore. Two days later I rose from the dining table but couldn't walk. The pain increased to the point that I couldn't ambulate without excruciating pain. Tears came to my eyes as I started up the stairs. I tried to ignore the pain and the symptoms. I tried to ignore the swelling. Finally, my uneven gait was noticed by my co-workers. I was sent to the doctor. He took X-rays. "Lucky," he said, "nothing is broken. All you have," he told me, "is degenerative arthritis. Bone on bone. It can only get worse."

I just looked at him, "How can that be, there wasn't any pain before I fell."

He offered pain medications and an anti-inflammatory, and told me to go home and live with it. "At your age you can only expect these problems to occur," he said.

And that's what pissed me off. I refused the steroids but took over-the-counter medications. Days, weeks passed, the pain continued. Finally, one day when I was alone, I screamed out to my mother, who had been gone for 10 years, "Why did you leave me! I need you!" I needed her to heal me. I want her to heal my pain. Couldn't she hear me crying? Couldn't she hear my heart begging for relief?

Nothing happened. Silence.

I wanted to feel her presence. I wanted to feel her touch. I asked the Great Spirit to help.

Once again silence. Or perhaps I just didn't hear.

We constantly hear that we make our own reality, so I started to try to direct healing toward myself. I asked others to pray. Nothing seemed to change.

And then one night I dreamed. I saw my mother as a young woman of 17 dancing in a field of wildflowers, laughing in a carefree manner. I tried to run to her, to stop her, just so she could touch me, and I touch her. I knew that if I could touch her I would be healed. She kept dancing just out of my reach.

When I woke up, I woke up to pain. Days passed. I constantly asked and prayed for help. I asked for the Great Spirit to intervene. And I asked that if my mother had any influence on her current plane of existence, to please help me. I dreamed of my mother again. As previously, she was just beyond my touch.

The next day while driving down the highway, I had to stop quickly, and tromped with my right leg on the brake. The pain ripped from my knee to my right hip. I had to pull over to the side of the road. I sat there for a few minutes. I said, "Great Spirit, Mother, help me!" In my head, or out of the air, I heard, "You don't need me. I taught you what you need to know."

The truths she had taught me began to enter my awareness: "No one can teach you the ways of the spirits/God. These things are only learned in your own silence. Look to your own spirituality." This is not what I wanted to hear. I wanted my mother to give me the magic formula that she had used 30 years ago. "What is my spirituality?" I asked.

Spirituality is a way of looking at and understanding this earth and yourself, a way of knowing what it is all about.

"I'm not looking for spirituality, Mother," I hollered out. "I'm looking for healing." Mother had always taught us that the spirit is everywhere: in the water, rocks, trees, birds. "How is this supposed to help now? I'm in a car. I can't go out into the woods, the forest." I sat there fighting with her voice in my head, because that's where it was. I finally was able to drive home.

I'm a nurse. But you cannot learn to work with Indian spirituality by going to medical school. An old holy person, a medicine person can teach you about herbs, and that everything must be in its proper place. They can teach you about using smoke, sweet grass, sage, and cedar for cleansing the environment and the air. They can teach you all of these things, but if the human spirit is not ready, the soul will not accept the teachings.

The native peoples believe that we were put on this earth with animals, plants, trees, and water. (I was taught this as a child, but I forgot this as an adult.) Native peoples believe that power comes from these things. Indian healers receive the power from spirit. Spirit is everywhere. You hear of animal helpers, but they don't give power; they are messengers that bring instructions from the spirit.

I continued to fight what Mother had said. How could my mother speak to me, a grown woman in a car going down the highway? And why did I keep calling to her? Because, deep in my heart, I knew that the spirituality my mother had taught me was still there.

After several days of fussing in my mind with how and why this was happening to me, I realized that I had to take control. I could almost sense my mother smirking in the corner: "So, finally you are going to do something about this. You have the qualities and abilities. You can heal yourself."

How could I take control? My body was controlling my every move, because of the pain. How could I take control? I couldn't even lean over to pick up a rock, smell the flowers. I could just see her saying, "You'll do it. You'll figure it out."

So I did. I began by taking an inventory of my being. I realized that I was overweight. My eating habits left a lot to be desired, and I always felt that exercise was self-abuse. So what could I do?

Once again I asked Great Spirit to help me. I realized that the task before me was more than I could handle alone. How could I change what had occurred over decades of life?

Then I had another dream. Mother always taught me that dreams are powerful things, almost like visions. In the dream I saw myself as I had seen my mother in a previous dream: not in a field of wildflowers, but as a young Indian girl running through the wooded hills of my childhood, barefoot, with the hair streaming down my back. In the dream the young girl turned and smiled at me, and I knew she was myself. What struck me most about my younger self was my smile and pain-free demeanor.

That weekend a dear friend came to visit. We stood back by the pond. I began telling her about the pain in my leg and my inability to walk and function. I told her about how I had been this way before, and how my mother had danced around my chair when I had received my healing 30 years earlier. Her face was puzzled, "How did she dance? Show me."

I began to do the two-step, slowly, as mother had done those years ago. I danced as she had danced the two-step to the spirit for my healing. My feet slipped naturally into the rhythm, my knees bent without pain, and I began the dance in the spirit of thanksgiving. My healing had begun. We went into the house and announced that I was able to dance without pain. I now knew without reservation that I was in charge of my healing.

My healing was and is spiritual. One must be ready to be healed. If our spirit is not ready, we will continue to live the role of sickness and pain. Sickness may be comforting to some. Many find their needs fulfilled in this way. I chose not to be sick or in pain. My spirit was willing to accept the healing. My spirit recognized that the time was right in a few traditional ritual dance steps. I know with the help of the Great Spirit, the loss of well over 50 pounds, the dietary changes to feed my soul, not just to satisfy my body, daily thanks to the Creator, and occasional thanks to my mother, I am now able to live as the spiritual being my mother taught and raised me to be with a much thinner body and lighter soul.

Bill's story.

"It happened so fast! Fire exploded out of the carburetor! My hands, head, chest, arms, my whole upper body was torched (50% of his body had third-degree burns) in the direct line of the flames, and I couldn't help but inhale the flames."

This began a life experience for Bill. Jeanne, his wife, was a nurse and rushed to his side with blankets to smother the flames that were frying her love. (She received second-degree burns on her hands and arms. Her hair was burned on the front of her head.)

The ambulance arrived and Bill was care-flown to the closest burn center, a 3-hour trip. The inhalation of the fire caused his throat to close, so he required intubation to survive the flight. Jeanne did not fly, but her nursing supervisor gave her a blanket and told her to go with Bill in the air ambulance, and sent her off to the plane.

Burns have to be the most painful experience, and third-degree burn, which is what Bill had experienced, the worst. If you have had the experience of burning your finger on a hot pan, you may remember what that feels like. Now multiply that feeling exponentially and begin to get a sense of what Bill was feeling. Two sets of skin grafts failed, due to infections and complications, and medical staff was concerned if the third graft would take.

Jeanne stayed by Bill's side. She is a woman of prayer and faith. Weeks passed, and with two failed skin grafts and concern that the third might not take, she prayed. That night when she had just gone to bed, she began to pray, "Oh God, I can't do this, I can't lose him, I can't face this. It is in your hands. I give up control." Almost immediately, the darkened room lit up with a bright blue light. The wall to her left opened up, and she could see into the burn unit. Bill was sitting in a recliner chair swathed in bandages: his arms, his chest, and his face. She saw a hand up to an elbow with thumb and index finger extended. The forefinger touched the fingers on Bill's right hand. Jeanne became frightened by what she saw. She thought, "I can't be seeing this, I must be crazy, I must be having a dream, I can't be seeing this," and the vision faded. Jeanne fell into a deep sleep that night. Prior to the vision she had slept very poorly since the day of the accident.

The next morning Jeanne was at the burn center as early as they allowed visitors. As she walked through the door, Bill was sitting in the recliner as in her vision, swathed in bandages, but the tips of his right hand were pink, whereas the day before they were black. She told him of her vision. Bill looked at her and said he had had a dream, her vision. Did they share a vision, a dream? They didn't question it. Jeanne took Bill home 2 weeks later.

"Does he have scarring? Yes. Does he have residuals? Yes. Daily he lives with the scarring, the external perceptions. Do we see the scars? No. What we see is a whole person, able to function with all the human deformities, at a high level."

From that day forward, Bill felt he was healed. He even told his nurses he was going to get well. Bill had accepted his healing and his healing process had begun.

When I asked Bill what he did to cooperate with the healing, all he would answer was, "I don't know."

What Jeanne tells is that the nurses in the burn unit told him to breathe deeply like a woman in childbirth. Breathe deeply, relax, and don't focus on the pain. He went into an altered state of consciousness. Bill did say that he had to go within and not focus on anything. In his words, he had to "clean his mind." A psychologist would say that he disassociated and detached from the pain. Jeanne said that when she changed the bandages at home, she, too, would go into an altered state, and disassociate from her perception of pain.

After the experience with the bright blue light, Bill was able to function on less medication than expected. When Bill was released from the hospital, he went home on ibuprofen. To this day, he only takes ibuprofen for pain.

"We always thought there was a greater power; now we know," were the couple's final words on the experience.

Randy's story.

Randy was born with a deformity, mild spinal bifida. He had lived with it all of his life. But with age the deformity grew more pronounced and visible. For example, you could tell if Randy was tired or had a bad day, because he would walk through the hospital corridors leaning to the right, and that leaning became more pronounced with time. It also became more

painful, to the degree that he needed a cane and couldn't climb stairs.

Surgery was his only alternative. In that surgery, they would fuse three vertebrae in his spine, making a paste of bone graft from his hip.

Randy was the head chaplain at the hospital, and always was there for anyone in need of prayer support. In his time of need and in preparation for his surgery, he asked the persons of prayer he trusted to pray with him for a successful outcome. In addition to Christians, his prayer team included those of Native American belief and Jewish, Buddhist, and Muslim traditions. This was his prayer team, and he related that he went into his surgery without fear. Even though this was a delicate surgery requiring the most skilled of surgeons, he had no fear.

Randy was no stranger to surgery. Previous post-surgical experiences of migraine and nausea could have presented a fear factor. He awoke out of the anesthesia with only a flash of nausea, which immediately dissipated.

Randy's wife, Joan, and one of his chaplain staff were waiting in his room as he was wheeled from recovery. He reported that he was so pain free and so hyped that he was unable to sleep until well past midnight. Nurses became concerned as he laid awake channel surfing and watching TV.

Surgery was on Tuesday. Wednesday morning Randy was standing, and that afternoon he walked with assistance. It did hurt and he did feel it, but there was no pain. He took an occasional pain shot the first couple of days.

Joan took Randy home on Saturday, and he walked up the stairs to the bedroom. He walked down those stairs Sunday and back up. He took hydrocodine every few hours for the first 10 days, as a prophylactic measure. But he just never had pain.

It was all pretty amazing. And Randy learned about the power of prayer over pain.

These four stories have four things in common. First, a power of the mind and heart existed to co-create the healing process. Second, each individual had medical involvement in his or her process. Third, each didn't hesitate to ask others to pray with and for his or her healing and highest good. These were persons who they knew could be objective and hold for the highest good without attachment to the outcome. And fourth, each was actively involved in his or her process. And unspoken, all learned to love themselves, forgive themselves for their parts in the health challenge (illness), accept that healing is possible, and trust the Universe for their learning and highest good.

What do these stories tell us as healthcare professionals committed to the healing arts and process? At some point, each patient makes a decision, consciously or unconsciously, what his or her healing process will be. As in the stories above, at some point the patients decided at the deep soul level that they wanted to experience healing. Each stated with feeling, he or she desired physical healing, and as that experience evolved, each healing meant alignment with the inner spirit. It wasn't instantaneous, although it could have been. Rather it was across time, possibly for the purpose of learning more about soul, spirit, and inner strength and power. Note, too, that the "illness-challenged" ones asked friends for prayer support. They chose persons who would be detached emotionally, and would hold for the highest good of the Universal plan.

While friends held for the highest good, the challenged person worked at what was his or her task for the healing. This included not only taking prescribed medications, but also practicing relaxation, losing weight, changing diet, using images to cooperate and facilitate with the process.

Also note that healing had to be accepted before it could occur. This brings up an interesting point: the challenged ones at some level came to terms, consciously or unconsciously, with what their contributions to the creation of the challenge was. They accepted responsibility and in that acceptance were able to take the next action step.

This brings us to the discussion of forgiveness. The author recalls asking the physician who diagnosed the shingles how this could have happened, as she was leading a wholesome lifestyle with good nutrition, exercise, etc. She had to come to terms with and forgive herself for not honoring the body's limitations before the pain could be managed. Until she could forgive herself for failing to recognize the body's needs and limitations, it would continue to give signals in the form of pain. Carolyn Myss' 1997 book on the power of forgiveness to heal indicates that forgiveness is the key to healing. Candice Pert's (1997) research suggests that the act and feeling of forgiveness send peptides along the neurotransmitters to the hurt part of the body, which helps create the healing. Forgiveness is a powerful energy experience, an act of self-love and self-responsibility with tremendous healing power.

WHAT IS THE HEALTHCARE PROFESSIONAL'S POSITION IN THIS PROCESS?

If we have done our own personal listening and learning, we will see more of these healing experiences in our practices. Awareness of our process helps us be more gentle and quiet, as well as better able to listen and hear what our patients are telling us. In the best way they can,

patients tell us what they want for healing. Professionals who have had their own challenges may know what is being said. Not that I advocate experiencing pain, but the experience of pain is a powerful teaching experience, emotionally, mentally, spiritually, and physically. The experience of pain makes us conscious of how powerful the body/mind/spirit is when it is in pain. It signals us to wake up and pay attention. And with help, it makes us grow. It teaches us how important our healthcare skill is in pain management. But it also teaches us that what is done on the outside to us is not the whole story in pain management. An inner quality to pain management exists that is the responsibility of patients, and they hold the key to the effectiveness of pain management and healing in whatever form it takes. We are to perform our skill, then step back, be aware, and listen, refraining from other than supportive comments. It is well documented that patients give power to the words we say about their process, which can be more potent than the medicines dispensed, or adjustments and manipulations made. To illustrate, while writing this chapter, my friend Joan telephoned. She had asked me to pray with her during a foot surgery. It was not an unusual surgery, but she knew the power of prayer. On the day she phoned, it was 3 months post-surgery and I inquired as to how she was doing. She replied that she had been to the doctor for a check-up and he had commented that her foot was healing nicely. He told her that she was actually 3 weeks ahead of schedule, and he was surprised. She chuckled as she responded, "I'm not."

Pain management and healing aren't new as we noted at the beginning of the chapter. Descartes began the scientific study of the body, which paved the way for learning how the body physical works. Pert provided us with the molecular level of understanding energy in the body. From the spiritual perspective, Jesus and the ancients were able to do healings, and with the help of Mesmer and the metaphysicians we learned the power of words and prayer for healing. These insights help us humbly acknowledge our limitations as healthcare professionals, encourage our respect, and recognize our patients and their power, immanent and transcendent, for pain management and healing. It reminds us that the management of pain is a cooperative process between patient and all levels of caregiving. Each of us is reminded that we are powerful beings, not by might or muscle, but by the power of our word and thought. Forgiveness is a powerful tool of pain management, as are healing and love. Forgiveness creates wholeness, and nonforgiveness keeps us separated. When something is separated or broken from the whole, there is pain. Forgiveness brings healing because there is wholeness and oneness again.

Finally, pain is the tool for teaching each of us to function as a whole person, and eventually a whole people — body, mind, and spirit. In the process we learn about and discover our whole selves. We learn the power of our thoughts and words to shape our life experiences. This is the ethics of care.

REFERENCES

Anon. (1999). A century of psychology. *APA Monitor, 30,* 11.

Cady, H.E. (1892). *Lessons in truth.* Unity Village, MO: Unity Books.

Chopra, D. (2000). *How to know God.* New York: Harmony Books.

Dalai Lama. (1999). *Ethics for the new millennium.* New York: Riverhead Books.

Dossey, L. (1999). *Reinventing medicine.* New York: Harper.

Myss, C. (1997). *Why people don't heal and how they can.* New York: Three Rivers Press.

Pert, C. (1997). *Molecules of emotion.* New York: Touchstone.

Shepherd, T. (1985). *Friends in high places.* Unity Village, MO: Unity Books.

Walsch, N. (1999). *Friendship with God.* New York: G.P. Putman's Sons.

Zukav, G. (1989). *Seat of the soul.* New York: Fireside.

78

Documenting Pain

Barbara L. Kornblau, J.D., O.T.R./L., F.A.O.T.A., D.A.A.P.M.
and Lori T. Andersen, Ed.D., O.T.R./L.

INTRODUCTION

Documenting pain presents unique challenges for pain practitioners. Because one cannot actually see pain as one can see a broken leg or a rib on X-ray, for example, documentation of the signs and symptoms plays a critical role in effective treatments.

Many stereotypes about individuals suffering from pain exist in the world of payers, insurance adjusters, defense attorneys, workers' compensation administrators, family members, and others. For example, often, when the patient in pain enters the world of litigation, the individual faces a world of nonbelievers. Pain patients often are dismissed as having psychiatric problems rather than physical problems. For example, some still argue that conditions such as fibromyalgia are not physical syndromes at all. Sometimes patients face accusations of malingering by nonbelievers rather than the reality of suffering from pain syndromes.

Some think an absence of objective evidence makes it impossible to diagnose pain. Others claim medical and rehabilitation providers cannot measure pain to prove its existence. The mistaken belief that patients with chronic pain cannot progress gives payers an excuse to deny reimbursement to therapists. Further, some payers accept the erroneous notion that occupational and physical therapy intervention with patients suffering from chronic pain falls short of the necessary skilled care required for reimbursement.

In addition to these stressors faced by the pain practitioner, in the 21st century, pain practitioners face increasing threats of malpractice, and managed care. Case managers and panel membership often limit access to pain practitioners. Obtaining payment from insurance companies seems to take more work and for less money. Workers' compensation seems to constantly reduce services it will cover and the amount it will pay for those services. Payers want second opinions and pain practitioners face more and more regulations from numerous government programs.

Though documentation presents challenges to pain practitioners, it also records our successes and presents them to the world. If done carefully, it helps grease the reimbursement wheel. The medical record almost always constitutes the only evidence payers, case managers, and others see to justify pain management treatment and payment.

On the other hand, the pain practitioner's documentation also can tout failures and/or lend credence to the failures of others. For example, when something goes wrong with a patient, the medical record serves as the key evidence the jury or judge sees to prove that the clinician met the standard of care.

Accurate documentation of pain in medical records can make a significant difference in the lives of patients. Often the contents of the medical record play a significant role in determining whether or not a pain patient receives workers' compensation, social security disability, or other important benefits (*Smollen v. Chater*, 1996)

One can define medical record documentation as a serial and legal record of the patient's condition and the course of the medical or therapeutic intervention from admission to discharge (Aquaviva, 1998). This record describes how the patient functioned and the behaviors the patient displayed at the time of initial evaluation, during the course of treatment, and at discharge. Essentially,

0-8493-0926-3/02/$0.00+$1.50
© 2002 by CRC Press LLC

the medical record should "tell the story" or "paint a picture" of the patient and the medical care provided.

REASONS FOR DOCUMENTATION

Documentation serves several purposes. First and foremost, accrediting bodies require it (Joint Commission on Accreditation of Healthcare Organizations, 2001a). To maintain accreditation status, hospitals, rehabilitation programs, outpatient programs, and others must maintain documentation according to the requirements of their accrediting bodies so they can maintain accreditation status. Accreditation is often required to qualify for reimbursement. Self-audits are performed as required by accreditation standards between surveys performed by the accreditation bodies themselves.

Documentation in the medical record provides a communication method for the members of the healthcare team. Healthcare clinicians may find themselves with little-to-no face-to-face contact. Other means of communication, such as telephone contact, prove difficult because of diverse schedules and the varied places where patients receive care. All healthcare clinicians have access to and should access the medical record. This access enables clinicians to read the documentation of other team members and thus keep apprised of the course of treatment, patient status, and progress from other viewpoints. This helps team members make appropriate decisions about patient course of treatment and facilitates coordination of patient care.

Looking ahead, documentation provides data for treatment innovations, research, and education. For example, a new type of pain treatment is administered to alleviate patients' pain. Documentation of the type of treatment rendered, the amount of treatment, the timing of treatment, and patient status and behaviors after treatment will demonstrate the efficacy and effectiveness of treatment. Data collected from all of those treated will provide researchers with outcomes data that clinicians also can use to justify the treatment to payers.

Outcomes data collected from documentation can be used for promoting or marketing one's program. For example, if an outpatient pain program has designed a specific program for returning injured workers to the workplace and the program succeeds in helping these injured workers return to work, the data available from the documentation will demonstrate the efficacy and effectiveness of the program. These data can be used to promote the program to case managers and others.

Documentation can be used for quality assurance and continuous quality improvement efforts to determine the effectiveness of specific treatment interventions or programs. The Joint Commission on Accreditation of Hospital Organizations (JCAHO), the Commission on Accreditation of Rehabilitation Facilities (CARF), and various other organizations all require monitoring of documentation to determine continuity of care and quality of services (Joint Commission on Accreditation of Healthcare Organizations, 2001a).

Documentation prevents clinicians and facilities from unsubstantiated claims of wrongdoing — in other words, "CYA." For this reason, hospitals usually include requirements for documentation in their policies and procedures. Physicians who fail to follow a hospital's documentation policy can lose their hospital privileges. (*Board of Trustees of Memorial Hospital of Sheridan County v. Pratt*, 1953). Accurate documentation can protect clinicians from erroneous charges of malpractice, or criminal charges of improper use of narcotics. Proper documentation can protect clinicians from civil and criminal penalties resulting from charges of Medicare and Medicaid fraud and abuse or other civil or criminal charges (McKessy, 1998).

Fiscal reviewers, auditors, intermediaries, and payers often review documentation to determine if services billed were, in fact, provided. These reviewers and auditors may also review documentation to determine if services were medically necessary. The Medicare program requires that services must be reasonable and medically necessary in order for coverage and reimbursement for the care of the patient under the Medicare Guidelines. As the saying goes, "In God We Trust, All Others Must Document."

Private insurance companies have similar requirements. Triggers that may start an audit or claims denial include overprescription of controlled substances; providing the wrong medication; providing treatment without pre-authorization, referral, or prescription; absence of a treatment plan; lack of patient compliance; using too many modalities; and continuing treatment without improvement or results. Proper and complete documentation can protect the practitioner from potential problems.

Finally, most licensure laws require that healthcare professionals keep written medical records justifying the course of treatment. Failure to do so can result in disciplinary action against the licensee. (See Table 78.1.)

TABLE 78.1
Reasons for Documentation

1.   To comply with accreditation requirements.
2.   To communicate with other members of the healthcare team.
3.   To provide data for treatment innovations, research, and education.
4.   To collect outcomes data to market programs.
5.   To provide data for quality assurance, continuous quality improvement and/or total quality management, peer review, and continued competency.
6.   To prevent unsubstantiated claims of wrongdoing (CYA).
7.   Payers review documentation to ensure treatment was performed as billed and medically necessary.
8.   Most licensure laws require documentation.

MEDICAL RECORD AS A LEGAL DOCUMENT

The medical record serves as a legal document. State and federal laws and regulations establish minimum standards for record keeping. These record-keeping standards serve as prerequisites to state licensure, receipt of federal funding, and participation in federal programs such as Medicare. As a legal document, medical records document the nature of the care provided, including the quantity and quality of care, and protocols used for treatment. The medical record also documents the charges for the care given. Above all, the medical record carries the signature of the clinician.

State and federal laws prescribe the contents of the medical records, and the ownership, access, and confidentiality requirements of medical records. Various laws also control how long clinicians must keep medical records following discharge. The length of time often is based upon the statute of limitations for various administrative, civil, and criminal laws. For example, participation in Medicare requires providers to keep medical records for a length of time to enable the government to conduct investigations for fraud and other matters.

Medical records that play a role as a "legal document" often come under scrutiny in administrative, civil, and criminal actions. For example, attorneys involved in administrative and civil cases such as divorce/custody, insurance fraud, medical malpractice, personal injury, workers' compensation, disability benefits, and licensure board discipline may subpoena medical records to present as evidence.

As a recognized legal document, pain practitioners should never destroy or alter records after the fact to conceal a mistake or error. Chances overwhelmingly point to the reality that someone already has a copy of the original records as they appeared before the clinician altered them. Further, these types of alterations are illegal and subject clinicians to disciplinary action and, in some cases, criminal action. We call this conduct "spoliation."

Black's Law Dictionary defines spoliation as "(t)he destruction of evidence" or "the destruction of, or the significant and meaningful alteration of a document or instrument" (Nolan, 1979). In *Bondu v. Gurvich*, the Florida Court of Appeals allowed a family member to proceed with an independent action for spoliation when the hospital was unable to produce the medical records needed as proof in a malpractice action. The patient died during the administration of anesthesia in a triple by-pass operation. Without the medical records as evidence, the malpractice action could not proceed (*Bondu v. Gurvich*, 1995). In another case involving spoliation, *State Board of Medical Examiners v. McCroskey*, the Court found that changing and backdating a note about a patient who bled to death cast doubt on the integrity of the medical record, violated the standard of care, and correctly subjected the physician to disciplinary action (*State Board of Medical Examiners v. McCroskey*, 1994).

In some jurisdictions, the jury can assume that missing evidence, if produced, would have been unfavorable to the spoiler. Other jurisdictions simply will exclude altered evidence while some courts will impose sanctions against the spoiler. Spoilers can also face criminal charges or dismissal of their case (Seigfreid, undated).

In addition to spoliation, clinicians must also watch out for falsification of documents. As a legal document, clinicians must never falsify anything in the medical record or face civil as well as criminal charges lest they do. In *People vs. Smithtown General Hospital,* a surgeon and a nurse falsified the medical record by omitting any reference to a prosthetic device salesman who assisted with hip replacement surgery. The surgeon and supervising nurse were criminally indicted for falsifying business records in the first degree, which was upheld by the court when the defended appealed to have the indictments dismissed (*People v. Smithtown General Hospital*, 1978).

CHARACTERISTICS OF GOOD DOCUMENTATION

Documentation must be clear, concise, objective, logically organized, legible, and contemporaneous. To communicate effectively, the documentation must be clear. To be clear, the healthcare professional must use terminology common to the people who will read the documentation. Know thy audience. Clinicians must assume someone else will read their records.

The pain practitioner's documentation often finds its way before the eyes of adjusters, attorneys, jurors, or others with little to no working knowledge of pain jargon. Medical records with pain jargon or other medical jargon lack clarity for a lay audience and lose much in translation. Clear, jargon-free, understandable documents can save clinicians a trip to court. In some jurisdictions, attorneys can subpoena medical records alone. If the attorney can understand the records, it ends there. If the records are not clear, the attorney may send a *subpoena duces tecum*, which requires the clinician to bring the documents to a deposition to read and explain them.

The use of abbreviations also renders medical records unclear. Facilities and agencies often develop an approved list of abbreviations for use in medical records. It is important that healthcare practitioners use the appropriate terminology or abbreviations, otherwise it will be like reading a foreign language for another healthcare practitioner. Even worse, miscommunication can occur with devastating results. The story of a physician who ordered ear drops for a patient is an example of miscommunication. The physician wrote in the medical record that the medication was to be administered t.i.d. in the patient's R ear. As there was no circle around the R, the recognized abbreviation for "right," the medication was administered elsewhere — not in the "ear."

Concise documentation presents the most important information about the patient without unnecessary distractors. It is much easier for one to read a concise record that gets to the point, as opposed to a lengthy note that one has to search for the relevant information. Most importantly, payers do not want to search for the information they need for payment. Those records will likely end up at the bottom of the payment pile in favor of another practitioner's concise records.

Avoid extraneous notes in the medical record that can confuse the reader or add unintended information. A notation in a chart referring to what another clinician reported with a handwritten "B.S." in the margin proved rather embarrassing for the clinician who, during her deposition was asked to explain the abbreviation.

Pain practitioners must use objective terms in their documentation. Pain behaviors and status should be described using measurable terms. Phrases such as "tolerated treatment well" or "patient doing well" provide no objective data. Payers and others in the medical record audience concern themselves with objective, functional changes the patient makes in response to treatment intervention. Clinicians should quantify pain measures and record objective changes in pain. Clinicians should describe the principles and methodologies used to reach their conclusions (*Daubert v. Merrell Dow Pharmaceuticals*, 1993). Objective records omit any pejorative comments about patients.

Clinicians must organize their records in a logical manner. No one wants to hunt through documentation to find specific information. Further, the time delay during the hunt may cause the patient harm. Categorizing information into sections and subsections easily identified by headings will assist readers in finding the information they seek. Clinicians should present data in an organized manner. In all cases, documentation should include a date and time of entry.

Clinicians should record their documentation contemporaneously and in a timely manner. Some clinicians find personal digital assistants (PDA) such as palm pilots helpful to write their documentation contemporaneously, while they examine their patients. By documenting when an event occurs, the clinician ensures a more accurate picture of what occurred. The more removed in time one writes the medical documentation, the more the medical record begins to look like a work of fiction. Furthermore, a late entry in the medical record attracts suspicion.

Finally, the documentation must be legible. Information written illegibly is considered to be undocumented or not written: "If I can't read it, you didn't write it." Illegible documentation will find its way to the bottom of the payer's payment pile in favor of easy-to-read documenta-

tion: "If I can't read it, I am not going to pay you." Like late entries, illegible documentation attracts suspicion: "What are they trying to hide?"

Illegible documentation does not provide protection (or CYA value) should the clinician face charges of malpractice, fraud, or disciplinary action. In fact, illegible documentation can lead to serious harm to the patient, and charges of malpractice, if other members of the healthcare team cannot read information. The classic problem arises when the pharmacist is unable to read the physician's illegible handwriting. In Texas, this problem led a jury to award almost a half million dollars to the family of a man who received the drug Plendil, used to treat high blood pressure, instead of the drug written on the prescription, Isordil, used to treat severe chest pain or angina (WebMD National News Center, 1999).

While the damage caused by illegible or sloppy documentation may not always lead to death of a patient, it can seriously damage one's reputation. Sloppy documentation can lead a jury, case manager, or insurance adjuster to believe the patient received sloppy care from the pain practitioner, which may lead to problems in the legal arena or a decrease in one's referral base.

The rules of documentation recognize that clinicians sometimes do make legitimate errors in writing their documentation. When clinicians make errors, they should draw a single line through the error, and write their initials and the date beside the error. Alternatively, clinicians may append the record with an explanation of the error. Erasures and correction fluid play no role in the medical record. Should clinicians not correct their errors, they live by the adage, "If it's in the chart, you did it."

TYPE AND FREQUENCY OF DOCUMENTATION

The type and frequency of documentation vary from facility to facility and are also affected by regulatory agencies such as JCAHO and CARF, state laws and regulations, and third-party payers. Agencies and facilities often have a procedure by which documentation forms are reviewed for possible inclusion in the medical record.

Clinicians perform the patient's initial evaluation upon the patient's admission to a service. Information documented in initial evaluations should include at a minimum medical history, current medications, allergies, drug sensitivities, presenting complaint, and assessment information. Initial evaluations may be written in longhand using a specific format, in a checklist format, dictated, written on a personal digital assistant (PDA), or some combination of methods. Oftentimes, regulations dictate the amount of time a healthcare practitioner has to complete and enter the initial evaluation into the medical record. In addition, in circumstances where a patient is transferred to another service, regulations or policies may require that clinicians complete a new initial evaluation on the patient and document it in the medical record.

Progress notes for each visit, daily or weekly, also are often required as part of the medical record documentation. The provider of pain management services determines the overall style of progress notes. Progress notes may also be written longhand, or in checklist format, dictated or written on a PDA, or combination again, depending on the department, type of service, practice, etc.

Many clinicians use S.O.A.P. note format for their progress notes. One should use care when using S.O.A.P. notes so to avoid writing "soapy" S.O.A.P. notes. Soapy S.O.A.P. notes skimp on the information provided so the reader loses the picture quality of treatment. These soapy notes include phases such as "Patient doing well," "Continue treatment," "Tolerated treatment well," "No Complaints," and the symbol ∅, instead of descriptive, functional information about the patient.

Some healthcare professionals such as physicians document a separate entry for every contact they have with the patient. In contrast, other healthcare professionals such as occupational therapists and physical therapists may not document a separate entry for each contact. Rather, the frequency of documentation may be determined by the frequency of change of status of a patient and/or treatment provided. For example, an acute-care facility would probably require more frequent documentation than a skilled nursing facility because status of patient may change more frequently. In another example, a rehabilitation therapist who consistently provides the same treatment each visit might only summarize the type of treatment provided and progress in a note documented each week. A contact note may be entered in the medical record to document phone contacts with other healthcare practitioners, the patient, and the patient's family members.

Discharge notes or summaries state what treatment has been rendered, improvement made, instructions given to the patient and/or significant others, and recommendations for further or future care. Copies or records of all should be kept and/or placed in the medical record. Discharge documentation should include the condition of the patient at discharge, and the reason for discharge. Reasons for discharge may include goals met, no further progress anticipated, or patient's care transferred to another agency or healthcare practitioner.

CONTENT OF MEDICAL RECORDS

The medical record consists of items dealing with the overall care of the patient. It may include correspondence, phone call transcripts, copies of prescriptions, billing records, personal digital assistant (PDA) records, email records, results of lab tests, X-rays, and others. The contents of the medical record may be determined by hospital policy (for inpatient records), accreditation bodies, state licensing regulations, federal regulations for various programs such as Medicare, and professional standards of practice.

Because many pain patients are involved in the court system in some way, pain practitioners need to prepare themselves for encounters they and their documentation may have with the legal system. Regardless of what the applicable law or regulation states, in practice, if subpoenaed for a deposition, everything becomes part of the medical record. Attorneys will send requests listing every possible item that might relate to the patient. This could encompass, for example, all items on your computer hard drive pertaining to the patient, including, but not limited to, emails, draft reports, etc.; handwritten notes pertaining to the patient; copies of telephone messages; appointment book entries for all of the patient's scheduled appointments; and any other documents pertaining to the patient.

The pain practitioner should include certain items in the medical record that will obviate the need to rely on memory 2 years down the road when the patient's case comes up before a judge. By preparing in advance with proper documentation, the pain practitioner can look thorough and professional when questioned about treatment that occurred in the distant past. Time spent answering questions regarding the patient or former patient's work status, disability status, and impairment rating is reduced if documentation is complete. Table 78.2 lists and describes minimal content of the pain practitioner's medical record. Statutory requirements, conditions of participation in federal or state programs and accreditation bodies will probably require additional items.

DOCUMENTATION OF PAIN

In the 1980s and early to mid-1990s, as a result of fear of addiction, public policy steered physicians away from prescribing narcotics for patients suffering from chronic pain. Physicians were disciplined or threatened with disciplinary action for overprescribing narcotics especially to patients with chronic pain (Angarola, 1994). Comprehensive documentation of the need for pain medication provided one of the tools for defending oneself from charges of overprescribing narcotics. However, documentation of the prescription of narcotics, if against state laws and regulations, also could work squarely against the physician.

Thus, the looming threat of discipline and the fear of addiction led to underprescribing of narcotics by many physicians (Angarola, 1994). With studies showing as many as one half of all patients in pain not provided with appropriate pain medication, public policy shifted away from the fear-based, underprescribing of pain narcotics to a realistic approach based upon the needs of the patient (Oregon Board of Medical Examiners, 1999; U.S. Agency for Health Care Policy and Research, 1994).

TABLE 78.2
Minimal Content of Pain Practice Medical Record*

Informed consent
History and physical examination
- Including history of drug substance abuse
Drug sensitivities or allergies
Document the pain with symptoms:
- Location
- Duration
- Frequency
- Intensity
- Precipitating or aggravating factors
Restrictions, limitations, and activity level
- Correlate pain to function
- How does the pain limit the ability to work or dress, etc.?
- How does the pain affect mental status?
- Is the patient depressed?
- Can the patient drive safely?
Evidence of impairment
- Pain itself is not an impairment
Subjective and objective measures of pain
Copies of prescriptions legibly written
Use of narcotics**
- Record dose, amount, and number of refills
- Document/contract, signed by the patient acknowledging
  - Use of controlled substances
  - Side effects and material risks
  - Method for dealing with
    - Exacerbations
    - Lost presciptions
    - Noncompliance with treatment
    - Misuse of medications
    - Substance abuse
Referrals to other professionals
Notation of reading consults and lab results
Compliance with treatment
Monitoring or other devices
Follow-up required?
Follow-up appointments scheduled and dated?
Signature and date on every entry
Discharge documentation
- Reason for discharge
- Referral upon discharge
- Condition upon discharge
- Conclusions
- Instructions given
Handouts given to patients — copies in charts
Time saving information (in case a request comes later)
- What information will workers' compensation want from you as a provider?
- What information will social security want from you as a provider?
- Is the person working now? If not, why not?
- What kind of impairment does the patient have?

---

* Check their state licensure laws to add state-mandated requirements and relevant accreditation bodies for their requirements. (From Joint Commission on Accreditation of Healthcare Organizations, Pain Standards for 2001, 2001a.)
** Recommended for physicians.

The acceptable contemporary approach to pain treatment emphasizes an assessment of the patient's pain, documentation of pain and management of the pain (Angarola, 1993; Oregon Board of Medical Examiners, 1999; U.S. Agency for Health Care Policy and Research, 1994). The key methodology to prove one's compliance with these basic elements lies in proactive comprehensive documentation using, at a minimum, the elements listed in Table 78.2.

Recognizing the controversy in prescribing pain medication that led to underprescribing of pain medications and the resulting unnecessary suffering of patients in pain, the JCAHO developed standards for pain management, enforceable through its accreditation process. These standards, effective for JCAHO surveys that occurred after January 1, 2001, state that all "patients have the right to appropriate assessment and management of pain" (Joint Commission on Accreditation of Healthcare Organizations, 2001b). Pursuant to the standards, the healthcare organization must take steps to ensure the pain of "all patients is recognized and addressed appropriately" (Joint Commission on Accreditation of Healthcare Organizations, 2001b). JCAHO standards require initial and regular reassessment of pain in patients. Proper documentation will demonstrate compliance with these standards.

According to the JCAHO standards, when documenting pain symptoms, the pain practitioner should include location, duration, frequency, intensity, quality, patterns, and precipitating, alleviating, or aggravating factors, and pain management history (Joint Commission on Accreditation of Healthcare Organizations, 2001b). However, the practitioner must realize that pain itself is not a disability. It is important to document how the pain restricts a patient's activity and his or her participation in life roles. The pain symptoms must be correlated to function. To document a pain patient's function, the pain practitioner may ask the following:

> Is the patient depressed?
> How has the pain affected his or her relationship with others?
> How is the pain affecting his or her mental status?
> Can the patient concentrate well enough to perform activities?
> Does the patient comply with the treatment regime?
> How does the pain limit the patient's ability to dress or care for him or herself? Can the patient drive safely?

The JCAHO standards delegate to each organization the responsibility to develop follow-up criteria for evaluation of patients in pain. The pain practitioner's documentation will be key to showing compliance with JCAHO's standards. Among the suggested criteria, the standards look at the need for information on the impact of pain on daily life, function, sleep, appetite, relationships with others, concentration, and others emotions. JCAHO surveyors will rely on the clinician's documentation to measure compliance with the standard. Therefore, documentation should reflect these areas. Clinicians who develop systems for documentation will assure they cover all of the bases.

THE SYSTEMS APPROACH TO DOCUMENTATION

Agency for Healthcare Research and Quality (AHRQ) (2001b) research shows that most medical errors are systems errors. For example, when a surgeon amputated Willie King's healthy leg, the system designed to track the proper body part through surgery failed (Institute of Medicine, 2000). Errors such as this are not the result of individual negligence or misconduct. The system failed and resulted in harm (Institute of Medicine, 2000).

Documentation plays a significant role in systems within healthcare. Peer reviewers and others can trace errors through documentation and documentation done properly can show an absence of errors, compliance with accreditation standards, or proof the system is properly working, resulting in error-free quality care.

The Institute of Medicine report (2000), "To Err is Human: Building a Safer System," suggests that the healthcare system look to ergonomic principles used in other industries but up to now ignored by the healthcare industry to improve efficiency and lower the error rate. Some of these methods that are successful in reducing errors in the medication process can be used to reduce errors and omission in documentation. These successful methods of prevention based on ergonomic principles include reducing reliance on memory which can be fallible and cause errors, simplifying of procedures, standardizing treatment processes, using standardized protocols and checklists, and decreasing reliance on multiple data entry (Institute of Medicine, 2000).

Pain practitioners can incorporate several of the ergonomic principles into their documentation systems to improve efficiency and decrease documentation errors, in other words, to streamline the process. To reduce reliance on memory, pain practitioners can use personal digital assistance (PDA) or handheld computers to write the documentation as the patient reports it to the clinician. This method also eliminates reliance on handwriting for ordering medication and other treatments, thereby eliminating potential errors (Agency for Healthcare Research and Quality, 2001a).

Standardizing and simplifying treatment policies and protocols and implementing checklists help the pain practitioner avoid confusion and reliance on memory. In essence, JCAHO's pain management standards spell out a standardized protocol for pain management, which gives practitioners a simplified process upon which to base treatment, policies, protocols, and checklists.

Avoiding the use of similar looking or sounding medications also lowers the likelihood of error. If physicians prefer to use certain specific medications on a regular basis, using preprinted prescription pads in a checklist format also can help eliminate errors.

Pain practitioners can eliminate other documentation errors by putting systems in place to document telephone calls with patients and consulting physicians. Systems for justifying and monitoring narcotics such as the contract listed in Table 78.2 provide one simplified method to document a potential problem on a consistent basis. Finally, pain practitioners should have systems to monitor the effectiveness of the systems they have put in place.

SUMMARY

Three rules of thumb to remember:

- If you charged for it, you did it.
- If the reader can't read it, you may not have done it.
- If you changed it after the case was filed in court or after you submitted a copy to the payer, you have a big problem.

Good medical record documentation can ensure quality care and protect the patient and practitioner.

REFERENCES

Agency for Healthcare Research and Quality. (2001a). Medical errors: The scope of the problem [On-line]. Available: http://www.ahcpr.gov/qual/errback.htm

Agency for Healthcare Research and Quality. (2001b). Reducing errors in healthcare [On-line]. Available: http://www.ahcpr.gov/research/errors.htm

Angarola, T. J., & Joranson, D.E. (1993). Wins and losses in pain control. *APS Bulletin, 4*(3), 8–9.

Angarola, T. J., and Joranson, D.E. (1994). Recent developments in pain management and regulation. *APS Bulletin, 4*(1), 9–11.

Aquaviva, J. (1998). Effective documentation for occupational therapy. Bethesda, MD: American Occupational Therapy Association.

Board of Trustees of Memorial Hospital of Sheridan County v. Pratt. 262 P.2d 682 (Wyoming Supreme Court 1953).

Bondu v. Gurvich, 473 So.2d 1307 (Fla App. 3 Dist. 1995).

Daubert v. Merrell Dow Pharmaceuticals, 509, 579 U.S. Supreme 1993).

Institute of Medicine. (2001). *To err is human: Building a safer health system* [On-line]. Available: http://books.nap.edu/books/0309068371/html/51.html#pagetop

Joint Commission on Accreditation of Healthcare Organizations. (2001a, February 4). *2001 Medical Record Review Summary Sheet* [On-line]. Available: http://jcprdw1.jcaho.org/accred/medrecs/im3211.html

Joint Commission on Accreditation of Healthcare Organizations. (2001b, February 6). *Pain Standards for 2001* [On-line]. Available: http://www.jcaho.org/standard/pm.html.

McKessy, A.S.I., & Sanner, R.J. (1998, July/August). *Protecting your practice with a Medicare and Medicaid compliance program* [On-line]. American Academy of Family Physicians. Available: http://www.aafp.org/fpm/980700fm/mckessy.html

Nolan, J. C., & Connolly, M.J. (1979). *Black's law dictionary*. St. Paul: West Publishing Co.

Oregon Board of Medical Examiners. (1999). *BME statement of philosophy on pain management* [On-line]. Available: http://www.bme.state.or.us/topics.html#Pain_Management

People v. Smithtown General Hospital. 402 N.Y.S.2d 318 Supreme Court, Suffolk County 1978.

Seigfreid, J. (Unknown). Spoliation of evidence. Baker, Sterchi, Cowden, & Rice LLC. Available: http://www.bscr-law.com/Seminars/Spoliation_of_Evidence/spoliation_of_evidence.html [2001, February 6,].

Smollen v. Chater. 80 F.3d 11273 (9th Cir. 1996.)

State Board of Medical Examiners v. McCroskey. 880 P.2d 1888 Colorado Supreme Court 1994.

U.S. Agency for Health Care Policy and Research. (1994). Management of cancer pain (clinical guide) [On-line]. Available: http://hstat.nlm.nih.gov/ftrs/default.browse?dbK=4&tocK=5&ftrsK=64273&tocm=00&lineK=0&t=981321719&collect=ahcpr

WebMD National News Center. (1999). Bad handwriting led to man's death [World Wide Web]. Available: http://onhealth.webmd.com/conditions/briefs/item,52258.asp

79

Motor Vehicle Accidents

Christopher R. Brown, D.D.S., M.P.S

In the last 30 years, there have been more than 10 million "moderate to severe" injuries and over 1.5 million deaths in the United States from motor vehicle accidents (MVAs). The National Safety Council reported in 1996 that 11.2 million traffic collisions occurred. Of those, 9.6 million were a combination of property damage only and/or nondisabling injury collisions. The economic cost to the United States was estimated to be $176.1 billion — a staggering amount of money.

In terms of the dollar costs involved, Evans (1991) in *Traffic Safety and the Driver* indicates property damage to top the list at 37%, with medical costs in fifth place at 6% of the total. Data from the National Highway Traffic Safety Administration (1987) estimate the following:

	$ (Billions)	% (Total Expenses)
Property	27.0	37.0
Insurance	21.0	28.0
Productivity	16.0	22.0
Legal and court	4.0	6.0
Medical	4.0	6.0
Emergency (transportation, diagnosis, and support)	0.7	0.9
Miscellaneous	0.45	0.6

Understanding what happens to humans in MVAs takes more than statistics, graphs, and charts. It requires a combination of learning tools, investigative procedures, and a thorough understanding of human anatomy and physiology.

From an engineering perspective, we need to know certain factors about the automobile such as weight, speed, and its vector (direction of motion). Other factors that may contribute to overall force need to be understood as well to fully appreciate and estimate the resulting forces that may contribute to human injury potential.

LOW SPEED VS. HIGH SPEED

For practical purposes, the working definition of a low-speed impact is a collision in which the change in velocity of the vehicles (usually the one that contains an occupant claiming an injury) is less than 10 mph. It must be emphasized that this definition of low speed is subjective. Clearly, no general consensus among experts exists.

Although it is commonly accepted to describe impact severity and injury potential as functions of change in velocity, caution should be used when considering impacts of grossly dissimilar durations. Comparison of impacts based solely on their respective changes in velocity inherently assumes the impacts occurred over a similar duration, typically 90 to 140 msec for low speed impacts. For the majority of accidents this is a reasonable assumption. However, in some collisions, such as underride or sideswipe collisions, the impact duration may be in excess of 300 msec. Given an equal change in velocity, a vehicle that undergoes a longer duration impact will be exposed to lower peak forces. For this reason, underride and override collisions, although sometimes involving very high dollar amounts of property damage, can be less severe than a "no damage" collision.

As an example of the effects of impact duration, consider skidding a vehicle to a stop. In theory, decelerating a vehicle from 30 mph to a stop by applying the brakes involves an impact between the tires and the roadway with a change in velocity of 30 mph, but with an impact duration of approximately 2.0 sec. The skidding vehicle is deceler-

0-8493-0926-3/02/$0.00+$1.50
© 2002 by CRC Press LLC

ated at approximately 0.7 gs. Although braking a vehicle to a stop involves a 30-mph change in velocity, this is a quite different event than a 30-mph front-to-barrier impact. The barrier impact occurs over a much shorter duration and typically involves decelerations of 30 to 50 gs.

A factor to consider in low-speed rear-end motor vehicle accidents (LSREMVAs) is impact forces concentrated over very small areas. As an everyday event, this may occur while backing into a small diameter pole in a parking lot or contacting a corner or small area of a bumper. Vehicle structures typically deform in proportion to the amount of force applied. In impacts with narrow objects or to the corners of vehicles, the contact forces are distributed over a very small area producing large local stresses (force per unit area). These large local stresses can damage bumper and vehicle components at changes in velocity below the strength of that area. Testing by the Insurance Institute for Highway Safety indicates that the amount of damage and costs of repair will vary dramatically from car to car and will even vary greatly for the same vehicle depending upon the type and angle of low speed collision (Kaufman, et al., 1993). These factors have to be taken into consideration to determine forces transferred.

In reality, though, the definition changes situationally according to needs. Low speed infers that the occupants can't be hurt. High speed infers they can. As a rule of thumb, engineering studies will routinely define low speed as less than 10 mph closing speed.

Can you draw the same conclusions? Are the collision biomechanics the same? Are the injury mechanisms the same?

In professions that deal with MVAs and human injury, an erroneous assumption often exists that "one size fits all." In other words, there is a mechanism of injury that either happens or does not happen — people get hurt or they don't. In the dental profession regarding TMJ injuries, it was assumed that for TMJs to become injured in a rear-end motor vehicle accident (REMVA), the mandible had to go through a full range of motion. Videos of LSREMVAs clearly indicate that in low speed collisions it is often not the case. A few authors, therefore, erroneously assume that because this particular mechanism of injury is not present the TMJs cannot be injured. That, of course, is false logic. All parts of the body no matter what the location can receive injuries from many sources. Clinicians need to be aware of these mechanisms to clearly understand, diagnose, and treat the injuries they see. Understanding leads to a more definitive diagnosis and more effective treatment.

Statistics themselves are not particularly significant when trying to predict individual occurrences. Statistics may be used as an academic yardstick but can't be used to predict how an individual or small group of occupants will respond in any given situation. Predicting or judging anything based on a population smaller than what is statistically significant in the measured population is erroneous.

There is no such thing as a *typical* REMVA. Most REMVAs are offset collisions producing torsion, tension, compression, and shear forces to the human body as a whole and to the individual parts.

In reality, actual numbers regarding REMVAs are impossible to track (fatal vs. nonfatal).

REAR-END MOTOR VEHICLE ACCIDENTS

While statistics on fatalities are easy to track, the statistics on injuries are not. This especially holds true when it comes to REMVAs. Take, for instance, the port of statistical entry for comparing the two. With a fatality, police are involved, certificates are signed — a definite traceable system exists. A definite path which societies have determined also needs to be followed.

With injuries, however, this is not the case. Take into consideration the possible portal of entry into the medical system of the United States. A victim of a MVA may very well start out at the emergency room with a description of minor injuries that do not need immediate attention. At that point, there may or may not be any type of follow through. The victim may be referred back to a family physician if he or she has one, or the victim may be left to find his or her own way.

The choices people have for treatment of pain are varied. For instance, for the treatment of headaches following a REMVA, the person may choose to visit a physician, a chiropractor, a dentist, a massage therapist, an acupuncturist, an optometrist, an ophthalmologist, and so on.

Statistics, as a result, are not accurate and there is no predetermined course of action as in fatalities. In fact, even the accepted terminology varies from source to source on how to even describe injuries as a result of REMVAs. They may be described as STI (Soft Tissue Injuries), MIST (Minimal Impact Soft Tissue), CAD (cervical acceleration deceleration) — all these descriptions are used to describe a pattern or type of injury as a result of "whiplash." Even with the difficulty of tracking these types of injuries, it has been estimated that 1 to 2 million CAD injuries occur per year from REMVAs (Evans, 1992). The 2 million per year estimates occur at rates roughly 5480/d, 1827/8 h, 228/h, 114/half h, and 4/min.

Not only are REMVA injuries substantial in number, they also can produce long-term residual effects. In fact, the rate of recovery in whiplash injuries is poor; 20 to 40% of whiplash injuries have debilitating symptoms that persist for years (Carette, 1994). Patients destined to recover will do so in the first 3 to 4 months after initial injury (Barnsley, et al., 1994). The consequences are both long term and far reaching, resulting in extended sick leave and increases in disability (Per-Olof, et al., 1998). Beyond that time period the probability of permanency increases.

While statistics vary greatly, it is safely assumed that up to 50% of all REMVAs will result in some type of neck injury. The risk of occupant disability is approximately 3 to 6%, a staggering number when one considers the number of motor vehicle accidents per year (Ono, et al., 1993). There is no truth to the assumption that injured people get better after some type of settlement or what is known as "green back poultice."

TESTING METHODS FOR PREDICTING HUMAN INJURY

Testing methods used to determine the kinds and types of injuries received in MVAs fall into five categories:

1. Humans (live)
2. Animals
3. Cadavers
4. Computer modeling
5. Anthropomorphic test dummies

The only totally accurate way to predict human response in REMVAs is to actually use living, breathing humans. Obviously, some restrictions apply for these types of situations.

First of all, humans get injured. A review of studies using live, human testing reveals that humans are brought to the bare minimum level of injuries and then no more. There are obviously good reasons for that! Therefore, the threshold of human injury is not totally statistically accurate.

Another drawback to the use of humans in crash tests is that although all test situations have very specific parameters small variables will cause a great change in human response to input forces. Variables such as occupant seating, anticipation of impact, the weight of apparatus strapped to the patient, helmet vs. no helmet, etc. greatly modify the parameters of human response, making each individual crash in truth anecdotal.

It also should be noted that crash tests are not designed to hurt human beings — they are designed to note human motion and/or response to energy input. All other testing sources, while providing great statistical information, provide no actual correlation to human injury. If one carefully reads published reports through the Society of Automobile Engineers (SAE), it will be obvious with a few biased exceptions that human motion studies do not predict injuries or lack thereof, but carefully note that they are individually dependent.

All other types of testing including cadavers are not accurate for the human response in low-impact REMVAs. In high speed crashes as the Delta V increases, the correlation between live human response and other factors increases. This is because all other testing measures purely mechanical response but no material response. Pain and dysfunction often result from the material response of viscoelastic human tissue. In other words, the quicker the impact, the higher the forces received, the more mechanical a human will respond and, therefore, mechanical/cadaver/computer modeling becomes more relevant. In low-impact REMVAs a few good studies with humans exist but virtually none with surrogates that correlate with human motion. As a result, while all crash test studies among living, nonliving, and nonhuman subjects yield good statistics for study and provide cost-effective ways to measure mechanical output, at best they provide unconfirmed approximate vague guidelines for human injury.

What crash and test studies won't do will give subjective information such as:

1. Pain
2. Central Nervous System (CNS) information
3. Biological information
4. Physiologic information
5. Kinetic dysfunction following impacts
6. Latent reaction

All information gathered from crash test studies is statistical in nature and can never be applied to an individual in a given situation.

BIOMECHANICS

Biomechanics is a very inexact science when it comes to human beings. While mathematical predictions are accurate and easily obtainable, human reactions under different stresses are not. How can one explain when a person's parachute fails to open, and he or she beats the odds and survives a multi-thousand foot fall while another person will trip coming down some stairs, fall several feet and die? Examples of human response to energy input quickly lead one to the conclusion that the predictability of individual response is based strictly upon the individual's response; nothing more, nothing less. It is important, however, to understand generalities so that a practicing clinician can approach human injury with logical sense.

There are four basis response modes for a body subjected to external forces:

1. Elasticity. Elasticity is defined as deformation induced during forced application, which is completely recovered when the load is recovered. An example of this is the perfect spring. This type of reaction is rarely found in the human body.
2. Plasticity. Plasticity results from deformation of the initial geometry when the load is released.

In other words, the loading and unloading path are different. The absorbed energy is the product of force × motion in the direction of motion. Plastic deformation in essence equals the permanently stored (absorbed) energy. A good example of plastic deformation is the human earlobe's response to weighted earrings or inserts. When pressure is applied over time, the soft tissue of the ear will bend and be permanently changed.

3. Viscoelasticity. Viscoelasticity is body deformation under a load such that it recovers its geometry upon load release, but it does so by following a different loading path. The initial geometry is recovered but the body absorbs some of the applied energy. In a mechanical sense, shock absorbers and tires are good examples. Human soft tissue responds in a viscoelastic manner unless force is applied to the point of actual tissue rupture.

4. Brittleness. A brittle body ruptures with negligent plastic flow. Up to the point of rupture, however, response is purely elastic. The best example of this is glass. While each part of the human body under various conditions can exhibit some of these properties, in the true sense of the word, the human soft tissues respond in a viscoelastic manner.

INSTANTANEOUS CENTER OF ROTATION (ICR)

ICR of a joint is the mathematical determination of a theoretical point on which all motions rotate. The concept of ICR in a kinematic and biomechanical sense is an important one. It can be considered under healthy conditions to be the physiological center upon which human motions of a given joint will move. Various ICRs have been measured and determined for different body parts. However, in an REMVA, the ICR may change within microseconds, causing a great change in load distribution of the human body. In a landmark study by Kaneoka, et al. (1999), the ICR of the spinal column was measured and found to change in as little as a sub-4-mph Delta V resulting in a pathological motion.

The term ICR has been misapplied and misunderstood in some instances of human motion. This is especially true in the TMJs. First of all, the motions of TMJs are not purely rotational and do not move around the fixed axis of rotation. The axis rotation of TMJs will vary in anatomical planes. When subsequent motion of the head and neck apparatus exists, or compressed tissue in the retrodiscal area, the TMJs translate from the first moment. In this instance, virtually no pure rotation occurs. Under normal circumstances, the initial axis of rotation and resulting translation can very well be different from one TMJ to another within one person, resulting in axes of rotations that are not coupled symmetrically with one another.

The surface of the TMJs can be nongeometric for many reasons, including degenerative joint disease, remodeling, growth, angles of eminentia, scar tissue, etc. The condition and surface of the articulating surfaces and supporting structures and the resulting musculature function determine the potential motions of the TMJs resulting in a very complex motion system.

For the ICR of the TMJs to be accurately determined, they would have to be rotating cylinders that remain stationary throughout the motion, which of course they do not. The mandible changes its position as it moves throughout the range of motion. The result is not just a change of the head of the mandible, but the mandible itself. As it translates, rotates, moves in a 3-dimensional position, the ICR changes as well. Studies also indicate that the trajectory of the condylar heads along the surfaces can be affected by velocity (distance/time) and is a multiplane vector that can be affected by muscle soreness, speed of forced opening, rotational forces, compressive forces, and shear forces. The ICR of the TMJ will change dramatically in a very slight, fractional opening. When the ICRs of the TMJs are not perfectly matched, the articulating surfaces of the joints can be either distracted or compressed, depending upon which moment in time is measured. Rapid acceleration, such as that experienced in an REMVA, can affect the standardization of motion of the TMJs, creating nonhabitual moment arms resulting in excessive forces not physiologically compatible with the human anatomy involved. These changing patterns from moment to moment will result in gross motor dysfunction, which will produce differing articular motions. The result is that the ICR of the TMJs is a mathematical theory only and not an accurate representation of reality. TMJs and their supporting structures can become excessively damaged from indirect trauma such as that received by whiplash. The following is a list of potential TMJ injury mechanisms:

Mechanisms Contributing to TMJ Injuries without Direct Impact to the Mandible as a Result of LSREMVAs

1. Coefficient of friction — change in fluid viscosity — fluid is different, rough, yielding more drag.

2. Blunt trauma due to linear condyle distalization compared to skull — bruising and tearing of soft tissues.

3. Slowness of muscles to react (seen in electromyographic studies) — Muscles and joints don't have to go through full range of motion (ROM) for injury to occur.

4. Morphology of articulating surfaces may not be smooth, especially under compression.

Mechanisms Contributing to TMJ Injuries without Direct Impact to the Mandible as a Result of LSREMVAs (continued)

5. Cellular ability to repair is altered.
6. ICR is altered and changes through ROM.
7. Fast and slow wave motion from headrest and condylar distalization resulting in tearing of soft tissues at hard tissue junctions.
8. Hydraulic differential between upper, lower joint space, and disc apparatus.
9. Set up for repetitive strain syndrome — change in posture of neck and mandible/upper jaw/skull. Occlusion doesn't change.
10. Sympathetically maintained pain syndrome may contribute to degenerative joint disease over time.
11. Tearing of pre-existing adhesions, fibrotic tissue.
12. Bleeding in the TMJs (hemarthrosis).
13. Referred pain patterns from other peripheral injuries.
14. Most TMJ diagnoses are inaccurate and/or misdiagnosed in the first place.

Common Soft Tissue Acceleration/Deceleration (STAD) MIST Injuries of the Head and Neck Resulting from LSREMVAs

1. Temporal tendinitis
2. Myofascial trigger points (MFTP)
3. Ernest syndrome
4. Occipital neuralgia (GON, LON)
5. Cervical facet joint inflammation
6. TMJ posterior capsulitis
7. TMJ lateral capsulitis
8. Myalgia

Note: These clinical injuries can occur as a result of the previously mentioned mechanisms.

COLLISION DYNAMICS

There are three different types of collisions in every REMVA:

1. Automobile to automobile
2. Occupant to automobile interior
3. Occupant body part to body part

AUTOMOBILE TO AUTOMOBILE

The easiest type of collision to understand is automobile to automobile. The motion is commonly divided into four different phases:

1. Contact
2. Vehicle at the peak of acceleration
3. Vehicle starting to slow down
4. Vehicle slowing to a stop

All such factors as bumper height, weight of the vehicle, angle of impact, and environmental factors may change the function of time and velocity resulting in an overlap of each phase.

OCCUPANT TO AUTOMOBILE

The second collision, occupant to automobile interior, can also be generalized into four separate phases:

1. 0 to 100 msec. The initial phase occurs at 0 to 100 ms. When the vehicle moves forward out under the test subject, initial forward and vertical motion of the hips and low back occurs. Simultaneously, the upper part of the seat begins to flex rearward under the load of the torso which remains stationary during this time period.
2. 100 to 200 msec. During the first 100 msec, the seatback reaches maximum rearward movement. The subject moves upward and forward resulting in neck compression, cervical spine straightening, and movement upward and rearward. The head is in a chin-up type of position and begins to rotate rearward. By 160 msec, the vertical motion of the torso begins to pull the neck forward as the head continues into the extension. During this phase, significant shearing forces and ramping may start (vertical rotation).
3. 200 to 300 msec. At 200 msec, maximum vertical motion has taken place. At 250 msec, the head starts a forward motion. The seatback returns to its original position while the torso extends back down the seatback.
4. 300 to 400 msec. At 300 msec, the descent of the torso is now complete and is moving at the same velocity as the vehicle. At 400 msec, active deceleration of the neck occurs. At 400 msec, all impact-related motions are virtually completed and the human body is moving at the vehicle's velocity.

The total time for human movement in REMVAs is between 0.1 to 0.2 sec. Whether the impact results from low or high velocity, the time of energy exchanged is virtually the same. This is due to the biomechanical properties of the elements involved and may vary only by a few fractions of a second.

OCCUPANT BODY PART TO BODY PART

Human injury comes not from the first collision, but from the second and third collisions. Obviously, contact from the human being to parts of the automobile can produce great amounts of soft tissue injury. These can come from movement of the body into the seat, the headrest, a seatbelt, steering wheel, dashboard, automobile pillars, windshield, etc. All are potential injury mechanisms for human beings. However, the third collision (body part to body part) has a great effect, especially in low impact situations. As the automobile goes through the motions, keeping in mind Newton's laws of motion, the occupants remain stationary relative to the automobile but seem to move toward the impact. The occupant lags behind the car, the torso lags behind the hips, the neck lags behind the torso, the head lags behind the neck, the vertebrae lag behind one another, the mandible lags behind the cranium, etc. As a result, the motion of the human during this time period is a non-physiological motion resulting in points of injury, which will almost always be at the connective tissue junctions between hard and soft tissues (as commonly seen in the TMJs and cervical vertebrae). The result is injuries to muscles, ligaments, and tendons. In an offset collision (which most are), a great amount of rotational forces will be placed on the body. The occupants will experience compression and shear forces, which cause great injury to the soft tissue. The differences in load variations to the human body during cycles of motion result in multiple stress and strain points. Each REMVA is unique and, accordingly, no such thing as pure forward and backward motion exists. Biomechanical forces applied in REMVAs are always multidimensional. As a result, there is no Delta V or closing speed under which a person cannot get hurt, nor is there a Delta V or closing speed over which all people will get hurt. The injuries are a result of individual response at a moment in time. These principles and conditions apply to soft tissue injuries and all body parts. The rate of acceleration of any given body part is of utmost importance (Newton's second law). The forces increase dramatically with an increase in acceleration. Soft tissue properties differ when applied with time variables.

Crushing of soft tissues can occur in blunt impact when body surface deforms and soft tissues get compressed between impact site and other hard tissues. Examples of these are

1. Tissues at the nuchal line and headrest (skull and headrest)
2. Tissues between spinal column and seatback
3. Tissues between vertebrae during ramping and submarining
4. Tissues between the condyles and skull (TMJ injuries)
5. Attachments of muscles (i.e., trapezius) during ramping and contact with friction of the seat, headrest, and body supports built into seats
6. Etc.

Because a moving body has inertia, when it collides a force is immediately produced on the impacted surface that starts to slow the body as a whole.

$$\frac{\text{Impacted Body Side}}{\text{Force Generated}} \rightarrow \frac{\text{Side Away from Impact}}{\text{Zero Force}}$$

The result is a net force that produces differential deceleration between body segments. The resulting biomechanical stresses (shear, compression, torque, etc.) acting simultaneously, and in opposite directions, often yield soft tissue damage.

WAVE MOTION

Stress waves travel at the speed of sound (square root of the ratio of the Young's modulus to the material density).

1. Travel through the body
2. Subject portions to local stresses and forces
3. Localized compressions
4. Localized tensions

Wave speeds for car material are approximately 9843 to 16,404 ft/sec (10 times the speed of sound). Time of energy transfer is 0.1 to 0.2 sec which means the energy travels the length of the car (15 ft) in 1.5 msec.

Elastic waves travel 67 times the car length (approximately 33 reverberations) in the energy transfer time of 0.1 to 0.2 sec.

Although viscoelastic for the most part at low forces, human soft tissue responds in an elastic manner. At high forces and as a function of time in which the force is applied, soft tissue may respond in a plastic manner resulting in permanent injury. Plastic waves travel much slower (slightly faster than the collapsing of impact surfaces) in automobiles and in human tissue as well. In MVAs, both waves are present due to crushed and uncrushed vehicle components. Not surprisingly, then, injuries often occur at locations remote from the impact site. The velocity (Newton's second law) of deformation is the predominant factor in determining the magnitude of wave created.

HIGH VELOCITY

Stress waves from impact site travel at the speed of sound in the surrounding tissues. Injuries occur at

1. Interfaces of unlike tissues (menenges, TMJs, muscle to bone attachments, facial linings, etc.).
2. Tissue/air interfaces (intestinal wall/gas, sinus cavities/linings).

A differentiation of tissue movement is contributed by the following mechanisms of injury:

1. Compression and expansion of the stressed tissues.

2. Production of pressure differential across a boundary.
3. "Spalling" energy is released as an energy wave attempts to go from a dense to less dense medium. (The wave is tensile, most human soft tissues can withstand more compression than tension.)

LOW VELOCITY (MOST COMMONLY EXPERIENCED IN MVAS)

Stress waves travel at less than 15 m/sec. Transverse waves of lower velocity and long duration (shear waves) are produced by displacements of body surfaces. The results are differentials created at

a. Sites of attachments
b. Sites of body part collisions

These forces will vary more when considering not only a difference in tissue viscosity but structural/architectural differences as well on both micro and macro levels.

HYDRAULIC PRESSURES

Tremendous amounts of pressure exerted within closed systems cause tearing at micro and macro levels. Fluid systems (i.e., shock absorbers) exhibit various mechanical characteristics under different rates of loading. Different types react in a dissimilar manner. The "containers" burst when loaded quickly. In other words, tissue reaction is time sensitive. The forces generated will be released through the path of least resistance. In humans, this path is often the point of connection between soft and hard tissues.

ENERGY INPUT AND FORCE × COMPRESSION: $F_{MAX} \times C_{MAX}$

This formula relates to how much energy is placed on a subject (or body part) during impact and how much is "lost" during the transfer. Tissues and organs can disrupt and dissipate energy transference. The larger the $F_{max} \times C_{max}$ the more energy loss will be experienced in the soft tissues and, therefore, more potential for destruction.

This relates back to Newton's first law (bodies at rest...). How much energy it takes to move tissues will determine injury potential. Tissues that slide over each other and don't resist won't absorb as much energy as those which cannot "get up and go" as fast as others. The lag time between body part motion due to differences in location, density, and reaction to forces plays a part in this phenomenon.

MUSCLE SPLINTING (PRE-TENSED)

Pre-tensing of the muscles can have an effect on injury in LSREMVAs in the following manners:

1. Increase injury potential
2. Decrease injury potential
3. Have no effect on injury potential

Contradictory? It is, but any or all of these can apply to each individual on any occasion or all at once and can apply to various body parts. For example:

1. Tighten neck
2. Lock knees anticipating impact
3. Pushing on the brake
4. Bracing with arms on the steering wheel anticipating impact

Any number of human responses can affect injury potential. The principles of movement are all the same.

All of the above can also relate directly or indirectly to cellular damage. Cell injury can occur when mechanical trauma damages the cell membrane, impairing its ability to act as a barrier to extra cellular calcium. Too much intra-cellular free calcium can overwhelm the mechanisms that normally maintain a relatively constant calcium concentration. The cell's inability to dispel the calcium can lead to an increase in osmotic pressure causing swelling, cell membrane damage, metabolic depletion, and cell death. This can occur in skeletal muscles, smooth muscles (blood vessel muscle lining), and nerve tissues. Mechanical cellular damage (from stretching) also can alter nerve tissue conduction. This cellular damage can result in muscle spasm, alteration of localized blood flow, hyperirritability, dysfunction, breakdown, and pain. All the aforementioned principles can apply to soft tissue injury on all levels simultaneously.

Common Soft Tissue Injuries Resulting from REMVAs

1. Cervical strain/sprain
2. Cervical facet joint inflammation
3. Occipital neuralgia
4. Myospasm
5. MFTPs
6. Temporal tendonitis
7. Stylomandibular ligament insertion tendinosis (Ernest Syndrome)
8. Injuries to the TMJs
   - Lateral capsulitis
   - Posterior capsulitis
   - Hemarthrosis
   - Disc displacement
     - Reducing
     - Nonreducing
   - Adhesions in the superior and inferior joint spaces

Principles Affecting Soft Tissue Injuries (How People Get Hurt): Thresholds for Soft Tissue Injuries

In The Real World (ITRW)

- There are no set thresholds for injuries to soft tissue.
- There are no set thresholds for injuries to hard tissues.
- Biomechanical trauma is unpredictable and anecdotal.
- Tissue strengths and tolerance will vary under different conditions.
- Body parts accelerate at different rates.
- Body parts move at rates different from the car and from one another.

ABBREVIATED INJURY SCALE (AIS)

The AIS was developed in 1971 by the Association for the Advancement of Automobile Medicine and the Society of Automobile Engineers to statistically track injury categories. Injuries for each body region area are placed into seven levels (0 to 6). The AIS level is based on the level of injury revealed by an examination shortly after the crash by doctors trained in its application (Gennarellii, et al., 1998).

0 No injury.
1 Minor (may not require professional treatment).
2 Moderate (nearly always requires professional treatment, but is not ordinarily life threatening or permanently disabling).
3 Serious (potential for major hospitalization and long-term disability, but normally not life threatening).
4 Severe (life-threatening and often permanently disabling, but survival is probable).
5 Critical (usually requires intensive medical care, survival uncertain).
6 Maximum (untreatable, virtually unsurvivable).

As the AIS increases, the cost of medical support greatly increases. However, the purpose of the AIS is for statistics only.

No level is supposed to be used as a predictor of final outcome nor to estimate the cost of treatment. It is possible for injuries at any AIS level to subsequently prove fatal, although the threat to life potential of the injury increases steeply with increasing AIS level (Evans, 1992).

INDIVIDUAL TOLERANCES AND RISK OF INJURY

OCCUPANT POSITION AT THE TIME OF IMPACT

Occupant position at the time of impact, one of the most important variables, is commonly overlooked and assumed in REMVAs. Occupant position will greatly reduce the Delta V required to surpass the soft tissue injury threshold. The Biomechanical Assessment Profile (BAP), a position assessment questionnaire developed by the author, allows the clinician and the occupant to help determine the true position at the time of impact. The slightest occupant position variation will greatly affect injury potential resulting in large increases of impact forces (SAE # 91294; SAE # 930211).

A normal position, such as that assumed by a crash test dummy, is not a normal position for most occupants (SAE # 700361). Being out of position is actually more normal for occupants than being in position, if normal is defined by the posture of crash test dummies at the time of impact. Positioning varies by occupants' driving habits, anatomy, seat comfort, and anticipation of a collision.

There are three common actions of bullet vehicle drivers prior to impact:

1. Braking
2. Swerving
3. Spinning/yawing

These motions will change the following:

1. Impact angles of vehicles
2. Closing speed
3. Vehicle contact
4. Will potentially negate built-in safety systems
5. Will potentially affect vehicle damage

These factors also greatly affect the passenger position at the time of impact. Virtually all rear impact testing with dummy and cadaver subjects has been conducted with properly positioned occupants (erect, backs firmly placed against the seat back) (SAE # 912914). Being out of position can dramatically change the occupant's reactions to forces and resulting kinematics. Humans react quite differently than crash test dummies especially in low speed accidents. Variations in occupant positioning may contribute little to injury potential in high-speed crashes but can greatly increase or decrease injury potential in low-speed collisions.

PRE-EXISTING CONDITIONS

"Pre-existing" is a term that is often misunderstood and abused. Susceptibility to injury does not negate the fact that damage can occur. In fact, a pre-existing condition can radically lower the amount of energy required to cause soft tissue damage. While there may be evidence of a condition radiographically, such as in localized bone breakdown of the cervical spine or the condylar head of the TMJs, the person may have been asymptomatic and remained so throughout his or her life if not for the large amount of energy transferred in such a short period of time as in a motor vehicle accident.

In fact, pre-existing conditions can make a person more susceptible to injury when forced to move faster or more than is habitually required. These conditions may include, but are not limited to:

Arthritis
Cervical disc disease
Fibromyalgia
TMD of many varieties
Myofascial disorders
Emotional disorders
Drug use
Chronic subluxation
Poor spinal alignment
Cranial lesions
Reaction time. The time span of energy input is rapid; total time is 0.1 to 0.2 sec. In contrast, human response time is slow (even healthy people's muscular reactions don't begin until .08 to .14 sec). Total personal response time has been estimated at 2.5 sec but will vary according to each individual and the circumstance at the time of impact.

Can an acute problem be superimposed over a chronic condition? Of course, this possibility can and should be taken into consideration when arriving at a differential diagnosis. It is crucial that the clinician have a thorough understanding of the patient's condition. A thorough health history is essential and may include contacting previous treating clinicians. Good diagnostic equipment and excellent diagnostic skills are also necessary.

Gender (Women Compared to Men):
Statistical Generalizations

Woman have:
Approximately two times more minor soft tissue injuries than men
Smaller neck diameters and longer necks
Higher frequency of spinal stenosis
Greater involvement in crashes/million miles driven (National Safety Council)
Higher frequency of injury claims
More severe injuries
More treatment
Higher healthcare bills
Slower recovery
Greater disability
Worse prognosis
More overall joint injuries (including TMJ)

Age (> 65 years):

Older drivers:
Are more prone to injury
Have decreased capacity for recovery
Have poorer recovery

Occupant Size

In general:
The larger the occupant's mass, the less likely an injury will occur.
Taller occupants have been shown to be at risk for higher neck injury (tall and thin vs. short and fat).
Size may correlate with age (child vs. adult; adult vs. old).
Size of body parts can influence injury potential.

Direct vs. Indirect Trauma

What is the difference between direct and indirect trauma? Can you separate the two when it comes to MVAs? Can you tell the difference clinically and with diagnostic testing? Actually, under the examination of an MRI or clinician's diagnostic exam, tissue reaction and dysfunction are the same.

Examples of direct trauma

1. Penetrating — puncture
2. Penetrating — laceration
3. Crush mechanisms (Yes and No)

Examples of indirect trauma

1. Coup–contra-coup brain injury
2. Concussion (football helmet blow, boxer sustaining blow to the mandible)
3. Fracturing a bone — direct or indirect?
4. Spraining a knee, elbow, wrist by abnormal/repetitive movement (tennis elbow)
5. Repetitive strain syndromes of all types (carpal tunnel)
5. TMJ injuries

As previously mentioned injuries commonly occur at the interfaces between unlike tissues due to the

1. Differential of speed of body parts (lagging behind)
2. Differential of tissue makeup yielding variance of wave transfer
3. Differential of hydraulic pressure
4. Hard tissue rebounding

5. Crush mechanism of hard tissues approximating each other
6. Cellular damage

Each connective tissue junction has potential for suffering stress/strain. These types of mechanisms rarely, if ever, occur by themselves. Biomechanical forces in the real world occur in multiple directions and conflicting degrees simultaneously. The delineation between direct and indirect trauma is not one of physiological origin but rather medicolegal only. Human tissues are limited in their ability to respond and are governed by the same laws of physics as the rest of the universe. To say that, for instance, the soft tissues of the TMJs or their supporting structures cannot be injured unless the mandible is directly struck indicates a lack of understanding, education, truthfulness, or all three. In fact, most injuries to the human body except at the exact point of impact are indirect in nature.

AUTOMOBILE COMPONENTS THAT CONTRIBUTE TO HUMAN INJURY POTENTIAL

HEADRESTS

Next to the position of the occupants at the precise time of impact, headrests are the most commonly overlooked contributors to head/neck injuries in REMVAs. They are often the silent contributors to occupant cervical injury. Federal law (FMVSS) requires that "head restraints must be at least 27.5 in. above the seating reference point in the highest position and not deflect more than 4 in. under a 120-lb load." Or, they must not allow the relative angle of the head and torso of a 95th percentile dummy to exceed 45° when exposed to an acceleration of 8 gs.

Vans and light trucks from 1991 have had to comply with standards. Studies show a 85-cm seatback height necessary to account for 95% of male occupants and 100% of female occupants. However, the generalization of headrest design does not allow for individual height differences and resulting cervical strain. The distance an occupant's head has to travel before impacting the headrest in a rear-end collision can greatly increase the forces applied to the head and neck (SAE # 670919). This distance can vary not only from structural design but also because of the occupant's build and seating preference. American consumers as a rule prefer adjustable headrests, but rarely have them adjusted to achieve maximum effectiveness. They are often set too low to protect the head/neck complex.

Transfer of energy (0.1 to 0.2 sec) and the slowness of human cervical muscles to respond (0.08 to 0.14 sec) result in almost no one being able to avoid direct contact with the headrest. Therefore, in almost every case involv-

ing a rear-end motor vehicle collision direct impact to the head, neck, and torso of the target vehicle occupants by the seatbacks/headrests occurs that can result in soft tissue injury.

Factors That Affect Headrest Protection of Occupants

1. Positioning
2. Ramping of the body
3. Flexion of the seatback
4. Head rides above and below
5. Distance the occupant's head travels to make initial contact (longer = more force)
6. Occupant positioning
7. Occupant's length of neck, arms, torso
8. Awareness of impact (bracing)
9. Virtually nonfunctional at best and detrimental at worse

Headrest design and position may contribute greatly to potential cervical/head injury. Due to occupant motion or pre-impact positioning, the headrest may even increase occupant injury.

SEAT CONSTRUCTION

Federal Standard FMVSS 207 advocates strength requirements of 20 times the weight of the seatback. Most seats weigh about 40 lb. The resulting strength would be 800 lb — not enough in a significant impact. In fact, impacts may produce forces beyond the seat's designed ability to rebound, resulting in seatback collapse that greatly affects the amount and direction of force to the occupant (SAE # 670919).

Seat construction is not uniform from one car to the next. It varies in:

1. Angle
2. Stiffness
3. Elasticity
4. Materials
5. Coefficient of friction

Seat design helps determine relative impact of each body part:

1. Can lead to large differential between head, spine, shoulders, pelvis, and supporting soft tissues.
2. Change angle of force vectors.
3. Compression of the spine in association with bending forces of the rotating pelvis.
4. Relative flexibility of the seat can help determine relative flexibility of the spine.
5. Can greatly affect shear, and rotational forces on the occupant.

6. Occupant rebound motion after the input of energy is greatly influenced by the seat design, and can increase these forces. The seatback's rebound velocity at up to 150% of the initial velocity.

7. If the torso rebounds before the head has reached its rearmost position, the relative velocity between the head and torso will produce unequal rebound speeds (SAE # 930211).

8. In LSREMVAs, the rebound of the occupants in the front seat may be due more to the elasticity of the seat back than to vehicle deceleration.

Lack of seat uniformity makes LSREMVA cervical studies difficult to standardize. As previously stated, any given study cannot be used to generalize or apply to a given individual.

RAMPING

The angle of the seat produces forces that may direct the occupant up the seatback. The target vehicle's rear may be deflected upward or downward depending upon the relative center of gravity between the target and bullet vehicles, resulting in the occupant traveling up the seat in a rearward position (relative to the car but stationary to the earth). The extent of ramping depends upon:

1. Angle of seatback deflection. Occupant ramping increases as seatback angle increases.

2. Slack of lap portion of the seatbelt — rearward deflection of the seat causes slack in the seatbelt. Use of a belt or no belt may affect occupant motion.

Four Important Factors of Body Motion Leading to Occupant Injury Related to Seat Construction

1. Head displacement, translation, rotation
2. Differential motion of head, neck, torso
3. Occupant ramping up seatback
4. Occupant rebound

No fully instrumented rear impact tests are required by law for seat design. In high impacts seatbacks cushion the occupants from great accelerations. In low impacts the same qualities account for greater occupant acceleration in the rebound phase. The seatback design and resulting ramping may increase injury potential to the struck automobile occupants during low-speed collisions. There is a design trade-off between comfort and function/occupant protection.

AIRBAGS

AIRBAG STATISTICS

- Over 103 million (50.3%) of the more than 206 million cars and light trucks on U.S. roads have driver airbags. Over 77 million (37.5%) of these also have passenger airbags. Another 1 million new vehicles with airbags are being sold each month.

- Through September 2000, driver airbags have inflated in over 3.3 million vehicles in crashes. More than 560,000 passenger airbags inflated when a passenger was occupying the right front seat.

- The National Highway Traffic Safety Administration estimates that more than 5899 people are alive today because of airbags.

- Of the 62 drivers killed by airbags (48 females, 14 males), 40 are believed to have been unbelted, 21 are believed to have been using lap/shoulder belts (5 of these may have misused their belts; 2 of these were unconscious and slumped over their steering wheels so they were on top of their airbags; 2 used the shoulder belt only; 1 used the lap belt only). Belt use is unknown for the remaining driver.

By 1995, 100% of passenger cars have driver systems, and 87% have passenger systems. A total of 85% of trucks have driver systems, and 23% have passenger systems (SAE # 960665).

AIRBAGS ARE DESIGNED TO SAVE LIVES

Overall, airbags have decreased belted fatalities overall by 12 and 27% of deaths in frontal crashes. It is estimated that 70% of frontal crash fatalities can be prevented by properly wearing safety belts and airbags (SAE # 922523).

Airbags save lives and decrease severity of *major* injuries in exchange for increasing the number of minor injuries. There is an increase in abrasions, contusions, and lacerations. The body regions most frequently injured are the head and neck, upper extremities, trunk, and lower extremities. Of injuries received 90% are AIS I (SAE # 960658). Airbags actually increase the total number of injuries from vehicle collisions, especially in the Delta V of 16 to 32 km/hr (10 to 20 mph) (SAE # 960658).

Occupant groups at risk from airbag deployment include

1. Unrestrained
2. Elderly
3. Small stature
4. Disabled

5. Children
6. Out of position
7. Compromised health status of occupants

Significant factors that may influence injuries in MVAs with airbag inflation:

1. Severity of crash
2. Interior compartment intrusion
3. Age of restrained occupant
4. Health status including medications, drug, and alcohol use
5. Occupant height, weight, and proportions
6. Occupant position at time of impact/inflation
7. Safety belt wearing including proper positioning
8. Other occupants in the vehicle affecting the restrained driver
9. Loose objects in the vehicle
10. Pre-crash factors including pre-crash cardiac arrest, drowning, fire, and suicide

AIRBAG SYSTEMS

Airbag inflation is an explosion (200 mph) capable of killing a person in which the force is stopped in time by a nylon bag. It has four elements:

1. Crash sensors and controls
2. Inflator
3. Air bag itself
4. Diagnostic circuitry

Sensors

A ball in a tube or spring mass sensors are mounted in the front of the vehicle, and are designed to activate airbag deployment when a sudden deceleration occurs in the vehicle's forward motion of approximately 16 to 19 km/h (9 to 11 mph). Deployment starts 15 to 20 msec after initial impact.

Inflator

A pyrotechnic device inflates a gas generant (sodium azide) in 18 to 23 msec; 21 to 27 msec after impact the burning sodium azide produces nitrogen gas that expands the nylon airbag. The actual inflation takes 20 to 40 msec. The force exits and inflates the airbag at approximately 200 mph.

Nylon Airbag

Nylon provides a high strength/weight ratio, and is abrasion resistant with good elongation properties allowing for uniform stress distribution along seams with equally distributed forces. The driver's side is smaller and circularly shaped. It has less time and distance in which to inflate due to the steering wheel. Passenger-side airbags are rectangular, and three to five times larger than those on the driver's side.

Airbag tethers limit intrusion of the airbag into the driver's space and allow for more lateral expansion (untethered bags extend 250 to 300 mm toward the driver and untethered bags extend 380 to 510 mm). Airbags deflate in about 80 to 100 msec through vent holes in the back of the bag.

Diagnostic Circuitry

The circuitry has three main functions:

1. Entire system is evaluated every time the vehicle is turned on.
2. Continuous monitoring.
3. Operates a backup power source for inflation should there be system power failure.

COMMON SOFT TISSUE INJURIES RESULTING FROM AIRBAG INFLATION

1. Abrasions, contusions to the head, neck and chest
2. Abrasions on the hands
3. Burns on the hands
4. Transient/permanent parasthesia of the chin
5. Injuries to the TMJs — external and internal
   a. Posterior capsulitis (damage to posterior lamina)
   b. Disc displacement
      1. Reducing
      2. Nonreducing
   c. Lateral capsulitis
   d. Adhesions in superior and inferior joint space
   e. Synovitis
   f. Hemarthrosis
6. Supporting structures
   a. Temporal tendons
   b. SM ligaments (Ernest syndrome)
   c. Teeth fractures and avulsions
7. Cervical strain/sprain
8. Cervical facet joint inflammation
9. Occipital neuralgia
10. Myospasm
11. MFTPs
12. Sphenopalatine ganglion neuralgia
13. Paresthesia at impact site
14. Compression neuropathies
15. Closed head injuries

Airbag Injuries Result from Both Direct and Indirect Trauma

"Smart" airbags that adjust their performance characteristics based upon the environment present at the time of the collision are in development. They are designed to "sense" the following:

1. Occupant seat position
2. Size of occupant
3. Child or infant
4. Severity of crash (closing speed)

There is a tremendous need for clinical case studies of injuries resulting from airbag deployment. Observations need to be documented and published by treating clinicians so engineers can have accurate information from the field.

SAFETY BELTS

Seatbelts are not perfect but nevertheless are among the most effective and simplest devices that help save lives. Although 49 states have seatbelt laws yet it is estimated that only 69% of U.S. citizens use seatbelts even when mandated. Seatbelts are designed to comfortably fit 80% of the U.S. population.

How Seatbelts Help Protect the Occupants

Seatbelts help in the following ways:

1. Controls ramping up the seat back.
2. May reduce the velocity of the occupant relative to the vehicle interior and thus reduce injuries resulting from occupant contacts.
3. Usage may minimize the potential of occupants to be out of position at the time of impact.
4. Allows the driver to be in position to remain in control of the vehicle after the impact.
5. May be effective in controlling forward rebound of the occupant.
6. Keeps occupant within the vehicle.
7. In frontal impacts, extends the time of "ride down," thus, effectively reducing the force on the occupant. This is accomplished by both structural design and stretching of the fabric.
8. Reduces the frequency and severity of occupant impact with the vehicle's interior (second collision). Occupants can still strike the vehicle's interior including dashboard, steering wheel, and windshield.

Most injuries from lap belts fall into the category of AIS I but can still cause permanent injury or death.

1. Increase in sternum fractures
2. Increase in neck sprains
3. Increase in thoracolumbar spine injuries
4. Increase in serious cervical spine injuries

All "increases" noted after mandatory seatbelt laws (Evans, 1992).

In addition, lap belts:

1. Can cause internal injuries upon frontal crashes or rebound from REMVA if the belt is positioned superior to the superior iliac crest of the pelvis.
2. Can cause severe strain on the lower back due to external forces.
3. Do not stop occupants from still striking the dashboard, steering wheel, or windshield with their heads.
4. Can cause "flailing" injuries of the lower extremities.
5. Can increase acceleration of the head/neck upon rebound in a REMVA.

A three-point shoulder harness (essential for airbag safety):

1. Can cause increased forces to the neck in a MVA even if properly positioned.
2. Can add rotational forces to the head/neck upon rebound (occupant rotates toward the door).
3. May actually increase likelihood of cervical injury in low speed collisions.
4. Reduce the incidence of serious injury by >57% (SAE # 912913).

Shoulder belts while very effective in saving lives can directly affect injury patterns and, in fact, cause injuries in low-speed accidents. Some common injuries include

1. Bruising and abrasions of shoulder, chest, neck, and abdomen
2. Cervical/head rotational and acceleration soft tissue damage

Even with seatbelts occupants can still directly contact the car's interior with their heads. This can vary according to the severity of the impact, location of the impact, and occupant body proportions.

VEHICLE DAMAGE AS A PREDICTION OF HUMAN INJURY

One of the most contentious areas of motor vehicle accident injuries is comparing the severity of injury to the cost of automobile repair. Although this argument at first seems logical, upon further examination it is revealed to be fallacious.

Facts about MVAs and the resulting biomechanics and kinematics:

1. Biomechanics is an unpredictable science. Mathematically, scenarios can be predicted via computer modeling, etc. and information can be gathered following an accident by extensively monitored crash test dummies or other surrogates, but one little change in an almost endless supply of variables can result in dramatically different resulting forces and injury potential. In fact, measurements may differ between individual test subjects in the same carefully monitored crash test rendering predictions of outcome totally inaccurate. Applying the measured outcomes from crash test studies to predict an individual's chance of physical harm in a completely different accident is impossible. In fact, valid scientific papers are all quick to point out that the gathered data cannot and should not be used in this manner (SAE # 930211).

2. If there is truly a cost/injury ratio, then the higher the cost of repair, the more extensive the injuries to the occupants. In fact, often the opposite is true. Whenever a non-bumper impact to a vehicle occurs, large amounts of upper body damage occur to the vehicles involved. Vehicular panels are meant to crush, dispersing energy transfer over a longer period of time, and thus reducing the forces applied to the occupants. In today's vehicles with computerized components the cost of repair can be quite high with very little energy transfer to the vehicle itself. In fact, a recent crash test demonstrated the cost of repair to the same vehicle at the same impact speed varied by over $1000, depending on the angle of impact. In bumper impacts a great amount of force can be transferred to the occupants with little or no vehicular damage. As has been previously discussed, bumpers are not designed to reduce impact to the occupants — they are meant to reduce the costs of repair in a collision (Kaufman, et al., 1993).

3. In no instances do the amount of energy transfer and resulting injury involving humans directly correlate with the cost of repair to plastic, metal, etc. This is easily demonstrated by watching a football game. When a player gets hit in the head, do the managers look at the helmet and determine if an injury has truly occurred based on the amount of damage to the plastic helmet?

On the other hand, when a person has an internal injury from a fall, is it correct to examine the floor upon which he or she landed and determine if an injury has occurred by the amount of damage to the floor? Of course not, yet this is attempted routinely in injuries resulting from MVAs.

4. Each accident must be analyzed as its own separate entity. The dollar amount to repair the involved automobiles cannot be correlated with injury potential.

When attempts are made to understand injuries that result from motor vehicle accidents many factors have to be included. The more the treating clinician understands about the forces involved, the more accurately treatment can be rendered. The cost of repair to the vehicles involved, however, is one factor that may be of interest for academic and epidemiological reasons but cannot be used as a yardstick for measuring the extent of injuries or the length of treatment time, or estimating the cost of service provided.

SUMMARY

Understanding the biomechanics and occupant kinematics in MVAs is essential for the clinician who treats soft tissue injuries. New car safety has dramatically decreased car accident fatalities in the United States. The result, however, is a new challenge to our healthcare system. People who would have died in the past are now living, but with extensive injuries. Soft tissue injuries are often dismissed as an annoyance or something that "you have to learn to live with." The truth is that they often can be debilitating and greatly affect the quality of life of victims and their families. "Learning to live with it" is not the answer. The answer lies in partnerships among victims, their families, treating clinicians, and third-party payers, partnerships based upon education and understanding. Too often a battleground is formed with experts representing vested interests lining up on each side. The result is a "double victim": one who was a victim of trauma from the automobile accident and also of the trauma of enduring medicolegal confrontations.

Treating clinicians can also become victims of sorts. It is commonly reported that carefully and thoroughly treating MVA victims is looked upon with distrust by third-party payers. Suggestions are being made that the practitioner cannot solely govern the formulation of a treatment plan (Farnham, 2001). Treating clinicians can become discouraged by the constant conflict of trying to help the patient heal and being castigated for trying to do so at the same time. As automobiles become more efficient in reducing deaths, the complexity of the injuries of the survivors will increase. Clinicians must strive continually to increase their diagnostic and treatment skills, keeping the best interests of the patient first and foremost.

> It is one of the most beautiful compensations in life that no person can sincerely try to help another without helping themselves.

Ralph Waldo Emerson

REFERENCES

Barnsley, L., et al. (1994). Clinical review: Whiplash. *Pain,* 283–307.

Carette, S. (1994). Whiplash injury and chronic neck pain. *New England Journal of Medicine, 330,* 1083–1084.

Evans, L. (1991). *Traffic safety and the driver* (p. 8). New York: Van Nostrand Reinhold.

Evans, R.W. (1992). Some observations on whiplash injuries. *Neurology Clinics, 10,* 975–979.

Farnham, E. (2001, April). Workers' comp abuse: Can we ever tip the scales? *Claims,* 56.

Gennarellii, T., et al. (1998). *The abbreviated injury scale.* Sonora, CA: AAPM.

Kaneoka, K., et al. (1999). Motion analysis of cervical vertebrae during whiplash loading. *Spine, 24,* 8, 763–770.

Kauffman, M., et al. (1993). Status report. (Vol. 3, pp. 2–7). Arlington, VA: Insurance Institute for Highway Safety.

Ono, K., et al. (1993). Influence of the physical parameters on the risk to neck injuries in low impact rear-end collisions. Presented at the International Conference on the Biomechanics of Impacts, Eindhoven, The Netherlands, Sept. 8–10.

Per-Olof, B., et al. (1998). Sick leave and disability pension among passenger car occupants injured in urban traffic. *Spine, 23,* 9, 1023, 1028.

Section XI

Future Trends

80

Achieving Insurance Independence in the Age of Managed Care

Christopher R. Brown, D.D.S., M.P.S.

INTRODUCTION

There has never been a better time to practice pain management in all of history!!! How many of you reading this book feel this in your heart and mind? Unfortunately, probably very few. The statement is absolutely true, however, and this chapter will help you start finding your path toward success in pain management.

In the history of the most common affliction, pain, there has never been greater opportunity for successful healing. The technology and knowledge are there for predictable individual success. Opportunities that did not exist even a few short years ago are commonplace today.

Yet in the midst of these opportunities lies a dark specter hovering over every field in the healing arts: Managed Care. The very name brings depression into the hearts of many practitioners no matter what their degrees. It seems the powers that be in our different professions have already given up and handed the mantle of control of patient care over to accountants and actuaries.

The following concepts can be the first steps in dealing with your life, your success, and healing the pain of your career.

These guidelines are not for everyone. In fact, only about 5% of those reading this will actually grasp and accept the concepts presented. It has been said that about 5% of the U.S. population make the decisions that dictate the other 95% of the population's lifestyles. The same percentage probably holds true in the healing arts as well. To those 5%ers the future lies in two main avenues:

1. Individual decisions. You have to develop the courage to take control of your future. This means in body, soul, mind, concept, and most importantly, actions. Without that commitment, you are doomed to stand in the breadline of healthcare delivery waiting for the crumbs that are left, especially in the area of managed care.

2. Working together. Each of us desires to become successful. Contrary to popular myth, there is no such thing as a "self-made" person. Highly successful people are always striving to establish relationships with their peers. One of the buzzwords of modern times is "networking." Networking is an essential aspect of success to the healthcare practitioner. The days of a solitary person isolating him- or herself within the confines of a practice without other professional contact are gone. We have to literally join hands to help each other or our ability to provide individual care tailored to each patient's needs will be gone.

- How many of you who once loved to practice now wish you had not chosen your profession?
- How many of you have given up on the idea of success and are just hanging on?
- How many of you feel alone and vulnerable?
- How many of you are tired of being scared?

If this sounds like you and you want things to change, then perhaps you are one of the 5% who will become the

0-8493-0926-3/02/$0.00+$1.50
© 2002 by CRC Press LLC

warriors of our professions. Our patients need our help. The rule of the day, however, is "physician heal thyself." In Micah 6:8, the author asks what God requires of His people. Is it the normal customs of the day? Is it rivers of oil or thousands of sheep? The answer, as is always the case, lies in simplicity: Seek justice, love kindness, walk humbly with your God.

All the techniques contained in this chapter are just means to help implement these ancient guidelines. Without these basic truths, all knowledge will be for nothing. These concepts are designed to lift those 5%ers to a level of practice few can imagine. The few who dare to take back their destiny. Success is a choice — so is failure. Which will you choose? There is no doubt in my mind that every person is a living, breathing, self-fulfilling prophecy. We become that upon which we dwell. In as much lie the attitude and fate of your practice.

Each day we redefine our office and create the environment in which we live. Each day holds the same potential as the next — no more, no less. Each day we choose to be happy, sad, mad, fulfilled, or empty. Each day has the potential of holding great achievement. We have the choice of processing the events of the day and deciding how to react. Events should not dictate our moods unless we make a choice to do so.

In II Timothy 2, Paul uses an illustration to demonstrate teamwork: In a house are many vessels: those of gold, silver, and pottery. All are different but all are used to enhance the household. Just like each vessel, each of us is different. We all feel, act, and react differently under any given circumstance. Also like each vessel, we are distinctly created and trained to serve a purpose. Each vessel uniquely made is designed to serve a purpose only it can fulfill; yet all work together for the common good. The purpose of this chapter is for each doctor and staff to find his or her unique position in the team to work for the common good of helping the patients whom we serve.

When I've been successful, I've been in control.

Katherine Hepburn

WHAT IS MANAGED CARE?

The concept of managed care has been around for quite some time. Historically, the industrial revolution is perhaps the best example of an actual "starting" point. Companies, along with the company store, had the company "doc" long before insurance was a concept in healthcare. If you were sick or injured, the company doctor took care of you. Costs were cheap and so were the results. In those limited days, that was the best that could be done. However, along the way, insurance companies decided they could make a large profit from illness, hence the concept of health insurance was born.

As a result of new technology, longer lives, new diseases, higher demand, etc., the costs and, more importantly, the risks involved dramatically changed the face of providing insurance coverage. As a result, the risk of predicting outgoing expenditures for the companies grew unpredictable. Insurance companies make money by accurate predictions balancing future risks with future income. That's the nature of the industry. Something in the formula had to change.

Make no mistake about it, capitalism is at the heart of our system. If insurance companies didn't make large sums of money with limited risk, then there would be no insurance. The days of any of us thinking insurance companies are altruistic in nature have fallen by the wayside, and really that's OK.

For a while, the formula changed by dumping huge sums of money into the funnel and adding some restrictions such as demanding out-patient surgery instead of the traditional in-hospital. The result? On paper it looked good, but in the good old American tradition, the marketplace responded. Out-patient surgery clinics sprang up all over the place. The costs? — Of course, they escalated.

Now the real culprit became predicting the future. In other words, if the future risks could be controlled along with costs, then true savings and control could be realized. That, in essence, is managed care: risk control. Instead of the insurance companies taking on the risk, they are now sharing the risks with the providers and the patients.

Actually, a pretty smart and pretty fair deal, in a way; that is, in concept. The problem is that there are other entanglements as well. At first glance, it would seem that the hardest thing for us as private practitioners is an apparent drop in income. While obviously that doesn't make one jump for joy, it is not really the problem. The true problem is taking the decision process out of the hands of the practitioners and patients and placing it in the arena of a third party in some far-off land. It also robs doctors of their most precious assets: freedom of choice and the resulting happiness. Money comes and goes. Money not spent can be saved, invested, and ultimately multiplied. Happiness not spent today does not lead to happiness tomorrow. Happiness is a fleeting commodity with no shelf life. It is important for the doctors, their staff, and patients served that the provider and the whole personal delivery system be happy and customized.

Pain patients are unique and have to be approached that way. Many of these problems don't fit into actuary tables with the means now used. Currently one way of dealing with patients in a managed situation is to ignore them, shift cost to someone else, and hope they go away, or better yet, deny them treatment because a certain procedure or ailment does not fit into their coverage. This policy is expensive and absurd. It is costing everyone untold millions of dollars, and lives are being destroyed. These new plans have been carefully marketed as the savior of our private system and for now, Congress and the American people for the most part are buying into it. Most practitioners are resigned to this story as their future, but if you want a different future, keep on reading. This is not the true story for our patients and us. A silver lining to this cloud exists and together we will find and live it. This chapter is not about insurance bashing, but rather taking control of our destiny.

What Does Managed Care Do for Patients?

Managed care provides a safety net of bottom line care for patients. It is, in essence, catastrophic coverage wrapped in the delusion of comprehensive care. It is the epitome of marketing. Promising something that cannot be delivered all the while convincing the recipients it's the best that can be done. If these principles were applied to you or me, it would be considered malpractice. Our society, however, has decided to grant special dispensation allowing for this misbehavior. The main drawback, to reiterate, is it leaves the patients out of the decision loop. Are people truly so stupid or misinformed that they should not be allowed to make their own healthcare decisions? In my opinion, the average individual is quite capable. I'm sure the people who devise these plans would whole-heartedly agree. In fact, they feel so strongly in that direction that they limit the patients' choices up front. As a result, the risk is reduced. If instead of three choices, the patient now only has two, then the risks are cut 33% right from the start. Now this is all well and good for someone with a runny nose or other predictable medical problems, but what about the pain patient who needs a multidisciplinary approach? It is hard to establish risk exposure so they are swept under the rug. Their choices are limited to the point of often not being able to get better within the system. This is where the 95%ers give up and throw in the towel. Guess what, though? Pain is one of the best motivators and people will continue to seek care from those who can heal them. Most patients who understand their problems and have hope are willing to own their health concerns and stop looking for a "big brother" to pay the bill. This is the area we will open your eyes to later. Don't give up — keep on reading; …people will continue to seek care from those who can heal them.

What Does Managed Care Do for the Practitioner?

Managed care when you boil it down is nothing more than a marketing scheme to assure you of patients in the future; nothing more and nothing less. It is a system built on the premise of "if you don't join our plan, someone else will and you'll be left out in the cold with no patients." In fact, one of the early marketing fliers sent to my office was a picture of a dental chair with cobwebs on it saying, "this will be you in the near future." No joke, it really was that blunt. For a moment, please try to get rid of the emotion joined with this issue and take a cold hard look at the programs in which you are involved or have been tempted to join.

In the healing arts, the marketing truism is that a healthy practice needs to reinvest 5% of its gross back into the practice in the form of marketing to attract new patients. Five percent! Does anyone out there belong to any plans that only drop your fees 5%? If you do, then it is probably a plan that is cost effective, if there is an equal drop in marketing costs to offset the decrease in earnings. If your fees are dropped more than 5%, then how much more? Most of the managed care plans reduce fees about 35%!

Many practitioners have an overhead of around 60%. If an office only has an estimated profit margin of 5%, how can the practitioner make any money? By volume? Come on. It'll never happen. Let's play a game. A new marketing firm comes along and says, "Doctor, have I got a deal for you. I have a group of patients who may or may not come to you, but I'm willing to market them with no upfront costs for you at all. However, I'm going to ask you to pay me 35% of the gross charges (before overhead) for every patient who walks in the door!!!" How long will those marketing firms last? Oh, they'd do quite well. In fact, they're called managed care organizations (MCO) and they are flourishing. The main problem is not the patients, their employers, or even the fact that insurance companies want to make money, it is the fact that doctors are willing to fall back on their heels and pay exorbitant rates for marketing. Let go of your fear, docs. That's all MCOs do for you — nothing more and nothing less. Why do thousands of doctors work for reduced fees? Strictly out of fear and lack of self-respect and self-confidence. Those are the only reasons I can come up with. It isn't for the lack of income. Heck, I was losing money on every patient as it was, so financially I was gaining nothing.

There are all sorts of formulas on how to determine if you can afford to be involved in an MCO. The invasion of Normandy on D-Day could not have been as complicated as some people try to make it. All it takes to arrive at an answer for you personally is to do the following: Ask yourself, your wife/husband, and your staff this simple question: Are you willing to spend up to 35% of your gross income to market new patients into your practice? In real overhead terms, that means if all things remain the same, you could lose almost half your patients at an MCO reimbursement of 65%, keep the other half at full pay and remain relatively the same in terms of net income. Think about it! If the answer to the above question is "no," then you need to consider your role in managed care.

YOUR WORST ENEMY — CREATING AND ACCEPTING FAILURE

Quick, without thinking, who is your practice's worst enemy? Make a list:

1. MCOs
2. Your front-desk person
3. The IRS
4. The ADA/AMA/ACA, etc.
5. Your patients
6. Anyone else but you…

Wrong!

Without question, the worst enemy with whom you have to deal is you, and your attitude. The first step toward getting your practice life together is confronting the true enemy. To quote the wise sage Pogo: "I have met the enemy and he is us." *We have blamed everyone but the one responsible for our failures.* Managed care? It's not the fault of the insurance companies. They are out to make a profit and are doing so at record rates. They have paid the price of millions of advertising dollars and are reaping the rewards.

We have no one to blame for our circle of fear and failure but ourselves by allowing negative thinking and poor planning to enslave us. The first step in any type of recovery program is to admit there's a problem and own up to it. You have a choice for the kind of future you desire and deserve. You no longer have to fear the future. Success or Failure — Which Do You Choose? Life is a choice; success is a choice. The first thing you have to do is choose where you want to be. Are you happy with your life? Are you happy with your circumstances? Are you happy with your income, level of patient care, etc.? If the answers to these questions are "no" then you need to make a decision about change. Don't wait for the next MCO contact to come down the road and hope it don't take anything else away from you and your patients.

If you continue to practice the way you do now, then don't be amazed when you get the same results? Remember, "What you sow so shall you reap." Don't plant weeds and expect roses. Things will only get worse. If your practice is losing ground, then what are you doing about it? Sitting around and complaining, drinking too much alcohol, running away to the golf course and pretending the problems aren't there, blaming others, getting an ulcer, self-destructing…what?

There are answers to all the problems you have in your practice. Most are easy, some are hard. Up until now, outside forces were calling the shots. You need to make a decision to dispel the circle of fear surrounding your practice and control your own destiny. Do you want things to change? Not back to the way things used to be but rather better than they used to be.

The first step starts with a desire for some internal modifications. You're the captain and you need to start making changes in your office to ensure your success. Only when you understand the problems within and without can you develop a strategy for practice that will properly reward your efforts. It's been said that if you keep on doing what you've been doing, you'll keep on getting what you've been getting. In the past, that was a true statement. In this day and age of information overload and increasingly rapid changes, if you keep on doing what you've been doing, you'll get less and less. The "less" I'm referring to is not just money, but less of life including

- Less time with your family and friends
- Less time in meditation and worship
- Less peace in your heart and mind
- Less enjoyment of your profession

In other words, you lose your balance of life. You only have so much time and energy to give to all your projects. If one area of your life pulls away all your attention, then another aspect suffers. Energy can be neither created or destroyed — it can only be changed into other kinds of energy. Our lives are the same way. Every ounce of energy we use takes away from something else. Your time and energy are limited. It's always easier to talk about what we ought to do and harder to do it. The first step to achieving success is allowing yourself the right to succeed. This is a very important step that is often missed. Walter Hailey of Planned Marketing Associates refers to this as the "Permission Statement." Allowing yourself and your office to succeed above your previous expectations is an important psychological barrier that you must break.

Breaking the 4-minute mile was thought to be impossible and was not accomplished until Roger Bannister did in 1954. But did you realize that the impossible barrier was broken seven times that same year by other runners after Bannister succeeded? The impossible became commonplace.

Don't expect permission for success to come from anyone but you and those who care about you. Do you think other practitioners (your loving colleagues) who are unhappy want to see you succeed? If you discuss this with them, they will be glorious naysayers and try to keep you from changing. After all, one definition of someone else's success is "someone who is slightly less advanced than I am." Don't rely on your colleagues to applaud your desire to change. If you and your staff agree that it is OK to succeed, then you will have taken the first step to success. Most professional practices never get this far along the road to freedom. Modern offices have been the victims of brilliant marketing. The doctor in our society, while still respected, used to be looked upon as the answer to our health problems. Through careful marketing and strategic positioning by third-party payers, the doctor's role has been perceptually altered to part of our healthcare system's problems. Healthcare deliverers "charge too much, test too much, pad expenses, etc." So begin at the beginning and let it be OK within you to achieve success. You can't fool the person in the mirror. If you feel good enough about yourself to allow success, then success can follow. Before you achieve, you must believe. Deserving success, however, is more than a slogan. All the motivational posters and cliches won't do you any good if it isn't in your heart.

The best way for you to be successful is to deserve success. Those who are willing to pay the price of success in blood, sweat, and tears over a long period of time will be successful. Hard work, in other words, is the foremost key to success. On the other hand, aimless hard work will serve no purpose. You must work hard in the right direction. Success in any profession is not achieved by winning the lottery or luck, but rather by working incredibly hard over a long period of time. Allowing your office to succeed means developing a work ethic that is second to none in your area of expertise. This means a no-compromise attitude toward working hard and doing the right things all the time. When your office affirms success, it also affirms a work ethic that will put others in second place. Managed care takes away the drive to succeed. Shedding that cloak and affirming your own destiny brings back the desire to work hard. Your practice once again becomes fun. Everybody wants to succeed but few people (5%ers) are willing to pay the price in terms of hard work. This step alone will help propel your office to the next level.

SELF-ESTEEM

Self-esteem is the value we place on the face in the mirror — ourselves. We all know people who would be willing to put in a job application as a speed bump and still feel inadequate. Feeling good about yourself is essential to your office's success. Constantly having a third party dictate your treatment of pain patients will wear you down over a period of time. The degradation of your clinical judgments by someone probably below your clinical skill level won't make him/her any smarter and will eventually bring you mentally down: the old "one bad apple…" scenario.

People who have low self-esteem are often unfocused, confused individuals who are easily frustrated. This is an almost fatal flaw in your position as a healthcare practice leader. People with low self-esteem create alibis for their failures. They also constantly blame others for their mistakes. People in this situation often think there's a "secret" out there somewhere that others know that they don't. It's difficult to work with these kinds of people in your office. It's even harder to deal with such a person over the phone dictating your clinical decision.

Individuals with great self-esteem will accomplish great things. Don't get this confused with the doctor who always argues with the speaker at meetings and always drives the most expensive car. Self-esteem allows for quiet control; one of the most self-destructive mechanisms is lack of control. Don't try to fool yourself. Self-esteem is something you must feel inside that you deserve. Developing a good work ethic and team effort will help fuel that inner engine that allows for success. Learning a self-esteem motto to be repeated over and over will not make success become a reality. If we keep telling ourselves we'll be successful, but not do the necessary mechanics, all we're doing is fantasizing. While positive verbal affirmations are important, unless they are linked with the mechanics necessary to bring success, we are only deceiving ourselves. Our words will be hollow and our self-esteem will never rise.

GOALS

Most successful people are dreamers: basically ordinary people who are not afraid to think big and dare to be different. Our dreams are our master plan, a direction in which we want to head. Yet dreams are often something so vague that they are nothing more than nebulous concepts with no definition. Goals, however, are our master plan, our step-by-step on how to live our dreams. Study any business success no matter what the field, and you'll find a common thread is having written, defined goals, and a plan on how to achieve them. What are your office dreams? Neither I nor anyone else can articulate them for you.

The first step is to have a clear vision of what you want: what you want to accomplish. For many people, this is the hardest step. Too many times our goals are built upon advice from others, what society thinks we should do, or plain old greed. None of the above will work for the long haul. At this point of your decision process, the details are not important. For those readers who love details, this concept will be difficult. The object is to determine where you want your life to go, not how to get there. It's often best at this point not to seek outside counsel unless your goals directly affect your family. Especially don't seek counsel from your professional peers. They often can be the worst naysayers in your life. Why would they want you to change? That may make them feel uncomfortable.

There's a line from an Amy Grant song "when the world around you sees you've changed, don't expect them to applaud…." Believe me, advice will come out of the woodwork at this stage and very little will be supportive. When the Wright brothers decided they wanted to make a flying machine, do you suppose the general consensus of their peers was supportive? I'm sure there would have been fellow bicycle makers lined up around the block with advice about how their plan would never work, how foolish they were, and how the bicycle industry would not accept a flying machine. History is rife with countless examples of people who set goals who were laughed at, cursed at, and discouraged in every way. Leave your trusted colleagues out of the decision loop entirely until you know your desired direction. Even with your friends and spouse, the danger is the instinctive reaction of many people to start discouraging you, even with the best of intentions. This is a private matter: what you want, what you need. The time for sharing comes later in the process.

You need to think, articulate, and write down the goals. If you do this, you are ahead of 98% of all practitioners. As previously stated, this step can be very difficult for some. For others, it may take 30 seconds. Don't aim toward an illusion. A goal is often confused with a wish. To "qualify" as a goal the accomplishment must be measurable. Wishes are not. Examples of wishes that have been presented to me as goals are

1. Having peace and harmony in the office
2. Be the best I can be
3. Achieving financial independence

While these are fine thoughts, they are totally lacking in measurability. How will you know if and when they are achieved? For instance, "being the best that you can be" is a fine slogan for Army recruiters, but what does it mean? Can we all not be "better" every day of our lives? How about achieving financial independence? I recently read a survey asking people what that meant. For those with net worths less than 1 million dollars, financial independence meant hitting the million-dollar mark. For those with net worths greater than 1 million dollars, the figure jumped to 5 million. For those with net worths of 5 million, the definition jumped to 15 million!!! The moral of the story is, don't aim toward an illusion. Make sure the goals you set are yardsticks that can be held up to the light of scrutiny so you can see instantly whether or not you have hit your mark.

As a bonus, those around you will catch the passion as well and your team will remain focused. Will you fail occasionally? Of course you will. There will be days, even weeks, where you seem to be going in reverse. Some people who read motivational books get pumped up until the first adversity comes along and "pop" goes the balloon and they fall back to where they started. In fact, they may fall back even farther becoming bitter in the process. We all know those who live their lives in defeat. Success and goal achievement always progress in fits and starts. That's normal. The difference between winners and losers is that the losers quit when adversity strikes. That's why it's important to establish goals you care about enough that you are willing to overcome the rough spots and keep moving forward. If a goal is not

worth working at, then it probably isn't really something your heart desires and your prophecy is true. It isn't worth your effort. So, in the process, be sure and match your goals to your gifts. That way each success builds toward the next. Disappointment in one area can actually motivate you to excel in another.

ESTABLISHING GOOD COMMUNICATION SKILLS

Communication is one of the toughest, most demanding, yet most rewarding skills you can acquire. Everyone needs to communicate better. The ability to communicate clearly is fundamental to success. Many people think good communicators are born, not made; that you either have it or you don't. Not true. Communication, both good and bad, is a habit that can be learned and mastered. Communication is interaction outside yourself with other people in a way that the right information is conveyed at the right time. It is, therefore, important not only to learn how to communicate, but when to do so. Content and time go hand in hand. Both aspects are essential. Communication involves much more than the practitioner lecturing to staff and patients. It also involves asking the right questions and patiently *listening* to the responses.

The first place to start with proper patient communication is where many practitioners make a fundamental error: asking patients what they expect as a result of seeking your care. In other words, what are their treatment goals? Sometimes you have to initially ignore your own preconceived notions of what the patient wants to achieve. *Don't assume — don't guess...Ask!!*

The object is not to cram your philosophy down patients' throats, but rather to make your goals and their goals the same. Asking, followed by listening, begins the building of a relationship with people that will overcome many barriers. By listening, you gain trust and make your patients more comfortable with you and your program. As a provider for an MCO, the relationship between you and your patient is initially based on the fact that you are willing to work more cheaply than the next guy. Patients are drawn to you because you are on a "preferred" list. Your communication with the patient is continually broken by the intervention of a third party. Communication is fundamentally flawed from the beginning.

If you fulfill patients' desires rather than dictate treatment, then everyone has the same agenda from the start. Too many times doctors try to dictate what pain patients should do rather than lead them in the direction that they already desire. This only propagates ingrained resistance from the word "go." It is a blueprint for failure.

One of the basic truths of any successful program is allowing the patient to "own" his or her problem. Until you and the patient are on the same side, how can you expect success? Also, how can you define success with a patient until you know what he/she even wants?

We all know that some patients want 100% success all the time or they are not satisfied — unrealistical to be sure, but it is what they expect. That behavior needs to be determined up front. We've all had the bad experience of finding out after the fact that a patient's expectations were impossible to achieve in the first place. Unfortunately, this is often discovered after treatment has been initiated. It is much better to tell patients what can and can't be achieved based on their desires before therapy has begun. Most patients have a more realistic approach and have reasonable expectations. Knowing this up front greatly reduces the stress of practice and allows for true healing to occur. The point is, how will you know what the patient wants unless you ask the patient?

Fulfilling a patient's desires will allow him or her to be a partner in the healing process and assures you of clinical success as defined by the patient, not you. Gone are the days of the doctor/dictator. They are replaced by the doctor/partner. When you replace your dictator role with that of a partner, you will without question experience the following:

1. Increase in case acceptance
2. Increase in case success
3. Increase in your income
4. Increase in your practice satisfaction
5. Increase in your enjoyment of life
6. Increase in self-esteem
7. Decrease in your stress

PERSISTENCE

We are in a society built on drive-through windows, electronic access, and instant gratification. Persistence and hard work are not fashionable. They are, however, the fabric from which success is woven. This is the part that determines if your office will be successful in the age of managed care. Persistence will make your office great. Persistence allows you to fulfill your dreams.

It is easy to read any book on success, get all pumped up, and start the next day to achieve your dreams. It is something else, however, to do things right a month, a year, 5 years from now. Many people dream of the home-run ball, winning the lottery, waiting for their ship to come, in, etc. You can compile all the get-rich-quick clichés you can think of, when, in actuality, financially successful people are the ones who make a plan and stick to it. That means, not only when it feels good, but also when there's major opposition. Persistence is what got us all through those long days of school. Dogged determination prevailed even when the days of practice seemed far away. We all remember waiting tables, driving cabs, or whatever helped make ends meet.

The fact that we successfully graduated and are in practice proves we all basically have what it takes to be successful, yet what has happened to our professions and us? For many, it has been a slow process of giving up a little of our practice at a time and persevering in the wrong areas, which have resulted in the erosion of private practice.

Many of us have just become sidetracked from all the distractions of modern practice life. Don't look to all of the excuses others use for their failures and for not achieving their dreams. Look within, forgetting excuses, and start looking instead for answers. Without dogged pursuit of your goals and dreams, you and your practice will never reach its full potential. How do you achieve a successful practice in the long run? How do you turn your practice around? How do you become the clinician you always dreamed you could be? You do the right things every day, day after day. Consistency and persistence will make all your plans fit together and reestablish your practice on your terms.

ESTABLISHING GOOD SYSTEMS

Without good systems, you will be like a car out of alignment. When you're going 15 mph, it seems to run pretty well, but when you're up to 80 mph the vehicle almost jumps off the road and you fight for control the whole time. With good systems come good habits. The old adage "practice makes perfect" is not true. Perfect practice makes perfect. Simply repeating the same mistakes over and over will not get you anywhere. Your systems need to be analyzed in light of your dreams and goals. Make your systems work for you and what you want to achieve, not vice versa. This is often a key to slavery in modern practices. Unless you have accomplished step one (asking permission to succeed with your staff), you will meet with major staff opposition. Don't let that happen or you will be taking a U-turn on the road to freedom. Watch out for a scary word — change.

Utilizing systems often conjures up thoughts of assembly-line healthcare delivery. In fact, however, developing good systems allows you to be more creative in your daily relationships with people. Good systems allow you more time to spend with your patients in an unhurried manner. Good systems allow you to utilize your time in a proper, effective manner, resulting in a more relaxed delivery of care. Your ability to properly serve your patients will increase while your stress will decrease.

POSITIONING YOURSELF FOR SUCCESS: THE ROAD NOT TAKEN

Positioning your practice for successful growth may go against conventional wisdom. It seems that nearly all the experts claim the future of healthcare delivery is a managed care model. Whether this will be true for society or not, no one can answer. Whether it is true for your individual practice only you can answer. When you and your staff can develop the ability to make patients feel better about themselves when they visit you than they do anywhere else, then you will have practice success no matter what direction society takes. The healing and loyalty of pain patients are more often directed by how you treat them rather than by strict methodology.

We live in a consumer age. People, regardless of how much they complain about costs, still want quality and are generally willing to pay for it. Notice, I said "quality". You can't charge for what you can't deliver. So don't ever be tempted not to do what's right for your patients. Unscrupulous behavior will always negate success in the long run. The best practice position is to make co-decisions with your patients without outside interference from third parties.

Looking at the buying habits of people indicates an interesting trend. Often, price is not the main obstacle when it comes to purchases. The main concern is how to pay for it! Fitting a purchase of any kind into the monthly budget is usually the deciding factor when making buying decisions for something that a person wants. Planning your office's successful financial future must include accommodating your patients' financial obligations and creating avenues for payment.

There are two ends of the spectrum, both of which are disasters for practice growth when it comes to financial planning for patient payment. They are opposite in nature yet identical in results.

The first is denying all patients' personal financial obligations and relying solely on third parties for financial responsibilities. Without that personal commitment, there is no pressure to get well. We all have examples of that in our office; two categories are welfare and cap programs. Across the nation in all disciplines of healthcare, these are generally the two groups of patients who don't show for their appointments, don't do what you ask, and generally feel no responsibility for their actions. The result is financial and case failure. Financial commitment often begets healing. It is just human nature.

The other end of the spectrum is putting all the obligations on the patients upfront. In a utopian society, that would be wonderful. I have heard of practitioners — perhaps you're one of them — who always demand payment in full, upfront from everyone all the time. I wish it could be that way, but realistically if you want to build a solid volume, you must make some accommodations.

The most predictable strategy is to provide reasonable avenues for payment on your terms. Let me repeat, on your terms. You can't let patients say, "just bill me, doc," or your practice will be swallowed up. It's amazing how in one billing cycle you go from being the patient's savior to the villain. It builds resentment from you, your staff,

and the patients. Everybody ends up stressed from the whole process. However, when established financial plans are in place and followed with persistence, the system will work and produce satisfied patients who are willing to pay for your services.

You can never provide healthcare for every person in your community. It physically can't be done. You have to make a choice. Which patient would you rather position your office to provide care for?

Most practitioners daily set themselves up to provide care for the patients with the least invested in their health — patients who tax you and your staff emotionally and financially. Why not choose to serve those who are willing to invest in their care and provide you with opportunities to provide treatment options that will give them a chance for true healing and a pain-free life? We as practitioners are faced with two basic choices:

1. Follow the crowd. Drop treatment goals so low that we give the cheapest form of care and fool our patients into thinking they are getting all our professional and personal skills can offer. The scenario will fill the model for managed care cost containment. The risk is placed on your shoulders and off those of third parties while letting someone else make your decisions for you and your patients. This is the road most healthcare practitioners are traveling. Is this what you want? Will this satisfy your life's dreams?

2. The road not taken. Develop high standards for your program, learn to properly communicate, carefully monitor its successes with outcome's measurement, skillfully market the type of patients you wish to treat, and provide reasonable avenues of payment for your patients. All decisions for your patient's treatment will be between you and your patient. Is this what you want? Will this satisfy your life's dreams?

Two roads diverged in the woods and,
I took the one less traveled by
And that has made all the difference.

Robert Frost

Most people (95%) will not take this road. That leaves endless opportunities for those of us who choose to place ourselves in the top 5% of our fields. There are lots of patients who want to get well and demand the best. In essence, there is very little competition when it comes to excellence. There is much competition for mediocrity. But how are patients to know the difference? Can we assume because we know ourselves that our patients should automatically be aware of our skills? In reality, what if our clinical skills are just mediocre? What if we are just another office? Let's face it, if patients perceive all practitioners as being equal, then why not choose the cheapest? If you want a shirt and see the exact one you want in two places, why not choose the cheaper of the two?

To free your professional life, you must be able to make it obvious to patients that your office is different. Different is good. People like different. The first step in becoming a different and unique office is to do the things you love. You have to develop uniqueness about your practice — a position that allows your talents and those of your staff to stand out in the crowd.

USP

In the business world, this is known as a USP (Unique Service Position). In the healthcare sense of the term, it can be thought of as a type of speciality determined and defined by your talents, desires, and state practice laws. In other words, what makes you different from any other office so that people are willing to become your patients. Setting your goals also involves identifying your gifts. Make your job your love, your hobby. Ask yourself and your staff, "What does our office do better than any other office?" Sifting through all the different procedures can be difficult and you can expect some false starts. That's fine. It's part of the process. Don't become obsessed with your failures, but rather focus on your strengths. It may help to actually list the procedures that you consider more fun than work and determine which ones you do better than anyone else you know. When you find that area, then that can become your USP — the aspect of your office that makes you so unique that people are willing to bypass other clinicians to come to you; aspects of your practice that people are willing to gladly pay for even if their insurance companies fail to do so.

Some examples of USP in different disciplines are:

1. Dentistry: pain management, cosmetics, time spent with the individual
2. Medicine: work-related injuries, pain management, time spent with the individual
3. Chiropractic: myofascial therapy, corrective therapy, time spent with the individual
4. Massage: sports injuries, therapeutic touch, time spent with the individual
5. All disciplines: nutritional counseling, vitamin and botanical complementary care

As you may have noticed, one theme is listed consistently: time spent with the individual. Managed care is forcing clinicians to become more cost effective. One of the most obvious ways to do that is to spend less time with each patient. In this world of being a number, and computerized telephone screenings and statistics, people crave attention. It's sad to say but in today's world of practice, spending time with your patients is indeed a USP. It also touches one of the most basic of human needs: the need to be loved and paid attention to. Have you ever heard of patients complaining that a healthcare deliverer spent too much time with them? Of course not. But how many times have you heard just the opposite? No matter what your USP, the element of spending time with your patients is the most valued trait of all.

You must not only find your USP, but also develop it to the best of your ability. That will mean staff support in the growth process. It also will probably mean furthering your education. An important aspect of change and growth is making technology a strategic resource. Learning the importance of strategic technology is an important step because it affects every aspect of your practice. You need to ask the right questions and be sure you are getting the right answers.

It means your practice will become a work in progress. Make sure your USP aligns directly with your goals and that of your staff so your life will grow in the process. It will also help you achieve the all-important balance needed between your professional and personal life. Balance doesn't come easy. Most successful, happy people lead a well-rounded life. In the long run, this provides more reserves of energy, depth of character, and a stress-free perspective on life.

It don't come easy.

Ringo Starr

PATIENT PROFILE

After you have determined your USP, you need to define what type of patient you want to serve and are able to serve best. This is the next logical step in your journey toward freedom of choice in today's healthcare environment. It is also one of the most important elements of a successful, happy career. You can't please everyone. You can't serve everyone. When first starting to practice, most clinicians try to be all things to everyone. It's impossible but it's also natural to try. After all, most people who go into healthcare fields sincerely want to help others.

That's the way it should be. However, those who are wise learn early in their careers that you can't be all things to everybody. Those who try end up exhausted, burned out, and bitter. Most providers learn this lesson slowly over a long period of time, eventually finding a niche from which to practice. Any healthcare provider by accident or by design will develop a patient profile. We are constantly reminded of situations that we often take for granted.

Let's look at a few examples in the business world. Did you know that McDonald's target market is only 15%

of the entire population in the United States? In other words, around 85% of American citizens don't go to McDonald's. Rather than be discouraged about the numbers, McDonald's markets to the people who will go to McDonald's. When you enter under those golden arches, you know what you will get. It's all the same wherever you go. So what do you get at McDonald's? You get predictable food (not necessarily good), fast, at a cheap price. You know what you'll get, how fast you'll get it, and how much it'll cost in a clean, well-lit environment. Cloth napkins and candlelight? Forget it. A clown, maybe, and a toy in a Happy Meal™, but that's about it. Don't expect a sirloin steak or a private chef. You won't find them there. There are those people who want steaks and private chefs. There's nothing wrong with that. However, how much success would McDonald's achieve if they, along with their Big Mac™ and fries, offered filet mignon, baked Alaska, and a sushi bar? More than likely, it would spend a lot of money and actually lose hamburger sales in the process. Yet with focused marketing, McDonald's has consistently been one of the fastest growing companies in the world, all the while relinquishing 85% of the market. It can't please everyone but is determined to please the customer who wants its products.

Most healthcare providers carry the mental image that they have to serve everyone all the time. No matter how hard you try, you just can't do it. You have to define your population. If you choose to accept a managed care program, you are already defining your patient population based upon price. In fact, your target market is chosen for you. You may compete somewhat with other offices within the provider network, but the defining paradigm is price based. You have to decide if that is the arena in which you want to compete. If you've made the decision not to go the managed care road, then you and your staff need to define what type of patient you want to serve.

There are many ways to define your patient population. Many practitioners opt to define their patient population by procedure. If a person needs a certain procedure(s), then he or she fits the profile. There are other ways, though, that may help define your patient base. The possibilities include:

1. People without insurance who pay with cash, credit card, or check
2. People with only certain types of insurance.
3. People with indemnity insurance
4. People who pay cash upfront regardless of insurance coverage
5. Patients in a certain age bracket
6. Patients who can come in at certain times of the day
7. Patients who always show up on time
8. Patients who don't cancel their appointments at the last moment

9. Walk-ins
10. Emergency service

Defining a patient population is as diverse as the wants of the practitioners. It may take some creative thinking and time to find out just what type of patient fits your practice's needs. Discuss this with your staff. Their input is of the utmost importance and is crucial to your office growth.

THE 80/20 PRINCIPLE

When beginning to define your patient population, keep in mind the 80/20 principle. In fact, this principle is a great yardstick with which to measure all procedures and activities. Train your office to think in terms of 80/20.

Thinking in terms of 80/20 allows you to compare relationships, time, and productivity. Because 80% of your income will come from 20% of your patient load, the first place to begin modifying your practice is to define who those patients are. Concentrating on those patients will bring the most effective results. What does concentrating mean? It can mean marketing, continuing education, or just scheduling extra time with them to help establish better relationships. As a result, if those same 20% give you 80% of your practice pleasure, then your personal satisfaction and that of your staff will increase as well. The line between work and pleasure will begin to blur and practicing will become fun again.

The second step is to do something about the weaker 80% of your practice that only accounts for 20% of your production and satisfaction. Eliminating your biggest source of irritation may be the best place to start. For instance, one of the biggest aggravations and revenue losses for many practices are last-minute cancellations and "no shows." The lost time literally adds days to your work schedule and can be the biggest overhead costs that you are forced to bear. Instead of the doctor storming up to the front desk and yelling at his receptionist, why not start a "no cancellation policy" for your patients? Might you lose some patients in the process? Yes, but guess what? They will now be messing up someone else's schedule and not yours. Not only will you drop the aggravation, but you will also become much more productive and regain control of your schedule. Now you guide the schedule. Before it was left up to the weakest part of the team, the patients who saw very little value in your services. In other words, utilizing this technique instead of being controlled, you are able to take control and guide your practice in the direction you choose. As a result, one of your patient profile attributes may be people who value your services enough to keep their appointments.

Some patients will really challenge your staff. After all, they have no control over their lives — why should you? That's why it's important to have defined goals with team members who back up one another. This especially includes the doctor. Nothing will break the morale of the staff more quickly than a doctor undercutting a staff member after he or she has gone through the trouble of enforcing a rule upon which you have all agreed. It takes courage at first to hold fast to the rules but it pays off rapidly. Your office collectively makes up its mind and collectively enforces it.

Unless you decide to change the direction of your office entirely, chances are 80% of your patients do not fit your desired profile and 20% cause you most (80%) of your aggravation. Changes must be made on purpose. Your office will not improve by accident. Your office must develop an 80/20 mentality to grow and regain your practice freedom. You must constantly ask yourself, "What is the 20% that is leading to the 80% and which 80% is it leading to?" You must never assume that your office is on automatic pilot and your problems are solved. 80/20 thinking is not linear but rather part logical and part intuitive. Your practice situation cannot be analyzed strictly by the numbers. Allow your creativity to bloom. You will be amazed at how rapidly and effectively implementation of shared changes will positively affect the office. You will certainly get more from less. More personal time, more fun, more income, more satisfaction, and more happiness. The less? Less stress, fewer patients to see every day with better results, less conflict, and less frustration. There are really no boundaries to your success. As you grow, the boundaries grow as well.

The first reaction of many clinicians is that there is little chance of escaping from the low yield activities. They feel these time wasters are an essential part of their service to others. "I have to do XYZ," or put another way, "my patients would leave if I don't…." If you catch yourself thinking this way, think again. There is a great deal more leeway in your practice than you are accustomed to believing. The point of successful utilization of the 80/20 principle begins when you begin to think unconventionally. Following the crowd will get you just what the crowd gets. Don't expect anything more. But even if dropping low-value activities does require a radical change in your practice, you can deal with it. The other alternative is to watch your practice diminish a little at a time. Success and happiness will never be achieved.

Can you entirely eliminate problem areas? More than likely not unless you somehow decide to not treat or hire human beings. You can minimize those most troublesome areas, however, maximizing your happiness and productivity in the process. When you have identified the activities that take 20% of your time and yield 80% of the desired results, make plans to turn the 80/20 around. A short-term goal that is achievable is to nudge the 20% of the time spent on productive activities up to 40% within a year. This one change can have a profound effect on your practice.

Another wonderful by-product is being able to take more time off. Instead of having your time stolen one appointment at a time, those hours turn into days, which you and your staff can utilize for continuing education, community service, or just rest. The result is a happy, stable staff with sufficient time away from the office to remain excited and cultivate a positive mental attitude.

The 80/20 Principle by Richard Koch lists several ways to implement this rule into your every day life:

- Celebrate productivity rather than raise average efforts.
- Look for the short cut rather than run the full course.
- Exercise control over our lives with the least possible effort.
- Be selective, not exhaustive.
- Strive for excellence in a few things, rather than good performances in many things.
- Delegate as much as possible.
- Choose employees with extraordinary care.
- Only do the things we enjoy the most and do the best.
- Look beyond the obvious to uncover the ironies and oddities.
- In every circumstance work out where 20% of the effort can lead to 80% of the positive results.
- Calm down, work less. Rather than pursue every possible opportunity, target a limited number of very valuable goals where the 80/20 principle will work.
- Make the most of those few "lucky" streaks in life when we are at our creative peaks.

Remember the quote from Arnold Palmer, "Golf is a game of luck. The more I practice, the luckier I get."

The greatest part about utilizing the 80/20 principle in your life is that you do not need to wait for someone else to do it for you. You have the ability to turn your life into the one dreams are made of. You remember the dream for which you worked all those hours in school? The one that somehow got lost in the daily struggle to survive?

You have the ability within you to multiply all your highs and subtract all your lows. Your life can take on more and more relevance and shed the energy-draining time wasters. You can isolate all the great aspects that make you unique both personally and professionally and climb out of your daily rut. As an even greater plus, you can help your staff and patients achieve more than they had expected. People will appreciate you more because you appreciate them more. If you want to get the most from 80/20 thinking, you have to integrate it into your life. Will it take some effort? Of course it will! Let's face it — like it or not, changes are coming down the road for healthcare providers. The choice is not if your practice will change but rather how it will change. The choice of how you will change and adapt for your benefit and those of your staff and patients is still up to you.

MASTERMIND ALLIANCES

A mastermind alliance is a relationship built when two or more minds work together toward common goals. The mastermind principle lets you utilize the full strength, experience, knowledge, and training of other people with similar desires. You can overcome any challenge or achieve any goal in your practice if you use the mastermind principle effectively. No one has ever achieved outstanding success in any field without applying the mastermind principle. All great minds are stimulated to creativity through contact with others of like desires. Without this contact, you will run out of creative energy and get off track. The steps of forming a mastermind group are

1. Determine your purpose. A group cannot determine a purpose if the individuals have not done so first. You must be sure the purpose of the group is the same as yours. This doesn't have to be down to the detail, but very close. Once you have decided what purpose a group will fulfill for you, then move on to step two.

2. Select members of your alliance who will help you attain your goals. Don't select members because you know and like them. Save those relationships for social settings, if desired. Make sure each member has the ability to work in harmony with others. A person who totally dominates meetings will adversely affect the group. Discord will destroy your alliance. There must be a complete meeting of the minds without hesitation from any member. In the mastermind setting, personal ambitions must be subordinate to the success of the goals and purposes of alliance. The harmony of your alliance is built upon mutual respect and honesty.

3. Determine your rewards for being involved with a mastermind group. They can be whatever you find is needed. These will vary according to each individual member's personal needs.

4. Set a time and place for regular meetings. Your alliance must be a priority or other commitments will get in the way.

Your professional mastermind alliance does not have to consist solely of others in the same profession. The beauty of these relationships is that most creative solutions to obstacles often come from outside your given area. Individual healthcare providers are often guilty of thinking they have the market cornered on problems, thinking other disciplines couldn't understand their problems "because they're not like me."

A problem that is unique to any given profession does not exist. The same challenges occur in chiropractic, dentistry, medicine, massage therapy, automobile repair, selling shoes, etc. As long as you are dealing with people and their money, the basic problems are all the same; only the individual circumstances and procedures change. Allow yourself the privilege of tapping into the minds of people with a common purpose but different perspectives. It is an exhilarating experience.

MARKETING

Once your USP and your 80/20 patient profile are defined, then the next step is to let others know about it, in other words, marketing. As you know, marketing carries many connotations, from sincere helper to used car salesman. Marketing should be a natural extension of your personal self. A multitude of excellent marketing courses, books, and tapes are available. The most important aspects of any marketing program for your USP are

1. It fits with your desires (goals/focus).
2. It's easy to implement.
3. It's cost effective.
4. It has measurable results (it works and you can prove it).

Note that one of the aspects not listed is "expensive." Some practitioners think if you throw a lot of money at a marketing program, it will be effective. Not so. Some of the most effective marketing programs are inexpensive. While it may be a good ego boost to see your smiling face plastered all over town, it may do nothing for your practice. Remember one true fact: people want to feel special. Despite all the problems in the modern healthcare delivery system, people still generally respect caregivers and want their personal attention. Which is better: working in five extra patients a day to pay for a super expensive marketing program so you can see even more patients or perhaps seeing five fewer patients and spending more time with each one individually so your overhead is less and your patients are happy with your care? Expensive and effective don't always go hand in hand.

When making paradigm shifts within your office, start with the simple marketing programs first before you get into expensive, extensive ones. Include your staff in marketing decisions. They will appreciate it and be able to provide creative ideas that can be tailored to your individual needs. Marketing should be fun and productive. If it is not, then your goals and desires are not in alignment. Our main obstacle is not managed care or third-party payers and other various programs, but rather our lack of self-esteem, lack of determination, and lack of desire to succeed. Positioning your office for success is a matter of doing the right things, at the right time, all the time, and developing a plan and sticking to it. There is no doubt about it. There has been no better time to practice in the history of mankind. Opportunities for greatness are all around you. The choice is yours.

FINAL THOUGHTS

One of the main problems as practitioners is that we feel we are facing the future alone. Make no mistake about it, private practice and clinicians being the decision-makers are under attack by well-financed organizations. Still, every crisis creates great opportunity. The fact that so many practitioners are willing to follow the winds that blow them in any direction leaves those who wish to develop happy productive lives almost unlimited opportunities. By nature of the trends, niche markets are being created for creative thinkers at a greater rate than ever before. The avenues for healthcare practitioners to be successful are virtually unlimited and growing more so every day.

Don't expect to do things the way you used to and get good results. It won't work. Don't expect our overseeing governing organizations to help us. Just as our patients fall into the cracks of the healthcare system, we, the creative thinking practitioners, fall in the cracks of our representative organizations. It's important to associate with people of like minds to recharge your batteries and allow the creative juices to flow. There's an old saying, "We grow too soon old and too late smart." If you wish to be successful, then make the choice to do so. Don't follow the crowd. It will take courage to take those first steps but the results as defined by your goals that lead to your dreams will be worth the effort. Proverbs 1 through 5 explain how to achieve happiness, the ultimate goal of everyone who is reading this book. The following are the essential keys to happiness:

1. Wisdom. The ability to know what is right, true, and enduring; good judgment; knowledge; to accept counsel, criticism, and instructions without anger; and to always keep learning.
2. Understanding. Being able to perceive with your senses. To be able to internalize your knowledge with total comprehension and apply that knowledge to your individual circumstances.
3. Discretion. The ability to break down information into specialized parts. To be able to digest information, categorize, and sort data so decisions can be made simpler in lieu of distinct circumstances and desired results.
4. Insight. Perception of the truth and hidden nature of things. Insight is developed as a result of the culmination of all achievements. It is the ultimate strength from which you may operate. Insight is the beginning and result of wisdom.

Surround all these gifts with vigilance. Be attentive. Always watch, work, and hone your skills. Be disciplined. Your practice life is like that of an athlete who must constantly work out to keep his/her physical attributes ready when opportunity for success presents itself. If you're attentive, then your insight will allow you to recognize opportunities and give you the skills to achieve them. It will take care of you far beyond measurable achievements. You will be successful even when logic says you can't. Like the old maxim, "Those who say it can't be done often get in the way of those doing it." Success doesn't happen by accident.

Developing wisdom, understanding, discretion, and insight takes hours, months, and years. Success is the point at which preparedness meets opportunity. If you wait for things to happen and only then get ready, you will meet with frustration and a sense of loss. Opportunity knocks all the time. The trick isn't being there to open the door at the precise moment but rather living in a state of preparedness with the ability to react. Success often comes disguised as a problem rather than being perceived at first as "golden." Surround yourself with people who are positive and believe in your mission. Apply these truths to your life and you will always be happy. Seek and develop these skills and, no matter what, your success will never be in question. You already have the tools to develop all the opportunities you will ever need. Your talents in conjunction with proven applied principles will assure your success. You have a choice for the kind of future you desire and deserve. You no longer have to fear the future. Success or failure — which do you choose?

—81—

A Practical Approach to Outcomes Measurement

Michael E. Clark, Ph.D. and Ronald J. Gironda, Ph.D.

INTRODUCTION

Outcomes assessment has become one of the "catch-words" of the 21st century among healthcare systems. With the advent of the Joint Commission for Accreditation of Healthcare Organizations (JCAHO) pain standards (2000), insurance company practice parameters, and state and/or federal practice guidelines (Agency for Health Care Policy Reform, 92-0032; 94-0592) outcomes assessment has become a necessary component of pain practice irrespective of practice setting. A multitude of pain outcomes instruments or outcomes systems exist, yet little guidance is offered as to how to choose an appropriate instrument or set of instruments. Indeed, a literature search on the topic of "pain treatment outcomes" yielded numerous articles reporting pain treatment results using a variety of outcome measures, but no articles focusing on how to select an appropriate outcomes method.

In the absence of specific selection criteria, practitioners' choices of outcomes methods may be determined more by happenstance than need. Often, instrument availability, economics, and marketing serve as the primary determinants of instrument selection rather than outcomes objectives or empirical findings. The end result may be the selection of an outcomes measurement system that has limited reliability or validity, fails to meet the needs of the practice setting, requires extensive financial or temporal investments, or, on occasion, overwhelms the practitioner with mountains of irrelevant or even inaccurate data.

This void in outcomes assessment guidance is remedied in the ensuing pages. We offer clinicians a practical means of selecting and using outcomes measures in an efficient and rational manner. In this regard, we first briefly review the recent history of healthcare outcomes assessment and the factors that contribute to its importance in today's pain practices. Next, we discuss issues that need to be considered in the selection of outcomes measures, and briefly review the most useful pain outcomes instruments. Finally, we outline a method for developing an appropriate outcomes methodology based on specific practice needs and outcomes interest. Note that our intent is not to promote any specific outcomes methodology or outcomes instrument. Instead, we hope to provide a method whereby any clinician can determine what available instruments best meet the needs of his or her practice and the limits of the setting.

DEFINITION OF OUTCOMES MEASUREMENT

Outcomes measurement refers to the systematic collection and analysis of information that is used to evaluate the efficacy of an intervention. *Systematic collection* requires that data are collected in a consistent, repetitive manner using the same outcomes measures or instruments. *Analysis* refers to the process of summarizing and reviewing the data to identify any meaningful trends. Often this second stage of outcomes measurement is underutilized. Data may be collected but are either filed away and not used,

0-8493-0926-3/02/$0.00+$1.50
© 2002 by CRC Press LLC

or data summaries are prepared but never reviewed by the most appropriate individual or body.

Outcomes measures usually are collected prior to and following an intervention. In healthcare systems, usually we assume that the changes in health status we observe are the results of our intervention efforts. However, although outcomes measurement may involve very sophisticated procedures that are grounded strongly in science, in most cases it lacks the rigor of more formal research endeavors. Thus, it is important to remember that without additional data gathered in more controlled settings we cannot be certain that the observed changes result directly from our treatment efforts.

HISTORICAL PERSPECTIVE

The first systematic use of outcomes measurement in healthcare dates to the early 1900s when Ernest Codman, a surgeon at Massachusetts General Hospital, introduced a method of monitoring surgical outcomes (Campassi & Lee, 1995; Tarlov, 1995). Subsequently, in 1950 healthcare outcomes were included as one of three medical quality management tiers (Tarlov, 1995; Iezzoni, 1997). However, not until the late 1980s and early 1990s did healthcare outcomes monitoring became commonplace. In 1988 Ellwood proposed that an outcomes management technology be implemented to monitor the quality of healthcare service delivery (Ellwood, 1988). With the proliferation of managed care organizations, the focus on enhanced service delivery quality inherent in the early outcomes management approaches has expanded to include cost containment, improved patient satisfaction, and increased quality of life as additional goals.

RATIONALE FOR OUTCOMES MEASUREMENT

There are numerous reasons why pain treatment outcomes monitoring has become an integral part of today's healthcare delivery systems. In some treatment settings outcomes management is mandated by regulatory bodies. For example, outcomes assessment is part of the State of Maine's Department of Public Health's standards for pain management (Dreyer, 1998). Similarly, major healthcare accreditation organizations now require that the components and results of pain treatment efforts of member facilities are monitored. The Rehabilitation Accreditation Commission (CARF) has been at the forefront of these efforts by developing elaborate outcomes standards for pain treatment programs (1999). JCAHO (2000) adopted standards for pain management in Acute Care and Behavioral Health settings that were implemented beginning January 2001. In addition, the American Academy of Pain Management (AAPM) pain treatment accreditation requirements mandate that an outcomes management system be in place (1997).

Other national and local bodies also have begun to recognize the necessity of monitoring the effects of pain treatment. Pain treatment guidelines, which include standards for pain outcomes monitoring, have been developed or adopted by the Agency for Health Care Policy and Research (1992, 1996) and the American Pain Society (1995). These guidelines incorporate recommendations for pain outcomes monitoring, as does the National Pain Management Strategy implemented by the Department of Veterans Affairs (2000).

With the increasing emphasis on medical care cost containment, healthcare insurers have become more interested in the cost effectiveness of pain treatment (Kulich & Lande, 1997). As a result, outcomes data may be required to justify charges for selected pain interventions. Marketing efforts also may benefit from developing an outcomes measurement system in that competition for the healthcare dollar is rampant and evidence of enhanced outcomes and treatment efficacy may increase patient referrals. Additionally, professional responsibilities and ethics may imply the necessity of monitoring outcomes. For example, many professions require that we not implement treatments that we know are harmful or ineffective. Yet, if we do not monitor outcomes we have no way to determine whether our efforts are effective. And finally, outcomes data, although they are not generally as reliable as data from laboratory studies, provide us with an empirical basis for treatment decisions where before we had only opinion based on anecdotal observations of the effectiveness of treatments.

BARRIERS TO PAIN OUTCOMES MONITORING

Although regulatory, accreditation, professional, consumer, and payor interest in pain outcomes has stimulated a rapid growth in the development of pain outcomes management systems, it is important to remember that the initial and primary purpose of outcomes management in general, and pain outcomes assessment specifically, is *quality improvement*. Unfortunately, numerous examples exist where pain outcomes data have been used in a punitive (e.g., denial of claims, denial of services) rather than a quality improvement fashion, particularly when cost containment is the ultimate goal. As a result, some providers are reluctant to adopt rigorous outcomes methodologies. Yet it is our opinion that implementation of an appropriate pain outcomes management system provides the best defense to the misuse of data cited above. For example, the data cited to deny claims or services typically originate from local, regional, or national practitioner databases. These data reflect considerable variability in treatment approach, practitioner experience, and effectiveness and rarely include pain-specific outcomes. In fact, they are not true outcomes data at all, but rather reflect patterns of professional practice. The collection of practice-based, pain-specific outcomes data using reliable and validated instruments provides an excellent means of challenging denial practices, particularly if the outcomes information also demonstrates reductions in medical utilization (i.e., cost savings) following pain treatment.

Of course, numerous other barriers to adoption of a pain outcomes methodology exist (Rudy & Kubinski, 1999). Staff time to collect, summarize, and review data is necessary, and training in instrument administration and scoring may be required. Administrative approval and support must be obtained, along with funds to cover related external costs (e.g., instrument purchase, trainer or consultant's time). Patient and staff resistance and burden (e.g., time to complete the measures) should be anticipated and minimized prior to implementation.

FACTORS AFFECTING THE SELECTION OF OUTCOMES MEASURES

Several factors influence the selection of appropriate pain outcomes measures. They include the objectives of outcomes measurement, the type of pain treated, and the characteristics of the pain service setting.

OBJECTIVES OF OUTCOMES MEASUREMENT

Pain outcomes methodologies differ in their objectives. Patient-focused outcomes approaches are concerned primarily with evaluating and improving patient treatment outcomes. Service delivery outcomes approaches focus on monitoring and enhancing pain service delivery systems. Professional association outcomes guidelines or standards (International Association for the Study of Pain, 1991) often address the former, while standards for service delivery outcomes tend to originate with accreditation organizations (e.g., JCAHO). It is important to note that these two approaches are not mutually exclusive. More elaborate outcomes systems may include aspects of each. Indeed, some pain accreditation bodies (AAPM and CARF) require that both types of pain-related outcomes be addressed.

Patient-Focused Outcomes

Outcomes methods that are patient focused primarily are concerned with treatment-related changes in patients' pain experience. These are the outcomes most familiar to pain practitioners. To assess treatment-related change, at least two administrations (pretreatment and posttreatment) of the relevant outcome measures are required. Often a series of measures collected at intervals during the individual's treatment provides the best picture of progress and may give more information regarding the efficacy of changes in treatment (e.g., altering the type or dosage of pain medications) occurring within the overall treatment episode.

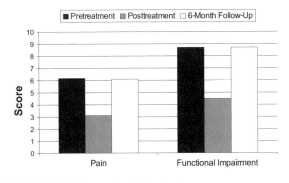

FIGURE 81.1 Effects of pain blockades.

Pain intensity is the most common patient-oriented measure, and typically is the outcome of greatest importance to the patient. Other key domains of patient functioning may include medication use, physical status (strength, flexibility), functional impairment, and emotional dysfunction, among others. Note, however, that the patients' primary interest will be pain relief. Numerous reliable and validated instruments are available to assess these other domains of pain outcomes (see "Pain Outcomes Instruments" for a limited review).

Patient-focused outcomes may be used in a number of ways. Information about average changes in pain measures following different treatment alternatives may assist the patient and the clinician in choosing which pain intervention best addresses the individual's pain problems and expectations. They also are a necessary component of *program evaluation* efforts that validate treatment effectiveness. The latter often are useful for marketing pain services or for increasing the likelihood of an insurer's payment for the services.

As an example, consider the hypothetical situation where providers at a university-based anesthesiology pain clinic decide to evaluate the effectiveness of their pain blockades. To accomplish this, they administer a multidimensional pain outcomes instrument to all patients with chronic nonmalignant pain undergoing the procedure prior to the first nerve block and again following the last nerve block. They also readminister the instrument 6 months after treatment to assess the short-term stability of any obtained changes. After 1 year of data collection (6 months of follow-up assessment) they graph their results, which are presented in Figure 81.1.

Based on these results, the providers conclude that the pain blockades appeared to provide some short-term pain relief and functional status improvement. However, they also conclude that the average benefits of the treatment were temporary, because after the 6 months following treatment the improvements had dissipated. As a result of these findings they decide to restrict their use of the procedure for the time being to individuals with severe acute pain or cancer pain, and to adopt other strategies for treating chronic nonmalignant pain.

Service Delivery-Focused Outcomes

Service delivery outcomes approaches are those that focus on the thoroughness and efficiency of the pain service delivery system rather than on patient outcomes per se. Service delivery outcomes measures are used to evaluate the performance of the service delivery system as it applies to the provision of pain treatment services. Performance measures may be compared to goals established by the service delivery organization, regulatory bodies, or to standards developed by accrediting bodies. Often this type of outcomes measurement approach is linked closely to quality improvement (QI) programs, where the ultimate goal is to improve the delivery of health services.

The recent dissemination of JCAHO pain standards has stimulated healthcare systems to develop measures to address service delivery outcomes. Unlike patient-oriented outcomes approaches where numerous reliable and validated outcomes instruments are available, data regarding service delivery outcomes generally are derived from compliance reviews of patient care documentation. Most often these reviews are conducted by randomly selecting and manually reviewing records to determine whether pain-related documentation is present, and if so, whether it meets the applicable standards. Standards may be those established by an external body (e.g., JCAHO) or those developed within the healthcare organization and adopted as policy.

Because the provision of pain services first requires the identification of individuals with a "pain problem," methods for differentiating between those with and without significant pain must be developed. Given that the JCAHO pain standards require that all patients be screened for pain (Joint Commission for the Accreditation of Healthcare Organizations, 2000), one way to identify those requiring further pain assessment and treatment is to define a pain intensity "trigger value." When a patient reports a pain intensity equaling or exceeding this value, the need for additional pain services is established. Service delivery outcomes measures then may be used to determine how well these pain services were delivered. Determining which specific outcomes measures to include depends on the objectives associated with the overall outcomes management program. Often selection of at least some of the measures will be determined by relevant outcomes standards or service delivery policies.

Consider the following example. A large tertiary care medical center that serves as a regional trauma center has identified reduction of debridement pain in its burn unit as a primary facility goal, motivated in part by concern over an upcoming JCAHO survey. An initial QI plan has been developed to monitor changes in debridement pain ratings as the first step in the process. Pain scores are collected every 15 minutes from all patients undergoing the procedure on each of four burn unit teams. Data are collected for 1 month. Results are presented in Figure 81.2.

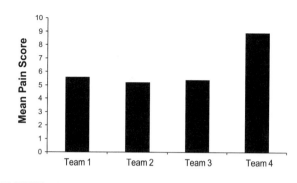

FIGURE 81.2 Mean pain ratings during burn debridement.

Based on these service delivery outcomes data, a QI plan is developed. Components of the plan include training staff to better assess and treat pain, educating patients regarding their pain treatment rights and the range of pain interventions that may be implemented, improving patient-controlled analgesia options, and reviewing Team 4's practices in detail to identify what factors (including chance effects) account for their lower levels of pain relief. During the QI process, pain ratings data will continue to be collected, and the interventions identified above will be implemented in steps to allow estimates of the relative impact of each.

Other examples of possible service delivery outcomes derived from the recent JCAHO standards include

- Percent of patients with significant pain who have a plan of pain care in their medical records.
- Percent of patients with significant pain where pain education was provided to the patient and family.
- Percent of patients with significant pain where evidence exists that pain interventions were provided.
- Patient satisfaction ratings of the service delivery system and service environment.

All of the above examples include a patient-focused pain measure (i.e., pain intensity) as the basis for identifying the patient population of interest. However, the primary intent of each is to evaluate the efficiency of the delivery of pain services rather than the effectiveness of pain treatments.

TYPE OF PAIN

Determining which patient outcomes domains to measure also depends on the type of pain typically treated in the setting of interest. For example, in a post-surgical unit, acute pain is likely to be the primary focus. Goals of pain treatment typically are limited to pain reduction. In this situation, pain intensity measures, collected over time (e.g., 1-hour periods), may be the only pain outcomes

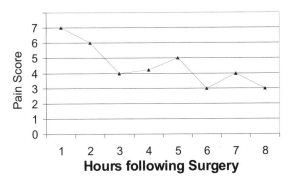

FIGURE 81.3 Pain scores over time on a postsurgical recovery unit.

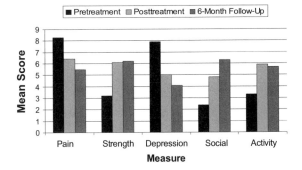

FIGURE 81.4 Changes in pain outcomes.

measure of importance. An example of the results of this type of outcomes evaluation is presented in Figure 81.3, and could be used to support the effectiveness of the pain treatment methods used in this setting.

Contrast this with a setting where chronic nonmalignant pain is the most frequent presenting problem. Chronic pain treatment goals generally encompass changes in many domains of function beyond pain reduction. Therefore, an appropriate outcomes measurement system should include multidimensional measures of pain-related functioning (International Association for the Study of Pain, 1991). Figure 81.4 illustrates some of the changes in these measures that might be expected following treatment. Note that the chronic pain outcomes include pretreatment, posttreatment, and follow-up measures of functioning. Changes in measures from pretreatment to posttreatment support the short-term efficacy of the interventions. However, the overarching goal of chronic pain treatment is to modify patients' long-term behaviors and adjustment. Therefore, readministration of the multidimensional measures at a point following treatment cessation is one way to assess the stability of treatment-related changes, and is required by some pain program accreditation bodies (American Academy of Pain Management, 1997; CARF, 1999). Table 81.1 summarizes suggested domains of outcomes relevant to specific types of pain.

TABLE 81.1
Recommended Outcomes Domains by Type of Pain

Acute Pain	Cancer Pain	Chronic Pain
Pain intensity	Pain intensity	Pain intensity
	Physical impairment	Physical impairment
	Interpersonal impairment	Interpersonal impairment
	Emotional dysfunction	Emotional dysfunction
	Activity level	Activity level
	Sleep difficulties	Pain-related fears
	Sexual impairment	Recreational impairment
		Sleep difficulties
		Vocational impairment
		Sexual impairment

PRACTICE SETTING

Practice setting refers to characteristics of the pain service delivery environment. Primary among these are the type and complexity of pain treatment services provided and the degree of administrative support.

Nature of Pain Services

Pain treatment encompasses a wide variety of interventions delivered in a multitude of settings. Some may involve minimal healthcare resources (medication management) while others may be highly technical (dorsal column stimulator implants) or lengthy (comprehensive multidisciplinary treatment). In general, the complexity of the outcomes system utilized should parallel that of the corresponding practice setting. That is, settings utilizing minimal treatment resources (total staff time and equipment) do not require, nor do they justify, elaborate outcomes measurement. In contrast, treatment settings with high resource demands (i.e., higher treatment costs) should utilize a broader spectrum of outcomes measures to detect change (or lack of change) in multiple outcomes domains.

A brief example may clarify this point. In an outpatient, single-provider pain clinic where the primary mode of pain treatment is pharmacological and resource demand is low, the associated patient-focused measures might be limited to pain intensity ratings and some brief measure of pain interference. A service delivery-focused measure, such as patient waiting times, also might be added. In contrast, an inpatient or outpatient pain surgical intervention practice, where resource demand is high, might be expected to monitor multiple patient-focused (pain intensity, functional impairment, changes in emotional status, return to work, etc.) and service delivery-focused (complication rates, surgical time, costs) over a longer timeframe.

Administrative Support

In the ideal practice setting, there would be no relationship between the type of outcomes system adopted and the degree of administrative support available. Unfortunately, in most cases, the degree of administrative support has a large impact on selection of an outcomes approach. Given the costs involved (i.e., supplies, contracts, and staff time), administrators may be reluctant to approve outlays for programs with no direct financial returns.

There are several steps a provider can take to maximize administrative support for pain outcomes measurement. First, identify all regulatory (state or federal), professional, and accreditation standards or guidelines that apply. Next, identify any local pain standards of practice that include pain outcomes requirements. Third, gather any available pain outcomes materials from local competing providers. Refer to these standards, regulations, and local outcomes data in the body of the pain outcomes proposal. It may be helpful to include some examples of consequences experienced by providers or settings that did not abide by the appropriate outcomes requirements as an additional means of persuasion. Last, meet with the administrative representative and present the basis and anticipated costs for the pain outcomes measurement program. Compromise may be necessary, but if the proposal is complete, well documented, and involves reasonable costs, the likelihood of approval will be maximized.

PAIN OUTCOMES INSTRUMENTS

Selection of appropriate instruments to use in a pain outcomes program requires some familiarity with basic measurement principals. Test *reliability* refers to the constancy of measurement; that is, the extent that the instrument yields similar results when administered under identical or very similar circumstances (Johnston, Keith, & Hinderer, 1992). If an instrument is unreliable, it is likely to generate inconsistent results that reflect the random effects of error rather than any systematic change attributable to treatment factors. Reliability is a necessary condition for *validity*, but adequate reliability does not ensure validity (Green, 1992). Validity generally refers to the degree to which the instrument measures what it was designed to measure (Johnston, Keither, & Hinderer, 1992). There are several types of validity which are assessed by different methods. In this review, we have chosen to emphasize *concurrent validity*, or how well the instrument or measure compares to other established ("gold standard") measures of the construct or variable. Measures with good concurrent validity exhibit relatively high and clinically significant correlations with established measures of the pain domain under study. Measures adopted for use as part of a patient-focused outcomes system should exhibit adequate reliability and validity (CARF, 1999). If they are to

be used in multidisciplinary settings, they also should conform to the Measurement Standards for Interdisciplinary Medical Rehabilitation established by the American Congress of Rehabilitation Medicine (Johnston, Keith, & Hinderer, 1992).

It is important to note that adequate test or measure validity and reliability do not ensure that a measure is appropriate for the outcomes context of interest. Although the determination of the appropriateness of a measure usually is a simple task (e.g., evaluating whether the education or knowledge requirements for completing the measure are consistent with the target population's abilities), occasions when the inappropriateness of a pain measure may not be immediately apparent do exist. For example, consider the situation where an outpatient, hospital-based pain treatment clinic wants to evaluate the effectiveness of its pain treatments. The clinic is in an urban area, with limited parking facilities, and caters mostly to elderly, inactive patients with multiple pain complaints. Clinic providers decide to use an 11-point (0 to 10) pain rating scale (a reliable and well-validated measure of pain intensity) as the primary effectiveness measure, administered prior to every visit. Patients are asked to report their current levels of pain using the 11-point scale. Data are collected and reported for a 6-month period. Results reveal no change in pain scores over time, and clinic staff members conclude that their efforts are not effective.

Are these conclusions justified? Probably not, as the question asked (current pain intensity) likely was not the best measure of pain intensity in this situation. Consider the difficulty this group of patients experiences in reporting for their appointments. They must prepare themselves for travel, arrange travel to the appointment, transport themselves to the clinic area, and sit in uncomfortable chairs waiting to be seen. As a result, their "current pain" rating may be closer to a "worst pain" rating, and may not accurately reflect the effectiveness of treatment. A better pain measure might instead be their "usual pain" which is less affected by the transient influences of the situation. Figure 81.5 presents hypothetical differences

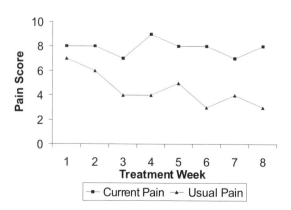

FIGURE 81.5 Pain scores over time.

TABLE 81.2
Domains of Outcome Assessed by Unidimensional Measures

Measure (Items)	Pain Intensity	Pain Interference	Emotional Distress	Pain-Related Fear
NRS/VAS (1)	Current, average, best, worst	—	—	—
MPQ (20)	Pain Rating Index	—	—	—
PDI (7)	—	Pain interference in role functioning	—	—
SIP (136)	—	Pain interference in physical, psychosocial, and overall functioning	—	—
BDI (21)	—	—	Depression	—
CES-D (20)	—	—	Depression	—
STAI (40)	—	—	Anxiety	—
PASS (40)	—	—	—	Pain-related fear and avoidance
TS (17)	—	—	—	Pain-related fear and avoidance

Note: NRS/VAS = Numeric Rating Scale/Visual Analog Scale; MPQ = McGill Pain Questionnaire; PDI = Pain Disability Index; SIP = Sickness Impact Profile; BDI = Beck Depression Inventory; CES-D = Center for Epidemiologic Studies-Depression Scale; STAI = State-Trait Anxiety Inventory; PASS = Pain Anxiety Symptoms Scale; TS = Tampa Scale.

between current and usual pain ratings gathered under these conditions, and clearly illustrates the desirability of carefully considering all aspects of a meas-ure when evaluating appropriateness.

There are several pain-specific self-report instruments that may be used to assess treatment outcome. The following review of selected pain treatment outcomes measures is limited to measures that have been validated with pain patient samples and were judged by the authors to have some utility for outcomes assessment. Absent from this review are several well-validated measures, such as the Coping Strategies Questionnaire (CSQ) (Rosensteil & Keefe, 1983), which tap important aspects of the pain experience and have been widely used in pain research, but lack significant evidence of utility for general pain outcomes assessment. For the reader who is interested in a wider range of pain measures, more comprehensive reviews may be found elsewhere (Bradely, Haile, & Jaworski, 1992; Jensen & Karoly, 1992; Tait, et al., 1987).

Both unidimensional and multidimensional pain outcomes measures are reviewed in the following pages. Criteria for inclusion in this review were (1) evidence of acceptable reliability; (2) data supporting instrument validity (particularly concurrent validity); (3) prior use as a pain outcomes instrument; and (4) high utility for pain outcomes assessment, as judged by the authors.

UNIDIMENSIONAL MEASURES

In contrast to standards for acute pain treatment, current chronic pain treatment standards necessitate the assessment of outcomes across multiple dimensions of functioning (CARF, 1999). Although specific standards vary by type of pain, treatment modality, and practice standards, comprehensive pain treatment outcomes measurement generally includes the assessment of pain intensity, pain interference, emotional distress, vocational functioning, patient satisfaction, and medical resource utilization. The most common approach to assessing multiple outcomes domains is to assemble a battery of unidimensional instruments, each of which measures a single pain outcomes domain. In the following sections, we attempt to provide readers with several choices of acceptable unidimensional outcomes instruments within each outcomes domain. A summary of key unidimensional instrument characteristics is presented in Table 81.2.

Pain Intensity

Pain intensity measures form the basis of all pain treatment outcomes measurement approaches and are essential for most pain service delivery outcomes measures as well. Luckily, the measurement of pain intensity is perhaps the simplest component of outcomes assessment, and there are several easy-to-administer, psychometrically sound scales available. The three broad categories of commonly used pain intensity measures include the Visual Analog Scale (VAS), Numeric Rating Scale (NRS), and Verbal Rating Scale (VRS). The VAS and NRS typically consist of a single item requiring the patient to quantify the intensity of his or her "current," "usual," "least," or "worst" pain. Empirical evidence suggests that the combination of "least" and "usual" pain ratings provide the best estimate of actual pain intensity, while "least" may be the single most accurate predictor (Jensen, et al., 1996). However, for practical purposes clinicians can have confidence in the choice of a single VAS or NRS rating of "usual" pain, which appears to provide a reasonably valid estimate of actual pain. Interestingly, "current" and "worst" pain ratings were found to have a weaker relationship with actual pain intensity (Jensen, et al., 1996).

A reliable and well-validated form of the VAS is a 10-cm line anchored with the phrases "no pain" and "worst possible pain" or "excruciating pain." Patients are instructed to bisect the line at the point that best represents their level of pain, and the score is simply the length of the segment to that point. The VAS has been found to be valid and sensitive to changes in acute, cancer, and chronic pain (Breivik, Bjornsson, & Skovlund, 2000; DeConno, et al., 1994; Ogon, et al., 1996), and it yields ratio level data (Jensen, et al., 1992). Although comparisons of horizontal and vertical line orientations yield mixed results, using the VAS horizontally may provide slightly higher sensitivity (Ogon, et al., 1996; Jensen, et al., 1999).

The NRS consists of a numeric range from 0 to 10 or 100 with anchors similar to those of the VAS, and can be administered in oral or written form. Individuals are asked to quantify their pain levels by choosing a single number from the 11- or 101-point scale. The NRS has been found to have good psychometric characteristics (Jensen, et al., 1999) and to be sensitive to changes in acute, cancer, and chronic pain (DeConno, et al., 1994; Paice & Cohen, 1997). The data provided by the NRS can be treated as ratio level (Jensen & Karoly, 1992).

Verbal rating scales typically consist of a list or lists of pain descriptors that are rank ordered along a continuum of severity. Patients are asked to select the most appropriate descriptor or set of descriptors, and a score is assigned based on the rank(s) of the chosen word(s) (Jensen & Karoly, 1992). The McGill Pain Questionnaire (MPQ) (Melzack, 1975a) is a well-validated, widely used VRS that consists of 20 lists of descriptors of the sensory, affective, and evaluative dimensions of pain (Melzack, 1975b). Support for the tripartite structure of the MPQ is mixed, and factor analyses generally reveal significant overlap among factors (Donaldson, 1995; Holroyd, et al., 1992; Turk, Rudy, & Saolovey, 1985). The standard scoring procedure yields a Pain Rating Index (PRI) for each of the three subscales, although in practice these subscales are often summed to create a single PRI. The PRI has been shown to be sensitive to change and valid for use among acute, cancer, and chronic populations (Davis, 1989; Lowe, Walker, & MacCallum, 1991; Sist, et al., 1998). However, as is true of other verbal scales, it only yields ordinal level data because questions have been raised about the assumption of equidistance between ranked descriptors (Choiniere & Amsel, 1996).

Practical considerations suggest that the VAS or the NRS may be preferred to the MPQ or other verbal scales for the clinical assessment of pain intensity as they provide psychometrically superior data that are relatively easy to collect and score. When ease of administration and scoring are of greatest concern, the 11-point NRS may be the best choice. In contrast, when greater measurement precision is desirable, the advantage goes to the VAS or to the 101-point NRS.

Pain Interference

A central goal of pain intervention is to reduce the extent to which pain impairs physical activity, emotional functioning, and psychosocial role fulfillment. Several unidimensional measures of pain interference are available to assess the degree and nature of pain-related limitations in one or more domains of functioning. It should be noted that although some of these measures, such as the Sickness Impact Profile (SIP), tap pain interference across multiple domains of functioning, the primary construct assessed is the single dimension of pain-related impairment. These measures of pain interference should not be confused with instruments that simply quantify functional status and do not attempt to account for the role of pain in an individual's level of impairment. This difference is illustrated by the contrast between the SIP psychosocial scale, which measures the extent of emotional and social difficulties that are attributed to the pain condition, and the Beck Depression Inventory (BDI) (Beck, 1987), which assesses depressive symptomatology without concern for etiology.

The Pain Disability Index (PDI) (Pollard, 1984) is a seven-item measure of pain interference in physical and psychosocial role performance. The PDI has good internal consistency ($\alpha = 0.87$) (Tait, et al., 1987) and 1-week test–retest reliability (intraclass $r = 0.91$) (Gronblad, et al., 1993), and it has been shown to effectively discriminate groups of pain patients with varying levels of disability (Tait, Chibnall, & Krause, 1990). The measure appears to be sensitive to change (Strong, Ashton, & Large, 1994), and it is valid for use with chronic and post-operative pain patients (Pollard, 1984). Factor analysis supports the classification of the PDI as a unidimensional measure of pain interference (Tait, Chibnall, & Krause, 1990). The PDI has practical appeal as a brief, easy-to-use, and psychometrically sound measure of general pain interference when less comprehensive assessment of pain-related disability is adequate.

The SIP is a widely used, 136-item measure of perceived impairment (Brown, 1995; Williams, 1988) with high test–retest reliability (0.92) and internal consistency (0.94) (Bergner, et al., 1981). The SIP administration instructions were altered by Turner and Clancy (Turner & Clancy, 1988) to reflect pain-related impairment rather than general physical impairment. The 14 SIP subscales assess pain interference across a wide range of functioning, and they are combined to form the Physical, Psychosocial, and Total scales. The SIP scales have been found to possess good concurrent validity in chronic pain and cancer pain patients (Beckham, et al., 1997; Watson & Graydon, 1989), and they are sensitive to change resulting from multidisciplinary inpatient treatment for chronic pain (Jensen, et al., 1992). From a practical standpoint, the main weaknesses of the SIP are its length and the relative difficulty of scoring the inventory. In addition, individuals with pain may find many SIP items to be less face valid and relevant to their conditions than those of measures developed specifically to tap pain-related disability. Nevertheless, the SIP remains the gold standard for detailed assessment of self-reported pain interference.

Emotional Distress

Although the measures of emotional distress presented here are not pain specific, they are widely used in pain intervention outcomes assessment. This reflects the considerable association between emotional distress and pain, the importance of treating concurrent depression and anxiety, and the recognition that psychological variables can have a significant impact on treatment outcome. The following emotional distress measures were selected based upon their brevity, convenience, and general acceptance among pain researchers for outcomes assessment.

The BDI is a 21-item measure of depressive symptomatology (Beck, 1987). This widely used instrument has been shown to have adequate psychometric properties (Beck, Steer, & Garbin, 1988), and it is sensitive to change resulting from multidisciplinary pain clinic treatment (Kleinke, 1991). The BDI discriminates well between chronic pain patients with and without depression (Geisser, Roth, & Robinson, 1997). However, researchers have raised questions about the appropriateness of using the BDI to detect depression among pain patients (de C. Williams & Richardson, 1993). Several BDI items contain somatic content (e.g., sleep disturbance, fatigability, and somatic preoccupation) that is confounded with commonly observed symptoms of chronic pain syndromes, and several studies have suggested that pain patients may produce higher scores on these items as a function of their pain-related physical symptomatology (Plumb & Holland, 1977; Wesley, et al., 1999). While this may limit total score comparisons with nonpain populations, removal of the somatic items has not been found to improve the accuracy of the measure for discriminating depressed from nondepressed chronic pain patients (Geisser, Roth, & Robinson, 1997). Consequently, clinicians may choose to use the BDI for treatment outcomes, although accurate classification of depressive symptomatology may require higher cutoffs.

An alternative measure of depression favored by some researchers for pain outcomes is the 20-item Center for Epidemiologic Studies-Depression Scale (CES-D) (Radloff, 1977). The CES-D has high internal reliability ($\alpha = 0.85$) in normal populations and good concurrent validity in chronic and cancer pain populations (Beckham, et al., 1997; Radloff, 1977). The CES-D may be somewhat more sensitive to change than the BDI (Turk & Okifuji, 1994). Normed on a normal population, the CES-D suffers from many of the same limitations as the BDI, potentially producing a high number of false positives among chronic and cancer pain patients. However, like the BDI, the CES-D has been shown to discriminate between chronic pain patients with and without depression, and removal of somatic items did not appreciably improve accuracy (Geisser, Roth, & Robinson, 1997; Turk & Okifuji, 1994). Nonetheless, higher cutoffs should be used in pain populations.

The impact of anxiety on pain treatment outcome has not been studied as extensively as that of depression. However, the existing evidence suggests a high concordance between pain and anxiety (Polantin, et al., 1993), and the need to address these symptoms in comprehensive pain intervention is well recognized. The State–Trait Anxiety Inventory (STAI) is a 40-item self-report inventory of state and trait anxiety that possesses adequate psychometric properties (Spielberger, et al., 1983), and is widely used for pain outcomes measurement. The STAI is sensitive to change (Mongini, Defilippi, & Negro, 1997) and is an adequate choice for the clinician wishing to quantify levels of both acute anxiety and the more stable tendency to perceive one's environment as threatening.

Pain-Related Fear

Recently, researchers have begun to focus on the role of pain-specific emotional distress in the experience of pain. Emerging data indicate that pain-specific emotional distress, particularly pain-related fear, may play a more important role than general levels of affective disturbance in the development and maintenance of pain-related physical disability (McCracken, Faber, & Janeck, 1998). The construct of pain-related fear may be defined broadly as the fear of pain and the avoidance of behaviors that are anticipated to produce painful sensation or injury. Although no evidence currently exists linking levels of pain-related fear to treatment outcome, the available data suggest that pain-related fear may seriously compromise an individual's willingness to initiate and persist in the degree of physical reactivation and restoration that is essential to reversing the progression of pain-related disability. Accordingly, clinicians and researchers are beginning to pay more attention to the role of pain-related fear in pain treatment outcome.

Of the few available unidimensional measures of pain-related fear, the Pain Anxiety Symptoms Scale (PASS) (McCracken, Zayfert, & Gross, 1992) and the Tampa Scale (TS) (Kori, Miller, & Todd, 1990) are the most promising. The PASS is the longer of the two measures, with 40 items assessing cognitive and pain-related physiological anxiety symptoms, escape and avoidance responses, and fearful appraisal of pain (McCracken, Zayfert, & Gross, 1992). The four PASS subscales have good internal consistency (McCracken, Zayfert, & Gross, 1993), and the total score has good predictive validity and appears to be adequate for

TABLE 81.3
Domains of Outcome Assessed by Multidimensional Measures

Outcome Dimensions	BPI (32)	MPI (52)	NPDB–VA v.2 (74)
Pain intensity	Right now, average, least, worst	Pain severity subscale	Usual (0–10 NRS)
Pain interference	Pain interference in physical functioning	Pain interference in physical functioning; activity level	Pain interference in physical functioning; activity level
Emotional distress	Pain interference in mood and interpersonal relations	Emotional distress; support/response from others	Emotional distress; pain interference in interpersonal activities
Pain–related fear	—	—	Pain-related fear
Vocational functioning	—	—	Employment status; pain work interference
Medical resource utilization	—	—	Inpatient and outpatient visits; surgeries
Patient satisfaction	—	—	Satisfaction with various treatment components

Note: BPI = Brief Pain Inventory; MPI = Multidimensional Pain Inventory; NPDB-VA v.2 = National Pain Data Bank-VA Version 2, NRS, Numeric Rating Scale.

outcomes assessment (McCracken, Faber, & Janeck, 1998). Scores on the PASS have been found to predict self-reported pain severity, disability, pain behavior, and range of motion on straight leg raise (McCracken, et al., 1993; McCracken, et al., 1996). In addition, pain patients classified as "dysfunctional" by the Multidimensional Pain Inventory (MPI) (Kerns, Turk, & Rudy, 1985) were more likely to produce high scores on the PASS than those classified as "interpersonally distressed" or as "adaptive copers" (Asmundson, Norton, & Allerdings, 1997).

Perhaps a better measure of the pain-related anxiety is the TS, a 17-item instrument developed to assess kinesiophobia, or the fear of movement and activity due to concerns about injury or reinjury (Kori, Miller, & Todd, 1990). Although limited, recent evidence suggests that the TS may possess greater predictive validity than the PASS and other measures of pain-related fear. The TS has been found to be a superior predictor of a range of pain symptoms and behaviors, even after controlling for known confounding factors such as pain intensity and duration, gender, and negative emotionality. For example, the TS was an incrementally valid predictor of self-reported disability and behavioral performance during a lifting task after controlling for pain onset, lower extremity radicular pain, and pain intensity, while the PASS was not (Crombez, et al., 1999). In addition, the TS has been found to be a superior predictor of disability as compared to pain intensity, biomedical signs and symptoms, and negative emotionality (Crombez, et al., 1999; Vlaeyen, et al., 1999). Although no data on the ability of either the TS or the PASS to capture treatment-related change exist, either measure may be appropriate. However, given its superior predictive validity and shorter length, the TS appears to be the instrument of choice for assessing treatment-induced changes in pain-related fear.

Advantages and Disadvantages of Unidimensional Instruments

Unidimensional pain outcomes instruments generally are easily available, inexpensive, and necessitate minimal administration training time. Additionally, they are an efficient means of collecting data when only a single or a few selected outcomes domains are to be assessed. Unfortunately, using unidimensional measures to assess multidimensional pain treatment outcomes requires assembling a battery of individual instruments. The idiosyncratic nature of these batteries often restricts or prevents comparisons between local outcomes data and community benchmarked data. In addition, some of these instruments are quite lengthy and may include items that are not directly relevant to pain. Thus, while unidimensional measures may be the most efficient means of collecting pain data for one or two selected pain outcomes domains, the use of many unidimensional measures to cover all key chronic pain outcomes domains may decrease the utility of the obtained data while increasing staff and patient burden.

MULTIDIMENSIONAL MEASURES

In response to the limitations associated with batteries of unidimensional instruments, a few multidimensional pain outcomes tools have been developed. Three of these are discussed below. Perhaps due to differences in the nature and extent of acute, cancer, and chronic pain conditions, two of these three instruments were developed to assess a specific type of pain. Validation of each of these three measures has been restricted largely to the types of pain for which the instrument was originally developed. Table 81.3 presents a comparison of the key features of these instruments, while Table 81.4 summarizes the strength of concurrent validity support for the instruments across acute, cancer, and chronic nonmalignant pain populations.

TABLE 81.4
Concurrent Validation Support
for Multidimensional Measures

Measure	Acute	Cancer	Chronic Nonmalignant
BPI	Moderate	Strong	None
MPI	None	Weak	Strong
NPDB-VA	None	None	Moderate

Brief Pain Inventory

The Brief Pain Inventory (BPI) (Cleeland & Ryan, 1994) is a 32-item instrument developed to assess pain history, pain intensity, perceived recent response to medication/treatment, and pain interference. The BPI is well validated among cancer and chronic disease pain patients, and it has been translated into several languages. Factor analytic studies consistently have revealed the two factors of pain severity and interference across samples and language versions (Caraceni, et al., 1996; Radbruch, et al., 1999; Saxena, Mendoza, & Cleeland, 1999; Wang, et al., 1996). However, empirical data are limited mostly to cancer and chronic disease samples, and little is known about the sensitivity to change or psychometric properties of the instrument when used with chronic pain populations.

Multidimensional Pain Inventory

The MPI, formerly the West Haven–Yale Multidimensional Pain Inventory, is a popular pain measure that was developed to facilitate the comprehensive assessment of chronic pain patients (Kerns, Turk, & Rudy, 1985). Designed to be used in conjunction with behavioral and psychophysiological measures, the 52 items comprise 12 subscales that are dispersed across three sections: (1) pain intensity, pain interference, dissatisfaction with current functioning, appraisal of support from others, perceived life control, and affective distress; (2) punishing, solicitous, and distracting responses from significant others to displays of pain behaviors; and (3) frequency of the performance of household chores, outdoor work, activities away from home, and social activities (Kerns, Turk, & Rudy, 1985). The 12 subscales possess good internal consistency (α = 0.70 to 0.90) and acceptable 2-week test–retest reliability (r = 0.62 to 0.91). Adequate levels of unique variance and concurrent validity have been demonstrated for most scales (Kerns, Turk, & Rudy, 1985). The MPI appears to be sensitive to change, but the utility of specific subscales may vary across levels of adaptation and functioning (Strategier, et al., 1997).

In addition to the measurement of treatment outcomes, the MPI has been used to classify chronic pain patients in order to identify major treatment needs. Cluster analyses have yielded a three-group typology of chronic pain

patients consisting of dysfunctional, interpersonally distressed, and adaptive copers or minimizers categories (Turk & Rudy, 1990). Clinicians may find this typology useful for purposes such as planning pain treatment or testing the effectiveness of different interventions or intervention components across MPI groups of patients.

National Pain Data Bank

The National Pain Data Bank (NPDB) is a software-driven, outcomes package consisting of intake, posttreatment, and follow-up questionnaires. The NPDB was developed specifically to assess treatment outcomes, and it is the only measure that encompasses all of the domains of functioning typically considered to be essential to comprehensive outcomes measurement. The outcomes package allows the clinician to track changes in pain intensity, pain interference, emotional distress, pain-related fear, vocational functioning, patient satisfaction, perceived improvement, and medical resource utilization from intake through follow-up, obviating the need to use more than one measure. In addition, a large database of benchmark data is available to allow comparisons with the outcomes of similar modalities across the nation, a requirement of many pain treatment standards (e.g., CARF). Selected subsets of NPDB items have been found to have moderate (0.73) to high (0.94) internal reliability (American Academy of Pain Management, 1997). A preliminary investigation of the psychometric properties of the instrument among a chronic pain impatient sample revealed that the NPDB demonstrated good concurrent validity in relation to a number of widely accepted gold standard measures of pain-related impairment (Clark & Gironda, 2000). Analysis of the final data set has confirmed the preliminary findings, and investigations of test–retest reliability, concurrent validity, and sensitivity to change are currently being conducted.

Advantages and Disadvantages of Multidimensional Measures

Multidimensional pain outcomes measures have several advantages relative to unidimensional measures. Because these instruments were specifically designed for pain populations, they often contain fewer total items than combinations of corresponding unidimensional measures and tend to be better integrated. Additionally, as the instruments are uniform, results can be compared across treatment settings or geographic regions, which may assist in the eventual development of universal pain outcomes benchmarks. Disadvantages of the multidimensional measures are that they may be more difficult to obtain, require additional administration or scoring training as well as more data entry and management time, are more costly in some cases and, with the exception of the NPDB, do not cover all of the key chronic pain outcomes domains. Nevertheless, when assessing multiple domains of outcomes in clinical settings, multidimensional measures generally are more practical.

A PRACTICAL APPROACH TO OUTCOMES MEASUREMENT

The process of designing a pain outcomes methodology consists of a series of discrete steps and requires that factors relevant to the outcomes system development process, such as those described above, be considered carefully. In the following pages we provide an outline of our suggested approach to this endeavor in the hope that it will assist the reader through this process.

IDENTIFY OUTCOMES OBJECTIVES

The first step in developing a pain outcomes measurement system consists of identifying goals, objectives, and scope of the outcomes program.

- Identify the basis for establishing the pain outcomes strategy. It may be a new hospital policy, legal opinion, or accreditation standard. Familiarity with the underlying rationale may make it easier to enlist administrative and staff support.
- Determine whether the outcomes objectives primarily focus on pain treatment issues or on the efficiency of pain service delivery. This distinction will have important implications for the eventual selection of outcomes measures.
- Define the scope of the outcomes plan. Are all available pain treatments to be included, or will only selected treatments be monitored? Does the plan cover every type of pain (acute, cancer, and chronic), or is it limited to only one or two?
- Choose which types of service settings will be included. Is it limited to outpatient areas, inpatient units, or specialty pain clinics? Are all providers working in the defined areas participating, or only some?
- Decide whether the outcomes data collection will be ongoing or limited to a preselected time interval.

IDENTIFY ADMINISTRATIVE SUPPORTS AND LIMITATIONS

Without sufficient administrative support, efforts to develop a pain outcomes system will fail. Staff will resent the added responsibilities in the absence of increased staff or concrete rewards. Presumably the basis for developing the pain outcomes system (JCAHO standards, insurer rec-

ommendations) will enhance administrative interest in the effort.

- Meet with the appropriate administrative representative to discuss anticipated costs and needed resources, citing any relevant local policies, local or national regulations, professional practice guidelines, or local competitors' outcomes practices and marketing data.
- Define the administrative limits (funds, positions) that are operative.
- Negotiate an agreement regarding support for the necessary resources.

SELECT THE RELEVANT OUTCOMES DOMAINS

Decisions regarding which pain outcomes domains to include often involve compromises between available resources and outcomes objectives. Yet outcomes efforts can be too ambitious as well. Collecting data for outcomes domains that are not central to the outcomes program objectives is a waste of staff resources and patient time.

- Select the relevant outcomes domains according to the focus of the outcomes program (treatment effects or service delivery), type of pain population involved (acute, cancer, or chronic), and setting.
- Avoid adding outcomes domains that are not directly relevant to the outcomes objectives. Additional domains may be added later if objectives change.
- Review any applicable guidelines, standards, or policies to ensure that all needed domains are included.

SELECT OR DESIGN THE NEEDED OUTCOMES MEASURES

Selecting Patient Outcomes Measures

If the objectives of the outcomes program involve evaluating the effects of pain treatment, it is likely that suitable pain outcomes instruments will be available for use. This will avoid the difficulties associated with designing and validating a new instrument and will minimize delays in implementing the outcomes programs.

- Identify potential instruments that assess the outcomes domains of interest (Tables 81.2 and 81.3 may be helpful when matching outcomes instruments to outcomes domains).
- Investigate the reported reliabilities and review the validation data available for the identified instruments.
- Review any available data concerning reading-level requirements, and determine whether

those requirements are consistent with the target population's reading abilities.
- Attend to instrument length, administration and scoring requirements, and costs so as to maximize value and minimize resource demands.
- Determine whether the instruments are available in other languages if this is desirable given the characteristics of the target population.
- Choose the instrument or battery of instruments to use based on the above information.

Designing Service Delivery Outcomes Measures

As indicated previously, service delivery outcomes measures generally are not available in the form of validated outcomes instruments. In fact, with the exception of generic customer satisfaction measures, pain service delivery measures typically need to be designed locally. Fortunately, these measures are relatively simplistic. Usually, they involve tracking whether required pain documentation is present or whether designated pain services were provided in an efficient and timely fashion. Thus, designing appropriate service measures may involve no more than developing pain-specific chart review forms or simple customer feedback tools.

- Identify the specific service delivery outcomes questions of interest.
- Design the necessary outcomes tools (e.g., chart review forms, customer satisfaction surveys).
- If patient surveys or questionnaires are involved, evaluate item wording, specificity, and reading level to meet the target population's abilities.

DEVELOP PROCEDURES NEEDED FOR IMPLEMENTATION

Once the scope of the outcomes project has been defined and the outcomes measures have been selected, specific procedures for implementing the outcomes system must be developed.

- Determine how the pain patients targeted for study will be identified.
- Identify the roles, responsibilities, and training needs of all involved staff.
- Develop a timeframe for implementing all aspects of the outcomes system.
- Decide on a sampling strategy (i.e., randomly sample from among all possible data sources or attempt to collect data from every source during the data collection phase) depending on the sample size desired and the projected timeframe.

DESIGN AND PREPARE THE OUTCOMES DATABASE

Preparation of the outcomes database prior to implementation of data collection requires reviewing every outcomes item or measure as well as all data entry and organization issues. Often this process yields valuable information that may streamline data collection and data management procedures.

- Decide what database and data analysis tools will be used.
- Design the necessary records storage and retrieval tools and conduct a "dry run" of data entry to identify any data collection problems.
- Make certain that the confidentiality of any patient information is maintained by discarding identifying information or by utilizing elaborate coding or encryption strategies.
- Develop a data analysis plan in advance of data collection efforts.

COLLECT THE OUTCOMES

- Provide training in outcomes measure administration and data collection routines to relevant staff.
- Test the data collection procedures using only a few patients (treatment outcomes project) or records (service delivery project) prior to full-scale implementation.
- Arrange for backup coverage for the individuals collecting the data in the event of unexpected absences.
- Periodically review the workflow and data collection procedures to identify and troubleshoot any problem areas.

ANALYZE, TREND, AND REPORT THE DATA

Unfortunately, it is common to find that elaborate outcomes data have been collected at significant expense but then are virtually ignored! Outcomes data analysis and trending are the cornerstones of an effective outcomes program. Analysis involves more than "eyeballing" the data. Although the level of statistical analysis will vary depending on the objectives of the outcomes plan and the psychometric sophistication of the staff involved, at the very least, it will be necessary to statistically summarize the data in a way that directly addresses the outcomes questions of interest. Ongoing review of the results by key personnel is critical and is mandated by some regulatory or accrediting bodies.

- For an ongoing outcomes program, establish a timeframe for systematically reviewing and reporting on the obtained data (monthly, quarterly, semiannually, or annually).

- Develop a report template that provides summary data regarding the outcomes questions and use that same template for each reporting period in order to allow comparisons over time.
- If performance improvement actions are instituted prior to or during a data collection period, note the nature of the changes implemented, along with the date, in the database so that the effects of the changes can be evaluated.
- After each reporting period, review data from all prior periods in concert with the current results in order to identify trends of change in the data.
- Provide each staff person involved in the project with copies of the analysis report and schedule a meeting after each data collection period for review and discussion of the data and any identified trends.
- Design and complete a brief version of the analysis report for distribution to key administrators to help maintain their support for the project.
- Use the obtained data to explore any additional outcomes questions or to investigate observed trends in the data.
- Implement treatment protocol changes based on the identified trends. Changes should be introduced sequentially in order to allow the effects of each change to be evaluated separately.
- Review the outcomes data following each change in treatment protocol and decide whether to accept or reject the change.

SUMMARY

Interest in outcomes monitoring in healthcare systems will only increase in the immediate future. Within the field of pain treatment, we will see growing demands for data supporting the effectiveness of our interventions. Regulatory and accreditation bodies increasingly will emphasize the importance of pain outcomes programs for providers across all treatment settings. Indeed, the recent development of JCAHO pain standards and the growing national interest in pain issues already have had a profound effect on the pain management field. Given these trends, it is only prudent that we anticipate these changes and enter the 21st century prepared to incorporate outcomes measures as a standard part of pain treatment efforts.

Some practitioners might portray the ever-increasing demands for pain documentation and treatment outcome data as a punitive, nonproductive exercise. We see it as both a challenge and an opportunity. It is a challenge in that it will require us to evaluate more closely our clinical practice of pain treatment, and perhaps reconsider some of our treatment biases. It is an opportunity in that it provides us with the motivation and the means to empirically justify that which we do, and to improve what we do or how we do it in order to increase our treatment effectiveness and efficiency.

In the preceding pages we attempted to summarize and briefly explore some of the key issues related to pain outcomes measurement endeavors. We also presented a general framework for designing and implementing outcomes measurement in pain treatment settings. In recognition of the wide variety of pain practitioner settings and outcomes objectives, we tried to maintain a generalist's approach to the topic. In this regard, we may have sacrificed precision to enhance utility. It is our hope that the information we provided will be of value to clinicians seeking to better understand and improve the effectiveness of their pain treatment interventions.

ACKNOWLEDGMENT

This material is the result of work supported in part by the Rehbilitation Research and Development Service, Office of Research and Development, Department of Veterans Affairs.

REFERENCES

Agency for Health Care Policy Reform. (1992). Acute pain management: Operative or medical procedures and trauma, Pub. No. 92-0032. Washington, D.C.: U.S. Department of Health and Human Services.

Agency for Health Care Policy Reform. (1996). Management of cancer pain, Pub. No. 94-0592. Washington, D.C.: U.S. Department of Health and Human Services.

American Academy of Pain Management. (1997). National Pain Data Bank reliability study. *Pain Program Standards*, Spring, 4–6.

American Academy of Pain Management. (1997). *Pain program accreditation manual* (p. 21). Sonora, CA: American Academy of Pain Management.

American Pain Society. (1995). Quality improvement guidelines for the treatment of acute pain and cancer. *Journal of the American Medical Association, 274,* 1874–1880.

Asmundson, G.J.G., Norton, G.R., & Allerdings, M.D. (1997). Fear and avoidance in dysfunctional chronic back pain patients. *Pain, 69,* 231–236.

Beck, A.T. (1987). *Beck Depression Inventory.* San Antonio, TX: The Psychological Corporation.

Beck, A.T., Steer, R.A., & Garbin, M.G. (1988). Psychometric properties of the Beck Depression Inventory: Twenty-five years of evaluation. *Clinical Psychology Review, 8,* 77–100.

Beckham, J.C., et al. (1997). Self-efficacy and adjustment in cancer patients: A preliminary report. *Behavioral Medicine, 23,* 138–142.

Bergner, M., et al. (1981). The Sickness Impact Profile: Development and final revision of a health status measure. *Medical Care, 19,* 787–805.

Bradely, L.A., Haile, J.M., & Jaworski, T.M. (1992). Assessment of psychological status using interview and self-interview instruments. (chap. 12). In D. C. Turk & R. Melzack (Eds.), *Handbook of pain assessment.* New York: Guilford Press.

Breivik, E.K. & Skoglund, L.A. (1998). Comparison of present pain intensity assessments on horizontally and vertically oriented visual analogue scales. *Methods and Findings in Experimental Clinical Pharmacology, 20,* 719–724.

Breivik, E.K., Bjornsson, G.A., & Skovlund, E. (2000). A comparison of pain rating scales by sampling from clinical trial data. *Clinical Journal of Pain, 16,* 22–28.

Brown, D. (1995). Quality assessment and improvement activities should be incorporated into our pain practices. *Pain Forum, 4,* 48–56.

Campazzi, E.J., & Lee, D.A. (1995). Quality is in the eye of the beholder: Patient satisfaction and outcomes management in physician practices. *American Health Consultants, 1,* 3336.

Caraceni, A., et al. (1996). A validation study of an Italian version of the Brief Pain Inventory (Breve Questionario per la Valutazione del Dolore). *Pain, 65,* 87–92.

CARF … (1999). The Rehabilitation Accreditation Commission, *2000 medical rehabilitation standards manual* (pp. 46–66). Tucson, AZ: CARF…The Rehabilitation Commission.

Choiniere, M., & Amsel, R. (1996). A visual analogue thermometer for measuring pain intensity. *Journal of Pain and Symptom Management, 11,* 299–311.

Clark, M.E., & Gironda, R.J. (2000). Concurrent validity of the National Pain Data Bank: Preliminary results. *American Journal of Pain Management, 10,* 25–33.

Cleeland, C.S. & Ryan, K.M. (1994). Pain assessment: Global use of the Brief Pain Inventory. *Annals Academy of Medicine (Singapore), 23,* 129–138.

Crombez, G., et al. (1999). Pain-related fear is more disabling than pain itself: Evidence on the role of pain-related fear in chronic back pain disability. *Pain, 80,* 329–339.

Davis, G.C. (1989). The clinical assessment of chronic pain in rheumatic disease: Evaluating the use of two instruments. *Journal of Advanced Nursing, 14,* 397–402.

De Conno, F., et al. (1994). Pain measurement in cancer patients: A comparison of six methods. *Pain, 57,* 161–166.

de C. Williams, A.C., & Richardson, P.H. (1993). What does the BDI measure in chronic pain? *Pain, 55,* 259–266.

Donaldson, G.W. (1995). The factorial structure and stability of the McGill Pain Questionnaire in patients experiencing oral mucositis following bone marrow transplantation. *Pain, 62,* 101–109.

Dreyer, P. (1998). Adoption of standards of the American Pain Society, Circular Letter #2–9–379. Augusta, ME: Department of Public Health, State of Maine.

Ellwood, P.M. (1988). Outcomes management: A technology of patient experience. *New England Journal of Medicine, 318,* 1549–1556.

Geisser, M.E., Roth, R.S., & Robinson, M.E. (1997). Assessing depression among persons with chronic pain using the Center for Epidemiological Studies-Depression Scale and the Beck Depression Inventory: A comparative analysis. *Clinical Journal of Pain, 13,* 163–170.

Green, B. (1992). A primer of testing. In A.E. Kazdin (Ed.), *Methodological issues & strategies in clinical research* (chap. 10). Washington, D.C.: American Psychological Association.

Gronblad, M., et al. (1993). Intercorrelation and test–retest reliability of the Pain Disability Index (PDI) and the Oswestry Disability Questionnaire (ODQ) and their correlation with pain intensity in low back pain patients. *Clinical Journal of Pain, 9,* 189–195.

Holroyd, K.A., et al. (1992). A multi-center evaluation of the McGill Pain Questionnaire: Results from more than 1700 chronic pain patients. *Pain, 48,* 301–311.

Iezzoni, L. I. (1997). Assessing quality using administrative data. *Annals of Internal Medicine, 127,* 666–673.

International Association for the Study of Pain. (1991). *Core curriculum for professional education in pain* (2nd ed.). Seattle: International Association for the Study of Pain.

Jensen, M.P. & Karoly, P. (1992). Self-report scales and procedures for assessing pain in adults. In Turk, D.C. and Melzack, R., Eds., *Handbook of pain assessment* (chap. 9). New York: Guilford Press.

Jensen, M.P., et al. (1992). Validity of the Sickness Impact Profile Roland scale as a measure of dysfunction in chronic pain patients. *Pain, 50,* 157–162.

Jensen, M.P., et al. (1996). The use of multiple-item scales for pain intensity measurement in chronic pain patients. *Pain, 67,* 35–40.

Jensen, M.P., et al. (1999). Comparative reliability and validity of chronic pain intensity measures. *Pain, 83,* 157–162.

Johnston, M.V., Keith, R.A., & Hinderer, S.R. (1992). Measurement standards for interdisciplinary medical rehabilitation. *Archives of Physical Medicine and Rehabilitation, 73*(Suppl.), S3–S23.

Joint Commission for the Accreditation of Healthcare Organizations. (2000). Pain assessment and management standards. http://www.jcaho.org/standard/pm_frm.html.

Kerns, R.D., Turk, D. C., & Rudy, T.E. (1985). The West Haven-Yale Multidimensional Pain inventory (WHYMPI). *Pain, 23,* 345–356.

Kleinke, C.L. (1991). How chronic pain patients cope with depression: Relation to treatment outcome in a multidisciplinary pain clinic. *Rehabilitation Psychology, 36,* 207–218.

Kori, S.H., Miller, R.P., & Todd, D.D. (1990). Kinisophobia: A new view of chronic pain behavior. *Pain Management, 3,* 35–43.

Kulich, R. & Lande, S.D. (1997). Managed care: The past and future of pain treatment. *APS Bulletin, 7,* 4–5.

Lowe, N.K., Walker, S.N., & MacCallum, R.C. (1991). Confirming the theoretical structure of the McGill Pain Questionnaire in acute clinical pain. *Pain, 46,* 53–60.

McCracken, L.M., et al. (1993). Prediction of pain in patients with chronic low back pain: Effects of inaccurate prediction and pain-related anxiety. *Behavior Research and Therapy, 31,* 647–652.

McCracken, L.M., et al. (1996). The assessment of anxiety and fear in persons with chronic pain: A comparison of instruments. *Behavior Research and Therapy, 34,* 927–933.

McCracken, L.M., Faber, S.D., & Janeck, A.S. (1998). Pain-related anxiety predicts non-specific physical complaints in persons with chronic pain. *Behavior Research and Therapy, 36,* 621–630.

McCracken, L.M., Zayfert, C., & Gross, R.T. (1992). The Pain Anxiety Symptoms Scale: Development and validation of a scale to measure fear of pain. *Pain, 50,* 67–73.

McCracken, L.M., Zayfert, C., & Gross, R.T. (1993). The Pain Anxiety Symptom Scale (PASS): A multimodal measure for pain specific anxiety symptoms. *Behavior Therapist, 16,* 183–184.

Melzack, R. (1975a). The McGill Pain Questionnaire. In Melzack, R. (Ed.) *Pain measurement and assessment* (pp. 41–47). New York: Raven Press.

Melzack, R. (1975b). The McGill Pain Questionnaire: Major properties and scoring methods. *Pain, 1,* 277–299.

Mongini, F., Defilippi, N., & Negro, C. (1997). Chronic daily headache, a clinical and psychological profile before and after treatment. *Headache, 37,* 83–87.

Ogon, M., et al. (1996). Chronic low back pain measurement with visual analogue scales in different settings. *Pain, 64,* 425–428.

Paice, J.A., & Cohen, F.L. (1997). Validity of a verbally administered numeric rating scale to measure cancer pain intensity. *Cancer Nursing, 20,* 88–93.

Plumb, M., & Holland, J. (1977). Comparative studies of psychological function in patients with advanced cancer. I: Self-reported depressive symptoms. *Psychosomatic Medicine, 39,* 264–276.

Polantin, P.B., et al. (1993). Psychiatric illness and chronic low back pain. *Spine, 18,* 66–71.

Pollard, C.A. (1984). Preliminary validity study of Pain Disability Index. *Perceptual and Motor Skills, 59,* 974.

Radbruch, L., et al. (1999). Validation of the German version of the Brief Pain Inventory. *Journal of Pain and Symptom Management, 18,* 180–187.

Radloff, L. (1977). The CES-D scale: A self-report depression scale for research in the general population. *Journal of Applied Psychology Measures, 1,* 385–401.

Rosensteil, A.K., & Keefe, F.J. (1983). The use of coping strategies in chronic low back pain patients: Relationship to patient characteristics and current adjustment. *Pain, 17,* 33–44.

Rudy, T.E., & Kubinski, J.A. (1999). Program evaluation methods for documenting pain management effectiveness. In J. Gatchel and D. Turk (Eds.), *Psychological approaches to pain management: A practitioner's handbook* (chap. 18). New York: Guilford Press.

Santor, D.A., et al. (1995). Examining scale discriminability in the BDI and CES-D as a function of depressive severity. *Psychology Assessment, 7,* 131–139.

Saxena, A., Mendoza, T., & Cleeland, C.S. (1999). The assessment of cancer pain in north India: The validation of the Hindi Brief Pain Inventory — BPI-H. *Journal of Pain and Symptom Management, 17,* 27–41.

Sist, T.C., et al. (1998). The relationship between depression and pain language in cancer and chronic non-cancer pain patients. *Journal of Pain and Symptom Management, 15,* 350–358.

Spielberger, C.D., et al. (1983). *Manual of the State-Trait Anxiety Inventory (Form Y)* (pp. 9–17). Palo Alto, CA: Consulting Psychologists Press.

Strategier, L.D., et al. (1997). Multidimensional assessment of chronic low back pain: Predicting treatment outcomes. *Journal of Clinical Psychology in Medical Settings, 4,* 91–110.

Strong, J., Ashton, R., & Large, R.G. (1994). Function and the patient with chronic low back pain. *Clinical Journal of Pain, 10,* 191–196.

Tait, R.C., Chibnall, J.T., & Krause, S. (1990). The Pain Disability Index: Psychometric properties. *Pain, 40,* 171–182.

Tait, R.C., et al. (1987). The pain disability index: Psychometric and validity data. *Archives of Physical Medicine and Rehabilitation, 68,* 438–441.

Tarlov, A.R. (1995). Multiple influences propel outcomes field. *Medical Outcomes Trust Bulletin, 3,* 1–3.

Turk, D.C., & Okifuji, A. (1994). Detecting depression in chronic pain patients: Adequacy of self-reports. *Behavior Research and Therapy, 32,* 9–16.

Turk, D.C., & Rudy, T.E. (1990). The robustness of an empirically derived taxonomy of chronic pain patients. *Pain, 43,* 27–35.

Turk, D.C., Rudy, T.E., & Salovey, P. (1985). The McGill Questionnaire reconsidered: Confirming the factor structures and examining appropriate uses. *Pain, 21,* 385–397.

Turner, J. A., & Clancy, S. (1988). Comparison of operant behavioral and cognitive-behavioral group treatment for chronic low back pain. *Journal of Clinical and Consulting Psychology, 56,* 261–266.

Veterans Health Administration. (2000). VHA national pain management strategy, Pain assessment: The 5th vital sign (pp. 27–29). Washington, D.C.: Veterans Health Administration.

Vlaeyen, J., et al. (1999). Fear of movement/(re)injury and muscular reactivity in chronic low back pain patients: An experimental investigation. *Pain, 82,* 297–304.

Wang, X.S., et al. (1996). The Chinese version of the Brief Pain Inventory (BPI-C): Its development and use in a study of cancer pain [see comments]. *Pain, 67,* 407–416.

Watson, J.H. & Graydon, J.E. (1989). Sickness Impact Profile: A measure of dysfunction with chronic pain patients. *Journal of Pain and Symptom Management, 4,* 152–156.

Wesley, A.L., et al. (1999). Toward more accurate use of the Beck Depression Inventory with chronic back pain patients. *Clinical Journal of Pain, 15,* 117–121.

Williams, R.C. (1988). Toward a set of reliable and valid measures for chronic pain assessment and outcome research. *Pain, 35,* 239–251.

82

Enhancing Adrenal Function

Arnold Sandlow, D.C. and Afshin Shargani, D.C.

INTRODUCTION

One of the most overlooked issues faced by the healthcare pain practitioner on a day-to-day basis is realizing and addressing the role of the adrenal gland and its dysfunction as related to the pain and nonpain patient alike. This chapter enables the practitioner to recognize, diagnose, and treat this common and underdiagnosed condition.

In our modern-day society we are barraged with various forms of stress on a daily basis. Some stressors are easy to adapt to, others can become seemingly insurmountable. Stress and stress-related disorders have been considered a significant cause of disease and may contribute to perhaps 75% of all illnesses. Pain subjects the patient to additional stress, which can potentially lead to stress-related disorders.

Thoughts about the adrenal gland automatically relate to thoughts of stress. They are inseparable. For the most part the lay public is familiar with the adrenal gland and its role in handling stress. From the perspective of the pain management practitioner the adrenal gland plays a major role, often unnoticed, and wholly underestimated. Understanding the relationship between the adrenal gland and the patient in pain can increase the ability of the practitioner to treat and manage the patient as a whole, addressing the underlying causes as well as the main causative factors.

Much of the healthcare in the United States is directed toward crisis care. Should we just wait until our patient has a full-blown organic dysfunction, or should we realize and be concerned with an adrenal gland that would allow us a higher level of health and well-being but is not functioning to meet the demands of the body? In the absence of gross pathology should any thought at all be placed on subtle, seemingly ubiquitous symptomatology?

"As the signs and symptoms of adrenal dysfunction are often relatively non-specific, adrenal disorders must be considered in the differential diagnosis of many common complaints" (Miller & Tyrell, 1996).

This chapter focuses on a continuum that exists somewhere between the likes of Addison's disease and Cushing's disease and is secondary to chronic maladaption. This chronic maladaption to stress leads to adrenal exhaustion and has been referred to by many different names. Dilman and Dean (1992) called it the Adrenal Maladaptation Syndrome, or hyperadaptosis. David Walther (1988), in *Applied Kinesiology-Synopsis,* calls it functional or relative hypoadrenia. Others call it adrenal insufficiency, exhaustion, or burnout (Table 82.1).

In contemporary society, long-term, never-ending emotional stress creates a tired or worn-out adrenal gland, principally because the adrenal gland does not have a chance to rebuild. Because stress is cumulative, stresses to which the body must react over time can cause mild to moderate adrenal insufficiency, the most common clinically observed entity. In this condition the individual can still react to stress; however, it will be done less efficiently and will take more time.

The goal of health is to maintain homeostasis. When the hypothalamic–pituitary–adrenal (HPAA) axis is disturbed, homeostasis is lost. A DHEA/cortisol balance (two hormones secreted by the adrenals) is considered to be a critical marker of overall hormonal health.

Also highlighted are diagnosis, laboratory testing, homeostasis, hormonal regulation, and feedback mechanisms, i.e., HPAA, and natural methods of controlling and

0-8493-0926-3/02/$0.00+$1.50
© 2002 by CRC Press LLC

TABLE 82.1
Common Causes of Adrenal Stress

- Anger
- Fear
- Worry/anxiety
- Depression
- Guilt
- Physical or mental strain
- Excessive exercise
- Sleep deprivation
- Light-cycle disruption
- Going to sleep late
- Surgery
- Trauma/injury
- Chronic inflammation
- Chronic infection
- Chronic pain
- Temperature extremes
- Toxic exposure
- Malabsorption
- Maldigestion
- Chronic illness
- Chronic/severe allergies
- Hypoglycemia
- Nutritional deficiencies

enhancing the function of the glands and the important hormones they produce.

ADRENAL GLANDS AND THEIR HORMONES

The adrenal glands (or suprarenal glands) are the major organs that deal with life's minor and major ups and downs. They are pyramidal-shaped structures located on top of each kidney. The adrenal glands are made of two distinct sections: the outer cortex and the inner medulla. They are essentially two different endocrine organs. The adrenal cortex is made of three distinct layers or zones, which produce different types of hormones. The zona glomerulosa is the outermost layer, which produces the mineralocorticoids (aldosterone). The zona fasiculata is the middle layer, which produces glucocorticoids (cortisol) and the zona reticularis is the innermost layer involved in the production of sex hormones, mainly androgens.

ALDOSTERONE

Aldosterone plays a vital role in the body, and its total absence, if untreated, can lead to death. Aldosterone stimulates the kidneys to excrete K and recapture Na, decreasing the blood K levels and increasing the Na levels. Increased levels of sodium, in turn, increase blood volume and pressure. Release of aldosterone is stimulated by increased blood K levels, decreased Na levels, loss of blood, and decreased blood pressure and volume. Control of blood pressure is in part achieved through the renin-angiotensin system with angiotensin II stimulating the release of aldosterone.

CORTISOL

Cortisol is the main hormone produced by the adrenal glands in response to various short- or long-term physical, psychological, and physiological stressful stimuli in conjunction with catecholamines from the adrenal medulla, or independently. Cortisol's main action is catabolism of fats and amino acids from their stores in adipose tissue, muscle, lymphatics, and bone, making them available for producing energy and the synthesis of other compounds including glucose and proteins. Cortisol promotes gluconeogenesis and protein synthesis by the liver, enhances the effects of glucagon and growth hormone and decreases glucose uptake by the peripheral tissues. This results in increasing blood sugar levels for use by brain and heart tissues.

Cortisol is also a well-known and potent anti-inflammatory agent exerting its effects by decreasing the permeability of capillary endothelium, stabilizing the liposomal membrane, and promoting production of arachadonic acid, a precursor of prostoglandins.

SEX HORMONES

Adrenal sex hormones are produced by the cells of the zona reticularis, the innermost layer of the adrenal cortex. The majority of these hormones are androgens, in the form of dehydroepiandrosterone (DHEA), which has one fifth of testosterone's potency. Other adrenal sex hormones, including estrogen and progesterone, are manufactured in very small amounts. Although they make up the main source of androgens in women, under normal conditions these hormones have a minor role in men mainly due to the presence of testosterone.

After the age of 25 a gradual decrease in DHT production is noted and at 75, it is 15 to 25% of its peak. DHEA levels have an indirect relationship with cortisol production. Therefore, a comparison of DHEA-S vs. cortisol levels can be used as an indicator of the patient's response to stress. DHEA also has been shown to act as a protective guard against stress in laboratory animals (Hornsby, 1997).

EPINEPHRINE AND NOREPINEPHRINE

The inner part of the adrenal gland, the medulla, is made of chromaffin cells and is essentially a part of the autonomic nervous system. It produces the catecholamines epinephrine (adrenaline) and norepinephrine (noradrenaline), as well as endorphins. These hormones play a major role in exciting the sympathetic nervous system for what is commonly known as the fight-and-flight response. The endorphins are natural painkillers and are secreted alongside epinephrine and norepinephrine.

HYPOTHALAMIC–PITUITARY–ADRENAL (HPA) AXIS AND BIOSYNTHESIS OF ADRENAL HORMONES

Stimulation and control of the hormonal production by the adrenal gland are orchestrated by a feedback mechanism

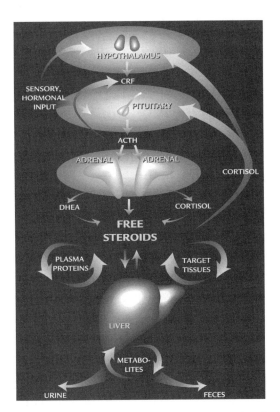

FIGURE 82.1 HPA axis and feedback loops. (Reprinted with permission of Great Smokies Diagnostic Laboratories.)

between the hypothalamus, pituitary, and adrenal glands. This is known as the HPA axis.

A healthy HPA axis (Figure 82.1) is one that involves an intricate interplay of positive and negative feedback loops that make up this marvelous homeostatic mechanism. The major players in this orchestra of hormones include cortisol, which is produced by the adrenal gland, adrenocorticotropic hormone (ACTH) produced by the pituitary, and the corticotropin-releasing factor (CRF) produced by the hypothalamus.

In addition to its regulation by the pituitary, ACTH is synchronized by counterregulation of CRF. A short-loop negative feedback on CRF by ACTH also emanates from the hypothalamic–pituitary region.

The process starts with the release of the CRF from the hypothalamus in response to physical, psychological, and physiologic stressors. CRF induces release of ACTH or corticotropin from the anterior pituitary directly into the blood. ACTH acts on the cells of the zona fasiculata, stimulating cortisol production and release.

Activation of the HPA axis due to a given stimulus leads to a stress response, which modulates the immune response. The interactions between the HPA and the immune system are characterized by a circuit, which includes activation of the HPA-axis and initiation of the stress response that, in turn, has immune-modulating properties, and a feedback mechanism derived from the immune system that regulates the HPA axis (Marx, Ehrhart-Bornstein, Scherbaum, & Bornstein, 1998).

The control of cortisol production is achieved by a negative feedback mechanism exerted by ACTH and cortisol. ACTH acts on the hypothalamus and decreases CRF production. Cortisol acts on both the hypothalamus and pituitary and decreases CRF and ACTH production. In the absence of stressful stimuli, cortisol production follows a normal circadian rhythm associated with sleep and wake cycles. Cortisol secretion is at its highest around 8 a.m. and gradually decreases, reaching its lowest point at midnight. Under prolonged stressful stimuli the brain overrides the normal negative feedback loop, constantly stimulating the adrenal cortex to produce cortisol. This disrupts the normal circadian rhythm of cortisol and results in a whole host of cortisol-related physiologic disorders, as well as hypertrophy of the adrenal glands. Increased cortisol levels are associated with accelerated aging, depression, schizophrenia, chronic fatigue syndrome, immune dysfunction, decreased REM sleep, obesity, hypertension, heart disease, and suppressed thyroid function.

Figure 82.2 shows the pathway of cortisol synthesis in the adrenal cortex. This synthesis begins with the conversion of cholesterol to pregnenolone, by the enzyme 20 α-hydroxylase, 22 hydroxylase, and 20,22 desmolase. In turn, pregnenolone (the mother of all hormones) may be converted into either sex hormones (androgens and estrogens) or mineral and glucocorticoids, more likely produced in the presence of chronic stress.

Pregnenolone's conversion to cortisol involves a series of enzymatic reactions, which are, in turn, controlled by ACTH and other stimulants of the adrenal gland as discussed earlier. A genetic deficiency of any of these enzymes can result in overproduction and underproduction of the dependent hormones.

ADRENAL GLAND DISORDERS

Adrenal gland disorders can be categorized into adrenocorticol hyper- or hypoactivity, resulting in severe excess or deficiency of adrenal cortex hormones, respectively. These conditions can be the result of pathological conditions within the gland itself, pituitary gland, supporting glands, or can be iatrogenic in nature.

ADRENOCORTICOL DEFICIENCY

Adrenocorticol deficiency is highlighted by a significant decrease in production of one or all adrenal hormones. This can be due to pathological conditions involving the adrenal gland itself or other causes. The patient's presentation varies, depending on the affected hormones.

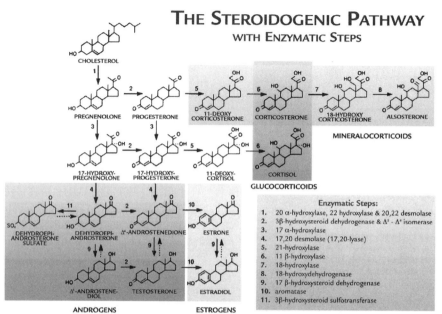

FIGURE 82.2 The steroidogenic pathway.

Addison's Disease

Primary adrenocorticol deficiency involves inherent disease of the adrenal cortex and is also known as Addison's disease. In Addison's disease all adrenal hormones are affected but most pronounced are the effects of decreased cortisol and aldosterone. Clinical findings include decreased weight, malaise, and gastrointestinal upset. Cortisol deficiency results in hypoglycemia and decreased ability to handle stress, while decreased aldosterone results in decreased blood pressure and electrolyte imbalance. Other findings include increased ACTH production by the pituitary; decreased blood levels of cortisol, aldosterone, and T4; and increased TSH. Increased pigmentation is another physical finding of adrenocorticol deficiency, which is due to increased production of ACTH and accompanying melatonin by the pituitary gland.

While Addison's disease is insidious, eventually it will result in severe deficiency of the adrenal hormones. This is known as Addison's crisis, a serious life-threatening emergency requiring immediate medical intervention.

Autoimmune and iatrogenic factors are the leading causes of Addison's disease in the Western countries, whereas tuberculosis is the leading causative factor worldwide. Other causes include metastases, adrenal hemorrhage, hemochromatosis, adrenomyeloneuropathy, and iatrogenic drug use.

Inherent Errors of Metabolism

Another cause of adrenocorticol deficiency is inherent errors of metabolism of the adrenal gland itself. It is also known as congenital adrenal hypertrophy. In this group of conditions the enzymes responsible for production of cortisol and aldosterone are deficient genetically, and depending on the severity of their deficiency can result in decreased production of cortisol and aldosterone that can be chronic or life threatening. The enzymatic deficiency also results in a buildup of aldosterone and cortisol precursors, which are converted to sex hormones, primarily androgens. This results in premature puberty in male children and virilism in female children. The decreased adrenal hormone production results in an overproduction of ACTH by the pituitary gland, which causes hypertrophy of the adrenal gland.

Secondary Adrenocorticol Deficiency

Secondary adrenocorticol deficiency is the group of disorders wherein the adrenal gland's function is intact but does not receive appropriate stimulation for production and release of its hormones. The most common cause of this type of condition is decreased function of the pituitary gland due to various causes, which results in decreased production of ACTH and, in turn, cortisol, while aldosterone's production remains intact.

Disorders of the renin and angiotensin system due to kidney disease and other causes are another rare type of secondary adrenocorticol deficiency, which results in decreased production of aldosterone while cortisol production remains intact.

Drug-induced adrenocorticol deficiency can occur as a result of treatment with pharmaceuticals including Metyrapone, opDDD (Metiotane), Aminoglutethemide, Ketocoazole, and Etomidate.

ADRENOCORTICOL EXCESS

This group of disorders is characterized by excess production of the adrenal hormones aldosterone and cortisol.

Cushing's Syndrome

Cushing's syndrome is characterized by excess cortisol in the circulation due to cortisol-producing adrenal tumors, ACTH-producing pituitary gland tumors, or iatrogenic causes. When the excess in cortisol production is due to adrenal tumors, excess androgens will also be present. When excess cortisol is due to ACTH-producing pituitary tumors the condition is known as Cushing's disease. Iatrogenic Cushing's is the most common type and is the result of treatment by glucocorticoids for their immunosuppressive or anti-inflammatory benefits.

Cushing's syndrome is characterized by a round or moon face, Buffalo hump, central obesity, thin arms and legs with muscle wasting, testicular atrophy and menstrual disturbances, high blood pressure, osteoporosis with increased risk of fractures, and immunosuppression resulting in increased susceptibility to infections. Mental changes may include depression, insecurity, uncertainty, and possible psychosis.

Conn's Syndrome

Conn's syndrome is characterized by elevated levels of aldosterone and is almost always the result of aldosterone-producing adrenal tumors, but on rare occasions it can also be due to renin-producing tumors. Elevated levels of aldosterone result in increased blood pressure and hypokalemia, which can lead to other clinical manifestations (Cotran, Jumar, & Robbins, 1989; Jeffcoate, 1993; Berkhow & Fletcher, 1987).

Pheochromocytoma

Pheochromocytoma is the only disease of the adrenal medulla that is caused by a tumor, which produces an excess of catecholamines. Symptoms of this disease include periodic high blood pressure, nausea, excessive sweats, pounding-type headache, anxiety, vomiting, and palpitations.

THE SCIENCE OF STRESS

A Canadian professor, Hans Selye, M.D., is responsible for pioneering the field of stress research. For this reason he was given the title "the father of stress." His writings on the subject date back to the 1930s, and he is credited with writing over 1700 papers and 39 books on the subject.

As the undisputed expert on the subject, he observed as early as 1925 that common symptoms are present in many diseases. He came to classify this as the syndrome of "just being sick." A triad was always present in this syndrome. After exposing rats to various types of stress they were sacrificed. Dissection revealed (1) adrenal cortex enlargement; (2) atrophy of the thymus, spleen, lymph nodes, and all other lymphatic structures; and (3) deep bleeding ulcers in the stomach and duodenum.

Selye classified the progression of stress on the body and its influence on the adrenal glands. The classification is called the "General Adaptation Syndrome" (GAS) (Selye, 1956). Three stages exist including alarm, resistance, and finally exhaustion.

Alarm Reaction: The alarm reaction is characterized by surprise and anxiety and is considered to be a general call to arms. The adrenal glands will secrete hormones, i.e., epinephrine, norepinephrine, and hydrocortisone. This phase is extremely rapid and the mechanism by which a seemingly petite mother lifts a car to get her child out from under it.

Resistance: With continuation of stress the body moves into this second phase, in which the body prepares to continue and adapt to the prolonged fight ahead. Adrenal hypertrophy and other factors of the stress triad are found in this stage. An individual can respond and meet the demands of the stress as long as this stage continues. If the adaptive stress is resolved, a rapid return to the resting state can be achieved.

Exhaustion: When the adrenal glands can no longer meet the demands placed on them due to prolonged stress, this stage is evident. This is then referred to as adrenal maladaptation, or hyperadaptosis, a term credited to Dilman and Dean (1992) (Dilman, you may recall, is responsible for the neuroendocrine theory of aging). Hyperadaptosis is considered by some to be a precursor to Cushing's syndrome. It is characterized by prolonged exposure to excess cortisol levels and is caused by the loss of hypothalamic sensitivity to the inhibitory effects of cortisol (Dilman, 1981). It is the chronically hyperactive HPA axis that causes these symptoms. These same high levels of stress have been shown by Selye (1976) to lead to many of the diseases of aging. Robert Sapolsky, the author of *Why Zebras Don't Get Ulcers* also recognizes the role of these hormones in disease (http://www-med.stanford.-edu/school/Neurosciences/faculty/sapolsky.html, 2000; Sapolsky, et al., 1987). Additionally, chronic health problems, long-term nutritional deficiencies, and long-term emotional problems can all lead to the state of adrenal exhaustion.

Researchers have identified eight physical indicators of an individual's stress load (McGwen, 1998). Stressful life events such as divorce, job loss, family arguments, and even traffic jams, in addition to daily maladaptation, all add to stress. Among the stress indicators are

1. Increased blood pressure
2. Suppressed immunity to disease
3. Increased fat around the abdomen
4. Weak muscles
5. Bone loss
6. Increases in blood sugar
7. Increases in cholesterol levels
8. Increases in steroid hormones, i.e., cortisol

How our bodies react by manufacturing stress hormones is ostensibly even more significant than how we feel about the events. When an episode of acute stress is experienced, cortisol is secreted to protect us by activating, through a complex chain of events, the body's defenses. Acute stress (in the sense of "fight" or "flight" or major life events) and chronic stress (the cumulative load of minor day-to-day stresses) can both have long-term consequences.

One of Selye's first observations of the general adaptation syndrome was that animals under extended stress developed sexual derangements. Intense stress causes young animals to cease to grow and lactating females to produce no milk. Prolonged stress may be partially or totally responsible for amenorrhea in female athletes who are under intense training (Brooks-Gunn, Warren, & Hamilton, 1987). Recent research reports that wounds heal more slowly when patients are under psychological stress (Kiecolt-Glaser & Glaser, 2000). With constant sympathetic activation the immune system becomes depressed. Years of scrutiny have revealed that never-ending stressors unfavorably influence brain development.

Current research finds that those women who have higher levels of cortisol (the stress hormone) tend to have more abdominal fat. Dr. Elissa Epel (2000) of UCLA stated, "Psychological stress may increase abdominal fat in healthy people who have normal resting levels of cortisol and are of average weight."

NEUROENDOCRINE THEORY OF AGING

DHEA

Dehydroepiandrosterone (DHEA), a 17 keto-steroid and DHEA-S, its more powerful sulfate, are the major adrenal androgens. Secreted by the adrenal cortex in the innermost layer, the zona reticulosa, this steroid, which is largely produced from the precursor pregnenalone, has been implicated as a possible anti-aging hormone. Serum concentrations of DHEA-S are 20 times that of serum cortisol and the concentration of DHEA is 1/20th that of cortisol. DHEA and its sulfate have been shown to be interconvertible. Testosterone is purported to be five times more potent than androgens. DHEA-S is primarily produced from DHEA in the adrenal gland and liver. Several organs that are targets of androgenic and estrogenic sex hormones convert DHEAS back to DHEA.

The plasma half-life of DHEA is relatively short, at just under 30 minutes. It is for this reason that over 95% of circulating DHEA is in the form of sulfate (Berdanier, Parenta, & McIntosh, 1993; Rosenfeld, Rosenberg, Fukushima, & Hellman, 1975).

In females, androgens are the main source of male sex steroids. In sexually mature humans, ACTH stimulates the secretion of adrenal sex steroids.

DHEA-S is the major source of androgens for the fetus before birth. DHEA-S is detectable by age 7 and serum concentrations of both DHEA and its sulfate appear to be highest in the third decade of life (Bonney, et al., 1984). Levels then begin to gradually decrease and continue to drop. By the age of 70 or 80 years, values have plummeted to approximately 20% of peak values in men and 30% in woman (Bonney, et al., 1984; Rotter, Wong, Lifrak, & Parker, 1985).

DHEA has a very short half-life (less than 30 minutes); therefore, it is stored as its sulfated form, DHEA-S, which makes up 95% of its circulating levels. DHEA-S can be readily converted to testosterone, estrione, and estradiol and plays a role in a variety of physiologic processes including protein synthesis and thyroid hormone function (Fitzgerald, 1992).

Adrenal insufficiency leads to a deficiency of DHEA. In a study published in the *New England Journal of Medicine* oral doses of 50 mg per day of DHEA or placebo were administered over a period of 4 months to women who were adrenal insufficient. They were evaluated for effects on well-being and sexuality, as well as on serum hormone and other biochemical values (Arlt, Callies, et al., 1999; Oelkers, 1999). When it came to scores of depression, anxiety, general well-being, and the physical and psychological aspects of sexuality, these adrenally deficient women were shown to have significant positive effects from DHEA supplementation (Oelkers, 1999). DHEA (12.5 to 50 mg/day taken in the a.m.) and pregnenolone (10 to 100 mg/day taken in the a.m.) have been recently propelled to the forefront by their over-the-counter availability and more is being published daily (Hornsby, 1997). DHEA has been touted as being effective for immune dysfunction, longevity, obesity, and depression. The verdict is not conclusive on all these possible usages, but they clearly are showing promise. The strongest evidence exists for its use with hormone replacement and for anti-aging. One marker of aging is a decrease in GnRH (gonadotrophin-releasing hormone) that may result in loss of reproductive function. This loss of function can

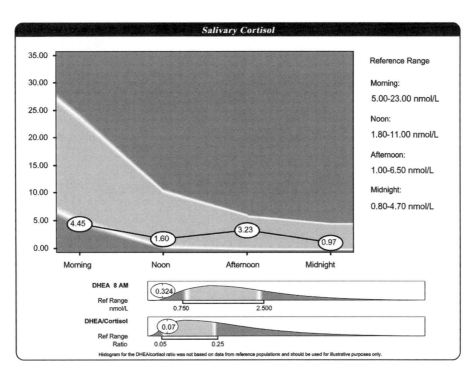

FIGURE 82.3 Lab report of salivary cortisol and DHEA. (Reprinted by permission of Great Smokies Diagnostic Laboratory.)

be reversed with a short administration of DHEA (Li, Givalois, & Pelletier, 1997).

DHEA is distinctive to primates. It is found in high levels only in humans, chimpanzees, and gorillas, and less so in monkeys.

Several articles talk about the anti-obesity effects of DHEA. "The anti-obesity function of DHEA is not simply one of inhibiting fat synthesis and deposition but is one of affecting a number of pathways that contribute to the maintenance of the isoenergetic state rather than the promotion of positive energy balance" (Berdanier, Parente, & McIntosh, 1993).

THE STRESS-IMMUNITY CONNECTION

It has long been proposed that the more stress on the body, irrespective of source, the more likely the immune system will be depressed. Elevated corticosteroids are known to have a significant effect in reducing immune defenses. In a recent study (Creuss, et al., 2000), 34 women with stage I and II breast cancer were divided into one of two randomized groups. One group received cognitive-behavioral stress management; the other group was placed on a waiting list. After 10 weeks of stress management, relaxation training, and cognitive therapy, patients from the treatment group noted significant changes that included a greater sense of purpose and meaning in their lives, better family relationships, and shifted priorities. Not surprisingly, their cortisol levels had dropped and were significantly lower ($p < 0.03$) when compared with the waiting-list patients who did not receive this care.

In a related study done by the National Cancer Institute (Sephton, Sapolsky, Kraemer, & Spiegel, 2000), salivary cortisol levels were checked four times daily in 104 patients with metastatic breast cancer for a period of 3 consecutive days. Patients with "flat" rhythms, an indication of a lack of normal variation, were found to have earlier mortality along with lower levels of natural killer (NK) cells and suppressed activity of those cells.

A nine-fold increased risk of recurrent breast cancer has been associated previously with extreme or severe stress (Ramirez, 1989).

LABORATORY TESTING

SALIVARY TESTING

A simple test to determine hormonal deficiency and imbalance is gaining widespread popularity. Saliva testing is unique in that it measures the unbound hormone, which is that portion available to the cells of the body. About 1 to 10% of the steroids in the blood are in unbound, or free form. Because only unbound steroids can freely diffuse into various target tissues in the body, they are the only hormones considered biologically active. Because it is the most active part of the hormone, saliva testing is a good way to analyze how hormones affect your health.

One of its main advantages is in the ease of collection. It is noninvasive, easy, convenient, painless, and can be done at home by the patient in the privacy of his or her own home. When blood work is utilized to ascertain adrenal hormonal levels, those same levels could easily become

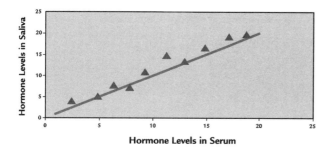

FIGURE 82.4 Linear correlation between salivary and serum hormones. (Reprinted with permission of Great Smokies Diagnostic Laboratory.)

elevated if the patient has any fear about injections, thus giving elevated and inaccurate information. Results retrieved in a stress-free environment will likely be the most sensitive. Figure 82.4 illustrates a comparison of hormone levels in saliva vs. serum, demonstrating a direct correlation.

When evaluating adrenal hormones, a 24-hour pattern of cortisol is examined at four different times, while DHEA is measured on two occasions in the same day.

Saliva samples are not just being utilized for DHEA and cortisol; they are being employed for measuring many hormones including estradiol, progesterone, testosterone and melatonin. Our hormones control many important psychological and physiological roles including our resistance, sleep patterns, and longevity. Thus, these tests provide physicians with accurate, dependable data that can be influential in prescribing hormones with confidence.

Mark Flinn, of the University of Missouri, has been studying the relationship that exists between health in children and stress. He maintains that the two best ways to measure stress are by measuring the adrenal hormone cortisol in saliva and by asking questions. This study has amassed data over the course of 13 years. In that time Flinn has collected more than 25,000 saliva samples from 287 children who live in the same rural Caribbean island village. An average of 96 separate samples were collected from each child. In addition, Flinn has tracked their growth, checked their health records, measured their levels of resistance, watched, listened, and asked questions in order to be very aware of what was happening in each of their lives.

He concludes that family matters more than anything else in a child's life. Stress hormones course through a child's system when a family has problems. "In the village, illness among children increases more than twofold following significant stress," says Flinn (Small, 2000).

Compilation of saliva subsequent to significant conflict within a group of children consistently failed to show high levels of cortisol, whereas one of those same children, returning home late from shopping a couple weeks later, had salivary cortisol levels that rose 60% above normal. This study gives scientific confirmation to the importance of how emotional stress contributes to physical illness.

During the Ceausescu regime in Romania thousands of children became orphaned as a by-product of his malevolence. Neglect that included being left alone in cribs or playpens, absent any stimulation and interaction, resulted in withdrawn, unpredictable children, who were prone to rocking in place and staring blankly at visitors. Harvard researchers have documented their later development, which included difficulty coping with normal human interaction and touch (Holden, 1996; DiPietro, 2000). Simply being touched and held throughout the first few years of infancy may well set up constructive stress-response patterns that last a lifetime.

OFFICE TESTING

RAGLAND'S SIGN

A simple test to help assess the status of the adrenal glands can be performed in an office-based setting as part of a thorough examination. Instead of simply taking a blood pressure reading while the patient is in the seated posture, begin by taking a reading while the patient is supine on the table. After recording the reading, immediately repeat the blood pressure in the standing position. Under normal circumstances, the systolic blood pressure should rise at least 8 mmHg. An abnormal drop in the systolic pressure is considered positive for adrenal hypofunction and this drop is referred to as postural hypotension.

NUTRITIONAL CONSIDERATIONS

In the context of this chapter it would be virtually impossible to enumerate and elucidate all the potentially beneficial supplements that aid in restoring a more properly functioning adrenal gland. We endeavor to discuss merely those that appear to be most advantageous and have the heaviest weight of published literature.

ADAPTOGENS

This group of substances helps the body adapt to stress, and has been shown to reduce the damage of the stress response, maintain homeostasis during chronic stress, reduce most evidence of the alarm stage, and delay the exhaustion phase. Royal Bee Jelly (one of the world's richest sources of pantothenic acid needed for the adrenal glands) is an adaptogen; however, the most widely researched are Siberian ginseng (*Eleutherococcus senticosus*) and licorice (*Glycyrrhiza*) (Ritchason, 1995).

Licorice

Licorice is a perennial herb native to the Mediterranean region, central to southern Russia, and Asia Minor to Iran, now cultivated throughout Europe, Asia, and the Middle

East (Bruneton, 1995; Karnick, 1994; Leung & Foster, 1996). It is one of the most widely used medicinal herbs and is found in numerous traditional formulas (Leung & Foster, 1996). Licorice is one of the most extensively researched medicinal and food plants. Licorice root has been used therapeutically for several thousand years in both Western and Eastern systems of medicine (Leung & Foster, 1996).

The Latin name for licorice is *Glycyrrhiza glabra.* Dioscorides, a 1st-century Greek physician is responsible for its genus name, *Glycyrrhiza,* which comes from *glukos* (sweet) and *riza* (root) (Foster & Tyler, 1999). The pharmacopeial name for licorice is Liquiritiae radix and it is known by other names including Liquorice, Gancao, sweet root, Yasti-madhu and Glycyrrhiza.

While the first recorded cultivation of the herb was in the 13th century by Piero de Cresenzi from Bologna, its use was first documented on Assyrian clay tablets ca. 2500 B.C.E for the treatment of coughs and relief of the unwelcome effects of laxatives. The Greeks used it ca. 372 to 287 B.C.E. for asthma, dry coughs, and all pectoral diseases. In China, first mention of the herb was in the *Shen Nong Ben Cao Jing* (ca. 25 C.E.). In addition to its advantageous properties as an expectorant and antitussive, the Chinese pharmacopeia notes its antispasmodic relief on gastrointestinal smooth muscle and its desoxycorticosterone-like action (Tu, 1992). Further to its other beneficial effects, the current ayurvedic pharmacopoeia reports it as an adrenal agent (Karnick, 1994). Licorice root and extracts as well as fluid and solid are in the U.S. *National Formulary* (1985). Studies have investigated and documented its favorable effects as an anxiolytic (Chen, Hsieh, & Lai, 1985). *The British Herbal Compendium* reported its actions as an anti-inflammatory, expectorant, demulcent, and adrenocorticotropic (Bradley, 1992).

Harvesting comes from cultivation of roots that are 3 to 4 years old. The roots and stolons contain glycyrrhizin, also called glycyrrhizic or glycyrrhizinic acid (5 to 9% by weight), which is believed to be some 50 times sweeter than sucrose. That same sweet taste is lost or reduced when in an acidic medium (Leung & Foster, 1996).

Licorice is a natural way to supplement the body's endogenous cortisol production, giving the adrenals a well-needed rest. Dosage is 25 to 100 mg/day. Pharmacopeial-grade licorice root must contain no less than 4% glycyrrhizic acid, calculated in the dried root.

Chemically speaking, licorice root contains triterpenoid saponins (4 to 24%), mostly glycyrrhizin, along with a mixture of potassium and calcium salts, flavonoids (1%), amines (1 to 2%), asparagines, choline, and betaine; amino acids; 3 to 15% glucose and sucrose; starch (2 to 30%); polysaccharides; sterols; resin and volatile oils. Research done by Heikens, Fliers, Endert, Ackermans, and van Montfrans (1995) proposes that the hydrolytic metabolite of glycyrrhizic acid, glycyrrhetenic acid, is the major dynamic element causing inhibition of peripheral metabolism of cortisol that binds to mineralocorticoid receptors in like fashion to aldosterone.

Two hypotheses for licorice's mechanism of action have been suggested by research:

1. The binding of glycyrrhetinic acid to mineralocorticoids receptors, and/or
2. Blocking the action of 11-beta-hydroxysteroid dehydrogenase.

Recent publications advocate that both hypotheses may be implicated, particularly with the substantiation that the blocking of 11-beta-hydroxysteroid dehydrogenase is short term and that subsequent to its occurrence, the pseudoaldosteronism is directly linked to increased plasma concentration of licorice metabolites and their binding to mineralocorticoids receptors. 11-beta-hydroxysteroid dehydrogenase usually metabolizes glucocorticoids into inactive compounds rapidly, thereby controlling glucocorticoids' access to mineralocorticoids and glucocorticoids receptors. Increased glucocorticoid concentration in mineralocorticoid responsive tissue results from the licorice thwarting inactivation of hydrocortisone. This results in glucocorticoids occupying mineralocorticoid receptors and producing a mineralocorticoid response that is demonstrated by hypertension and increased sodium retention (Chandler, 1997).

Extreme quantities of licorice consumption (more than 20 g per day) have elevated concerns about the potential for glycyrrhizin in licorice producing pseudoaldosteronism (excess levels of aldosterone), which may cause symptoms of headache, hypertension, lethargy, potassium loss that upsets the balance of sodium and potassium and possible cardiac arrest. The pseudoaldosterone-like effects are generally attributed to the glycyrrhizic acid. Of note, within several weeks of cessation any symptoms of hyperaldosteronism disappear (Mantero, 1981). A deglycyrrhizinated licorice (DGL) preparation has been developed that provides most of the therapeutic benefits while reducing risk.

Usage should be limited to no more than 4 to 6 weeks at a time to prevent potentiation of glucocorticoids and mineralcorticoids. Prolonged use with high doses may result in water and Na retention and K loss. This may be accompanied by edema, hypertension, and hypokalemia. It is not recommended while pregnant and is contraindicated with liver cirrhosis, hypertonia, hypokalemia, severe kidney insufficiency, and cholestatic liver disorders.

Ginseng

The Latin name for ginseng is *Panax ginseng.* Its pharmacopeial name is Ginseng radix. Other names for it include Chinese ginseng, Korean ginseng, true ginseng and Asian ginseng. The genus name *Panax* is derived from the Greek *pan* (all) and *akos* (cure), meaning cure-all. Like licorice, ginseng's therapeutic uses were recorded over 2000 years ago in the oldest comprehensive material medica, *Shen Nong Ben Cao Jing*.

Ginseng is a slow-growing perennial herb native to the northeastern mountain forests of China, Korea, and the far eastern portions of Russia. It is cultivated extensively in these same countries. Flowering of the plant begins in the fourth year and its roots take 4 to 6 years until the plant reaches full maturity. Many types and grades of the herb exist.

Pharmacopoeia grade ginseng from both China and Japan should be collected from the dried matured root in the autumn. The rootlets must be removed. Confirmation of botanical identity is confirmed by thin-layer chromatography (TLC) in addition to micro- and macroscopic examination.

Asian medicine uses dried ginseng as a tonic to revitalize and replenish vital energy (qi). Traditional uses include as a prophylactic aid to restore resistance, reduce vulnerability to sickness, and encourage health and longevity.

The origins of its activity are based on whole body effects rather than specific organs and systems, which provides support to the time-honored view that ginseng is a tonic that can invigorate the functioning of the organism as a whole. Ginseng is in the national pharmacopoeias of several European countries, Russia, and China. In the United States, it has been used as a stand-alone herb or as the main ingredient in a wide range of tonics, and energy and immunostimulant supplements. Over the course of the last half-century, numerous scientific studies of varying quality have been published on ginseng (Foster & Chongxi, 1992). Ten clinical trials have investigated the efficacy of ginseng on physical stress and psychomotor functions.

One such study by Caso Marasco et al. reported on its ability to improve quality-of-life in persons subjected to high stress (Caso Marasco, Vargas Ruiz, Salas Villagomex, & Begona Infante, 1996). This same study found that when ginseng was added to the base of a multivitamin it improved subjective parameters in a population exposed to high physical and mental stress. This suggests an adaptogenic effect to this combination.

The biologically active constituents in *P. ginseng* are made up of a fusion of triterpene saponins known as ginsenosides. Ginsenosides are found nowhere else in nature. The two main ginsenosides, Rb1 and Rg1, correspondingly suppress and stimulate the central nervous system. It is proposed that these contrasting actions may contribute to the adaptogenic portrayal of this herb and its ostensible capacity to balance corporal functions.

The Commission E monographs from Germany noted that the resistance of rodents was enhanced when various stress models such as coldness and immobilization tests were performed.

Siberian ginseng (*Eleutherococcus senticosus*) is in the same family but contains eleutheros instead of ginsenosides. It is also considered to be adaptogenic.

Use is contraindicated in hypertension. The *British Herbal Compendium* contraindicates use during pregnancy; however, the Commission E report fails to corroborate that. Ginseng is known to have estrogenic activity. It could negatively affect estrogen-dependent diseases in woman, i.e., endometriosis, fibrocystic breasts, or breast cancer.

Dosage for the root is between 1 and 2 g/day for as long as 3 months at a time. Tinctures, fluid extracts, standardized extracts, and decoctions are also available and dosage is dependent upon the source. Ginseng needs to be taken for at least 1 month before any positive effects are likely to be felt.

Ginseng along with another adaptogenic herb, ashwagandha, has been suggested to influence adrenal hormone activity by helping to support normal HPA function (Brown, 1996).

Other herbs shown to be of benefit to the adrenal glands include astragalas, bayberry, borage, burdock, kava, kelp, parsley, and rose hips (Leung & Foster, 1996).

VITAMINS AND NUTRIENTS

Vitamin C reduces the effects of chronic stress by decreasing cortisol production (American Chemical Society, 1999; Nathan, van Droux, & Feiss, 1991). A high dietary intake of vitamin C may even help reduce the effects of chronic stress by inhibiting the release of stress hormones. Ascorbic acid when given orally (1 g twice daily) also buffered exogenous ACTH-induced increases in cortisol. An additional function of ascorbate in the adrenal glands is as a protective compound for cytochrome (Hornsby, Harris, & Aldern, 1985).

Evidence indicates adrenal cortex function is compromised in the event of a deficiency of vitamin B5 derivatives and metabolites (Gregory & Kelly, 1999). Alternatively, the administration of pantethine in several experimental animal models appears to enhance adrenal function (Kosaka, Okida, Kaneyuki, et al., 1973; Onuki & Hoshino, 1970).

Lipoic acid, known as the universal antioxidant, appears to prevent the accretion of catecholamines in cardiac tissue secondary to stress. It also augments the abolition of catecholamine degradation products (Fomichev & Pchelintsev, 1993).

Other nutrients that demonstrate possible effects include tyrosine, phosphotidylserine (PS), and plant sterols and sterolins.

TABLE 82.2
Associated Symptoms and Consequences
of Impaired Adrenals

• Low body temperature	• Alternating diarrhea and constipation
• Weakness	• Osteoporosis
• Unexplained hair loss	• Auto-immune hepatitis
• Nervousness	• Auto-immune diseases
• Difficulty building muscle	• Lightheadedness
• Irritability	• Palpitations (heart fluttering)
• Mental depression	• Dizziness that occurs upon standing
• Difficulty gaining weight	• Poor resistance to infections
• Apprehension	• Low blood pressure
• Hypoglycemia	• Insomnia
• Inability to concentrate	• Food and/or inhalant allergies
• Excessive hunger	• PMS
• Tendency toward inflammation	• Craving for sweets
• Moments of confusion	• Dry and thin skin
• Indigestion	• Headaches
• Poor memory	• Scanty perspiration
• Feelings of frustration	• Alcohol intolerance

BIOFEEDBACK

Biofeedback utilizes audiovisual input to teach patients to control their own reactions to pain, stress, and similar noxious stimuli. Patients are able to visualize graphic representations of the effects of noxious stimuli on various physiologic responses such as blood pressure, heart rate, skin temperature, and sweating on computer monitors or auditory input. Then through trial and error subjects learn to control these physiological responses in order to decrease the negative effects of the noxious stimuli on their bodies.

Biofeedback has had particular success when utilized in the treatment of chronic pain and stress management (Kong, Lim, & Oon, 1989). Typically, a series of five to ten treatments are given.

IMPROVING ADRENAL HEALTH WITH LIFESTYLE

The most common reason why the adrenals are impaired is unresolved emotional stress. Attend to this first. Recognize concealed causes of stress. These could include toxins from solvents, pesticides, yeast, dysbiosis, parasites, structural misalignments, etc.

Optimize the diet. Also, get appropriate amounts of sleep. Because repair and rest occur between 11 p.m. and 1 a.m. these tools should be optimized. From an acupuncture point of view, the gallbladder releases toxins between these same 2 hours. If you are awake, they can back up into the liver.

In a recent study in the *Journal of Behavioral Medicine,* progressive relaxation was shown to be the most effective means of reducing the stress response when compared to music, attention control, and silence, which were found to be effective, but less so (Scheufele, 2000).

Sleep is an often overlooked piece of the health puzzle that has recently been shown to be of major significance. A new study in the *Journal of the American Medical Association* (*JAMA*) reports that sleep-related hormone imbalances often start to surface in the mid-1930s (Cauter, Leproult, & Plat, 2000) 149 healthy men between the ages of 16 and 83 were involved in this sleep study. By the time the men reached 36 to 50 years of age the amount of sleep spent in the most restful state (slow wave) had decreased by almost 80% from the late teens and early 20s. Sleep deprivation on any given night results in increased levels of cortisol and decreased growth hormone secretion the subsequent night. The relationship between sleep quality and hormone function may very well be a two-way street: lack of adequate sleep may interrupt hormonal equilibrium and at the same time hormonal imbalances can trigger sleep difficulties.

In a related editorial in the same *JAMA* issue, Blackman (2000) notes that early intervention (with hormonal testing) is the best method for screening.

When it comes to dealing with stress, humor plays a significant role that should be acknowledged and encouraged. Humor helps us make sense of, understand, and cope with reality and serves as nature's biofeedback, stress-control system (Woodhouse, 1993).

Massage, avoidance of food allergies and hypersensitivities, proper diet, and changed attitudes are just some of the positive tools that can be utilized in an effort to improve lifestyle. Learning stress management is a quintessential tool in reducing adrenal tension.

EXERCISE

The positive effect exercise plays in reducing daily stress cannot be overemphasized (Carmack, et al., 1999). Among working adults, physical activity performed during leisure time was found to decrease perceived stress (Aldana, Sutton, Jacobson, & Quirk, 1996).

Exercise is a great stimulator of positive mental and physical well-being. It increases oxygen uptake by red blood cells, lymphatic circulation, excretion of toxins, and has a profound positive effect on one's self-image. Exercise also increases endorphin production, which can indirectly reduce stress and pain throughout the body. Caution should always be exerted not to over exercise, which will overstress the body, thus reversing the beneficial effects.

Clinical experience strongly suggests that exercise is an effective way for stressed individuals to enhance their sense of self-control and coping self-worth (ACSM). The importance of regular aerobic activity as a means of dealing with stress is well documented. In addition to several positive effects already mentioned, it has been shown to reduce the cardiovascular impact of emotional stressors (Sotile, 1996).

Other forms of exercise that increase relaxation and mental focus include yoga and Tai Chi Chuan. The term "relaxation training" has been used to describe these types of intervention. Other relaxation training techniques are self-hypnosis, meditation, breathing exercises, and biofeedback.

Many believe that combining more than one type of relaxation training increases their effectiveness.

CONCLUSIONS

In the absence of serious disease, tumors, or other pathology, there exists a state of adrenal overuse that is brought on by difficulty dealing with the increasing stresses of life. Every human has a different adaptational capacity (i.e., tolerance to stress). Irrespective of the stressor, the response they elicit from the body is very similar, the most common being from emotional stimuli.

Recent advances in laboratory tests utilizing saliva that are both easy and convenient have been developed to help with diagnosis. Early testing, as promulgated by Blackman (Scheufele, 2000), is the first line of defense in maintaining a stronger endocrine system.

A healthy endocrine system starts essentially at the embryologic level. From the time of birth the simplest of things including cuddling, touching, and holding signal the beginnings of a healthy adrenal gland. Experiments with rat pups that had especially attentive mothers found they have more of a certain type of receptor on the surface of the hippocampus than in the relatively neglected group of rats. These specific receptors responded to a cortisol-like hormone. The fact that more of these corticosterone-receptors were present presages that the brain would be more sensitive and efficient in utilizing this hormone to terminate the stress response.

The conventional medical establishment has frowned upon natural approaches to managing adrenal function, generally because there has been no apparent relationship established between many illnesses and waning adrenal function. More often than not, adrenal decline is perceived as a side effect of the disease process instead of as the direct cause. It may be borne out that the decline of the adrenal gland is, in fact, both an indirect cause and a side effect of numerous persistent and acute infirmities.

The sum of all the stresses during the course of a lifetime can contribute to the aging process. The neuro-endocrine theory of aging validates the paralleling decline of the endocrine glands and the aging process. It further bears out that restoring more youthful hormonal levels to these same organs can slow down, and in many instances reverse, some of the effects of that same aging process.

Profoundly potent herbs, along with certain vitamins including ascorbic acid, vitamins B1 and B6, the co-enzyme forms of vitamin B5 (pantethine) and B12 (methylcobalamin), the amino acid tyrosine, and other nutrients such as lipoic acid, phosphotidylserine, and plant sterol/sterolin combinations (Kelly, 1999; Shelygina, Spivak, Zaretskii, et al., 1975). DHEA and pregnenalone supplementation, and a healthy lifestyle that includes regular exercise, proper rest, humor, de-stressing the nervous system and energy flows of the body through chiropractic and acupuncture, progressive relaxation, and biofeedback-make up the foundation of a prescription for a strong and vibrant adrenal gland.

REFERENCES

6/18/2000 http://www-med.stanford.edu/school/Neurosciences/faculty/sapolsky.html.

ACSM's resource manual for guidelines for exercise testing and prescription (3rd ed., p. 550). Philadelphia: Lippincott Williams & Wilkens.

Adrenal maladaptation syndrome. (1998). *VRP Nutritional News, 12*, 5.

Aldana, S.G., Sutton, L.D., Jacobson, B.H., & Quirk, M.G. (1996). Relationships between leisure time physical activity and perceived stress. *Perceptual Motor Skills, 82*(1), 315–321.

Arlt, W., et al. (1999). Dehydroepiandrosterone replacement in women with adrenal insufficiency. *New England Journal of Medicine, 30*, 341(14), 1013–1020.

Berdanier, C.D., Parente, J.A., Jr., & McIntosh, M.K. (1993). Is dehydroepiandrosterone an anti-obesity agent? *Federation of American Societies for Experimental Biology Journal, 7*(5), 414–419.

Berkhow, R., & Fletcher, A.J. (1987). *The Merck manual* (15th ed.). Whitehouse Station, NJ: Merck.

Blackman, M.R. (2000). Age-related alterations in sleep quality and neuroendocrine function: Interrelationship and implications. *Journal of the American Medical Association, 284*(7), 861–868.

Bonney, R.C., et al. (1984). The interrelationship between plasma 5-ene adrenal androgens in normal women. *Journal of Steroid Biochemistry, 20*(6A), 1353–1355.

Bradley, P.R. (Ed.). (1992). *British herbal compendium* (Vol. 1.) Bournemouth: British Herbal Medicine Association.

Brooks-Gunn, J., Warren, M.P., & Hamilton, L.H. The relation of eating problems and amenorrhea in ballet dancers. *Medicine and Science in Sports and Exercise, 19*, 1.

Brown, D. (1996, Summer). Licorice root: Potential early intervention for chronic fatigue syndrome. *Quarterly Review Nature and Medicine*, 95–97.

Bruneton, J. (1995). *Pharmacognosy, phytochemistry, medicinal plants*. Paris: Lavoisier Publishing.

Carmack, C.L. (1999). *Annals of Behavioral Medicine, 21*(3), 251–257.

Caso Marasco, A., Vargas Ruiz, R., Salas Villagomez, A., & Begona Infante, C. (1996). Double-blind study of a multi-vitamin complex supplemented with ginseng extract. *Drugs under Experimental and Clinical Research, 22*(6), 323–329.

Cauter, E., Leproult, R., & Plat, L. (2000). Age-related changes in slow wave sleep and REM sleep and relationship with growth hormone and cortisol levels in healthy men. *Journal of the American Medical Association, 284*(7), 861–868.

Chandler, R.F. (1997). Glycyrrhiza glabra. In P.A. De Smet, K. Keller, & R. Hansel, *Adverse effects of herbal drugs* (Vol. 3). New York: Springer Verlag.

Chen, H.C., Hsieh, M.T., & Lai, E. (1985). Studies on the suanzaorentang in the treatment of anxiety. *Psychopharmacology* (Berlin), *85*(4), 486–487.

Cotran, R.S., Kumar, V., & Robbins, S.L. (1989). *Robbins pathologic basis of disease* (4th ed.). W.B. Saunders.

Creuss, D.G., et al. (2000). Cognitive-behavioral stress management reduces serum cortisol by enhancing positive contributions among women being treated for early stage breast cancer. *Psychosomatic Medicine, 62*(3), 304–308.

Dilman, V. (1981). The law of deviation of homeostasis in diseases of aging, John Wright. PSG.

Dilman, V., & Dean, W. (1992). *The neuroendocrine theory of aging and degenerative disease*. Pensacola, FL: The Center for Bio-Gerontology.

DiPietro, J.A. (2000). Baby and the brain: Advances in child development. *Annual Review of Public Health, 21*, 455–471.

Fitzgerald, P.A. (1992). Adrenal cortex physiology. *Current medical diagnosis and treatment* (p. 982). MA Lange Publishers.

Fomichev, V.I., & Pchelintsev, V.P. (1993). The neurohumoral systems of patients with ischemic heart disease and under emotional pain-stress: The means for their pharmacological regulation. *Kardiologiia, 33*, 15–18.

Foster, S., & Tyler, V.E. (1999). *Tyler's honest herbal: A sensible guide to the use of herbs and related remedies*. New York: Haworth Herbal Press.

Foster, S., & Chongxi, Y. (1992). *Herbal emissaries: Bringing Chinese herbs to the West* (pp. 102–112). Rochester, VT: Healing Arts Press.

Gregory, S., & Kelly, N.D. (1999). Nutritional and botanical interventions to assist with the adaptation to stress. *Alternative Medicine Review, 4*(4), 249–265.

Heikens, J., Fliers, E., Endert, E. Ackermans, M., & van Montfrans, G. (1995). Liquorice-induced hypertension — a new understanding of an old disease: Case report and brief review. *Netherlands Journal of Medicine, 47*(5), 230–234.

Holden, C. (1996). Child development: Small refugees suffer the effects of early neglect. *Science, 274*, 1076–1077.

Hornsby, P.J. (1997). DHEA: A biological perspective. *Journal of the American Geriatrics Society, 45*, 1395–1401.

Hornsby, P.J., Harris, S.E., & Aldern, K.A. (1985). The role of ascorbic acid in the function of the adrenal cortex: Studies in adrenocorticol cells in culture, *Endocrinology, 117*(3), 1264–1271.

Ipel, E. (2000, September). *Psychological Medicine, 62*, 623–632.

Jeffcoate, W. (1993). *Lecture notes on endocrinology*, 5th ed. Blackwell Scientific Publications.

Karnick, C.R. (1994). *Pharmacopoeial standards of herbal plants* (Vols. 1–2). Delhi: Sri Satguru Publications.

Kelly, G.S. (1999). Nutritional and botanical interventions to assist with the adaptation of stress. *Alternative Medicine Review, 4*(4), 249–265.

Kiecolt-Glaser J., & Glaser, R. (2000, April 15). Presentation to the British Psychological Society.

Kong, D.S., Lim, L.J., & Oon, C.H. (1989). Biofeedback and stress management strategies, *Annals of the Academy of Medicine, Singapore, 18*(3), 261–265.

Kosaka, C., Okida, M., Kaneyuki, T., et al. (1973). Action of pantethine on the adrenal cortex of hypophysectomized rats. *Horumon to Rinsho, 21*, 517–525.

Leung, A.Y., & Foster, S. (1996). *Encyclopedia of common natural ingredients used in food, drugs, and cosmetics* (2nd ed.). New York: John Wiley & Sons, Inc.

Li, S., Givalois, L., & Pelletier, G. (1997). Dehydroepiandrosterone administration reverses the inhibitory influence of aging on gonadotropin-releasing hormone expression in the male and female rat brain. *Endocrine, 6*(3), 265–270.

Mantero, F. (1981). Exogenous mineralocorticoid-like disorders. *Clinical Endocrinology and Metabolism, 10*(3), 465–478.

Marx, C., Ehrhart-Bornstein, M., Scherbaum, W.A. & Bornstein, S.R. (1998). Regulation of adrenocortical function by cytokines relevance for immune-endocrine interaction. *Hormone and Metabolism Research, 6–7*, 416–20.

McGwen, B.S. (1998). Protective and damaging effects of stress mediators. *New England Journal of Medicine, 338*, 3, 171–179.

Miller, W.L., & Tyrell, J.B. (1996). The adrenal cortex. In *Endocrinology and metabolism.* New York: McGraw-Hill.

Nathan, N., van Droux, J.C., & Feiss, P. (1991). *American and French Anesthesiologie et Reanimation, 10*(4), 329–332.

National Formulary (NF) (16th ed.) (1985). Washington, D.C.: American Pharmaceutical Association.

Oelkers, W. (1999). Dehydroepiandrosterone for adrenal insufficiency. *New England Journal of Medicine, 30*, 341(14), 1073–1074.

Onuki, M., & Hoshino, H. (1970). Effects of pantethine on the adrenocorticol function. *Horumon to Rinsho, 18*, 601–605.

Ramirez, A.J. (1989). *British Medical Journal, 298*(6669), 291–293.

Ritchason, N.D. (1995). *The little herb encyclopedia.* Sacramento, CA: Woodland Health Books.

Rosenfeld, R.S., Rosenberg, B.J., Fukushima, D.K., & Hellman, L. (1975). 24-hour secretory pattern of dehydroepiandrosterone and dehydroepiandrosterone sulfate. *Journal of Clinical Endocrinology and Metabolism, 40*(5), 850–855.

Rotter, J.I., Wong, F.L., Lifrak, E.T., & Parker, L.N. (1985). A genetic component to the variation of dehydroepiandrosterone sulfate. *Metabolism, 34*(8), 731–736.

Sapolsky, R., et al. (1987). Stress and glucocorticoids in aging. *Endocrinology and Metabolism Clinics of North America, 16*(4), 965–980.

Scheufele, P.M. (2000). Effects of progressive relaxation and classical music on measurements of attention, relaxation, and stress responses. *Journal of Behavioral Medicine, 23*(2), 207–228.

Selye, H. (1956). *The stress of life.* New York: McGraw-Hill Book Co.

Selye, H. (1976). *The stress of life* (rev. ed.). New York: McGraw-Hill Book Co.

Sephton, S.E., Sapolsky, R.M., Kraemer, H.C., & Spiegel, D. (2000). Diurnal cortisol rhythm as a predictor of breast cancer survival. *Journal of the National Cancer Institute, 92*(12), 994–1000.

Shelygina, N.M., Spivak, Ria., Zaretskii, M.M., et al. (1975). Influence of Vitamin C, B1 and B6 on the diurnal periodicity of the glucocorticoid function of the adrenal cortex in patients with atherosclerotic cardiosclerosis. *Voprosy Pitaniya, 2*, 25–29.

Small, M. (2000, August), *Discover,* 66–71.

Sotile, W.M. (1996). *Psychosocial interventions for cardiopulmonary patients: A guide for health professionals.* Champaign IL: Human Kinetics.

Tu, G. (Ed.). (1992). *Pharmacopoeia of the People's Republic of China,* 118–119. (English Ed., 1992). Beijing: Guangdong Science and Technology Press.

Walther, D. (1988). *Applied kinesiology,* Colorado: Synopsis Systems DC.

Woodhouse, D.K. (1993). The aspects of humor in dealing with stress. *Nursing Administration Quarterly, 18*(1), 80–89.

83

Aromatherapy for Pain Relief

A.R. Hirsch, M.D.

In explaining the persuasive attraction of alternative medicine, Kaptchuk and Eisenberg (1998) note, "The fundamental premises are an advocacy of nature, vitalism, science, and spirituality." With this in mind, the science underpinning aromatherapy will be explored.

DEFINITIONS

One of the difficulties in understanding aromatherapy is that it means different things to different people. One part of its definition that is agreed upon is that aromatherapy uses odorous compounds to promote health and healing (Kaptchuk & Eisenberg, 1998). Beyond this, opinions differ. Aromachologists speak of using odors not to treat disease, but to promote wellness. Aromatologists believe in ingestion of the substance being used as well as its inhalation (Price & Price, 1995). Many aromatherapists believe in using massage coincident with inhalation (Tisserand, 1977). In this chapter, aromatherapy is defined as the use of odorants as inhalants to treat underlying medical or psychiatric conditions. This definition excludes any effects of ingestion or percutaneous absorption, although they may be significant depending upon the method of application (Weyers & Brodbeck, 1989). As defined, aromatherapy use is also independent of any effects of coincident, noninhalational therapy, such as massage, interpersonal interaction, or bathing.

This definition is consistent with the literature indicating that real aromatherapy involves the uptake of fragrant compounds only through inhalation, not by other methods (Buchbauer, 1993).

Many in the aromatherapy community believe that natural or essential oils are effective and that artificial synthesized compounds are not. However, in the treatment of neurologic and psychiatric diseases, literature does not differentiate between them (King, 1994). No distinction will be made herein between the use of synthesized as opposed to naturally occurring oils.

BACKGROUND

Why is the concept of aromatherapy under consideration today? One reason is its history. Throughout history, odorants have been used to treat various diseases. More than 5000 years ago the Egyptians treated disease using odors (Lindsay, Pitcaithly, & Geelen, 1997), and 3500 years ago the Babylonians used odors to exorcise demons of disease (Roebuck, 1988). The ancient Aztecs also used odors to treat disease. Aromatherapy has known no cultural or geographic boundaries. Virtually all cultures have fumigated the sick (Buchbauer, 1993).

ANATOMY OF OLFACTION

Neuroscience provides insight into the mechanisms by which odors may impact behavior and neurologic functioning.

There is an anatomic basis for the belief that odors can affect the brain and behavior (Brodal, 1969). Once an odor passes through the olfactory epithelium, it must stimulate the olfactory nerve, which consists of unmyelinated olfactory fila. The olfactory nerve has the slowest conduction rate of any nerve in the body. The olfactory fila pass through the cribiform plate of the ethmoid bone and enter the olfactory bulb. During trauma, much damage occurs

0-8493-0926-3/02/$0.00+$1.50
© 2002 by CRC Press LLC

in this bulb (Hirsch & Wyse, 1993). Different odors localize in different areas of the olfactory bulb.

Inside the olfactory bulb is a conglomeration of neuropil called the glomeruli. Approximately 2000 glomeruli reside in the olfactory bulb. Four different cell types make up the glomeruli: processes of receptor cell axons, mitral cells, tufted cells, and second-order neurons that give off collaterals to the granule cells and to cells in the periglomerular and external plexiform layers. The mitral and tufted cells form the lateral olfactory tract and establish a reverberating circuit with the granule cells. The mitral cells stimulate firing of the granule cells, which, in turn, inhibit firing of the mitral cells.

A reciprocal inhibition exists between the mitral and tufted cells. This results in a sharpening of olfactory acuity. The olfactory bulb receives several efferent projections, including the primary olfactory fibers, the contralateral olfactory bulb and the anterior nucleus, the prepiriform cortex (inhibitory), the diagonal band of Broca (with neurotransmitters acetylcholine and GABA), the locus coeruleus, the dorsal raphe, and the tuberomamillary nucleus of the hypothalamus.

The olfactory bulb's efferent fibers project into the olfactory tract, which divides at the olfactory trigona into the medial and lateral olfactory stria. These project to the anterior olfactory nucleus; the olfactory tubercle; the amygdaloid nucleus (which, in turn, projects to the ventral medial nucleus of the hypothalamus, a feeding center); the cortex of the piriform lobe; the septal nuclei; and the hypothalamus, in particular the anterolateral regions of the hypothalamus, which are involved in reproduction. The neurotransmitters by which the olfactory bulb conducts its information include glutamate, aspartate, NAAG, CCK, and GABA.

The anterior olfactory nucleus receives afferent fibers from the olfactory tract and projects efferent fibers, which decussate in the anterior commissure and synapse in the contralateral olfactory bulb. Some of the efferent projections from the anterior olfactory nucleus remain ipsilateral, and synapse on internal granular cells of the ipsilateral olfactory bulb.

The olfactory tubercle receives afferent fibers from the olfactory bulb and the anterior olfactory nucleus. Efferent fibers from the olfactory tubercle project to the nucleus accumbens as well as the striatum. Neurotransmitters of the olfactory tubercle include acetylcholine and dopamine.

The area on the cortex where olfaction is localized, that is, the primary olfactory cortex, includes the prepiriform area, the periamygdaloid area, and the entorhinal area. Afferent projections to the primary olfactory cortex include the mitral cells, which enter the lateral olfactory tract and synapse in the prepiriform cortex (lateral olfactory gyrus) and the corticomedial part of the amygdala. Efferent projections from the primary olfactory cortex extend to the entorhinal cortex (area 28), the basal and lateral amygdaloid nuclei, the lateral preoptic area of the hypothalamus, the nucleus of the diagonal band of Broca, the medial forebrain bundle, the dorsal medial nucleus and submedial nucleus of the thalamus, and the nucleus accumbens.

It should be noted that the entorhinal cortex is both a primary and a secondary olfactory cortical area. Efferent fibers from the cortex project via the uncinate fasciculus to the hippocampus, the anterior insular cortex (next to the gustatory cortical area), and the frontal cortex. (This may explain why temporal lobe epilepsy that involves the uncinate often produces parageusias of burning rubber, known as uncinate fits (Acharya, Acharya, & Luders, 1996).

Some of the efferent projections of the mitral and tufted cells decussate in the anterior commissure and form the medial olfactory tract. They then synapse in the contralateral parolfactory area and contralateral subcallosal gyrus. The exact function of the medial olfactory stria and tract is not clear. The accessory olfactory bulb receives afferent fibers from the bed nucleus of the accessory olfactory tract and the medial and posterior corticoamygdaloid nuclei. Efferent fibers from the accessory olfactory bulb project through the accessory olfactory tract to the same afferent areas, for example, the bed nucleus of the accessory olfactory tract and the medial posterior corticoamygdaloid nuclei. It should be noted that the medial and posterior corticoamygdaloid nuclei project secondary fibers to the anterior and medial hypothalamus, the areas associated with reproduction. Therefore, the accessory olfactory bulb in humans may be the mediator for human pheromones (Hirsch, 1998a).

Some unique aspects of the anatomy of the olfactory system are worth mentioning. Smell is the only sensation to reach the cortex before reaching the thalamus. The only sensory system that is primary ipsilateral in its projection, olfaction does not depend upon the cortex, as has been demonstrated in decorticated cats.

Neurotransmitters of the olfactory cortex are multiple, including glutamate, asparatate cholcystekinin, LHRH, and somatastatin.

Furthermore, perception of odors causes modulation of olfactory neurotransmitters within the olfactory bulb and the limbic system. Virtually all known neurotransmitters are present in the olfactory bulb. Thus, odorant modulation of neurotransmitter levels in the olfactory bulb, tract, and limbic system intended for transmission of sensory information may have unintended secondary effects on a variety of different behaviors and disease states that are regulated by the same neurotransmitters. For instance, odorant modulation of dopamine in the olfactory bulb/limbic system may affect manifestations of Parkinson's disease. Mesolimbic override to many of the components of Parkinson's disease have been well documented, for example, motoric activation associated with emotional distress and fear of injury in a fire.

EMOTIONAL AND BEHAVIORAL EFFECTS OF ODORS

Odors can affect behavior by acting as alternative sensory stimuli. The phenomena of visual system mediation of the movements of Parkinsonian gait through the visual stimuli of lines placed on the floor (Dietz, Goetz, & Steddings, 1990) is an example of alternative stimuli. Other sensory input, including pain, has been shown to inhibit the Jacksonian march in epilepsy (Gowers, 1881 in Efron, 1957). Similarly, odors may act as competing sensory stimuli during an uncinate seizure (Efron, 1957). It seems possible that other sensory input, including odors, could modify Parkinson's disease as well as other neurologic conditions by acting as competing sensory stimuli.

Using another mechanism of action, odors can affect behavior and mood by producing secondary effects on the emotions of the individual. This is different from a direct neurophysiologic effect of the limbic system. Rather, the odor can change the mood of the individual, which then has secondary neurologic effects. For instance, mood or level of alertness can affect a variety of neurologic conditions, including the perception of pain. A soldier who is severely wounded in battle may continue to fight and not feel pain until the battle is over. Studies also suggest that persons in a positive state of mind are less bothered by pain (Fields, 1967).

Substantial evidence exists that odors can affect mood. As early as 1908, Freud stressed the importance of olfaction on emotion in his description of a patient with an obsessional neurosis.

> By his own account, when a child, he recognized everyone by their smell, like a dog, and even when he was grown up he was more susceptible to sensations of smell than other people … and I have come to recognize that a tendency towards osphresiolagnia which has become extinct since childhood may play a part in the genesis of neuroses.

> In a general way I should like to raise the question whether the inevitable shunting of the sense of smell as a result of man's turning away from the earth and the organic repression of smell pleasure produced by it does not largely share in his predisposition to nervous diseases. It would thus furnish an explanation for the fact that with the advance of civilization it is precisely the sexual life which must become the victim of repression. For we have long known what an intimate relation exists in the animal organization between the sexual impulse and the function of the olfactory organs.

Of all the sensations, olfaction is the one most intertwined with limbic system functioning (MacLean, 1973). The profuse anatomic and physiologic interconnections through the olfactory bulb, stria, and nuclei to the olfactory tubercle, and from there to the prepiriform cortex, the amygdala, and numerous other limbic system structures support this (Brodal, 1969).

Smells are described differently from other sensory modalities, adding credence to their connection to emotion. Other sensory modalities are first described cognitively; a picture, for instance, is identified as being of a ship, a woman, or a house and only secondarily is it described affectively: "I like," or "I dislike it" (Ehrlichman & Halpern, 1988). But odors are first and foremost described affectively: "I like," or "I dislike" it.

The olfactory/limbic/hippocampal connections help to explain olfactory-evoked nostalgia, the phenomena whereby an odor induces a vivid recall of a scene from the distant past (Hirsch, 1992). In 86% of 989 subjects queried, certain odors triggered vivid associations analogous to a flashbulb memory. Classically, an event must induce strong emotions for deposition of such memories to occur (Squire, 1987; Brown & Kulik, 1977). By directly stimulating the limbic system, odors likewise can act as the inducing agent. This phenomenon was vividly described by Proust (1934), who wrote that the aroma of madeleine dipped in tea evoked a flood of memories and nostalgic feelings. Olfactory-evoked recall is usually a positive experience, but it can be negative, as in the olfactory flashbacks of posttraumatic stress disorder (Kline & Rausch, 1985). Hence, it seems possible that olfactory-evoked nostalgia may affect behavior because approximately 90% of these memories are associated with strong affective tones (Laird, 1988).

The facts brings to the forefront the question of how odors impact behavior or mood. The answer can be represented by either of two constructs: the Lock and Key Theory or the General Affective Theory of Odors.

THE LOCK AND KEY THEORY OF ODORS

The lock and key theory of odors (also called the systemic effect theory) (Buchbauer, 1993) suggests that odor acts very much like a specific neurotransmitter, a drug, or an enzyme. In this paradigm, an odorant has a specific effect on behavior or emotion — one odor for one emotion or one odor for, at most, a few emotions. Thus, an odor could be viewed like a medication in the pharmacopeia. For instance, in the world of neurology, propranolol is used for modulation of essential tremor, migraine headache, and anxiety. However, one would not use propranolol as a treatment for insomnia, dementia, or multiple sclerosis. The lock and key theory suggests that specific odors have specific effects. This theory has been proposed in virtually every book about aromatherapy in which specific odors are recommended for specific health effects (Damien & Damien, 1995; Cunningham, 1995; Feller, 1997; Price, 1991; Price & Price, 1995; Schnaubelt, 1995; Keville & Green, 1995).

An argument supporting the Lock and Key Theory is that odorants exert central nervous system (CNS) effects outside a subject's conscious awareness. In test animals, the more lipophilic an odor is, the greater its sedative effect. In addition, steric differences in odors create different effects despite similarities in perceived odor and volatility (Buchbauer, 1993; Buchbauer, et al., 1993).

According to the Lock and Key Theory, odors act as a drug (Buchbauer, 1993) with a potentially pharmacologic mechanism of action. The odorants are integrated in the membrane of the cells causing an increase in membrane volume due to disruption of the membrane lipids. This leads to electrical stabilization of the membrane, thus blocking the inflow of calcium ions and suppressing permeability for sodium ions. As a result, action potential production is inhibited, which induces narcosis or local anesthesia. At higher concentrations of odorant, the conductivity of potassium ions is reduced. It also is possible that the odorants act on protein kinase C, which could impact upon the spontaneous rhythm of nerve cells (Buchbauer, 1993).

This mechanism of action is further supported by established physiology for the action of an odor on the target organ, in this case, the brain. Inhalation of an odorant would have to produce measurable levels in the blood, sufficient to pass through the blood–brain barrier. Stimpfl et al. (1995) demonstrated that this does occur. One subject inhaled 1,8-cineol for 20 minutes, which produced a linear increase of 1,8-cineol in the blood, up to 275 ng/ml, a level high enough to allow penetration of the blood–brain barrier (Stimpfl, et al., 1995).

THE GENERAL AFFECTIVE THEORY OF ODORS

An alternative theory, the General Affective Theory of Odors, also called the Reflectorial Effect Theory (Buchbauer, 1993), holds that an odor experienced as hedonically positive induces a positive, happy mood and when in a happy mood, an individual does almost everything better. For instance, when a person feels happy, it is easier to learn and to sleep, and headaches are less frequent. According to the General Affective Theory, a single odor could have a multitude of diverse effects, thus affecting virtually all behaviors.

The major premise that hedonically positive odors induce happier moods was demonstrated by Alaoui-Ismaili, et al. (1997); 44 subjects inhaled five odorants, namely, vanillin, menthol, eugenol, methyl methacrylate, and propionic acid. Six autonomic nervous system parameters were recorded: skin potential, skin resistance, skin temperature, skin blood flow, instantaneous respiratory frequency, and instantaneous heart rate. Evaluation of these parameters demonstrated a pattern consistent with known emotional states. Hedonically pleasant odors evoked mainly happiness and surprise, and unpleasant ones induced mainly disgust and anger (Alaoui-Ismaili, et al., 1997).

Milter, et al. (1994) also showed that exposure to odors could change emotions in the same direction as the hedonic valence of the odor. Using the startle reflex amplitude as a physiologic indicator of emotional valence, he found that the odor of hydrogen sulfide (H₂S) increased the startle reflex amplitude and the odor of vanillin reduced it.

Aromatherapists recognize the affective impact of odors as the mechanism of action. Buchbauer notes, "A pleasant odor has always been, and still is, an important factor for people to feel good, and feeling well is synonymous with good health. Therefore, we can conclude that all substances which are able to create a certain amount of well-being and well-feeling possess therapeutic properties and, therefore, can be called therapeutic agents" (Buchbauer, 1990). The General Affective Theory of Odors might be extended to include nonodorants in the pharmacologic arena such as valium. Valium may be useful for virtually all medical conditions because reducing anxiety makes conditions such as chronic pain, movement disorders, or insomnia less bothersome. Hence, an entire branch of medicine could be built around Valium: "Valiotherapy." If one ascribes aromatherapeutic results to the General Affective Theory as the mechanism of action, it follows that any odor that one likes induces a happier state and, hence, would have a positive effect on any disease. Again, the concept could be expanded beyond odors to any environmental stimuli, for example, a bird singing or a pretty landscape. A *Star Wars* movie might induce happiness in some observers and could be seen as inducing a positive mood state. The positive mood might lead to a reduction in pain, anxiety, and negative feelings. One could then categorize this as a form of alternative therapy: "Lucastherapy."

Reliance on the General Affective Theory of Odors implies that virtually any sensory stimulus could be used as a therapeutic tool. This largely trivializes the definition of therapy.

Another problem with the General Affective Theory of Odors is that the same odor, in different contexts, may induce opposite emotional tones (Sugawara, Hino, & Kawasaki, 1999). In *The Invalid's Story*, Mark Twain compares the disgust at the odor of a rotting corpse to the delight at the smell of cheese. The odors were the same but perceived to be from different sources. This suggests that an odor that is contextually appropriate in one situation might be considered totally inappropriate in another. Smelled in a positive context, it would be appreciated as hedonically positive and would enhance a positive affective state; smelled in a negative context, it would be perceived as hedonically negative and would, thus, induce a negative affective state. Therefore, the same odor could produce opposite mood states and opposite effects.

A variant of the General Affective Theory is that odors may induce a mood more congruent with the demands of the external environment. For instance, if the external environment requires that the individual be alert, the odor induces awareness of this; therefore, the individual responds by becoming more alert. Alternatively, if the external environment is such that it is more appropriate to be relaxed, the odor induces that awareness and the individual responds by becoming more relaxed. Evidence for the validity of this variant comes from studies of muguet odor. Where the external demand is for a greater degree of relaxation, individuals do become more relaxed, and in an environment where they are required to be more alert and vigilant, they become more alert. Warm, Dember, and Parasuraman (1991) demonstrated this effect of odorant-induced recognition of affective demands. A total of 40 subjects underwent vigilance tasks for 40 minutes during which they received periodic 30-second whiffs of air or one of two hedonically positive fragrances: muguet (independently judged as relaxing) or peppermint (independently judged as alerting). Those who received either the relaxing or alerting fragrance detected more signals during the vigilance task than the unscented air controls ($p = 0.05$).

This odorant-induced congruence of mood may also be applied to the pharmacologic agent, valium. Valium can induce opposite mood states in the same individual at different times. It can reduce anxiety to enhance concentration on a test, or it can reduce concentration to act as a soporific when the same individual is suffering with insomnia.

A corollary to the General Affective Theory is that hedonically negative odors or malodors have a negative effect on mood. If this is true, the simple elimination or masking of malodors with neutral or hedonically positive odors would induce positive effects.

Literature supports the negative effects of hedonically negative odors. Miner (1980) described some effects of exposure to the odor of livestock waste. They included annoyance, depression, nausea, vomiting, headache, shallow breathing, coughing, insomnia, and impaired appetite.

One of the malodorous pollutants that has been studied, trichloroethylene, a universally present air pollutant, can cause cephalgia (Hirsch & Rankin, 1993). Acute exposure to nitrogen tetroxide can cause cephalgia (Hirsch, 1995a) and chronic neurotoxicity (Hirsch, 1995b). Acute exposure to chlorine gas can cause neurotoxicity (Hirsch, 1995c). In 1991, Neutra, et al. (1991) reported that people living near hazardous waste sites suffer more physical symptoms during times when they can detect malodors than when they are unaware of them. Shusterman (1992) demonstrated that even at levels considered nontoxic, chemical effluviums can cause physical symptoms.

HEALTH EFFECTS OF MALODORS

Health effects of malodors can be divided into six categories: respiratory, chemosensory, cardiovascular, immune, neurologic, and psychologic.

Respiratory. Asthmatics are especially affected by malodors. Any strong odor may induce an attack in persons with unstable asthma and, even in nonasthmatics, malodors have been demonstrated to affect the cardiorespiratory system. Increased ambient oxidant levels correlate with slower cross-country running times in high school students (Wayne, Wehrle, & Carroll, 1967).

Chemosensory. Chronic exposure to malodors from pulp mills can cause permanent olfactory loss (Maruniak, 1995).

Cardiovascular. Certain malodors can induce an adrenocortic and adrenomedullary response leading to elevated blood pressure and a subsequent increase in stroke and heart disease (Evans, 1994).

Immune. Immune function may be compromised either directly, as a result of olfactory/neural projections to lymphoid tissue (Evans, 1994), or indirectly, as a result of malodor-induced depression or other negative mood states (Weisse, 1992).

Neurologic. Chronic exposure to intermittent malodors from a U.S. Navy dump site in Port Orchard, Washington induced cortical and subcortical dysfunction, which was manifested by encephalopathy: limbic encephalopathy and cephalgia (Hirsch, 1995d). Both ambient NO_2 and SO_2 impair visual adaptation to darkness and sensitivity to brightness, and increase alpha wave desynchronization on EEG (Izmerov, 1971).

Psychologic. Recognized for centuries and noted by Freud and others, psychologic effects of odors vary widely among individuals. Persons under major stress are particularly vulnerable to the psychologic effects of ambient malodors (Evans, 1994). Persons with a distorted or impaired olfactory sense may be annoyed by odors that other persons usually consider pleasant (Evans, 1994).

Certain bad odors irritate nasal passages. Resultant trigeminal stimulation releases adrenaline, leading to a tense and angry state. Thus, bad odors can trigger aggression that may then be covertly expressed. For example, in one experiment college men were instructed to apply electric shocks of varying intensity to their colleagues, supposedly for the purpose of training them. When bad odors were present, the subjects chose to inflict greater degrees of pain upon their colleagues (Rotton, et al., 1979). Another example involves air pollution. On days when malodorous air pollution is high, the number of motor vehicle accidents increases, indicating that people drive more aggressively in a polluted environment (Ury, Perkins, & Goldsmith, 1972).

Various studies show how mood and well-being suffer in the presence of malodors. Residents exposed to the effluvium from nearby commercial swine operations reported that they suffered increased tension, fatigue, confusion, depression, and anger, and that their vigor decreased (Schiffman, et al., 1995). According to one study (Rotton, et al., 1978) ambient pollutants decreased personal attraction. In a German urban area, the moods of young adults fluctuated in synchrony with the daily fluctuations in quality of environmental air, a pattern especially marked among more emotionally unstable individuals (Brandstatter, Fuhrwirth, & Kitchler, 1988). Further, daily diary entries of women in Bavaria showed that variations in their psychologic well-being coincided with variations in ambient air quality. The correlation was particularly marked among women suffering from chronic diseases such as diabetes (Bullinger, 1989a; 1989b). In Israel, negative health effects were significantly associated with levels of urban pollution (Zeidner & Schecter, 1988).

The number of family disturbances and the number of 911 emergency psychiatric calls also were linked to malodors in the environment, as determined by ozone levels (Rotton & Frey, 1985). In several cities, the number of psychiatric admissions paralleled the quality of environmental air (Briere, Downes, & Spensley, 1983).

In a study of the malodorous emanations from a mulching site southeast of Chicago, it was found that on days when the miasma wafted from the site to the school across the street, children at the school demonstrated increased behavioral problems (Hirsch, 1998b).

Malodorous ambient SO_2 levels correlate with psychiatric admissions, child psychiatric emergencies (Valentine, et al., 1975), and behavioral difficulties with decreased cooperation (Cunningham, 1979). Ambient NO_2 levels covary with psychiatric emergency room visits (Strahilevitz, Strahilevitz, & Miller, 1979).

In nonsmokers, the odor of cigarette smoke has been demonstrated to exacerbate aggressive behavior (Jones & Bogat, 1978).

The fatigue and annoyance caused by ambient malodors undoubtedly reduce individuals' capacities to function normally. Their abilities to tolerate frustration, to learn, and to cope with other stressors are impaired. In one laboratory study, subjects exposed to unpleasant odors experienced increased feelings of helplessness (Rotton, 1983).

CONTRADICTORY THEORIES

If the General Affective Theory of Odors is true, a single odor can induce a positive mood in one person and a negative mood in another. This negates the Lock and Key Theory in which odors' effects are produced outside of conscious awareness. Robin, et al. (1999) demonstrated this using eugenol. Eugenol, which is often associated with the smell of dental cement, was rated pleasant by nonfearful dental subjects and unpleasant by fearful subjects ($p = 0.036$). Changes in subjects' autonomic nervous system measurements were consistent with their emotional states; (Robin, et al., 1998; 1999) 19 subjects were exposed to eugenol while recording six autonomic nervous system parameters, including two electrodermal, two thermovascular, and two cardiorespiratory. The results of seven subjects with high dental fear were compared with those of 12 without such fear. Those with dental fear had a stronger electrodermal response ($p = 0.006$), suggesting that eugenol triggered different emotional responses depending upon the unpleasantness of the subject's past dental experiences. Thus, the same odor can have different effects depending upon the past experience of the individual (Robin, et al., 1998).

On the other hand, if the Lock and Key Theory is true, and an odor's behavioral effects are produced outside of awareness and independent of affective reaction, this negates the General Affective Theory of odors. Ludvigson and Rottman do just that, demonstrating that the scent of lavender enhances mood state while impairing arithmetic reasoning ($p = 0.01$) (Ludvigson & Rottman, 1989).

Given the previous information, several factors must be taken into account in reviewing the literature regarding efficacy of aromatherapy in the treatment of neurologic disease. Can odors elevate mood as the general affective theory maintains or do they act in lock and key fashion? Were the odors tested considered hedonically positive by each subject? This question is essential because what is hedonically positive for one person can be hedonically negative for another, and an odor that is hedonically positive at one concentration may be hedonically negative at another (Distel, et al., 1999). Was an associated change in mood independent of the desired effect? Was there a control group? Was it a single-blind or double-blind procedure? Was the subject size sufficient to obviate falsely positive test results? Did the subjects of the experiment have a normal or near-normal sense of smell?

Could suggestion have an effect? This is particularly relevant because various studies suggest that, as in traditional pharmacologic intervention (Flaten, Simonsen, & Olsen, 1999), odors have both placebo and nocebo effects as demonstrated by Knasko, Gilbert, and Sabini, (1990). Knasko subjected 90 people to water vapor sprayed in a room; 30 subjects were told that the water vapor odor was pleasant, 30 that it was unpleasant, and 30 that it was neutral. Those who had been told that the odorant was pleasant reported being in a better mood than did the other two groups ($p = 0.05$). Subjects who had been told the odor was unpleasant reported having more health symptoms ($p < 0.0003$).

Were the experiments controlled not only for the effect of suggestion, but also for the effect of expectation of outcome? It seems possible that persons with a positive view of aromatherapy who believe that odors can have a positive effect will experience a positive effect because of their bias.

The effect of expectation has been demonstrated neurophysiologically by Lorig and Roberts (1990) who measured the contingent negative variation (CNV) of the EEG in 18 subjects presented with a mixed odor of lavender, jasmine, and galbanium. They found CNV amplitude for the mixed odors varied depending on what the subjects were told about it ($p = 0.05$).

Did the experimenter consider the effect of social desirability whereby subjects try to please the examiner by biasing their answers? (Visser, 1999)·

In light of such questions, one must be circumspect regarding articles touting aromatherapeutic efficacy in the treatment of neurologic disease. Because the basic physiologic mechanism of aromatherapy intervention has not been fully established, skepticism seems all the more appropriate.

AROMATHERAPY FOR VARIOUS NEUROLOGIC DISEASES

As a general rule, neurologic diseases can be positively influenced by improving the patient's mood or allaying anxiety. Virtually all neurologic diseases are made worse with depression and/or high anxiety. If moods can be ameliorated by aromatherapy, it would suggest that aromatherapy could have a positive role in treating neurologic disease.

With this in mind, let us review the literature discussing the effects of aromatherapy in specific neurologic complaints and diseases.

HEADACHE

Nontraditional therapies are frequently used in the management of headache, such as acupuncture, massage, and biofeedback.

Historically, odors have been recognized to have analgesic effects. When Roman soldiers returned from battle, they placed bay leaves in their baths to reduce their pains (Genders, 1972). In ancient Greece, the Corinthian physician, Philonides, recommended pressing cool, scented flowers against the temples to relieve headaches (Genders, 1972).

In contemporary lay literature, a multitude of unsupported claims are made for headache and pain reduction using specific odorants. These claims do not indicate whether the mechanism of action is primarily analgesic, soporific, or anxiolytic. Suggested odorants include cloves for dental pain (Price & Price, 1995); wintergreen for muscle pain (Price & Price, 1995; Gobel, et al., 1995); menthol, ginger, lemon grass, rosewood, clary sage (Damien & Damien, 1995), cajeput, tea tree, juniper, pepper, and rose (Walji, 1996), for headaches (Price & Price, 1995); lavender (Passant, 1990) *lavandula angustifolia, chamaemelum mobile, ocimum basilicum, origanum majorana, rosmarinus officinalis* (Price & Price, 1995), eucalyptus (Damien & Damien, 1995), and true melissa (Price, 1991) for migraine; *mentha × piperita* for "headache caused by digestive disorder" (Price & Price, 1995); peppermint and eucalyptus for tension headache (Saller, Hellstein, Hellenbrecht, 1988).

Experimental studies of odors for pain management are few. Hirsch and Kang (1998) studied 50 chronic sufferers whose headaches met International Headache Society criteria. Upon olfactory testing, only 31 demonstrated normal olfactory ability. Green apple odor was given in an aromatherapy inhaler. Only 15 subjects found the odor hedonically pleasant. In this open label, nonblinded study, subjects served as their own controls. The control condition consisted of resting in a dark, quiet room, and the experimental condition involved inhaling the green apple odor while resting in the same dark, quiet room. Results indicated that green apple odor produced no statistically significant improvement over simple resting in a dark, quiet room. However, in the subgroup of 15 subjects who liked the odor, there was a statistically significant reduction in the severity of the headache ($p < 0.03$). Therefore, the efficacy of the green apple odor was hedonically dependent. Subjects who liked the smell experienced a statistically significant reduction in the severity of the headaches, but patients who disliked the smell experienced no significant improvement.

The mechanism of the odor's action in reducing headaches in these 15 patients is subject to speculation. The odor may have induced a variety of psychologic effects. The therapeutic result may have been mediated through Pavlovian conditioning. For example, the respondents may have consciously or unconsciously associated (Kirk-Smith, Van Toller, & Dodd, 1983) the green apple odor with past anxiolytic or pain-alleviating experiences so that the association reproduced this same effect during the headache episodes. The odor also might have worked through olfactory-evoked recall, because olfactory-evoked recall is usually pleasant and associated with a positive mood state. The green apple scent, by inducing a positive mood state in the 15 patients, could thus have reduced perception of pain (Fields, 1967). This corresponds with the General Affective Theory of Odors described previously.

The lack of response in those who found the green apple scent unpleasant indicates that hedonics were more important than the particular odor used. This does not preclude the possibility of a neurophysiologic effect of the odor, including a change in serotonin, dopamine, acetylcholine, norepinephrine, GABA, gastrin, beta endorphin, or substance P, all of which are known to be modulators of headache, including migraine. Because these neurotransmitters exist within the olfactory bulb, they could, theoretically, be influenced by odors (Anselmi, et al., 1980; Appenzeller, Atkinson, & Standefer, 1981; Foote, Bloom, & Aston-Jones, 1983; Gall, et al., 1987; Haberly & Price, 1978; Halasz & Shepherd, 1983; Hardebo, et al., 1985; Igarashi, et al., 1987; Leston, et al., 1987; Macrides & Davis, 1983; Mair & Harrison, 1991; Moskowitz, 1984; Nattero, et al., 1985; Shipley, Halloran, & Torre, 1985; Sjaastad, 1986; Zaborsky, et al., 1985).

Green apple odor may have worked somewhat like pharmacologic agents used in the treatment of headache, for example, amitriptyline or propranolol, by modifying the neurotransmitters in the pain pathway. In patients who disliked the odor, a strong negative mood state may have been induced that overwhelmed the odor's neurophysiologic effect. Therefore, the pain was not alleviated.

Gobel also studied the effects of odors on headaches (Gobel, et al., 1995; Gobel, Schmidt, & Soyka, 1994). In that study, 32 healthy subjects underwent a double-blind, placebo-controlled, randomized crossover study of the effects of peppermint oil, eucalyptus, and ethanol. The odors were used in different combinations on various measures of headache pain, including the relaxation of peri-cranial muscles and contingent negative variation. In this study, three applications of odorant were placed on the skin of the forehead and temples at 15-minute intervals using a small sponge. After 45 minutes, parameters were assessed. To avoid factors of circadian rhythm, all testing took place between 3 and 6 p.m. To prevent subjects from recognizing the presence vs. the absence of odors and thereby breaking the double-blind nature of the study, "traces" of peppermint oil and eucalyptus oil were added to all applications.

Eucalyptus had no effect. Peppermint combined with eucalyptus and ethanol relaxed pericranial muscles ($p < 0.05$) as did a combination of peppermint and ethanol. The most reduction of pain sensitivity as measured by algesimetry was from a combination of peppermint oil and ethanol. Regulation of pericranial muscles was a postulated mechanism of action of the peppermint.

This study has several potential problems. Because the traces of peppermint and eucalyptus were sufficient to cause olfactory response, they also may have been sufficient to produce an effect, although they were described as inert. Hence, the authors may not have tested the particular odors they thought they tested. Furthermore, no parameter was measured to determine whether the effect was based on hedonics, to eliminate any influence of the general affective theory of odors. No assessment was made of subjects' olfactory abilities, nor was the anticipation effect (belief vs. nonbelief in aromatherapy) addressed.

The author postulated that the odors, through a peripheral mechanism in the gate control theory of pain, acted by segmental inhibition of the posterior horn (Gobel, et al., 1995). However, this same pathway could have been activated totally independently of the odors. The experimental procedure of applying the odors by rubbing cold oils on the skin may, in and of itself, have influenced the pain pathway. The cold stimuli could have induced firing of A delta fibers, which would have increased blood flow in the skin and created a counterstimulus to reduce the headache pain. Alternatively, the inhalation of odors may have affected central serotonergic systems leading to a change in mood state and, thus, a reduction in pain (General Affective Theory of Odors).

In another study, Gobel and colleagues found aromatherapy with peppermint oil was effective in treating tension headaches meeting IHS classification (Gobel, et al., 1996). Peppermint oil was applied locally in a randomized, placebo-controlled, double-blind, crossover fashion; 10 g of peppermint oil and 90% ethanol was used. The placebo was 90% ethanol solution to which traces of peppermint oil were added for blinding purposes. During their headache attacks, peppermint oil was applied across the foreheads and temples of 41 patients. The application was repeated after 15 and 30 minutes. Compared with the placebo, peppermint oil significantly reduced headache intensity after 15 minutes ($p < 0.01$). The analgesic effect equaled that of 1000 mg of acetaminophen. Very few studies that claim to have demonstrated efficacy of aromatherapy have been as carefully performed (Woolfson & Hewitt, 1992).

Another possible mechanism by which peppermint may relieve headache is by noncompetitive inhibition of serotonin and substance P (Saller, Hellstein, & Hellenbrecht, 1988). Odors may inhibit headaches by acting as calcium channel blockers. *Romarinus officinalis*, for example, has been demonstrated to relax tracheal smooth muscle by way of its calcium antagonistic property (Aqel, 1991).

OTHER CHRONIC PAIN

Opinion regarding relief of nonheadache pain is mixed. In a blinded study by Dale & Cornwell (1994) of 635 postpartum women, use of lavender in the daily bath was compared with an aromatic placebo consisting of 2-methyl-3-isobutyl tyrosine diluted in distilled water. Of the women, 217 received lavender, 213 synthetic, and 205 control. This study demonstrated no statistically significant effect of using lavender in treating peroneal pain. In a study that was not randomized, not double-blinded, and not age-controlled, Woolfson and Hewitt (1992) gave aromatherapy and massage in 20-minute sessions twice a week to 12 patients. Another 12 patients received massage only. The aromatherapy patients were massaged with lavender oil in an almond oil base. The other patients were massaged with almond oil only. Observations were recorded at the beginning and end of each 20-minute session and 30 minutes after treatment. All sessions were conducted in midafternoon. Approximately 50% of the patients were in the coronary care unit and the others were in intensive-care units; 50% of the patients were artificially ventilated. The authors state that 50% of the aromatherapy patients and 41% of massage-only patients reported a decrease in pain. This could be misleading, however. That six patients responded to aromatherapy and five patients responded to massage without aromatherapy is clearly not a statistically significant difference. If anything, these results indicate that aromatherapy was no better than massage alone. Given their selection of patients, however, one would not anticipate that aromatherapy would be effective, because the pathway for olfactory input was compromised by artificial ventilation.

In a study by Burns and Blamey (1994) of 585 women, no statistically significant effects were described, but analgesia was noted in four women who inhaled lavender, one who inhaled eucalyptus, three who inhaled clary sage, one who inhaled jasmine, two who inhaled chamomile, and one who inhaled lemon.

In 100 patients with pain of the periarticular system (Krall & Krause, 1993), treatment of from 10 to 20 days compared the efficacy of mint oil with that of hydroxyethylsalicylate gel. The mint oil was put into a gel and applied topically. Of the patients and physicians, 78% thought that mint therapy was highly effective and 50% of patients and 34% of physicians thought that hydroxyethylsalicylate gel was highly effective. None of the confounding parameters previously mentioned, such as olfactory ability, expectation, and hedonics, were addressed in this study.

COMMON SUSCEPTIBILITIES

Before using aromatherapy in neurologic conditions, consideration must be given to the potential risks of the treatment. Adverse reactions can occur among patients with diseases that predispose them to the development of side effects, and among the population as a whole as well.

Certain diseases make their sufferers particularly susceptible to adverse effects of aromatherapy. Approximately 40% of migraineurs report osmophobia, whereby an odorant induces a migraine headache (Blau & Solomon, 1985). A wide range of odorants can act as such triggers, depending on the individual. These triggers include perfume, cigarette smoke, and food odors (Hirsch & Kang, 1998).

Asthmatics, upon exposure to common odors, can suffer a worsening of their respiratory status independent of their olfactory ability. In a survey of 60 asthmatic patients, 57 (95%) described respiratory symptoms upon exposure to common odors including insecticide (85%), household cleaning agents (78%), perfume and cologne (72%), cigarette smoke (75%), fresh paint (73%), automobile exhaust or gas fumes (60%), and cooking aromas (37%). Room deodorant and mint candy also could cause respiratory distress (Shim & Williams, 1986). Four subjects who underwent an odor challenge with four squirts of a popular cologne all had an immediate decline in 1-second forced expiratory volume (18 to 58% reduction) (Shim & Williams, 1986).

Among persons who suffer complaints consistent with multiple chemical sensitivities, 24% of the men and 39% of the women note that odors precipitate their complaints (Miller, 1996). However, double-blind studies fail to demonstrate odorant-induced multiple chemical sensitivity symptoms (Ross, et al., 1999).

Inhalation of odorants can produce measurable levels in the blood (Stimpfl, et al., 1995), and because many common fragrances contain naphthalene-related compounds (including menthol and camphor), persons with G6PD deficiency may be at risk from aromatherapeutic exposures (Olowe & Ransome-Kuti, 1980). In neonates, dermal application has demonstrated this, but in adults, it remains only a theoretic risk for inhalational aromatherapy.

A variety of essential oils are said to be able to precipitate seizures in epileptics. Whether these effects can occur by inhalation alone as opposed to ingestion or by percutaneous absorption is unclear. Proconvulsant odorants include rosemary (Betts, 1994; Tisserand, 1977), fennel, hyssop, sage, and wormwood (Tisserand, 1977).

Because aromatherapeutic inhalation of essential oils can produce detectable levels of the oils in the blood, these compounds, like any pharmacologic agents, could induce adverse drug–drug interactions in persons on medication. Such interactions could enhance metabolism of anticonvulsants or pain medications, for example, thus predisposing an epileptic to have a seizure or a chronic pain patient to withdraw from medication. Jori, Bianchetti, and Prestini (1969) demonstrated this potential. Inhalation of eucalyptol by rats increased microsomal enzyme systems, thus decreasing the effect of pentobarbital.

Odorants can produce harmful side effects not only among persons predisposed to disease, but among the healthy population as well. Airborne-induced allergic contact dermatitis is a recognized result of aromatherapeutic inhalation of tea tree oil (melaleuca oil) (DeGroot, 1996). Examples of common melaleuca oil allergens include d-limonene, aromadendrene, alpha-terpinene, 1,8-cineole (eucalyptol), terpinen-4-ol, p-cymene, and alpha-phellandrene. Because of the highly volatile nature of essential oils, their common constituents and cross-sensitization, DeGroot postulated that the same airborne-induced contact dermatitis could occur with several other essential oils including lavender and a mixture of eucalyptus, pine, and peppermint (DeGroot, 1996). Bridges suggested that if odorants can sensitize the respiratory system as they do the skin, they might not only exacerbate asthma, but might actually precipitate asthma (Bridges, 1999).

CONCLUSION

With aromatherapy, just as with any therapeutic tool, practitioners must weigh the relative risk/benefit ratio in deciding upon its use in the treatment of pain.

Having spent the last decade and a half investigating the scientific basis of aromatherapy and having published more than 100 peer-reviewed articles in this area, the author does not believe that scientific literature supports, nor the risk/benefit ratio justifies, use of aromatherapy in pain management at present. This is a fluid position and as more studies are performed delineating the efficacy of aromatherapy, the author expects to endorse and use aromatherapy as part of the therapeutic armamentarium. Until such time, this form of alternative medicine in the treatment of pain cannot be recommended.

REFERENCES

Acharya, V., Acharya, J., & Luders, H. (1996). Olfactory epileptic auras. *Neurology, 46,* A446.

Alaoui-Ismaili, O., et al. (1997). Basic emotions evoked by odorants: Comparison between autonomic responses and self-evaluation. *Physiology and Behavior, 62,* 713–720.

Anselmi, B., et al. (1980). Endogenous opioids in cerebrospinal fluid and blood in idiopathic headache sufferers. *Headache, 20,* 294–299.

Appenzeller, O., Atkinson, R.A., & Standefer, J.C. (1981). Serum beta endorphin in cluster headache and common migraine. In F.C. Rose & E. Zikha (Eds.), *Progress in migraine.* London: Pitman.

Aqel, M.B. (1991). Relaxant effect of the volatile oil of *Romarinus officinalis* on tracheal smooth muscle. *Journal of Ethnopharmacology, 33,* 57–62.

Benton, D. (1982). The influence of androstenol — a putative human pheromone — on mood throughout the menstrual cycle. *Biological Psychology, 15,* 249–256.

Betts, T. (1994). Sniffing the breeze. *Aromatherapy Quarterly, 1,* 19–22.

Betts, T., et al. (1995). An olfactory countermeasure treatment for epileptic seizures using a conditioned arousal response to specific aromatherapy oils. *Epilepsia, 36*(3), S130–S131.

Blau, J.N., & Solomon, F. (1985). Smell and other sensory disturbances in migraine. *Journal of Neurology, 232,* 275–276.

Brandstatter, H., Furhwirth, M., & Kitchler, E. (1988). Effects of weather and air pollution on mood: Individual difference approach. In D. Canter, et al. (Eds.), *NATO advanced research workshop on social and environmental psychology in the European context: Environmental social psychology.* Boston: Kluwer.

Bridges, B. (1999). Fragrances and health. *Environmental Health Perspectives, 107*(7), A340.

Briere, J., Downes, A., & Spensley, J. (1983). Summer in the city: Urban weather conditions and psychiatric-emergency room visits. *Journal of Abnormal Psychology, 92,* 77–80.

Brodal, A. (1969). *Neurological anatomy in relation to clinical medicine,* (Vol. 10), (3rd ed.). New York: Oxford University Press.

Brown, R., & Kulik, J. (1977). Flashbulb memories. *Cognition, 5,* 73–99.

Buchbauer, G. (1990). Aromatherapy: Do essential oils have therapeutic properties? *Perfumer and Flavorist, 15,* 47–50.

Buchbauer, G. (1993). Biological effects of fragrances and essential oils. *Perfumer and Flavorist, 18,* 19–24.

Buchbauer, G., et al. (1993). Fragrance compounds and essential oils with sedative effects upon inhalation. *Journal of Pharmaceutical Sciences, 82*(6), 660–664.

Bullinger, M. (1989a). Psychological effects of air pollution on healthy residents: A time series approach. *Journal of Environmental Psychology, 9,* 103–118.

Bullinger, M. (1989b). Relationships between air-pollution and well-being. *Zeitschrift Sozial und Praventivmedizin, 34,* 231–238.

Burns, E., & Blamey, C. (1994). Using aromatherapy in childbirth. *Nursing Times, 90*(9), 54–60.

Cunningham, M. (1979). Weather, mood, and helping behavior: Quasi-experiments with the sunshine samaritan. *Journal of Personality and Social Psychology, 37,* 1947–1956.

Cunningham, S. (1995). *Magical aromatherapy: The power of scent.* St Paul: Llewellyn Publications.

Dale, A., & Cornwell, S. (1994). The role of lavender oil in relieving perineal discomfort following childbirth: A blind randomized clinical trial. *Journal of Advanced Nursing, 19,* 89–96.

Damian, P., & Damian K. (1995). *Aromatherapy scent and psyche.* Rochester: Healing Arts.

DeGroot, A.C. (1996). Airborne allergic contact dermatitis from tea tree oil. *Contact Dermatitis, 35,* 304–305.

Dietz, M.A., Goetz, C.J., & Steddings, G.T. (1990). Evaluation of visual cues as a modified inverted walking stick in the treatment of Parkinson's disease freezing episodes. *Movement Disorders, 5,* 243–247.

Distel, H., et al. (1999). Perception of everyday odors — correlation between intensity, familiarity and strength of hedonic judgement. *Chemical Senses, 24,* 191–199.

Efron, R. (1957). The effect of olfaction stimuli in arresting uncinate fits. *Brain, 79,* 267–281.

Ehrlichman, H., & Halpern, J.N. (1988). Affect and memory: effects of pleasant and unpleasant odors on retrieval of happy and unhappy memories. *Journal of Personality and Psychology, 55,* 769–779.

Evans, G.W. (1994). Psychological costs of chronic exposure to ambient air pollution. In R.I. Isaacson & K.F. Jensen (Eds.), *The vulnerable brain and environmental risks* (Vol. 3). New York: Plenum Press.

Feller, R.M. (1997). *Practical aromatherapy: Understanding and using essential oils to heal the mind and body*. New York: Berkeley Books.

Fields, H. (1967). *Pain*. New York: McGraw-Hill.

Flaten, M.A., Simonsen, & T., Olsen, H. (1999). Drug-related information generates placebo and nocebo responses that modify the drug response. *Psychosomatic Medicine, 61*, 250–255.

Foote, S., Bloom, F., & Aston-Jones, G. (1983). Nucleus locus coeruleus: New evidence of anatomical and physiological specificity. *Physiological Reviews, 86*, 844–914.

Freud, S. (1908). Bemerkungen uber einen Fall von Zwangs neurosa. *German Healthcare, VIII*, 350.

Gall, C.M., et al. (1987). Events for co-existence of GABA and dophamine in neurons of the rat olfactory bulb. *Journal of Comparative Neurology, 266*, 307–318.

Genders, R. (1972). *Perfume through the ages*. New York: G. Putnam and Sons.

Gobel, H., et al. (1995). Essential plant oils and headache mechanisms. *Phytomedicine, 2*(2), 93–102.

Gobel, H., et al. (1996). Effectiveness of peppermint oil and paracetamol in the treatment of tension headache. *Nervenarzt, 67*, 672–681.

Gobel, H., Schmidt, G., & Soyka, D. (1994). Effect of peppermint and eucalyptus oil preparations on neurophysiological and experimental algesimetric headache parameters. *Cephalalgia, 14*, 228–234.

Haberly, L.B., & Price, J.L. (1978). Association and commissural fiber systems of the olfactory cortex in the rat. II. Systems originating in the olfactory peduncle. *Journal of Comparative Neurology, 178*, 781–808.

Halasz, N., & Shepherd, G.M. (1983). Neurochemistry of the vertebrate olfactory bulb. *Neuroscience, 10*, 579–619.

Hardebo, J.E., et al. (1985). CSF opioid levels in cluster headache. In F.C. Rose (Ed.), *Migraine*. Basel: Karger.

Hirsch, A.R. (1992). Nostalgia: Neuropsychiatric understanding. *Advanced Consumer Research, 19*, 390–395.

Hirsch, A.R., & Wyse, J.P. (1993). Posttraumatic dysosmia: Central vs. peripheral. *Journal of Neurological, Orthopedic, and Medical Surgery, 14*, 152–155.

Hirsch, A.R. (1995a). Cephalgia as a result of acute nitrogen tetroxide exposure. *Headache, 35*, 310.

Hirsch, A.R. (1995b). Neurotoxicity as a result of acute nitrogen tetroxide exposure. International Congress on Hazardous Waste: Impact on human and ecological health. Atlanta: U.S. Department of Health and Human Services, Public Health Agency for Toxic Substances and Disease Registry.

Hirsch, A.R. (1995c). Chronic neurotoxicity of acute chlorine gas exposure. Thirteenth International Neurotoxicity Conference, Hot Springs, Arkansas.

Hirsch, A.R. (1995d). Chronic neurotoxicity as a result of landfill exposure in Port Orchard, Washington: International Congress on Hazardous Waste: Impact on human and ecological health. Atlanta: U.S. Department of Health and Human Services: Public Health Agency for Toxic Substances and Disease Registry.

Hirsch, A.R. (1998a). *Scentsational sex*. Boston: Element Books.

Hirsch, A.R. (1998b). Negative health effects of malodors in the environment: A brief review. *Journal of Neurological, Orthopedic and Medical Surgery, 18*, 43–45.

Hirsch, A.R., & Kang, C. (1998). The effect of inhaling green apple fragrance to reduce the severity of migraine: A pilot study. *Headache Quarterly, 9*, 159–163.

Hirsch, A.R., & Rankin, K.M. (1993). Trichloroethylene exposure and headache. *Headache, 33*, 275.

Igarashi, H., et al. (1987). Cerebrovascular sympathetic nervous activity during cluster headaches. *Handbook of Clinical Neurology, 7*(6), 87–89.

Izmerov, N. (1971). Establishment of air quality standards. *Archives of Environmental Health, 22*, 711–719.

Jones, J.W., & Bogat, G.A. (1978). Air pollution and human aggression. *Psychological Reports, 43*, 721–722.

Jori, A., Bianchetti, A., & Prestini, P.E. (1969). Effect of essential oils on drug metabolism. *Biochemical Pharmacology, 18*(9), 2081–2085.

Kaptchuk, T.J., & Eisenberg, D.M. (1998). The persuasive appeal of alternative medicine. *Annals of Internal Medicine, 129*, 1061–1065.

Keville, K., & Green, M. (1995). *Aromatherapy: A complete guide to the healing art*. Santa Cruz, CA: Crossing Press.

King, J.R. (1994). Scientific status of aromatherapy. *Perspectives in Biology and Medicine, 37*(3), 409–415.

Kirk-Smith, M.D., Van Toller, C., & Dodd, G.H. (1983). Unconscious odour conditioning in human subjects. *Biological Psychology, 17*, 221–231.

Kite, S.M., et al. (1998). Development of an aromatherapy service on a cancer center. *Palliative Medicine, 12*, 171–180.

Kline, N., & Rausch, J. (1985). Olfactory precipitants of flashbacks in post traumatic stress disorders: Case reports. *Journal of Clinical Psychiatry, 46*, 383–384.

Knasko, S.C., Gilbert, A.N., & Sabini, J. (1990). Emotional state, physical well-being, and performance in the presence of feigned ambient odor. *Journal of Applied Social Psychology, 20*(16), 1345–1357.

Krall, B., & Krause, W. (1993). Efficacy intolerance of mentha arvensis aetheroleum. Program abstracts, Twenty-fourth International Symposium of Essential Oils.

Laird, D.A. (1988). What can you do with your nose? *Scientific Monthly, 1*, 319–322.

Leston, J., et al. (1987). Free and conjugated plasma catecholamines in cluster headache. *Cephalagia, 7*(6), 331.

Lindsay, W.R., Pitcaithly, D., & Geelen, N. (1997). A comparison of the effects of four therapy prodedures on concentration and responsiveness in people with profound learning disabilities. *Journal of Intellectual Disability Research, 41* (3), 201–207.

Lorig, T.S., & Roberts, M. (1990). Odor and cognitive alteration of the contingent negative variation. *Chemical Senses, 15*(5), 537–545.

Ludvigson, H.W., & Rottman, T.R. (1989). Effects of ambient odors of lavender and cloves on cognition, memory, affect and mood. *Chemical Senses, 14,* 525–536.

Macht, D.I., & Ting, G.C. (1921). Experimental inquiry into the sedative properties of some aromatic drugs and fumes. *Journal of Pharmacology and Experimental Therapeutics, 18,* 361–372.

MacLean, P.D. (1973). *Triune concept of the brain and behavior.* Toronto: University of Toronto Press.

Macrides, F., & David, B.J. (1983). Olfactory bulb. In P.C. Emson (Ed.), *Chemical Neuroana.* New York: Raven Press.

Mair, R.G., & Harrison, L.M. (1991). Influence of drugs on smell function. In Laing, D.G., Doty, R.L., & Briephol, W, (Eds.). *Human sense of smell.* Berlin: Springer-Verlag.

Markopoulou, K., et al. (1977). Olfactory dysfunction in familial Parkinsonism. *Neurology, 49,* 1262–1267.

Maruniak, J.A. (1995). Deprivation and the olfactory system. In R.L. Doty (Ed.), *Handbook of olfaction and gustation.* New York: Marcel Dekker.

Miller, C.S. (1996). Chemical sensitivity: Symptom, syndrome or mechanism for disease? *Toxicology, 111,* 69–86.

Miltner, W., et al. (1994). Emotional qualities of odorants and their influence on the startle reflex in humans. *Psychophysiology, 31,* 107–110.

Miner, J.R. (1980). Controlling odors from livestock production facilities: State-of-the-art. In *Livestock waste: Renewable resource.* St. Joseph: American Society of Agricultural Engineers.

Mobert, R.J., & Doty, R.L. (1997). Olfactory function in Huntington's disease patients and at-risk offspring. *International Journal of Neuroscience, 89,* 133–139.

Moskowitz, M.A. (1984). Neurobiology of vascular head pain. *Annals of Neurology, 16,* 157–158.

Nattero, G., et al. (1985). Serum gastrin levels in cluster headache and migraine attacks. In V. Pfaffenrath, P.O. Lundberg, & O. Sjaastad (Eds.), *Updating in headache.* Berlin: Springer-Verlag.

Neutra, R., et al. (1991). Hypotheses to explain the higher symptom rates observed around hazardous waste sites. *Environmental Health Perspectives, 94,* 31–38.

Olowe, S.A., & Ransome-Kuti, O. (1980). The risk of jaundice in glucose-6-phosphate dehydrogenase deficient babies exposed to menthol. *Acta Paediatrica Scandinavica, 69,* 341–345.

Passant, H. (1990). A holistic approach in the ward. *Nursing Times, 86*(4), 26–28.

Price, S. (1991). *Aromatherapy for common ailments.* New York: Fireside Book.

Price, S., & Price, L. (1995). *Aromatherapy for health professionals.* New York: Churchill Livingstone.

Proust, M. (1934). *Remembrance of things past* (Vol. 1). New York: Random House (Translated by C.D. Scott Moncrieff).

Robin, O., et al. (1998). Emotional responses evoked by dental odors: An evaluation from autonomic parameters. *Journal of Dental Research, 77*(8), 1638–1646.

Robin, O., et al. (1999). Basic emotions evoked by eugenol odor differ according to the dental experience: A neurovegetative analysis. *Chemical Senses, 24,* 327–335.

Roebuck, A. (1988). Aromatherapy: Fact or fiction. *Perfumer and Flavorist, 13,* 43–45.

Ross, P.M., et al. (1999). Olfaction and symptoms in the multiple chemical sensitivities syndrome. *Preventive Medicine, 28,* 467–480.

Rotton, J. (1983). Affective and cognitive consequences of malodorous pollution. *Basic Applied Social Psychology, 4,* 171–191.

Rotton, J., et al. (1978). Air pollution and interpersonal attraction. *Journal of Applied Social Psychology, 8,* 57–71.

Rotton, J., et al. (1979). Air pollution experience and physical aggression. *Journal of Applied Social Psychology, 9,* 347–412.

Rotton, J., & Frey, J. (1985). Air pollution, weather, and violent crimes: Concomitant time series analysis of archival data. *Journal of Personality and Social Psychology, 49,* 1207–1220.

Saller, R., Hellstein, A., & Hellenbrecht, D. (1988). Klinische Pharmakologie und Therapeutische Anwendung von Cineol (eukalyptus) und Menthol als Bestandteil Atherischer ole. *Internistische Praxis 28*(2), 355–364.

Schnaubelt, K. (1995). *Advanced aromatherapy: The science of essential oil therapy.* Rochester: Healing Arts.

Shakespeare, W. *Hamlet,* Act IV, Scene VI.

Schiffman, S.S., et al. (1995). The effect of environmental odors emanating from commercial swine operations on the mood of nearby residents. *Brain Research Bulletin, 37,* 369–375.

Shim, C., & Williams, M.H., Jr. (1986). Effect of odors in asthma. *American Journal of Medicine, 80,* 18–22.

Shipley, M., Halloran, F., & Torre, J. (1985). Surprisingly rich projection from locus coeruleus to the olfactory bulb in the rat. *Brain Research, 329,* 294–299.

Shusterman, D. (1992). Critical review: Health significance of environmental odor pollution. *Archives of Environmental Health, 47,* 76–87.

Sjaastad, O. (1986). Cluster headaches. In P.J. Vinken, G.W. Bruyn, & H.L. Klawans (Eds.), *Handbook of clinical neurology headache* (Vol. 48). New York: Elsevier Science.

Squire, L.R. (1987). *Memory and brain.* New York: Oxford University Press.

Stimpfl, T., et al. (1995). Concentration of 1,8-cineol in human blood during prolonged inhalation. *Chemical Senses, 20*(3), 349–350.

Strahilevitz, M., Strahilevitz, A., & Miller, J.E. (1979). Air pollutants and the admission rate of psychiatric patients. *American Journal of Psychiatry, 136*(2), 205–207.

Sugawara, Y., Hino, Y., & Kawasaki, M. (1999). Alteration of perceived fragrance of essential oils in relation to type of work: A simple screening test for efficacy of aroma. *Chemical Senses, 24,* 415–421.

Tanner, B.A., & Zeiler, M. (1975). Punishment of self-injurious behavior using aromatic ammonia as the aversive stimulus. *Journal of Applied Behavior Analysis, 8,* 53–57.

Tisserand, R.B. (1977). *The art of aromatherapy.* Rochester: Healing Arts.

Ury, H.K., Perkins, M.A., & Goldsmith, J.R. (1972). Motor vehicle accidents and vehicular pollution in Los Angeles. *Archives of Environmental Health, 25,* 314–322.

Valentine, J.H., et al. (1975). Human crises and the physical environment. *Man–Environmental Systems, 5*(1), 23–28.

Visser, A. (1999). Social desirability in health research. *Psychosomatic Medicine, 61,* 106.

Walji, H. (1996). *The healing power of aromatherapy.* Rocklin: Prima Publishing.

Warm, J.S., Dember, W.N., & Parasuraman, R. (1991). Effects of olfactory stimulation on performance and stress in a visual sustained attention task. *Journal of the Society of Cosmetic Chemists, 42,* 199–210.

Wayne, W., Wehrle, P., & Carroll, R. (1967). Oxidant air pollution and athletic performance. *Journal of the American Medical Association, 199,* 901–904.

Weisse, C.S. (1992). Depression and immunocompetence: Review of the literature. *Psychological Bulletin, 111,* 475–489.

Weyers, W., & Brodbeck R. (1989). Hautdurchdringung atherischer ole (Skin absorption of volatile oils). *Pharmazie in unserer Zeit, 18*(3), 82–86.

Woolfson, A., & Hewitt, D. (1992). Intensive aromacare. *International Journal of Aromatherapy, 4*(2), 12–13.

Zaborsky, L., et al. (1985). Cholinergic and GABA-ergic projections to the olfactory bulb in the rat. *Journal of Comparative Neurology, 243,* 468–509.

Zeidner, M., & Schechter, M. (1988). Psychological responses to air pollution: Some personality and demographic correlates. *Journal of Environmental Psychology, 8,* 191–208.

84

Objective Evaluation and Treatment Outcome Measurements in Soft Tissue Injury

Gabriel E. Sella, M.D., M.P.H., M.Sc, Ph.D. (Hon. C.),
F.A.A.D.E.P., S.D.A.B.D.A., F.A.C.F.E., F.A.C.F.M., D.A.A.P.M.

Bones forget, muscles remember.

Old English Proverb

DEFINITION

SOFT TISSUE INJURY

This type injury or traumatic pathological condition involves the soft tissues of the body as compared to the skeleton (Cailliet, 1988b). This chapter refers exclusively to injuries affecting muscles and fascia.

Skeletal muscle and overlying fascia form a continuum through the body (Busquet, 1998). The myofascial train comprises of fascial attachments and a continuum over bones, muscles, and connecting ligaments, capsules, tendons, and fascia covering individual muscular fasciculi and fibers (Cailliet, 1988a; 1993; Busquet, 1998). Thus, muscular or myofascial injuries have to be considered together both on an anatomic basis and on a functional basis (Anchor & Felicetti, 1999; Cailliet, 1988a; Sella & Donaldson, 1998).

Injuries may vary in etiology from an acute sharp or blunt form to acute hyperextension types (Cailliet, 1992a; 1991a; 1992b; 1991b; 1988b; 1994; Maigne, 1996; Pope, Anderson, Frymoyer, & Chaffin, 1991).

Any myofascial or muscular injury may affect the development of localized inflamation and consequent dysfunction (Maigne, 1996; Pope, Anderson, Frymoyer, & Chaffin, 1991; Travell & Simons, 1983).

Because muscles/fascia function in myotatic units, an injury affecting one muscle or the fascial envelope of one muscle is reflected to a relative dysfunction of the whole myotatic unit around the pertinent joint(s) movable by the affected muscle (Busquet, 1998; Sella, 2000a; 2000b). Consequently, homolateral myotatic units proximal or distal to the affected unit may become relatively dysfunctional (Busquet, 1998; Cailliet, 1988a; Travell & Simons, 1983). Because the contralateral myotatic unit may need to pick up at least part of the work of the affected unit, functional changes may occur in time in the contralateral unit as well (Busquet, 1998; Cailliet, 1988a; Travell & Simons, 1983).

It is very important for the investigator of soft tissue injury to realize that there is a complex myofascial relationship between the locus of injury and the rest of the myofascial envelope of the body (Busquet, 1998; Maigne, 1996; Pope Anderson, Frymoyer, & Chaffin, 1991). Whereas acute injuries may be followed by localized splinting, the chronic phase of such injuries is evidenced by protective guarding, which may be quite complex (Cailliet, 1988a; 1993). The investigator and/or treating clinician needs to be fully aware of the protective guarding pattern involving the case.

From this standpoint, it is far more complex to evaluate and treat soft tissue injuries than bony injuries such as fractures (Cailliet, 1988a).

THE OBJECTIVE EVALUATION

In order to evaluate adequately soft tissue injury, one must understand the main parameters of symptoms/signs of such injury (Sella, 1995; 1998a; 1998b; 2000c; Sella & Donaldson, 1998). These parameters are usually a combination of any of the following:

Pain
Relative loss of strength
Relative loss of range of motion (ROM)
Relative loss of adequate function
Radiation of symptoms and dysfunction to the contralateral side of the injury site
Relative early or late development of myofascial pain syndrome exemplified by trigger points
Late development of muscular hypotrophy/atrophy and relative shortening

Whereas bone injuries can be evaluated with radiologic means such as X-rays, CT scans, or MRI, soft tissue injury involving skeletal muscles and fascia usually cannot be evaluated properly with any of these radiologic means (Cailliet, 1988a; 1993).

Therefore, the investigator and treating clinician have to rely not only on the clinical experience of evaluation/treatment of soft tissue injuries but also on other objective tools (Anchor & Felicetti, 1999; Galen, 1979; Sella & Donaldson, 1998;).

A prime concept regarding objective evaluation in the clinical sciences in general is that any methodology has to rely on epidemiologic and statistical criteria compatible with scientific and medicolegal requirements of today's society (Galen, 1979; Sella & Donaldson, 1998;). The primary parameter of such methodologies requires validity of clinical and objective measurement. Validity depends on a number of criteria, most particularly the following:

1. Internal consistency of any number of repetitions of the testing, with particular regard to any methodology used;
2. Test/re-test repeatability of any methodology utilized;
3. Reliability of results not only on clinical grounds but also in terms of measurements and/or comparisons against known databases or normative values;
4. Specificity, sensitivity, and predictive values of the clinical measurements according to the statistical requirements of epidemiologic tests;
5. Functional use of the results of the tests of different methodologies in clear clinical terms, especially involving the direction of the rehabilitation process (if the results of some tests have no clinical value in directing treatment,

the results may be valid statistically but not in terms of clinical utilization);
6. Functional use of the results of different methodologies in terms of during, pre-, and post-evaluation of the treatment outcome.

Pain practitioners must become aware that the time-honored clinical opinion on diagnostic evaluation and treatment outcome has little value in the medicolegal eyes of the *Daubert* requirements for objective evaluation with new technologies (Sella, 2000c).

The pain practitioner dealing with soft tissue injury evaluation and treatment needs to utilize objective methodologies appropriate for each one of the major parameters of soft tissue injury symptoms/signs (Sella & Donaldson, 1998).

The discussion below details each methodology, including major strengths and limitations (Sella & Donaldson, 1998).

It may be relevant to note *a priori* that any such limitations of any given investigative modality may be countered by the strengths of another given modality. Thus, it is most usually advisable to utilize complementary investigative/treating modalities in order to obtain more robust results.

OBJECTIVE TREATMENT OUTCOME MEASUREMENT

Each subject discussed below includes this section as it applies to it.

The clinician must use objective methods of rehabilitation to evaluate the resolution of symptoms and optimization of function. This may comprise questionnaires to be utilized during each visit, dynamometry or inclinometry utilized at regular intervals during the rehabilitation period, etc. As such, the outcome measure may contain not only the final quantitative values but also the chronology of symptom resolution and functional improvement.

SOFT TISSUE INJURY/DYSFUNCTION PARAMETERS

PAIN

Acute soft tissue pain is most usually localized to the area of injury. It may involve direct or indirect trauma to the skin, subcutaneous tissue, blood vessels, nerves, fascia, and skeletal muscle as well as tendons, ligaments and bursae, periosteum, and bone (Cailliet, 1988a; 1993). As stated, only pain involving the muscles and fascia are discussed in this presentation (Anchor & Felicetti, 1999; Travell & Simons, 1983).

The acute pain is reflected by the body's reflex of splinting, part of the old survival complex of "fight or flight."

The injured part is "splinted," i.e., defended by the surrounding area of muscles, joints, and fascia as well as the contralateral area and the appropriate myotatic units of either side.

If the acute pain is not resolved properly in terms of investigation and treatment, it may result in the development of myofascitis and protective guarding (Travell & Simons, 1983).

Pain assessment of soft tissue injury is difficult to perform using the statistical requirements described above. Nonetheless, it is the duty of the modern pain practitioner to do so (Sella & Donaldson, 1998). It is relevant to perform any test a number of times (i.e., at least five times) and measure the internal consistency of performance of the evaluee or patient (Sella, 2000a; 2000c). Any methodology or diversity of methodologies utilized should show a good measure of repeatability of pain assessment or reduction (Sella, 2000a; 2000c). When normative values or databases of objective measurements are known, the results of the pain investigation and/or treatment should be measured against those normative values for reliability (Sella, 2000a; 2000c). When the specificity, sensitivity, and predictive values of any pain investigative methodology are known, the clinical results may be comparable to such data (Sella, 2000a).

The functional utilization of any pain investigative methodology is only as good as the results obtained in relation to it. Therefore, the clinician may want to describe the validity of the application of the pain investigative tool in terms of the results obtained (Sella & Donaldson, 1998).

Because it is necessary to evaluate treatment results before, during, and post-treatment, any methodology for pain investigation/treatment needs to be objective and numerical in terms of the overall outcome measurement (AMA, 1993; Sella & Donaldson, 1998).

The following methodologies for soft tissue pain measurement are considered below.

Pain Questionnaires

There are a variety of soft tissue injury pain questionnaires. The McGill questionnaire is perhaps the best known and most commonly utilized (Melzack, 1975; 1987).

Any pain questionnaire utilization in soft tissue injury evaluation may have to be validated in terms of the statistical and functional criteria described above. Thus, the following may need to apply in order for the clinician or the investigator to be able to state that there is objective validity to the results of the pain questionnaire:

1. The questionnaire testing may be repeated at least five times within 1 month of testing or beginning treatment. The responses may be validated by showing internal consistency of coefficients of variation (CV < 10%) among the 5

or more repetitions for each question and response.

2. The test/re-test repeatability questionnaire tests can be evaluated in terms of the consistency of the response to the pain inquiry. The repeatability validation may be considered if the responses vary within 10%.

3. The reliability of the questionnaire results may need to be evaluated in comparison with known databases for the same kind of injury/response.

4. If available, the pain questionnaire may be considered in terms of specificity, sensitivity, and predictive values.

5. As the treatment is initiated, repeated pain questionnaire tests may show improvements in the overall symptoms/signs, especially with regard to the overall intensity/frequency of the soft tissue injury pain.

For the clinician who cannot afford the effort and luxury of repeated pain inquiry questionnaires in order to satisfy the objectivity criteria defined above, it is advisable to use such questionnaires no less than three times in the course of the clinical relationship. Thus, the patient/evaluee may have to respond to an original pain inquiry questionnaire during (1) the diagnostic evaluation, at the (2) beginning of the treatment period, and (3) at the end of the treatment period. Ideally, the responses should show a decrease or disappearance of the pain symptoms in time with treatment.

The Pain Visual Analogue

This is a visual format that allows the patient/evaluee to describe on a line or graph the intensity and/or frequency of the pain. It also may describe graphically the type of pain of soft tissue injury that one perceives.

The visual analogue is usually formatted on a "___/10" scale where 10/10 represents the highest degree of pain perceived in intensity/frequency and 0/10 represents a complete lack of pain in any region before or after treatment. The visual analogue is easy to perform and takes very little time to accomplish. The application of the visual analogue testing for soft tissue injury pain perception is rather similar to the pain questionnaire.

1. The pain visual analogue may be repeated at least 5 times within 1 month of testing or beginning of treatment. The responses may be validated by showing internal consistency of coefficients of variation (CV < 10%) among the 5 or more repetitions for each test.

2. The test/re-test repeatability pain visual analogues can be evaluated through the consistency of the response to the pain inquiry. The

repeatability validation may be considered if the responses vary within 10%. This holds true for the variables of pain intensity, frequency, or quality (e.g., burning, dull, etc.).

3. The reliability of the pain visual analogue results for adequacy of treatment may need to be evaluated in comparison with known databases for the same kind of injury/response.
4. If such results are available, the pain visual analogue may be considered in terms of specificity, sensitivity, and predictive values.
5. As the treatment is initiated, repeated pain visual analogue testing may show improvements in the overall numerical values representing the pain parameters.

For the clinician who cannot afford the effort and luxury of repeated pain inquiry visual analogues to satisfy the objectivity criteria defined above, it is advisable to use such pain visual analogues no less than three times in the course of the clinical relationship. Thus, the patient/evaluee may have to respond to an original pain inquiry pain visual analogue during (1) the diagnostic evaluation, at the (2) beginning of the treatment period, and (3) at the end of the treatment period. Ideally, the responses should show a decrease or disappearance of the pain symptoms in time with treatment.

The Pain Perception Threshold (P.P.T.)

The P.P.T. is a methodology whereby a pressure gauge is applied and pressed with a determined force on a trigger point or on a traumatized area until the evaluee/patient acknowledges the presence of pain rather than a perception of pressure (Fischer, 1977a, 1987a, 1990, 1994, 1997b; Sella & Donaldson, 1998). It can be used further (with the patient/evaluee's permission) to press until the evaluee states that the pain perception is that maximally tolerated. This tool objectively identifies the number of millimeters of pressure that differentiate the pressure perception from that of pain and/or that of pain recognition vs. maximal pain tolerance.

In forensic terms, it may be relevant to identify any degree of symptom magnification of pain perception/tolerance by applying the P.P.T. gauge on several areas, homolateral and contralateral and identify pain perception in areas that have not suffered from soft tissue injury.

1. The P.P.T. may be repeated at least five times on the affected area and on the contralateral area within of 1 month of testing or the beginning of treatment. The responses may be validated by showing internal consistency of coefficients of variation (CV < 10%) among the five or more repetitions for each test.

2. The test/re-test repeatability of such repeated P.P.T. can be evaluated through the response consistency to the pressure gauge. The repeatability validation may be considered if the responses vary within 10%. This holds true for the variables of pain perception at given pressures and perception of maximal pain.
3. The reliability of the P.P.T. results may need to be evaluated for treatment adequacy in comparison with known databases for the same kind of injury/response.
4. If such results are available, the P.P.T. may be considered in terms of specificity, sensitivity, and predictive values.
5. As the treatment is initiated, repeated P.P.T. testing may show improvements in the overall numerical values of millimeters of pressure required to elicit the pain response.

For the clinician who cannot afford the effort and luxury of repeated P.P.T. to satisfy the objectivity criteria defined above, it is advisable to use P.P.T. no less than three times in the course of the clinical relationship. Thus, the patient/evaluee may have to be tested with P.P.T. during (1) the diagnostic evaluation, at the (2) beginning of the treatment period, and (3) at the end of the treatment period. Ideally, the responses should show a decrease or disappearance of the pain symptoms in time with treatment, i.e., an increase in the number of millimeters required to perceive pain or maximal pain. The eventual responses should be quite similar on the affected soft tissue injury site and on the contralateral site.

The Tissue Compliance Measurement (T.C.M.)

This methodology is particularly applicable to soft tissue injury where there is tissue edema and/or chronic myofascitis (Fischer, 1977a, 1977b, 1984, 1987b, 1987c; Sella & Donaldson, 1998). The same criteria that apply to the P.P.T. methodology apply to the T.C.M. methodology.

S-EMG

Surface electromyography is a valid methodology for the investigation and treatment of soft tissue injury pain where skeletal muscles are affected. S-EMG reflects the degree of muscular electrical activity and effort during rest and dynamic action (Fischer & Chang, 1985; Sella, 2000a; 1995).

A number of S-EMG amplitude potentials (V RMS) parameters are particularly applicable to muscular dysfunction including (electrical) spasm, hypertonus, hypotonus, co-contraction, myokymia, fasciculations, elevated resting potential values, and abnormal laterality values differences between the affected sites and the nonaffected contralateral sites (Sella, 1995).

The S-EMG methodology has been described before in terms of specificity, sensitivity, predictive values, laterality, internal consistency, repeatability, and reliability by the author (Sella, 2000a). It involves dynamic protocols of bilateral myotatic units, at least one of which is affected by a soft tissue injury site (Sella, 1993).

1. The S-EMG dynamic protocol testing may be repeated at least five times for each segment of ROM on the affected area and on the contralateral area at any particular time. The responses may be validated by showing internal consistency of coefficients of variation (CV < 10%) among the five or more repetitions for each test. If the CV > 10% for the injured muscle but not for the unaffected muscles, the result is relevant for treatment follow-up.

2. The test/re-test repeatability of repeated S-EMG dynamic protocol testing can be evaluated if clinically necessary by at least three repetitions during at least 1 month of testing or treatment. The repeatability validation may be considered if the responses vary within 10%. This holds true for the S-EMG normal or pathological variables.

3. The reliability of the S-EMG dynamic protocol testing results may need to be evaluated for treatment adequacy in comparison with known databases for the same kind of injury/response.

4. Because such results are available for most skeletal muscles, the S-EMG dynamic protocol testing may be considered in terms of specificity, sensitivity, and predictive values.

5. As the treatment is initiated, repeated S-EMG dynamic protocol testing may show improvements in the overall pattern of change from pathological electric curves to normal curves during activity and rest.

For the clinician who cannot afford the effort and luxury of repeated S-EMG dynamic protocol testing to satisfy all the objectivity criteria defined above, it is advisable to use such S-EMG dynamic protocol testing no less than three times in the course of the clinical relationship. Thus, the patient/evaluee may have to be tested with S-EMG dynamic protocol testing during (1) the diagnostic evaluation, at the (2) beginning of the treatment period, and (3) at the end of the treatment period. Ideally, the responses should show a decrease or disappearance of the pathological curve variables described above. The eventual responses should be quite similar on the affected soft tissue injury site and on the contralateral site.

Current Perception Threshold (C.P.T.)

The C.P.T. is a valid methodology that evaluates individual perception of pain via electrical stimulation of the peripheral pain fibers at the fingertip site (Sella & Donaldson, 1998). In addition to the perception of pain in A and C fibers, the C.P.T. also evaluates the perception of touch/pressure fibers of the A type.

Whereas such perception of any type of fiber, i.e., either touch/pressure or pain, may be considered subjective, repeated testing with the current on or off allows the investigator to distinguish quite easily between a patient with consistent responses vs. a symptom magnifier. Thus, even though the pain or touch perception may be an individual factor, testing may allow the investigator to address the issue of consistency vs. functional overlay. Individuals with soft tissue injury may or may not have nerve damage. When such nerve damage is of the sensory type and involves the A, Aα, and Cδ fibers, the C.P.T. evaluation is an excellent tool for exclusion of nervous lesion vs. myofascial or other type of soft tissue pathology (Liu, Kopacz, & Carpenter, 1995; Masson & Boulton, 1991).

For the clinician who cannot afford the effort and luxury of repeated S-EMG dynamic protocol testing in order to satisfy all the objectivity criteria defined above, it is advisable to use such S-EMG dynamic protocol testing no less than three times in the course of the clinical relationship.

Thus, the patient/evaluee may have to be tested with S-EMG dynamic protocol testing during (1) the diagnostic evaluation, at the (2) beginning of the treatment period and (3) at the end of the treatment period.

Ideally, the responses should show a decrease or disappearance of the pathological curve variables described above. The eventual responses should be quite similar on the affected soft tissue injury site and on the contralateral site.

Objective Treatment Outcome Measurement

Objective treatment refers to numerical modalities involved in the pain rehabilitation process. Such modalities may be analgesics, in which case one would have to know the type of "pain killer" and the posology given in time. The objective outcome could be a linear follow-up of the pain level at the beginning of the treatment, at each visit, and at the end of the treatment period. For instance, the initial soft tissue injury pain level intensity may be 9/10; in time it may show a decrease pattern to 7/10, 5/10 and eventually reach 1/10 at the end of the treatment period. The example given above is pertinent to one pain treating modality or to a combination of modalities. The main object is to demonstrate a framework of pain level measurement that is consistent, numerical, and spans the beginning to the end of the treatment period.

Strengths and Limitations of Pain Investigation Methodologies

Every scientific methodology has inherent strengths and limitations. Therefore, it is incumbent upon the researcher, investigator or clinician to utilize multiple modalities or methodologies. The choice of combination(s) must be such that the strength of one modality can overcome the limitation of another modality. Furthermore, while theoretically any result derived from any individual modality may have artifact properties, results deriving from a battery of modalities cannot be considered technical artifacts.

In terms of pain investigation, pain questionnaires have the strength of consistency if they are given repeatedly. At the same time, responses are subjective because pain is a subjective phenomenon, thus the limitation of questionnaires. The same criteria apply to the pain picture or visual analogue.

The strength of the pain perception threshold methodology is that it helps to differentiate the perception of pressure from that of pain. Furthermore, it helps to assess individual perception of maximal tolerable pain threshold at the point of pressure. The limitation of the modality is that the subject could state, without any check for consistency, that he or she has pain or maximal pain. This inherent limitation was modified with the test of consistency (Sella & Donaldson, 1998) that modifies the original procedure which required testing of the injured or symptomatic site. The contralateral and other sites are tested at least three to five times for consistency of the numerical value of pain perception. If the responses are statistically consistent, especially with regard to pain perception of the symptomatic site, then the test can be considered valid.

The same considerations apply to the tissue compliance measurement (T.C.M.).

The strength of the S-EMG modality in the investigative mode is that it measures the consistency of effort of any muscular activity. If the amplitude of contraction pattern is abnormal related to pain or other dysfunction, it will remain so as an autonomous factor. The same applies to the parameter of spectral frequency. Specificity and sensitivity studies have shown that the likelihood of amplitude curve abnormality is high in myofascial pain, when tested with S-EMG (Sella, 2000a). The limitation of the S-EMG modality is that it cannot measure the intensity of the pain; to date no studies have been done on the subject so far.

S-EMG can be utilized concomitantly with other modalities. It can strengthen the reliability of the results of the pain questionnaire, pain visual analogue, P.P.T., and T.C.M. by the demonstration of internal consistency, because S-EMG has been shown to demonstrate internal consistency well (Sella, 2000c).

The current perception threshold modality investigates the perceptual threshold of electric stimulation of (close to the surface) nerve endings of peripheral nerves. Its

strength may be that of the pain recognition at rather similar micro-electrical stimulation intensities, if the test is done repeatedly.

Its limitation is that recognition is a subjective perception and expression. However, repeated C.P.T. testing and statistical analysis of the results can demonstrate consistency or rule out inconsistency. Performance of this test as part of the battery described above can validate the pain symptom/perception, because the presence of pain should be paralleled by the consistent response pattern in all the tests.

Thus, one can investigate pain of soft tissue injury with several modalities and counter the limitations of one with the strength of another.

RELATIVE LOSS OF STRENGTH (L.O.S.)

Acute soft tissue injury is often followed by loss of strength of the injured muscle or myotatic unit (Anchor & Felicetti, 1999; Sella & Donaldson, 1998). The L.O.S. may involve direct or indirect trauma to the skin, subcutaneous tissue, blood vessels, nerves, fascia, and skeletal muscle as well as periosteum and bone. As stated, only L.O.S. involving the muscles and fascia is discussed in this presentation.

Acute L.O.S. is reflected by the body's reflex of splinting. The injured part is "splinted," i.e., defended by the surrounding area in terms of muscles, joints, and fascia as well as the contralateral area and the appropriate myotatic units of either side. The deconditioning maintained by pain and tissue inflamation results in relative L.O.S. If the acute L.O.S. is not resolved properly through investigation and treatment, it may result in the development of myofascitis and protective guarding L.O.S.

L.O.S. assessment of soft tissue injury is easy to perform in terms of the statistical requirements described above. Loss of strength can be measured objectively with dynamometry. A variety of dynamometers are on the market. They may refer to several areas of the body. For consistency, dynamometric testing must be performed at least through five repetitions and measure the internal consistency of strength performance of the evaluee or patient.

For repeatability, the dynamometry or other methodologies utilized to assess strength should show a good measure of repeatability for L.O.S. assessment and rehabilitation of strength. When normative values or databases of objective measurements are known, the results of the L.O.S. investigation and/or treatment should be measured against those normative values for reliability.

When the specificity, sensitivity and predictive values of any L.O.S. investigative methodology are known, the clinical results may be comparable to such data. The functional utilization of any L.O.S. investigative methodology is as good as the results obtained in relation to it. Therefore, the clinician may want to describe the validity of the application of the L.O.S. investigative tool in terms of the results obtained from knowledge of the treatment.

Because it is necessary to evaluate the treatment results before, during, and post-treatment, any methodology for L.O.S. investigation/treatment needs to be objective and numerical for the overall outcome measurement.

Methodologies for soft tissue L.O.S. measurement are considered below.

L.O.S. Questionnaires

Questionnaires can be used to assess the event and presence of L.O.S. The evaluee/patient needs to be asked about the perception of L.O.S. before the injury as well as at the time of examination. L.O.S. questionnaires also may assess strength rehabilitation through the treatment period. Any L.O.S. questionnaire utilization in soft tissue injury evaluation may have to be validated through the statistical and functional criteria described above. Thus, the following may need to be applied in order for the clinician or investigator to be able to state that objective validity to the results of the L.O.S. questionnaire exists:

1. The questionnaire may be repeated at least five times within 1 month of testing or beginning of treatment. The responses may be validated by showing internal consistency of coefficients of variation (CV < 10%) among the five or more repetitions for each question and response.
2. The test/re-test repeatability of such repeated questionnaires can be evaluated for the response consistency to the L.O.S. inquiry. The repeatability validation may be considered if the responses vary within 10%.
3. The reliability of the questionnaire results may need to be evaluated in comparison with known databases for the same kind of injury/response.
4. If available, the L.O.S. questionnaire may be considered in terms of specificity, sensitivity, and predictive values.
5. As the treatment is initiated, repeated L.O.S. questionnaires may show improvements in the overall symptoms/signs, especially with regard to the overall intensity of the soft tissue injury L.O.S.

For the clinician who cannot afford the effort and luxury of repeated L.O.S. inquiry questionnaires to satisfy the objectivity criteria defined above, it is advisable to use such questionnaires no less than three times in the course of the clinical relationship. Thus, the patient/evaluee may have to respond to an original L.O.S. inquiry questionnaire during (1) the diagnostic evaluation, at the (2) beginning of the treatment period, and (3) at the end of the treatment period. Ideally, the responses should show in time a decrease or disappearance of L.O.S. symptoms with treatment.

The L.O.S. Visual Analogue

This is a visual format that allows the patient/evaluee to describe on a line or graph the intensity of the L.O.S. The visual analogue is usually formatted on a "___/5" scale where 0/5 represents the highest functional degree of L.O.S. perceived in intensity and 5/5 represents full strength.

The visual analogue is easy to perform and takes very little time to accomplish. In terms of the parameters described above for the L.O.S. questionnaire, the application is rather similar to the visual analogue testing for soft tissue injury L.O.S. perception.

1. The L.O.S. visual analogue may be repeated at least five times within 1 month of testing or beginning of treatment. The responses may be validated by showing internal consistency of coefficients of variation (CV < 10%) among the five or more repetitions for each test.
2. The test/re-test repeatability of L.O.S. visual analogues can be evaluated by the response consistency to the L.O.S. inquiry. The repeatability validation may be considered if the responses vary within 10%.
3. The reliability of L.O.S. visual analogue results for adequacy of treatment may need to be evaluated by comparison with known databases for the same kind of injury/response.
4. If such results are available, the L.O.S. visual analogue may be considered in terms of specificity, sensitivity, and predictive values.
5. As the treatment progresses, repeated L.O.S. visual analogue testing may show improvements in the overall numerical values representing the L.O.S. parameter.

For the clinician who cannot afford the effort and luxury of repeated L.O.S. visual analogues to satisfy the objectivity criteria defined above, it is advisable to use such L.O.S. visual analogues no less than three times in the course of the clinical relationship.

Thus, the patient/evaluee may have to respond to an original L.O.S. inquiry or L.O.S. visual analogue during (1) the diagnostic evaluation, at the (2) beginning of the treatment period, and (3) at the end of the treatment period. Ideally, over time the responses should show a decrease or disappearance of the L.O.S. symptoms with treatment.

DYNAMOMETRY

Dynamometry is the most useful methodology for measuring strength (Sella & Donaldson, 1998). It measures the sum total of myotatic unit strength rather than individual muscle. Therefore, soft tissue injury to one muscle and probable L.O.S. in that muscle are reflected by L.O.S. on the dynamometric testing. However, the testing involves several groups of muscles and it is likely that all the other muscles involved in the testing try to "protectively guard" the injured muscle and put out more effort than they would have done otherwise.

Dynamometry involves mechanical or electronic gauges. The numbers obtained for the various degrees of effort tested represent the overall strength of voluntary contractions of the muscular groups that are active in the testing.

In forensic terms, it may be relevant to identify any degree of symptom magnification of L.O.S. perception by applying the dynamometric instrument to several muscle groups (homolateral and contralateral) and identify L.O.S. perception in areas which have not suffered from soft tissue injury.

1. Dynamometry may be repeated at least five times on the affected and contralateral areas 1 month of testing or beginning of treatment. The responses may be validated by showing internal consistency of coefficients of variation (CV < 10%) among the five or more repetitions for each test.
2. The test/re-test repeatability of such dynamometry can be evaluated for response consistency. Repeatability validation may be considered if strength testing results vary within 10%.
3. The reliability of dynamometry results may need to be evaluated for adequacy of treatment through comparison with known databases for the same kind of injury/response.
4. If such results are available, the dynamometry may be considered in terms of specificity, sensitivity, and predictive values.
5. As the treatment is initiated, repeated dynamometric testing may show improvements (kilos or pounds) in the overall numerical values representing L.O.S. perception.

For the clinician who cannot afford the effort and luxury of repeated dynamometry to satisfy the objectivity criteria defined above, it is advisable to use dynamometry no less than three times in the course of the clinical relationship. Thus, the patient/evaluee may have to be tested with dynamometry during (1) the diagnostic evaluation, at the (2) beginning of the treatment period, and (3) at the end of the treatment period. Ideally, in time and with treatment the responses should show a decrease or disappearance of the L.O.S. symptoms i.e., an increase in the number of kilos or pounds.

S-EMG

Surface electromyography is a valid methodology for the investigation and treatment of soft tissue injury L.O.S. where skeletal muscles are affected (Sella, 1993, 1995, 1998a, 1998b). S-EMG reflects the degree of muscular electrical activity and effort during rest and dynamic action (Basmajian & DeLuca, 1985). The S-EMG methodology has been described in terms of specificity, sensitivity, and predictive values, laterality, internal consistency, repeatability, and reliability.

S-EMG involves dynamic protocols of bilateral myotatic units, at least one of which is affected by a soft tissue injury site. The S-EMG amplitude parameter is useful as an indicator of muscular effort and ability to proceed with a determined effort. The affected muscle will show a higher amplitude of activity potentials (V RMS) by comparison with the nonsymptomatic contralateral muscle (Sella, 1995, 2000a). This may be because it needs to use and elicit utilization of an increased number of contractile elements in order to obtain and achieve the same strength requirement end result.

However, injured muscle strength is usually lower than that of the asymptomatic muscle and at a certain point of effort requirement, it can no longer sustain the effort and increase the amplitude of contraction. Clinically, that occurs when the evaluee/patient gets rather severe muscular pain and states that he/she can no longer sustain the effort of contraction.

As compared to dynamometry, S-EMG does not reflect exactly strength but rather effort and ability to elicit effort (Kumar & Mital, 1996). On the other hand, it is specific to any given muscle in the myotatic unit, including the injured muscle. As stated above, dynamometry is not specific to a given muscle but to the whole myotatic unit or to the sum total of the myotatic units involved in the effort of strength testing (Sella & Donaldson, 1998).

1. The S-EMG dynamic protocol testing may be repeated at least five times for each ROM segment on the affected area and on the contralateral area at any particular time. The responses may be validated by showing internal consistency of coefficients of variation (CV < 10%) among the five or more repetitions for each test. If the CV > 10% for the injured muscle and its loss of strength but not for the unaffected muscles, such a result is relevant of treatment follow-up.
2. The test/re-test repeatability of such S-EMG dynamic protocol testing can be evaluated if

clinically necessary by at least three repetitions during at least 1 month of testing or treatment. The repeatability validation may be considered if the responses vary within 10%. This holds true for the S-EMG normal or pathological variables.

3. The reliability of S-EMG dynamic protocol testing results treatment adequacy may need to be evaluated in comparison with known databases for the same kind of injury/response.

4. Because results are available for most skeletal muscles, the S-EMG dynamic protocol testing may be considered in terms of specificity, sensitivity, and predictive values.

5. As the treatment is initiated, repeated S-EMG dynamic protocol testing of L.O.S. may show improvements in the overall pattern of change from pathological electric curves to normal curves during activity and rest.

For the clinician who cannot afford the effort and luxury of repeated S-EMG dynamic protocol testing in order to satisfy all the objectivity criteria defined above, it is advisable to use such S-EMG dynamic protocol testing no less than three times in the course of the clinical relationship.

Thus, the patient/evaluee may have to be tested with S-EMG dynamic protocol testing during (1) the diagnostic evaluation, at the (2) beginning of the treatment period, and (3) at the end of the treatment period. Ideally, the L.O.S. responses should show a normalization of the S-EMG amplitude curve described above.

The eventual responses should be quite similar on the affected soft tissue injury site and on the contralateral site. The S-EMG spectral analysis parameter mirrors the element of fatigue. Muscles which have been injured and suffer from L.O.S. are easily fatigable in clinical terms. Improvement of strength and stamina may be mirrored by the S-EMG spectral analysis results which show the decremental curve of the affected/treated muscle to parallel that of the asymptomatic muscle.

Objective Treatment Outcome Measurement

Objective treatment refers to numerical modalities involved in the L.O.S. rehabilitation process. Such modalities may include physical therapy aimed at muscle strengthening, agility, and increased endurance. The objective outcome could be a linear follow-up of the L.O.S. level at the beginning of the treatment, at each visit, and at the end of the treatment period. For instance, the initial soft tissue injury L.O.S. level may be 50% of the contralateral strength. With therapy, the strength may increase and normalize in time to 95% of the expected level in terms of the contralateral strength. This is pertinent

to one L.O.S. treating modality or to a combination of modalities.

It is most relevant to demonstrate of measurement of strength regained through therapy which is consistent and numerical and spans from the beginning to the end of the treatment period.

Strengths and Limitations of Loss of Strength (L.O.S.) Investigation Methodologies

In terms of L.O.S. investigation, the L.O.S. questionnaires are consistent if they are given repeatedly. At the same time, the responses are subjective because L.O.S. is a subjective phenomenon, thus the limitation of questionnaires. The same criteria apply to the L.O.S. picture or visual analogue.

The strength of the S-EMG modality in the investigative mode is that it measures the consistency of effort for any muscular activity. If the amplitude of the contraction pattern is abnormal, it will remain so as an autonomous factor. As described above, in general, the amplitude of muscular contraction (at the minimal voluntary contraction level of effort) is higher in a muscle affected by loss of strength, probably because of the need to recruit more contractile elements for the activity (Sella, 1995).

The limitation of the S-EMG modality is that it cannot measure the intensity of the L.O.S. (Kumar & Mital, 1996).

S-EMG can be utilized concomitantly with dynamometry. Thus, it can demonstrate internal consistency in itself and also validate the statistical demonstration of the internal consistency of dynamometry (Sella & Donaldson, 1998; Sella, 2000c).

Thus, one can investigate L.O.S. of soft tissue injury with several modalities and counter the limitations of one with the strength of another.

RELATIVE LOSS OF RANGE OF MOTION (L. ROM)

Acute soft tissue injury is often followed by L. ROM related to functional shortening of the injured muscle, myotatic unit or joint components (Anchor & Felicetti, 1999; Sella & Donaldson, 1998). The L. ROM may involve direct or indirect trauma to the skin, subcutaneous tissue, blood vessels, nerves, fascia and skeletal muscle, articular components, as well as periosteum and bone. As stated, only L. ROM involving the muscles and fascia are discussed in this chapter. Acute L. ROM is reflected by the body's reflex of splinting. The injured part is "splinted," i.e., defended, by the surrounding area in terms of muscles, joints, and fascia as well as the contralateral area and the appropriate myotatic units of either side. The loss of range of motion maintained by pain and tissue inflamation results in relative L. ROM. If the acute L. ROM is not resolved properly by investigation and treatment, it may result in the development of myofascitis and protective guarding of L. ROM-related features.

L. ROM assessment of soft tissue injury is easy to perform using the statistical requirements described above. L. ROM can be measured with goniometry (inclinometry) objectively. A variety of goniometers and inclinometers are on the market (AMA, 1993; Gerhardt, 1992). They may be applicable to several areas of the body. It is very important to utilize the right instrument with the appropriate consistency of methodology (Gerhardt, 1992).

For consistency, goniometric testing should be performed at least through five repetitions measuring the internal consistency of joint motion performance of the evaluee or patient. For repeatability, the goniometry or other methodologies utilized to assess joint motion should show a good measure of repeatability for L. ROM assessment and rehabilitation of joint motion. For reliability, when normative values or databases of objective measurements are known, the results of the L. ROM investigation and/or treatment should be measured against those normative values in terms of reliability.

There are several consensus ROM speciality tables. However, the human joint ROM needs further studies in terms of normative data acquisition.

When the specificity, sensitivity and predictive values of any L. ROM investigative methodology are known, clinical results may be comparable to such data. The functional utilization of any L. ROM investigative methodology is only as good as the results obtained in relation to it. Therefore, the clinician may want to describe the validity of the application of the L. ROM investigative tool in comparison to the results obtained from knowledge of other treatment.

Because it is necessary to evaluate treatment results of joint motion rehabilitation before, during, and after treatment, any methodology for L. ROM investigation/treatment needs to be objective and numerical in terms of the overall outcome measurement.

The following methodologies for soft tissue L. ROM measurement are considered.

L. ROM Questionnaires

Questionnaires can be used to assess the cause and presence of loss of joint range of motion. The evaluee/patient needs to be asked about his or her perception of L. ROM before the injury as well as at the time of examination. L. ROM questionnaires also may assess joint motion rehabilitation through the period of treatment. Any L. ROM questionnaire utilization in soft tissue injury evaluation may have to be validated in terms of the statistical and functional criteria described above. Thus, the following may need to apply for the clinician or the investigator to be able to state that the L. ROM questionnaire's results are objectively valid.

1. The questionnaire may be repeated at least five times within 1 month of testing or beginning of treatment. The responses may be validated as showing internal consistency in terms of coefficients of variation (CV < 10%) among the five or more repetitions for each question and response.

2. The test/re-test repeatability of such questionnaires can be evaluated for consistent response to the L. ROM inquiry. Repeatability validation may be considered if the responses vary within 10%.

3. The reliability of questionnaire results may need to be evaluated in comparison with known databases for the same kind of injury/response.

4. If available, the L. ROM questionnaire may be considered in terms of specificity, sensitivity, and predictive values.

5. As the treatment progresses, repeated L. ROM questionnaires may show improvements in joint ROM overall symptoms/signs, especially with regard to the overall intensity of the soft tissue injury.

For the clinician who cannot afford the effort and luxury of repeated L. ROM questionnaires to satisfy the objectivity criteria defined above, it is advisable to use such questionnaires no less than three times in the course of the clinical relationship. Thus, the patient/evaluee may have to respond to an original L. ROM questionnaire during (1) the diagnostic evaluation, at the (2) beginning of the treatment period, and (3) at the end of the treatment period. Ideally, with treatment and time the responses should show a decrease or disappearance of the L. ROM symptoms.

The L. ROM Visual Analogue

This is a visual format which allows the patient/evaluee to describe on a line or graph the extent of joint ROM loss. The visual analogue may be formatted on a ___/X° scale where 0/0° represents the highest functional degree of L. ROM perceived (ankylosis) and X°/X° represents full joint motion.

The visual analogue is easy to perform and takes very little time to accomplish. In terms of the parameters described above for the L. ROM questionnaire, the application is rather similar to visual analogue testing for soft tissue injury L. ROM perception.

1. The L. ROM visual analogue may be repeated at least five times within 1 month of testing or the beginning of treatment. The responses may be validated by showing internal consistency using coefficients of variation (CV < 10%) among the five or more repetitions for each test.

2. The test/re-test repeatability of such L. ROM visual analogues can be evaluated for response consistency to the L. ROM inquiry. Repeatability validation may be considered if the responses vary within 10%.

3. Reliability of the L. ROM visual analogue results may need to be evaluated in comparison with known databases for adequacy of treatment for the same kind of injury/response.

4. If such results are available, the L. ROM visual analogue may be considered in terms of specificity, sensitivity, and predictive values.

5. As treatment is initiated, repeated L. ROM visual analogue testing may show improvements in the overall numerical values representing the L. ROM parameter.

For the clinician who cannot afford the effort and luxury of repeated inquiry using L. ROM visual analogue to satisfy the objectivity criteria defined above, it is advisable to use the methodology no less than three times in the course of the clinical relationship. Thus, the patient/evaluee may have to respond to an original L. ROM visual analogue during (1) the diagnostic evaluation, at the (2) beginning of the treatment period, and (3) at the end of the treatment period. Ideally, with time and treatment the responses should show a decrease or disappearance of the L. ROM symptoms.

Goniometry (Inclinometry)

Goniometry is the most useful methodology for measuring joint motion (Cailliet, 1994). It measures the sum total of myotatic unit and joint motion rather than individual muscles or joint components. Therefore, soft tissue injury to one muscle and probable L. ROM in that muscle are reflected by goniometric testing. However, the testing involves several groups of muscles and the joint. It is likely that the other muscles involved in the testing try to protectively guard the injured muscle and suffer from functional L. ROM as a consequence. Inflamation of the joint may reduce the ability to achieve full motion. Goniometry involves mechanical or electronic gauges. The numbers obtained with various degrees of tested effort represent the overall joint motion of the muscular groups that are active in the testing.

In forensic terms, it may be relevant to find any degree of symptom magnification of L. ROM perception by applying the goniometric instrument to several muscle groups and joints, homolateral and contralateral, and identify the L. ROM perception in areas that have not suffered from soft tissue injury.

1. Goniometry may be repeated at least five times on the affected area and on the contralateral area within 1 month of testing or the beginning of treatment. The responses may be validated by showing internal consistency with coefficients of variation (CV < 10%) among the five or more repetitions for each test.

2. The test/re-test repeatability of such goniometry can be evaluated through the consistency of the response. Repeatability validation may be considered if the joint motion testing results vary within 10%.

3. Reliability of the goniometry results may need to be evaluated in comparison with known adequacy of treatment databases for the same kind of injury/response.

4. If such results are available, the goniometry may be considered in terms of specificity, sensitivity and predictive values.

5. As the treatment is initiated, repeated goniometric testing may show improvements in the overall numerical values representing L. ROM perception of degrees of motion.

For the clinician who cannot afford the effort and luxury of repeated goniometry in order to satisfy the objectivity criteria defined above, it is advisable to use such goniometry no less than three times in the course of the clinical relationship. Thus, the patient/evaluee may have to be tested with goniometry during (1) the diagnostic evaluation, at the (2) beginning of the treatment period, and (3) at the end of the treatment period. Ideally, responses should show a decrease or disappearance of the L. ROM symptoms in time with treatment, i.e., normalization of the degrees of joint motion.

S-EMG

Surface electromyography is a valid methodology for the investigation and treatment of soft tissue injury L. ROM where skeletal muscles are affected. S-EMG reflects the degree of muscular electrical activity and effort during rest and dynamic action. The S-EMG amplitude curve of a joint motion may be different if that motion is partial or complete. In other words, the amplitude curve of the biceps during 50% of full elbow flexion will be different than that of 100% of full elbow flexion.

The S-EMG methodology has been described already in terms of specificity, sensitivity, predictive values, laterality, internal consistency, repeatability, and reliability. It involves dynamic protocols of bilateral myotatic units, at least one of which is affected by a soft tissue injury site.

The S-EMG amplitude parameter is useful as an indicator of muscular effort and the ability to proceed with a determined effort through full joint ROM. As compared to goniometry, S-EMG does not reflect exactly joint motion but rather effort and ability to elicit effort. On the other hand, it is specific to any given muscle in the myotatic unit, including the injured muscle. As stated above, goniometry is not specific to a given muscle but to the whole myotatic unit or to the sum total of the myotatic units and joint(s) involved in the effort of joint motion testing.

1. S-EMG dynamic protocol testing may be repeated at least five times for each segment of ROM on the affected area and on the contralateral area at any particular time. The responses may be validated by showing internal consistency of coefficients of variation (CV < 10%) among the five or more repetitions for each test. If the CV > 10% for the injured muscle and its L. ROM but not for the unaffected muscles, such a result is relevant treatment follow-up.

2. The test/re-test repeatability of such S-EMG dynamic protocol testing can be evaluated if clinically necessary by at least three repetitions during at least 1 month of testing or treatment. Repeatability validation may be considered if the responses vary within 10%. This holds true for the S-EMG normal or pathological variables.

3. Reliability of the S-EMG dynamic protocol testing results may need to be evaluated in comparison with known databases for the same kind of injury/response for treatment adequacy of L. ROM.

4. Since such results are available for most skeletal muscles, the S-EMG dynamic protocol testing may be considered in terms of specificity, sensitivity, and predictive values.

5. After treatment is initiated, repeated S-EMG dynamic protocol testing of L. ROM may show improvements in the overall pattern of change from pathological electric curves to normal curves during activity and rest.

For the clinician who cannot afford the effort and luxury of repeated S-EMG dynamic protocol testing to satisfy all the objectivity criteria defined above, it is advisable to use such S-EMG dynamic protocol testing no less than three times in the course of the clinical relationship. Thus, the patient/evaluee may have to be tested with S-EMG dynamic protocol testing during (1) the diagnostic evaluation, at the (2) beginning of the treatment period, and (3) at the end of the treatment period. Ideally, the responses of L. ROM should show a normalization of the S-EMG amplitude curve described above. The eventual responses should be quite similar on the affected soft tissue injury site and on the contralateral site.

Objective Treatment Outcome Measurement

Objective treatment refers to numerical modalities involved in the L. ROM rehabilitation process. Such modalities may include physical therapy aimed at muscle stretching and lengthening as well as joint ROM. The objective outcome could be a linear follow-up of the L. ROM level at the beginning of the treatment, at each visit, and at the end of the treatment period. For instance, the initial soft tissue injury L. ROM level may be 50% of the contralateral joint motion. With therapy, the joint motion may increase and normalize in time to 95% of the expected level of contralateral joint motion.

The example given above is pertinent to one L. ROM treating modality or to a combination of modalities. It is relevant to demonstrate a framework of measurement of joint motion normalization through therapy which is consistent and numerical and spans the beginning to the end of the treatment period.

Strengths and Limitations of Loss of Range of Motion (L. ROM) Investigation Methodologies

For L. ROM investigation, L. ROM questionnaires have the strength of consistency if they are given repeatedly. At the same time, the responses are subjective because active L. ROM is a subjective phenomenon, thus the limitation of questionnaires. The same criteria apply to the L. ROM picture or visual analogue.

The strength of the S-EMG modality in the investigative mode is that it measures the consistency of effort of any muscular activity at any given point or curve of joint ROM. If the amplitude of the contraction pattern is abnormal related to L. ROM, it will remain so as an autonomous factor. The limitation of the S-EMG modality is that it cannot measure the extent of active L. ROM (Kumar & Mital, 1996; Sella, 2000b).

S-EMG can be utilized concomitantly with goniometry. Thus, it can demonstrate internal consistency and also validate the statistical demonstration of goniometry's internal consistency (Sella, 2000c; Sella & Donaldson, 1998).

Thus, one can investigate L. ROM of soft tissue injury with several modalities and counter the limitations of one with the strength of another.

RELATIVE LOSS OF ADEQUATE FUNCTION (L.A.F.)

Acute soft tissue injury is often followed by loss of adequate function of the injured muscle or myotatic unit (Sella, 1995; 1998a; 1998b). The L.A.F. may involve direct or indirect trauma to the skin, subcutaneous tissue, blood vessels, nerves, fascia, and skeletal muscle as well as periosteum and bone. Only L.A.F. involving the muscles and fascia are discussed in this chapter.

Acute L.A.F. is reflected by the body's reflex of splinting. The injured part is splinted, i.e., defended by the surrounding area of muscles, joints, and fascia as well as the contralateral area and the appropriate myotatic units of either side. De-conditioning may be maintained by pain, tissue inflamation, and resulting relative loss of strength and range of motion. If the acute L.A.F. is not resolved properly through investigation and treatment, it may result in the development of myofascitis and protective guarding.

L.A.F. assessment of soft tissue injury can be performed according to the components described above. However, because function is very variable in different individuals, there may be a need for further testing for pain, loss of range of motion, or loss of strength. Functional testing needs to follow the same procedural and statistical principles described above.

For consistency, it is important to perform any test as many times as possible and measure internal performance consistency of the evaluee or patient. Repeatability, any methodology or diversity of methodologies utilized should show a good measure of repeatability for L.A.F. assessment or reduction. Normative values or databases of objective measurements of loss of function related to soft tissue injury are not available because of the diversity of such losses. Nonetheless, the clinician needs to be on guard for consistency of performance or lack of performance of individual functional activities, e.g., typing on a computer.

When the specificity, sensitivity and predictive values of any L.A.F. investigative methodology are known, the clinical results may be comparable to such data. The functional utilization of any L.A.F. investigative methodology is only as good as the results obtained in relation to it. Therefore, the clinician may want to describe the validity of the application of the L.A.F. investigative tool in terms of the results obtained from knowledge of the treatment.

Because it is necessary to evaluate the treatment results before, during, and after treatment, any methodology for L.A.F. investigation/treatment needs to have objective and numerical overall outcome measurement.

The following methodologies for soft tissue L.A.F. measurement are considered.

L.A.F. Questionnaires

No soft tissue injury loss of function questionnaires exist. Therefore, the clinician needs to use models of questionnaires utilized for L. ROM and L.O.S., and modify them for each individual loss of function case. Any L.A.F. questionnaire utilization in soft tissue injury evaluation may have to be validated using the statistical and functional criteria described above. Thus, the following may need to apply for the clinician or the investigator to be able to state that there is objective validity to the results of the L.A.F. questionnaire:

1. The questionnaire may be repeated at least five times within 1 month of testing or beginning of treatment. The responses may be validated by showing internal consistency of coefficients of

variation (CV < 10%) among the five or more repetitions for each question and response.
2. The test/re-test repeatability of such questionnaires can be evaluated for response consistency to the L.A.F. inquiry. The repeatability validation may be considered if the responses vary within 10%.
3. The reliability of the questionnaire results may need to be evaluated in comparison with known databases for the same kind of injury/response.
4. If available, the L.A.F. questionnaire may be considered in terms of specificity, sensitivity and predictive values.
5. The treatment progresses, repeated L.A.F. questionnaires may show improvements in the overall symptoms/signs, especially with regard to the overall intensity/frequency of the soft tissue injury L.A.F.

For the clinician who cannot afford the effort and luxury of repeated L.A.F. inquiry questionnaires to satisfy the objectivity criteria defined above, it is advisable to use such questionnaires no less than three times in the course of the clinical relationship. Thus, the patient/evaluee may have to respond to an original L.A.F. inquiry questionnaire during (1) the diagnostic evaluation, at the (2) beginning of the treatment period, and (3) at the end of the treatment period. Ideally, with time and treatment the responses should show a decrease or disappearance of the L.A.F. symptoms.

The L.A.F. Visual Analogue

This is a visual format which allows the patient/evaluee to describe on a line or graph the intensity and/or frequency of the L.A.F. It also may describe graphically the type of L.A.F. that one perceives. The visual analogue is usually formatted on a ___/10 scale where 10/10 represents the highest degree of L.A.F. perceived in intensity/frequency and 0/10 represents a complete lack of L.A.F. of any region before or after treatment.

The visual analogue is easy to perform and takes very little time to accomplish. In terms of the parameters described above for the L.A.F. questionnaire, the application is rather similar for the visual analogue testing of soft tissue injury L.A.F. perception.

1. The L.A.F. visual analogue may be repeated at least five times within 1 month of testing or the beginning of treatment. The responses may be validated by showing internal consistency of coefficients of variation (CV < 10%) among the five or more repetitions for each test.
2. The test/re-test repeatability of such L.A.F. visual analogues can be evaluated for response

consistency to the L.A.F. inquiry. The repeatability validation may be considered if the responses vary within 10%. This holds true for the variables of L.A.F. intensity, frequency, or quality.

3. The reliability of the L.A.F. visual analogue results may need to be evaluated in comparison with known databases of adequacy of for the same kind of injury/response treatment.

4. If such results are available, the L.A.F. visual analogue may be considered in terms of specificity, sensitivity and predictive values.

5. After treatment is initiated, repeated L.A.F. visual analogue testing may show improvements in the overall numerical values representing the L.A.F. parameters.

For the clinician who cannot afford the effort and luxury of repeated inquiry of L.A.F. visual analogue to satisfy the objectivity criteria defined above, it is advisable to use such L.A.F. visual analogues no less than three times in the course of the clinical relationship. Thus, the patient/evaluee may have to respond to an original L.A.F. visual analogue inquiry during (1) the diagnostic evaluation, at the (2) beginning of the treatment period, and (3) at the end of the treatment period. Ideally, with time with treatment the responses should show a decrease or disappearance of the L.A.F. symptoms.

Multiple Modalities

A number of objective tests such as dynamometry, goniometry etc. may be applicable on a case-by-case basis loss of functional activity. No example can be given since each loss of function may include different components.

S-EMG

This technology is probably the only soft tissue injury methodology applicable to most, if not all, losses of functional activity. The parameters of utilization during investigation and treatment have been described above.

OBJECTIVE TREATMENT OUTCOME MEASUREMENT

Objective treatment refers to numerical modalities involved in the L.A.F. rehabilitation process. Such modalities are usually multiple. The objective outcome could be a linear follow-up of the L.A.F. level at the beginning of the treatment, at each visit, and at the end of the treatment period. For instance, the initial soft tissue injury L.A.F. intensity level may be 9/10, in time it may show a decrease pattern to 7/10, 5/10, and eventually reach 1/10 at the end of the treatment period. It is important to demonstrate measurement of the L.A.F. level which is consistent and numerical and spans the beginning to the end of the treatment period.

STRENGTHS AND LIMITATIONS OF LOSS OF ADEQUATE FUNCTION (L.A.F.) INVESTIGATION METHODOLOGIES

In terms of L.A.F. investigation, the L.A.F. questionnaires have the strength of consistency if they are given repeatedly. At the same time, the responses are subjective because L.A.F. is a subjective phenomenon, thus the limitation of questionnaires. The same criteria apply to the L.A.F. picture or visual analogue.

The strength of the S-EMG modality in the investigative mode is that it measures the consistency of effort of any muscular activity, be it normal or related to dysfunction. If the amplitude of the contraction pattern is abnormal related to L.A.F., it will remain so as an autonomous factor. The limitation of the S-EMG modality is that it cannot measure the L.A.F. level (Kumar & Mital, 1996). S-EMG can be utilized concomitantly with dynamometry, goniometry, or other modalities described above (Sella & Donaldson, 1998). Thus, one can investigate L.A.F. of soft tissue injury with several modalities and counter the limitations of one with the strength of another.

RADIATION OF SYMPTOMS AND DYSFUNCTION TO THE CONTRALATERAL SIDE OF THE INJURY SITE

Acute soft tissue injury is often followed by loss of adequate function of the injured muscle or myotatic unit (Anchor & Felicetti, 1999). The contralateral and related sites are called into action. The general pattern and process as known as "protective guarding." It is important to note that the protective guarding has an immediate positive and beneficial effect of sparing the injured site.

A problem ensues if the injured site does not get immediate investigative and rehabilitative attention. In the latter case, protective guarding regresses from functional benefit to a dysfunctional process. Only symptoms and dysfunctions involving the contralateral side of the injury site muscles and fascia are discussed in this chapter.

The contralateral side is overworked, and muscular effort and imbalance are reflected shortly by the symptom of fatigue. Eventually, there may be functional loss of strength and even joint inflammation. The muscles and the fascia may develop primary or secondary myofascitis (Busquet, 1998; Cailliet, 1988a; 1992a; Travell & Simmons, 1983).

If the initial dysfunction related to protective guarding and indirect radiation of symptoms is not resolved properly during investigation and treatment, it may result in the development of chronic pain and further dysfunction. It is likely that for muscular function, an engram change exists, with the engram of the contralateral side becoming dysfunctional. Therefore, in addition to the investigation and treatment of the various symptoms such as described above, there is need for S-EMG biofeedback (neuromuscular reeducation) to redress the chronic functional disequilibrium.

The assessment of the symptom radiation to the contralateral side may be performed using the components described above. However, since function is very variable in different individuals, there may be an additional need for testing for pain, loss of range of motion, or loss of strength. Functional testing needs to follow the same procedural and statistical principles described above.

For consistency, it is important to perform any test as many times as possible and measure the internal consistency of the evaluee's or patient's performance. For repeatability, any methodology or diversity of methodologies utilized should show a good measure of repeatability in terms of symptoms radiation assessment or reduction.

Normative values or databases of objective measurements of contralateral loss of function related to soft tissue injury are not available because of the diversity of such losses. Nonetheless, the clinician needs to be on guard for consistency of performance or lack of performance of individual functional activities, e.g., typing at a computer.

When the specificity, sensitivity and predictive values of any contralateral investigative methodology are known, the clinical results may be comparable to such data. The functional utilization of any contralateral investigative methodology is only as good as the results obtained in relation to it. Therefore, the clinician may want to describe the validity of the application of the contralateral investigative tool in terms of the results obtained from the knowledge of the treatment.

Because it is necessary to evaluate treatment results before, during, and after treatment, any methodology for contralateral radiation of symptoms/signs and investigation/treatment needs to be an objective and numerical overall outcome measurement.

The following methodologies for soft tissue contralateral radiation measurement are considered:

Questionnaires of Contralateral Symptom Radiation

No soft tissue injury symptoms radiation to the contralateral side questionnaires exists. Therefore, the clinician needs to use the model of questionnaires utilized for L. ROM and L.O.S., and modify such a model for each individual case of contralateral radiation/loss of function. Any such questionnaire utilization in soft tissue injury evaluation may have to be validated according to the statistical and functional criteria described above.

The Contralateral Symptoms Radiation Visual Analogue

This is a visual format which allows the patient/evaluee to describe on a line or graph the intensity and/or frequency of contralateral symptoms radiation. It also may describe graphically the type of symptoms of soft tissue injury perceived. The visual analogue may be formatted on a ___/10 scale where 10/10 represents the highest degree of contralateral dysfunction/radiation perceived in intensity/frequency and 0/10 represents a complete lack of such dysfunction before or after treatment. The visual analogue is easy to perform and takes very little time to accomplish. In terms of the parameters described above for other symptoms questionnaires, the application is rather similar for the visual analogue testing for soft tissue injury radiation to the contralateral side.

Objective Tests

A number of objective tests such as dynamometry, goniometry, etc. may be applicable from case to case of functional activity losses. No example can be given because each loss of function may include different components.

S-EMG

This technology is probably the only soft tissue injury methodology applicable to most, if not all, losses of functional activity related to symptom/signs radiation to the contralateral side. The parameters of utilization during investigation and treatment have been described above.

Objective Treatment Outcome Measurement

Objective treatment refers to numerical modalities involved in the rehabilitation process of radiation of symptoms to the contralateral side. Such modalities are usually multiple. The objective outcome could be a linear follow-up of the dysfunction level at the beginning of the treatment, at each visit, and at the end of the treatment period. For instance, the initial soft tissue injury contralateral dysfunction intensity level may be 9/10, in time it may show a decrease to 7/10, 5/10, and eventually reach 1/10 at the end of the treatment period. The main thing is to demonstrate a framework of measurement of the dysfunctional level which is consistent and numerical and spans the beginning to the end of the treatment period.

RELATIVE EARLY OR LATE DEVELOPMENT OF MYOFASCIAL PAIN SYNDROME EXEMPLIFIED BY TRIGGER POINTS

Myofascitis, exemplified by the presence of trigger points and associated pain and dysfunction usually develops early in the chronology of soft tissue injury (Anchor &

Felicetti, 1999). The symptoms are usually a combination of the following:

1. The presence of exquisitely tender trigger points with or without radiation
2. The presence of tenderness on the involved muscle
3. The presence of loss of strength, time dependent on the same muscle
4. The eventual functional shortening of the affected muscle and possibly of the primary myotatic unit followed by loss of strength of the subtended joint(s)
5. The presence of pain that may become chronic and dysfunctional in itself
6. The radiation to the contralateral side with possible dysfunction in terms of secondary development of trigger points and myofascitis to that region
7. Development of symptoms in the radiation area

Radiation of myofascial dysfunction to the contralateral side is usually referred to as a late development in the chronology of myofascitis. It is important for the clinician to understand whether a muscle affected by trigger points is a primary muscle or a secondary muscle. In terms of treatment, a muscle which has secondary myofascial involvement needs treatment not only for itself, but also for the contralateral muscle/myotatic unit that was originally affected by the soft tissue injury.

The questionnaires and investigative modalities described above are valid within the framework of the symptoms/signs which develop and present themselves in primary or secondary myofascitis. The objective identification of a reduction of symptoms/signs needs to follow the same numerical pattern described above for each major soft tissue injury.

LATE DEVELOPMENT OF MUSCULAR HYPOTROPHY/ATROPHY AND RELATIVE SHORTENING

Muscular hypotrophy has to be identified as resulting from structural or functional etiologies (AMA, 1993; Sella, 1995). The clinician needs to rule out neurological pathology from myofascial dysfunction. This presentation does not involve muscular or fascial diseases such as genetic, metabolic, endocrine or toxic myopathies, and related conditions.

The hypotrophy related to untreated myofascial conditions is a functional one, in the sense that the muscle may regain its normal size as the rehabilitative treatment progresses (Bousquet, 1998; Calilliet, 1992a). A finding of muscular hypotrophy and functional shortening is clinically a sign of lack of appropriate treatment for at least 2 months after the original injury event.

Muscular hypotrophy can be investigated with circumferential measurements (AMA, 1993). The limitation of this technique is that it measures the whole myotatic unit of the muscle, i.e., for biceps brachii hypotrophy, the circumferential measurement also assesses the other arm muscles such as the triceps, brachialis, and brachioradialis.

Nonetheless, this is an objective technique. As such it can be utilized within the statistical framework described above. Muscular shortening of functional origin may produce pain with motion and functional loss of joint ROM. These features can be investigated with the means discussed earlier.

S-EMG testing of the hypotrophic/shortened muscle can be done within the framework of the S-EMG ROM protocols. A hypotrophic muscle usually shows loss of strength and increased amplitude of contraction (μV RMS). Therefore, the S-EMG statistical techniques and the dynamometric statistical techniques are valid within this context.

In terms of treatment, physical therapy aimed at muscular agility, strengthening, and endurance in conjunction with S-EMG neuromuscular rehabilitation helps redress the hypotrophy/shortening of the dysfunctional muscles, even if applied late in the history of the pathologic event. The same statistical criteria for objectively follow-up of the treatment results described above apply within this context.

SOFT TISSUE INJURY: IMPAIRMENT MEASUREMENT

If there is a forensic or medicolegal issue with the etiology and post-treatment results of soft tissue injury, the clinician may be asked to perform an impairment evaluation. The clinician needs special training for this task. On the assumption that one can perform such an evaluation, the following parameters are paramount to the granting of any impairment-related percentage:

1. The affected part or system must have attained the state of "maximal medical improvement" (AMA, 1993; Sella & Donaldson, 1998). This means that the intensity/frequency/quality of any present symptom/sign must have a rather constant value within at least 6 months prior to the evaluation, and presumably stay within the same range for the foreseeable 24 months. This excludes, of course, terminal events such as amputations or other surgeries which preclude return to the *status quo ante* function without the help of prostheses, etc.
2. The impairment needs to be considered within medical technology knowledge to be permanent rather than temporary in nature (AMA, 1993). A temporary impairment cannot be granted the

status of permanency as with a given degree of permanent disability.

3. The examinee needs to use approved impairment percentages granted according to legal criteria, which may apply differently from state to state. The degree of impairment may be granted according to the consensus process and utilization of the *AMA Guides* or other criteria texts (AMA, 1993), as may be found in the Social Security, Workers' Compensation, or federal guidelines, legislative rules, etc.

4. All permanent percentages depend on an objective evaluation process with the statistical input described above.

SUMMARY

This chapter described criteria for the objective evaluation of parameters of dysfunction related to soft tissue injury and tissue response. The methodologies described may be utilized in a specific or focused manner as they pertain to specific dysfunctions. For instance, dynamometry may be appropriate in strength testing. Utilizing the strengths of different methodologies to counter the limitations of others is part of the arsenal of diagnostic investigation and follow-up through rehabilitation.

REFERENCES

AMA. (1993). *AMA guides to evaluation of permanent impairment* (4th ed.). Chicago: American Medical Association.

Anchor, K., & Felicetti, T.C. (Eds.) (1999). *Disability analysis in practice* (chap. 15, pp. 279–314). Dubuque, Iowa: Kendall/Hunt Publishing Co.

Basmajian, J.V. & DeLuca, C.J. (1985). *Muscles alive, their functions revealed by electromyography* (5th ed.). Baltimore: Williams & Wilkins.

Busquet., L. (1998). *Les chaines musculaires* (Tomes I, II, III, IV). Paris: Frison Roche.

Cailliet, R. (1988a). *Low back pain syndrome*. Rene Cailliet Pain Series, Edition 4, Philadelphia: Davis Co,

Cailliet, R. (1988b). *Soft tissue pain and disability*. Rene Cailliet Pain Series, Edition 2. Philadelphia: Davis Co.

Cailliet, R. (1991a). *Neck and arm pain*. Rene Cailliet Pain Series, Edition 3. Philadelphia: Davis Co.

Cailliet, R. (1991b). *Shoulder pain*. Rene Cailliet Pain Series, Edition 3. Philadelphia: Davis Co.

Cailliet, R. (1992a). *Head and face pain syndromes*. Rene Cailliet Pain Series, Edition 1. Philadelphia: Davis Co.

Cailliet, R. (1992b). *Knee pain and disability*. Rene Cailliet Pain Series, Edition 3. Philadelphia: Davis Co.

Cailliet, R. (1993). *Pain: Mechanism and management*. Rene Cailliet Pain Series, Philadelphia: Davis Co.

Cailliet, R. (1994). *Hand pain and impairment*. Rene Cailliet Pain Series, Edition 4. Philadelphia: Davis Co.

Fischer, A.A. (1977a). New developments in diagnosis of myofascial pain and fibromyalgia. *Physical Medicine and Rehabilitation Clinics of North America, 8,* 1–21.

Fischer, A.A. (1977b). New approaches in treatment of myofascial pain. *Physical Medicin and Rehabilitation Clinics of North America, 8,* 153–169.

Fischer, A.A. (1984). Diagnosis and management of chronic pain in physical medicine and rehabilitation. In A.P. Ruskin (Ed.). *Current therapy in physiatry* (pp. 123–145). Philadelphia: W.B. Saunders.

Fischer, A.A. (1987a). Pressure algometry over normal muscles. Standard values, validity and reproducibility of pressure threshold. *Pain, 30,* 115–126.

Fischer, A.A. (1987b). Pressure threshold measurement for diagnosis of myofascial pain and evaluation of treatment results. *Clinical Journal of Pain, 2,* 207–214.

Fischer, A.A. (1987c). Muscle tone in normal persons measured by tissue compliance. *Journal of Neurological and Orthopaedic Medicine and Surgery, 8,* 227–233.

Fischer, A.A. (1990). Application of pressure algometry in manual medicine. *Journal of Manual Medicine, 5,* 145–150.

Fischer, A.A. (Summer, 1994). Quantitative and objective documentation of soft tissue abnormalities: Pressure algometry and tissue compliance recording. *Spinal Manipulation,* 1–4.

Fischer, A.A. (1997). Clinical use of tissue compliance meter for documentation of soft tissue pathology. *Clinical Journal of Pain, 3,* 23–30.

Fischer, A.A., & Chang, C.H. (1985). Electromyographic evidence of paraspinal muscle spasm during sleep in patients with low back pain. *Clinical Journal of Pain, 27,* 203–210.

Galen, R.S. (1979). Selection of appropriate laboratory tests. In D.S. Young, et al. (Eds.). *Clinician and Chemist: The Relationship of the Laboratory to the Physician.* Washington, D.C.: Association for Clinical Chemistry.

Gerhardt, J.J. (1992). *Documentation of joint motion* (rev. 3rd ed.). Portland, OR: Oregon Medical Association.

Kumar, S., & Mital, A. (1996). *Electromyography in ergonomics.* Toronto: Taylor & Francis.

Liu, S., Kopacz, D.J., & Carpenter, R.L. (1995). Quantitative assessment of differential sensory nerve block after lidocaine spinal anesthesia. *Anesthesiology, 82*(1), 60–63.

Maigne, R. (1996). *Diagnosis and treatment of pain of vertebral origin.* Baltimore: Williams & Wilkins.

Masson, E.A., & Boulton, A.J.M. (1991). The neurometer: Validation and comparison with conventional tests for diabetic neuropathy. *Diabetic Medicine, 8,* S63–S66.

Melzack, R. (1975). The McGill pain questionnaire: Major properties and scoring methods. *Pain, 1,* 277–299.

Melzack, R. (1987). The short form McGill pain questionnaire. *Pain, 30,* 191–197.

Pope, M., Anderson, G., Frymoyer, J., & Chaffin, D. (Eds.). (1991). *Occupational low back pain. Assessment, treatment and prevention.* St. Louis: Mosby Year Book.

Sella, G.E. (1993). *Muscles in motion: The S-EMG of the range of motion of the human body.* Martins Ferry, OH: GENMED Publishing.

Sella, G.E. (1995). *Neuromuscular testing with S-EMG.* Martins Ferry, OH: GENMED Publishing,

Sella, G.E. (1997). Daubert and new technologies: An independent medical examiner's view (Parts 1 & 2). *Forensic Examiner, The Official Journal of the American College of Forensic Examiners, 6*(8), 5–8.

Sella, G.E. (1998a). The utilization of S-EMG in neuromuscular rehabilitation, Proceedings 9th European Congress of Clinical Neurophysiology, Ljubljana, Slovenia, June 4–7, pp. 357–359.

Sella, G.E. (1998b). S-EMG Utilization in low back pain investigation and rehabilitation. *Kinesitherapie Scientifique, 383,* 35.

Sella, G.E. (2000a). *Muscular dynamics: Electromyographic assessment of energy and motion.* Martins Ferry, OH: GENMED Publishing,

Sella, G.E. (2000b). *Graphics of motion: The electromyography of muscular dynamics.* Martins Ferry, OH: GENMED Publishing.

Sella, G.E. (2000c). Internal consistency, reproducibility & reliability of S-EMG testing. *Europa Medicophysica, 36,* 1, 31–38.

Sella, G.E. (2000d). *Guidelines for neuro-muscular reeducation: The electromyographic approach.* Martins Ferry, OH: GENMED Publishing,

Sella, G.E., & Donaldson, C.C.S. (1998). *Soft tissue injury evaluation: Forensic criteria: A practical manual.* Martins Ferry, OH: GENMED Publishing,

Travell, J., & Simons, D. (1983). *Myofascial pain and dysfunction: A trigger point manual* (Vol. I & II). Baltimore: Williams & Wilkins.

85

From Psychics of the Body to Clinical Outcome via Neurochemistry

Gary W. Jay, M.D., F.A.A.P.M., D.A.A.P.M.

The title of this chapter was given to me. At first I didn't like it: "Psychics of the body"? Then I realized that this is, more times than we'd like to think and far more frequently than we would like to admit, an accurate description of what may pass for medicine, particularly pain management.

Looking at the way we were trained, anatomically biased for the most part, we have become a group of physicians who think we know what is going on when seeing a patient purely on the basis of where the pain is located. The differential diagnosis then becomes a matter of which nerves connect to which nerves and the spinal cord, and then the brain, and how we can stop the pain from peripheral nervous system response to injury.

We have begun to develop a significant armamentarium in our treatment options. Almost always, it begins with analgesics. Good primary care physicians recognize that they need to ameliorate a patient's pain. That is what they were trained to do. So, unless there are reasons for doing any tests, the vast majority of which look at anatomy (plain X-rays, CAT scans, MRI scans), analgesic medications are utilized.

Then there are the pain management specialists who are trained to do blocks. They do them very well. Unfortunately, some are satisfied in knowing that a patient's pain is in his or her neck. Like any carpenter with a hammer, everything is a nail. The patient, therefore, will undergo a series of epidural blocks. If these don't stop the patient's pain, he or she is trundled off to another type of specialist, frequently a psychiatrist or psychologist.

When I began to practice pain management in 1980, interdisciplinary pain management programs were coming into their own. Patient outcomes were good. Over the last 2 decades, the business people controlling the application of medicine, good or bad, realized that while these types of patient treatment programs did work, they were expensive. So, getting reimbursed for applying inter- or transdisciplinary pain treatment was lost, because of monetary interests rather than patient care interests.

Anatomical, mechanistic algorithms were developed and placed into the practice setting. Physicians didn't need to be told what they could or couldn't do. They were just stymied by their inability to receive payment for services that the insurers didn't feel like reimbursing. Some insurers went even further, independent of medical realities, determining which disorders were, to them, real, and which ones were not. Those that insurers did not want to recognize as real were *a priori* not real and medical treatment for them did not justify reimbursement.

Today business people who are involved in running pain centers ask, "You tell me that psychological or psychiatric input is necessary in the treatment of chronic pain patients. Well, how come I can't find any multidisciplinary pain centers that have psychologists in them?"

Unfortunately, they are correct.

Some of these folk have looked at the nonmedical realities and determined that a real interdisciplinary pain center now consists of a physician and a physical therapist. Why? Both can receive reimbursement, however poor it may be.

0-8493-0926-3/02/$0.00+$1.50
© 2002 by CRC Press LLC

A lot of psychologists are driving cabs, it seems.

So, where does that leave us? It seems to this author that it leaves us with four choices. First, pain management specialists should band together for the sake of their patients and fight this administrative determination of "appropriate care" of chronic pain patients. This needs to be done locally, regionally, and nationally, at the various levels of the insurance companies, the HMOs, the PPOs, and, of course, in Washington. However, until three physicians in a room can come to a single consensus, this probably won't happen. More importantly, if an insurance company doesn't want something to be done, it has the clout (read: Money) to not only assure that it doesn't get done, but also to destroy those physicians who care enough about their patients to persistently try to do it.

Second, we can meekly continue to do things the way they are now. Incredibly intelligent pain management physicians are losing their livelihoods as well as their self-respect because they can't band together effectively to enable the best patient care to be used. The national physician organizations appear to be too mired in their own internal politics to help.

Third, we can do our best to teach the patients, the folks who have lost their ability to receive the care they need and deserve, and enlist their help in trying to change the way things are. Unfortunately, if the layperson isn't sick, he or she seems to find no reason to fight for something not needed. At least not yet.

Finally, we, as physicians, can make the best of what we have left to use to help our pain patients. Anatomical, mechanistic treatments are going to have to take second place to a better understanding of neurochemistry: the physiology and the pathophysiology of the "software" of both the peripheral and the central nervous systems.

As the insurance companies, HMOs, and PPOs have determined, it costs only 1.2 cents for a generic acetaminophen and codeine tablet. Cheap enough to allow hundreds and thousands to be prescribed. This makes some sense to them, as an hour of hands-on physical therapy costs far more. In their minds, stopping the pain is fine, and drugs, especially inexpensive ones, are good ways to do this.

As pain management physicians, we should be the most knowledgeable regarding the pathophysiology of neurotransmitter systems in the brain, and how to use this information for the betterment of our patients.

However, looking at the original premise of how we were taught, we tend to look at the anatomy first. Patient Jones is in a motor vehicle accident. His spleen is ruptured; this is verified by a CAT scan, so we surgically remove it. His arm is broken. Radiographic studies show us the break. Orthopedists are called in and the appropriate treatment is performed. Mr. Jones' headaches secondary to the acceleration/deceleration, or whiplash injury he received, are treated with NSAIDS. He is out of the hospital in a week. Medical rechecks with his orthopedist

reveal that his broken arm is healing well. His general surgeon is happy with the way the abdominal wounds from surgery have healed. His primary care physician gives him more medication, "mild" opiates, for his continued complaints of headache.

Six months later, Mr. Jones is complaining about continued headache as well as pain in the abdomen around the scar tissue and continued pain in the arm.

Tests are done; CAT scans, MRI scans, blood work, all are normal. Mr. Jones is now a chronic pain patient, with no anatomical or mechanistic explanations of any of his pain complaints.

The initial injuries were clear, "exact" problems with ramifications directly to the periphery. Pain from Mr. Jones' injuries was transmitted via the peripheral nervous system to the spinal cord and then to the central nervous system via neuroanatomic pathways that are understood: Pain, via C- and A-delta fibers, comes into the spinal cord dorsal horns, some decussate and travel rostrally via the spinothalamic tract, among other pathways. The question, 6 months later, is simply put: Mr. Jones' arm is healed, he had no complications from surgery for his ruptured spleen, and no anatomical lesions exist in the cervical spine. Yet, he still has pain.

The peripheral nervous system has no reason to be ringing the pain bell, no reasons for nociception to be continuing.

Many physicians stop there in their analysis and begun to look for secondary gain issues or other motivations for Mr. Jones to have pain. Does he like his narcotics too much? Does he want to stay home and not return to work?

The obvious fact is that peripheral mechanisms of pain may affect central mechanisms. These central mechanisms may essentially take on a nociceptive life of their own. At this point, treating the peripheral end organ does not help the pain, as the pain is now central in nature, with continuous central nervous system input that is no longer a function of the first initiating peripheral mechanisms.

Most commonly, the surgeon looks at Mr. Jones' belly and can't find a reason for the pain. The orthopedist cannot find a reason for continued arm pain, which is now associated with edema, hyperesthesia, and even allodynia. The primary care physician cannot find a reason for Mr. Jones' headache, except possibly some minimal spasm in the cervical paravertebral muscles and the bilateral trapezius musculature.

In general, physicians tend to look for the primary anatomical reasons for pain, acute or chronic. When they are not found, the ability to give further aid is uncertain.

The pain is a pathophysiological problem that cannot be found on examination. Windup phenomena, whereby continuous C-fiber stimulation of the wide dynamic range neurons in the spinal cord, which turns these "on-off" cells on, full time, cannot be anatomically located via any standard testing. Pain derived from the sympathetic nervous system secondary to such a physiological problem cannot be seen with any anatomical test currently used.

There are no blood tests for pain, nor are any other anatomic, mechanistic tests of chronic benign pain feasible at this time. Greater levels of information must be obtained and used by the pain management specialist. Before one can utilize a test for selective tissue conductance (sudomotor, or sweat testing), the physician must have determined a basis for looking.

Pathological changes of the central nervous system do exist in patients with chronic pain if it is of neuropathic or sympathetic origin. Neuroma formation, deafferentation, Wallerian degeneration do occur, with cell death in the periphery as well as the spinal cord. Gliosis following such neuronal cell death has been found on autopsy to occur in the spinal cord, as well as in the thalamus. However, there are no tests available to the clinician that show this.

When pain becomes centralized, techniques must be used to deal with aberrant, dysmodulated neurotransmitter systems. Anticonvulsant medications which function by increasing inhibitory neurotransmitter functions (such as gabapentin working to increase GABA, gamma aminobutyric acid, an inhibitory neurotransmitter; or clonazepam, which increases GABA in the internuncial neurons of the spinal cord) become very useful, despite the fact that no seizures are occurring.

However, one must know the pathophysiology of the problem on a neurochemical level to knowing what medications to use, and why.

Unfortunately, again, some clinicians treat by rote. They have read in a journal that gabapentin helped, anecdotally, several patients with reflex sympathetic dystrophy/complex regional pain syndrome-I and so they use it at the dosages that they read were used. I think this is bad only insofar as the clinicians are doing something that they have read about to help a patient without fully understanding the pathophysiological problem they are attempting to treat, or more importantly, why it may help.

Of course, with so much to read and so many specialties and subspecialties to read it for, I certainly would not expect all physicians who use gabapentin (again, only an example) to have such a deep understanding of its neuropharmacology. But, this is an area that the pain specialist should be accountable for learning; in reality, any and all pain specialists who are responsible for the diagnosis and treatment of chronic pain should be highly conversant with this information.

This is an area of extreme import, a place where we, as pain specialists, can and should excel.

Turning to Mr. Jones' headaches, the applied treatment has been analgesics, starting with simple analgesics and then climbing the WHO (World Health Organization) ladder to narcotics. This is a simplistic, knee jerk response to the complaint of pain, in this case, chronic headache.

The pathophysiology of chronic (posttraumatic) tension-type headache has been described in detail in another chapter in this volume. To summarize: initial myofascial nociception secondary to the acceleration/deceleration injury will, if not treated appropriately in the first 2 to 6 weeks postinjury (via physical therapy, NSAIDS, and for some patients a muscle relaxant) will develop into a myofascial pain syndrome, with continuous nociceptive information going to the cervical aspects of the trigeminal nucleus and then rostrally. Continued nociception will induce changes in the serotonergic system via loss of metabolic ability to maintain homeostasis and the development of "empty neurons" as well as serotonergic receptor hypersensitivity. Affective disorders secondary to these same neurochemical changes of the serotonergic, noradrenergic, and endogenous opiate systems occur. The primary locus of pain from chronic tension-type headache then becomes central, secondary to dysmodulation of such neurotransmitter systems, while the initiating peripheral mechanisms become secondary.

At this point, physical therapy will be palliative, as the pain problem is central, not peripheral.

To treat this entity one must return the central neurotransmitter systems to a homeostatic norm. Treatment should thus be geared to this goal. The use of neuropharmacological entities that can do this is mandatory. Serotonergics and GABAnergic medications, possibly with others, are necessary. The use of other types of medications such as the alpha-II agonist tizanidine, which acts as a muscle relaxant and also works to diminish muscle pain via noradrenergic system manipulation, also may be effective, but only if used by physicians who recognize the problem for what it is and utilize neuropharmacological manipulations that can appropriately affect central neurotransmitter systems.

All that stated, the clinician must remember that while trying to return the dysmodulated central neurotransmitter systems to normal pharmacologically, the associated sleep disorder must be dealt with (again, serotonergically), along with physical therapy to stop any further continuation of peripheral nociception, and psychological care, to prevent the affective problems of depression and/or anxiety (both with a neurochemical basis) from persisting and, therefore, preventing the return of central neurotransmitter system(s) homeostasis.

Then there is the issue of chronic analgesic usage. This problem creates a separate headache entity, analgesic rebound headache. The continuous use of analgesics, narcotic or not, will further depress the innate, endogenous opiate system via a negative feedback loop. Until this headache form, which is purely neurochemical/neurophysiological in nature, is dealt with by stopping all exogenous analgesics in a safe, physiological manner, no other form of treatment for any of the headache problems Mr. Jones is enduring will be effective.

Finally, there is the continued abdominal pain that is bothering Mr. Jones. His pain is described as lancinating, with electrical-like jolts. These pain attributes speak for neuropathic pain, most commonly from the cutting of sensory nerves during the surgery. These nerves may develop neuromas, with ectopic electrogenesis inducing continuous nociceptive information. This continuous afferent nociceptive stimulation can induce central changes, first at the level of the spinal cord, and later in the brain.

Once again, the clinician is forced to think about central neurochemical changes as well as, at least initially, peripheral changes. The use of tricyclic antidepressant (TCA) medications to help with the nerve-generated (neuropathic) pain may work both centrally as well as peripherally, with the TCAs also acting as local anesthetics at the site of nerve injury/ectopic electrogenesis and/or via the peripheral sodium pumps. Anticonvulsant medications also may work both centrally and possibly peripherally. Mexiletine Hcl, essentially an oral form of lidocaine, has been used for its ability to diminish abnormal nerve impulses. Again, the use of specific medications for their specific abilities to deal with the specific pathophysiological problems associated with a particular form of pain is appropriate and of extreme import.

The use of narcotics for central and neuropathic pain has been felt only recently to be useful. The logic, over the last several years, is that all pain must be eradicated. This is surely a worthy goal. I have found that narcotics are useful, but only in combination with other appropriate neuropharmacological treatments, specifically to maximize function.

The use of narcotics with N-methyl-D-aspartate (NMDA) receptor antagonists is an area of burgeoning research. To date, none are clinically helpful. Oral dosing of dextromethorphan creates significant side effects. Ketamine, in several forms, is being investigated. These medications are being tested to see if their use will decrease problems with narcotic tolerance as well as possibly allow a lesser dosage of narcotic to be utilized, again, very worthy goals.

Some clinicians are pushing the use of chronic narcotics for chronic benign headache. In my 2 decades of treating thousands of headache patients, I have never had to use this tactic to ameliorate or eradicate chronic headache. However, I was able to utilize an interdisciplinary treatment protocol to effectively treat headache patients. Now, with the inability to be reimbursed for appropriate interdisciplinary treatment of chronic headache patients, this may become the surrogate treatment of choice because fewer and fewer of the appropriate modalities are being reimbursed when used to treat these patients.

We appear to be at some sort of crossroad. Pain is now the "fifth vital sign" in the VA hospital system. JCAHO (Joint Commission on Accreditation of Hospital Organizations) has decided to come out with specific guidelines for the treatment of pain. CARF (Commission on Accreditation of Rehabilitation Facilities) has been doing this for years.

What is most confusing is that the CARF guidelines stress and demand an interdisciplinary treatment team. What I have seen of the JCAHO guidelines echoes this. Some states even tie reimbursement to being CARF accredited. I would certainly think this reasonable, if not for the fact that we clinicians who go the extra mile to achieve such accreditation lose money every time, as we must (and wish to) bring in psychological care, biofeedback for stress reduction, and more, as the guidelines indicate we must.

Yet, the vast majority of insurance companies, HMOs, and PPOs, along with Medicare and Medicaid, will not pay for (reimburse) these services — the same ones we must have to meet accreditation standards.

This all leaves us to do what we can, in spite of the moneyed forces arrayed against us.

We should be gathering information regarding the various treatment modalities, single or multiple, that are used effectively, or not so effectively, for specific pain problems. Clinical outcomes measurement is important and all pain specialists should focus more on this. Evidence-based medicine is important, and will hopefully become more important as time passes. Money saved by pain specialists who use proper treatments and who can document their outcomes, monetarily and from other aspects such as degree of pain relief, degree of functional return, and return to work data, is important information to document. The data may eventually have some impact on the insurers.

Nonfunding of treatment by insurers and employers appears to be bad judgment, as they do not save costs, just put them off into the future, where a patient may need several times the initial amount of capital for care than would have been necessary had it been done appropriately at the onset of the patient's pain problem.

What we as clinicians also can do is work to understand the pathophysiology of chronic pain in enough detail to use the tools, the medications we do have, in the best way possible. This may be, for now at least, the best we can do to help our chronic pain patients. We should be the best at doing it, and have the greatest understanding of the intrinsic reasons for using specific medications to deal with specific CNS neuropharmacological abnormalities.

It is the least, or the most, we can do.

86

Musculoskeletal Ultrasound

John Porter, M.D. and Michael S. Jablon, M.S.T.

BRIEF HISTORY

According to leading radiologist Barry Goldberg, in an article published in the May 1998 issue of *Diagnostic Imaging,* "…in ten years ultrasound will account for more than half of all soft-tissue imaging studies." Ultrasound, which is the first study of choice in obstetrics and cardiology, will become the primary imaging study for all soft-tissue abnormalities, with CT, MR, nuclear medicine, and angiography relegated to a secondary position when, in rare instances, ultrasound cannot provide adequate diagnostic information.

The history of ultrasound dates back to 1912 when Lewis Fry Richardson in England patented two schemes for obstacle avoidance as a response to the sinking of the *Titanic.* The outbreak of World War I in 1914 and the menace of the submarine focused new attention on ultrasound as a way to detect objects underwater.

Since ultrasound's potential value in clinical medicine was first realized in the late 1940s and early 1950s, a slow but steady advance in its use has occurred. This process has been spurred by improvements in technology that have enabled ultrasound systems to obtain increasingly refined anatomical detail and to detect flow in increasingly smaller vessels.

The utilization of ultrasound has progressed to the point at which almost 25% of all imaging studies worldwide are ultrasound exams. The World Health Organization recommends the use of ultrasound after basic X-ray, and not CT or MR, due to wide availability of scanners.

The merits of ultrasonography as a diagnostic study are obvious. It is noninvasive and has no know risk. It can be done quickly, with little discomfort to the patient, and the capacity for bilateral imaging makes comparison with the asymptomatic, contralateral limb possible. In most centers, it is much less expensive than other imaging studies. Disadvantages, such as a learning curve, ease of interpretation, and variable image quality, seem to be diminishing as technology and experience increase.

Ultrasound is the ideal modality for the examination of soft tissue because of its multiplanar and real-time capabilities. Sonography yields anatomic information during active and passive mobilization that is unattainable with other modalities. In addition, synovial and cartilage thickness can be accurately quantitated, providing an objective means of following patients with inflammatory arthritides. Ultrasound examination of deep-seated joints such as the hip and shoulder is especially valuable. Joint effusions, loose bodies, tendonitis, and tendon and muscle ruptures can all be demonstrated sonographically. The noninvasive nature of the examination and lack of ionizing radiation make it very well accepted by patients, especially children.

ULTRASOUND — THE NEW GOLD STANDARD FOR SHOULDERS

In the April 2000 issue of the *Journal of Bone and Joint Surgery,* Sharlene A. Teefey M.D., et al., in an article entitled "Ultrasonography of the Rotator Cuff," concluded that "Ultrasonography was highly accurate for detecting full-thickness rotator cuff tears, characterizing their extent, and visualizing dislocations of the biceps tendon." The article also revealed the results…"Ultrasonography correctly identified all sixty-five full thickness rotator cuff tears (a sensitivity of 100 percent). There were seventeen true-negative and three false-positive ultrasonograms (a specificity of 85 percent). The overall accuracy was 96 percent."

0-8493-0926-3/02/$0.00+$1.50
© 2002 by CRC Press LLC

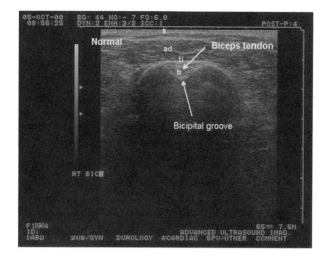

FIGURE 86.1 A normal biceps tendon in a transverse imaging plane. (s) skin surface; (ad) anterior deltoid; (tl) transverse humeral ligament; (b) biceps tendon.

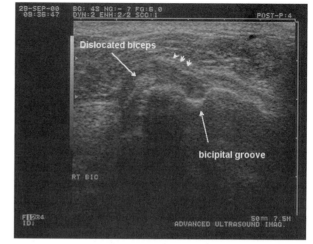

FIGURE 86.2 A complete medial dislocation of the biceps tendon. The transverse humeral ligament (small arrows) appears markedly distended.

MUSCULOSKELETAL ULTRASOUND VS. MRI

BENEFITS OF MRI

MRI use in medicine dates back to the early 1970s, and it has several advantages over diagnostic ultrasound. First, MR images, because of the similarity to actual anatomy, are familiar to both radiologists and referring physicians. Second, MR images can be acquired at distant sites 24 hours a day and interpreted in a timely and cost-efficient manner. Third, MR images provide a comprehensive evaluation of an extremity, including abnormalities of bone, cartilage, and soft tissues. Finally, standard MRI protocols have been systematized to the point that they are mostly operator independent.

BENEFITS OF ULTRASOUND

Sonography, which has been used in medicine for more than 30 years, has a different set of benefits. First, new and continuously improving high-frequency transducers allow detailed visualization of superficial structures. Second, sonography is portable, more available, and less expensive. Third, because sonography works in real time, procedures such as joint aspiration can be guided with sonography once an abnormality is detected. Fourth, because sonography measures motion, a dynamic examination may detect abnormalities that are present only with joint positioning and not obtainable with MRI.

Sonography should be the modality of choice when a tendon abnormality is clinically suspected. It is likely that because of the new high-resolution transducers differentiation between full-thickness and partial-thickness tendon tears can be identified with greater ease than with MRI. In addition, when evaluating the biceps brachii long head tendon for subluxation, the sonogram

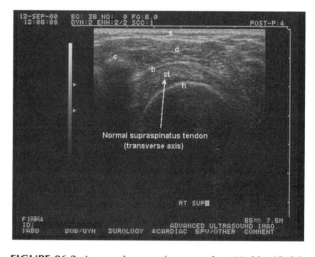

FIGURE 86.3 A normal supraspinatus tendon. (s) skin; (d) deltoid; (c) coracoid process; (b) bursa; (st) supraspinatus tendon; (h) humerus.

allows for evaluation in the neutral position and during external rotation. This view is important as transient medial subluxation of the long head of the biceps brachii tendon may occur only in this position. Because MRI is utilizing static pictures, if transient biceps brachii tendon dislocation is not present in the neutral position it will remain undetected (Jacobson, 1998) (Figures 86.1 and 86.2).

Another abnormality that may be identified better by sonography than by MRI is calcium hydorxyapatite crystal deposition or calcific tendonitis. Because calcifications, like tendons, appear as low signal on MRI images, their intratendonous presence may go unrecognized (Figures 86.3 and 86.4).

The Achilles tendon can be quickly and accurately evaluated. Sonography, like MRI, is useful in demon-

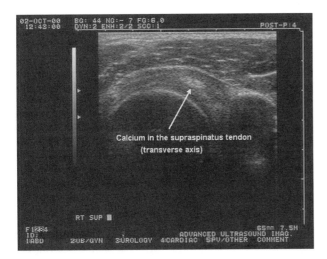

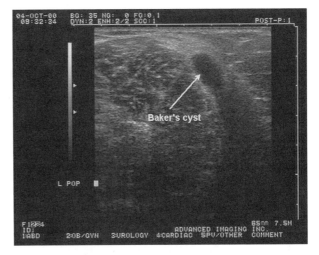

FIGURE 86.4 The area of increased echo signal within the interstitial fibers of the supraspinatus tendon is consistent with calcification (arrow).

FIGURE 86.6 An enlarged gastrocnemius-semimembranosis bursa, consistent with a Baker's cyst.

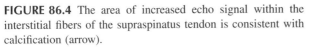

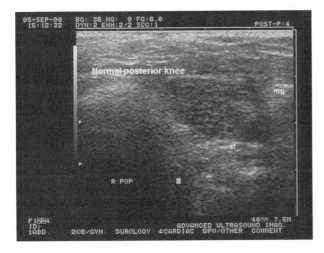

FIGURE 86.5 A normal posteriomedial aspect of the popliteal fossa. (mg) medial head of the gastrocnemius muscle; (st) semimembranosis tendon.

strating full-thickness tendon tear, partial-thickness tear, and tendonitis. High-resolution sonography allows detection of an intact plantaris tendon, difficult at best to identify with MRI imaging. When a full-thickness Achilles tendon tear is identified by sonography, passive plantar flexion is used to determine if the torn tendon ends become approximated. Obtaining similar results with MRI imaging would require patient repositioning and generally is not done. Accurate sonographic information regarding the plantaris tendon and the torn Achilles tendon approximation can assist the surgeon in deciding between surgical and conservative treatment. Cost savings and patient convenience will become major considerations in the near future.

A palpable mass within the medial aspect of the posterior knee suggests the possibility of gastrocnemius-

semimembraneous bursa, or Baker cyst. Sonography can confirm the presence of a cystic mass between the semimembraneous and the medial head of the gastrocnemius tendons. The diagnosis of Baker cyst, however, requires demonstration of a communicating neck between the posterior knee joint and the semimembraneous-medial gastrocnemius cyst. Other cystic masses can essentially be excluded once this communication is identified (Figures 86.5 and 86.6).

For patients with contraindications for MRI sonography is recommended as an alternative imaging method. Potential contraindications for MRI include the presence of certain metal implants or metal foreign bodies, cardiac pacemakers or other implanted electronic devices, pregnancy, and claustrophobia.

GENERAL APPLICATIONS OF SONOGRAPHY

SONOGRAPHY OF MUSCLE

Fifteen years before the development of MRI, ultrasound was the first real time imaging modality available for the evaluation of muscle pathology. Sonography can provide all of the information available with MRI and more with regard to muscle pathology. Its spatial resolution and definition of muscle structure are usually superior to that provided by MRI.

Numerous muscular pathologies can be readily detected with sonography. Small intramuscular lesions, localized inflammation and edema within the tissue (myositis), and detection of intramuscular lesions are readily detected with sonography. Sonography provides the functional capability of evaluating an area in motion; therefore, even the most obscure of intramuscular pathology can be detected. Overstretching (distraction) lesions, which most often occur in runners, ballet dancers, and gymnasts, are also routinely identified with sonography.

SONOGRAPHY OF TENDONS

Prior to the application of ultrasound to the evaluation of the musculoskeletal system, clinicians relied on low-kilo voltage radiography and xeroradiography to aid in the diagnosis of tenomuscular injury (Bock, et al., 1981). These techniques provided little information beyond indicating the site of soft tissue swelling. Ultrasound provides detailed information about the involved anatomy and nature of the pathology.

Chronic tendonitis is easily diagnosed by an experienced musculoskeletal ultrasound sonographer. Frequently an increase in synovial fluid does not exist. The most common finding is thickening of the tendon itself (Middleton, et al., 1985; 1986). Ultrasonic comparisons with the asymptomatic side are essential to make the diagnosis of chronic tendonitis (Bruce et al., 1982; Crass et al., 1984, 1986; Demarais et al., 1984; Dillehay et al., 1984; Blei et al., 1986; Fornage, 1986).

Tendonitis is almost always attributable to chronic trauma and a high level of athletic activity (Roels & Martens, 1978; Feretti, Puddu, & Mariani, et al., 1985). The sonographic findings are identical in all locations. Focal thickening of the tendon and increased distance between the longitudinal collagen fibers are invariably present. Focal hypoechoic areas within the tendon are also present. The longitudinal tendon fibers are seen to be intact. In some patients, tendonitis continues for years with intermittent flare-ups. Calcification is most common at the distal tendon insertion.

TENDON RUPTURE

Rotator cuff tears are a frequent finding in the elderly and may be entirely asymptomatic. Autopsy studies of individuals more than 55 years old have discovered rotator cuff tears in 32% (Peterson & Gentz, 1983). However, a true traumatic tear is a rare finding. These lesions are most common in athletes, such as baseball pitchers, javelin throwers, and football quarterbacks.

The principal sonographic findings (Bretzke, Crass, Craig, 1985; Linnen et al., 1985) are fluid-filled defects in the supraspinatus tendon and increased fluid in the subacromial deltoid bursa. In some chronic cases of rotator cuff tear, the supraspinatus muscle layer may be completely absent (Mack, Matsen, Kolcoyne, et al., 1985). The diameter of the tear measured sonographically is always smaller than that observed with arthroscopy, plain film arthrography, or CT arthrography (Beltran, Gray, Bools, et al., 1986). In all of these invasive diagnostic modalities the joint is distended with fluid, air, or both. This leads to an exaggeration of the dimensions of the tear and the degree of muscle retraction (Ahovuo, Poavolaine, & Slatis, 1984).

Tendon tears can be isolated to the intrasubstance fibers. Often, they will not communicate with the capsule or subacromial deltoid bursa.

These intrasubstance tears cannot be repaired surgically. Sonography demonstrates the full extent of the lesion. This allows the surgeon to prepare most accurately in a pre-operative setting.

Three other disease processes are included in the differential diagnosis of soft tissue lesions of the shoulder. These are biceps tendonitis, biceps tendon dislocation, and edema of the rotator cuff (Jobe & Jobe, 1983).

SONOGRAPHY OF LIGAMENTS

Traumatic injury of ligaments in the knee and ankle are very common, usually involving athletes participating in contact sports. Clinical examination is usually difficult to perform immediately following an injury. Chronic ligamentous injuries and cartilage defects associated with either acute or chronic trauma are difficult to evaluate clinically. Arthroscopy is an excellent tool to evaluate the cruciate ligaments and menisci, but extracapsular ligaments cannot be visualized. Computed tomography (CT) lacks appropriate contrast resolution to delineate ligamentous structures. Ultrasound and magnetic resonance imaging (MRI) are the best diagnostic modalities utilized today for the examination of ligaments. Both of these imaging techniques provide multiplanar capability and demonstrate ligamentous anatomy well (van Holsbeeck & Introcaso, 1991).

The advantages of ultrasound over MRI are ambulatory diagnostic capabilities, along with dynamic examination, cost, and patient compliance. The test also can be performed in the locker room, bedside, or in a physician's office. Often, rapid diagnosis allows for prompt therapy and rehabilitation, thus giving a better diagnosis.

SONOGRAPHY OF BURSAE

The word *bursa* is derived from the Greek, meaning a wine skin. In modern usage, bursa refers to a variety of structures that have several features in common. They are all saclike structures with a lining similar to that found in diarthrodial joints. In addition, they are situated to facilitate movement of musculoskeletal structures (Canoso, 1981). Bursae are found in areas where a significant amount of motion can be expected, yet not necessarily isolated to synovial joints.

The analogy of a wine skin is quite appropriate; both have their greatest dimensions in length and width. This provides a large surface area that occupy little volume under normal circumstances (Codman, 1931). When positioned between two structures, this alignment allows mobility and gliding of one structure on the other.

Some anatomists (Gray, Piersol) believe that bursae are sacs filled with fluid. This is a misconception resulting from studies performed by injecting bursae with various materials.

Physicians who perform bursography and bursocopy often share this misconception because they distend the bursae with contrast material or irrigation fluid. In reality, bursae contain only a thin film of viscous fluid, which serves as a lubricant. The walls are separated by a fluid film approximately 1 mm thick. There fore, bursae are really potential spaces, only becoming fluid-filled sacs under pathological conditions (van Holsbeeck & Introcaso, 1989).

Bursae are divided into two groups, communicating and noncommunicating, depending on their relationship to a joint space. Noncommunicating bursae are more common in humans. Further categorization of bursae may be made based on their location: subcutaneous or deep (Canoso, 1981). Subcutaneous bursae are located between a bone and the overlying skin, such as the pre-patellar and olecranon bursae. Bursae are located in many places deep in the fascia. They separate the joint capsule, tendons, ligaments, and fascial planes (iliotibial tract).

Ultrasound provides the clinician with a noninvasive means of examining the bursae. In acute traumatic bursitis the primary value of sonography is to confirm that disease is limited to the bursa. Associated tendons, ligaments and joint space are easily examined to exclude bursitis secondary to pathology originating in these structures (Figures 86.7 and 86.8).

SONOGRAPHY OF THE SHOULDER

In the 1960s, clinicians called the shoulder the "forgotten joint" (Golding, 1962). There were no diagnostic modalities other than plain radiography for shoulder evaluation. Plain films are normal in more than 90% of patients with chronic shoulder pain. Tendon calcifications are present in some of these patients; others have ossified tendon insertions or cystic lesions around the anatomical neck. The significance of all these plain film findings is still debated in literature (Depalma, 1983; Refior, Krodel, & Melzer, 1987). There is, as yet, no proof of the relationship of these findings to certain types of shoulder disease, such as hydroxyapatite deposition disease, impingement, and rotator cuff disease. More recently, finding ossification in the coracoacromial ligament, acromioclavicular osteoarthritis, and narrowing of the subacromial space have been cited as signs of rotator cuff disease (Peterson and Gentz, 1983; Resnick & Niwayama, 1988; Gielen, van Holsbeeck, Hauglustaine, et al., 1990).

Both arthrography and arthroscopy of the shoulder were introduced during the 1970s. Arthroscopy of the shoulder is, without doubt, the most complete examination of the rotator cuff (Ogilvie Harris & Wiley, 1986). The orthopaedic surgeon examines the articular surface of the rotator cuff through the joint. Then a new incision is made to examine the bursal surface of the cuff through the subacromial deltoid bursa. Not only are rotator cuff tears seen, but tears of the labrum also are visualized. The orthopaedic surgeon has a clear view of the synovial cavity and can, therefore, diagnose synovial disease at an early stage. Arthroscopic surgery may be performed during the same session (Van Holsbeeck & Introcaso, 1989).

A disadvantage of arthroscopy is the invasive character of the procedure. Numerous complications such as neurovascular complications, damage to the labrum, considerable muscle injury, infection, and hemarthrosis have been described (Jeffries, Gainor, & Allen, et al., 1987; Lindenbaum, 1981). Chronic draining fistulas and leaking of synovial fluid are often cited as the most common complications (Henderson & Hoson, 1982).

Not all shoulder pathology is detectable with an arthroscope (Jobe & Jobe, 1983). Rotator cuff lesions communicating with the joint or subacromial-subdeltoid bursa are detected arthroscopically (Refior, Krodel, & Melzer, et al., 1987). Rotator cuff edema and fibrosis, generally regarded as the precursor of a rotator cuff tear, are not an arthroscopic

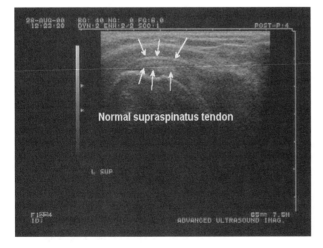

FIGURE 86.7 A normal supaspinatus tendon and overlying SA-SD bursa (arrows).

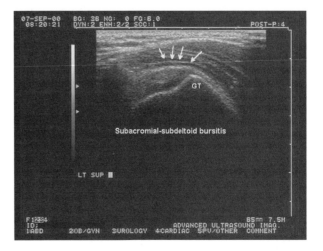

FIGURE 86.8 Inflammation and thickening in the bursa consistent with bursitis.

diagnosis (Neer, 1983). Orthopedic surgeons refer to these abnormalities as impingement syndrome.

Arthrography of the shoulder is less invasive than arthroscopy (Ahovuo, 1984). This procedure identifies full-thickness tears of the rotator cuff and tears involving the articular surface of the supraspinatus tendon. Detection of incomplete tears to the superior surface of the rotator cuff requires injection of the subacromial deltoid bursa (Neer, 1983). This type of tear is less common, and represents less than 5% of all rotator cuff tears. Most of the interventional radiologists, therefore, rarely perform an injection of the subacromial deltoid bursa. Arthrography has not been found to be effective in the evaluation of edema and interstitial defects of the rotator cuff. Like arthroscopy, arthrography is costly, invasive, and usually uncomfortable for the patient.

Impingement is the most common pathology causing chronic shoulder pain (Neer, 1983). It is caused by compression of the anterior cuff against the anterior acromial edge and coracoacromial ligament. The initial developments are edema and hemorrhage, which progress to tendonitis and fibrosis. Partial and full-thickness tears of the rotator cuff are the end stage of the disease spectrum referred to as "impingement syndrome." Unfortunately, no clinical tests exist that will differentiate impingement from rotator cuff disease. The persistence of symptoms may help the clinical diagnosis, depending on the patient's age and history. The majority of patients will experience 10 to 15 years of chronic shoulder pain before impingement progresses to rotator cuff tear.

Treatment for the early stages of impingement syndrome is often drastically different from the treatment for rotator cuff tears. Tendonitis of the rotator cuff is generally treated conservatively for as long as possible. This usually entails avoidance of painful elevation of the arm, anti-inflammatory medication, and injections of anti-inflammatory drugs into the subacromial space. Rotator cuff tears are treated differently. Surgery is usually recommended when large full-thickness tears exist. Early intervention is important before the tear becomes too large, grossly retracted and subsequently nonrepairable (Figures 86.9 to 86.12).

In a patient with impingement syndrome and rotator cuff tendonitis, a conservative, noninvasive approach is optional.

The ideal technique should be readily available for screening a large population with chronic shoulder pain and be able to distinguish tears from edema of the cuff in the majority of cases. Ultrasound is the ideal technique. It is noninvasive and widely available for screening on a large scale (Crass, 1987; Mack et al., 1985). Reported sensitivity is more than 90% (Van Holsbeeck 1991).

WORKUP OF SHOULDER DISEASE

The estimated frequency of rotator cuff tears in people more than 60 years old is approximately 30% (Cofield, 1985).

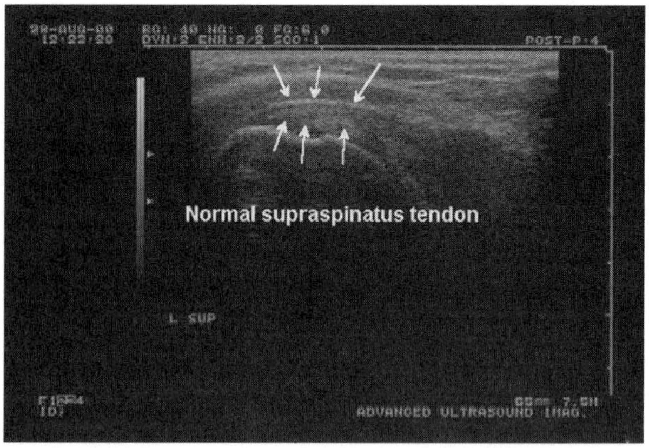

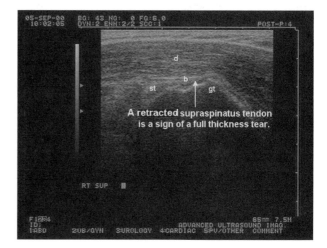

FIGURE 86.9 The normal distal supraspinatus tendon along the greater tuberosity.

FIGURE 86.10 A grossly retracted supraspinatus tendon (st). A complete absence of the supraspinatus tendon is a reliable indicator of a full thickness tear. (d) = deltoid; (b) = bursa; (gt) = greater tuberosity.

With such a large potential group of patients, ultrasound is preferred to more invasive, expensive, and time-consuming techniques, such as arthrography, arthroscopy, and magnetic resonance imaging (MRI). The cost effectiveness of the technique and its noninvasive capability make ultrasound the first choice when evaluating soft tissue injuries.

Every examination of the shoulder should begin with a plain radiograph. The most detailed examination of the bony anatomy is still the conventional radiograph. Substantial narrowing of the subacromial space with an acromiohumeral distance equal to or less than 5 mm is due to large rotator cuff tears. In these cases, no further investigations are necessary (Cofield, 1985). Radiographs also can exclude referred pain to the shoulder due to a lesion in the adjacent structures or a neurovascular syndrome secondary to a Pancoast tumor (Batemen, 1983).

When chronic shoulder symptoms persist and normal plain films and positive clinical test results indicating cuff

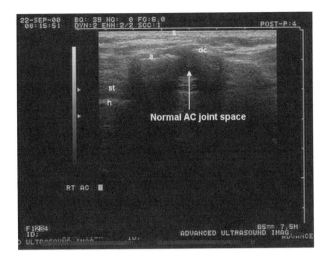

FIGURE 86.11 Coronal view of the AC joint. (a) = acromion; (dc) = distal clavicle; (st) = supraspinatus tendon; (h) = humerus; (s) = skin.

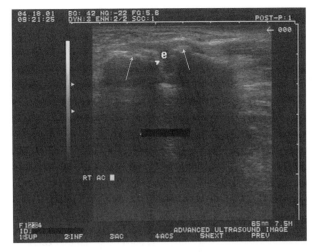

FIGURE 86.12 Degenerative changes involving the acromion process and distal clavicle (arrows). ≤ developing spur is identified (small arrowhead). Effusion is present within the joint (e).

disease exist, ultrasound is the tool of choice for establishing a diagnosis. Arthroscopy should be considered when patients present with normal radiograph and a normal sonogram of the shoulder, but with an unequivocal clinical examination (limited abduction).

SONOGRAPHY OF LARGE SYNOVIAL JOINTS

Large synovial joints are difficult to evaluate clinically; therefore, ultrasound examinations are often requested. Ultrasound is broadening our approach to the evaluation of joint disease. Even the smallest joints can be examined sonographically, i.e., interphalyngeal joints in the hands and feet. Arthroscopy is limited to the intra-articular structures. It allows the orthopaedic surgeon to evaluate the cartilage and perform corrective surgery in the same procedure. However, arthroscopy is an invasive technique with the possibility of risk to the patient.

The main advantage of ultrasound over arthroscopy is its ability to examine the extra-articular soft tissues. Many pain syndromes do not originate in bone or articular cartilage. Until now, these were strictly clinical diagnoses. Sonography can be used to diagnose disease of the extra-articular tissues with high sensitivity and specificity. Sonography can be tendonous, ligamentous, and muscular lesions. It can differentiate scar, granulation tissue, and complete and incomplete tears. In addition, ultrasound is completely non-invasive and requires no anesthesia or pre-medication.

Intra-articular pathology also can be accurately diagnosed utilizing sonography. It can routinely identify intra-articular effusion. In addition, ultrasound can locate synovial inflammation, hemarthrosis, and loose bodies within the joint. Cartilage and synovial thickness can be measured accurately, providing an excellent method to evaluate

the effectiveness of treatment and the progression of disease (Aisen, McCune, McGuire et al., 1984).

In summary, sonography is a valuable diagnostic tool for both extra-articular and intra-articular pathologies. If the intra-articular examination is normal, no additional imaging studies are needed. Abnormal sonographic examination is an indication for evaluation with MRI, arthrography, or arthroscopy.

SONOGRAPHY OF THE ELBOW, WRIST, AND HAND

Clinical examination of the elbow, wrist, and hand is less complex than examination of the shoulder, knee, and hip. These joints are much more accessible due to their superficial nature. Ultrasound is valuable in the diagnosis of muscle, tendon, and ligament pathology, as well as cortical abnormalities, i.e., stress fractures, bone cysts, and arthritis. When radiographic examination is normal, ultrasound is indicated to evaluate persistent pain and swelling.

THE ELBOW

The most common soft tissue disorder of the elbow is epicondylitis. Tendonitis of the common extensor tendons (tennis elbow) and common flexor tendons (golfer's elbow) are often mistaken for intra-articular pathology, due to their close proximity.

Lateral epicondylitis is most frequent in elbow disorders. Biceps and triceps tendonitis also may be mistaken for joint pathology. These problems are best evaluated with ultrasound because calcifications are seen only in chronic disease. At the same time, the examiner also can evaluate for intra-articular loose bodies or cartilaginous defects. Joint effusion is a clear indicator of

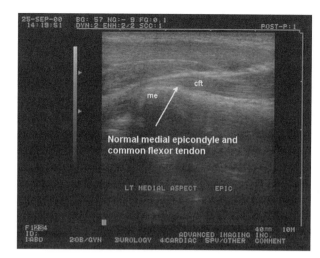

FIGURE 86.13 A normal common flexor tendon insertion (cft) along the medial epicondyle (me).

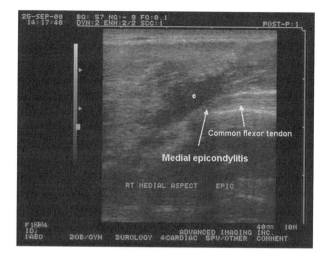

FIGURE 86.14 Inflammation of the common flexor tendon and adjacent soft tissues. Note the large effusion (e).

joint pathology. The most frequently observed joint pathology in the absence of radiographic findings is cartilaginous loose bodies. These loose bodies will be found in the anterior joint recess (Figures 86.13 and 86.14).

THE WRIST AND HAND

The initial indications for ultrasound examination of the wrist and hand are evaluation of tendon disorders and identification of the origin of swelling. Tendon ruptures are easily detected with ultrasound. A motion evaluation helps to identify tendon dislocations and entrapment. Tenosynovitis of the flexor tendons of the wrist and carpal tunnel syndrome are diagnosed easily with ultrasound. Identification of synovial cysts and specification of their origin are easily diagnosed with ultrasound. A cyst arising from a tendon sheath differs from that of a cyst originating from the joint. This can help in surgical management. Often these cysts feel solid during clinical assessment and may be mistaken for boney hypertrophy. The triangular fibrocartilage of the wrist also may be examined.

SONOGRAPHY OF THE KNEE, HIP, AND ANKLE

KNEE

Sonographic examination of the knee is a commonly requested study of the lower extremity. The knee is a bicondylar joint stabilized by soft tissue structures: ligaments, tendons, menisci, and the joint capsule. These structures are all easily injured by trauma, particularly sports-related trauma. Ultrasound is the only readily available nonsurgical technique for the examination of soft tissue injuries at the time the patient presents for clinical evaluation. Normal plain film examination following injury is a definite indication for sonographic examination.

Intra-articular and extra-articular pathologies are equally common causes of knee pain. Pain and swelling of the knee accompanied by a normal radiographic examination are a clear indication for an ultrasound examination. Arthrography and arthroscopy are invasive techniques that evaluate only the intra-articular pathology. Sonography has the capability of demonstrating noninvasively both intra-articular and extra-articular pathologies. Ultrasound can provide information about a joint during a real-time examination. No other diagnostic imaging modality has this capability. In addition, the risk, discomfort, high cost, and delay that may be expected with other diagnostic procedures do not exist.

Tendonitis is a common cause of knee pain. Most frequently involved are the quadriceps, biceps, and patellar tendons. Increased edema and decreased acoustic signal within the involved tendon are visualized. Calcifications often are seen in cases with chronic tendonitis.

Bursitis also may be the cause of knee pain. Traumatic, septic, and hemorrhagic etiologies may cause bursitis. Rupture of Baker's cyst is almost always associated with pain and swelling of the knee, which may extend to involve the entire lower extremity. Ultrasound also is valuable in evaluating ligamentous injuries, synovial cysts, ganglia, muscle tears, aneurysms, and venous thrombosis.

Examination of intra-articular pathology can demonstrate synovial thickening, meniscal tears, articular cartilage defects, loose bodies, and cruciate ligament tears. Several limitations must be kept in mind. Tears of the posterior horn of the meniscus are diagnosed more easily than tears of the mid-body and anterior horn. The only absolute limitation of the intra-articular examination is that the cartilage surface of the patella and tibial plateau cannot be examined due to the lack of an acoustic window. Technical advances, such as new transducers and the further development of transmission ultrasound, will reduce

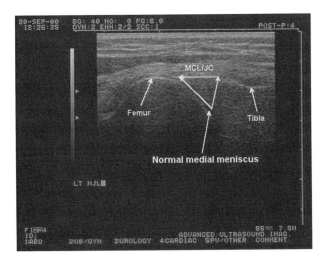

FIGURE 86.15 The normal triangular "wedge" representing the medial meniscus. Note the deep layer of the MCL and joint capsule appears intact (MCL/JC).

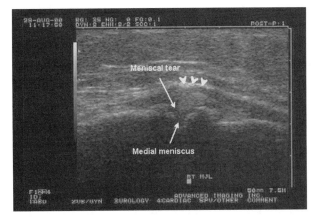

FIGURE 86.16 A torn meniscus with distention of the medial joint capsule along with herniation of the medial meniscus (arrowheads).

or eliminate these limitations. However, a normal sonographic examination demonstrating no effusion indicates that the source of pain lies outside of the joint (Figures 86.15 and 86.16).

HIP

Trauma to the hip results in bony injury almost exclusively. This is due to the protection and stabilization inherent in its ball-in-socket configuration. Often, the trauma is the result of a motor vehicle accident or sports-related injury. Plain radiograph and computed tomography (CT) are the best diagnostic modalities for evaluating these injuries. However, when radiographs and CT are normal, ultrasound examination is an excellent diagnostic tool to consider.

Ultrasound is highly sensitive in the identification of joint effusion. Joint effusions may be seen in infection, inflammatory arthritis, osteonecrosis, trauma, and tumoral diseases.

ANKLE

The most common ankle injury is a sprain/strain. Most frequently, the lateral ligament complex is involved and the anterior talofibular ligament is damaged. The peroneal tendons and medial flexor tendons are beautifully imaged sonographically. These structures usually are completely exposed for sonographic examination. A motion evaluation is recommended to assess integrity and function. Cortical irregularities also can be detected in the ankle, i.e., stress fractures, bone chips, and osteochondral defects. In addition, joint effusions are easily identified. The plantar fascia can be viewed along the medial tubercle of the calcaneus. The normal measurement for this location is 3.5 mm thick. Any inflammatory change increasing the

thickness of the fascia at this location may be indicative for plantar fascitis.

HEMATOMA

Hematoma formation is a hallmark of muscle rupture. The degree of the hematoma is an excellent indicator of the extent of the underlying pathology. Intramuscular hematoma is characterized by blood dissecting within the fascial planes between muscles. More extensive injury will result in formation of intramuscular fluid collections easily identified on ultrasound images.

The evolution and resolution of intramuscular hematoma do not differ from hematoma anywhere in the body. Their initial sonographic appearance is that of a homogenous hypoechoic fluid collection.

HEALING MUSCLE RUPTURE

Ultrasound is an excellent diagnostic tool for the evaluation of the various stages of muscle healing which often can take between 3 to 16 weeks to complete.

The role of sonography in the identification of muscle rupture healing lies in three areas. First is the identification of the extent of injury and measurement of the separation of wound margins. The larger the percentage of muscle tissue involved and the greater the distance of retraction, the larger proportion of scar tissue. This information will help the clinician in determining what steps are necessary, and if any are indicated. Ultrasound-guided aspiration of a hematoma may be desirable at the time of examination to reduce the distraction gap (van Holsbeeck & Intracosa, 1991).

The availability, ease of examination, no contraindications to its use, and low cost relative to MRI make follow-up of healing lesions practical. The majority of patients referred for evaluation of muscle lesions are athletes. Several studies have demonstrated that approximately 30% of all sports injuries are muscular in origin (Peterson & Renstrom, 1986). In these patients the decision of when to return to training or competition is extremely important. Recurrent injury resulting from early resumption of activity can be costly for both the individual athlete and the team. Repeated sonographic examinations can evaluate accurately the stage of healing, significantly decreasing the likelihood of recurrent damage.

Because of the low cost of ultrasound and no contraindications or patient discomfort, sonography can be used repeatedly to evaluate the various stages in muscle healing.

MYOSITIS/MYOSITIS OSSIFICANS

Myositis is a general term used to specify inflammation of muscle. Myositis ossificans, muscular contusion with intramuscular hematoma, may calcify and then ossify. These lesions are frequent findings in athletes involved in contact sports such as rugby or football.

The progression of myositis ossificans is easily followed with ultrasound. Maturation of these lesions takes approximately 5 to 6 months. Initially, within 3 weeks of injury, the lesion is identified as a soft tissue mass with disorganized inhomogeneous internal architecture. At this stage, the lesion is indistinguishable sonographically from a soft tissue neoplasm. Clinicians may refer to this lesion as gleosis, a palpable firm mass within muscle. This term comes from the Latin *gelare,* to freeze.

SONOGRAPHY OF RHEUMATOID DISEASES

Early diagnosis, assessment of inflammation, and detection of complications of rheumatoid disease are problems that can be addressed using ultrasound. The use of noninvasive techniques is especially important in patients with rheumatoid disease. Joint aspiration and arthrography are extremely painful when performed on an inflamed joint. In addition, these procedures are associated with significant risk of infection in this population due to immune suppression from chronic steroid therapy. Arthrography, arthroscopy, and joint aspiration must be kept to an absolute minimum in these patients (Moore, Sarti, & Lovie, et al., 1975).

Over the past 20 years, many noninvasive techniques have been proposed to evaluate cartilaginous involvement of rheumatoid disease. Most recently, magnetic resonance imaging (MRI) and sonography have come to the forefront in the noninvasive evaluation of rheumatoid disease. Given a perfect world scenario, both of these diagnostic studies are equally suitable for the diagnosis and follow-up of rheumatoid disease. Sonography has a major advantage over MRI in that the test can be conducted on the spot. Rheumatoid patients usually cannot tolerate lying motionless on a hard table for the 60 to 90 minutes required for an MRI examination. In addition, during sonographic examination the patient may move other extremities rela-

tively freely, and it does not require sedation. Cost and availability factors also strongly favor ultrasound.

EVALUATION OF FOREIGN BODIES

One of the most frequent requests made of musculoskeletal radiologists in the emergency setting is the identification and localization of foreign bodies. The patient can give an indication of the likelihood of the presence of a foreign body, the material involved, and the general location. However, many of these patients may be children and difficult to evaluate clinically. Barefoot children possess a magnetic attraction to foreign bodies. All inquiries by the physician or parent about the accident are answered with screaming and tears. Another challenge is the evaluation for foreign bodies in patients involved in motor vehicle accidents. Commonly, they are under the influence of alcohol, received intravenous (IV) analgesics, lost consciousness during the accident, or have numerous injuries. Frequently, foreign bodies in these patients go unidentified. Unrecognized foreign bodies will result in chronic draining wounds, abscesses, and persistent pain. Surrounding infection can lead to devitalization of large amounts of tissue, joint destruction, and even limb loss (Gooding, Hardiman, & Sumers, et al., 1987).

In looking for foreign bodies, radiographs alone are not adequate (Gooding, Hardiman, Sumers, et al., 1987; Anderson, Newmeyer, & Kilgore, 1982). A retrospective study of foreign bodies showed that the average time between injury and detection was 7 months; 38% of retained foreign bodies were overlooked on initial examination (Anderson, Newmeyer, & Kilgore, 1982). Nonradiopaque foreign bodies and patients with orthopedic implants pose the greatest challenge. These are the cases in which ultrasound is the most beneficial. In general, the use of ultrasound will increase the rate of success of identifying and localizing foreign bodies by at least 20%.

CONCLUSION

Sonography has demonstrated its cost-effective reliability in the evaluation of numerous musculoskeletal disorders. The techniques are difficult to perform; however, this can be minimized with proper training and standardized technique. The role of sonography in the evaluation of the musculoskeletal system is evolving. As technology continues to improve and experience with this imaging modality increases, sonography will establish itself as the gold standard for the diagnosis of musculoskeletal disorders (Jacobson, 1998).

ACKNOWLEDGMENTS

We would like to thank Marnix van Holsbeeck, M.D., Joseph H. Introcaso, and John Jacobson, M.D. of the

Henry Ford Hospital/University of Michigan's Radiology Department, for their efforts in advancing the global availability of information on the topic of musculoskeletal ultrasound. We have made numerous references to their work and tried to make the appropriate references at all times. For more information from the Henry Ford Hospital/University of Michigan, you may contact its website @ www.med.umich.edu/rad/muscskel/mskus/index.html

REFERENCES

Ahovuo, J., (1984). Single and double contrast arthrography in lesions of the gleohumeral joint. *European Journal of Radiology, 4,* 237–240.

Ahovuo, J., Paavolaine, P., & Slatis, P. (1984).The diagnostic value of arthrography in rotator cuff tears. *Acta Orthopaedica Scandinavica, 55,* 220–223.

Aisen, A.M., McCune, W.J., McGuire, A., et al. (1984). Sonographic evaluation of cartilage of the knee. *Radiology, 153,* 781–784.

Anderson, M.A., Newmeyer, W.L., & Kilgore, E.S. (1982). Diagnosis and treatment of retained foreign bodies in the hand. *American Journal of Surgery, 144,* 63.

Batemen, J.E. (1983). Neurologic painful conditions affecting the shoulder. *Clinical Orthopaedics, 173,* 44–54.

Beltran, J., Gray, L.A., Bools, J.C., et al. (1986). Rotator cuff lesions of the shoulder: Evaluation by direct sagittal CT arthrography. *Radiology, 160,* 161–165.

Blei, C.L., Nirschl, R.P., & Grant, E.G. (1986). Achilles tendon: Ultrasound diagnosis of pathologic conditions. *Radiology, 159,* 765–767.

Bock, E., Cotroneo, A.R., et al. (1981). Xeroradiography of tendomuscular traumatic pathologic conditions of the limbs. *Diagnostic Imaging in Clinical Medical, 50,* 235–248, 89.

Bretzke, L.A., Crass, J.R., Craig, E.V., et al. (1985). Ultrasonography of the rotator cuff: Normal and pathologic anatomy. *Investigative Radiology, 20,* 311–315.

Bruce, B.K., Hale, T.L., & Gilbert, S.K. (1982). Ultrasonograph evaluation for ruptured Achilles tendon. *Journal of the American Pediatric Medical Association, 72,* 15–17.

Canoso, J.J. (1981). Bursae, tendons and ligaments. *Clinics in Rheumatic Diseases, 7,* 189–221.

Codman, E.A. (1931). *The shoulder: Rupture of the supraspinatus tendon and other lesions in or about the subacromial bursa.* Boston: Thomas Todd Co.

Cofield, R.H. (1985). Rotator cuff disease of the shoulder. *Journal of Bone and Joint Surgery (U.S.A.), 67,* 974–979.

Crass, J.R. (1987). Ultrasonography of rotator cuff tears: A review of 400 diagnostic studies (abstract*).* Presented at the American Roentgen Ray Society Annual Meeting, Miami Beach, Fl.

Crass, J.R., Craig, E.V. (1984). Thompson, R.C., et al. Ultrasonography of the rotator cuff: Surgical correlation. *Journal of Clinical Ultrasound, 12,* 487–491.

Demarais, Y., Houles, J.P., Parier, J.H., et al. (1984). Echoscannographie dans les tendinites achilleennes et rotuliennes specialement chez le sportif. *Cinesiologie, 23,* 249–256.

Depalma, A.F. (1983). Biologic aging of the shoulder. In A.F. De Palma (Ed). *Surgery of the shoulder.* Philadelphia: J.B. Lippincott Co.

Dillehay, G.L., Deschler, T., Rogers, L.F., et al. (1984). The ultrasonographic characterization of tendons. *Investigative Radiology, 19,* 338–341.

Feretti, A., Puddu, G., Mariani, P.P., et al. (1985). The natural history of jumper's knee. Patellar or quadriceps tendonitis. *International Orthopaedics, 8,* 239–242.

Fornage, B. (1986). Achilles tendon: U.S. examination. *Radiology, 159,* 759–764.

Gielen, J., van Holsbeeck, M., Hauglustaine, D., et al. (1990). Growing bone cysts in long-term hemodialysis. *Skeletal Radiology, 19,* 43–49.

Goldberg, B. (1997, December). Contrast-enhanced ultrasound to become dominant. Radiology in the 21st century, *Supplement to Diagnostic Imaging.*

Golding, F.C. (1962). The shoulder, the forgotten joint. *British Journal of Radiology, 35*(41), 149–158.

Gooding, G.A.W., Hardiman, T., Sumers, M., et al. (1987). Sonography of the hand and foot in foreign body detection. *Journal of Ultrasound in Medicine, 6,* 441–447.

Henderson, C.E., & Hopson, C.N. (1982). Pneumoscrotum as a complication of arthroscopy. *Journal of Bone and Joint Surgery (U.S.A.), 64,* 1238–1240.

Jacobson, J. (1998, May). Sonography: Ultrasound takes on musculoskeletal MRI. *Diagnostic Imaging,* 49–57.

Jeffries, J.T., Gainor, B.J., Allen, W.C., et al. (1987). Injuries to the popliteal artery as a complication of arthroscopic surgery. *Journal Bone and Joint Surgery (U.S.A.), 69,* 783–785.

Jobe, F.W., & Jobe, C.M. (1983). Painful athletic injuries of the shoulder. *Clinical Orthopaedics, 173,* 117–124.

Jobe, F.W., & Jobe, C.M. (1983). Painful athletic injuries of the shoulder. *Clinical Orthopaedics, 173,* 117–124.

Lindenbaum, B.L. (1981). Complications of knee joint arthroscopy. *Clinical Orthopaedics, 160,* 158.

Mack, L.A. (1988). Sonographic evaluation of the rotator cuff. *Radiology Clinics of North America, 26*(1), 161–177.

Mack, L.A., Matsen, F.A., Kolcoyne, H.F., et al. (1985). U.S. evaluation of the rotator cuff. *Radiology, 157,* 205–209.

Middleton, W.D., Reinus, W.R., Totty, W.G., et al. (1986). Ultrasonic evaluation of the rotator cuff and biceps tendon. *Journal of Bone and Joint Surgery (U.S.A.) 68,* 440–450.

Moore, C.P., Sarti, D.A., & Lovie, S.S. (1975). Ultrasonographic demonstration of popliteal cysts in rheumatoid arthritis: A noninvasive technique. *Arthritis and Rheumatism, 18,* 557–580.

Neer, C.S. (1983). Impingement lesions. *Clinical Orthopaedics, 173,* 70–73.

Ogilvie Harris, D.J., & Wiley, A.M. (1986). Arthroscopic surgery of the shoulder. *Journal of Bone and Joint Surgery (U.S.A.), 68,* 201–207.

Peterson, C.J., & Gentz, C.F. (1983). Ruptures of the supraspinatus tendon. *Clinical Orthopaedics, 174,* 143–148.

Peterson, L., & Renstrom, P. (1986). *Sports injuries.* Chicago: Yearbook Medical Publishers.

Refior, H.F., Krodel, A., & Melzer, C. (1987). Examinations of the pathology of the rotator cuff. *Archives of Orthopaedic and Traumatic Surgery, 106,* 301–308.

Resnick, D., & Niwayama, G. (1988). *Diagnosis of bone and joint disorders* (2nd ed.). Philadelphia: W.B. Saunders.

Roels J., & Martens, M. (1978). Patellar tendonitis (jumper's knee). *American Journal of Sports Medicine, 6,* 362–368.

Teefey, S., Ashhfaq, H., Middleton, W., et al. (2000). Ultrasonography of the rotator cuff. *Journal of Bone and Joint Surgery, 82-A,* 498–504.

van Holsbeeck, M., & Introcaso, J. (1989). Sonography of the postoperative shoulder. *American Journal of Roentgenology,* 152–202.

van Holsbeeck, M., & Introcaso, J.H. (1989). *Musculoskeletal ultrasound.* St. Louis: Mosby Yearbook.

van Holsbeeck, M., & Introcaso, J.H. (1991). *Musculoskeletal ultrasound.* St. Louis: Mosby Yearbook.

87

Minimally Invasive Endoscopic Surgery for the Treatment of Lumbar Discogenic Pain

Anthony T. Yeung, M.D. and John Porter, M.D.

INTRODUCTION

The history of low back pain and sciatica dates back to ancient times. Domenico Cotugno first described "sciatica" in its classic terminology in 1764 and believed that pain was generated by the nerve itself. The big three Vs — Valliex, Virchow, and Von Luschka — introduced the possibility of structure-referred pain (i.e., vertebral, body, disc, or nerve) in the 1800s. With the advent of X-rays 100 years ago, imaging of spinal anatomy allowed correlation of anatomic findings to conditions that explained the origin of low back pain.

The "Dynasty of Disc" began in the 1930s when Mixter and Barr demonstrated that radicular pain was associated with disc herniation (Farlan, 1973). Attempts were made later to minimize the paradoxical effects of invading the spinal canal by utilizing smaller incisions and image magnification. Although the overall result was not altered, minimal invasiveness did reduce the morbidity of traditional approaches.

Each change required a learning curve that initially was more difficult for the surgeon, but ultimately was embraced by surgeons because it was better for the patient. Endoscopic spine surgery continues this trend, but recent experience has revealed a much greater benefit that will ensure and secure the role of endoscopic spine surgery for the diagnosis and treatment of discogenic back pain.

This quantum leap from open decompression (lumbar laminectomy) to micro-decompression with endoscopic spinal surgery finally solved the problem of traumatizing spinal muscle and ligament, destabilizing the spine, and creating epidural and perineural scarring. This rapid advance was further aided by the parallel evolution of radiologic imaging such as CT and MRI.

ENDOSCOPIC SPINE SURGERY: WHAT IS ITS ROLE?

Few physicians question arthroscopic surgery's role in advancing our understanding of knee and shoulder pain and the treatment options arthroscopy affords. Endoscopic spinal surgery is poised to serve the same role (Kirkaldy). Introduced in the United States by Kambin, the procedure has evolved from a nucleotomy and targeted fragmentectomy to a surgical technique with the potential to offer a minimally invasive approach to spinal conditions currently without a viable surgical alternative.

The favorable efficacy of endoscopic lumbar discectomy compared to open discectomy, in a prospective randomized study, was published by Hermantin, Peters, Quartararo and Kambin in 1999. Endoscopic spine surgery, through the selective endoscopic discectomy technique, expands the endoscopic restrictions described in the article and does not exclude difficult cases at L5-S1 or extruded, migrated, recurrent, or sequestrated disc herniations. The technique also provides minimally invasive access to degenerative conditions of the lumbar spine.

0-8493-0926-3/02/$0.00+$1.50
© 2002 by CRC Press LLC

ENDOSCOPIC SPINE SURGERY: THE POSTEROLATERAL APPROACH

The posterolateral approach allows access to spinal structures such as the superior articular process, the pedicle of the superior and inferior vertebra, the traversing and exiting nerve root, and the annulus in the area of the foramen.

A newly developed spinal endoscopy system by Richard Wolf Surgical Instrument Company, the Yeung Endoscopic Spine System (Y.E.S.S.), features a multichannel scope and special access cannulas that allow spinal probing in a conscious patient, diagnostic endoscopy, and "tube surgery" with very little surgical morbidity. This technique revolutionizes the old concept that all disc surgery is really decompressive nerve surgery. It brings in a new era that will allow true "disc surgery" and a more focused surgery at the tissue level such as contracting and sealing annular tears, annular reinforcement, and artificial discs.

The recent introduction of IDET (Intradiscal Electrothermal Annuloplasty) provides another tool for treating patients who suffer from back pain caused by annular tears, but IDET is another nonvisualized technique that will be noted for historical purposes as we now have the ability to do a "visualized IDET" under direct visual control. The history of minimally invasive spine surgery supports the view that a visualized endoscopic procedure will eventually advance a "blind" technique whose success is dependent on very strict inclusion criteria, and its eventual demise through overutilization by less experienced and lesser trained clinicans. The role of IDET may be defined further by data gathered from visual imaging of annular tears and correlating it with our current imaging studies.

TEAM APPROACH

Due to the complexity of back pain, it is important to treat the whole person. The medical team interfaces with the surgical team to obtain the best possible response and outcome for the patient (Yeung, 1999a). With the endoscopic spinal techniques described, the ability to identify the tissue pain generator is available through spinal probing. Furthermore, a multidimensional treatment algorithm can be devised that will lead to improved outcomes and better patient selection for surgery.

Patients not responding to standard conservative methods who may or may not be candidates for invasive surgery now have an opportunity for pain relief with endoscopic spine surgery. The endoscopic procedure, coupled with discography and spinal probing under local anesthesia, allows the patient to participate in his or her care (Kuslich, 1990; Yeung, 1999b).

CURRENT IMAGING METHODS

When compared with conditions diagnosed by spinal endoscopy, imaging studies are only about 70% accurate and specific (Yeung, 1999a; Kuslich, 1990). Conditions such as annular tears, rim tears with associated endplate separation, and various other discogenic pathologies are missed almost a third of the time. Tears that are in the ventral aspect of the disc are routinely missed by MRI studies. Small disc herniations that protrude beyond the outer fibers of the annulus may be missed. This is because the fragment may be flattened against the posterior longitudinal ligament or nerve, looking like a swollen or enlarged nerve. On the MRI, subligamentous herniations may appear as a thickened or bulged annulus. When the nerve is inflamed, the MRI may not be able to distinguish the enlarged nerve from a conjoined nerve, an anomalous branch, or a nerve with an adherent piece of disc.

Spinal endoscopy has allowed the endoscopic surgeon to identify the actual pathologic lesion, correlating it with the imaging study, and making the clinician more aware of the pitfalls of relying too much on imaging alone. It is imperative that the patient be examined with all these possibilities in mind to avoid labeling the patient a "head case."

CLINICAL PRESENTATIONS CORRELATED WITH ENDOSCOPIC FINDINGS

When the disc tissue is in direct contact with the nerve, chemical irritation occurs and an inflammatory membrane forms. Even a large epidural venous plexus that is inflamed can contribute to back pain and sciatica. When an inflammatory membrane is present ventral to the traversing and/or exiting nerve root, the clinical picture may not be clear.

Spinal endoscopy has confirmed nondermatomal pain in multiple patients with proximal thigh, buttock, and groin pain at levels distal to the root origin of the anatomic area. These also include patients who are considered to have spine pain by nonorganic physical signs.

INCLUSION CRITERIA

All disc herniations are amenable to selective endoscopic discectomy in a skilled endoscopic surgeon's hands. Each surgeon will select his or her patient dependent on his level of skill. Discogenic pain from internal disc disruption and annular tears may benefit from thermal and chemical modulation of the disc.

IDEAL INDICATION

Perhaps the ideal lesion for selective endoscopic discectomy is the far lateral, extra-foraminal disc herniation.

This type of herniation is the most difficult for the majority of spinal surgeons. A skilled spinal surgeon can access the lateral zone of the disc with a paramedian incision, but the posterior approach utilized by most traditional surgeons requires the removal of a significant amount of facet to actually reach the herniation. This approach also causes extensive tissue trauma due to the dissection, which is quite vascular.

Our experience suggests that it is easier to access the extraforaminal zone with the endoscope. Endoscopically it is also more difficult than a contained herniation, but the approach is much less traumatic for the patient. It is very important to remember that the success of any surgical procedure depends on proper patient selection, surgeon skill, the correct use of treatment modalities, as well as the combined diagnostic and surgical skills of the treatment team.

We have found that for the team diagnostic endoscopy confirms valuable information on predicted pain generators to actual sites. This approach also may alleviate the need for a surgical approach that is potentially destructive to muscle and adjacent soft tissue when a less invasive or conservative treatment is available.

Other validated indications include excisional biopsy of spinal structures and tissue. A prime example is discitis. Currently treated with long-term antibiotics, discitis is much more effectively treated with endoscopic debridement and excisional biopsy of infected tissue. The initial clinical data results are promising, suggesting endoscopic excisional biopsy and debridement offer the optimal treatment option for this condition.

ALTERNATIVES TO FUSION

Fusion has traditionally been reserved for spinal instability and deformity. More recently with the development of fusion cages, patients have been offered fusion for discogenic back pain without leg pain. The pain generators have been discovered to arise primarily from the annulus, but also can involve the endplates and facet joints.

Patients with debilitating lumbar pain are currently being offered surgical fusion as a treatment option to stabilize the motion segment. Pain nociceptors from the annulus which are innervated by branches of the sinu-vertebral nerve, have been shown to be deformed by heat at least 42°C. When the heat is increased to 65°C, type one collagen of the annulus contracts and thickens (Saal, Saal, and Ashley, 1997). Thermal therapy has been utilized to tighten stretched ligaments and unstable joints.

This approach is being applied to annular tears with favorable results. This type of lesion cannot always be imaged, even with the most sophisticated techniques; however, provocative discography has demonstrated its ability to diagnose such pathologies. Furthermore, when imaging studies identify these lesions as a high intensity zone (HIZ), there is a high incidence of positive confirmation by provocative discography.

Spinal endoscopy allows direct visualization of annular tears, identifying interpositional disc tissue as the single most common finding preventing annular tears from healing. This approach may provide a possible alternative to fusion as a first line of surgical treatment for discogenic pain with its origin from annular tears.

PROVOCATIVE DISCOGRAPHY

Our clinic utilizes discography as an integral part of the surgical workup. The literature supporting discography is currently considered controversial in some circles. The controversy presents because of the high inter-observer variability by discographers in reporting the patient's subjective pain. However, if the surgeon works closely on a team with an experienced discographer, and there is ongoing communication, we have found the two can help decrease the variability in the interpretation of the patient's response.

It is ideal for the surgeon to perform his or her own discography, as he or she is the one who must take the responsibility for deciding whether the patient will respond to endoscopic spine surgery. Furthermore, the surgeon always repeats the discogram at the time of surgery if the Selective Endoscopic Protocol that emphasizes vital dye staining of targeted tissue is used.

The discogram can be used to predict the presence of a collagenized disc fragment vs. a soft herniation, and the extrusion of a disc fragment as a noncontained herniation. In addition, discography can diagnose the presence of the type, grade, and location of painful vs. nonpainful annular tears (Yeung, 1995).

The senior author follows a classification for discograms based on Adams, et al. (1986), Osti (1992), and Sachs, et al. (1987). According to Adams, the basic pattern is grades I to V. The radial extensions are per Dallas where grade III is the extension to the inner annulus, grade IV up to the outer annulus, and grade V beyond the outer annulus. The extension of circumferential tears is described per Osti. When this classification is used, the number of quadrants of involvement can be determined by discography alone, and it is not necessary to do a post-discogram CT scan to get enough information to determine the efficacy of endoscopic surgery.

The Revised Discogram Classification

1. Cotton ball nucleus (normal cotton ball pattern).
2. Oval nucleus and painless extension of fragmentation beyond center.

3. Radial fissured extension to the inner annulus with no circumferential extension and no disc protrusion.
4. Radial extension to the outer annulus and circumferential component to 1 to 4 quadrants and disc protrusion.
5. Radial tear past outer annulus, circumferential 1 to 4 quadrants, most variable and definite disc protrusion with possible extruded fragment.

Clinically

- Grades 1 and 2 give no pain.
- Grade 3: Pain present at moderate pressure.
- Grade 4: Predominately back pain. Leg pain associated with central and far lateral protrusion, inflammatory membrane may be present.
- Grade 5: MRI can only detect in Zones I and II, the central and foraminal zones (may be associated with herniation). Possible prolonged healing time up to 9 months, depending on the size of the tear.

The Technique Incorporates Adjunctive Modalities

1. Flexible probes
2. Flexible mechanical instruments
3. Thermomodulation
   a. Radio frequency
   b. Laser

Since 1991 the senior author has treated over 1000 patients with a wide spectrum of disc herniations endoscopically. These include extruded and sequestered fragments. The success rate in the first 500 patients is an overall 86% good/excellent by MacNab Criteria. The success rate has continued to rise concurrent with diligence in the refinement of indications, techniques, and adjunctive therapy.

With the addition of a focused multidisciplinary team that enjoys working together, it is our hope that with a coordinated team approach we can easily reach the 90% plus good/excellent outcome and avoid the failed spine surgery syndrome so prevalent in today's surgical environment.

INTRADISCAL THERMAL THERAPY

As of July, 2000, only one published study on the treatment of back pain using Electrothermal Therapy (IDET) has been published. Electrothermal Annuloplasty (IDET) involves the insertion of an electrothermal catheter into a putatively painful disc under fluoroscopic guidance. Thermal energy delivered by the catheter

results in a breakdown and restructuring of collagen fibers in the annulus. Proponents offer several explanations as to why this procedure might relieve pain attributed to the disc. It may be due to a stiffening of the disc itself, possibly alter the annular tears or, in fact, it may ablate nerve endings. Nevertheless, Saal, Saal, and Ashley (1997) report that 80% of the patients treated with IDET noted a significant decrease in their back pain of at least 2 points on a 10-point analog scale, improvement in sitting tolerance, and reduction in medication usage. An SF-36 Questionnaire revealed a positive change of at least 7 points.

Recent information from the International Society for the Study of the Lumbar Spine (ISSLS) was critical of IDET. They cited the lack of high-quality scientific evidence exists in favor of this treatment. Furthermore, no evidence in favor of IDET from randomized controlled trials, or from other published controlled studies about long-term safety, yet reports suggest over 20,000 patients have undergone this procedure. Caution is advised as with any procedure. These patients present with back pain without severe radiculopathy. Patients with severe radicular symptoms due to frank disc herniations are not candidates. If there is any amount of disc protrusion or herniation, selective endoscopic discectomy would be the treatment of choice.

VISUALIZED THERMAL ANNULOPLASTY

The author's choice of a visualized technique over the blind technique of a thermal resistive catheter is supported by his success in converting failed IDET procedures to successful ones using the selective discectomy and visualized thermal annuloplasty technique. In our experience one of the most common findings with failed IDET is the presence of a disc fragment or interpositional disc tissue fragment preventing shrinkage of the annular tear. On rare occasions one is able to find necrotic disc tissue (confirmed by pathology slides) in patients who have undergone IDET treatment.

We feel strongly that direct visualization overcomes both conditions when visual control of tissue reaction to thermal energy allows the surgeon to avoid carbonization of tissue and target the annular tear directly. In the Y.E.S.S. technique, inclusion of a side firing Ho:Yag laser also serves as the energy source that offers a tool that affects tissue shrinkage to the ablation of bone, just by controlling the laser setting.

Further advancement and application of these techniques will help expand the surgical capabilities of this procedure, allowing for treatment of conditions in a degenerative spine that are painful, but not responding to conservative treatment.

CHYMOPAPAIN

Low-dose chymopapain 500 units help "digest" the soft herniation and treat the collagenized fragment for ease of removal. The senior author uses chymopapain when disc fragments are found to be extruded and migrated behind the vertebral body. Other applications are when a recurrent herniation exists. Chymopapain is used to decrease the recurrence rate and dissolve the missed fragments. Chymopapain is injected and left in the nucleus pulposus for up to 5 minutes before endoscopic discectomy.

When chymopapain is used as adjunctive therapy, we have had no adverse effects or allergic reactions, even when the discogram identifies leakage beyond the annular fibers into the epidural space. If the discogram demonstrates uptake by the venous plexus, if it is absorbed as soon as it is injected, or if it communicates in any way with the thecal sac, demonstrating a communication with the disc space, we have not injected chymopapain. As a precaution against an allergic reaction, we routinely administer Benadryl™, 50 mg, and cimetidine, 300 mg IV, before injecting the chymopapain.

INTRAOPERATIVE STEROIDS

Whenever an inflammatory membrane was observed, stimulation of the nerve and surrounding tissue elicited pain. When there is no inflammatory membrane, the nerve and annulus can be manipulated without eliciting pain. When an inflammatory membrane is present, the patient's pain is often considered out of proportion to the imaged pathology. When there is significant inflammation noted, Depo-medrol® is placed intradiscally at the conclusion of the procedure.

RISKS AND COMPLICATIONS

Surgical risks and complications are real issues that need to be weighed before considering any invasive procedure. These include dural tear, nerve root damage, bleeding, or infection. The authors have seen variations of nerve anatomy and distribution on the annulus, including conjoined nerves not appreciated by imaging studies and accessory nerve branches that often connect the traversing with the exiting nerve. Removal of these branches usually do not affect the patient's clinical course.

The most common adverse effect of the use of electrothermal therapy is dysesthesia. Fortunately, most dysesthesia will resolve completely, as in a second-degree controlled burn. Occasionally, there will be severe sympathetic pain that will challenge post-operative pain management. A multidisciplinary team is extremely helpful in assisting the patient to cope with the pain. Usually good pain management with selective epidurals or nerve root block, the use of long-acting oral analgesics, and judicious use of gabapentin (Neurontin™) will mitigate this condition.

We have noted the presence of dysesthesia as a delayed response days and weeks after the procedure. Therefore, while we blame the use of laser and electrothermal therapy, the actual cause of this regional sympathetic condition is still unknown. The incidence of dysesthesia is about 5%. Complications of discitis, nerve injury, dural tear, and psoas hematoma total less than 1 to 2% overall.

REFERENCES

Adams, M.A., Dolan, P., & Hutton, W.C. (1986). The states of disc degeneration as revealed by discograms. *Journal of Bone and Joint Surgery (Britain), 68*(1), 36–41.

Choy, D.S. (1992). Percutaneous laser disc decompression. A new therapeutic modality. *Spine, 17*, 949–956.

Cresswell, C.C. (1992). Introduction to electrosurgery. *Journal of British Podiatric Medicine*, 47, 11–15.

Farlan, H.F. (1973). *Mechanical disorder of the low back.* Philadelphia: Lea & Febiger.

Fritsch, E.W., Heisel, J., & Rupp, S. (1996). The failed back surgery syndrome: Reasons, intraoperative findings, and long-term results. A report of 182 operative treatments. *Spine, 21*, 626–633.

Hermantin, F.U., Peters, T., Quartararo, L., & Kambin, P. (1999). A prospective, randomized study comparing the results of open discectomy with those of video-assisted arthroscopic microdiscectomy. *Journal of Bone and Joint Surgery, 81*(A), 958–965.

Jacobson, J.H. (1997). The early days of microsurgery in Vermont. *Mt. Sinai Journal of Medicine, 64*, 160–163.

Kambin, P., O'Brien, E., Zhou, L., & Schaffer, J.L. (1998). Arthroscopic microdiscectomy and selective fragmentectomy. *Clinical Orthopedics, 347*, 150–167.

Kirkaldy, W.W. (1983). *Managing low back pain.* New York: Churchill.

Kuslich, S.D. Microsurgical lumbar nerve root decompression utilizing progressive local anesthesia. In W. Williams, J. McCulouch, & P. Young (Eds.). *Microsurgery of the lumbar spine.* Rockville, MD: Aspen.

Osti, O.L., Vernon-Roberts, B., Moore, R., & Fraser, R.D. (1992). Annular tears and disc degeneration in the lumbar spine. A post mortem. *Journal of Bone and Joint Surgery (Britain), 74*(5), 678–682.

Saal, J.A., & Saal, J.S. The use of a thermal resistive coil for the treatment of discogenic pain. A preliminary report. *Spine* (in press).

Saal, J.A., Saal, J.S., & Ashley, J. (1997). Targeted intradiscal thermal therapy: Preliminary feasibility studies. Issls conference, June 2–3.

Sachs, B., Vanharanta, H., Spivey, M.A., et al. (1987). Dallas discogram description: A new classification of CT/discography in low back pain disorders. *Spine, 12*(3), 287–294.

Sauguaro, T., Oegeme, R.T., & Bradford, D.S. (1986). The effects of chymopapain on prolapsed human intervertebral disc: A clinical and correlate histochemical study. *Clinical Orthopedics, 213,* 223–231.

Yeung, A.T. (1995, March). *The intraoperative discogram: Its role in arthroscopic microdiscectromy.* La Jolla, CA: International Intradiscal Therapy Society, Inc.

Yeung, A.T. (2000). The evolution of percutaneous spinal endoscopy and discectomy: State of the art. *Mt. Sinai Journal of Medicine, 67,* 327–332.

Yueng, A.T. (1999). Minimally invasive disc surgery with the Yeung Endoscopic Spine System (Y.E.S.S.). *Surgical Technology International VIII,* 1–11.

88

Phytomedicinal Approaches to Pain Management

James Giordano, Ph.D.

Recent medical practice has seen a phenomenal increase in the utilization of alternative and complementary approaches by patients as well as physicians. One of the most dynamic and rapidly growing areas of complementary medical care involves herbal or phytomedicinal intervention. In the United States, herbs and phytomedicinals are commercially available in accordance with the Dietary Supplement and Health Education Act (DSHEA) of 1994. This act offers the proviso that herbs sold as supplements cannot be marketed for diagnostic, therapeutic, or preventive interventions for disease, and relegates them to the status of foods stuffs, additives, or (as the name would imply) nutritional supplements (or nutriceuticals). In this country, official governmental standards are not provided for the production of herbal products and, therefore, purity, potency, and viability can vary highly with regard to level of extract, contaminates, co-substances, and dose provided. Certainly this is not the case worldwide. Of particular note are the actions of Germany's "Commission E," a subgroup of the German Federal Health Agency. This organization has conducted an exhaustive study of over 350 common and medicinally used botanical preparations, and has amassed basic scientific and clinical data that identify active constituents, chemical profiles, clinical applications, side effects, and contraindications for these herbs. Thus, the Commission E monographs stand alone as the most comprehensive and efficacious review of medicinal herbs currently available. Of equal importance is the current *Physician's Desk Reference for Herbal Medicines*. This volume provides a review of over 700 herbs

as assembled by PhytoPharm, U.S. Institute of Phytopharmaceuticals. The U.S. *PDR for Herbal Medicines* provides easy access for practitioners in an easy-to-read format for herbs that are commercially available, as well as enhanced research data on adverse effects, formulation, and safety.

Taken together, these documents demonstrate that many herbs contain potent ingredients capable of exerting powerful biological effects. Also, active principal ingredients coupled with numerous constituent co-factors may set the stage for herb–drug interactions. Although consumers may view herbs as simple nutritional supplements, the potencies of these pharmacologic actions are medically important. When properly utilized, herbs can serve as adjunctive or perhaps primary agents in pain management. It is important for the practitioner to recognize that herbs often contain heterogeneous combinations of active principles. These can affect indication and use and may warrant pharmacologic contraindications. Although many herbs possess few or no notable side effects, a knowledge of the possible range of effects is critical. Similarly, a clinician must be aware that patients often maintain a "microwave mentality," in which the assumption is erroneously made that an herb is a "natural" product, therefore, "a little is good…more must be better." In accordance with the aforementioned information, it is exceedingly possible that overdosing even relatively benign herbs can have serious consequences. It is important for practitioners to be aware of not only active principles and constituents, but also to recognize viable dose ranges to maintain clinical effects. It should be noted, however, that both Commission

0-8493-0926-3/02/$0.00+$1.50
© 2002 by CRC Press LLC

E and the U.S. *PDR for Herbal Medicines* offer very well-defined caveats regarding the dosage of commercially available herbs. Clinicians and consumers must be cautious in their utilization of herbs, because these substances are not under direct governmental control for quality assurance, and doses of active and subconstituents can vary widely among preparations.

This being the case, clinicians who look to integrate herbal and phytomedicinal agents into their practice must be very specific when questioning patients about herbs (with precise inquiry regarding brand, dose, frequency, and combinations during initial assessments, follow-ups, and discharge planning). It may be useful, if considering integrating herbal preparations into practice, to procure the collaborative services of a compounding pharmacist to assist in the acquisition of superior quality, "pure herbs," that are as close to pharmaceutical grade extract as conceivably possible. For allopathic, osteopathic, and chiropractic practitioners, many medical associations offer ongoing continuing education in herbal treatments and nutriceuticals that provides information on effects, indications/contraindications, and use of herbs for specific disorders. Interactive recruitment of a naturopathic physician also may be of critical benefit if an expanded, integrative herbal practice is to be considered.

The herbs considered in this chapter fall into the category of "occidental" herbal preparations, and it is beyond the scope of this writing to address those herbs utilized in traditional Chinese, Indian, and various folk medicinal practices to treat pain. The U.S. *PDR for Herbal Medicines* addresses compounds that fall within these categories, and the reader is referred to that document for appropriate review. Thus, while many herbs are capable of affecting some component of pain symptoms, the following group represents those with specific well-documented actions on specific processes that mediate pain. These are presented alphabetically for ease of access and readability.

BLACK COHOSH (*CIMICIFUGA RACEMOSA*)

A native plant of the North American continent, black cohosh is specifically cultivated as a medicinal herb in Europe. Alcohol-aqueous extract of icopropenolic extract of the plant yields the active constituents of several types of triterpenes including triterpene glycoside, 27-deoxiactein, and simifugoside. Active quinolizidine alkaloids include cytisines and methyl cytisine and the phenyl propane derivatives including isoferulic acid.

The active constituents of the plant appear to be the triterpene glycosides that affect the activity of central and peripheral estrogen receptors. Although equivocal evidence reports that LH levels are also affected by cohosh, studies demonstrate the major action is through either a direct effect on estrogen receptors or an indirect estrogenic-like activity of triterpene glycoside on smooth muscle of the female

genital urinary tract. In this regard, black cohosh has been highly touted as an agent to relieve pain of premenstrual dysmenorrhea and perimenopausal discomfort.

In general, no overt side effects have been demonstrated or reported with use of black cohosh within the therapeutic dose range, although some initial dyspepsia may occur in sensitive individuals. Of particular note, however, is the activity of black cohosh in altering uterine smooth muscle motility; this agent is contraindicated during pregnancy due to a high potential for inducing uterine contractility and evoking spontaneous abortion. The actions of the tripertene glycosides can synergize the effect of antihypertensive medications through relaxant effects on peripheral vascular smooth muscle. Thus, the herb is contraindicated for use in individuals who are pharmacologically maintained on antihypertensive medication (due to the risk of profound hypotension). Overdose in excess of 5 to 10 g per day has been reported to result in dizziness, orthostatic hypotension, disorientation, headache, and vomiting, all apparently attributable to its vaso-relaxant mechanism and resultant central and peripheral hypotensive sequelae.

BLACK PEPPER (*PIPER NIGRUM*)

Black pepper is an indigenous plant to the Indian continent and is commercially cultivated in Asia and throughout the Caribbean. Berries of the pepper plant that have been liberated from the pericarp and berry-like fruit parts are utilized internally for stomach pain and are externally applied as a salve or ointment for neuralgia. Preparation yields a volatile oil whose chief constituents include sabineine, limonene, caryophyllene, α- and β-pinene and Δ-3 carene. Acidic amides include piperine, piperylin, piperolein A and B, and coumaperine. The plant also yields fatty oils and polysaccharides. The mechanism of action involves both volatile oils and acid amides, although certain glycosides (3,4-dyhydroxy phenyl ethanol glycoside, considered a substrate for enzymes responsible for producing the color of the plant) may have some activity as well. Taken internally, black pepper activates buccal high-intensity thermal receptors and increases salivation. Within the alimentary tract, pepper increases secretion of gastric mucosal cells. When topically applied, volatile oils and acid amides act at A-Δ and perhaps C-thermosponsive and polymodal afferents, either as a counterirritant or (indirect) secretogogue.

Adverse side effects and contraindications have not been reported for black pepper, nor have herb–drug interactions; black pepper appears to be safe and effective when used as an adjunctive agent in the treatment of dyspeptic gastric pain (including NSAID-induced dyspepsia due to decreased secretion of gastric mucosal cells) and as a topically applied agent for mild to moderate pain of neuropathic etiology.

BORAGE (*BORAGO OFFICINALIS*)

The borage plant is indigenous to Central and Eastern Europe where it is also cultivated commercially for culinary and medicinal purposes. Explants of borage are now grown throughout Europe and in the United States and Canada. The medicinal components of the plant consist of dried flowers, leaves, stems, and seeds. Borage oil is the fatty extract derived from the seeds. The chief constituent of the fatty oil is γ-linolenic acid, although linoleic acid is found in lesser quantities. The borage leaf yields several active constituents including numerous pyrrolizidine alkaloids (including supinin, lycopsamin, intermedin, amabiline, and thesinine), a variably water-soluble silicic acid, tannins, and mucilages. The oil is used in either liquid or capsular form for the treatment of neurodermatitis, its therapeutic effect due to the activity of alkaloids and tannins. The leaf is used as an external astringent, attributable to the tannins and mucilage.

Of note is that the borage leaf contains hepatotoxic alkaloids, which although present in nominal quantities, warrant against its internal use. An added caveat is that the borage leaf should be used as an external astringent for only brief periods of time, to lessen possible effects of the transdermal absorption of toxic alkaloids. Borage oil has not been shown to be contraindicated when used within the therapeutic dose ranges and duration, and no known herb–drug interactions have been reported for the oil preparation.

CAJUPUT (*MELALEUCA LEUCADENDRA*)

This large tree is originally from southeastern Asia and the Australian continent, and grown commercially elsewhere for medicinal purposes. The medicinal component is the oils of the fresh twigs and leaves, which are extracted, air dried, and steam distilled. This process yields active constituents of sineol, ± alpha terpineols, ± α-terpineols valerates, α-pinenes, and bicyclic sesquiterpenes. The oil is used externally as a salve or linament for sprains, myofascitis, tendonous and ligamentous over-exertion injury, and may be applied topically over arthritic joints. Mechanism of action appears to involve direct activity of the terpineols with both anti-inflammatory and perhaps mild muscular relaxant effects. The high sineol content yields toxicity if the drug is taken internally or is allowed to contact mucus membranes of the lips, eyes, or nose. This latter effect is particularly viable in young children, in whom wherein facial application has been documented to induce glottal, bronchial, and diaphragmatic spasm. As well, the high sineol content may induce rapid overdose following internal consumption by adults. Profound hypotension, vascular and respiratory failure, myoclonus and spasm, and electrolyte disruption have all been reported. Other than contraindications against internal use or accidental contact with viable mucus membranes facilitating internal absorption, no direct contraindications for this substance exist. Health hazard and/or side effects for moderate external use of cajuput oil have not been reported, although some individuals report an initial irritative dermatitis that subsequently dissipates.

CAYENNE (*CAPSICUM VARIANTS*)

Capsicum is native to Mexico, Central America, and the southern United States and is grown in numerous locations for both medicinal and culinary purposes. The active ingredients are the capsacinoids (vanillyl amine amides), principally capsaicin and dihydrocapsaicin. Cayenne also contains carotinoids including violaxanthine, flavoniods (apiin and luteolin-7-0-glucoside), and steroid saponins. The principal utility of capsicum is as a topical analgesic. The active moiety capsaicin, when afforded transdermal access (characteristically via delivery in a pluronic lecithin organogel), binds to a vanilloid calcium-channel receptor on peripheral nociceptive C-fiber afferents. Capsicum binding to this site facilitates an inward flux of calcium leading to a rapid membrane depolarization and release of these fibers' primary neurotransmitter, substance-P (please refer to Chapter 89 on the neurobiology of pain). Thus, capsicum acts as a secretogogue at peripheral C-fiber afferents. Capsicum binding appears to be long lasting, thereby blocking the channel, depleting the C-fiber of substance-P, and producing a rightward shift in the stimulation-response curve of C-fiber afferents to thermal, mechanical, and chemical noxious input. Commission E has approved the use of capsicum for pain of muscular (myoscitis, myofascitis) and rheumatic origin.

Of note is that use should be limited to 2 days, with a 10- to 14-day interval between applications. Prolonged use of topical capsicum may cause festering dermatitis and ulceration. Capsicum should not be used on the periorbital skin, and should be discontinued should hypersensitivity, rhinoconjunctivitis, or dermatitis occur. It has been suggested that hypersensitivity to capsicum is due infrequently to direct sensitization, but rather is a result of a generalized pollen hypersensitivity with cross-reactivity to cayenne.

ENGLISH CHAMOMILE (*CHAMAEMELUM NOBILE*)

English chamomile, also known as Roman chamomile, grows naturally in southern Europe and northern Africa, and is cultivated throughout Europe and the American continent. The medicinal oil extracted from the fresh or dried flower heads contains volatile oils including the esters of angelic and tiglic acid. Sesquiterpine lactones, including nobilin, epinobilin and 4-α hydroperoxy manolide. Flavoniods include anfemoside, cosmosioside, and caffeic and ferulic acid esters. The mechanism of action is not well documented; however, the sesquiterpine lactones appear to act in the central nervous system, perhaps inducing the release of inhibitory neurotransmitters for central modulation of pain. English chamomile has been used for treatment of general headache, somatic distress, and premenstrual pain.

It has been suggested that use of English chamomile may result in sensitization reactions; however, no known side effects or herb interactions have been documented. In light of the sparse documentation of potential interactions and effects, the drug is not indicated for use during pregnancy.

GERMAN CHAMOMILE (*MATRICARIA RECUTITA*)

Growing naturally throughout western Europe and cultivated in North America, the flowers and entire herb are used as an infusion for inflammatory pain and pain-related anxiety. Active ingredients include the volatile oil consisting of (−) −α-bisabolor, chanazulene, and spathulenol. Bioactive flavonoids include flavone glycosides, apigenin, luteolin, flavinol glycosides including quercetin, and methoxylized flavoniods including chrysosplenetin. German chamomile also contains phytomedicinal hydroxycoumarins and mucilages. Analgesic effects are centrally mediated and are due to the activity of flavoniods: apigenin is an agonist at CNS benzodiazepine receptors, and may potentiate binding at the benzodiazepine–chloride ion channel complex. Apigenin also appears to exert activity as a monoamine oxidase inhibitor, with specific activity at monoamine oxidase A, and lesser activity at monoamine oxidase B. Thus, both norepinephrine and serotonin concentrations may be transiently elevated through the use of chamomile. These latter effects subserve spinal and supraspinal mechanisms of analgesia.

Patients who are hypersensitive to grass and mudwort pollen may exhibit cross-reactivity and sensitization to chamomile. Co-administration of CNS sedative agents including benzodiazepines, barbiturates, and ethanol should be avoided due to potentiation of central activity at benzodiazepine-binding sites and GABA potentiation. Concomitant use of monoamine oxidase inhibiting drugs should be avoided due to the potential for sympathomimetic and hypertensive effects.

GINSENG (AMERICAN AND KOREAN *PANAX* GINSENG)

A native plant of China, Korea, and Japan, it is also cultivated for nutriceutical purposes in the United States. The powdered preparation is used as either an infusion or in capsule form and is prepared from the dried root of the native plant. Active ingredients include the triterpene saponins; aglycone (20S)-protopanaxadiols including numerous ginsenosides (Ra1, Ra2, Ra3, Rb1, Rb2, and Rb3); aglycone (20S) propanax triols including ginsenosides Re, Rf, and Rg, aglycone oneanolic acids of ginsenosides Ro, saponin V, Rb1 and Rb2, the water-soluble polysaccharides panaxane (subtypes A-U) and several polyynes. The most active ingredients are the ginsenosides, which act as steroidal saponins. One reported mechanism of ginseng's analgesic effect is through the reduction in platelet-derived serotonin. The ginsenosides Ro, Rg1, and Rg2 inhibit platelet release reaction and thromboxane formation, thereby reducing platelet contribution to inflammatory and nocisponsive events. Saponin glycosides have been shown to stimulate corticotropin release, which may mediate, at least in part, a component of neuroendocrine analgesia. Although conflicting studies exist, data exist that illustrate the direct CNS activity of ginsenosides Rg2 and Rg3 at nicotinic ACh receptors. It is unclear whether this constituent functions as a partial agonist or mixed agonist-antagonist. By acting through central nicotinic ACh receptors, these ginsenosides appear to mediate a limbic component of pain processing, and thereby affect pain perception. Ginsenosides Rg2 and 3 may have activity at central GABA receptors, acting as partial agonists or mixed agonist-antagonists, to mediate a component of nociceptive modulation.

In general, care should be taken when considering use of ginseng in patients with cardiovascular disease (due to nicotinic stimulation) and/or diabetes (due to stimulation of insulin release and adrenergically mediated hypoglycemia). Thus, patients taking insulin or hypoglycemic agents should not employ ginseng as an adjunct analgesic. The use of nonsteroidal anti-inflammatory agents may be problematic due to the combined and potentiated anti-platelet and thrombolytic activity of NSAIDs and ginseng. The use of monoamine oxidase inhibitors with ginseng is contraindicated due to increased potential for sympathomimetic events (headache, tremor, hypertension).

SIBERIAN GINSENG (*ELEUTHEROCOCCUS SENTISOSUS*)

This plant is native to the Siberian regions of Russia, Northern China, Mongolia, and Korea. It is grown in Japan and North America. The dried roots and rhizomes are extracted for the production of the active compounds caffeic acid, hydroxycoumerins, several lignans including sasamine, eleutheroside-d phytosterols including β-sitosterol-3-O-β-D glucoside, rephinal acrylic acid eleutheroside B, several polysaccharides including eleutherane A-G, steroid glycosides, and triterpene saponins (eleutherosides I, K, L, and M). Siberian ginseng is used as an analgesic against kidney pain, rheumatoid pain (primarily due to its immune modulating effect on T-lymphocytes induced by the eleutherane polysaccharides), and inflammatory pain. The latter effect is modulated by platelet-inhibiting actions mediated by hydroxycoumarins and triterpene saponins. The anti-platelet activity may reduce peripheral concentrations of platelet-derived serotonin that activate peripheral C-fibers in inflammatory pain.

Due to the stimulating effects of caffeic acid and the plant steroids, the herb is contraindicated for patients with hypertension. Possible interactions include a potentiated thrombolytic effect when used with nonsteroidals, salicylates, or anticoagulant agents. In addition, the hypoglycemic activity of the herb contraindicates its use for patients on hypoglycemic agents or insulin.

JAPANESE MINT
(*MENTHA ARVENSIS PIPERASCENS*)

Indigenous to Europe, Asia, and commercially grown in North America, the mint oil is obtained through distillation of the flowering herb and removal of the active menthol ingredient. Chief components include menthol, menthone, limonene, neomenthol, and α and β pinene. It is used in Indian and Chinese medicine as a topical application of the essential oil for joint pain, headache, myalgia, and peripheral neuralgia.

Although Japanese mint, mint oil, and menthol can be used internally for the treatment of gastrointestinal pain, dyspepsia, and relief of respiratory congestion, the possibility of hepatic insult and hepatotoxicity contraindicates long-term internal use. As well, the cholagogic effect may precipitate and worsen cholestatic disease in patients with this comorbidity. Topically applied, precautions and contraindications are few; however, asthmatic patients may have exacerbation of airway or bronchiolar spasm upon initiation of menthol application. Facial, perioral, and perinasal use of menthol oil is contraindicated in pediatric patients because of increased risk of glottal and bronchial spasm. The anti-myospastic and neurotropic effects of topically applied menthol are due to the actions of menthol and menthone, perhaps as a counterirritant or through a direct mechanism not completely understood.

KAVA KAVA (*PIPER METHYSTICUM*)

A native plant of Polynesia and the South Sea Islands, kava kava is harvested for the dried rhisome and roots. Active ingredients are the kava lactones including (+)-kavain, yangonin, desmethoxy yangonin, kava pirones, and chalcones including flavokavain A and B. Used orally, kava lactones and pirones act at central GABA synapses to potentiate GABA release or facilitate GABA binding (primarily in brain). Kavain and dihydrokavain inhibit voltage-dependent sodium and calcium channels, thus

exerting both a central and peripheral muscle relaxant and neural inhibitory effect. Desmethoxy yangonin, yangonin, and kavain reversibly antagonize monoamine oxidase B, resulting in increased availability of synaptic serotonin at spinal and supraspinal sites. This increase in serotonin subserves the analgesic effect via inhibition of nociceptive neurons in the spinal cord. Additional analgesic properties are attributed to kavain, which can inhibit cyclo-oxygenase 1 and perhaps cyclo-oxygenase 2 in peripheral tissues, as well as the CNS. By inhibiting formation of the principal initiating enzyme of the archidonic acid cascade, kavain thus attenuates the formation of prostaglandins and thromboxane which act as potent inflammatory and nociceptive mediators.

As a mild depressant, the drug is contraindicated for patients with a history or current presentation of depression. Initially, administration may lead to mild allergic hypersensitivity and dyspepsia; however, this appears to dissipate with repeated use. Some initial lethargy has also been reported but this side effect also decreases with repetitive use. Based upon mechanism of actions, kava should not be used with alcohol due to reciprocal potentiation of effect, with benzodiazepines because of potentiation of benzodiazepine activity at GABA receptors, or with CNS depressants (e.g., barbiturates) due to potentiated depressant effects. Patients taking SSRIs, tri- or heterocylic antidepressants should use kava with caution because of the potential for enhanced psychotropic effects. There are reports of dopaminergic antagonism occurring with kava; thus, use of kava in Parkinsonian patients is contraindicated. Similarly, cardiac patients should use kava with caution due to variable effects of kava on dopaminergic control of the heart. Although these contraindications and caveats are applicable to specific patient populations, a more general precaution is that patients should use care when operating heavy machinery or engaging in fine motor tasks, particularly during the initial phase of kava therapy because of decreased motor coordination, increased reaction time, and sedative effects. While these may be transient, the early phase of therapy produces the most salient side effects for which the greatest precautions are warranted.

MARIJUANA (*CANNABIS SATIVA*)

Originating as a hashish derivative in the Near and Middle East, *cannabis* is cultivated throughout Europe, Asia, and North and South America as a substrate for illicit recreational drug use. The active ingredients are the cannaboids, mainly 9-tetrahydracanabinol and other bioactive cannabinoids. The flavoniods canniflavone-1 and -2 are also present. The analgesic actions of the cannabinoids appear to be due to binding at a discrete CNS receptor present in the thalamic, limbic, and cortical regions of the brain. Additionally, the effect of cannabinoids and flavoniods on membrane lipid metabolism, specifically, the diversion of fatty acid metabolism against archidonic acid, appears to be a mechanism by which peripheral analgesic effects may be mediated. The legal implications of cannabis use are obvious. It warrants mention that this agent has seen licit use as an analgesic, and may have utility as a marketed compound (dronabinol) for the treatment of pain, AIDS-induced anorexia, and as an anti-emetic for use during chemotherapy. Characteristically, cannabis is smoked (in cigarette or water-pipe form), ingested (either directly or incorporated into sweets), or taken in capsular form. Multiple effects are attributed to cannabis including vacillation of mood, lethargy, altered concentration, increased reaction time, and alteration of sensations. Physiologically, cannabis induces bronchial dilation, mild to moderate immunosuppression, increased cardiac chronotropy, and mild hypothermia.

Although specific contraindications do not exist, the aforementioned side effects limit its utility and caveats against operating a motor vehicle or heavy equipment or engaging in complex tasks are afforded. Although regional interest in legalizing cannabis use for general purposes (both medicinal and recreational) exists, marijuana still remains an illegal substance with often dire penal consequences for possession and use. Thus, its use is limited to prescription dosing (dronabinol, marketed under the brand name Marinol™) for appetite stimulation, anti-emetic action, and as an analgesic adjuvant (generally employed in end-stage terminal disease pain).

SCOTCH PINE (*PINUS*)

Native species are found in Europe, Siberia, the near East, and Scotch pine is cultivated worldwide. Medicinal components include tar extracted from the trunk and branch, oil extracted from needles, and pine tips from dried shoots. Active compounds include a volatile oil containing bornyl acetate, cadinene, and α tinnene, ascorbic acid and several resins. The pine needle oil contains Δ-3-carene and α- and β-pinenes. A subspecies of pine, *pinus sylvesteris*, contains camphene, limonene, and terpinolene yielded from the raw turpentine oil from the plant. Pine shoots are advocated by Commission E for the treatment of neuralgia and oral inflammation. Pine needle oil and turpentine oil are externally used in the treatment of neuralgia and rheumatoid pain. These effects are due to its enzymatic actions that inhibit prostaglandin formation in peripheral tissues.

No specific precautions are noted for external use of pine oils; however, patients with extensive skin injuries, acute burns, and open wounds should avoid application. Prolonged and extensive use of pine-based turpentine oils may have nephrotoxic and peripheral neurotoxic potential.

SPRUCE (SPECIES OF *PICEA*)

Indigenous to north, central, and western Europe, spruce is grown worldwide. Medicinal oils are extracted from needles, branches, and shoots. These yield needle oil containing bornoachinate, limonene, camphene, and pinene. Spruce shoots yield a volatile oil containing primarily limonene, borniol, bornyl acetate, and ascorbic acid. Spruce needle oil and spruce shoots are sanctioned by Commission E for topical application in the treatment of neuralgia and rheumatic-type pain. Mechanism of action appears to be due to a secretolytic and tonic inhibitory effect on peripheral nociceptive afferents.

As with scotch pine oils, patients with skin trauma and injury should avoid use of spruce oil or use it cautiously. Pediatric use is not recommended due to the enhanced possibility of absorption and toxicity.

ST. JOHN'S WORT (*HYPERICUM PERFORATUM*)

Growing natively throughout Europe and North Africa, the plant has been introduced to Asia, the Australian continent, New Zealand, and is currently cultivated in North America. The specific medicinal utilization is of buds and flowers. These yield several active constituents; anthrosene derivatives include hypericin and pseudo-hypericin. Active flavoniods include hyperosides, querciterin, rutin, and amentoflavone. Hypericum also contains zanthones, catechintannins, caffeic acid derivatives, and a volatile oil whose main constituents are aliphatic hydrocarbons and mono- and sesquiterpenes. The herb is Commission E approved for treatment of depression, anxiety, and may be used as an adjunct analgesic. These properties are related to the activity of the flavone and flavinol derivatives. Hypericin has been shown to inhibit reuptake of serotonin, norepinepherine, and dopamine and may evoke pineal release of melatonin. The reuptake blocking effects of hypericum increase the synaptic availability of serotonin and norepinepherine within the brain and spinal cord, mechanisms that facilitate supraspinal and centrifugal pain modulation.

Although no specific precautions are rendered against the use of St. John's Wort, numerous side effects warrant discussion. Some patients experience paradoxical restlessness (initially thought to be a hypomanic effect somewhat similar to that seen with SSRIs), while others experience fatigue and lethargy. Transient headache is also a reported side effect, although this occurs in less than 10% of patients. Initially, patients may experience dyspepsia or GI pain with St. John's Wort use; this effect is transient. Of note is that hypericum produces photosensitivity, particularly with higher doses, and patients should be cautioned regarding ultraviolet light exposure (i.e., sun tanning and/or tanning beds). The documented neurotropic action of hypericum warrants precaution against several drug interactions. Certainly, SSRIs used concomitantly with St. John's Wort increase the potential for facilitated serotonergic availability and the occurrence of serotonin syndrome ("wet dog shakes," diaphoresis, tremor, agitation, flushing). Similarly, the use of monoamine oxidase inhibitors is contraindicated due to increased adrenergic neurotransmission and the possibility for hypertensive crisis and other sympathomimetic effects on the cardiovascular system. St. John's Wort induces hepatic cytochrome P450 enzyme activity; other drugs metabolized through this pathway may have significant disruption of hepatic transformation. Specifically, these include cyclosporine (decreased serum concentration of cyclosporine following concomitant use of St. John's Wort), indinavir (greater than 50% reduction in plasma concentration of indinavar with concomitant use of St. John's Wort), theophylline and digoxin (decreased area-under-the-curve serum concentration digoxin with decreased digoxin efficacy and anticipation of rising digoxin levels approaching toxicity after discontinuation of St. John's Wort).

TURMERIC (*CURCUMA DOMESTICA*)

Native to India, turmeric is grown throughout south east Asia and privately cultivated in the southern United States. Medicinally, the rhizome is stewed and dried to yield the active volatile oils α- and β-tumerone, artumerone, α- and γ-atlantone, zingiberene, and curcumol. The plant contains curcumoids including curcumin, demethoxycurcumin, and bidemethoxycurcumin. Turmeric is approved by Commission E for dyspepsia, loss of appetite, and abdominal pain. Prepared as a tea or in capsular form, it is taken internally after meals. Additionally, tincture of turmeric is used for anti-inflammatory effects and analgesia against inflammatory pain. It is believed that the tumerones, zingiberene and curcumin, are the active moities in reducing the inflammatory cascade through direct stabilization of membrane fatty acid content (thereby preventing biosynthesis of arachidonic acid and, subsequently, prostaglandins). This action may subserve analgesic effects as well.

Although frank precautions or adverse effects are not known for tumeric, the use of this agent has been found to potentiate cholecystic disease in patients with premorbid cholecystic pathology.

VALERIAN (*VALERIANA OFFICINALIS*)

Native to Europe and Asia, it is also cultivated in Japan and the United States for phytomedicinal purposes. The dried roots are utilized to yield the iridoids including the valepotriates, isovaltrate, and acevalterate. The volatile oil contains bornyl isovalerenate and valerenic acid. The plant yields the sesquiterpenes of valerenic acid, 2-hydroxyvalerenic acid,

and 2-acetoxy-valerenic acid. Additionally, pyridine alkaloids including valerianine and α-methyl tyrrylketone are present. The valerenic acids inhibit the enzymatic degradation of GABA, thereby making this inhibitory neurotransmitter more viable at supraspinal and spinal postsynaptic binding sites. Nonselective GABA-A and GABA-B receptor effects are achieved through the use of valerian. Valerian also has a high content of glutamine, a metabolic precursor to the glial GABA shunt for the biosynthesis of GABA. This ultimately increases neuronal GABA content and potentiates post-synaptic GABA-ergic effects further. The anxiolytic, muscle relaxant, and sedative effects are similar to those seen with administration of other GABA receptor agonists (e.g., the benzodiazepines). However, unlike benzodiazepines, tolerance, dependence, and withdrawal are rarely seen when utilizing therapeutic doses of valerian.

The activity at central GABA receptors contraindicates the use of valerian with benzodiazepines or barbiturate agents that are also agonists at this multimolecular receptor site. As well, a caveat (particularly during the initial use of valerian) against the operation of complex machinery or complex motoric tasks due to the spinal motor inhibition, muscle relaxant, and CNS sedative effects should be noted.

WHITE FIR (*ABIES ALBA*)

Indigenous to the Balkans, it is cultivated throughout Europe and in the United States as a domestic plant and for phytomedicinal purposes. The timber yields an essential oil through extraction, with active compounds of limonene, α-pinene, champhene, bornyl acetate, and santene. These oils may act as mild counter irritants initially, and perhaps as secretogogues to nociceptive afferents. White fir oil is approved by Commission E for topical application in treatment of neuralgia and rheumatic pain.

Like other essential oils of pine and fir trees, over exposure to volatile oils may yield glottal and bronchial spasm. Thus, application to the face, periorbital, and perinasal regions and use in pediatric patients are contraindicated.

WHITE WILLOW (*SALIX*)

Native to central Europe, the plant also is cultivated in the North American continent where the bark yields the active glycosides and salicylic acid. Additionally, white willow contains tannins and flavoniods. White willow is approved by Commission E for general treatment of pain and inflammatory states. This is directly attributable to plant esters and glycosides that yield salicin, the metabolic precursor of salicylic acid. Salicylate is a potent inhibitor of cyclo-oxygenase (both 1, and to a lesser extent, 2), thereby disrupting the

TABLE 88.1
Suggested Dose, Utility and Precautions of Herbs with Pain-Modulating Activity

Herb	Dose	Utility/Precautions
Black cohosh	40–60 mg qd/bid or 60mg (2) bid	Not to exceed 1–3 g/d Possible abortifacient
Borage	500 mg qd/bid as a capsule	Short-term internal use (1 week) Possibly hepatotoxic
Cajuput	1 g/cc topical oil	Not for facial use Not for pediatric use Use sparingly
Cayenne	0.25%, 0.75% cream or topical transdermal gel (not to exceed 10 g/d)	Short-term (2–3 days) use only Avoid oral, occular contact Avoid genital contact
English chamomile	1.5 g bid/tid Infusion 50–200 ml	Not for use during pregnancy
Ginseng		
Korean	1–2 g/d as capsule (100–1250 mg available) or liquid (3 mg/ml)	Not to exceed 3 g/d Contraindicated in cardiovascular, hypertensive diabetic patients Not for use during pregnancy
Siberian	2–3 g/d root as extract (or capsule)	Not for use in hypertensive or diabetic patients
Japanese mint	2–3 drops extracted oil topically applied	Not to exceed 3 times daily Not for orofacial use Not for pediatric use
Kava kava	150–300 mg extract (capsular form) bid	Best taken with food Not to exceed 600 mg/d Not for use in excess of 3 months without supervision Not for use during pregnancy/nursing
Marijuana	2.5, 5.0, 10 mg capsules (Dronabinol: Marinol) 2.5–10 mg bid-qid	Legal ramifications Not for prolonged use Precaution in motoric tasks/coordination-dependent activity
Scotch pine	100 g alcohol extract bid; 20–50% topical cream, ointment, gel (1cc) tid	Not for orofacial use Not for pediatric use Not for use in asthmatic patients
Spruce	20–30% oil ointment (1cc) tid	Not for orofacial use Not for pediatric use Not for use in asthmatic patients
St. John's Wort	125–500 mg (0.3% hypericin) capsules; 200–300 mg tid	Initial 6-week trial recommendation Not for use with MAO-inhibitors, TCA, or SSRI/SNRI agents (potentiated effects) Photosensitizing: avoid UV exposure during use Induces hepatic microsomal P450 enzymes
Turmeric	1.5–3.0 g/d	Not for use in patients with premorbid or active cholecystic disease Not for use during pregnancy
Valerian	100–1000 mg capsules; 100–1000 mg qhs	Titrate dose to effect Not for use with alcohol, benzodiazepines, barbiturates May cause daytime drowsiness/lethargy Not for use during pregnancy or nursing

membrane arachidonic acid cascade that yields pro-inflammatory and pro-nocisponsive prostaglandins.

Although direct hazards and adverse side effects are not reported for therapeutic doses, patients who are hypersensitive to salicylates should not utilize white willow. As well, pediatric use of white willow should be cautious due to possible occurrence of Reyes syndrome. Long-term use and/or dose escalation may yield salicylate toxicity (typically characterized by tinnitus and metabolic acidosis). In light of the salicylate content of white willow, concomittant use of nonsteroidal anti-inflammatories or aspirin is contraindicated. This is to avoid possible adverse hepatic effects, concentration-induced toxic effects, and unwanted thrombolytic effects. There is equivocal evidence to suggest the utility and contraindication of white willow bark in patients with premorbid gastritis and/or history of peptic ulcer disease. Certainly, the use of this compound should be cautious in patients with co- or pre-morbid ulcer due to the systemic action of salicylate on prostaglandin-induced mucus secretion in the stomach, thereby exacerbating ulcerative symptomology. However, studies suggest the direct action of white willow on the gastric mucosa may be considerably less than that of aspirin or other nonsteroidals. Regardless, it is best to be prudent in the use of this compound in patients with peptic or duodenal ulcerative disease.

SUMMARY

The information contained in this chapter is provided as an overview of those herbs identified to have viable, clinically researched evidence for treatment of pain. Their use as primary and/or adjunctive analgesics requires considerable expertise and caution on the part of practitioners. Unfortunately, precise pharmacokinetic parameters of each herbal preparation are not completely understood. A single herbal preparation may contain numerous active principles that are differentially yielded based upon type of preparation. Also, the actual concentration of the active principles may vary widely based upon preparation, quality of herb, season of herbal harvesting, as well as other factors. Accurate prediction of dose–response relationships, time course of effects, specific parameters for interaction and pharmacodynamic mechanisms and actions are somewhat difficult to assess given available information. For the clinician considering integrating phytomedicinals to clinical practice, a working maxim would be to "start low and go slow" utilizing the purest form of the herb commercially available, at the lowest viable dose, incrementally increasing that dose to effect, while observing for putative side effects and potential drug interactions.

To reiterate, recruiting the aid of a compounding pharmacist (to assist in obtaining the purest commercial form of herb), a naturopathic physician, and receiving specific (advanced) training in phytomedicinal practice are strongly advocated. Clinicians must be aware that simply because a substance is "natural" does not guarantee its safety. Although herbs often provide a reasonable alternative to commercially manufactured pharmaceutical products, a complete understanding of their chemistry, pharmacologic mechanisms and effects, and potential physiologic and pharmacologic side effects and interactions is mandatory.

ACKNOWLEDGMENT

The author wishes to thank Connie Parker for her assistance in preparation of all phases of this manuscript.

REFERENCES

Almeida, J.C., & Grimsley, E.W. (1996). Coma from the health food store: interaction between kava and alprazolam. *Annals of Internal Medicine, 125,* 940.

Ammon, H.P., & Wahl, M.A. (1991). Pharmacology of curcuma longa. *Planta Medica, 57,* 1.

Araya, O.S., & Ford, E.J. (1981). An investigation of the type of photosensitization caused by the ingestion of St. John's Wort (hypericum perforatum) by calves. *Journal of Comparative Pathology, 91,* 135.

Attele, A.S., Wu, J.A., & Yuan, C.S. (1999). Ginseng pharmacology: Multiple constituents and multiple actions. *Biochemical Pharmacology, 1,* 58(11), 1685.

Baldt, S., & Wagner, H. (1994). Inhibition of MAO by fractions and constituents of hypericum extract. *Journal Geriatric Psychiatry and Neurology, 7*(1), 57.

Bennett, D. A., Phun, L., & Polk, J.F. (1998). Neuropharmacology of St. John's Wort (hypericum). *Annals of Pharmacotherapy, 32*(11), 1201.

Biro, T., Acs, G., Acs, P., et al. (1997). Receptor advances and understanding of vanilloid receptors, a therapeutic target for treatment of pain and inflammation in the skin. *Journal of Investigative Dermatology, 2,* 56.

Bonte, F., Noel-Hudson, M.S., Wepierre, J., & Meybeck, A. (1997). Protective effect of curcuminoids on epidermal skin cells under oxygen-free radical stress. *Planta Medica, 8,* 265.

Bradley, P.R. (Ed.). (1992). *British herbal compendium,* Dorset, U.K.: British Herbal Medicine Assn.

Cowan, R.A., Heartnel, G., Lowdell, C., Baird, I., & Leak, A. (1984). Metabolic acidosis induced by carbonic anhydrase inhibitors and salicylates in patients with normal renal function. *British Medical Journal, 289,* 6441, 347.

Daiber, W. (1983). Klimakterishe Beschwerden: Ohne Capital Hormone zum Erfolg. *Artzl. Praxis, 35,* 1946.

Davies, L.P., Drew, C.A., Duffield, P., et al. (1992). Kava pirones and resin: Studies on GABA-A, GABA-B, and benzodiazepine binding in rodent brain. *Pharmacology and Toxicology, 71*(2), 120.

Duke, J.A. (1985). *CRC handbook of medicinal herbs.* Boca Raton: CRC Press.

Duker, E.M., Kopanski, L., Jarry, H., & Wattke, W. (1991). Effects of extracts from *simicifuga racemosa* on gonadotropin release in menopausal women and ovariectomized rats. *Planta Medica, 57,* 420.

Faure-Raynaud, M. (1970). Study of volatile oil from abies alba miller. I. Study of raw material. *Acta Poloniae Pharmaceutica, 132*(B), 71.

Furst, D.E., Sarkissian, E., Blocka, K., et al. (1987). Serum concentration of salicylate and naproxen during concurrent therapy in patients with rheumatoid arthritis. *Arthritis and Rheumatism, 30*(10), 1157.

Fusco, B. M., Fiore, G., Gallo, F., et al. (1994). Capsaicin-sensitive sensory neurons in cluster headache: Pathophysiological aspects and therapeutic indication. *Headache, 34*(3) 132.

Gleits, J., Beile, A., Peters, T., et al. (1995). (+/-)-kavain inhibits veratridine-activated voltage-dependent Na^+-channels in synaptosomes prepared from rat cerebral cortex. *Neuropharmacology, 34*(9), 1133.

Hasmeda, M., & Polya, G.M. (1996). Inhibition of cyclic AMP-dependent protein kinase by curcumin. *Phytochemistry, 42,* 599.

Hernandez, M.L., Garcia-Gile, L., Berrendero, F., Ramos, J.A., and Fernandez-Ruiz, J.J. (1997). Delta 9-tetrahydrocanapinol increases activity of tyrosine hydroxylise in cultured fetal mesencephalic neurons. *Journal of Molecular Neuroscience, 8,* 83.

Hiller, K.O., & Zetler, G. (1996). Neuropharmalogical studies on ethanol extracts of *valeriana officinalis*: Behavioral, anti-convulsive properties. *Phytotherapy Research, 10,* 145.

Hoffman, D. (1988). *The herbal handbook: A user's guide to medicinal herbalism.* Rochester, VT: Healing Arts Press.

Huang, H.C., Jan, T.R., & Yeh, S.F. (1992). Inhibitory effect of curcumin, an anti-inflammatory agent on vascular smooth muscle cell proliferation. *European Journal of Pharmacology, 54,* 381.

Ippen, H. (1995). Gamma-linolensure besser aus nachtkerzen-oder aus borretschol? *Zeitschrift Pflanz u Phytotherapie, 16*(3) 167.

Isaacs, O. (1993). Chamaemelum nobile. *Zeitschrift Pflanz u Phytotherapie, 14*(4) 212.

Jamieson, D.D., & Duffield, P.H. (1990). The anti-nociceptive actions of kava components in mice., *Clinical and Experimental Pharmacology and Physiology, 17*(7), 495.

Kohane, D., Kuang, Y., Lou, N., et al. (1999). Vanilloid receptor agonists potentiate the *in vivo* local anesthetic activity of percutaneously injected type-1 sodium channel blockers. *Anesthesiology, 90*(2), 524.

Kuo, S.C., Teng, C.M., Lee, J.C., et al. (1990). Anti-platelet components in panax ginseng. *Planta Medica, 56* (2) 164.

Leung, A.Y. (1980). *Encyclopedia of common natural ingredients used in food, drug and cosmetics.* New York: John Wiley and Sons, Inc.

Lewis, R., Wake, G., Court, G., et al. (1999). Non-ginsenoside nicotinic activity in ginseng species. *Phytotherapy Research, 13*(1), 59.

Liske, E. (1998). Therapeutic efficacy and safety of *simicifuga racemosa* for gynecologic disorders. *Advanced Therapeutics, 15*(1), 45.

Mackie, K., & Hille, B. (1992). Cannabinoids inhibit N-type calcium channels in neuroblastoma-glioma cells. *Proceedings of the National Academy of Science (U.S.A.), 89,* 3825.

Muller, W.D., & Rossol, R. (1994). Effects of hypericum extract on the expression of serotonin receptors. *Journal Geriatric Psychiatry and Neurology, 7*(1), 63.

Newall, C.A., Anderson, L.A., & Phillipson, J.D. (1996). *Herbal medicine: A guide for healthcare professionals.* London: Pharmaceutical Press.

Physician's desk reference for herbal medicines. (2000). Montvale, NJ: Medical Economics Co.

Ridel, E., Hansel, R., & Ehrke, G. (1982). Hemmung des Gamma-aminobuttersaureabbaus durch Valerensaurederivate. *Planta Medica, 46,* 219.

Ruh, N.F., Taylor, J.A., Howlett, A.C., & Welshons, W.V. (1996). The volatile oil composition of fresh and air-dried buds of *cannabis sativa. Journal of Natural Products, 53,* 49.

Schirrmacher, K., Busselberg, D., Langlasch, J.M., et al. (1999). Effects of (+/-)-kavain on voltage-activated inward currents of dorsal root ganglion cells from neonatal rats. *European Neuropsychopharmacology, 9*(1–2), 171.

Schmidt, B., & Heide, L. (1995). The use of salicis cortex in rheumatic disease: Phytotherapy with known mode of action? *Phytomedicine, 61,* 94.

Seizt, U., Schule, A., and Gleitz, J. (1997). [3H]-Monoamine uptake inhibition properties of kava pirones. *Planta Medica, 63*(6), 548.

Srivastava, K.C., Bordia, A., & Verma, S.K. (1995). Curcumin: A major component of food spice turmeric (*curcuma longa*) inhibits aggregation and alters eicosanoid metabolism in human blood platelets. *Prostaglandins Leukotrienes and Essential Fatty Acids, 52,* 232.

Steinegger, E., & Hanscl, R. (1980). *Pharmakognosie* (p. 258). Heidelberg: Springer-Verlag.

Teng, C.M., Kuo, S.C., Ko, F.N., et al. (1989). Anti-platelet actions of panaxynol and ginsenosides isolate from ginseng. *Acta Biochemica et Biophysica, 990*(3), 315.

Teuscher, E. & Lindquist, U. (1994). *Biogene gifte: Biologie Chemie, Pharmakologie.* Stuttgard: Fischer Verlag.

Thomas, D.F., Adams, I.B., Mascareloa, S.W., Martin, B.R., & Razdan, R.K. (1996). Structure-activity analysis of anandamide analogs: Relationship to a cannabinoid pharmacophore. *Journal of Medicinal Chemistry, 58,* 471.

Tyler, V.E. (1994). *Herbs of choice: The therapeutic use of phytomedicinals.* Binghamton: Pharmaceutical Products Press.

Uebelhick, R., Frank, L., & Schewe, H.J. (1998). Inhibition of platelet MAO-B by kava pirone-enriched extract from *piper methysticum forster* (kava kava). *Pharmacopsychiatry, 31*(5), 187.

Wheatley, D. (1998). Hypericum extract: Potential in the treatment of depression. *CNS Drugs, 9,* 431.

Wichtl, M. (1994). *Herbal drugs and phytopharmaceuticals.* Boca Raton: CRC Press.

Yamamoto, I., Matsunaga, T., Kobayashi, H., Watanabe, K., & Yoshimura, H. (1991). Analysis and pharmacotoxicity of feruloyltyramine as a new constituent and p-coumaroyltyramine in cannabis sativa. *Pharmacology, Biochemistry, and Behavior, 40,* 465.

Yun-Choi, H.S., Kim, J.H., & Lee, J. (1987). Potential inhibitors of platelet aggregation from plant sources. *Journal Natural Products, 50*(6), 1059.

89

The Neurobiology of Pain

James Giordano, Ph.D.

Pain is a most beguiling clinical problem. With both subjective and objective components, pain becomes a unique experience for each individual. The neural substrates that are involved in processing noxious input contribute to both the sensation and perception of pain. By understanding the components of the pain transmitting and modulating systems we may gain insight toward the development of therapeutic strategies against chronic pain.

NOCICEPTORS

The first step in the nociceptive sensory pathway is the transduction of noxious stimuli to a relevant neural signal. In cutaneous, muscle, and visceral tissues, free nerve endings of nocisponsive primary afferents are responsible for this transduction step. It remains somewhat unclear whether the free nerve endings respond to the actual noxious stimulus or to evoked changes in the tissues which they innervate. In the latter case, noxious stimuli incur a cascade of cellular damage evoking the release of fatty acids and free ions from cell membranes. Among the fatty acids, arachidonic acid serves as the initiative substrate for induction of the enzymes cyclooxygenase 1 and 2 to catalyze the inflammatory cascade (subsequently mediated by prostaglandins and leukotrienes). Change in local tissue pH and the concentration of various ions, such as potassium (K^+), serves to directly affect membrane polarity of free nerve endings in the affected tissue as well as altering vascular permeability and mast cell degranulation. Degranulation of mast cells causes release of histamine and serotonin, which exacerbate vasodilatory and inflammatory effects.

Serotonin may work directly upon the terminals of free nerve endings to initiate a sodium (Na^+) and/or calcium (Ca^{++}) current leading to heightened excitation.

The burning sensation that often accompanies high-intensity mechanical and thermal stimulation may be indicative of the sequential activation of discrete populations of differentially sensitive nociceptor nerve endings (and their associated primary afferents): first by the stimulus directly, followed by the resultant chemical changes in the affected tissue.

The free nerve endings subserving the transduction of noxious stimuli are responsive to high-intensity mechanical input (i.e., pinch, squeeze, intense pressure), high-intensity thermal input (e.g., noxious heat in excess of 45°C), mixed high-intensity mechanothermal input, and chemical stimulation (disturbance of the local chemical or ionic environment and presence of various pro-nociceptive substances). Transduction occurs as these stimuli evoke changes in the neural membrane integrity, producing a inward sodium and/or calcium current. The receptor potential for free nerve endings appears to be a graded response, with time- and intensity-dependence of the membrane polarity. Subsequent to transduction, the nociceptive signal is transmitted from free nerve endings in the periphery (or viscera) along what appears to be stimulus-specific, labeled lines of nociceptive primary afferent fibers. There are two type of primary nociceptive afferents, A-delta and C-fibers. These subtend distinct types of noxious input (e.g., thermal, mechanical, polymodal) and are responsible for differing subjective qualities of fast (i.e., "first") and slow (i.e., "second") pain, respectively.

0-8493-0926-3/02/$0.00+$1.50
© 2002 by CRC Press LLC

PRIMARY AFFERENTS

A-DELTA FIBERS

These fibers are small, thinly myelinated neurons 1 to 5 μm in diameter, with conduction velocities in the range of 5 to 30 m/sec. The rapid rate of conduction is responsible for the initial sensation of pain (first pain) typically described as sharp, localized, and well defined. A-delta fibers have small receptive fields and are relatively modality specific. A-delta thermosponsive fibers respond to extremes of temperature. One population is activated by noxious heat, with an initial response threshold in the range of 40 to 45°C. Response function increases directly, although not necessarily linearly, as a consequence of temperature elevation, with maximal responses occurring at temperatures of 46 to 53°C. These responses subserve both the rapid, demonstrably painful response to an initial presentation of noxious heat and the ability to quickly discriminate the extent of thermal pain as a function of heat intensity. A second population, high-threshold cold afferents, respond to cold temperatures at or below a threshold of approximately 20°C.

A-delta mechanoreceptive afferents are activated by high-intensity mechanical stimulation (deep pressure, stab, pinch), although these fibers may be sensitized by and become secondarily responsive to noxious heat. Unlike A-delta thermal afferents, sensitized A-delta mechanoreceptive afferents respond to suprathreshold heat (usually in excess of 50 to 55°C) and/or repetitive presentation of noxious heat, rather than to a singular exposure to a heat stimulus at or above the nociceptive threshold. The sensitization of this second population to nociceptive A-delta afferents is thought to underlie clinical patterns of hyperalgesia (increased sensation of pain) seen following heat and burn injury.

C-FIBERS

C-fibers are small, unmyelinated afferents. With fiber diameters ranging from 0.25 to 1.5 μm, the absence of myelin leads to slower conductance velocities that vary from 0.5 to 2 m/sec. This slower conductance subserves "second pain," a diffuse, poorly localized burning, throbbing, and/or gnawing sensation that follows, and is temporally and qualitatively distinct from the initial sensation of first pain. Numerically, C-fibers constitute the majority of primary nociceptive afferents found in cutaneous tissue. C-fibers are polymodal, and can be activated by thermal, mechanical, and chemical stimuli. In addition to responding to noxious (thermal, mechanical, and chemical) stimuli, C-fiber polymodal afferents may be activated by certain types of non-noxious, low-intensity stimulation. C-fiber thresholds to such non-noxious stimuli can be sensitized by high-intensity heat, pressure, or chemical disturbance. Similarly, C-fibers may be sensitized to lower

thresholds for mechanical and chemical stimuli by noxious heat. However, unlike thermal sensitization of mechanosponsive A-delta fibers, C-fibers are sensitized by noxious heat of lower intensity (48 to 50°C). This may account for both the persistent second pain and hyperalgesia that occur following a milder burn injury. In this light, C-fibers may contribute to multiple sensations from a painful region. C-fibers also innervate muscle tissue, localized to the intrafibril matrix, tendons, and areas surrounding the vascular walls. C-fiber muscle afferents are polymodal, and are responsible for the nociceptive response to intense mechanical stimulation, numerous chemicals (including lactic acid), and heat. Although not directly activated by muscular contraction or the stretch reflex, intramuscular C-fibers can be sensitized (under ischemic conditions) to respond to even small myofibril contraction, and may respond vigorously to excessive stretch. This sensitization helps to explain the diffusely painful response to both passive and active movement of over-exerted, traumatized, or ischemic skeletal muscle.

VISCERAL PRIMARY NOCICEPTIVE AFFERENTS

Primary afferent innervation of the viscera is not completely understood. Conflicting evidence exists regarding the potential for nociceptive transmission from the viscera. Numerous stimuli are capable of producing visceral pain. Distention, compression, and chemical and tactile irritation of several visceral structures have all been shown to elicit distinct and quantifiable pain responses in humans that are often accompanied by reports of localized somatic and cutaneous pain. The diversity of responsiveness to various types of noxious stimuli suggests the presence of afferents with polymodal qualities. Taken with the diffuse, poorly localized quality that often accompanies visceral pain, such findings implicate the involvement of C-fiber-type innervation. C-fiber-type afferents innervate several visceral structures, although studies also have demonstrated the presence of A-delta fibers with polymodal sensitivity, particularly in the testes and structures surrounding the heart. As well, a small, unmyelinated J-fiber has been identified in the parenchyma of the lung. J-fibers have structural properties, receptive fields, and conductance velocities similar to C-fibers and respond to high-intensity mechanical changes in lung volume (i.e., distention and compression), inflammation, and exogenous chemical irritants (e.g., acidic and basic substances).

Nociceptive afferent innervation of visceral structures has several characteristics that are markedly distinct from those in cutaneous and muscle tissues. First, nociceptive afferent innervation of the viscera is relatively sparse, with considerable diffusion at projection sites at second-order neurons within the spinal dorsal horn. Thus, nociceptive input from the viscera may not evoke strong, well-localized volleys of excitation capable of spatially and/or temporally summating at spinal relays. Second, the nature of visceral afferents is such that sensitization by chemical mediators and/or sympathetic activity (see below) appears to be required for their sustained firing. Given the sparse distribution of these fibers throughout the viscera and the diffuse connections with nociceptive units of the spinal cord, it appears that this sustained firing is responsible for the activation of second-order spinal afferents, and ultimately the transmission of visceral nociceptive signals. The perception of visceral nociception is vague, becoming more intense (and better localized) as increased painful activity in the innervated structure(s) sensitizes the involved afferents. Third, nociceptive afferent innervation of the viscera is often structurally co-localized with sympathetic afferent (and perhaps efferent) neurons. Noxious stimulation from the viscera can lead to concurrent excitation of both visceral nociceptive afferents and sympathetic innervation, capable of producing retrograde sympathetic outflow and sympathetically maintained regional hyperalgesia. Last, visceral nociceptive afferents are often integrated anatomically with somato-cutaneous nociceptive afferents within dorsal root ganglia or within the neuropil of second-order afferents of the spinal cord. Reciprocal sensitization within the dorsal root ganglion and the overlap of second-order receptive fields for visceral and somato-cutaneous input subserve the somatic referred component that is characteristic of much of visceral pain. In this regard it becomes clinically relevant to understand the convergence of visceral and somato-cutaneous afferents when attempting to predicting involvement of visceral structures in patterns of referred somatic pain.

PROJECTIONS TO THE SPINAL DORSAL HORN

Although a small number of nociceptive afferents synapse within the ventral spinal cord, the vast majority of somato-cutaneous and visceral nociceptive primary afferent fibers project to defined areas of the superficial dorsal horn. This area has been anatomically distinguished into discrete zones, known as the laminae of Rexed. The laminae, or layers, are numbered consecutively from dorsal to ventral regions. Both A-delta and C-fibers have been shown to terminate on specific populations of second-order spinal neurons in laminae I, II, IIa, and V, which are the origins of the ascending spinal pathways critical to pain transmission.

NEUROCHEMISTRY OF PRIMARY AFFERENT PAIN TRANSMISSION

The principal neurochemical mediator at the synaptic cleft between primary afferent nociceptors and dorsal horn cells appears to be glutamate. Post-synaptically, glutamate is capable of binding to two sets of discrete receptors. The AMPA (α-amino-3-hydroxy-5-methyl-isoxazole-4 propionic acid) receptor appears to be the initial or first molecular

target for glutamate binding. Glutamate-induced AMPA receptor activation evokes a ligand-gated sodium current in post-synaptic second-order neurons of the dorsal horn that produces a rapid, depolarization. Glutamate is also capable of binding to a second site, the NMDA (N-methyl-D-aspartate) receptor. It appears that AMPA receptors either directly or indirectly modulate activation of NMDA receptors by glutamate through allosteric modulation of magnesium binding to a shared or cooperative domain of the NMDA receptors. With persistent AMPA receptor activation, the rise in intracellular sodium displaces a magnesium "gate" from the NMDA receptor, thereby increasing its sensitivity or releasing it from an inaccessible configuration to actively bind glutamate. It is hypothesized that this molecular change on the receptor level subserves a component of the altered neurological responses from acute to chronic pain. Glutamate binding at the NMDA receptor is responsible for mediating an inward calcium current that initiates a protein kinase-C to catalyze the induction of the enzyme nitric oxide (NO) synthase required for the intracellular production of NO.

Protein kinase-C is also capable of catalyzing other intracellular enzymatic reactions that stimulate protein synthesis in the second-order neuron. These glutamate-dependent protein kinase-C related reactions may be responsible for the production of new membrane-bound calcium channels and "new" NMDA receptors that may mediate or prolong sensitization of second-order afferents to input from nociceptors. It also has been posited that these molecular changes subserve, at least in part, second-order afferent sensitization to subthreshold primary afferent input, thereby producing hyperalgesic and perhaps allodynic responses. There is further evidence to suggest that prolonged activation of newly synthesized NMDA receptors may instigate protein kinase-C mediated nuclear reactions that may affect cell vitality and viable function (i.e., induction of apoptotic mechanisms of programmed cell degeneration and death).

Primary afferent nociceptors also release the undecapeptide substance-P. It is unclear whether substance-P is released directly following depolarization of primary afferents or as a consequence of feedback stimulation following glutamate release. Substance-P binds post-synaptically to neurokinin-1 (NK-1) receptors on second-order dorsal horn neurons. Prolonged activation of neurokinin receptors has been shown to result in the initiation and accumulation of a stimulatory proto-oncogene, *c-fos* and its protein product. *c-fos* proto-oncogene appears to be responsible for mediating increased metabolic activity within the second-order neuron. Also, *c-fos* may interact on a molecular level to induce or increase the production of other proto-oncogenes, namely, *ras* and perhaps *jun*. Together, these proto-oncogenes may be responsible for promoting nuclear mechanisms that code for novel (and perhaps aberrant) structural and functional proteins involved in remodeling second-order neurons that are actively processing chronic pain.

In addition, sensitized primary afferents are capable of anti-dromic or retrograde release of neurochemical mediators of the inflammatory response. Prolonged activation of primary afferent A-delta, and particularly C-fibers, has been shown to evoke an anti-dromic release of substance-P. Substance-P provokes degranulation of mast cells in peripheral tissue leading to the release of several potent vasoactive and pro-inflammatory mediators including histamine and serotonin. Substance-P also may act directly as a vasodilator. In addition to anti-dromic release of substance-P, primary afferent nociceptors release calcitonin gene-related peptide (CGRP) from terminal branches to affect distal peripheral (and/or visceral) tissues. CGRP activates the enzyme NO synthase from the vascular endothelium leading to an increase production of nitric oxide and, ultimately, vasodilatation. Taken together, the effects of histamine, mast cell-derived serotonin, substance-P, and CGRP produce potent peripheral vasodilatory effects that lead to extravasation of chemical mediators that both propagate the inflammatory response and are directly pro-nocisponsive. These include vasoactive intestinal peptide (VIP), bradykinin, and platelet-derived serotonin. Of particular interest is the effect of rising concentrations of serotonin in extra-vascular tissue from mast cells and degranulated platelets. Our research has demonstrated that as peripheral serotonin concentrations rise, serotonin 5-HT$_3$ receptors on terminals of C-fiber primary afferents become directly stimulated, facilitating an increase in C-fiber depolarization and continuity of this cycle. These mechanisms help to explain how prolonged primary afferent activity can transform acute and subacute pain into a chronic condition with distinct neurologic and neurochemical properties.

SECOND-ORDER AFFERENTS

The dorsal horn of the spinal cord is a critical site for the convergence and neural processing of nociceptive information from peripheral primary afferent fibers. A-delta and C-fibers form synaptic connections upon distinct classes of wide dynamic range (WDR) and nociceptive-specific (NS) neurons within the spinal cord whose functional properties contribute to spatial and temporal transformations of the afferent input. These second-order neurons aggregate in the dorsal horn, project contralaterally, and ascend within the anterolateral quadrant(s) as the spinothalamic tract (STT) to sites within the brainstem, midbrain, and thalamus. The unique physiologic characteristics of WDR and NS neurons encode specific qualities of intensity, modality, and localization to the nociceptive signal that is transmitted to supraspinal targets.

WIDE DYNAMIC RANGE NEURONS

Wide dynamic range (WDR) neurons are localized with the highest concentrations in laminae I, II, V, and VI, with greatest numbers found in the latter levels. Although WDR neurons receive input from low-threshold cutaneous mechanoreceptor afferents (A-β type), they are also a site of convergence for both A-delta and C-fiber nociceptive afferents. WDR neurons that are driven by nociceptive input are organized hierarchically within the dorsal horn, with the majority of primary A-delta and C-fiber afferent input occurring in laminae V. The size and responsivity of WDR neuron receptive fields increases progressively from laminae I to V: WDR units in laminae I and II have smaller receptive fields that are sensitive to gentle mechanical stimuli, those of laminae V have larger, overlapping receptive fields with graded sensitivities containing small, discrete regions excited by non-nociceptive input and broad regions that are maximally sensitive to high-threshold nociceptive stimulation.

WDR neurons are not individually sensitive to specific types of stimuli. Rather, individual WDR neurons, based upon response properties within their receptive fields, function to discriminate stimulus intensity. Increases in stimulus intensity activate coexistent areas of receptive fields of numerous WDR neurons. This pattern of engagement would involve slight differences in temporal activation, with individual WDR responses becoming phase-shifted. The activation of greater numbers of WDR neurons by high-intensity nociceptive stimuli would, therefore, result in spatial and temporal summation of these responses.

NOCICEPTIVE SPECIFIC (NS) NEURONS

In contrast to the anatomical distribution of WDR neurons, nociceptive specific (NS) neurons are found in highest concentrations in laminae I and II, with lesser numbers in laminae V. NS neurons receive excitatory input from A-delta fibers and polymodal C-fiber afferents. Generally, NS neurons have small, non-overlapping receptive fields with a well-defined, center-surround organization. The central region is maximally excited by high intensity stimuli, while the outer region is differentially excited by frequency-based repetitive stimulation. This outer region may be inhibited by non-noxious input. The homogeneity of input from nocisponsive primary afferents and the small size and nociceptive selectivity of their receptive fields provide evidence that NS neurons appear to function in localization, and perhaps qualitative discrimination of particular types of noxious input (i.e., noxious pressure and/or heat).

Although painful sensations and responses can be evoked by WDR neuron excitation alone, WDR and NS activity appears to be necessary for the constellation of spatial and temporal qualities ascribed to pain. This becomes apparent when the convergent inputs of A-delta and C-fibers upon WDR and NS neurons are considered.

The unique properties of the primary afferents and the second-order neurons essentially assemble the neurologic pain signal. For example, the sensation of first pain as punctate, well-localized, and temporally well-defined is a function of the response characteristics of both rapidly conducting A-delta primary afferents and their excitation of WDR and NS neurons. In contrast, second pain, a more diffuse, long-lasting nociceptive sensation that follows the initial stimulus is the result of the threshold, firing and conduction properties of C-fibers sustained by local tissue damage and/or chemical change, as well as patterns of temporal and spatial summation of C-fiber inputs by WDR and NS neurons. Both WDR and NS neurons are capable of after-responses that persist as a consequence of nociceptive afferent volley number and frequency; factors related to nociceptive stimulus intensity and continuity.

The anatomic and physiologic properties of second-order afferents also subserve the phenomenon of referred pain. As previously discussed, primary afferent innervation of visceral and deep muscular structures is organized so that these fibers converge upon WDR and NS neurons that also receive input from primary nociceptive (and non-nociceptive) afferents from specific somato-cutaneous regions. The convergence of visceral and cutaneous afferents from a given somatotome upon second-order WDR and NS neurons underlies patterns of clinical referred pain syndromes. Thus, sensory information from the viscera is often interpreted subjectively as afferent information from a cutaneous structure within the corresponding somatotome.

SPINOTHALAMIC TRACT(S)

The majority of WDR and NS neurons project contralaterally within the spinal cord and ascend within the anterolateral quadrant, forming the spinothalamic tract(s) (STT). A minority of fibers remain ipsilateral, and ascend outside of the STT within the ventrolateral white matter to supraspinal sites that correspond to the contralateral anterolateral quadrant projections. Anatomically, axons from second-order neurons in the superficial dorsal horn (laminae I and II) are segregated from those of deeper laminae (lamina V). This provides anatomical separation between the neospinothalamic (NSTT) and paleo-spinothalalmic (PSTT) tracts. While both the NSTT and PSTT may be considered "labeled-lines" for the transmission of pain signals, the differential localization of NS neurons to laminae I and II, in contrast to a greater abundance of WDR neurons in lamina V, subserves functional distinctions in the type of nociceptive information that is transmitted in these pathways.

The NSTT projects directly to the ventroposterior lateral (VPL) nuclei of the thalamus and is composed predominately of NS neurons from lamina I and II. WDR neurons are in smaller numbers within these laminae and they comprise only a minority of NSTT fibers. Recall that NS neurons receive almost completely homogeneous input from A-delta and high-threshold polymodal C-fiber afferents, and encode stimulus localization and modality. Therefore, the main role of the NSTT appears to involve transmission of these signal qualities to the thalamus.

The PSTT is composed of axons from second-order neurons arising in lamina V of the spinal cord. WDR neurons constitute the majority of cells from this lamina, with only a smaller number of NS neurons contributing to the axonal pool of the PSTT. Heterogeneous input to lamina V WDR neurons from both nocisponsive and non-nocisponsive primary afferents contributes to the transmission of some non-nociceptive signals along the PSTT. WDR neurons of lamina V also send axons ipsilaterally to ascend within the dorsal column medial lemniscal tract. This latter pathway is responsible for the transmission of light touch, vibration, and other low-threshold stimuli. Given the role of lamina V WDR neurons to encode noxious stimulus intensities, the co-localized transmission of nociceptive and non-nociceptive afferent information within the PSTT appears to serve a stimulus discriminatory function. This is further supported by the properties of PSTT WDR neurons to accumulate strong after-responses following nociceptive input. Such after-responses override weaker impulses evoked by non-nociceptive afferent stimuli, and produce temporally summated volleys within the PSTT. These events are correlated to, and appear to subserve the qualities and subjective characteristics of clinically relevant, second, and/or chronic pain.

Unlike the NSTT, the PSTT is not a direct thalamic pathway. PSTT fibers project to several supraspinal sites that are involved in (nociceptive) sensory processing and that may exert pain modulatory control. The PSTT may be divided into spinoreticular, spinotectal, and ultimately spinothalamic projections. Spinoreticular pathways project to areas of the brainstem reticular formation. These include the raphe nuclei of the rostroventral medulla and the nuclei reticularis gigantocellularis (NRGC) and para-gigantocellularis (NRpG) of the caudal pons.

Spinotectal projections terminate within the tectum and periaqueductal grey (PAG) region of the midbrain. The spinoreticular and spinotectal circuits function in centrifugal pain control and ascending neurons from these sites serve as relays between spinal pathways and higher centers that mediate the perceptual and affective dimensions of pain. Of particular note are defined tracts from the reticular formation to several regions of the limbic forebrain, and a reciprocal neuraxis involving the PAG, the periventricular gray region (PVG), and hypothalamus. Thalamic projections of the PSTT differ from those of the NSTT; PSTT fibers project diffusely to the thalamus, with terminations at several intralaminar nuclei. (See Figure 89.1.)

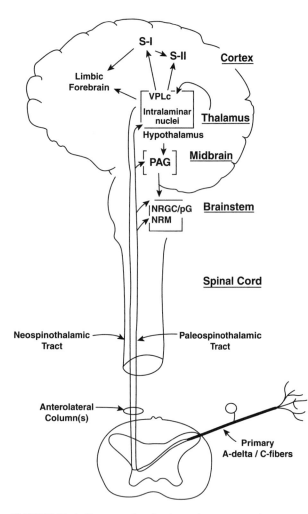

FIGURE 89.1 Cross-sectional schematic representation (not to scale) of spinothalamic tracts projecting to supraspinal loci involved in nociceptive processing.

BRAINSTEM NOCICEPTIVE NEURAXES

PSTT neurons differentially project to specific sites within the brainstem. Some stimulus specificity exists in PSTT activation of raphe and/or NRGC/NRpG neurons. Input from NS and/or WDR units excited by thermosponsive primary afferents appears to evoke greater excitation of raphe circuitry, while WDR and NS neurons driven by mechanosponsive input elicit somewhat greater activation of the NRGC/NRpG. Both circuits are apparently engaged by chemosponsive or polymodal C-fiber afferent activation of WDR or NS neurons. It has been suggested that such stimulus specificity is maintained at the midbrain level, and may be involved in the differential activation of PAG-raphe or PAG-NRGC centrifugal analgesic systems. The former system involves a release of opioids from the PAG that disinhibits serotonergic cells of the raphe nuclei, thereby causing an increased turnover and release of serotonin in pathways that descend in the dorsal lateral funiculi. These serotonergic fibers synapse heterogeneously in laminae I, II, and V, where

serotonin may bind to serotonin 5-HT1$_b$ receptors on processes of second-order nociceptive neurons. As well, serotonin may bind to 5-HT1$_b$ receptors on an interneuron pool in several laminae of the dorsal horn to disinhibit the release of the inhibitory transmitter gamma-amino-butyric acid (GABA) and enkephalin to produce graded inhibition of second-order pain-transmitting afferents. PAG-NRGC connections involve a release of opioids from the periacqueductal grey that disinhibit noradrenergic neurons of the reticular formation (whose axons similarly descend in the dorsal lateral funiculi) to evoke a release of norepinephrine in laminae II and V. Norepinephrine binds to α_2 receptors on primary (and perhaps second-order afferents) to produce a graded hyperpolarizing inhibitory current, thereby toning down these neurons and producing an analgesic response. Whether these distinctions actually subserve modality specificity or reflect differential activation based upon stimulus intensity remains speculative. Although stimulus or intensity differences in the involvement of particular reticular nuclei exist, it is unlikely that any further discriminative processing of the nociceptive signal occurs at the reticular level. PSTT excitation of reticular neurons also activates neural systems involved in pain-related aversive and arousal responses.

MIDBRAIN NOCICEPTIVE MECHANISMS

Anatomical evidence demonstrates that PSTT fibers project to the midbrain PAG both directly and through interneuronal pathways from the reticular formation. Studies suggest that the PAG is somatotopically and perhaps stimulus-specifically organized. Somatotopic organization corresponds to the ascending hierarchy of PSTT afferents from progressively rostral somatotomes: the posterior PAG receives input from PSTT fibers of the caudal spinal cord while the anterior PAG receives PSTT projections from more rostral regions.

Stimulus-specific organization of the PAG seems to be a function of the population characteristics of PSTT WDR or NS neurons that are selectively excited by mechanical, thermal, or polymodal primary afferents. While it is difficult to determine whether absolute stimulus-specific organization exists, it is likely that regions of the PAG respond to somatotopic innervation of the periphery and would thus be maximally excited by input from a particular modality or intensity.

Although the function of the PAG in centrifugal pain control is clear, the role of the PAG in afferent processing of the nociceptive signal remains more enigmatic. Pathways exist between the PAG and hypothalamus and several structures of the forebrain. Stimulation of the PAG or fibers within this pathway elicit an array of arousal and behavioral activation responses that have distinct aversive or frightening emotional content. It is not completely understood whether the PAG mediates these responses alone, or acts in concert with reticular structures, higher brain structures of the limbic system, or both.

THE THALAMUS

The NSTT and PSTT project to different nuclei within the thalamus. NSTT neurons project to a caudal area of the ventroposterior lateral nucleus (VPLc). Nociceptive inputs from the NSTT are arranged in columnar zones that are somatotopically organized. Thalamic neurons within these zones retain many response characteristics of WDR and NS units. Thalamic wide-range neurons have center-surround receptive fields with distinct, small areas sensitive to low-threshold excitation and a broad area that is excited by high-threshold nociceptive input. Thalamic NS neurons, like their spinothalamic counterparts, have smaller receptive fields that are excited by high-intensity mechanical or thermal input.

WDR and NS neurons of the VPLc summate responses as a function of stimulus frequency and intensity. Slow temporal and spatial summation is accompanied by a prolonged firing phase that exceeds the actual noxious stimulus and primary and secondary afferent discharges. This transformation parallels the time-course for the human experience of pain. It is probable that the temporal aspects of pain *perception* reflect serial processing of afferent information from the peripheral to the thalamic levels, with progressive extension of after-discharges along the pathway. It is tempting to speculate that such effects may "match" sensory, arousal, and environmental cues in establishing conditioned responses to circumstances surrounding painful stimuli.

The PSTT projects to several intralaminar thalamic nuclei, including the nucleus centralis lateralis and medialis dorsalis. Most of the neurons within these thalamic areas are of the wide-range type, sensitive to both nociceptive and non-nociceptive activation and with extensive overlapping input from cutaneous and visceral innervation. These units do not have the adaptive properties of neurons of the VPLc; intralaminar neurons summate responses, but response patterns do not reflect direct spatial or temporal transformation of increments in stimulus frequency or intensity. Unlike neurons of the VPLc, intralaminar neurons appear to be arranged in a "looser" somatotopic pattern and project diffusely to several regions of the cortex. The response patterns of individual intralaminar neurons, together with their anatomic distribution and cortical projections, suggest that thalamic connections of the PSTT act more as a relay to engage cortical systems involved in behavioral activation associated with nociception.

CORTICAL PROJECTIONS

Neurons from the NSTT project to the VPLc of the thalamus; thalamo-cortical fibers from this region terminate in S-I (and to a lesser extent S-II areas) of the somatosensory cortex. Thalamo-cortical fibers from the intralaminar nuclei, driven by the PSTT, project more diffusely, with only a small number terminating in S-I or S-II. The somatotopic organization of the thalamus is preserved in cortical projections, and nociceptive input contributes to distinct regions of somatosensory dominance within the cortex (i.e., the so-called sensory "homunculus," the spatial representation of bodily structures across the cortical sensory field). Somatosensory cortical regions are arranged in vertical dominance columns in which hierarchical processing of afferent input occurs. Only a small percentage of nociceptive input constitutes each given cortical column. Nociceptive thalamo-cortical input is distributed differentially within each column. Superficial cortical layers receive thalamic input from non-nociceptive pathways, while WDR- and NS-activated inputs are concentrated throughout the deeper cortical layers. Thus, for any given bodily region represented in a cortical column there is an array of non-noxious information (relayed through medial lemniscal tracts) and nociceptive information (relayed through the STTs) that creates the "depiction" of sensations that determines the subjective sensory experience. The integrity of the pain signal, and the unique qualities of its duration and intensity are a function of the additive transformation of afferent volleys from primary nociceptors through multiple processing ultimately terminating in cortical neurons. The slow adaptation, long after-discharges, and spatial summation of cortical S-I and S-II neurons represent the final and most direct contribution to the temporal and intensity dimensions of pain perception. Therefore, the experience of pain is not only individually variant, but may vary according to myriad combinations of exteroceptive circumstances for each individual.

The multiple intra-cortical projections from S-I/S-II to other parietal, frontal, and temporal regions most probably engage these brain areas in discriminatory, cognitive, and affective dimensions of pain.

PAIN MODULATING SYSTEMS

CORTICAL INHIBITORY PROCESSING

Neurons of the sensory cortex are capable of inhibitory control over the thalamo-cortical units of STT origin that project to them (although cortico-thalamic inhibition can also occur over neurons of the medial lemniscal tract that are non-nocisponsive). The extent of inhibition appears to vary with the frequency and intensity of thalamo-cortical input. For nociceptive input that is both rapidly temporally and spatially summating, a greater level of inhibition exists. Cortical inhibition involves "normalization" or "stabilization" of afferent volleys. This compensates for differences in response characteristics between thalamic and cortical neurons and ultimately enhances the input-response function of thalamically driven nociceptive cortical inputs. In this way, a more direct transformation of the incoming signal is generated without over-summation. Cortical neurons also can excite thalamo-cortical fibers and STT units directly. This inhibition and excitation serve a modulatory role over afferent information that affects cortical circuitry. Cortical neurons can discriminately amplify or reduce the extent of nociceptive input. Such modifications strengthen the signal-to-noise ratio of particular afferent volleys and facilitate discrimination of sensory input. As well, this alternate excitation/inhibition may subserve changes in the nociceptive sensorium as a consequence of levels of cortical activity (e.g., sleep, hypnosis, biofeedback, etc.).

MIDBRAIN PAIN MODULATION

There is considerable evidence to show that the midbrain PAG is a principal site for endogenous pain control. Efferent projections from mesolimbic structures and the hypothalamus are capable of exciting PAG opioid neurons, as do inputs from the PSTT. The PAG exerts pain modulation by centrifugal inhibition of the PSTT and NSTT via disinhibition of bulbospinal projections from the raphe nuclei and NRGC/NRpG. Defined pathways from the PAG to the raphe nuclei and NRGC/NRpG are activated by high-threshold, high-frequency afferent volleys from the PSTT. Mechanical, thermal, or polymodal nocisponsive units of the PSTT appear to differentially stimulate discrete areas of the PAG to activate the raphe nuclei, NRGC/NRpG, or both. It is not fully understood whether selective PAG engagement of raphe-spinal or NRGC/NRpG-spinal neuraxes is dependent upon the modality, frequency, or intensity of the evoking afferent input.

The connections between the PAG and brainstem are polysynaptic, involving one or more pools of interneuronal relays. These multiple circuits function in levels of modulation that have the capacity for both serial and concomitant activation. This type of "volume control" is a function of the nature of the afferent nociceptive stimulus, the extent of PAG activation by PSTT (and perhaps hypothalamic and mesolimbic) neurons, and the excitation or inhibition of specific neural circuits to the brainstem. Thus, the PAG can discriminately recruit bulbospinal substrates whose net output determines the extent and properties of centrifugal pain modulation.

BULBOSPINAL PAIN MODULATION

Projections from the PAG synapse upon interneurons with terminations in the ventromedial pons and rostro-ventral medulla of the brainstem. These are the subcerulear nuclear group of the pons, consisting of the nucleus reticularis gigantocellularis (NRGC), nucleus reticularis paragigantocellularis (NRpG), and the nucleus paragigantocellularis lateralis (NpGL). These sites are often referred to as the reticular magnocellular nuclei (RMC). In the rostro-ventral medulla. PAG-originating interneurons synapse on neurons of the raphe nuclei, including the nuclei raphe alatus and raphe lateralis. These sites are combined when referring to the nucleus raphe magnus (NRM). The NRM and RMC directly receive efferent input from the PAG and afferent input from the PSTT. Both neuraxes are capable, either alone or in concert, of exciting NRM or RMC neurons to elicit centrifugal pain modulation. Inhibitory connections between these groups of brainstem nuclei exist as well. This inter-brainstem inhibition appears to determine the relative participation of NRM, RMC, or both groups in bulbospinal analgesia; moderate levels of activity within the RMC inhibit the NRM. In contrast, higher levels of RMC activity excite certain NRM neurons. Projections from the NRM and RMC descend in the dorsolateral funiculi (DLF) of the spinal cord and terminate in dense synaptic fields within laminae I, II, and V of the dorsal horn. Synaptic connections within these layers involve polysynaptic circuits of multiple spinal interneurons, as well as monosynaptic contacts with wide dynamic range, nociceptive-specific and primary afferent neurons.

Spinal interneurons receiving efferent projections from the brainstem synapse on WDR and NS second-order neurons as well as the terminals of primary afferent fibers. These interneurons are neurochemically heterogeneous, many release the inhibitory transmitter glycine, while others release the opioids enkephalin and/or dynorphin. These interneuronal contacts provide selective, multi-focal inhibition of specific groups of nociceptive afferents.

Synaptic connections between bulbospinal and WDR, NS, and perhaps primary afferent neurons exist in laminae I, II, and V. A single fiber from the brainstem may synapse on several second-order afferents within a given lamina. The differential projection of NRM or RMC terminals onto discrete populations of mechanosponsive, thermosponsive, or polymodally driven WDR and NS neurons in laminae I, II, and V further suggests that some stimulus- or modality-specificity may exist in the analgesic axis that originates from these brainstem nuclei. Figure 89.2 provides a schematic representation of this possible organization.

INTRASPINAL PAIN MODULATION

In addition to descending analgesic systems from the brainstem, pain modulation can occur through the activation of local circuits within the spinal dorsal horn. Interneurons that receive collateral projections from primary A-delta and C-fibers are found in laminae I, II,

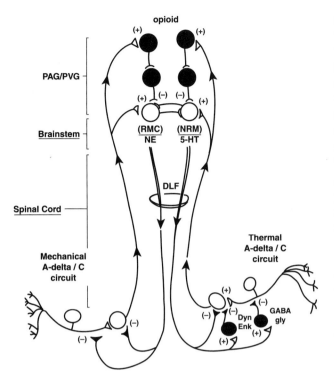

FIGURE 89.2 Schematic depiction of putative analgesic neuraxes modulating thermal and mechanical noxious input. Thermosponsive A-delta and C-fiber afferents may engage a descending serotonergic circuit (either directly or via activation of opioid neurons in the PAG/PVG that inhibit interneurons to disinhibit raphe-spinal mechanisms). 5-HT released from raphe-spinal neurons may (a) directly inhibit pain-transmitting afferents; (b) act at (excitatory) 5-HT$_3$ receptors on spinal opioid, GABA, and glycine interneurons to evoke release of the transmitters and modulate activity of primary or secondary nociceptive afferents. Mechanosponsive A-delta and C-fibers appear to engage a descending noradrenergic neuraxis (from the magnocellular reticular formation) either directly or indirectly via PAG/PVG activation. Norepinephrine released from reticulo-spinal neurons acts at α_2 receptors to modulate activity of primary and second-order nociceptive afferents. DLF = dorso-lateral funiculus; Dyn = dynorphin; Enk = leu/met-enkephalin; GABA = γ-amino butyric acid; gly = glycine; (+) = excitatory synapse(s); (−) = inhibitory synapse(s).

and V. These interneurons form reciprocal synapses upon primary afferent(s) and, in certain cases, second-order WDR and NS neurons. The majority of such interneuronal connections are found within a given horizontal section of the spinal cord, although some interneurons have terminal fields that are trans-segmental. Pharmacologic and electrophysiologic evidence has demonstrated that these interneurons are inhibitory. Many produce and release the inhibitory transmitter glycine, as well as the opioid peptide dynorphin. The pharmacology of this latter compound has been exten-

sively studied. Dynorphin binds post-synaptically with κ-opioid receptors. There is some heterogeneity in κ-receptor populations; however, most found in the spinal cord are negatively coupled to N-type calcium ionic channels. Dynorphin binding at these κ-sites on primary or second-order afferents closes the calcium channel thereby producing a hyperpolarizing inhibitory current, essentially "tuning down" or "shutting off" the transmission of nociceptive information along this neuraxis. This local circuit inhibition modulates firing of primary A-delta and C-fibers afferents; a particular pattern of primary afferent firing may excite populations of local interneurons to exert recurrent inhibition. Similarly, primary afferent activity may evoke local spinal inhibition of certain populations of WDR and NS neurons.

Low-threshold mechanosponsive dorsal column afferents, driven by a A-β mechanoreceptors, also exert modulatory influence over WDR and NS neurons that comprise the STT. Interneurons in laminae IIa, III, and IV with synaptic fields linking the dorsal columns and STT evoke brief inhibitory post-synaptic potentials (IPSPs) in STT cells following dorsal column excitation by low-intensity mechanical stimuli. These IPSPs persist after termination of the low intensity stimulus, and cause a brief, rightward shift in both the time- and threshold-based stimulus response function of the affected WDR and NS cells within the STT. In other words, low-level mechanical stimulation of the dorsal column tract is capable of overriding or de-sensitizing WDR and NS activity within the STT. This phenomenon subserves the clinical efficacy of low-frequency transcutaneous electrical nerve stimulation (TENS), and helps to explain the somewhat beneficial effect of rubbing a painful area.

SUMMARY

The anatomical and physiologic systems that subserve pain and analgesia are complex. Heterogeneous populations of neurons from the periphery, through the spinal cord, brainstem, thalamus, and ultimately the cortex with discrete neurochemical and physiological properties, all contribute to the amalgam of sensations that compromise the constellation of features known as pain. By understanding the structure and function of this system, we may develop enhanced therapeutic approaches to acute and chronic pain that target these substrates more effectively and selectively, thereby reducing deleterious side effects while facilitating an enhanced quality of life.

ACKNOWLEDGMENTS

The author wishes to acknowledge the untiring assistance of Connie Parker in the preparation of this manuscript.

TABLE 89.1
Physiologic and Pharmacologic Properties of Primary Afferent Nociceptors

Type	Stimulus	Anatomy	Diameter	Conduction/Properties	Chemistry
A-delta	High threshold Mechanical Thermal (>45°C) (<20°C) Mixed-sensitized	Free endings Myelinated Punctate fields	1–5 μm	10–30 m/sec Fast; first pain; well localized	Glutamate Subs-P CGRP (?) VIP Post-synaptic activation of AMPA receptors Short-term NK-1 receptor activation
C-fiber	High threshold Polymodal Thermal Mechanical Chemical Sensitized	Free endings Unmyelinated Diffuse receptive fields	0.5–1.5 μm	0.5–2 m/sec Slow; second pain; chronic; poorly localized	Glutamate Subs-P CGRP CGRP (?) CCK (?) Post-synaptic activation of NMDA receptors Potentiated NK-1 receptor activation May induce neural plasticity (?)

TABLE 89.2
Physiologic and Pharmacologic Properties of Selected Pain Modulating Systems

System	Anatomy	Chemistry	Physiology/Properties
<u>Intraspinal</u> Segmental	Interneurons, laminae II, V Synaptic contact with recurrent processes of A-delta fibers	Opioid Dynorphin Leu/met-enkephalin GABA Glycine	 Acts upon κ-receptors Acts upon δ (and perhaps μ) receptors Acts upon $GABA_B$ receptors: potentiates chloride flux hyperpolarization Stabilization of membrane fatty acid metabolism Glycine binding site modulation
<u>Bulbospinal</u> NRM	Descending fibers from NRM of medulla Fibers descend via DLF Mono- and polysynaptic contacts with primary and second-order units of dorsal horn Synapse upon interneurons	5-HT	Acts upon post-synaptic 5-HT$_{1b}$ receptors on (pre- synaptic) primary afferents and (post-synaptic) second-order neurons Hyperploarizing; inhibitory Acts upon post-synaptic 5-HT$_3$ receptors on GABA, glycine, and opioid spinal interneurons; excitatory; evokes release of inhibitory modulators
RMC	Descending fibers from NRGC/NRpG of pons Fibers descend via DLF Mono- and polysynaptic contacts with primary and second-order afferents of dorsal horn	NE	Acts upon post-synaptic α$_2$-receptors on (pre- synpatic) primary afferents and second-order afferents Graded hyperpolarization, inhibitory
<u>Midbrain</u> PAG PVG	Multilevel connections: inputs from hypothalamus, limbic system, cortex Activated by STT Polysynaptic contact with brainstem to disinhibit centrifugal modulatory systems	Opioid Leu/met-enkephalin endorphin	 Acts upon μ and δ sites Acts upon μ-receptor subtypes (perhaps ε-receptors) Some direct opioid release into CSF Graded slow hyperpolarization; inhibitory

REFERENCES

Albe-Fessard, D., Condes-Lara, M., Kesar, S., & Sanderson, P. (1983). Tonic cortical controls acting on spontaneous and evoked thalamic activity. In G. Machi, A. Rustioni, & R. Sperafico (Eds.), *Somato-sensory integration in the thalamus* (p. 273). Amsterdam: Elsevier.

Basbaum, A.I., & Fields, H.L. (1978). Endogenous pain control mechanisms: Review and hypothesis. *Annals of Neurology, 4,* 451.

Basbaum, A.I., & Fields, H.L. (1979). The origin of descending pathways in the dorsolateral funiculus of the spinal cord of the cat and rat: Further studies of the anatomy of pain modulation. *Journal of Comparative Neurology, 187,* 513.

Brookoff, D. (2000). Chronic pain: 1. A new disease? *Hospital Practice, 35*(7), 45.

Burbut, D., Polak, J.M., & Wall, P.D. (1981). Substance-p in spinal cord dorsal horn decreases following peripheral nerve injury. *Brain Research, 205,* 289.

Devor, M., & Wall, P.D. (1981). Plasticity in the spinal cord sensory map following peripheral nerve injury in rats. *Journal of Neuroscience, 1*(7), 679.

Dickenson, A.H. (1994). NMDA receptor antagonists as analgesics. In H.L. Fields, & J.C. Liebeskind (Eds.), *Progress in pain research* (Vol. 1, p. 173). Seattle: IASP Press.

Dickenson, A.H., Oliveras, J.L., and Besson, J.M. (1979). Role of the nucleus raphe magnus in opiate analgesia as studied by the microinjection technique in the rat. *Brain Research, 170,* 95.

Dong, W.K., Ryu, H., & Wagman, I.H. (1978). Nociceptive responses of neurons in the medial thalamus and their relationship to spinothalamic pathways. *Journal of Neurophysiology, 41,* 1592.

Dubner, R. (1985). Specialization in nociceptive pathways: Sensory discrimination, sensory modulation and neural connectivity. In H.L. Fields, R. Dubner, and F. Cervero (Eds.), *Advances in pain research and therapy,* (Vol. 9, p. 285). New York, Raven Press.

Dubner, R., & Bennett, G.J. (1983). Spinal and trigeminal mechanisms of nociception. *Annual Review of Neuroscience, 6,* 381.

Fields, H.L., & Basbaum, A.I. (1978). Brainstem control of spinal pain transmission neurons. *Annual Review of Physiology, 40,* 193.

Gebhart, G.F. (1982). Opiate and opioid peptide effects on brainstem neurons: Relevance to nociception and antinociceptive mechanisms. *Pain, 12,* 93.

Giordano, J. (1991). Analgesic profile of centrally administered 2-methylserotonin against acute pain in rats. *European Journal of Pharmacology, 199,* 223.

Giordano, J., & Barr, G.A. (1987). Morphine and ketocyclazocine-induced analgesia in the developing rat; differences due to type of noxious stimulus and body topography. *Developmental Brain Research, 32,* 247.

Giordano, J., & Barr, G.A. (1988). Possible role of spinal 5-HT and μ- and κ-opioid receptor-mediated analgesia in the developing rat. *Developmental Brain Research, 33,* 121.

Gobel, S. (1976). Principles of organization in the substantia gelatinosa layer of the spinal trigeminal nucleus. In J.J. Bonica & D. Albe-Fessard (Eds.), *Advances in pain research and therapy* (Vol. 1, p. 165). New York: Raven Press.

Jessell, T.N. (1982). Substance-p in nociceptive primary sensory neurons. In R. Porter & M. O'Connor (Eds.), *Substance-P in the nervous system, Ciba Foundation Symposium 91* (p. 225). London: Pitman.

King, J.S., Gallant, P., Myerson, V., & Perl, E.R. (1976). The effects of anti-inflammatory agents on the responses and sensitization of unmyelinated C-fiber polymodal nociceptors. In Y. Zotterman (Ed.), *Sensory functions of the skin in primates* (p. 441). Oxford: Pergamon Press.

Kumazawa, T. & Perl, E.R. (1976). Differential excitation of dorsal horn marginal and substantia gelatinosa neurons by primary afferents units with fine a-delta and C-fibers. In Y. Zotterman (Ed.), *Sensory functions of the skin in primates* (Vol. 27, p. 67). Oxford: Pergamon Press.

LaMotte, R.H., Thalhammer, J.G., Torebjork, H.E. & Robinson, C.J. (1982). Peripheral neural mechanisms of cutaneous hyperalgesia following mild injury by heat. *Journal of Neuroscience, 2,* 765.

Lavene, J.D., Lane, S.R., Gordon, N.C., & Fields, H.L. (1982). A spinal opioid synapse mediates the interaction of spinal and brainstem sites in morphine analgesia. *Brain Research, 236,* 85.

Lumbard, N.C., Nashold, B.S., & Pelissier, T. (1979). Thalamic recordings in rats with hyperalgesia. In J.J. Bonica, J. Liebeskind, and D. Albe-Fessard (Eds.), *Advances in pain research and therapy* (Vol. 3, p. 767). New York: Raven Press.

Lynn, B. (1977). Cutaneous hyperalgesia. *British Medical Bulletin, 33,* 103.

Macchi, G., & Bentivoglio, M. (1979). The use of axonal transport in the neural anatomical study of subcortical projections to the neocortex. *Archivio Italiano di Anatomia e di Embriologia, 84,* 35.

Melzack, R., & Casey, K.L. (1968). Sensory, motivational and central control determinance of pain. In D.R. Kenshalo (Ed.), *The skin senses.* Springfield, IL: Charles C Thomas Press,

Melzack, R., & Wall, P.D. (1965). Pain mechanisms: A new therapy, *Science, 150,* 971.

Mense, S., Light, A.R., & Perl, E.R. (1981). Spinal terminations of subcutaneous high-threshold mechanoreceptors. In A.G. Brown & M. Rethelyi (Eds.), *Spinal cord sensation* (p. 79). Edinburg: Scottish Academic Press.

Ochoa, J., & Torebjork, H.E. (1981). Pain from skin and muscle. *Pain,* (Suppl.) *1,* 87.

Price, D.D., & Dubner, R. (1977). Neurons that subserve the sensory-discriminative aspects of pain, *Pain, 3,* 307.

Price, D.D., Hayes, R.L., Ruda, M., & Dubner, R. (1978). Spatial and temporal transformation of input to spinothalamic tract neurons and their relation to somatic sensations. *Journal of Neurophysiology, 41,* 933.

Raj, P.P. (1996). Pain mechanisms. In P.P. Raj (Ed.), *Pain medicine: A comprehensive review* (p. 12). St. Louis: Mosby.

Rexed, B. (1952). The cytoarchitectonic organization of the spinal cord in the cat. *Journal of Comparative Neurology, 96*, 415.

Rogers, L., & Giordano, J. (1990). Effects of systemically administered monoamine re-uptake blocking agents on patterns of buspirone-induced analgesia in rats. *Life Science, 47*(2), 961.

Rolston, H.J. (1983). The synaptic organization of ventrobasal thalamus in the rat, cat and monkey. In G. Macchi (Ed.), *The somatosensory thalamus* (p. 241). Amsterdam: Elsevier.

Ruda, M.A. (1982). Opiates and pain pathways: Demonstration of enkephalin synapses on dorsal horn projection neurons. *Science, 215*, 1523.

Ruda, M.A., Bennett, G.J., & Dubner, R. (1986). Neurochemistry and neurocircuitry in the dorsal horn. *Progressive Brain Research, 66*, 219.

Rustinoni, A., Hayes, N.L., & O'Neill, S. (1979). Dorsal column nuclei and ascending spinal afferents in macaques. *Brain, 102*, 95.

Sapienza, S., Talbi, B., Jacquemin, J., & Albe-Fessard, D. (1981). Relationship between input and output of cells in motor and somatosensory cortices of the chronic awake rat, *Experimental Brain Research, 43*, 47.

Satoh, M., Akaike, A., Nakazawa, T., & Takagi, H. (1980). Evidence for involvement of separate mechanisms in the production of analgesia by electrical stimulation of the nucleus reticularis paragigantocellularis and nucleus raphe magnus in the rat. *Brain Research, 194*, 525.

Sufka, K., Schomburg, F., & Giordano, J. (1992). Receptor mediation of 5-HT-induced inflammation and nociception in rats. *Pharmacology, Biochemistry, and Behavior, 41*(1), 53.

Takagi, H., Satoh, M., Akaike, A., Shibata, T., & Kuraishi, Y. (1977). The nucleus reticularis gigantocellularis of the medulla oblongata is a highly sensitive site in the production of morphine analgesia in the rat. *European Journal of Pharmacology, 45*, 91.

Torebjork, H.E. (1974). Afferent c-units responding to mechanical, thermal and chemical stimuli in human non-glabrous skin. *Acta Physiologica Scandinavica, 92*, 374.

Torebjork, H.E., & Ochoa, J. (1981). Pain and itch from c-fiber stimulation. *Society for Neuroscience Abstracts, 7*, 228.

Urban, M.O., & Gebhart, G.F. (1999). Central mechanisms in pain. *Medical Clinics of North America, 83*, 585.

Van Hees, J., & Gybels, J. (1981). C-nociceptor activity in human nerve during painful and non-painful skin stimulation. *Journal of Neurology, Neurosurgery, and Psychiatry, 44*, 600.

Willis, W.D., Kenshalo, D.R., & Lenoard, R.B. (1979). The cells of origin of the primate spinothalamic tract. *Journal of Comparative Neurology, 188*, 543.

Yaksh, T.L. & Noueihed, R. (1985). The physiology and pharmacology of spinal opiates. *Annual Review of Pharmacology and Toxicology, 25*, 433.

Yaksh, T.L., & Tyce, G.M. (1979). Micro injection of morphine into the periaqueductal grey evokes the release of serotonin from the spinal cord. *Brain Research, 171*, 176.

Zemlan, F.P., Corrigan, S.A., & Pfaff, D.W. (1980). Noradrenergic and serotonergic mediation of spinal analgesia mechanisms. *European Journal of Pharmacology, 61*, 111.

Zieglgansberger, W., & Tulloch, I.F. (1979). The effects of methionine- and leucine-enkephalin on spinal neurons of the cat. *Brain Research, 167*, 53.

Appendices

APPENDIX A

Code of Ethics

PREAMBLE

The American Academy of Pain Management recognizes the many facets and problems that pain patients experience. For this reason, the American Academy of Pain Management endorses and reaffirms the benefit of the interdisciplinary and multidisciplinary commitment which professionals from a variety of disciplines can make to the field of pain management.

The conduct of the individuals credentialed by the American Academy of Pain Management shall be consistent with all applicable local, state, and federal regulations, and with codes of conduct as established by the credentialed individual's primary discipline. Individuals who are credentialed by the American Academy of Pain Management are committed to increasing their knowledge of the mechanisms of pain, and its respondent behavior. Every effort will be made to safeguard the health and welfare of patients who seek the services of individuals credentialed by the American Academy of Pain Management.

PROFESSIONAL CONDUCT BY SPECIALTY

The credentialed individuals are obligated to maintain their skill competency such that it conforms to the standards of conduct to the individual's community, practice, and discipline. The treatment of pain, and the implementation of a patient's plan is a multidisciplinary/interdisciplinary effort. Credentialed individuals will conduct their professional behavior so that it facilitates the services of all team members for maximum benefit to the patient.

RESPONSIBILITY

The credentialed individuals shall be responsible for determining that standards are applied evenly and fairly to all individuals who receive services. Individuals who are employed by an institution, agency, or clinic have responsibility to be alert for institutional pressure which may be counter to the best interest of the patient, and shall make every effort to improve those conditions.

Credentialed individuals provide thorough documentation and timely feedback to members of the team, employers, carriers, and other interested parties in order to assure coordinated, managed care. All reports will be objective and based upon an independent professional opinion, within the credentialed individual's expertise. Credentialed individuals will provide only those services for which the individual is competent and qualified to perform. Credentialed individuals will refrain from providing services which are counter to the ethical standards of their discipline, or which would be a violation of standards established by applicable regulatory boards governing service to pain patients.

CONFIDENTIALITY

Credentialed providers are obligated to safeguard information obtained in the course of their involvement with a patient. Information may be released with a patient's permission; in circumstances where there is a clear and imminent danger to the patient, or others; and, where required by court or subpoena. Individuals who seek the services of a credentialed provider shall also be advised, that in some jurisdictions, insurance companies and regulatory boards may also have access to collected information, test results, and opinions. Patients have the privilege to the extent that is feasible and practical, and in those cases where there would be no legal or clinical contraindications, to see their chart when this can be arranged at a mutually convenient time.

EDUCATION, TRAINING, AND COMPETENCE

Credentialed providers shall maintain high standards of professional competence. They shall recognize the limits of their skills and license. They shall offer services consistent with the standards of their profession.

Credentialed individuals have an obligation to accurately represent and disclose their training, education, and experience to the public. Credentialed providers shall engage in continuing education. This will minimally include 100 hours of relevant education in pain management every 4 years. Credentialed providers recognize that the field of pain management is rapidly developing and shall be open to evaluate and consider new procedures and approaches to pain management. Credentialed providers should refrain from any activity which may result in harm to a patient without first considering alternatives to such an approach, seeking services which may achieve the same benefit without the associated risk, obtain consultations from other providers, and inform the patient of any risks inherent to any procedure or approach.

BUSINESS PROCEDURES

Credentialed providers will abide by all prevailing community standards. They will adhere to all federal, state, and local laws regulating business practice. Competitive advertising must be honest, factual, and accurate. Such advertising shall avoid exaggerated claims. Credentialed providers will not enter into any arrangement where fees are exchanged that would be likely to create conflict of interest or influence their opinion about services rendered.

Credentialed providers shall engage in behavior which conforms to high standards of moral, ethical, and legal behavior. Credentialed providers will not engaged in sexual contact with patients.

RESEARCH

Credentialed providers may engage in research about the management of pain. In doing so, they shall have the safety of their subjects as a priority. Investigation shall be consistent with the traditions and practices of the credentialed individual's discipline. Credit is given to all individuals who participate in a study.

APPENDIX

B

Patient's Bill of Rights

The American Academy of Pain Management endorses a Patient's Bill of Rights. It is an expectation that compliance with patient's rights can contribute to an effective patient care program. A modification of the American Hospital Association's statement on a Patient's Bill of Rights has been incorporated as part of the framework of the American Academy of Pain Management's Bill of Rights. The modifications consist of the following:

1. The patient has the right to considerate and respectful care.
2. The patient has the right to obtain from his or her credentialed provider, complete current information concerning their diagnosis, treatment, and prognosis in terms the patient can reasonably be expected to understand. When it is not advisable to give such information to the patient, the information should be made available to an appropriate person on his/her behalf.
3. The patient has the right to receive from his/her credentialed provider, information to make informed consent prior to the start of any procedure and/or treatment. This shall include such information as the medically significant risks involved with any procedure and probable duration of incapacitation. Where medically appropriate, alternatives for care or treatment should be explained to the patient.
4. The patient has the right to refuse any and all treatment, to the extent permitted by law, and to be informed of any of the medical consequence of his/her action.
5. The patient has a right to every consideration of privacy concerning his/her own medical care program, limited only by state statues, rules, regulations, or imminent danger to the individual or others.
6. The patient has the right to be advised if the clinician, hospital, clinic, etc. proposes to engage in or perform human experimentation affecting his/her care or treatment. The patient has the right to refuse to participate in such research projects.
7. The patients has the privilege to examine and receive an explanation of the bill.

All activities of pain management are to be conducted with an overriding concern for the patient and above all, the recognition of their dignity as a human being.

APPENDIX
C

American Academy
of Pain Management Credentialing

The American Academy of Pain Management is a nonprofit organization whose members are committed to increasing their knowledge of mechanisms of pain and its respondent behavior. The Academy is the largest organized association of multidisciplinary pain practitioners in any country. The Academy serves as the official Board for Credentialed Practitioners.

Problems associated with pain and attempts to control pain have historically been the principal reasons individuals seek healthcare. In recent years, the medical community has made great strides in its ability to treat pain patients.

Along with this progress has come a considerable change in pain management. Multidisciplinary pain facilities have demonstrated a new service delivery approach to pain management. Added to this phenomenal growth are a number and variety of inpatient and outpatient pain clinics.

With increasing frequency, the topic of pain management is on the agenda of discussion at clinical conferences. Insurance carriers and employment/governmental bodies have begun to focus great attention of this topic. Credentialed practitioners listed in the Academy's Registry have found increased referrals and have provided expert testimony about pain.

The Academy offers a credentialing process for individuals who treat pain patients. The Academy was founded and organized by individuals with years of relevant experience in treating acute, recurrent acute, cancer, and chronic pain sufferers. All respective disciplines are interested in furthering the knowledge and management of pain.

Pain management is not best delivered by any one profession or specialty, and for this reason the Academy represents a comprehensive, interdisciplinary membership. Credentialing is offered to professionals from a wide variety of disciplines who meet high standards for the practice of pain management. The Academy has developed a Model Code of Ethical Practice and continues to develop the standard of care in pain management. To the extent that standards are rigorously adhered to, it will be the intent of the Academy to include various disciplines.

When applying for credentialing, applicants must submit three professional letters of reference, copies of their license, official academic transcripts, application form, and curriculum vitae. The Credential Review Committee evaluates this material. The Academy has a written evaluation for new applicants.

Individuals who are credentialed receive a registered certificate, listing in the *National Registry of Multidisciplinary Pain Practitioners,* notice of conferences with reduced fees, and periodic educational publication.

The Academy presently publishes quarterly, *The Pain Practitioner,* containing hands-on information regarding pain management. The association also publishes a peer review journal, *American Journal of Pain Management.* Members will have an opportunity to serve on committees that will help shape the discipline. The American Academy of Pain Management is the only multidisciplinary pain management credentialing body.

COMMONLY ASKED QUESTIONS

Q: What is the American Academy of Pain Management?

A: The Academy is a nonprofit organization established to provide credentialing for individuals who treat patients suffering from chronic pain.

Q: Who is the Academy's Board of Advisors?

A: The board of the Academy is national in scope and blends both academicians and practitioners for the purpose of establishing rigorous standards for the treatment of pain patients.

Q: How does one become a member of the American Academy of Pain Management?

A: Healthcare providers may apply for membership. Credentialing is dependent upon the level of education and work experience in fields related to pain management.

Q: What are the benefits of membership with the Academy?

A: There are many, including a certificate registered by the Academy noting your status; listing in, and copy of the *National Registry of Multidisciplinary Pain Practitioners;* notices of conferences with reduced fees; periodic publications; and continuing education opportunities.

Q: What education and training are available?

A: An annual clinical meeting provides pain practitioners with the latest state-of-the-art treatment methods.

Q: How does one apply for membership to the American Academy of Pain Management?

A: An application packet, which includes the Statement of the Purpose of the Academy, the Code of Ethics, The Patient's Bill of Rights, a listing of the Board of Directors, and the biographical application dossier are available by contacting:

American Academy of Pain Management
13947 Mono Way #A
Sonora, CA 95370
(209) 533-9744

APPENDIX
D

Overview of Academy Services and Products

It is the goal of the Academy to bring together the many clinicians who work with individuals in pain and to assist in the creation of quality services for those individuals. The intent of the Academy is to be inclusionary, and not restrictive to any specialty. The Academy has developed many services and products which can help clinicians reduce pain and improve quality of life for their patients. Please take your time and learn more about the American Academy of Pain Management. Visit our website at www.aapainmanage.org, ask questions, make suggestions and invite your friends and colleagues to visit as well.

MEMBERSHIP

Membership is available to clinicians, individuals, and students for a $150 annual fee. As a benefit of membership you are listed in the *Directory of Pain Practitioners* on the Academy web site and you may link your web page to this Directory. You will also receive a membership card, the quarterly journal and newsletter, as well as discounts on Academy services and products.

CREDENTIALING

The purpose of credentialing is to establish a professional Code of Ethics and Patient's Bill of Rights; to promote professional accountability and visibility; to identify those pain practitioners who have met specific professional standards; to advance cooperation among the various specialties that treat individuals suffering pain; and to encourage continued professional growth and development of pain practitioners and the field of pain management. The Academy offers three levels of credentialing to clinicians: Diplomate, Fellow, and Clinical Associate.

PUBLICATIONS

The Academy publishes a peer-reviewed, quarterly journal, *The American Journal of Pain Management,* which provides valuable clinical research information in a multidisciplinary format. The Academy also publishes a quarterly newsletter, *The Pain Practitioner,* which features useful clinical topics, monitors trends, and reports important Academy news.

The Academy also has a best-selling multidisciplinary textbook titled *Pain Management: A Practical Guide for Clinicians.* This textbook is a very comprehensive overview of multidisciplinary pain management.

INTERNET

The award winning Academy web site provides diverse and meaningful information. Browse through informational pages, search Citeline for medical topics, join the on-line pain management community in the Open Forum, read the latest newsletters, access current research on outcome measurement in pain management, read the Patient's Bill of Rights and much, much more.

ANNUAL CLINICAL MEETING

In September of each year, the Academy holds a clinical meeting which has over 100 nationally known faculty and offers CME/CEU credit in many disciplines. This meeting is designed for clinicians who are interested in providing state-of-the-art multidisciplinary pain management, and who are looking for information, answers, and solutions to the issues and dilemmas confronting clinicians in pain management.

CONTINUING EDUCATION

The Academy is approved by ACCME to provide category 1 MD credit. The Academy is also approved to provide continuing education by The American Psychological Association (APA), The American Dental Association (ADA), The American Association of Oriental Medicine (AAOM), The National Board for Certified Counselors (NBCC), American Association of Nurse Anesthetists (AANA), and the American Podiatric Medical Association (CPME). The Academy also provides continuing education to nurses and pharmacists in cooperation with the University of the Pacific School of Pharmacy and Health Services and to chiropractors in association with Cleveland Chiropractic College.

PAIN PROGRAM ACCREDITATION

Pain Program Accreditation is a voluntary process that gives pain management programs an opportunity to demonstrate compliance with peer-reviewed quality treatment standards established by pain practitioners. The Academy has a long history of accrediting pain programs based on published standards and onsite review. A broad cross-section of pain programs is eligible for accreditation.

NATIONAL PAIN DATA BANK

The purpose of the National Pain Data Bank is to collect information about patient demographics, history, pain profile, functional status, quality of life and daily living, return to work, treatment satisfaction, and cost of care. A quarterly report of the data is sent to all participating programs. Participating programs have found this data useful in determining treatment outcomes, in creating more cost-effective treatment protocols, in creating marketing strategies, and in working with third-party payers.

The National Pain Data Bank has been featured twice at the American Medical Association (AMA) Practice Parameter Forum as a demonstration of how to conduct and analyze outcome measurement in pain management.

SECOND OPINION UTILIZATION REVIEW

The purpose of Second Opinion Utilization Review is to create unbiased reports for clinicians that would be available for use in record review, institutional privileges, arbitration, medicolegal matters, reimbursement disputes, malpractice, and licensing disputes. Experts are available for depositions and trials. Contact the Academy at (209) 533-9744 if you are interested in learning more about this program.

UNIVERSITY OF INTEGRATED STUDIES

The University of Integrated Studies offers Master of Arts and Doctor of Philosophy degrees in Integrated Studies, with disciplines in Pain Studies, Anti-Aging, and Mind/Body/Spirit, through a distance learning format. Visit the University web site at www.univintegratedstudies.edu to learn more about this exciting offering. The Academy was given initial temporary approval to operate a degree-granting university on July 2, 2000 by the State of California.

WORKING TOGETHER

As a leader in pain management with a vast infrastructure we can assist you with creative pain management solutions, conflict resolution, continuing education, life-long graduate university learning, accreditation, and measuring outcomes in pain management. Join the Academy's dynamic pain management team!

For information about any area of the above, please contact:

American Academy of Pain Management
13947 Mono Way #A
Sonora, CA 95370
(209) 533-9744
richard@aapainmanage.org

APPENDIX
E

Definition of Pain Management

PAIN MANAGEMENT

- The systematic study of clinical and basic science and its application for the reduction of pain and suffering.
- The blending of tools, techniques, and principles taken from discrete healing art disciplines and reformulated as a holistic application for the reduction of pain and suffering.
- A newly emerging discipline emphasizing an interdisciplinary approach with a goal of the reduction of pain and suffering.

Richard S. Weiner, Ph.D.
Executive Director
American Academy of Pain Management

Kathryn A. Weiner, Ph.D.
Associate Director
American Academy of Pain Management

Index

A

Abbreviated Injury Scale, 970
Abdominal pain, 421
  upper, 451
Abies alba, 1085
Abstinence syndromes, 865
Academy for guided imagery, 843
Accidents. *See also* Motor vehicle accidents
  low impact, 86
Acetaminophen, 114, 409, 436–437
  dosage guidelines, 437, 919
  opioids and, 487
  pediatric use, 488
  rectal administration, 488
  toxicity, 437
  tramadol and, 430
Acetylsalicylic acid, 114, 403
Achilles tendon calcification, 80–81
Achilles tendonitis, 81
Acupuncture, 9, 12, 150–152, 626–627
  body, 151, 153
  distal release points, 610, 676, 683
  ear, 152, 153, 604–605
  hand, 605–608
    Chinese, 606–607
    Korean, 607–608
  head, 608–609
  "jing well" points, 676
  myofascial, 241, 611–612
  pilot study, 150–151
  points, 610, 669–670, 735
    meridian numbering system, 669–670
  practitioners' guide, 154
  prolotherapy *vs.,* 386
Acute pain, 29, 415–416, 435
  characteristics, 917
  chronic *vs.,* 28, 30, 834
  low back, 745, 746
  orofacial, 140
  pediatric, 856
  pelvic, 453
  recurrent, 30
  of tension-type headache, 113–116
Adaptogens, 1018
Addison's disease, 99, 1014
Adrenal glands, 1012–1022

disorders, 1013–1015
  Addison's disease, 1014
  adrenocorticol deficiency, 1013–1014
    secondary, 1014
  adrenocorticol excess, 1015
  Conn's syndrome, 1015
  Cushing's syndrome, 1015
  inherent errors of metabolism, 1014
  laboratory testing for, 1017–1018
  office testing for, 1018
  pheochromocytoma, 1015
enhancing function, 1018–1021
  adaptogens for, 1018
  biofeedback, 1021
  exercise for, 1022
  ginseng for, 1019–1020
  licorice for, 1018–1019
  lifestyle changes for, 1021–1022
  vitamins and nutrients for, 1020
hormones, 1012
  HPA axis and biosynthesis of, 1012–1013
stress and, 1015
Adrenal maladaptation syndrome, 1011
Adrenocorticol deficiency, 1013
  secondary, 1014
ADVIL, 409. *See also* Ibuprofen
Agency for Healthcare Policy and Research, 19, 285, 289
Agency for Healthcare Policy Reform, 995
Aging, neuroendocrine theory of, 1016–1017
Ajulemic acid, 366–367
Alcohol
  cluster headache and, 203
  opioids and, 441
Alcohol Use Disorders Identification Test (AUDIT), 829
Alcoholism, 868–870
  abuse of other drugs and, 870
  costs, 868
  diagnostic criteria, 868
  genetic factors, 869
  hallucinations associated with, 869
  long-term effects, 869
  physiological mechanisms, 868
  treatment, 869–870
  withdrawal symptoms, 868
Aldosterone, 1012
ALEVE, 409
Allodynia, 221